Advances in HFpEF Management (AHM)
(CKM Navigation)
A Textbook of Cardiology

Advances in HFpEF Management (AHM)
(CKM Navigation)
A Textbook of Cardiology

Editors-in-Chief

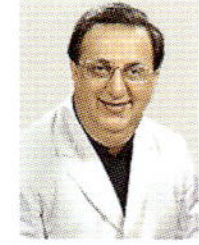

HK Chopra
Senior Consultant Cardiologist
Medanta–Moolchand Heart Institute, New Delhi, India
Chairman, CME, Moolchand Medcity
National Awardee, DST, Government of India
Chairman, World Wellness Foundation, WHA
Country Head, AHA
Former National President, CSI and IAE
Former National Editor-in-Chief, IHJ, JIAE
Editor-in-Chief, Top 14 Textbooks of Cardiology
Chief Advisor, Health Committee SCOPE

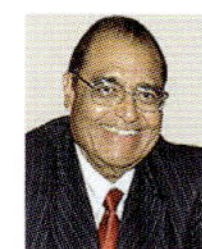

Navin C Nanda
Distinguished Professor
Department of Medicine and Cardiovascular Disease
University of Alabama at Birmingham
Birmingham, Alabama, USA
Editor-in-Chief, Echocardiography: A Journal of Cardiovascular Ultrasound and Allied Techniques
President, International Society of Cardiovascular Ultrasound (ISCU)

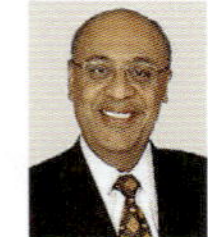

Jagat Narula
Executive Vice President
Chief Academic Officer
UTHealth Houston
Houston, Texas, USA
President, World Heart Federation

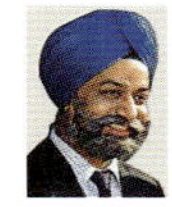

GS Wander
Professor and Head
Department of Cardiology
Dayanand Medical College and Hospital
Unit of Hero DMC Heart Institute
Ludhiana, Punjab, India
Past President, API

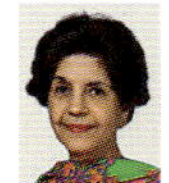

Sarita Bajaj
Senior Consultant Endocrinologist
Former Director-Professor and Head
Department of Medicine
MLN Medical College
Prayagraj, Uttar Pradesh, India

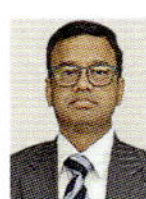

Viveka Kumar
Principal Director and Chief
Catheter Laboratories
(Pan Max)—Cardiac Sciences
Max Super Speciality Hospital (East Block)
Saket, New Delhi, India

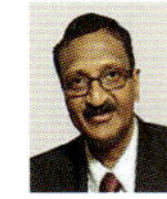

Tiny Nair
Head
Department of Cardiology
PRS Hospital
Thiruvananthapuram
Kerala, India

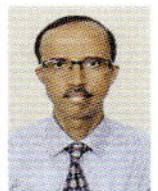

CK Ponde
Chief, Noninvasive Cardiac Laboratory and Associate Director of Cardiac Catheter Laboratory
PD Hinduja National Hospital and Medical Research Center
Mumbai, Maharashtra, India
Past President, IAE

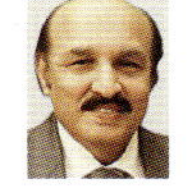

AK Pancholia
Head
Department of Medicine
Clinical and Preventive Cardiology
Arihant Hospital
Indore, Madhya Pradesh, India

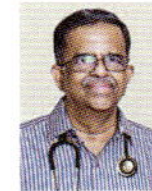

S Shanmugasundaram
Senior Consultant Cardiologist
Billroth Hospitals
Chennai, Tamil Nadu, India

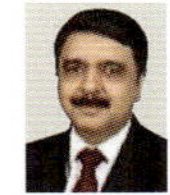

Dinesh Khullar
Chairman and Head
Department Nephrology and Renal Transplant Medicine
Max Super Speciality Hospital
Saket, New Delhi, India

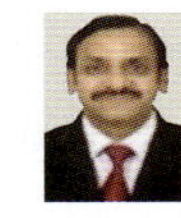

Satyendra Tewari
Professor
Department of Cardiology
Sanjay Gandhi Postgraduate Institute of Medical Sciences
Lucknow, Uttar Pradesh, India

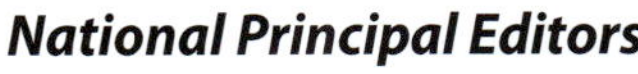

National Principal Editors

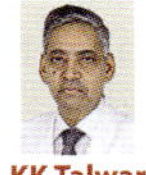 **KK Talwar**, New Delhi

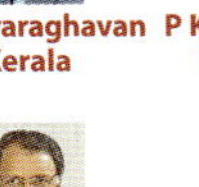 **G Vijayaraghavan**, Kerala

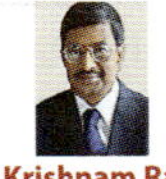 **P Krishnam Raju**, Hyderabad

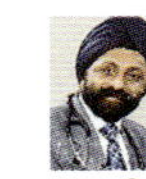 **JPS Sawhney**, New Delhi

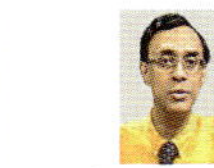 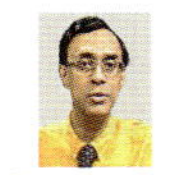 **Saumitra Ray**, Kolkata

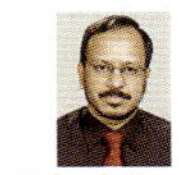 **Rakesh Gupta**, New Delhi

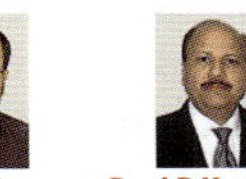 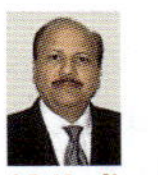 **Ravi R Kasliwal**, Gurugram

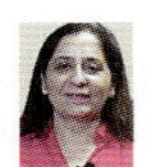 **Poonam Malhotra Kapoor**, New Delhi

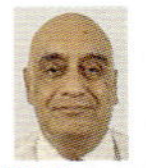 **KK Kapur**, New Delhi

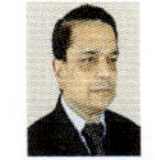 **Vinod Sharma**, New Delhi

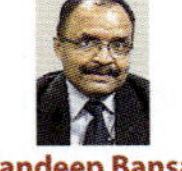 **Sandeep Bansal**, New Delhi

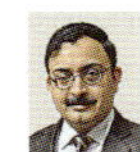 **NN Khanna**, New Delhi

Rajeev Gupta, Jaipur

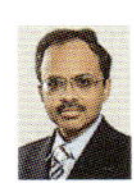 **Nitin Burkule**, Mumbai

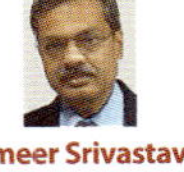 **Sameer Srivastava**, New Delhi

SC Govind, Bengaluru

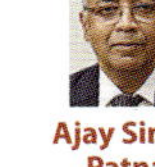 **Ajay Sinha**, Patna

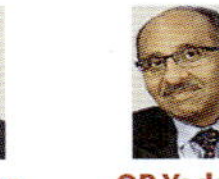 **OP Yadava**, New Delhi

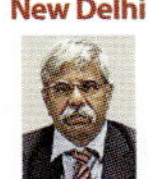 **V Amuthan**, Madurai

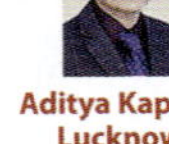 **Aditya Kapoor**, Lucknow

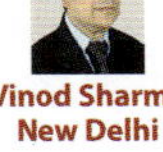 **SS Mishra**, Cuttack

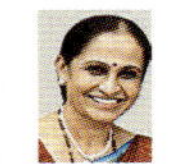 **IB Vijayalakshmi**, Bengaluru

Asha Moorthy, Chennai

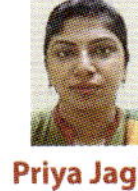 **Priya Jagia**, New Delhi

Mona Bhatia, New Delhi

Roopali Khanna, Lucknow

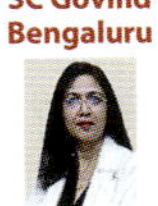 **Sarita Rao**, Indore

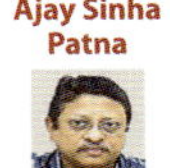 **SN Routray**, Cuttack

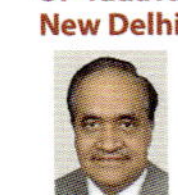 **Harshwardhan**, New Delhi

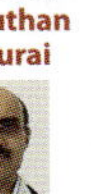 **Sanjay Mittal**, Gurugram

Ashwin Mehta, New Delhi

Manish Bansal, Gurugram

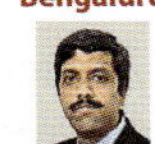 **S Ramakrishan**, New Delhi

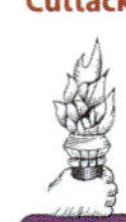

JAYPEE BROTHERS MEDICAL PUBLISHERS
The Health Sciences Publisher
New Delhi | London

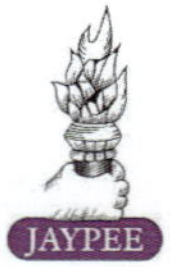

JAYPEE **Jaypee Brothers Medical Publishers (P) Ltd**

Headquarters
Jaypee Brothers Medical Publishers (P) Ltd
EMCA House, 23/23-B
Ansari Road, Daryaganj
New Delhi 110 002, India
Landline: +91-11-23272143, +91-11-23272703
+91-11-23282021, +91-11-23245672
Email: jaypee@jaypeebrothers.com

Corporate Office
Jaypee Brothers Medical Publishers (P) Ltd
4838/24, Ansari Road, Daryaganj
New Delhi 110 002, India
Phone: +91-11-43574357
Fax: +91-11-43574314
Email: jaypee@jaypeebrothers.com

Overseas Office
JP Medical Ltd.
83, Victoria Street, London
SW1H 0HW (UK)
Phone: +44 20 3170 8910
Fax: +44 (0)20 3008 6180
Email: info@jpmedpub.com

Website: www.jaypeebrothers.com
Website: www.jaypeedigital.com

Inquiries for bulk sales may be solicited at: jaypee@jaypeebrothers.com

Advances in HFpEF Management (AHM) (CKM Navigation): A Textbook of Cardiology

First Edition: **2025**

ISBN: 978-93-6616-747-3

Printed at: Samrat Offset Pvt. Ltd.

Dedicated to

The world and Cardiological Society of India (CSI), our parents, our teachers, all the members of CSI, our colleagues, patients, students, and our families.

Contributors

A George Koshy
Senior Consultant
Department of Cardiology
Cosmopolitan Hospital, Thiruvananthapuram
Former Professor and Head
Department of Cardiology
Government Medical College
Thiruvananthapuram, Kerala, India

Aafreen Naik
Senior Manager
Medical Affairs
JB Chemicals and Pharmaceuticals Ltd.
Mumbai, Maharashtra, India

Aarya A Naik
University of Tennessee Medical Center
Memphis, Tennessee, USA

Aashish Jain
Senior Consultant (Cardiac Anesthesia)
Medanta Institute of Critical Care
and Anesthesiology
Medanta—The Medicity
Gurugram, Haryana, India

Aatish Rengan
Department of Cardiology
All India Institute of Medical Sciences
New Delhi, India

Aayushi Gupta
Senior Resident
Lok Nayak Jai Prakash Narain Hospital
New Delhi, India

Abdirahman Wardhere
Division of Cardiovascular Medicine
University of Texas Medical Branch
Galveston, TX, USA

Abdul Subhan Talpur
Liaquat University of Medical and
Health Sciences
Jamshoro, Pakistan

Abdullah AS Majumder
Professor of Cardiology and Former Director
National Institute of Cardiovascular Diseases
Dhaka, Bangladesh

Abhishek
Department of Nephrology and Renal
Transplant Medicine
Max Super Speciality Hospital
New Delhi, India

Abhishek Garg
Department of Cardiology
Dayanand Medical College and Hospital
Unit of Hero DMC Heart Institute
Ludhiana, Punjab, India

Abhishek Rathore
Consultant Cardiologist and Electrophysiologist
Department of Cardiology
Apollo Hospitals
Indore, Madhya Pradesh, India

Achukatla Kumar
Research Consultant
Department of Cardiology
Apollo Hospitals
Indore, Madhya Pradesh, India

Aditi A Naik
Smt NHL Medical College and VS Hospital
Ahmedabad, Gujarat, India

Aditi Tanwar
Department of Radiation Oncology
Dharamshila Narayana Superspecialty Hospital
New Delhi, India

Aditya Kapoor
Professor and Head
Department of Cardiology
Sanjay Gandhi Postgraduate Institute of
Medical Sciences
Lucknow, Uttar Pradesh, India

Agam Vora
Medical Director
Brahma Kumaris' Global Hospital and
Research Centre
Manager
BSES MG Hospital
Mumbai, Maharashtra, India

Ajay Kumar Sinha
Medanta Hospital
Patna, Bihar, India

Ajay M Naik
Cardiac Electrophysiologist
Marengo CIMS Hospital
Ahmedabad, Gujarat, India

AK Omar
Director and Head
Non-invasive Cardiology and
Heart Command Centre
Fortis Escorts Heart Institute
New Delhi, India

AK Pancholia
Head
Department of Medicine
Clinical and Preventive Cardiology
Arihant Hospital
Indore, Madhya Pradesh, India

Akash Jain
Consultant
Aku92 Clinics
Yamunanagar, Haryana, India

AKM Monwarul Islam
Associate Professor and Head
Department of Noninvasive Cardiology
National Institute of Cardiovascular Diseases
Dhaka, Bangladesh

Ameet G Sattur
Director (Cath Lab)
KLE Suchirayu Hospital and Sattur Heart Care
Hubballi, Karnataka, India

Amit Garg
Senior Consultant
Department of Imaging
Fortis Escort Heart Institute
New Delhi, India

Amit Malik
Senior Director and Coordinator
Cardiac Sciences
Max Super Speciality Hospital
Ghaziabad, Uttar Pradesh, India

Amrish Agrawal
Senior Consultant and Cardiologist
Associate Professor of Medicine
Fujairah Hospital, Emirates Health Services (EHS)
Fujairah, UAE

Anamika Roy
Resident (General Medicine)
Holy Family Hospital
New Delhi, India

Anil Pareek
President
Medical Affairs and Clinical Research
IPCA Laboratories Ltd
Mumbai, Maharashtra, India

Aniruddha De
Consultant
Suraksha Diagnostics Private Limited
Kolkata, West Bengal, India

Anish Kumar Gupta
Department of Nephrology and Renal Transplant Medicine
Max Super Speciality Hospital
New Delhi, India

Ankit Tandon
Dr DY Patil Medical College, Hospital and Research Centre
Pune, Maharashtra, India

Ankush Sachdeva
Senior Consultant (Noninvasive Cardiology)
Fortis Escorts Heart Institute
New Delhi, India

Anshika Gulati
Consultant Radiologist
National Heart Institute
New Delhi, India

Anu Gaur
Consultant
US and Global Regulatory Affairs for Medical Devices
Massachusetts (MA), USA

Anu Grover
Director
Scientific Communication
Mangrove Creations
New Delhi, India

Aparajita Kumar
Associate Consultant
Clinical and Preventive Cardiology
Medanta—The Medicity
Gurugram, Haryana, India

Arati Dave Lalchandani
Former Principal and Dean
Ganesh Shankar Vidyarthi Memorial (GSVM) Medical College
Kanpur, Uttar Pradesh, India
Member Board of Governors
All India Institute of Medical Sciences, Gorakhpur

Archit Dahiya
Senior Interventional Cardiologist
Holy Heart Hospital
Rohtak, Haryana, India

Arijit Ghosh
Consultant Cardiologist and Cath Lab In-charge
Manipal Hospitals
Kolkata, West Bengal, India

Arindam Pande
Senior Consultant and Cardiologist
Medica Superspecialty Hospital
Kolkata, West Bengal, India

Arshad Nazir
Assistant Professor
Department of Cardiology
Sanjay Gandhi Postgraduate Institute of Medical Sciences
Lucknow, Uttar Pradesh, India

Arunkumar S
Associate Professor
Department of Nephrology
All India Institute of Medical Sciences
New Delhi, India

Arup Dasbiswas
Emeritus Professor of Cardiology
PKG Medical College and Hospital, Kolkata
Former Director, Head and Professor
Department of Cardiology
ICVS—Institute of Postgraduate Medical Education and Research (IPGMER)
Kolkata, West Bengal, India

Asesh Haldar
Consultant Cardiologist
Medica Superspecialty Hospital
Kolkata, West Bengal, India

Asharam Panda
Assistant Professor
Department of Cardiology
Dhaneswar Rath Institute of Engineering and Medical Sciences
(DRIEMS University) and Padmini Care Hospital
Cuttack, Odisha, India

Ashokan Nambiar
Head
Department of Cardiology
Baby Memorial Hospital
Kozhikode, Kerala, India

Atit A Gawalkar
Assistant Professor
Department of Cardiology
All India Institute of Medical Sciences
New Delhi, India

Atul Kaushik
Department of Cardiology
Fortis Escorts Heart Institute
New Delhi, India

Ayan Kar
Consultant and Interventional Cardiologist and Lead in Heart Failure Services
Narayana Hospital—RN Tagore Hospital
Kolkata, West Bengal, India

Bagirath Raghuraman
Senior Interventional Cardiologist
Director of Heart Transplant
Department of Cardiology
Narayana Institute of Cardiac Sciences
Bengaluru, Karnataka, India

Bhagwan Mantri
Head
Department of Pulmonology and Sleep Medicine
Emirates Health Services (EHS)
Dubai, UAE

Bhanu Duggal
Professor and Head
Department of Cardiology
All India Institute of Medical Sciences
Rishikesh, Uttarakhand
Grant Medical College and Sir JJ Group of Hospitals
Mumbai, Maharashtra, India

Bhavik Shah
Department of Cardiology
Seth GS Medical College and KEM Hospital
Mumbai, Maharashtra, India

Bhavna Mastebhakti
Fortis Escorts Heart Institute
New Delhi, India

Bhawna Mathur
Department of Cardio Thoracic and Vascular Surgery (CTVS)
Max Superspecialty Hospital
New Delhi, India

Biaus Samanta
Department of Cardiology
NRS Medical College
Kolkata, West Bengal, India

Bijay Yadav
National Institute of Medical Sciences and Research
NIMS University
Jaipur, Rajasthan, India

BR Mishra
Senior Consultant and Cardiologist
Max Diagnostics
Cuttack, Odisha, India

C Venkata S Ram
Apollo Hospitals and Medical College
Hyderabad, Telangana, India
University of Texas Southwestern Medical Center
Dallas, Texas, USA

Chanchal Pal
Senior Consultant
ENT and Head and Neck Surgery
Indraprastha Apollo Hospital
New Delhi, India

CK Ponde
Chief, Noninvasive Cardiac Lab
Associate Director, Cardiac Cath Lab
PD Hinduja National Hospital and
Medical Research Center
Mumbai, Maharashtra, India

Dayasagar Rao V
Consultant Cardiologist
KIMS Hospital
Secunderabad, Telangana, India

Debabrata Roy
Senior Consultant Cardiologist and
Academic Co-ordinator
Narayana Hospital—RN Tagore Hospital
Kolkata, West Bengal, India

Debopom Goswami
Consultant Interventional Cardiologist
Manipal Broadway Hospital
Kolkata, West Bengal, India

Debopriyo Mondal
Consultant Cardiologist
Manipal Group of Hospitals
Kolkata, West Bengal, India

Deepak Panigrahi
Department of Nephrology and
Renal Transplant Medicine
Max Super Specialty Hospital
New Delhi, India

Deepika Misra
Attending, Clinical Cardiology
Columbia University
Division of Cardiology
Mount Sinai Medical Center, USA

Dennis Fong
Department of Cardiology
Sarver Heart Centre
University of Arizona
Tucson, Arizona, USA

Deodatta Chafekar
Director and Consultant Nephrologist
Supreme Kidney Care, Nashik
Professor and Head of Nephro Division
Dr Vasantrao Pawar Medical College Hospital
and Research Centre
Nashik, Maharashtra, India

Devesh Kumar
Assistant Professor
Department of Cardiology
Vardhman Mahavir Medical College
and Safdarjung Hospital
New Delhi, India

Dharmendra Jain
Professor
Department of Cardiology
Institute of Medical Sciences
Banaras Hindu University
Varanasi, Uttar Pradesh, India

Dhiman Kahali
Director
Department of Interventional Cardiology
CK Birla Heart Hospital
Kolkata, West Bengal, India

Dinesh Khullar
Chairman and Head
Department of Nephrology and
Renal Transplant Medicine
Max Super Speciality Hospital
Saket, New Delhi, India

DP Sinha
Consultant and Head (Cardiology)
ILS Hospitals
Kolkata, West Bengal, India

Durlabh Debbarma
Medica Super Specialty Hospital
Kolkata, West Bengal, India

Dushyant Singh Gaur
Professor and Head
Immunohematology and Blood Transfusion
Himalayan Institute of Medical Sciences
Dehradun, Uttarakhand, India

Esha Choudhary
Maharishi Markandeshwar Medical College
Ambala, Haryana, India

Franz H Messerli
Professor
University of Bern, Switzerland
Jagiellonian University
Krakow, Poland

Ganesan Manohar
Director
Department of Cardiology
MGM Malar Hospital, Chennai
Former Professor
Rajiv Gandhi Government General Hospital
and Madras Medical College
Chennai, Tamil Nadu, India

Garima Aggarwal
Consultant Nephrologist
Manipal Hospitals
Bengaluru, Karnataka, India

Gautam Singal
Associate Professor
Department of Cardiology
Dayanand Medical College and Hospital
Unit of Hero DMC Heart Institute
Ludhiana, Punjab, India

Geetha Subramanian
Head and Professor (Retd)
Department of Cardiology
Institute of Medical Sciences
Banaras Hindu University, Varanasi
Former Head and Professor
Institute of Cardiology
Madras Medical College and Rajiv Gandhi
Government General Hospital
Emeritus Professor (Cardiology)
The Tamil Nadu Dr MGR Medical University
Tamil Nadu, India

Geevar Zachariah
Chairman
Mother Heart Care and Mother Hospital
Thrissur, Kerala, India

Girish Sabnis
Department of Cardiology
Seth GS Medical College and KEM Hospital
Mumbai, Maharashtra, India

Gulshan B Tolani
Vijan Hospital and Research Centre
Nashik, Maharashtra, India

Gurpreet Singh Wander
Professor and Head
Department of Cardiology
Dayanand Medical College and Hospital
Unit of Hero DMC Heart Institute
Ludhiana, Punjab, India
Past President, API

GV Senthilnathan
Clinical Lead and Senior Interventional
Cardiologist
Sugam Hospital
Chennai, Tamil Nadu, India

Hala Elmarsafawy
Professor of Pediatrics and Pediatric Cardiology
Director, Cardiac Catheterization Laboratory
Children Hospital
Mansoura University, Egypt

Hansa Gupta
Senior Consultant Cardiologist
Paras Hospital
Gurugram, Haryana, India

Harikrishnan S
Professor and Head
Department of Cardiology
Sree Chitra Tirunal Institute for
Medical Sciences and Technology
Thiruvananthapuram, Kerala, India
Editor-in-Chief, Heart Failure Journal of India

Harinder K Bali
Chairman (Cardiac Sciences) and
Dean (Academics and Research)
Livasa Hospital
Mohali, Punjab, India

Harmesh Aggarwal
Senior Physician and Cardiologist
Director, Aggarwal Centre for Diabetes
and Cancer Care
Gurugram, Haryana, India

Harsh Mahajan
Founder and Chief Radiologist
Mahajan imaging and Labs
Chairman, Department of Nuclear Medicine
and PET-CT
Sir Ganga Ram Hospital
Chairman
Centre for Advanced Research in Imaging,
Neurosciences and Genomics
New Delhi, India

Harsh Wardhan
Principal–Director
Cardiac Sciences
Supreme Hospital
Faridabad, Haryana, India

Harshit Khare
Assistant Professor
Department of Cardiology
Sanjay Gandhi Postgraduate Institute
of Medical Sciences
Lucknow, Uttar Pradesh, India

Hemant Bareth
NIMS Institute of Pharmacy
NIMS University
Jaipur, Rajasthan, India

Himanshu Jain
Clinical Assistant
Indraprastha Apollo Hospital
New Delhi, India

Himanshu Verma
Professor and Head
Department of Nephrology
Vardhman Mahavir Medical College and
Safdarjung Hospital
New Delhi, India

HK Chopra
Senior Consultant Cardiologist
Medanta–Moolchand Heart Institute
New Delhi, India
Chairman, CME, Moolchand Medcity
National Awardee, DST, Government of India
Chairman, World Wellness Foundation, WHA
Country Head, AHA
Former National President, CSI and IAE
Former National Editor-in-Chief, IHJ, JIAE
Editor-in-Chief, Top 14 Textbooks of Cardiology
Chief Advisor, Health Committee SCOPE

IB Vijayalakshmi
Professor Emeritus
Former Professor and Head
Department of Pediatric Cardiology
Sri Jayadeva Institute of Cardiovascular Sciences
and Research
Bengaluru, Karnataka, India

Ilayaraja Uthirapthi
Cardiologist
Billroth Hospitals
Chennai, Tamil Nadu, India

Indu Bansal
Group Director and Head
Department of Radiation Oncology
Paras Hospital
Gurugram, Haryana, India

Iniya Rajendran
Department of Cardiology
Sarver Heart Center
University of Arizona
Tucson, Arizona, USA

Isha Nandal
Assistant Professor
Department of Obstetrics and Gynecology
World College of Medical Sciences and
Research and Hospital
Jhajjar, Haryana, India

J Cecily Mary Majella
Professor
Department of Cardiology
Senior Interventional Cardiologist
Tamil Nadu Government Multi Super
Speciality Hospital
Chennai, Tamil Nadu, India

Jabir Abdullakutty
Senior Consultant and
Director of Clinical Research (Cardiology)
Lisie Hospital
Ernakulam, Kerala, India

Jai Bharat Sharma
Consultant Cardiology
Himachal Heart Institute
Mandi, Himachal Pradesh, India

Jasmine Sethi
Assistant Professor
Department of Nephrology
Postgraduate Institute of Medical Education
and Research
Chandigarh, India

Jayagopal PB
Director and Senior Interventional Cardiologist
Lakshmi Hospital
Palakkad, Kerala, India

Jishnu Prem
Department of Radiation Oncology
Dharamshila Narayana Superspeciality
Hospital
New Delhi, India

Johann Christopher
Director of Cardiac Imaging
CARE Hospitals
Hyderabad, Telangana, India

Jostol Pinto
Associate Professor
Department of Cardiology
Father Muller Medical College
Mangaluru, Karnataka, India

JPS Sawhney
Chairperson
Department of Cardiology
Dharma Vira Heart Centre
Sir Ganga Ram Hospital
New Delhi, India

Juhi Singh
Department of Cardiology
Dharma Vira Heart Center
Sir Ganga Ram Hospital
New Delhi, India

Kajal Ganguly
Consultant Interventional Cardiologist
Department of Cardiology
Manipal Broadway Hospital
Kolkata, West Bengal, India

Kanika Sood Sharma
Department of Radiation Oncology
Dharamshila Narayana Superspeciality
Hospital
New Delhi, India

Karishma Suri
Department of Cardiology
Maharishi Markandeshwar Institute
of Medical Sciences and Research
Ambala, Haryana, India

Karthika Gopal D
Department of Imaging
Fortis Escorts Heart Institute
New Delhi, India

Karthikaa Saminathan
Assistant Professor
Department of Cardiology
Sri Muthukumaran Medical College Hospital and Research Institute
Chennai, Tamil Nadu, India

Kartikeya Bhargava
Senior Director
Cardiac Electrophysiology and Pacing
Medanta—The Medicity
Gurugram, Haryana, India

Kavita Tyagi
Associate Consultant
Dharma Vira Heart Center
Sir Ganga Ram Hospital
New Delhi, India

Kiran Rao Kanjerla
Consultant Cardiologist and Cardiac Electrophysiologist
KIMS–SUNSHINE Hospitals
Hyderabad, Telangana, India

Kiron Varghese
Professor
Department of Cardiology
St John's Medical College and Hospital
Bengaluru, Karnataka, India

KK Kapur
Chief and Senior Consultant
Noninvasive Cardiology
Apollo Hospitals
New Delhi, India

Kousalya Rajendran
Division of Cardiology
Sri Ramakrishna Hospital
Coimbatore, Tamil Nadu, India

Krishna Vaitheeswaran
Senior Consultant Ophthalmologist
Moolchand Kharaiti Ram Hospital
(Moolchand Medcity)
New Delhi, India

Kulwant Singh
Department of Nephrology and Renal Transplant Medicine
Max Super Specialty Hospital
New Delhi, India

Kunal Mahajan
Consultant Cardiology
Himachal Heart Institute
Mandi, Himachal Pradesh

Kushal Madan
Cardiac Rehabilitation Consultant
Dharma Vira Heart Center
Sir Ganga Ram Hospital
New Delhi, India

Lakshmi Nalini Kopalle
Associate Professor and Senior Consultant Endocrinologist
Ayaan Institute of Medical Sciences
Fernandez Foundation Apollo Clinics
Hyderabad, Telangana, India

Leyla Kedir Bereka
Senior Physician and Intensivist
Emirates Health Services
UAE

M Edwin Fernando
Professor and Head
Department of Nephrology
Government Stanley Medical College
Chennai, Tamil Nadu, India

M Karthikeyan
Government Stanley Medical College
Chennai, Tamil Nadu, India

M Somasundaram
Senior Consultant Cardiologist
Meenam Medicare Center
Chennai, Tamil Nadu, India

Madhu Mary
Principal Consultant Cardiology
Medanta—The Medicity
Gurugram, Haryana, India

Madhuri Matta
Head
Department of Medicine
INHS Kalyani Hospital
Visakhapatnam, Andhra Pradesh, India

Mainak Mukhopadhyay
Consultant Cardiologist
Department of Cardiology
Manipal Hospital
Kolkata, West Bengal, India

Manbir Singh
Senior Interventional Cardiologist
Deep Hospital
Ludhiana, Punjab, India

Mangesh Tiwaskar
Mumbai, Maharashtra, India
Editor-in-Chief
Journal of the Association of Physicians of India

Manish Bansal
Senior Director
Clinical and Preventive Cardiology
Medanta—The Medicity
Gurugram, Haryana, India

Manisha Sahay
Professor and Head
Department of Nephrology
Osmania Medical College and Osmania General Hospital
Hyderabad, Telangana, India

Manisha Sharma
Consultant Noninvasive Cardiology
Mediversal Super Speciality Hospital
Patna, Bihar, India

Manna Bhattacharya
National Institute of Medical Sciences and Research
NIMS University
Jaipur, Rajasthan, India

Manoranjan Mandal
Department of Cardiology
NRS Medical College
Kolkata, West Bengal, India

Manpreet Singh Brar
PG Resident
Department of ENT
Krishna Mohan Medical College and Hospital
Mathura, Utter Pradesh, India

Mark Hellerman
Stony Brook University Hospital

Masood Ahmad
Division of Cardiovascular Medicine
University of Texas Medical Branch
Galveston, TX, USA

Md Inamul Haque
Moolchand Kharaiti Ram Hospital
(Moolchand Medcity)
New Delhi, India

Meemansa Kashyap Buch
Department of Cardiology
Narayana Institute of Cardiac Sciences
Bengaluru, Karnataka, India

Megha Saigal
Department of Nephrology
All India Institute of Medical Sciences
Patna, Bihar, India

Meghna Gupta
Assistant Professor
Department of Psychiatry
Krishna Mohan Medical College
Mathura, Utter Pradesh, India

Mitendra Yadav
Department of Cardiac Sciences
Max Super Specialty Hospital
New Delhi, India

Mohamad Akram
Department of Cardiology
Fortis Escorts Heart Institute
New Delhi, India

Mohan Bhargava
Director Cardiology
Max Super Specialty Hospital
New Delhi, India

Mohit M Bhagwati
In-charge
Acute Cardiac Care and HF Clinic
Holy Family Hospital
New Delhi, India

Mohit Tayal
Fellow in Noninvasive Cardiology
Dayanand Medical College and Hospital
Unit of Hero DMC Heart Institute
Ludhiana, Punjab, India

Mohsin Raj Mantoo
Department of Cardiology
Cardiothoracic and Neurosciences Center
All India Institute of Medical Sciences
New Delhi, India

Mohsin Wali
Senior Physician and Consultant
Sir Ganga Ram Hospital
New Delhi, India

Mona Bhatia
Principal Director and Head
Department of Imaging
Fortis Escorts Heart Institute
New Delhi, India

Monashis Sahu
Consultant (Endocrinology)
Max Hospitals
New Delhi, India

Monika Nadar
Senior Consultant Ophthalmologist
Moolchand Kharaiti Ram Hospital
(Moolchand Medcity)
New Delhi, India

Mrinal Kanti Das
Consultant Cardiologist
CK Birla Hospitals
[BM Birla Heart Research Centre/
The Calcutta Medical Research Institute (CMRI)]
Kolkata, West Bengal, India

Mukesh Sharma
Professor and Head
Department of Cardiology
Rabindranath Tagore Medical College and
Maharana Bhupal Government Hospital
Udaipur, Rajasthan, India

Mustafa Sajjad Cheema
CMH Lahore Medical College and
Institute of Dentistry
Lahore, Pakistan

Muthu Jayaraman
Former Professor of Nephrology
Stanley Medical College
Chennai, Tamil Nadu, India

N Ramachandran
Assistant Professor
Department of Nephrology
Pondicherry Institute of Medical Sciences (PIMS)
Puducherry, India

Nakul Sinha
Chairman
Department of Cardiology
Max Hospital
Lucknow, Uttar Pradesh, India

Namrata Gaur
Additional Professor and Head Unit-2
Department of Cardiothoracic and
Vascular Surgery
All India Institute of Medical Sciences
Rishikesh, Uttarakhand, India

Narendra Kumar
Heartbeats Z Academy
Norfolk, UK

Narinder Pal Singh
Department of Nephrology and
Renal Transplant Medicine
Max Super Specialty Hospital
New Delhi, India

Navdeep S Sidhu
Assistant Professor
Department of Cardiology
All India Institute of Medical Sciences
Bilaspur, Himachal Pradesh, India

Naveen Garg
Senior Medical Officer and
In-charge Clinical Cardiology
Civil Hospital
Palwal, Haryana, India

Naveen Sharma
Consultant
Accord Superspecialty Hospital
Faridabad, Haryana, India

Navin C Nanda
Distinguished Professor
Department of Medicine and
Cardiovascular Disease
University of Alabama at Birmingham
Birmingham, Alabama, USA
Editor-in-Chief, Echocardiography: A Journal
of Cardiovascular Ultrasound and
Allied Techniques
President, International Society of
Cardiovascular Ultrasound (ISCU)

Neelima Chafekar
Professor and Head
Department of Medicine
Dr Vasantrao Pawar Medical College Hospital
and Research Centre
Nashik, Maharashtra, India

Neeru Gera
Director Endocrinology
Max Hospitals
New Delhi, India

Neha Chaudhary
Department of Anesthesia and
Pain Management
Moolchand Medcity
New Delhi, India

Nidhi Dhawan
Director
Department of ENT
Moolchand Kharaiti Ram Hospital
(Moolchand Medcity)
New Delhi, India

Nilashish Dey
Fortis Escorts Heart Institute
New Delhi, India

Nilay S Nimbalkar
Director of Cardiac Imaging
Precision Scan and Research Centre
Nagpur, Maharashtra, India

Nilufar Fatema
Assistant Professor
Department of Cardiology
Bangabandhu Sheikh Mujib Medical University
Dhaka, Bangladesh

Nirmal Ghati
Assistant Professor
Department of Cardiology
Cardiothoracic Sciences Centre
All India Institute of Medical Sciences
New Delhi, India

Nirmal Kumar Mohanty
Professor
Department of Cardiology
Srirama Chandra Bhanja Medical College
and Hospital
Cuttack, Odisha, India

Nitish Kumar Parmar
Senior Consultant and In-charge
Department of Critical Care Medicine
Moolchand Kharaiti Ram Hospital
(Moolchand Medcity)
New Delhi, India

Nitish Naik
Department of Cardiology
Cardiothoracic and Neurosciences Center
All India Institute of Medical Sciences
New Delhi, India

NN Khanna
Senior Consultant
Department of Cardiology
Indraprastha Apollo Hospital
New Delhi, India

NR Shastry
Consultant Cardiologist
Medanta Moolchand Heart Centre
New Delhi, India

OP Yadava
CEO and Chief Cardiac Surgeon
National Heart Institute
New Delhi, India

Pallavi Prasad
Assistant Professor
Department of Nephrology
Vardhman Mahavir Medical College and
Safdarjung Hospital
New Delhi, India

Parveen Gulati
Director and Consultant Radiologist
Dr Gulati Imaging Institute
New Delhi, India

Pavithra Arumugam
Department of General Medicine
Sri Muthukumaran Medical College Hospital
and Research Institute
Chennai, Tamil Nadu, India

Payal Gupta
Consultant Dermatologist
Moolchand Kharaiti Ram Hospital
(Moolchand Medcity)
New Delhi, India

PC Manoria
Director
Manoria Heart and Critical Care Hospital
Bhopal, Madhya Pradesh, India

Peeyush Jain
Director, Noninvasive Cardiology
Head, Department of Preventive Cardiology
Fortis Escorts Heart Institute
New Delhi, India

Piyush Tak
Department of Cardiology
Rabindranath Tagore Medical College and
Maharana Bhupal Government Hospital
Udaipur, Rajasthan, India

Poonam Malhotra Kapoor
Professor (Cardiac Anesthesia and Critical Care)
Cardio Thoracic Centre
All India institute of Medical Sciences
New Delhi, India

Prabhakar Dorairaj
Preventive Interventional Cardiologist
Ashwin Clinic
Chennai, Tamil Nadu, India

Pradeep Jain
Senior Interventional Cardiologist
Indraprastha Apollo Hospital
New Delhi, India

Prashuka Jain
Consultant
Aku92 Clinics
Yamunanagar, Haryana, India

Prasit Maity
Attending Consultant
Department of Imaging
Fortis Escorts Heart Institute
New Delhi, India

Prayaag Kini
Senior Consultant Cardiologist
Sri Sathya Sai Superspecialty Hospital
Bengaluru, Karnataka, India

Preetinder Kaur
Senior Consultant Ophthalmologist
Moolchand Kharaiti Ram Hospital
(Moolchand Medcity)
New Delhi, India

Prerna Goyal
Deputy Medical Superintendent and
Senior Consultant Physician
RG Stone—Urology and Laparoscopy Hospital
Ludhiana, Punjab, India

Priti Meena
Department of Nephrology
All India Institute of Medical Sciences
Bhubaneswar, Odisha, India

Priya Jagia
Professor and Head
Department of Cardiovascular Radiology
All India Institute of Medical Sciences
New Delhi, India

Purshotam Lal
Director, Interventional Cardiology
Chairman
Metro Group of Hospitals
Noida, Uttar Pradesh, India

R Divya
Meenam Medicare Centre
Chennai, Tamil Nadu, India

Rabindra Nath Chakraborty
Senior Vice Chairman
Senior Consultant and Head of Cardiology
Manipal Group of Hospitals
Kolkata, West Bengal, India

Raghuram A Krishnan
Senior Consultant
Department of Cardiology
Baby Memorial Hospital
Kozhikode, Kerala, India

Rahul Grover
Department of Nephrology and
Renal Transplant Medicine
Max Super Specialty Hospital
New Delhi, India

Rahul Mehrotra
Chief—NIC and Clinical Cardiology
Artemis Hospital
Gurugram, Haryana, India

Rajeev Chawla
Senior Consultant Diabetologist and Director
North Delhi Diabetes and Cardiac Centre
New Delhi, India

Rajeev Garg
Senior Interventional Cardiologist and Head
Gleneagles AWARE Hospital
Hyderabad, Telangana, India

Rajeev Gupta
Department of Preventive Cardiology and Medicine
Eternal Heart Care Centre and Research Institute
Jaipur, Rajasthan, India

Rajeevalochana Parthasarathy
Consultant Nephrologist
Madras Medical Mission
Chennai, Tamil Nadu, India

Rajesh Janardhanan
Professor of Medicine and Medical Imaging
Medical Director, Noninvasive Cardiac Imaging
Director of Echocardiography
Sarver Heart Center
University of Arizona
Tucson, Arizona, USA

Rajesh Meena
Department of Medicine
Moolchand Kharaiti Ram Hospital (Moolchand Medcity)
New Delhi, India

Rajiv Passey
Department of Cardiology
Dharma Vira Heart Centre
Sir Ganga Ram Hospital
New Delhi, India

Rajneesh Malhotra
Vice Chairman and Head
Department of Cardio Thoracic and Vascular Surgery (CTVS)
Max Superspecialty Hospital
New Delhi, India

Rajpal Prajapati
Associate Professor
Department of Cardiology
Institute of Medical Sciences
Banaras Hindu University
Varanasi, Uttar Pradesh, India

Rakesh Varma
Professor and Chief Cardiologist
Former Director General of Health Services (Addl)
Former Physician to The Prime Minister of India

Ramesh Daggubati
Heart and Vascular Disease
West Virginia University
Morgantown, WV, USA

Ranabrata Sen
Consultant Cardiologist
Narayana Hospital—Rabindranath Tagore International Institute of Cardiac Sciences (RTIICS)
Kolkata, West Bengal, India

Ranjan Kumar
Consultant Cardio-Physician
Ranjan Heart Clinic
Patna, Bihar, India

Ranjan Modi
Senior Consultant Interventional Cardiologist
Sarvodaya Health Care
Faridabad, Haryana, India

Ratna Malika Kumar
Principal Consultant
Department of Cardio Thoracic and Vascular Surgery (CTVS)
Max Superspecialty Hospital
New Delhi, India

Ravi Prakash
Senior Consultant
Pushpawati Singhania Research Institute (PSRI)
New Delhi, India

Ravi R Kasliwal
Chairman—Clinical and Preventive Cardiology
Medanta—The Medicity
Gurugram, Haryana, India

Rekha Mishra
Consultant and Noninvasive Cardiologist
Indraprastha Apollo Hospital
New Delhi, India

Richa Kothari
Consultant Radiologist
Narayana Hrudayalaya
Bengaluru, Karnataka, India

Richard Raj R
Department of Cardiology
Sree Chitra Tirunal Institute for Medical Sciences and Technology
Thiruvananthapuram, Kerala, India

RJ Cecily Mary Majella
Professor
Department of Cardiology
Senior Interventional Cardiologist
Tamil Nadu Government Multi Super Specialty Hospital
Chennai, Tamil Nadu, India

Rohan Patel
Department of Cardiology
Dharma Vira Heart Centre
Sir Ganga Ram Hospital
New Delhi, India

Rohit Tandon
Consultant Physician
Dayanand Medical College and Hospital
Unit of Hero DMC Heart Institute
Ludhiana, Punjab, India

Rohit Walia
Head
Department of Cardiology
Maharishi Markandeshwar College of Medical Sciences and Research
Ambala, Haryana, India

Roopali Khanna
Professor
Department of Cardiology
Sanjay Gandhi Postgraduate Institute of Medical Sciences
Lucknow, Uttar Pradesh, India

Roshan Rao
Senior Interventional Cardiologist and Head
Department of Cardiology
Apollo Hospitals
Indore, Madhya Pradesh, India

Ruhani Bali
Senior Consultant Cardiologist
Deepak Heart Institute
Ludhiana, Punjab, India

Ruman Kugashiya
Senior Resident and DNB Fellow
Batra Hospital and Medical Research Centre
New Delhi, India

Rupender Saha
Department of Cardiology
All India Institute of Medical Sciences
Rishikesh, Uttarakhand, India

RVA Ananth
Department of Cardiology
Government Virudhunagar Medical College
Virudhunagar
Consultant Cardiologist
Jeyalakshmi Heart Centre
Madurai, Tamil Nadu, India

S Shanmugasundaram
Cardiologist
Billroth Hospitals
Chennai, Tamil Nadu, India

Sabarish Sankaran
Department of Cardiology
Narayana Institute of Cardiac Sciences
Bengaluru, Karnataka, India

Sachin Raiya
Department of Imaging
Fortis Escort Heart Institute
New Delhi, India

Sadanand Shetty
Sadanand Healthy Living Centre Ltd
Mumbai, Maharashtra, India

Sahil Garg
Consultant Nephrologist and
Transplant Physician
Amritdhara—My Hospital
Karnal, Haryana, India

Sameer Gupta
Senior Interventional Cardiologist
Group Director
Metro Group of Hospitals
Noida, Uttar Pradesh, India

Samuel Jebavaram
Consultant Cardiologist
Billroth Hospitals
Chennai, Tamil Nadu, India

Sanchita Sen
Loyola University Chicago
Stritch School of Medicine
Maywood, Illinois, USA

Sandeep Mahajan
Professor
Department of Nephrology
All India Institute of Medical Sciences
New Delhi, India

Sandeep Seth
Professor
Department of Cardiology
All India Institute of Medical Sciences
New Delhi, India
President, Indian Society for Heart and
Lung Transplantation
Fellow, European Society of Cardiology
Founder Editor-in-Chief, Journal of Practice
of Cardiovascular Sciences

Sandipta Ray
Consultant Interventional Cardiologist
Department of Cardiology
Manipal Broadway Hospital
Kolkata, West Bengal, India

Sangeeta Dhir
Department of Cardiac Sciences
Max Super Specialty Hospital
New Delhi, India

Sanil Omar
Resident Medical Officer
Fortis Escorts Heart Institute
New Delhi, India

Sanjay Mittal
Vice Chairman
Clinical and Preventive Cardiology and Research
Medanta—The Medicity
Gurugram, Haryana, India

Santanu Guha
Former Professor and Head
Government Medical College, Kolkata
Senior Consultant Interventional Cardiologist
Nightingale Hospital
Kolkata, West Bengal, India

Sarita Bajaj
Senior Consultant Endocrinologist
Former Director-Professor and Head
Department of Medicine
MLN Medical College
Prayagraj, Uttar Pradesh, India

Sarita Rao
Senior Interventional Cardiologist
Director, Cath Lab
Apollo Hospitals
Indore, Madhya Pradesh, India

Satish C Govind
Chief of Noninvasive Cardiology
Narayana Institute of Cardiac Sciences
Narayana Health City
Bengaluru, Karnataka, India

Satyanarayan Routray
Professor
Department of Cardiology
SCB Medical College and Hospital
Cuttack, Odisha, India

Satyendra Tewari
Professor
Department of Cardiology
Sanjay Gandhi Postgraduate Institute
of Medical Sciences
Lucknow, Uttar Pradesh, India

Saumitra Ray
Consultant Cardiologist
Manipal Hospitals and Woodlands Hospital
Kolkata, West Bengal, India

Saurabh Bagga
Consultant Cardiology
Fortis Hospital
New Delhi, India

Saurabh Bhardwaj
Junior Consultant
Indraprastha Apollo Hospital
New Delhi, India

SB Gupta
Ex-Consultant Physician Cardiologist
Asian Heart Institute, Mumbai
Former Head, Department of Medicine and
Cardiology
Central Railway Headquarters Hospital
Mumbai, Maharashtra, India

Shachi Kalyani
Moolchand Kharaiti Ram Hospital
(Moolchand Medcity)
New Delhi, India

Shaima Khaled Zakaria
Consultant
Department of Adult and Congenital Cardiology
Mahalla Cardiac Center
Ministry of Health
Teaching Stuff, Medical School
New Mansoura University
Mansoura, Egypt

Shashank Joshi
Senior Endocrinologist
Joshi Clinic, Lilavati Hospital
Mumbai, Maharashtra, India

Shashank Mohanty
Attending Consultant
Pushpawati Singhania Research Institute
(PSRI Hospital)
New Delhi, India

Sheikh Ubair Nabi
Consultant (Critical Care)
Moolchand Kharaiti Ram Hospital
(Moolchand Medcity)
New Delhi, India

Shibba Takkar Chhabra
Professor
Department of Cardiology
Dayanand Medical College and Hospital
Unit of Hero DMC Heart Institute
Ludhiana, Punjab, India

Shilpa Deshmukh Kadam
Interventional Cardiologist
Department of Cardiology
MGM New Bombay Hospital
Professor and Faculty
MGM Institute of Health Sciences
Mumbai, Maharashtra, India

Shoma Mukerjee Sharma
Senior Consultant Radiodiagnosis
Department of Radiology
Mahajan Imaging and Labs
Fortis Hospital
New Delhi, India

Shraddha Ranjan
Senior Consultant (Cardiology)
Jay Prabha Medanta Super Specialty Hospital
Patna, Bihar, India

Shradha Ranjan
Medanta Hospital
Patna, Bihar, India

Shruti Hegde
Division of Cardiovascular Medicine
University of Massachusetts Chan
Medical School
Worcester, MA, USA

Siddant Trehan
North Delhi Diabetes and Cardiac Centre
New Delhi, India

Siddhant Passey
Department of Internal Medicine
University of Connecticut Health Center
Connecticut, USA

Simit V Shah
Interventional Cardiologist
Smt SR Mehta and Sir KP Cardiac Institute
Mumbai, Maharashtra, India

Simmi Manocha
Director (Cardiology)
Accord Superspecialty Hospital
Faridabad, Haryana, India

Simran Kaur
Department of Nephrology and
Renal Transplant Medicine
Max Super Specialty Hospital
New Delhi, India

Simran Thakkar
Trainee/Registrar
Department of Endocrinology
Indraprastha Apollo Hospital
New Delhi, India

SK Kaushik
Chairman, Cardiac Sciences
GBH American Hospital
Udaipur, Rajasthan, India

SK Parashar
Senior Consultant Cardiologist and Director
Noninvasive Cardiac Laboratory
Heart Centre
New Delhi, India

SK Wangnoo
Senior Consultant
Department of Endocrinology
Indraprastha Apollo Hospital
New Delhi, India

Smadar Kort
Stony Brook University Hospital

Smita Mishra
Head
Department of Pediatric Cardiology
Human Care Medical Charitable Trust (HCMCT)
Manipal Hospital
New Delhi, India

SN Pathak
Senior Consultant Interventional Cardiology
Indraprastha Apollo Hospital
New Delhi, India

Sneha Garg
Associate Consultant
Max Super Specialty Hospital
New Delhi, India

Soneil Guptha
Adjunct Faculty
Department of Medicine
Rocky Vista University
Ivins, Utah, USA

Sonia El-Saiedi
Professor of Pediatric Cardiology
Cairo University Children Hospital
Director, Pediatric Cardiac ICU
Director, Cardiomyopathy Clinic, Egypt

Soumik Ghosh
Associate Professor
Department of Cardiology
Institute of Medical Sciences
Banaras Hindu University
Varanasi, Uttar Pradesh, India

Soumit Sharma
Medical Officer
Central Government Health Scheme
New Delhi, India

Sourabh Agstam
Assistant Professor
Department of Cardiology
All India Institute of Medical Sciences
New Delhi, India

Sreejith Parameswaran
Professor and Head
Department of Nephrology
Jawaharlal Institute of Postgraduate Medical
Education and Research
Puducherry, India

Sreelal Variar
Academic Senior Resident
Department of Cardiovascular Radiology
All India Institute of Medical Sciences
New Delhi, India

Srikanta Sharma
Senior Consultant (Medicine)
Kalinga Institute of Medical Sciences
Bhubaneswar, Odisha, India

SS Iyengar
Senior Consultant Cardiologist
Manipal Hospitals
Bengaluru, Karnataka, India

SS Mishra
Professor and Director
SOA University, Bhubaneswar
Professor and Director
Dhaneswar Rath Institute of Engineering
and Medical Sciences
(DRIEMS University) and Padmini Care Hospital
Cuttack
Director, Med-n-Heart Clinic
Cuttack, Odisha, India

Subhashis Chakraborty
Department of Cardiology
NRS Medical College
Kolkata, West Bengal, India

Subhasis Roy Chowdhury
Consultant Cardiologist and
Cath Lab In-charge
Manipal Hospitals
Kolkata, West Bengal, India

Sugandhi Gopal
Interventional Cardiologist
Founder Director
Carditek Medical Devices
Bengaluru, Karnataka, India

Suman Bhandari
Director
Department of Cardiology
Fortis Escorts Heart Institute
New Delhi, India

Sundeep Mishra
Vice Chancellor (President)
Director and Head
Department of Cardiology
National Institute of Medical Sciences
and Research
NIMS University
Jaipur, Rajasthan, India

Sunil Modi
Senior Consultant Cardiologist
Indraprastha Apollo Hospital
New Delhi, India

Sunil Prakash
Principal Director and Head
Department of Nephrology and
Renal Transplant Service
BLK Max Super Specialty Hospital
New Delhi
Max Hospital, Gurugram, Haryana, India

Sunil Raheja
Clinical Director and Director
(Internal Medicine)
Moolchand Kharaiti Ram Hospital
(Moolchand Medcity)
New Delhi
Former Director, General Health Services
Medical Superintendent
GB Pant Hospital Affiliated Maulana
Azad Medical College
New Delhi, India

Sunil Roy Thottuvelil
Consultant Interventional Cardiologist
Department of Cardiology
Aster Medcity
Kochi, Kerala, India

Sunil S Bohra
Senior Consultant
Apollo Hospitals
Bengaluru, Karnataka, India

Surender Himral
Consultant Cardiology
Himachal Heart Institute
Mandi, Himachal Pradesh, India

Suriyakanth
Assistant Professor of Cardiology
Interventional Cardiologist
Tamil Nadu Government Multi Super
Specialty Hospital
Chennai, Tamil Nadu, India

Sutapa Chaudhuri
Senior Consultant and Head
Department of Critical Care Medicine
Indian Spinal Injury Centre
New Delhi, India

Suyash Tripathi
Associate Professor
Department of Cardiology
Institute of Medical Sciences
Banaras Hindu University
Varanasi, Uttar Pradesh, India

Tanay Malla
The University of Pittsburgh
Dietrich School of Arts and Sciences

Tanymol Saju
Senior Physician
Emirates Health Services
UAE

Tapan Ghose
Senior Director and Head of Cardiology
Head (Clinical Research and Academics)
Research Advisor, Fortis CSR Foundation
Flt Lt Rajan Dhall Hospital
New Delhi, India

Thair Al Jumaily
Consultant Interventional Cardiologist
Fujairah Hospital, EHS
Fujairah, UAE

Tiny Nair
Head
Department of Cardiology
PRS Hospital
Thiruvananthapuram, Kerala, India

Uday M Jadhav
Cardiology, Cardiac CT and Cardiac MRI
Department
MGM New Bombay Hospital
Navi Mumbai, Maharashtra, India

Umesh K Pandey
Associate Professor
Department of Cardiology
Institute of Medical Sciences
Banaras Hindu University
Varanasi, Uttar Pradesh, India

Upendra Kaul
Dean (Academics and Research)
Batra Hospital and Medical Research Centre
New Delhi, India

V Amuthan
Emeritus Professor of Cardiology
The Tamil Nadu Dr MGR Medical University
Formerly Professor and Head
Department of Cardiology
Madurai Medial College, Madurai
Director, 4D Echo Lab
Jeyalakshmi Heart Center, Madurai
Senior Interventional Cardiologist
Vadamalayan Hospital
Madurai, Tamil Nadu, India

Vaibhav Shukla
Senior Interventional Cardiologist
Department of Cardiology
Apollo Hospitals
Indore, Madhya Pradesh, India

Vaidehi Mendpara
Division of Internal Medicine
Cleveland Clinic
Cleveland, OH, USA

Vaishnavi Venkatasubramanian
Consultant Physician and Transplant Physician
Asian Institute of Nephrology and Urology
Visakhapatnam, Andhra Pradesh, India

Vardhini Vijaykumar
Consultant Periodontist
Independent Consultant
Hyderabad, Telangana, India

Varun Anil Damle
Dr Mohan's Diabetes Specialities Centre
Chennai, Tamil Nadu, India

Venugopal Krishnan Nair
Senior Consultant Cardiologist
Department of Cardiology
SP Fort Hospital
Thiruvananthapuram, Kerala, India

Vidushi Bangia
Director
Department of Anesthesia
Moolchand Kharaiti Ram Hospital
(Moolchand Medcity)
New Delhi, India

Vijay Kumar
Department of Cardiology
All India Institute of Medical Sciences
Rishikesh, Uttarakhand, India

Vijay Kumar
Medanta Hospital
Patna, Bihar, India

Vijayadithyan Jaganathan
Division of Cardiovascular Medicine
University of Massachusetts Chan
Medical School
Worcester, MA, USA

Vijin Joseph
Consultant Cardiologist
Lisie Hospital
Ernakulam, Kerala, India

Vikas Goyal
Senior Cardiologist
Department of Cardiology
Paras Hospital
Gurugram, Haryana, India

Vikash K Maurya
DM Research Scholar
Department of Cardiology
Institute of Medical Sciences
Banaras Hindu University
Varanasi, Uttar Pradesh, India

Vikrant V Vijan
Vijan Hospital and Research Centre
Nashik, Maharashtra, India

Vineet Behera
Consultant Nephrologist
Professor (Medicine)
INHS Kalyani
Visakhapatnam, Andhra Pradesh, India

Vinodkumar BG
Physician
Billroth Hospitals
Chennai, Tamil Nadu, India

Vinod M Vijan
Senior Interventional Cardiologist
Department of Cardiology
Vijan Hospital and Research Centre
Nashik, Maharashtra, India

Vinod Mittal
Senior Consultant Diabetologist and Head
Centre for Diabetes and Metabolic Diseases
Delhi Heart and Lung Institute
New Delhi, India

Vinod Sharma
Senior Consultant Cardiologist
National Heart Institute
New Delhi, India

Vishal Agrawal
Specialty Registrar
Warrington and Halton Hospitals
NHS Foundation Trust, UK

Vishwas Gulati
Consultant
Department of Nephrology and
Renal Transplant Service
BLK Max Superspecialty Hospital
New Delhi and
Max Hospital
Gurugram, Haryana, India

Viswanathan Mohan
Dr Mohan's Diabetes Specialities Centre
Department of Diabetology
Madras Diabetes Research Foundation
Chennai, Tamil Nadu, India

Vitull K Gupta
Senior Consultant
Kishori Ram Hospital and Diabetes Care Centre
Bathinda, Punjab, India

Viveka Kumar
Principal Director and Chief
Catheter Laboratories
(Pan Max)—Cardiac Sciences
Max Super Speciality Hospital (East Block)
Saket, New Delhi, India

Vivudh Pratap Singh
Senior Consultant
Department of Cardiology
Fortis Escorts Heart Institute
New Delhi, India

VK Shah
Senior Interventional Cardiologist
SR Mehta Cardiac Institute, Mumbai
Sir HN Reliance Foundation Hospital
and Research Centre
Mumbai, Maharashtra, India

Wissam I Khalife
Division of Cardiovascular Medicine
University of Texas Medical Branch
Galveston, TX, USA

Yasser Sedky
Consultant Pediatric Cardiologist
Egypt

Yatin Mehta
Chairman
Medanta Institute of Critical Care
and Anesthesiology
Medanta—The Medicity
Gurugram, Haryana, India

Zakia Khan
Senior Consultant Cardiologist
Fortis Hospital
Mumbai, Maharashtra, India

Foreword

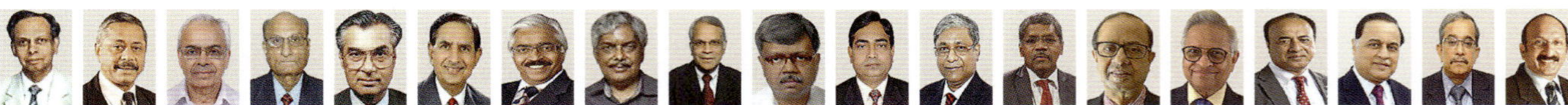

We are honored and have a great pleasure to write the foreword for the state-of-art *Advances in HFpEF Management (AHM) (CKM Navigation): Textbook of Cardiology*. The textbook on HFpEF was long due considering the wealth of data, new strategies of management, advances in diagnostic, prognostic and therapeutic technology based in the clinical practice in Cardio Kidney Metabolic Disorders. It is one of the most needed, comprehensive, illustrative, and well-structured book, published with enormous information about advances in clinical approach, imaging including echocardiography, multimodality imaging, drug, mechanical and surgical interventions for better patient's care in HFpEF-inflicted morbidity and mortality reduction in various clinical situations.

The book is an excellent and outstanding educational initiative by the joint efforts of 12 Editors-in-Chief, 33 National Principal Editors, 18 International Editors, 112 National Editors and over 300 contributing authors. This book comprises 21 sections, 169 chapters including Clinical Spectrum, Diagnostic Biomarkers, Echo and Imaging, Coronary Artery Disease, Arrhythmia, Hypertension, Congenital Heart Disease, Renal Disease, Critical and Emergency Care, Cardio-obstetrician and Gynecology, Cardio-ophthalmology, Cardiodermatology, Cardio-ENT and Cardiopulmonary Disease, Cardiodiabetes and Metabolic Disease, Cardiolipidology, Cardionutrition, Cardio-oncology, ECMO, Therapeutics including ARNI, SGLT2i, β-blockers, MRA, FCM, Semaglutide, Finerenone, Device Therapy; Rehabilitation, and Future Direction, etc.

The chapters are well outlined, structured, well written, and referenced. The writing style of every chapter is vivid, concise and practical. There are excellent graphics, tables, figures, and flowcharts that present the relevant information. The printing and binding are of excellent quality. This book represents a milestone for HFpEF management strategies, one of its kind from India to the world.

We congratulate the Editors-in-Chief Drs HK Chopra, Navin C Nanda, Jagat Narula, GS Wander, Sarita Bajaj, Viveka Kumar, Tiny Nair, CK Ponde, AK Pancholia, S Shanmugasundaram, Dinesh Khullar, Satyendra Tewari; National Principal Editors, International Editors, National Editors, and the Contributors for accomplishing this prodigious achievement of great clinical relevance in cardiology practice today for meticulous HFpEF management.

M Khalilullah
Director and Senior
Consultant Cardiologist
The Heart Centre
New Delhi, India
Past President, National CSI

Naresh Trehan
Chairman and
Managing Director
Medanta—The Medicity
Gurugram, Haryana, India

SC Manchanda
Senior Consultant
Department of Cardiology
Dharma Vira Heart Center
Sir Ganga Ram Hospital
New Delhi, India

SK Parashar
Senior Consultant Cardiologist
The Heart Centre
New Delhi, India
Past President, CSI, IAE

DB Pahlajani
Head, Department of
Interventional Cardiology
Breach Candy Hospital
Research Centre
Mumbai, Maharashtra, India
Past President, CSI

Kamal K Sethi
Chairman and
Managing Director
Director of Cardiology
Delhi Heart and Lung Institute
New Delhi, India
Past President, CSI

Ashok Seth
Chairman
Fortis Escorts Heart Institute
New Delhi, India
President, APSIC
Past President, National CSI

PK Deb
Former Chief, Cardiologist
ESI PG Institute of
Medical Sciences
Kolkata, West Bengal, India
Past President, National CSI

C Venkata S Ram
Director, Apollo Institute for
Blood Pressure Management
World Hypertension League/
South Asia Office
Apollo Hospitals
Hyderabad, Telangana, India
Texas Blood Pressure Institute
Dallas, Texas, USA

Santanu Guha
Professor and Head
Department of Cardiology
Medical College
Kolkata, West Bengal, India
Past President, National CSI

KC Goswami
Former Professor
Department of Cardiology
All India Institute of
Medical Sciences
New Delhi, India
Past President, National CSI

MK Das
Senior Consultant and
Interventional Cardiologist
CK Birla Hospital
Kolkata, West Bengal, India
Past President, National CSI

PP Mohanan
Director and Head
Department of Cardiology
Westfort Hi-Tech Hospital
Thrissur, Kerala, India
Past President, National CSI

Partha Sarathi Banerjee
Senior Consultant
Interventional Cardiologist
Columbia Asia Hospital
Kolkata, West Bengal, India
Past President, National CSI

Vijay Bang
Senior Interventional
Cardiologist
Lilavati Hospital and
Research Centre
Mumbai, Maharashtra, India
Past President, National CSI

PC Rath
Senior Consultant
Cardiologist and Head
Department of Cardiology
Apollo Hospitals
Hyderabad, Telangana, India
Immediate Past President
National CSI

Sanjay Tyagi
Senior Consultant
Cardiologist and Clinical Lead
Department of Cardiology
Apollo Hospitals Group
Northern Region
President, CSI

Dhiman Kahali
Director, Interventional Cardiology
BM Birla Heart Hospital
Kolkata, West Bengal, India
President-Elect, CSI and
Scientific Committee
Chair, CSI 2025
Editor, Cardiology Update 2025

Praveen Chandra
Chairman
Department of Cardiology
Medanta—The Medicity
Gurugram, Haryana, India

Preface

"Science knows no country, because knowledge belongs to humanity, and is the torch that illuminates the world."

—Louis Pasteur

Heart failure with preserved ejection fraction (HFpEF) has emerged as one of the most complex cardiovascular syndromes of the 21st century, challenging clinicians and researchers alike with its elusive pathophysiology and diverse clinical presentations. Once thought to be a less severe form of heart failure, HFpEF is now recognized as a distinct entity with its own diagnostic criteria, mechanisms, and therapeutic challenges. This textbook, *Advances in HFpEF Management (AHM) (CKM Navigation): A Textbook of Cardiology*, seeks to provide a comprehensive understanding of HFpEF, encompassing its history, evolving definitions, global and Indian scenarios, associated comorbidities, clinical spectrum, and therapeutic advancements.

The term HFpEF was first delineated to describe patients with clinical features of heart failure but preserved left ventricular ejection fraction (≥50%). Initially, this condition was often underdiagnosed due to the lack of clear criteria. With time, consensus guidelines from major societies such as the European Society of Cardiology (ESC) and the American Heart Association (AHA) have established diagnostic frameworks, including the use of echocardiographic parameters, biomarkers like N-terminal pro-B-type natriuretic peptide (NT-proBNP), and the HFpEF-specific diagnostic algorithms that incorporate scoring systems.

Globally, HFpEF accounts for nearly half of all heart failure cases. In India, the burden is steadily increasing due to a growing aging population and the rising prevalence of lifestyle diseases such as hypertension, obesity, and diabetes mellitus. In contrast to heart failure with reduced ejection fraction (HFrEF), HFpEF disproportionately affects older adults, particularly women, and is often characterized by a complex interplay of comorbidities such as atrial fibrillation (AF), chronic kidney disease (CKD), cardiovascular–kidney–metabolic syndrome (CKMS). These comorbidities not only contribute to its pathogenesis but also complicate its clinical course and management.

The clinical spectrum of HFpEF is broad, ranging from mild exertional dyspnea to acute decompensated heart failure. At its core lies diastolic dysfunction, but the underlying mechanisms extend far beyond impaired ventricular relaxation. Atriopathy, systemic inflammation, endothelial dysfunction, and the interplay of neurohormonal and metabolic factors have all been implicated. Emerging evidence also highlights the pivotal role of AF in precipitating HFpEF-related complications such as stroke.

Diagnosis requires a multimodal approach, combining clinical assessment with advanced imaging techniques including echocardiography, cardiac magnetic resonance imaging, CT scan, PET scan, etc., biomarkers, and invasive hemodynamic studies wherever necessary. The ESC and AHA guidelines provide detailed diagnostic echocardiographic and clinical algorithms, which emphasize the importance of diastolic stress testing and the identification of structural heart disease or elevated filling pressures.

HFpEF's complications, particularly atriopathy, contribute significantly to morbidity and mortality. The connections between AF, stroke, CKD, and HFpEF are becoming increasingly recognized, forming a vicious cycle that exacerbates outcomes. Prognosis remains poor, with high rates of hospitalization and mortality, underscoring the need for effective therapeutic strategies.

In recent years, therapeutic advancements have brought new hope for HFpEF patients. Sodium–glucose cotransporter-2 inhibitors (SGLT2is), such as dapagliflozin and empagliflozin, have demonstrated significant benefits in HFpEF populations, improving symptoms and reducing hospitalizations. SGLT2is are iconic molecules of the century and are game changers with enormous morbidity and mortality benefits. Recently, SGLT2is have documented lifelong benefits, thereby enhancing longevity. Similarly, glucagon-like peptide-1 receptor agonists (GLP-1 RA) such as semaglutide and dual agonists such as tirzepatide show promise in addressing the metabolic aspects of HFpEF, especially in obesity and metabolic syndrome as documented in the recent ESC algorithm. Established agents such as nonsteroidal mineralocorticoid receptor antagonists (NS-MRA), angiotensin receptor–neprilysin inhibitors (ARNis), and loop diuretics remain vital components of the treatment algorithm, complemented by lifestyle modifications, exercise training, and management of comorbidities.

The field of HFpEF management continues to evolve with ongoing research into novel pathways, including inflammatory modulators and endothelial stabilizers. This textbook aims to provide a holistic understanding of these advancements, guided by evidence-based algorithms and expert perspectives.

The contributors to this volume have brought together their expertise and experience to create a resource rich in knowledge and practical insights. Their dedication and efforts have made this textbook a repository of information, tailored to meet the needs of clinicians, researchers, and healthcare professionals striving to optimize patient care.

We extend our heartfelt gratitude to all the authors whose contributions have enriched this work. Your meticulous efforts, clinical acumen, and commitment to advancing the understanding of HFpEF have culminated in a textbook that we hope will serve as a valuable reference for years to come.

As you explore the pages of *Advances in HFpEF Management (AHM) (CKM Navigation): A Textbook of Cardiology*, we trust that this compendium will not only enhance your understanding of this complex condition but also inspire further research and innovation in its management. Together, let us illuminate the path to better care for patients with HFpEF, improving not only their survival but also their quality of life.

Our sincere gratitude extends to all the contributors and editors whose unwavering dedication and expertise have culminated in the realization of this edition. Their commitment to advancing the realm of cardiology is commendable, setting an exemplary standard for forthcoming endeavors.

We earnestly hope that *Advances in HFpEF Management (AHM) (CKM Navigation): A Textbook of Cardiology*, the first of its kind from India to the world, will serve as a catalyst for the progression and development of effective and innovative methodologies in managing HFpEF, thereby contributing to the betterment of the lives of innumerable individuals globally.

We have made every possible effort to maintain the quality and standard of advances in HFpEF management (AHM). We are sure that this book will serve as an important reference guide for postgraduate students, fellows, internists, cardiologists, neurologists, critical care specialists, pulmonologists, pediatricians, pediatric surgeons, cardiovascular surgeons, imaging experts, and nutritionists. Bringing up *Advances in HFpEF Management (AHM) (CKM Navigation): A Textbook of Cardiology* was a phenomenal task and requires well-structured team efforts with immense dedication, devotion, and coordination.

We express our gratitude to all the eminent cardiologists, including M Khalilullah, Naresh Trehan, GS Sainani, SC Manchanda, SK Parashar, DB Pahlajani, KK Sethi, Ashok Seth, PK Deb, C Venkata S Ram, Santanu Guha, KC Goswami, MK Das, PP Mohanan, Partha Sarathi Banerjee, Vijay Bang, PC Rath, Sanjay Tyagi, Dhiman Kahali, and Praveen Chandra for writing the foreword for this book.

We also express our thanks to each and every member of the Cardiological Society of India (CSI), manuscript contributors, industry, and our National Principal Editors, KK Talwar, G Vijayaraghavan, P Krishnam Raju, JPS Sawhney, Saumitra Ray, Rakesh Gupta, Ravi R Kasliwal, Poonam Malhotra Kapoor, KK Kapur, Vinod Sharma, Sandeep Bansal, NN Khanna, Rajeev Gupta, Nitin Burkule, Sameer Srivastava, SC Govind, Ajay Sinha, OP Yadava, V Amuthan, Aditya Kapoor, SS Mishra, IB Vijayalakshmi, Asha Moorthy, Priya Jagia, Mona Bhatia, Roopali Khanna, Sarita Rao, SN Routray, Harshwardhan, Sanjay Mittal, Ashwin Mehta, Manish Bansal, S Ramakrishan, and all the editors for their constant support.

We also express our thanks to M/s Jaypee Brothers Medical Publishers (P) Ltd, New Delhi, India, for publishing this book so well. We also thank Shri Jitendar P Vij (Group Chairman), Mr Ankit Vij (Managing Director), Mr MS Mani (Group President), Ms Pooja Bhandari [Director—Production (Books and Journals)], Ms Nikita Chauhan (Publishing Manager), Mr Ashwani Kumar Singh (Senior Manager), Ms Seema Dogra (Cover Visualizer), Mr Ashwani Kumar (Quality Controller), Mr Mohd Iqbal (InDesign Operator), and Mr Gopal Singh Kirola (Graphic Designer) for their help, guidance, and timely active intervention in composing, designing, and editing of the book.

Our sincere thanks go to Soban Singh, who worked really hard to keep the record of every minor and finer communication.

HK Chopra (India), Navin C Nanda (USA), Jagat Narula (USA)
GS Wander, Sarita Bajaj, Viveka Kumar, Tiny Nair, CK Ponde (India)
AK Pancholia, S Shanmugasundaram, Dinesh Khullar, Satyendra Tewari (India)

Preface

It is a great pleasure and honor to write the preface for the book *Advances in HFpEF Management (AHM) (CKM Navigation): A Textbook of Cardiology*, which is the brainchild of Dr HK Chopra. Because left ventricular ejection fraction is normal in practically half of patients with heart failure, not only the diagnosis but also the management of heart failure with preserved ejection fraction (HFpEF) patients have presented a unique challenge in the past. However, many recent advances in diagnosis and therapeutic aspects have occurred which have shone a new light in the management of these patients.

As many as 28 chapters in this book deal with echocardiography and HFpEF. Assessment of HFpEF using echocardiographic techniques such as three-dimensional echocardiography and more recent advances such as speckle tracking of echocardiography for assessment of left ventricular, left atrial, right ventricular, and right atrial strain are well covered in the book. Echocardiographic ventricular and atrial remodeling reversal with various therapeutic agents including sodium-glucose cotransporter-2 (SGLT2) inhibitors, angiotensin receptor–neprilysin inhibitor (ARNI), and bisoprolol is given due prominence. In addition, the use of echocardiography in guiding therapy and evaluating prognosis in HFpEF is well described. An interesting chapter deals with exercise-induced left atrial hypertension in HFpEF. The effect of various therapeutic agents on left atrial stiffness index, left atrial function, and other left ventricular diastolic parameters is also well discussed. The section also focuses on specific disease entities such as hypertrophic cardiomyopathy, amyloidosis, and sarcoidosis that lead to HFpEF.

All-in-all, this book provides a comprehensive coverage of recent advances in the use of various echocardiography modalities in the assessment of HFpEF.

Navin C Nanda (USA)

Preface

Preserved yet Puzzling: Puzzle of the Pandora's Pot of HFpEF

Pandora was created by the Olympian gods and her curiosity led her to open the forbidden box, and the story mirrors that of the Biblical Eve. In the grammatical terms, we have also used it not only as a symbolization of what happens when human curiosity gets in the way. However, the more we try to know, the more complex it starts to get. Heart failure with preserved ejection fraction (HFpEF) has emerged as one of the most complex challenges in cardiovascular medicine. Unlike heart failure with reduced ejection fraction (HFrEF), HFpEF is characterized by normal or near-normal left ventricular ejection fraction (LVEF) but significant clinical symptoms. Even though some progress has been made in therapeutic recommendations for HFpEF, substantial gaps remain in pathophysiology and management. We have year after year brought you a volume addressing the advances in a contemporary clinical problem and felt it to be a high time to gather all that is new in the HFpEF field, the remaining gaps, and the future directions. We were fortunate to bring together a galaxy of investigators from far and wide and believe that we have an offering that will provide you an interesting read and you would be as keen to open the pot as Pandora was!

It is not a unique disease, but HFpEF is a syndrome of heterogeneous origin with an interplay of systemic inflammation, endothelial dysfunction, microvascular dysfunction, and myocardial stiffness in an inexorable progression, invoked by a variety of comorbidities including obesity, diabetes, hypertension, and chronic kidney disease. It is being increasingly understood that the presence of systemic inflammation might play a central role linking adipose tissue inflammation, heightened cytokinemia, endothelial dysfunction, and impaired nitric oxide bioavailability with reduced microvascular coronary reserve and myocardial remodeling and stiffness, all culminating in diastolic dysfunction. It is a syndrome with diverse phenotypes, and a simple classification based on the presence or absence of LV dysfunction does not fully capture the complexity precluding the development of precision therapeutics. For instance, a patient with obesity and systemic inflammation may require altogether a different approach than one with postmenopausal hypertensive heart disease.

The therapeutic advancements in HFpEF have lagged those for HFrEF, until the introduction of sodium–glucose cotransporter 2 (SGLT2) inhibitors, when clinical trials such as EMPEROR-Preserved and DELIVER demonstrated substantial relief from repeated risk of hospitalization with worsening heart failure. The recent success of glucagon-like peptide-1 (GLP-1) agonists has fortified the fledgling hope. Although encouraging, the effect size of these interventions is modest, the impact on harder endpoints is at best minimal, and many patients continue to experience significant symptoms. Other pharmacological interventions, such as mineralocorticoid receptor antagonists (MRAs) and angiotensin receptor blocker and neprilysin inhibitors (ARNIs), have also shown only modest improvements. The role of device therapies has failed to live up to expectations.

Diagnosis of HFpEF remains challenging due to the lack of a definitive diagnostic test. We currently rely on a combination of clinical features, echocardiographic findings, and natriuretic peptide levels. These markers do overlap with other conditions, and there remains a need for greater consensus on diagnostic thresholds, especially in those with borderline LVEF or atypical presentations. The diagnostic algorithms have also witnessed progress in diagnostic approaches including cardiac magnetic resonance (CMR) with direct T1 mapping targeted at better definition of interstitial myocardial fibrosis and tissue characterization. The biomarkers such as soluble suppression of tumorigenesis-2 (sST2) and galectin-3 have allowed for somewhat better risk stratification. In addition, the use of machine-learning algorithms has promised to help integrate clinical, imaging, and biomarker repertoires to improve diagnostic accuracy. Future research is likely to focus on developing a more nuanced definition of HFpEF phenotypes, integrating multiomics to decipher molecular underpinnings and advanced artificial intelligence to help identify patient subgroups paving the way for precision medicine.

There is a need for interventions that target the underlying pathophysiology such as anti-inflammatory agents (e.g., IL-6 inhibitors), agents restricting myocardial fibrosis (e.g., galectin-3 inhibitors), and therapies aimed at improving mitochondrial function and hence myocardial metabolic efficiency. It is important that we investigate novel biomarkers and imaging techniques to better characterize HFpEF phenotypes and disease progression. Further refinement of CMR parametric mapping and automated echocardiographic analyses should improve diagnostic accuracy. Clinical trials would need to prioritize patient phenotyping and stratification to identify responders to specific therapies, especially incorporating real-world data and inclusion of in-silico and digital twin technologies to help bridge the gap between clinical research and routine practice.

In conclusion, HFpEF represents a persistently growing global health problem, underscoring the need for aggressive attention to care delivery. While SGLT2 inhibitors and GLP-1 agonists offer hope, much work remains to probe the Pandora's pot of multifaceted complexities. By hailing precision medicine, advanced diagnostic platforms, and targeted therapy, we must make strides in improving the lifestyle of patients suffering from this challenging problem.

Jagat Narula (USA)

The Editorial Board of
Advances in HFpEF Management (AHM) (CKM Navigation): A Textbook of Cardiology
Express their gratitude and thanks to the following Academic Partners

Platinum Academic Partner

IPCA Laboratories Ltd.

Gold Academic Partners

JB Chemicals and Pharmaceuticals Ltd.
Merck Ltd.

Silver Academic Partners

Eris Lifesciences Ltd.
Micro Labs Ltd.
Healthy Heart Society

Bronze Academic Partners

USV Pvt. Ltd.
Zydus Cadila Healthcare Ltd.
Mankind Pharma Limited
Marico Ltd.
Bayer India
KRBL Limited
Lupin Limited
Zydus Lifesciences Limited
Boehringer Ingelheim India Pvt. Ltd.
Osren Healthcare Pvt. Limited
Diabetes Education Foundation

Supporters

Emcure Pharmaceutical Ltd.
Apichem Healthcare
United Drilling Tools Ltd.
Triumph Technologies
Nutrabuff Nutraceuticals
Optimal Pharmtech
Lakshmi Medical Devices

For rendering unrestricted education support which made this book possible in its current enhanced form as "*Global Education Initiative in Cardiology*".

Contents

SECTION 1: HFpEF: CLINICAL SPECTRUM

1. **Regional Variation of Mortality in HFpEF Across Asia: Outcomes in the ASIAN-HF Registry** 3
   Abhishek Garg, Gautam Singal, Gurpreet Singh Wander
2. **Indian Heart Failure Registries: Focusing on HFpEF** 10
   Richard Raj R, Harikrishnan S
3. **Epidemiology of Heart Failure** 15
   Zakia Khan
4. **Cellular and Molecular Differences Between HFpEF and HFrEF: A Step Ahead in an Improved Pathological Understanding** 20
   Rohan Patel, Saurabh Bagga, JPS Sawhney
5. **Differentiation between HFpEF and HFrEF** 23
   Manoranjan Mandal, Biaus Samanta, Subhashis Chakraborty
6. **Advances in HFpEF Management** 30
   Mrinal Kanti Das
7. **Prevalence of Coronary Microvascular Dysfunction in HFpEF: A Systematic Review and Meta-analysis** 37
   Arijit Ghosh, Subhasis Roy Chowdhury, Arup Dasbiswas
8. **Evaluation and Management of HFpEF: New Dimensions** 43
   Ajay Kumar Sinha, Narendra Kumar, Vijay Kumar, Shradha Ranjan
9. **Diagnosis of HFpEF: Novel Insights** 53
   Soneil Guptha, Rajeev Gupta
10. **Diagnosis of HFpEF Among Patients with Unexplained Dyspnea** 60
    Harsh Wardhan, Isha Nandal, Archit Dahiya
11. **Application of Diagnostic Algorithms for HFpEF to Community** 64
    Kiran Rao Kanjerla, Dayasagar Rao V
12. **Diving into Diagnostic Score Algorithms of HFpEF** 72
    HK Chopra, Shachi Kalyani, Rajesh Meena, Neha Chaudhary
13. **HFpEF and COVID** 76
    Satyanarayan Routray, Nirmal Kumar Mohanty
14. **Vascular Biology in HFpEF** 80
    SS Mishra, BR Mishra, Asharam Panda
15. **Bendopnea in HFpEF: A Narrative Review** 85
    Tiny Nair
16. **Aging and HFpEF: Is There a Difference?** 87
    Sheikh Ubair Nabi
17. **Prognosticating and Palliating in Older Adults with HFpEF** 90
    SN Pathak
18. **Fat, Female, Fatigued: Features of the Obese HFpEF Phenotype** 94
    Vitull k Gupta, Meghna Gupta, Manpreet Singh Brar

19. **Mechanisms of HFpEF in Diabetes Mellitus** 100
Lakshmi Nalini Kopalle

20. **Nonpharmacological Therapies for HFpEF** 105
Dharmendra Jain, Vikash K Maurya, Umesh K Pandey, Suyash Tripathi, Soumik Ghosh, Rajpal Prajapati

21. **HFpEF Management: What are Newer Advances?** 111
Mohsin Raj Mantoo, Nitish Naik

22. **Role of Amyloidosis in HFpEF Trials** 115
Saumitra Ray, Ayan Kar

23. **Updates on HFpEF** 118
Sanchita Sen, Tanay Malla, Deepika Misra

24. **HFpEF: Scenario and Therapeutic Strategies** 125
Rakesh Varma

25. **Risk Stratification of SCD in HFpEF** 134
Ravi Prakash, Shashank Mohanty

26. **Guideline Update in HFpEF Pharmacotherapy** 137
Arindam Pande, Durlabh Debbarma

27. **HFpEF: Advances in Pharmacological Therapy and Clinical Trials** 147
Hemant Bareth, Manna Bhattacharya, Bijay Yadav, Sundeep Mishra

28. **HFpEF: New Guidelines are Pertinent for Primary Care** 165
Geevar Zachariah

29. **Advances in Optimizing HFpEF Management** 170
Santanu Guha, Debopom Goswami

30. **HFpEF Management: Recent Strategies** 178
PC Manoria

31. **Recent Advances in Management of HFpEF** 182
CK Ponde, HK Chopra

32. **Impaired Pressure Natriuresis and Its Clinical Implications: From Uncontrolled Hypertension to Heart Failure** 188
Anil Pareek, Franz H Messerli, C Venkata S Ram, HK Chopra, Mohsin Wali

33. **Exercise-induced Left Atrial Hypertension in HFpEF** 199
Jayagopal PB

34. **HFpEF and Left Atrial Cardiomyopathy: Advanced Therapeutic Navigation** 202
HK Chopra, Viveka Kumar, CK Ponde, Aafreen Naik

35. **Hypertrophic Cardiomyopathy: As a Mimicker of HFpEF in Consideration of ACC 2023 Expert Consensus Decision Pathway for HFpEF** 209
S Shanmugasundaram, Ilayaraja Uthirapthi, Samuel Jebavaram, Vinodkumar BG

36. **Management of HFpEF: Normalizing the Apparently Normal Heart** 214
Sarita Rao, Roshan Rao, Vaibhav Shukla, Abhishek Rathore, Achukatla Kumar

37. **HFpEF: Definition, Pathology and Newer Management Strategies** 221
Vinod Sharma

38. **Advances in Management of HFpEF: Chasing the Elusive "Jigsaw"** 233
Prayaag Kini

39. **HFpEF: As Multimorbidities Disease— Advances in Management** 255
Prabhakar Dorairaj, Samuel Jebavaram

40. **HFpEF to Acute Heart Failure: What is It? Management Strategies** 259
Tapan Ghose, Sutapa Chaudhuri

41. **Advances and New Dimensions in HFpEF Management** 265
Ranabrata Sen, Debabrata Roy

SECTION 2: HFpEF AND DIAGNOSTIC BIOMARKERS

42. **NT-proBNP: Diagnostic, Prognostic, and Therapeutic Implications** 275
Srikanta Sharma, Aayushi Gupta, Soumit Sharma, HK Chopra

43. **Multiple Plasma Biomarkers for Risk Stratification in Patients with HFpEF in Emergency** 279
Nitish Kumar Parmar, Sheikh Ubair Nabi

44. **Use of Color Scalograms in the Diagnosis of HFpEF** 284
Sugandhi Gopal

SECTION 3: HFpEF, ECHO AND IMAGING

45. **Role of Three-dimensional Echocardiography in the Assessment of HFpEF** 291
Vijayadithyan Jaganathan, Vaidehi Mendpara, Kousalya Rajendran, Shruti Hegde, Navin C Nanda, HK Chopra

46. **Effect of ARNI on Left Atrial and Left Ventricular Strain by Speckle Tracking Echocardiography in Heart Failure** 295
Vijayadithyan Jaganathan, Vaidehi Mendpara, Kousalya Rajendran, Navin C Nanda, HK Chopra

47. **Echocardiographic Evaluation of Atrial Function in HFpEF** 300
Mark Hellerman, Smadar Kort

48. **3D Echocardiography and BNP Screening in HFpEF** 305
V Amuthan, RVA Ananth

49. **Echocardiographic Evaluation of Atrial Fibrillation with Atriopathy and Thromboembolism** 319
Manish Bansal, Ravi R Kasliwal, HK Chopra

50. **Echocardiographic Remodeling Reversal with SGLT2i and ARNI in HFpEF** 327
Abdirahman Wardhere, Wissam I Khalife, Masood Ahmad

51. **Echocardiographic-guided Therapy in HFpEF** 332
Iniya Rajendran, Dennis Fong, Rajesh Janardhanan

52. **Echocardiographic Evaluation of Diastolic Functions Beyond Guideline** 339
Rohit Tandon, SK Parashar

53. **Echocardiography Evaluation of the Left Atrial Strain on Patients with SGLT2i and ARNI with HFpEF** 349
Amrish Agrawal, Vishal Agrawal, Thair Al Jumaily

54. **Echocardiographic Evaluation of Left Atrium and Mitral Annulus in HFpEF Patients on ARNI and SGLT2i Therapy** 355
Satish C Govind

55. **Atrial Strain: A Piece of the HFpEF Puzzle Found, but is It Yet in Place** 360
Aniruddha De

56. **Echocardiographic Evaluation of HFpEF in Emergency** 371
Rekha Mishra, Manisha Sharma

57. Echocardiographic Diagnostic, Prognostic, and Therapeutic Indications of E/e' and LAVI in HFpEF **383**
Naveen Garg, KK Kapur

58. Effect of E/e' in HFpEF Management on SGL2i, ARNI, and Beta-blocker Therapy **391**
Simmi Manocha, Naveen Garg, Naveen Sharma

59. Echocardiographic Variables on Cardiac Atrial and Ventricular Remodeling Reversal by ARNI and SGLT2i in HFpEF **399**
Ankush Sachdeva, Sanil Omar, AK Omar

60. Effect of SGLT2 Inhibitors and ARNI on Increased Left Atrial Stiffness Index in HFpEF **406**
Rahul Mehrotra, Mohit M Bhagwati, Anamika Roy

61. Atrial Dysfunction: Echocardiographic Evaluation in Patients with HFpEF and AF **411**
Hansa Gupta, Madhu Mary, Ranjan Kumar

62. Deciphering the Dilemma: Anticoagulation for HFpEF with AF **417**
Jabir Abdullakutty, Vijin Joseph

63. The Evolving Role of Nonimplant Interatrial Shunts in Managing HFpEF **419**
S Shanmugasundaram, Ilayaraja Uthirapthi, Samuel Jebavaram, Vinodkumar BG

64. Deterioration in RV Structure and Function in HFpEF Echocardiographic Evaluation **425**
Sunil S Bohra, Akash Jain, Prashuka Jain

65. Echocardiographic Evaluation of HFpEF in Oncology **432**
Manish Bansal, Ravi R Kasliwal, HK Chopra

66. Echocardiographic Evaluation of Left Atrial Stiffness Index and Right Ventricular and Right Atrial Strain in HFpEF **437**
Nilufar Fatema

67. HFpEF and Left Atrial Atriopathy: Advanced Therapeutic Navigation **447**
HK Chopra, Viveka Kumar, Anil Pareek, Anu Grover, Ruhani Bali

68. Computed Tomography Angiography in HFpEF **452**
Priya Jagia, Sreelal Variar

69. CMR Evaluation on Cardiac Remodeling Reversal after ARNI in HF **459**
Mona Bhatia, Karthika Gopal D, Prasit Maity, Amit Garg, Sachin Raiya

70. Cardiac Magnetic Resonance to Enhance Phenotypic Characterization of HFpEF **464**
Johann Christopher, Nilay S Nimbalkar, Richa Kothari

71. Focal and Diffuse Fibrosis in HFpEF: Cardiac Magnetic Resonance Evaluation and Outcomes **471**
Shoma Mukerjee Sharma, Harsh Mahajan

72. Role of CT Evaluation for Transcatheter Aortic Valve Implantation in HFpEF **480**
Anshika Gulati, Parveen Gulati

SECTION 4: HFpEF AND CORONARY ARTERY DISEASE

73. Dapagliflozin after AMI: Cardiometabolic Benefits (With or Without HFpEF) **489**
Jai Bharat Sharma, Kunal Mahajan, Surender Himral

74. Treatment of STEMI with HFpEF: Focusing on Mortality Benefits **494**
VK Shah, Simit V Shah

75. **ARNI Postpercutaneous Coronary Intervention in STEMI to Prevent HFpEF** 498
Sameer Gupta, Purshotam Lal

76. **CABG in LV Dysfunction and Heart Failure** 502
OP Yadava

SECTION 5: HFpEF AND ARRHYTHMIA

77. **HFpEF and Atrial Fibrillation: A Dual Challenge** 515
Arshad Nazir, Aditya Kapoor

78. **SGLT2i in HFpEF with AF with Stroke, Peripheral Vascular Disease** 519
NN Khanna, Saurabh Bhardwaj

79. **Lower Heart Rate Associated with Lower All-cause Mortality in HFpEF** 525
Shraddha Ranjan, Kartikeya Bhargava

SECTION 6: HFpEF AND HYPERTENSION

80. **Resistant Hypertension and HFpEF: Management Strategies** 533
Jostol Pinto, A George Koshy

81. **Role of ARNI in Resistant Hypertension with HFpEF** 539
Rohan Patel, Rajiv Passey, Siddhant Passey

SECTION 7: HFpEF AND PEDIATRICS

82. **HFpEF in Congenital Cyanotic Heart Diseases** 545
Yasser Sedky, Sonia El-Saiedi

83. **Pediatric HFpEF** 550
Hala Elmarsafawy, Shaima Khaled Zakaria

84. **Prevention of HFpEF in Children** 559
Smita Mishra

85. **HFpEF Management in Children** 567
IB Vijayalakshmi

SECTION 8: HFpEF AND RENAL DISEASE

86. **Sodium-glucose Cotransporter 2 Inhibitors in Chronic Kidney Disease and HFpEF** 581
Vishwas Gulati, Sunil Prakash

87. **Cardiovascular–Kidney–Metabolic Syndrome: Management Strategies** 587
Deodatta Chafekar, Neelima Chafekar

88. **Efficacy and Safety of Spironolactone in Patients with HFpEF and CKD** 592
Muthu Jayaraman, Rajeevalochana Parthasarathy

89. **Current Management of HFpEF in Chronic Kidney Disease: An Overview** 598
Dinesh Khullar, Narinder Pal Singh, Kulwant Singh, Simran Kaur, Anish Kumar Gupta

90. **Renal Safety and Efficacy of ARNI in HFpEF** 604
M Edwin Fernando, M Karthikeyan

91. **Cardiorenal Syndrome in HFpEF** 607
Vineet Behera, Madhuri Matta

92. SGLT2i in HFpEF in Patient with Diabetes and Chronic Kidney Disease 611
Garima Aggarwal, Amit Malik

93. Heart Failure in Chronic Kidney Disease: Conclusions from a KDIGO Controversies Conference 616
Arunkumar S, Sandeep Mahajan

94. Role of New Antihyperkalemic Agents in the Treatment of Patients with HFpEF and Chronic Kidney Disease 621
N Ramachandran, Sreejith Parameswaran

95. Efficacy and Safety of Steroidal MRAs in Patients with HFpEF and Chronic Kidney Disease 625
Vaishnavi Venkatasubramanian, Sahil Garg, Jasmine Sethi

96. Efficacy and Safety of Novel Nonsteroidal MRAs in Patients with HFpEF and Chronic Kidney Disease 629
Dinesh Khullar, Rahul Grover, Abhishek, Deepak Panigrahi, Anish Kumar Gupta

97. Role of IV Iron in Management of Patients with HFpEF and Chronic Kidney Disease 634
Megha Saigal, Priti Meena

98. Emerging Strategies in the Management of HFpEF in CKD: What does the Future Hold? 637
Manisha Sahay

SECTION 9: HFpEF, CRITICAL AND EMERGENCY CARE

99. Role of ARNI in Critical Care Patients with HFpEF 647
Aashish Jain, Yatin Mehta

100. HFpEF Care in an Intensive Care Unit 653
Bhavik Shah, Girish Sabnis, Sadanand Shetty

SECTION 10: HFpEF: CARDIO-OBSTETRICIAN AND GYNECOLOGY

101. Role of the ARNI and SGL2i in Women with HFpEF 659
Mohan Bhargava, Sneha Garg

102. Estrogen Deficiency in Postmenopausal Women: Harbinger to HFpEF 663
Shibba Takkar Chhabra, Prerna Goyal

103. Gender Differences in HFpEF Pathophysiology 668
Rupender Saha, Vijay Kumar, Bhanu Duggal

104. Obesity is Culprit in Heart Failure: Do not Miss HFpEF especially in Obese Women 675
RJ Cecily Mary Majella, Suriyakanth, Geetha Subramanian

105. HFpEF Risk Decreased with More Physical Activity Among Older Women 679
Geetha Subramanian, J Cecily Mary Majella, Karthikaa Saminathan, Pavithra Arumugam, Ganesan Manohar

106. Heart Failure in Women 683
Harshit Khare, Roopali Khanna

SECTION 11: HFpEF: CARDIO-OPHTHALMOLOGY

107. Retinal Microvascular Impairment in HFpEF 691
Krishna Vaitheeswaran, Preetinder Kaur, Monika Nadar

108. **Impact of Diabetic Retinopathy on Prognosis of Patients with HFpEF** 695
Monika Nadar, Krishna Vaitheeswaran, Preetinder Kaur

SECTION 12: HFpEF AND CARDIODERMATOLOGY

109. **Skin Autofluorescence as a Predictor of First Heart Failure Hospitalization in Patients with HFpEF** 699
Payal Gupta

SECTION 13: HFpEF, CARDIO-ENT AND CARDIOPULMONARY DISEASE

110. **Pulmonary Hypertension in HFpEF: Management Strategies** 705
Bhagwan Mantri, Tanymol Saju, Leyla Kedir Bereka

111. **Pulmonary Hypertension in HFpEF: Current Challenges and Promising New Therapies** 712
Agam Vora, Mangesh Tiwaskar

112. **Obstructive Sleep Apnea and Hypertension to HFpEF: Management Strategies** 718
Chanchal Pal

113. **Noise Pollution, Hypertension, and HFpEF** 721
Nidhi Dhawan, HK Chopra

SECTION 14: HFpEF, CARDIODIABETES AND METABOLIC DISEASE

114. **Metabolic Syndrome and HFpEF: Management Strategies** 729
Sarita Bajaj

115. **Diabetes and HFpEF: New Insights** 734
Varun Anil Damle, Viswanathan Mohan

116. **SGLT2i and Semaglutide in Cardiometabolic Syndrome with HFpEF** 739
Simran Thakkar, SK Wangnoo

117. **Obesity and HFpEF** 743
SS Iyengar

118. **Management of HFpEF: A Recent Approach** 748
Siddant Trehan, Rajeev Chawla

119. **Interplay Between HFpEF and Hypothyroidism** 752
Vinod M Vijan, Vikrant V Vijan, Gulshan B Tolani

120. **Role of Sodium–Glucose Cotransporter-2 Inhibitors in Patients with HFpEF** 758
Vinod Mittal

121. **Effect of SGLT2i on Cardiovascular Outcomes and Mortality in Type 2 DM with HFpEF** 766
Namrata Gaur, Dushyant Singh Gaur, Anu Gaur

122. **Cardiovascular Outcome Studies with SGLT2 Inhibitors on HFpEF** 772
Neeru Gera, Monashis Sahu

SECTION 15: HFpEF AND CARDIOLIPIDOLOGY

123. **HFpEF and Cardiolipidology** 777
Juhi Singh, Rohan Patel, JPS Sawhney

SECTION 16: HFpEF AND CARDIONUTRITION

124. Iron Deficiency and HFpEF with Atrial Fibrillation **785**
Rabindra Nath Chakraborty, Debopriyo Mondal

125. Malnutrition and HFpEF **789**
Preetinder Kaur, Krishna Vaitheeswaran, Monika Nadar

126. Ideal Edible Oil for Heart Health Among Indians **791**
Shashank Joshi

SECTION 17: HFpEF AND CARDIO-ONCOLOGY

127. The Role of ARNI in Doxorubicin-induced Cardiotoxicity and HFpEF **799**
Indu Bansal, Vikas Goyal, Harmesh Aggarwal

128. HFpEF After Chemotherapy: Management Strategies **804**
Kanika Sood Sharma, Aditi Tanwar, Jishnu Prem

SECTION 18: HFpEF AND ECMO

129. Extracorporeal Membrane Oxygenation and HFpEF **811**
Poonam Malhotra Kapoor

SECTION 19: HFpEF AND THERAPEUTICS

HFpEF and ARNI

130. Angiotensin Receptor Blocker and Neprilysin Inhibitor in HFpEF **825**
Bhavna Mastebhakti, Nilashish Dey, Peeyush Jain

131. Top 10 Take-home Messages from the ACC/AHA and HFSA on SGLT2 Inhibitor/ ARN Inhibitor in HFpEF **831**
Satyendra Tewari, Harshit Khare

132. Angiotensin Receptor-Neprilysin Inhibitor in HFpEF: Outcome Data **834**
Venugopal Krishnan Nair, Sunil Roy Thottuvelil

133. Patiromer in Hyperkalemia in HF and CKD and ARNI Use in HFpEF **839**
Asesh Haldar, DP Sinha

134. ARNI as In-hospital Therapy in HFpEF **844**
Uday M Jadhav, Shilpa Deshmukh Kadam

135. ARNI and MRA Combination in PARAGON-HF: Odd Couple or Dynamic Duo in HFpEF **849**
Suman Bhandari, Mohamad Akram

HFpEF and SGLT2i

136. Role of SGLT2 Inhibitors in HFpEF **853**
Nakul Sinha

137. SGLT2 Inhibitors in Acute HFpEF: Is It Time to Broaden the Horizon? **858**
Harshit Khare, Aditya Kapoor

138. Role of SGLT2 Inhibitors in HFpEF with Diabetes Mellitus **864**
Saumitra Ray, Mainak Mukhopadhyay

139. **Indication, Contraindication and Uniqueness of SGLT2i and ARNI in HFpEF** 871
HK Chopra, Md Inamul Haque, Sunil Raheja, Vidushi Bangia, NR Shastry

140. **Role of SGLT2i in HFpEF with Takotsubo Syndrome** 879
Sandipta Ray, Mainak Mukhopadhyay, Kajal Ganguly

141. **SGLT2i in HFpEF: Fighting the Enemy with a Newly Crafted Weapon** 882
Ashokan Nambiar, Raghuram A Krishnan

142. **Dapagliflozin with Sitagliptin in HFpEF and Diabetes** 886
Mohit Tayal, Ankit Tandon, Rohit Tandon

143. **SGLT2 Inhibitor and DPP-4 Inhibitor Combination in Diabetes Mellitus with HFpEF** 890
Sunil Modi, Ranjan Modi

144. **Left Atrial Failure in HFpEF: The Role of SGLT2is, ARNI, Bisoprolol, and MRAs** 894
Harinder K Bali, Navdeep S Sidhu

145. **Development of Treatment Selection Algorithm for SGLT2 Inhibitors in HFpEF** 898
Devesh Kumar, Nirmal Ghati

146. **Role of SGLT2 Inhibitors in Cardiac Remodeling Reversal: Beyond Glycemic Control in HFpEF** 902
Mukesh Sharma, Piyush Tak, SK Kaushik

147. **Role of SGLT2i in all Spectrum of HFpEF Management** 906
Arati Dave Lalchandani

HFpEF and Beta-blockers

148. **ACC/AHA Guidelines on Beta-blocker Use in HFpEF** 908
Ruman Kugashiya, Upendra Kaul

149. **Role of Bisoprolol in HFpEF with AF, Stroke, and Hypertension** 912
Pradeep Jain, Himanshu Jain, SN Pathak

150. **Morbidity and Mortality Benefits of SGLT2i, ARNI, and Bisoprolol in HFpEF with Atrial Fibrillation** 915
Dhiman Kahali

151. **Promise of Bisoprolol in HFpEF: Present Status** 919
Ameet G Sattur

152. **Role of Bisoprolol in Patients with HFpEF** 922
Kiron Varghese

153. **Beta-blockers in the Management of HFpEF: What is the Consensus?** 925
M Somasundaram, GV Senthilnathan, R Divya

154. **Use of Beta-blockers in Patients with HFpEF and Comorbidities** 929
Abdullah AS Majumder, AKM Monwarul Islam

HFpEF and MRA

155. **Mineralocorticoid Receptor Antagonist in HFpEF and Atrial Fibrillation** 935
Esha Chaudhary, Karishma Suri, Rohit Walia

HFpEF and FCM

156. **Global Data on Ferric Carboxymaltose in HFpEF** 939
SB Gupta

HFpEF and Semaglutide

157. **Semaglutide in Patients with Obesity and HFpEF with or without Diabetes and Prespecified Pooled Analysis of STEP-HFpEF and STEP-HFpEF-DM Trials** 942
AK Pancholia, HK Chopra

158. **Semaglutide in Obesity, HFpEF, and Diabetes Mellitus: STEP-HFpEF Trial** 949
Sanjay Mittal, Aparajita Kumar

HFpEF and Finerenone

159. **Finerenone in HFpEF with Chronic Kidney Disease: Hope or Hype** 957
Himanshu Verma, Pallavi Prasad

HFpEF and Device Therapy

160. **Heart Support Devices in HFpEF** 962
Atul Kaushik, Manbir Singh, Vivudh Pratap Singh

161. **MitraClip in Heart Failure in Patients on Angiotensin Receptor Neprilysin Inhibitors: When and How?** 967
Ramesh Daggubati, Abdul Subhan Talpur, Mustafa Sajjad Cheema

162. **Stage D HFpEF, Heart Transplantation, and Mechanical Circulatory Support** 972
Bhawna Mathur, Ratna Malika Kumar, Rajneesh Malhotra

163. **Drug Switch or Device: How do I Decide in HFpEF?** 977
Sabarish Sankaran, Meemansa Kashyap Buch, Bagirath Raghuraman

164. **Implant or No-implant, Interatrial Shunt for HFpEF Patients** 984
Ajay M Naik, Aarya A Naik, Aditi A Naik

165. **Renal Denervation: A Novel Treatment for Hypertension** 989
Viveka Kumar, Sangeeta Dhir, Mitendra Yadav

SECTION 20: HFpEF AND REHABILITATION

166. **Exercise Training and Rehabilitation in HFpEF** 995
Kushal Madan, Kavita Tyagi, JPS Sawhney

SECTION 21: HFpEF AND FUTURE DIRECTION

167. **Recent Advances in HFpEF** 1001
Aatish Rengan, Sourabh Agstam, Atit A Gawalkar, Sandeep Seth

168. **Ongoing Drugs and Device Trials in HFpEF** 1006
Rajeev Garg, Vardhini Vijaykumar

169. **Emerging Epidemic of HFpEF: Issues and Challenges in 2025 and Beyond** 1011
Abhishek Garg, Gautam Singal, Gurpreet Singh Wander

Index *1019*

SECTION 1

HFpEF: Clinical Spectrum

1. Regional Variation of Mortality in HFpEF Across Asia: Outcomes in the ASIAN-HF Registry
2. Indian Heart Failure Registries: Focusing on HFpEF
3. Epidemiology of Heart Failure
4. Cellular and Molecular Differences Between HFpEF and HFrEF: A Step Ahead in an Improved Pathological Understanding
5. Differentiation between HFpEF and HFrEF
6. Advances in HFpEF Management
7. Prevalence of Coronary Microvascular Dysfunction in HFpEF: A Systematic Review and Meta-analysis
8. Evaluation and Management of HFpEF: New Dimensions
9. Diagnosis of HFpEF: Novel Insights
10. Diagnosis of HFpEF Among Patients with Unexplained Dyspnea
11. Application of Diagnostic Algorithms for HFpEF to Community
12. Diving into Diagnostic Score Algorithms of HFpEF
13. HFpEF and COVID
14. Vascular Biology in HFpEF
15. Bendopnea in HFpEF: A Narrative Review
16. Aging and HFpEF: Is There a Difference?
17. Prognosticating and Palliating in Older Adults with HFpEF
18. Fat, Female, Fatigued: Features of the Obese HFpEF Phenotype
19. Mechanisms of HFpEF in Diabetes Mellitus
20. Nonpharmacological Therapies for HFpEF
21. HFpEF Management: What are Newer Advances?
22. Role of Amyloidosis in HFpEF Trials
23. Updates on HFpEF
24. HFpEF: Scenario and Therapeutic Strategies
25. Risk Stratification of SCD in HFpEF
26. Guideline Update in HFpEF Pharmacotherapy
27. HFpEF: Advances in Pharmacological Therapy and Clinical Trials
28. HFpEF: New Guidelines are Pertinent for Primary Care
29. Advances in Optimizing HFpEF Management
30. HFpEF Management: Recent Strategies
31. Recent Advances in Management of HFpEF
32. Impaired Pressure Natriuresis and Its Clinical Implications: From Uncontrolled Hypertension to Heart Failure
33. Exercise-induced Left Atrial Hypertension in HFpEF
34. HFpEF and Left Atrial Cardiomyopathy: Advanced Therapeutic Navigation
35. Hypertrophic Cardiomyopathy: As a Mimicker of HFpEF in Consideration of ACC 2023 Expert Consensus Decision Pathway for HFpEF
36. Management of HFpEF: Normalizing the Apparently Normal Heart
37. HFpEF: Definition, Pathology and Newer Management Strategies
38. Advances in Management of HFpEF: Chasing the Elusive "Jigsaw"
39. HFpEF: As Multimorbidities Disease—Advances in Management
40. HFpEF to Acute Heart Failure: What is It? Management Strategies
41. Advances and New Dimensions in HFpEF Management

CHAPTER

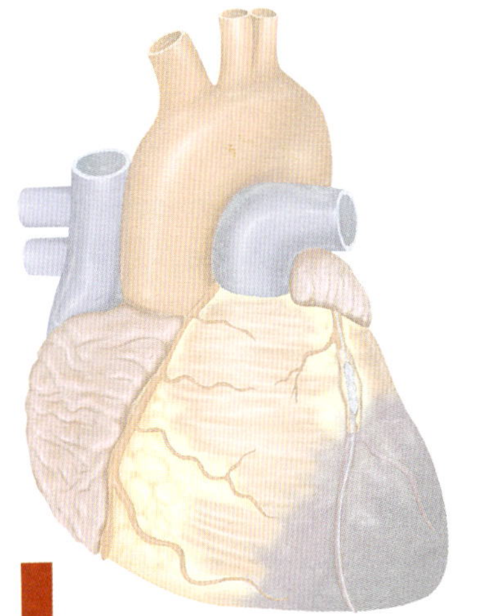

Regional Variation of Mortality in HFpEF Across Asia: Outcomes in the ASIAN-HF Registry

Abhishek Garg, Gautam Singal, Gurpreet Singh Wander

INTRODUCTION

Heart failure (HF) with preserved ejection fraction (HFpEF) is emerging as a critical global public health issue and is becoming the more prevalent form of HF in the aging population adding significantly to mortality and morbidity.[1] The high prevalence of cardiovascular risk factors throughout Asia is a harbinger of the upcoming HFpEF epidemic in the continent. Currently, there is a lack of extensive data on the Asian HFpEF phenotype.[1] This chapter aims to outline the baseline clinical and mortality variation of HFpEF patients within the prospective multinational Asian Sudden Cardiac Death in Heart Failure (ASIAN-HF) registry, which is the first comprehensive pan-Asian registry for HF data. Additionally, this study showed that Asian HFpEF patients are different from their Western counterparts.

SUBJECTS IN ASIAN-HF STUDY

ASIAN-HF was a prospective observational registry of Asians aged more than 18 years of patients with symptomatic HF which was defined by at least one episode of decompensated HF in the preceding 6 months resulting in hospitalization or outpatient treatment.[2] The recruitment of Asian patients occurred in two phases. In the first stage, patients with heart failure and reduced ejection fraction (HFrEF; EF <40%) were recruited. Patients with HFpEF (EF ≥50%) were recruited during the second phase, which overlapped with the first.[2] In this chapter, we primarily focus on HFpEF. A total of 1,204 patients with HFpEF were recruited from 46 medical centers across 11 Asian regions, grouped as Northeast Asia (China, Hong Kong, Japan, Korea, Taiwan), Southeast Asia (Malaysia, Singapore, Thailand, Philippines, Indonesia), and South Asia (India) with informed consent and included both private and public hospitals, as well as university, tertiary, and cardiovascular specialty hospitals in the capital and provincial cities.[2] Patients were excluded if they had significant valve disease as the main reason for heart failure, had any critical comorbidity with a life expectancy of less than 1 year, were unable or unwilling to provide consent, or were simultaneously enrolled in a clinical therapeutic trial.

Outcome data were available for 1,112 patients (92%), while 92 patients (8%) were lost to follow-up.[2] For patients with outcome data available for less than 1 year, their data were censored at the date of their last known visit. An independent committee was responsible for adjudicating the outcomes.[2]

Results

Demographic Results

Among 1,204 patients with HFpEF, 543 (45%) were from Northeast Asia, 252 (21%) were from South Asia, and 409 (34%) were from Southeast Asia **(Table 1)**. The average age was 68.4 ± 12.3 years, with 37% of patients being under 65 years.[2] Nearly half of the patients (49.6%) were women. The mean BMI was 27.1 ± 6.0 kg/m^2, with 34% classified as overweight, 26% as obese, and 3% as underweight. Most patients (59%) were classified as NYHA class II, while 24% were in NYHA class III/IV. The average systolic blood pressure was 132 ± 22 mm Hg. The most common

TABLE 1: Variable of patients with HFpEF in ASIAN-HF.[1]

	Overall	*Northeast Asia*	*South Asia*	*Southeast Asia*	*p-value*
n	*1,204*	*543*	*252*	*409*	
Demographics Age (years)	68.4 (12.3)	71.6 (11.7)	63.4 (12.5)	67.4 (11.6)	<0.001*
Women	597 (49.6)	275 (50.6)	118 (46.8)	204 (49.9)	0.6
NYHA class					<0.001*
I	163 (16.6)	37(9.3)	51 (27.9)	75 (18.7)	
II	582 (59.4)	240(60.6)	87 (47.5)	255 (63.6)	
III	209 (21.3)	102 (25.8)	42 (23.0)	65 (16.2)	
IV	26 (2.7)	17 (4.3)	3 (1.6)	6 (1.5)	
Body mass index (kg/m^2)	27.1 (6.0)	25.7(5.5)	28.1 (6.1)	28.2 (6.2)	<0.001*
LVEF (%)	60 (55–65)	63 (56–69)	60 (55–60)	60 (55–65)	<0.001*
Inpatients	457 (38.0)	125 (23.0)	103(40.9)	229 (56.0)	<0.001*
Previous hospitalization	691 (57.4)	239(44.0)	134(53.2)	318 (77.8)	<0.001*
Symptoms and signs of HF					
Orthopnea	182 (15.1)	66 (12.2)	22 (8.8)	94 (23.0)	<0.001*
Paroxysmal nocturnal dyspnea	125 (10.4)	47 (8.7)	19 (7.6)	59 (14.5)	0.004*
Elevated JVP	123 (10.3)	34 (6.3)	14 (5.6)	75 (18.4)	<0.001*
Peripheral edema	386 (32.2)	166 (30.6)	37 (14.9)	183 (45.0)	<0.001*
Pulmonary rales	183 (15.3)	55 (10.1)	19 (7.7)	109 (26.7)	<0.001*
Previous medical history					
CAD	347 (29.3)	144 (26.5)	54 (22.9)	149 (36.7)	<0.001*
Diabetes	536 (45.1)	214 (39.4)	68 (28.8)	254 (62.1)	<0.001*
Stroke	96 (8.1)	46 (8.5)	4 (1.7)	46 (11.2)	<0.001*
Atrial fibrillation	338 (28.5)	193 (35.5)	17 (7.2)	128 (31.3)	<0.001*
Hypertension	843 (71.0)	409 (75.3)	95 (40.3)	339 (82.9)	<0.001*
Smoker (current/former)	275 (23.2)	133 (24.5)	11 (4.7)	131 (32.1)	<0.001*
Alcohol (current/former)	180 (15.2)	94 (17.3)	11 (4.7)	75 (18.4)	<0.001*
CKD (eGFR <60 mL/min)	481 (50.4)	207 (44.3)	45 (41.3)	229 (60.4)	<0.001*

*Significant after correction for multiple comparisons using a false discovery rate of 0.05.

presenting symptoms of HF were shortness of breath on exertion (59.7%) and decreased exercise tolerance (58.5%). Prevalence of comorbidities was high with 70% of patients having two or more comorbid conditions. The most common comorbidities included hypertension (71%), anemia (57%), CKD (50%), diabetes (45%), CAD (29%), a history of AF (29%), and obesity (26%). Natriuretic peptide levels were measured in a subset of 455 patients, and 90% of these had values above the guideline-recommended cutoff points. There was no significant difference in levels of measured natriuretic peptides among geographic regions ($p = 0.261$). Baseline ECGs revealed atrial fibrillation in 23.6% of cases, with a mean QRS duration of 97.8 ms and left bundle branch block in 3.3% of patients. Medications included the use of diuretics in 70.9% of patients, angiotensin-converting enzyme (ACE) inhibitors or angiotensin II receptor blockers (ARBs) in 66.4%, beta-blockers in 67.7% and mineralocorticoid receptor antagonists (MRAs) were prescribed to 21.5% **(Table 1)**.

Patient Profiles by Region

Patients from South Asia were the youngest with a mean age of 63.4 ± 12.5 years, while those from Northeast Asia were the oldest, averaging 71.6 ± 11.7 years. Southeast Asians had an intermediate average age of 67.4 ± 11.6 years ($p < 0.001$). Systolic blood pressure was lowest among

Northeast Asians (131 ± 21 mm Hg) and highest among Southeast Asians (135 ± 24 mm Hg; $p = 0.021$). The mean BMI was lowest in Northeast Asians (25.7 ± 5.5 kg/m^2) and highest in Southeast Asians (28.2 ± 6.2 kg/m^2; $p < 0.001$). Southeast Asians exhibited significantly more symptoms such as dyspnea at rest, orthopnea, and peripheral edema as compared to South Asians and Northeast Asians. The use of ACE inhibitors/ARBs, beta-blockers, and diuretics was least common among South Asians and most frequent among Southeast Asians. Hypertension was most prevalent in Southeast Asians (82.9%) and least prevalent in South Asians (40.3%). The prevalence of CAD was more in Southeast Asians (36.7%) and least frequent in South Asians (22.9%). CKD was most common in Southeast Asians (60.4%), followed by Northeast Asians (44.3%) and South Asians (41.3%) ($p < 0.001$). Anemia was present in 57.4% of the total cohort, with the highest prevalence among South Asians (60.0%) and Southeast Asians (63.6%) ($p = 0.002$). Obesity (BMI ≥ 30 kg/m^2) was most prevalent in South Asia (36.2%) and least prevalent in Northeast Asia (16.5%; $p < 0.001$).

REGIONAL MORTALITY DIFFERENCES IN HFpEF ACROSS ASIA

One-year crude all-cause mortality due to HFpEF was 60 (5.4%), including deaths from cardiovascular, noncardiovascular, and unknown causes (53.3 and 23.3%, respectively). Mortality at 1 year was higher in hospitalized patients compared to outpatients (8.3 vs. 3.7%). In Southeast Asia, the mortality rate was the highest at 10.3%, with more than half of the deaths attributed to cardiovascular causes **(Fig. 1 and Table 2)**. Both South Asia and Northern Asia had a mortality rate of 2%. Further analysis of cardiovascular deaths revealed **(Table 3)** that in Southeast Asia, the most common cause was acute myocardial infarction (13.6%), followed by sudden death and heart failure, both with an incidence of 9.1%. In Northeast Asia, heart failure was the leading cause of cardiovascular death (71.4%). In South Asia, heart failure, acute myocardial infarction, and stroke each contributed equally to cardiovascular deaths (33.3%).

After multivariable analysis, it was found that regional differences influenced the relationship between key factors and mortality. Enrolments as an inpatient were associated with significantly worse outcomes in Northeast and South Asia, but not in Southeast Asia. This could suggest that inpatients in Southeast Asia may not be as critically ill as those in Northeast and South Asia, or it could be attributed to the higher enrolment of inpatients from Singapore and Malaysia, where advanced tertiary care is available. Importantly, in South Asia, AF was linked to a significantly higher risk of death compared to other regions. This finding is exciting given the much lower prevalence of AF in South Asia.

Mortality and Hospitalized for Heart Failure

Among the 891 patients who completed the 1-year follow-up, 129 (14.5%) either died or were hospitalized due to HF.[1] The rate of deaths and hospitalization for heart

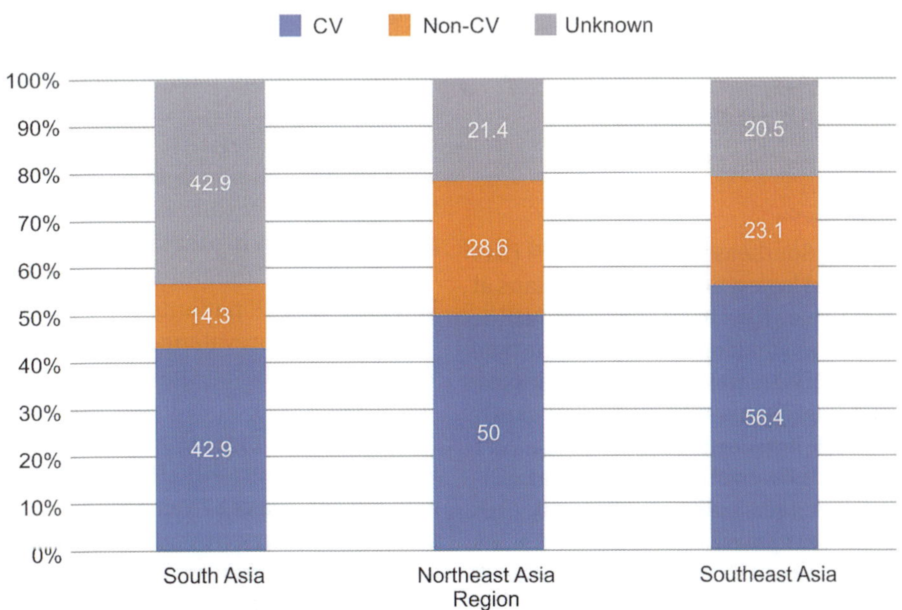

Fig. 1: Regional 1-year specific mortality rates.[2]

TABLE 2: 1-year mortality rates in ASIAN-HF for HFpEF.[2]

HFpEF					
All-cause death			*CV death*	*Non-CV death*	*Unknown*
n		*n (%)*	*n (%)*	*n (%)*	*n (%)*
ASIAN-HF	1,114	60 (5.4)	32 (53.3)	14 (23.3)	14 (23.3)
By region					
South Asia	242	7 (2.9)	3 (42.9)	1 (14.3)	3 (42.9)
Northeast Asia	495	14 (2.8)	7 (50.0)	4 (28.6)	3 (21.4)
Southeast Asia	377	39 (10.3)	22 (56.4)	9 (23.1)	8 (20.5)
By enrolment status					
Inpatient	410	34 (8.3)	17 (50.0)	9 (26.5)	8 (23.5)
Outpatient	704	26 (3.7)	15 (5.7)	5 (19.2)	6 (23.1)

(CV: cardiovascular)

TABLE 3: 1-year-specific mortality rates in ASIAN-HF for HFpEF.[2]

HFpEF			
No. of cardiovascular death	South Asia	North Asia	Southeast Asia
	3	7	22
Specific cause of cardiovascular death			
Sudden death	0	2 (28.6)	2 (9.1)
HF death	1 (33.3)	5 (71.4)	2 (9.1)
AMI death	1 (33.3)	0	3 (13.6)
Stroke death	1 (33.3)	0	1 (4.6)
Cardiovascular hemorrhage death	0	0	2 (9.1)
Other cardiovascular death	0	0	12 (55.5)

(AMI: acute myocardial infarction; HF: heart failure)

failure was highest among Southeast Asians at 25.4% (345 per 1,000 person-years) and lowest among South Asians at 4.5% (55 per 1,000 person-years) ($p < 0.001$).[1] After adjusting for age, sex, previous HF hospitalization, enrolment type (inpatient or outpatient), NYHA class, AF, CAD, diabetes, and hypertension, Southeast Asians still had a significantly higher risk of death or HF hospitalization within 1 year [hazard ratio (HR) 2.68, 95% confidence interval (CI) 1.72–4.17], while South Asians had a similar risk (HR 0.77, 95% CI 0.36–1.66) compared to Northeast Asians **(Figs. 2A and B)**.[1] For all-cause mortality alone, Southeast Asians had significantly worse outcomes (HR 3.86, 95% CI 2.00–7.46) compared to East Asians. South Asians were hospitalized less frequently for HF (HR 0.14, 95% CI 0.14–0.22) but did not exhibit lower mortality rates (HR 1.32, 95% CI 0.49–3.57).[1] When examining ethnic differences, Malays had the poorest outcomes (HR 2.13, 95% CI 1.34–3.37) compared to Chinese even after adjusting comorbidities as mentioned above.[1]

ALIGNMENT WITH PRIOR RESEARCH

This study was the first prospective, multinational examination of HFpEF patients across Asia. Compared to their Western counterparts, Asian HFpEF patients were generally younger (with over a third under 65 years) and less obese (only 20% were obese) **(Box 1)**.[1] Despite their relative youth and lower obesity rates, they had a high burden of comorbidities, with 70% having two or more comorbidities.[1] Significant regional differences were observed in comorbidity types, cardiac remodeling, and HFpEF outcomes across Asia. South Asians were the youngest group and more frequently obese, but they had the lowest incidence of AF despite showing the most concentric LV hypertrophy.[1] Southeast Asians were slightly older and had the highest rates of comorbidities (excluding AF), the most LV hypertrophy, and the worst outcomes.[1] Northeast Asians were the oldest, had the highest prevalence of AF, and exhibited eccentric LV hypertrophy.[1] In terms of ethnicity, Indian and Malay patients with HFpEF were markedly younger than their Chinese and Japanese/Korean counterparts. Despite their youth, Malay patients had very high rates of obesity, CKD, diabetes, and anemia, resulting in the worst outcomes compared to other ethnic groups **(Box 2)**.[1]

Previous research from the ADHERE Asia Pacific registry showed that Asian patients were younger and had lower rates of CAD and AF than their American counterparts in the US ADHERE registry; however, specific data on HFpEF were lacking.[3] Research by Guo et al.[4] in Northeast China found a 3.5% prevalence of HFpEF among the general population, with higher rates of obesity and hypertension. A study from Kumamoto region, Japan, revealed that Japanese HFpEF patients were significantly younger, yet had a similar prevalence of hypertension compared to Western patients.[5] Despite the age differences, rates of key comorbidities such as hypertension, CKD, and diabetes mellitus were comparable between ASIAN-HF patients and Western patients with HFpEF. Southeast Asian patients, with a mean age of 67 years, had a striking 62% prevalence of diabetes. In contrast, the prevalence of AF was notably lower in Asian patients compared to Western cohorts,[6-8] likely due to the younger age and lower obesity rates in the ASIAN-HF population. The highest prevalence of AF was

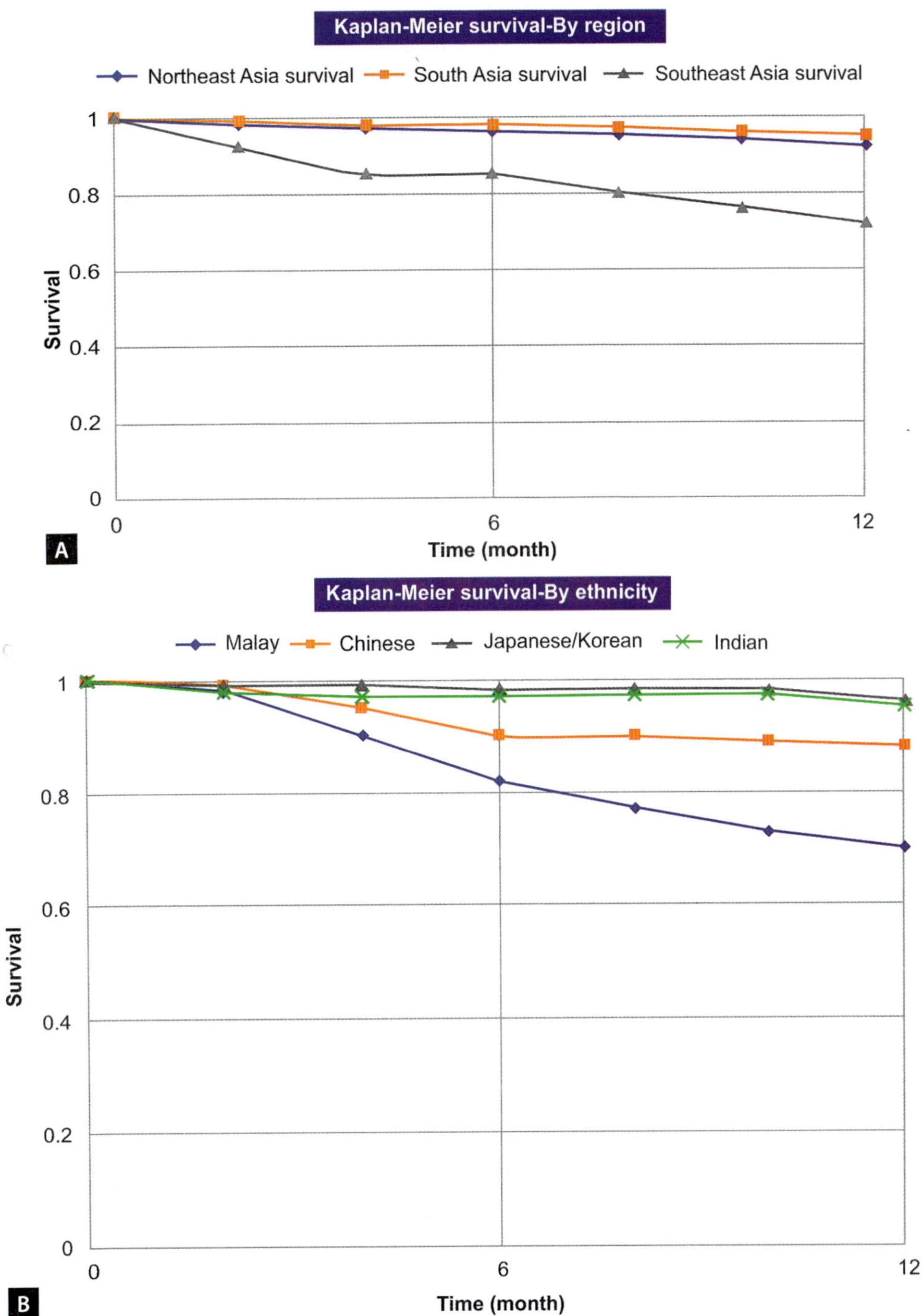

Figs. 2A and B: The trends of mortality and heart failure by (A) Region and (B) Ethnicity.[1]

observed among Japanese/Korean patients, while Indians had the lowest prevalence despite having the highest rates of obesity and concentric LV hypertrophy. This low prevalence of AF among Indians aligns with previous reports and suggests that Indian ethnicity may offer some protection against AF. Studies from the UK have shown that South Asians have a 70% lower risk of developing AF despite a higher burden of risk factors. Furthermore, research from Trivandrum, India,[9] demonstrated very low rates of AF among HF patients.

Compared to Western registries (e.g., SWEDE-HF,[6] ADHERE-HF,[7] and GWTG-HF[8]) Asian HFpEF patients are nearly a decade younger **(Table 4)**. Despite their younger age, Asian HFpEF patients had a high prevalence

BOX 1: Unique aspect of heart failure in Asians.

- Younger onset (a decade earlier)
- Less obese
- High burden of comorbidities: Diabetes, CKD
- Underdiagnosis of HFpEF
- Low awareness, treatment

BOX 2: Peculiar aspect of South Asians relative to other regions in Asia.

- Younger
- More obese
- Low prevalence of AF
- Least prevalence of hypertension, diabetes mellitus, smoking
- Less frequent hospitalization for heart failure
- Less use of guideline-directed medical therapy

TABLE 4: Comparison of ASIAN-HF with global registries of HF.[1]

Study	*n*	*Type of study*	*Age (years)*	*Men (%)*	*NYHA Class I/II/III/IV (%)*	*LVEF (%)*	*SBP (mm Hg)*	*BMI (kg/m²)*	*HTN (%)*	*CAD (%)*	*DM (%)*	*CKD (%)*	*AF (%)*	*Type of outcome*
ASIAN-HF[2]	1,204	Registry	68.4	50.4	17/59/21/3	60	132.2	27.1	71	29	45	50	29	Composite
SWEDE-HF[6]	9,140	Registry	77.5	45.4	16/45/35/3	NA	133.4	27.5	64	44	26	55	60	NA
ADHERE-HF[7]	26,322	Registry	73	38	NA	NA	152.5	NA	77	50	45	26	21	In-hospital mortality
GWTG-HF[8]	18,897	Registry	82	32.7	NA	60	126	27.4	81	45	41	20	41	Composite

(ADHERE-HF: acute decompensated heart failure; GWTG-HF: get with the guidelines; SWEDE-HF: swedish heart failure)

of comorbidities, particularly CKD, diabetes, and hypertension. The outcomes for Asian HFpEF patients were generally better than those observed in Western HFpEF populations from the GWTG-HF registries. It is important to note that GWTG-HF primarily involved patients hospitalized for acute heart failure or exacerbations of symptoms, which suggests that these groups were more severely ill compared to the ASIAN-HF cohort. Within the Asian cohort, Southeast Asian HFpEF patients had notably worse outcomes compared to those from Northeast Asia. A recent analysis from the INTER-CHF registry,[10] which mainly included HFrEF patients, found that Chinese HF patients had better outcomes than their Southeast Asian counterparts, which aligns with the ASIAN-HF registry for HFpEF. On the other hand, the INTER-CHF study reported poorer outcomes for Indian patients, likely due to their inclusion from more rural settings compared to the ASIAN-HF cohort and the predominance of HFrEF patients in the INTER-CHF registry.[10]

CONCLUSION

The marked differences in mortality observed in ASIAN-HF can only be partially attributed to variations in patient demographics, comorbidities, and treatment approaches. After multivariable adjustment, these measurable factors explain less than half of the differences in mortality risk. The bulk of regional mortality variation is likely due to unmeasured factors, including disparities in healthcare infrastructure, delays in seeking medical attention, and inconsistencies in healthcare access and quality. This is evident from the fact that countries with the weakest healthcare systems exhibit the highest mortality rates. Genetic, environmental, and cultural influences may also play significant roles. Therefore, focusing on addressing and identifying these unmeasured factors, along with enhancing regional and national healthcare infrastructure and organization, could significantly improve survival outcomes for patients with heart failure in Asia.

REFERENCES

1. Tromp J, Teng TH, Tay WT, et al. Heart failure with preserved ejection fraction in Asia. Eur J Heart Fail. 2019;21(1):23-36.
2. MacDonald MR, Tay WT, Teng TH, et al. Regional variation of mortality in heart failure with reduced and preserved ejection fraction across Asia: outcomes in the ASIAN-HF registry. J Am Heart Assoc. 2020;9(1):e012199.
3. Kociol RD, Krum H; ADHERE International–Asia Pacific Scientific Advisory Committee. Patient characteristics from a regional multicenter database of acute decompensated heart failure in Asia Pacific (ADHERE International–Asia Pacific). J Card Fail. 2012;18:82-8.
4. Guo L, Guo X, Chang Y, et al. Prevalence and risk factors of heart failure with preserved ejection fraction: a population-based study in Northeast China. Int J Environ Res Public Health. 2016;13:E770.

5. Shimokawa H, Miura M, Nochioka K, et al. Heart failure as a general pandemic in Asia. Eur J Heart Fail. 2015;17:884-92.
6. Alehagen U, Benson L, Edner M, et al. Association between use of statins and mortality in patients with heart failure and ejection fraction of ≥50%. Circ Heart Fail. 2015;8:862-70.
7. Yancy CW, Lopatin M, Stevenson LW, et al.; ADHERE Scientific Advisory Committee and Investigators. Clinical presentation, management, and in-hospital outcomes of patients admitted with acute decompensated heart failure with preserved systolic function. J Am Coll Cardiol. 2006;47:76-84.
8. Cheng RK, Cox M, Neely ML, et al. Outcomes in patients with heart failure with preserved, borderline, and reduced ejection fraction in the Medicare population. Am Heart J. 2014;168:721-30.e3.
9. Harikrishnan S, Sanjay G, Anees T, et al. Clinical presentation, management, in-hospital and 90-day outcomes of heart failure patients in Trivandrum, Kerala, India: the Trivandrum Heart Failure Registry. Eur J Heart Fail. 2015;17:794-800.
10. Dokainish H, Teo K, Zhu J, et al. Global mortality variations in patients with heart failure: results from the International Congestive Heart Failure (INTER-CHF) prospective cohort study. Lancet Glob Health. 2017;5(7):e665-72.

CHAPTER

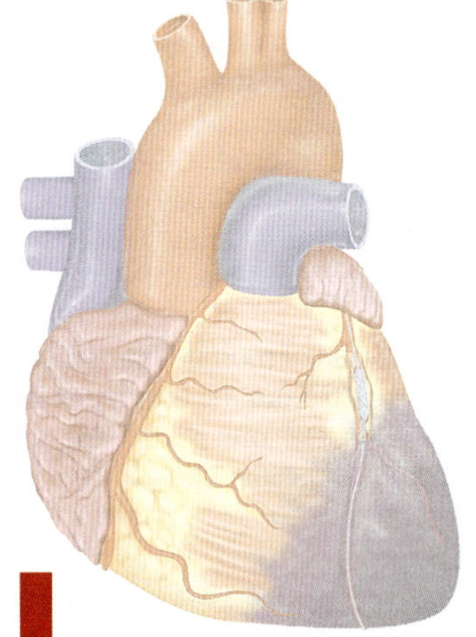

Indian Heart Failure Registries: Focusing on HFpEF

Richard Raj R, Harikrishnan S

INTRODUCTION

The heart failure with preserved ejection fraction (HFpEF) burden is rising probably due to an increase in prevalence and possibly due to increased case detection rates. We know that the diagnostic criteria for HFpEF is constantly evolving and yet to get settled.[1] However, in countries like India, many cases may be missed due to a lack of awareness about the condition among both patients and healthcare providers.

The clinical presentation of HFpEF makes routine diagnostic approaches less yielding as the symptoms are very atypical and nonspecific. We also now have the information that there are different phenotypic spectra in HFpEF which actually are yet to be characterized clearly. So, there is an increasing focus on individualized medicine in HFpEF, considering the varying patient characteristics and comorbidities. The refinement of algorithms for diagnosis and treatment plans has been ongoing for a long time. Moreover, the epidemiological data on HFpEF from India is scarce. Here is a look at HFpEF in the Indian context, focusing on its prevalence, unique challenges, and considerations.

HFpEF IN INDIA—EPIDEMIOLOGY—ARE WE MISSING CASES? WHY?

All the major registries from India have shown the prevalence of HFpEF is <20% **(Table 1)**. The first HF registry from India, the Trivandrum HF registry which recruited patients in 2013 showed a prevalence of 16%.[2] The Kerala HF registry which recruited patients in 2018 showed a prevalence of 15% and the National HF registry (2019–20) showed a prevalence of 13% only. In contrast, the *Indus (India-UKieri) study* by Vivek Chaturvedi et al.,[3] screened just over 10,000 adults across six villages which were the peripheral centers of the All-India Institute of Medical Sciences (AIIMS), New Delhi. Those who had shortness of breath for >6 months were included and the heart failure burden amounted to 1.2/1,000 population, out of which two-thirds were HFpEF.

TABLE 1: Heart failure with preserved ejection fraction (HFpEF) prevalence across various registries in India.

	HFrEF <40%	*HFmrEF 40–49%*	*HFpEF = ≥50%*
NHFR (*n* = 10,851)	65%	22%	13%
THFR (*n* = 1,205)	62%	22%	16%
KHFR (*n* = 7,512)	67%	18%	15%
ICC-HF registry (*n* = 5,269)	68%		32% (>40%)

(HFmrEF: heart failure with mid-range or mildly reduced ejection fraction; HFrEF: heart failure with preserved ejection fraction; ICC-HF: Indian College of Cardiology-Heart Failure; KHFR: Kerala Acute Heart Failure Registry; NHFR: National Heart Failure Registry; THFR: Trivandrum HF registry)

The reasons for the low prevalence of HFpEF could be manyfold. The most important is that probably many cases are missed. The lack of awareness among patients and physicians might also contribute to this issue. Since HFpEF has nonspecific symptoms such as pedal edema and dyspnea, patients may be treated for asthma, and many with diuretics alone. The lack of awareness among physicians when patients are labeled as normal when seeing normal ejection fraction also may contribute to the issue. The elaborate and not-so-easy diagnostic criteria is another factor that adds to the missing of cases. Even experienced echocardiographers find it difficult to assess the patient with all the recommended parameters. In a busy echo room in India, it is not practically possible to perform such an elaborate and time-consuming echo evaluation. It is high time that we develop some simple echo criteria to diagnose HFpEF. The diastolic stress test which is recommended is difficult to perform and facilities for such evaluation are limited in Indian hospitals. Invasive cardiac catheterization facilities are not available in most of the hospitals and those who have the facility do not have trained people to accurately assess the patient and interpret the results. The universal definition of HF has mandated natriuretic peptide (NP) levels in the diagnosis of HF. As we know NP tests are not available in all health facilities in India, and it is too costly. That also may be a factor in missing the cases.

HFpEF "A DISEASE OF COMORBIDITIES"

Most of the patients with HFpEF present with the backdrop of one or more comorbidities, often poorly controlled with medications due to various reasons **(Fig. 1)**. The higher baseline blood pressure (BP) levels in the aging population as studied by Agrawal et al., from Odisha, based on the insights from SAGE wave-2 (Study on global aging and adult health) (2015–16) study[4] aggravated by poor adherence to medications, and more importantly, by the failure to monitor the BP periodically to dose adjust these medications to target levels. In addition to these, the higher body mass index (BMI) associated

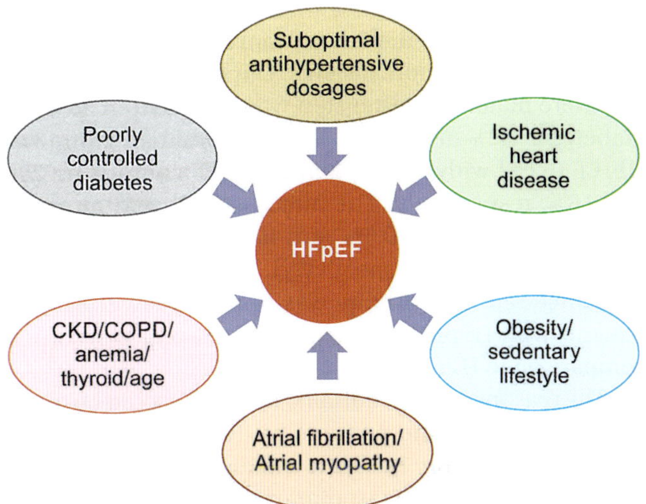

Fig. 1: Causative factors of heart failure with preserved ejection fraction (HFpEF) in Indian background.

with the aging Indian population was shown in a meta-analysis by Daniel et al. from the All-India Institute for Medical Science, New Delhi, which comprised a total of 60,006 participants.[5] The pooled prevalence of overweight/obesity among elderly persons in India was 21.5% (95% confidence interval: 17.1–26.2%) which significantly worsened their functional status, probably as a result of the sedentary lifestyle with a lack of regular physical activity and poor diet habits, although this does not correlate exactly with the NT-proBNP levels that might remain falsely low despite worsening symptoms.[6]

PHENOTYPES OF HFpEF

The HFpEF represents a heterogeneous syndrome with different clinical phenotypes which will help in identifying patients at a higher risk of HF hospitalizations and in tailoring the follow-up for that individual. HFpEF clinical phenogroups from the TOPCAT (Treatment of Preserved Cardiac Function Heart Failure with an Aldosterone Antagonist Trial) participants were classified into three.[7] Phenogroup 1 exhibited younger age, higher smoking prevalence, preserved functional class, and the least evidence of left ventricular (LV) hypertrophy, and arterial stiffness. Phenogroup 2 was older, with normotrophic concentric LV remodeling, atrial fibrillation, left atrial enlargement, large-artery stiffening, and innate immunity and vascular calcification biomarkers. Phenogroup 3 demonstrated more functional impairment, obesity, diabetes, chronic kidney disease, concentric LV hypertrophy, high renin, and biomarkers of tumor necrosis factor-alpha–mediated inflammation, liver fibrosis, and tissue remodeling. Compared with phenogroup 1, phenogroup 3 exhibited the highest risk of the primary endpoint of cardiovascular death, heart failure hospitalization, or aborted cardiac arrest. Phenogroups 2 and 3 demonstrated similar all-cause mortality. Spironolactone randomized therapy was associated with a more pronounced reduction in the risk of HF hospitalization and mortality in phenogroup 3 comparatively.

Similarly, a cluster model from the Swedish Heart Failure Registry (Swede HF)[8] identified five distinct clusters: cluster 1 (10% of patients) were young patients with a low comorbidity burden and the highest proportion of implantable devices; cluster 2 (30%) patients had atrial fibrillation, hypertension without diabetes; cluster 3 (25%) patients were the oldest with many cardiovascular comorbidities and hypertension; cluster 4 (15%) patients had obesity, diabetes and hypertension; and cluster 5 (20%) patients were older with ischemic heart disease, hypertension, and renal failure and were most frequently prescribed diuretics. Patients in cluster 1 had the best prognosis, while patients in clusters 3 and 5 had the worst age- and sex-adjusted prognosis.

Interestingly, Shah et al., have also classified HFpEF into seven phenotypes based on the etiology.[9] (1) "garden variety" HFpEF, associated with a lot of comorbidities; (2) CAD-associated HFpEF; (3) atrial fibrillation-predominant HFpEF; (4) right heart failure-predominant HFpEF; (5) hypertrophic cardiomyopathy-induced or hypertrophic-cardiomyopathy-like HFpEF; (6) multi-valvular HFpEF; and (7) restrictive cardiomyopathies such as cardiac amyloidosis.

All the aforementioned studies have inferred that the higher the comorbidity burden, as commonly seen in the Indian population, the higher the mortality and heart failure hospitalization. Also, the effectiveness of spironolactone in reducing the risk is of notable importance.

MORTALITY WITH HFpEF

The Western data had shown that HFpEF and HFrEF mortality are similar, especially by Tsao et al. from Boston who studied the temporal trends in the incidence and mortality-associated with heart failure with preserved and reduced ejection fraction.[10] Across the two decades, the HF incidence rate ratio was similar. During follow-up after HF, 67.4%; died [HFrEF (33%), HFpEF (29%)]. There were no significant differences in mortality rates (overall, CVD, and non-CVD) across decades within HF subtypes, nor between HFrEF and HFpEF within the decade. But the data from India showed different numbers.

Short-term Mortality

The Cardiology Society of India-Kerala Acute Heart Failure Registry (CSI-KAHFR)[11] published in the year 2021, the majority of whom were HFrEF (67.5%), while a nearly equal number of patients have HFmrEF (17.6%) and HFpEF (14.9%). The mean age was 64 ± 12.9 years (males 63 ± 12.5 and females 66 ± 13.5) with an overall male predominance (63%), which was marked in HFrEF and HFmrEF groups, while no significant sex difference was noted in the HFpEF group. Coronary artery disease (CAD) being the most common etiology (65.5%). The majority had diabetes mellitus (61.5%) and hypertension (53%). Patients with HFrEF had higher mortality rates (7.7%) compared to those with HFmrEF (5.2%) and HFpEF (5.6%). The 90-day mortality was marginally higher in HFrEF (12.3%; 95% CI: 11.4–13.2) than in HFpEF (10.6%; 95% CI: 8.8–12.5) or HFmrEF (9.9%; 95% CI: 8.5–11.3) (log-rank 0 = 0.022). The mortality per 100 person-days

TABLE 2: Mortality differences between heart failure with reduced ejection fraction (HFrEF) and heart failure with preserved ejection fraction (HFpEF) from Indian registries.

	HFrEF	*HFpEF*
CSI-KHFR 90-Day	12.3%	10.6%
NHFR—India	15.7%	12.5%
Asian HF Registry—1 year	10.6	5.4%

(CSI-KHFR: Cardiology Society of India-Kerala Acute Heart Failure Registry; NHFR: National Heart Failure Registry)

was 15.5% with HFrEF, 12% with HFmrEF, and 13% with HFpEF.

Then came the National Heart Failure Registry (NHFR),[12] which included 10,851 patients from 54 centers across 24 states and 2 union territories. This study assessed the clinical profile and 90-day outcome of heart failure patients across various parts of the country and the numbers revealed that the most common presentation was HFrEF in two-thirds (65.2%) of the study population, followed by HFmrEF (22%) and HFpEF (12.7%). Ischemic heart disease was the predominant etiology for HF (72%). Hypertension and diabetes were the most frequently comorbid conditions (48.9% and 42.3%, respectively). Atrial arrhythmia was prevalent in 9.5% of the study population. Chronic kidney disease, stroke, and chronic obstructive pulmonary disease (COPD) were reported in 8.5%, 3.0%, and 6.9% of the study population, respectively. Overall, 90-day mortality was 14.2, it was highest in HFrEF (15.7%) and in HFpEF it was 12.5% **(Table 2)**.

Long-term Mortality

The 5-year data from the Trivandrum Heart Failure Registry (THFR)[2] provided more insights. Out of the 1,205 patients, 59% were males. Hypertension was prevalent in 55% and diabetes in 52% of patients. The predominant group was HFrEF (62%) with HFpEF and HFmrEF comprising 20% and 18%, respectively. The unadjusted 5-year mortality rate was 59% (61.3%, 60.5%, and 46.8% in HFrEF, HFmrEF, and HFpEF groups, respectively). The lowest cumulative incidence rate of mortality was in patients with HFpEF. Patients with HFpEF had a 28% lower 5-year mortality in comparison to HFrEF.

The reasons for low mortality in HFpEF could be many. The lower age of the patients by 10 years may be one factor. The mortality in THFR is mainly cardiovascular—96%—and noncardiovascular mortality is pretty low. HFpEF patients are older, and they may have many comorbidities. They have many patients dying of noncardiovascular causes, which may not be the case in this relatively younger cohort from India.

PHARMACOLOGICAL FACETS

Compared to the treatment options available in managing HFrEF, the pharmacological options when it comes to HFpEF are evolving and will continue to evolve in the coming years. The five pillars of managing HFpEF are: treating circulatory congestion by diuretics, controlling comorbidities, using evidence-based drugs, identifying and managing secondary etiologies, and cardiopulmonary rehabilitation, which is not well utilized in the Indian context. When it comes to the Indian population, after adequate optimization of medications in controlling the comorbidities, patients have to be started on the new evidence-based drugs—sodium-glucose co-transporter-2 (SGLT2) inhibitors, mineralocorticoid receptor antagonists (MRAs)—with the recent evidence for Finerenone) provided there are no contraindications for the same. Beyond medications, advanced interventional procedures targeting autonomic modulation, respiratory modulation, electrophysiological modulation, structural interventions targeting interatrial shunting,[13] etc., the data is evolving and is yet to come to regular practice.

WHAT DO THE HEART FAILURE REGISTRIES IN INDIA TEACH US?

The patients with HF were younger than the patients in the high-income countries (HIC) by a decade (mean age; ADHERE registry 74 years, European HFS registry 70 years, and ATTEND registry 73 years). The younger age of onset of illness also points toward the socioeconomic impact of the disease at an individual and community level. Acute HF patients in the subcontinent are predominantly HFrEF. While there are measures that are effective in controlling factors that result in HFrEF, treatment of HFpEF is largely linked to symptomatic measures and management and control of risk factors **(Fig. 2)**.

CONCLUSION

Continued research into the versatile mechanisms of HFpEF and the development of new treatment modalities is vital. Indeed, the past few decades have seen significant improvement in diagnosing and managing HFpEF. The continued research on the complex pathophysiology and advances in molecular biology is likely to identify the key mechanisms in HFpEF development and progression. Research is now strongly focusing on the phenotyping of HFpEF and understanding regional differences in HFpEF prevalence and pathology among different ethnic and socioeconomic subgroups. In most parts of the country, particularly in low-resource settings, access to advanced diagnostic tools and therapies is often limited. Addressing these disparities will be crucial for improving the diagnosis and betterment of outcomes for HFpEF patients in India.

Clinical assessment:
- Functional class
- JVP/Crepitations/S3/ Pedal edema
- 6-minute walk distance
- NT-ProBNP

Comorbidities:
- BMI
- ECG, HbA1C
- BP/Antihypertensives
- Hb, lipids, TFT, PFT, creatinine

Echocardiogram:
- LV ejection fraction
- Septal and PW thickness
- LA volume index
- E/A, septal and lateral e', E/e' ratio
- TR jet velocity/RVSP

Management:
- Lifestyle measures comorbidity control
- SGLT2i, MRA, Diuretics
- Drug compliance
- Nonpharmacologic interventions

Fig. 2: Heart failure with preserved ejection fraction (HFpEF) evaluation and management algorithm. (BP: blood pressure; ECG: electrocardiography; HbA1C: hemoglobin A1c; JVP: jugular venous pressure; LV: left ventricular; MRA: mineralocorticoid receptor antagonists; NT-proBNP: N-terminal pro B-type natriuretic peptide; RVSP: right ventricular systolic pressure; SGLT2i: sodium-glucose co-transporter-2 inhibitors; THT: thyroid function test; TR: tricuspid regurgitation)

REFERENCES

1. Pillai HS, Ganapathi S. Heart failure in South Asia. Curr Cardiol Rev. 2013;9(2):102-11.
2. Harikrishnan S, Jeemon P, et al. Five-year mortality and readmission rates in patients with heart failure in India: Results from the Trivandrum heart failure registry. Int J Cardiol. 2021;326:139-43.
3. Chaturvedi V, Parakh N, Seth S, et al. Heart failure in India: The INDUS (INDia Ukieri Study) study. J Pract Cardiovasc Sci. 2016;2:28-35.
4. Agrawal R, Murmu J, Sinha A, et al. Association of dietary sodium intake and hypertension among older adults in India: Insights from (Study on global AGEing and adult health) SAGE wave-2, Clinical Epidemiology and Global Health. 2023;23(4):101358.
5. Daniel RA, Kalaivani M, Aggarwal P, et al. Prevalence of overweight/obesity among elderly persons in India: A systematic review and meta-analysis. J Prim Care Spec. 2024;5(1):22-35.

6. Obokata M, Reddy YNV, Pislaru SV, et al. Evidence supporting the existence of a distinct obese phenotype of heart failure with preserved ejection fraction. Circulation. 2017;136(1):6-19.
7. Cohen JB, Schrauben SJ, Zhao L, et al. Clinical Phenogroups in Heart Failure with Preserved Ejection Fraction. JACC Heart Fail. 2020;8(3):172-84.
8. Uijl A, Savarese G, Vaartjes I, et al. Identification of distinct phenotypic clusters in heart failure with preserved ejection fraction. Eur J Heart Fail. 2021;23(6):973-82.
9. Shah SJ, Katz DH, Deo RC, et al. Phenotypic Spectrum of Heart Failure with Preserved Ejection Fraction. Heart Fail Clin. 2014;10(3):407-18.
10. Tsao CW, Lyass A, Enserro D, et al. Temporal Trends in the Incidence of and Mortality Associated with Heart Failure with Preserved and Reduced Ejection Fraction. JACC Heart Fail. 2018;6(8):678-85.
11. Joseph S, Panniyammakal J, Abdullakutty J, et al. The Cardiology Society of India-Kerala Acute Heart Failure Registry: poor adherence to guideline-directed medical therapy. Eur Heart J. 2022;43:908-15.
12. Harikrishnan S, Bahl A, Roy A, et al. Clinical profile and 90-day outcomes of 10,851 heart failure patients across India: National Heart Failure Registry. ESC Heart Fail. 2022;9(6):3898-908.
13. Shah SJ, Borlaug BA, Chung ES, et al. Atrial shunt device for heart failure with preserved and mildly reduced ejection fraction (REDUCE LAP HF II): a randomized, multicentre, blinded, sham-controlled trial. Lancet. 2022;399(10330):1130-40.

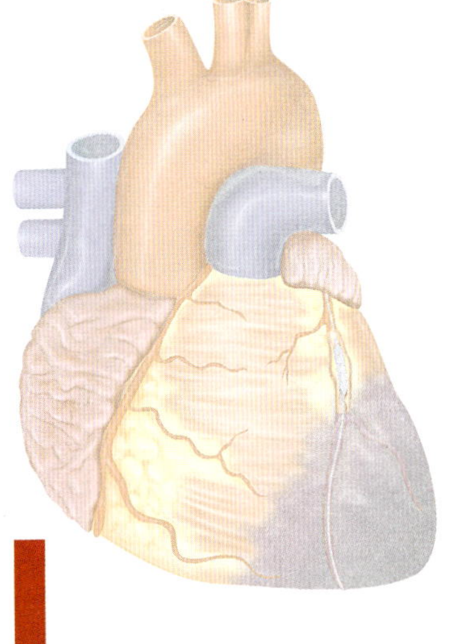

Epidemiology of Heart Failure

Zakia Khan

INTRODUCTION

In the past, epidemiology of heart failure was focused primarily on heart failure with reduced ejection fraction. However, recognition of heart failure syndrome has expanded the number of cases included in heart failure definition. It is projected that heart failure prevalence will increase by 46% and the total population affected will increase from 2.42 to 2.97% despite significant advances in therapy.[1]

Heart failure carries a high mortality, and 1 year mortality after heart failure hospitalization ranges between 20 and 36%. Three out of four patients died between 2005 and 2009 within 5 year of diagnosis, regardless of their EF. The survival rates are lower than some of the chronic cancers.[2-3]

PREVALENCE AND INCIDENCE

As the population ages and the heart failure therapies continue to improve, the prevalence of heart failure is expected to increase. Based on the National Health and Nutrition Examination Survey (NHANES 2013-2016), prevalence of heart failure in US overall is 2%, and expected to increase significantly after the age of 60. The highest prevalence was observed after the age of 80 where 12.8% of males and 12% of females had a diagnosis of heart failure. The following table summarizes the prevalence of heart failure around the world **(Table 1)**.

PATIENT CHARACTERISTICS

Impact of Demographics and Socioeconomic Status, Age, and Sex

Age and Sex

Age is a major contributor to the development of heart failure. Due to higher incidences of coronary artery disease in men at a younger age, male preponderance is seen with reduced ejection fraction compared to females at that age. However, worsening diastolic dysfunction leads to more women being affected at a higher age. Men are more likely to develop HFrEF whereas women are more prone to HFpEF.[4,5]

Socioeconomic Status

It is a key determinant of Heart Failure risk in the UK among persons of similar age and sex. Those in the most deprived socioeconomic quintile were the most likely to develop heart Failure. (IR 1.61, 95% CI 1.58–1.64). This distinction was more apparent in the younger age groups. The patients from the deprived sections of society were 3.5 years younger at diagnosis compared to those from the affluent sections.

ETIOLOGY OF HEART FAILURE

Ischemic Heart Disease

In a Swedish National registry, primary percutaneous coronary intervention increased from 6.0 to 91.5%

TABLE 1: Population Prevalence of heart failure (HF) in registries and surveys across the world.

Country	*Population sample*	*Study period*	*Ascertainment of heart failure cases*	*Total (%)*	*Men (%)*	*Women (%)*
Sweden (Zarrinkoub, Wettermark et al. 2013)	2.1 million	2010	Primary or secondary diagnosis of HF (ICD-10 code 150 in primary care (2003 to 2010), secondary care 1997 to 2010), or during hospitalization (1997 to 2010)	2.2*	2.2	2.2
Spain (Farre, Vela et al. 2017)	7.5 million	2012	Hospital diagnosis of HF (ICD-9-CM codes 402.X1, 404. X1, 404.X3, 428.X) or outpatient diagnosis followed by loop diuretic prescription between 2011 and 2012	1.2 (among age >15)		
United States (Streng, Nauta et al. 2018)	5,761	2013-2014	National Health and Nutrition Examination Survey, multi-stage probability sampling, self-reported HF*	1.9*	1.8	2.0
United Kingdom (Conrad, Judge et al. 2018)	4.0 million	2002-2014	ICD-10 codes (I50.X, I42.0 I42.9, I11.0, I13.0, I13.2, I25.5) for in hospital and NHS Read codes for primary care diagnosis of HF in any diagnostic position	1.6	1.8	1.2
South Korea (Lee, Oh et al. 2016)	1.4 million	2014	Adult patients with any outpatients or inpatients services with a primary or secondary diagnosis of HF (ICD-10 code I50.X, I11.0, I13.0, I13.2, I42.0, I42.5, I25.5) in 2014	1.2 (among age >18)		

*Estimated prevalence in the national population
(HF: heart failure; ICD-10: International Classification of Diseases, Version 10; NHS: National Health Service)
Source: ICD-9-CM International Classification of Diseases, Ninth Revision, Clinical Modification.

between 1996 and 2008, accompanied by a decrease in the incidence of HF during first admission from 46 to 28%. The decrease was more distinct for ST-segment elevation AMI. Notably, reduction in post-AMI HF rates has been reported for HFrEF but not HFpEF.

Among patients discharged without HF, 12.6%% were admitted or died because of HF after a median of 3.2 years and the risk of HF was higher during the first 6 months post AMI. The annual incidence of heart failure per 1,000 person-years was 31% in men and 46% in women (p <0.01) **(Fig. 1)**.

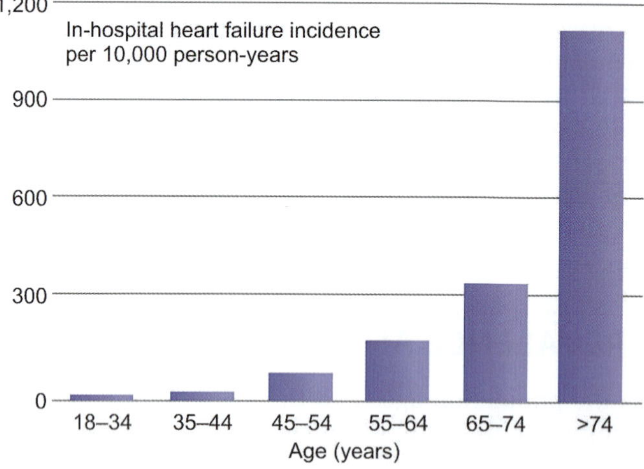

Fig. 1: Incidence of in-hospital heart failure diagnosis among adults in Denmark, 2012.
Source: Christiansen MN, Kobel L, Weeke P, et al. Age-Specific Trends in Incidence, Mortality, and Comorbidities of Heart Failure in Denmark, 1995 to 2012. Circulation. 2017;135:1214-23.

Comorbidities

Over 80% of patients have at least two concomitant chronic conditions. The most common comorbidities are hypertension, ischemic heart disease, diabetes mellitus, cerebral and peripheral vascular disease atrial fibrillation, chronic kidney disease, chronic obstructive lung disease, anemia, and depression. In the UK, the number of comorbidities in patients with HF increased from 3.4 ± 1.9 in 2002 to 5.4 ± 2.5 in 2014, and the percentage of patients with >3 additional conditions increased from 68 to 87%. Overall, there has been a shift from a model where HF was mainly a consequence of CAD with male preponderance to a disease of older adults equally affection both sexes and accompanied by a complex medical profile.

Hypertension

The impact of SBP control on HF risk was effectively demonstrated in the landmark SPRINT trial which compared intensive (<120 mm Hg) with conventional (<140 mm Hg) target SBP. Intensive SBP target reduced the risk of HF by 37% consistently across all subgroups.

Diabetes

Heart failure was approximately two-fold higher among patients with diabetes (type 1 + type 2) versus those without it. There is a higher short-term mortality (30 days) in those with type 1 diabetes.

Atrial Fibrillation

It is a negative prognostic factor in heart failure and increases risk of HF especially HFpEF. In the Framingham heart study, among 1,737 individuals, patients with new AF (mean age 75 ± 12 years; 48% women), more than one-third had HF. Conversely among 1,166 individuals with new HF (mean age 79 ± 11 years; 53% women), more than half had AF. In the community based ORBIT-AF registry, among approximately 6,500 OPD patients with AF in the US (median age 74 years; 43.6% females), annualized HF incidence was 1.5% over a 2 year follow-up period with a higher proportion of HFpEF compared with HFrEF. It is also important to note that, in contrast to general heart failure cases, the incidence of heart failure after AF does not seem to declining.[6]

Renal Disease

Renal impairment imparts a poor prognosis in heart failure. The annualized incidence of heart failure is 2.2% among those with CKD versus 0.62% without. Incidence was higher in African Americans and Hispanics. AKI also carries an increased risk of HF. In a cohort of 300,000 hospitalized US veterans without HF, a 0.3 mg/dL or 50% increase in serum creatinine from the baseline, was associated with a 23% increased 2 year risk of heart failure. In a cohort of over 3,500 patients with CKD, cystatin-C based eGFR and albuminuria predicted risk of heart failure better than creatinine based eGFR; anemia, insulin resistance, inflammation, and poor glycemic control were additional risk factor.[7]

OUTCOMES

Despite advances in heart Failure therapy in the past 20 years, heart failure related mortality and rehospitalization rates at the population level have become difficult to curb.[8] This is secondary to:

- Increasing patient age and comorbidities.
- Negative results of trials with pharmaceuticals/devices targeting non-neurohormonal pathways.
- Lack of effective treatment for patients with acute HF and HFpEF.

Mortality Trends

In the large paradigm HF study, a landmark trial in HFrEF, 81% deaths were attributed to vascular causes. Of these 45% were due to sudden cardiac death, and 26% due to HF. Even in the early stages of heart failure, patients are at a higher risk of sudden cardiac death, making the case for aggressive treatment of stage B and mildly symptomatic stage C HF patients extremely crucial. Currently, 1 year mortality for outpatients with HF in observational studies in developed countries ranges between 5 and 10%. However, it is considerably higher (10–20%) in national registries, developing countries and in older patients.

For hospitalized patients, 1 year mortality is generally >20% and exceeds 30% in several national registry.

Heart Failure Rehospitalization

Readmission rates after a hospitalization for HF remains high with 20–30% of patients in US, readmitted in the first 1 month and half to two-thirds readmitted within the first year. However, overall length of stay in hospital has reduced with optimum use of GDMT. Despite decreasing mortality trends, 5 year survival after HF diagnosis in population studies does not exceed 50% in most systems, regardless of setting (outpatient vs. inpatient) and is as low as 25% in older patients, regardless of EF.[9] In contrast to hospitalized patients in the ESC-HF-LT registry, mortality at 1 year was 8.8% among outpatients with HFrEF, 7.6% with mid-range EF and 6.3% with HFpEF. Adherence to GDMT was associated with lower mortality at 1 year **(Fig. 2)**.[10]

Mortality significantly decelerated among patients with HFrEF after 1 year. Age and sex-adjusted 3 year mortality was 16.3%, 13.2%, and 4.8% in patients with HFrEF, HFpEF, and HFrecEF, respectively. Patients with HFrecEF had overall lower all-cause, cardiovascular, heart failure related mortality as well as lower sudden cardiac death rates and fewer HF hospitalizations.

CONCLUSION

Public awareness regarding control of risk factors such as hypertension, diabetes, ischemic heart disease, and smoking has curbed the incidence of HF in the more

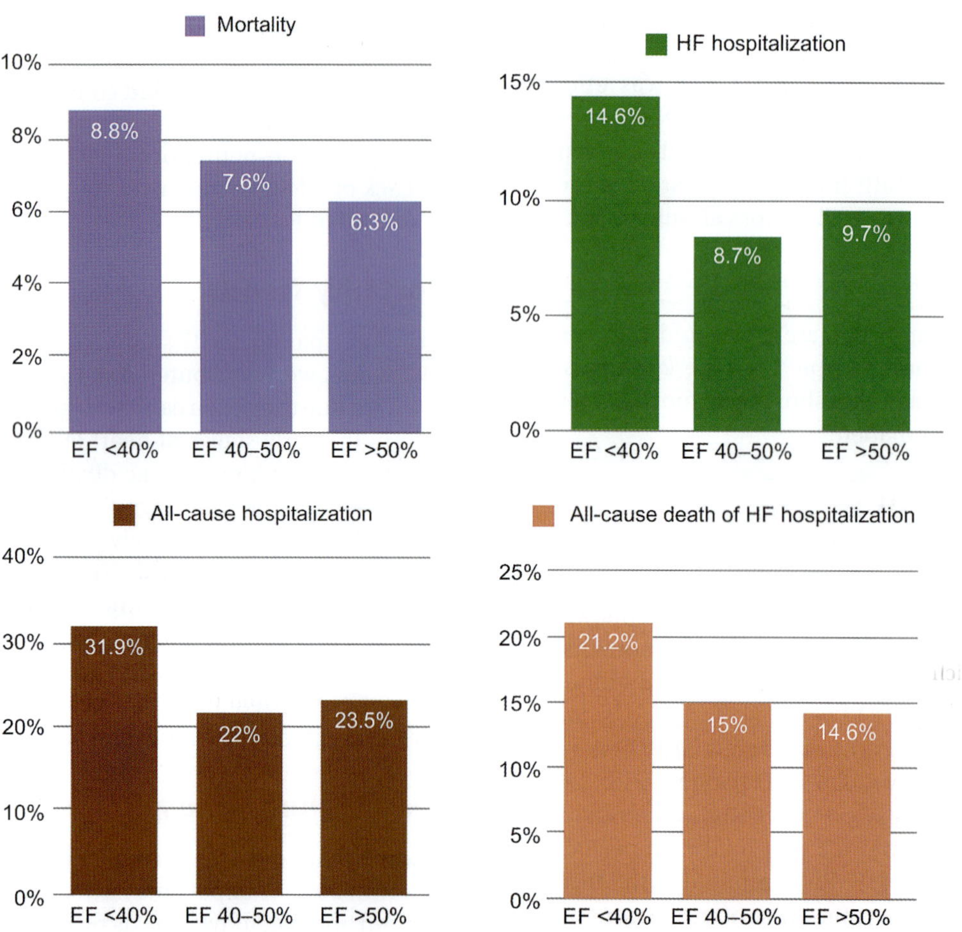

Fig. 2: Outcomes at 1 year in outpatients with heart failure in the ESC heart failure long-term registry. (EF: ejection fraction: HF: heart failure)
Source: Chioncel O, Lainscak M, Seferovic PM, et al. Epidemiology and one-year outcomes in patients with chronic heart failure and preserved, mid-range and reduced ejection fraction: an analysis of the ESC Heart Failure Long-Term Registry. Eur J Heart Fail. 2017;19:1574-85.

developed countries. However, the overall prevalence of heart failure continues to increase because of aging population. Mortality after a diagnosis of HF is still high despite advances in GDMT and devices. Therefore, intensification of mass education and early diagnosis of metabolic diseases is warranted. Unfortunately, in developing countries the disease burden is increasing and affecting younger population a decade earlier.

CLINICAL FEATURES OF HEART FAILURE WITH PRESERVED EJECTION FRACTION

The clinical features of HFpEF are generally similar to other forms of heart failure. Dyspnea on exertion, paroxysmal nocturnal dyspnea and orthopnea, and fatigue are the most common symptoms of HFpEF **(Table 2)**.

TABLE 2: Symptoms and signs in patients with HFpEF enrolled in PARAGON-HF.

Symptoms and signs of heart failure	*Percentage of patients (%)*
DOE	98
Fatigue	59
Edema	45
Orthopnea	22
JVD	17
Rales	11
PND	7.60
Dyspnea at rest	4.60

(HFpEF: heart failure with preserved ejection fraction; DOE: dyspnea on exertion; JVD: jugular vein distention; PND: paroxysmal nocturnal dyspnea)
Source: Solomon SD, Rizkala AR, Lefkowitz MP, et al. Baseline characteristics of patients with heart failure and preserved ejection fraction in the PARAGON-HF trial. Circ Heart Fail. 2018;11:e004962.

Exertional chest pain is also a commonly reported symptom in HFpEF. In general, signs and symptoms cannot be used to distinguish between HFpEF and HFrEF.

When to suspect HFpEF: When a patient presents with history or physical examination which reveal at least 1 symptom from the above table that is not sufficiently explained by another diagnosis. The presence of certain conditions increases the likelihood that HFpEF is present:

- Age >60 years
- Obesity
- Hypertension
- Coronary artery disease
- Atrial fibrillation
- Diabetes
- Chronic kidney disease

REFERENCES

1. Heidenreich PA, Albert NM, Allen LA, et al. Forecasting the impact of heart failure in the United States: a policy statement from the American Heart Association. Circ Heart Fail. 2013;6:606-19.
2. Shah KS, Xu H, Matsouaka RA, et al. Heart failure with preserved, borderline, and reduced ejection fraction: 5-year outcomes. J Am Coll Cardiol. 2017;70:2476-86.
3. Mamas MA, Sperrin M, Watson MC, et al. Do patients have worse outcomes in heart failure than in cancer? A primary care-based cohort study with 10 year follow up in Scotland. Eur J Heart Fail. 2017;19:1095-104.
4. Pandey A, Omar W, Ayers C, et al. Sex and race differences in lifetime risk of heart failure with preserved ejection fraction and heart failure with reduced ejection fraction. Circulation. 2018;137:1814-23.
5. Stolfo D, Uijl A, Vedin O, et al. Sex-based differences in heart failure across the ejection fraction spectrum: phenotyping, and prognostic and therapeautic implications. JACC Heart Fail. 2019;7:505-15.
6. Pandey A, Kim S, Moore C, et al. Predictors and prognostic implications of incident heart failure in patients with prevalent atrial fibrillation. JACC Heart Fail. 2018;5:44-52.
7. He J, Shlipak M, Anderson A, et al. Risk factors for heart failure in patients with chronic kidney disease: the CRIC study. J Am Heart Assoc. 2017;6:e005336.
8. Crespo-Leiro MG, Anker SD, Maggioni AP, et al. European Society of Cardiology Heart Failure Long-term registry (ESC-HF-LT): 1-year follow-up outcomes and differences across regions. Eur J Heart Fail. 2016;18:613-25.
9. Park CS, Park JJ, Mebazaa A, et al. Characteristics, outcomes, and treatment of heart failure with improved ejection fraction. J Am Heart Assoc. 2019;8:e011077.
10. Pandey A, Golwala h, Xu H, et al. Association of 30-day readmission metric for heart failure under the hospital readmissions reduction program with quality of care and outcomes. JACC Heart Fail. 2016;4:935-46

Cellular and Molecular Differences Between HFpEF and HFrEF: A Step Ahead in an Improved Pathological Understanding

Rohan Patel, Saurabh Bagga, JPS Sawhney

INTRODUCTION

Heart failure (HF) is one of the leading causes of hospitalization in the world. Globally, 3.6 million patients are diagnosed with HF resulting in significant socioeconomic burden.[1] HF can be divided into three main categories depending upon LVEF: (1) HF with reduced ejection fraction (HFrEF)—LVEF is ≤40%; (2) HF with mildly reduced ejection fraction (HFmrEF)—LVEF is 41–49%; and (3) HF with preserved ejection fraction (HFpEF)—LVEF is ≥50%.[2] There are certain cellular, molecular, and pathophysiological differences in HFpEF and HFrEF. HFpEF is often associated with or preceded by comorbidities such as type-2 diabetes mellitus (T2DM), obesity, hypertension, and renal failure. HFrEF is often preceded by acute or chronic loss of cardiac myocytes due to ischemia, infarction, myocarditis, valvular disease, and genetic mutation.[3] Drugs acting on neurohormonal pathways have been shown to reduce cardiovascular mortality and HF hospitalization significantly in HFrEF. However, these drugs have shown less benefit in HFpEF as compared to HFrEF. This differential response may also be due to different cellular, molecular, and pathophysiological mechanisms associated with HFrEF and HFpEF.[4]

DIFFERENCES IN RISK FACTORS AND COMORBIDITIES ASSOCIATED WITH HFrEF AND HFpEF

Certain risk factors and comorbidities are similar between HFpEF and HFrEF. However, there are some risk factors and comorbidities that differ between HFpEF and HFrEF. HFpEF is more common in elderly, females, and obese. HFrEF is more common in males due to their increased susceptibility to myocardial infarction.[5] Patients with HFpEF have a higher prevalence of noncardiac comorbidities (i.e., T2DM, hypertension, CKD, anemia, pulmonary disease, liver disease, sleep apnea, gout, and cancer) than HFrEF patients.[6]

DIFFERENCES IN SYSTEMIC AND CARDIAC INFLAMMATION IN HFpEF AND HFrEF

Inappropriate inflammation is an important factor causing damage to the heart in both HFrEF and HFpEF but has different roles in the onset and propagation. Inflammation can be classified into three groups: (1) Sterile, (2) metabolic risk, and (3) nonsterile-induced inflammation.

Sterile inflammation occurs due to ischemic or toxic necrosis, massive trauma, hemorrhage, and/or resuscitation. It is more commonly seen in the HFrEF condition. During this response, sterile endogenous stimuli trigger inflammation by various pathways such as pathogen recognition receptor (PRR) pathway, cytokines mediated pathways, and CD36 mediated pathways. Dying cells release matrix metalloproteinases, which degrade extracellular matrix and oxidize macromolecules.[7] Excessive adrenergic stimulation leads to overproduction of neutrophils in bone marrow.[8] Neutrophils are rapidly released in the blood and go to heart, where they phagocytose the damaged cells. The serum neutrophil-to-lymphocyte ratio is considered a useful marker for the prediction of mortality in patients admitted for ST-segment elevation MI (STEMI).[9] Within 24 hours after MI, the splenic monocytes accumulate in heart. Monocytes subsequently infiltrate and produce growth factors, which repress inflammatory signaling, promote new blood vessel formation by endothelial cells and vascular smooth muscle cells, and scar formation by myofibroblast activation.[10]

Inflammation in HFpEF is the result of a cluster of metabolic and inflammatory risk factors, including obesity, diabetes, anemia, hypertension, chronic obstructive pulmonary disease, autoimmune diseases, and renal failure. Obese and type 1 and 2 diabetic patients have, for example, elevated levels of advanced glycation end products (AGEs). These AGEs interact with their receptors and activate secondary proinflammatory cytokines, chemokines, and adhesion molecules. This leads to development of low-grade chronic systemic inflammation causing microvascular changes in HFpEF.[4] HFpEF patients also had elevated circulating levels of neutrophils and monocytes. In patients with HFpEF, echocardiographic indices of diastolic dysfunction (E/e') correlate with monocyte recruitment in the spleen.[11]

Nonsterile inflammation can be induced by a viral infection. In viral myocarditis, there is exaggerated immune response in immune-susceptible persons. The initial acute phase is characterized by increased circulating and cardiac neutrophils and monocytes, while in later phases, increased circulating T-cells, specifically cytotoxic T-cells and B-cells can be detected. This results in scar tissue formation and a reduced contractile function in the chronic phase.[12]

In short, regardless of the cause of HFrEF, inflammation results in cardiac remodeling driven by cardiomyocyte damage or loss, which causes cardiomyocyte autophagy, apoptosis, and necrosis. In contrast, metabolic risk factors in HFpEF drive the chronic low-grade systemic inflammation along with the increased expression of adhesion molecules on the endothelial cells, leading to systemic and local cardiac inflammation.[4]

CARDIOMYOCYTE DEATH IN HFrEF

Cardiomyocyte damage in HFrEF patients, indicated by increased circulating levels of troponin-T, leads to a reduction in functioning cardiomyocyte mass in combination with excessive fibrotic tissue.[4] Recent evidence has suggested that cardiomyocyte autophagy and necroptosis (a controlled form of necrosis) play a larger role than apoptosis. In contrast, circulating troponin-T, which indicates elevated levels of cardiomyocyte cell death, is not detected in HFpEF patients. Thus, cardiomyocyte cell death is a characteristic observed in HFrEF and not in HFpEF.[13]

ENDOTHELIAL DYSFUNCTION: DIFFERENCES IN HFpEF AND HFrEF

Structural and/or functional abnormalities of endothelial cells strongly affect cardiac function. Endothelial dysfunction is seen in early stages of cardiovascular diseases such as HF. It is an important indicator of cardiovascular mortality. It is seen in both HFpEF and HFrEF. However, in HFpEF, multiple comorbidities lead to more pronounced and earlier microvascular dysfunction than in HFrEF.[14] Microvascular dysfunction is seen at a later stage in HFrEF.[4] Increased oxidative stress, imbalanced nitric oxide (NO) bioavailability, neurohormonal activation, and vasoconstriction in response to reduced cardiac output (CO) are central mechanisms causing endothelial dysfunction. Interestingly, in patients with chronic HFrEF, endothelium-mediated vasodilation is an independent predictor of cardiac death and hospitalization.[15] In HFpEF, despite the microvascular paradigm, endothelial dysfunction is not sufficiently well evaluated.[4]

CARDIOMYOCYTE ALTERATIONS IN HFrEF AND HFpEF: ECCENTRIC VERSUS CONCENTRIC HYPERTROPHY

During HFrEF, remodeling is driven by cardiomyocyte damage and loss causing eccentric remodeling, with left ventricular dilation, but a normal or reduced wall thickness. In contrast, HFpEF patients reveal concentric cardiomyocyte hypertrophy, where the left ventricle wall thickens. Remodeling differences in HFrEF and HFpEF can be explained by differences in stimuli and altered cellular signaling observed in HFrEF and HFpEF.[16]

DIFFERENT TYPES OF CARDIAC FIBROSIS IN HFrEF AND HFpEF

In a healthy heart, the ECM is mainly composed of thicker collagen type I fibers (~85%), which confer tensile strength, and thin collagen type III fibers (~11%), which maintain the elasticity of the matrix network. In HFrEF, cardiac fibrosis is mainly the consequence of cardiomyocyte loss and may contribute to systolic dysfunction via several mechanisms such as the loss of fibrillar collagen leading to impairment in conversion of cardiomyocyte contraction into myocardial force, uncoordinated contraction of cardiac myocytes, and disruption of cardiac mass and systolic reserve. This contrasts with HFpEF, where excessive collagen deposition and a reduction of the more flexible collagen III results in increased cardiac stiffness.[17] The effects of cardiac fibrosis are also determined by its location. Perivascular fibrosis is the consequence of systemic and cardiac inflammation in both HFpEF and HFrEF but is significantly greater in HFpEF. In the healing phase after MI, a collagen-based mature scar that is devoid of cardiomyocytes develops. This type of replacement fibrosis is only present in HFrEF. Thus, differences in the location, composition, and cross-linking of the cardiac fibrous tissue contribute to the differences in HFrEF and HFpEF.[18]

CONCLUSION

There are substantial differences in molecular, cellular, and pathophysiological mechanisms underlying HFpEF and HFrEF. Systemic inflammation, cardiac remodeling (endothelial function, hypertrophy, and cardiomyocyte cell death), and stiffness (fibrosis and levels) differ between HFpEF and HFrEF. HFrEF, mostly, occurs as the consequence of cardiomyocyte loss. In contrast, HFpEF is often diagnosed in elderly patients, who suffer from (a cluster of) noncardiac comorbidities, such as hypertension, T2DM, stroke, anemia, pulmonary disease, liver disease, sleep apnea, gout, and CKD. HFpEF is characterized by low-grade chronic systemic inflammation and capillary dysfunction, with consequential low-grade cardiac inflammation. In HFrEF, systemic and cardiac inflammation are secondary to the causes of cardiomyocyte loss. Whereas in HFpEF endothelial dysfunction mainly precedes its progression, in HFrEF endothelial dysfunction may rather be the consequence. Depending on the stimulus, perivascular (metabolic risks in HFpEF), interstitial (e.g., aging and hypertension in both HFpEF and HFrEF), or replacement (e.g., MI in HFrEF) fibrosis occurs and is differentially managed between the two conditions.

REFERENCES

1. Ambrosy AP, Fonarow GC, Butler J. et al. The global health and economic burden of hospitalizations for heart failure: lessons learned from hospitalized heart failure registries. J Am Coll Cardiol. 2014;63:1123-33.
2. Arbelo E, Protonotarios A, Gimeno JR, et al. 2023 ESC Guidelines for the management of cardiomyopathies. Eur Heart J. 2023;44(37):3503-626.
3. Borlaug BA, Melenovsky V, Russell SD, et al. Impaired chronotropic and vasodilator reserves limit exercise capacity in patients with heart failure and a preserved ejection fraction. Circulation. 2006;114(20):2138-47.
4. Paulus WJ, Tschöpe C. A novel paradigm for heart failure with preserved ejection fraction: comorbidities drive myocardial dysfunction and remodeling through coronary microvascular endothelial inflammation. J Am Coll Cardiol. 2013;62:263-71.
5. Ho JE, Lyass A, Lee DS, et al. Predictors of new-onset heart failure: differences in preserved versus reduced ejection fraction. Circ Heart Fail. 2013;6:279-86.
6. Ergatoudes C, Schaufelberger M, Andersson B, et al. Non-cardiac comorbidities and mortality in patients with heart failure with reduced vs. preserved ejection fraction: A study using the Swedish Heart Failure Registry. Clin Res Cardiol. 2019;108:1025-33.
7. Van Linthout S, Tschöpe C. Inflammation: cause or consequence of heart failure or both? Curr Heart Fail Rep. 2017;14(4):251-65.
8. Katayama Y, Battista M, Kao WM, et al. Signals from the sympathetic nervous system regulate hematopoietic stem cell egress from bone marrow. Cell. 2006;124:407-21.
9. Núñez J, Núñez E, Bodí V, et al. Usefulness of the neutrophil to lymphocyte ratio in predicting long-term mortality in ST segment elevation myocardial infarction. Am J Cardiol. 2008;101:747-52.
10. van der Laan AM, Nahrendorf M, Piek JJ. Republished: Healing and adverse remodelling after acute myocardial infarction: role of the cellular immune response. Postgrad Med J. 2013;89(1047):52-8.
11. Hulsmans M, Sager HB, Roh JD, et al. Cardiac macrophages promote diastolic dysfunction. J Exp Med. 2018;215:423-40.
12. Pollack A, Kontorovich AR, Fuster V. Viral myocarditis–diagnosis, treatment options, and current controversies. Nat Rev Cardiol. 2015;12(11):670-80.
13. Corsetti G, Chen-Scarabelli C, Romano C, et al. Autophagy and oncosis/necroptosis are enhanced in cardiomyocytes from heart failure patients. Med Sci Monit Basic Res. 2019;25:33-44.
14. Wander GS, Sawhney JPS, Yap J, et al. Microvascular disease in patients with diabetes with heart failure and reduced ejection versus preserved ejection fraction. Diabetes Care. 2019;42:1792-9.
15. Fischer D, Rossa S, Landmesser U, et al. Endothelial dysfunction in patients with chronic heart failure is independently associated with increased incidence of hospitalization, cardiac transplantation, or death. Eur Heart J. 2005;26(1):65-9.
16. Zile MR, Gottdiener JS, Hetzel SJ, et al. I-PRESERVE Investigators. Prevalence and significance of alterations in cardiac structure and function in patients with heart failure and a preserved ejection fraction. Circulation. 2011;124:2491-501.
17. Echegaray K, Andreu I, Lazkano A, et al. Role of myocardial collagen in severe aortic stenosis with preserved ejection fraction and symptoms of heart failure. Rev Esp Cardiol (Engl Ed). 2017;70:832-40.
18. Dai Z, Aoki T, Fukumoto Y, et al. Coronary perivascular fibrosis is associated with impairment of coronary blood flow in patients with non-ischemic heart failure. J Cardiol. 2012;60:416:21.

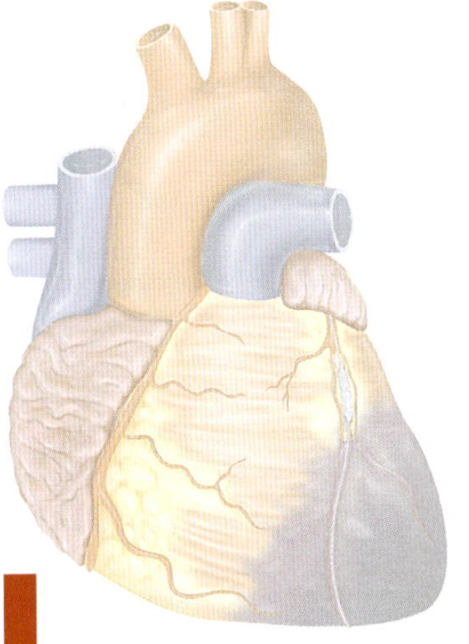

Differentiation between HFpEF and HFrEF

Manoranjan Mandal, Biaus Samanta, Subhashis Chakraborty

INTRODUCTION

Heart failure remains most prevalent cause of cardiovascular morbidity and mortality around the globe. CDC estimates around 6.7 million individuals to be affected by heart failure in USA only. Due to lack of surveillance studies reliable estimates of heart failure is missing on Indian population but according to Huffman et al. conservative prediction is 1.3 million to 22.7 million, with an annual incidence of 0.5–1.8 million in India.[1,2]

Heart failure is a clinical entity rather than just a disease, as etiology, risk factors, and symptoms vary. The critical measure that classifies heart failure if left ventricular ejection fraction (LVEF), heart failure with reduced ejection fraction (HFrEF) is defined as LVEF <40%, heart failure with mid-range ejection fraction (HFmrEF) defined as LVEF 40–50%, HFpEF when LVEF is 50% or more with compelling signs and symptoms of heart failure and increased natriuretic peptide.

In this article we will discuss similarities and juxtaposition between HFrEF and HFpEF on various aspects.

CONTENTS AND DESCRIPTION

Epidemiology

Heart failure (HF) with mid-range ejection fraction and heart failure with preserved ejection fraction (HFpEF) constitute substantial portions of the HF patient population across various registries and clinical trials. These subgroups represent 8.1–24% and 11–43% of HF patients, respectively.[3-7]

For instance, the HF-PATHWAYS study in Spain identified 19,762 HF patients, among them, 51.7% had HFrEF, 8.1% had HFmrEF, and 40.2% had HFpEF.[6] Similarly, the ESC HF long-term registry encompassing European and Mediterranean countries reported HFmrEF and HFpEF as comprising 24.2 and 16.0% of patients, respectively, out of 9,134 cases.[3] A Chinese trial involving 35.54% HFrEF, 21.7% HFmrEF, and 42.97% HFpEF patients further highlights the prevalence of these subgroups.[5] A Swedish registry observed HFpEF, HFmrEF, and HFrEF in 18, 19, and 63% of patients, respectively (Frohlich H). Lastly, a pooled analysis of Northwestern European cohorts included 7,080 HFrEF, 1,146 HFpEF, and 2,086 HFmrEF patients among 10,312 with stable HF.[4] As per Trivandrum heart failure registry which included 1,205 HF patients had 74.19% patient who have LVEF <45 and 25.81% had LVEF >45%.

These findings underscore the importance of recognizing HFmrEF and HFpEF as distinct patient populations requiring tailored management strategies.

Comorbidities/Risk Factors in Heart Failure with Reduced Ejection Fraction and Heart Failure with Preserved Ejection Fraction

While acute cardiovascular events affecting both HFrEF and HFpEF patients share numerous risk factors, certain comorbidities distinguish between these two groups **(Table 1, Fig. 1)**. HFpEF is more prevalent in older individuals, with women outnumbering men by a factor of two. Conversely, men are more likely to develop HFrEF,

TABLE 1: Comorbidities and risk factors of HFpEF and HFrEF.

	HFpEF	*HFrEF*
Sex	Women (62%)	Men (60%)
Age	74 years	70 years
Obesity	41%	35%
Hypertension	77%	69%
Diabetes	45%	40%
Chronic kidney disease	56%	45%
Coronary artery disease	50%	59%
Prior MI	24%	36%
LV remodeling	Concentric	Eccentric
Atrial fibrillation at hospitalization	65%	59%
Ventricular arrythmia	3%	11%
HF hospitalization	Increasing	Decreasing

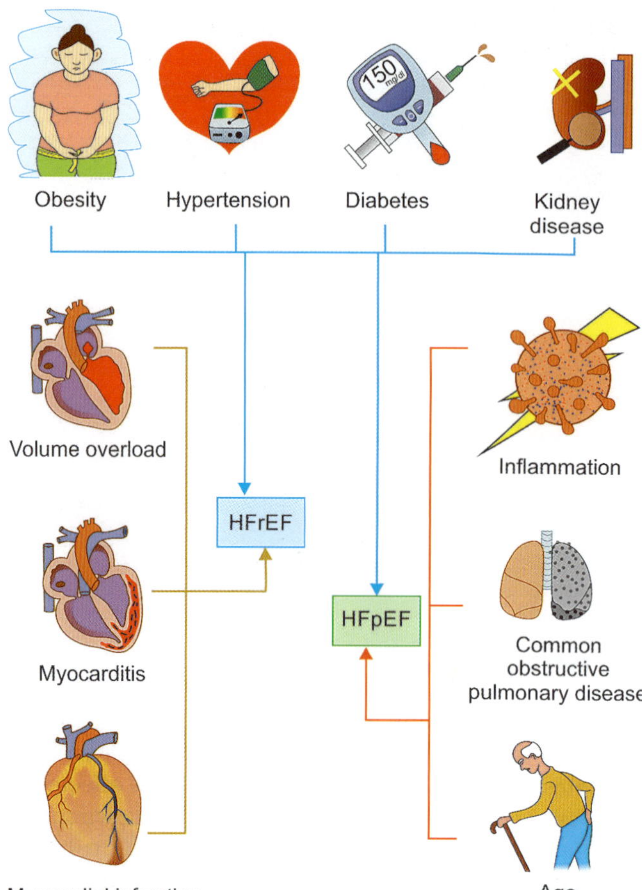

Fig. 1: Risk factors and comorbidities involved in the development of either heart failure with reduced ejection fraction, heart failure with preserved ejection fraction or both.

potentially due to a higher susceptibility to myocardial infarction. Additionally, men tend to experience eccentric left ventricular hypertrophy in response to pressure overload, while women are more prone to concentric hypertrophy.

Patients with HFpEF exhibit a higher incidence of noncardiac comorbidities, including hypertension, type 2 diabetes, stroke, anemia, pulmonary disease, liver disease, sleep apnea, gout, and cancer compared to those with HFrEF. Although the mortality risk associated with these comorbidities is similar in both HF types, HFpEF patients experience more hospitalizations related to comorbidity-induced illnesses.

Cellular and Molecular Similarities and Differences in Heart Failure with Reduced Ejection Fraction and Heart Failure with Preserved Ejection Fraction (Table 2)

Inflammation

HFrEF is associated with sterile inflammation when it is occurring due to massive ischemia. Some HFrEF inflammation is also associated with nonsterile inflammation when HF occurs because of viral infection, viral myocarditis. Sterile inflammation is associated with increased cardiac neutrophils followed by cytotoxic T cells in later phase. In HFpEF inflammation is associated with extracardiac metabolic risk-induced inflammation (obesity, diabetes, anemia, hypertension, chronic obstructive pulmonary disease (COPD), auto-immune diseases, and renal insufficiency)[8] **(Fig. 2)**.

Endothelial Dysfunction

Endothelial dysfunction although present both in HFrEF and HFpEF, presence of comorbidities leads to profound and early onset dysfunction in HFpEF. In HFrEF endothelial dysfunction is of late onset and when patient is already symptomatic. In HFpEF endothelial dysfunction develops much earlier than symptoms.[9,10]

Cardiomyocyte Cell Death

Myocyte loss is a typical feature of HFrEF. In ischemic HF activation of FAS and caspase pathway leads to myocyte apoptosis and necrosis. In viral myocarditis excessive inflammatory response causes apoptosis. Exposure of lipid, i.e., steatosis causes apoptotic pathway activation, which occurs in diabetic and other metabolic causes of cardiomyopathy. On the contrary HFpEF generally is Troponin I negative, which is a marker of cell death.[11-15]

TABLE 2: Summary of cellular, and molecular similarities, and differences between heart failure with preserved ejection fraction (HFpEF) and heart failure with reserved ejection fraction (HFrEF).

	HFpEF	*HFrEF*
Inflammation	Metabolic risk induced	• Sterile • Nonsterile
Cardiac hypertrophy	Concentric	Eccentric
Cardiomyocyte cell death	Present	Absent
Cardiac fibrosis	• ↑↑ Perivascular fibrosis • Interstitial fibrosis • ↑ Collagen crosslinking *Fibrotic signaling:* • ↑↑ Serum TGFβ1 • ↑ MCP-1	• ↑ Perivascular fibrosis • Interstitial fibrosis • Replacement fibrosis • Collagen crosslinking? *Fibrotic signaling:* • ↑ Serum TGFβ1 • ↓ MCP-1
Left ventricular stiffness	• ↑ Left ventricular stiffness *Titin:* • ↑ Cardiomyocyte F passive • N2BA → N2B • N2B hypophosphorylation • N2Bus hyperphosphorylation at S4185 • PEVK hyperphosphorylation at S11878 *Cardiac calcium signaling:* • ↑ Myocardial Ca2+ levels	• Left ventricular stiffness? *Titin:* • Cardiomyocyte F passive? • ↑ N2BA • Titin dephosphorylation • Titin aggregation • Titin cleavage *Cardiac calcium signaling:* • ↑ Myocardial [Na+]I • ↓ SERCA2a activity
Endothelial dysfunction	• Early-stage symptom • ↑ Prevalence • ↓ Microvascular density • ↓↓ NO bioavailability	• Late-stage symptom • ↓ Prevalence • ↓ Microvascular density • ↓ NO bioavailability

Cardiac Fibrosis in HFrEF and HFpEF

In HFrEF, cardiac fibrosis primarily results from cardiomyocyte loss. This can lead to systolic dysfunction through several mechanisms. For instance, the loss of fibrillar collagen might impair the transmission of cardiomyocyte contractions into myocardial force, causing uncoordinated contractions.[16] Additionally, fibrosis can disrupt the connections between cardiomyocytes and capillaries, hindering their interactions and reducing systolic reserve. This is different from HFpEF, where excessive collagen deposition and a decrease in flexible collagen III led to increased cardiac stiffness.[17,18]

Left Ventricular Stiffness in HFrEF and HFpEF

Left ventricular stiffness is one of the hallmark features of HFpEF.[19] HFrEF patients can have increased left ventricular stiffness to normal and up to reduced stiffness. Several factors play critical role in maintaining left ventricular stiffness such as titin modification and cardiac calcium levels.[20]

Pathophysiological Differences between Heart Failure with Reduced Ejection Fraction and Heart Failure with Preserved Ejection Fraction

LV Diastolic Dysfunction

A key characteristic of HFpEF is increased pressure in the left ventricle (LVFP). In severe cases, this pressure is high even when the person is resting. However, in early stages, LVFP only rises significantly during physical activity. This increased pressure can lead to difficult breathing, changes in breathing patterns, and reduced exercise capacity. In HFrEF conditions like ischemic heart disease LV diastolic dysfunction is a late feature when there is fibrosis. A significant challenge in diagnosing diastolic dysfunction in heart failure with preserved ejection fraction (HFpEF) is the age-related changes in noninvasive measures of diastolic function. Distinguishing between pathological and benign changes can be difficult. Using current guideline-based criteria, over 90% of people over 65 have at least one abnormal diastolic measure. By employing

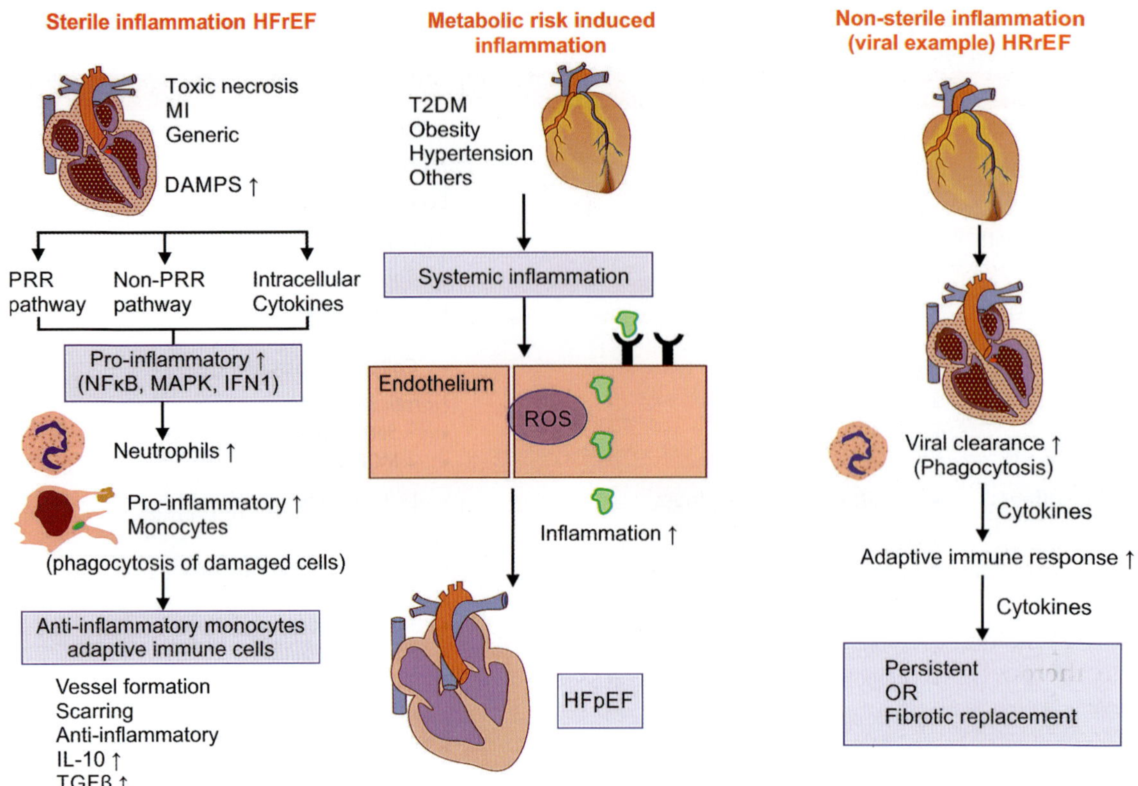

Fig. 2: Schematic of sterile-, metabolic risk-, and non-sterile-induced inflammation in the development of heart failure with reduced ejection fraction and heart failure with preserved ejection fraction. (HFpEF: heart failure with preserved ejection fraction; HFrEF: heart failure with reduced ejection fraction; HSC: hemopoietic stem cell; IFN1: interferon 1; IL-10: interleukin 10; MAPK: mitogen-activated protein kinase; NFκB: nuclear factor kappa B; PRR: pathogen recognition receptor; T2DM: type 2 diabetes mellitus; ROS: reactive oxygen species, TGFβ: transforming growth factor beta)
Note: Image created using artwork from Servier medical art.

age-appropriate reference limits derived from healthy elderly individuals, we can reduce the misclassification of diastolic abnormalities in older people. This approach improves risk prediction for heart failure or death. Even with these adjusted criteria, nearly 54% of older individuals still exhibit diastolic abnormalities.[21]

LV Systolic Dysfunction

While HFpEF is defined by a preserved left ventricular ejection fraction (LVEF), the heart's systolic function is not always normal. Both myocardial and chamber-level impairments exist at rest, but they become significantly worse during exercise. This limits the heart's ability to increase stroke volume, hindering the body's response to physical activity.[22-25] HFrEF reduced systolic function is cornerstone of diagnosis.

LA Function

HFpEF can lead to secondary remodeling and dysfunction of the left atrium (LA). Preservation of LA function might be a protective mechanism in HFpEF, to protect lungs and right heart. Impaired LA function is linked to worse exercise capacity, more severe pulmonary vascular disease, and a higher risk of death. Atrial fibrillation, a common complication in HFpEF, is further associated with LA remodeling and dysfunction. In HFrEF LA function and remodeling is much more late feature along with AF, primarily due to secondary MR.[26]

Pulmonary Hypertension

HFrEF patients present with pulmonary hypertension mainly because of passive LA hypertension. Whereas HFpEF patients are present with pulmonary hypertension (PH) more commonly due to various overlapping metabolic risk factors. Apart from passive LA hypertension pulmonary vasoconstriction and structural remodeling of pulmonary vasculature remains important contributor of PH in HFpEF.[27] Presence of PH is a poor prognostic marker regarding CV mortality in both HFrEF and HFpEF.

Large Vessel and Microvascular Dysfunction

HFpEF is associated with abnormal systemic vascular function. The aorta and other major arteries become stiffer, leading to excessive blood pressure fluctuations, and increased afterload, especially during exercise. This is partly due to endothelial dysfunction, as evidenced by impaired flow-mediated dilation and improved vascular function with nitric oxide supplementation.[28] Large vessel disease occurs in both HFrEF and HFpEF.

Diagnostic Dilemma

According to universal definition HF failure is defined as clinical syndrome with symptoms and/or signs caused by a structural and/or functional cardiac abnormality and corroborated by elevated natriuretic peptide levels and/or objective evidence of pulmonary or systemic congestion.[29]

HF is often subclassified by ejection fraction into HFrEF, HFpEF, HFmrEF, and HFimpEF.[28] Diagnosis of HFrEF is simple but HFpEF identification requires keen clinical insight and thorough investigation as it can be easily missed. Several prognostic scores like H2FPEF score have been utilized to better screening of HFpEF among patients with unexplained dyspnea. Several echocardiography parameters have been used to increase sensitivity and specificity of diagnosis of HFpEF but still many patients require advanced functional testing for diagnosis[30] **(Table 3)**.

Treatment

The HFrEF patients have robust treatment options at disposal that significantly decrease CV mortality and hospitalization targeting specific pathology. In HFpEF patients until recently treatment is focused on management of risk factors only, which is still mainstay of treatment of HFpEF.

Mortality and Morbidity

Regardless of LVEF, heart failure (HF) is associated with higher mortality compared to individuals without HF. Epidemiological studies consistently show a greater risk of all-cause and cardiovascular death in HF with preserved ejection fraction (HFpEF) compared to those without HF. While some studies have found similar mortality rates between HFpEF and HF with reduced ejection fraction (HFrEF), this is not always true. Other studies report lower mortality rates in HFpEF.[31-33]

Epidemiological evidence suggests that cardiovascular mortality is lower, but noncardiovascular mortality is higher, in HFpEF compared to HFrEF. These findings are consistent with the observations from clinical trials. Importantly, hospitalization rates, duration of hospital stays, and patient-reported outcomes like quality of life appear similar between HFpEF and HFrEF.[34,35]

TABLE 3: Echocardiographic and natriuretic peptide criteria for heart failure with preserved ejection fraction patients in sinus and atrial fibrillation.[30]

	Functional	*Morphological*	*Biomarker (SR)*	*Biomarker (AF)*
Major	Septal e' <7 cm/s or Lateral e' <10 cm/s or Average E/e' ≥15 or TR velocity >2.8 m/s (PASP >35 mm Hg)	LAVI >34 mL/m² or LVMI ≥149/122 g/m² (m/w) and RWT 0.42	NT-proBNP >220 pg/mL or BNP >80 pg/mL	NT-proBNP >660 pg/mL or BNP >240 pg/mL
Minor	Average E/e' 9–14 or GLS <16%	LAVI 29–34 mL/m² or LVMI >115/95 g/m² (m/w) or RWT >0,42 or LV wall thickness >12 mm	NT-proBNP 125–220 pg/mL or BNP 35–80 pg/mL	NT-proBNP 365–660 pg/mL or BNP 105–240 pg/mL
Major criteria: 2 points		*≥5 points: HFpEF*		
Minor criteria: 1 point		*2–4 points: Diastolic stress test or invasive hemodynamic measurements*		

(GLS: global longitudinal strain; NT-proBNP: N-terminal pro b-type natriuretic peptide; PASP: pulmonary arterial systolic pressure; LAVI: left atrial volume index; LVMI: left ventricular mass index; RWT: relative wall thickness; TR: tricuspid regurgitation)

LIMITATION

Despite enormous advancement of diagnostic modalities and better access to health care heart failure is still underdiagnosed and underreported particularly in developing countries. HFpEF is still not addressed properly due to overlapping symptoms with comorbid condition. Also HFpEF and HFrEF is not static condition as HFpEF patient can develop HFrEF in future and HFrEF patients may have improvement of ejection fraction with guideline directed treatment.

CONCLUSION

Early diagnosis and treatment are necessary for all patients with heart failure. Early initiation of treatment significantly reduces heart failure hospitalization and economic burden particularly in developing countries.

REFERENCES

1. Huffman MD, Prabhakaran D. Heart failure: Epidemiology and prevention in India. Natl Med J India. 2010;23(5):283-8.
2. Harikrishnan S, Bahl A, Roy A, et al. National Heart Failure Registry, India: Design and methods. Indian Heart J. 2019;71(6):488-91.
3. Chioncel O, Parissis J, Mebazaa A, et al. Epidemiology, pathophysiology and contemporary management of cardiogenic shock - a position statement from the Heart Failure Association of the European Society of Cardiology. Eur J Heart Fail. 2020;22(8):1315-41.
4. Fröhlich H, Rosenfeld N, Tager T, et al. Epidemiology and long-term outcome in outpatients with chronic heart failure in Northwestern Europe. Heart. 2019;105(16):1252-9.
5. Wang H-J, Rozanski GJ, Zucker IH. Cardiac sympathetic afferent reflex control of cardiac function in normal and chronic heart failure states. J Physiol. 2017;595(8):2519-34.
6. Simmonds SJ, Cuijpers I, Heymans S, et al. Cellular and molecular differences between HFpEF and HFrEF: a step ahead in an improved pathological understanding. Cells. 2020;9(1):242.
7. Savarese G, Becher PM, Lund LH, et al. Global burden of heart failure: a comprehensive and updated review of epidemiology. Cardiovasc Res. 2023;118(17):3272-87.
8. Paulus WJ, Tschöpe C. A novel paradigm for heart failure with preserved ejection fraction. J Am Coll Cardiol. 2013;62(4):263-71.
9. Mohammed SF, Hussain S, Mirzoyev SA, et al. Coronary microvascular rarefaction and myocardial fibrosis in heart failure with preserved ejection fraction. Circulation. 2015;131(6):550-9.
10. Seferović PM, Coats AJS, Ponikowski P, et al. European Society of Cardiology/Heart Failure Association position paper on the role and safety of new glucose-lowering drugs in patients with heart failure. Eur J Heart Fail. 2020;22(2):196-213.
11. Cheng RK, Cox M, Neely ML, et al. Outcomes in patients with heart failure with preserved, borderline, and reduced ejection fraction in the Medicare population. Am Heart J. 2014;168(5):721-30.e3.
12. Hamblin M, Smith HM, Hill MF, et al. Dietary supplementation with vitamin E ameliorates cardiac failure in type I diabetic cardiomyopathy by suppressing myocardial generation of 8-iso-prostaglandin F2a and oxidized glutathione. J Card Fail. 2007;13(10):884-92.
13. Fuentes-Antrás J, Picatoste B, Gómez-Hernández A, et al. Updating experimental models of diabetic cardiomyopathy. J Diabetes Res. 2015; 2015:1-15.
14. Wei F-F, Xue R, Thijs L, et al. Associations of left ventricular structure and function with blood pressure in heart failure with preserved ejection fraction: Analysis of the TOPCAT Trial. J Am Heart Assoc. 2020;9(15).
15. Brown DA, Perry JB, Allen ME, et al. Mitochondrial function as a therapeutic target in heart failure. Nat Rev Cardiol. 2017;14(4):238-50.
16. Weber KT. Heart failure: Lessons learned over the past 25 years. Clin Cardiol. 1995;18(3):123-30.
17. Henning RJ. Diagnosis and treatment of heart failure with preserved left ventricular ejection fraction. World J Cardiol. 2020;12(1):7-25.
18. Wang J, Kurrelmeyer KM, Torre-Amione G, et al. Systolic and diastolic dyssynchrony in patients with diastolic heart failure and the effect of medical therapy. J Am Coll Cardiol. 2007;49(1):88-96.
19. Westermann D, Lindner D, Kasner M, et al. Cardiac inflammation contributes to changes in the extracellular matrix in patients with heart failure and normal ejection fraction. Circ Heart Fail. 2011;4(1):44-52.
20. van Heerebeek L, Paulus WJ. Understanding heart failure with preserved ejection fraction: where are we today? Neth Heart J. 2016;24(4):227-36.
21. Shah AM, Claggett B, Kitzman D, et al. Contemporary assessment of left ventricular diastolic function in older adults: The Atherosclerosis Risk in Communities study. Circulation. 2017;135(5):426-39.
22. Obokata M, Reddy YNV, Melenovsky V, et al. Myocardial injury and cardiac reserve in patients with heart failure and preserved ejection fraction. J Am Coll Cardiol. 2018; 72(1):29-40.
23. Maeder MT, Karapanagiotidis S, Dewar EM, et al. Accuracy of echocardiographic cardiac index assessment in subjects with preserved left ventricular ejection fraction. Echocardiography. 2015;32(11):1628-38.
24. Reddy YNV, Kaye DM, Humdoko LM, et al. Diagnosis of heart failure with preserved ejection fraction among patients with unexplained dyspnea. JAMA Cardiol. 2022;7(9):891.
25. Borlaug BA, Sharma K, Shah SJ, et al. Heart failure with preserved ejection fraction. J Am Coll Cardiol. 2023;81(18):1810-34.

26. Mohammed SF, Hussain I, AbouEzzeddine OF, et al. Right ventricular function in heart failure with preserved ejection fraction: A community-based study. Circulation. 2014;130(25):2310-20.
27. Fayyaz AU, Edwards WD, Maleszewski JJ, et al. Global pulmonary vascular remodeling in pulmonary hypertension associated with heart failure and preserved or reduced ejection fraction. Circulation. 2018;137(17):1796-810.
28. Reddy YNV, Andersen MJ, Obokata M, et al. Arterial stiffening with exercise in patients with heart failure and preserved ejection fraction. J Am Coll Cardiol. 2017;70(2):136-48.
29. Bozkurt B, Coats AJS, Tsutsui H, et al. Universal definition and classification of heart failure. J Card Fail. 2021;27(4):387-413.
30. Pieske B, Tschöpe C, Boer RA, et al. How to diagnose heart failure with preserved ejection fraction: the HFA–PEFF diagnostic algorithm: a consensus recommendation from the Heart Failure Association (HFA) of the European Society of Cardiology (ESC). Eur Heart J. 2019;40(40):3297-317.
31. Bursi F, Weston SA, Redfield M, et al. Systolic and diastolic heart failure in the community. JAMA. 2006;296(18):2209-16.
32. Owan TE, Hodge DO, Herges RM, et al. Trends in prevalence and outcome of heart failure with preserved ejection fraction. N Engl J Med. 2006;355(3):251-9.
33. Bhatia RS, Tu JV, Lee DS, et al. Outcome of heart failure with preserved ejection fraction in a population-based study. N Engl J Med. 2006;355(3):260-9.
34. Lewis EF, Lamas GA, O'Meara E, et al. Characterization of health-related quality of life in heart failure patients with preserved versus low ejection fraction in CHARM. Eur J Heart Fail. 2007;9(1):83-91.
35. Loop MS, Van Dyke MK, Chen L, et al. Comparison of length of stay, 30-day mortality, and 30-day readmission rates in medicare patients with heart failure and with reduced versus preserved ejection fraction. Am J Cardiol. 2016;118(1):79-85.

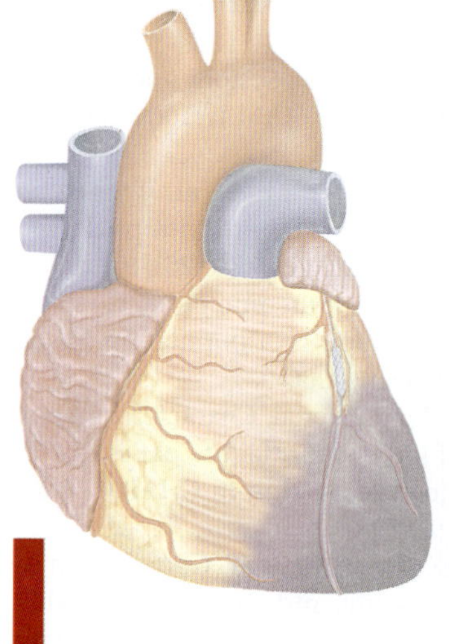

Advances in HFpEF Management

Mrinal Kanti Das

INTRODUCTION

Heart failure (HF) is a major public health problem, affecting 26 million people worldwide. It is a major cause of morbidity and mortality. A number of guidelines have been formulated over many years by the physicians to guide the principles of treatment of HF, based on the conception about the pathophysiology, availability of the drugs at the particular point of time, and the personal real-life and real-world experiences. However, with changing time, the evidence-based medicine evolved, and the stakeholders of health imposed the guideline with the help of evidence and routinized the clinical practice. From time to time, the guidelines have been updated and published on the diagnostic and management principles, which have changed the paradigm of therapy for HF with huge geoeconomic and secular effects, resulting in lowering of morbidity and mortality.[1,2] Conforming with the title of the topic, only the latest concept will be dealt with, without repeating the standard echocardiographic pictures of diastolic HF, which is many a time synonymously used for Heart failure with preserved ejection fraction (HFpEF).

HISTORICAL PERSPECTIVE

EH Starling brought physics into the mechanism of heart function in 1910 and opined that as the muscles get elongated or dilated up to certain extent, the contractile function increases. This was referred to as Starling's law of the heart. This gave way to the principle that as the heart gets filled and end-diastolic volume increases, cardiac performance increases to a point. This explained the HF with dilated heart with abnormal contractile function but could not explain the HF in patients without dilation of the ventricle.[3] In 1940–1960, the journey of cardiac catheterization and surgery revealed many aspects of HF in rheumatic and congenital heart diseases, in terms of hemodynamic abnormalities, but they also failed to explain HF with obstructive coronary arteries or hypertension or without any evidence of so-called obvious cause.[4,5] From these inputs, the concept of remodeling came into the picture, which can happen in different ways such as concentric or eccentric hypertrophy of the heart without external dilatation and dilated heart with an increase in length of the muscles at the cost of strength and width. Remodeling and reverse remodeling are considered very important in the progression or deterioration of HF, treatment responses, and further consequences.[6] The concept of remodeling later on enthused workers to propose different names of the HF. This concept of remodeling and prior and postremodeling events at heart and cellular levels is depicted in **Flowchart 1 and Figure 1**. In the meantime, the concept of ejection fraction (EF) developed over a period of time starting with the idea of dilatation of the left ventricle by Sir William Harvey[7] and later on by various workers with the help of cardiac catheterization and other tests, including echocardiography, which formed the stellar procedure for diagnosis of HF. **Figures 2 and 3** are suggestive of the pathways to the concept of EF, including the timeline.

But the EF could not explain many aspects related to HF. There were heterogeneous responses to medications. Some were responders, and some were nonresponders. This led to the concept of "clusters" based on phenotyping and phenomapping. The guideline-directed treatments

Flowchart 1: Preremodeling.

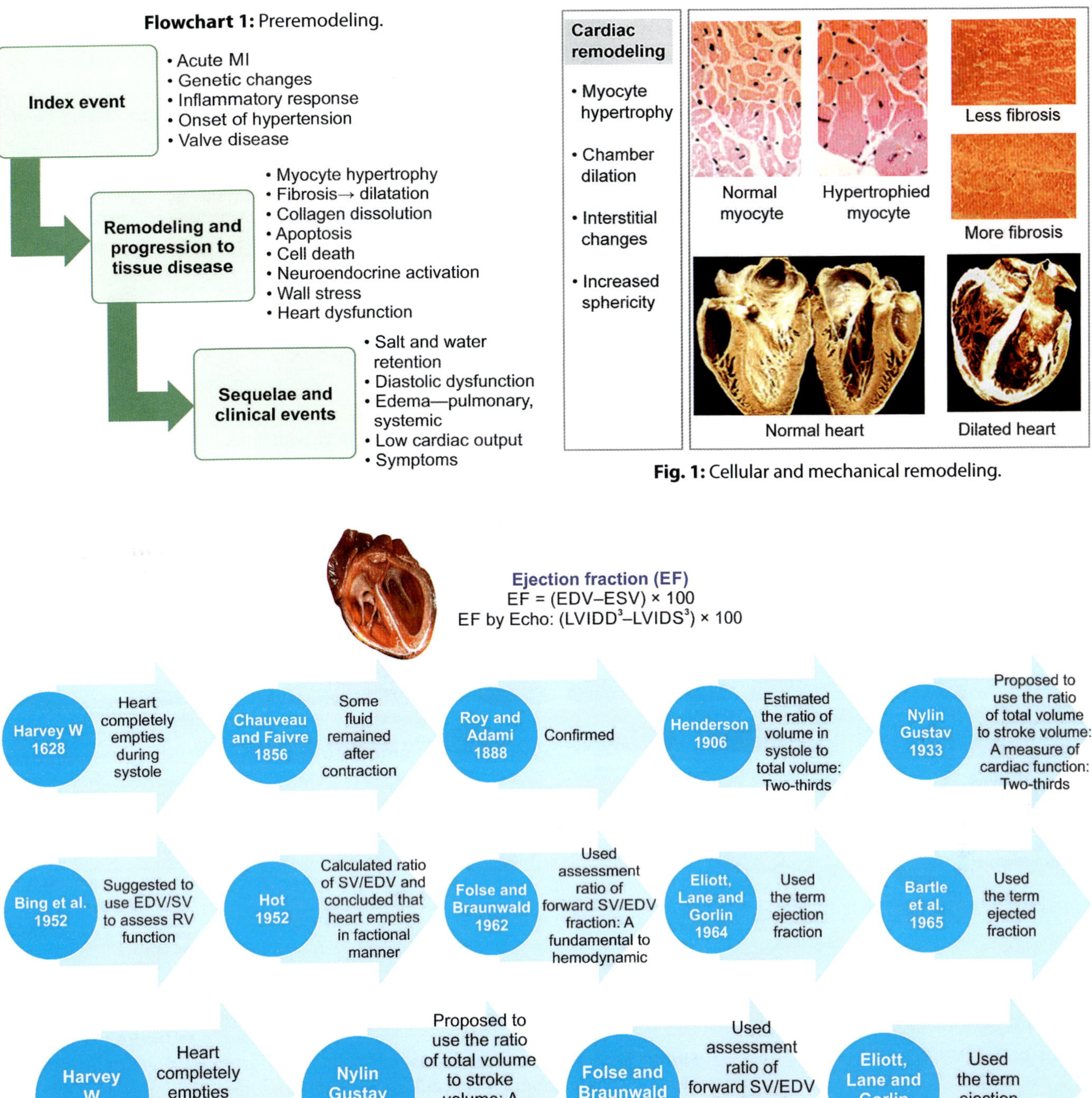

Fig. 1: Cellular and mechanical remodeling.

Fig. 2: Conceptualization of EF.

were proposed toward the specific cluster, which offered personalized care of HF patients. The HFpEF was clustered into three types based on environmental factors, comorbidities, and genetic susceptibility:

1. *Type 1:* Exercise-induced increase in LA pressure
2. *Type 2:* Volume overload
3. *Type 3:* Pulmonary hypertension and RV failure

The concept of clusters is still evolving and is shown in **Figure 4**. It highlights Kaplan–Meier curve for the composite of clinical events of different clusters on the

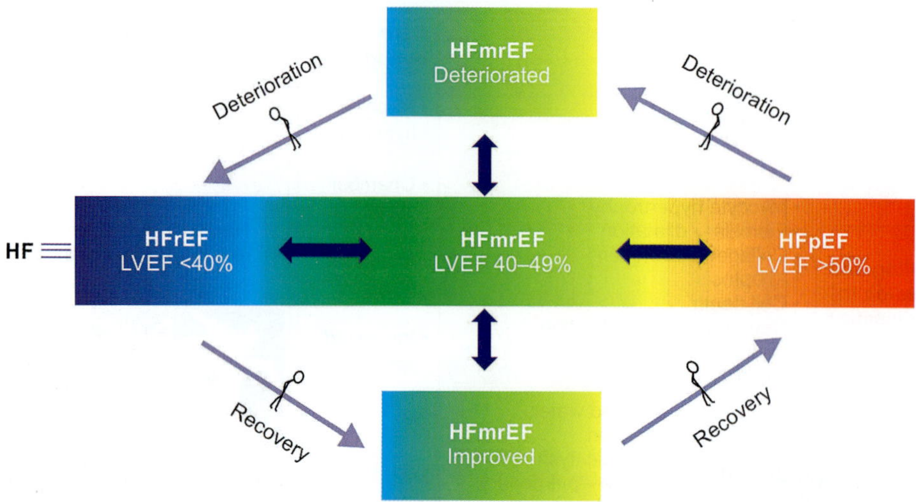

Fig. 3: Continuum and evolution of classification of LVEF-based HFEF with time.

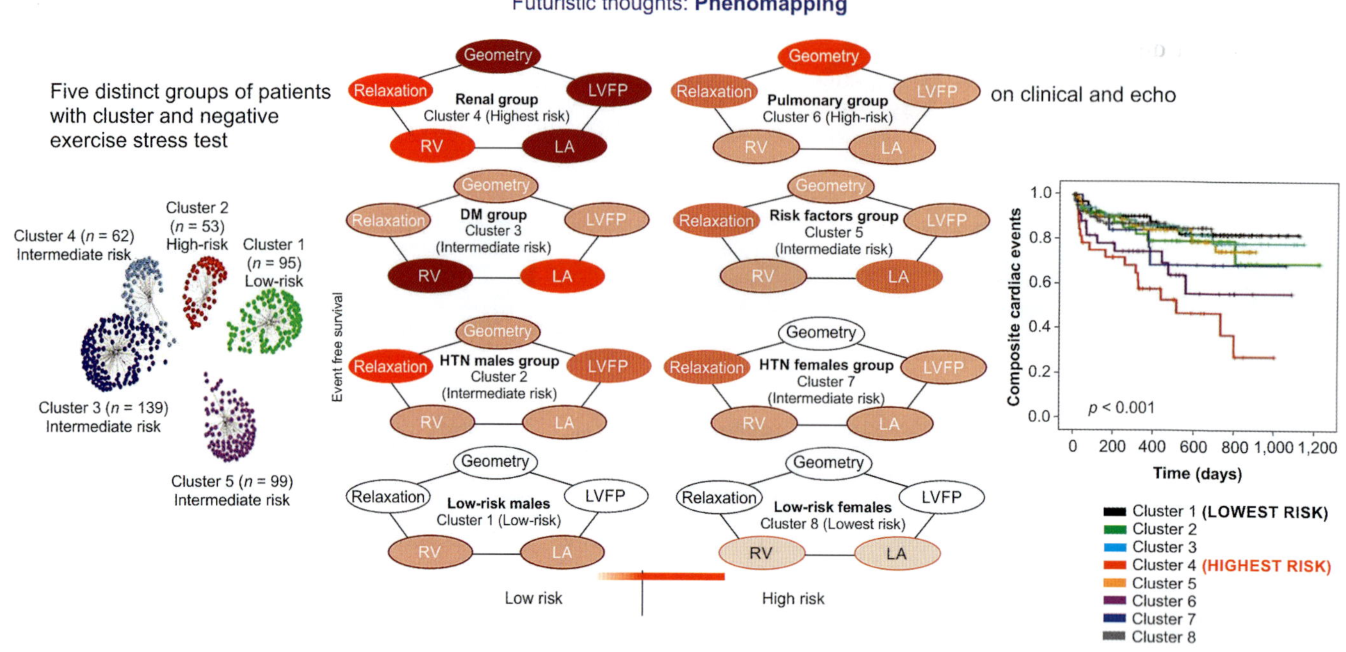

Fig. 4: Clusters of HF and risk status.
Source: Adapted from Omar et al.[8]

right side of **Figure 4** along with various clinical clusters in the middle.[8]

GUIDELINE-DIRECTED DIAGNOSIS AND MANAGEMENT OF HFpEF

Let us embark on the similarities or dissimilarities in different guidelines.[9,10] Since HF has been conceived as a continuum, the management principles are also continuum, and similar group of drugs are used in HFrEF, HFmrEF, HFpEF, or HFnEF with different recommendation levels. This will cover both the diagnostic approach and therapeutic consideration combining the guidelines of different cardiac societies such as the European Society of Cardiology (ESC) and the American College of Cardiology/American Heart Association/Heart Failure Society of America (ACC/AHA/HFSA).

Both the groups agree on various diagnostic and therapeutic approaches on the following fronts and highlight these:

- The importance of history and examination in the diagnosis of HF and its etiology as well as in the setting of decompensation to identify the cause of clinical deterioration.
- All patients with a new diagnosis of HF should have a three-generation pedigree analysis to assess family history of cardiomyopathy.
- The investigations need to be carried out are given as follows:
    - Electrocardiogram (ECG)
    - *Blood tests:* Natriuretic peptides (BNP or NT-proBNP), serum urea and electrolytes, creatinine, complete blood count, lipid profile, iron studies, and liver and thyroid function tests are recommended to differentiate HF from other conditions, provide prognostic information, and guide potential therapy.
    - *Transthoracic echocardiography (TTE):* This aids in determining the left ventricular ejection fraction (LVEF) and identifying the underlying etiology of HF.
    - *Chest X-ray:* This provides supportive evidence of HF and aids in ruling out alternative causes of breathlessness.
- The ESC recommends that CMR may be useful for the assessment of myocardial ischemia in patients with dilated cardiomyopathy who would be suitable for coronary revascularization [class of recommendation (CoR): 2b]. In comparison, the ACC/AHA/HFSA guidelines recommend the same may be reasonable (CoR: 2b).
- The ESC and ACC/AHA/HFSA guidelines both suggest noninvasive stress imaging [such as CMR, stress echocardiography, and single-photon emission computed tomography (SPECT)] to assess inducible ischemia and viability for patients with coronary artery disease (CAD) who are suitable for coronary revascularization. For patients with a low to intermediate pretest probability of CAD or those with inconclusive noninvasive stress tests, computed tomography coronary angiography (CTCA) may be considered to rule out the diagnosis of CAD. Invasive coronary angiography is recommended for patients with persistent angina despite pharmacological therapy and those with an intermediate to high pretest probability of CAD and heart failure with reduced ejection fraction (HFrEF) who are deemed suitable for coronary revascularization.
- Endomyocardial biopsy should be considered as per both guidelines and performed when a specific diagnosis is sought, and when that diagnosis would significantly impact management, particularly in cases of rapidly progressive HF or worsening ventricular function despite treatment. This approach ensures that the risks of the procedure are justified by the potential impact on guiding the appropriate management decisions.
- Both the guidelines recommend all four drugs in asymptomatic HF stages A and B to prevent them from transiting to stages C and D.

    In patients with a recent or remote history of MI or acute coronary syndrome and LVEF <40%, statins should be used to prevent symptomatic HF and adverse CV events, and evidence-based beta-blockers should be used to reduce mortality.
- In stage C, all the measures for stages A and B should be followed and along with them, all the four drugs should be strongly recommended, initiated, and dosage optimized. Both the ACC/AHA/HFSA 2022 HF guideline and the ESC 2021 HF guideline recommend diuretics to reduce congestion and improve symptoms. The diuretics furosemide/bumetanide or chlorthalidone/chlorothiazide may be used. The latter should be specially considered in cases of furosemide failure.
- Both guidelines agree that implantable cardioverter defibrillators (ICDs) are effective at reducing sudden cardiac death (SCD), and improving cardiac function and quality of life, in selected patients with HF.
- Both the ACC/AHA/HFSA and ESC guidelines support the use of inotropes in the palliative setting for symptom relief (CoR: 2b). These recommendations are echoed in the ESC guideline; however, the evidence has not been assessed.
- Both the ACC/AHA/HFSA and ESC guidelines emphasize the critical role of a multidisciplinary team (MDT) approach in the management of HF.

There are few disagreements as shown below and they also define the different groups of HF, which are not complicated:

- The *ESC* guidelines recommend CMR for characterization of myocardial tissue in suspected infiltrative disease, Fabry disease, inflammatory disease (e.g., myocarditis), left ventricular (LV) noncompaction, amyloid, sarcoidosis, and hemochromatosis (CoR: 1). The *ACC/AHA/HFSA* guidelines find that CMR is reasonable in patients with nonischemic cardiomyopathy if the diagnosis is uncertain based on the recent OUTSMART-HF trial, although with a lower strength of recommendation than the ESC guidelines (CoR: 2a).
- The classification of HF by LVEF is shown in **Table 1**.

TABLE 1: Classification of HF by LVEF.

Types of HF	ACC/AHA/HFSA	ESC
HFrEF	<40%	<40%
HF improved EF	<40% improved to >40%	Not mentioned
HFmrEF	41–49% + Evidence of spontaneous or provokable increased LV filling pressures (e.g., elevated natriuretic peptide, noninvasive and invasive hemodynamic measurement)	41–49%
HFpEF	>50% + Evidence of spontaneous or provokable increased LV filling pressures (e.g., elevated natriuretic peptide, noninvasive and invasive hemodynamic measurement such as combination of echocardiographic parameters such as an elevation in the ratio of mitral inflow velocity to mitral annular excursion (E/e' ≥15), or a reduction in the latter, as well as increased LA volume or pulmonary hypertension)	>50% Objective evidence of cardiac structural and/or functional abnormalities consistent with the presence of LV diastolic dysfunction/raised LV filling pressures, including raised natriuretic peptides

- The *H2FPEF score*, described in the ACC/AHA/HFSA guideline, and *HFA-PEFF score*, described in the ESC guideline, have been proposed to aid diagnosis, although the ESC suggests a simplified diagnostic approach that is yet to be critically assessed or compared to the score-based algorithms.
- *In stage A, which encompasses most of the cases of HFpEF*, the ACC/AHA/HFSA guidelines provide detailed recommendations on management for patients at risk for HF (stage A). While not strictly categorized as a stage of HF, the ESC guidelines also provide a guide to prevention of HF for those with risk factors.
- *SGLT2i therapy in patients with diabetes:* The ACC/AHA/HFSA guidelines recommend that patients with type 2 diabetes mellitus (T2DM) and either established CV disease or at high risk of CV disease should be commenced on SGLT2i therapy (CoR: 2A) to improve survival and prevent HF hospitalizations irrespective of diabetes status. SGLT2 inhibitors could be canagliflozin, empagliflozin, or dapagliflozin, all of which showed benefits as per the different trials (CANVAS, EMPA-REG OUTCOME, DAPA-HF, and DAPA-PRESERVE). The ESC, on the other hand, recommends SGLT2i for HFpEF with DM[2] (CoR: 1). Recently, the updated version of the ACC/AHA/HFSA has dealt with HFpEF in some more detail.
- *In stage B, which also encompasses most of the cases of HFpEF*, all recommendations for patients with stage A HF also apply to those with stage B HF. The ESC guidelines do not distinguish between stage A and stage B in their recommendations for the prevention of HF.
- *Telemonitoring:* The guidelines differ slightly on the recommendations for telemonitoring. The ACC/AHA/HFSA guidelines suggest that telemonitoring is not recommended, and further research is required. The ESC guidelines suggest that telemonitoring may be reasonable to reduce the risk of recurrent CV and HF hospitalizations and CV death (CoR: 2b).

  Emerging data have shown promise in smartphone-based options for telemonitoring, and this is likely to be a focus in *future guidelines*.

Flowchart 2: Algorithm of the drug therapy for HFpEF.[10]

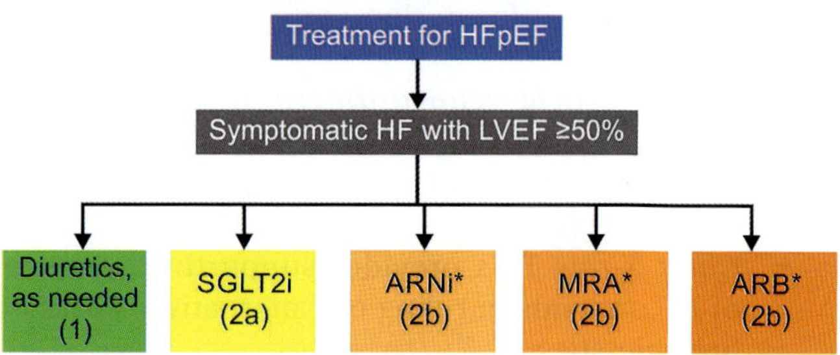

Note: *Greater benefit in patients with LVEF closer to 50%.
Source: Adapted from Heidenreich et al.[11]

- The ACC/AHA/HFSA guidelines recommend that all patients with HF should receive palliative and supportive care to improve quality of life (CoR: 1), with the suggestion that patients who have stage D HF, uncontrolled symptoms, multimorbidity, frailty, or cognitive impairment should be referred to specialist palliative care (CoR: 2a). There is no such suggestion in the ESC guidelines.

Algorithms for the advanced therapy of HFpEF are shown in **Flowcharts 2 and 3; Figures 5 and 6.** These include overall drug management for HFpEF, followed by special management principles of a correctable cause of the disease, namely amyloidosis and comorbidities, and lastly the recommendations for atrial fibrillation in HF, which influences the course

Flowchart 3: Algorithm of the diagnosis and drug therapy for HFpEF with transthyretin cardiac amyloidosis.

Diagnosis and treatment of transthyretin cardiac amyloidosis

History, ECG, echocardiogram, cardiac MRI suggestive of cardiac amyloidosis

Check for monoclonal light chains (1)

Presence of monoclonal light chain?

Yes

Hematology–oncology consultation and consider heart or other biopsy

Amyloid on heart biopsy?

No evidence of amyloid

Cardiac amyloidosis unlikely

Evidence of amyloid

AL-CM

Treatment by hematologist-oncologist

ATTR-CM

No

Check Tc-99m-PYP scan (1)

Tc-99m-PYP abnormal?

No

Cardiac amyloidosis unlikely

Yes

Perform TTR gene sequencing (1)

ATTRwt-CM

ATTRv-CM

Treatment

Atrial fibrillation → Anticoagulation regardless of CHA2DS2-VASc score (2a)

NYHA I-III symptoms → Tafamidis (1)

HFrEF → Individualized therapy

- Referral to genetic counselor
- Potential screening of family members
- TTR silencer therapy if neuropathy

At 2020 list prices, tafamidis provides low economic value (>$180,000 per QALY gained) in patients with HF with wild type or variant transthyretin cardiac amyloidosis

Value statement:
Low value (B-NR)

Source: Adapted from Heidenreich et al.[11]

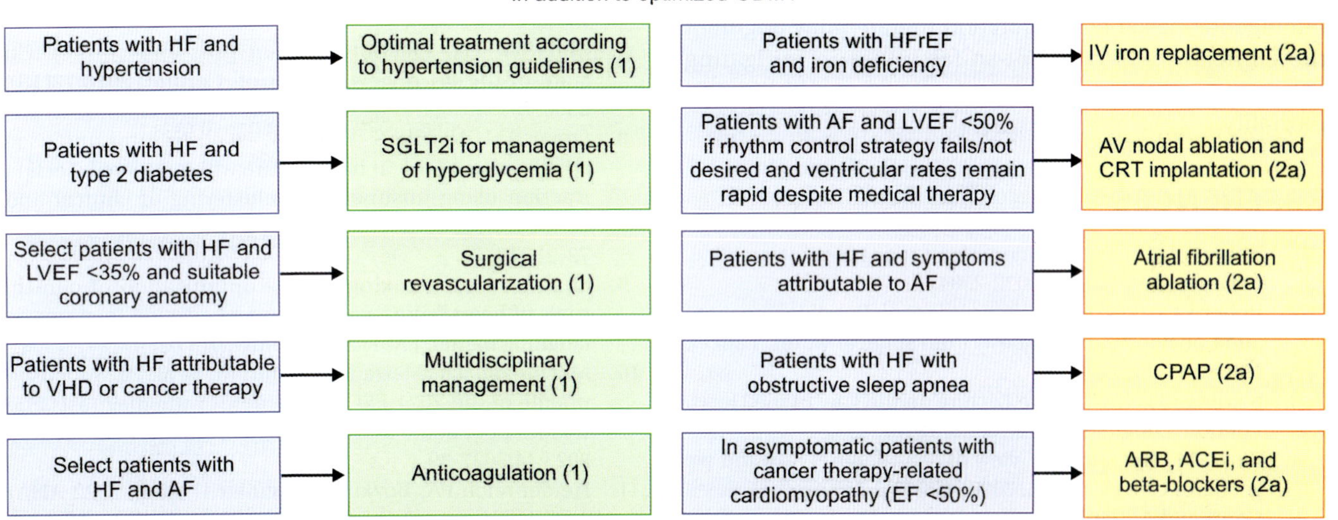

Fig. 5: Algorithm of the additional therapy for comorbidities.
Source: Adapted from Heidenreich et al.[11]

of events in most of the patients. Since the algorithms themselves are self-explanatory, so if the readers wish, they have the choice to explore them further from the references appended below.[11]

CONCLUSION

Heart failure is a complex syndrome with failure to either maintain cardiac output and fill the ventricles and thus the understanding of the disease took so much time over centuries of researches and studies. The HFpEF is more complex because of interaction between epigenetics (environmental factors), comorbidities, genomics, cytokines inducing inflammation, and remodeling of the heart, which loses its normal function of supplying oxygen and nutrition to tissues and organs and, thus, generates a precarious situation with multiple symptoms and clinical, mechanical, and biochemical changes in the body.

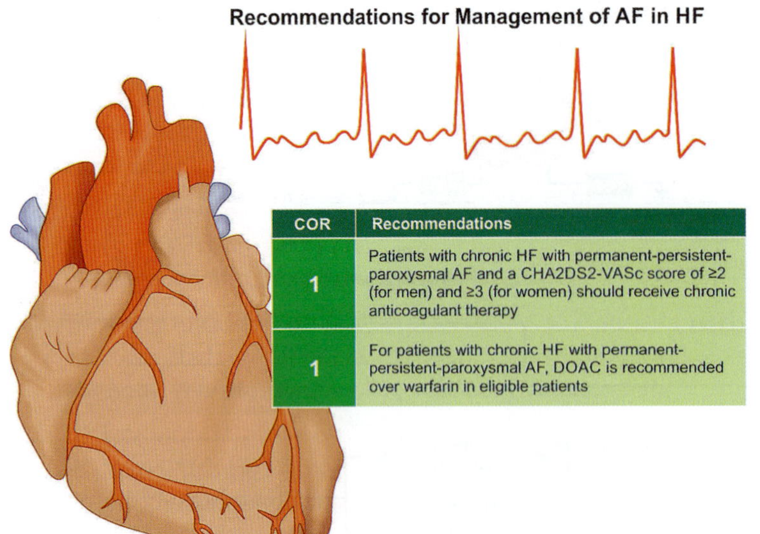

COR	Recommendations
1	Patients with chronic HF with permanent-persistent-paroxysmal AF and a CHA2DS2-VASc score of ≥2 (for men) and ≥3 (for women) should receive chronic anticoagulant therapy
1	For patients with chronic HF with permanent-persistent-paroxysmal AF, DOAC is recommended over warfarin in eligible patients

COR	Recommendations
2a	For patients with HF and symptoms caused by AF, AF ablation is reasonable to improve symptoms and QOL
2a	For patients with AF and LVEF ≤50%, if a rhythm control strategy fails or is not desired, and ventricular rates remain rapid despite medical therapy, AV nodal ablation with implantation of a CRT device is reasonable
2a	For patients with chronic HF and permanent-persistent-paroxysmal AF, chronic anticoagulant therapy is reasonable for men and women without additional risk factors

Fig. 6: Recommendation of the drug therapy for atrial fibrillation in HFpEF.
Source: Adapted from Heidenreich et al.[11]

Being complex in nature, "one-size-does-not fit-all" may be the reality of life in this condition, and artificial intelligence-based evaluation and therapy may augment the clinician's effort in not-so-far future in mitigating the menacing disease both in terms of morbidity and mortality.

REFERENCES

1. Roberts J. The moral character of management practice. J Manag Stud. 1984;21:0022-2384.
2. Roberts CJ, Fowkes FG, Ennis WP, et al. Possible impact of audit on chest X-ray requests from surgical wards. Lancet. 1983;2(8347):446-8.
3. Starling EH. The Linacre Lecture on the Law of the Heart. London: Longmans Green & Co; 1918.
4. Katz AM. The 'modern' view of heart failure: how did we get here? Circ Heart Fail. 2008;1:63-71.
5. Cournand A. Cardiac catheterization; development of the technique, its contributions to experimental medicine, and its initial applications in man. Acta Med Scand Suppl. 1975;579:3-32.
6. Coats AJS. Left ventricular remodelling—concepts and pathophysiology: current understanding. Heart Fail J India. 2024;2:50-4.
7. Marwick TH. Ejection fraction pros and cons: JACC state-of-the-art review. J Am Coll Cardiol. 2018;72(19): 2360-79.
8. Omar AM, Narula S, Yugay A, et al. Natural unbiased stratification of risk in heart failure with preserved ejection fraction using unsupervised clustering of clinical and echocardiographic variables. J Am Coll Cardiol. 2019; 73(9):973.
9. Shah SJ. Matchmaking for the optimization of clinical trials of heart failure with preserved ejection fraction: no laughing matter. J Am Coll Cardiol. 2013;62.
10. McDonagh TA, Metra M, Adamo M, et al. 2023 focused update of the 2021 ESC guidelines for the diagnosis and treatment of acute and chronic heart failure. Eur Heart J. 2023;44:3627-39.
11. Heidenreich PA, Bozkurt B, Aguilar D, et al. 2022 AHA/ ACC/HFSA guideline for the management of heart failure: a report of the American College of Cardiology/American Heart Association Joint Committee on Clinical Practice Guidelines. Circulation. 2022;145:e895-1032.

Prevalence of Coronary Microvascular Dysfunction in HFpEF: A Systematic Review and Meta-analysis

Arijit Ghosh, Subhasis Roy Chowdhury, Arup Dasbiswas

INTRODUCTION

The worldwide incidence of heart failure (HF) is on the rise, and heart failure with preserved ejection fraction (HFpEF) accounts for over half of the newly diagnosed HF in the community.[1] HFpEF is associated with increasing age and is the most common HF phenotype in those above 65 years.[2] However, the rising incidence of HFpEF cannot be explained by aging alone, and obesity and type 2 diabetes (T2D) are the two comorbidities strongly associated with HFpEF.[3] HFpEF is also associated with other comorbidities, such as chronic obstructive pulmonary disease, atrial fibrillation (AF), chronic kidney disease, and hypertension.[4]

In a paradigm shift from the traditional model of excessive afterload leading to diastolic dysfunction, an inflammatory hypothesis of HFpEF has been put forward, with coronary microvascular dysfunction (CMD) taking the center stage of its pathophysiology.[5] In the inflammatory hypothesis, chronic comorbidities are thought to induce a systemic proinflammatory state, resulting in endothelial dysfunction (cardiac and extracardiac) leading to impaired vasodilatory capacity and microvascular dysfunction (MVD), which leads to the downstream sequelae of hypertrophy, fibrosis, and stiffening of the myocardium, along with LA dilation and abnormal LV relaxation.[5]

This chapter explores the importance of MVD in HFpEF pathophysiology.

PATHOPHYSIOLOGY OF MICROVASCULAR DYSFUNCTION

Myocardial coronary blood flow (CBF) is governed by a complex interplay of aortic pressure, epicardial coronary arterial vessel patency, and microvascular resistance. The phasic compression and decompression of the coronary microvasculature by surrounding cardiac myocytes during myocardial contraction and relaxation further influences coronary flow, so-called "cardiac-coronary coupling."[6]

In the healthy heart, the lion's share of coronary flow occurs during diastole, with the backward expansion wave (BEW) reflecting decompression of the microvasculature during early diastole. In MVD, during exercise and pharmacologically induced microvascular dilation, blunting of the BEW (which ordinarily accelerates flow) and accentuation of the backward compression wave (which ordinarily decelerates flow) have been noted.[7] Therefore, in HFpEF, impaired lusitropy (i.e., the degree of LV relaxation and diastolic dysfunction) may attenuate the BEW and thereby cause impaired myocardial perfusion.[8]

Microvascular dysfunction is defined as an abnormality in the myocardial microcirculation, leading to an inadequate vasodilatory response following physiological or pharmacological stress.[9] It has predominantly two endotypes such as structural and functional. Though both endotypes exhibit impaired myocardial perfusion reserve (MPR) in response to adenosine, the mechanisms are different. Structural MVD is associated with elevated minimal microvascular resistance; in functional MVD, the microvascular resistance remains normal, with reduced vascular tone at rest, but during stress, there is an attenuated vasodilatory reserve.[7,10] Again, structural MVD exhibits normal resting myocardial blood flow but with an impaired ability to augment blood flow in response to stress and diminished peripheral endothelium-dependent dilatation, which can precipitate exercise-induced hypertension. Both endotypes have a similar core phenotype, with a high prevalence of inducible ischemia and inefficient cardiac–coronary coupling during physical exercise. However, their pathophysiology differs at the endothelial and microvascular levels.

PATHOPHYSIOLOGY OF MICROVASCULAR DYSFUNCTION IN HFpEF

Microvascular dysfunction may contribute to the progression of HFpEF and has been proposed as a precursor of HF in otherwise asymptomatic individuals (e.g., those with T2D).[11-13] Recognizing the clinical and prognostic significance of these early cardiomyopathic changes, the American College of Cardiology/American Heart Association (ACC/AHA) has classified such individuals as having stage B HF **(Flowchart 1)**.

Microvascular Dysfunction in Established Heart Failure with Preserved Ejection Fraction

Microvascular dysfunction in HFpEF arises from a combination of microvascular structural alterations (e.g., rarefaction), endothelial dysfunction (endothelium-dependent MVD), and/or vascular smooth muscle dysfunction (endothelium-independent MVD). Nitric oxide (NO) is crucial to endothelial and smooth muscle function and is synthesized by NO synthase (NOS).[10] Patients with functional MVD have a heightened resting microvascular blood flow and NOS reactivity, reflecting a near-maximal vasodilatory state at rest (reduced resting microvascular tone), leading to attenuated vasodilatory responses to stress.[7,10]

Endothelial NOS (eNOS) dysfunction is thought to be integral in the pathogenesis of HFpEF.[5] A systemic inflammatory state induced by comorbidities such as T2D, obesity, and chronic obstructive pulmonary disease may lead to the increased production of endothelial reactive oxygen species (ROS).[14] The reaction between ROS and eNOS cofactors diminishes NO production and bioavailability. The resulting decline in NO availability reduces levels of protein kinase G, which is essential for the phosphorylation of titin, a cytoskeletal protein responsible for myocardial diastolic recoil and distensibility.[15] Therefore, impaired titin phosphorylation due to the

Flowchart 1: Proposed pathophysiological mechanisms behind heart failure with preserved ejection fraction, including contributions from microvascular dysfunction and fibrosis.

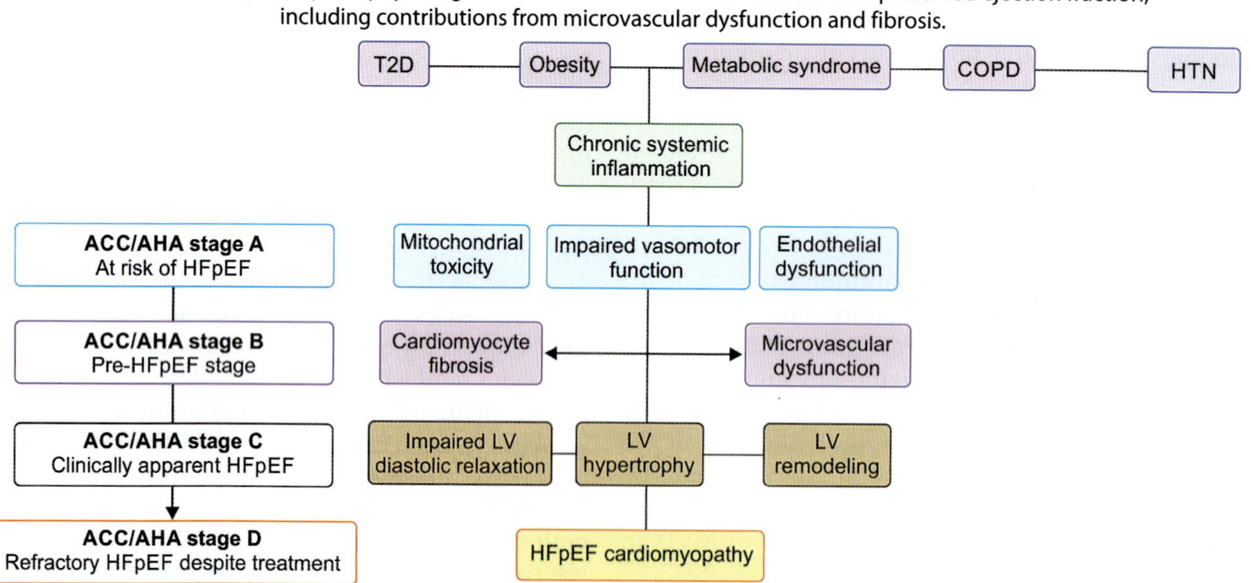

(ACC/AHA: American College of Cardiology/American Heart Association; COPD: chronic obstructive pulmonary disease; HFpEF: heart failure with preserved ejection fraction; HTN: hypertension; LV: left ventricle; T2D: type 2 diabetes)

Source: Adapted from Bilak et al.[28] Used with permission from Sage under a Creative Commons CC BY 4.0 license.

dysregulation of the NO-protein kinase G axis may contribute to impaired lusitropy and LV diastolic reserve in HFpEF.[15]

Biopsy studies in HFpEF have previously demonstrated deficiencies in NO signaling and altered collagen homeostasis, with increased titin phosphorylation.[15] This has further been implicated as a potential mechanism underlying the transition from hypertensive heart disease to HFpEF.[16] In a murine model of HFpEF, pharmacological inhibition of eNOS enhanced inducible NOS (iNOS) activity, resulting in subsequent dysregulation of protein control within cardiomyocytes, with the accumulation of misfolded proteins, cardiomyocyte dysfunction, and, again, impaired lusitropy.[17] Importantly, pharmacological inhibition of iNOS also resulted in improved lusitropy and exercise tolerance.[17] Although impaired lusitropy has an adverse impact on coronary flow, resulting in ischemia exacerbated by physiological stress (e.g., exercise), ischemia may itself precipitate exertion-related diastolic dysfunction.[8] Therefore, conclusive ascertainment of causality between MVD, ischemia, and diastolic dysfunction remains challenging.

In humans, autopsy data have previously shown that HFpEF subjects have greater microvascular rarefaction, lower microvascular density, and myocardial fibrosis compared with controls of a similar age and regardless of epicardial CAD severity, with the authors proposing microvascular endothelial inflammation as the possible trigger for MVD and fibrotic development.[18]

IMPACT OF CORONARY MICROVASCULAR DYSFUNCTION IN HFpEF: A META-ANALYSIS

A meta-analysis evaluating the prevalence of CMD in patients with HFpEF has recently been published. This meta-analysis was performed according to the Meta-analysis of Observational Studies in Epidemiology (MOOSE) guidelines and the current PRISMA guidelines for meta-analyses. The protocol was registered in the International Prospective Register of Systematic Reviews (PROSPEROCRD42022361360).[19] Relevant articles published in PubMed, Scopus, and Wiley Online Library up to May 1, 2023 were searched using the following keywords: "heart failure," "preserved ejection fraction," "HFpEF," "microvascular dysfunction," and "coronary microcirculation." The inclusion criteria were as follows: (a) studies reporting the prevalence of CMD in HFpEF patients and/or (b) comparing HFpEF patients with and without CMD in terms of echocardiographic variables included in the current HFA-PEFF score, adverse clinical outcomes, and prevalence of AF. A total of 14 studies involving 1,138 individuals were analyzed.[20-33]

Definition of Coronary Microvascular Dysfunction

Reduction in the CFR was the most frequently used parameter in comparison studies. Notably, slightly different thresholds were employed to define the presence of CMD across the various studies, as shown in **Table 1**. A broader definition of CMD, including both structural (endothelial independent) and functional (endothelial dependent) microvascular dysfunctions, was also reported.

Echocardiographic Variables

Three different echocardiographic variables were considered important in this meta-analysis [i.e., left atrial volume index (LAVi), left ventricular mass index (LVMi), and E/e′ ratio derived from averaged septal and lateral mitral annular diastolic velocities] to assess whether the presence of CMD affects the echocardiographic phenotype of HFpEF patients. HFA-PEFF, one of the most validated diagnostic scores of HFpEF, also includes these echocardiographic criteria.

Clinical End Points

A composite clinical end point of death and hospitalization due to HF was chosen for the meta-analysis because it was the most adopted end point in the included studies. Finally, the prevalence of AF was also considered for meta-analysis. Four out of the 14 studies provided only prevalence data, and four studies delivered time-to-event data suitable for meta-analysis. The mean follow-up time for the clinical end point was 2.4 years.

RESULTS

Prevalence of Coronary Microvascular Dysfunction in HFpEF

Among 14 studies, the pooled prevalence of any type of CMD was 58% (95% CI, 42–74%), with a high-grade heterogeneity. In the sensitivity analysis performed using the inverse-variance method after Freeman–Tukey double arcsine transformation, a consistent prevalence value was found [57% (95% CI, 43–71%)]. In the meta-regression analysis, hypertension was found to be a stronger predictor of CMD when compared to diabetes. The high heterogeneity of prevalence proportions among the included studies was limited to the subgroup studies where CFR was estimated using noninvasive methods.

TABLE 1: Definition of CMD in different studies with duration of follow-up.

Author	Study design	Method	Cutoff	Median follow-up
Srivaratharajah et al.[20]	Retrospective/observational	PET-derived MFR after dipyridamole administration	MFR <2	NA
Shah et al.[21]	Prospective/observational	CFR measured with adenosine stress transthoracic Doppler echocardiography	CFR <2.5	NA
Dryer et al.[22]	Prospective/observational	CFR measured invasively after adenosine administration	CFR <2.0	NA
Yang et al.[23]	Prospective/observational	CFR measured invasively after adenosine administration	CFR <2.5	12.5 years
Allan et al.[24]	Prospective/observational	CFR measured invasively after adenosine administration	CFR <2.0	1 year
Löffler et al.[25]	Prospective/observational	CMR-derived MPR with adenosine infusion	MPR <2.5	NA
Mahfouz et al.[26]	Prospective/observational	CFR measured with adenosine stress transthoracic Doppler echocardiography	CFR <2.0	NA
Hage et al.[27]	Prospective/observational	CFR measured with adenosine stress transthoracic Doppler echocardiography	CFR <2.5	388 days
Kato et al.[28]	Retrospective/observational	CMR-derived CFR with adenosine infusion	CFR <2.0	4.1 years
Rush et al.[29]	Retrospective/observational	CFR measured invasively after adenosine administration	CFR <2.0	18 months
Ozcan et al.[30]	Prospective/observational	CFR measured invasively after adenosine administration	CFR <2.0	NA
Ahmad et al.[31]	Prospective/observational	CFR measured invasively after adenosine administration	CFR <2.5	NA
Arnold et al.[32]	Prospective/observational	CMR-derived MPR with adenosine infusion	MPR <2.0	3.1 years
Mohammed et al.[33]	Retrospective/observational	IMR	IMR >25	NA

Methodological features of included studies, CMD definitions, and median follow-up.
(CBF: coronary blood flow; CFR: coronary flow reserve; CMD: coronary microvascular dysfunction; CMR: cardiac magnetic resonance; IMR: index of microvascular resistance; MFR: myocardial flow reserve; MPR: myocardial perfusion reserve; NA: not applicable; PET: positron emission tomography)

Echocardiographic Variables

In the pooled analysis, two of the three echocardiographic variables were significantly higher in patients with CMD than in patients without CMD: LAVi (MD 3.85, CI 1.19–6.5; $p < 0.01$) and E/e′ ratio (MD 2.76, CI 1.54–3.97; $p < 0.01$). LVMi did not significantly differ between the groups (MD 6.33, CI 2.31–14.9; $p = 0.15$). Moderate heterogeneity across studies was observed for each echocardiographic variable. These echocardiographic parameters, which are markers of increased LV filling pressure, have been included in two clinically validated diagnostic criteria (H2FPEF and HEF-PEFF) of HFpEF recommended by the ESC 2021.[34]

Clinical Outcomes

In the pooled analysis of reconstructed HRs, patients with HFpEF showed a significantly higher rate of the composite clinical end point of death and hospitalization for HF (HR 3.19, CI 1.04–9.57, $p = 0.04$) **(Fig. 1)**. Moderate-to-severe heterogeneity across the included studies was observed (I^2 81%; Q test, $p < 0.01$). In the leave-one-out analysis, the removal of three studies influenced the outcome measure.

The present study has several limitations.[19] First, the meta-analysis was based on observational studies, five of which are only retrospective. Hence, the association between CMD and both echocardiographic variables and clinical outcomes cannot be determined to be causative. Second, the statistical method used for the composite clinical end point analysis provided an approximation of patient-level time-to-event data. Third, the reliability of the pooled results was weakened by the high variability of the definitions and thresholds adopted for the diagnosis of CMD and HFpEF across the included studies. Fourth, the included studies differed in their definitions of HFpEF, possibly affecting the pooled results. Fifth, among the

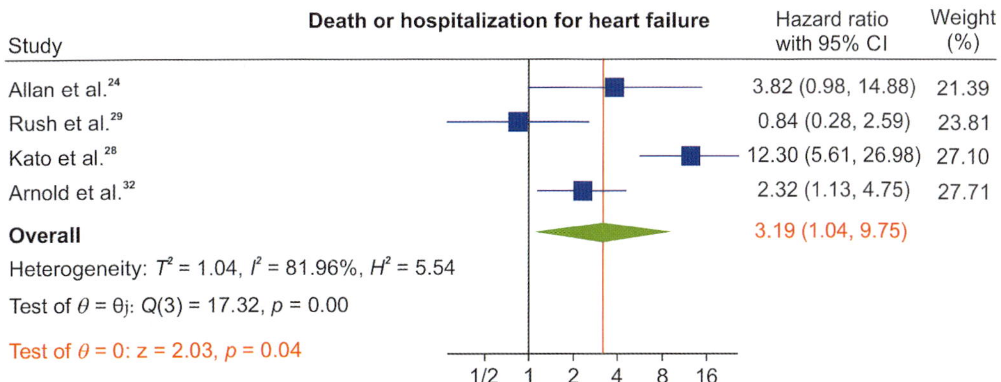

Fig. 1: Forest plots of pooled analysis for the clinical end points. Patients with HFpEF and CMD have a higher mortality and hospitalization for heart failure compared to HFpEF without CMD.

echocardiographic variables, we did not include the global longitudinal strain.

CONCLUSION

The prevalence of structural or functional CMD or both in HFpEF patients was 58% in the meta-analysis, whereas the pooled prevalence of structural CMD (i.e., impaired CFR) was only 50%, suggesting that structural MVD is the primary type of CMD in HFpEF patients.[19] The natural consequence of CMD is the occurrence of areas of chronic ischemia and fibrosis. Several studies have proposed that repeated subclinical episodes of microischemia cause focal areas of fibrosis, ultimately promoting diastolic dysfunction. The pathophysiological mechanisms behind CMD-related HFpEF probably lie on three pillars, feeding each other in a vicious cycle: (1) Inflammatory-mediated reduction of NO bioavailability, (2) structural changes in the microcirculatory bed (i.e., capillary rarefaction and fibrosis), and (3) diastolic dysfunction. CMD in HFpEF increases interstitial fibrosis without increasing the LV mass, so the meta-analysis revealed higher E/e′ ratio and LAVi values but with similar LVMi values. It can be assumed that CMD represents the common soil between atrial dysfunction and HFpEF.[33] This meta-analysis also substantiated an increased association of increased mortality and HF hospitalization in CMD-HFpEF endotype. Finally, systemic inflammation and CMD may be a target for novel interventions in HFpEF in the future.

REFERENCES

1. Savarese G, Lund LH. Global public health burden of heart failure. Card Fail Rev. 2017;3:7-11.
2. Lam CSP, Fat CC. Fat, female, fatigued: features of the obese HFpEF phenotype. JACC Heart Fail. 2018;6:710-3.
3. Gulsin GS, Athithan L, McCann GP. Diabetic cardiomyopathy: prevalence, determinants and potential treatments. Ther Adv Endocrinol Metab. 2019;10:2042018819834869.
4. Lam CS, Donal E, Kraigher-Krainer E, et al. Epidemiology and clinical course of heart failure with preserved ejection fraction. Eur J Heart Fail. 2011;13:18-28.
5. Paulus WJ, Tschope C. A novel paradigm for heart failure with preserved ejection fraction: comorbidities drive myocardial dysfunction and remodeling through coronary microvascular endothelial inflammation. J Am Coll Cardiol. 2013;62:263-71.
6. Perera D. Cardiac–coronary coupling. J Am Coll Cardiol. 2016;68:1661-3.
7. Rahman H, Ryan M, Lumley M, et al. Coronary microvascular dysfunction is associated with myocardial ischemia and abnormal coronary perfusion during exercise. Circulation. 2019;140:1805-16.
8. Sinha A, Rahman H, Webb A, et al. Untangling the pathophysiologic link between coronary microvascular dysfunction and heart failure with preserved ejection fraction. Eur Heart J. 2021;42:4431-41.
9. Cannon RO, Epstein SE. "Microvascular angina" as a cause of chest pain with angiographically normal coronary arteries. Am J Cardiol. 1988;61:1338-43.
10. Rahman H, Demir OM, Khan F, et al. Physiological stratification of patients with angina due to coronary microvascular dysfunction. J Am Coll Cardiol. 2020;75:2538-49.
11. Athithan L, Gulsin GS, McCann GP, et al. Diabetic cardiomyopathy: pathophysiology, theories and evidence to date. World J Diabetes. 2019;10:490-510.
12. Gulsin GS, Henson J, Brady EM, et al. Cardiovascular determinants of aerobic exercise capacity in adults with type 2 diabetes. Diabetes Care. 2020;43:2248-56.
13. Gulsin GS, Swarbrick DJ, Athithan L, et al. Effects of low-energy diet or exercise on cardiovascular function in working-age adults with type 2 diabetes: a prospective, randomized, open-label, blinded end point trial. Diabetes Care. 2020;43:1300-10.

14. Franssen C, Chen S, Unger A, et al. Myocardial microvascular inflammatory endothelial activation in heart failure with preserved ejection fraction. JACC Heart Fail. 2016;4:312-24.
15. van Heerebeek L, Hamdani N, Falcao-Pires I, et al. Low myocardial protein kinase G activity in heart failure with preserved ejection fraction. Circulation. 2012;126: 830-9.
16. Zile MR, Baicu CF, Ikonomidis JS, et al. Myocardial stiffness in patients with heart failure and a preserved ejection fraction: contributions of collagen and titin. Circulation. 2015;131:1247-59.
17. Schiattarella GG, Altamirano F, Tong D, et al. Nitrosative stress drives heart failure with preserved ejection fraction. Nature. 2019;568:351-6.
18. Mohammed SF, Hussain S, Mirzoyev SA, et al. Coronary microvascular rarefaction and myocardial fibrosis in heart failure with preserved ejection fraction. Circulation. 2015;131:550-9.
19. D'Amario D, Laborante R, Bianchini E, et al. Impact of coronary microvascular dysfunction in heart failure with preserved ejection fraction: a meta-analysis. ESC Heart Fail. 2024;11(4):2063-75.
20. Srivaratharajah K, Coutinho T, deKemp R, et al. Reduced myocardial flow in heart failure patients with preserved ejection fraction. Circ Heart Fail. 2016;9: e002562.
21. Shah SJ, Lam CSP, Svedlund S, et al. Prevalence and correlates of coronary microvascular dysfunction in heart failure with preserved ejection fraction: PROMIS-HFpEF. Eur Heart J. 2018;39:3439-50.
22. Dryer K, Gajjar M, Narang N, et al. Coronary microvascular dysfunction in patients with heart failure with preserved ejection fraction. Am J Physiol Heart Circ Physiol. 2018;314: H1033-42.
23. Yang JH, Obokata M, Reddy YNV, et al. Endothelium-dependent and independent coronary microvascular dysfunction in patients with heart failure with preserved ejection fraction. Eur J Heart Fail. 2020;22:432-41.
24. Allan T, Dryer K, Fearon WF, et al. Coronary microvascular dysfunction and clinical outcomes in patients with heart failure with preserved ejection fraction. J Card Fail. 2019;25:843-5.
25. Löffler AI, Pan JA, Balfour PC, et al. Frequency of coronary microvascular dysfunction and diffuse myocardial fibrosis (measured by cardiovascular magnetic resonance) in patients with heart failure and preserved left ventricular ejection fraction. Am J Cardiol. 2019;124:1584-9.
26. Mahfouz RA, Gouda M, Abdelhamid M. Relation of microvascular dysfunction and exercise tolerance in patients with heart failure with preserved ejection fraction. Echocardiography. 2020;37:1192-8.
27. Hage C, Svedlund S, Saraste A, et al. Association of coronary microvascular dysfunction with heart failure hospitalizations and mortality in heart failure with preserved ejection fraction: a follow-up in the PROMIS-HFpEF study. J Card Fail. 2020;26:1016-21.
28. Kato S, Fukui K, Kodama S, et al. Cardiovascular magnetic resonance assessment of coronary flow reserve improves risk stratification in heart failure with preserved ejection fraction. J Cardiovasc Magn Reson. 2021;23:112.
29. Rush CJ, Berry C, Oldroyd KG, et al. Prevalence of coronary artery disease and coronary microvascular dysfunction in patients with heart failure with preserved ejection fraction. JAMA Cardiol. 2021;6:1130-43.
30. Ozcan C, Allan T, Besser SA, et al. The relationship between coronary microvascular dysfunction, atrial fibrillation and heart failure with preserved ejection fraction. Am J Cardiovasc Dis. 2021;11:29-38.
31. Ahmad A, Corban MT, Toya T, et al. Coronary microvascular dysfunction is associated with exertional haemodynamic abnormalities in patients with heart failure with preserved ejection fraction. Eur J Heart Fail. 2021;23:765-72.
32. Arnold JR, Kanagala P, Budgeon CA, et al. Prevalence and prognostic significance of microvascular dysfunction in heart failure with preserved ejection fraction. JACC Cardiovasc Imaging. 2022;15:1001-11.
33. Mohammed AQ, Abdu FA, Su Y, et al. Prognostic significance of coronary microvascular dysfunction in patients with heart failure with preserved ejection fraction. Can J Cardiol. 2023;39:971-80.
34. Coats AJS, Heymans S, Farmakis D, et al. Atrial disease and heart failure: the common soil hypothesis proposed by the Heart Failure Association of the European Society of Cardiology. Eur Heart J. 2021:ehab834.

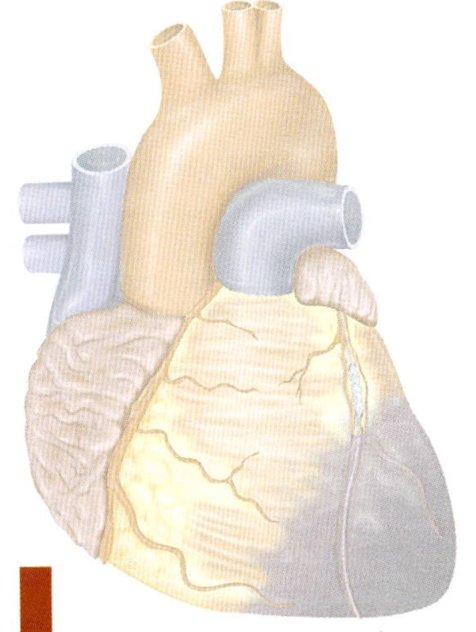

Evaluation and Management of HFpEF: New Dimensions

Ajay Kumar Sinha, Narendra Kumar, Vijay Kumar, Shradha Ranjan

INTRODUCTION

Heart failure (HF) is a clinical syndrome, not a disease.[1] HF is broadly divided into three main subtypes: (1) HF with reduced ejection fraction (HFrEF), (2) HF with mildly reduced ejection fraction (HFmrEF), and (3) HF with preserved ejection fraction (HFpEF).[2] Over the last decade, the incidence of HFpEF has increased due to the aging population and multiple comorbidities.

The clinical signs and symptoms overlap grossly between these HF types; however, HFpEF continues to raise pertinent questions concerning diagnosis, clinical assessment, and treatment. From a pathophysiological standpoint, HFpEF develops when the left ventricle (LV) is unable to accept an adequate volume of blood during diastole at normal diastolic pressures and at volumes sufficient to maintain an appropriate stroke volume. These abnormalities are caused by a decrease in ventricular relaxation and/or an increase in ventricular stiffness.[1]

The prevalence of HFpEF is about 1.1–1.5% in the general population (~32 million worldwide) and accounts for 50% of all HF cases. Every year the HFpEF prevalence is rising by 1% due to the aging population and ongoing epidemics of hypertension, obesity, and diabetes mellitus (DM). HFpEF is also characterized by high morbidity and mortality.[3]

Data from the Trivandrum Heart Failure Registry and ASIAN-HF reveal that the proportion of HFpEF in India is approximately 19–25%, which is much lower than that of the Western population.[4]

Although patients with HFpEF comprise nearly half of those with HF, evidence-based treatment options have historically been limited.

In practice, the management of HFpEF is based on the following principles:

- Establish the diagnosis of HF and exclude potentially treatable alternatives
- Institute general measures to manage congestion and address comorbidities/precipitating factors
- Initiate evidence-based medical therapy[5]

The graph indicates the following trends over the years: The proportion of HFpEF (blue line) shows an increasing trend, particularly after 2010. The proportion of HFrEF (red line) shows a decreasing trend. The proportion of HFmrEF (black line) appears to remain stable over time.

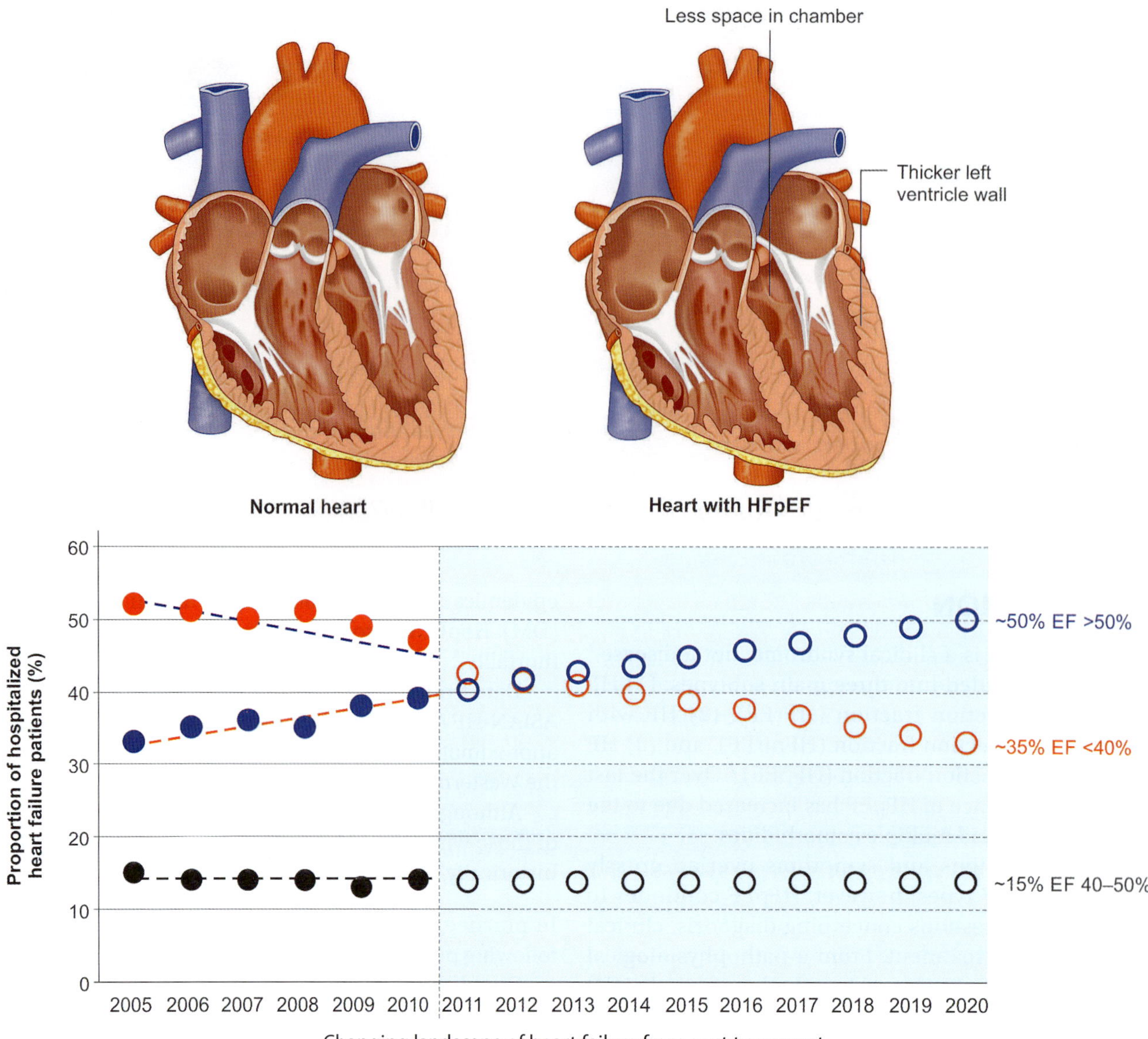

Changing landscape of heart failure from past to present.

PATHOPHYSIOLOGY OF HFpEF

Figure 1 shows the pathophysiological progression of HFpEF.

EVALUATION OF HFpEF

Exertional dyspnea is a common clinical complaint in HFpEF.[6]

The clinical diagnosis of HFpEF remains challenging due to its heterogeneous etiology. Of late, it has been speculated that different HFpEF phenotypes may require different treatment strategies with much focus on patient's comorbidities **(Fig. 2)**.[1]

Other challenges faced during the diagnosis of HFpEF are as follows.

- The first challenge in the diagnosis of HFpEF is determining what ejection fraction (EF) threshold constitutes HFpEF.
- The second challenge in the diagnosis of HFpEF is using the correct terminology as HFpEF is not synonymous with diastolic dysfunction.
- The third major diagnostic challenge with HFpEF is that there is no single test that definitively establishes the diagnosis of HFpEF.[7]

However, the introduction of two different *diagnostic tools* has greatly enhanced the ability to diagnose HFpEF in recent years.

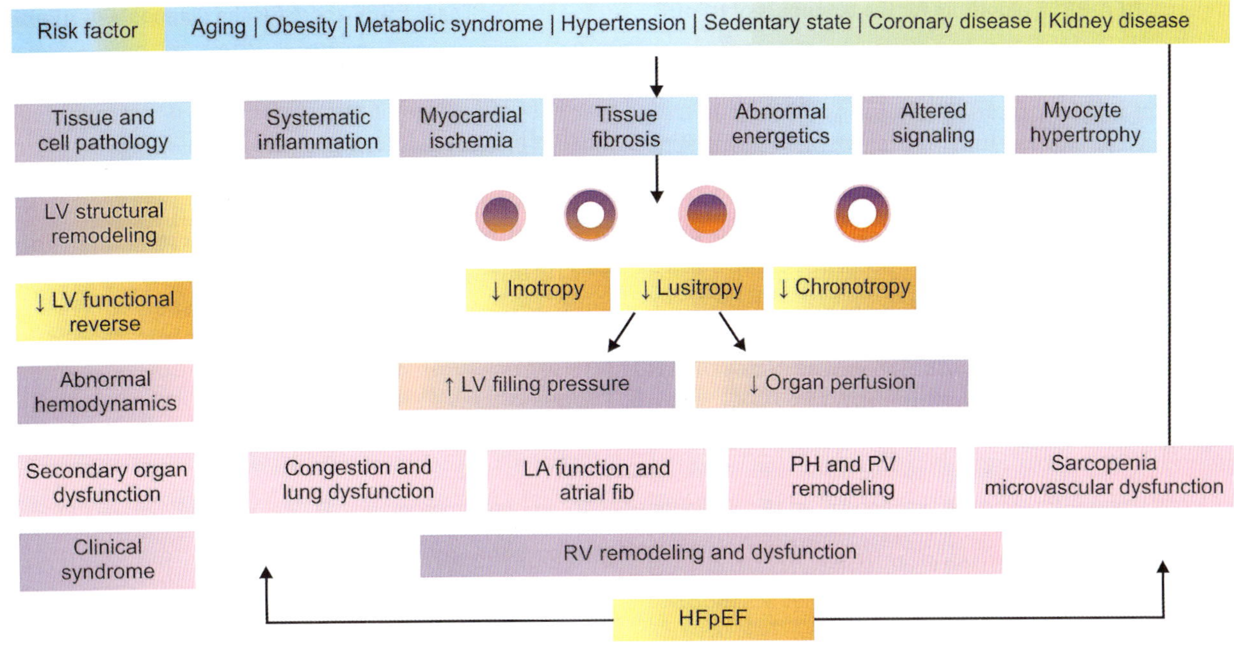

Fig. 1: The pathophysiological progression of HFpEF.

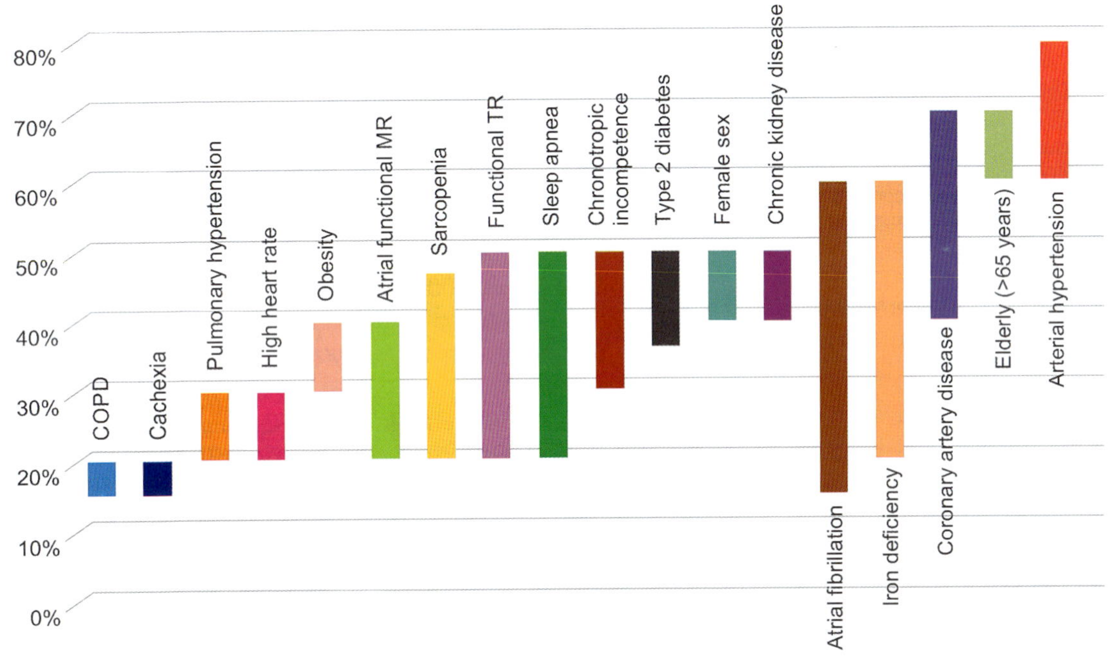

Fig. 2: HFpEF phenotypes with the upper and lower boundary of the estimated prevalence values. (COPD: chronic obstructive pulmonary disease; MR: mitral regurgitation; TR: tricuspid regurgitation)
Source: Adapted from von Haehling et al.[1]

1. The HFA-PEFF algorithm offers a structured approach to the diagnosis of HFpEF by assessing predisposing risk factors, clinical signs and symptoms, objective evidence of cardiac dysfunction, and functional and structural abnormalities. Each criterion is assigned a score, reflecting the probability of HFpEF and its impact on prognosis.
2. A recently proposed diagnostic tool is the H_2FPEF score.

Both algorithms are summarized in **Figure 3.**[1]

HFA-PEFF algorithm for the diagnosis of HFpEF

P	Initial workup [Step 1 (P): Pretest assessment]	Symptoms and/or signs of HF: • Comorbidities/risk factors ECG • Standard echocardiography • Natriuretic peptides • Ergometry/6 minutes walking test or cardiopulmonary exercise testing
E	Diagnostic workup [Step 2 (E): Echocardiographic and natriuretic peptide score]	• Comprehensive echocardiography • Natriuretic peptides, if not measured in step 1
F1	Advanced workup [Step 3 (Fl): Functional testing in case of uncertainty]	• Diastolic stress test: Exercise stress echocardiography • Invasive hemodynamic measurements
F2	Actiological workup [Step 4 (F2): Final etiology]	• Cardiovascular magnetic resonance • Cardiac or noncardiac biopsies • Scintigraphy/CT/PET • Genetic testing • Specific laboratory tests

The H_2EPEF score for the diagnosis of HFpEF

	Clinical variable	Values	Points
H_2	Heavy	Body mass index >30 kg/m²	2
	Hypertensive	2 or more antihypertensive medicines	1
F	Atrial Fibrillation	Paroxysmal or persistent	3
P	Pulmonary hypertension	Doppler echocardiographic estimated pulmonary artery systolic pressure >35 mm Hg	1
E	Elder	Age >60 years	1
F	Filling pressure	Doppler echocardiographic E/e' >9	1
		H_2FPEF score	Sum (0–9)

Total points	0	1	2	3	4	5	6	7	8	9
Probability of HFpEF	0.2	0.3	0.4	0.5	0.6	0.7	0.8	0.9	0.95	

Fig. 3: Clinical scores estimating the likelihood of an HFpEF diagnosis. (CT: computed tomography; ECG: electrocardiogram; PET: positron emission tomography)
Source: Adapted from von Haehling et al.[1]

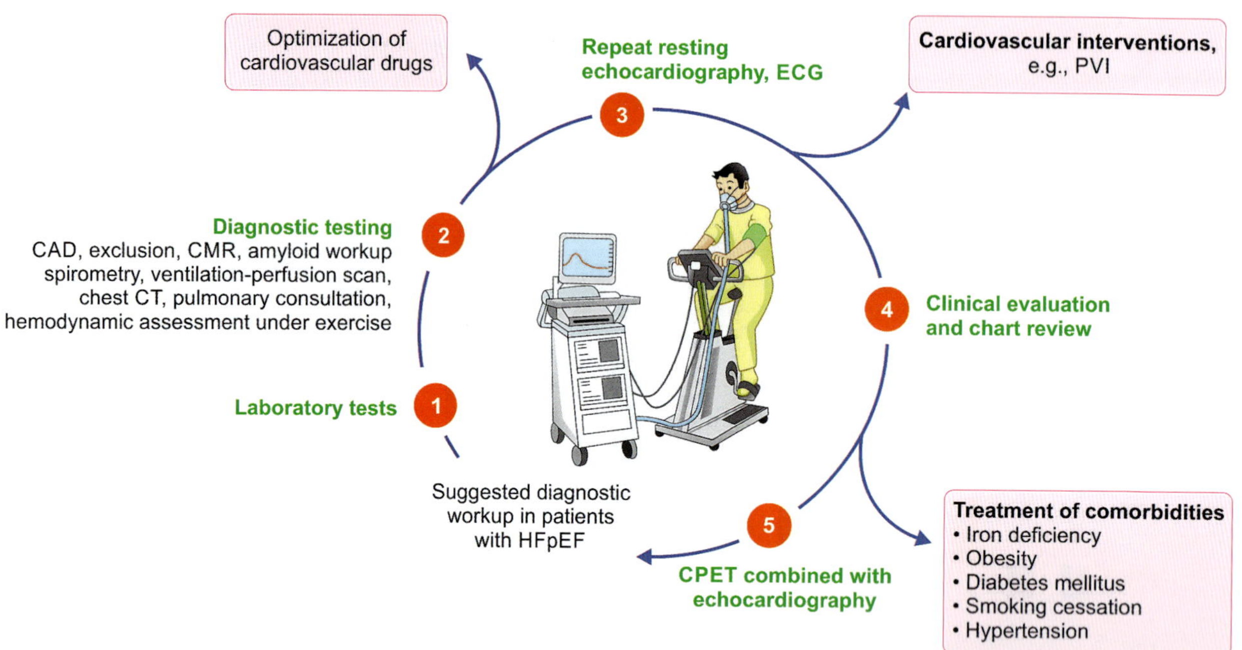

Fig. 4: Components of assessing the contributors to dyspnea in patients with confirmed diagnosis of HFpEF according to the HFA-PEFF or the H_2FPEF score. Cutoff values were ≥5 and ≥6, respectively. (CAD: coronary artery disease; CMR: cardiac magnetic resonance imaging; CPET: cardiopulmonary exercise test; CT: computed tomography; ECG: electrocardiogram; PVI: pulmonary vein isolation)
Source: Adapted from von Haehling et al.[1]

A recently proposed diagnostic algorithm for patients with HFpEF helps to identify comorbidities involved in the development of dyspnea and/or other symptoms suggestive of HFpEF **(Fig. 4)**.[1]

Thus, the *diagnostic approach to HFpEF* should focus on evaluating the differential diagnosis of dyspnea and edema, excluding noncardiac causes and cardiac mimics, and establishing diagnostic probability with the H_2FPEF score before establishing the likely diagnosis of HFpEF **(Flowchart 1)**.[7]

HFA-PEFF DIAGNOSTIC ALGORITHM

HFA-PEFF diagnostic algorithm is shown in **Flowchart 2**.

The first cluster is that of young patients with an average age <60 years and a reduced burden of comorbidities, including arterial hypertension and obesity. This group of patients also includes those with HF with improved EF. Weight loss and blood pressure control using renin-angiotensin-aldosterone system (RAAS) inhibitors (RAASi) are central to these patients. Inflammation is responsible for remodeling the left atrial muscle and conduction tissue, promoting the progression of these patients toward "left atrial myopathy," associated with increased pulmonary pressures and right ventricular dysfunction, defining a subtype of this first phenotype.

Flowchart 1: The diagnostic approach to HFpEF.

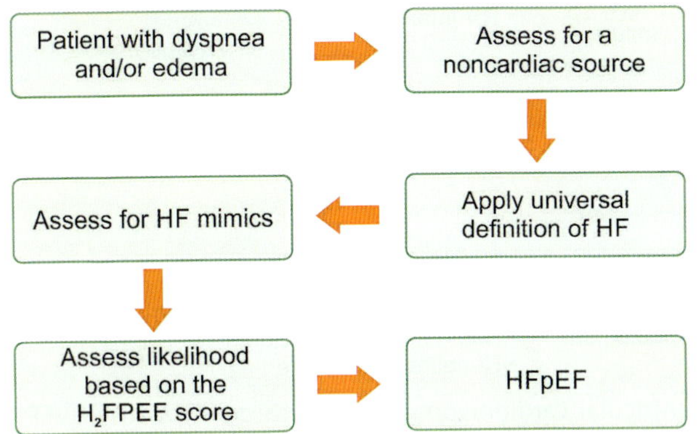

Source: Adapted from Kittleson et al.[7]

Although dyspnea is a common presenting symptom of HFpEF, it is imperative to consider other causes of dyspnea before assigning the diagnosis. A similar approach can be taken to the differential diagnosis of edema although the first step should be to differentiate edema from lymphedema.[7]

Figure 5 outlines the *differential diagnosis of HFpEF.*[5]

Flowchart 2: HFA-PEFF diagnostic algorithm.

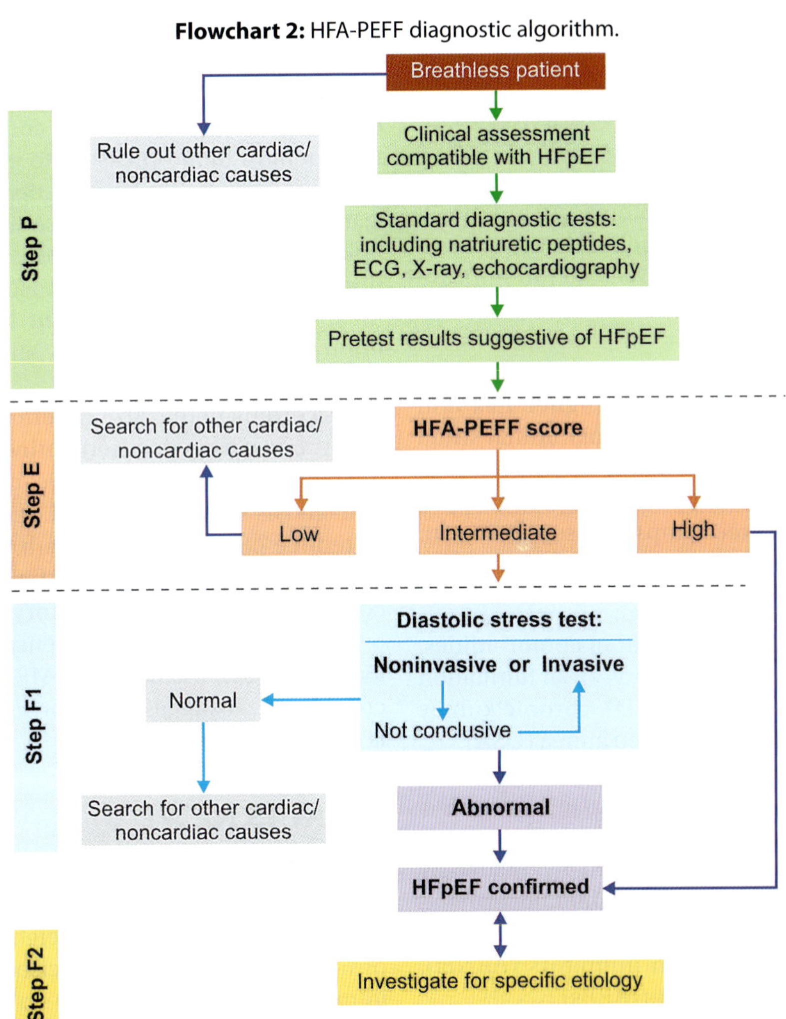

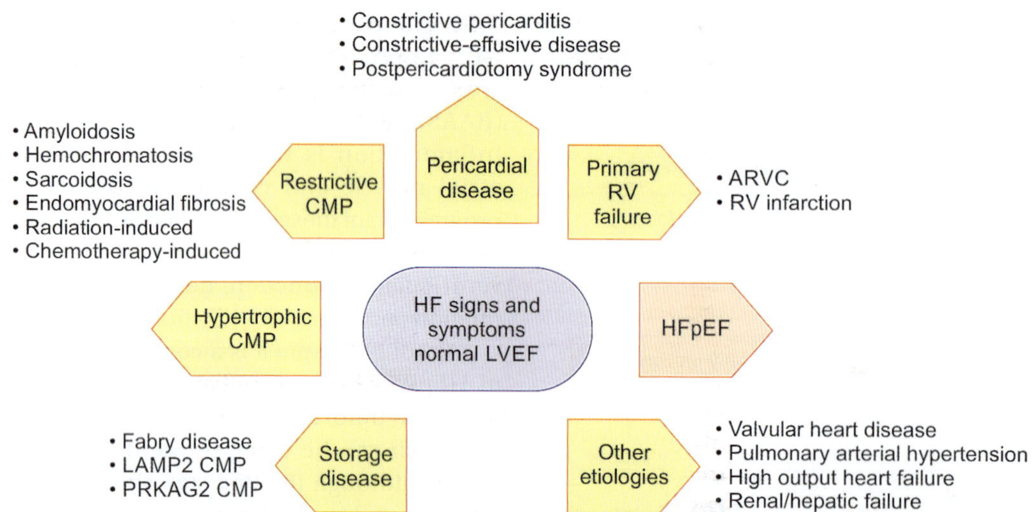

Fig. 5: Differential diagnosis of HFpEF. (ARVC: arrhythmogenic right ventricular cardiomyopathy; CMP: cardiomyopathy; LVEF: left ventricular ejection fraction)
Source: Adapted from Desai et al.[5]

MANAGEMENT OF HFpEF

Even if the diagnosis of HFpEF is confirmed, therapeutic challenges remain. Clinicians should set up a multidisciplinary collaboration to consider the role of comorbidities that contribute to symptoms and prognosis, nonpharmacological options to ameliorate symptoms, guideline-directed medical therapy (GDMT) to improve quality of life (QoL) and reduce HF as well as non-HF hospitalizations.

The diagnosis and management of HFpEF are more challenging in women. Women have higher EFs and more preserved left ventricular global longitudinal strain compared with men and therefore may be less likely to develop a reduced EF. A careful history of pregnancy is important as the history of preeclampsia is associated with an increased risk of subsequent HFpEF hospitalization.[7]

Management of HFpEF should focus on:

- Risk stratification and management of comorbidities, including hypertension, DM, obesity, atrial fibrillation (AF), coronary artery disease (CAD), chronic kidney disease (CKD), and obstructive sleep apnea (OSA)
- Nonpharmacological management, including the role of exercise and weight loss and the use of wireless, implantable pulmonary artery monitors
- Symptom management and disease-modifying therapy with loop diuretic agents, SGLT2is, mineralocorticoid receptor antagonists (MRAs), especially finerenone, angiotensin receptor–neprilysin inhibitors (ARNIs), and angiotensin receptor blockers (ARBs).[7]

Once the diagnosis of HFpEF is confirmed, treatment should focus on decongestion and optimal management of cardiac and noncardiac comorbidities. Aggressive treatment of blood pressure to guideline-recommended targets is appropriate for all patients. Coronary revascularization is appropriate for those with ischemic symptoms, and a trial of sinus rhythm maintenance/restoration may be indicated for those with AF. Guidance for lifestyle modification, weight loss, conditioning, and improved functional capacity should be provided to the patients.

According to the 2023 American College of Cardiology expert consensus decision pathway on the management of HFpEF, barring contraindication, all individuals with a diagnosis of HFpEF should be treated with an SGLT2i to reduce cardiovascular death/HF hospitalization and improve health status. Initiation of an SGLT2i may be considered for either ambulatory individuals with HFpEF or those with acutely decompensated HF. In those with an LVEF <55–60%, the use of an MRA, ARNI, or ARB may be considered. A suggested *algorithm for HFpEF* treatment is outlined in **Flowchart 3.**[5,7]

WHAT IS NEW?

STEP-HFpEF trial has recently demonstrated in obese HFpEF patients that semaglutide versus placebo significantly reduced body weight, improving symptoms, physical limitations, and exercise function, with a positive impact on QoL, inflammatory status, and survival.[8]

MANAGEMENT OF COMORBIDITIES IN HFpEF

There is a complex interplay between comorbidities, which influences the genesis of HFpEF and outcomes of individuals with HFpEF. Hypertension, DM, and obesity can result in CAD, AF, sleep apnea, and CKD. CKD and sleep apnea can, in turn, worsen hypertension. All these factors influence the pathogenesis and outcomes of individuals with HFpEF **(Fig. 6)**.[7]

Although a majority of HFpEF cases are attributable to common CV risk factors and comorbidities such as hypertension, DM, and obesity, a possibility of non-CV systemic etiology should be considered in situations outlined in **Box 1**, in which secondary HFpEF may be present.

Comorbidities and secondary HFpEF as a result of systemic disease should be assessed using a structured approach as outlined in **Figure 4**.[1]

Flowchart 3: Algorithm for GDMT in HFpEF.

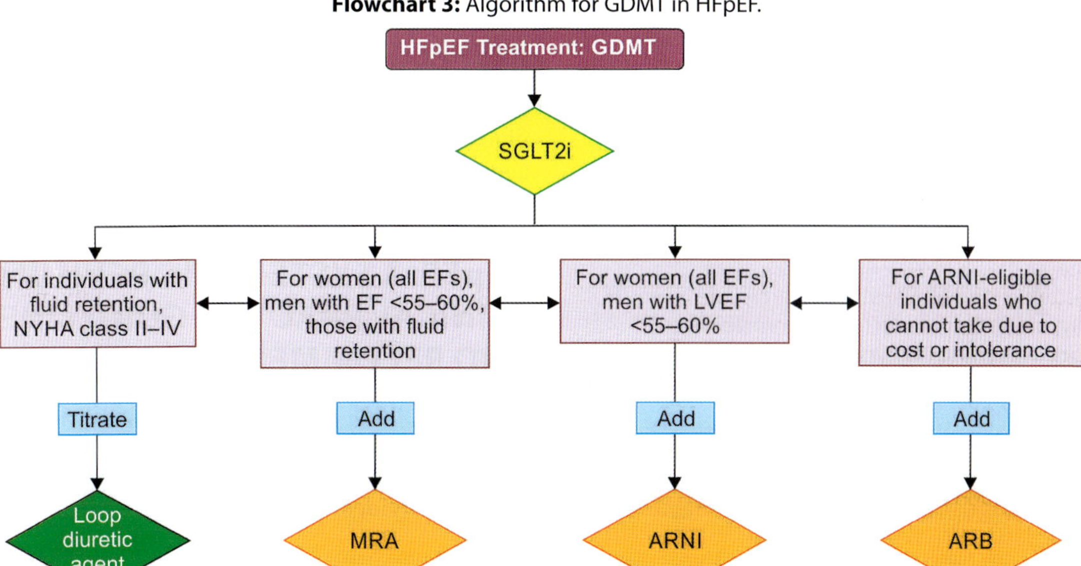

Green color identifies a class 1 therapy from clinical practice guidelines, yellow color indicates a class 2a therapy, and orange color denotes class 2b therapy. SGLT2is received a class 2a indication in the 2022 AHA/ACC/HFSA HF guidelines, but the benefit, now confirmed in two randomized trials, suggests that SGLT2is may receive a stronger class of recommendation in future guidelines, and thus the box is shaded yellow with a green border.

(ARB: angiotensin receptor blocker; ARNI: angiotensin receptor–neprilysin inhibitor; EF: ejection fraction; GDMT: guideline-directed medical therapy; LVEF: left ventricular ejection fraction; MRA: mineralocorticoid antagonist; NYHA: New York Heart Association; SGLT2i: sodium–glucose cotransporter 2 inhibitor)

Source: Adapted from Kittleson et al.[7]

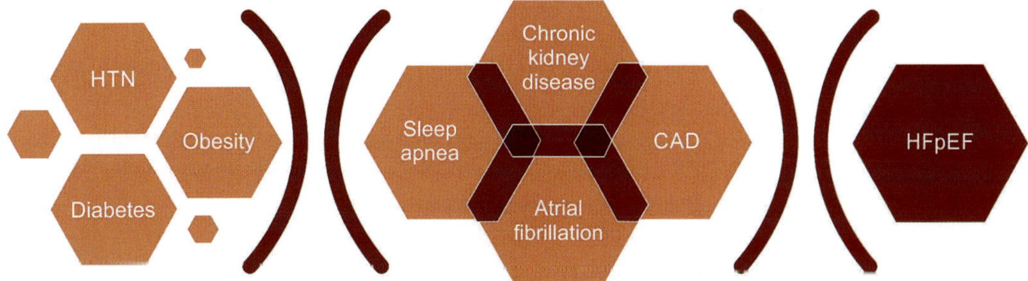

Fig. 6: Interplay of HFpEF comorbidities. (CAD: coronary artery disease; HTN: hypertension)
Source: Adapted from Kittleson et al.[7]

Appropriate management of key noncardiac and cardiac comorbidities in HFpEF patients is outlined in **Table 1**.[5]

DEVICE-BASED THERAPIES FOR HFpEF

Using devices to treat patients with HFpEF aims to reduce pressure in the LA. The devices used in clinical and preclinical studies are as follows:

- Interatrial shunt devices work by forming a shunt between the LA and another cavity to reduce LA pressure and, consequently, retrograde pressure toward the pulmonary circulation.
- Left ventricular expander devices that assist early ventricular filling by optimizing elastic energy during systole and releasing during diastole
- Mechanical circulatory support devices, predominantly the continuous flow rotodynamic blood pumps, aim to decompress the left atrium and restore arterial pulsatility and cardiac output.
- Neurohumoral devices are used to control the autonomic nervous system response in these patients.[9]

BOX 1: Criteria for considering a noncardiovascular cause of HFpEF.

- Young age
- Family history of cardiomyopathies/heart failure
- No or only minor classical risk factors/comorbidities
- Inadequate left ventricular hypertrophy (>13 mm)
- Specific echocardiographic strain patterns (e.g., amyloidosis)
- Significant ventricular arrhythmias
- Severe right heart dilatation
- Significant scar tissue (in cardiac MRI)
- Regional wall motion abnormalities

ATRIAL FIBRILLATION NEEDS A SPECIAL PLACE

Figure 7 illustrates the clinical significance of atrial fibrillation in HFpEF.

INEFFECTIVE THERAPIES

Organic nitrates, phosphodiesterase-5 inhibitors, and digoxin are ineffective for the treatment of HFpEF. These agents may be used to treat other conditions (e.g., angina in chronic coronary syndrome, rate control in AF).

HFpEF: A SYSTEMATIC REVIEW OF CLINICAL PRACTICE GUIDELINES AND RECOMMENDATIONS

Multiple guidelines exist for the diagnosis and management of HFpEF. A recently published systematic review of clinical practice guidelines and recommendations of HFpEF provides a summary of the areas of agreement,

TABLE 1: Management of key noncardiac and cardiac comorbidities in patients with HFpEF.

Condition	*Recommended strategies*
Hypertension	BP management to guideline-recommended targets, typically <130/80 mm Hg
Diabetes/dysglycemia	• Prioritize SGLT2 inhibitors (as in all patients) • ACE inhibitor/ARB for CKD/proteinuria • Finerenone for ongoing proteinuria despite ACE inhibitor/ARB
Obesity	• Calorie restriction, aerobic exercise training • Screening and treatment of OSA • Consider GLP-1 agonists, tirzepatide, bariatric surgery
CKD	• ACE inhibitor/ARB for proteinuria • SGLT2 inhibitors • Finerenone (if diabetes and ongoing proteinuria despite ACE inhibitor/ARB)
Coronary artery disease/coronary microvascular dysfunction	• Antiplatelet therapy • Moderate-to-high intensity statin therapy for those with elevated LDL • Revascularization for patients with angina or ischemia on provocative testing
Atrial fibrillation	• Anticoagulation for stroke prophylaxis • Consider a trial of rhythm control
Chronotropic incompetence	Avoid routine use of beta-blockers in the absence of compelling indication

(ACE: angiotensin-converting enzyme; ARB: angiotensin receptor blocker; BP: blood pressure; CKD: chronic kidney disease; GLP: glucagon-like peptide; LDL: low-density lipoprotein; OSA: obstructive sleep apnea; SGLT2: sodium–glucose cotransporter-2)
Source: Adapted from Desai et al.[5]

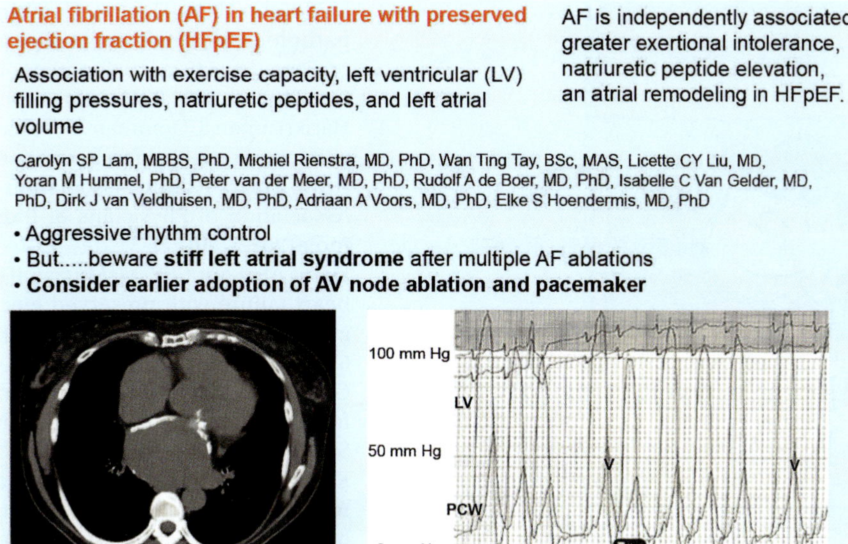

Fig. 7: Clinical significance of atrial fibrillation in HFpEF. (AV: atrioventricular; PCW: personal care worker)

TABLE 2: Management of key noncardiac and cardiac comorbidities in patients with HFpEF.

Condition	*Recommended strategies*
Hypertension	BP management to guideline-recommended targets, typically <130/80 mm Hg
Diabetes/ dysglycemia	• Prioritize SGLT2 inhibitors (as in all patients) • ACE inhibitor/ARB for CKD/proteinuria • Finerenone for ongoing proteinuria despite ACE inhibitor/ARB
Obesity	• Calorie restriction, aerobic exercise training • Screening and treatment of OSA • Consider GLP-1 agonists, tirzepatide, bariatric surgery
CKD	• ACE inhibitor/ARB for proteinuria • SGLT2 inhibitors • Finerenone (if diabetes and ongoing proteinuria despite ACE inhibitor/ARB)
Coronary artery disease/ coronary microvascular dysfunction	• Antiplatelet therapy • Moderate to high intensity statin therapy for those with elevated LDL • Revascularization for patients with angina or ischemia on provocative testing
Atrial fibrillation	• Anticoagulation for stroke prophylaxis • Consider a trial of rhythm control
Chronotropic incompetence	Avoid routine use of beta-blockers in the absence of compelling indication

(ACE: angiotensin-converting enzyme; ARB: angiotensin receptor blocker; BP: blood pressure; CKD: chronic kidney disease; GLP: glucagon-like peptide; LDL: low-density lipoprotein; OSA: obstructive sleep apnea; SGLT2: sodium–glucose cotransporter-2)
Source: Adapted from Desai et al.[5]

disagreement, and potential gaps in evidence requiring future clarification **(Table 2)**.[2]

CONCLUSION

Accurate diagnosis of HFpEF is essential to guide management and treatment strategies, ultimately improving patient outcomes. The clinical diagnosis of HFpEF is a multifaceted process and remains a challenge to manage due to its heterogeneous etiology. However, the introduction of HFA-PEFF algorithm and H_2FPEF score has greatly enhanced the ability to diagnose HFpEF in recent years. In addition, accurate identification and treatment of comorbidities contributing to the HFpEF syndrome is also very important. The development of future tools holds great promise for improving the diagnosis and management of HFpEF. As the understanding of HFpEF evolves, so too will the ability to harness these cutting-edge technologies to benefit patients and optimize care. In conclusion, among the three clinical phenotypes, there is a gradient of age, inflammation, diagnostic tools, and poor prognosis, which is highest in the "older, vascular aging" phenotype and gradually decreases from the "metabolic, obese" to the "younger, low BNP" phenotype.

In all cases, patients should be provided with guidance for lifestyle modification and an exercise prescription to facilitate weight loss, conditioning, and improved functional capacity. Based on the cumulative evidence of efficacy, all patients with symptomatic HFpEF should be treated with SGLT2 inhibitors in the absence of contraindications or previous intolerance.

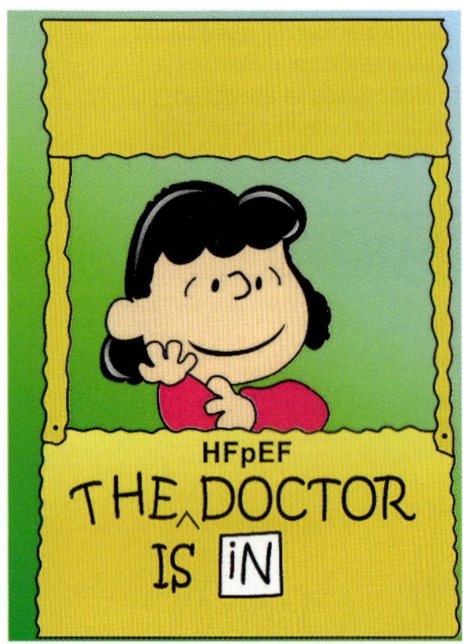

REFERENCES

1. von Haehling S, Assmus B, Bekfani T, et al. Heart failure with preserved ejection fraction: diagnosis, risk assessment, and treatment. Clin Res Cardiol. 2024;113(9):1287-305.
2. Mahmood A, Dhall E, Primus CP, et al. Heart failure with preserved ejection fraction management: a systematic review of clinical practice guidelines and recommendations. Eur Heart J Qual Care Clin Outcomes. 2024;10(7):571-89.
3. Li Y, Kubo H, Yu D, et al. Combining three independent pathological stressors induces a heart failure with preserved ejection fraction phenotype. Am J Physiol Heart Circ Physiol. 2023;324(4):H443-60.
4. Harikrishnan S, Oomman A, Jadhav UM, et al. Heart failure with preserved ejection fraction: management guidelines (from Heart Failure Association of India, endorsed by Association of Physicians of India). J Assoc Physicians India. 2022;70(8):71-3.
5. Desai AS, Lam CSP, McMurray JJV, et al. How to manage heart failure with preserved ejection fraction: practical guidance for clinicians. JACC Heart Fail. 2023;11(6):619-36.
6. Golla MSG, Shams P. Heart failure with preserved ejection fraction (HFpEF). In: StatPearls [Internet]. Treasure Island: StatPearls Publishing; 2024.
7. Kittleson MM, Panjrath GS, Amancherla K, et al. 2023 ACC expert consensus decision pathway on management of heart failure with preserved ejection fraction: a report of the American College of Cardiology Solution Set Oversight Committee. J Am Coll Cardiol. 2023;81(18):1835-78.
8. Kosiborod MN, Abildstrom SZ, Bourlag BA, et al. Semaglutide in patients with heart failure with preserved ejection fraction and obesity. N Engl J Med. 2023;389:1069-84.
9. Parra-Lucares A, Romero-Hernández E, Villa E, et al. New opportunities in heart failure with preserved ejection fraction: from bench to bedside... and back. Biomedicines. 2022;11(1):70.

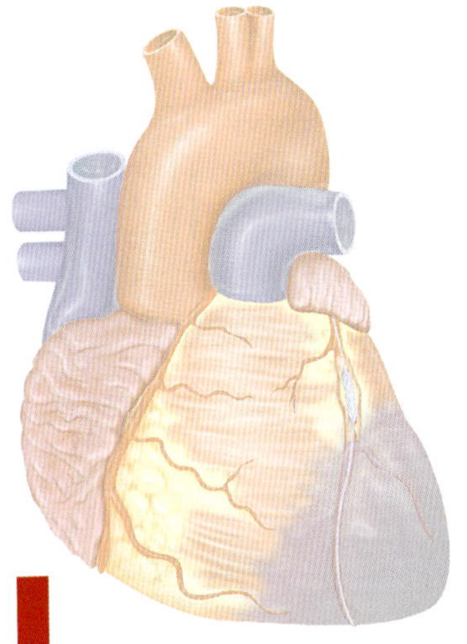

Diagnosis of HFpEF: Novel Insights

Soneil Guptha, Rajeev Gupta

INTRODUCTION

Heart failure with preserved ejection fraction (HFpEF) is classified in ICD-10 as a distinct condition. This clinical diagnosis is marked by inadequate pumping despite a normal or nearly normal left ventricular ejection fraction (LVEF). Clinicians refer to HFpEF as "diastolic heart failure," characterized by the left ventricle's inability to relax adequately during the diastolic (filling) phase, resulting in symptoms and signs of heart failure (HF). Individuals with current or past HF symptoms, (LVEF of 50% or greater, and elevated natriuretic peptides[1] are considered indicative. Additionally, there is evidence of increased intravascular volume load, indicated by elevated left ventricular filling pressures and pulmonary capillary wedge pressures exceeding 15 mm Hg at rest and 25 mm Hg during exercise.[1]

EPIDEMIOLOGY

Community-based studies suggest that 30–50% of patients with HF predominantly have HFpEF.[2] In the Framingham Heart Study (FHS), the prevalence ranged from 8 to 66 per 1,000 in men and 8 to 79 per 1,000 in women among those aged 50–89 years.[3] Data on the prevalence of HF is not available in the Global Burden of Disease (GBD) study.[4] A recent systematic review reported that HF affects more than 64 million people worldwide.[5] The prevalence rates of HFpEF in 2017 in Central Europe and the Middle East ranged from 1,133 to 1,196 per 100,000 population, with lower rates in Eastern Europe and Southeast Asia at 499–595 per 100,000 population. In the European Society of Cardiology registry, 16% of HF cases were classified as HFpEF, while in the USA-based registries, higher rates were reported in both OPTIMIZE-HF (24%)[6] and GWTG-HF (47%).[7] In the multicountry Asian HF registry, proportions similar to those in the USA were reported in Japan (43%) and China (36%).[8] In the INTERCHF registry from low-income countries, including India, HFpEF among HF was 15%.[9] In the G-CHF registry in lower-middle and middle-income countries, HFpEF was reported in 24%.[10] In India, the high burden of HF is indicated by a prevalence of 1.3–4.6 million cases, affecting 1.3–6.7% of adults.[11] Minor registries in India indicate that approximately 25% of HF patients have HFpEF.[12-14] Recent registries, such as the Trivandrum HF Registry,[15] Medanta HF Registry,[16] Kerala Heart Failure Registry,[17] multisite Indian College of Cardiology,[18] and Indian Council of Medical Research registries,[19] reported figures ranging from 15 to 30%. As we gain more insights into this syndrome, the epidemiological prevalence and incidence rates are expected to evolve, particularly due to the rising risk factors for HFpEF both globally and in India.[20] Early diagnosis of HFpEF using classical clinical criteria and recent biomarker-based methods is essential. In this chapter, we briefly discuss both.

PATHOPHYSIOLOGY AND BIOCHEMICAL DIAGNOSIS

A key pathophysiological factor in HFpEF is diastolic relaxation abnormality, which results from delayed myocardial relaxation and the passive stiffening of the left ventricle.[21] In HFpEF, diastolic dysfunction does not alter the final filling volume. However, filling necessitates

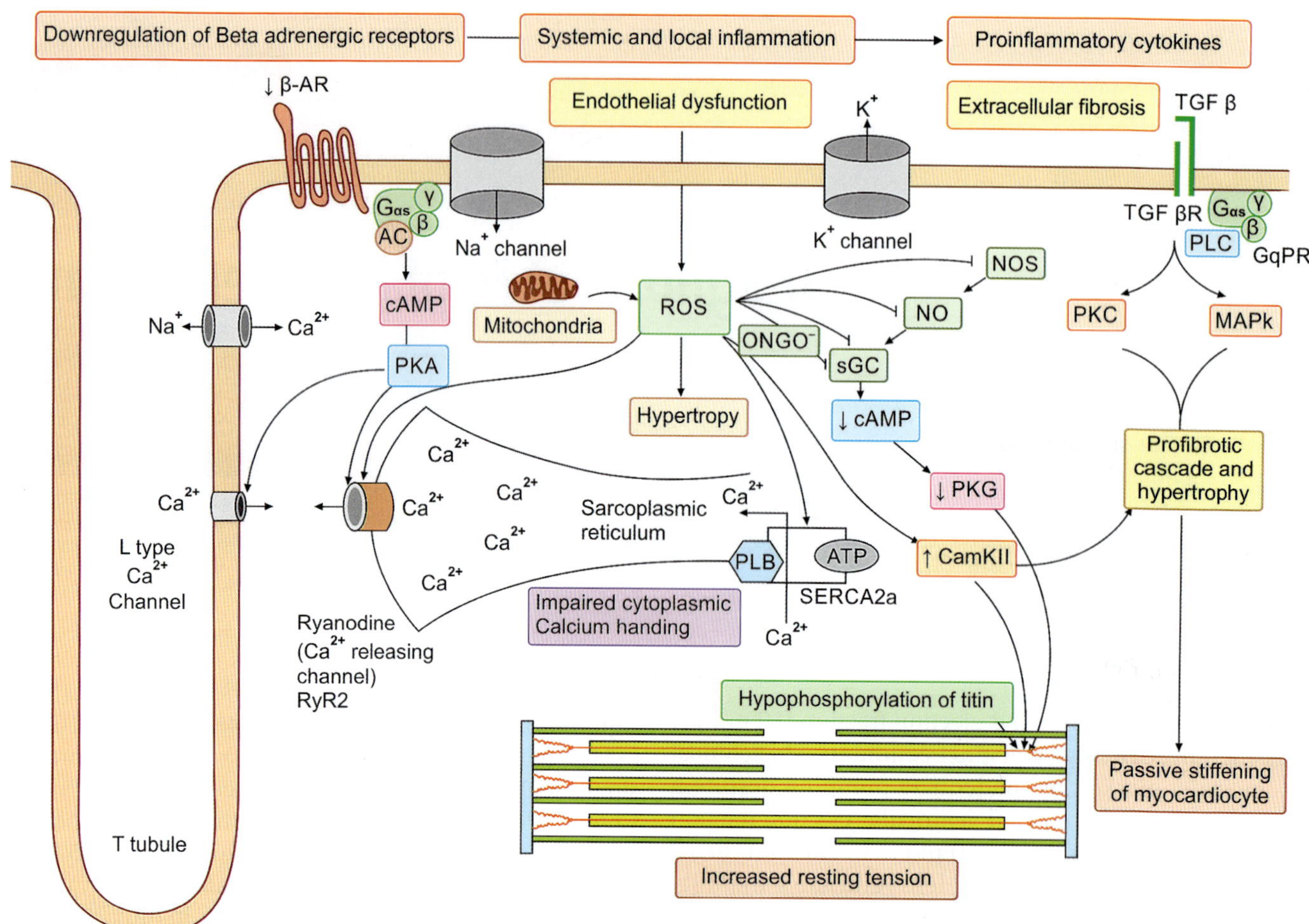

Fig. 1: Basic cellular pathophysiology of HFpEF. (AC: adenyl cyclase; ATP: adenosine triphosphate; B-AR: beta-adrenergic receptor; cAMP: cyclic adenosine monophosphate; CamKII: Calcium/calmodulin-dependent protein kinase II; GqPR: Gq-protein coupled receptor; MAPk: mitogen-activated protein kinase; NO: nitric oxide; NOS: nitric oxide synthase; ONOO: peroxynitrite; PKA: protein kinase A; PKC: protein kinase C; PKG: protein kinase G; PLC: phospholipase C; PLIB: phospholamban; ROS: reactive oxygen species; SERCA: sarco(endo)plasmic reticulum Ca^{2+}-ATPase; sGC: soluble guanylate cyclase)

increased effort and elevated filling pressure because of the diminished suction capability of both the right and left ventricles. This heightened effort becomes more noticeable in specific vascular loading conditions and during elevated heart rates, contributing to exercise intolerance and other HF symptoms.[22-26] Left atrial remodeling is common in HFpEF. Besides being a reservoir and conduit to the left ventricle, the left atrium maintains LV stroke volume through contraction. To sustain normal LV filling and stroke volume, the left atrium contracts, resulting in hypertrophy, a key risk factor for atrial fibrillation (AF). **Figure 1** shows microlevel biochemical changes in HFpEF. All these factors should be considered when developing a diagnostic algorithm for HFpEF. Inflammation is implicated in initiating various cascades at the cellular level, contributing to cardiac remodeling and the development of HFpEF.[25] Systemic and regional inflammation affects coronary microvascular endothelial cells, increasing adhesion molecules that attract leukocytes. Activated leukocytes release proinflammatory cytokines, generating reactive oxygen species and reducing nitrous oxide. Conditions such as diabetes, chronic kidney disease, obesity, and chronic obstructive pulmonary disease exacerbate microvascular inflammation and endothelial dysfunction. Inflammation alters the myocardium's extracellular matrix; monocytes release TGF-beta, which promotes fibroblast differentiation into myofibroblasts and collagen deposition, resulting in interstitial fibrosis.[25] Dysfunction and inflammation lead to cardiomyocyte hypertrophy and fibrosis, causing diastolic dysfunction and myocardial stiffening.[21,24,25]

The HFpEF and HFrEF have distinct pathophysiological differences: HFpEF often arises from comorbidities, while HFrEF is linked to cardiomyocyte loss due to ischemia, myocarditis, valvular disorders, or genetic mutations. These variations indicate potentially different molecular mechanisms.[26] Literature on cellular and molecular differences between HFpEF and HFrEF shows that cardiac remodeling in HFpEF, coupled with noncardiac comorbidities and low-grade inflammation, characterizes HFpEF. While inflammation is prevalent in both, endothelial dysfunction typically precedes HFpEF but follows cardiomyocyte loss in HFrEF. This dysfunction, resulting from reduced Ca^{2+} signaling and titin modification, causes ventricular stiffness and increased fibrosis linked to HFpEF.

In contrast, in HFrEF, titin switching is less consistent, and ventricular stiffness may be unaffected, increased, or even reduced.[26] HFpEF pathophysiology encompasses various interrelated mechanisms **(Fig. 1)** influenced by systemic or regional diseases that initiate or exacerbate HFpEF pathogenesis.[21,24-26] Diastolic relaxation abnormalities, proinflammatory state, endothelial dysfunction, oxidative stress, left atrial dysfunction, pulmonary hypertension, right ventricular dysfunction, ventricular dyssynchrony, aging, and comorbidities like obesity, diabetes, and chronic kidney disease are crucial underlying risk factors of HFpEF.[21-26] Multiple biomarkers could be used for the diagnosis of HFpEF. However, this area is still being researched and precision medicine techniques for HFpEF diagnosis are still in the early stages.

Some biomarkers and their possible candidates are given in **Table 1**.

B-type natriuretic peptide or NT-proBNP for diagnosis, severity assessment, and prognosis: NT-proBNP is a biologically inactive form of BNP. The predominant secretion of BNP is from the ventricular myocardium as a prohormone, which is cleaved to vasoactive BNP (half-life 22 minutes) and inactive NT-proBNP, BNP (half-life to minutes). Secretion of BNP reflects myocardial stretch. High BNP or NT-proBNP (both) are directly correlated to elevated filling pressure and are robust predictors of outcome. NT-proBNP, though sensitive, is not specific to the diagnosis of HFpEF as it can be influenced by tachycardia, AF, obesity, renal dysfunction, and ischemic myocardium.[27] Additionally, low or mildly elevated filling pressures can present with normal NT-proBNP, suggesting that low NT-proBNP measures are not recommended to exclude HFpEF, nor do elevated NT-proBNP levels suggest isolated evidence of diastolic dysfunction.[27,28] Finally, for patient management, can BNP concentrations help guide therapy in the whole spectrum of HF, including the group of patients with HFpEF? Current evidence does not support the routine measurement of BNP or NT-proBNP to guide the titration of therapy.[28-30]

TABLE 1: Biomarker-based diagnosis of HFpEF.

Biomarkers	*Possible candidates*
Standard biochemical markers	*Natriuretic peptides:* • B-type natriuretic peptide (BNP) • N-terminal pro-B-type natriuretic peptide (NT-proBNP)
Cardiac injury markers	High sensitivity troponins
Inflammatory markers	• Soluble suppression of tumorigenesis-2 (ST-2) • Galectin-3 • Neutrophil–lymphocyte ratio • Interleukin-6 • Lipocalin-2 (LCN-2) • Uric acid • Fatty acid binding proteins (FABP-4) • Growth differentiation factor-15 (GDF-15)
Genetic markers	• Specific SNPs and genes • Multiple genes and polygenic risk scores (PRS)

CLINICAL DIAGNOSIS AND DIFFERENTIAL DIAGNOSES

Until recently, international guidelines defined HFpEF as a syndrome indicated by symptoms and either (a) elevated natriuretic peptides (BNP, pro-BNP, or NT-pro-BNP) or (b) objective evidence of cardiogenic congestion. Echocardiographic evaluation remained central to HFpEF diagnosis, correlating well with cardiac catheterization indexes.[22,23] Key criteria are summarized in **Table 2**.

The 2023 ACC Consensus Pathway for HFpEF management[23] and other guidelines[27-29] cover diagnostics, differential diagnoses, investigations, comorbidities, gender-specific issues, and classification of HF based on EF and are summarized in **Table 3**.

The ESC Focused Update[30] emphasizes the significance of addressing comorbidities. Both updates complement each other and propose the following points that are pertinent to clinical practice.

- HFpEF is diagnosed when EF >50%. EF of 40–50% is HFmrEF, a nonhomogeneous category that includes patients with improved HFrEF and worsening HFpEF. HFmrEF is therapeutically closer to HFrEF than HFpEF.
- Standardization of echocardiography is essential for measuring ejection fraction (EF). Echocardiographic performance varies, and the cutoffs likely represent local variability.

TABLE 2: Diagnostic criteria for HFpEF in international practice guidelines.

	Guidelines		
	ACCF/ AHA (2013)[27]	ESC 2016[28]	CCS [2017][29]
Clinical	*Symptoms and signs of HF*		
LV ejection fraction	≥50%		
Bio-markers		BNP >35 pg/mL or NT-proBNP >125 pg/mL	BNP >50 pg/mL or NT-proBNP >125 pg/mL
Imaging	LV diastolic dysfunction	• LV diastolic dysfunction • LA volume index >34 mL/m² • LV mass index (men/women) >115/95 g/m² • E/e' >13 • Mean e' <9 cm/sec • LV Hypertrophy and/or LA enlargement	LV diastolic dysfunction

(BNP: brain natriuretic peptide; HF: heart failure; NT-proBNP: n-terminal pro-BNP; LA: left atrium; LV: left ventricle)

TABLE 3: Classification of heart failure (HF) by left ventricular ejection fraction (EF).

HF subgroup	*Symptoms*	*Ejection fraction*
HFpEF	*Heart failure with preserved ejection fraction:* Clinically diagnosed symptomatic HF	≥50%
HFmREF	*Heart failure with mildly reduced ejection fraction:* Clinically diagnosed symptomatic HF	41–49%
HFrEF	*Heart failure with reduced ejection fraction:* Clinically diagnosed symptomatic HF	≤40%
HFimpEF	*Heart failure with improved ejection fraction:* Clinically diagnosed symptomatic HF	Baseline EF <40%; 10-point increase in EF at repeat measurement or EF >40%
HFpEF mimics	Clinically diagnosed symptomatic HF with primary noncardiac cause (kidney or liver disease) or an underlying cardiac cause (infiltrative, hypertrophic, valvular disease, pericardial disease, and high-output HF	≥50%

- Cardiac conditions like constrictive pericarditis, hypertrophic cardiomyopathy, infiltrative diseases (e.g., amyloidosis and sarcoidosis), valvular heart diseases, and high-output heart failure must be ruled out. This is also true for noncardiac conditions mimicking HFpEF, such as acute asthma, exacerbation of chronic obstructive pulmonary disease, kidney or liver diseases, and metabolic disorders.[23]
- The ACC[23] and ESC[28] now advise against using diastolic dysfunction, as other factors can cause it without HF.[22] Although this conclusion seems significant, it is essential to remain open-minded until the pathophysiology and causes are more clearly understood within the context of the Indian population.[31]
- The ACC statement[23] emphasizes noncardiac factors that can imitate HF. **Table 4** presents key differential diagnoses for dyspnea and edema, which are the main symptoms of HF.

TABLE 4: Differential diagnoses of dyspnea and edema.

Symptoms	*Major causal group*	*Clinical conditions*
Dyspnea	Cardiac causes	• Cardiomyopathy • Coronary artery disease • Valvular heart disease • Pericardial disease • Arrhythmias
	Pulmonary causes	• Obstructive lung disease • Restrictive lung disease • Pleural disease • Pulmonary embolism
	Other causes	• Anemia • Neuromuscular diseases • Deconditioning • Anxiety
Edema	↑Capillary hydrostatic pressure	• Cardiac causes (cardiomyopathy, valvular disease, and pericardial disease) • Cirrhosis with portal hypertension • Renal failure • Others (venous insufficiency, pregnancy, and medications such as CCBs, NSAIDs, and steroids)
	↓Capillary oncotic pressure	• ↓Protein intake (malnutrition) • ↓Protein production (cirrhosis) • Protein loss (malabsorption and nephrotic syndrome)

HEART FAILURE WITH PRESERVED EJECTION FRACTION DIAGNOSTIC SCORING SYSTEMS

The universal definition of HF serves as a helpful guide for clinicians when diagnosing HFpEF. The H_2FPEF score includes six accessible factors, while HFA-PEFF follows a more complex algorithm involving clinical features, echocardiographic assessments, and serum NT-ProBNP levels.[22,23]

In Indian clinical practice, the universal definition of HF aids in diagnosing HFpEF. However, diagnosis is challenging due to the lack of easily detected cardiac abnormalities and the ambiguous nature of the syndrome, along with the unavailability of natriuretic peptide testing.[31] In this context, the ACC Expert Consensus scoring systems H_2FPEF and HFA-PEFF **(Table 5)** serve as valuable tools for the diagnosis of suspected HFpEF patients, facilitating guidelines-directed medical therapy (GDMT), as illustrated in the diagnostic algorithm **(Flowchart 1)**.

CRITERIA FOR REFERRALS TO SPECIALIST UNITS

A fundamental component of the ACC and ESC guidelines[23,30] pertaining to the management of HFpEF is the recommendation that a clinical cardiologist should oversee the care of each patient diagnosed with HFpEF in collaboration with both a primary-care physician and an HF specialist. Moreover, emphasis is placed on identifying barriers to the effective delivery of care. The guidelines present indicators and checklists to facilitate referrals from primary-care physicians to both general cardiology specialists and HF specialists. To assist in the referral process from primary-care physicians to cardiovascular specialists, the acronym CHECK-IN has been proposed and encompasses several key components:

- *Collaboration:* Need for specialist care to manage comorbidities such as AF, hypertension, diabetes, CAD, etc.
- *High-risk features:* Hospitalizations, pulmonary hypertension, and right ventricular dysfunction
- *Extensive evaluation needed:* Exercise testing, invasive hemodynamic or cardiac MRI.
- Cardiorenal syndrome
- Knowledge of HFpEF mimics
- Increased need for diuretics
- NYHA Class III or IV symptoms

An additional acronym, INNHALE, has been proposed for referral to specialists in HF as well as multidisciplinary teams.[23]

- *In need of diagnosis:* Lack of conventional HFpEF risk factors and exercise intolerance phenotype
- Nonresponsive to diuretic agents or medical therapy

TABLE 5: HFpEF diagnostic scoring systems in ACC consensus decision pathway.

Scoring system	*Acronym*	*Clinical criteria*	*Points*
H_2FPEF score (≥6 points is highly diagnostic)	H_2	• Heavy BMI ≥30 kg/m^2 • ≥2 antihypertensives	2 1
	F	Atrial Fibrillation	3
	P	Pulmonary hypertension (PASP >35 mm Hg on Doppler echocardiography	1
	E	Elder (age >60 years)	1
	F	Filling pressures (E/e' >9 on doppler echocardiography)	1
HFA-PEEF score (≥5 points is highly diagnostic)	P	• Symptoms or signs of heart failure • Comorbidities/risk factors • Standard echocardiography	1 1 1
	E	• Comprehensive echocardiography • *Functional measures:* Septal e' <7 cm/s, lateral e' <10 cm/s, average E/e' ≥15. TR velocity >2.8 m/s, GLS <16%) • *Morphological:* LAVI >34 mL/m^2, or LVMI ≥149/122 (M/F), and RWT >0.42 or LVWT ≥12 mm • *Natriuretic peptides:* NT ProBNP >220 pg/mL or BNP >80 pg/mL • *Natriuretic peptides (AFib):* NT ProBNP >660 pg/mL or BNP >240 pg/mL	1 1 1 1
	F_1	• Diastolic stress test (exercise echocardiography) • Invasive hemodynamic measurements	1 1
	F_2	• Special imaging (CMR, CT, PET, and scintigraphy) • Biopsies • Genetic testing	1 1 1

Flowchart 1: Diagnostic algorithm.

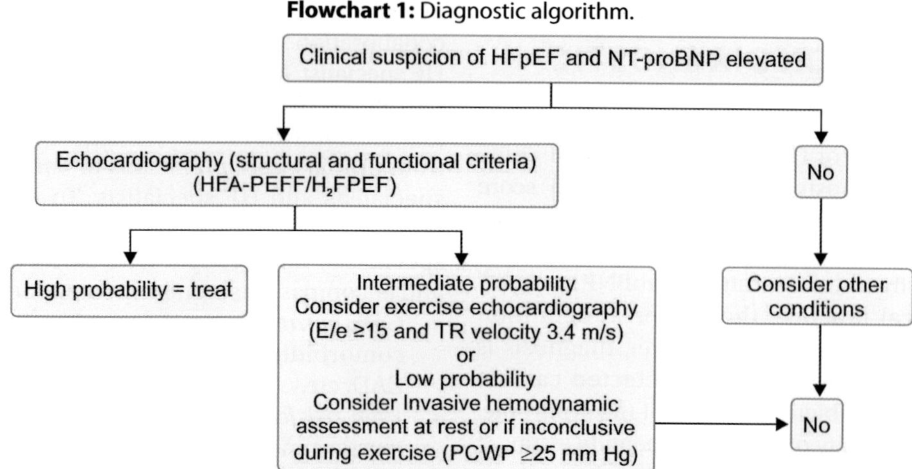

- *Natriuretic peptides are extremely high:* NT-ProBNP >3,000 pg/mL or BNP >1,000 pg/mL
- *Hospitalized frequently for heart failure:* More than or equal to hospitalizations in the past year
- *Acute or chronic end-organ dysfunction:* Worsening liver or kidney function and cardiac cachexia
- *Low blood pressure:* Systolic BP <100 mm Hg.
- Evidence of HFpEF mimics and rare or unusual cardiomyopathies

CONCLUSION

Heart failure with preserved ejection fraction presents a significant challenge in clinical medicine due to its rising prevalence, frequent underdiagnosis, poor outcomes, and limited treatment options. Addressing the missed diagnosis that often leads to an unfavorable prognosis of HFpEF is a formidable challenge, making it crucial to prioritize algorithm-based diagnosis.[32] In the future, artificial intelligence-led strategies could be important for early diagnosis and precision therapy.

REFERENCES

1. Redfield MM. Heart failure with preserved ejection fraction. N Engl J Med. 2017;376(19):1868-77.
2. Gladden JD, Linke WA, Redfield MM. Heart failure with preserved ejection fraction. Pflugers Arch. 2014; 466(6):1037-53.
3. Ho KK, Pinsky JL, Kannel WB, et al. The epidemiology of heart failure: The Framingham Study. J Am Coll Cardiol. 1993;22(Suppl A):6A-13A.
4. Vaduganathan M, Mensah GA, Turco JV, et al. The global burden of cardiovascular diseases and risk: a compass for future health. J Am Coll Cardiol. 2022;80(25):2361-71.
5. Savarese G, Becher PM, Lund LH, et al. Global burden of heart failure: a comprehensive and updated review of epidemiology. Cardiovasc Res. 2023;118(17):3272-87.
6. Fonarow GC, Stough WG, Abraham WT, et al. Characteristics, treatments, and outcomes of patients with preserved systolic function hospitalized for heart failure: a report from the OPTIMIZE-HF Registry. J Am Coll Cardiol. 2007;50(8):768-77.
7. Vaduganathan M, Greene SJ, Zhang S, et al. Applicability of US Food and Drug Administration labeling for dapagliflozin to patients with heart failure with reduced ejection fraction in US clinical practice: The Get With the Guidelines-Heart Failure (GWTG-HF) Registry. JAMA Cardiol. 2021;6(3):267-75.
8. Asian HF Registry. Regional variation of mortality in heart failure with reduced and preserved ejection fraction across Asia: Outcomes in the Asian-HF Registry. J Am Heart Assoc. 2020;9:e014512.
9. Dokainish H, Teo K, Zhu J, et al. Global mortality variations in patients with heart failure: Results from the International Congestive Heart Failure (INTERCHF) prospective cohort study. Lancet Glob Health. 2017;5(7):e665-672.
10. G-CHF Investigators; Joseph P, Roy A, Lonn E, et al. Global variations in heart failure etiology, management, and outcomes. JAMA. 2023;329(19):1650-61.
11. Huffman MD, Prabhakaran D. Heart failure: epidemiology and prevention in India. Natl Med J India. 2010;23(5): 283-8.
12. Gupta R, Pathak V. Left ventricular failure in elderly: an echocardiographic study highlighting normal left ventricle size and mitral stenosis. Indian J Gerontol. 1993;7:13-8.
13. Dhingra A, Garg A, Kaur S, et al. Epidemiology of heart failure with preserved ejection fraction. Curr Heart Fail Rep. 2014;11(4):354-65.
14. Gupta R, Grover V, Roy S, et al. Heart failure etiologies, management, and short-term outcomes in hospitalized and clinic-based patients in India. RUHS J Health Sci. 2018;3:5-10.

15. Harikrishnan S, Sanjay G, Agarwal A, et al. One-year mortality outcomes and hospital readmissions of patients admitted with acute heart failure: Data from the Trivandrum Heart Failure Registry in Kerala, India. Am Heart J. 2017;189:193-9.
16. Chopra VK, Mittal S, Bansal M, et al. Clinical profile and one-year survival of patients with heart failure with reduced ejection fraction: The largest report from India. Indian Heart J. 2019;71(3):242-8.
17. Joseph S, Jeemon P, Abdullakutty J, et al. Cardiology Society of India-Kerala Acute Heart Failure registry: Poor adherence to guidelines directed medical therapy. Eur Heart J. 2022;43:908-15.
18. Jayagopal PB, Sastry SL, Nanjappa V, et al. Clinical characteristics and 30-day outcomes in patients with acute decompensated heart failure: Results from Indian College of Cardiology National Heart Failure Registry. Int J Cardiol. 2022;356:73-8.
19. Harikrishnan S, Bahl A, Roy A, et al. Clinical profile and 90 days outcomes of 10,851 heart failure patients across India: National Heart Failure Registry. ESC Heart Fail. 2022;9(6):3898-908.
20. Kalra A, Jose AP, Prabhakaran P, et al. The burgeoning cardiovascular disease epidemic in Indians: Perspectives on contextual factors and potential solutions. Lancet Reg Health Southeast Asia. 2023;12:100156.
21. Rao VN, Parikh KS. The pathophysiology of heart failure with preserved ejection fraction. In: Kalogeropoulos AP, Skopicki HA, Butler J (Eds). Heart Failure: An Essential Clinical Guide. New Delhi: CRC Press;2022.
22. Borlaug BA, Sharma K, Shah SJ, et al. Heart failure with preserved ejection fraction: JACC Scientific Statement. J Am Coll Cardiol. 2023;81:1810-34.
23. Kittleson MM, Panjrath GS, Amancherla K, et al. 2023 ACC expert consensus decision pathway on management of heart failure with preserved ejection fraction: A report of the American College of Cardiology Solution Set Oversight Committee. J Am Coll Cardiol. 2023;81(18): 1835-78.
24. Packer M. Leptin-aldosterone-neprilysin axis: Identification of its distinctive role in the pathogenesis of the three phenotypes of heart failure in people with obesity. Circulation. 2018;137(15):1614-31.
25. Budde H, Hassoun R, Mügge A, et al. Current understanding of molecular pathophysiology of heart failure with preserved ejection fraction. Frontiers Physiol. 2022; 13:928232.
26. Simmonds SJ, Cuijpers I, Heymans S, et al. Cellular and molecular differences between HFpEF and HFrEF: a step ahead in an improved pathological understanding. Cells. 2020;9(1):242.
27. Yancy CW, Jessup M, Bozkurt B, et al. 2013 ACCF/AHA guideline for the management of heart failure: A report of the American College of Cardiology Foundation/American Heart Association Task Force on Practice Guidelines. J Am Coll Cardiol. 2013;62(16):e147-239.
28. Ponikowski P, Voors AA, Anker SD, et al. 2016 ESC guidelines for the diagnosis and treatment of acute and chronic heart failure: the task force for the diagnosis and treatment of acute and chronic heart failure of the European Society of Cardiology (ESC). Developed with the special contribution of the Heart Failure Association (HFA) of the ESC. Eur J Heart Fail. 2016;37(27):2129-200..
29. Ezekowitz, Justin A. 2017 comprehensive update of the CCS guidelines for the management of heart failure. Can J Cardiol. 2017;33(11):1342-433.
30. McDonough TA, Metra M, Adamo M, et al. 2023 focused update of the 2021 ESC guidelines for the diagnosis and treatment of acute and chronic heart failure. Eur Heart J. 2023;44(37):3627-39.
31. Harikrishnan S, Oommen A, Jadhav UM, et al. Heart failure with preserved ejection fraction: Management guidelines from Health Failure Association of India endorsed by Association of Physicians of India. J Assoc Physicians India. 2022;70:71-3.
32. Brownell NK, Fonarow GC. Hospitalization for heart failure requires a PROMPT response. Eur Heart J. 2023; 44(40):4243-45.

10
CHAPTER

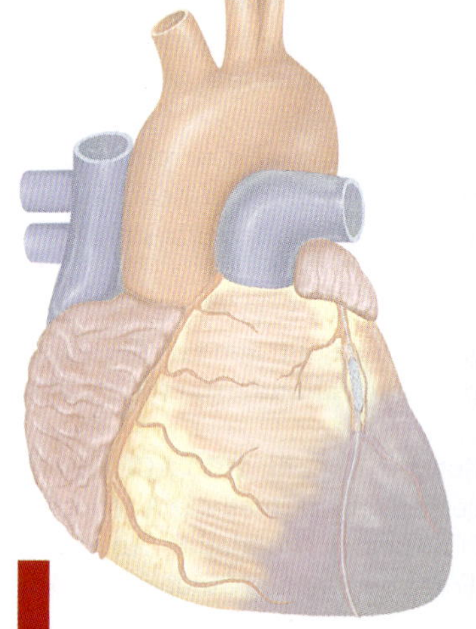

Diagnosis of HFpEF Among Patients with Unexplained Dyspnea

Harsh Wardhan, Isha Nandal, Archit Dahiya

INTRODUCTION

Unexplained dyspnea is one of the most important factors interfering with quality of life. On echocardiogram, finding of normal left ventricular ejection fraction (LVEF) can sometimes mislead the physicians to exclude heart failure and thus missing the possibility of heart failure with preserved ejection fraction (HFpEF).

HFpEF is defined as heart failure symptoms with/without heart failure signs, LVEF ≥50%, and objective evidence of cardiac structural and/or functional abnormalities, including raised natriuretic peptide levels.[1] HFpEF accounts for more than half of patients with heart failure and is associated with high morbidity and mortality.[2,3] Therefore, early diagnosis is essential for reducing the heart failure burden in this population.

There is a lack of clear consensus on the HFpEF definition including the LVEF value. Classical symptoms include shortness of breath, orthopnea, PND (paroxysmal nocturnal dyspnea), reduced exercise capacity, fatigue, and lower limb swelling while classical signs include peripheral edema, lung crepitations, elevated jugular venous pressure (JVP), or third heart sound.

Dyspnea is the major HFpEF symptom. However, these patients are usually elderly and may have other conditions mimicking heart failure such as coronary artery disease (CAD), chronic obstructive airway disease, anemia, obesity, diabetes, and atrial fibrillation (AF).

HEART FAILURE WITH PRESERVED EJECTION FRACTION DIAGNOSIS

Electrocardiogram

An electrocardiogram (ECG) helps in diagnosing the underlying etiology of heart failure. In heart failure patients, normal ECG is an unusual finding. Some of the common ECG findings in heart failure are left ventricular hypertrophy (LVH), ST-T alterations, pathological Q waves, AF/flutter, conduction abnormalities, and left bundle branch block (LBBB).[4]

Chest X-ray and Lung Ultrasound

Pulmonary congestion or cardiomegaly are the usual findings on a chest X-ray in heart failure patients.[5] Lung ultrasound can help both in the diagnosis and prognosis of heart failure patients as the more the number of B-lines on ultrasound, the worse is the adverse outcome.

NATRIURETIC PEPTIDES

Natriuretic peptides are hormones that regulate body fluid homeostasis and blood pressure. The levels of these peptides are raised not only in heart failure but also in other conditions such as myocardial infarction, arrhythmias, pulmonary embolism, acute and chronic kidney injury, sepsis, elderly, left ventricular hypertrophy, chronic obstructive airway disease, and AF.[6] The levels may be falsely low in obese patients and thus do not rule out the diagnosis of HFpEF in this subset of the population.

Brain natriuretic peptide (BNP) is a slightly poorer marker for HFpEF than N-terminal pro-B-type natriuretic peptide (NT-proBNP) and it is recommended to use NTproBNP ≥300 pg/mL if normal sinus rhythm and ≥600 pg/mL if AF for HFpEF diagnosis.[7,8]

Regarding other natriuretic peptides, the use of midregional proatrial natriuretic peptide (MR-proANP) as a biomarker has not yet been fully studied for HFpEF diagnosis. Some recent studies show that raised MR-proANP levels in HFpEF patients are associated with a higher risk of cardiovascular events.[9]

OTHER BIOMARKERS

For HFpEF diagnosis, other biomarkers include high-sensitivity troponins (hs-TnT), soluble suppression of tumorigenesis-2 (sST2), growth differentiation factor 15 (GDF-15), galectin-3 (Gal-3), carbohydrate antigen 125 (CA125), soluble glycoprotein 130 and heat shock protein 27 (hsp27).[10-12]

Troponin

Troponins correlate well with the severity of acute as well as chronic heart failure. It is raised in heart failure mainly due to myocardial inflammation and stretch, hypoxia, neurohormonal activation, and cytotoxicity. However, for HFpEF, high-sensitivity troponins hold a lesser prognostic value as compared to HFrEF.[13]

Soluble Suppression of Tumorigenesis-2

Soluble suppression of tumorigenesis-2 belongs to the toll-like/interleukin-1 receptor superfamily, which is released after myocardial stretch and cardiovascular injury. In HFpEF patients, sST2 levels were found to be associated with right ventricular (RV) pressure overload, systemic congestion, and proinflammatory comorbidities but not with left ventricular geometry or function.[14]

In a study on acute decompensated HFpEF, sST2 was found to be a significant predictor of noncardiovascular mortality during a median follow-up of 14 months.[15] Also, sST2 and not NT-proBNP, had emerged as an independent predictor of intermediate-term mortality in 200 HFpEF patients with acute dyspnea.[16]

Growth Differentiation Factor 15

Growth differentiation factor 15 belongs to the transforming growth factor-β (TGF-β) cytokine superfamily and is produced as an inactive precursor that undergoes proteolytic activation leading to the release of the N-terminal pro-peptide from the mature GDF-15 protein, which is then secreted as a dimer. Unlike the NT-proBNP, GDF-15 levels are not affected by AF. GDF-15 levels act as a prognostic marker for heart failure. In another study of 380 patients, GDF-15, Gal-3, and sST2 were able to predict the two-year mortality risk in acute HFpEF patients.[17,18]

Galectin-3

It is a type of soluble β-galactoside binding lectin, and it promotes cardiovascular inflammation, fibroblast proliferation, and fibrosis leading to the development of HFpEF. Gal-3 levels in plasma are increased in patients with HFpEF and are also associated with indices of diastolic dysfunction left ventricular stiffness, and heart failure severity.[19] Gal-3 can help in determining long-term outcomes in HFpEF patients and the predictive value of Gal-3 seems higher in HFpEF than in HFrEF, as shown by a subanalysis of data from the Coordinating study evaluating Outcomes of Advising and Counseling in Heart Failure (COACH) study.[20]

ECHOCARDIOGRAPHY

Echocardiography is one of the key diagnostic investigations for HFpEF. It is used to determine the LVEF and RV ejection fraction, LV chamber size, and valvular function, as well as the presence of regional wall motion abnormalities (RWMA), LVH, pulmonary hypertension, and diastolic function markers. The various criteria for HFpEF diagnosis by echocardiography are mentioned in **Table 1**.

STRESS ECHOCARDIOGRAPHY

It is done to unmask LV systolic and diastolic dysfunction, and this is mainly a submaximal exercise stress test, whereas the maximal exercise stress test is generally used to exclude ischemia. Stress echocardiography criteria used for HFpEF are mitral E/e′ ratio and tricuspid regurgitation (TR) peak velocity and these are closely linked with mean pulmonary capillary wedge pressure (PCWP) and pulmonary artery systolic pressure (PASP) respectively. The lack of increased cardiac output during exercise at peak stress levels, average E/e′ ratio ≥15, and a TR velocity >3.4 m/s helps in the diagnosis of HFpEF.[20]

RIGHT HEART CATHETERIZATION

It is needed only in rare cases of unexplained dyspnea. HFpEF diagnosis can be there if invasively measured

PCWP ≥15 mm Hg or left ventricular end-diastolic pressure (LVEDP) ≥16 mm Hg at rest is present in these patients.[21]

DIAGNOSTIC SCORES[22,23]

The two scores for HFpEF diagnosis are H2FPEF **(Table 2)** and HFA-PEFF **(Table 3)**. The use of both scores in the same patient is more beneficial as these scores may identify different HFpEF phenotypes. Uncertainty in the diagnosis is the main indication for the use of these diagnostic scores. The scores are valid for patients with unexplained dyspnea and suspected heart failure and should not be used in asymptomatic patients or patients with symptoms clearly due to another cause of dyspnea.

H2FPEF >5 or HFA-PEFF >4 is highly suggestive of HFPEF while a lower score virtually rules out HFpEF.

TABLE 1: HFpEF diagnosis by echocardiography.[19]

	Functional criteria	*Structural criteria*
Major	• Septal e′ <7 cm/s or lateral e′ <10 cm/s or • Average E/e′ ≥15 or tricuspid regurgitation velocity >2.8 m/s (PA systolic pressure >35 mm Hg)	LA volume index >34 mL/m^2 Or LV mass index ≥149/122 g/m^2 (male/female) and relative wall thickness >0.42
Minor	Average E/e′ ≥9–14 or global longitudinal strain <16%	LA volume index 29–34 mL/m^2 Or LV mass index >115/95 g/m^2 (male/female) Or Relative wall thickness >0.42 Or Left ventricular wall thickness ≥12 mm

(HFpEF: heart failure with preserved ejection fraction; LA: left atrial; LV: left ventricular; PA: pulmonary artery)

TABLE 2: H2FPEF score.

Parameter	*Characteristic*		*Points*
H_2	Heavy	BMI >30 kg/m^2	2
	Hypertension	≥2 antihypertensive medications	1
F	Atrial Fibrillation	Persistent or paroxysmal	3
P	Pulmonary hypertension	PASP >35 mm Hg*	1
E	Elderly	Age >60 years	1
F	Filling pressures	E/e′ >9*	1
H2FPEF score			Sum (0–9)
Interpretation		• 0–1: Low probability (unlikely HFpEF) • 2–5: Intermediate probability • 6–9: High probability (likely HFpEF)	

*Measured by echocardiogram

(BMI: body mass index; HFpEF: heart failure with preserved ejection fraction)

TABLE 3: HFA-PEFF score.

Domain	*Major criteria (two points)*	*Minor criteria (1 point)*	*Score (maximum two points per domain)*
Functional	• Septal e′ <7 or Lateral e′ <10 • Average E/e′ ratio ≥15 • TR velocity >2.8 m/s (PASP >35 mm Hg)	• Average E/e′ ratio 9–14 • GLS <16%	
Morphological	• LAVI >34 mL/m^2 or • LVMI >149/122 g/m^2 (m/w) and RWT >0.42	• LAVI 29–34 mL/m^2 • LVMI >115/95 g/m^2 (m/w) • RWT >0,42 • LVWT ≥12 mm	
Biomarker (Sinus Rhythm)	NT-proBNP >220 pg/mL BNP >80 pg/mL	NT-proBNP 125–220 pg/mL or BNP 35–80 pg/mL	
Biomarker (Atrial fibrillation)	NT-proBNP >660 pg/mL or BNP >240 pg/mL	NT-proBNP 365–660 pg/mL or BNP 105–240 pg/mL	
HFA-PEFF score			Sum (0–6)
Interpretation		• 0–1: Low probability (unlikely HFpEF) • 2–4: Intermediate probability • 5–6: High probability (HFpEF diagnosis)	

(BNP: B-type natriuretic peptide; GLS: global longitudinal strain; HFpEF: heart failure with preserved ejection fraction; LAVI: left atrial volume index; LVMI: left ventricular mass index; m: men; NT-proBNP: N-terminal B-type natriuretic peptide; PASP: pulmonary artery systolic pressure; LVWT: left ventricular wall thickness; RWT: relative wall thickness; TR: tricuspid regurgitation; w: women)

CONCLUSION

Heart failure with preserved ejection fraction is a very common condition that is associated with high morbidity and mortality. However, confirming a diagnosis of HFpEF is challenging, as affected patients have many comorbidities that can mimic the condition. Additionally, HFpEF is not defined based on a single criterion but on a cluster of parameters, mainly increased natriuretic peptide levels and specific echocardiographic alterations. Newer biomarkers are being studied to help diagnose patients of HFpEF. The use of diagnostic scores may be helpful in diagnosis. Compared with the HFA-PEFF score, the H2FPEF score uses a simpler approach and seems to be more accurate in detecting HFpEF defined by the hemodynamic criteria.

REFERENCES

1. McDonagh TA, Metra M, Adamo M, et al. 2021 ESC Guidelines for the diagnosis and treatment of acute and chronic heart failure. Eur Heart J. 20201;42(36):3599-726.
2. Escobar C, Palacios B, Varela L, et al. Prevalence, characteristics, management and outcomes of patients with heart failure with preserved, mildly reduced, and reduced ejection fraction in Spain. J Clin Med. 2022;11(17):5199.
3. Escobar C, Palacios B, Varela L, et al. Healthcare resource utilization and costs among patients with heart failure with preserved, mildly reduced, and reduced ejection fraction in Spain. BMC Health Serv Res. 2022;22(1):1241.
4. Bjerkén LV, Rønborg SN, Jensen MT, et al. Artificial intelligence enabled ECG screening for left ventricular systolic dysfunction: a systematic review. Heart Fail Rev. 2023;28(2):419-30.
5. Morvai-Illés B, Polestyuk-Németh N, Szabó IA, et al. The prognostic value of lung ultrasound in patients with newly diagnosed heart failure with preserved ejection fraction in the ambulatory setting. Front Cardiovasc Med. 2021;8:758147.
6. Mueller C, McDonald K, de Boer RA, et al. Heart Failure Association of the European Society of Cardiology practical guidance on the use of natriuretic peptide concentrations. Eur J Heart Fail. 2019;21(6):715-31.
7. Formiga F, Nuñez J, Moraga MJC, et al. Diagnosis of heart failure with preserved ejection fraction: a systematic narrative review of the evidence. Heart Fail Rev. 2024; 29(1):179-89.
8. Shah SJ. BNP: Biomarker Not Perfect in heart failure with preserved ejection fraction. Eur Heart J. 2022; 43(20):1952-54.
9. Jensen J, Schou M, Kistorp C, et al. MR-proANP and incident cardiovascular disease in patients with type 2 diabetes with and without heart failure with preserved ejection fraction. Cardiovasc. Diabetol. 2020;19(1):180.
10. Morfino P, Aimo A, Castiglione V, et al. Biomarkers of HFpEF: natriuretic peptides, high-sensitivity troponins and beyond. J Cardiovasc Dev Dis. 2022;9(8):256.
11. Trippel TD, Mende M, Düngen H-D, et al. The diagnostic and prognostic value of galectin-3 in patients at risk for heart failure with preserved ejection fraction: results from the DIASTCHF study. ESC Heart Fail. 2021;8(2):829-41.
12. Liu S, Iskandar R, Chen W, et al. Soluble glycoprotein 130 and heat shock protein 27 as novel candidate biomarkers of chronic heart failure with preserved ejection fraction. Heart Lung Circ. 2016;25(10):1000-6.
13. Ledwoch J, Kraxenberger J, Krauth A, et al. Prognostic impact of high-sensitive troponin on 30-day mortality in patients with acute heart failure and different classes of left ventricular ejection fraction. Heart Vessel. 2022; 37(7):1195-202.
14. AbouEzzeddine OF, McKie PM, Dunlay SM, et al. Suppression of Tumorigenicity 2 in Heart Failure With Preserved Ejection Fraction. J Am Heart Assoc. 2017; 6(2):e004382.
15. Sugano A, Seo Y, Ishizu T, et al. Soluble ST2 and brain natriuretic peptide predict different mode of death in patients with heart failure and preserved ejection fraction. J Cardiol. 2019;73(4):326-32.
16. Shah KB, Kop WJ, Christenson RH, et al. Prognostic utility of ST2 in patients with acute dyspnea and preserved left ventricular ejection fraction. Clin Chem. 2011;57(6): 874-82.
17. Gao Y, Bai X, Lu J, et al. Prognostic value of multiple circulating biomarkers for 2-year death in acute heart failure with preserved ejection fraction. Front Cardiovasc Med. 2021;8:779282.
18. Mendez Fernandez AB, Ferrero-Gregori A, Garcia-Osuna A, et al. Growth differentiation factor 15 as mortality predictor in heart failure patients with non-reduced ejection fraction. ESC Heart Fail. 2020;7(5):2223-9.
19. Beltrami M, Ruocco G, Dastidar AG, et al. Additional value of Galectin-3 to BNP in acute heart failure patients with preserved ejection fraction. Clin Chim Acta. 2016; 457:99-105.
20. de Boer RA, Lok DJ, Jaarsma T, et al. Predictive value of plasma galectin-3 levels in heart failure with reduced and preserved ejection fraction. Ann Med. 2011;43(1):60-8.
21. Pieske B, Tschöpe C, de Boer RA, et al. How to diagnose heart failure with preserved ejection fraction: the HFA-PEFF diagnostic algorithm: a consensus recommendation from the Heart Failure Association (HFA) of the European Society of Cardiology (ESC). Eur Heart J. 2019; 40(40):3297-317.
22. Guazzi M, Wilhelm M, Halle M, et al. Exercise testing in heart failure with preserved ejection fraction: an appraisal through diagnosis, pathophysiology and therapy - a clinical consensus statement of the Heart Failure Association and European Association of Preventive Cardiology of the European Society of Cardiology. Eur J Heart Fail. 2022;24(8):1327-45.
23. Baratto C, Caravita S, Soranna D, et al. Current limitations of invasive exercise hemodynamics for the diagnosis of heart failure with preserved ejection fraction. Circ Heart Fail. 2021;14(5):e007555.

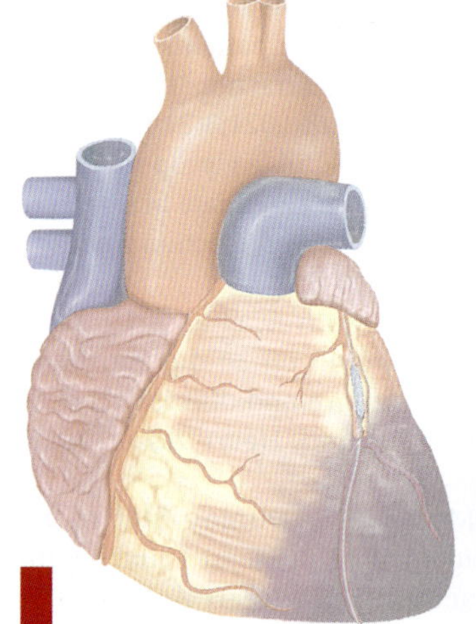

CHAPTER

Application of Diagnostic Algorithms for HFpEF to Community

Kiran Rao Kanjerla, Dayasagar Rao V

INTRODUCTION

Heart failure (HF) is associated with significant morbidity and mortality in adult population. It is a common cause of repeated hospitalizations globally. HF is defined as clinical syndrome with symptoms and/or signs caused by a structural and/or functional cardiac abnormality and corroborated by elevated natriuretic peptide levels and/or objective evidence of pulmonary or systemic congestion. HF has been classified into subgroups according to left ventricular ejection fraction (LVEF) at HF diagnosis. HF with reduced EF (HFrEF) is defined by an EF of 40% or less, HF with mildly reduced EF (HFmEF) is defined by an EF of 41–49%, and HF with preserved EF (HFpEF) is defined by an EF of 50% or greater.[1] Currently, HFpEF accounts for approximately 50% of all diagnoses of HF.[2,3] HFpEF is more complex to diagnose and therapeutic options are limited as compared to HFrEF.

Heart failure with preserved EF is a systemic syndrome triggered by combination of risk factors and comorbidities[4] and is diagnosed by presence of signs and symptoms of CHF with preserved LVEF >50% and left ventricular end-diastolic volume index (LVEDVI) <97 mL/m^2 with evidence of LV diastolic dysfunction. The current paradigm proposes that comorbidities drive structural and functional remodeling through systemic endothelial inflammation. Comorbidities associated with HFpEF lead to systemic and coronary endothelial inflammation, which reduce the bioavailability of nitric oxide by endothelium and cyclic guanosine monophosphate (cGMP) by cardiac myocyte. This process leads to hypophosphorylation of titin leading to increased myocardial hypertrophy, myofibroblast activation, and interstitial fibrosis, which leads to increased myocardial stiffness. Although, diastolic dysfunction is predominant abnormality, other mechanism such as ventricular-vascular stiffening, impaired systemic vasodilatory reserve, chronotropic incompetence, pulmonary hypertension (PH) and RV dysfunction, contribute to clinical syndrome of HFpEF. Thus, HFpEF is a heterogeneous clinical syndrome with multiple, associated comorbidities, thus no single therapy is effective in all cases of HFpEF.

Different phenotypes of HFpEF differ in prognosis and optimal management. Attempt is made to identify phenotypes using artificial intelligence (AI) from medical information database, using clinical variables and echo data, which revealed four different phenotypes of HFpEF having differing prognosis. This data can be used to assess risk and target therapy that may improve clinical outcomes.[5]

CLINICAL PRESENTATION

The most common presenting symptom of HF is dyspnea, either on exertion or at rest. Majority of HF patients show either systemic or pulmonary venous congestion like peripheral edema, ascites, jugular venous distention, and S_3 gallop on physical examination. Other patients (approximately 35%) present with dyspnea on exertion but do not have evidence of congestion on physical examination. These patients with unexplained dyspnea and no evidence of congestion require additional testing to diagnose HFpEF.[6,7] Assessment of presence of risk factors such as age, obesity, hypertension, CAD, and AF increase the pretest probability of HFpEF. The key diagnostic tests include chest X-ray (for pulmonary venous congestion), biomarkers (BNP and NT-Pro BNP), and transthoracic echocardiography. Any ambiguity in diagnosis of HFpEF, after the primary data and investigation is resolved by functional testing; noninvasively by diastolic stress testing using echo or invasively (LVEDP >15 mm Hg at rest or >25 mm Hg during exercise) by cardiac catheterization, which is the gold standard.

Diastolic Stress Echo Test

Diastolic stress echo test (DiSE) is an indirect test for measuring LV filling pressures during exercise, which does not increase in patients without heart disease. This test is indicated in patients suspected with HFpEF, but with no evidence of elevated filling pressures at rest. The LV filling pressure is indirectly estimated by ratio of mitral flow, early velocity (E wave) to annular early diastolic velocity ("e") and has been endorsed as surrogate marker of LV filling pressures. Ramped exercise protocol in semisupine position, using bicycle ergometer, starting at 25 watts of work and measuring changes from basal echo Doppler parameters, E/'e ratio [lateral (>14), medial >15 RVSP (using TR jet velocity) is helpful in diagnosis of HFpEF. During exercise in those with normal diastolic function, e' velocity increase to similar extent (diastolic reserve) as mitral flow "E" velocity and over all E/'e ratio, essentially, remains unchanged. DiSE is considered abnormal in the presence of all these three parameters.

1. *e' velocity:* Mitral annular by TDI using speckle tracking method
   a. e' <7 cm/s medial or lateral <10 cm/s at rest
2. Average E/e' velocity >14 or E/e' ratio >15 with exercise septal
3. TR jet velocity >2.8 m/s (reflection of elevated LA pressure)

Addition of E/e' ratio improves sensitivity and negative predictive value, suggesting that diastolic stress test helps to rule out HFpEF.

Left atrial (LA) dysfunction is key component in pathophysiology of HFpEF. Recently, LA strain in reservoir phase (LASr strain) has been found to have role not only in diagnosis but also in prognostication of HFpEF. In 2019, one study[8] has shown that LA strain (reservoir phase) outperformed traditional echo parameters such as e' velocity—E/e' and TR velocity. In this study, HFpEF was diagnosed by invasive measurement and found that LASr had highest diagnostic utility (AUC 0.719, *p* value <0.0001) than other echo parameters suggested by European Society of Cardiology 2019. Recent meta-analysis involving 1,906 patients from 20 studies demonstrated that LASr had greater sensitivity in diagnosing elevated LV filling pressures than E/e' and Left atrial volume index (LAVI).

The LASr strain quantifies the deformation of LA during LA filling—where in less deformation (lower strain) has been associated with adverse LA remodeling and LA fibrosis. This is thought to reflect cumulative impact of adverse LA and LV remodeling over time from high filling pressure, mediated through systemic inflammation, and AV uncoupling. LASr may offer technical advantages, over other indices particularly, in patients where mitral annular motion is altered such as BBB, cardiac pacing, and mitral annular calcification (MAC). LASr strain (29 + 16% abnormal vs. 40 + 13%) and conduit strain (18 + 10% normal 22 + 10%) were significantly impaired in patients with HFpEF compared to noncardiac causes of dyspnea (NCD). Out of all echo parameters, LASr best discriminated HFpEF from NCD, outperforming E/e' ratio, LA enlargement, TR velocity, and GLS. Stiffness index LA (compliance), derived as ratio of reservoir strain to LA pressure (E/e') (E/e'/LA strain) improved diagnostic performance, compared to LA reservoirs strain. in some studies,[8] further LASr is easy to perform and highly reproducible.

Peak atrial longitudinal stain of <19% performs better than LAVI >34 mL/m^2 for identifying elevated LV filling pressures. Further, these parameters of reduced LA longitudinal strain, also predict elevated LA pressures during exercise in patients with intermediate probability of HFpEF (using pretest risk score).

DIAGNOSIS

All patients with suspected HFpEF require pretest probability of the disease and two most common scoring models have been developed to estimate probability of HFpEF in patients with unexplained dyspnea. These include H_2FPEF and HFA-PEFF algorithm in clinical practice for the diagnostic evaluation HFpEF.

A diagnosis of HFpEF requires evidence of increased cardiac filling pressures (right atrial pressure, pulmonary capillary wedge pressure, or left ventricular end-diastolic pressure) at rest or with exercise.[1] In addition to structural abnormalities of ventricles, increased cardiac filling pressures can be detected by direct measurement at right heart catheterization (RHC) or can be inferred by findings on physical examination, chest radiography, echocardiography, or natriuretic peptide assays. Patients may have electrocardiographic features of LVH (such as a Sokolov–Lyon Index ≥3.5 mV; abnormal repolarization) and/or LA enlargement. There is no specific EKG finding diagnostic of HFpEF.[6] Atrial fibrillation is common in patients of HFpEF.[7,9]

In addition to routine assessment, specific diagnostic testing and evaluation is often necessary to identify specific cause and other comorbidities in patients with HF.

All patients with HF symptoms should undergo transthoracic echocardiography to assess LV and RV systolic function, diastolic function, atrial and ventricular size, ventricular wall thickness (global or regional wall thickening), valve disease, or wall motion abnormalities suggesting prior myocardial infarction.[10]

Assessment of pretest probability of HFpEF can be ascertained by any one of following scores.

- H_2FPEF algorithm
- HFA-PEFF algorithm

HFA-PEFF Score

The Heart Failure Association (HFA) of the European Society of Cardiology (ESC) published HFA-PEFF diagnostic algorithm for diagnosis of HFpEF **(Flowchart 1)**.

It is a four-step algorithm to diagnose patients with suspected HFpEF.

Step 1: (P = Pretest Assessment)

Initial workup is typically performed in the clinic setting and includes assessment for HF symptoms and signs, typical clinical demographics (obesity, hypertension, diabetes mellitus, elderly, and atrial fibrillation), and diagnostic laboratory tests such as electrocardiogram, and echocardiography. 20% of patients with invasively proven HFpEF have natriuretic peptides below the diagnostic thresholds, which represents a limitation to the use of natriuretic peptides.[11,12]

Step 2: Diagnostic Workup (Table 1)

If the preassessment is suggestive of HFpEF, comprehensive echocardiography and brain natriuretic peptide/ N-terminal natriuretic peptide levels should be obtained.

Patients are classified using major (2 points) and minor (1 point) criteria.

Flowchart 1: HFA-PEFF diagnostic algorithm.

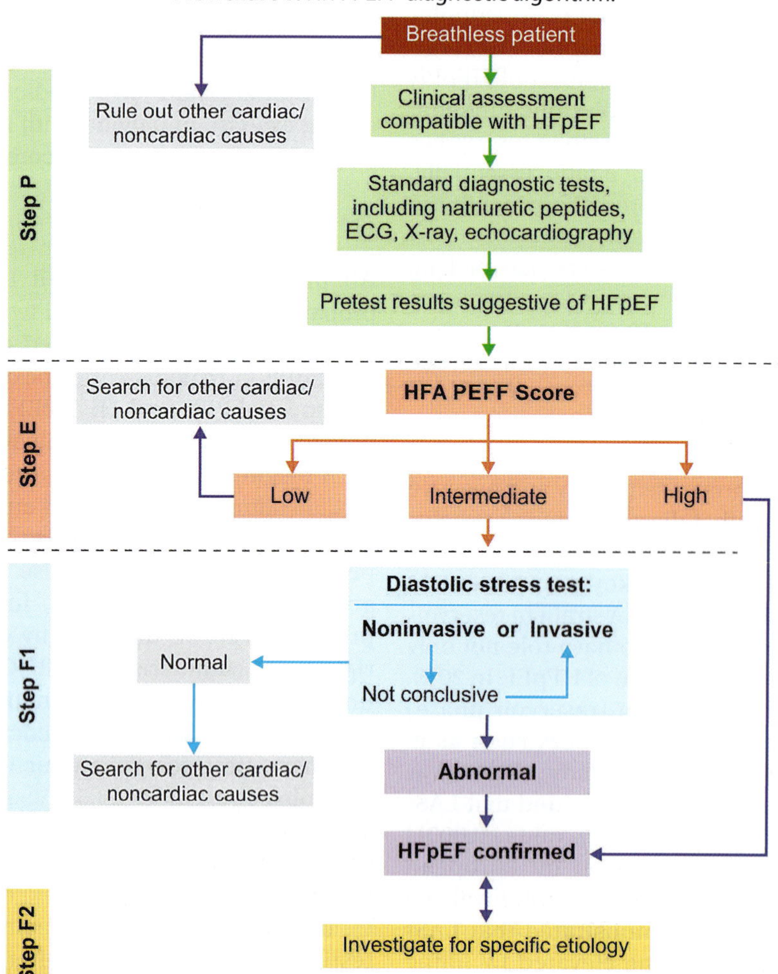

TABLE 1: Echocardiographic and natriuretic peptide heart failure with preserved ejection fraction workup and scoring system (Diagnostic workup—HFpEF).

	Functional	*Morphological*	*Biomarker (SR)*	*Biomarker (AF)*
Major	Septal e' <7 cm/s or Lateral e' <10 cm/s or Average E/e' ≥15 or TR velocity >2.8 m/s (PASP >35 mm Hg)	LAVI >34 mL/m² Or LVMI ≥149/122 g/m² (m/w) and RWT > 0.42	NT-proBNP >220 pg/mL or BNP >80 pg/mL	NT-proBNP >660 pg/mL or BNP >240 pg/mL
Minor	Average E/e' 9–14 or GLS <16%	LAVI 29–34 mL/m² or LVMI >115/95 g/m² (m/w) or RWT >0.42 or LV wall thickness >12 mm	NT-proBNP 125–220 pg/mL or BNP 35–80 pg/mL	NT-proBNP 365–660 pg/mL or BNP 105–240 pg/mL
Major criteria: 2 points		≥5 *points:* HFpEF		
Minor criteria: 1 point		*2–4 points:* Diastolic stress test or invasive hemodynamic measurements		

A score of ≥5 indicates a high probability of HFpEF, while ≤1 indicates a low probability. When there is a diagnostic doubt, an intermediate score of 2-4 points indicates that step 3 (F1—functional testing) together with invasive hemodynamic exercise stress tests or echocardiograms should be advised.

Step 3 (F1): Functional Testing

Step 3 (F): Functional tests in cases of diagnostic uncertainty

If step E is inconclusive, Step F1 ought to be carried out. An invasive or noninvasive stress test is advised, depending on the clinical facilities and the health status of the patient. If the results of the noninvasive stress test are inconclusive, there is still an alternative to use the invasive stress test, which has a greater validity **(Flowcharts 2A and B)**.

An average E/e′ ratio of ≥15 during exercise raises the HFA-PEFF score by two points. A peak TR velocity of >3.4 m/s and an average E/e′ ratio of ≥15 add 3 points to the preceding step 2 (E) score. When the sum of the scores from steps 2 (E) and 3 (F1) is greater than or equal to 5, HFpEF can be diagnosed. If the score remains <5 points or if exercise echocardiography cannot be performed, invasive hemodynamic stress test in any case of doubt, especially if a therapeutic decision depends on the results.

Invasive demonstration of elevated LV filling pressures at rest (LVEDP ≥16 mm Hg) confirms definite evidence of HFpEF.[13] RHC should be considered for the suspected HFpEF, especially when left heart pressures are not available. Resting mean pulmonary capillary wedge pressure (PCWP) ≥15 mm Hg confirms definite evidence of HFpEF. However, normal LVEDP or mean PCWP levels at rest do not exclude HFpEF. In compensated HFpEF, hemodynamic alterations may be detected only during exercise or when the patient health deteriorates.[14-16] If resting filling pressures are normal, exercise RHC is recommended for the definite workup of unexplained exertional dyspnea,[15] especially, if the patient has an intermediate score in step 2(E) or if exercise echocardiography is inconclusive or not feasible. Specialized centers may perform exercise RHC upfront in the absence of exercise echocardiography, depending on the individual experience of the site.

Step 4 (F2): Final Etiology (Flowcharts 3A and B)

The fourth step, step F_2 is to identify a specific etiology of HFpEF to tailor targeted therapies. Apart from traditional risk factors and comorbidities associated with HFpEF, uncommon conditions leading to HFpEF should be identified. Specific heart muscle diseases that may present with the HFpEF phenotype include hypertrophic cardiomyopathies, myocarditis and chronic inflammatory cardiomyopathy, autoimmune diseases, noninfiltrative and infiltrative cardiomyopathies, idiopathic or acquired endomyocardial fibrosis, storage diseases, and other genetic disorders including early stages of cardiomyopathies associated with muscular dystrophy. Rare causes, such as toxicity from drugs or heavy metals, radiation, and metabolic causes related to hormonal or nutritional disease, should also be considered.

Flowcharts 2A and B: Advanced HFpEF workup: Echo stress test and invasive hemodynamic measurements.

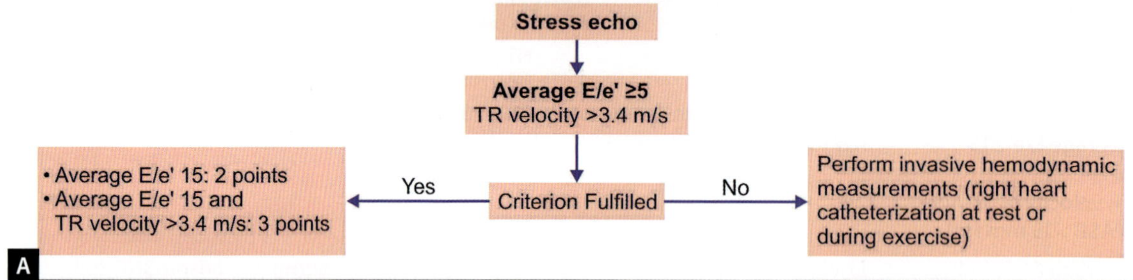

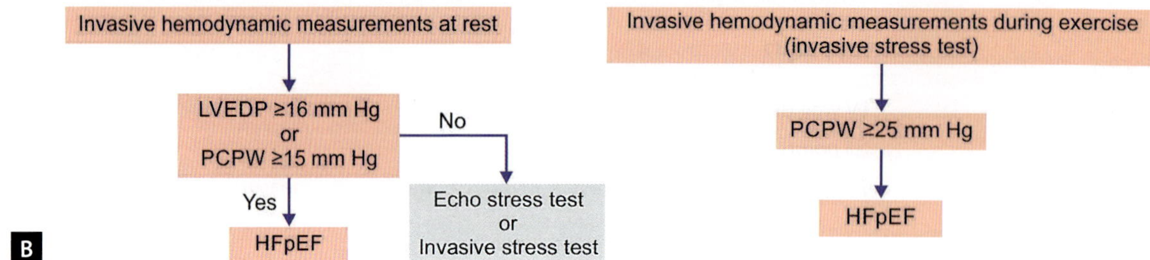

Flowcharts 3A and B: Step 4 (F_2)—final etiological workup.

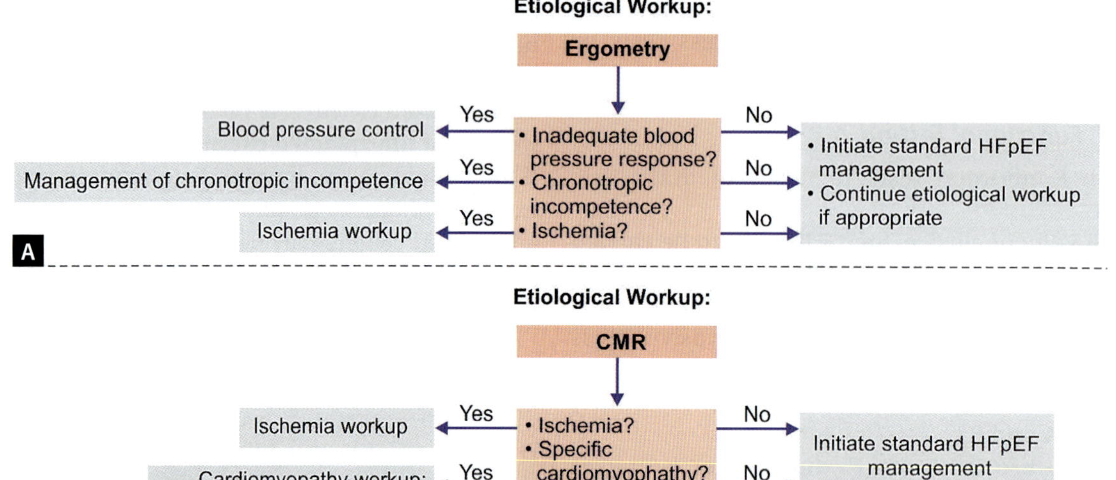

Nonmyocardial etiologies that may mimic HFpEF, such as constrictive pericarditis, primary valvular heart disease, or high output failure should not be considered part of the HFpEF syndrome.

H_2FPEF Score

This is noninvasive scoring system developed to discriminate noncardiac cause of dyspnea from HFpEF using the invasive hemodynamic assessment, the gold standard for diagnosis. The score ranges from 1–9 and provides estimated probability of diagnosis of HFpEF. A score of 6 or more has been suggested as diagnostic of HFpEF whereas score of 0 or 1 excludes diagnosis.

The H_2FPEF score (**Table 2**; range 0–9)[6] is recommended by the 2022 ACC/AHA HF guidelines to estimate the likelihood of HFpEF in patients with unexplained dyspnea. H2FPEF score relies on simple clinical characteristics

TABLE 2: Description of the H_2FPEF score. Description of the H2FPEF score and point allocations for each clinical characteristic (top), with associated probability of having heart failure with preserved ejection fraction (HFpEF) based on the total score as estimated from the model (bottom).

	Clinical Variable	*Values*	*Points*
H_2	Heavy	Body mass index >30 kg/m^2	2
	Hypertensive	Two or more antihypertensive medicines	1
F	Atrial fibrillation	Paroxysmal or persistent	3
P	Pulmonary hypertension	• Doppler echocardiographic estimated • Pulmonary artery systolic pressure >35 mm Hg	1
E	Elder	Age >60 years	1
F	Filling pressure	Doppler echocardiographic E/e' >9	1
	H_2FPEF score		Sum (0–9)

Total points:	0	1	2	3	4	5	6	7	8	9
Probability of HFpEF:	0.2	0.3	0.4	0.5	0.6	0.7	0.8	0.9	0.95	

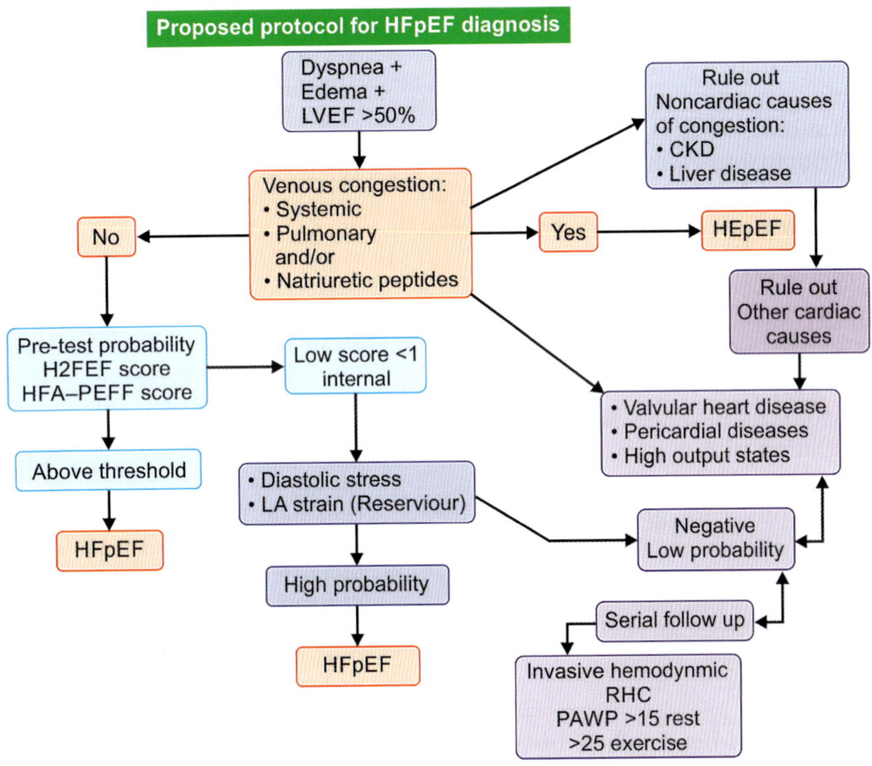

Flowchart 4: HFpEF diagnostic algorithm.

and echocardiography, enables discrimination of HFpEF from noncardiac causes of dyspnea, and can assist in determination of the need for further diagnostic testing in the evaluation of patients with unexplained exertional dyspnea. Although the predictive values of risk score vary with disease prevalence, in a consecutive series of patients with normal EF and unexplained dyspnea (HFpEF prevalence of 50–60%),[6,7] a score of 6 or higher was associated with >95% probability of HFpEF, whereas a score of 0 or 1 was associated with <25% probability of HFpEF. Additional testing (rest/exercise RHC or rest/exercise Doppler echocardiography) is required in patients with intermediate (2–5) scores.[6,7] The use of NT-proBNP levels did not incrementally add diagnostic ability to the H_2FPEF score.

On comparison of two scores HFA-PEFF and H_2FPEF in estimating the likelihood of HFpEF amongst 4,892 community-based participants of atherosclerosis risk in community (ARIC),[17] participants aged 67–90 years without other cardiopulmonary causes of dyspnea revealed that scores above threshold (H2FpEF >6-HFA-PEFF >5) had equivalent risk of hospitalization with HF and mortality compared to patients with known HFpEF. In 28% patients, the scores were discordant (i.e., high risk by one algorithm) while 4% were high risk by both scores. In another comparative study using invasive hemodynamics as gold standard in patients with atrial fibrillation, the diagnostic accuracy was similar (AUC 0.663 vs. 0.707). In another study of 736 patients in community with unexplained dyspnea, H2FPEF performed better with AUC of 0.845 compared to with HFA-PEFF score.

AI model[18] was recently developed to identify patients with HFpEF using single apical four-chamber video clip from standard TTE. This retrospective study assessed the association between model output with HF biomarkers, risk for HHF, and cardiac mortality, and compared the performance with two other scores H_2FpEF and HFA-PEFF. The following conclusions were arrived using beforementioned AI model for diagnosis of HFpEF.

- Positive model output was associated with increased risk for hospitalization for heart failure (HHF-HR: 3.76) and cardiac mortality.
- Patients with uncertain outputs demonstrated intermediate risk for HHF and cardiac mortality.
- This AI model reclassified HHF risk in nondiagnostic clinical scores—91% for H2FPEF and 92% HFA-PEFF
- It shows linear correlation with machine output and clinical events for HHF and cardiac mortality. The higher the machine output score, greater the events rates.

The diagnostic algorithm for HFpEF is given in **Flowchart 4**.

CONCLUSION

The HFpEF accounts for half of heart failure hospitalizations. In hospitalized patients, overt congestive signs on physical examination, chest radiography, and transthoracic echocardiography showing elevated filling pressures with normal systolic function and elevated natriuretic peptide assays help in diagnosis of HFpEF. However, in outpatients with exertional dyspnea, overt congestion is often absent at rest, and the diagnosis may be challenging. Right-sided heart catheterization, with exercise if resting filling pressures are normal, is the gold standard for HFpEF diagnosis but is not universally available, and noninvasive estimates of cardiac filling pressures lack sensitivity. Diagnostic algorithms for HFpEF have robust specificity but sensitivity is poor. Therefore, HFpEF remains under diagnosed in the community. Invasive hemodynamic testing is not routinely available and expensive. The H_2FPEF and HFA-PEFF algorithms may be used to effectively rule out disease among patients with low scores, to establish the diagnosis with reasonably high confidence at higher scores, and to identify patients for whom additional testing is needed with intermediate scores. All individuals diagnosed with HFpEF should undergo further diagnostic assessment to identify causes, for which there are disease-specific therapies. In future, AI models will be used more frequently both for diagnosis and classification of phenotypes, which will improve therapy an prognosis.

REFERENCES

1. Heidenreich PA, Bozkurt B, Aguilar D, et al. 2022 AHA/ACC/HFSA guideline for the management of heart failure: A report of the American College of Cardiology/American Heart Association Joint Committee on Clinical Practice Guidelines. Circulation. 2022;145(18): e895-1032.
2. Dunlay SM, Roger VL, Redfield MM. Epidemiology of heart failure with preserved ejection fraction. Nat Rev Cardiol. 2017;14(10):591-602.
3. Roger VL. Epidemiology of heart failure: a contemporary perspective. Circ Res. 2021;128(10):1421-34.
4. Heidenreich PA, Albert NM, Allen LA, et al.; American Heart Association Advocacy Coordinating Committee; Council on Arteriosclerosis, Thrombosis and Vascular Biology; Council on Cardiovascular Radiology and Intervention; Council on Clinical Cardiology; Council on Epidemiology and Prevention; Stroke Council. Forecasting the impact of heart failure in the United States: A policy statement from the American Heart Association. Circ Heart Fail. 2013;6(3):606-19.
5. Morgane Pierre-Jean, BMarut B, Curtis E, et al. Phenotyping of heart failure with preserved ejection faction using electronic health records and echocardiography. EHJ Open. 2024:4(1).
6. Reddy YNV, Carter RE, Obokata M, et al. A simple, evidence-based approach to help guide diagnosis of heart failure with preserved ejection fraction. Circulation. 2018;138(9):861-70.
7. Reddy YNV, Kaye DM, Handoko ML, et al. Diagnosis of heart failure with preserved ejection fraction among patients with unexplained dyspnea. JAMA Cardiol. 2022;7(9):891-9.
8. Reddy YNV, Obokata M, Egbe A, et al. Left atrial strain and compliance in the diagnostic evaluation of heart failure with preserved ejection fraction. Eur J Heart Fail. 2019;21(7):891-900.

9. Reddy YNV, Obokata M, Gersh BJ, et al. High prevalence of occult heart failure with preserved ejection fraction among patients with atrial fibrillation and dyspnea. Circulation. 2018;137:534-5.
10. Lang RM, Badano LP, Mor-Avi,V, et al. Recommendations for cardiac chamber quantification by echocardiography in adults: An update from the American Society of Echocardiography and the European Association of Cardiovascular Imaging. J Am Soc Echocardiogr. 2015; 28:1-39.e14.
11. Meijers WC, Hoekstra T, Jaarsma T, et al. Patients with heart failure with preserved ejection fraction and low levels of natriuretic peptides. Neth Heart J. 2016;24(4):287-95.
12. Ponikowski P, Voors AA, Anker SD, et al.; ESC Scientific Document Group.2016 ESC Guidelines for the diagnosis and treatment of acute and chronic heart failure: The Task Force for the diagnosis and treatment of acute and chronic heart failure of the European Society of Cardiology (ESC). Developed with the special contribution of the Heart Failure Association (HFA) of the ESC. Eur Heart J. 2016;37(27):2129-200.
13. Borlaug BA, Kass DA. Invasive hemodynamic assessment in heart failure. Heart Fail Clin 2009;5:217-28.
14. Obokata M, Kane GC, Reddy YN, et al. Role of diastolic stress testing in the evaluation for heart failure with preserved ejection fraction: a simultaneous invasive-echocardiographic study. Circulation. 2017;135(9):825-38.
15. Borlaug BA, Nishimura RA, Sorajja P, et al. Exercise hemodynamics enhance diagnosis of early heart failure with preserved ejection fraction. Circ Heart Fail. 2010;3(5):588-95.
16. Paulus WJ. H2FPEF score. At last, a properly validated diagnostic algorithm for heart failure with preserved ejection fraction. Circulation 2018;138:871-3.
17. Selvaraj, S, Myhre, P, Vaduganathan, M. et al. Application of diagnostic algorithms for heart failure with preserved ejection fraction to the community. JACC Heart Fail. 2020;8(8):640-53.
18. Akerman AP, Porumb M, Scott CG, et al. Automated echocardiographic detection of heart failure with preserved ejection fraction using artificial intelligence. JACC: Advances. 2023;2(6):100452.

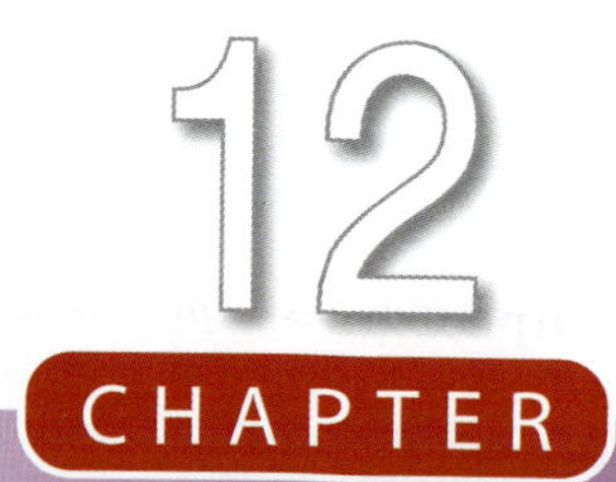

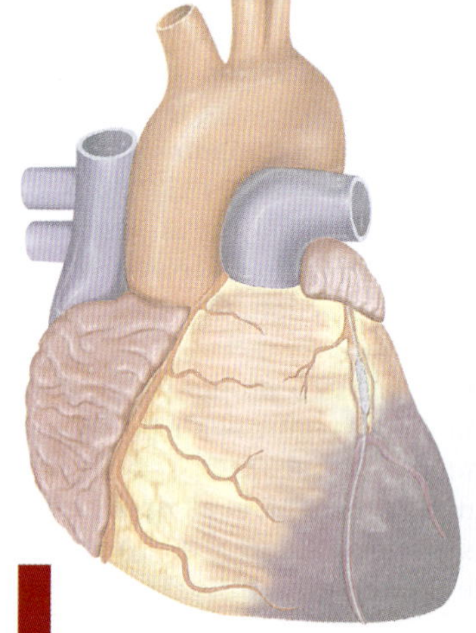

Diving into Diagnostic Score Algorithms of HFpEF

HK Chopra, Shachi Kalyani, Rajesh Meena, Neha Chaudhary

INTRODUCTION

Heart failure with preserved ejection fraction (HFpEF) is a complex clinical ailment which has vague clinical symptoms such as dyspnea (includes paroxysmal nocturnal dyspnea, orthopnea), fatigue, these symptoms can be presentation of many other disorders.[1] Structurally, it causes left atrial enlargement (LAE), left ventricular hypertrophy (LVH), diastolic dysfunction which is also seen in HFrEF. Thus, it is usually misdiagnosed, mistreated, and hence requires detailed physical examination, review of comorbidities, and risk factors. To conquer this, various diagnostic score algorithms have been developed to facilitate the diagnosis of HFpEF. This chapter focuses on various diagnostic scores algorithms.

Several scoring systems in the diagnosis of HFpEF are as follows:

HEART FAILURE ASSOCIATION-PRESERVED EJECTION FRACTION SCORE (TABLE 1)

The Heart Failure Association-Preserved Ejection Fraction (HFA-PEFF) score: This score has functional,

TABLE 1: The HFA-PEFF algorithm for the diagnosis of HFpEF. Overview of the diagnostic HFpEF steps 1–4 (P–F).[3]

P	Initial workup [*Step 1 (P):* Pretest assessment]	• Symptoms and/or signs of heart failure (HF) • Comorbidities/risk factors • Electrocardiogram (ECG) • Standard echocardiography • Natriuretic peptides • Ergometry/6-minute walking test or cardiopulmonary exercise testing
E	Diagnostic workup [*Step 2 (E):* Echocardiographic and natriuretic peptide score]	• Comprehensive echocardiography • Natriuretic peptides, if not measured in step 1
F1	Advanced workup [*Step 3 (F_1):* Functional testing in case of uncertainty]	• *Diastolic stress test:* Exercise stress echocardiography • Invasive hemodynamic measurements
F2	Etiological workup [*Step 4 (F_2):* Final etiology]	• Cardiovascular magnetic resonance • Cardiac or noncardiac biopsies • Scintigraphy/computed tomography (CT)/positron emission tomography (PET) • Genetic testing • Specific laboratory tests

(HFpEF: heart failure with preserved ejection fraction; HFA-PEFF: heart failure association-preserved ejection fraction)

morphological, and biomarker domains. Each major criteria—2 points, minor criteria—1 point.[2] According to the HFA-PEFF score, the patients were divided into three risk groups for HFpEF probability: Low (0–1 points, HFpEF unlikely), intermediate (2–4, HFpEF uncertain), and high (5–6, HFpEF diagnostic).

1. Step 1 (P: Pretest assessment) is typically performed in the ambulatory setting and includes assessment for heart failure symptoms and signs, typical clinical demographics (obesity, hypertension, diabetes mellitus, elderly, and atrial fibrillation), and diagnostic laboratory tests, electrocardiogram, and echocardiography. In the absence of overt noncardiac causes of breathlessness, HFpEF can be suspected if there is a normal left ventricular (LV) ejection fraction, no significant heart valve disease or cardiac ischemia, and at least one typical risk factor. Elevated natriuretic peptides support, but normal levels do not exclude a diagnosis of HFpEF.
2. Step 2 (E: Echocardiography and natriuretic peptide score) requires comprehensive echocardiography and is typically performed by a cardiologist. Measures include mitral annular early diastolic velocity (E′), LV filling pressure estimated using E/E′, left atrial volume index, LV mass index, LV relative wall thickness, tricuspid regurgitation velocity, LV global longitudinal systolic strain, and serum natriuretic peptide levels. Major (2 points) and Minor (1 point) criteria were defined from these measures. A score ≥5 points implies definite HFpEF; ≤1 point makes HFpEF unlikely.
3. An intermediate score (2–4 points) implies diagnostic uncertainty, in which case step 3 (F_1: Functional testing) is recommended with echocardiographic or invasive hemodynamic exercise stress tests.
4. Step 4 (F_2: Final etiology) is recommended to establish a possible specific cause of HFpEF or alternative explanations. Further research is needed for a better classification of HFpEF.[3]

H_2FPEF SCORE (TABLE 2)

This score is based on clinical characteristics and echocardiography, it differentiates HFpEF from other noncardiac disorders causing similar symptoms. Thus, it can determine further line of evaluations in patients of dyspnea and fatigue.

This score does not include NT-proBNP as according to formative body states "rather, our data suggest that NT-proBNP may not add incremental information to clinical variables and echocardiography in diagnosing HFpEF among patients with unexplained dyspnea. This is in contrast to patients presenting with acute dyspnea that is present at rest, for which the diagnostic performance of the natriuretic peptides is well established."[4-6]

Description of the H_2FPEF Score

Description of the H_2FPEF score and point allocations for each clinical characteristic (top), with associated probability of having HFpEF based on the total score as estimated from the model.[6]

H_2FPEF score enables robust discrimination of HFpEF from noncardiac causes of dyspnea at low and high scores while identifying patients at intermediate probability in whom additional testing is needed to refine the diagnosis.

TWO-STEP GUIDELINE[7]

2024 guidelines of Taiwan Society of Cardiology for the Diagnosis and Treatment of Heart Failure with Preserved

TABLE 2: H_2FPEF score.

	Clinical variable	*Values*	*Points*
H_2	Heavy	Body mass index >30 kg/m^2	2
	Hypertensive	Two or more antihypertensive medicines	1
F	Atrial fibrillation	Paroxysmal or persistent	3
P	Pulmonary hypertension	Doppler echocardiographic estimated pulmonary artery systolic pressure >35 mm Hg	1
E	Elder	Age >60 years	1
F	Filling pressure	Doppler echocardiographic E/e′ >9	1
		H_2FPEF score	Sum (0–9)

Total points	0	1	2	3	4	5	6	7	8	9
Probability of HFpEF	0.2	0.3	0.4	0.5	0.6	0.7	0.8	0.9	0.95	

Flowchart 1: Two-step diagnosis of HFpEF.

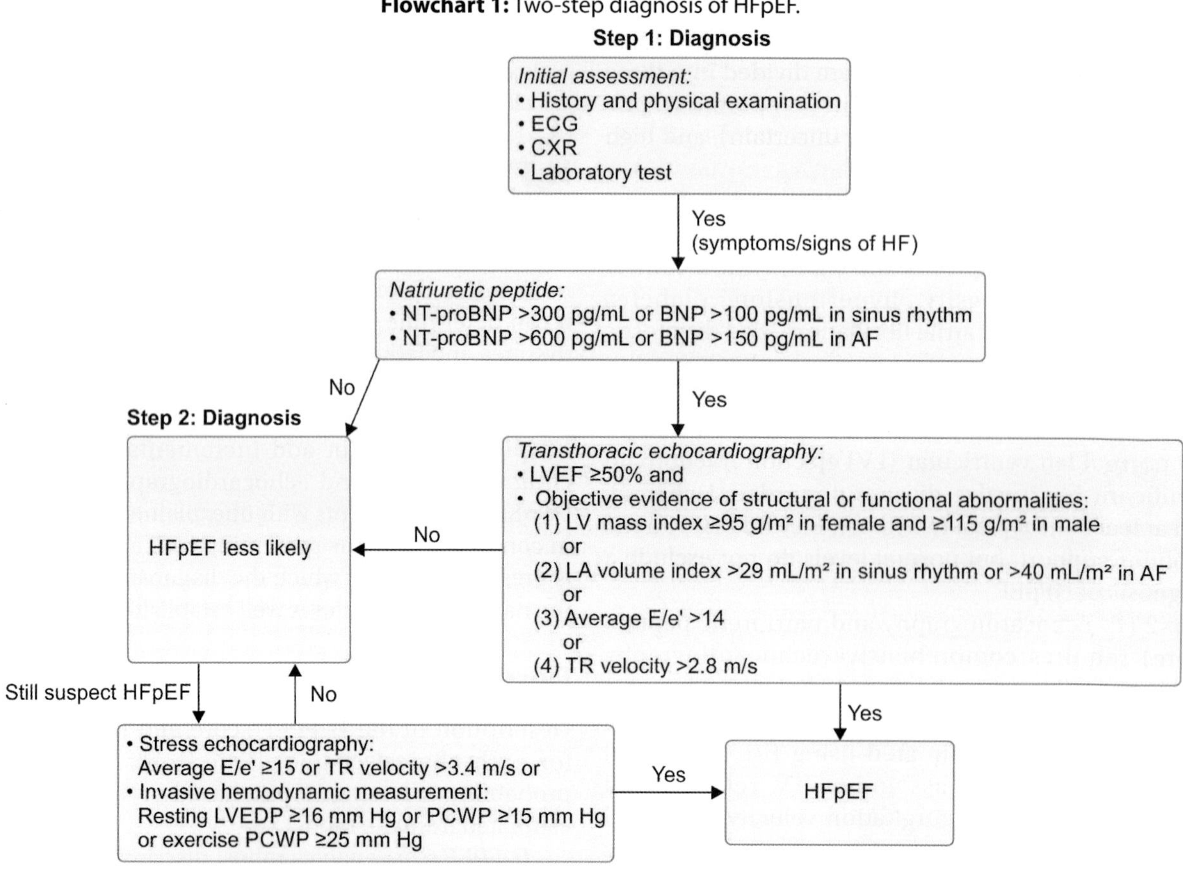

(AF: atrial fibrillation; ECG: electrocardiogram; CXR: chest X-ray; HFpEF: heart failure with preserved ejection fraction; HF: heart failure; LA: left atrium; LV: left ventricular; LVEF: left ventricular ejection fraction; LVEDP: left ventricular end-diastolic pressure; NT-proBNP: N-terminal prohormone of brain natriuretic peptide; PCWP: pulmonary capillary wedge pressure; TR: tricuspid regurgitation)

Ejection Fraction. In the first step, the diagnosis of HFpEF can be made if patients have symptoms and/or signs of heart failure, left ventricular ejection fraction ≥50%, increased natriuretic peptide, and objective evidence of left atrial or left ventricular abnormalities, or raised left ventricular filling pressure. If diagnosis is still uncertain, invasive or noninvasive stress test can be performed in the second step **(Flowchart 1)**.

LIMITATIONS

In spite of these scores and guidelines on HFpEF after many years of researches, consensus its diagnosis remains complex:

- Similar clinical presentation of many other disorders.
- Inadequate sensitivity and specificity of biomarkers and imaging modalities.
- Discordance in different scorings and diagnostic criteria.
- Subjectivity of the investigator in imaging, experience of physicians in evaluating different symptoms, and scoring them.

UPCOMING POSSIBILITIES

Ongoing researches emphasis on following:

- Developing more sensitive and specific biomarkers.
- Advanced imaging techniques.
- Individualized approach for evaluation and management (including study of genetic composition of patients, treating patient at biochemical levels).
- Researches emphasizing on HFpEF pathophysiology, structural, biochemical development, and progression of disease in end-stage heart disease.

CONCLUSION

Diagnostic score algorithms, biomarkers, and imaging modalities help in the diagnosis of HFpEF. However, education of physician about the critical analysis of clinical evaluation of HFpEF is a paramount importance for cardiologists, intensivists, nephrologists, diabetalogists, and imaging experts. The correct algorithms diagnosis has tremendous diagnostic, prognostic, and therapeutic implications in short-term and long-term morbidity and mortality reduction.

REFERENCES

1. Heidenreich PA, Bozkurt B, Aguilar D, et al. 2022 American College of Cardiology/American Heart Association/Heart Failure Society of America Guideline for the Management of Heart Failure: Executive Summary. J Card Fail. 2022; 28(5):810-30.
2. Egashira K, Sueta D, Komorita T, et al. HFA-PEFF scores: prognostic value in heart failure with preserved left ventricular ejection fraction. Korean J Intern Med. 2022; 37(1):96-108.
3. Pieske B, Tschöpe C, de Boer RA, Fraser AG, Anker SD, Donal E, et al. How to diagnose heart failure with preserved ejection fraction: the HFA-PEFF diagnostic algorithm: a consensus recommendation from the Heart Failure Association (HFA) of the European Society of Cardiology (ESC). Eur J Heart Fail. 2020;22(3):391-412.
4. Steinhart B, Thorpe KE, Bayoumi AM, Moe G, Januzzi JL, Mazer CD. Improving the diagnosis of acute heart failure using a validated prediction model. J Am Coll Cardiol. 2009;54:1515-21
5. Januzzi JL, Chen-Tournoux AA, Christenson RH, Doros G, Hollander JE, Levy PD et L; ICON-RELOADED Investigators. N-terminal pro-B-type natriuretic peptide in the emergency department: the ICON-RELOADED Study. J Am Coll Cardiol. 2018;71:1191-200
6. Reddy YNV, Carter RE, Obokata M, et al. A simple, evidence-based approach to help guide diagnosis of heart failure with preserved ejection fraction. Circulation. 2018;138:861-70.
7. Li YH, Wang CC, Hung CL, et al. 2024 Guidelines of the Taiwan Society of Cardiology for the Diagnosis and Treatment of Heart Failure with Preserved Ejection Fraction. Acta Cardiologica Sinica. 2024;40(2):148-71.

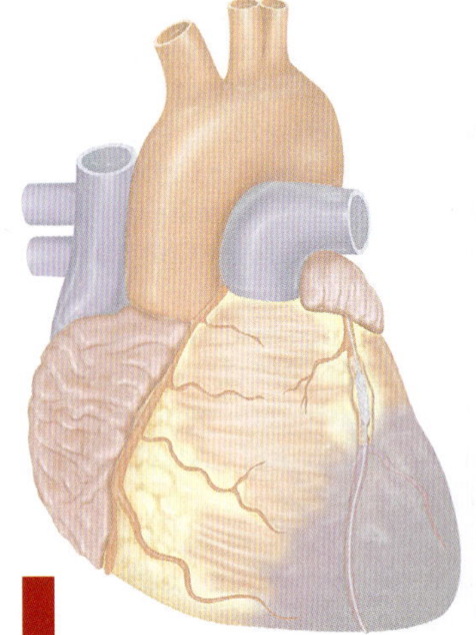

HFpEF and COVID

Satyanarayan Routray, Nirmal Kumar Mohanty

INTRODUCTION

Heart failure with preserved ejection fraction (HFpEF) is a form of heart failure where the patient present with symptoms and signs of heart failure but the ejection fraction (EF) is normal. In this condition diastolic function is abnormal in the form of impaired ventricular relaxation, distensibility, and filling. COVID-19 pandemic has highlighted a significant connection between HFpEF and COVID. Observation suggests existence of an association between COVID and diastolic dysfunction, systolic dysfunction and heart failure.[1,2]

EPIDEMIOLOGY

Approximately 1–2% of world population are suffering from heart failure and half of them have HFpEF. COVID-19 has exacerbated this epidemic with the studies showing:

- HFpEF patients 2–3 times more likely to develop severe COVID.
- Shared comorbidities are hypertension (70%), diabetes (40%), chronic kidney disease (30%), and obesity (25%).
- Mortality rate is higher among HFpEF and COVID-19 (20–30%).

COVID in patients with HFpEF results in increased risk of cardiac arrhythmias, hospitalization, worsening heart failure, and mortality. Prevalence of HFpEF in patients of COVID-19 varies from 2.5 to 9.5% in most studies, some other studies have shown prevalence up to 20%.[1-5] In patients of long COVID heart failure develops in about 2% of cases maturity being HFpEF.

PATHOPHYSIOLOGY

Adverse cardiac events are higher in patients of cardiovascular disease with COVID-19. Several mechanisms are hypothesized relating cardiac injury in patients of COVID. Immune response of viral host and its relationship and effects on cardiovascular system is extremely important for our understanding. HFpEF can also develop in a patient of COVID-19 as a result of hyperimmune response and cytokine storm. Mechanisms of myocardial injury are direct myocardial invasion, microvascular injury, acute coronary syndrome, stress cardiomyopathy, systemic inflammatory response, and organs supply demand mismatch. Several associated comorbidities such as obesity, diabetes mellitus, hypertension, chronic kidney disease (CKD), anemia, and chronic pulmonary disease aggravate cardiac condition particularly in elderly and women **(Fig. 1)**.[1,6-8]

KEY MECHANISMS[1,9,10] (FLOWCHART 1)

- Direct myocardial injury by the virus.
- Cytokine storm (raised IL 6 and TNF-α) promotes vascular inflammation, fibrosis, and cardiac remodeling.
- Endothelial injury causes endothelial dysfunction leading to impaired vasodilation and increased vascular resistance.
- Reduced capillary density and microvascular resistance impair myocardial perfusion and lead to myocardial dysfunction.

- Activated immune cells (T cells and macrophases) contribute to myocardial injury and fibrosis.
- Transforming growth factor beta (TGF-β) mediated myocardial fibrosis stiffens the heart reducing compliance.
- Autonomic dysfunction secondary to sympathetic and parasympathetic imbalance affects heart rate and blood pressure regulation.
- Systemic inflammation and oxidative stress.
- Endothelial activation and thrombosis.

CLINICAL PRESENTATION

Patient of HFpEF and COVID may present with features suggestive of heart failure or worsening dyspnea, increased fatigue, weight gain, edema, decreased exercise tolerance, and palpitation. Symptoms may be shared one (both HFpEF and COVID) such as dyspnea, fatigue, edema, cough, chest discomfort, or specific for each condition. Physical findings are usually raised JVP, edema, tachypnea, tachycardia, systolic murmur, crepitations both lung bases, hepatomegaly, ascites, and hypoxemia.[2,9,11,12]

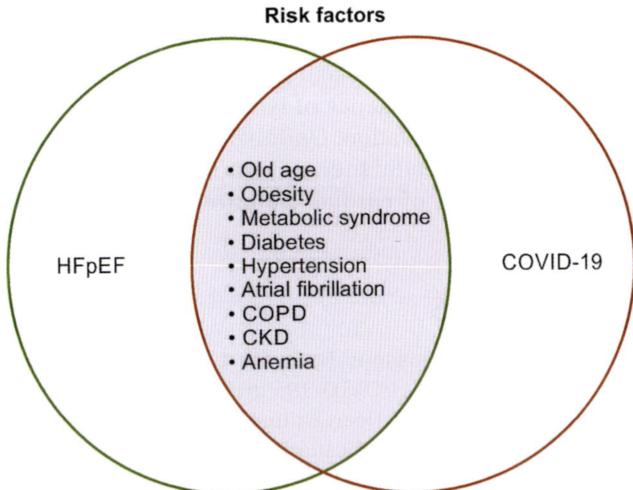

Fig. 1: Overlapping risk factors for heart failure with preserved ejection fraction (HFpEF) and COVID-19. (COVID-19: coronavirus disease; CKD: chronic kidney disease; COPD: chronic obstructive pulmonary disease)

DIAGNOSIS

COVID-19 is diagnosed according to WHO criteria. HFpEF is diagnosed by echocardiography with LVEF ≥50% and features of diastolic dysfunction. NT-ProBNP is high in nearly 90% of cases. Routine hematological, biochemical tests, biomarkers such as NT-ProBNP, troponin, CRP, IL-6, TNF-α, imaging like chest X-ray, CT/MRI of thorax may be done to assess severity and help in management.[13-16]

MANAGEMENT

Management of both conditions are done according to guidelines (ACC/AHA, ESC, and WHO). General principle consists multidisciplinary care in acute and subacute cases involving primary care physicians, infectious disease specialists, intensivist and cardiologist. There are several therapeutic challenges such as balancing fluid management, managing hypertension, optimizing RAAS inhibition, and preventing cardiovascular complications. Special consideration in therapy will be for elderly, obese, diabetic, hypertensive, and patients with preexisting CVD, COPD, and CKD. Such patients should be followed up with ECHO, cardiac MRI, etc., as and when required.[13-16]

PROGNOSIS

- *Short term (30 days) prognosis:* Mortality 5–10%, hospitalization 20–30%.
- *Long term (1 year) prognosis:* Mortality 15–30%, hospitalization 40–60%.

Predictors of poor prognosis are:[16,17]

- Advanced age
- Comorbidities (hypertension, diabetes, and CKD)

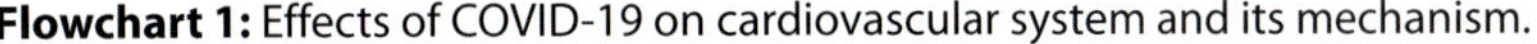

Flowchart 1: Effects of COVID-19 on cardiovascular system and its mechanism.

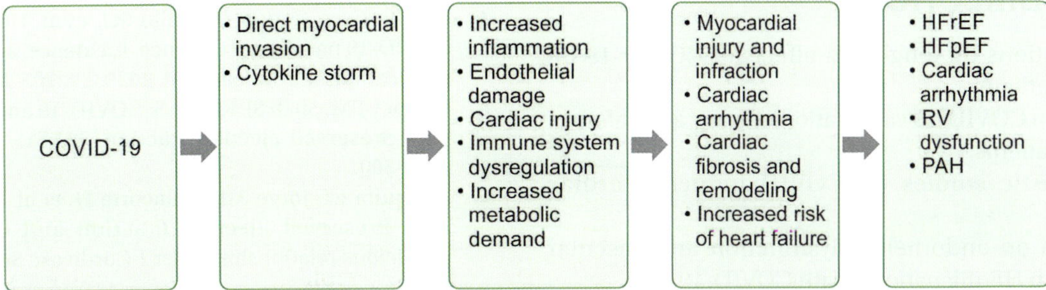

(HFpEF: heart failure with preserved ejection fraction; HFrEF: heart failure with reduced ejection fraction; PAH: pulmonary arterial hypertension; RV: right ventricular)

- NYHA class III and IV
- Elevated NT-ProBNP and troponin
- Anemia
- Hypotension
- Renal dysfunction
- Pulmonary hypertension
- Left ventricular dysfunction

HFA-PEFF score is a diagnostic tool developed by Heart Failure Association (HFA) of European Society of Cardiology (ESC) used to identify patients with HFpEF. Symptoms (4 points), signs (4 points), echocardiography (4 points), biomarkers (2 points), and comorbidities (2 points) are taken into consideration for scoring and according to points it is HFpEF unlikely (0–4 points), possible (5–7 points), probable (8–10 points), and definite (11–14 points).[13,14] HFA-PEFF score is used to diagnosis, risk stratification, and predicting mortality and hospitalization in patients of HFpEF.[16] HFA-PEFF score ≥8 points associated with increased mortality risk in HFpEF patients with COVID (HR 2.51, 95% CI 1.94–3.25) and increased hospitalization risk (HR 2.51, 95% CI 1.94–3.25).

HEART FAILURE WITH PRESERVED EJECTION FRACTION AND LONG COVID

Long COVID refers to persistent symptoms lasting ≥4–6 weeks after initial COVID-19 infection. Prevalence of long COVID in HFpEF is high, 30.8% in the study by Wang et al. and 43.8% in the study by Patel et al.; and may be due to persistent inflammation, endothelial dysfunction, immune system dysregulation, and ongoing fibrosis and unmasking of preexisting HEpEF. Long COVID is a significant concern in HFpEF patients with persistent symptoms and biomarker changes. Further studies required to understand pathophysiological mechanism and develop effective management strategies.[18,19]

FUTURE DIRECTION

- Investigations on long-term effects of COVID-19 on HFpEF patients.
- Studies on COVID-19 vaccination efficacy and safety in HFpEF patients.
- Mechanistic studies on COVID induced cardiac fibrosis.
- Research on endothelial dysfunction and vascular stiffness in HFpEF patients with COVID-19.
- Studies on potential therapeutic targets for HFpEF in COVID-19 patients.

LIMITATION

As most studies are of retrospective design, it may not be free of bias. Many studies are of small sample size and from single center; reducing statistical significance and limiting its general liability. It is difficult to establish causality as many studies lack control groups. There are chances of selection bias, incomplete data, ethnic diversity, and other methodological limitations in certain studies. Most studies lack proper monitoring and follow-up. Prospective randomized multicenter studies could have given better information.

CONCLUSION

The HFpEF patients are at increased risk of severe COVID-19, higher rate of hospitalization and mortality. COVID exacerbates inflammation, endothelial dysfunction, and cardiac fibrosis in HFpEF patients. Biomarkers (NT-ProBNP, troponin, and CRP) can predict adverse outcome and guide treatment. Patients who had COVID in the past, can present with acute systolic or diastolic heart failure and higher incidence of HFpEF compared to non-COVID general population. Optimizing HFpEF treatment and COVID-19 specific therapy can improve outcomes. Close monitoring of cardiac function and biomarkers are crucial.

REFERENCES

1. Zacconea, Tomasoni D, Italia L, et al. Myocardial Involvement in COVID-19: an Interaction between Comorbidities and Heart Failure with Preserved Ejection Fraction. A Further Indication of the Role of Inflammation. Curr Heart Fail Rep. 2021;18:99-106.
2. Nasrullah A, Gansu K, Cannon HR, et al. COVID-19 and heart failure with preserved and reduced ejection fraction clinical outcomes among hospitalized patients in the United States. Virusen. 2023;15:600.
3. Yonas E, Alwi I, Pranata R, et al. Effect of heart failure on the outcome of COVID19—A meta-analysis and systematic review. Am J Emerg Med. 2021;46:204-11.
4. Rey JR, Caro-Codón J, Rosillo SO, et al. Heart failure in COVID-19 patients: prevalence, incidence, and prognostic implications. Eur J Heart Fail. 2020;22:2205-15.
5. Freaney PM, Shah SJ, Khan SS. COVID-19 and heart failure with preserved ejection fraction. JAMA. 2020;324(15): 1499-500.
6. Mesquita ET, Jorge AJL, Villacorta H, et al. Heart Failure with Preserved Ejection Fraction and COVID-19: a pernicious relationship. Inter I Cordivasc Sci. 2020;33(4): 412-8.
7. Tomasoni D, Italia L, Adamo M, et al. COVID-19 and heart failure: from infection to inflammation and angiotensin II

stimulation. Searching for evidence from a new disease. Eur J Heart Fail. 2020;22(6):957-66.

8. Glezeva N, Baugh JA. Role of inflammation in the pathogenesis of heart failure with preserved ejection fraction and its potential as a therapeutic target. Heart Fail Rev. 2014;19:681-94.
9. Akbari H, Tabrizi R, Lankarani KB, et al. The role of cytokine profile and lymphocyte subsets in the severity of coronavirus disease 2019 (COVID-19): a systematic review and meta-analysis. Life Sci. 2020;258: 118167.
10. Mehta P, McAuley DF, Brown M, et al. HLH Across Speciality Collaboration, UK. COVID-19: consider cytokine storm syndromes and immunosuppression. Lancet. 2020;395(10229):1033-4.
11. Bhatt AS, Jering KS, Vaduganathan M, et al. Clinical outcomes in patients with heart failure hospitalized with COVID-19. JACC Heart Fail. 2021;9:65-73.
12. Targher G, Mantovani A, Wang XB, et al. Patients with diabetes are at higher risk for severe illness from COVID-19. Diabetes Metab. 2020;46:335-7.
13. Pieske B, Tschöpe C, de Boer RA, et al. How to diagnose heart failure with preserved ejection fraction: the HFA-PEFF diagnostic algorithm: a consensus recommendation from the Heart Failure Association (HFA) of the European Society of Cardiology (ESC). Eur J Heart Fail. 2020;22:391-412.
14. Reddy YNV, Carter RE, Obokata M, et al. A simple, evidence-based approach to help guide diagnosis of heart failure with preserved ejection fraction. Circulation. 2018;138: 861-70.
15. Bhatt AS, Kosiborod MN, Claggett BL, et al. Impact of COVID-19 in patients with heart failure with mildly reduced or preserved ejection fraction enrolled in the DELIVER trial. Eur J Heart Fail. 2023;25(12):2177-88.
16. Hadzibegovic S, Lena A, Churchill TW, et al. Heart failure with preserved ejection fraction according to the HFA-PEFF score in COVID-19 patients: clinical correlates and echocardiographic findings. Eur J Heart Fail. 2021; 23(11):1891-902.
17. Zhu H, Rhee JW, Cheng P, et al. Cardiovascular complications in patients with COVID-19: consequences of viral toxicities and host immune response. Curr Cardiol Rep. 2020;22(5):32.
18. Zuin M, Rigatelli G, Roncon L, et al. Risk of incident heart failure after COVID-19 recovery: a systematic review and meta-analysis. Heart Fail Rev. 2023;28:859-64.
19. Siripanthong B, Asatryan B, Hanff TC, et al. The pathogenesis and long-term consequences of COVID-19 cardiac injury. JACC Basic Trans Sci. 2022;7(3_Part_1):294-308.

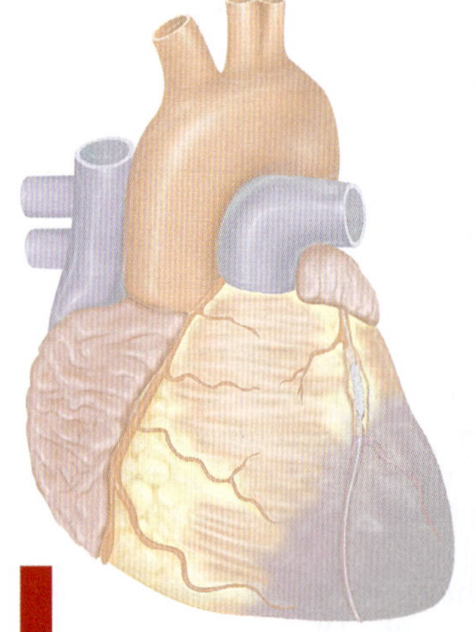

Vascular Biology in HFpEF

SS Mishra, BR Mishra, Asharam Panda

INTRODUCTION

The heart failure with preserved ejection fraction (HFpEF) represents nearly half of all heart failure cases, and its prevalence continues to rise, particularly among the elderly.[1] The pathophysiology of HFpEF is multifactorial, involving complex interactions between the heart, vasculature, and other organ systems.[2] Unlike HFrEF, where myocardial systolic dysfunction predominates, HFpEF is characterized by diastolic dysfunction, often accompanied by systemic hypertension, obesity, diabetes, and chronic kidney disease **(Fig. 1)**. A growing body of evidence suggests that vascular dysfunction is central to the pathogenesis of HFpEF, contributing to both the initial development of the disease and its subsequent progression.[3] In adults vessels are about 72, 000–100,000 km long out of which about 500 km are in heart perfusing in diastole in contrast to systemic vessel which perfuse other organs in systole. The structural and functional derangement is contributed by multiple risk factors to diastolic dysfunction in spite of normal ejection fraction.[4]

Currently, there are limited therapeutic options for HFpEF within compared to HFrEF with similar outcome. Pathophysiology of HFpEF is poorly understood and needs further exploration. Although ventricular diastolic dysfunction recognized to play a central role, alteration in vascular biology of both cardiac and systemic vessels has also been attributed as major contributing factor. Clinical heart failure results from complex interplay between ventricular diastolic dysfunction and vascular changes in the form of structure and function. Although specific vascular changes such as endothelial dysfunction, autonomic imbalance, decreased nitric oxide (NO) activity, microvascular dysfunction, and oxidative stress contribute to major vascular alteration in HFpEF.[5]

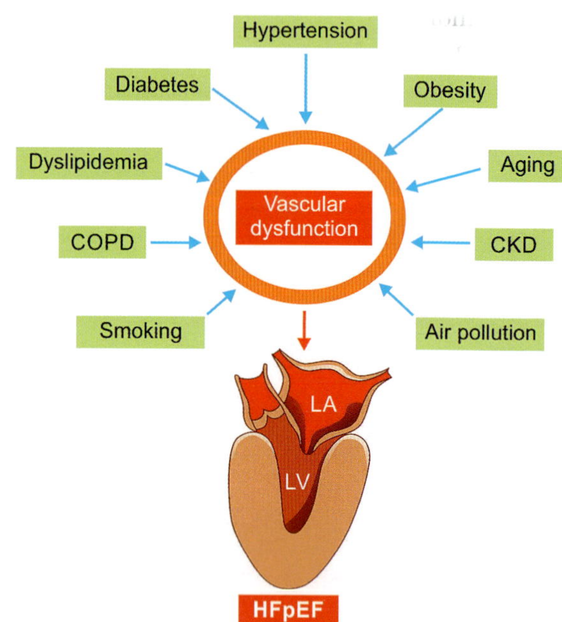

Fig. 1: Schematic diagram showing interaction of several factors in the pathogenesis of vascular dysfunction which ultimately leads to heart failure with preserved ejection fraction (HFpEF). (COPD: chronic obstructive pulmonary disease; CKD: chronic kidney disease; LA: left atrium; LV: left ventricle)

ENDOTHELIAL DYSFUNCTION

Endothelial dysfunction is a hallmark of HFpEF and plays a critical role in its pathophysiology. The endothelium regulates vascular tone, platelet aggregation, leukocyte adhesion, and smooth muscle cell proliferation, etc. In HFpEF, endothelial dysfunction is characterized by impaired NO bioavailability, increased oxidative stress, and heightened inflammatory response. Reduced NO availability leads to vasoconstriction, increased arterial stiffness, and impaired coronary microcirculatory function, all of which contribute to diastolic dysfunction and the clinical manifestations of HFpEF.[6,7]

Mechanisms of Endothelial Dysfunction in Heart Failure with Preserved Ejection Fraction

Oxidative stress: Reactive oxygen species (ROS) generated by NADPH oxidase, uncoupled endothelial NO synthase (eNOS), and mitochondrial dysfunction play a significant role in reducing NO bioavailability. This oxidative environment fosters vascular inflammation and stiffness.[6]

Inflammation: Chronic low-grade inflammation, often driven by comorbid conditions such as obesity diabetes, hypertension, air pollution, smoking, nano-plastic pollution leading to endothelial activation, increased expression of adhesion molecules, and infiltration of inflammatory cells, which modify vascular structure and function.[8]

Arterial stiffness: Arterial stiffness is a key contributor to the increased afterload observed in HFpEF. The stiffening of large arteries, particularly the aorta, leads to increased systolic blood pressure, left ventricular hypertrophy, and impaired diastolic filling. Arterial stiffness also contributes to microvascular dysfunction, as the increased pulsatile load is transmitted to the microcirculation, causing *capillary rarefaction* and further impairing tissue perfusion. The factors that contribute to arterial stiffness in HFpEF are aging, hypertension, and metabolic factors, age-related changes in the extracellular matrix, such as increased collagen deposition and elastin fragmentation, contribute significantly to arterial stiffening. Hypertension accelerates arterial stiffening through mechanical stress, which induces vascular smooth muscle cell hypertrophy and fibrosis. Metabolic factors such as hyperglycemia, insulin resistance and dyslipidemia are associated with increased glycation end-products and oxidative stress, both of which contribute to arterial stiffness.[9,10]

MICROVASCULAR DYSFUNCTION

Microvascular dysfunction in HFpEF is characterized by impaired vasodilation, capillary rarefaction, and increased vascular permeability. These changes lead to inadequate tissue perfusion and contribute to the symptoms of HFpEF, such as exercise intolerance and dyspnea.[9] Microvascular dysfunction is also associated with increased myocardial fibrosis, which impairs diastolic relaxation and contributes to the progression of HFpEF. Capillary rarefaction cause loss of capillaries reducing the surface area for oxygen exchange, leading to tissue hypoxia which exacerbates myocardial and skeletal muscle dysfunction. Increased vascular permeability results from interaction of inflammatory cytokines and oxidative stress leading to interstitial edema, that further impairs myocardial and skeletal muscle function.[11] Reduced microcirculation of the intestine with altered microbiota stimulate the inflammatory markers such as leptins and IL-6 contributing to systemic vasoconstriction and altered vascular biology. This area needs further research and evaluation.

Macrovascular Changes and Arterial Stiffness

Macrovascular changes in the form of increase in stiffness of large conduit vessels is commonly seen in HFpEF. Stiff conduit arteries lead to increase in pulse pressure and pulse wave velocity, which ultimately adversely affect downstream microvasculature. Stiff arteries cannot absorb pulse energy of cardiac systole causing high systolic pressure. This excess pressure gets transmitted to downstream delicate microvascular bed. This also causes reflected wave return fast and poses load to ventricle during mid-late systole. Early reflected wave cannot contribute to diastolic pressure and therefore leading to impaired coronary perfusion during diastole.[12] In this way arterial stiffness ultimately cause myocardial ischemia and tissue damage.

Elastic property of vascular wall is determined by its composition such as extracellular matrix, smooth muscle cells, cell-cell and cell-matrix connections. Deposition of extracellular matrix in aortic wall was initially considered to be mainly responsible for aortic thickening and stiffness. However, recent evidence suggest activation of vascular smooth muscle with increased contractility also appears to play important role in arterial stiffness.[13] Focal adhesions (connection between extracellular matrix and smooth muscle cytoskeleton) in smooth muscle has been described as another mechanism of arterial stiffness and this is well-regulated.[13] Increased focal adhesions leads to better transmission of contractile force of smooth muscles to arterial wall contributing stiffness. Src-FAK signaling enhance these focal adhesions and can be targeted for therapy.[13,14] Active vasoconstriction has also been attributed to abnormal myosin expression in smooth muscle. Smooth muscle contains two types of myosin, nonmuscle (NM), and smooth muscle (SM). NM myosin release from actomyosin slower than SM myosin and spends more time in crossbridge with actin. Overexpression of NM myosin has been suggested in HFpEF and hypertension, responsible for aortic stiffness and subsequent ventricular remodeling.[15,16]

Few studies also propose macrovascular stiffness as a consequence of microvascular dysfunction, which is the primary driving force for overall pathophysiology.[17] Current evidence suggests both microvascular and macrovascular changes associated with HFpEF. However, whether these are consequence/adaptive response to heart failure or primary mechanism leading to heart failure is yet to be understood.

AUTONOMIC IMBALANCE

Sympathetic and parasympathetic system innervate vascular smooth muscle and regulate vasomotor tone. Vascular smooth muscle express β and α receptor responsible for vasodilation and vasoconstriction, respectively. Muscarinic receptors over smooth muscle cell activated by parasympathetic system are also responsible for vasoconstriction. Endothelial cells also express β and α2 receptor. Role of β receptor is not clear and α2 receptor activation leads to release of NO causing vasodilation. Autonomic imbalance leads to overall vasoconstrictive state. Long standing elevated levels of catecholamines is associated with adverse long-term outcome in heart failure both HFrEF and HFpEF.[18] Autonomic imbalance also leads to maladaptive vascular response by inducing endothelial NO synthase (eNOS) isoform. This in turn leads to reduced NO availability and increased oxidative stress.

NITRIC OXIDE SIGNALING

Vascular nitric oxide (NO) secreted from endothelium act mainly on vascular smooth muscle and circulating platelets, causing vasodilation and inhibition of platelet aggregation, respectively. It also has antifibrotic, antiapoptotic, anti-inflammatory, and proangiogenic properties.[18,19] NO diffuses into vascular smooth muscle and stimulates soluble guanylate (sGC) cyclase producing cyclic GMP (cGMP). This in turn activates protein kinase G (PKG). PKG phosphorylates many proteins causing decrease in intracellular calcium and actin-myosin binding. This pathway underlies vasodilation of majority of microvascular beds. NO diffuse into myocardium from adjacent microvascular bed modulating cardiac function.[20] In HFpEF endothelial dysfunction leads to alteration in NO-cGMP-PKG pathway and impaired vasodilation. Autonomic imbalance also contributes decreased NO availability in microvasculature. Normally β-adrenergic stimulation activates endothelial NO synthase isoform (eNOS) stimulating NO synthesis. Increased sympathetic activity in HFpEF leads to chronic activation of eNOS. However, overexpression of eNOS usually result in maladaptive response with increased production of super oxide anion and reduced NO availability. Oxygen free radicals (superoxide anion) combine with NO forming reactive nitrogen species, which has prothrombotic and proinflammatory effect on microvasculature. NO-cGMP-PKG pathway has been recognized as central dogma of pathophysiology of HFpEF forms basis of both vascular and myocardial dysfunction.[21,22]

Alteration in NO-cGMP-PKG pathway affect myocardium in terms of delayed relaxation, increased stiffness, ventricular hypertrophy, and interstitial fibrosis.[21] cAMP-PKA pathway is considered to regulate myocardial hypertrophy and lusitropy and cGMP/PKG counteract PKA mediated hypertrophy and diastolic dysfunction. NO and natriuretic peptide stimulate guanylyl cyclase to produce cGMP and in turn activate PKG. Phosphodiesterase (PDE) metabolizes cGMP and its blockade might increase levels of circulating cGMP. Based on this, benefit of sildenafil (PDE 5 inhibitor) was evaluated in HFpEF.[23] However, there was no clinical benefit. Lack of clinical benefit was attributed to decreased expression of PDE5 in cardiac tissue.

VASCULAR INFLAMMATION AND OXIDATIVE STRESS

Common risk factors for HFpEF such as diabetes mellitus, hypertension, obesity, and CAD trigger a systemic proinflammatory state. This is characterized by elevated circulatory levels of leukocyte adhesion molecules (ICAM-1 and VCAM-1), corresponding leukocyte ligands and increased infiltration of CD45+ and CD3+ T-lymphocytes.[24] In patients with HFpEF, reduced flow mediated dilation (FMD) closely associated with elevated CRP, IL-6, TNF-α and NFG15.[25] Inflammation of coronary vasculature partly mediated by nuclear factor-kappa B (NFκB) signaling pathway.[26]

Vascular Dysfunction in the Development of Heart Failure with Preserved Ejection Fraction

Vascular dysfunction plays a critical role in the initiation of HFpEF by contributing to diastolic dysfunction and systemic inflammation. Endothelial dysfunction and arterial stiffness increase left ventricular afterload and impair relaxation, leading to increased left atrial pressure and pulmonary congestion. These changes are often exacerbated by comorbidities such as hypertension,

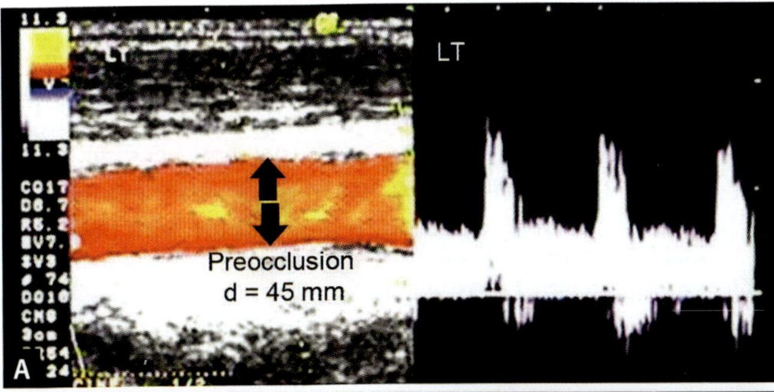

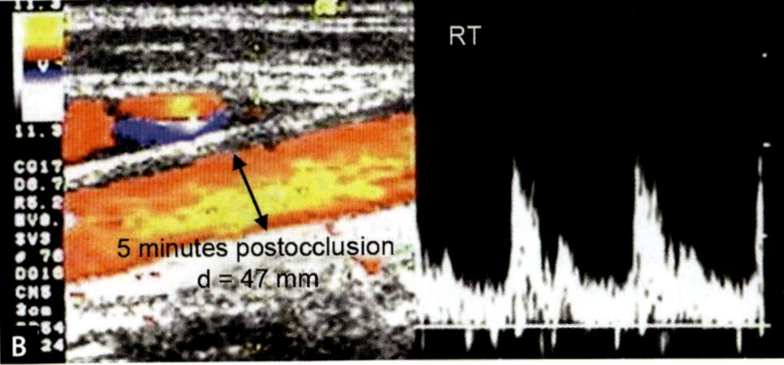

Figs. 2A and B: (A) Preocclusion brachial artery dimension 45 mm; (B) Postocclusion dimension 47 mm, flow mediated dilation (FMD) = 47–45/45 = 4.4% indicating severe endothelial dysfunction.

obesity, and diabetes, which are prevalent in patients with HFpEF.[27] Clinically endothelial dysfunction can also be diagnosed by measuring FMD in brachial artery by ultrasound methods **(Figs. 2A and B)**.[28]

Vascular Dysfunction in the Progression of Heart Failure with Preserved Ejection Fraction

Once established, vascular dysfunction perpetuates the HFpEF phenotype through a vicious cycle of increased afterload, myocardial stiffening, and systemic inflammation. The interplay between vascular and myocardial dysfunction leads to progressive diastolic dysfunction, increased filling pressures, and symptomatic heart failure. Moreover, microvascular dysfunction contributes to myocardial ischemia, fibrosis, and further deterioration of cardiac function.[29]

As HFpEF progresses, the ongoing vascular dysfunction contributes to worsening symptoms and increased morbidity. The progression of arterial stiffness and microvascular dysfunction leads to further increases in left ventricular filling pressures, pulmonary hypertension, and right ventricular dysfunction. This progression is often accelerated by worsening comorbid conditions, particularly those that exacerbate vascular inflammation and oxidative stress.[30]

Therapeutic Implications of Vascular Dysfunction in Heart Failure with Preserved Ejection Fraction

Understanding the role of vascular dysfunction in HFpEF opens the door to novel therapeutic strategies. Current treatments for HFpEF focus primarily on symptom management and control of comorbid conditions. However, targeting vascular dysfunction may offer additional benefits in slowing disease progression.

Therapeutic approaches targeting endothelial function improvement such as phosphodiesterase-5 inhibitors and soluble guanylate cyclase stimulators increase NO bioavailability which has the potential of improving endothelial function and reduce vascular stiffness.

Anti-inflammatory therapies targeting systemic inflammation with agents such as interleukin-1 blockers or novel anti-inflammatory drugs may reduce vascular inflammation and improve outcomes in HFpEF.

Antioxidant therapies have shown limited success in clinical trials, targeting specific sources of oxidative stress, such as NADPH oxidase inhibitors, may offer more targeted benefits.

Arterial stiffness reduction by pharmacologic agents such as aldosterone antagonists and angiotensin receptor-neprilysin inhibitors, may improve hemodynamics and reduce the burden on the left ventricle.[31]

CONCLUSION

Vascular dysfunction both structural and functional in systemic as well as cardiac vessels are central players in the pathophysiology of HFpEF, contributing to the development, maintenance, and progression of the disease. The complex interplay between endothelial dysfunction, arterial stiffness, and microvascular inflammation underscores the importance of a comprehensive approach to managing HFpEF. Future research should focus on identifying novel therapeutic targets within the vascular system to improve outcomes for patients with HFpEF. Understanding the underlying mechanisms of vascular dysfunction in HFpEF not only provides insights into the disease process but also highlights potential therapeutic avenues that could change the current treatment paradigm. As our knowledge of HFpEF continues to evolve, addressing vascular dysfunction may prove to be a key strategy in reducing the growing burden of this challenging condition.

REFERENCES

1. Tsao CW, Lyass A, Enserro D, et al. Temporal trends in the incidence of and mortality associated with heart failure

with preserved and reduced ejection fraction. JACC Heart Fail. 2018;6(8):678-85.

2. Heidenreich PA, Bozkurt B, Aguilar D, et al. 2022 AHA/ACC/HFSA Guideline for the Management of Heart Failure: A Report of the American College of Cardiology/American Heart Association Joint Committee on Clinical Practice Guidelines. Circulation. 2022;145(18):E895-E1032.
3. Alem MM. Endothelial dysfunction in chronic heart failure: assessment, findings, significance, and potential therapeutic targets. Int J Mol Sci. 2019;20(13):3198.
4. Mishra SS, Pradhan PK, Routray SN, et al. Chapter 11. In: PK Deb (Ed). Endothelium and Coronary artery Disease-Clinical Applications, Cardiological Society of India, Cardiology Update, 2012. President-Elect, CSI and Chairman, Scientific Committee, 64th Annual CSI Conference & SAARC Cardiac Congress; 2012. pp. 65-74.
5. Mohammed SF, Hussain S, Mirzoyev SA, et al. Coronary microvascular rarefaction and myocardial fibrosis in heart failure with preserved ejection fraction. Circulation. 2015;131(6):550-9.
6. Yang JH, Obokata M, Reddy YNV, et al. Endothelium-dependent and independent coronary microvascular dysfunction in patients with heart failure with preserved ejection fraction. Eur J Heart Fail. 2020;22(3):432-41.
7. Shah SJ, Lam CSP, Svedlund S, et al. Prevalence and correlates of coronary microvascular dysfunction in heart failure with preserved ejection fraction: PROMIS-HFpEF. Eur Heart J. 2018;39(37):3439-50.
8. Dridi H, Santulli G, Gambardella J, et al. IP3 receptor orchestrates maladaptive vascular responses in heart failure. J Clin Invest. 2022;132(4).
9. van de Wouw J, Sorop O, van Drie RWA, et al. Perturbations in myocardial perfusion and oxygen balance in swine with multiple risk factors: a novel model of ischemia and no obstructive coronary artery disease. Basic Res Cardiol. 2020;115:1-18.
10. Wang J, Du Y, Rio R Del. Vascular dysfunction in HFpEF: potential role in the development, maintenance, and progression of the disease. Front Cardiovasc Med. 2022; 9:1070935.
11. Bennett J, van Dinther M, Voorter P, et al. Assessment of microvascular disease in heart and brain by MRI: application in heart failure with preserved ejection fraction and cerebral small vessel disease. Medicina (Lithuania). 2023;59(9).
12. Reddy YNV, Andersen MJ, Obokata M, et al. Arterial stiffening with exercise in patients with heart failure and preserved ejection fraction. J Am Coll Cardiol. 2017; 70(2):136-48.
13. Gao YZ, Saphirstein RJ, Yamin R, et al. Aging impairs smooth muscle-mediated regulation of aortic stiffness: a defect in shock absorption function? Am J Physiol-Heart Circulatory Physiol. 2014;307(8):H1252-61.
14. Saphirstein RJ, Gao YZ, Jensen MH, et al. The focal adhesion: a regulated component of aortic stiffness. PLoS One. 2013;8(4):e62461.
15. Zhang W, Gunst SJ. Non-muscle (NM) myosin heavy chain phosphorylation regulates the formation of NM myosin filaments, adhesome assembly and smooth muscle contraction. J Physiol. 2017;595(13):4279-300.
16. Contard F, Sabri A, Glukhova M, et al. Arterial smooth muscle cell phenotype in stroke-prone spontaneously hypertensive rats. Hypertension. 1993;22(5):665-76.
17. Lee JF, Barrett-O'Keefe Z, Garten RS, et al. Evidence of microvascular dysfunction in heart failure with preserved ejection fraction. Heart. 2016;102(4):278-84.
18. Lymperopoulos A, Rengo G, Koch WJ. Adrenergic nervous system in heart failure: pathophysiology and therapy. Circ Res. 2013;113(6):739-53.
19. Cyr AR, Huckaby L V, Shiva SS, et al. Nitric oxide and endothelial dysfunction. Crit Care Clin. 2020;36(2):307-21.
20. Wang P, Wei M, Zhu X, et al. Nitric oxide down-regulates voltage-gated Na+ channel in cardiomyocytes possibly through S-nitrosylation-mediated signaling. Sci Rep. 2021; 11(1):11273.
21. Greene SJ, Gheorghiade M, Borlaug BA, et al. The cGMP signaling pathway as a therapeutic target in heart failure with preserved ejection fraction. J Am Heart Assoc. 2013; 2(6):e000536.
22. Chirinos JA, Akers SR, Trieu L, et al. Heart failure, left ventricular remodeling, and circulating nitric oxide metabolites. J Am Heart Assoc. 2016;5(10):e004133.
23. Redfield MM, Chen HH, Borlaug BA, et al. Effect of phosphodiesterase-5 inhibition on exercise capacity and clinical status in heart failure with preserved ejection fraction: a randomized clinical trial. JAMA. 2013;309(12): 1268-77.
24. Westermann D, Lindner D, Kasner M, et al. Cardiac inflammation contributes to changes in the extracellular matrix in patients with heart failure and normal ejection fraction. Circ Heart Fail. 2011;4(1):44-52.
25. Collier P, Watson CJ, Voon V, et al. Can emerging biomarkers of myocardial remodelling identify asymptomatic hypertensive patients at risk for diastolic dysfunction and diastolic heart failure? Eur J Heart Fail. 2011;13(10):1087-95.
26. Forrester SJ, Kikuchi DS, Hernandes MS, et al. Reactive oxygen species in metabolic and inflammatory signaling. Circ Res. 2018;122(6):877-902.
27. Degen C V, Bishu K, Zakeri R, et al. The emperor's new clothes: PDE5 and the heart. PLoS One. 2015;10(3): e0118664.
28. Mishra SS, Mishra B, Routray SN, et al. Chapter 9. In: Chopra HK, Joshi SR, warder GS (Eds.). Endothelial Dysfunction in Atrial Fibrillation with Type 2 Diabetes, Cardiovascular Update A Text Book of Cardiology, 1st edition. New Delhi: Jaypee Brothers Medical Publisher (P) Ltd; 2018, pp. 49-54.
29. Redfield MM, Anstrom KJ, Levine JA, et al. Isosorbide mononitrate in heart failure with preserved ejection fraction. New Engl J Med. 2015;373(24):2314-24.
30. Reddy YNV, Lewis GD, Shah SJ, et al. INDIE-HFpEF (Inorganic Nitrite Delivery to Improve Exercise Capacity in Heart Failure With Preserved Ejection Fraction) Rationale and Design. Circ Heart Fail. 2017;10(5):e003862.
31. Lyle MA, Brozovich FV. HFpEF, a disease of the vasculature: a closer look at the other half. Mayo Clin Proc. 2018; 93(9):1305-14.

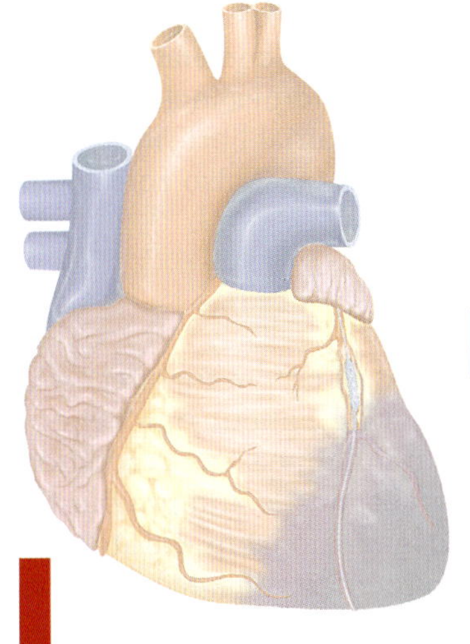

Bendopnea in HFpEF: A Narrative Review

Tiny Nair

INTRODUCTION

The symptoms of heart failure range from totally asymptomatic (echocardiographic LV dysfunction) to severely symptomatic patients with breathlessness at rest (orthopnea in advanced heart failure). Symptoms could also range from fatigue to dizzy spells and pedal edema to altered sleep patterns and palpitations, which could be easily confused with pulmonary or other comorbid systemic disease (anemia and thyrotoxicosis) leading to missed diagnosis. Effort intolerance with breathlessness still remains the dominant symptom in most cases.[1,2]

QUANTIFYING BREATHLESSNESS

Quantifying a symptom is not easy. During early 90's, physicians in New York found an easy way out—asking patients how many blocks they are able to walk without symptoms. A typical New York block measured 80 meters between streets; a patient able to walk 2 blocks (160 meters) without symptoms was labeled as class 1, those who completed but had symptoms were class 2, those who were unable to complete 2 blocks were labeled class 3, and those unable to do anything, class 4. Over time this NYHA class became the gold standard for assessment of CV disease (especially heart failure) symptoms worldwide.

Other objective tools for breathlessness quantification include a simple 6-minute-walk test and a standard treadmill test (modified Bruce protocol for those with significant limiting symptoms).[3]

ORTHOPNEA

Dyspnea on attaining supine posture is termed orthopnea. Elevation of diaphragm, coupled with increased venous return to the right heart on attaining supine posture, increases pulmonary congestion and the patient tends to sit up to relieve the symptoms. Attaining a propped-up posture is more comfortable for some, while others tend to sleep on a cardiac table. Orthopnea is a clear indication of severe underlying cardiopulmonary disease.[1,2]

PAROXYSMAL NOCTURNAL DYSPNEA

Paroxysmal nocturnal dyspnea (PND) results from a complex hemodynamic interaction similar to orthopnea, but not severe enough to cause symptoms, but the symptoms tend to worsen after a period of sleep and then the patient gets up and sits up with cough and breathlessness akin to early pulmonary edema. The mechanism of trigger is supposed to be absorption of edema fluid, resulting in increase in the circulatory volume, coupled with depression of respiratory center during sleep.[3]

Bendopnea is a newly described symptom where the patient complains of "breathlessness" "uneasiness" or "discomfort" in activities involving bending down like tying a shoelace or putting on a pair of socks or trying to pick up objects from floor. Bendopnea could be documented by a drop of oxygen saturation on bending down (by at least 3% or more). Though initially described in HFpEF, this symptom has been noted in the entire spectrum of heart failure, including both HFrEF and HFpEF.

Bendopnea has also been described in pulmonary hypertension and abdominal obesity.[2,3]

REVIEW OF LITERATURE

Karauzum et al. studied 53 patients of pulmonary hypertension presenting with bendopnea. They documented worse NYHA class and a poorer 6-minute-walk test. In fact, 83% with bendopnea belonged to class III and class IV NYHA compared to 17% without bendopnea. Surprisingly, patients with and without bendopnea had similar elevations of NT-proBNP and LVEF. They had a higher PA pressure and a higher PVR.[1]

Martínez Cerón et al. studied 633 patients and tried to compare bendopnea in heart failure versus COPD. They documented that heart failure had a much higher chance of harboring heart failure (HR 2.42, 95% CI 1.10–4.04), while not significantly related to COPD and CAD.[3]

Espriella et al. looked into bending oxygen saturation and bendopnea. 21% of their 440 studied patients had bendopnea while 27% had a bending oxygen saturation drop by 3% or more. There was moderate degree of agreement between subjective bendopnea, and objective saturation drop on bending down. Bending down drop of oxygen saturation by 3% or more correlated to hospital admission with worsening heart failure (WHF) events but a symptom of bendopnea did not.[4]

Thibodeau et al. tried to look into the hemodynamic changes in bendopnea. In 102 patients of heart failure, subjected to cardiac catheterization, 28% had bendopnea, with an average time of appearance of symptoms being 8 seconds of bending. Bendopnea correlated with a higher RAP and higher PCWP and elevated filling pressures but similar cardiac index (CI).[2,5]

A meta-analysis of all studies (Pranata et al.) analyzed data from 42 studies and a total of 601 patients with heart failure. They found bendopnea in 283 patients (prevalence 31%). Patients with bendopnea had worse functional status, more symptoms, more PND (OR 2.76) more orthopnea (OR 3.02), and a higher all-cause mortality (OR 2.24).[6]

Data from 457 patients of heart failure with mid-range ejection fraction (HFmrEF) showed correlation with bendopnea symptoms with comorbidities including old age, chronic kidney disease (CKD), atrial fibrillation (AF) and diabetes. Bendopnea in this dataset also correlated with higher all-cause mortality.[7]

CONCLUSION

Bendopnea is a newly described symptom that needs to be recognized and elicited during patient interaction. From an interesting caveat, bendopnea has graduated to a major symptom that has diagnostic and prognostic therapeutic implications. Close relationship with HFpEF makes this symptom even more interesting. More clarity on its sensitivity and specificity is awaited.

REFERENCES

1. Karauzum K, Karauzum I, Kilic T, et al. Bendopnea and its clinical importance in outpatient patients with pulmonary arterial hypertension. Acta Cardiol Sin. 2018; 34(6):518-25.
2. Thibodeau JT, Turer AT, Gualano SK, et al. Characterization of a novel symptom of advanced heart failure: Bendopnea. JACC Heart Fail. 2014;2(1):24-31.
3. Martínez Cerón DM, Garcia Rosa ML, Lagoeiro Jorge AJ, et al. Association of types of dyspnea including 'bendopnea' with cardiopulmonary disease in primary care. Rev Port Cardiol. 2017;36(3):179-86.
4. de la Espriella R, Amiguet M, Miñana G, et al. Bending oxygen saturation index and risk of worsening heart failure events in chronic heart failure. Eur J Heart Fail. 2022;24(11):2108-17.
5. Akaslan D, Aslanger E, İsmail Basa C, et al. Bendopnea predicts right ventricular energy failure in patients with pulmonary hypertension. Turk Kardiyol Dern Ars. 2023;51(7):440-6.
6. Pranata R, Yonas E, Chintya V, et al. Clinical significance of bendopnea in heart failure—Systematic review and meta-analysis. Indian Heart J. 2019;71(3):277-83.
7. Liu Z, Zhu Y, Zhang L, et al. Impact of signs and symptoms on the prognosis of patients with HFmrEF. BMC Cardiovasc Disord. 2023;23(1):420.

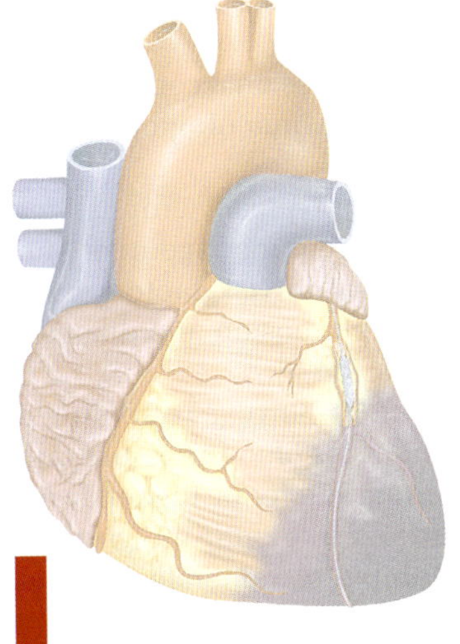

Aging and HFpEF: Is There a Difference?

Sheikh Ubair Nabi

INTRODUCTION

Aging itself is not the cause of heart failure; still, it is a contributing factor in the manifestation of heart failure due to the decline of the cardioprotective system making it an important risk factor for all cardiovascular diseases.[1,2]

Age-related changes occur in cardiovascular structure and function along with other organs. This essentially leads to a progressive increase in cardiovascular disease in the elderly.[3,4]

When it comes to patients with younger age, heart failure with preserved ejection fraction (HFpEF) is a rare entity and cardiac remodeling is a major factor with obesity as the major driver.[5]

In this chapter, we will be defining HFpEF and whether there is any difference in pathophysiology and management related to age, especially with age groups: 40–50 years, 50–60 years, and >65 years.

PATHOPHYSIOLOGY OF HFpEF

The relation of HFpEF to aging is related to physiological changes that occur in different age groups. These changes can be due to structural changes, functional alterations, and cellular modifications within the heart.[6,7]

In individuals aged 40–50 years, HFpEF may often arise from a combination of lifestyle factors and emerging comorbidities and is due to diastolic dysfunction attributed to:

- Obesity causes metabolic syndrome and insulin resistance, adversely affecting myocardial function.[8,5]
- Early-stage hypertension can result in diastolic dysfunction.[1,7]

Individuals in the 50–60 years age group can develop age-related cardiac changes like:

- *Increased arterial stiffness:* As a person ages, the elasticity of the arterial wall diminishes, leading to higher systolic blood pressure with increased afterload.[1,6]
- *Myocardial fibrosis:* As aging happens, this phenomenon contributes to impaired diastolic filling.[7,9]

In those over 65 years of age, HFpEF is usually the result of cumulative structural and functional changes, including:

- *Advanced fibrosis:* Extensive myocardial fibrosis significantly impairs diastolic function.[3,9]
- Multiple chronic conditions (e.g., diabetes and chronic kidney disease) further complicate the clinical picture.[4,6]

CLINICAL PRESENTATION

The clinical manifestations of HFpEF can vary widely across age groups, influencing diagnosis and treatment approaches.

- In younger adults (40–50 years), symptoms may be subtle and easily overlooked. They are commonly present with exertional dyspnea, fatigue, and weakness, which is often triggered by physical activity.[5]
- But when it comes to the age between 50 and 60 years, the symptoms mentioned above become more prominent along with orthopnea.[4,10]

- And for >65-year-old adults, they often present with classic and debilitating symptoms such as:
  - *Severe dyspnea (modified medical research council—March grade IV):* This can occur even at rest significantly impacting the quality of life.[8,10]
  - *Paroxysmal nocturnal dyspnea:* Sudden nighttime breathlessness that awakens patients is common.[8,10]

DIAGNOSTIC CHALLENGES

The diagnosis of HFpEF requires a careful assessment that includes clinical history, physical examination, biomarker tests, echocardiography (used to confirm preserved ejection fraction (>50%) with an assessment of diastolic function, chamber sizes, and left ventricular filling pressures), and sometimes additional imaging like magnetic resonance imaging (MRI) and computed tomography (CT).

- *40–50 years:* Early signs of HFpEF may be subtle. Echocardiography and exercise testing play a key role in diagnosis, with less credence on biomarkers like brain natriuretic peptide (BNP) and N-terminal brain natriuretic peptide (NT-proBNP).[7,8]
- *50–60 years:* There is greater reliance on BNP/NT-proBNP, and stress testing becomes crucial for diagnosing HFpEF. Imaging such as echocardiography or cardiac MRI/CT is important for assessing cardiac structure.[3,9]
- *>65 years:* Echocardiography, biomarkers, and comorbidity management are key. Advanced imaging and hemodynamic testing are used selectively, with care taken due to the risks with invasive procedures in elderly patients.[7,10]

RISK FACTORS

The risk factors for HFpEF vary significantly by age group, influencing prevention and management strategies.

- Common risk factors in 40–50 years demography include obesity, sedentary lifestyle, and early-onset hypertension.[5,6]
- For individuals crossing 50 years of life, the picture of risk factors changes with worsening comorbidities like hypertension, diabetes, and hyperlipidemia, which becomes more prevalent. And also, psychosocial factors like stress and depression can impact lifestyle choices and treatment adherence.[8,9]
- In older adults >65 years, the presence of multiple chronic conditions creates a complex interplay of risk factors including frailty and polypharmacy that can lead to adverse effects, further complicating HF management.[3,10]

TREATMENT APPROACHES

The management of HFpEF often relies on a combination of lifestyle modifications and pharmacological interventions, tailored to each age group.

- For younger patients, treatment typically emphasizes lifestyle modifications with weight management and dietary modifications. Control of risk factors with aggressive management of hypertension and diabetes is essential to prevent progression.[5,9]
- Patients in the age group of 50–60 years often need more aggressive management for blood pressure and comorbidities, and they generally tolerate higher doses of medications. Medications like sodium-glucose cotransporter-2 (SGLT2) inhibitors, mineralocorticoid receptor antagonists (MRAs), and angiotensin receptor-neprilysin inhibitors (ARNIs) can be used more liberally due to fewer concerns about renal function and electrolyte imbalances within this individualized age.[2,6,7,8]
- Elderly patients of >65 years require more cautious dosing and closer monitoring due to increased risk of hypotension, renal dysfunction, and electrolyte disturbances. The focus is on symptom relief, avoiding adverse effects and minimizing polypharmacy. SGLT2 inhibitors and ARNIs can still be beneficial, but their use requires careful titration.[2,8]

PROGNOSIS AND OUTCOMES

The prognosis for patients with HFpEF varies significantly across age groups, influenced by comorbidities, functional capacity, and treatment adherence.

- *40–50 years:* Younger patients typically have a better prognosis as with earlier diagnosis and recognition, younger patients can implement lifestyle changes that positively impact outcomes. Also, the absence of multiple chronic conditions often correlates with a better overall outlook.[5,6]
- *50–60 years:* In this demographic, prognosis begins to worsen due to the presence of conditions like diabetes and hypertension complicating treatment and outcomes. Along with deteriorating functional capacity, physical limitations may begin to affect daily activities and quality of life.[7,9]
- *>65 years:* Older adults face the most significant challenges regarding prognosis with higher mortality rates as advanced age and multiple comorbidities contribute to increased mortality associated with HFpEF.[3,10]

Older patients often experience recurrent hospital visits for acute exacerbations, leading to a cycle of worsening health.

CHALLENGES

The challenges include the following:

- HFpEF in young patients can present with unique challenges. It can be misdiagnosed in younger individuals as symptoms can mimic other conditions such as anxiety or obesity.[5,7]
- Younger patients often have different comorbid conditions (like obesity, hypertension, or diabetes) that can complicate the clinical picture and management of HFpEF.
- The underlying mechanisms of HFpEF in younger patients may differ from those in older adults, often involving more structural or functional heart issues, such as diastolic dysfunction or valvular disease.
- As most studies on HFpEF focus mostly on older populations, evidence-based guidelines and management strategies for younger patients are limited.[9]
- Treatment options are not well-defined for young patients who face challenges with adherence to lifestyle modifications and medications, which can affect their quality of life and can lead to psychological impact due to a heart failure diagnosis at a young age.[8,10]
- There is limited data on the long-term prognosis of young patients with HFpEF, making it difficult to predict outcomes and tailor long-term care strategies.[2,9]
- Addressing these limitations requires a more comprehensive and individualized approach to diagnosis, management, and sociopsychological support for young patients with HFpEF.

CONCLUSION

Heart failure with preserved ejection fraction presents with a clinical challenge that alters at different age groups and understanding the differences between various age groups is important for optimizing diagnosis, treatment, and overall management.

Though younger adults often present with lifestyle-related risk factors, the older age group has more complex age-related changes and underlying comorbidities that complicate their clinical status. Much ongoing research is essential to redefine treatment strategies and improve the quality of care for all patients living with HFpEF.[3,8]

REFERENCES

1. Yancy CW, Jessup M, Bozkurt B, et al. 2013 ACCF/AHA Guideline for the management of heart failure: A report of the American College of Cardiology Foundation/American Heart Association Task Force on Practice Guidelines. Circulation. 2013;128(16):1810-52.
2. Solomon SD, et al. Heart failure with preserved ejection fraction: A scientific statement from the American Heart Association. Circulation; 2019.
3. McMurray JJV, et al. Heart failure with preserved ejection fraction: a clinical dilemma. Eur Heart J. 2015.
4. Bhatia RS, Tu JV, Lee DS, et al. The impact of age on the clinical presentation of heart failure. J Card Fail; 2006.
5. Ait-Aissa, K., et al. Obesity-induced cardiac dysfunction in young adults: symptomless but not harmless. Heart Fail Rev; 2019.
6. Paulus WJ, Tschöpe C. A novel paradigm for heart failure with preserved ejection fraction: comorbidities drive myocardial dysfunction and remodeling through coronary microvascular endothelial inflammation. J Am Coll Cardiol. 2013;62(4):263-71.
7. Borlaug BA, Redfield MM. Diastolic and systolic heart failure are distinct phenotypes within the heart failure spectrum. Circulation. 2011;128(18):2006-13; discussion 2014.
8. Lam CSP, Solomon SD. The expanding burden of heart failure with preserved ejection fraction in a changing demographic. Circulation Research. 2014
9. Zile MR, Brutsaert DL. New concepts in diastolic dysfunction and diastolic heart failure: Part I: Diagnosis, prognosis, and measurements of diastolic function. Circulation. 2002;105(11):1387-93.
10. Kitzman DW, Upadhya B. Heart failure with preserved ejection fraction in older adults. Heart Fail Clin. 2017;13: 485-502.

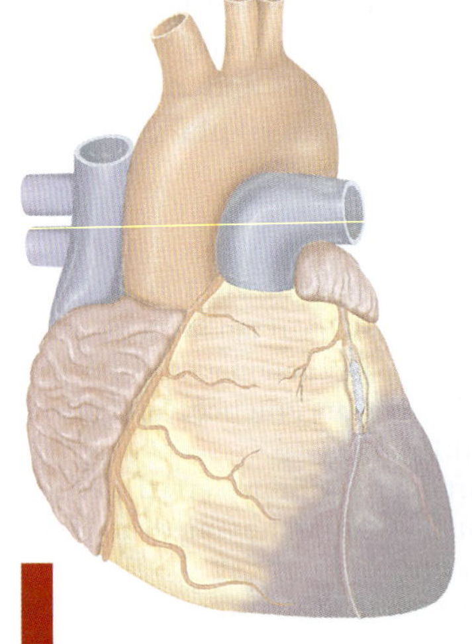

Prognosticating and Palliating in Older Adults with HFpEF

SN Pathak

INTRODUCTION

Heart failure with preserved ejection fraction (HFpEF) is a clinical syndrome characterized by symptoms and signs of heart failure with elevated left ventricular filling pressures at rest or during exercise. It is the most common type of heart failure in the elderly and its prevalence increases with age and is higher in females at any given age. HFpEF is frequently accompanied by comorbid conditions such as diabetes mellitus, obesity, atrial fibrillation, and renal dysfunction. HFpEF is associated with significant morbidity and mortality that may benefit from incorporation of palliative care. The estimated 1-year and 5-year mortalities after the diagnosis of HFpEF are 20% and 50%, respectively.[1]

Heart failure with preserved ejection fraction is defined, in the recent 2022 American Heart Association (AHA)/American College of Cardiology (ACC)/Heart Failure Society of America (HFSA) heart failure guidelines, as ejection fraction ≥50% with evidence of spontaneous or provokable increased left ventricular filling pressures.[2]

PATHOPHYSIOLOGY

Ventricular-arterial stiffening is an important element of HFpEF pathophysiology. A stiff ventricle has lower contractile and stroke volume reserve. The stiff artery will increase total afterload. Left atrium (LA) enlargement is a marker of chronically elevated LV filling pressures and is frequently present in patients with HFpEF. More recently, the importance of LA mechanical dysfunction has been recognized as another key player in the HFpEF pathophysiology. Increased left ventricular end-diastolic pressure leads to increased left atrial pressure, increased pulmonary venous pressure, and pulmonary hypertension. Chronotropic incompetence defined as an inadequate heart rate response to exercise has been detected in >30% of patients with HFpEF. In addition, abnormal heart rate recovery is also frequent, affecting approximately 20% of patients with HFpEF. Careful analysis of exercise stress testing may help to detect these abnormalities.[3]

PALLIATIVE CARE

Palliative care (PC) is an interdisciplinary field that seeks to maximize quality of life, optimize goals of care, manage complex symptoms, coordinate care services, and provide psychological and spiritual support for patients with chronic illnesses.[4] Prior studies have demonstrated the benefit of PC in patient populations with heart failure in terms of quality of life, physical and emotional symptom burden, quality of death, and healthcare utilization.[5-8] Contrary to common physician misconceptions,[9,10] PC has been shown to benefit patients throughout their disease course, not only at end of life.

Guidelines and Recommendations for Palliative Care in Heart Failure

In the 2022 update to the ACC/AHA/HFSA guidelines, it is suggested that primary palliative and supportive care should be provided to all patients with heart failure, but the specific criteria for specialist PC referral are unclear.[11] To address this uncertainty, a Delphi study developed consensus criteria for heart failure and PC specialists for PC referral.[12] However, many of these metrics focus on patients with reduced ejection fraction or who are at end-of-life **(Table 1)**, leaving limited guidance for PC referral for patients with HFpEF throughout the disease course.

In the PARAGON-HF trial (Prospective Comparison of ARNI with ARB Global Outcomes in Heart Failure With Preserved Ejection Fraction), patients with an ejection fraction <57% were more likely to die of cardiovascular death, whereas patients with an ejection fraction >57% were more likely to die from noncardiovascular causes.[13] Although cardiovascular death still represents the majority of HFpEF deaths (50–70% in various trials) either from sudden cardiac death or worsening heart failure, this patient population is more likely to die from cancer, infection/sepsis, respiratory illness, or other organ failure than patients with HFrEF.[13,14]

CHALLENGES IN HEART FAILURE WITH PRESERVED EJECTION FRACTION PROGNOSTICATION

In addition to limited data, one of the greatest challenges in HFpEF care is prognostic uncertainty. Despite similar rates of morbidity and mortality to HFrEF, HFpEF does not have validated risk-prediction models to guide prognostication for physicians to know when to incorporate PC.[16] Some of the validated prognostic models for HFrEF have been studied in the HFpEF population, although no single model has been widely adopted **(Table 2)**. In addition to physician challenges to prognostication, patients are also often unaware of the severity of their illness.

Palliative care is underutilized for patients with HFpEF, despite evidence of improved quality of life, quality of death, and health care utilization metrics in small, randomized trials. To improve incorporation of PC into HFpEF care, we have the following recommendations **(Fig. 1)**.

- To develop evidence-based practice, there should be dedicated trials of PC interventions specific to the needs of an HFpEF population.
- To improve provider prognostication, we need further study to validate HFpEF prognostic tools, including incorporation of noncardiac multimorbidity.
- To facilitate specialist PC referral, expert opinion is needed to develop clear consensus criteria for PC referral for heart failure, irrespective of ejection fraction and specific to HFpEF patient needs.
- To improve provider's understanding of PC, comfort with providing primary PC, ACGME competencies for cardiology fellowship training, and training for

TABLE 1: Delphi criteria for specialist palliative care referral based on ejection fraction.[15]

Referral criteria	*Applicable to HFpEF*	*Applicable before end-of-life*
Criteria applicable regardless of ejection fraction		
Dependent on ≥3 basic ADLs	•	•
≥2 ER visits within the past 3 months	•	•
≥2 hospitalizations within the past 3 months	•	•
Severe physical symptoms	•	•
Severe emotional symptoms	•	•
Severe spiritual or existential symptoms	•	•
Patient/family/care team request	•	•
Assistance with goals of care/decision-making/care planning	•	•
Presence of ≥1 noncardiac life-threatening disease in addition to heart failure	•	•
Cardiorenal syndrome	•	•
Clinician-estimated life expectancy of ≤6 months	•	
Refractory symptoms requiring palliative sedation	•	
Cardiac cachexia	•	
Multiorgan failure	•	
Discussion regarding withdrawal/de-escalation of life-prolonging interventions	•	
Request for hastened death/assisted suicide	•	
Hospice referral/discussion	•	
Criteria mostly applicable to HFrEF		
Persistent LVEF <20%		•
Persistent malignant arrhythmias		•
Implantable cardioverter defibrillator shocks		•
Inability to tolerate or resistance to guideline-directed therapies		•
Eligible for, but did not receive for a specified reason, advanced heart failure therapies		
Chronic inotropes		
Mechanical circulatory support		
Chronic inotropes		
Cardiac transplant evaluation		

(ADL: activities of daily living; ER: emergency room; HFrEF: heart failure with reduced ejection fraction; LVEF: left ventricular ejection fraction)

TABLE 2: Prognostic score of heart failure mortality.

Score	Predictor
SHFM	• Cardiovascular mortality • Composite cardiovascular mortality and heart failure hospitalization
MAGGIC heart failure risk score	Composite cardiovascular mortality and heart failure hospitalization
H_2FPEF score	• Composite cardiovascular events (cardiovascular death, nonfatal myocardial infarction, unstable angina, HF hospitalization, and nonfatal stroke) • Heart failure hospitalization
EFFECT Score	• 28-day all-cause mortality • 1-year all-cause mortality

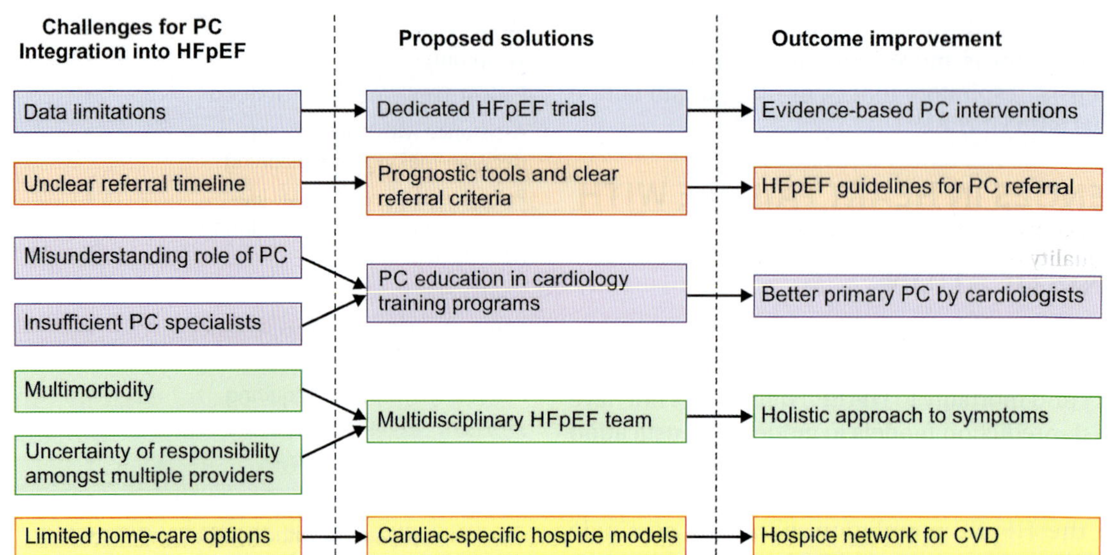

Fig. 1: Framework for incorporating palliative care (PC) into heart failure with preserved ejection fraction (HFpEF) care.

cardiology advanced practice, providers should include measurable PC principles, including communication skills and advance care planning education.

- To address the complex needs of multimorbidity, we should develop a multidisciplinary team approach to HFpEF care that incorporates PC principles.
- To ensure appropriate end-of-life care that aligns with patient goals of care, hospice programs should develop cardiac-specific models to address the unique symptoms and needs of heart failure patients.

CONCLUSION

As HFpEF is becoming the predominant form of heart failure worldwide, more patients are faced with the complex symptoms, significant comorbidities, and limited quality of life associated with this disease process. PC has been shown to enhance important patient-centered outcomes for patients with heart failure, regardless of ejection fraction. Providing accurate prognostication and guidance to patients with HFpEF is challenging in current practice, and as a result, many patients are never referred to specialty PC despite the potential improvement in quality of life and goal-concordant care. There are significant barriers to PC integration into HFpEF care; however, we propose important steps to establish an evidence-based, multidisciplinary framework that addresses the complex physical, psychosocial, spiritual, and end-of-life needs of patients with HFpEF.

REFERENCES

1. Dunlay SM, Roger VL, Redfield MM. Epidemiology of heart failure with preserved ejection fraction. Nat Rev Cardiol. 2017;14(10):591-602.
2. Heidenreich PA, Bozkurt B, Aguilar D, et al. 2022 AHA/ ACC/ HFSA guideline for the management of heart failure: A report of the American College of Cardiology/American

Heart Association Joint Committee on clinical practice guidelines. J Am Coll Cardiol. 2022;79(17):1757-80.
3. Phan TT, Shivu GN, Abozguia K, et al. Impaired heart rate recovery and chronotropic incompetence in patients with heart failure with preserved ejection fraction. Circ Heart Fail. 2010;3(1):29-34.
4. Morrison RS, Meier DE. Palliative care. N Engl J Med. 2004;350:2582-90.
5. Diop MS, Rudolph JL, Zimmerman KM, et al. Palliative Care Interventions for Patients with Heart Failure: A Systematic Review and Meta-Analysis. J Palliat Med. 2017; 20(1):84-92.
6. Sahlollbey N, Lee CKS, Shirin A, et al. The impact of palliative care on clinical and patient-centred outcomes in patients with advanced heart failure: a systematic review of randomized controlled trials. Eur J Heart Fail. 2020;22(12):2340-6.
7. Kavalieratos D, Gelfman LP, Tycon LE, et al. Palliative care in heart failure: rationale, evidence, and future priorities. J Am Coll Cardiol. 2017;70(15):1919-30.
8. Quinn KL, Shurrab M, Gitau K, et al. Association of Receipt of Palliative Care Interventions with Health Care Use, Quality of Life, and Symptom Burden Among Adults with Chronic Noncancer Illness: A Systematic Review and Meta-Analysis. JAMA. 2020;324(14):1439-50.
9. Ziehm J, Farin E, Seibel K, et al. Health care professionals' attitudes regarding palliative care for patients with chronic heart failure: an interview study. BMC Palliat Care. 2016;15:76.
10. Crousillat DR, Keeley BR, Buss MK, et al. Palliative care education in cardiology. J Am Coll Cardiol. 2018; 71(12):1391-4.
11. Hill L, Prager Geller T, Baruah R, et al. Integration of a palliative approach into heart failure care: A European Society of Cardiology Heart Failure Association position paper. Eur J Heart Fail. 2020;22(12):2327-39.
12. Chang YK, Allen LA, McClung JA, et al. Criteria for referral of patients with advanced heart failure for specialized palliative care. J Am Coll Cardiol. 2022;80(4):332-44.
13. Vaduganathan M, Patel RB, Michel A, et al. Mode of death in heart failure with preserved ejection fraction. J Am Coll Cardiol. 2017;69(5):556-69.
14. Manolis AS, Manolis AA, Manolis TA, et al. Sudden death in heart failure with preserved ejection fraction and beyond: an elusive target. Heart Fail Rev. 2019;24: 847-66.
15. Evangelista LS, Lombardo D, Malik S, et al. Examining the effects of an outpatient palliative care consultation on symptom burden, depression, and quality of life in patients with symptomatic heart failure. J Card Fail. 2012; 18:894-9.
16. Oktay AA, Rich JD, Shah SJ. The emerging epidemic of heart failure with preserved ejection fraction. Curr Heart Fail Rep. 2013;10:401-10.

18

CHAPTER

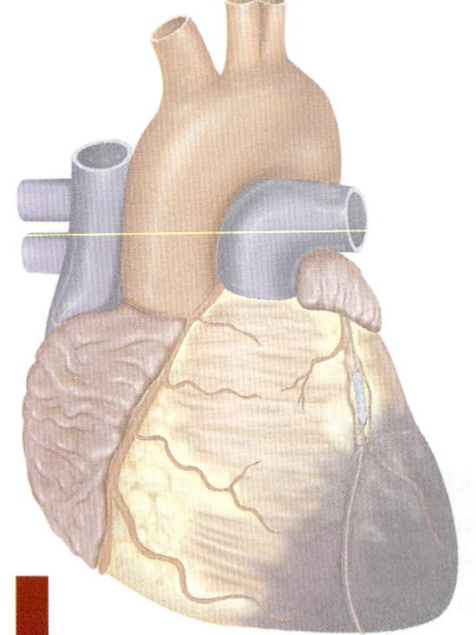

Fat, Female, Fatigued: Features of the Obese HFpEF Phenotype

Vitull K Gupta, Meghna Gupta, Manpreet Singh Brar

INTRODUCTION

Heart failure (HF) is considered to be a clinical syndrome rather than a disease, increasingly being recognized as a global occurrence adversely affecting more that 60 million people worldwide.[1] There is paucity of modern population-based prospective studies to document the true prevalence of HF with preserved ejection fraction (HFpEF). Most of the current estimates are largely based on electronic health records showing the prevalence of known HF to be 1–2% the adult population and it is estimated that 50% are HFpEF.[2] However, a meta-analysis documented calculated prevalence of 4.2% of all-type HF in the general population and about 3% for HFpEF.[3]

Epidemiological evidence show that prevalence of HFpEF relative to HF with reduced ejection fraction (HFrEF) is increasing at a rate of 1% per year, suggesting that HFpEF is becoming the most common type of HF.[2]

DEFINITION AND CLASSIFICATION OF HEART FAILURE[4]

In 2021, universal definition and classification of HF was suggested, defining HF as a clinical syndrome with signs and/or symptoms caused by functional and/or cardiac abnormality, corroborated by increased natriuretic peptide (NP) levels with or without objective evidence of systemic or pulmonary congestion. The stages were also revised defining state A as at risk for HF, stage B as pre-HF, stage C as symptomatic HF, and stage D as advanced HF. Recently the classification based on LVEF was also revised, including categories of HF with reduced LVEF (HFrEF; EF ≤40%), mildly reduced LVEF (HFmrEF; EF 41–49%) and HF with preserved LVEF (HFpEF; EF ≥50%). A new category of HF with improved LVEF (HFimpEF; baseline LVEF ≤40%, a ≥10 point increase from baseline LVEF, and a second measurement of LVEF >40%) was included to explain the dynamic clinical picture of HF syndrome and patients showing substantial improvement in LVEF with therapy.

HEART FAILURE WITH PRESERVED EJECTION FRACTION

In the CHARM program "preserved ejection fraction" term was first mentioned.[5] International guidelines took decades to agree on the nomenclature of HFpEF. First the European Society of Cardiology (ESC) in 2008 used the term HFpEF instead of "diastolic HF."[6] HFpEF is recognized as a dominant form of HF, and presently, about 50% of all diagnosed HF are HFpEF.[7] Various studies and registries estimated the prevalence of HFpEF to be between 19 and 55% of all HF cases. Presently, it is estimated that HFpEF represents about one-third to one-half of all individuals suffering from HF.[8]

In India there is paucity of studies documenting the prevalence of HFpEF but acute HF registry of 7,507 patients documented 67.5% patients of HFrEF, 17.6% patients with HFmrEF and 14.9% patients with HFpEF of all patients of HF.[9] The National Heart Failure Registry including 10,851 acute HF patients from 53 tertiary hospitals from 21 Indian states between 2019 and 2020 and documented the prevalence of 65.2% patients of HFrEF, 22% HFmrEF and 12.7% patients with HFpEF.[10] A South Indian registry including 449 patients documented prevalence of 65.9% HFrEF, 20% HFmrEF, and 14.03% HFpEF.[11]

PATHOPHYSIOLOGY

Previously, HFpEF was seen as solely a LV diastolic dysfunction but with more evidence HFpEF is now considered to be a heterogeneous multisystem entity with complex pathophysiology partly triggered by inflammation with contributions from genetic predisposition, aging, lifestyle factors, and multiple comorbidities along with multisystem structural and functional abnormalities.[7]

Alterations in HFpEF including endothelial dysfunction, LV hypertrophic remodeling, prolonged myocardial relaxation, ventricular dyssynchrony, increases in chamber stiffness, atrial dysfunction and atrial fibrillation (AF), right ventricle (RA) dysfunction, pulmonary vascular disease, pericardial restraint, chronotropic incompetence, altered myocardial energetic, reduced myocardial ATP availability, altered substrate utilization, mild systolic ventricular dysfunction, volume expansion, systemic inflammation, neurohormonal activation, and multiple noncardiac organ dysfunction.[12,13]

HEART FAILURE WITH PRESERVED EJECTION FRACTION PHENOTYPES: COMPLEX CLINICAL PUZZLE

Pathophysiological complexity and clinical heterogeneity of HFpEF have lead researchers to propose specific phenotypes. Shah et al., one of the first research groups identified phenotypes based on comorbidities related to obesity, metabolic syndrome (MS), and pulmonary hypertension (PH).[14]

Uijil et al. suggested five clusters of HFpEF based on age and comorbidities induced from recorded of the Swedish Heart Failure Registry externally validating it with the Chronic Heart Failure European Society of Cardiology guideline-based Cardiology Practice Quality project registry.[15] Review by Peters et al. identified the three most recurrent HFpEF phenotypes, "older, vascular aging,' "metabolic, obese" and "NP deficiency" phenotype.[16]

Presently six major phenotypes of HFpEF are described according to distinct clinical features, aging phenotype, obesity or cardio metabolic phenotype, arterial hypertension phenotype, pulmonary arterial hypertension phenotype, coronary artery disease (CAD) phenotype, and left atrial myopathy phenotype.[8]

This chapter explores the obese HFpEF phenotype, focusing on the triad of obesity, female gender, and fatigue.

Obesity Phenotype

Various epidemiological studies have documented a strong association between HFpEF and obesity. About 80% of patients with HFpEF are obese or overweight. More than half of all HF patients of HFpEF are associated with comorbidity of obesity and heterogeneous MS including HTN, insulin resistance (IR), diabetes, and hyperlipidemia.[8]

PATHOPHYSIOLOGY OF OBESE HEART FAILURE WITH PRESERVED EJECTION FRACTION[13,17,18]

Pathophysiology of obese HFpEF is suggested to be multifactorial involving complex association between inflammatory, hemodynamic, and metabolic pathways, though still pathophysiology is incompletely understood. Chronic inflammatory state is suggested to activate the fibrotic pathways causing cardiomyocyte stiffening, microvascular, and endothelial dysfunction causing pulmonary vasoconstriction, insufficient skeletal muscle perfusion, and renal hyperfiltration along with other organ dysfunctions. Multiorgan dysfunction observed in HFpEF is suggested to be mediated by autonomic dysfunction, neurohormonal activation, and increased production of reactive oxygen species (ROS). Higher body mass especially visceral fat deposition via metabolic dysfunctions such as IR, impaired free fatty acid storage, expanded total blood volume, increases cardiac filling pressures and ventricular remodeling contributes to adverse cardiac, and extracardiac manifestations. There is strong evidence to support excess of proinflammatory epicardial adipose tissue as an independent risk factor for HFpEF and is responsible for both systolic and diastolic cardiac dysfunction.[8,19]

Obesity and diabetes are the main cause of systemic microvascular inflammation, adversely affecting cardiomyocyte and increase in fibrosis.[19] Evidence from USA and European cohorts suggest critical role of regional, abdominal visceral, and/or epicardial adiposity in pathophysiology and outcomes of patients with HFpEF as compared to simply total body mass index.[16]

Obstructive sleep apnea (OSA) has high prevalence among obese individuals and is considered as another factor responsible for HFpEF. Multiple mechanisms triggered by hypoxia increases oxidative stress are implicated in the pathophysiology of HFpEF in patients of OSA.[8]

Obokata et al. documented that obese HFpEF patients showed increased plasma volume expansion, more profound RV dysfunction, more concentric biventricular remodeling, elevated pericardial restraint, worse exercise competence, more severe disarrangements in hemodynamics with exercise and weaker pulmonary vasodilation as compared to nonobese HFpEF, and control group without HF.[20] Obesity may cause neurohormonal stimulation such as renin-angiotensin-aldosterone system (RAAS) activation, sympathetic nervous system (SNS), and activation of adipokines causing fluid retention, increased sodium reabsorption causing shifting of blood from splanchnic circulation to the central circulation, HTN and cardiac remodeling.[21]

New pathophysiological mechanisms continue to emerge exploring the association as well as interplay between HFpEF and obesity.

Fat, Female, Fatigued: Clinical Characteristics

The obese HFpEF phenotype more commonly seen in females is associated with clinically unique cardinal HF symptom of fatigue. Savji et al. provided epidemiologic insights into triad of "Fat, Female and Fatigued" which is increasingly being recognized as a significant and distinct clinical subset and a cardinal risk feature for future development of HFpEF.[3]

Clinical Characteristics of Being Fat

Hemodynamic studies comparing obese, nonobese HFpEF, and controls demonstrated worse exercise capacity, depressed PA vasodilatory reserve, and more biventricular filling pressures in obese HFpEF. Moreover, RV dysfunction, cardiomegaly due to increased epicardial adiposity causing enhanced pericardial restraint and ventricular interaction was observed in obese HFpEF.[12,20]

Posthoc analysis of the RELAX trial also showed similar results of worse peak oxygen consumption and 6-minute walk distance in obese HFpEF as compared with nonobese HFpEF.[22]

Clinical Characteristics of Being Female

Gender differences are present in many aspects of HFpEF but because of paucity of gender specific studies, our understanding is largely limited. Evidence suggests that globally the prevalence of obesity is higher in females and every one standard deviation increase in BMI leads to 34% increase risk of HFpEF.[23] Epidemiological data suggest that HFpEF is more common in females than in males. A study showed 67% females had HFpEF as compared to 42% men.[2] Swede-HF registry reported 55% HFpEF as compared to 29% HFrEF among all HF patients.[24] This gender difference is particularly pronounced in the obese HFpEF phenotype as higher prevalence of HFpEF in females has been shown as compared to males.[12]

A study showed HFpEF hospitalizations were double in females than males. Moreover among females, the lifetime risk of HFpEF is almost double (10.7 vs. 5.8%), than that of HFrEF among females whereas the lifetime risk of HFrEF and HFpEF was similar among men.[25] A study from four community-based cohorts showed strong association of obesity and related cardiometabolic traits with risk of future HFpEF as compared to HFrEF, moreover, results documented pronounced differential risk of HFpEF with obesity especially among females that may underlie gender differences in HF subtypes.[3]

Several female-specific risk factors such as neurogenically triggered coronary dysfunction such as takotsubo cardiomyopathy, metabolic and autoimmune disorders such as rheumatoid arthritis and SLE, peripartum cardiomyopathy, and radiotherapy-induced cardiomyopathy in breast cancer may trigger endothelial inflammation and microvascular dysfunction increasing the risk of HFpEF. Systemic and pulmonary endothelial impairment is more in females, an important pathophysiological mechanism of HFpEF.[26]

Clinical Characteristics of Fatigue[8,27,28]

Chronic fatigue is a debilitating and prominent symptom in obese HFpEF patients and 59% patients with HFpEF typically exhibit fatigue. The mechanisms causing fatigue are multifactorial including reduced cardiac output, skeletal muscle abnormalities, sleep-disordered breathing issues, and psychosocial factors. Obesity itself as well as because of IR and chronic inflammation is associated with reduced muscle mass, muscle wasting, weakness and muscle dysfunction termed as sarcopenic obesity further exacerbate fatigue in patients of HFpEF. Sarcopenic obesity is characterized by the loss of muscle mass in spite of high body fat. OSA in obese HFpEF is responsible for intermittent hypoxia and disturbed fragmented sleep resulting in daytime sleepiness causing fatigue. Moreover, obesity-related symptoms in patients of HFpEF including physical limitations and chronic fatigue are more as compared to nonobese patients and adversely affect quality of life in obese female population with HFpEF.

Obesity Paradox in Heart Failure with Preserved Ejection Fraction

Obesity is a well-established risk factor for HFpEF and like most chronic diseases, obesity paradoxically provides protection against adverse outcomes in established HFpEF patients.[13]

These observations are largely based on cross-sectional studies, which are limited by reverse causation that is patients of severe HF may lose weight due to cachexia and survival bias that increasingly sick obese patients die before assessment. A Mendelian randomization study has raised questions with the obesity paradox in HF after overcoming the limitations of cross-sectional analyses.[29] An observational cohort suggested a relatively minor risk showing the hazard ratio of 1.04 (95% CI, 1.03–1.06) for HF mortality per 1 kg/m^2 increase in BMI. In contrast, with

Mendelian randomization a potentially stronger causal relationship (causal risk ratio 1.18; 95% CI, 1.00–1.38) between high BMI and HF mortality was shown for the same 1 kg/m^2 increase in BMI, though the differential relationships may have been because of differences in population characteristics.[29] Other studies have shown no paradox and continuous increase in risk of all-cause and CV mortality with greater body fat measured by more specific measures of adiposity like weight circumference instead of BMI.[30] A longitudinal multinational study, demonstrated the value of different adiposity parameters in assessing the outcomes in established HF showing better outcomes with higher BMI, yet in patients with HF, higher waist circumference was associated with worse outcomes.[31]

DIAGNOSIS

The diagnosis of HFpEF in fat, female, and fatigued involves a combination of clinical evaluation, imaging, and laboratory tests used routinely in diagnosis of HF with symptoms of breathlessness and fatigue along with objective evidence of congestion and an EF ≥50% including detailed assessment of obesity-related comorbidities such as diabetes, HTN, and OSA.

Typically, in patients with overt symptoms and signs of breathlessness and congestion, the diagnosis might be straightforward in patients fulfilling the ESC criteria of NT-proBNP >125 pg/mL in sinus rhythm, >365 pg/mL in AF, brain natriuretic peptide (BNP) of >35 pg/mL in sinus rhythm or >105 pg/mL in AF, evidence of congestion on radiological investigation or of elevated filling pressures on echocardiography.[2]

Echocardiography is the cornerstone of diagnosis, staging, and classification of HF and evidence of diastolic dysfunction help in diagnosis of HFpEF. But absence evidence of congestion or diastolic dysfunction does not exclude diagnosis of HFpEF because LV filling pressures are normal at rest and only increase during exercise in about one-third of patients with HFpEF so exercise testing is needed to diagnose or exclude HFpEF. For diagnosis of HFpEF the new universal definition requires presence of objective evidence of congestion and for that gold standard diagnostic test is hemodynamic assessment with right heart catheterization during rest and exercise. Since invasive testing is costly and not universally available, exercise stress echocardiography can be used as an alternative but is often limited by the ability to get quality imaging during stress and false-negative results.[12]

BNP or NT-proBNP is useful in HFpEF diagnosis but due to increased clearance and lower secretions because of other factors such as IR, NPPB polymorphisms, and increased androgenicity in females, the levels may be lower in obese patients in spite of elevated LV filling pressures, so normal levels cannot be used to rule out HFpEF.[12]

Diagnostic scoring systems, the H_2FPEF, and HFA-PEFF (Heart Failure Association Pre-test assessment, Echocardiography and NP, Functional testing, Final etiology) scores have been used to evaluate patients with possible HFpEF, with low or high scores are used to exclude or diagnose HFpEF, respectively, and intermediate scores patients are referred for exercise testing. But in patients with signs and symptoms of overt HF, elevated NPs, a low H_2FPEF score does not exclude HFpEF, but may suggest atypical causes of HFpEF like infiltrative cardiomyopathies.[12]

Cardiac MRI can evaluate extent of myocardial fibrosis and subtle abnormalities not picked up by echocardiography. Cardiac CT may be used to diagnose CAD often associated with obese HFpEF patients.

MANAGEMENT

Management options are limited for patients with HFpEF as compared to well established guideline based quadruple therapy including renin-angiotensin system inhibitors (RASis), sodium-glucose cotransporter 2 inhibitors (SGLT2is), β-blockers, and mineralocorticoid receptor antagonists (MRAs) for management of HFrEF. Since HFpEF is a complex syndrome, it is difficult to identify a specific pharmacological treatment, so identification of clinical phenotype may play an important role in selecting specific strategies to treat specific pathophysiological alterations and comorbidities, both cardiac and noncardiac.

NONPHARMACOLOGICAL MANAGEMENT[32]

The nonpharmacological or life style management is similar in all HF including weight loss, heart-healthy diet and nutrition, physical activity in form of regular resistance or aerobic exercise, tobacco or smoking cessation, and abstinence or moderation of alcohol intake can improve symptoms, CV health, muscle strength, overall fitness, well-being, and improves prognosis in HFpEF.

PHARMACOLOGICAL MANAGEMENT

Evidence suggests differential gender responses to pharmacological management of HF because of differences in the pharmacodynamics and pharmacokinetics drugs.[23] Considering the cardinal pathophysiological mechanisms of the obese phenotype, SGLT2i, RAASi, MRAs, diuretics, and neprilysin inhibitors (ARNI) are increasingly being used in management of HFpEF.[33]

Diuretics[13]

Diuretics effectively reduce filling pressures and congestion as obese HFpEF often show volume expansion, but obese HFpEF patients may poorly tolerate diuresis as compared to nonobese HFpEF, with increased risk of worsening renal function in spite of marked volume expansion. Therapy is initiated with loop diuretics, if insufficient diuresis is observed, addition of a thiazide or thiazide like diuretic or MRAs is suggested individually or in combination.

Mineralocorticoid Antagonists[8,13]

Evidence suggests greater benefit of MRAs in obese HFpEF. A meta-analysis including three randomized trials (TOPCAT, Aldo-DHF, and HOMAGE) showed improvement in patients with HFpEF with spironolactone, but failed to show reduction in all-cause mortality and only showed reduction hospitalization rates in HFpEF, as compared to HFrEF patients. Posthoc analyses of TOPCAT showed greater benefit from MRA in patients with lower NT-proBNP levels and more prominent central adiposity, whereas HFrEF patients with greater waist circumference showed more favorable results with eplerenone as compared to patients without central obesity.

Neprilysin Inhibitors[13]

Neprilysin is expressed on adipocytes and degrades BNP and other vasoactive peptides, suggesting beneficial effect on obese HFpEF. Results of PARAGON-HF trial narrowly missed statistical significance in reduction in the rate of HF hospitalizations or CV death, (rate ratio, 0.87; $p = 0.06$) with treatment of the dual neprilysin/ARB, sacubitril valsartan, but subgroup analysis showed clinical benefit in females and patients with LVEF <57%.

STATINS[13]

Statins reduce systemic inflammation, which is implicated in pathogenesis of obese HFpEF. Nochioka et al. observed that there is some evidence of reduced mortality in patients with HFpEF with statin. Observational studies have shown association of statins with lower event rates in HFpEF, though data from RCTs is lacking.

Sodium–Glucose Cotransporter 2 Inhibitors[2,8,13]

First positive outcome trials in HFpEF were published in 2021 and 2022. SGLT2i reduced the composite of CV death and HF hospitalizations by 20% [hazard ratio (HR) 0·80; 95% CI 0·73–0·87; p <0·0001] in the EMPEROR Preserved and DELIVER trials. The ESC 2023 Heart Failure Guideline update has given class 1a recommendation for SGLT2i use in HFpEF. SGLT2i improves patients with HF along the entire spectrum, from HFrEF to HFpEF.

GLP-1 Receptor Agonists

In the STEP-HFpEF trial, GLP-1RA semaglutide showed greater reduction in symptoms and physical limitations with marked improvement in exercise function, weight reduction, and health status in HFpEF patients. Reduction in levels of NT-proBNP was about 15% more with semaglutide as compared to placebo indicating reduction in LV filling pressures. Semaglutide also reduced C-reactive protein levels.[34] This trial will in future define the role of GLP-1RA in management of obese HFpEF phenotype.

MANAGEMENT OF COMORBIDITIES

Management of underlying comorbidity and modifiable risk factors for HF forms the core of therapeutic recommendations in management of HFpEF. Commonly associated comorbidities with HFpEF such as HTN, CAD, obesity, sleep apnea, anemia, diabetes, CKD, AF, and chronotropic incompetence might accelerate disease progression and contribute to increased morbidity and mortality. Pragmatic strategies for management of comorbidities are addressed in various international and national guidelines.

CONCLUSION

Present chapter provides insight in to the triad of "fat, female, fatigued" which constitute the cardinal features of obese HFpEF phenotype. Obese HFpEF phenotype presents unique challenges in understanding pathophysiology, clinical presentation, diagnosis, and management. A comprehensive, multidisciplinary approach is suggested to manage the complex interaction of factors contributing to obese HFpEF phenotype. Since there is no universally accepted management approach for patients with HFpEF and its phenotypes particularly obese phenotype, the ideal strategy is to focus on lifestyle modifications, optimal management of risk factors and comorbidities, and incorporating personalized therapeutic strategies including SGLT2i, RAASi, β-blockers, MRAs, neprilysin inhibitors (ARNI), and GLP-1RA to improve outcomes and quality of life for patients of obese HFpEF phenotype. In spite of important advances in understanding of obese HFpEF phenotype, several gaps still persist in our knowledge of HFpEF in females, as females are underrepresented in trials and male predominant studies are represented in guidelines, necessitating further studies to fill the gaps in our knowledge about obese HFpEF phenotype especially in female population.

REFERENCES

1. Savarese G, Becher PM, Lund LH, et al. Global burden of heart failure: a comprehensive and updated review of epidemiology. Cardiovasc. 2023;118(17):3272-87.
2. Campbell P, Rutten FH, Lee MM, et al. Heart failure with preserved ejection fraction: everything the clinician needs to know. Lancet. 2024;403(10431):1083-92.
3. Savji N, Meijers WC, Bartz TM, et al. The association of obesity and cardiometabolic traits with incident HFpEF and HFrEF. JACC Heart Fail. 2018;6(8):701-09.
4. Shahim B, Kapelios CJ, Savarese G, et al. Global Public Health Burden of Heart Failure: An Updated Review. Card Fail Rev. 2023;9:e11.
5. Swedberg K, Pfeffer M, Granger C, et al. Candesartan in heart failure: assessment of reduction in mortality and morbidity (CHARM): rationale and design. Charm-Programme Investigators. J Card Fail. 1999;5(3):276-82.
6. von Haehling S, Assmus B, Bekfani T, et al. Heart failure with preserved ejection fraction: diagnosis, risk assessment, and treatment. Clin Res Cardiol. 2024;113(9):1287-305.
7. Redfield MM, Borlaug BA. Heart failure with preserved ejection fraction: a review. JAMA. 2023;329:827-38.
8. Stoicescu L, Crişan D, Morgovan C, et al. Heart Failure with Preserved Ejection Fraction: The Pathophysiological Mechanisms behind the Clinical Phenotypes and the Therapeutic Approach. Int J Mol Sci. 2024;25(2):794.
9. Joseph S, Panniyammakal J, Abdullakutty J, et al. The Cardiology Society of India-Kerala Acute Heart Failure Registry: poor adherence to guideline-directed medical therapy. Eur Heart J. 2022;43(9):908-15.
10. Harikrishnan S, Bahl A, Roy A, et al. Clinical profile and 90 day outcomes of 10851 heart failure patients across India: national Heart Failure Registry. ESC Heart Fail. 2022;9:3898-908.
11. Shukkoor AA, George NE, Radhakrishnan S, et al. Clinical characteristics and outcomes of patients admitted with acute heart failure: insights from a single-center heart failure registry in South India. Egypt Heart J. 2021;73(1):38.
12. Borlaug B, Sharma K, Shah SJ, et al. Heart Failure with Preserved Ejection Fraction: JACC Scientific Statement. JACC. 2023;81(18):1810-34.
13. Borlaug BA, Jensen MD, Kitzman DW, et al. Obesity and heart failure with preserved ejection fraction: new insights and pathophysiological targets. Cardiovascular Research. 2022;118:3434-50.
14. Shah SJ, Katz DH, Selvaraj S, et al. Phenomapping for novel classification of heart failure with preserved ejection fraction. Circulation. 2015;131:269-79.
15. Uijl A, Savarese G, Vaartjes I, et al. Identification of distinct phenotypic clusters in heart failure with preserved ejection fraction. Eur J Heart Fail. 2021;23:973-82.
16. Peters AE, Tromp J, Shah SJ, et al. Phenomapping in heart failure with preserved ejection fraction: insights, limitations, and future directions. Cardiovascular Research. 2022;118(18):3403-15.
17. Nanni M, Hu V, Eriksson MJ, et al. Phenotypic differences in obese patients with heart failure with preserved ejection fraction (HFpEF)-a mini review. New Insights. Obes Gene Beyond. 2024;8:001-5.
18. Koepp KE, Obokata M, Reddy YNV, et al. Hemodynamic and functional impact of epicardial adipose tissue in Heart Failure With Preserved Ejection Fraction. JACC Heart Fail. 2020;8(8):657-66.
19. Kitzman DW, Lam CSP. Obese heart failure with preserved ejection fraction phenotype: from pariah to central player. Circulation. 2017;136:20-3.
20. Obokata M, Reddy YNV, Pislaru SV, et al. Evidence Supporting the Existence of a Distinct Obese Phenotype of Heart Failure With Preserved Ejection Fraction. Circulation. 2017;136(1):6-19.
21. Da Young Lee. Obesity and heart failure with preserved ejection fraction: pathophysiology and clinical significance. Cardiovascular Prevention and Pharmacotherapy. 2022; 4(2):70-4.
22. Reddy YNV, Lewis GD, Shah SJ, et al. Characterization of the obese phenotype of heart failure with preserved ejection fraction: a RELAX trial ancillary study". Mayo Clin Proc. 2019;94:1199-209.
23. Maddury J. Heart failure in women. Indian J Cardiovasc Dis Women. 2022;7(3):162-74.
24. Savarese G, Vasko P, Jonsson A, et al. The Swedish heart failure registry: a living, ongoing quality assurance and research in heart failure. Ups J Med Sci. 2019;124(1): 65-9.
25. Pandey A, Omar W, Ayers C, et al. Sex and race differences in lifetime risk of heart failure with preserved ejection fraction and heart failure with reduced ejection fraction. Circulation. 2018;137(17):1814-23.
26. Teramoto K, Teng TK, Chandramouli C, et al. Epidemiology and clinical features of heart failure with preserved ejection fraction. Card Fail Rev. 2022;8:e27.
27. Kirkman DL, Bohmke N, Billingsley HE, et al. Sarcopenic obesity in heart failure with preserved ejection fraction. Front Endocrinol (Lausanne). 2020;11:558271.
28. Golla MSG, Shams P. Heart failure with preserved ejection fraction (HFpEF). In: StatPearls. Treasure Island (FL): StatPearls Publishing; 2024.
29. Benn M, Marott SCW, Tybjaerg-Hansen A, et al. Obesity increases heart failure incidence and mortality: observational and Mendelian randomization studies totalling over 1 million individuals. Cardiovasc Res. 2022; 118(18):3576-85.
30. Tsujimoto T, Kajio H. Abdominal obesity is associated with an increased risk of all-cause mortality in patients with HFpEF. J Am Coll Cardiol. 2017;70(22):2739-49.
31. Chandramouli C, Tay WT, Bamadhaj NS, et al.; ASIAN-HF Investigators. Association of obesity with heart failure outcomes in 11 Asian regions: a cohort study. PLoS Med. 2019;16:e1002916.
32. Tah S, Valderrama M, Afzal M, et al. Heart failure with preserved ejection fraction: an evolving understanding. Cureus. 2023;15(9):e46152.
33. Balestrieri G, Limonta R, Ponti E, et al. The therapy and management of heart failure with preserved ejection fraction: new insights on treatment. Cardiac Failure Review. 2024;10:e05.
34. Kosiborod MN, Abildstrøm SZ, Borlaug BA, et al. Semaglutide in patients with heart failure with preserved ejection fraction and obesity. N Engl J Med. 2023;389:1069-84.

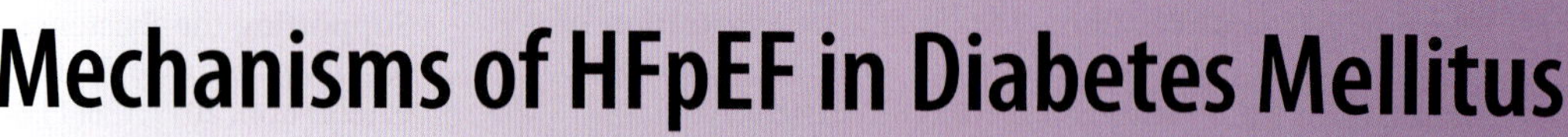

Mechanisms of HFpEF in Diabetes Mellitus

Lakshmi Nalini Kopalle

INTRODUCTION

Heart failure with preserved ejection fraction (HFpEF) is a common and serious complication of diabetes. Evidence from epidemiological data suggests that HFpEF occurs in about half of the patients with heart failure (HF). A preserved ejection fraction (EF) in heart failure is especially common in patients with diabetes mellitus (DM). 20–40% of people with HF have DM (T2D). The burden of DM as well as HF are on rise. According to IDF 2021, there are about 537 million individuals between the ages of 20 and 79 years, living with DM.[1]

DEFINITION

The HF defined based on EF can be categorized primarily into three categories. HF with reduced ejection fraction (HFrEF) where in EF <40%, HF with preserved ejection fraction (HFpEF), EF>50%, and the third type called borderline or HF with mildly reduced ejection fraction (HFmrEF), EF between 40–50%.

MECHANISMS OF HEART FAILURE WITH PRESERVED EJECTION FRACTION IN DIABETES MELLITUS

The diabetic heart undergoes structural as well as functional changes that often evolve into HF. Although the primary cause of HF is development of coronary disease, patients with diabetes can also develop HF independent of coronary artery disease and hypertension. There is increasing evidence that diabetes-associated heart disease is mediated, at least in part, by the direct action of excess glucose on cardiomyocytes, cardiac glucotoxicity. The pathophysiological mechanisms linking diabetes to HFpEF are complex and multifactorial, involving metabolic, neurohormonal, vascular, cellular, structural, and functional alterations in the heart. Diabetic heart is at an increased risk of fibrosis leading to heart failure.[2,3]

Metabolic Abnormalities

Reduction in cardiac insulin metabolic signaling due to insulin resistance is being increasingly identified as a major factor for the development of HF-the cardiometabolic syndrome.[3] Additionally, insulin resistance and chronic hyperglycemia in diabetes lead to alterations in myocardial energy metabolism. The heart shifts from utilizing glucose to increased fatty acid oxidation, which is less efficient and produces toxic intermediates, contributing to myocardial dysfunction. In insulin sensitive individuals, insulin acts via phosphatidylinositol 3 kinase (PI3- kinase)/protein kinase B (Akt) signaling pathway to elicit metabolic response causing uptake of glucose in myocardial tissue and skeletal muscle. Additionally, there is nitric oxide (NO)-mediated coronary vasodilation, metabolic flexibility, and energy homeostasis occurring in normal individuals.[4,5]

Oxidative stress in obese individuals induces activation of kinases including JNK and S6 kinase, via the mTor pathway. This results in "serine phosphorylation" of IRS-1 instead of tyrosine phosphorylation thus inhibiting insulin metabolic signaling. Additionally, insulin resistance causes accumulation of advanced glycation end-products (AGEs) in the myocardium, causing stiffness and impaired relaxation by cross-linking collagen and affecting extracellular matrix (ECM) proteins.

Microvascular Dysfunction

Endothelial dysfunction is the major component and causative factor of microvascular dysfunction. Multiple, interrelated mechanisms contribute to endothelial cell dysfunction in the presence of insulin resistance. The exact mechanism by which dyslipidemia contributes to endothelial dysfunction is unknown. Evidence from animal studies and in vitro studies point toward dysfunction of nitric oxide synthase (NOS) which is exaggerated by circulating oxidized LDL.[6,7] HDL cholesterol donates cholesterol and can prevent the oxidized LDL-mediated decrease in cholesterol in caveolae, prevent the translocation of endothelial NOS.[8] It is likely that many of the components of the metabolic syndrome directly alter endothelial vasoreactivity.

The presence of hypertension and other atherosclerotic risk factors is associated with increased RAAS activity. As discussed earlier, increased RAAS activity leads to oxidative stress and subsequent serine phosphorylation of IRS1 and decreased flexibility of endothelium.

Together, hyperglycemia and insulin resistance impair endothelial function, reducing NO availability and leading to microvascular rarefaction and ischemia **(Fig. 1)**.

Structural Factors

The obesity-LV concentric remodeling association was first reported in observational studies and later confirmed in several community-based cohorts.[9-11]

There is a loose correlation between obesity-induced LV concentric remodeling and left ventricular diastolic dysfunction (LVDD) suggesting other mechanisms than obesity heightened cardiac pre- and afterload.[12] Not unexpectedly, obesity is now a recognized risk factor for incident HFpEF.[13,14] Evidence from I-PRESERVE,[15,16] RELAX,[17] PARAGON-HF trials[18] clearly show the occurrence of HFpEF in obese individuals particularly women.

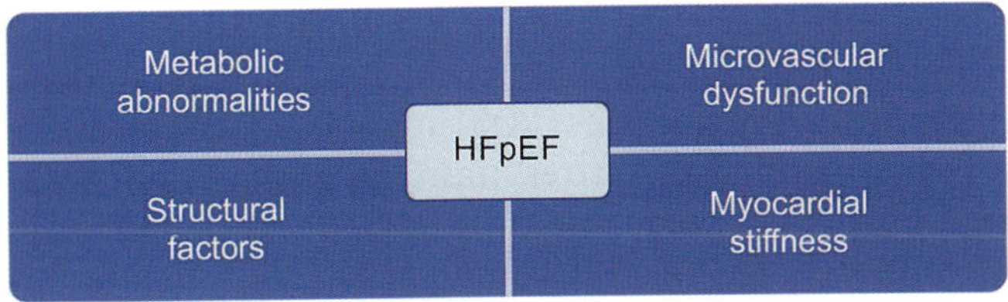

Fig. 1: Causes of HFpEF in diabetes.
(HFpEF: heart failure with preserved ejection fraction)

Myocardial Stiffness and Fibrosis (Box 1)

At the pathophysiological confluence of several vascular, neurohormonal, and cellular mechanisms lies myocardial fibrosis which is a hallmark of HFpEF. The myocardial stiffness arising out of the fibrosis along with diastolic dysfunction are the ultimate causes of HFpEF. Extensive evidence of presence of myocardial fibrosis in patients with diabetes and studies in diabetic patient employing cardiac magnetic resonance imaging (CMRI) identifies myocardial scars (replacement fibrosis) in diabetics with no history suggestive of myocardial infarction; these findings most likely reflect silent coronary events. Multiple signaling pathways exist for such an occurrence, most common of those are hyperglycemia induced activation of profibrotic pathways, neurohormonal activation, increase in proinflammatory cytokines and chemokine, formation of AGES, and ECM remodeling. A growing body of evidence suggests role microRNA (miRNA) in cardiac fibrosis.[19]

Hyperglycemia-induced Activation of Profibrotic Pathways

The role of hyperglycemia in mediating fibrotic remodeling of the diabetic heart remains unclear. The changes found in in vitro studies has not been observed in clinical data. Additionally, randomized controlled trials do not support the notion that intensive glycemic control reduces the incidence of heart failure in diabetics. Also, correction of hyperglycemia does not consistently attenuate diabetes-associated fibrosis in extracardiac tissues. High glucose stimulates fibroblast proliferation, promotes myofibroblast transdifferentiation, and activates transcription and secretion of ECM proteins in in vitro studies.[20,21] This effect of excess glucose is attributed to several interlinked mechanisms including activation of angiotensin II and transforming growth factor-beta (TGF-β) signaling, ROS generation and subsequent stimulation of Erk pathways.[20,22,23] Diabetes activates several profibrotic signaling pathways, including TGF-β and connective

BOX 1: Mechanisms of myocardial fibrosis.

- Hyperglycemia induced activation of profibrotic pathways
- Increase in proinflammatory cytokines and chemokines
- Formation of advanced glycation end products (AGES)
- Neurohormonal activation
- Extracellular matrix remodeling
- Autonomic dysfunction
- Renal dysfunction
- Mitochondrial dysfunction
- miRNA

tissue growth factor (CTGF), leading to increased collagen deposition and myocardial fibrosis.

Increase in Proinflammatory Cytokines and Chemokines

Activation of immune pathways and increased production of proinflammatory cytokines such as tumor necrosis factor-α (TNF-α), and interleukin (IL)-1β are associated with modulation of fibroblast phenotype and subsequently cardiac fibrosis. In cardiac fibroblasts, TNF-α stimulation induces proliferation and enhances collagen synthesis.[24] IL-1β on the other hand, delays myofibroblast conversion, promoting α matrix-degrading proinflammatory fibroblast phenotype.[25] The cellular targets of TNF-α and the molecular signals responsible for activation of a profibrotic program in the diabetic heart still remain unknown. Chemokines may also be implicated in cardiac fibrosis through direct actions on fibroblasts or through recruitment of fibro genic monocyte subsets.[26]

Formation of Advanced Glycation End Products

Due to prolonged exposure to glucose, proteins, and lipids undergo nonenzymatic glycation and oxidation, leading to formation of AGEs. In diabetic tissues, accelerated accumulation of AGEs may mediate inflammation and fibrosis. AGEs accumulate in both intracellular and extracellular space and may play a key role in diabetes-associated cardiac fibrosis through multiple mechanisms. These mechanisms range from simple accumulation of AGEs to direct receptor binding or via increasing the oxidative stress or macrophage mediated activation of profibrotic pathways.[27-31]

Neurohormonal Activation

Activation of neurohormonal systems (RAAS system) plays an important pathophysiological role in HF.[32] Increased activation of these systems has often been demonstrated in diabetes and is associated with adverse ventricular remodeling, arrhythmias, and cardiac death, mostly sudden. Additionally, a vicious self-promoting neurohormonal activation is often observed in diabetes which leads to more insulin resistance which further heightens the neurohormonal activity.[33]

RAAS system hyperactivation in diabetes has a multipronged effect that eventually causes cardiac fibrosis. Firstly, there is an increase in angiotensin-mediated AT1 signaling which promotes fibroblast activation via increased formation of reactive oxygen species (ROS). It also increases TGF-β expression and activation by stimulating both Smad-dependent and independent pathways.[34] Secondly, angiotensin II may additionally also accentuate TGF-β responses by inducing expression of the endoglin. Endoglin is a profibrotic TGF-β coreceptor.[35]

Extracellular Matrix Remodeling

The hallmarks of HFpEF include increased passive myocardial stiffness and diastolic dysfunction. The former depends mainly on two components: the ECM and the cardiomyocytes. Quantitative and qualitative changes in collagen metabolism leading to myocardial fibrosis determine the ECM-based stiffness of the myocardium. The imbalance between matrix metalloproteinases (MMPs) and their inhibitors (TIMPs) results in excessive extracellular matrix remodeling, contributing to diastolic dysfunction. AGEs along with increased oxidative stress and other mechanisms increases myocardial stiffness due either to collagen crosslinking and/or fibroblast activation.[36]

Autonomic Dysfunction

Diabetes-related autonomic neuropathy affects heart rate variability and impairs autonomic regulation of cardiac function, contributing to diastolic dysfunction and HFpEF. Sympathetic neural excitation has been assumed to contribute to the pathophysiology of HFpEF by impairing left ventricular relaxation and increasing diastolic left ventricular stiffness.[37,38]

Renal Dysfunction

Long standing uncontrolled blood sugars can cause diabetic microvascular injury leading to diabetic kidney disease. Subsequent to impaired renal function there is impaired sodium handling and volume overload. This exacerbates hypertension and contributes to myocardial stiffening and HFpEF.[39,40]

Mitochondrial Dysfunction and Formation of Reactive Oxygen Species

The increase in the plasma concentration of glucose causes overfueling of the mitochondria which results in production of reactive oxygen species (ROS) and subsequent oxidative stress. This oxidative stress inhibits glyceraldehyde-3-phosphate dehydrogenase (GAPDH). Alternate pathways of glucose metabolism become predominant due to this rerouting of glucose thus reducing the redox potential of the cardiac myocyte and further increasing ROS at cellular levels.

Additionally, hyperglycemia also promotes ROS production in a mitochondria-independent manner, via stimulation of the sodium-myoinositol cotransporter 1/ reduced nicotinamide adenine dinucleotide phosphate oxidase isoform 2 (SMIT1/NOX2) pathway. NOX2 is a multiprotein complex composed of the NOX isoform, Rac1, p91phox, and p47phox, and relaxation. Mitochondrial dysfunction contributes to energy deficit and myocardial stiffness.[41]

MicroRNAs

MicroRNAs (miRNAs) are short noncoding RNAs that regulate gene expression and are involved in virtually all cellular responses. A growing body of evidence suggests a critical role for miRNAs in cardiac fibrosis.[42] miRNAs have multiple targets, including cytokines and growth factors, extracellular matrix proteins, proteases, and even matricellular macromolecules, all of these are implicated directly and indirectly in the pathophysiology of HFpEF. Although we have limited evidence of role of miRNA in diabetes-associated cardiac fibrosis, evidence from mouse models of type 1 diabetes strongly points toward their role of type 1 diabetes.[43,44] Diabetic hearts had alterations, both up regulation of "profibrotic miRNA" as well as downregulation of "fibrosis inhibiting miRNA" in levels of several miRNAs. The up regulation of miR-125b and miR-199a, and downregulation of miR-150, miR-29b, and miR-30a has been observed. This, dysregulated expression of fibrosis-associated miRNAs remained altered despite receiving insulin therapy to achieve intensive glycemic control.[44] Over expression of miR-133 overexpression attenuated the fibrotic response attenuating Erk and Smad activation. Indirect evidence points toward downregulation of this miR-133 in a diabetic heart.[45] The role of miRNA in diabetic heart is still in its incipient phases and more information is required to identify the role of miRNA specific to diabetic cardiac fibrosis and subsequent HFpEF.

CONCLUSION

Heart failure with preserved ejection fraction remains a therapeutic conundrum. The obese-T2D phenotype has distinct pathophysiology encompassing inflammation, coronary microvascular dysfunction, and LV remodeling. Myocardial fibrosis and diastolic dysfunction are at the confluence of various mechanisms that lead to HFpEF. Knowledge of the underlying mechanisms causing HFpEF gives us insights into potential therapeutic possibilities and improve outcomes in HFpEF.

REFERENCES

1. Jia G, Whaley-Connell A, Sowers JR. Diabetic cardiomyopathy: a hyperglycaemia- and insulin-resistance-induced heart disease. Diabetologia. 2018;61(1):21-8.
2. Rodrigues B, Cam MC, McNeill JH. Metabolic disturbances in diabetic cardiomyopathy. Molecular and Cellular Biochemistry. 1998;180(1-2):53-7.
3. Aroor AR, Mandavia CH, Sowers JR. Insulin resistance and heart failure: molecular mechanisms. Heart Fail Clin. 2012;8(4):609-17.
4. Bertrand L, Horman S, Beauloye C, et al. Insulin signaling in the heart. Cardiovasc Res. 2008;79(2):238-48.
5. Saha AK, Xu XJ, Balon TW, et al. Insulin resistance due to nutrient excess: is it a consequence of AMPK downregulation? Cell Cycle. 2011;10(20):3447-51.
6. Rizzo V, McIntosh DP, Oh P, et al. In situ flow activates endothelial nitric oxide synthase in luminal caveolae of endothelium with rapid caveolin dissociation and calmodulin association. J Biol Chem. 1998;273(52): 34724-9.
7. Blair A, Shaul PW, Yuhanna IS, et al. Oxidized low-density lipoprotein displaces endothelial nitric-oxide synthase (eNOS) from plasmalemmal caveolae and impairs eNOS activation. J Biol Chem. 1999;274(45):32512-19.
8. Uittenbogaard A, Shaul PW, Yuhanna IS, et al. High-density lipoprotein prevents oxidized low-density lipoprotein-induced inhibition of endothelial nitric-oxide synthase localization and activation in caveolae. J Biol Chem. 2000; 275(15):11278-83.
9. Peterson LR, Waggoner AD, Schechtman KB, et al. Alterations in left ventricular structure and function in young healthy obese women: assessment by echocardiography and tissue Doppler imaging. J Am Coll Cardiol. 2004;43:1399-404.
10. Reis JP, Allen N, Gibbs BB, et al. Association of the degree of adiposity and duration of obesity with measures of cardiac structure and function: the CARDIA study. Obesity. 2014;22:2434-40.
11. Yan Y, Li S, Guo Y, et al. Life-Course Cumulative Burden of Body Mass Index and Blood Pressure on Progression of Left Ventricular Mass and Geometry in Midlife: the Bogalusa Heart Study. Circ. Res. 2020;126:633-43.
12. Russo C, Jin Z, Homma S, et al. Effect of obesity and overweight on left ventricular diastolic function: a community-based study in an elderly cohort. J Am Coll Cardiol. 2011;57(12):1368-74.
13. Savji N, Meijers WC, Bartz TM, et al. of Obesity and Cardiometabolic Traits With Incident HFpEF and HFrEF. JACC Heart Fail. 2018;6(8):701-9.
14. Pandey A, Patel KV, Vaduganathan M, et al. Physical Activity, Fitness, and Obesity in Heart Failure With Preserved Ejection Fraction. JACC Heart Fail. 2018;6(12):975-82.
15. Massie BM, Carson PE, McMurray JJ, et al. Irbesartan in patients with heart failure and preserved ejection fraction. N Engl J Med. 2008;359:2456-67.

16. Haass M, Kitzman DW, Anand IS, et al. Body mass index and adverse cardiovascular outcomes in heart failure patients with preserved ejection fraction: results from the Irbesartan in Heart Failure with Preserved Ejection Fraction (I-PRESERVE) trial. Circ. Heart Fail. 2011;4(3):324-31.
17. Reddy YNV, Lewis GD, Shah SJ, et al. Characterization of the Obese Phenotype of Heart Failure With Preserved Ejection Fraction: a RELAX Trial Ancillary Study. Mayo Clin Proc. 2019;94(7):1199-209.
18. McMurray JJV, Jackson AM, Lam CSP, et al. Effects of Sacubitril-Valsartan Versus Valsartan in Women Compared With Men With Heart Failure and Preserved Ejection Fraction: insights From PARAGON-HF. Circulation. 2020; 141(5):338-51.
19. Russo I, Frangogiannis NG. Diabetes-associated cardiac fibrosis: Cellular effectors, molecular mechanisms and therapeutic opportunities. J Mol Cell Cardiol. 2016;90: 84-93.
20. Han DC, Isono M, Hoffman BB, et al. High glucose stimulates proliferation and collagen type I synthesis in renal cortical fibroblasts: mediation by autocrine activation of TGF-beta. J Am Soc Nephrol. 1999;10(9):1891-9.
21. Shamhart PE, Luther DJ, Adapala RK, et al. Hyperglycemia enhances function and differentiation of adult rat cardiac fibroblasts. Can J Physiol Pharmacol. 2014;92(7):598-604.
22. Fiaschi T, Magherini F, Gamberi T, et al. Hyperglycemia and angiotensin II cooperate to enhance collagen I deposition by cardiac fibroblasts through a ROS-STAT3-dependent mechanism. Biochim Biophys Acta. 2014;1843(11): 2603-10.
23. Tang M, Zhang W, Lin H, et al. High glucose promotes the production of collagen types I and III by cardiac fibroblasts through a pathway dependent on extracellular-signal-regulated kinase 1/2. Mol Cell Biochem. 2007;301:109-14.
24. Venkatachalam K, Venkatesan B, Valente AJ, et al. WISP1, a pro-mitogenic, pro-survival factor, mediates tumor necrosis factor-alpha (TNF-alpha)-stimulated cardiac fibroblast proliferation but inhibits TNF-alpha-induced cardiomyocyte death. J Biol Chem. 2009;284:14414-27.
25. Saxena A, Chen W, Su Y, et al. IL-1 induces proinflammatory leukocyte infiltration and regulates fibroblast phenotype in the infarcted myocardium. J Immunol. 2013;191(9): 4838-48.
26. Dobaczewski M, Frangogiannis NG. Chemokines and cardiac fibrosis. Front Biosci (Schol Ed). 2009;1(2):391-405.
27. Goldin A, Beckman JA, Schmidt AM, et al. Advanced glycation end products: sparking the development of diabetic vascular injury. Circulation. 2006;114:597-605.
28. Zhao LM, Zhang W, Wang LP, et al. Advanced glycation end products promote proliferation of cardiac fibroblasts by upregulation of KCa3.1 channels. Pflugers Arch. 2012; 464:613-21.
29. Oldfield MD, Bach LA, Forbes JM, et al. Advanced glycation end products cause epithelial-myofibroblast transdifferentiation via the receptor for advanced glycation end products (RAGE) J Clin Invest. 2001;108(12):1853-63.
30. Yamazaki KG, Gonzalez E, Zambon AC. Crosstalk between the renin-angiotensin system and the advance glycation end product axis in the heart: role of the cardiac fibroblast. J Cardiovasc Transl Res. 2012;5(6):805-13.
31. Singh R, Barden A, Mori T, et al. Advanced glycation end-products: a review. Diabetologia. 2001;44(2):129-46.
32. Levine TB, Francis GS, Goldsmith SR, et al. Activity of the sympathetic nervous system and renin-angiotensin system assessed by plasma hormone levels and their relation to hemodynamic abnormalities in congestive heart failure. Am J Cardiol. 1982;49(7):1659-66.
33. Miller JA, Floras JS, Zinman B, et al. Effect of hyperglycaemia on arterial pressure, plasma renin activity and renal function in early diabetes. Clin Sci (Lond). 1996; 90(3):189-95.
34. Zhou Y, Poczatek MH, Berecek KH, et al. Thrombospondin 1 mediates angiotensin II induction of TGF-beta activation by cardiac and renal cells under both high and low glucose conditions. Biochem Biophys Res Commun. 2006; 339(2): 633-41.
35. Chen K, Mehta JL, Li D, et al. Transforming growth factor beta receptor endoglin is expressed in cardiac fibroblasts and modulates profibrogenic actions of angiotensin II. Circ Res. 2004;95:1167-73.
36. Franssen C, González Miqueo A. The role of titin and extracellular matrix remodelling in heart failure with preserved ejection fraction. Neth Heart J. 2016;24(4):259-67.
37. van der Horst IC, de Boer RA, Hillege HL, et al. Neurohormonal profile of patients with heart failure and diabetes. Neth Heart J. 2010;18(4):190-6.
38. Vinik AI, Ziegler D. Diabetic cardiovascular autonomic neuropathy. Circulation. 2007;115(3):387-97.
39. Patel RB, Mehta R, Redfield MM, et al. Renal Dysfunction in Heart Failure With Preserved Ejection Fraction: Insights From the RELAX Trial. J Card Fail. 2020;26(3):233-42.
40. Kolset SO, Reinholt FP, Jenssen T. Diabetic nephropathy and extracellular matrix. J Histochem Cytochem. 2017; 65(4):229-39.
41. Bugger H, Abel ED. Mitochondria in the diabetic heart. Cardiovascular Res. 2010;88(2):229-40.
42. Thum T. Noncoding RNAs and myocardial fibrosis. Nat Rev Cardiol. 2014;11(11):655-63.
43. Diao X, Shen E, Wang X, et al. Differentially expressed microRNAs and their target genes in the hearts of streptozotocin-induced diabetic mice. Mol Med Rep. 2011; 4(4):633-40.
44. Costantino S, Paneni F, Luscher TF, et al. MicroRNA profiling unveils hyperglycaemic memory in the diabetic heart. Eur Heart J. 2016;37(6):572-6.
45. Chen S, Puthanveetil P, Feng B, et al. Cardiac miR-133a overexpression prevents early cardiac fibrosis in diabetes. J Cell Mol Med. 2014;18:415-21.

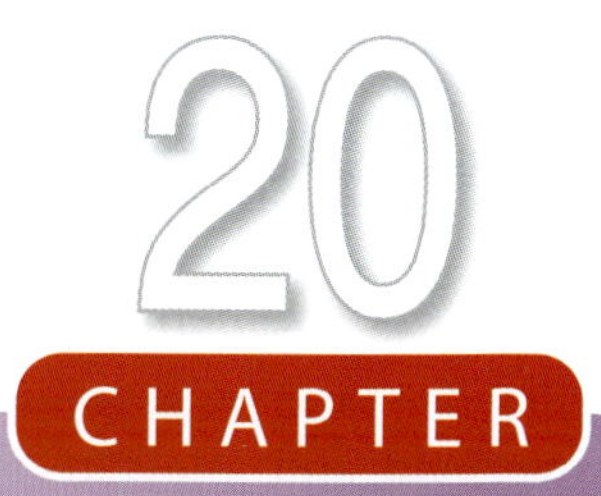

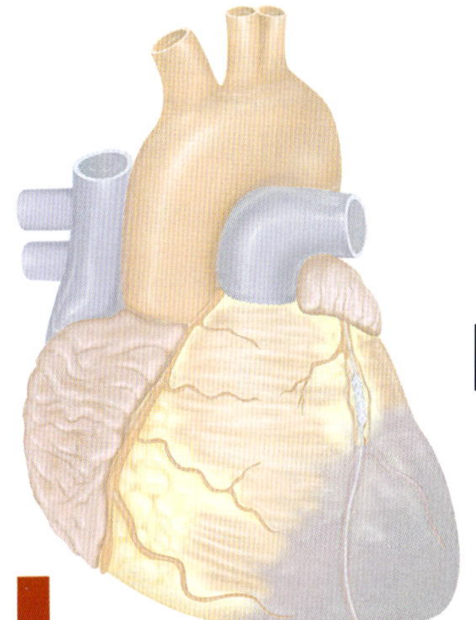

Nonpharmacological Therapies for HFpEF

Dharmendra Jain, Vikash K Maurya, Umesh K Pandey, Suyash Tripathi, Soumik Ghosh, Rajpal Prajapati

INTRODUCTION

Heart failure with preserved ejection fraction (HFpEF) constitutes a substantial portion of heart failure cases, making up nearly half of all HF hospitalizations. HFpEF is characterized by heart failure symptoms alongside a normal or nearly normal left ventricular ejection fraction (LVEF), presenting unique challenges for effective treatment. While pharmacological approaches have shown limited success in improving outcomes for HFpEF patients, nonpharmacological therapies offer promising alternatives for enhancing quality of life and clinical outcomes. Various nonpharmacological interventions for HFpEF includes lifestyle changes, exercise regimens, device-based therapies, and emerging methods under research.

PATHOPHYSIOLOGY OF HEART FAILURE WITH PRESERVED EJECTION FRACTION

The HFpEF is a multifaceted clinical syndrome stemming from structural and functional abnormalities in the myocardium, vasculature, and other organ systems. Understanding these mechanisms is essential for developing effective nonpharmacological therapies. Key mechanisms include:

- *Diastolic dysfunction:* Impaired relaxation and increased stiffness of the left ventricle.
- *Endothelial dysfunction:* Reduced nitric oxide bioavailability, leading to impaired vasodilation.
- *Inflammation and oxidative stress:* Chronic systemic inflammation contributing to myocardial fibrosis and dysfunction.
- *Comorbidities:* Conditions such as obesity, hypertension, diabetes, and atrial fibrillation, which are often associated with HFpEF and exacerbate its progression.

NONPHARMACOLOGICAL THERAPIES FOR HEART FAILURE WITH PRESERVED EJECTION FRACTION

Lifestyle Modifications

Dietary Interventions

Dietary management is a fundamental aspect of HFpEF therapy. Key dietary recommendations include:

- *Sodium restriction:* Reducing sodium intake to lower fluid retention and blood pressure.
- *Balanced diet:* Emphasizing the intake of fruits, vegetables, whole grains, and lean proteins to improve overall cardiovascular health.
- *Weight management:* Achieving and maintaining a healthy weight to decrease the burden on the heart.

Several studies have demonstrated the benefits of dietary interventions for HFpEF patients. For instance, the dietary approaches to stop hypertension (DASH) diet has been shown to lower blood pressure and improve symptoms in HF patients.[1]

Fluid Management

Effective fluid management is crucial to prevent volume overload and alleviate symptoms in HFpEF patients. Recommendations include:

- *Monitoring fluid intake:* Tracking daily fluid intake to avoid excessive fluid retention.
- *Daily weighing:* Monitoring weight changes to detect early signs of fluid accumulation.

Exercise Training

Exercise training is among the most effective non-pharmacological interventions for HFpEF, improving cardiovascular fitness, enhancing quality of life, and reducing symptoms. Key components of exercise training include:

- *Aerobic exercise*

Aerobic exercises such as walking, cycling, and swimming have been shown to improve peak oxygen uptake (VO_2 peak) and exercise tolerance in HFpEF patients. Regular aerobic exercise also enhances endothelial function and reduces inflammation.[2]

- *Resistance training*

Resistance training, which involves weight lifting or resistance bands, helps improve muscle strength and endurance. Combining resistance training with aerobic exercise has shown synergistic effects on functional capacity and quality of life in HFpEF patients.[3]

- *High-intensity interval training*

High-intensity interval training (HIIT) involves short bursts of intense exercise followed by periods of rest or low-intensity exercise. HIIT has gained attention for its ability to improve cardiovascular fitness more efficiently than continuous moderate-intensity exercise. Studies have demonstrated significant improvements in VO_2 peak and endothelial function with HIIT in HFpEF patients[3-8] **(Table 1)**.

Device-based Therapies

Several device-based therapies have been explored for managing HFpEF, targeting different aspects of the disease pathophysiology.

Continuous Positive Airway Pressure

Sleep-disordered breathing, particularly obstructive sleep apnea (OSA), is common in HFpEF patients and contributes to disease progression. Continuous positive airway pressure (CPAP) therapy has been shown to improve sleep quality, reduce blood pressure, and enhance left ventricular function in patients with HFpEF and OSA.[9]

Implantable Hemodynamic Monitors

Implantable hemodynamic monitors, such as the CardioMEMS™ device, provide continuous monitoring of pulmonary artery pressures. This allows for early detection of fluid overload and timely adjustment of therapy. The role of one implantable pulmonary artery sensor, CardioMEMS (Abbott, Abbott Mark, and Illinois) was evaluated in the CHAMPION (CardioMEMS Heart Sensor Allows Monitoring of Pressure to Improve Outcomes in NYHA Class III Heart Failure Patients) trial. Clinical trials have demonstrated reduced HF hospitalizations

TABLE 1: Studies for nonpharmacological intervention in heart failure with preserved ejection fraction (HFpEF).

Study	Sample size	Intervention	Outcome
Edelmann et al.[3]	64	3 months of endurance/resistance training	• Peak VO_2 increased by 3.3 mL/kg/min • Improved quality of life • Improvement in E/e' and left atrial volume index
Mueller et al.[5]	176	12 weeks of high-intensity interval training and moderate continuous training	Improved peak VO_2 at 3 months
Kitzman et al.[6]	63	16 weeks of exercise training	• Peak VO_2 increased by 2 mL/kg/min • Improved quality of life
Kitzman et al.[7]	100	20 weeks of caloric restriction, aerobic exercise, or both	Increase in peak VO_2 by: • *Exercise:* 1.2 mL/kg/min • *Diet:* 1.3 mL/kg/min • *Both (additive):* 2.5 mL/kg/min
Brubaker et al.[8]	88	20 weeks of (caloric restriction and aerobic exercise) ± resistance training	• Addition of resistance training to caloric restriction and aerobic exercise • Increase in leg strength and muscle quality • No additive increase in peak VO_2 or quality of life (QOL)

TABLE 2: Studies for nonpharmacological intervention in heart failure with preserved ejection fraction (HFpEF).

Study	Sample size	Intervention	Outcome
Adamson et al.[15]	119	Implantable pulmonary artery monitor	50% reduction in HF hospitalization with mean follow-up of 17.6 months
Lindenfeld et al.[16]	795	Implantable pulmonary artery monitor	No reduction in all-cause mortality, HF hospitalizations, and urgent HF visits

and improved quality of life with the use of implantable hemodynamic monitors in HF patients[10] **(Table 2)**.

Baroreflex Activation Therapy

Baroreflex Activation Therapy (BAT) involves electrical stimulation of the carotid sinus to activate the baroreflex, resulting in reduced sympathetic activity and improved cardiovascular function. Preliminary studies have shown promising results in reducing blood pressure and improving quality of life in HFpEF patients.[11]

Other device interventions for HFpEF such as blood volume analysis, interatrial shunting devices, splanchnic nerve ablation, or cardiac contractility modulation are under evaluation; their benefits remain ambiguous. Such procedures should be considered only within the context of clinical trials.[12-14]

Novel Approaches and Future Directions

Cardiac Rehabilitation

Cardiac rehabilitation programs offer comprehensive management, including exercise training, education, and psychological support. Participation in cardiac rehabilitation has been associated with improved functional capacity, reduced hospitalizations, and enhanced quality of life in HF patients.[17]

Yoga and Mind-body Interventions

Yoga and other mind-body interventions, such as Tai Chi and meditation, have been explored for their potential benefits in HFpEF. These interventions can reduce stress, improve exercise tolerance, and enhance overall well-being.[18]

Nutritional Supplements

- Several nutritional supplements, including omega-3 fatty acids, coenzyme Q10, and vitamin D, have been investigated for their potential benefits in HFpEF. While some studies have shown promising results, further research is needed to establish their efficacy and safety in this patient population.[19]

LIMITATIONS OF NONPHARMACOLOGICAL THERAPIES FOR HEART FAILURE WITH PRESERVED EJECTION FRACTION

Lifestyle Modifications

Adherence Challenges

One of the main limitations of lifestyle modifications, such as dietary changes and sodium restriction, is patient adherence. Long-term adherence to dietary recommendations can be challenging due to the habitual nature of eating patterns, cultural food preferences, and the availability of healthier food options. Many patients find it difficult to sustain these changes over the long term, which can limit the effectiveness of these interventions.

Variable Impact

The impact of lifestyle modifications can vary significantly among individuals. Factors such as age, comorbidities, socioeconomic status, and baseline dietary habits can influence the degree of benefit patients receive from dietary interventions and other lifestyle changes. This variability makes it difficult to standardize recommendations and predict outcomes.

Exercise Training

Patient Limitations

Exercise training is a cornerstone of nonpharmacological therapy for HF, but it has limitations related to patient-specific factors. Patients with severe HF symptoms, advanced age, or multiple comorbidities may find it difficult to engage in and sustain regular exercise programs. Additionally, physical limitations such as joint problems or other musculoskeletal issues can hinder participation in exercise training.

Supervision and Accessibility

Effective exercise training often requires supervision by healthcare professionals, especially in the initial stages, to ensure safety and proper technique. This need for supervision can limit the accessibility of exercise programs, particularly for patients in rural or underserved areas.

Moreover, the costs associated with supervised exercise programs can be a barrier for some patients.

Device-based Therapies

Cost and Accessibility

Device-based therapies, such as CPAP for sleep-disordered breathing and implantable hemodynamic monitors, can be expensive and may not be accessible to all patients. The cost of these devices and the associated medical procedures can be prohibitive, especially for patients without adequate health insurance coverage.

Invasive Nature

Some device-based therapies involve invasive procedures, which carry inherent risks such as infection, bleeding, and complications related to device implantation. The invasive nature of these treatments can be a significant drawback, particularly for older patients or those with multiple comorbidities who are at higher risk for procedural complications.

Novel Approaches and Future Directions

Limited Evidence

Many novel nonpharmacological approaches, such as yoga, mind-body interventions, and nutritional supplements, have limited evidence supporting their efficacy in HF management. While preliminary studies may show promise, larger, well-designed clinical trials are needed to establish their effectiveness and safety conclusively. The lack of robust evidence can limit the acceptance and implementation of these therapies in clinical practice.

Individual Response Variability

The response to novel interventions can vary widely among individuals. Factors such as genetics, baseline health status, and environmental influences can affect how patients respond to these therapies. This variability poses a challenge in predicting which patients will benefit the most from specific interventions, making it difficult to tailor treatments effectively.

Comprehensive Management and Coordination

Need for Multidisciplinary Approach

Effective nonpharmacological management of HF often requires a multidisciplinary approach involving cardiologists, dietitians, physical therapists, and other healthcare professionals. Coordinating care among these providers can be challenging, particularly in healthcare systems with fragmented services. Ensuring that patients receive comprehensive, coordinated care is crucial for optimizing outcomes but can be difficult to achieve in practice.

Patient Education and Engagement

Educating patients about the importance of nonpharmacological therapies and engaging them in their care is essential for success. However, this requires significant time and resources from healthcare providers. Patients may also face barriers to engagement, such as low health literacy, lack of motivation, or competing life priorities, which can limit the effectiveness of these interventions.

GUIDELINES

2022 AHA/ACC/HFSA Guideline for the Management of Heart Failure[20] (Tables 3 to 6)

TABLE 3: Recommendations for nonpharmacological interventions: Self-care support in heart failure (HF).

COR	*LOE*	*Recommendation*
1	A	Patients with HF should receive care from multidisciplinary teams to facilitate the implementation of GDMT, address potential barriers to self-care, reduce the risk of subsequent rehospitalization for HF, and improve survival
1	B-R	Patients with HF should receive specific education and support to facilitate HF self-care in a multidisciplinary manner
2a	B-NR	In patients with HF, vaccinating against respiratory illnesses is reasonable to reduce mortality
2a	B-NR	In adults with HF, screening for depression, social isolation, frailty, and low health literacy as risk factors for poor self-care is reasonable to improve management

TABLE 4: Recommendation for dietary sodium restriction.

COR	*LOE*	*Recommendation*
2a	C-LD	For patients with stage C HF, avoiding excessive sodium intake is reasonable to reduce congestive symptoms

TABLE 5: Recommendations for management of stage C heart failure (HF): Activity, exercise prescription, and cardiac rehabilitation.

COR	LOE	Recommendation
1	A	For patients with HF who are able to participate, exercise training (or regular physical activity) is recommended to improve functional status, exercise performance, and QOL
2a	B-NR	In patients with HF, a cardiac rehabilitation program can be useful to improve functional capacity, exercise tolerance, and health-related QOL

TABLE 6: Recommendation for wearables and remote monitoring (including telemonitoring and device monitoring).

COR	LOE	Recommendation
2b	B-R	In selected adult patients with NYHA class III HF and history of a HF hospitalization in the past year or elevated natriuretic peptide levels, on maximally tolerated stable doses of GDMT with optimal device therapy, the usefulness of wireless monitoring of PA pressure by an implanted hemodynamic monitor to reduce the risk of subsequent HF hospitalizations is uncertain

CONCLUSION

Nonpharmacological therapies play a vital role in managing HFpEF, offering significant benefits in symptom relief, functional improvement, and quality of life enhancement. Lifestyle modifications, exercise training, and device-based therapies are key components of a comprehensive management plan for HFpEF patients. Additionally, novel approaches such as cardiac rehabilitation, yoga, and nutritional supplements hold promise for future therapeutic strategies. Continued research and clinical trials are essential to further refine these interventions and develop personalized treatment plans for HFpEF patients.

REFERENCES

1. Sacks FM, Obarzanek E, Windhauser MM, et al. Rationale and design of the Dietary Approaches to Stop Hypertension trial (DASH). A multicenter controlled-feeding study of dietary patterns to lower blood pressure. Ann Epidemiol. 1995;5(2):108-118.
2. Kitzman DW, Brubaker PH, Morgan TM, et al. Exercise training in older patients with heart failure and preserved ejection fraction: a randomized, controlled, single-blind trial. Circ Heart Fail. 2010;3(6):659-67.
3. Edelmann F, Gelbrich G, Düngen HD, et al. Exercise training improves exercise capacity and diastolic function in patients with heart failure with preserved ejection fraction: results of the Ex-DHF (Exercise training in Diastolic Heart Failure) Pilot Study. J Am Coll Cardiol. 2011;58(17):1780-91.
4. Angadi SS, Mookadam F, Lee CD, et al. High-intensity interval training vs. moderate-intensity continuous exercise training in heart failure with preserved ejection fraction: a pilot study. J Appl Physiol (1985). 2015;119(6): 753-8.
5. Mueller S, Winzer EB, Duvinage A, et al. Effect of high-intensity interval training, moderate continuous training, or guideline-based physical activity advice on peak oxygen consumption in patients with heart failure with preserved ejection fraction: a randomized clinical trial. JAMA. 2021;325:542-51.
6. Kitzman DW, Brubaker PH, Herrington DM, et al. Effect of endurance exercise training on endothelial function and arterial stiffness in older patients with heart failure and preserved ejection fraction: a randomized, controlled, single-blind trial. J Am Coll Car-diol. 2013;62:584-92.
7. Kitzman DW, Brubaker P, Morgan T, et al. Effect of caloric restriction or aerobic exercise training on peak oxygen consumption and quality of life in obese older patients with heart failure with preserved ejection fraction: a randomized clinical trial. JAMA. 2016;315:36-46.
8. Brubaker PH, Nicklas BJ, Houston DK, et al. A randomized, controlled trial of resistance training added to caloric restriction plus aerobic exercise training in obese heart failure with preserved ejection fraction. Circ Heart Fail. 2023;16:e010161.
9. Oldenburg O, Lamp B, Faber L, et al. Sleep-disordered breathing in patients with symptomatic heart failure: a contemporary study of prevalence in and characteristics of 700 patients. Eur J Heart Fail. 2007;9(3):251-7.
10. Abraham WT, Adamson PB, Bourge RC, et al. Wireless pulmonary artery haemodynamic monitoring in chronic heart failure: a randomised controlled trial. Lancet. 2011;377(9766):658-66.
11. Zile MR, Lindenfeld J, Weaver FA, et al. Baroreflex activation therapy in patients with heart failure with reduced ejection fraction. J Am Coll Cardiol. 2020;76(1):1-13.
12. Shah SJ, Feldman T, Ricciardi MJ, et al. One-year safety and clinical outcomes of a transcatheter interatrial shunt device for the treatment of heart failure with preserved ejection fraction in the Reduce Elevated Left Atrial Pressure in Patients With HeartFailure (REDUCE LAP-HF I) trial: a randomized clinical trial. JAMA Cardiol. 2018;3: 968-77.
13. Feldman T, Mauri L, Kahwash R, et al. Transcatheter interatrial shunt device for the treatment of heart failure with preserved ejection fraction [REDUCELAP-HF I (Reduce Elevated Left Atrial Pressure in Pa-tients with

Heart Failure)]: a phase 2, randomized, sham-controlled trial. Circulation. 2018;137:364-75.

14. Shah SJ, Borlaug BA, Chung ES, et al. Atrial shunt device for heart failure with preserved and mildly reduced ejection fraction (REDUCE LAP-HF II): a randomised, multicentre, blinded, sham-controlled trial. Lancet. 2022;399:1130-40.
15. Adamson PB, Abraham WT, Bourge RC, et al. Wireless pulmonary artery pressure monitoring guides management to reduce decompensation in heart failure with preserved ejection fraction. Circ Heart Fail. 2014;7:935-44.
16. Lindenfeld J, Zile MR, Desai AS, et al. Haemodynamic-guided management of heart failure (GUIDE-HF): a randomized controlled trial. Lancet. 2021;398:991-1001.
17. Taylor RS, Walker S, Ciani O, et al. Exercise-based cardiac rehabilitation for chronic heart failure: the EXTRAMATCH II individual participant data meta-analysis. Health Technol Assess. 2019;23(25):1-98.
18. Yeh GY, McCarthy EP, Wayne PM, et al. Tai Chi exercise in patients with chronic heart failure: a randomized clinical trial. Arch Intern Med. 2011;171(8):750-7.
19. Butler J, Teng TK, Bao H, et al. Clinical course of patients with heart failure and preserved ejection fraction. J Am Coll Cardiol. 2019;73(5):579-89.
20. Heidenreich, P, Bozkurt, B, Aguilar, D. et al. 2022 AHA/ACC/HFSA Guideline for the Management of Heart Failure: A Report of the American College of Cardiology/American Heart Association Joint Committee on Clinical Practice Guidelines. JACC. 2022;79(17):e263-e421.

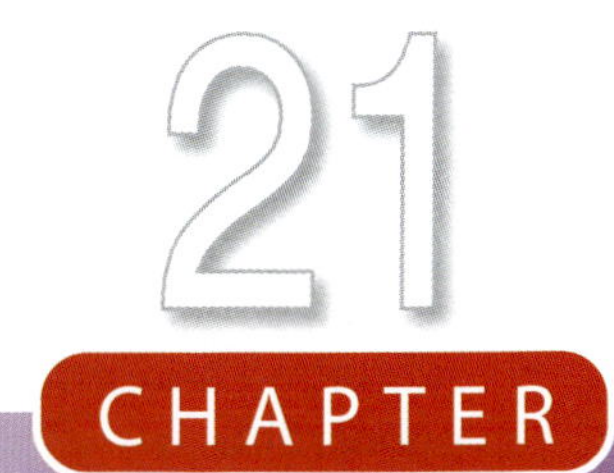

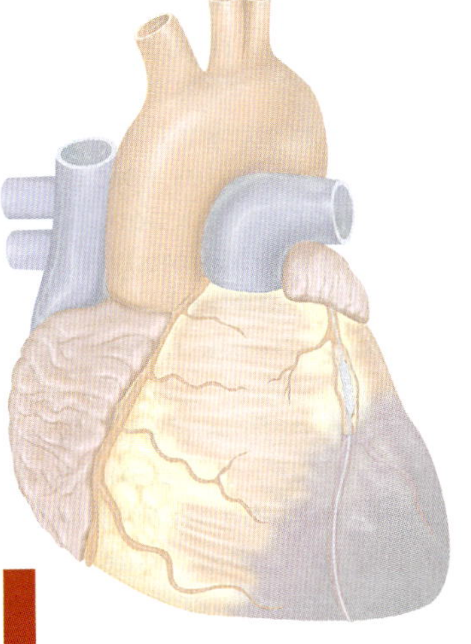

HFpEF Management: What are Newer Advances?

Mohsin Raj Mantoo, Nitish Naik

INTRODUCTION

Heart failure (HF) is a clinical syndrome characterized by symptoms and/or signs (like dyspnea, orthopnea, fatigue, edema, rales, etc.) attributed to a structural and/or functional cardiac abnormality like reduced ejection fraction or impaired diastolic filling. The contemporary "universal definition of HF" also impresses upon the objective evidence of systemic or pulmonary congestion like rales, jugular venous distention, or edema on physical examination, raised natriuretic peptide levels, raised E/e′ on echocardiography or raised ventricular filling pressures on invasive hemodynamic assessment.[1] Subsequently, the presence of a preserved left ventricular (LV) ejection fraction (LVEF ≥50%) is required for making a diagnosis of HFpEF. HF is a clinical diagnosis; however, history and physical exam alone cannot differentiate HFrEF from HFpEF. The prevalence of HFpEF has increased over years so it now accounts for almost 50% of overall HF population.[2] Heart failure with preserved ejection fraction (HFpEF) is the most common type of HF in elderly (age >65 years).

The symptoms of HFpEF are nonspecific and can be explained by a myriad of comorbidities that are common in this patient population. To aid in the diagnosis of HFpEF, various societal guideline documents have come up with HFpEF diagnostic scoring systems (H_2FPEF score in the American guidelines and HFA-PEFF score in the European guidelines) that have been validated against the gold standard—"exercise invasive hemodynamics".[3,4] The H_2FPEF score is based on clinical and echocardiographic parameters including age, body mass index (BMI), hypertension, atrial fibrillation (AF), and echocardiographic evidence of pulmonary hypertension (estimated PASP >35 mm Hg), and raised filling pressures (E/e′ >9). A weighted score based on these six variables is used to generate the H_2FPEF score ranging from 0 to 9. Scores <2 and >5 predict low and high likelihood of HFpEF, respectively. A score between 2 and 5 requires further testing like exercise echocardiography or invasive hemodynamic assessment for clarification of diagnosis. HFA-PEFF score is more elaborate and incorporates pretest clinical likelihood of HFpEF, laboratory parameters like natriuretic peptide levels as well as echocardiographic pointers of structural and functional ventricular abnormality [like E/e′, LV wall thickness, LV mass, left atrium (LA) volume, global longitudinal strain, etc.].

RULING OUT THE NONHEART FAILURE WITH PRESERVED EJECTION FRACTION CAUSES

Heart failure signs and symptoms with a normal LVEF are not always just HFpEF. Clues from clinical evaluation as well as multimodality imaging may point to specific etiologies with entirely different treatments.

Clues from history:

- Atypical epidemiology (young, lean, and male)
- Atypical comorbidities (absence of hypertension, diabetes, and obesity)
- *Classic patterns:*
  - *Bilateral carpal tunnel syndrome, dysautonomia:* Amyloidosis
  - *Acroparesthesias, kidney disease:* Fabry disease

  - *Diabetes, bronze skin:* Hemochromatosis
  - *Radiation and prior cardiac surgery:* Constrictive pericarditis
  - *Heart blocks, ventricular arrhythmias:* Sarcoidosis
- *Clues from physical examination:*
  - *Periorbital ecchymoses, macroglossia:* Amyloidosis
  - *Dysautonomia:* Amyloidosis
  - *Kussmaul's sign and pericardial knock:* Constrictive pericarditis
- *Clues from imaging:*
  - *Thick walls with sparkling echotexture, biatrial enlargement, and atrial septal hypertrophy:* Amyloidosis
  - *Asymmetric septal hypertrophy with outflow obstruction and mitral valve abnormalities:* Hypertrophic cardiomyopathy
  - *Apical sparing pattern on GLS imaging:* Amyloidosis
  - *Biatrial enlargement and markedly reduced tissue Doppler velocities (medial and lateral e'):* Restrictive cardiomyopathy
  - *Diffuse subendocardial late gadolinium enhancement on MRI:* Amyloidosis

MANAGEMENT OF COMORBIDITIES

Treatment of the comorbidities (hypertension, diabetes, obesity, etc.) is the mainstay of therapy in HFpEF. It is important to stick to the established guidelines for these comorbidities. Treatment of hypertension to a target <130/80 mm Hg using the guideline-recommended antihypertensive agents is important. Obesity is highly prevalent in HFpEF and has been implicated in the evolution of this disease phenotype as well as key outcomes. Diet and lifestyle modifications targeting weight loss are recommended in these patients. There is evidence from randomized trial data that weight loss through calorie restriction improves exercise capacity (peak VO_2) and reduces markers of inflammation in obese patients with HFpEF.[5] As discussed below, various antiobesity drugs have been shown to improve the functional status and adverse HF events in this population subset. Treatment of diabetes to target HBA1C values (<7%) is recommended with preferential use of agents like Sodium-glucose cotransporter 2 (SGLT2) inhibitors and glucagon-like peptide-1 (GLP-1) receptor agonists.

Atrial fibrillation is common in HFpEF and its management should focus on prevention of stroke and systemic embolism (HFpEF patients need anticoagulation, irrespective of $CHA_2DSVASc_2$ score) and rate and rhythm control according to the latest available guidelines. There are no dedicated randomized trials of AF ablation in HFpEF. Some observational data and HFpEF subsets of studies like EAST AFNET-4 and CABANA do point to a significant clinical benefit of aggressive rhythm control strategy in this subgroup.[6]

Coronary artery disease (CAD) is present in nearly two-thirds of HFpEF patients. This includes epicardial CAD as well as coronary microvascular dysfunction. There is data from observational studies that demonstrate the benefit of coronary revascularization in HFpEF patients with significant angina or demonstrable myocardial ischemia.[7,8]

Patients with concomitant iron deficiency (defined as serum ferritin <100 ng/mL or 100–300 ng/mL with transferrin saturation <20%) should be treated with intravenous iron therapy to improve their functional capacity and quality of life (although this stems from the data done in patients with reduced ejection fraction).

GUIDELINE-DIRECTED MEDICAL THERAPY FOR HEART FAILURE WITH PRESERVED EJECTION FRACTION

There has been a paradigm shift in how we approach management of HFpEF with new therapies showing promising results in large, randomized studies.

Diuretics

Loop diuretics are recommended to relieve congestive symptoms in HFpEF, just like HFrEF (class I recommendation). Thiazide diuretics (e.g., hydrochlorothiazide) may be added for synergistic effects, particularly in patients with resistant edema. However, diuretics only produce symptom relief and do not modify the natural history of HF. Paradoxically, diuresis can result in amplification of neurohormonal pathways implicated in HF progression.

Sodium–Glucose Cotransporter 2 Inhibitors

For the first time in history, we now have agents like empagliflozin and dapagliflozin that reduce HF events in patients with HFpEF. These agents, initially developed for diabetes management, have demonstrated favorable effects on HF outcomes. The mechanisms underlying these benefits include diuresis, natriuresis, and improved myocardial metabolism. EMPEROR-Preserved trial randomized 5,988 HFpEF patients (defined as LVEF >40%) to empagliflozin versus placebo. At around 2 years follow-up, empagliflozin was associated with a 21% relative risk reduction in the primary composite endpoint of cardiovascular (CV) death or HF hospitalization

(HR 0.79, 95% CI 0.69–0.90, $p < 0.001$). This was driven by a reduction in HF hospitalizations and there was no statistically significant reduction in CV deaths.[9] Similarly, DELIVER trial for dapagliflozin enrolled 6,263 HFpEF (LVEF >40%) patients and demonstrated a significant 18% reduction in composite endpoint of worsening HF or CV death (HR: 0.82, 95% CI 0.73–0.92, $p < 0.001$). There was no statistically significant difference in deaths due to CV cause (HR: 0.88, 95% CI: 0.74–1.05).[10] In a subsequent meta-analysis, SGLT2i use reduced the composite endpoint of CV death or first HF hospitalization (HR 0.80, 95% CI 0.73–0.87) including a significant reduction of CV death (HR: 0.87, 95% CI: 0.79–0.95).[11] Based on these data, guidelines now recommend use of SGLT2i in all HFpEF patients, irrespective of diabetes status (class IIa recommendation in ACC guidelines and class I in European guidelines).[3,12]

Renin–Angiotensin–Aldosterone System Inhibitors

The ACEi/ARBs/ARNI and mineralocorticoid receptor antagonists (MRAs) are given class IIb recommendations in ACC and ESC HFpEF guidelines. The studies evaluating the efficacy of these agents were largely negative like CHARM-preserved (candesartan), I-PRESERVE (irbesartan), and PEP-CHF (perindopril).

Sacubitril-valsartan, an ARNI, was compared against valsartan in HFpEF population (defined as LVEF >45%) in the PARAGON-HF trial. The primary composite endpoint of total HF hospitalizations and CV death was numerically in favor of ARNI, but it barely missed statistical significance (HR: 0.87, 95% CI 0.75–1.01, $p = 0.06$).[13] Following these results, the US FDA expanded the indication of ARNI to include HFpEF patients as well.

Mineralocorticoid receptor antagonists such as spironolactone and eplerenone, have shown promise in HFpEF management. Even though the trial for spironolactone (TOPCAT) was a negative trial, there was some evidence of benefits in favor of spironolactone like reduced HF hospitalizations or benefits in female subgroup. MRAs help mitigate fibrosis and inflammation, contributing to improved diastolic function. However, their use requires careful monitoring of renal function and potassium levels due to the risk of hyperkalemia.

A recent trial, FINEARTS-HF trial, evaluated the safety and efficacy of nonsteroidal MRA (finerenone) in patients with HF and mildly reduced or preserved ejection fraction. Finerenone produced a statistically significant reduction in the primary composite outcome of CV death or worsening HF event.[14]

Newer Therapies

Heart failure with preserved ejection fraction and obesity often coexist. Obesity-related HFpEF (compared to nonobese HFpEF) is characterized by younger age, expanded plasma volume, lower NTproBNP levels, more inflammation (higher CRP levels), worse symptoms and functional status as well as impaired response to decongestion. Recently, drugs that specifically target obesity have been tested in HFpEF population and have shown promising results. Semaglutide, GLP-1RA, was recently studied in a randomized trial (STEP-HFpEF) that enrolled 529 HFpEF patients who were obese (body mass index of 30 or higher) to receive once-weekly subcutaneous semaglutide or placebo for 52 weeks. Semaglutide use was associated with greater weight loss (absolute difference of −10.7 percentage points) and a greater improvement in quality of life as assessed by Kansas City cardiomyopathy questionnaire (KCCQ-CSS).[15] Another study (STEP-HFpEF DM trial) randomized patients with HFpEF, obesity, and type 2 diabetes and found a greater improvement in KCCQ-CSS as well as weight loss in semaglutide arm.[16] Hence, semaglutide is emerging as yet another agent to improve symptoms in obese HFpEF patients. However, its impact on hard endpoints like CV death and HF hospitalizations is unclear.

Tirzepatide, a dual glucose-dependent insulinotropic polypeptide (GIP) and GLP-1RA, has recently shown promise in HFpEF as demonstrated by the SUMMIT trial. This trial enrolled obese HFpEF patients ($n = 731$) and demonstrated a statistically significant reduction in the primary composite endpoint of CV death or a worsening HF event, driven by reduced rates of HF events.[17]

Interventional and Device Therapies

Emerging device-based therapies offer new avenues for HFpEF management. HFpEF is essentially characterized by elevated LV and LA filling pressures, which rise further on exercise. This is basic hemodynamic mechanism responsible for symptoms in HFpEF patients. Atrial shunt device theoretically allows decompression of LA and prevents the rise of LA filling pressure on exercise. However, such a strategy using Corvia Medical interatrial shunt device system in the recently published REDUCE LAP-HF II trial failed to show any significant clinical benefit. There was no difference in the composite primary endpoint of CV death, stroke, and HF events.[18]

Another such approach is the use of CardioMEMS™, a pulmonary artery pressure monitoring system, that allows for real-time hemodynamic assessment and titration of therapy. This device has shown promise in reducing HF hospitalizations by enabling timely interventions based on pressure changes.[19]

KNOWLEDGE GAPS IN HEART FAILURE WITH PRESERVED EJECTION FRACTION

Despite significant improvements in the available GDMT for HFpEF (especially SGLT2i and GLP-1RA), there is still a large unmet need in this field. HFpEF is underdiagnosed and its mechanisms are less understood. There is a need for better noninvasive tests for diagnosis of HFpEF that should offer similar accuracy as the gold standard invasive hemodynamics. The exact mechanisms that connect the root cause (obesity and insulin resistance) to the cardiometabolic abnormalities like HFpEF are not completely understood. The role of inflammation and extracardiac perturbations needs to be explored and addressed. There is also a need for dedicated randomized trials for comorbidities in HFpEF like CAD, AF, iron deficiency, and obesity.

CONCLUSION

Heart failure signs and symptoms with a normal LVEF are not always just HFpEF; we need to rule out HFpEF mimics that have treatment implications. Different HFpEF diagnostic scoring systems are available which increase the accuracy of our diagnosis. Treatment of the comorbidities (hypertension, diabetes, obesity, etc.) is the mainstay of therapy in HFpEF and needs to be according to the latest available guidelines for same. SGLT2i and GLP-1RA therapies have been demonstrated to decrease HF events in this difficult-to-treat population.

REFERENCES

1. Bozkurt B, Coats AJ, Tsutsui H, et al. Universal definition and classification of heart failure: A Report of the Heart Failure Society of America, Heart Failure Association of the European Society of Cardiology, Japanese Heart Failure Society and Writing Committee of the Universal Definition of Heart Failure. J Card Fail. 2021;27(4):387-413.
2. Pfeffer MA, Shah AM, Borlaug BA. Heart failure with preserved ejection fraction in perspective. Circ Res. 2019; 124(11):1598-617.
3. Heidenreich PA, Bozkurt B, Aguilar D, et al.; ACC/AHA Joint Committee Members. 2022 AHA/ACC/HFSA Guideline for the Management of Heart Failure: A Report of the American College of Cardiology/American Heart Association Joint Committee on Clinical Practice Guidelines. Circulation. 2022;145(18):e895-1032.
4. Pieske B, Tschöpe C, de Boer RA, et al. How to diagnose heart failure with preserved ejection fraction: the HFA-PEFF diagnostic algorithm: a consensus recommendation from the Heart Failure Association (HFA) of the European Society of Cardiology (ESC). Eur Heart J. 2019; 40(40): 3297-317.
5. Kitzman DW, Brubaker P, Morgan T, et al. Effect of Caloric Restriction or Aerobic Exercise Training on Peak Oxygen Consumption and Quality of Life in Obese Older Patients with Heart Failure with Preserved Ejection Fraction: A randomized clinical trial. JAMA. 2016;315(1):36-46.
6. Reddy YNV, Borlaug BA, Gersh BJ. Management of atrial fibrillation across the spectrum of heart failure with preserved and reduced ejection fraction. Circulation. 2022;146(4):339-57.
7. John JE, Claggett B, Skali H, et al. Coronary artery disease and heart failure with preserved ejection fraction: The ARIC Study. J Am Heart Assoc. 2022;11(17):e021660.
8. Fu M, Wang Y, Han X, et al. Revascularization for patients with heart failure with preserved ejection fraction and coronary artery disease. Am J Cardiol. 2024;213:86-92.
9. Anker SD, Butler J, Filippatos G, , et al. Empagliflozin in heart failure with a preserved ejection fraction. N Engl J Med. 2021;385(16):1451-61.
10. Solomon SD, McMurray JJV, Claggett B, et al. Dapagliflozin in heart failure with mildly reduced or preserved ejection fraction. N Engl J Med. 2022;387(12):1089-98.
11. Vaduganathan M, Docherty KF, Claggett BL, et al. SGLT2 inhibitors in patients with heart failure: a comprehensive meta-analysis of five randomised controlled trials. Lancet. 2022;400(10354):757-67.
12. McDonagh TA, Metra M, Adamo M, et al.; ESC Scientific Document Group. 2023 Focused Update of the 2021 ESC Guidelines for the diagnosis and treatment of acute and chronic heart failure. Eur Heart J. 2023;44(37):3627-39.
13. Solomon SD, McMurray JJV, Anand IS, et al. Angiotensin-neprilysin inhibition in heart failure with preserved ejection fraction. N Engl J Med. 2019;381(17):1609-20.
14. Solomon SD, McMurray JJV, Vaduganathan M, et al.; FINEARTS-HF Committees and Investigators. Finerenone in Heart Failure with Mildly Reduced or Preserved Ejection Fraction. N Engl J Med. 2024;391(16):1475-85.
15. Kosiborod MN, Abildstrøm SZ, Borlaug BA, et al. Semaglutide in patients with heart failure with preserved ejection fraction and obesity. N Engl J Med. 2023;389(12): 1069-84.
16. Kosiborod MN, Petrie MC, Borlaug BA, et al. Semaglutide in patients with obesity-related heart failure and type 2 diabetes. N Engl J Med. 2024;390(15):1394-407.
17. Packer M, Zile MR, Kramer CM, et al. Tirzepatide for heart failure with preserved ejection fraction and obesity. N Engl J Med. 2024.
18. Gustafsson F, Petrie MC, Komtebedde J, et al. 2-Year outcomes of an atrial shunt device in HFpEF/HFmrEF. JACC Heart Fail. 2024;12(8):1425-38.
19. Abraham WT, Adamson PB, Bourge RC, et al. Wireless pulmonary artery haemodynamic monitoring in chronic heart failure: a randomised controlled trial. Lancet. 2011; 377(9766):658-66.

CHAPTER

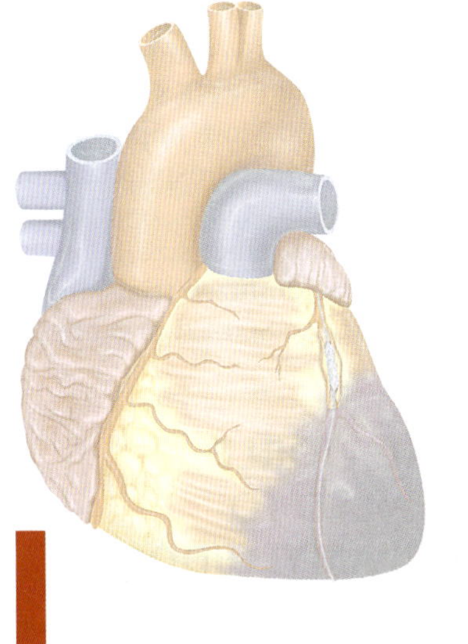

Role of Amyloidosis in HFpEF Trials

Saumitra Ray, Ayan Kar

INTRODUCTION

Heart failure with preserved ejection fraction (HFpEF) happens to be a common and difficult form of heart failure to treat, compromising almost 50% of all hospital admissions.[1] Unlike, heart failure with reduced ejection fraction, which has the fabulous four pillars of therapy, treatment for HFpEF remains more elusive with a strong recommendation for treatment of associated comorbidities in addition to loop diuretics for congestion and SGLT2 inhibitors, in the absence of standard guideline-directed medical therapy.[2,3] The repeated failure of well-researched and established drugs borrowed from heart failure with reduced ejection fraction subsets tells us that the pathophysiology is often unique and heterogeneous. As clinicians, our clinical experiences are often mirrored in the outcomes of comprehensive large-scale contemporary clinical trials of patients with HFpEF where time-tested drugs do not give favorable results in HFpEF.[4] Apart from the heterogeneity, there is a possibility that we are including cases of undiagnosed cardiac amyloidosis, which could significantly affect the overall outcomes of such trials.

CARDIAC AMYLOIDOSIS: A HFpEF MASQUERADER

Cardiac amyloidosis (CA), typically transthyretin (TTR) amyloidosis, is a progressive infiltrative cardiomyopathy manifested by the deposition of misfolded amyloid proteins in the myocardium and valvular tissues.[5] Several single-center trials peg the prevalence of CA in HFpEF cohorts between 5 and 20% depending on selection criteria.[6] The most Common presentations are heart failure with preserved or mildly reduced function, aortic stenosis, and rhythm disorders.

Our evolving knowledge of CA today has made it easier to diagnose cases of amyloidosis with robust algorithms.[5] However, it entails ordering incremental diagnostic investigations and imaging, which is often not a part of traditional heart failure workup and often not a part of standard exclusion criteria of contemporary trials of HFpEF.

Given the heterogeneity of presentation of CA, consecutive trials in heart failure have resorted to increasingly stringent exclusion criteria, for example, CHARM-Preserved had 8 exclusion criteria and PARAGON HF had 33 exclusion criteria suggesting the increasing attention paid to the prevalence of CA as an active masquerader in patients presenting with HFpEF.[7] In a very eloquent state-of-art review by Oghina et al., it was shown that when exclusion criteria for major HFpEF trials were applied to diagnosed CA cohorts, their ability to diagnose CA was limited to 16–65% of the cases, allowing undiagnosed cases of CA to affect outcomes of such trials.[7]

Since incremental testing is not easy, it may be prudent to discuss common nonhistologic features that should raise suspicion of ATTR CA.[5]

Clinical features:

- History of carpal tunnel syndrome
- Spontaneous biceps tendon rupture
- Spinal stenosis

- Isolated right heart failure
- Elderly and male gender
- Disproportionately high pro-B-type natriuretic peptide (proBNP) compared to left ventricular (LV) dysfunction

Electrocardiographic features:
- Atrial fibrillation
- Conduction abnormalities
- ECG-echocardiography mismatch (low voltage to mass or wall thickness ratio)

Echocardiographic features:
- Concentric LV hypertrophy
- Reduce S' velocity on the mitral annulus
- Reduced global longitudinal strain with apical sparing
- Paradoxically low stroke volume relative to LV function

CARDIAC AMYLOIDOSIS IN CONTEMPORARY HFpEF TRIALS

Although most trials of HFpEF have historically excluded diagnosed cases of infiltrative cardiomyopathy including CA, undiagnosed cases of CA have always remained difficult to exclude. Depending on echo and clinical criteria discussed above, an enriched subset from the TOPCAT trial showed the prevalence of CA to be close to 23%. It used simple echo measures like a reduced S' velocity <6 cm/s of the mitral annulus and interventricular septum (IVS) thickness >1.2 cm to identify patients with suspected CA.[8] This subgroup had worse outcomes compared to the rest of the patients.

Similarly, in the PARAGON trial, male gender and high LVEF, the two subsets where the efficacy of valsartan sacubitril was conspicuously diminished, are typically seen in patients with wild-type ATTR CA.[9] More so, the difference in geographic responses of ARNI to CA in Western Europe and America compared to the rest of Asia is possibly a reflection of earlier identification of CA given the availability of robust referral centers.

As transthyretin amyloid cardiomyopathy (ATTR-CM) was an exclusion criterion in randomized clinical trials of sodium-glucose cotransporter 2 inhibitors (SGLT2i), it is difficult to assess the role of the latter in ATTR-CM. A study was published recently to assess the efficacy and tolerability of SGLT2i in patients with ATTR-CM. A total number of 2,356 consecutive ATTR-CM patients (2014–2022) were analyzed, of whom 260 (11%) were found to have received SGLT2i. After a thorough comparison done between the groups according to the treatment, 14 variables were found to be significantly different including age and N-terminal proBNP. A propensity score reflecting the likelihood of being treated with SGLT2i for each patient was determined using 16 variables. The study concluded that SGLT2i was well tolerated by ATTR-CM patients and was beneficial for HF symptoms, renal function, and need for diuretics. More importantly, SGLT2i treatment reduced the risk of HF hospitalization and cardiovascular and all-cause mortality, regardless of the ejection fraction, despite the effect size is likely overestimated. In the absence of randomized trials, these data may encourage clinicians to use SGLT2i in patients with ATTR-CM.[10]

PROGNOSIS OF REAL-WORLD PATIENTS AND THE NEED TO DIAGNOSE CARDIAC AMYLOIDOSIS

The overwhelming need to identify such cases is that they often tend to have worse prognoses and are notorious for their poor response to standard guideline-directed medical therapy. It is important also to note that novel therapies for ATTR CA work only in subsets where patients are diagnosed in the early stage of disease. Current medial survival of patients with diagnosed CA stands at 51% at 40 months portending a dismal prognosis.[7]

PROPOSED PATHWAY FOR EXCLUDING CARDIAC AMYLOIDOSIS PATIENTS FROM HFpEF TRIALS

Patients with previously mentioned nonhistologic criteria also known as "red flags", suspicious of CA should undergo a technetium 99m pyrophosphate (PYP) scan along with serum light chain assay, which has a sensitivity of 100%[11] to diagnose CA. Certain pitfalls in PYP screening need to be highlighted but may be beyond the scope of this chapter.

CONCLUSION

Cardiac amyloidosis in particular ATTR is not a common subset of infiltrative cardiomyopathy but is often difficult to diagnose due to the lack of clinical suspicion and expensive diagnostic testing. However, its overall poor prognosis and refractoriness to standard guideline-directed therapy, suggest the need not just only to diagnose, but to diagnose them early and start on disease-modifying therapy at the earliest. By doing so, we will also prevent them from jeopardizing further clinical trials of HFpEF. Using clinical red flags, echo Doppler with global longitudinal strain, and Tc PYP scan along with light chain assay is extremely useful in confidently diagnosing patients of CA.

REFERENCES

1. Pfeffer MA, Shah AM, Borlaug BA. Heart failure with preserved ejection fraction in perspective. Circ Res. 2019;124(11):1598-617.
2. Solomon SD, McMurray JJ, Anand IS, et al. Angiotensin–neprilysin inhibition in heart failure with preserved ejection fraction. New Eng J Med. 2019;381(17):1609-20.
3. Anker SD, Butler J, Filippatos G, et al. Empagliflozin in heart failure with a preserved ejection fraction. New Eng J Med. 2021;385(16):1451-61.
4. Lam CS, Voors AA, de Boer RA, et al. Heart failure with preserved ejection fraction: from mechanisms to therapies. Eur Heart J. 2018;39(30):2780-92.
5. Ruberg FL, Grogan M, Hanna M, et al. Transthyretin amyloid cardiomyopathy: JACC state-of-the-art review. J Am Coll Cardiol. 2019;73(22):2872-91.
6. García-Pavía P, García-Pinilla JM, Lozano-Bahamonde A, et al. Prevalence of transthyretin cardiac amyloidosis in patients with heart failure with preserved ejection fraction: The PRACTICA study. Rev Esp Cardiol (Eng Ed). 2024.
7. Oghina S, Bougouin W, Bézard M, et al. The impact of patients with cardiac amyloidosis in HFpEF trials. JACC Heart Fail. 2021;9(3):169-78.
8. Sperry BW, Hanna M, Shah SJ, et al. Spironolactone in patients with an echocardiographic HFpEF phenotype suggestive of cardiac amyloidosis: results from TOPCAT. JACC Heart Fail. 2021;9(11):795-802.
9. González-López E, Gallego-Delgado M, Guzzo-Merello G, et al. Wild-type transthyretin amyloidosis as a cause of heart failure with preserved ejection fraction. Eur Heart J. 2015;36(38):2585-94.
10. Porcari A, Cappelli F, Nitsche C, et al. SGLT2 inhibitor therapy in patients with transthyretin amyloid cardiomyopathy. J Am Coll Cardiol. 2024;83(24):2411-22.
11. Treglia G, Glaudemans AWJM, Bertagna F, et al. Diagnostic accuracy of bone scintigraphy in the assessment of cardiac transthyretin-related amyloidosis: a bivariate meta-analysis. Eur J Nucl Med Mol Imaging. 2018;45(11):1945-55.

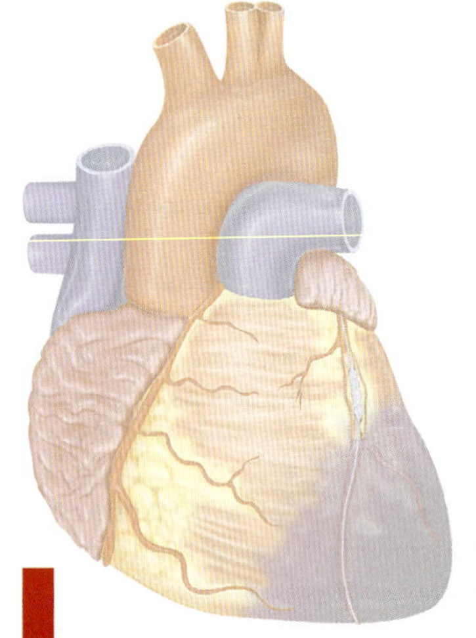

Updates on HFpEF

Sanchita Sen, Tanay Malla, Deepika Misra

INTRODUCTION

Heart failure with preserved ejection fraction (HFpEF) is defined as heart failure (HF) in the presence of left ventricular ejection fraction (LVEF) ≥50%. Patients with HFpEF are hospitalized approximately 1.4 times per year and have a mortality rate of approximately 15% per year.[1] The prevalence of HFpEF is expected to increase over time.

Uijil et al. proposed a model consisting of five HFpEF phenotypic clusters obtained from patients within the Swedish Heart Failure (SwedeHF) Registry and validated externally using the Chronic Heart Failure European Society of Cardiology Guideline-Based Cardiology Practice Quality project registry **(Fig. 1)**. Overall, heterogeneity of HFpEF was considerable. The five clusters identified included: (1) Young-low comorbidity burden cluster; (2) atrial fibrillation-hypertensive cluster; (3) older-atrial

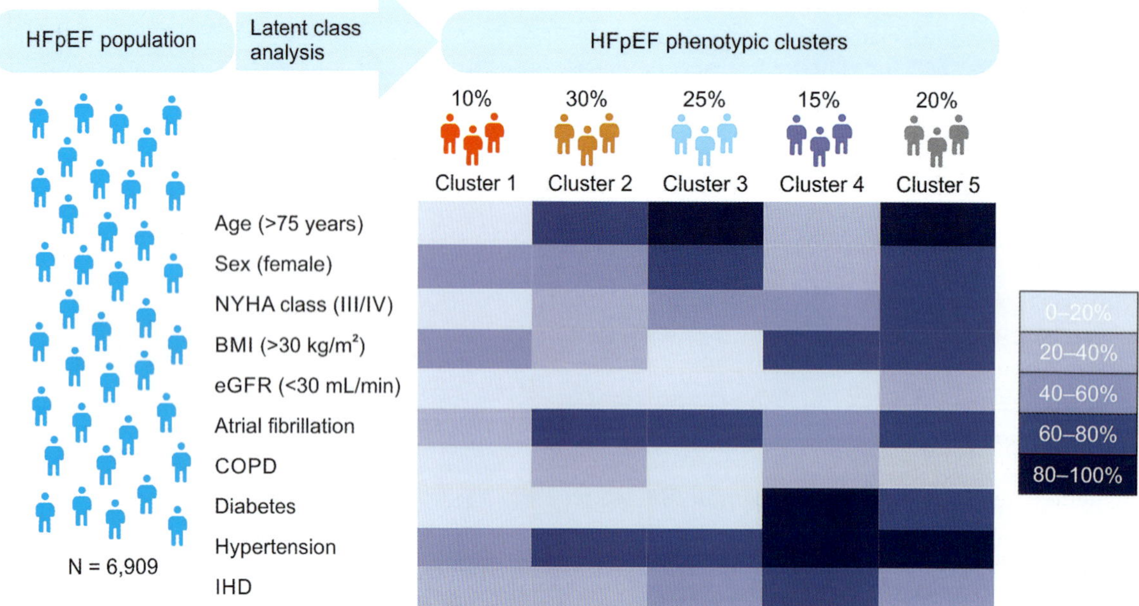

Fig. 1: Cluster model of HFpEF phenotypic presentation.
Source: Uijl et al. (2021).

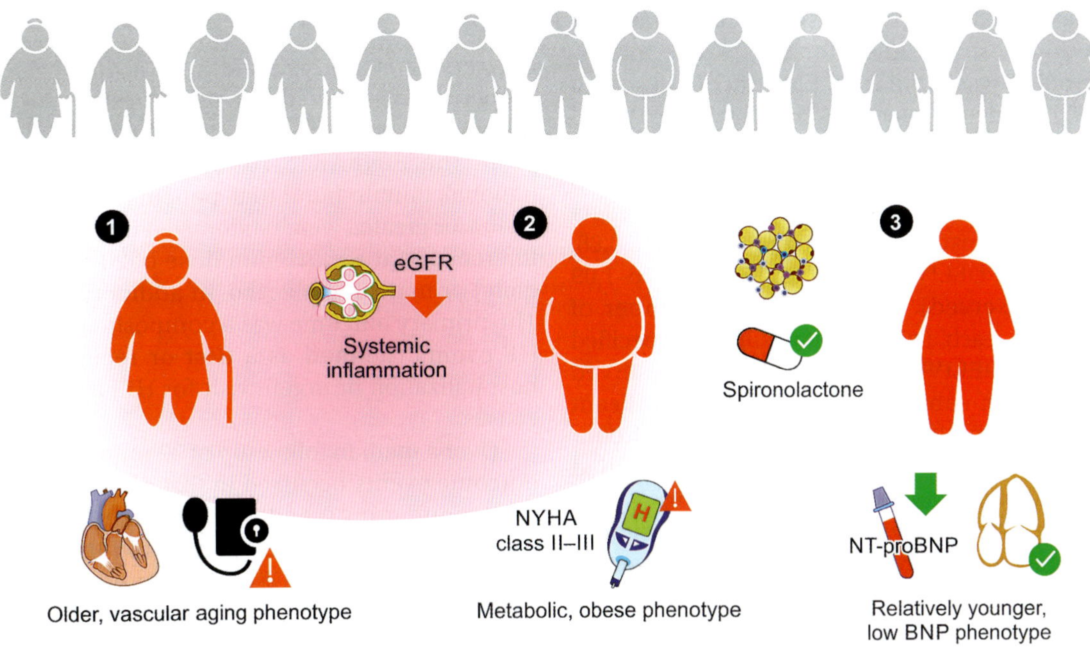

Fig. 2: Phenomapping in heart failure with preserved ejection fraction. The first phenotype is "older, vascular aging", characterized by arterial stiffness, leading to arterial hypertension and left ventricular hypertrophy. It is associated with significant systemic inflammation and often coexists with chronic kidney disease, which is also observed in the second phenotype, the "metabolic, obese", where type 2 diabetes mellitus is the prevalent comorbidity and patients often report dyspnea and reduced tolerance to physical activity, which can also be attributed to deconditioning. The last phenotype is the "younger, low BNP", which overlaps with the previous one due to the frequent presence of excess body weight and, notably, responsiveness to spironolactone. (BNP: B-type natriuretic peptide; eGFR: estimated glomerular filtration rate; NT-proBNP: N-terminal pro-B-type natriuretic peptide; NYHA: New York Heart Association)
Source: Peters et al. (2023).

fibrillation cluster; (4) obese-diabetic cluster; and (5) cardiorenal cluster. Patients in the young-low comorbidity burden cluster had the lowest, while patients in the older-atrial fibrillation and cardiorenal cluster demonstrated the highest event rates. These distinct clusters were validated using an external validation cohort.[2]

Recently, a review conducted by Peters et al. identified the three most recurrent HFpEF phenotypes in studies investigating specific characteristics through statistical analysis of large datasets, a technique known as "phenomapping" **(Fig. 2)**. They included: (1) Older, vascular aging phenotype; (2) metabolic and obese phenotype; and (3) relatively younger, low BNP phenotype. These three phenotypes were additionally identified in studies where researchers did not employ this static strategy, demonstrating the robustness of the results.[3]

While older HFpEF patients often experience classic symptoms, such as dyspnea and fatigue, younger patients with low BNP levels may present with other symptoms, including exercise intolerance, unexplained dyspnea on exertion, or other nonspecific complaints. Medications, lifestyle modifications, and interventions that have been shown to benefit older HFpEF patients may need to be better tailored to this younger cohort.

TREATMENT

New and effective treatments for HFpEF, including sodium-glucose cotransporter-2 (SGLT2) inhibitors, angiotensin receptor-neprilysin inhibitors (ARNIs), and mineralocorticoid receptor antagonists (MRAs) have proven to be efficacious. These treatments can improve symptoms, quality of life (QoL), and reduce the risk of hospitalization and death.[4]

Sodium–Glucose Cotransporter-2 Inhibitors

The SGLT2 inhibitors have an important role in the treatment optimization of HFpEF patients. In two trials investigating empagliflozin (EMPEROR-Preserved trial) and dapagliflozin (DELIVER trial), SGLT-2 inhibitors demonstrated positive results, with a significant reduction in the primary outcome [a composite of cardiovascular (CV) death and hospitalization for HF].[5,6] The magnitude of the effect was similar in EMPEROR-Preserved [HR 0.79, 95% confidence interval (CI) 0.69–0.90, $p < 0.001$] and in DELIVER (HR 0.82, 95% CI 0.73–0.92, $p < 0.001$). The positive result was driven primarily by a lower risk of hospitalization for HF and worsening HF events. The effect on CV deaths was almost significant in both trials (HR 0.88, 95% CI 0.74–1.05 in DELIVER; HR 0.91, 95% CI 0.76–1.09 in EMPEROR-Preserved). Given the large number of patients needed to reach a significant result, a prespecified meta-analysis of DELIVER and EMPEROR-Preserved was planned, which subsequently proved a significant reduction in CV mortality (HR 0.88, 95% CI 0.77–1.00).[7] SGLT2i also improved health status and QoL, as measured by the Kansas City Cardiomyopathy Questionnaire.

In summary, empagliflozin and dapagliflozin significantly reduced the incidence of CV events and worsening HF in HFpEF, demonstrating that SGLT2 inhibitors improve HF prognosis irrespective of ejection fraction status. As per American College of Cardiology (ACC)/American Heart Association (AHA) HF guidelines, diuretics remain class I and SGLT2 inhibitors are class IIa for use in HFpEF. The ESC, however, has approved SGLT2 inhibitors as class I across all types of HF.

Mineralocorticoid Receptor Antagonists

Spironolactone

The efficacy and safety of MRAs as an HFpEF treatment have been tested in a large, multicenter, randomized, double-blind, placebo-controlled clinical trial. The TOPCAT trial enrolled patients aged >50 years with at least one sign or symptom of HF, LVEF >45%, history of HF hospitalization in the previous 12 months, or elevated natriuretic peptide (NP) level.[8]

The overall result on the primary outcome of composite CV death and HF hospitalization was neutral (HR 0.89, 95% CI 0.77–1.04, $p = 0.14$) as only HF hospitalizations were significantly reduced in the treatment arm (HR 0.83, 95% CI 0.69–0.99, $p = 0.04$). A post hoc analysis proved that the outcome was met in patients enrolled in countries other than Russia and Georgia, suggesting variations in drug adherence or distribution in these regions.[9]

The TOPCAT trial shaped much of our knowledge around the use of MRA in HFpEF, as it is the only large-scale clinical trial with clinically relevant outcomes. Smaller studies found beneficial effects of MRA on echocardiographic measures (improvement in diastolic dysfunction, induction of reverse remodeling, and decreased natriuretic peptide) but not on QoL, symptoms, and exercise capacity measures.[10,11]

Finerenone

Finerenone is a nonsteroidal MRA. Its physicochemical properties are distinct from those of steroidal MRAs, such as spironolactone.

In the FINEARTS-HF study, which was an international, double-blind trial, patients with HF and an LVEF of 40% or greater, were randomized in a 1:1 ratio, to receive finerenone (at a maximum dose of 20 mg or 40 mg once daily) or matching placebo, in addition to usual therapy. The primary outcome was a composite of total worsening HF events (defined as a first or recurrent unplanned hospitalization or urgent visit for HF) and death from CV causes.

Over a median follow-up of 32 months, 1,083 primary-outcome events occurred in 624 of 3,003 patients in the finerenone group, and 1,283 primary-outcome events occurred in 719 of 2,998 patients in the placebo group (rate ratio 0.84, 95% CI 0.74–0.95; $p = 0.007$). The total number of worsening HF events was 842 in the finerenone group and 1,024 in the placebo group (rate ratio 0.82, 95% CI 0.71–0.94, $p = 0.006$). The percentage of patients who died from CV causes was 8.1 and 8.7%, respectively (hazard ratio 0.93, 95% CI 0.78–1.11). Finerenone was associated with an increased risk of hyperkalemia and a reduced risk of hypokalemia.

In this study, SGLT2i and GLP1 receptor agonist use was low; dedicated studies are underway to assess whether concomitant use of finerenone has clear additional benefits and safety in HF.[12]

The SPIRRIT-HFpEF (Spironolactone Initiation Registry Randomized Interventional Trial in Heart Failure with Preserved Ejection Fraction) is an RRCT under development within the SwedeHF registry. It is prospective randomized, multicenter, safety/efficacy, parallel assignment, intention-to-treat, open-label treatment, phase-4, event-driven interventional trial in HFpEF, testing spironolactone and usual care versus usual care alone in patients with HF and EF ≥40%.

The 2022 guidelines from the AHA, ACC, and HF Society of America assigned MRAs a class 2b recommendation for reducing HF hospitalizations, particularly in LVEF patients. In contrast, the European guidelines do not include MRAs as a recommended treatment for HFpEF.

Antagonist Receptor–Neprilysin Inhibitors

The PARAGON-HF trial randomized 4,822 patients with NYHA class II–IV, EF >45%, elevated NP, and structural heart disease to valsartan alone or sacubitril/valsartan (ARNI).[13] The primary endpoint was a composite of total HF hospitalization or CV death and was not found significant in this study. Analyzing the components of the outcomes separately demonstrated no effect on CV mortality (HR 0.95, 95% CI 0.79–1.16) and a modest positive effect on HF hospitalizations (rate ratio 0.85, 95% CI 0.72–1.00), though the confidence interval reached 1. Other important secondary outcomes (NYHA class improvement, change in QoL assessed by the Kansas City Cardiomyopathy Questionnaire, and renal function preservation) showed benefit from ARNI treatment compared with valsartan alone. Prespecified subgroups analysis underscored a higher treatment benefit in women than in men, with treatment efficacy up to an EF of 57%.[14]

Recently, the PARAGLIDE study randomized 466 patients with LVEF >40% and a recent event of worsening HF to sacubitril/valsartan versus valsartan was reported. The primary endpoint of N-terminal fraction of pro-BNP reduction was greater in the sacubitril/valsartan group ($p = 0.0049$). Despite experiencing greater symptomatic hypotension, sacubitril/valsartan was associated with the additional clinical benefit of reduced renal failure progression in contrast to the valsartan cohort.[15]

A pool analysis of PARAGLIDE and PARAGON showed that in a population of 5,262 patients, sacubitril/valsartan versus valsartan alone significantly reduced CV death and total worsening HF events ($p = 0.027$).[16] Overall, these data suggest the clinical benefits of ARNI use in heart failure patients over the use of an angiotensin receptor blocker, such as valsartan, alone.

Glucagon-like Peptide-1 Agonists

In the STEP-HFpEF trial, 529 patients with HFpEF and a body-mass index ≥30 received either once-weekly semaglutide (2.4 mg) or placebo treatment for 52 weeks.[17] The dual primary endpoints included change from baseline in the Kansas City Cardiomyopathy Questionnaire Clinical Summary Score (KCCQ-CSS) (scores range from 0 to 100, with higher scores indicating fewer symptoms and physical limitations) and change in body weight. The semaglutide cohort demonstrated significantly better outcomes than placebo in the primary endpoint measure.

In patients with HFpEF and obesity, treatment with semaglutide (2.4 mg) led to larger reductions in symptoms and physical limitations, greater improvements in exercise function, and greater weight loss than placebo.

One limitation of this trial was that very few patients were on SGLT2 inhibitor treatment at baseline. It is additionally unclear whether improvements in HF-related QoL measures were driven by weight loss (suggesting that other weight loss measures could be considered and potentially beneficial) or were independent of this metric.

Devices for Heart Failure with Preserved Ejection Fraction

Transcatheter Interatrial Shunt Device

One of the key hemodynamic features of HFpEF is elevated left atrial and pulmonary venous pressure at rest or on exertion, resulting in dyspnea and reduced exercise capacity. The REDUCE LAP-HF II trial was conducted to test whether a transcatheter interatrial shunt device to unload the left atrium could translate into reductions in CV death, nonfatal ischemic stroke, and HF events, or produce a change in QoL as measured by the KCCQ overall summary score.[18] The trial enrolled 1,072 patients, of which 314 underwent an atrial shunt device procedure and 312 a sham procedure. The overall population results were neutral both for the composite primary endpoint (win ratio 1.0, 95% CI 0.8–1.2, $p = 0.85$) and for the single components of the outcome. In the analysis of pre-specified subgroups demonstrated in the highest tertiles of exercise pulmonary artery pressure (pulmonary pressure >70 mm Hg) and right atrial volume (>29.7 mL/m^2), the HF events rate was higher in the device-treated patients compared to those in the sham procedure arm. This suggests a detrimental effect of the implanted interatrial shunt device. Several clinical trials are ongoing or awaiting initiation to investigate the role of interatrial devices, with the goal of shedding light on the net clinical benefit of this strategy in HFpEF (FROST-HF study, NCT05136820).

At 2 years of follow-up in REDUCE LAP-HF II, **(Fig. 3)** there was no difference in efficacy between the atrial shunt and sham groups in the overall trial group. The potential clinical benefit identified in the responder group after 1 and 2 years of follow-up is currently being evaluated in the RESPONDER-HF trial.[19]

Cardiac Contractility Modulation

Cardiac contractility modulation (CCM) is a new device that functions by stimulating myocytes during the absolute refractory period of the action potential, leading to an increase in peak calcium concentration and inducing positive inotropism. It may help with atrial and ventricular remodeling. CCM has been shown to improve tolerance to exercise and outcomes in HFrEF patients, and growing data exist on the benefits in HFmrEF in terms of functional status and QoL. A prospective, multicenter, single-arm study (CCM-HFpEF) was designed to assess the impact of CCM in a bigger HFpEF cohort. Over a 24-week follow-up period in a population of 47 patients in NYHA II and III with LVEF >50%, CCM demonstrated improvements in health status and KCCQ with no impact on safety outcomes.[20] Larger randomized clinical trials are needed to better

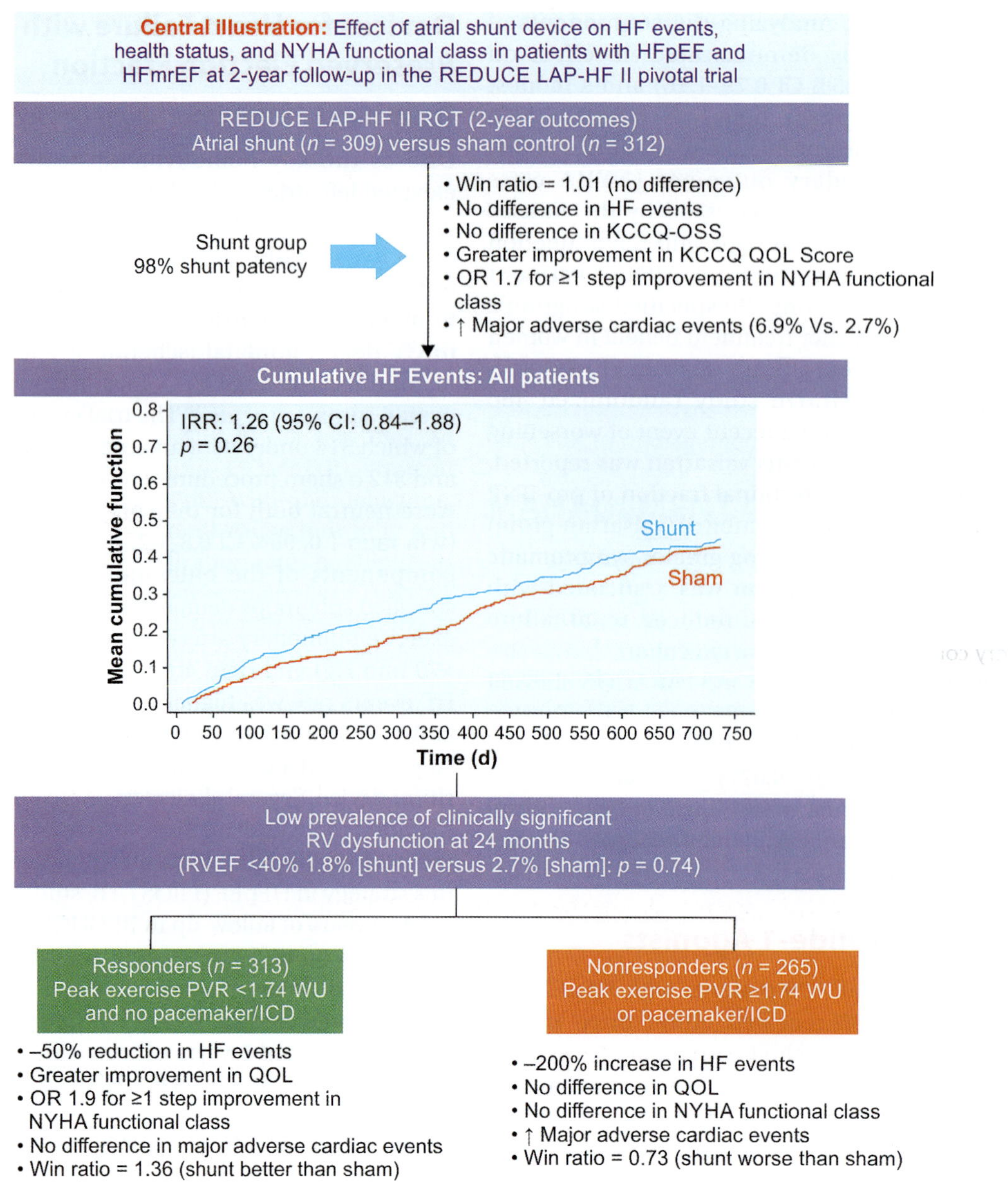

Fig. 3: Reevaluation of the Corvia atrial shunt device in a precision medicine trial to determine efficacy in mildly reduced or preserved ejection fraction heart failure.
Source: Gustafsson et al. (2024).

define the potential impact on outcome and prognosis of this innovative device in HFmrEF and HFpEF.

CONCLUSION

While diuretics have been the mainstay of therapy for HFpEF, the advent of new medications such as SGLT2 inhibitors, GLP-1 agonists, ARNIs, and MRAs show promise for the treatment of this complex condition. However, addressing comorbidities that contribute to the burden of disease is additionally important in improving outcomes for this patient population **(Fig. 4)**.[21] A multipronged approach, which incorporates these therapies in addition to comorbidity treatment, may further optimize outcomes in HFpEF patients.

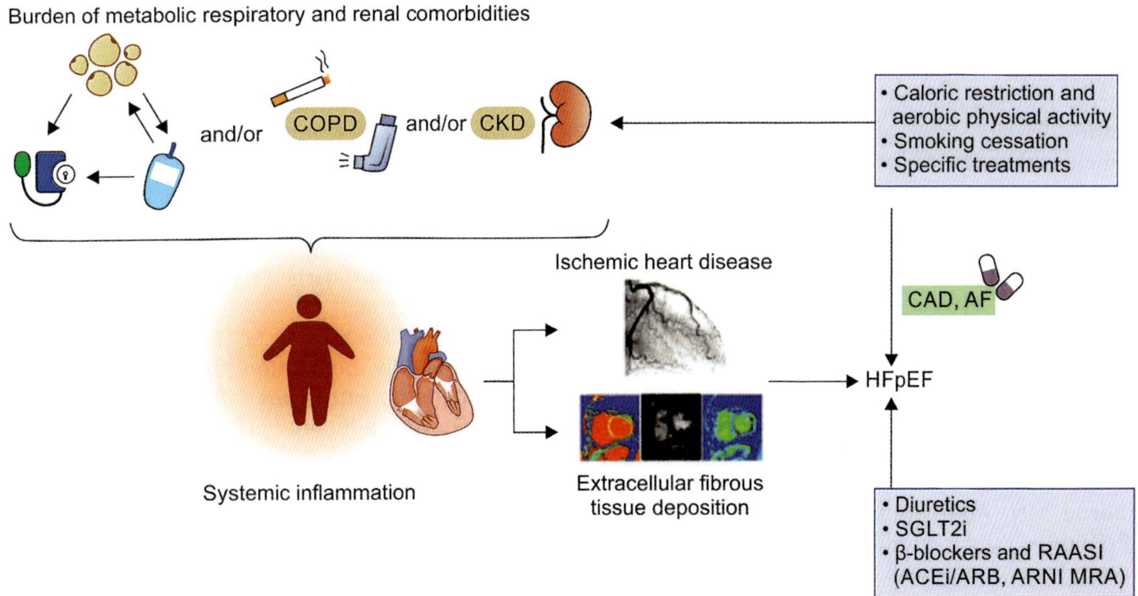

Fig. 4: Contributions of metabolic, respiratory, and renal comorbidities to HFpEF disease burden. The global burden of renal–metabolic and respiratory comorbidities increases systemic inflammation, which in turn promotes endothelial dysfunction, atherosclerosis, and fibrocollagen deposition in the myocardial interstitium following fibroblast activation. Weight control, achieved through both calorie restriction and regular aerobic physical activity (which also improves conditioning and reduces exercise intolerance), smoking cessation, and treatment of individual noncardiac comorbidities play a central role. At the cardiac level, early identification and equally intensive treatment of comorbidities, such as ischemic heart disease (coronary artery disease) and AF, are mandatory. Furthermore, all patients should be offered a loop diuretic to reduce congestive symptoms and an SGLT2i to improve cardiovascular and renal prognosis in patients with HFpEF. (ACEi: angiotensin-converting enzyme inhibitors; ARB: angiotensin receptor blockers; ARNI: antagonist receptor–neprilysin inhibitors; CAD: coronary artery disease; CKD: chronic kidney disease; COPD: chronic obstructive pulmonary disease; HFpEF: heart failure with preserved ejection fraction; MRA: mineralocorticoid receptor antagonists; RAASi: renin–angiotensin–aldosterone system inhibitors; SGLT2i: sodium–glucose cotransporter type 2 inhibitors)
Source: Giulio et al. (2024).

REFERENCES

1. Redfield MM, Borlaug BA. Heart failure with preserved ejection fraction: A review. JAMA. 2023;329(10):827-38.
2. Uijl A, Savarese G, Vaartjes I, et al. Identification of distinct phenotypic clusters in heart failure with preserved ejection fraction. Eur J Heart Fail. 2021;23(6):973-82.
3. Peters AE, Tromp J, Shah SJ, et al. Phenomapping in heart failure with preserved ejection fraction: Insights, limitations, and future directions. Cardiovasc Res. 2023;118(18):3403-415.
4. Peikert A, Solomon SD. Contemporary treatment options in heart failure with preserved ejection fraction. Eur Heart J Cardiovasc Imaging. 2024;25(11):1517-24.
5. Butler J, Filippatos G, Siddiqi TJ, et al. Empagliflozin, health status, and quality of life in patients with heart failure and preserved ejection fraction: The EMPEROR-Preserved trial. Circulation. 2022;145(3):184-93.
6. Kosiborod MN, Bhatt AS, Claggett BL, et al. Effect of dapagliflozin on health status in patients with preserved or mildly reduced ejection fraction. J Am Coll Cardiol. 2023;81(5):460-73.
7. Vaduganathan M, Docherty KF, Claggett BL, et al. SGLT-2 inhibitors in patients with heart failure: A comprehensive meta-analysis of five randomised controlled trials. Lancet. 2022;400(10354):757-67.
8. Pitt B, Pfeffer MA, Assmann SF, et al. Spironolactone for heart failure with preserved ejection fraction. N Engl J Med. 2014;370:1383-92.
9. De Denus S, O'Meara E, Desai AS, et al. Spironolactone metabolites in TOPCAT–new insights into regional variation. N Engl J Med. 2017;376(17):1690-2.
10. Edelmann F, Wachter R, Schmidt AG, et al. Effect of spironolactone on diastolic function and exercise capacity in patients with heart failure with preserved ejection fraction: The Aldo-DHF randomized controlled trial. JAMA. 2013;309(8):781-91.
11. Boccanelli A, Mureddu GF, Cacciatore G, et al. Anti-remodelling effect of canrenone in patients with mild chronic heart failure (AREA IN-CHF study): Final results. Eur J Heart Fail. 2009;11(1):68-76.
12. Solomon SD, McMurray JJ, Vaduganathan M, et al.; FINEARTS-HF Committees and Investigators. Finerenone in heart failure with mildly reduced or preserved ejection fraction. N Engl J Med. 2024;391(16):1475-85.

13. Solomon SD, McMurray JJV, Anand IS, et al. Angiotensin-neprilysin inhibition in heart failure with preserved ejection fraction. N Engl J Med. 2019;381:1609-20.
14. McMurray JJV, Jackson AM, Lam CSP, et al. Effects of sacubitril-valsartan versus valsartan in women compared with men with heart failure and preserved ejection fraction: Insights from PARAGON-HF. Circulation. 2020; 141(5):338-51.
15. Mentz RJ, Ward JH, Hernandez AF, et al. Angiotensin-neprilysin inhibition in patients with mildly reduced or preserved ejection fraction and worsening heart failure. J Am Coll Cardiol. 2023;82(1):1-12.
16. Vaduganathan M, Mentz RJ, Claggett BN, et al. Sacubitril/valsartan in mildly reduced or preserved ejection fraction: A pre-specified participant-level pooled analysis of PARAGLIDE-HF and PARAGON-HF. Eur Heart J. 2023; 44(31):2982-93.
17. Kosiborod MN, Abildstrøm SZ, Borlaug BA, et al.; STEP-HFpEF Trial Committees and Investigators. Semaglutide in patients with heart failure with preserved ejection fraction and obesity. N Engl J Med. 2023;389: 1069-84.
18. Shah SJ, Borlaug BA, Chung ES, et al.; REDUCE LAP-HF II investigators. Atrial shunt device for heart failure with preserved and mildly reduced ejection fraction (REDUCE LAP-HF II): A randomised, multicentre, blinded, sham-controlled trial. Lancet. 2022;399(10330):1130-40.
19. Gustafsson F, Petrie MC, Komtebedde J. et al. 2-year outcomes of an atrial shunt device in HFpEF/HFmrEF: Results from REDUCE LAP-HF II. JACC Heart Fail. 2024; 12(8):1425-38.
20. Linde C, Grabowski M, Ponikowski P, et al. Cardiac contractility modulation therapy improves health status in patients with heart failure with preserved ejection fraction: A pilot study (CCM-HFpEF). Eur J Heart Fail. 2022;24(12):2275-84.
21. Balestrieri G, Limonta R, Ponti E, et al. The therapy and management of heart failure with preserved ejection fraction: New insights on treatment. Cardiac Fail Rev. 2024;10:e05.

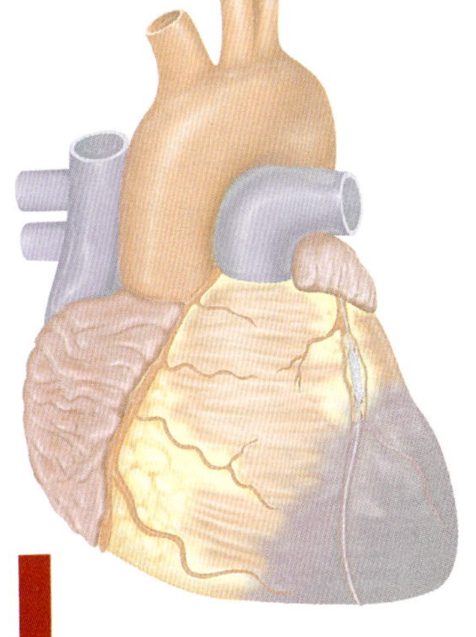

HFpEF: Scenario and Therapeutic Strategies

Rakesh Varma

INTRODUCTION

Heart failure is prevalent *across the globe, be it developed countries or underprivileged populations of Africa or Asia,* more so in almost all countries, with aging populations. Fortunately, *advances in therapeutic modalities* have led to new treatments and improved prognosis. This chapter elucidates these with a focus on the diagnosis and medical management of heart failure with preserved ejection fraction (HFpEF). The main changes include (1) the four foundational drug classes now recommended for patients with heart failure and reduced left ventricular ejection fraction (LVEF), (2) use of sodium-glucose cotransporter-2 inhibitors for those with a higher ejection fraction, and (3) the importance of rapid initiation of life-prolonging therapies. Device management and other nondrug management have also been dealt with in this chapter.

EPIDEMIOLOGY OF HEART FAILURE

The *Global Burden of Disease Study*[1] estimated that 57 million people were living with heart failure in 2019. Large differences in prevalence are noted for both men and women. The region with the highest prevalence of heart failure includes the high-income countries of North America, and the lowest prevalence was found in central Asia.

POSSIBLE SURVIVAL AFTER DIAGNOSIS

Survival following a diagnosis of heart failure is poor and is highly influenced by age. In the UK, survival approaches *80%* at 5 years for people *aged 45–64 years* but is closer to *20%* at 5 years for those aged.[2] Fortunately, survival rates have improved since *2000*, particularly among younger patients.[3]

Overall, while survival is important, it is the outcome of the combined effects of all the conditions of a patient. Moreover, years of life lost, due to heart failure, can be estimated with difficulty. Data from the UK have shown that heart failure is associated with a *2.4*-fold greater loss of time alive than observed in the age- and sex-matched general population—over 10 years.[4] The length of life lost with heart failure varies from *5 months* (women) to *1 year* (men) for people with no *comorbidities* and from *3 years* (women) to *4.5 years* (men) for those with three or more *comorbidities.*[5]

DIAGNOSIS

The diagnosis of heart failure requires the presence of symptoms consistent with cardiac dysfunction along with evidence of either:

- Significantly reduced left ventricular systolic function (≤40%) and/or
- Increased filling pressures.

This is now incorporated into the recently published universal definition of heart failure.

Heart failure is categorized into *three groups* based on the LVEF:

1. Heart failure with reduced ejection fraction (*HFrEF*) if the LVEF is ≤40%
2. Heart failure with mildly reduced ejection fraction (*HFmrEF*) if the LVEF is 41–49%

3. Heart failure with preserved ejection fraction (*HFpEF*) if the LVEF is ≥50%

Patients with LVEF >40% require additional evidence of increased filling pressures (at rest or with exercise) to establish a diagnosis of heart failure.

Diagnosis of HFpEF

The diagnosis of HFpEF is particularly challenging, as determining increased filling pressure can be difficult. Most definitions of HFpEF *exclude* patients with heart failure symptoms due to valve disease, arrhythmia, pericardial constraint, or high cardiac output. Although invasive testing with cardiac catheterization is the gold standard for determining *elevated left ventricular filling pressures*, the diagnosis can be made noninvasively. However, unfortunately, no single noninvasive test result has both a high sensitivity and a high specificity.

Accordingly, clinical scores have been created using the results from multiple tests to diagnose *HFpEF*.

These include:

- *H2FPEF:*
  - *H*eavy
  - *2* or more hypertensive drugs
  - *A*trial fibrillation
  - *P*ulmonary hypertension (pulmonary artery systolic pressure >35 mm Hg)
  - *E*lder age >60 years
  - *E*levated filling pressures (*E/e′* >9)[6]
- *HFA-PEFF* means:
  - *H*eart *f*ailure *a*ssociation
  - *P*retest assessment
  - *E*chocardiography and natriuretic peptide score
  - *F*unctional testing
  - *F*inal etiology[7]

These two scores have similar prognostic value, although 28% of patients had discordant findings.

It is important to make the diagnosis of heart failure but more important is to determine whether the patient will benefit from therapy for *HFpEF*.

FOUR MEDICATIONS—MAIN PILLARS OF HFpEF THERAPY

For patients with heart failure and a reduced LVEF to ≤40% (HFrEF), four classes of drugs are now known to improve survival. These are **(Table 1)**:

1. Renin-angiotensin system inhibitors including angiotensin converting enzyme (ACE) inhibitors and angiotensin receptor blockers (ARBs) or angiotensin receptor/neprilysin inhibitors (ARNI)
2. β blockers

TABLE 1: Life-prolonging medications for heart failure with reduced left ventricular ejection fraction.

Treatment	*Background therapy for treatment and control groups*	*Relative risk reduction (death)*	*NNT to prevent 1 death at 3 years*
ACEi/ARB	No other life prolonging medication	17	26
β blocker	ACEi (>90%)	34	9
MRA	ACEi (≥90%); β blockers 10%	30	6
ARNI	ACEi (100%: active control); p blockers (>90%); MRAs (>50%)	16	27
SGLT2i	ACEi/ARB/ANRI (90%); p blockers (>90%); MRAs (>70%)	17	22

(ACEi: angiotensin converting enzyme inhibitor; ARB: angiotensin receptor blocker; ARNI: angiotensin receptor/neprilysin inhibitor; MRA: mineralocorticoid receptor antagonist; NNT: number needed to treat; SGLT2i: sodium–glucose cotransporter-2 inhibitor)

Source: Reproduced from Bassi et al. (2020).[8]

3. Mineralocorticoid receptor antagonists (MRAs)
4. Sodium–glucose cotransporter-2 (SGLT2) inhibitors

It has been estimated that the combination of the four pillars of *HFrEF* therapy will lead to a *73%* relative risk reduction in mortality and a number needed to treat of *4* to *prevent a death* compared with no treatment. Similar results are expected for HFpEF.

TREATMENT OF HFmrEF AND HFpEF

As noted above, an LVEF of 41–49% is mildly reduced (*HFmrEF*) whereas patients with an LVEF ≥50% are considered to have preserved ejection fraction (*HFpEF*). These labels apply only to patients who have not previously had an LVEF ≤40% (*these are referred to as heart failure with improved ejection fraction*). SGLT2 inhibitors are recommended as the *first-line* medication for patients with mildly reduced or preserved LVEF on the basis of the two trials that enrolled many patients with an LVEF >40%.

Of the other treatments for HFrEF, *ARNI, ACE inhibitors, ARBs, and MRAs* are *second-line therapies* for HFpEF as the evidence for benefit is much weaker than for patients with HFrEF. Accordingly, MRAs and ACE inhibitors/ARBs/ARNI have a class 2B recommendation for *HFmrEF and HFpEF* in guidelines.[9]

Left Ventricular Ejection Fraction and Benefit of Medical Therapy

Left ventricular ejection fraction can be difficult to quantify with echocardiography, but it has been routinely used to determine the eligibility for clinical trials in heart failure. Given the growing evidence for treatment benefit in patients with higher LVEF levels, some authors have questioned the continued use of the LVEF to classify patients with heart failure. Multiple drug therapies have been tested across the ejection fraction spectrum: β blockers, ACE inhibitors/ARBs, ARNI, MRAs, and SGLT2 inhibitors. Traditionally, trials have stratified patients on the basis of LVEF ≤40 or >40%. However, most therapies have shown a benefit at higher thresholds than the traditional cutoff of reduced LVEF at 40%. For β blockers, a reduction in cardiovascular mortality was observed with LVEF <50%. For MRA therapy, a larger treatment benefit is more likely for patients with LVEF 41–49% than with LVEF ≥50%. The treatment benefit of *sacubitril/valsartan* was observed with LVEF <60%. For SGLT2 inhibitor therapy, the relative treatment effect was similar across the LVEF spectrum. Overall, these results suggest that the LVEF thresholds for systolic dysfunction used in treatment trials may benefit from reclassification but that LVEF will remain important for determining optimal management.

The association of LVEF with the benefit of early initiation and titration was evaluated in a substudy of the *STRONG-HF trial.*[10] This study showed the consistency of the rapid implementation of guideline-based medical therapy across the entire spectrum of LVEF after an admission for heart failure.

Angiotensin Receptor/Neprilysin Inhibitor

The combination of an ARB and a neprilysin inhibitor is now recommended as one of the pillars of HFrEF therapy. The *PARADIGM-HF*[11] (*Prospective Comparison of ARN Inhibitors with ACE Inhibitors to Determine Impact on Global Mortality and Morbidity in HF*) trial randomized *8,442 patients* with *HFrEF*. It found a *20%* reduction in cardiovascular death or admission to hospital for heart failure with sacubitril and valsartan compared with enalapril (*hazard ratio 0.80, 95% confidence interval 0.73–0.87*). Sacubitril/valsartan was also associated with a significant reduction in symptoms, as measured by the *Kansas City Cardiomyopathy Clinical Summary Score*[11] (*hazard ratio 1.64, 95% confidence interval 0.63–2.65*). A second RCT was conducted in patients admitted to hospital with heart failure—*PIONEER-HF58* [Comparison of Sacubitril-Valsartan vs. Enalapril on Effect of N-Terminal Pro-Brain Natriuretic Peptide (*NTproBNP*) in Patients

Flowchart 1: Schematic of treatment of heart failure with reduced ejection fraction.

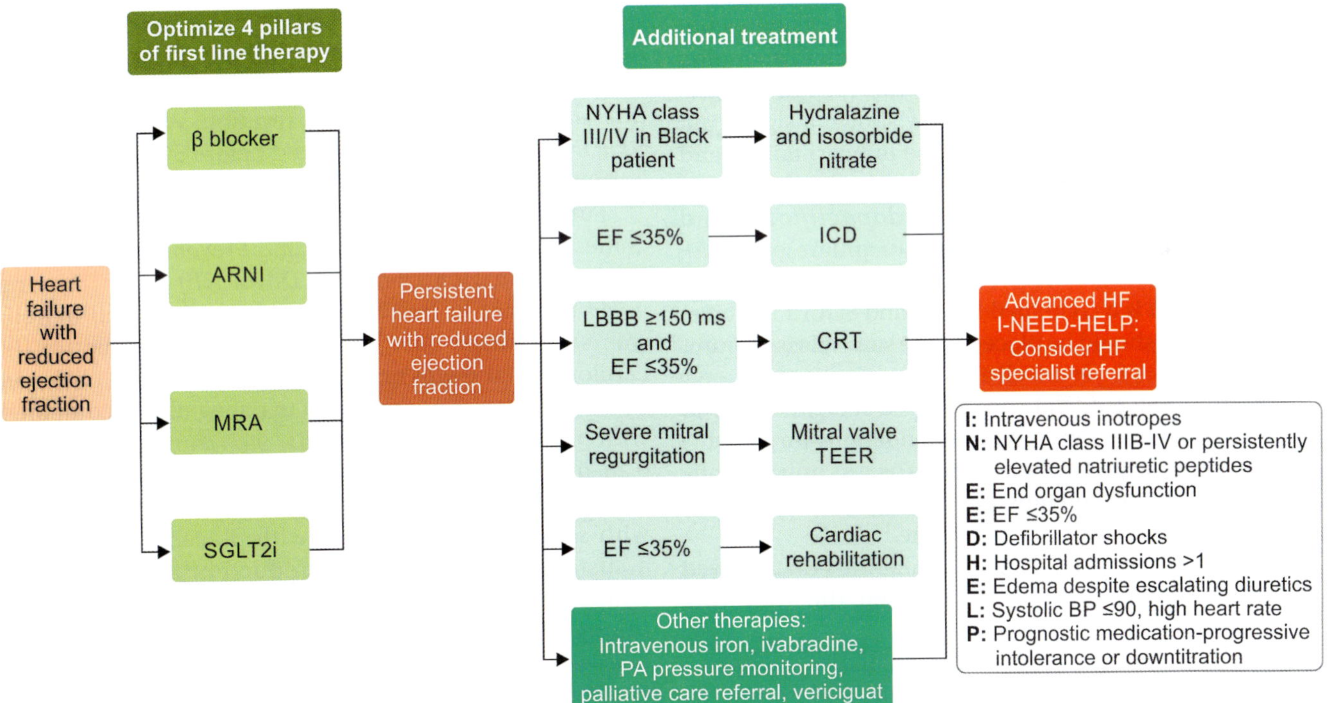

(ARNI: angiotensin receptor/neprilysin inhibitor; BP: blood pressure; CRT: cardiac resynchronization therapy; EF: ejection fraction; HF: heart failure; ICD: implantable cardiac defibrillator; LBBB: left bundle branch block; MRA: mineralocorticoid receptor antagonist; NYHA: New York Heart Association; PA: pulmonary artery; SGLT2i: sodium–glucose-linked cotransporter 2 inhibitor; TEER: transcatheter edge-to-edge repair)

Source: Reproduced from Heidenreich P, Sandhu A. Advances in management of heart failure. BMJ. 2024;385:e077025.

Stabilized From an Acute HF Episode]. This trial consisting of 881 patients showed a reduction in *NT-proBNP* concentrations (*ratio of change 0.71, 95% confidence interval 0.63–0.81*) for patients starting *sacubitril/valsartan* during hospital admission compared with those treated with enalapril. Safety was also demonstrated, with no significant differences in worsening renal function, hyperkalemia, and symptomatic hypotension.

The 2022 US Heart Failure Guideline now recommends ARNI as the *first-line* agent with ACE inhibitor or ARB alone for patients unable to take ARNI.

Use of ARNI along with an ACE inhibitor is not advisable but contraindicated.

No benefit with ARNI was observed, for patients with advanced heart failure falling in NYHA class IV nor in patients taking chronic inotropic therapy. The *LIFE*[12] (*LCZ696 in Advanced HF*) study randomized 335 patients with advanced heart failure and found that after 24 weeks of treatment, changes in *NT-proBNP* were not clearly different between patients treated with *sacubitril/valsartan* and those treated with valsartan alone (*ratio of change 0.95, 95% confidence interval 0.84–1.08*).

Sodium–glucose Cotransporter-2 Inhibitors

This new class of drugs (*SGLT2 inhibitors*) was originally designed to improve glycemic regulation in diabetes but was found to also improve cardiac outcomes, including the prevention of heart failure. Several trials in patients with reduced LVEF have consistently shown a significant reduction in hospital admissions due to heart failure and also a reduction in cardiovascular mortality.

Accordingly, this class (e.g., *dapagliflozin* and *empagliflozin*) is now one of the four pillars of *HFrEF* therapy.

Sotagliflozin is a combined SGLT1 and SGLT2 inhibitor, and whether it should be placed in the same class as purer SGLT2 inhibitors is yet not clear.

The 2021 ESC guideline has grouped sotagliflozin with the SGLT2 inhibitors in its recommendations for patients with heart failure and diabetes. The drug was only recently approved in the US and thus was not eligible for inclusion in the ACC/AHA/HFSA 2022 guideline.[13,14]

The two clinical trials of SGLT2 inhibitors that showed benefit for patients with *HFpEF* used the following enrolment criteria:

- New York Heart Association (NYHA) II–IV symptoms
- Treatment with a diuretic, an NT-BNP >300 pg/mL
- If sinus rhythm (*>600 or >900 pg/mL if atrial fibrillation*)
- Evidence of structural heart disease (*left atrial enlargement, left ventricular hypertrophy*)

In the *DELIVER* (Dapagliflozin Evaluation to Improve the Lives of Patients with Preserved Ejection Fraction Heart Failure) trial[15] or a recent hospital admission for heart failure.

β Blockers

It is important to note that β blockers are *not recommended* for patients with *HFpEF* (2B recommendation for *HFmrEF*). Lack of benefit for *HFpEF* was noted in a meta-analysis of randomized trials of β blockers, which reported a nonsignificant trend toward increased cardiovascular and all-cause mortality in patients with preserved LVEF and sinus rhythm (*hazard ratio 1.70, 95% confidence interval 0.78–4.10*).[16]

Importance of Rapid Initiation of Therapy

The importance of rapid initiation of life-prolonging heart failure medication is now recognized owing to results from the Safety, Tolerability and Efficacy of Rapid Optimization, Helped by *NT-proBNP* Testing, of Heart Failure Therapies (*STRONG-HF*) trial. This multicenter study with 1,078 patients from 87 hospitals in 14 countries examined rapid uptitration of guideline-directed medication after an admission for acute heart failure. The intervention group had their medications uptitrated to 100% of recommended doses within 2 weeks of discharge.

The primary endpoint of *180*-day readmission to hospital due to heart failure or all-cause death was reduced by an absolute percentage of *8.1%* (*95% confidence interval 2.9–13.2%*) with rapid titration. We note that the *STRONG-HF trial* was conducted before SGLT2 inhibitors became standard of care for *HFrEF* therapy.

Further evidence of the benefit of rapid initiation comes from the Dapagliflozin and Prevention of Adverse Outcomes in Heart Failure (*DAPA-HF*) trial.[17] Among *4,744* patients in this trial, the time to clinical benefit was surprisingly fast with a significant reduction in cardiovascular death or worsening heart failure observed by 28 days after randomization to dapagliflozin compared with placebo (*hazard ratio 0.51, 95% confidence interval 0.28–0.94*).

Similar results were observed in 1,222 patients treated with *sotagliflozin* compared with placebo; the time to a sustained and significant reduction in the primary endpoint was 27 days (*hazard ratio 9.62, 95% confidence interval 0.39–0.99*). However, the time to benefit was *twice* as long for patients with heart failure and preserved ejection fraction.

Though the goal is to initiate all four drug classes in a rapid, timely manner, the optimal order and timing of initiation remain uncertain. Investigators have modeled the potential benefit of different strategies based on how quickly benefits were observed in clinical trials.

It was observed that the strategy of starting treatment with SGLT2 inhibitors and MRAs leads to the greatest improvement in outcome. Other authors propose for a more rapid approach, starting all four drugs together at low doses. Starting drugs rapidly in combination may be the quickest way to reach recommended doses, keeping in mind a possible increase in the risk of temporary side effects such as hypotension or elevated creatinine.

Side effects may lead clinicians and patients to assume a permanent drug intolerance and reduce the chance that the patient is ultimately treated with all four recommended classes. The patient's condition may indicate the appropriate drug to use first. For example, an SGLT2 inhibitor or MRA may be the first appropriate drug in those with borderline low blood pressure.

There is an ongoing review of strategies for implementation of guideline-directed medical therapy which shall suggest newer guidelines.

Diuretics

Although diuretics are a mainstay of treatment for patients with signs or symptoms of congestion, they *do not improve mortality*. The efficacies of two loop diuretics were compared in the *TRANSFORM-HF trial*[18] of 2,859 patients who were randomized to *furosemide* or *torsemide*. The primary outcome of all-cause death was similar for the two loop diuretics (*hazard ratio with torsemide treatment 1.02, 95% confidence interval 0.89–1.18*).

The efficacy of intravenous *acetazolamide* in addition to intravenous loop diuretics was examined in the – *ADVOR (Acetazolamide in Decompensated Heart Failure with Volume Overload) trial.*[19] Among 519 patients with heart failure, greater decongestion was seen in the group randomized to *acetazolamide* (*successful decongestion within 3 days: 42.2 vs. 30.5%; p < 0.001*). In the *Safety and Efficacy of the Combination of Loop with Thiazide-type Diuretics in Patients with Decompensated Heart Failure—CLOROTIC trial,*[20] 239 patients were randomized to a *thiazide* diuretic or placebo in addition to a loop diuretic. The addition of the thiazide significantly increased decongestion but with an increase in serum creatinine. Together, the *ADVOR* and *CLOROTIC trials* suggest that add-on diuretic therapy can improve decongestion compared with loop diuretics alone, while long-term safety is uncertain.

Other Drug Treatments

Several additional medications can be used to improve outcomes among patients with HFrEF. This section discusses several of these therapies: *Hydralazine/isosorbide dinitrate therapy, ivabradine, vericiguat, intravenous iron,* and *glucagon-like peptide-1 receptor agonists (GLP1RA).* We discuss their evidence and contemporary role.

Hydralazine/Isosorbide Dinitrate Therapy[23]

The combination of *hydralazine* and *isosorbide dinitrate* is a guideline-recommended therapy for self-identified Black patients with *HFrEF* with NYHA class III or IV heart failure despite treatment with optimal medical therapy as described above. The combination therapy causes both arterial and venous vasodilation in addition to nitrous oxide augmentation that may have remodeling benefits. The benefits in HFpEF are not documented significantly.

Ivabradine

Ivabradine inhibits the channel responsible for the cardiac pacemaker current, I(f), in the sinus node. In *SHIFT* (Systolic Heart failure treatment with the If inhibitor ivabradine Trial),[24] among 6,558 patients with HFrEF with sinus rhythm and a heart rate ≥70 bpm, ivabradine led to an 18% relative reduction (*hazard ratio 0.82, 95% confidence interval 0.75–0.90*) compared with placebo. There are no recommendations for the use of ivabradine in HFpEF patients.

Vericiguat

Vericiguat is a novel heart failure medication that stimulates soluble guanylate cyclase and uptitrates the nitric oxide signaling pathway promoting vasodilation and reduced cardiac remodeling. In the *VICTORIA*[25] (*Vericiguat Global Study in Subjects with Heart Failure with Reduced Ejection Fraction*) trial, it was found that the risk of cardiovascular death or hospital admission for heart failure reduced in patients with HFrEF only. But there are no authentic recommendations for HFpEF patients.

Intravenous Iron Infusion[26]

Multiple studies have shown that iron deficiency and anemia are associated with increased mortality and decreased exertional capacity. Several trials have shown that intravenous iron reduces the risk of hospital admission for heart failure and improves patient-reported health status among patients with HFrEF only.

Glucagon-like Peptide-1 Receptor Agonists

Similar to SGLT2 inhibitors, GLP1RA were initially developed to improve glycemic control among patients with diabetes mellitus. In a meta-analysis of eight trials with cardiovascular outcomes evaluating *GLP1RA* among patients with type 2 diabetes mellitus, GLP1RA reduced the risk of cardiovascular death (hazard ratio 0.87, 95% confidence interval 0.80–0.94) and hospital admission for heart failure (0.89, 95% confidence interval 0.82–0.98). However, the prevalence of heart failure at baseline was between only 9 and 24% across these trials.

Glucagon-like peptide-1 receptor agonists were subsequently shown to be potent therapies for weight loss among obese patients without diabetes mellitus. In the Semaglutide Effects on Cardiovascular Outcomes in People with Overweight or *Obesity SELECT trial,*[27,28] semaglutide versus placebo was found to significantly reduce the composite outcome of cardiovascular death, nonfatal myocardial infarction, or nonfatal stroke among patients with existing atherosclerotic cardiovascular disease who were overweight or obese but without diabetes mellitus. 24% had chronic heart failure at baseline.

The effect of STEP-HFpEF (Semaglutide 2.4 mg once weekly on function and symptoms in subjects with obesity-related heart failure with preserved ejection fraction) trial[27,29] evaluated the effect of semaglutide versus placebo on patient-reported health status among 529 nondiabetic patients with ejection fraction ≥45%, obesity, and evidence of impaired health status [*Kansas City Cardiomyopathy Questionnaire (KCCQ) score of* <*90*] at baseline. Participants treated with semaglutide had on average a 7.8 (*95% confidence interval 4.8–10.9*) greater increase in their KCCQ score than patients treated with placebo, in addition to a significant 20.3 m larger improvement in their 6-minute walk distance.

Mitral Transcatheter Edge-to-edge Repair

Repair of the mitral valve via transcatheter edge-to-edge repair (TEER) is a well-accepted and useful therapy in patients of HFrEF.

Revascularization

Coronary artery bypass grafting (CABG) for patients, with severe coronary artery disease, has been shown to improve outcomes compared with medical therapy in patients of heart failure but HFrEF only.

NONDRUG, NONDEVICE THERAPIES

- *Restricting dietary sodium intake* is commonly recommended to reduce symptoms of heart failure. However, limited data are available to support such restriction. The *SODIUM-HF* (*Study of Dietary Intervention under 100 mmol in Heart Failure*) *trial*[30] randomized 806 patients to a low-sodium diet of <1,500 mg/day or usual care. It found similar rates of cardiovascular hospital admission, cardiovascular emergency department visits, or all-cause death (*hazard ratio 0.89, 95% confidence interval 0.63–1.26*). However, patients with a low-sodium diet had higher/better patient-reported health status. The US cardiovascular disease guidelines continue to recommend dietary sodium restriction. However, excessive sodium restriction may contribute to poor nutrition or may exacerbate deleterious neurohormonal activation.
- *Fluid restriction* heart failure has also been tested in several randomized trials. A meta-analysis of six trials found that liberal fluid consumption *did not* increase readmissions due to heart failure or all-cause mortality. Accordingly, heart failure guidelines now state that the benefit of fluid restriction is uncertain.

MEASURING PATIENT-REPORTED OUTCOMES IN HEART FAILURE

Without treatment, heart failure not only substantially increases the risk of mortality but also impairs the quality of life. Improving health-related quality of life is an important goal of heart failure treatment. Multiple therapies have been shown to significantly improve quality of life on the basis of patient-reported health status.

The two most commonly used measures of patient-reported health status in treatment trials have been the (1) *KCCQ*[31] and (2) *Minnesota Living with Heart Failure Questionnaire,*[32] which are not being elaborated herein.

DIFFERENT OUTCOMES DESPITE SIMILAR TREATMENT

- Inequitable outcomes for health conditions among different groups often exist within societies; obviously, heart failure is no exception.
- Data from the US suggest differences in the incidence of and survival with heart failure depending upon race and ethnicity.
- The cause of disparities in outcome is multifactorial, and these are often driven as much or more by social determinants of health than by differences in patient management.
- Recent studies found similar use of drug treatments to prolong survival for patients with heart failure, across race and ethnicity groups.
- A focus beyond treatment differences is needed if the overall health is to be improved.
- Including subjects from different/various races and ethnicities in clinical trials is important to improve our ability to provide appropriate customized care to all patients with heart failure.

CURRENT GUIDELINES FOR TREATMENT OF HFpEF

Several clinical guidelines have been published recently including the ESC (2021) and ACC/AHA/HFSA (2022) guidelines.

Important differences in guideline recommendations are rare and largely due to differences in the published evidence that occurred between publication.

- The 2022 ACC/AHA/HFSA guideline includes a 2A recommendation for *SGLT2* inhibitors for patients with *HFmrEF* and *HFpEF* following the publication of a large clinical trial showing outcome benefit.
- Important studies that were published after these guidelines include a second randomized trial showing benefit of *SGLT2* inhibitors in patients with an LVEF >40%.
- The *STRONG-HF* trial showed benefit of rapid initiation and titration of medications for those with *HFrEF*.
- A trial showed that pulmonary pressure monitoring using the *CardioMEMS* device improved outcome.
- Future guidelines will likely incorporate the trial results into revised recommendations.

Box 1 summarizes new evidence published since the 2022 ACC/AHA/HFSA and 2021 ESC heart failure guidelines.

An update to the 2021 ESC guideline incorporates new clinical trials of SGLT2 inhibitors, finerenone, and intravenous iron therapy.

EMERGING TREATMENTS

Continued progress in treatment remains critical given the residual morbidity for patients with heart failure.

- *Omecamtiv mecarbil* is a cardiac myosin activator that improves cardiac contractility. In the *GALACTIC-HF*[33,34] (*Global Approach to Lowering Adverse Cardiac Outcomes through Improving Contractility in Heart Failure*) trial, 8258 patients with *HFrEF* who received Omecamtiv Mecarbil showed an 8% relative reduction (*0.92, 95% confidence interval 0.86–0.99*) in the risk of cardiovascular death or heart failure event (*hospital admission or urgent visit*).

Omecamtiv mecarbil is not available freely.

- The *VICTOR trial* is evaluating the efficacy of *vericiguat* among patients with heart failure who have not had a recent worsening heart failure event.
- The *DECISION trial*[35] is testing the efficacy and safety of *digoxin* at low serum concentrations.
- The *TOPCAT trial*[36] findings further ignited controversy about spironolactone. Two ongoing trials are evaluating the efficacy of *spironolactone* among patients with heart failure with LVEF ≥40%.

BOX 1: Updates in heart failure since the 2022 American College of Cardiology/American Heart Association/Heart Failure Society of America and 2021 European Society of Cardiology heart failure guidelines. Of note, angiotensin receptor/neprilysin inhibitor (ARNI) may not be beneficial in patients with a left ventricular ejection fraction >60%.

SGLT2 inhibitors
- DELIVER trial confirmed benefit of SGLT2 inhibitors for patients with HFmrEF and HFpEF
- Sotagliflozin approved for HF treatment in US

ARNI for HFpEF
- Pooled PARAGLIDE-HF and PARAGON trials show that ARNI reduces worsening HF events and CV death in patients with HFmrEF/HFpEF

Intravenous iron for HFrEF
- Meta-analyses of intravenous iron find reduction in hospital admissions for HF and improved HRQOL

Diuretic therapy
- Adjunctive diuresis with acetalozamide improved decongestion without improving clinical outcomes in ADVOR trial
- Outpatient torsemide and furosemide have similar outcomes in TRANSFORM-HF trial

HF medical management
- Rapid uptitration of HF therapy reduced composite of all-cause death and HF readmissions in STRONG-HF trial

PA pressure monitoring
- PA pressure monitoring led to improvement in HRQOL and reduction in hospital admission for HF In MONITOR-HF trial

Sodium restriction
- Dietary sodium restriction did not improve clinical outcomes in SODIUM-HF trial

Coronary revascularization
- Percutaneous coronary revascularization for ischemic cardiomyopathy did not improve clinical outcomes in REVIVED-BCIS2 trial

Advanced HF
- Heart donation after circulatory death had similar survival rates to donation after brain death

(CV: cardiovascular; HF: heart failure; HFmrEF: heart failure with mildly reduced ejection fraction; HFpEF: heart failure with preserved ejection fraction; HFrEF: heart failure with reduced ejection fraction; HRQOL: health-related quality of life; PA: pulmonary artery; SGLT2: sodium–glucose cotransporter-2)

Source: Reproduced from Heidenreich P, Sandhu A. BMJ. 2024; 385:e077025.

Many *novel therapies* for heart failure are under evaluation in clinical trials:

- These include multiple trials of *finernone*[37] among patients with heart failure across the ejection fraction spectrum.

- The *SUMMIT trial*[38] is evaluating the effect of *tirzepatide*, another *GLP1RA*, among patients with *HFpEF* and *obesity*.
- Other ongoing studies are testing *anti-inflammatory therapies* among patients with *HFmrEF/HFpEF*.

Nondrug care of patients with heart failure also continues to evolve.

- The *CABA-HFPEF trial* is testing *catheter ablation* among patients with heart failure with LVEF ≥40% and atrial fibrillation (NCT05508256).
- Multiple ongoing trials are evaluating *tricuspid valve interventions* among patients with severe tricuspid regurgitation.

Several ongoing trials will help to clarify the role of existing heart failure therapies.

CONCLUSION

Management of patients with heart failure has improve markedly, with evidence for four life-prolonging classes of drugs for patients with reduced LVEF and the benefit of SGLT2 inhibitors for those with mildly reduced and preserved LVEF. Device management and other nondrug management have evolved as results from new clinical trials are published. Identification of appropriate candidates for treatment requires accurate diagnosis, which can be challenging for patients with heart failure and preserved ejection fraction. Additional questions remain—in particular, how best to implement these new treatment recommendations into clinical practice.

POINTS—REMAINING UNANSWERED

- Does the order of initiation of medications for heart failure with reduced LVEF affect the ability to achieve sustained treatment with all four pillars of therapy?
- Does the simultaneous initiation of medications increase or decrease the probability of sustained drug treatment?
- What are the benefits of medications in addition to sodium-glucose cotransporter-2 inhibitors for patients with heart failure with preserved LVEF?
- Which patients should receive a trial of medication withdrawal if their symptoms resolve and their left ventricular function becomes normal?

REFERENCES

1. GBD 2019 Diseases and Injuries Collaborators. Global burden of 369 diseases and injuries in 204 countries and territories, 19902019: a systematic analysis for the Global Burden of Disease Study 2019. Lancet. 2020;396:1204-22.
2. Yan T, Zhu S, Yin X, et al. Burden, Trends, and Inequalities of Heart Failure Globally, 1990 to 2019: A Secondary Analysis Based on the Global Burden of Disease 2019 Study. J Am Heart Assoc. 2023;12:e027852.
3. Jain V, Minhas AMK, Khan SU, et al. Trends in HF Hospitalizations Among Young Adults in the United States From 2004 to 2018. JACC Heart Fail. 2022;10:350-62.
4. Taylor CJ, Ordóñez-Mena JM, Jones NR, et al. National trends in heart failure mortality in men and women, United Kingdom, 2000-2017. Eur J Heart Fail. 2021;23:3-12.
5. Drozd M, Relton SD, Walker AMN, et al. Association of heart failure and its comorbidities with loss of life expectancy. Heart 2021;107:1417-21.
6. Folsom AR, Shah AM, Lutsey PL, et al. American Heart Association's Life's Simple 7: Avoiding Heart Failure and Preserving Cardiac Structure and Function. Am J Med 2015;128:970-6.e2.
7. Heidenreich PA, Albert NM, Allen LA, et al., American Heart Association Advocacy Coordinating Committee Council on Arteriosclerosis, Thrombosis and Vascular Biology Council on Cardiovascular Radiology and Intervention Council on Clinical Cardiology Council on Epidemiology and Prevention Stroke Council. Forecasting the impact of heart failure in the United States: a policy statement from the American Heart Association. Circ Heart Fail. 2013;6:606-19.
8. Bassi NS, Ziaeian B, Yancy CW, et al. Association of optimal implementation of sodium-glucose cotransporter 2 inhibitor therapy with outcome for patients with heart failure. JAMA Cardiol. 2020;5:948-51.
9. Pieske B, Tschöpe C, de Boer RA, et al. How to diagnose heart failure with preserved ejection fraction: the HFA-PEFF diagnostic algorithm: a consensus recommendation from the Heart Failure Association (HFA) of the European Society of Cardiology (ESC). Eur Heart J. 2019;40:3297-317.
10. Mebazaa A, Davison B, Chioncel O, et al. Safety, tolerability and efficacy of up-titration of guideline-directed medical therapies for acute heart failure (STRONG-HF): a multinational, open-label, randomised, trial. Lancet. 2022;400:1938-52.
11. McMurray JJ, Packer M, Desai AS, et al., PARADIGM-HF Investigators and Committees. Angiotensin-neprilysin inhibition versus enalapril in heart failure. N Engl J Med. 2014;371:993-1004.
12. Mann DL, Givertz MM, Vader JM, et al., LIFE Investigators. Effect of Treatment With Sacubitril/Valsartan in Patients With Advanced Heart Failure and Reduced Ejection Fraction: A Randomized Clinical Trial. JAMA Cardiol. 2022; 7:17-25.
13. Bhatt DL, Szarek M, Steg PG, et al., SOLOIST-WHF Trial Investigators. Sotagliflozin in patients with diabetes and recent worsening heart failure. N Engl J Med 2021; 384:117-28.
14. Bhatt DL, Szarek M, Pitt B, et al. SCORED Investigators. Sotagliflozin in Patients with Diabetes and Chronic Kidney Disease. N Engl J Med. 2021;384:129-39.

15. Solomon SD, McMurray JJV, Claggett B, et al., DELIVER Trial Committees and Investigators. Dapagliflozin in heart failure with mildly reduced or preserved ejection fraction. N Engl J Med. 2022;387:1089-98.
16. Cleland JGF, Bunting KV, Flather MD, et al. Beta-blockers in Heart Failure Collaborative Group. Beta-blockers for heart failure with reduced, mid-range, and preserved ejection fraction: an individual patient-level analysis of double-blind randomized trials. Eur Heart J. 2018;39: 26-35.
17. Kosiborod MN, Jhund PS, Docherty KF, et al. Effects of Dapagliflozin on Symptoms, Function, and Quality of Life in Patients With Heart Failure and Reduced Ejection Fraction: Results From the DAPA-HF Trial. Circulation. 2020;141:90-9.
18. Mentz RJ, Anstrom KJ, Eisenstein EL, et al., TRANSFORM-HF Investigators. Effect of Torsemide vs Furosemide After Discharge on All-Cause Mortality in Patients Hospitalized With Heart Failure: The TRANSFORM-HF Randomized Clinical Trial. JAMA. 2023;329:214-23.
19. Mullens W, Dauw J, Martens P, et al., ADVOR Study Group. Acetazolamide in acute decompensated heart failure with volume overload. N Engl J Med 2022;387:1185-95.
20. Trullàs JC, Morales-Rull JL, Casado J, et al., CLOROTIC trial investigators. Combining loop with thiazide diuretics for decompensated heart failure: the CLOROTIC trial. Eur Heart J. 2023;44:411-21.
21. Nallamshetty S, Castillo A, Nguyen A, et al. Clinical predictors of improvement in left ventricular ejection fraction in U.S. veterans with heart failure. Am Heart J Plus. 2022;19:100183.
22. Lewis GD, Malhotra R, Hernandez AF, et al. NHLBI Heart Failure Clinical Research Network. Effect of Oral Iron Repletion on Exercise Capacity in Patients With Heart Failure With Reduced Ejection Fraction and Iron Deficiency: The IRONOUT HF Randomized Clinical Trial. JAMA. 2017;317:1958-66.
23. Khazanie P, Liang L, Curtis LH, et al. Clinical Effectiveness of Hydralazine-Isosorbide Dinitrate Therapy in Patients With Heart Failure and Reduced Ejection Fraction: Findings From the Get With The Guidelines-Heart Failure Registry. Circ Heart Fail. 2016;9:e002444.
24. Swedberg K, Komajda M, Böhm M, et al., SHIFT Investigators. Ivabradine and outcomes in chronic heart failure (SHIFT): a randomised placebo-controlled study. Lancet. 2010;376:875-85.
25. Senni M, Lopez-Sendon J, Cohen-Solal A, et al. Vericiguat and NTproBNP in patients with heart failure with reduced ejection fraction: analyses from the VICTORIA trial. ESC Heart Fail. 2022;9:3791-803.
26. Salah HM, Savarese G, Rosano GMC, et al. Intravenous iron infusion in patients with heart failure: a systematic review and study-level meta-analysis. ESC Heart Fail. 2023;10:147380.
27. Wilding JPH, Batterham RL, Calanna S, et al. STEP 1 Study Group. Once-Weekly Semaglutide in Adults with Overweight or Obesity. N Engl J Med 2021;384:989-1002.
28. Neves JS, Packer M, Ferreira JP. Increased Risk of Heart Failure Hospitalization With GLP-1 Receptor Agonists in Patients With Reduced Ejection Fraction: A Meta-Analysis of the EXSCEL and FIGHT Trials. J Card Fail. 2023;29:1107-9.
29. Jastreboff AM, Aronne LJ, Ahmad NN, et al. SURMOUNT-1 Investigators. Tirzepatide Once Weekly for the Treatment of Obesity. N Engl J Med. 2022;387:205-16.
30. Ezekowitz JA, Colin-Ramirez E, Ross H, et al. SODIUM-HF Investigators. Reduction of dietary sodium to less than 100 mmol in heart failure (SODIUM-HF): an international, open-label, randomised, controlled trial. Lancet. 2022; 399:1391-400.
31. Spertus JA, Jones PG, Sandhu AT, et al. Interpreting the Kansas City Cardiomyopathy Questionnaire in Clinical Trials and Clinical Care: JACC State-of-the-Art Review. J Am Coll Cardiol. 2020;76:2379-90.
32. Bilbao A, Escobar A, García-Perez L, et al. The Minnesota living with heart failure questionnaire: comparison of different factor structures. Health Qual Life Outcomes. 2016;14:23.
33. Teerlink JR, Diaz R, Felker GM, et al. GALACTIC-HF Investigators. Cardiac Myosin Activation with Omecamtiv Mecarbil in Systolic Heart Failure. N Engl J Med 2021; 384:105-16.
34. Docherty KF, McMurray JJV, Claggett BL, et al. Efficacy of omecamtiv mecarbil in heart failure with reduced ejection fraction according to N-terminal pro-B-type natriuretic peptide level: insights from the GALACTIC-HF trial. Eur J Heart Fail 2023;25:248-59.
35. Lewis EF, Kim HY, Claggett B, et al. TOPCAT Investigators. Impact of Spironolactone on Longitudinal Changes in Health-Related Quality of Life in the Treatment of Preserved Cardiac Function Heart Failure With an Aldosterone Antagonist Trial. Circ Heart Fail. 2016;9:e001937.
36. Bakris GL, Agarwal R, Anker SD, et al. FIDELIO-DKD Investigators. Effect of Finerenone on Chronic Kidney Disease Outcomes in Type 2 Diabetes. N Engl J Med. 2020;383:2219-29.
37. Jastreboff AM, Aronne LJ, Ahmad NN, et al. SURMOUNT-1 Investigators. Tirzepatide Once Weekly for the Treatment of Obesity. N Engl J Med. 2022;387:205-16.
38. Arnold SV, Chinnakondepalli KM, Spertus JA, et al. COAPT Investigators. Health Status After Transcatheter Mitral-Valve Repair in Heart Failure and Secondary Mitral Regurgitation: COAPT Trial. J Am Coll Cardiol. 2019;73:2123-32.

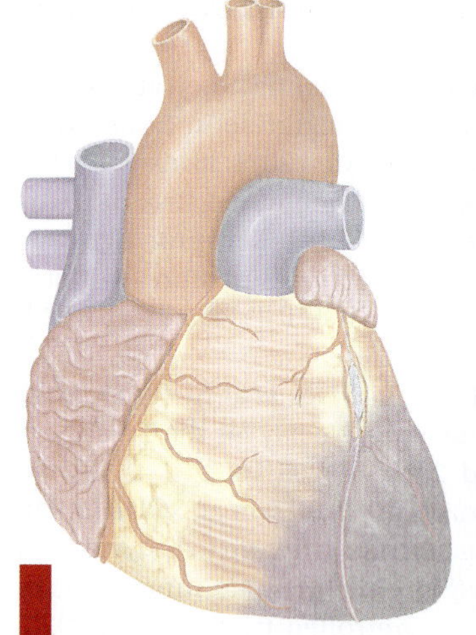

Risk Stratification of SCD in HFpEF

Ravi Prakash, Shashank Mohanty

INTRODUCTION

Heart failure (HF) is a complex clinical syndrome in which structural or functional myocardial abnormalities result in symptoms and signs of hypoperfusion and/or pulmonary or systemic congestion at rest or during exercise.[1,2]

Heart failure with preserved ejection fraction (HFpEF) represents half of HF patients, who are more likely older, women, hypertensive, and with atrial fibrillation. HFpEF poses a significant clinical challenge, with sudden cardiac death (SCD) emerging as one of the leading causes of mortality. Despite significant advancements in cardiovascular medicine, predicting and preventing SCD in HFpEF remains complex due to multifactorial pathophysiological mechanisms and patient heterogeneity. Unlike heart failure with reduced ejection fraction (HFrEF), where impaired contractility and ventricular remodeling predominate, HFpEF pathophysiology involves heavy burden of comorbidities such as hypertension, obesity, and diabetes. Diverse mechanisms, including diastolic dysfunction, microvascular abnormalities, and inflammation, also contribute to SCD risk profiles. Various parameters such as clinical factors, electrocardiogram features, advanced imaging modalities, and biomarkers offer promise in risk prediction, yet comprehensive risk stratification models specific to HFpEF are lacking.

The definition of SCD by World Health Organization (WHO) in 1985 referred to "sudden unexpected death occurring either within 1 hour of symptom onset (witnessed), or within 24 hours of having been observed alive and symptom-free (unwitnessed)."[3]

Currently, SCD accounts for about 40–45% of all deaths in HFrEF patients, and the proportion of SCD is higher in patients with milder symptoms [New York Heart Association (NYHA) class II–III].[4-7] Two-thirds of patients with NYHA functional class II experience SCD, compared with only one-third of those with NYHA functional class IV symptoms, who died preponderantly for advanced HF.[8]

Limited epidemiological data are available exploring the landscape of SCD in patients with HFpEF, however recent trials reported that SCD occurs in about 20% of patients with HFpEF. There is a great unmet need in the field of SCD in HFpEF regarding risk stratification and appropriate device therapy with ICD implantation.

SUDDEN CARDIAC DEATH IN PATIENTS WITH HEART FAILURE WITH PRESERVED EJECTION FRACTION

Although patients with HFpEF were less prone to SCD compared to patients with HFrEF, patients with HFpEF did account for a significant proportion of all HF patients who encountered SCD. An observational study in Netherland showed that the incidence of SCD in patients with a LVEF >50% and a previous HF history was 19%, while the incidence of SCD was 61% in patients with a LVEF >50% but without HF history.[9] Another study by Stecker et al. assessed 121 SCD patients who had LVEF data before SCD. They found that 48% of these SCD patients have a normal (≥55%) LVEF.[3] The incidence of SCD in patients with HFpEF remains unknown in these two studies. In the TOPCAT, I-PRESERVE, and CHARM-Preserved trials, SCD consistently accounted for around one-fourth of total death in HFpEF patients in these trials.[10] In the I-PRESERVE trial, the annual SCD rate was 1.35% in patients with HFpEF.[10]

MECHANISMS OF SUDDEN CARDIAC DEATH IN HEART FAILURE WITH PRESERVED EJECTION FRACTION

Myocardial substrate remodeling, including myocardial scars, left ventricular hypertrophy (LVH), cardiac fibrosis, and collagen deposition, might enhance anisotropic ventricular conduction and facilitate re-entrant ventricular arrhythmia.[11]

RISK STRATIFICATION OF SUDDEN CARDIAC DEATH IN HEART FAILURE WITH PRESERVED EJECTION FRACTION

In the Oregon Sudden Unexpected Death Study (Oregon SUDS), LVH was reported to have a statistically significant impact on SCD prediction in multivariate analyses.[10] Despite employing different echocardiographic criteria of LVH among several studies, LVH was consistently shown to be a robust predictor of SCD in HFpEF patients.

Other conditions at high risk of SCD with preserved ejection fraction are idiopathic dilated cardiomyopathy, hypertrophic cardiomyopathy (HCM), arrhythmogenic right ventricular cardiomyopathy (ARVC), channelopathies, and valvular diseases.

In the I-PRESERVE trial, patients with age ≥75 years, NT-proBNP ≥339 pg/mL, presence of diabetes mellitus, previous hospitalization for HF, and NYHA class IV showed a significant increase in event rate, including SCD. Women had significantly lower rates of events, compared to men. Diabetes mellitus seems to play an important role in the SCD risk of patients with HFpEF.

Using the Duke University databank for cardiovascular disease, Al-Khatib et al.[12] found that five clinical variables were predictors of SCD in patients with isolated diastolic HF: diabetes mellitus, mitral regurgitation, severity of symptoms as assessed by NYHA class, history of myocardial infarction (MI), and severity of coronary artery disease (number of diseased coronary arteries). In a subanalysis of the I-PRESERVE trial, the following variables were associated to a ≥10% risk of SCD over 5 years at multivariable analysis: age, gender (male), history of diabetes mellitus, history of MI, left bundle branch block (LBBB), and $\log_e$ NT-proBNP.

Recently, an impaired LV global longitudinal strain was also found to be an independent predictor of SCD. Finally, in the JCARE-CARD registry, the only predictor of SCD in HFpEF was lower eGFR.

Risk stratification for SCD in patients with previous MI and preserved LVEF has been explored in the PEACE study,[13,14] where clinical variables associated with a higher proportional risk of SCD were angina pectoris, LVEF >40% but <50% (as opposed to >50%), diuretics use, digitalis use, prior coronary revascularization, and being female or Caucasian. These variables were confirmed to a certain extent in the PRE-DETERMINE study,[15,16] with age <60 years, LVEF 30–49% and diabetes mellitus being associated to SCD.

In a prospective multicenter study, 301 patients with non-ST-elevation myocardial infarction (NSTEMI) and 268 patients with ST-elevation myocardial infarction (STEMI) with preserved LVEF were enrolled to receive baseline echocardiographic evaluation. During a median 30 months of follow-up, decreased global longitudinal strain (GLS), increased mechanical dispersion, and increased postsystolic strain index (PSSI) were associated with increased arrhythmias risk in both the NSTEMI and STEMI groups.[17] This finding indicated that regional myocardial motion impairment on echocardiography could be predictors for SCD in patients with ischemic heart disease and HFpEF.

The ECG also serves as a simple tool to identify the proarrhythmic state. T wave alternans (TWA), defined by beat-to-beat variation in T wave morphology, have been found to be associated with lethal arrhythmia.[18] TWA has been validated in some clinical trials of ischemic cardiomyopathy with HFrEF to predict SCD.[19] In a prospective observational study, TWA analyzed after acute MI in patients with HFpEF (an LVEF ≥ 40%) was associated with increased SCD risk.[20,21]

Thus, unlike the risk predictors for SCD in patients with ischemic cardiomyopathy and HFrEF, the risk predictors for SCD in nonischemic HFpEF patients remain inconclusive. Anatomical remodeling, autonomic dysfunction, electrical remodeling, and genetic characteristics could be equally important and will serve as the four pillars to determine the SCD risks in patients with HF.

PREVENTION AND RISK REDUCTION IN HEART FAILURE WITH PRESERVED EJECTION FRACTION

Since ICD trials enrolling patients with systolic dysfunction (LVEF ≤35%), including both ischemic and nonischemic causes showed benefit in reducing SCD from ICD primary prevention.[18] SCD prevention by ICD implantation in HFrEF is therefore a well-established treatment. Other backbone drugs or device therapy for HFrEF, including angiotensin-converting enzymes inhibitors (ACEi), β-blockers, mineralocorticoid receptor antagonists (MRA), neprilysin inhibitors, and CRT, also showed a trend toward SCD reduction in subgroups in the randomized controlled trials.

Due to the limited data, prevention of SCD in HFpEF is still inconclusive. Considering heterogeneity in HFpEF and complex comorbidities in these patients, priority should be placed at treating the disease-causing mechanisms, such as ischemia, valvular heart diseases, hypertension, or diabetes, and preventing any precipitating factor such as electrolyte imbalance.

CONCLUSION

Researches regarding SCD in patients with systolic dysfunction has been well studied. As the new HF classification has been established, and epidemiologic data highlighted the large number of SCD cases in HFpEF, more attention is attracted to the risk of SCD in this group. When trying to extrapolate the well-established HF management concepts from HFrEF to HFpEF, heterogeneity in HFpEF remains a major challenge in defining an integral framework for risk stratification. Multi-pronged approaches to prevent anatomic remodeling, autonomic dysfunction, electrical remodeling, and identify genetic characteristics are essential. Effective prevention such as ICD implantation could thereafter be implemented only if we can predict SCD in HFpEF precisely.

REFERENCES

1. Metra M, Teerlink JR. Heart Failure. Lancet. 2017; 390:1981-95.
2. Gupta R, Joshi P, Mohan V, et al. Epidemiology and causation of coronary heart disease and stroke in India. Heart. 2008;94:16-26.
3. WHO. Sudden cardiac death. Report of a WHO Scientific Group. World Health Organ Tech Rep Ser. 1985;726:5-25.
4. Yusuf S, Sleight P, Pogue J, et al. Effects of an angiotensin-converting-enzyme inhibitor, ramipril, on cardiovascular events in high-risk patients. The Heart Outcomes Prevention Evaluation Study Investigators. N Engl J Med. 2000;342:145-53.
5. Uretsky BF, Sheahan RG. Primary prevention of sudden cardiac death in heart failure: Will the solution be shocking? J Am Coll Cardiol. 1997;30:1589-97.
6. Klein L, Hsia H. Sudden cardiac death in heart failure. Cardiol Clin. 2014;32:135-44.
7. Rosanio S, Schwarz ER, Vitarelli A, et al. Sudden death prophylaxis in heart failure. Int J Cardiol. 2007;119:291-6.
8. Saour B, Smith B, Yancy CW. Heart failure and sudden cardiac death. Card Electrophysiol Clin. 2017;9(4):709-23.
9. Gorgels APM, Gijsbers C, de Vreede-Swagemakers J, et al. Out-of-hospital cardiac arrest-the relevance of heart failure. The Maastricht Circulatory Arrest Registry. Eur Heart J. 2003;24(13):1204-9.
10. Pitt B, Pfeffer MA, Assmann SF, et al. Spironolactone for heart failure with preserved ejection fraction. N Engl J Med. 2014;370:1383-92.
11. Zile MR, Gaasch WH, Anand IS, et al. Mode of death in patients with heart failure and a preserved ejection fraction: results from the Irbesartan in Heart Failure With Preserved Ejection Fraction Study (I-Preserve) trial. Circulation. 2010;121(12):1393-405.
12. Al-Khatib SM, Shaw LK, O'Connor C et al. Incidence and predictors of sudden cardiac death in patients with diastolic heart failure. J Cardiovasc Electrophysiol. 2007; 18:1231-5.
13. Gatzoulis KA, Tsiachris D, Arsenos P, et al. Arrhythmic risk stratification in post-myocardial infarction patients with preserved ejection fraction: the PRESERVE EF study. Eur Heart J. 2019;40(35):2940-9.
14. Hsia J, Jablonski KA, Rice MM, et al. Sudden cardiac death in patients with stable coronary artery disease and preserved left ventricular systolic function. Am J Cardiol. 2008;101(4):457-61.
15. Sfairopoulos D, Zhang N, Wang Y, et al. Association between sodium-glucose cotransporter-2 inhibitors and risk of sudden cardiac death or ventricular arrhythmias: a meta-analysis of randomized controlled trials. Europace. 2022;24(1):20-30.
16. Chatterjee NA, Moorthy MV, Pester J, et al. Sudden Death in Patients with Coronary Heart Disease Without Severe Systolic Dysfunction. JAMA Cardiol. 2018;3(7):591-600.
17. Haugaa KH, Grenne BL, Eek CH, et al. Strain echocardiography improves risk prediction of ventricular arrhythmias after myocardial infarction. JACC Cardiovasc Imaging. 2013;6(8):841-50.
18. Saour B, Smith B, Yancy CW. Heart failure and sudden cardiac death. Card Electrophysiol Clin. 2017;9(4): 709-23.
19. Chow T, Kereiakes DJ, Onufer J, et al. Does microvolt T-wave alternans testing predict ventricular tachyarrhythmias in patients with ischemic cardiomyopathy and prophylactic defibrillators? The MASTER (Microvolt T Wave Alternans Testing for Risk Stratification of Post-Myocardial Infarction Patients) trial. J Am Coll Cardiol. 2008;52(20): 1607-15.
20. Ikeda T, Yoshino H, Sugi K, et al. Predictive value of microvolt T-wave alternans for sudden cardiac death in patients with preserved cardiac function after acute myocardial infarction: results of a collaborative cohort study. J Am Coll Cardiol. 2006;48(11):2268-74.
21. Buxton AE, Lee KL, DiCarlo L, et al. Electrophysiologic testing to identify patients with coronary artery disease who are at risk for sudden death. Multicenter unsustained tachycardia trial investigators. N Engl J Med. 2000;342(26): 1937-45.

Guideline Update in HFpEF Pharmacotherapy

Arindam Pande, Durlabh Debbarma

INTRODUCTION

Heart failure (HF) remains a leading cause of morbidity and mortality globally. The 2022 HF guideline provides recommendations based on contemporary evidence for the treatment of these patients. The recommendations present an evidence-based approach in managing patients with HF, with the intent to improve quality of care and align with patients' interests. Many recommendations from the earlier HF guidelines have been updated with new evidence, and new recommendations have been made based on newly published data.[1,2]

Despite advances in therapy, HF continues to be a major cause of morbidity and mortality worldwide, with a lifetime risk of approximately 20% at age 40 years.[3] Although the incidence of overall HF in the United States appears to be stable or even declining, the incidence of heart failure with preserved ejection fraction (HFpEF) continues to rise.[4,5] HFpEF now accounts for >50% cases of HF,[6] with outcomes comparable to heart failure with reduced ejection fraction (HFrEF).[7] HFpEF is often underrecognized and results in substantial resource utilization. Historically, treatment options were limited to managing comorbidities; however, revolutionary advances in the past decade regarding the pathophysiology of HFpEF, improved methods of diagnosis, and insights into prognostic predictions now yield novel, effective management strategies. With many recent clinical trial results, there is an increasing urgency for accurate diagnosis and timely implementation of guideline-directed medical therapy (GDMT).

CLASSIFICATION AND STAGES

Classification of Heart Failure by Left Ventricular Ejection Fraction

The classification of HF by left ventricular ejection fraction (LVEF) is given in **Table 1**.

TABLE 1: Classification of HF by LVEF.

Type of HF according to LVEF	*Criteria*
HFrEF (HF with reduced EF)	LVEF ≤ 40%
HFimpEF (HF with improved EF)	Previous LVEF ≤ 40% and a follow-up measurement of LVEF > 40%
HFmrEF (HF with mildly reduced EF)	LVEF = 41–49% Evidence of spontaneous or provokable increased LV filling pressures (e.g., elevated natriuretic peptide, noninvasive and invasive hemodynamic measurement)
HFpEF (HF with preserved EF)	LVEF ≥ 50% Evidence of spontaneous or provokable increased LV filling pressures (e.g., elevated natriuretic peptide, noninvasive and invasive hemodynamic measurement)

Flowchart 1: ACC/AHA stages of HF.

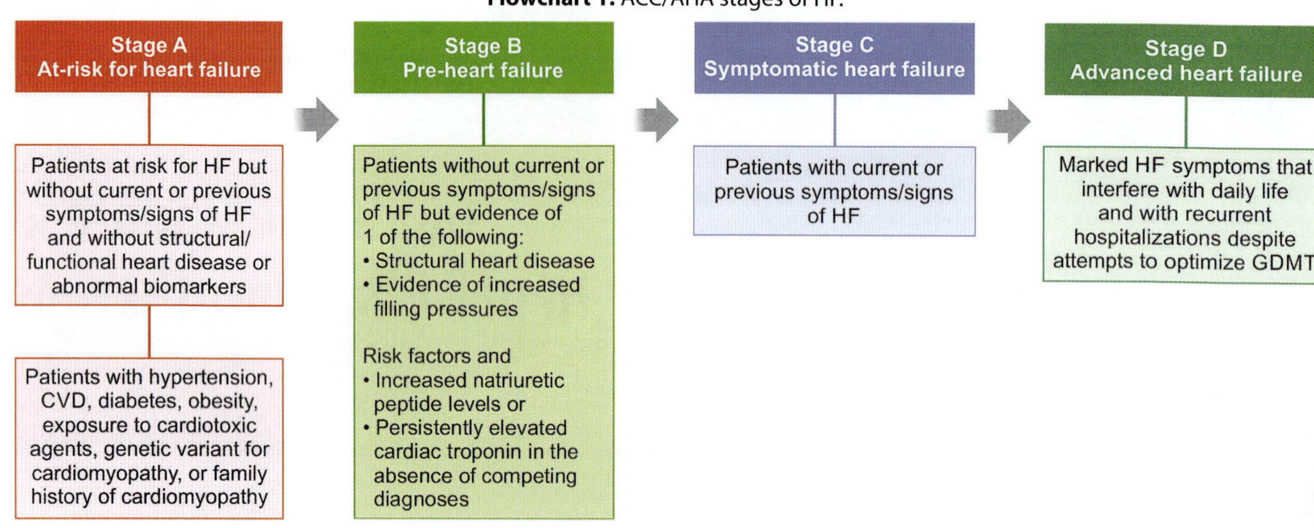

(ACC: American College of Cardiology; AHA: American Heart Association; CVD: cardiovascular disease; GDMT: guideline-directed medical therapy; HF: heart failure)

Stages of Heart Failure

The ACC/AHA stages of HF are shown in **Flowchart 1**.

DEFINITIONS

- *GDMT:* Treatment options supported for use by clinical practice guidelines
- *HF:* Defined as per the universal definition of HF;[8] symptoms and/or signs of HF caused by structural/ functional cardiac abnormalities and at least one of: (1) Elevated natriuretic peptides or (2) objective evidence of cardiogenic pulmonary or systemic congestion. An HF event, including hospitalization, is defined by the criteria outlined by the 2014 ACC/AHA Key Data Elements and Definitions for Cardiovascular Endpoint Events in Clinical Trials.[9]
- *HFrEF:* Clinical diagnosis of HF and LVEF < 40%.[10]
- *HFmrEF:* Clinical diagnosis of HF and LVEF 41–49%.[10]
- *HF with improved EF:* Previous LVEF < 40% and a follow-up measurement > 40%.
- *HFpEF:* Clinical diagnosis of HF and LVEF > 50%.[10] not attributable to an underlying cause such as an infiltrative cardiomyopathy, hypertrophic cardiomyopathy, valvular disease, pericardial disease, or high-output HF.
- *HFpEF mimics:* Clinical diagnosis of HF and LVEF > 50% with a primary noncardiac cause (kidney or liver disease) or an underlying cardiac cause (infiltrative cardiomyopathy, hypertrophic cardiomyopathy, valvular disease, pericardial disease, or high-output HF).
- The *New York Heart Association (NYHA)* functional classification is given as follows:
  - *Class I:* No limitation of physical activity. Ordinary physical activity does not cause symptoms of HF.
  - *Class II:* Slight limitation of physical activity. Comfortable at rest, but ordinary physical activity results in symptoms of HF.
  - *Class III:* Marked limitation of physical activity. Comfortable at rest but less than ordinary activity causes symptoms of HF.
  - *Class IV:* Unable to perform any physical activity without symptoms of HF or symptoms of HF at rest.

DIAGNOSIS OF HEART FAILURE WITH PRESERVED EJECTION FRACTION

The universal definition of HF is given in **Figure 1**.

Heart Failure with Preserved Ejection Fraction Diagnostic Scoring Systems

The HFpEF diagnostic scoring systems are shown in **Table 2**.

The H_2FPEF score includes six clinically accessible factors.

The HFA-PEFF score is shown in **Figure 2**.

Heart Failure with Preserved Ejection Fraction Mimics

The HFpEF mimics is shown in **Table 3**.

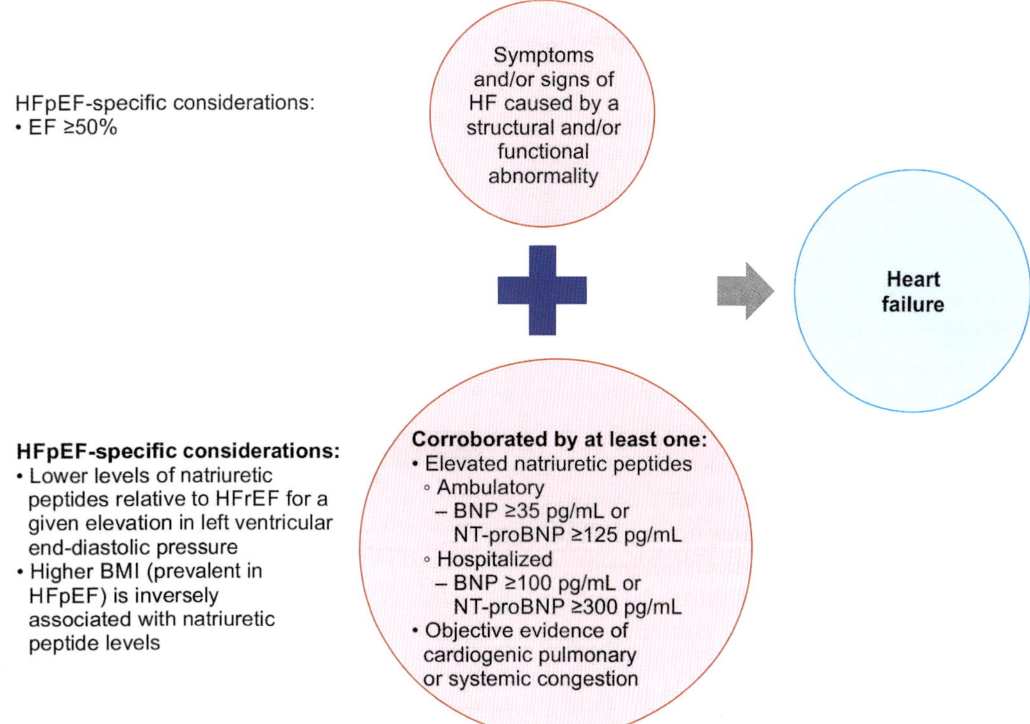

Fig. 1: Universal definition of HF.
Note: The universal definition of HF requires symptoms and/or signs caused by structural/functional cardiac abnormalities *and* at least one of: (1) Elevated natriuretic peptides *or* (2) objective evidence of cardiogenic pulmonary or systemic congestion. In HFpEF, specific additional criteria include EF 50% or greater and consideration of pitfalls as described in the assessment of natriuretic peptide levels.
(BMI: body mass index; BNP: B-type natriuretic peptide; HF: heart failure; HFpEF: heart failure with preserved ejection fraction; HFrEF: heart failure with reduced ejection fraction; NT-proBNP: N-terminal pro-B-type natriuretic peptide)

TABLE 2: HFpEF diagnostic scoring systems.

	H_2FpEF	
H_2	*H*eavy (BMI > 30 kg/m^2) On ≥2 anti*H*ypertensives	2 1
F	Atrial *F*ibrillation	3
P	*P*ulmonary hypertension (PASP > 35 mm Hg on Doppler echocardiography)	1
E	*E*lder (age > 60 years)	1
F	*F*illing pressure (E/é >9 on Doppler echocardiography)	1
	≥6 points: highly diagnostic of HFpEF	

MANAGEMENT OF HEART FAILURE WITH PRESERVED EJECTION FRACTION

Management of HFpEF focuses on: (1) Risk stratification and management of comorbidities, including hypertension, DM, obesity, atrial fibrillation (AF), CAD, CKD, and obstructive sleep apnea; (2) nonpharmacological management, including the role of exercise and weight loss and the use of wireless, implantable pulmonary artery monitors; and (3) symptom management and disease-modifying therapy with loop diuretic agents, SGLT2is, mineralocorticoid receptor antagonists (MRAs), angiotensin receptor-neprilysin inhibitors (ARNIs), and angiotensin receptor blockers (ARBs) **(Flowchart 2)**.

Guideline-directed Medical Therapy for Heart Failure with Preserved Ejection Fraction

Historically, medical therapy for HFpEF resulted in a discouraging array of negative trials with no demonstrated benefit in HFpEF, including trials of perindopril,[11] irbesartan,[12] beta-blockers,[13,14] nitrates,[15] digoxin,[16] ivabradine,[17] sildenafil,[18] and serelaxin.[19] However, recent clinical trials have demonstrated the benefit of GDMT in individuals with HFpEF, and initiation of key agents is essential to improve symptoms and functional capacity

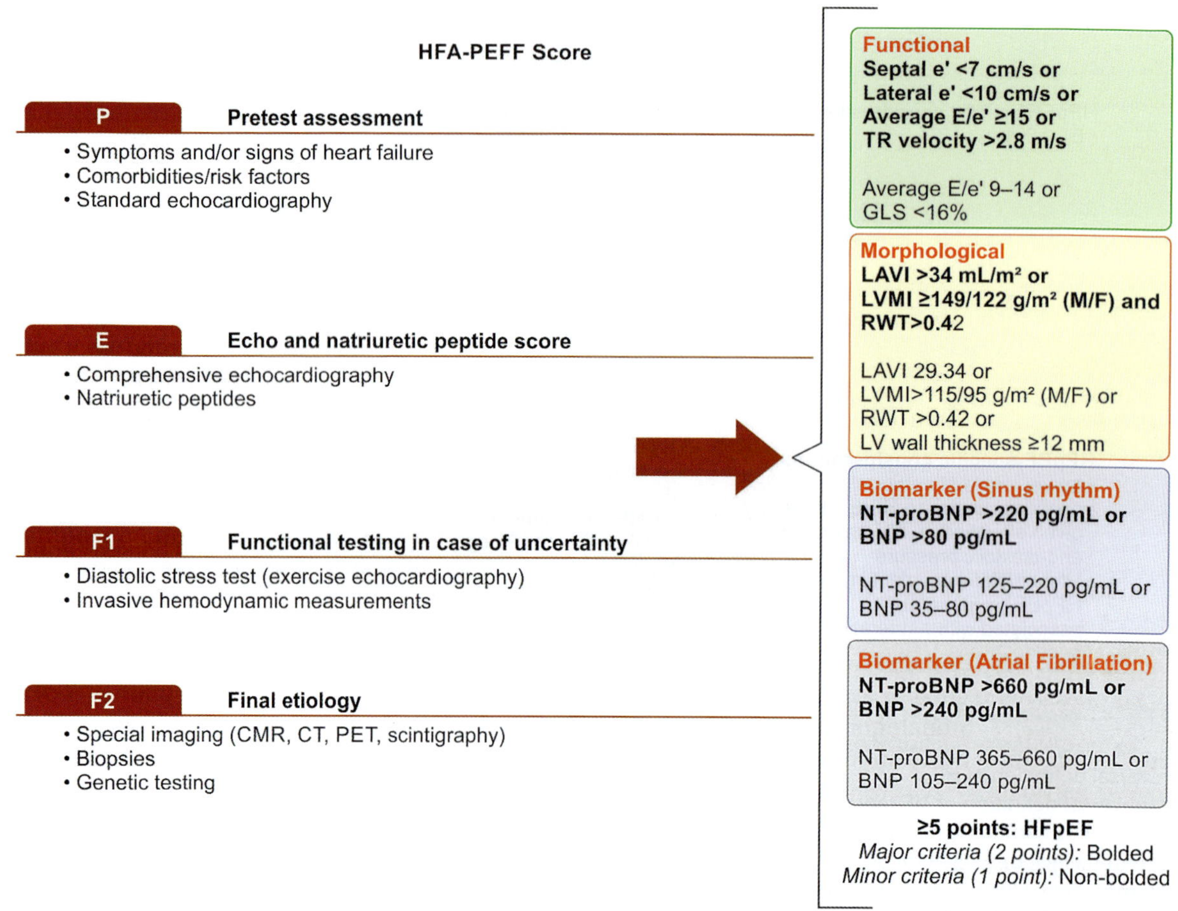

Fig. 2: HFA-PEFF score. HFA-PEFF includes a more involved diagnostic algorithm starting with pretest assessment, echocardiographic and natriuretic peptide score, functional testing for an advanced evaluation, and final etiology assessment. (BMI: body mass index; BNP: B-type natriuretic peptide; CMR: cardiac magnetic resonance; CT: computed tomography; GLS: global longitudinal strain; HFpEF: heart failure with preserved ejection fraction; LAVI: left atrial volume index; LVMI: left ventricular mass index; NT-proBNP: N-terminal pro-B-type natriuretic peptide; PASP: pulmonary artery systolic pressure; PET: positron emission tomography; RWT: relative wall thickness; TR: tricuspid regurgitation)

TABLE 3: Diagnostic clues and recommended testing for HFpEF mimics.

HFpEF mimics	*Clinical clues*	*Diagnostic testing*
Cardiac amyloidosis	• Increased IV wall thickness • Musculoskeletal issues (carpal tunnel syndrome, lumbar spinal stenosis) • Neuropathy (sensory or autonomic)	• Monoclonal protein screen (serum/urine immunofixation electrophoresis and serum-free light chains) • Technetium pyrophosphate scan interpreted in the context of a negative monoclonal protein screen • Endomyocardial biopsy if monoclonal protein screen is positive
Hypertrophy cardiomyopathy	• Unexplained LV hypertrophy • LV outflow tract obstruction • Family history	CMR if diagnosis is uncertain based on echocardiogram
Cardiac sarcoidosis	• Extracardiac disease (pulmonary, ocular, dermatologic) • High-degree atrioventricular block (especially if age < 60 years) • Ventricular arrhythmias	• CMR • FDG-PET scan • Tissue biopsy (cardiac or extracardiac)

Contd...

Contd...

HFpEF mimics	*Clinical clues*	*Diagnostic testing*
Hemochromatosis	• Family history or history of frequent blood transfusions • Diabetes • Erectile dysfunction	• Ferritin and transferrin • MFE genetic testing • CMR with T2* imaging
Fabry disease	• Angiokeratomas • Sensory neuropathy • Proteinuria • X-linked inheritance	• Serum alpha-galactosidase level (in men) • *GLA* genetic testing • Biopsy of affected tissue
High-output HF	Echocardiogram with four-chamber enlargement and/or increased LV outflow tract VTI	Investigate and treat underlying cause: Anemia, arteriovenous malformations, cirrhosis, fistulas, and thiamine deficiency
Myocarditis	• Antecedent viral infection • Elevated troponin in the absence of coronary artery disease • Heart block and/or ventricular arrhythmias	• CMR • Endomyocardial biopsy
Pericardial disease	• Prior cardiac surgery, chest radiation, or pericarditis • Right-sided HF symptoms	• CMR • Right and left heart catheterization to demonstrate discordance in LV/RV pressure tracings during inspiration

(CMR: cardiac magnetic resonance; FDG-PET: fluorodeoxyglucose-positron emission tomography; HF: heart failure; HFE: hereditary hemochromatosis gene; HFpEF: heart failure with preserved ejection fraction; LV: left ventricular; RF: radiofrequency; RV: right ventricular; VTI: velocity time integral)

Flowchart 2: Treatment algorithm for guideline-directed medical therapy in HFpEF.

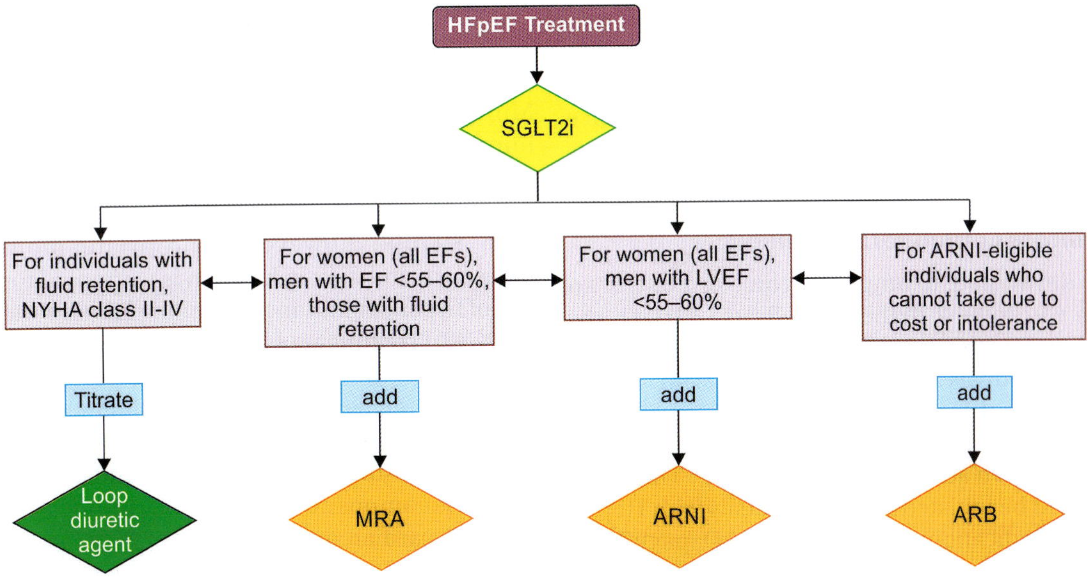

HFpEF Treatment

SGLT2i

For individuals with fluid retention, NYHA class II-IV

For women (all EFs), men with EF <55–60%, those with fluid retention

For women (all EFs), men with LVEF <55–60%

For ARNI-eligible individuals who cannot take due to cost or intolerance

Titrate

add

add

add

Loop diuretic agent

MRA

ARNI

ARB

Note: Green color identifies a class 1 therapy from clinical practice guidelines, yellow color indicates a class 2a therapy, and orange color denotes a class 2b therapy. SGLT2is receive a class 2a indication in the 2022 AHA/ACC/HFSA HF guidelines, but the benefit, now confirmed in two randomized trials, suggests that SGLT2is may receive a stronger class of recommendation in future guidelines, and thus the box is shaded yellow with a green border.

(AF: atrial fibrillation; ARB: angiotensin receptor blocker; ARNI: angiotensin receptor neprilysin inhibitor; EF: ejection fraction; GDMT: guideline-directed medical therapy; HFpEF: heart failure with preserved ejection fraction; LVEF: left ventricular ejection fraction; MRA: mineralocorticoid receptor antagonist; NYHA: New York Heart Association; SGLT2i: sodium–glucose cotransporter-2 inhibitor)

TABLE 4: Starting and target doses of select GDMTs for HFpEF.

Drug class	Starting dose	Target dose
SGLT2is		
Dapagliflozin	10 mg daily	10 mg daily
Empagliflozin	10 mg daily	10 mg daily
Aldosterone antagonists		
Spironolactone	25 mg daily	50 mg daily
ARNIs		
Sacubitril/valsartan	24/26 mg twice daily	97/103 mg twice daily
ARBs		
Candesartan	4–8 mg daily	32 mg daily

(ARB: angiotensin receptor blocker; ARNI: angiotensin receptor-neprilysin inhibitor; GDMT: guideline-directed medical therapy; HFpEF: heart failure with preserved ejection fraction; SGLT2is: sodium–glucose cotransporter-2 inhibitors)

and reduce the morbidity and mortality associated with HF.[10] Initiation of GDMT is safe and effective in both acute and chronic care settings.[20-22] Clinicians should also consider relevant cautions and contraindications when prescribing GDMT and also the approach to GDMT initiation and titration **(Table 4)**.

Diuretics have remained the mainstay of HFpEF management as they help mitigate volume overload. Diuretic agents should be used judiciously as needed to reduce congestion and improve symptoms.[10] Beta-blockers may be used in individuals with HFpEF who have specific indications, including prior myocardial infarction (for up to 3 years),[23] angina, or AF, but exercise tolerance should be monitored due to the potential for chronotropic incompetence.[10]

Sodium–glucose Cotransporter-2 Inhibitors

Originally developed to improve glucose control in individuals with type 2 diabetes mellitus (T2DM), the SGLT2is have demonstrated significant cardiovascular benefits in individuals with and without T2DM. This is particularly evident in individuals with HF, as SGLT2is significantly reduce the risk of hospitalization for HF and cardiovascular death across all EF subgroups.[24] Therefore, SGLT2is should be initiated in all individuals with HFpEF lacking contraindications. The *DELIVER* (Dapagliflozin Evaluation to Improve the LIVEs of Patients with PReserved Ejection Fraction Heart Failure)[25] and *EMPEROR-Preserved* (Empagliflozin Outcome Trial in Patients with Chronic Heart Failure with Preserved Ejection Fraction)[26] trials specifically evaluated the effects of dapagliflozin and empagliflozin, respectively, on clinical outcomes in individuals with HF and LVEF > 40%. A significant decrease in hospitalization for HF was observed in both trials; a meta-analysis also suggests reduction in cardiovascular death with SGLT2is in individuals with HFmrEF/HFpEF (HR: 0.88; 95% CI: 0.77–1.00).[24] Improvements in health status related to use of SGLT2is were also observed in both trials, with the greatest benefit in those with baseline symptomatic impairment.[27] Additional evidence for improvement in health status and quality of life with SGLT2i use in HFpEF was observed in the PRESERVED-HF (Dapagliflozin in PRESERVED Ejection Fraction Heart Failure) trial.[28]

Mineralocorticoid Antagonists

Mineralocorticoid receptor antagonists significantly improve measures of diastolic function in individuals with HFpEF.[29,30] Spironolactone may reduce the risk of hospitalizations for HF in specific subsets of individuals with HFpEF; however, appropriate monitoring of potassium and kidney function is warranted to reduce the risk of hyperkalemia and worsening kidney function.[30] The TOPCAT (Treatment of Preserved Cardiac Function Heart Failure with an Aldosterone Antagonist) trial[30] enrolled 3,445 individuals with HF and LVEF > 45% and randomized to spironolactone (15–45 mg daily) or placebo. The initially published results did not show a significant benefit in the primary composite outcome of cardiovascular death, aborted cardiac arrest, or hospitalization for HF (HR: 0.89; 95% CI: 0.77–1.04), although there was a significant reduction in the individual component of hospitalization for HF (HR: 0.83; 95% CI: 0.69–0.99). Notably, within the TOPCAT trial, the benefit of spironolactone was most evident in patients within the lower tertile of natriuretic peptide levels, corresponding to a B-type natriuretic peptide <166 pg/mL and an N-terminal pro-B-type natriuretic peptide (NT-proBNP) level < 682 pg/mL,[31] among those with an LVEF < 60%[32] and in women,[33] where reductions in events were similar across all LVEF strata.

Although MRAs have not been shown to improve quality of life or exercise tolerance in individuals with HFpEF,[29] most individuals with HFpEF will still benefit from MRAs to provide balanced diuresis with sequential nephron blockade, control hypertension, and reduce HF hospitalizations.

Angiotensin Receptor–Neprilysin Inhibitors

Sacubitril inhibits neprilysin, an enzyme that inactivates several important vasoactive peptides that contribute to the pathogenesis and progression of HF, including natriuretic peptides, bradykinin, and substance P. Combination with valsartan is necessary because neprilysin inhibition increases angiotensin levels, which could offset the vasodilatory effect of sacubitril unless also inhibited. Sacubitril/valsartan provides the modest additional benefit compared with valsartan in individuals with HFpEF. Although serum creatinine elevations and hyperkalemia occur less frequently with ARNI therapy, hypotension and angioedema, albeit rare, occur more frequently with ARNIs.[34]

The role of an ARNI in individuals with HFpEF was evaluated in the PARAGON-HF (Prospective Comparison of ARNI With ARB Global Outcomes in HF With Preserved Ejection Fraction) trial,[19] which enrolled 4,822 study participants with LVEF ≥ 45%, elevated natriuretic peptides, and evidence of structural heart disease, and randomized them to sacubitril/valsartan (target dose of 97/103 mg twice daily) or valsartan (target dose of 160 mg twice daily). The primary composite endpoint of total hospitalizations for HF and cardiovascular death was numerically lower with sacubitril/valsartan but was not statistically significant (HR: 0.87; 95% CI: 0.75–1.01).

Recently hospitalized study participants showed substantially greater reduction in risk from treatment with an ARNI compared with valsartan.[35]

Angiotensin Receptor Blockers

Although an ARNI is likely more effective than an ARB, an ARB may be used when an ARNI is contraindicated (e.g., history of angioedema) or lack of affordability impedes access. Angiotensin-converting enzyme (ACE) inhibitors are not considered a reasonable alternative due to lack of benefit with perindopril in the PEP-CHF (Perindopril in Elderly People with Chronic Heart Failure) trial, which enrolled 850 older adults (aged > 70 years) with LVEF >40%.[11]

The CHARM (Candesartan in Heart Failure Assessment of Reduction in Mortality and Morbidity)-Preserved trial[36] randomized 3,023 study participants with LVEF > 40% to candesartan (target dose of 32 mg daily) or placebo, and although the primary composite of hospitalization for HF and cardiovascular death was borderline significant (adjusted HR: 0.86; 95% CI: 0.74–1.00), there was a moderate reduction in the individual component of hospitalizations for HF (adjusted HR: 0.84; 95% CI: 0.70–1.00) **(Table 5)**.

Sex-specific Differences in Heart Failure with Preserved Ejection Failure Guideline-directed Medical Therapy

Important differences between response to therapies for HFpEF exist between women and men. Thus, although the use of SGLT2 inhibitors is an expected component of treatment for both sexes, barring contraindication, the use of sacubitril/valsartan,[37] as well as spironolactone[33] should be considered across the entire LVEF spectrum for women with HFpEF. The reason why women with HFpEF may respond more favorably to these therapies at a relatively higher EF may be because women tend to

TABLE 5: Contraindications and cautions for SGLT2i, MRAs, ARNIs, and ARBs.

Drug class	*Contraindications*	*Cautions*
SGLT2i	• Type 1 diabetes mellitus (limitation to use) • Lactation • On dialysis • Known hypersensitivity	*Kidney impairment:* • For dapagliflozin, eGFR < 25 mL/min/1.73 m^2 • For empagliflozin, eGFR < 20 mL/min/1.73 m^2 *Pregnancy:* • Increased risk of mycotic genital infections • May contribute to volume depletion or hypotension • Ketoacidosis (including euglycemic) in individuals with poorly controlled diabetes, dehydration, or fasting • Acute kidney injury • Necrotizing fasciitis of the perineum (Fournier's gangrene) is rare but can be serous and life-threatening

Contd...

Contd...

Drug class	*Contraindications*	*Cautions*
MRAs	• Potassium ≥ 5.0 mmol/L • Addison's disease • Pregnancy • Known hypersensitivity	*Kidney impairment:* • Avoid if eGFR < 30 mL/min/1.73 m^2 or serum creatinine 2.5 mg/dL • Initiate at half dose if eGFR 30–50 mL/min/1.73 m^2 • Concomitant use with drugs and supplements that increase serum potassium, such as potassium supplementation, ACE inhibitors, ARBs, ARNIs, NSAIDs, trimethoprim, gynecomastia (consider use of eplerenone), and lactation
ARNIs	• Coadministration within 36 hours of ACE inhibitor use • History of any angioedema • Pregnancy/lactation • Severe (Child–Pugh C) hepatic impairment • Known hypersensitivity • Use of aliskiren in individuals with diabetes mellitus	*Reduce the starting dose to half the usually recommended starting dose if:* • Not currently taking an ACE inhibitor or ARB or taking a low dose of an ACE inhibitor or ARB • Moderate (Child–Pugh B) hepatic impairment • Renal artery stenosis • Hypotension
ARBs	• Pregnancy/lactation • Avoid concomitant use with an ACE inhibitor, aliskiren, or ARNI • Known hypersensitivity • Renal artery stenosis	History of any angioedema, hyperkalemia, hypotension, and cute kidney injury

(ACE: angiotensin-converting enzyme; ARB: angiotensin receptor blocker; ARNI: angiotensin receptor-neprilysin inhibitor; eGFR: estimated glomerular filtration rate; MRA: mineralocorticoid receptor antagonist; NSAIDs: nonsteroidal anti-inflammatory drugs; SGLT2i: sodium–glucose cotransporter-2 inhibitor)

have smaller LV chamber size and are thus more prone to demonstrate higher LVEFs when compared to men.[38] Although simplistic, this means an LVEF of 50–55% in a woman may be abnormally low compared with a man and identifies potential differential response to therapies with effects on the neurohormonal system.

APPROACH TO GUIDELINE-DIRECTED MEDICAL THERAPY INITIATION AND TITRATION

Barring contraindication, all individuals with a diagnosis of HFpEF should be treated with an SGLT2i, with the goal of reducing cardiovascular death/HF hospitalization and improving health status. Initiation of an SGLT2i may be considered for either ambulatory individuals with HFpEF or those with acutely decompensated HF. In those with an LVEF < 55–60%, use of an MRA, ARNI, or ARB (when an ARNI is not feasible based on the strength of evidence and more contemporary evidence of ARNI vs. ARB as described earlier) may be considered.

Angiotensin receptor-neprilysin inhibitors and MRAs should be titrated to the maximum tolerated dosages based on symptoms, blood pressure, potassium, and creatinine, as confirmed in the STRONG HF (Safety, Tolerability, and Efficacy of Up-Titration of Guideline-Directed Medical Therapies for Acute Heart Failure) trial.[39] This trial randomized individuals hospitalized with HF, regardless of LVEF, to usual care or high intensity care, consisting of initiation of GDMT at one-half of the target dosages before hospital discharge with the goal of titration to target dosages over the next 2 weeks, with frequent follow-up visits over the 2 months following discharge.

Management of Comorbidities

The management of comorbidities associated with HFpEF is shown in **Flowchart 3**.

CONCLUSION

All individuals with a diagnosis of HFpEF should be treated with an SGLT2i, with the goal of reducing cardiovascular death/HF hospitalization and improving health status. Initiation of an SGLT2i may be considered for either ambulatory individuals with HFpEF or those with acutely decompensated HF. In those with an LVEF < 55–60%, use of an MRA, ARNI, or ARB (when an ARNI is not feasible based on the strength of evidence and more contemporary evidence of ARNI vs. ARB as described earlier) may be considered.

Flowchart 3: HFpEF comorbidities.

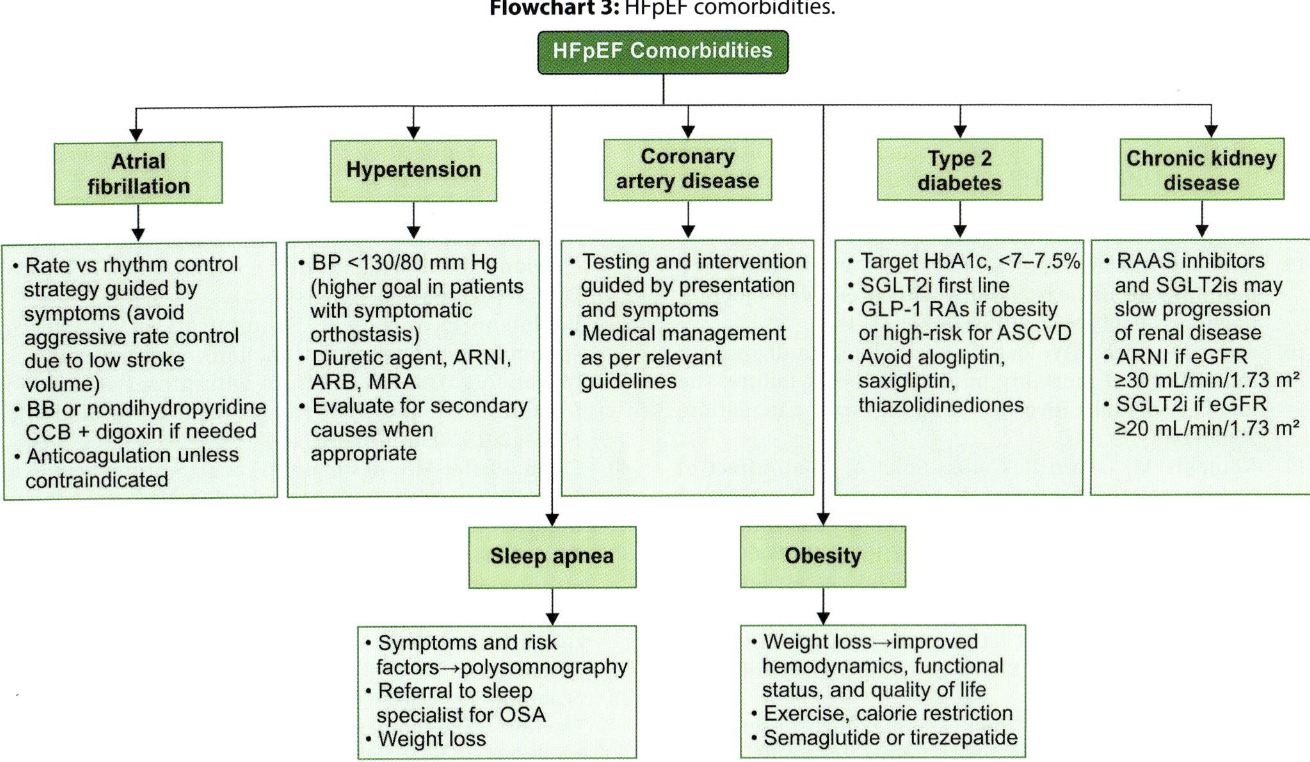

(ARB: angiotensin receptor blocker; ARNI: angiotensin receptor-neprilysin inhibitor; ASCVD: atherosclerotic cardiovascular disease; BB: beta-blockers; BP: blood pressure; CCB: calcium-channel blocker; CPAP: continuous positive airway pressure; eGFR: estimated glomerular filtration rate; GLP1-RA: glucagon-like peptide 1 receptor agonist; HbA1c: glycosylated hemoglobin; MRA: mineralocorticoid receptor antagonist; OSA: obstructive sleep apnea; RAS: renin–angiotensin system; SGLT2i: sodium–glucose cotransporter-2 inhibitor)

REFERENCES

1. Gevaert AB, Kataria R, Zannad F, et al. Heart failure with preserved ejection fraction: recent concepts in diagnosis, mechanisms and management. Heart. 2022; 108(17):1342-50.
2. Shah SJ, Borlaug BA, Kitzman DW, et al. Research priorities for heart failure with preserved ejection fraction: National Heart, Lung, and Blood Institute Working Group Summary. Circulation. 2020;141(12):1001-26.
3. Lloyd-Jones DM, Larson MG, Leip EP, et al. Lifetime risk for developing congestive heart failure: the Framingham Heart Study. Circulation. 2002;106(24):3068-72.
4. Gerber Y, Weston SA, Redfield MM, et al. A contemporary appraisal of the heart failure epidemic in Olmsted County, Minnesota, 2000 to 2010. JAMA Intern Med. 2015;175(6):996-1004.
5. Tsao CW, Lyass A, Enserro D, et al. Temporal trends in the incidence of and mortality associated with heart failure with preserved and reduced ejection fraction. JACC Heart Fail. 2018;6(8):678-85.
6. Virani SS, Alonso A, Benjamin EJ, et al. Heart disease and stroke statistics-2020 update: a report from the American Heart Association. Circulation. 2020;141(9):e139-596.
7. Shah KS, Xu H, Matsouaka RA, et al. Heart failure with preserved, borderline, and reduced ejection fraction: 5-year outcomes. J Am Coll Cardiol. 2017;70(20): 2476-86.
8. Bozkurt B, Coats AJ, Tsutsui H, et al. Universal definition and classification of heart failure: a report of the Heart Failure Society of America, Heart Failure Association of the European Society of Cardiology, Japanese Heart Failure Society and Writing Committee of the Universal Definition of Heart Failure. J Card Fail. 2021;S1071-9164(21):00050-6.
9. Hicks KA, Tcheng JE, Bozkurt B, et al. 2014 ACC/AHA key data elements and definitions for cardiovascular endpoint events in clinical trials: a report of the American College of Cardiology/American Heart Association Task Force on Clinical Data Standards (Writing Committee to Develop Cardiovascular Endpoints Data Standards). J Am Coll Cardiol. 2015;66(4):403-69.
10. Heidenreich PA, Bozkurt B, Aguilar D, et al. 2022 AHA/ ACC/HFSA guideline for the management of heart failure: a report of the American College of Cardiology/American Heart Association Joint Committee on Clinical Practice Guidelines. J Am Coll Cardiol. 2022;79(17):e263-421.
11. Cleland JGF, Tendera M, Adamus J, et al. The perindopril in elderly people with chronic heart failure (PEP-CHF) study. Eur Heart J. 2006;27(19):2338-45.
12. Massie BM, Carson PE, McMurray JJ, et al. Irbesartan in patients with heart failure and preserved ejection fraction. N Engl J Med. 2008;359(23):2456-67.

13. Fonarow GC, Abraham WT, Albert NM, et al. Factors identified as precipitating hospital admissions for heart failure and clinical outcomes: findings from OPTIMIZE-HF. Arch Intern Med. 2008;168(8):847-54.
14. Hernandez AF, Hammill BG, O'Connor CM, et al. Clinical effectiveness of beta-blockers in heart failure: findings from the OPTIMIZE-HF (Organized Program to Initiate Lifesaving Treatment in Hospitalized Patients with Heart Failure) registry. J Am Coll Cardiol. 2009;53(2):184-92.
15. Redfield MM, Anstrom KJ, Levine JA, et al. Isosorbide mononitrate in heart failure with preserved ejection fraction. N Engl J Med. 2015;373(24):2314-24.
16. Ahmed A, Rich MW, Fleg JL, et al. Effects of digoxin on morbidity and mortality in diastolic heart failure: the ancillary digitalis investigation group trial. Circulation. 2006;114(5):397-403.
17. Komajda M, Isnard R, Cohen-Solal A, et al. Effect of ivabradine in patients with heart failure with preserved ejection fraction: the EDIFY randomized placebo-controlled trial. Eur J Heart Fail. 2017;19(11):1495-503.
18. Redfield MM, Chen HH, Borlaug BA, et al. Effect of phosphodiesterase-5 inhibition on exercise capacity and clinical status in heart failure with preserved ejection fraction: a randomized clinical trial. JAMA. 2013;309(12):1268-77.
19. Metra M, Teerlink JR, Cotter G, et al. Effects of serelaxin in patients with acute heart failure. N Engl J Med. 2019;381(8):716-26.
20. Bhagat AA, Greene SJ, Vaduganathan M, et al. Initiation, continuation, switching, and withdrawal of heart failure medical therapies during hospitalization. JACC Heart Fail. 2019;7(1):1-12.
21. Hollenberg SM, Stevenson LW, Ahmad T, et al. 2019 ACC expert consensus decision pathway on risk assessment, management, and clinical trajectory of patients hospitalized with heart failure: a report of the American College of Cardiology Solution Set Oversight Committee. J Am Coll Cardiol. 2019;74(15):1966-2011.
22. Bhatt DL, Szarek M, Steg PG, et al. Sotagliflozin in patients with diabetes and recent worsening heart failure. N Engl J Med. 2021;384(2):117-28.
23. Fihn SD, Gardin JM, Abrams J, et al. 2012 ACCF/AHA/ACP/AATS/PCNA/SCAI/STS guideline for the diagnosis and management of patients with stable ischemic heart disease: a report of the American College of Cardiology Foundation/American Heart Association Task Force on Practice Guidelines, and the American College of Physicians, American Association for Thoracic Surgery, Preventive Cardiovascular Nurses Association, Society for Cardiovascular Angiography and Interventions, and Society of Thoracic Surgeons. J Am Coll Cardiol. 2012;60(24):e44-164.
24. Vaduganathan M, Docherty KF, Claggett BL, et al. SGLT-2 inhibitors in patients with heart failure: a comprehensive meta-analysis of five randomised controlled trials. Lancet. 2022;400(10354):757-67.
25. Solomon SD, McMurray JJV, Claggett B, et al. Dapagliflozin in heart failure with mildly reduced or preserved ejection fraction. N Engl J Med. 2022;387(12):1089-98.
26. Anker SD, Butler J, Filippatos G, et al. Empagliflozin in heart failure with a preserved ejection fraction. N Engl J Med. 2021;385(16):1451-61.
27. Kosiborod MN, Bhatt AS, Claggett BL, et al. Effect of dapagliflozin on health status in patients with preserved or mildly reduced ejection fraction. J Am Coll Cardiol. 2023;81(5):460-73.
28. Nassif ME, Windsor SL, Borlaug BA, et al. The SGLT2 inhibitor dapagliflozin in heart failure with preserved ejection fraction: a multicenter randomized trial. Nat Med. 2021;27(11):1954-60.
29. Edelmann F, Wachter R, Schmidt AG, et al. Effect of spironolactone on diastolic function and exercise capacity in patients with heart failure with preserved ejection fraction: the Aldo-DHF randomized controlled trial. JAMA. 2013;309(8):781-91.
30. Pitt B, Pfeffer MA, Assmann SF, et al. Spironolactone for heart failure with preserved ejection fraction. N Engl J Med. 2014;370(15):1383-92.
31. Anand IS, Claggett B, Liu J, et al. Interaction between spironolactone and natriuretic peptides in patients with heart failure and preserved ejection fraction: from the TOPCAT trial. JACC Heart Fail. 2017;5(4):241-52.
32. Solomon SD, Claggett B, Lewis EF, et al. Influence of ejection fraction on outcomes and efficacy of spironolactone in patients with heart failure with preserved ejection fraction. Eur Heart J. 2016;37(5):455-62.
33. Merrill M, Sweitzer NK, Lindenfeld JA, et al. Sex differences in outcomes and responses to spironolactone in heart failure with preserved ejection fraction: a secondary analysis of TOPCAT trial. JACC Heart Fail. 2019;7(3):228-38.
34. Solomon SD, McMurray JJV, Anand IS, et al. Angiotensin-neprilysin inhibition in heart failure with preserved ejection fraction. N Engl J Med. 2019;381(17):1609-20.
35. Vaduganathan M, Claggett BL, Desai AS, et al. Prior heart failure hospitalization, clinical outcomes, and response to sacubitril/valsartan compared with valsartan in HFpEF. J Am Coll Cardiol. 2020;75(3):245-54.
36. Yusuf S, Pfeffer MA, Swedberg K, et al. Effects of candesartan in patients with chronic heart failure and preserved left-ventricular ejection fraction: the CHARM-Preserved trial. Lancet. 2003;362(9386):777-81.
37. McMurray JJV, Jackson AM, Lam CSP, et al. Effects of sacubitril-valsartan versus valsartan in women compared with men with heart failure and preserved ejection fraction: insights from PARAGON-HF. Circulation. 2020;141(5):338-51.
38. Addetia K, Miyoshi T, Amuthan V, et al. Normal values of left ventricular size and function on three-dimensional echocardiography: results of the World Alliance Societies of Echocardiography Study. J Am Soc Echocardiogr. 2022;35(5):449-59.
39. Mebazaa A, Davison B, Chioncel O, et al. Safety, tolerability and efficacy of up-titration of guideline-directed medical therapies for acute heart failure (STRONG-HF): a multinational, open-label, randomised, trial. Lancet. 2022;400(10367):1938-52.

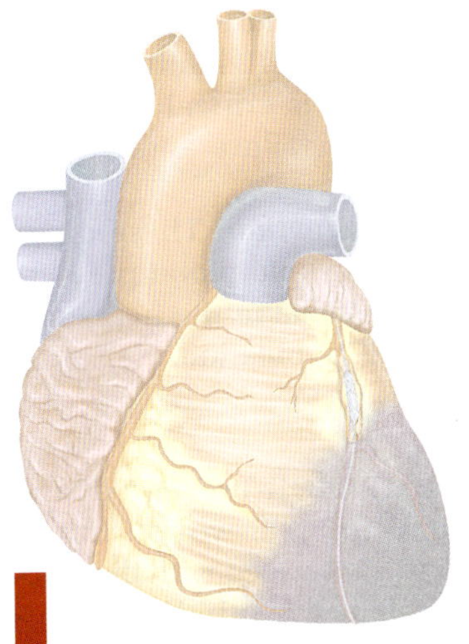

HFpEF: Advances in Pharmacological Therapy and Clinical Trials

Hemant Bareth, Manna Bhattacharya, Bijay Yadav, Sundeep Mishra

INTRODUCTION

Heart failure with preserved ejection fraction (HFpEF) has long been a challenging clinical entity, partly because its pathophysiology differs significantly from heart failure with reduced ejection fraction (HFrEF). While HFrEF management has seen considerable progress with guideline-directed therapies, HFpEF remained without a definitive treatment for many years. However, recent advancements in understanding the complex mechanisms underlying HFpEF have opened the door to innovative pharmacologic, device-based, and personalized approaches. Here is an expanded discussion of these developments.

PHARMACOLOGIC THERAPIES

Sodium–Glucose Cotransporter-2 Inhibitors

Sodium–glucose cotransporter-2 (SGLT2) inhibitors were originally developed for the treatment of type 2 diabetes mellitus by inhibiting glucose reabsorption in the proximal tubules of the kidney, thus promoting glucose excretion through urine. However, their utility has expanded significantly in cardiovascular medicine, particularly in the management of heart failure, including *HFpEF*.

Mechanism of Action in Heart Failure with Preserved Ejection Fraction

While SGLT2 inhibitors' primary action relates to glucose excretion, their benefits in heart failure appear to be largely independent of blood sugar control. The exact mechanisms by which SGLT2 inhibitors exert their cardioprotective effects in HFpEF are complex and multifactorial. Key mechanisms include:

- *Osmotic diuresis and natriuresis:* SGLT2 inhibitors reduce plasma volume through osmotic diuresis, which lowers both preload and afterload, leading to reduced cardiac filling pressures. This can be particularly beneficial in HFpEF, where elevated filling pressures are a hallmark.
- *Reduction in interstitial volume:* SGLT2 inhibitors preferentially reduce interstitial fluid rather than intravascular volume, which may help alleviate the symptoms of congestion (e.g., dyspnea) in HFpEF patients without triggering significant drops in blood pressure.
- *Improved myocardial energy efficiency:* SGLT2 inhibitors may promote a shift in myocardial metabolism from glucose to ketone bodies, which are more efficient energy substrates for the failing heart. This metabolic adaptation may enhance myocardial function and reduce ischemic injury, which is critical in HFpEF where myocardial stiffness and poor relaxation are often seen.
- *Anti-inflammatory and antifibrotic effects:* HFpEF is increasingly recognized as a condition associated with systemic inflammation and myocardial fibrosis. SGLT2 inhibitors may reduce inflammation and inhibit pathways involved in cardiac fibrosis, improving left ventricular (LV) relaxation and compliance.
- *Vascular effects:* SGLT2 inhibitors improve endothelial function, reduce vascular stiffness, and promote nitric

oxide bioavailability, all of which can contribute to better peripheral and coronary circulation in HFpEF patients.

Clinical Trials in Heart Failure with Preserved Ejection Fraction

The most pivotal clinical trials investigating SGLT2 inhibitors in HFpEF are the *EMPEROR-Preserved* trial (with empagliflozin) and the *DELIVER* trial (with dapagliflozin).

- EMPEROR-Preserved trial (empagliflozin)
    - *Study design:* This randomized, double-blind, placebo-controlled trial enrolled over 5,000 patients with HFpEF [left ventricular ejection fractions (LVEF) ≥40%]. Patients were randomized to receive either empagliflozin or placebo.
    - *Results:* Empagliflozin significantly reduced the composite endpoint of cardiovascular death or heart failure hospitalizations by 21%. The benefit was primarily driven by a 29% reduction in heart failure hospitalizations. Importantly, the trial demonstrated that these benefits were consistent across various subgroups, including patients with and without diabetes.
    - *Conclusion:* Empagliflozin became the first therapy to show a statistically significant benefit in a broad HFpEF population, marking a major milestone in HFpEF treatment.
- DELIVER trial (dapagliflozin)
    - *Study design:* Similar to EMPEROR-Preserved, DELIVER enrolled over 6,000 patients with HFpEF (LVEF ≥40%), randomized to dapagliflozin or placebo.
    - *Results:* Dapagliflozin also demonstrated a significant reduction in the primary composite endpoint of cardiovascular death or worsening heart failure. The reduction in heart failure hospitalizations was a prominent feature, and the benefits were seen regardless of diabetes status.
    - *Conclusion:* Dapagliflozin, like empagliflozin, became a key therapeutic option for HFpEF patients, further solidifying the role of SGLT2 inhibitors as a cornerstone of HFpEF management.

Benefits Beyond Hospitalization Reduction

In addition to reducing heart failure hospitalizations, SGLT2 inhibitors improve other important clinical outcomes in HFpEF:

- *Quality of life (QoL):* SGLT2 inhibitors have been shown to significantly improve patients' symptoms and exercise capacity, as measured by patient-reported outcomes using tools such as the *Kansas City Cardiomyopathy Questionnaire (KCCQ).*
- *Kidney function:* In both HFrEF and HFpEF, kidney function is often compromised. SGLT2 inhibitors help preserve renal function, which is critical given the strong interplay between heart failure and chronic kidney disease.
- *Weight and blood pressure reduction:* These drugs have mild effects on weight loss and blood pressure reduction, which may be beneficial in the frequently obese and hypertensive HFpEF population.

Real-world Applications

The implications of the EMPEROR-Preserved and DELIVER trials are profound for real-world clinical practice. Historically, HFpEF was managed with diuretics and treatments aimed at controlling comorbid conditions [e.g., hypertension and atrial fibrillation (AF)]. However, SGLT2 inhibitors have shifted the paradigm by directly targeting heart failure pathophysiology:

- *Wide applicability:* Unlike previous therapies, which only benefited narrow subgroups of HFpEF patients, SGLT2 inhibitors have shown efficacy across a broad spectrum of patients, making them suitable for general use in the HFpEF population.
- *Synergistic use with other therapies:* SGLT2 inhibitors can be safely combined with other heart failure medications such as mineralocorticoid receptor antagonists (MRAs) and angiotensin receptor-neprilysin inhibitors (ARNIs), potentially providing additive benefits.

Mineralocorticoid Receptor Antagonists

Mineralocorticoid receptor antagonists (MRAs), including *spironolactone* and *eplerenone*, are well-established therapies in HFrEF due to their ability to block the effects of *aldosterone*. Aldosterone, a hormone in the renin-angiotensin-aldosterone system (RAAS), contributes to sodium retention, potassium excretion, vascular stiffness, and myocardial fibrosis—pathophysiological processes highly relevant to *HFpEF*. Given these effects, MRAs have been investigated as a potential treatment option in HFpEF, where fibrosis and diastolic dysfunction are prominent features.

Mechanisms of Action in Heart Failure with Preserved Ejection Fraction

Mineralocorticoid receptor antagonists target multiple mechanisms that contribute to the pathophysiology of HFpEF:

- *Inhibition of myocardial fibrosis:* Aldosterone promotes myocardial fibrosis, which stiffens the heart muscle and impairs its ability to relax properly during diastole, a hallmark feature of HFpEF. By blocking aldosterone, MRAs reduce fibrosis, improving LV compliance and diastolic function.

- *Reduction in vascular stiffness:* MRAs have been shown to reduce vascular stiffness and improve endothelial function. This is critical in HFpEF, where increased vascular resistance and arterial stiffness contribute to elevated afterload and impaired ventricular relaxation.
- *Anti-inflammatory effects:* Aldosterone also drives inflammation, which plays a role in the progression of heart failure. MRAs help mitigate inflammation, reducing cardiac remodeling and improving overall cardiac function.
- *Prevention of sodium retention:* By blocking aldosterone's effects in the kidneys, MRAs reduce sodium and water retention, lowering plasma volume and reducing heart failure-related congestion.

Clinical Evidence: The TOPCAT Trial

The most significant study investigating the role of MRAs in HFpEF is the *TOPCAT (Treatment of Preserved Cardiac Function Heart Failure with an Aldosterone Antagonist* trial.

- *Study design:* The TOPCAT trial was a large, randomized, placebo-controlled study that enrolled over 3,400 patients with HFpEF (LVEF ≥45%). Patients were assigned to receive either spironolactone or placebo.
- *Primary endpoint:* The primary composite endpoint was cardiovascular death, aborted cardiac arrest, or heart failure hospitalization.

Overall results: The overall results of the TOPCAT trial were mixed. While spironolactone did not significantly reduce the primary composite endpoint across the entire study population, important findings emerged in post hoc analyses:

- *Reduction in heart failure hospitalizations:* Spironolactone significantly reduced the rate of heart failure hospitalizations (by 17%) in patients with HFpEF, indicating a benefit in preventing worsening heart failure events. This was particularly noted in patients with higher baseline levels of *natriuretic peptides*, which are biomarkers of heart failure severity.
- *Geographic variability:* One of the key findings from post-hoc analyses was the substantial regional variation in outcomes. Patients enrolled in *the Americas* (the U.S., Canada, Brazil, and Argentina) showed more pronounced benefits from spironolactone than those enrolled in *Eastern Europe*. It was suggested that some of the Eastern European data may have been confounded by poor drug adherence or misclassification of heart failure status. In contrast, patients from the Americas who had elevated natriuretic peptide levels derived significant benefits from spironolactone.
- *Patient subgroup analysis:* Post hoc analyses indicated that *patients with elevated natriuretic peptides* (a marker of elevated cardiac filling pressures) experienced more favorable outcomes with spironolactone, particularly in reducing heart failure hospitalizations. This suggests that careful patient selection based on clinical characteristics and biomarkers can optimize the benefits of MRAs in HFpEF.

Key conclusions from TOPCAT:

- *Heart failure hospitalization benefit:* Despite mixed overall results, spironolactone significantly reduced hospitalizations for heart failure, which is a critical endpoint in managing HFpEF patients who frequently suffer from recurrent hospital admissions due to fluid overload and dyspnea.
- *Geographic variability and patient selection:* The variability in response based on geographic region and natriuretic peptide levels underscores the importance of patient selection. MRAs may provide the greatest benefit in HFpEF patients with elevated filling pressures or congestion markers, such as natriuretic peptides.

Real-world Implications and Use

The findings from the TOPCAT trial have influenced clinical practice, particularly in the following ways:

- *Patient selection:* Clinicians are more cautious in selecting HFpEF patients who are likely to benefit from MRAs. Those with elevated natriuretic peptides or evidence of fluid retention are considered ideal candidates for spironolactone therapy. This targeted approach helps optimize outcomes and minimize adverse effects such as hyperkalemia and renal dysfunction, which are common concerns with MRA use.
- *Combination therapy:* MRAs are often used in combination with other therapies such as diuretics and, more recently, *SGLT2 inhibitors* in HFpEF. The combination of therapies may have complementary effects, particularly in reducing hospitalizations and managing symptoms.
- *Monitoring and safety:* Due to the risk of hyperkalemia and worsening renal function, close monitoring of electrolyte levels and kidney function is essential when using MRAs, especially in older adults and those with chronic kidney disease.

Future Directions

While the TOPCAT trial provided valuable insights, there remains a need for more robust clinical trials to better define the role of MRAs in HFpEF, particularly in combination with other emerging therapies like SGLT2 inhibitors and *ARNIs.*

Angiotensin Receptor–Neprilysin Inhibitors

Angiotensin receptor–neprilysin inhibitors, particularly sacubitril/valsartan (brand name *Entresto*), have made significant strides in the treatment of HFREF. However, their role in HFpEF has been more ambiguous and remains a topic of active research and clinical debate.

PARAGON-HF Trial Overview

The PARAGON-HF trial was designed to evaluate the effects of sacubitril/valsartan in patients with HFpEF. HFpEF is characterized by symptoms of heart failure but with a preserved ejection fraction (typically ≥50%). In contrast to HFrEF, where pharmacological treatments such as ARNIs have shown consistent benefit, HFpEF has proven to be more challenging to treat, likely due to its heterogeneous pathophysiology.

In the PARAGON-HF trial:

- *Study population:* The trial enrolled over 4,800 patients with HFpEF, defined as those with an ejection fraction ≥45%, who were symptomatic (NYHA Class II–IV) and had evidence of elevated filling pressures.
- *Study objective:* The trial aimed to assess whether sacubitril/valsartan could reduce the composite primary endpoint of heart failure hospitalizations and cardiovascular deaths in this population.
- *Primary endpoint:* The trial did *not* meet its primary endpoint, as the reduction in heart failure hospitalizations and cardiovascular deaths in the sacubitril/valsartan group did not reach statistical significance compared to the control group (those receiving valsartan alone).

Key findings and subgroup analyses:

Despite not meeting the primary endpoint, the PARAGON-HF trial provided important insights into specific patient subgroups that may benefit from ARNIs:

- *Ejection fraction spectrum:*
  - Patients on the *lower end* of the ejection fraction spectrum (40–55%) showed a more favorable response to sacubitril/valsartan, with a reduction in heart failure hospitalizations.
  - This suggests that the benefit of ARNIs in HFpEF may be more pronounced in patients whose ejection fraction is closer to the borderline between HFrEF and HFpEF, a group sometimes referred to as "mid-range" or "borderline" HFpEF. These patients may share more similarities with those who have HFrEF, including structural heart changes such as LV dilation and systolic dysfunction.
- *Sex differences:* Women appeared to derive greater benefit from sacubitril/valsartan compared to men in terms of reduced heart failure hospitalizations. This finding is of particular interest, as HFpEF is more prevalent in women, and prior studies have suggested that women may experience different pathophysiological mechanisms of heart failure compared to men.
- *Renal function and blood pressure:* Patients with *better preserved renal function* and those with *higher baseline blood pressures* also seemed to benefit more from sacubitril/valsartan. This is relevant because elevated blood pressure is a common risk factor in HFpEF, and neprilysin inhibition (a mechanism of sacubitril) may help modulate blood pressure and reduce the burden on the heart.

Mechanistic Insights

The theoretical benefit of ARNIs in HFpEF lies in their dual mechanism of action:

- *Neprilysin inhibition* increases levels of natriuretic peptides, bradykinin, and other vasoactive substances that have favorable effects, such as vasodilation, natriuresis, and reduced fibrosis. These effects could be beneficial in HFpEF, where stiffness of the heart and high filling pressures contribute to symptoms.
- *Angiotensin receptor blockade* (via valsartan) reduces the negative effects of the RAAS, including vasoconstriction, sodium retention, and maladaptive cardiac remodeling.

Clinical Implications and Future Directions

The results of the PARAGON-HF trial, while not definitive, have led to several important discussions about the management of HFpEF:

- *Targeted therapy in HFpEF:* HFpEF is a heterogeneous condition with varying underlying causes, such as hypertension, AF, obesity, and diabetes. Sacubitril/valsartan may offer particular benefits to subsets of patients with certain characteristics (e.g., lower ejection fractions or higher blood pressures). This underscores the need for a more personalized approach to HFpEF treatment.
- *Role of ejection fraction:* The findings from PARAGON-HF blur the line between HFpEF and HFrEF in some patients, especially those with ejection

fractions in the 40–55% range. This has led some experts to advocate for reclassifying heart failure into more nuanced categories [e.g., "heart failure with mildly reduced ejection fraction" (HFmrEF)].

- *Guideline changes:* Based on the trial's subgroup analyses, sacubitril/valsartan is now recommended for certain patients with HFpEF in the 2022 AHA/ACC/HFSA heart failure guidelines, particularly those with ejection fractions on the lower end of the HFpEF spectrum. However, its use is not yet universally accepted for all patients with HFpEF.

Soluble Guanylate Cyclase Stimulators

Vericiguat is an emerging therapy that stimulates soluble guanylate cyclase (sGC), enhancing the nitric oxide (NO) signaling pathway. This pathway is often dysregulated in HFpEF due to endothelial dysfunction:

- Although vericiguat is currently more established for use in HFrEF, ongoing research suggests potential benefits in HFpEF by improving myocardial relaxation, vascular compliance, and reducing pulmonary pressures, which could alleviate symptoms and improve exercise capacity.

Mechanism of Action of Vericiguat

Vericiguat is an oral sGC stimulator that enhances the activity of sGC, the enzyme responsible for converting guanosine triphosphate (GTP) to cyclic guanosine monophosphate (cGMP). This action is crucial because cGMP plays a significant role in various physiological processes, including vasodilation, inhibition of smooth muscle contraction, and modulation of cellular signaling pathways. Here's how vericiguat may benefit patients with HFpEF:

- *Enhanced nitric oxide signaling:* In HFpEF, the endothelial cells often exhibit dysfunction, leading to reduced bioavailability of nitric oxide (NO). Vericiguat compensates for this by directly stimulating sGC, even in the absence of NO, thereby increasing cGMP levels. This enhancement can lead to improved vasodilation and reduced vascular stiffness, crucial for alleviating symptoms of HFpEF.
- *Myocardial relaxation and vascular compliance:*
  - Elevated cGMP levels contribute to improved myocardial relaxation. In HFpEF, impaired relaxation is a significant contributor to diastolic dysfunction, leading to symptoms such as shortness of breath and exercise intolerance. Vericiguat may improve diastolic function by enhancing myocardial compliance and reducing filling pressures.
  - Increased cGMP also promotes vascular compliance, which helps maintain appropriate blood flow and reduces afterload on the heart. This can be particularly beneficial in patients experiencing elevated pulmonary pressures, a common issue in HFpEF.
- *Pulmonary pressure reduction:* One of the hallmark features of HFpEF is elevated pulmonary capillary wedge pressure (PCWP) due to left atrial pressure overload. Vericiguat's vasodilatory effects can lead to a reduction in pulmonary pressures, improving symptoms of exertional dyspnea and right heart function.
- *Symptom relief and improved exercise capacity:* By targeting the underlying pathophysiology of HFpEF, including endothelial dysfunction and impaired myocardial relaxation, vericiguat may help alleviate symptoms such as fatigue, dyspnea, and edema. Improved vascular function can also enhance exercise tolerance and overall quality of life for patients with HFpEF.

Clinical Evidence and Ongoing Research

While vericiguat is currently more established in the treatment of HFrEF, ongoing research is exploring its potential in HFpEF. Key points include:

- *VITALITY-HF Study:* This trial examines the efficacy and safety of vericiguat in patients with HFpEF. Early results suggest that vericiguat can improve clinical outcomes, such as reducing hospitalizations and improving quality of life, particularly in patients with significant comorbidities.
- *Targeted patient populations:* Research is also focusing on identifying patient populations within the HFpEF spectrum that may derive the most benefit from vericiguat. Factors such as baseline pulmonary pressures, renal function, and severity of diastolic dysfunction are being evaluated to optimize treatment strategies.

Potential Benefits and Considerations

Benefits:

- *Combination therapy:* Vericiguat may be particularly effective when used in combination with other therapies, such as ARNIs, diuretics, or beta-blockers, to provide a comprehensive approach to managing HFpEF.
- *Reduced hospitalizations:* The ability of vericiguat to lower pulmonary pressures and improve vascular dynamics may result in fewer heart failure hospitalizations, a key goal in managing HFpEF patients.

Considerations:

- *Monitoring:* Patients on vericiguat may require regular monitoring for potential side effects, including hypotension, particularly if combined with other vasodilators or diuretics.
- *Long-term data:* While early studies show promise, more long-term data is needed to fully understand the safety and efficacy profile of vericiguat in HFpEF.

NONPHARMACOLOGIC THERAPIES

Exercise Training and Rehabilitation

Background

Heart failure with preserved ejection fraction is marked by exercise intolerance, which significantly affects patients' QoL. This symptom is multifactorial and arises from:

- *Impaired ventricular relaxation:* This contributes to diastolic dysfunction, leading to symptoms such as shortness of breath and fatigue during exertion.
- *Systemic vascular stiffness:* Reduced compliance in blood vessels elevates afterload and impairs the heart's ability to pump effectively during physical activity.
- *Reduced peripheral oxygen extraction:* This limitation hampers the muscles' ability to utilize oxygen efficiently during exercise, contributing to fatigue and decreased exercise capacity.

Given these challenges, exercise training has emerged as a vital nonpharmacologic intervention for managing HFpEF.

Benefits of Exercise Training

Benefits of exercise training include:

- *Improved peak oxygen consumption (VO_2 max):*
  - *Enhanced aerobic capacity:* Supervised aerobic exercise programs can significantly increase peak VO_2 max, a key measure of cardiovascular fitness. Improvements in VO_2 max translate into a greater ability to perform physical activities and reduce the burden of symptoms.
  - *Mechanisms of improvement:* Enhanced VO_2 max is attributed to improved cardiac output, increased muscle oxidative capacity, and enhanced capillary density in peripheral tissues.
- *Reduction of symptoms:*
  - *Symptom relief:* Regular exercise training is associated with a decrease in symptoms like dyspnea, fatigue, and exercise-related discomfort. Patients often report feeling less breathless during daily activities, leading to a more active lifestyle.
  - *Mechanistic insights:* Exercise may improve ventilatory efficiency and lower the threshold for lactic acid production, reducing the sensation of breathlessness during exertion.
- *Enhanced QoL:*
  - *Psychosocial benefits:* Participating in structured exercise programs positively impacts mental health, leading to lower levels of anxiety and depression. Many patients express increased satisfaction with their lives, better mood, and a stronger sense of control over their health.
  - *Holistic impact:* Improved QoL is not just about physical capability; it also encompasses psychological and social well-being, allowing patients to engage more fully in their communities and family activities.
- *Muscle strength and function:*
  - *Strength training benefits:* Incorporating resistance training into exercise regimens can enhance muscle strength and endurance, which are often diminished in patients with HFpEF. Increased muscle strength allows patients to perform daily activities more efficiently.
  - *Functional capacity:* Enhanced muscle function directly correlates with improved performance in activities of daily living, such as climbing stairs, carrying groceries, or engaging in recreational activities.
- *Improvement in cardiovascular and pulmonary function:*
  - *Vascular health:* Exercise training can improve endothelial function, reducing systemic vascular stiffness and contributing to better overall cardiovascular health. Improved endothelial function enhances vasodilation and reduces afterload on the heart.
  - *Pulmonary pressure management:* In many patients with HFpEF, pulmonary hypertension (PH) is common. Exercise training may help attenuate the rise in pulmonary pressures during physical activity, contributing to improved exercise tolerance and functional capacity.

Mechanisms behind Exercise Benefits

- *Metabolic adaptations:*
  - *Increased mitochondrial density:* Exercise promotes adaptations at the cellular level, including increased mitochondrial density in muscle tissues, leading to improved energy production and utilization.
  - *Enhanced glycogen storage:* Regular training increases the muscles' ability to store glycogen, providing more readily available energy during physical activity.

- *Improved muscle oxygenation: Capillary growth*—Exercise induces angiogenesis, which increases the number of capillaries in muscles. More capillaries facilitate better oxygen delivery and nutrient exchange, enhancing muscle performance and endurance.
- *Neurohormonal regulation:*
  - *Reduced sympathetic overactivity:* Exercise training may help modulate the sympathetic nervous system, reducing sympathetic overactivity commonly seen in heart failure. This can lead to improved heart rate control and lower blood pressure.
  - *Hormonal changes:* Regular physical activity can alter levels of hormones such as catecholamines and natriuretic peptides, which play crucial roles in cardiovascular health and fluid balance.

Considerations for Implementation

- *Supervision and safety:*
  - *Tailored programs:* Supervised exercise programs are recommended to ensure safety and efficacy. Individualized exercise prescriptions based on patient assessment can optimize outcomes.
  - *Monitoring during exercise:* Continuous monitoring of vital signs and symptoms during exercise sessions helps prevent adverse events and ensures that training remains within safe limits.
- *Multidisciplinary approach:*
  - *Team involvement:* Successful rehabilitation programs often involve a multidisciplinary team, including cardiologists, physical therapists, dietitians, and exercise physiologists, to address all aspects of patient care.
  - *Education and support:* Providing education about heart failure management, nutrition, and lifestyle changes is essential for fostering long-term adherence to exercise and improving overall health.
- *Motivation and adherence:*
  - *Goal setting:* Establishing realistic and achievable exercise goals can enhance motivation and promote adherence to exercise programs.
  - *Behavioral strategies:* Incorporating behavioral strategies, such as group exercise or community support, can help sustain motivation and foster a supportive environment for patients.

Diet and Weight Management

Background

Obesity is a prevalent risk factor for HFpEF, where excess body weight exacerbates the disease's pathophysiology. In particular, the obesity-related HFpEF phenotype is characterized by increased LV filling pressures, impaired diastolic function, and heightened systemic vascular resistance. As such, effective diet and weight management strategies are crucial for improving patient outcomes and alleviating symptoms in HFpEF.

Benefits of Weight Management

- *Improved exercise tolerance:*
  - *Mechanisms of improvement:* Weight loss interventions have been shown to enhance exercise tolerance by reducing the metabolic and hemodynamic burden on the cardiovascular system. As body weight decreases, there is a corresponding reduction in heart rate and oxygen demand during physical activity, allowing patients to engage in exercise more comfortably.
  - *Increased functional capacity:* Enhanced exercise tolerance leads to increased functional capacity, which is essential for daily activities. This improvement often results in a greater QoL, allowing patients to participate in social and physical activities they may have previously avoided due to symptoms.
- *Lower blood pressure:*
  - *Hypertension management:* Effective weight management is closely linked to better control of blood pressure. Studies have demonstrated that losing weight can lead to significant reductions in systolic and diastolic blood pressure levels, thereby decreasing the risk of cardiovascular complications. This is particularly relevant in HFpEF, where hypertension is a common comorbidity.
  - *Long-term blood pressure control:* Maintaining a healthy weight is critical for the long-term management of hypertension, which helps prevent the progression of heart failure and other cardiovascular diseases.
- *Reduced LV filling pressures:*
  - *Diastolic function improvement:* Weight loss can lower LV filling pressures, enhancing diastolic function. In HFpEF, where impaired ventricular relaxation is prevalent, improving this aspect can alleviate symptoms and improve overall cardiac function.
  - *Symptom reduction:* As diastolic function improves, patients often experience a reduction in classic heart failure symptoms such as dyspnea, fatigue, and edema. This symptom relief can lead to a better overall QoL.

Weight Loss Interventions

- *Caloric restriction:*
  - *Effective strategies:* Caloric restriction, when combined with regular physical activity, has been shown to be effective in promoting weight loss among obese HFpEF patients. Creating a negative energy balance through reduced caloric intake can lead to significant weight loss and subsequent improvements in cardiovascular health.
  - *Impact on diastolic function:* Research indicates that caloric restriction can directly improve diastolic function and reduce LV filling pressures, which are critical aspects of managing HFpEF.
- *Behavioral and lifestyle modifications:*
  - *Structured programs:* Implementing structured weight loss programs, often facilitated by healthcare professionals, can help patients set achievable goals, track their progress, and make sustainable lifestyle changes.
  - *Support systems:* Support from dietitians, exercise physiologists, and peer groups can enhance adherence to dietary and exercise recommendations, fostering a sense of community and motivation among participants.
- *Exercise integration:*
  - *Aerobic exercise:* Incorporating aerobic exercise, such as walking, cycling, or swimming, into daily routines can enhance weight loss efforts while simultaneously improving cardiovascular fitness and functional capacity.
  - *Strength training:* Resistance training can also be beneficial in preserving muscle mass during weight loss. It helps improve muscle strength, which can enhance overall physical performance and reduce the risk of frailty.

Nutritional Interventions

- *Dietary approaches to stop hypertension (DASH) diet:*
  - *Nutritional composition:* The DASH diet emphasizes fruits, vegetables, whole grains, lean proteins, and low-fat dairy products while minimizing saturated fats, cholesterol, and sodium. This diet is designed to manage hypertension and improve overall cardiovascular health.
  - *Health benefits:* Adopting the DASH diet can lead to significant reductions in blood pressure and improvements in heart health. In HFpEF patients, the anti-inflammatory properties of a diet rich in fruits and vegetables can also contribute to better outcomes.
- *Mediterranean diet:*
  - *Heart-healthy choices:* This diet is characterized by high consumption of fruits, vegetables, whole grains, legumes, fish, and healthy fats such as olive oil, along with moderate intake of dairy and limited red meat. The Mediterranean diet has been associated with a reduced risk of cardiovascular disease and may benefit HFpEF patients by promoting weight loss and improving metabolic health.
  - *Anti-inflammatory effects:* The Mediterranean diet's emphasis on anti-inflammatory foods can help mitigate the systemic inflammation often present in obese HFpEF patients, further improving heart function and symptoms.
- *Personalized nutrition plans:*
  - *Individualized approaches:* Developing personalized nutrition plans that account for individual preferences, cultural factors, and nutritional needs can enhance adherence and success in weight management. A tailored approach can help patients find sustainable dietary changes that fit their lifestyles.
  - *Monitoring and support:* Regular follow-ups with nutritionists or dietitians can help monitor progress, adjust dietary plans as needed, and provide ongoing support to encourage healthy eating habits.

DEVICE-BASED INTERVENTIONS

Interatrial Shunt Devices

Background

Heart failure with preserved ejection fraction is a complex syndrome characterized by elevated left atrial pressures, particularly during exertion. This increase in pressure is primarily due to impaired ventricular relaxation and elevated systemic vascular resistance, which leads to congestion and a range of debilitating symptoms, including dyspnea, fatigue, and reduced exercise tolerance. Conventional therapeutic approaches have primarily focused on managing symptoms and associated comorbidities. However, they may not effectively address the underlying hemodynamic issues present in HFpEF. Interatrial shunt devices (IASDs) offer a novel strategy to mitigate elevated left atrial pressures, potentially improving patient outcomes.

Mechanism of Action

- *IASD:*
  - The IASD is a minimally invasive device implanted between the left atrium and the right atrium to

create a small, controlled shunt. This allows for blood to flow from the high-pressure left atrium to the lower-pressure right atrium during diastole.
  - The primary purpose of this shunt is to reduce left atrial pressure, especially during exertion when pressure levels typically spike.
- *Hemodynamic benefits:*
  - By facilitating blood flow from the left atrium to the right atrium, the IASD can effectively lower left atrial pressures. This reduction may help alleviate pulmonary congestion and the associated symptoms of dyspnea, especially during physical activity.
  - Lower left atrial pressures may also lead to improved diastolic function and reduced ventricular filling pressures, thereby enhancing overall cardiac efficiency.

Clinical Evidence

- *REDUCE left atrial pressure in heart failure (LAP-HF) trials:*
  - The REDUCE LAP-HF trials were pivotal studies designed to assess the safety and efficacy of the IASD in patients with HFpEF.
  - Results indicated significant improvements in exercise tolerance and hemodynamics among patients with elevated left atrial pressures who received the IASD. Specifically, these studies demonstrated:
    - *Increased exercise capacity:* Patients showed improvements in exercise capacity measured through the 6-minute-walk test and peak oxygen consumption (VO_2 max).
    - *Reduction in dyspnea symptoms:* Many participants reported fewer episodes of dyspnea and an overall improvement in their QoL.
    - *Lower left atrial pressures:* Hemodynamic measurements showed significant reductions in left atrial pressures post-implantation, contributing to the symptomatic relief observed.
- *Patient selection:*
  - While IASDs may offer benefits, they are not suitable for all HFpEF patients. Ideal candidates typically exhibit:
    - Persistent symptoms despite optimal medical management
    - Elevated left atrial pressures as demonstrated by echocardiography or invasive hemodynamic monitoring
    - No significant structural heart disease that would contraindicate the procedure

Potential Advantages

- *Symptom relief:* By directly targeting the hemodynamic abnormalities responsible for HFpEF symptoms, IASDs may offer more substantial relief than conventional therapies, which primarily focus on symptom management.
- *Minimally invasive approach:* The implantation of IASDs is typically performed via a catheter-based approach, making it less invasive than surgical options. This method reduces recovery times and hospital stays compared to traditional surgical interventions.
- *Long-term benefits:* Although long-term data are still emerging, the potential for sustained improvements in symptoms and exercise capacity could significantly enhance the QoL for patients living with HFpEF.

Considerations and Challenges

- *Risk of complications:* As with any interventional procedure, there are risks associated with IASD implantation, including device-related complications, arrhythmias, and the potential for paradoxical embolism. Careful patient selection and monitoring are essential to minimize these risks.
- *Need for further research:* While initial trials have demonstrated promising results, ongoing research is required to better understand the long-term efficacy and safety of IASDs in HFpEF patients. Larger, multicenter studies will be critical to validate these findings and establish guidelines for clinical practice.
- *Integration with other therapies:* IASDs should not be viewed as standalone treatments. Instead, they may be most effective when used in conjunction with comprehensive management strategies that include lifestyle modifications, pharmacotherapy, and exercise training. A multidisciplinary approach will ensure that patients receive the most effective care tailored to their unique needs.

Cardiac Resynchronization Therapy

Background

Cardiac resynchronization therapy (CRT) has become a standard treatment for patients with HFrEF, particularly those who have evidence of ventricular dyssynchrony, such as left bundle branch block (LBBB). CRT employs a specialized pacemaker to coordinate contractions between the left and right ventricles, improving heart efficiency and alleviating heart failure symptoms. The application of CRT in HFpEF is an evolving area of research, raising the possibility that certain HFpEF patients could benefit from this technology, especially those with associated conduction abnormalities.

Understanding Dyssynchrony in Heart Failure with Preserved Ejection Fraction

- *Ventricular dyssynchrony:*
  - *Definition:* Ventricular dyssynchrony refers to the asynchronous contraction of the left and right ventricles. In HFpEF patients, this can stem from conduction delays, leading to poor mechanical performance.
  - *Mechanism:* Dyssynchrony affects the timing of ventricular filling and ejection, which can impair cardiac output and lead to symptoms of heart failure, particularly during physical activity.
- *Characteristics of HFpEF patients:*
  - Patients with HFpEF typically present with normal LVEF but have underlying diastolic dysfunction characterized by impaired relaxation and elevated left atrial pressures.
  - Some HFpEF patients exhibit conduction abnormalities such as intraventricular conduction delays or LBBB, which can lead to significant ventricular dyssynchrony.

Mechanism of Action of Cardiac Resynchronization Therapy in HFpEF

- *Improved synchrony:*
  - *Electrical synchrony:* CRT restores coordinated electrical activation of the ventricles by delivering pacing impulses that synchronize their contractions, potentially improving diastolic filling times and reducing left atrial pressure.
  - *Mechanical synchrony:* By improving the timing of ventricular contractions, CRT may enhance myocardial perfusion and optimize stroke volume, thus improving functional capacity and alleviating symptoms.
- *Hemodynamic benefits:*
  - CRT has the potential to lower left atrial pressures and improve diastolic function, particularly in patients who exhibit mechanical dyssynchrony. This is crucial in HFpEF, where elevated pressures often lead to pulmonary congestion and associated symptoms.
  - Enhanced cardiac output from improved synchrony can lead to better oxygen delivery to tissues and improved exercise tolerance.

Clinical Evidence Supporting Cardiac Resynchronization Therapy in HFpEF

- *Emerging studies:*
  - Recent studies have suggested that a subset of HFpEF patients with evidence of ventricular dyssynchrony may experience improvements in symptoms and functional status with CRT.
  - For instance, a study found that patients with HFpEF and LBBB demonstrated a significant reduction in heart failure symptoms and improved exercise capacity following CRT implantation.
  - The presence of significant conduction disturbances in HFpEF may indicate a better likelihood of response to CRT.
- *Challenges in study design:*
  - While some studies have shown promising results, research in this area is complicated by the heterogeneous nature of HFpEF and the multifactorial causes of symptoms.
  - Larger, multicenter randomized controlled trials are necessary to definitively establish the efficacy and safety of CRT in HFpEF, including optimal patient selection criteria.
- *Patient selection:*
  - Identifying HFpEF patients who might benefit from CRT requires careful assessment of their conduction status and symptoms.
  - Patients with documented evidence of dyssynchrony via echocardiographic assessment (such as a prolonged QRS duration) may be more likely to benefit from CRT.

Potential Benefits of Cardiac Resynchronization Therapy in HFpEF

- *Symptomatic relief:*
  - Many patients report improvements in symptoms such as fatigue and dyspnea, potentially leading to enhanced QoL and exercise capacity.
  - The reduction in heart failure hospitalizations may represent a significant clinical benefit for these patients.
- *Exercise capacity:*
  - CRT may enhance exercise tolerance, as evidenced by improvements in metrics such as the 6-minute-walk test and peak oxygen consumption (VO_2 max).
  - Improved functional capacity is critical for HFpEF patients, who often experience significant limitations in daily activities due to symptoms.

- *QoL:* Studies have indicated that CRT can positively impact health-related QoL scores in patients with HFpEF, helping them engage more fully in daily activities and reducing the burden of heart failure symptoms.

Considerations and Challenges

- *Patient characteristics:*
  - Not all HFpEF patients are candidates for CRT. Those with significant structural heart disease, severe comorbidities, or who do not meet specific criteria for dyssynchrony may not benefit.
  - Understanding the underlying mechanisms of heart failure symptoms in individual patients is crucial for determining CRT candidacy.
- *Complications:* Although CRT is generally safe, potential complications include infection, lead displacement, and arrhythmias. Close monitoring and follow-up care are essential to manage these risks.
- *Need for further research:*
  - Continued research is needed to better define the role of CRT in HFpEF, including exploring different patient populations, optimizing device settings, and identifying biomarkers that predict response.
  - Investigating the long-term effects of CRT on morbidity and mortality in HFpEF patients will be essential for establishing its clinical utility.

UNDERSTANDING HFpEF PHENOTYPES: A TAILORED THERAPEUTIC APPROACH

As we continue to advance our understanding of HFpEF, it has become clear that it is not a single, homogenous condition. HFpEF represents a spectrum of underlying pathologies, each of which manifests with different clinical features, comorbidities, and therapeutic responses. Identifying these specific *phenotypes* has important implications for personalized treatment approaches, as it allows clinicians to target the key drivers of the disease in individual patients. An expanded discussion on the major HFpEF phenotypes and their tailored management strategies are as follows.

Obesity-related Heart Failure with Preserved Ejection Fraction

Pathophysiology: Obesity is a common comorbidity in HFpEF and often contributes to the development of the syndrome. Excess body fat leads to systemic inflammation, altered metabolic profiles, and increased cardiac workload. Obesity can also impair ventricular relaxation and increase LV filling pressures, exacerbating symptoms of HFpEF.

Clinical features:
- Patients tend to present with significant exercise intolerance, high blood pressure, and higher levels of circulating inflammatory markers.
- Increased body mass index (BMI) is often linked to more severe symptoms and a higher burden of comorbidities such as diabetes.

Therapeutic implications:
- *Weight loss:* Intentional weight loss through caloric restriction and exercise has been shown to improve functional capacity, reduce LV filling pressures, and decrease symptoms in obese HFpEF patients.
- *Exercise training:* Supervised aerobic exercise programs can enhance cardiorespiratory fitness (VO_2 max), improve diastolic function, and alleviate symptoms of fatigue and dyspnea.
- *Bariatric surgery:* In morbidly obese patients, bariatric surgery may offer additional benefits by significantly reducing body weight and improving cardiovascular outcomes.

Hypertensive Heart Failure with Preserved Ejection Fraction

Pathophysiology: Chronic hypertension leads to LV hypertrophy and stiffening of the ventricular walls, contributing to impaired relaxation and diastolic dysfunction, both hallmark features of HFpEF. In hypertensive HFpEF, elevated afterload increases myocardial wall stress, driving symptoms of heart failure.

Clinical features:
- These patients often have a history of poorly controlled or long-standing hypertension, with concentric LV hypertrophy and thickened ventricular walls observed on echocardiography.
- Symptoms typically include exertional dyspnea and fatigue, and there is often evidence of left atrial enlargement due to elevated LV filling pressures.

Therapeutic implications:
- *Aggressive blood pressure control:* Controlling blood pressure is crucial in hypertensive HFpEF. Antihypertensive agents such as angiotensin-converting enzyme (ACE) inhibitors, angiotensin receptor blockers (ARBs), and calcium channel blockers can help reduce afterload and improve diastolic function.

- *MRAs:* Agents such as spironolactone may offer benefits by reducing fibrosis and improving diastolic properties of the heart.
- *SGLT-2 inhibitors:* Emerging evidence suggests that SGLT-2 inhibitors, like empagliflozin, may improve outcomes in HFpEF, potentially by reducing blood pressure and myocardial stress.

Atrial Fibrillation-related Heart Failure with Preserved Ejection Fraction

Pathophysiology: Atrial fibrillation (AF) is common in HFpEF due to elevated left atrial pressure and volume overload. AF worsens diastolic dysfunction, reduces cardiac output, and contributes to increased heart failure symptoms.

Clinical features: Patients with AF-related HFpEF often have a history of AF, with intermittent or persistent episodes of rapid and irregular heartbeats. They frequently experience palpitations, fatigue, and worsening dyspnea, especially during AF episodes.

Therapeutic implications:
- *Rhythm control:* Maintaining sinus rhythm may improve symptoms and exercise capacity. Strategies include antiarrhythmic drugs (e.g., amiodarone) and catheter ablation, depending on the patient's AF burden and heart failure severity.
- *Rate control:* If rhythm control is not feasible or successful, managing the ventricular rate during AF episodes using beta-blockers, calcium channel blockers, or digoxin can alleviate symptoms and improve functional capacity.
- *Anticoagulation:* Patients with AF-related HFpEF are at an increased risk of stroke, making anticoagulation therapy critical to preventing thromboembolic events.

Coronary Artery Disease-related Heart Failure with Preserved Ejection Fraction

Pathophysiology: Myocardial ischemia from coronary artery disease (CAD) can worsen diastolic function, impair relaxation, and elevate LV filling pressures. CAD-related HFpEF is driven by the interaction between ischemic heart disease and the impaired ability of the myocardium to fill properly during diastole.

Clinical features: Patients with this phenotype often have a history of angina, myocardial infarction, or significant coronary artery stenosis. They may present with exertional chest pain or shortness of breath, and diagnostic tests may reveal evidence of ischemia on stress testing or coronary angiography.

Therapeutic implications:
- *Anti-ischemic therapies:* Medications such as nitrates, beta-blockers, and calcium channel blockers can reduce myocardial oxygen demand and alleviate ischemia-related symptoms.
- *Revascularization:* For patients with significant coronary artery stenosis, revascularization via percutaneous coronary intervention (PCI) or coronary artery bypass grafting (CABG) may improve myocardial perfusion, reduce symptoms, and potentially improve heart failure outcomes.
- *Statin therapy:* Aggressive lipid management with statins is essential to stabilize atherosclerotic plaques and reduce the risk of future cardiovascular events.

Diabetes-related Heart Failure with Preserved Ejection Fraction

Pathophysiology: Diabetes is a significant contributor to HFpEF through mechanisms such as microvascular dysfunction, increased myocardial fibrosis, and metabolic derangements that impair both systolic and diastolic function.

Clinical features: Diabetic HFpEF patients often have a constellation of other metabolic risk factors, including obesity, hypertension, and dyslipidemia. They may also exhibit signs of autonomic dysfunction, such as resting tachycardia and orthostatic hypotension.

Therapeutic implications:
- *Glycemic control:* Tight blood sugar control with medications such as SGLT-2 inhibitors or glucagon-like peptide-1 (GLP-1) receptor agonists has been shown to reduce heart failure hospitalizations and improve cardiovascular outcomes in diabetic patients with HFpEF.
- *SGLT-2 inhibitors:* Emerging evidence, particularly from trials like EMPEROR-Preserved, suggests that SGLT-2 inhibitors can reduce the risk of heart failure hospitalization and improve symptoms in patients with diabetes-related HFpEF.

Pulmonary Hypertension-related Heart Failure with Preserved Ejection Fraction

Pathophysiology: Pulmonary hypertension (PH) often accompanies HFpEF, resulting from chronic elevations in left atrial pressure, leading to pulmonary vascular remodeling and increased pulmonary artery pressures.

Clinical features: These patients typically present with severe dyspnea on exertion and signs of right heart failure, including peripheral edema and jugular venous distention. Echocardiography often shows elevated pulmonary artery pressures and right ventricular dysfunction.

Therapeutic implications:

- *Targeted PH therapies:* In selected patients, pulmonary vasodilators (e.g., phosphodiesterase-5 inhibitors or sGC stimulators like vericiguat) may help reduce pulmonary pressures and improve right ventricular function.
- *Diuretics:* Aggressive management of volume overload with diuretics can alleviate symptoms and reduce pulmonary congestion.
- *Exercise training:* Pulmonary rehabilitation and supervised exercise programs can improve functional capacity and alleviate symptoms in patients with PH-related HFpEF.

TARGETING COMORBIDITIES: A COMPREHENSIVE APPROACH

In HFpEF, comorbidities play a central role in both the progression of the disease and the worsening of symptoms. Unlike HFrEF, where heart muscle dysfunction is the predominant issue, HFpEF is characterized by a more complex interplay of multiple systemic conditions that exacerbate heart failure. Addressing these comorbidities is a key strategy for improving both symptoms and prognosis in HFpEF patients. An expanded discussion on the management of some of the most impactful comorbidities in HFpEF is as follows.

Atrial Fibrillation in Heart Failure with Preserved Ejection Fraction

Pathophysiology: AF is particularly common in HFpEF, affecting around 40–60% of patients. The atria play a critical role in helping fill the stiff left ventricle in HFpEF, so when AF occurs, the loss of atrial contraction (atrial kick) leads to reduced LV filling. This contributes to worsening of heart failure symptoms, including fatigue and exercise intolerance, as well as increased risk of hospitalization. Additionally, the rapid, irregular heart rates often seen in AF can exacerbate diastolic dysfunction and further increase left atrial pressures.

Management:

- *Rate control:* For patients with AF, managing heart rate can help reduce symptoms, but it may not completely resolve the issue of poor filling and hemodynamics.
- *Rhythm control:* Strategies to maintain sinus rhythm, such as antiarrhythmic drugs or catheter ablation, have shown promise in reducing heart failure symptoms and improving QoL. Particularly in younger patients or those with recent-onset AF, restoring sinus rhythm can significantly improve outcomes.
- *Anticoagulation:* Due to the high risk of thromboembolic events (e.g., stroke) in HFpEF patients with AF, anticoagulation therapy is essential. Direct oral anticoagulants (DOACs) are often preferred over warfarin for stroke prevention in this population, given their safety and ease of use.

Emerging therapies: Catheter ablation has shown positive outcomes in restoring and maintaining sinus rhythm in selected patients with HFpEF and AF. Ongoing studies are evaluating its long-term benefits for HFpEF patients, especially in reducing hospitalization and mortality.

Obstructive Sleep Apnea in Heart Failure with Preserved Ejection Fraction

Pathophysiology: Obstructive sleep apnea (OSA) is prevalent in HFpEF patients, especially those who are obese, and can contribute to worsening heart failure through mechanisms like intermittent hypoxia, increased sympathetic nervous system activity, and elevated pulmonary and systemic blood pressures. These changes lead to increased LV filling pressures and diastolic dysfunction. Untreated OSA also contributes to daytime fatigue, further limiting exercise capacity in HFpEF patients.

Management:

- *Continuous positive airway pressure (CPAP) therapy:* It is the mainstay of OSA treatment and has been shown to improve nocturnal oxygenation, reduce sympathetic overactivity, and lower blood pressure. For HFpEF patients, CPAP may help reduce LV filling pressures and improve heart failure symptoms.
- *Lifestyle modifications:* Weight loss and sleep hygiene improvements are also crucial for managing OSA, as they can reduce the severity of the condition and improve overall cardiovascular health.

Clinical evidence: While CPAP therapy is commonly used in patients with OSA, its impact on long-term outcomes like mortality in HFpEF patients is still being investigated. However, it has shown benefits in terms of improving exercise capacity and reducing symptoms in HFpEF.

Hypertension in Heart Failure with Preserved Ejection Fraction

Pathophysiology: Hypertension is one of the most common comorbidities in HFpEF, contributing to LV hypertrophy, increased myocardial stiffness, and elevated filling pressures. In HFpEF, controlling blood pressure is critical because even small increases in systolic blood pressure can significantly worsen diastolic dysfunction and lead to heart failure exacerbations.

Management:

- *Aggressive blood pressure control:* Optimal blood pressure management is essential to prevent further LV remodeling and progression of diastolic dysfunction. First-line treatments often include ACE inhibitors, ARBs, or calcium channel blockers. Diuretics are used to manage volume overload.
- *Targeted therapies:* In patients with specific HFpEF phenotypes, like those with preserved systolic function and concentric LV hypertrophy, therapies like MRAs and ARNIs may offer additional benefits in reducing heart failure hospitalizations.

Emerging evidence: The PARAGON-HF trial has provided insights into the potential benefits of ARNI therapy (sacubitril/valsartan) in hypertensive HFpEF patients, particularly in those with lower ejection fractions (40–55%). This suggests that certain subsets of hypertensive HFpEF patients may benefit from ARNI therapy.

Coronary Artery Disease in Heart Failure with Preserved Ejection Fraction

Pathophysiology: While CAD is a primary cause of heart failure in HFrEF, it also plays a significant role in HFpEF by causing myocardial ischemia, which worsens diastolic dysfunction and LV stiffness. Patients with HFpEF and CAD may experience recurrent ischemic episodes, leading to further deterioration in cardiac function and increased risk of heart failure exacerbations.

Management:

- *Anti-ischemic therapy:* Optimizing anti-ischemic therapies, including beta-blockers, nitrates, and calcium channel blockers, is important to reduce myocardial oxygen demand and improve coronary blood flow. Statins are also recommended to manage atherosclerosis and prevent future ischemic events.
- *Revascularization:* In selected HFpEF patients with significant CAD, revascularization (through PCI or CABG) may improve symptoms and exercise capacity. However, the benefits of revascularization in this population are still under investigation.

Clinical insights: CAD-related HFpEF represents a distinct phenotype where targeting ischemia with optimal medical therapy and revascularization (when indicated) may help alleviate heart failure symptoms and improve QoL.

Diabetes Mellitus in Heart Failure with Preserved Ejection Fraction

Pathophysiology: Diabetes is a key contributor to HFpEF by promoting systemic inflammation, endothelial dysfunction, and myocardial fibrosis. Diabetic patients with HFpEF often have worse outcomes due to these mechanisms, which increase LV stiffness and impair relaxation.

Management:

- *Glycemic control:* Tight glucose control is crucial in reducing cardiovascular complications in diabetic HFpEF patients. SGLT2 inhibitors, such as empagliflozin and dapagliflozin, have emerged as promising treatments for HFpEF, showing benefits in reducing heart failure hospitalizations and improving QoL, even in nondiabetic patients.
- *Metformin and other therapies:* Metformin is typically the first-line therapy for managing diabetes in HFpEF patients, while GLP-1 receptor agonists are also considered for cardiovascular protection.

Emerging evidence: SGLT2 inhibitors are now being evaluated in large trials specifically for their benefits in HFpEF patients, including improvements in exercise capacity and reductions in hospitalization.

Chronic Kidney Disease in Heart Failure with Preserved Ejection Fraction

Pathophysiology: Chronic kidney disease (CKD) is a common comorbidity in HFpEF, contributing to fluid retention, increased LV filling pressures, and worsening diastolic function. The interplay between the kidneys and heart (cardiorenal syndrome) complicates management, as both organs affect each other negatively.

Management:

- *Renal protection:* Managing fluid overload with diuretics is essential, but care must be taken to avoid worsening renal function. RAAS inhibitors (ACE inhibitors and ARBs) and MRAs are often used to help protect renal function while managing heart failure. Careful adjustment of dosages is required in patients with advanced CKD.
- *SGLT2 inhibitors:* These drugs are increasingly recognized for their dual benefit in both reducing HFpEF symptoms and slowing the progression of CKD.

Emerging insights: Ongoing trials are exploring the role of novel agents, such as SGLT2 inhibitors and MRAs, in better managing both heart failure and CKD in patients with HFpEF.

EMERGING BIOMARKERS

Biomarkers are gaining prominence in the management of *HFpEF* due to their ability to reflect critical underlying processes like *inflammation, fibrosis,* and *myocardial stress*. Since HFpEF is a heterogeneous syndrome, biomarkers can help tailor treatment by identifying specific pathophysiological drivers. Here's a detailed look at key emerging biomarkers and their potential applications in HFpEF:

N-terminal pro-B-type Natriuretic Peptide

N-terminal pro-B-type natriuretic peptide (NT-proBNP) is widely recognized as a biomarker of *myocardial stress* and *volume overload*. It is released in response to increased ventricular wall stretch and pressure. In HFpEF, NT-proBNP levels can help:

- *Confirm the diagnosis* of heart failure, particularly when clinical signs are ambiguous.
- *Guide therapy,* especially when tailoring diuretic use to reduce congestion.
- *Predict prognosis,* as elevated NT-proBNP levels are associated with a higher risk of heart failure hospitalization and mortality.

However, *NT-proBNP* levels tend to be lower in HFpEF compared to HFrEF, potentially reflecting differences in hemodynamic stress between these conditions. This makes interpretation more nuanced in HFpEF patients.

Galectin-3

Galectin-3 is a biomarker associated with *fibrosis* and *inflammation*, both of which are crucial in the pathophysiology of HFpEF. Galectin-3 plays a role in the activation of fibroblasts, which leads to excessive collagen deposition and myocardial stiffening. In HFpEF:

- Elevated *galectin-3* levels correlate with *worsening cardiac remodeling* and *fibrotic burden*.
- Higher levels are linked with *adverse outcomes*, including hospitalization and death.
- *Antifibrotic therapies* targeting galectin-3 pathways could be explored as future treatment avenues.

Galectin-3 levels may also be valuable in differentiating between *cardiac* and *noncardiac* causes of symptoms in patients with dyspnea, potentially offering additional diagnostic precision.

Suppression of Tumorigenicity-2

Suppression of tumorigenicity-2 (ST2) is another biomarker involved in the regulation of *myocardial fibrosis* and *remodeling*. It exists in two forms: Soluble ST2 (sST2), which is released in response to mechanical strain on the heart, and a transmembrane form that mediates inflammation. In HFpEF:

- Elevated *sST2* levels are indicative of *adverse remodeling* and *increased myocardial stress*.
- ST2 levels can predict *poor clinical outcomes*, such as hospitalization and cardiovascular mortality, similar to NT-proBNP.
- Monitoring sST2 levels can help *gauge the effectiveness of therapy*, especially in reducing cardiac stress and improving diastolic function.

The combination of *NT-proBNP* and *ST2* offers a complementary approach, as they reflect different mechanisms of heart failure.

High-sensitivity C-reactive Protein

High-sensitivity C-reactive protein (hsCRP) is a well-known marker of systemic *inflammation*, which plays a role in the progression of HFpEF. Inflammatory states are closely linked to endothelial dysfunction and the development of myocardial stiffening. In HFpEF:

- Elevated *hsCRP* levels correlate with *worse functional capacity* and *increased symptom burden*.
- High hsCRP levels are associated with *worse outcomes*, including heart failure progression and death.
- Targeting the inflammatory pathways in HFpEF could open avenues for novel therapies.

Cardiac Troponins (Troponin T and I)

Although *troponins* are more commonly used as markers of myocardial injury in acute coronary syndromes, they have prognostic utility in HFpEF as well:

- *Elevated troponin levels* in HFpEF indicate ongoing *myocardial injury*, which may be due to factors such as *microvascular ischemia* or *pressure overload*.
- Persistent low-level elevation of troponins is associated with *worse prognosis* in HFpEF patients.
- Regular monitoring may help identify high-risk patients who might benefit from *more aggressive therapy*.

Potential Applications of Biomarkers in Heart Failure with Preserved Ejection Fraction

- *Risk stratification:* Biomarkers like NT-proBNP, Galectin-3, and ST2 can help identify patients who are at high risk of adverse outcomes and require closer monitoring or more intensive therapy.
- *Guiding therapy:* By tracking biomarker levels, clinicians can tailor treatments such as diuretics, vasodilators, or even emerging therapies like *SGLT2*

inhibitors in response to changes in myocardial stress or fibrosis markers.

- *Personalized medicine:* As more biomarkers are identified, there is a potential to better match therapeutic strategies to specific *HFpEF phenotypes*, such as *inflammation-driven* or *fibrosis-dominant* subtypes.
- *Prognosis and monitoring:* Regular assessment of biomarkers can help gauge the progression of HFpEF and predict long-term outcomes, allowing for timely intervention when levels worsen.

FUTURE RESEARCH DIRECTIONS

The evolving landscape of HFpEF research reflects the complexity and heterogeneity of the condition. As therapeutic needs grow and current treatments prove insufficient for many patients, new approaches are being investigated to better understand and address HFpEF pathophysiology. Here are some of the most promising areas of future research:

Inflammation and Myocardial Fibrosis

Inflammation and fibrosis are central to the pathophysiology of HFpEF, contributing to myocardial stiffness, impaired relaxation, and diastolic dysfunction. Novel therapies targeting these processes are being explored:

- *Anti-inflammatory agents:* As chronic low-grade inflammation is a hallmark in many HFpEF patients, particularly those with obesity or metabolic syndrome, researchers are investigating anti-inflammatory therapies to mitigate this inflammatory response. These therapies may help reduce myocardial damage and improve heart function.
- *Anti-fibrotic therapies:* Since myocardial fibrosis leads to stiffening of the heart muscle, new drugs are being developed to directly target and reduce fibrosis. Some research is exploring the potential of *pirfenidone*, an anti-fibrotic agent, to reverse cardiac fibrosis in HFpEF patients.

Metabolic Modulation

Many HFpEF patients have metabolic disorders such as obesity, diabetes, or insulin resistance, which can contribute to myocardial dysfunction. Targeting these metabolic pathways presents an exciting area of research:

- *SGLT2 inhibitors:* These drugs, initially developed for diabetes management, have shown promise in heart failure, including HFpEF. They work by improving myocardial metabolism and reducing oxidative stress, which can improve cardiac efficiency.
- *Mitochondrial-targeted therapies:* Mitochondrial dysfunction plays a role in HFpEF, particularly in patients with metabolic syndrome. Therapies aimed at improving mitochondrial function could enhance energy utilization in the myocardium, alleviating symptoms and improving outcomes.

Targeting Comorbidities

Heart failure with preserved ejection fraction is characterized by a high burden of comorbidities such as *AF*, *OSA*, and *hypertension*. Treating these comorbid conditions effectively may help alleviate heart failure symptoms:

- *AF management:* Rhythm control strategies, including catheter ablation and antiarrhythmic drugs, may be particularly useful for symptom relief in HFpEF patients with AF.
- *OSA treatment:* CPAP is being investigated for its potential to reduce heart failure symptoms in HFpEF patients with sleep apnea by lowering sympathetic activity and improving oxygenation.
- *Obesity-related HFpEF:* Given the strong link between obesity and HFpEF, weight loss through caloric restriction and bariatric surgery is being studied for its long-term impact on cardiac function and exercise tolerance.

Precision Medicine

With HFpEF being a heterogeneous condition, a one-size-fits-all approach is unlikely to be effective. Advances in machine learning and *artificial intelligence (AI)* are enabling researchers to identify unique phenotypes within HFpEF:

- *Phenotype-guided therapy:* By recognizing distinct HFpEF subgroups (e.g., obesity-related HFpEF and hypertensive HFpEF), clinicians can tailor treatment strategies to target the underlying causes of heart failure in each subgroup.
- *Biomarker-driven treatment:* The use of biomarkers such as *NT-proBNP*, *ST2*, and *galectin-3* may help stratify HFpEF patients based on their risk profile and treatment responsiveness, allowing for more personalized therapeutic approaches.

Cardiac and Vascular Stiffness

The stiffness of both the myocardium and the vasculature contributes significantly to HFpEF pathophysiology.

Ongoing research is investigating how to improve vascular compliance and reduce myocardial stiffness:

- *sGC stimulators*: Drugs like *vericiguat*, which target the NO pathway, are being explored for their potential to improve vascular relaxation and myocardial compliance in HFpEF patients.
- *Pirfenidone:* Studies show that exercise training can improve vascular stiffness and endothelial function, which could provide symptomatic relief in HFpEF patients by improving functional capacity and reducing pulmonary pressures.

Device-based Therapies

Interatrial shunt devices and other novel technologies are being explored for their ability to mechanically reduce the pressures that drive HFpEF symptoms:

- *IASDs:* These devices create a small, controlled shunt between the left and right atria to relieve elevated left atrial pressure, which is a common feature in HFpEF. Trials like the *REDUCE LAP-HF* have shown improvements in exercise capacity and QoL in HFpEF patients with elevated left atrial pressure.
- *CRT:* Though primarily used in HFrEF, CRT is being explored in HFpEF patients with evidence of ventricular dyssynchrony. Early studies suggest CRT may improve LV function and reduce heart failure symptoms in select HFpEF patients.

Emerging Biomarkers

Biomarkers reflecting inflammation, fibrosis, and myocardial stress are gaining attention in HFpEF for their potential to guide therapy and predict outcomes:

- *Galectin-3, ST2, and NT-proBNP:* These biomarkers are being investigated for their ability to identify high-risk patients and monitor response to therapies, helping clinicians tailor interventions and potentially improve prognoses in HFpEF.

Clinical Trials and Drug Development

Several new therapies and interventions are in clinical trials, investigating the efficacy of novel drugs targeting distinct HFpEF mechanisms:

- *PARALLAX trial:* Evaluating the effects of sacubitril/valsartan on various clinical outcomes in HFpEF patients with different phenotypes
- *VITALITY-HFpEF:* Investigating *vericiguat* in improving functional capacity in HFpEF patients

CONCLUSION

Recent advancements in the management of HFpEF have brought new hope to patients facing this difficult condition. SGLT2 inhibitors, such as empagliflozin and dapagliflozin, have emerged as pivotal therapies, reducing hospitalizations and improving QoL, even in nondiabetic populations. The EMPEROR-Preserved and DELIVER trials highlight the value of these drugs, which are now central to HFpEF management. MRAs like spironolactone also show promise, particularly in patients with elevated natriuretic peptides, though their benefits require further clarification.

Nonpharmacologic interventions, such as exercise training and weight management, are increasingly recognized for improving symptoms and enhancing QoL. Device-based therapies, like IASDs and CRT, are showing potential for select patients, though additional research is needed to refine their use.

A more nuanced understanding of HFpEF phenotypes and comorbidities allows for personalized treatment strategies, addressing factors like obesity, hypertension, and AF. Emerging therapies, such as vericiguat, aim to improve myocardial function, while ongoing research into biomarkers and novel treatments continues to drive progress. Ultimately, these advances in both pharmacologic and nonpharmacologic strategies offer hope for better outcomes and more individualized care for HFpEF patients.

SUGGESTED READING

1. Anker SD, Butler J, Filippatos G, et al.; EMPEROR-Preserved Trial Investigators. Empagliflozin in heart failure with preserved ejection fraction. N Engl J Med. 2021;385(16):1451-61.
2. Armstrong PW, Pieske B, Anstrom KJ, et al. Vericiguat in patients with heart failure and reduced ejection fraction. N Engl J Med. 2020;382(20):1883-93.
3. Bayes-Genis A, Januzzi JL. Galectin-3 and soluble ST2 in heart failure. Cardiol Clin. 2015;33(4):681-90.
4. Bitter T, Westerheide N, Prinz C, et al. Cheyne–Stokes respiration and obstructive sleep apnea are independent risk factors for malignant arrhythmias in patients with congestive heart failure. Eur Heart J. 2011;32(1):61-74.
5. Borlaug BA, Paulus WJ. Heart failure with preserved ejection fraction: pathophysiology, diagnosis, and treatment. Eur Heart J. 2011;32(6):670-9.
6. Campbell DJ. Neprilysin inhibition in the context of dual renin–angiotensin system inhibition. Circ Res. 2017;120(5):755-7.
7. Desai AS, Lewis EF, Solomon SD, et al. Effect of spironolactone on hospitalization for heart failure in

patients with preserved ejection fraction: The TOPCAT trial. J Am Coll Cardiol. 2016;68(8):1331-32.

8. Dorn GW, Vega RB. Mitochondrial dynamism and dysfunction in HFpEF and heart failure with reduced ejection fraction. JACC Basic Transl Sci. 2021;6(8):760-75.
9. Ezekowitz JA, O'Connor CM, Troughton RW, et al. Vericiguat in patients with heart failure and preserved ejection fraction: VITALITY-HFpEF study. JACC Heart Fail. 2020;8(10):710-24.
10. Feldman T, Mauri L, Kahwash R, et al. A transcatheter interatrial shunt device for heart failure with preserved ejection fraction (REDUCE LAP-HF I [Reduce Elevated Left Atrial Pressure in Patients With Heart Failure]): A phase 2, randomized, sham-controlled trial. Circulation. 2018;137(4):364-75.
11. Gaggin HK, Januzzi JL Jr. Biomarkers and diagnostics in heart failure. Biochim Biophys Acta. 2013;1832(12):2442-50.
12. Kitzman DW, Brubaker PH. Exercise training in heart failure with preserved ejection fraction: mechanisms and future directions. Circulation. 2019;139(4):247-9.
13. Kitzman DW, Shah SJ. The HFpEF obesity phenotype: the elephant in the room. J Am Coll Cardiol. 2016;68(2):200-3.
14. Kosiborod M, Cavender MA, Fu AZ, et al.; CVD-REAL Investigators and Study Group. Lower risk of heart failure and death in patients initiated on sodium-glucose cotransporter-2 inhibitors versus other glucose-lowering drugs: The CVD-REAL study. Circulation. 2017; 136(3):249-59.
15. Kotecha D, Piccini JP. Atrial fibrillation in heart failure: What should we do? Eur Heart J. 2015;36(46):3250-7.
16. Lopéz B, Ravassa S, Gonzalez A, et al. Myocardial collagen cross-linking is associated with heart failure hospitalization in patients with hypertensive heart failure. J Am Coll Cardiol. 2016;67(3):251-60.
17. McMurray JJV, Packer M, Desai AS, et al.; PARADIGM-HF Investigators and Committees. Angiotensin-neprilysin inhibition versus enalapril in heart failure. N Engl J Med. 2014;371(11):993-1004.
18. McMurray JJV, Solomon SD, Inzucchi SE, et al.; DAPA-HF Trial Committees and Investigators. Dapagliflozin in patients with heart failure and reduced ejection fraction. N Engl J Med. 2019;381(21):1995-2008.
19. Packer M, Anker SD, Butler J, et al.; EMPEROR-Reduced Trial Investigators. Cardiovascular and renal outcomes with empagliflozin in heart failure. N Engl J Med. 2020;383(15):1413-24.
20. Pandey A, Patel KV, Vaduganathan M, et al. Physical activity, fitness, and obesity in heart failure with preserved ejection fraction. JACC Heart Fail. 2018;6(12): 975-82.
21. Paulus WJ, Tschöpe C. A novel paradigm for heart failure with preserved ejection fraction: comorbidities drive myocardial dysfunction and remodeling through coronary microvascular endothelial inflammation. J Am Coll Cardiol. 2013;62(4):263-71.
22. Pitt B, Pfeffer MA, Assmann SF, et al.; TOPCAT Investigators. Spironolactone for heart failure with preserved ejection fraction. N Engl J Med. 2014;370(15):1383-92.
23. Shah AM, Claggett B, Loehr LR, et al. Obesity and heart failure with preserved ejection fraction: a population-based study. J Am Coll Cardiol. 2017;70(15):1877-88.
24. Shah SJ, Katz DH, Deo RC, et al. Phenomapping for novel classification of heart failure with preserved ejection fraction. Circulation. 2015;131(3):269-79.
25. Solomon SD, McMurray JJV, Anand IS, et al.; PARAGON-HF Investigators and Committees. Angiotensin-neprilysin inhibition in heart failure with preserved ejection fraction. N Engl J Med. 2019;381(17):1609-20.
26. Solomon SD, Rizkala AR, Gong J, et al. Angiotensin receptor neprilysin inhibition in heart failure with preserved ejection fraction: rationale and design of the PARALLAX trial. JACC Heart Fail. 2020;8(4):345-56.
27. Verma S, McMurray JJV. SGLT2 inhibitors and mechanisms of cardiovascular benefit: a state-of-the-art review. Diabetologia. 2018;61(10):2108-17.
28. Zannad F, Ferreira JP, Pocock SJ, et al. Sodium-glucose cotransporter-2 inhibitors in heart failure with reduced ejection fraction: a systematic review and meta-analysis of randomized controlled trials. Lancet. 2020;396(10254): 819-29.

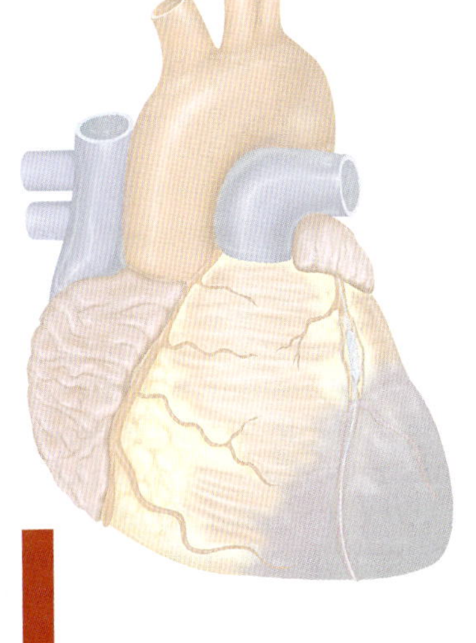

HFpEF: New Guidelines are Pertinent for Primary Care

Geevar Zachariah

INTRODUCTION

The incidence of heart failure with preserved ejection fraction (HFpEF) is increasing all over the world. However, this entity is underrecognized. Correct and timely diagnosis is important because, presently, we have evidence-based treatment modalities that have been shown to improve outcomes. When patients with HFpEF present in the emergency care settings, diagnosis is relatively straightforward. However, most cases of HFpEF are encountered in primary care. When they are present in the community, diagnosis is much more challenging, and there is often the risk of misdiagnosis or underdiagnosis. This is because patients may underreport symptoms or may present with atypical symptoms such as fatigue, reduced exercise tolerance, or ankle swelling. Other causes of misdiagnosis are lack of awareness of heart failure (HF) as a cause of respiratory symptoms, presence of mimicking comorbidities, lack of facilities for testing for natriuretic peptide or performing echocardiography, and uncertainty on how to diagnose HFpEF. Guidelines are important tools to help clinicians decide the best course of action for an individual patient with a given condition. They summarize the available evidence, and this is especially important in conditions such as HF, where so many randomized controlled trials are being published every year. HFpEF has remained an enigma in terms of its definition, classification, and approach to treatment. Over the past 3 years, we have seen several advances in managing this elusive disease. Four major guidelines were published: the 2021 ESC guidelines for the diagnosis and treatment of HF, the 2022 AHA/ACC/HFSA guideline on heart failure, the 2023 focused update of the 2021 ESC guideline for heart failure, and the 2023 ACC Expert Consensus Decision Pathway on the management of HFpEF. These new guidelines will help update the current recommendations in the management of HFpEF. However, to be useful, the recommendations offered should be applicable in the primary care settings where most cases of HFpEF will be encountered and managed. We should also remember that guidelines are roadmaps and should not replace clinical judgment.

DEFINITION AND DIAGNOSIS OF HEART FAILURE WITH PRESERVED EJECTION FRACTION

The 2022 AHA/ACC/HFSA guidelines for the management of HF consider classification based on ejection fraction (EF) to be important because most clinical trials enroll patients with HF based on EF. HFpEF is usually defined as those with symptoms and signs of HF and an LVEF ≥50%. However, signs and symptoms of HF are often nonspecific and overlap with other clinical conditions. Hence, diagnosis of HFpEF should be supported by objective measures of increased left ventricular (LV) filling pressures at rest, exercise, or on provocation. These can be elevated levels of natriuretic peptides, echocardiographic diastolic parameters such as an E/e′ >15 or other evidence of elevated LV filling pressures, or invasive hemodynamic measurement at rest or exercise. The presence of structural heart disease, as evidenced by the increase in left atrial size and volume (left atrial volume index) and/or an increase in LV mass (LV mass index), may be useful to further support the diagnosis. If the diagnosis remains uncertain, exercise testing with echocardiographic evaluation of diastolic parameters may be helpful. Alternatively, invasive hemodynamic parameters at rest or with exercise with an assessment of filling pressures (pulmonary capillary wedge pressures, pulmonary artery pressures, stroke volumes, and cardiac output) can support the diagnosis of HFpEF.[1]

The 2021 ESC guidelines also recommended EF of ≥50% to define HFpEF.[2] The diagnosis should include the following three components, namely (1) symptoms and signs of HF, (2) an LVEF ≥50%, and (3) objective evidence of cardiac structural and/or functional abnormalities consistent with the presence of LV diastolic dysfunction/raised LV filling pressures. These include an LV mass index ≥95 g/m^2 in females and >115 g/m^2 in males, relative wall thickness >0.42 (absence of LV hypertrophy does not exclude HFpEF), LA volume index >34 mL/m^2 if in sinus rhythm or >40 mL/m^2 if in atrial fibrillation (AF), an E/e′ ratio at rest >9 (sensitivity 78% and specificity 59%), NT-proBNP >125 pg/mL in sinus rhythm or >365 pg/mL in AF, PA systolic pressure >35 mm Hg, and TR velocity at rest >2.8 m/s. Additional confirmatory tests will be required when diagnosis is uncertain. The ESC 2021 guidelines emphasize the value of noninvasive markers of raised LV filling pressures. Greater the number of these objective markers, higher the probability of diagnosis of HFpEF.[2]

As can be seen, the major guidelines do not differ substantially in the diagnosis and classification of HFpEF. However, these complicated definitions make it more difficult to diagnose HFpEF than HF with reduced EF.[3] There is no simple definition combining imaging or natriuretic peptides that help to rule in or rule out whether a person has HFpEF. This creates problems in managing patients at the primary care level.

Further, it should be remembered that approximately 20% of patients with HFpEF have normal natriuretic peptide levels.[4] This is because natriuretic peptide release occurs due to diastolic wall stress, which may not be high in the presence of LV hypertrophy seen commonly in HFpEF.[3] Another possible explanation is the coexistence of obesity. Obese patients with HF have lower levels of natriuretic peptide due to rapid degradation by fat tissue and increased expression of receptors involved in their clearance.[5]

Heart failure with preserved ejection fraction, as a chronic condition, presents with effort-related breathlessness. Signs of pulmonary or systemic venous congestion may not be evident. Often, effort intolerance is attributed to other common comorbidities such as obesity, diabetes, chronic obstructive pulmonary disease, frailty, and deconditioning. Hence, diagnosis is often missed in primary care. In a Dutch study among elderly patients with diabetes, imaging studies revealed new HF in 27.7% of patients, and the majority of them had HFpEF.[6]

DIAGNOSTIC WORKUP

All patients with suspected HFpEF should have an evaluation of BNP/NT-proBNP, 12-lead ECG, transthoracic echocardiogram, chest X-ray, and routine blood tests for comorbidities, including full blood count, urea, electrolytes, thyroid function, fasting glucose, HbA1C, lipids, and iron status (class 1, LOE C, ESC 2021 guidelines).[2] Many authors recommend ergometry/6-minute walk test or cardiopulmonary exercise testing as part of the initial workup.[3] In the second step, a comprehensive echocardiography should be carried out. If the diagnosis is uncertain, the next step should be a diastolic stress test (exercise stress echocardiography). Finally, in selected cases, an etiological evaluation should be carried out with advanced investigations such as cardiovascular magnetic resonance, cardiac or noncardiac biopsies, scintigraphy/CT/PET, genetic testing, and other specific laboratory tests.

HEART FAILURE WITH PRESERVED EJECTION FRACTION SCORES

There are two accepted scoring systems to diagnose HFpEF: (1) HFA-PEFF score and (2) H_2FPEF score. The HFA-PEFF score has functional, morphological, and biomarker domains. In each domain, a major criterion is given 2 points, and a minor criterion is given 1 point. A total score of ≥5 points is considered to be diagnostic, while a low score of ≤1 indicates a low likelihood of HFpEF. Patients with an intermediate score (2–4) will require further investigations.[4]

H_2FPEF score gives 2 points for heavy (BMI >30 kg/m^2), 1 point for hypertensive on two or more medications, 1 point for pulmonary hypertension (Doppler echocardiographic estimated pulmonary artery systolic pressure >35 mm Hg), 1 point for elderly (age >60 years), and 1 point for filling pressures (Doppler echocardiographic E/e′ >9). H_2FPEF score ranges from 0 to 9. Odds of having HFpEF increase by a factor of 2 for every one unit increase in the score. The use of NT-proBNP levels does not add to the diagnostic utility of the score.[7]

DIAGNOSTIC ALGORITHM

An algorithm has been proposed based on the ESC HF guidelines and risk scores for the diagnosis of HFpEF.[7]

Step 1 is to identify a defining characteristic of HFpEF, such as congestion or elevated natriuretic peptide, in patients presenting with dyspnea with or without signs and EF ≥50%. If, in addition, at least one of the echocardiographic criteria is satisfied, we can confidently diagnose HFpEF. Step 1 can diagnose HFpEF in about 80% of the patients. At the primary care level, when the diagnosis is uncertain after step 1 and if there is a high index of suspicion, it is better to seek guidance from an HF specialist. In step 2, the probability of HFpEF is assessed by one of the two scores, HFA-PEFF or H_2FPEF. A low score will practically exclude, and a high score will favor a diagnosis of HFpEF. If the score is intermediate, go to step 3 where patients undergo invasive or noninvasive study of exercise hemodynamics.

The ACC/AHA Expert Decision Pathway 2023 discusses a practical diagnostic approach to a patient presenting with dyspnea and/or edema at the primary care level.[8] The first step will be to consider all noncardiac causes and then look for HFpEF mimics such as valvular heart disease, infiltrative cardiomyopathy, pericardial disease, hypertrophic cardiomyopathy, and high output HF. The next step is to apply the universal definition of HF, which consists of symptoms and/or signs of HF caused by a structural and/or functional abnormality corroborated by elevated natriuretic peptide and/or objective evidence of cardiogenic pulmonary edema or systemic venous congestion. Then, assess the likelihood of HFpEF based on the H_2FPEF score.

MANAGEMENT OF HEART FAILURE WITH PRESERVED EJECTION FRACTION

As per the ESC 2023 focus update to 2021 HF guidelines, management of HFpEF revolves around three class 1 recommendations: (1) diuretics for fluid retention, (2) SGLT2 inhibitors (dapagliflozin/empagliflozin) and treatment for etiology, and (3) cardiovascular (CV) and non-CV comorbidities.[9] These are simple recommendations that are easy to follow at the primary care level. Both the ESC and ACC/AHA guidelines recommend the use of diuretics to reduce symptoms of congestion (class 1) for HF in general, along with other nonpharmacological management.

The 2022 AHA/ACC/HFSA guidelines give class 2a recommendations for the use of SGLT inhibitors in reducing HF hospitalizations and CV death (2a B-R).[1] This is based on the EMPEROR-Preserved trial, which showed significant benefits in symptomatic patients with HFpEF (EF >40%) and elevated natriuretic peptide.[10] The 2023 focused update of the 2021 ESC guidelines gives class 1, LOE A recommendations for the use of dapagliflozin or empagliflozin in patients with HFpEF to reduce the risk of HF hospitalization or CV death.[9] Apart from the EMPEROR-Preserved trial, they considered the DELIVER trial, which reported the effects of dapagliflozin compared with placebo in >6,000 patients.[11] Dapagliflozin reduced the primary end point of CV death or worsening HF by 18%. The 2023 ESC focused update also quotes a meta-analysis of the two trials, which confirmed a 20% reduction in the composite end point of CV death or first hospitalization for HF.[12] CV death was not reduced significantly. However, HF hospitalization was reduced by 26%.

Apart from SGLT2 inhibitors, the 2022 ACC/AHA/HFSA guidelines recommend the consideration of MRAs in selected patients to decrease hospitalizations, especially if LVEF is on the lower side (2b B-R).[1] The recommendation was based on the TOPCAT trial, which investigated the effects of spironolactone in patients with HFpEF.[13] In this trial, even though the reduction of primary end point of composite of death, aborted cardiac death, and HF hospitalization was not statistically significant (HR 0.89), reduction of HF hospitalization was significant (HR 0.83). Hence, an MRA can be considered in symptomatic patients with HFpEF with LVEF ≥45%, elevated BNP level or HF admission within 1 year, eGFR >30 mL/min/1.73 m^2, creatinine <2.5 mg/dL, and potassium <5.0 mEq/L. Careful monitoring of serum potassium and a close watch on renal function are important. They also recommend consideration of using ARB or ARNI in selected patients with HFpEF, to decrease hospitalizations, especially if LVEF is on the lower side (2b B-R).[1]

The guidelines also recommend the management of comorbidities in HFpEF. CV comorbidities include AF, coronary artery disease (CAD), hypertensive heart disease, and stroke. Non-CV comorbidities include diabetes, obesity, chronic kidney disease (CKD), lung disease, obstructive sleep apnea, and miscellaneous disorders such as thyroid disorders, frailty, cachexia, anemia, iron deficiency, electrolyte disturbances, gout, arthritis, erectile dysfunction, depression, cancer, and systemic infection. The 2022 ACC/AHA/HFSA guidelines stress the importance of the management of hypertension in HFpEF. Medications titrated to attain blood pressure targets should be instituted (1C-LD). The optimal blood pressure goal and preferred antihypertensive drugs for HFpEF are yet to be elucidated. Management of AF will help improve symptoms (2aC-EO).

When managing patients with HFpEF at the primary care level, we should know when to refer a patient for a more detailed evaluation. Referring to a CV specialist is to be considered when there is a need to manage comorbidities such as AF, hypertension, diabetes, or CAD; the presence of high-risk features such as recurrent hospitalizations, pulmonary hypertension, or RV dysfunction; need for exercise hemodynamic testing (invasive or noninvasive); cardiorenal syndrome; presence of HFpEF mimics such as valvular disease, HCM, amyloid disease, or pericardial disease; increased need for diuretics; and patients with the NYHA class 3 or 4 symptoms.[8]

PRIMARY PREVENTION OF HEART FAILURE WITH PRESERVED EJECTION FRACTION

In the 2021 ESC HF guidelines, the treatment of hypertension is a class 1A recommendation to prevent or delay the onset of HF and to prevent HF hospitalization. Treatment with statins in patients at high risk of CV disease or with CV disease to prevent or delay the onset of HF and to prevent HF hospitalization is also a class 1A recommendation. Also, it is the use of SGLT2 inhibitors in patients with diabetes at high risk of CV disease or with CV disease to prevent HF hospitalization. Counseling against a sedentary lifestyle, obesity, cigarette smoking, and alcohol abuse is important to prevent or delay the onset of HF (class 1C).[2]

In the 2023 ESC focused update, fresh recommendations were given to prevent HF in patients with diabetes and CKD. They gave class 1A recommendations for the use of SGLT2 inhibitors in patients with diabetes and CKD to reduce the risk of HF hospitalization or CV death.[9] This was based on two trials: (1) DAPA-CKD and (2) EMPA-KIDNEY.[14,15] In a meta-analysis that included four major trials, the reduction in HF hospitalization and CV death was similar, irrespective of history of diabetes.[16]

The 2023 ESC 2023 focused update also recommends the use of finerenone in patients with CKD and T2DM to reduce the risk of HF hospitalization (class 1A).[9] This was based on the FIDELIO-CKD trial and the FIGARO-DKD trial.[17,18]

CONCLUSION

Diagnosis of HFpEF is challenging, and underdiagnosis and misdiagnosis are common in the primary care settings where it is commonly encountered. Major guidelines give recommendations on how to diagnose and manage this often elusive disease. However, the diagnostic workup suggested is sometimes complicated and requires sophisticated investigative tools. Hence, at the primary care level, it is important to understand the initial evaluation of the patients presenting with dyspnea and or edema and how to exclude HFpEF mimics. A simple diagnostic algorithm derived from the guidelines will help to evaluate these patients and to decide when to refer suspected patients for more detailed investigations. The management of HFpEF revolves around nonpharmacological management, diuretics for congestion, SGLT2 inhibitors for all, MRA and ARNI/ARB in selected patients, management of comorbidities, cardiac and noncardiac, and treatment of etiological factors. Prevention of HFpEF is equally important, and control of hypertension and the use of newer agents in patients with diabetes and kidney disease are promising.

REFERENCES

1. Heidenreich PA, Bozkurt B, Aguilar D, et al. 2022 AHA/ACC/HFSA guideline for the management of heart failure: a report of the American College of Cardiology/American Heart Association Joint Committee on clinical practice guidelines. J Am Coll Cardiol. 2022;79(17):e263-421.
2. McDonagh TA, Metra M, Adamo M, et al. 2021 ESC guidelines for the diagnosis and treatment of acute and chronic heart failure. Eur Heart J. 2021;42(36):3599-726.
3. Campbell P, Rutten FH, Lee MM, et al. Heart failure with preserved ejection fraction: everything the clinician needs to know. Lancet Lond Engl. 2024;403(10431):1083-92.
4. Pieske B, Tschöpe C, de Boer RA, et al. How to diagnose heart failure with preserved ejection fraction: the HFA-PEFF diagnostic algorithm: a consensus recommendation from the Heart Failure Association (HFA) of the European Society of Cardiology (ESC). Eur J Heart Fail. 2020;22(3):391-412.
5. Obokata M, Reddy YNV, Pislaru SV, et al. Evidence supporting the existence of a distinct obese phenotype of heart failure with preserved ejection fraction. Circulation. 2017;136(1):6-19.
6. Winter LJM, Rutten FH, Cramer MJM, et al. High prevalence of previously unknown heart failure and left ventricular dysfunction in patients with type 2 diabetes. Diabetologia. 2012;55(8):2154-62.
7. Reddy YNV, Carter RE, Obokata M, et al. A simple, evidence-based approach to help guide diagnosis of heart failure with preserved ejection fraction. Circulation. 2018;138(9):861-70.
8. Kittleson MM, Panjrath GS, Amancherla K, et al. 2023 ACC Expert Consensus Decision Pathway on management of heart failure with preserved ejection fraction: a report of the American College of Cardiology Solution Set Oversight Committee. J Am Coll Cardiol. 2023;81(18):1835-78.
9. McDonagh TA, Metra M, Adamo M, et al. 2023 focused update of the 2021 ESC guidelines for the diagnosis and treatment of acute and chronic heart failure. Eur Heart J. 2023;44(37):3627-39.
10. Anker SD, Butler J, Filippatos G, et al. Empagliflozin in heart failure with a preserved ejection fraction. N Engl J Med. 2021;385(16):1451-61.

11. Solomon SD, McMurray JJV, Claggett B, et al. Dapagliflozin in heart failure with mildly reduced or preserved ejection fraction. N Engl J Med. 2022;387(12):1089-98.
12. Vaduganathan M, Docherty KF, Claggett BL, et al. SGLT-2 inhibitors in patients with heart failure: a comprehensive meta-analysis of five randomised controlled trials. Lancet Lond Engl. 2022;400(10354):757-67.
13. Pitt B, Pfeffer MA, Assmann SF, et al. Spironolactone for heart failure with preserved ejection fraction. N Engl J Med. 2014;370(15):1383-92.
14. Heerspink HJL, Stefánsson BV, Correa-Rotter R, et al. Dapagliflozin in patients with chronic kidney disease. N Engl J Med. 2020;383(15):1436-46.
15. Herrington WG, Staplin N, Wanner C, et al. Empagliflozin in patients with chronic kidney disease. N Engl J Med. 2023;388(2):117-27.
16. Impact of diabetes on the effects of sodium glucose co-transporter-2 inhibitors on kidney outcomes: collaborative meta-analysis of large placebo-controlled trials. Lancet. 2022;400(10365):1788-801.
17. Pitt B, Filippatos G, Agarwal R, et al. Cardiovascular events with finerenone in kidney disease and type 2 diabetes. N Engl J Med. 2021;385(24):2252-63.
18. Bakris GL, Agarwal R, Anker SD, et al. Effect of finerenone on chronic kidney disease outcomes in type 2 diabetes. N Engl J Med. 2020;383(23):2219-29.

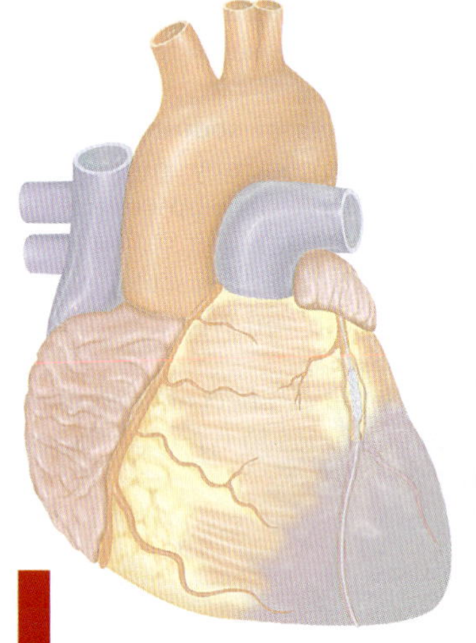

Advances in Optimizing HFpEF Management

Santanu Guha, Debopom Goswami

INTRODUCTION

Heart failure can be classified into: (1) *Heart failure with reduced ejection fraction (HFrEF):* Left ventricular ejection fraction (LVEF) ≤40%; (2) *HF with mildly reduced ejection fraction:* LVEF 41–49%; (3) *Heart failure with preserved ejection fraction (HFpEF):* LVEF ≥50%; and (4) *HF with improved ejection fraction:* Baseline LVEF ≤40%, LVEF increase ≥LVEF >40% at the second measurement. Despite the availability of evidence-based pharmacological treatments, the management of HFpEF remains challenging. From a hemodynamic perspective, a hallmark of this syndrome is a pulmonary capillary wedge pressure of ≥15 mm Hg (at rest) or ≥25 mm Hg (after exercise), or LV end-diastolic pressure ≥16 mm Hg (at rest).

EPIDEMIOLOGY

Multiple community-based studies performed in vast populations across United States and Europe have showed that HFpEF accounts for close to 50% of patients presenting with HF. As per the Trivandrum Heart Failure Registry[1] and Asian-HF, among the heart failure patients, HFpEF comprises only 19–25%. In developing countries like India many cases can go undiagnosed. The mean age of detection of HFpEF subset in India is also 10 years younger than the data reported from the west. Globally the prevalence of HFpEF is on the rise, a phenomenon related to aging of the population.

PHENOTYPES OF HEART FAILURE WITH PRESERVED EJECTION FRACTION

The HFpEF patients have varying presentations and clinical trajectories which prompted cardiologists to use artificial intelligence and machine learning techniques in categorizing patients based on pathophysiologic phenotypes. This strategy helps in providing more targeted and efficacious therapies.

More recently, Uijil et al.[2] proposed a model consisting of five clusters obtained from HFpEF patients.

1. The first cluster is that of young patients (<60 years) and a reduced burden of comorbidities.
2. The second cluster is the most represented and consists of patients with an average age of 77 years who have AF, without diabetes.
3. The third cluster consists of the oldest patients, with an average age of 88 years, the highest burden of comorbidities and the highest concentration of natriuretic peptides (NPs). These patients present with frank congestion, which must be attenuated using diuretics, including antialdosterone agents.
4. The fourth cluster consists of patients with an average age of 71 years, AF, and diabetes. In this group of patients, in addition to glycemic control, the introduction of an SGLT2 inhibitor appears to be beneficial.
5. The fifth cluster is the fusion of the second and fourth clusters because it includes elderly patients with an average age of 82 years, diabetes and AF.

Flowchart 1: Pathophysiology.

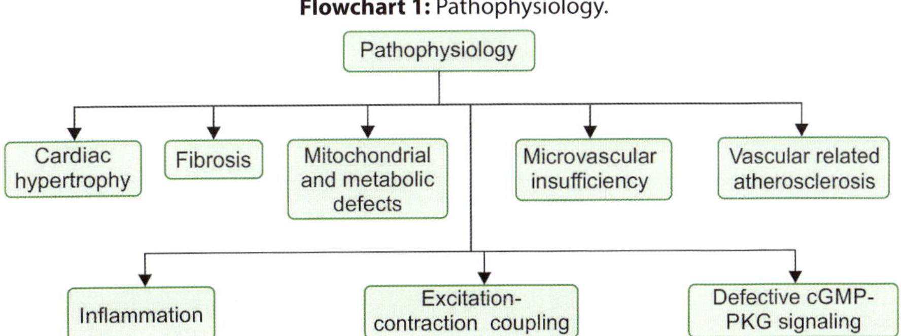

PATHOPHYSIOLOGY

The HFpEF usually affects older women with comorbidities such as anemia, metabolic syndrome, hypertension, and diabetes. The underlying interactions contribute to the complexity of the pathogenesis of HFpEF and at least partially contribute to the lack of effective therapies for HFpEF.

Numerous cellular and molecular abnormalities such as improper calcium handling, oxidative stress, cell death, inadequate angiogenesis, mitochondrial dysfunction, and myocardial interstitial fibrosis result in cardiac hypertrophy—the common phenotypic characteristic in HFpEF which results in diastolic dysfunction. Extracardiac abnormalities such as vascular-related atherosclerosis and decreased vascular responsiveness to nitric oxide have also been shown to contribute to the pathophysiology of HFpEF **(Flowchart 1)**.

DIAGNOSIS[3]

Refer to **Flowchart 2**.

TREATMENT OF HEART FAILURE WITH PRESERVED EJECTION FRACTION

General Considerations

As signs and symptoms of HFpEF are nonspecific, before diagnosing a patient to have HFpEF, it is important to recognize that there are several differential diagnoses which need to be ruled out.

EXCLUSION OF OTHER CAUSES OF SIGNS/SYMPTOMS

Refer to **Table 1**.

OPTIMIZING MANAGEMENT OF COMORBIDITIES

Cardiovascular and noncardiovascular comorbidities are common in patients with HFpEF, and are responsible for the burden of morbidity and mortality in this population. Comorbidities such as obesity, hypertension, diabetes, COPD, and chronic kidney disease contribute in the pathophysiology of HFpEF and accelerate disease progression. A systematic evaluation of these comorbidities is essential in planning out the therapeutic strategy **(Table 2)**.

PHARMACOLOGICAL MANAGEMENT

Diuretics

Although all patients with HFpEF are not congested at rest, signs and symptoms of volume overload are frequently present in HFpEF. Use of diuretics for symptomatic relief of fluid retention in chronic HFpEF is well-established. Loop diuretics, conventionally furosemide, are the drugs of choice. Loop diuretics are the backbone of acute fluid overload management, and when initially ineffective there is preference for initial dose up-titration over combination diuresis strategies. With regard to the choice of loop diuretics, the results of the TRANSFORM-HF[4] trial did not suggest a difference between furosemide and torsemide with regard to all-cause mortality or all-cause hospitalization among HFpEF patients discharged after hospitalization for HF.

- In refractory edema, addition of a thiazide or thiazide-like diuretic such as metolazone can be considered to maximize diuretic synergy through sequential nephron blockade.
- Adjunctive tolvaptan was another option provided by various guidelines.
- Addition of acetazolamide alongside loop diuretics has recently been shown to increase incidence of successful decongestion across the LVEF spectrum.

Flowchart 2: Diagnosis.

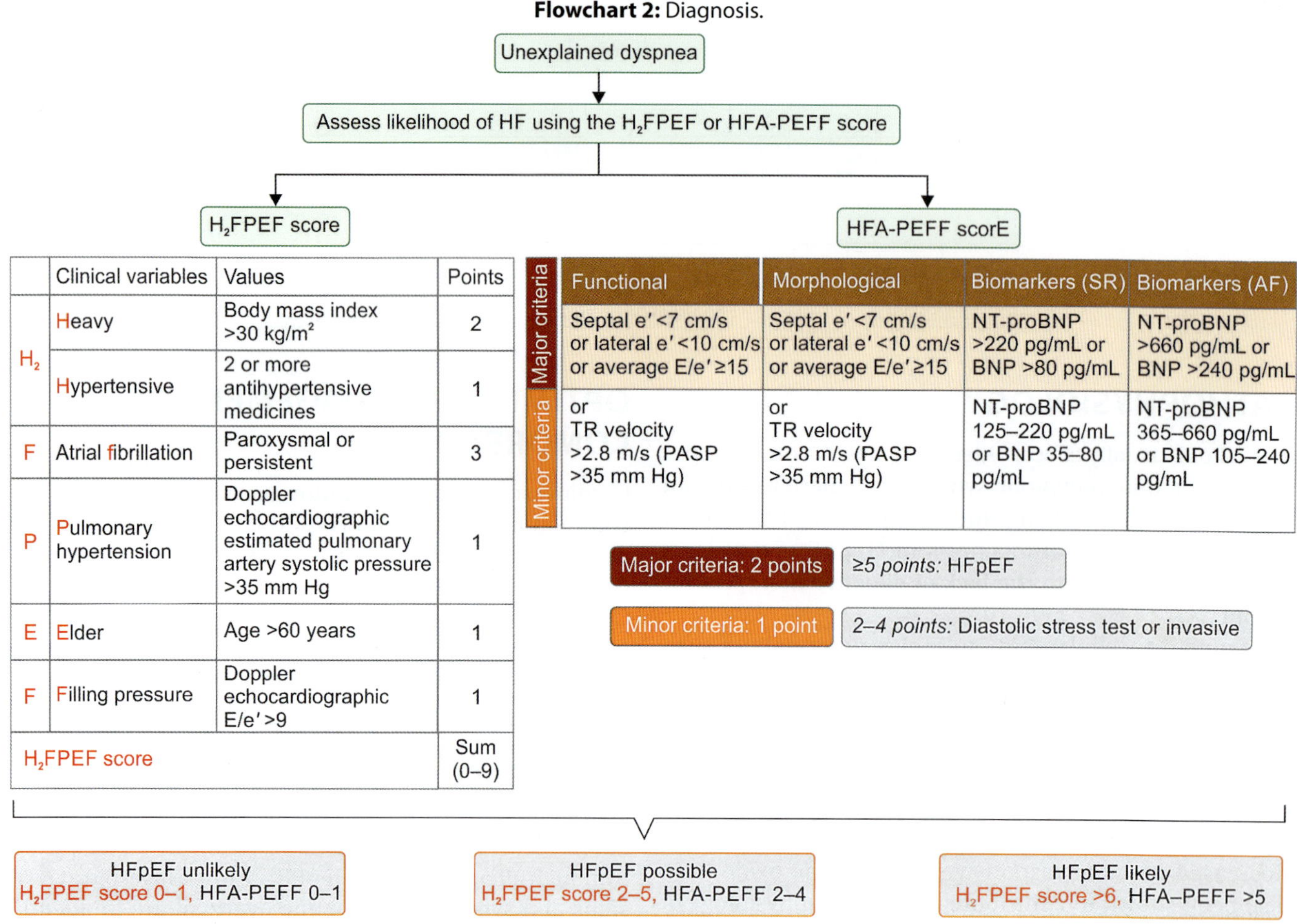

	Clinical variables	Values	Points
H_2	Heavy	Body mass index >30 kg/m^2	2
	Hypertensive	2 or more antihypertensive medicines	1
F	Atrial fibrillation	Paroxysmal or persistent	3
P	Pulmonary hypertension	Doppler echocardiographic estimated pulmonary artery systolic pressure >35 mm Hg	1
E	Elder	Age >60 years	1
F	Filling pressure	Doppler echocardiographic E/e′>9	1
H_2FPEF score			Sum (0–9)

	Functional	Morphological	Biomarkers (SR)	Biomarkers (AF)
Major criteria	Septal e′<7 cm/s or lateral e′<10 cm/s or average E/e′≥15	Septal e′<7 cm/s or lateral e′<10 cm/s or average E/e′≥15	NT-proBNP >220 pg/mL or BNP >80 pg/mL	NT-proBNP >660 pg/mL or BNP >240 pg/mL
Minor criteria	or TR velocity >2.8 m/s (PASP >35 mm Hg)	or TR velocity >2.8 m/s (PASP >35 mm Hg)	NT-proBNP 125–220 pg/mL or BNP 35–80 pg/mL	NT-proBNP 365–660 pg/mL or BNP 105–240 pg/mL

Sodium-glucose Cotransporter-2 and Sodium-glucose Cotransporter-1 Inhibitors

In HFpEF, SGLT2 inhibitors act via multiple mechanism:

- Cause improvements in blood sugar, blood pressure, and attenuation of kidney disease progression.
- Induce a nutrient-deprivation and hypoxic-like transcriptional paradigm, with increased ketosis, erythropoietin, and autophagic flux in addition to altering iron homeostasis.
- Reduce epicardial adipose tissue and alter adipokine signaling.
- Impact cardiomyocyte ionic homeostasis.
- Reduce myofilament stiffness as well as extracellular matrix remodeling/fibrosis in the heart, improving diastolic function.

In the EMPEROR-Preserved trial,[5] 5,988 patients with chronic HF, LVEF >40%, NYHA functional class II–IV HF symptoms, and elevated NPs were randomly assigned to treatment with empagliflozin or placebo. Patients assigned to empagliflozin experienced a 21% reduction in rates of the primary composite outcome of cardiovascular death or HF [*HR:* 0.79 (95% CI: 0.69–0.90)]; $p < 0.001$. Based on these data the 2022 American College of Cardiology (ACC)/American Heart Association (AHA) guidelines now suggest that use of SGLT2 inhibitors o treat patients with HF and LVEF >50% is reasonable.

More recently, in the DELIVER trial,[6] 6,263 patients with chronic HF, LVEF >40%, NYHA functional class II–IV HF symptoms, and evidence of structural heart disease by echocardiography were randomized to treatment with dapagliflozin. Patients assigned to dapagliflozin experienced an 18% reduction in the primary composite outcome with a significant reduction of 21% in worsening HF events.

The SOLOIST-WHF trial[7] of sotagliflozin, a composite SGLT1/2 inhibitor, highlights that treatment benefits are robust in higher-risk HFpEF patients initiated on treatment during HF hospitalization or early after hospital discharge,

TABLE 1: Exclusion of other causes of signs/symptoms.

Etiology	*Diagnostic tools*	*Management*
Cardiac amyloidosis	Monoclonal proteins, radionuclide scintigraphy, biopsy	Tafamidis (for transthyretin amyloidosis) or chemotherapy (for light-chain amyloidosis); avoid neurohormonal antagonists
Hypertrophic cardiomyopathy	Echocardiography, cardiac MRI	Beta blockers, calcium channel blockers, or septal reduction therapies (for obstructive cardiomyopathy); avoid vasodilators
Cardiac sarcoidosis	Cardiac MRI, FDG-PET, biopsy	Immunosuppressive agents
Constrictive pericarditis	Echocardiography, cardiac MRI or CT imaging, invasive hemodynamic measurements	Pericardiectomy
Valvular heart disease	Echocardiography, invasive hemodynamic measurements with ventriculography	Surgical or percutaneous valve interventions
Coronary artery disease	Invasive coronary angiography, stress imaging or CT imaging	Revascularization, aspirin, statins, beta blockers, and nitrates
High-output heart failure	Evaluate for arteriovenous shunts and liver disease	Treatments directed at the cause of high cardiac output (such as fistula ligation for shunts, liver transplantation for cirrhosis)
Myocarditis	Cardiac MRI, endomyocardial biopsy	Immunosuppressive agents for some types (such as giant cell myocarditis or eosinophilic myocarditis)

(CT: computed tomography; FDG-PET: fluorodeoxyglucose-positron emission tomography; MRI: magnetic resonance imaging)

supporting the rationale for predischarge initiation of these agents in eligible patients.

Collectively, these data support the efficacy of SGLT2 inhibitors as a treatment for HFpEF.

TABLE 2: Management of comorbidities.

Conditions	*Recommended strategies*
Hypertension	Management of BP to guideline-recommended targets, typically <130/80 mm Hg
Diabetes	• Prioritize SGLT2 inhibitors (as in all patients) • ACE inhibitor/ARB for CKD/proteinuria • Finerenone for ongoing proteinuria despite ACE inhibitor
Obesity	Routine recommendation for calorie restriction, aerobic exercise training • Screening and treatment of obstructive sleep apnea • Consider GLP-1 agonists, tirzepatide, bariatric surgery
Chronic kidney disease	• ACE inhibitor/ARB for proteinuria; SGLT2 inhibitors • Finerenone (if diabetes and ongoing proteinuria despite ACE inhibitor/ARB)
Coronary artery disease	• Antiplatelet therapy • Moderate-high intensity statin therapy for those with elevated LDL • Revascularization for patients with angina or ischemia on provocative testing
Atrial fibrillation	• Anticoagulation for stroke prophylaxis • Consider trial of rhythm control
Chronotropic incompetence	Avoid routine use of β-blockers in absence of compelling indication

(ACE: angiotensin-converting enzyme; ARB: angiotensin-receptor blocker; BP: blood pressure; CKD: chronic kidney disease; GLP-1: Glucagon-like peptide-1; LDL: low-density lipoprotein; SGLT2: sodium-glucose cotransporter-2)

Glucagon-like Peptide-1 Receptor Antagonists

The relationship between elevated BMI and risk of incident heart failure has been well described: Studies have suggested that each progressive 1-point increase in BMI above normal is associated with 5–7% increase in incident HF. Up to two-thirds of patients with HFpEF are overweight or have obesity. Currently, use of emerging antiobesity medications which support intentional weight loss may improve heart failure status.

GLP-1 receptor antagonists are emerging as a new pillar in the management of HFpEF patients. Several trials have been conducted recently in HFpEF patients.

The recently published STEP-HFpEF[8] and STEP-HFpEF DM trials concluded that semaglutide treatment resulted in fewer symptoms, improved exercise function, and increased weight loss compared with placebo.

However, the effect of semaglutide on HF hospitalization or mortality was only investigated as a composite secondary endpoint. Furthermore, these trials predate the advent of SGLT2 inhibitors as key therapeutics, and the effects of combination therapy remains unknown.

The SUMMIT trial[9] included 731 patients with obesity and HFpEF. They were randomized to receive tirzepatide up to 15 mg subcutaneously weekly or placebo. There were fewer worsening HF events in the tirzepatide group with no difference in cardiovascular death.

Among patients with established HFpEF, obesity is associated with poor quality of life, higher symptom burden, and greater risk of heart failure hospitalization. Emerging antiobesity medications may offer an opportunity to reduce the burden of heart failure symptoms with obesity.

Neurohormonal Antagonism

In HFpEF, renin-angiotensin-aldosterone system (RAAS) inhibition acts via the following mechanism:

- Lowering blood pressure
- Improvement of diastolic function, and
- Reduction of myocardial fibrosis

There is reduced activation of the renin-angiotensin system in HFpEF patients, which might account for the limited therapeutic success of these agents.

Three large-scale randomized clinical trials tested the safety and efficacy of angiotensin-converting enzyme inhibitors in HFpEF. Two of them, the CHARM-Preserved and the I-PRESERVE used an angiotensin receptor blocker (ARB), the PEP-CHF trial used an angiotensin-converting enzyme inhibitor.

- CHARM-preserved[10] included patients with LVEF >40%, New York Heart Association (NYHA) class II–IV and previous hospital admission for HF. The primary outcome of composite CV death and HF admission was not met [HR 0.89; (95% CI 0.77–1.03); $p = 0.118$]. Based on this evidence, the 2022 American Heart Association/American College of Cardiology/Heart Failure Society of America guidelines give a class 2b recommendation for ARB use with the aim of reducing HF hospitalization, especially in the lower end of the LVEF.
- The I-PRESERVE trial[11] did not show a benefit comparing irbesartan to placebo in patients with HF and an LVEF above 45%. The primary outcome of all-cause death or cardiovascular hospitalization was similar between treatment groups (HR 0.95, 95% CI 0.86–1.05; $p = 0.35$).
- PEP-CHF trial[12] which compared ACE inhibitor perindopril with placebo, included 850 patients with HF and LVEF >45%. The hazard ratio for the primary endpoint, a composite of all-cause mortality and unplanned HF hospitalization was 0.92.

Sacubitril/valsartan comprises of the ARB valsartan and sacubitril, a prodrug neprilysin inhibitor. Neprilysin is responsible for breaking down vasoactive peptides, ANP, BNP, and CNP; adrenomedullin; endothelin; and angiotensin II; pairing both a neprilysin inhibitor with an ARB, blocks the RAS, and augments the endogenous vasoactive peptide system. Two clinical trials the PARAGON-HF trial and the PARAGLIDE trial have tested the safety and efficacy of ARNI in HFpEF.

The PARAGON-HF[13] trial randomized 4,822 patients with NYHA class II–IV, EF >45%, elevated NP and structural heart disease to valsartan alone or sacubitril/valsartan. The primary endpoint was a composite of total HF hospitalization or CV death. Among patients with HFpEF, sacubitril valsartan was not effective at reducing the incidence of cardiovascular death or hospitalization for heart failure compared to valsartan.

Recently, the PARAGLIDE study[14] randomized 466 patients with LVEF >40% and a recent event of worsening heart failure to sacubitril/valsartan versus valsartan. The primary endpoint of N-terminal fraction of pro-BNP reduction was greater in the sacubitril/valsartan group ($p = 0.0049$), and was associated with clinical benefit as reduced worsening renal failure compared with valsartan alone, despite a more symptomatic hypotension.

Mineralocorticoid Receptor Antagonists

Two large, multicenter, randomized, double-blind, placebo-controlled clinical trial and other smaller studies have tested the efficacy and safety of MRA in HFpEF.

The TOPCAT trial[15] enrolled patients with at least one sign or symptom of HF and LVEF >45%, history of HF hospitalization in the previous 12 months or NP level. The primary outcome of a composite CV death and HF hospitalization was neutral.

Finearts-HF trial[16] randomized 6,001 patients with HF and a LVEF of 40% or greater to receive finerenone at a maximum dose of 20 mg or 40 mg once daily ($n = 3{,}003$) or matching placebo ($n = 2{,}998$), in addition to usual therapy. The primary outcome was a composite of total worsening HF events or death from cardiovascular causes over a medium of follow-up of 32 months. Overall results showed that finerenone resulted in a significantly lower rate of composite of total worsening HF events and death from cardiovascular causes than placebo. Researchers noted that finerenone was associated with an increased risk of hyperkalemia and a reduced risk of hypokalemia.

The 2022 American Heart Association/American College of Cardiology/Heart Failure Society of America guidelines give a class 2b recommendation for MRA use, with the aim of reducing HF hospitalization, especially in the lower LVEF range.

However, the European guidelines do not mention MRA for HFpEF.

β-blockers

While β-blockers are considered the cornerstone of treatment for HFrEF the same may not apply to patients with HFpEF. A meta-analysis performed on 13,189 records showed that β-blocker therapy has the potential to reduce all-cause mortality in patients with HFpEF based on observational studies. Nevertheless, it did not affect rehospitalization for heart failure or it is composite with all-cause mortality. Large scale randomized trials are needed to clarify this uncertainty.

NONPHARMACOLOGICAL MANAGEMENT[17]

Nonpharmacological approaches encompass a diverse array of techniques, ranging from physical therapies and invasive procedures to targeted treatments for comorbidities. The exploration and development of these innovative strategies have the potential to significantly advance patient care for those with HFpEF and contribute to a better understanding of the condition's complex nature. In the following sections, we will discuss various nonpharmacological management approaches, highlighting their potential benefits and applications in the treatment of HFpEF.

Vagal Nerve Stimulation (Flowchart 3)

Vagal nerve stimulation (VNS) is a neuromodulation technique that regulates the functional activity of the vagus nerve via chronic microcurrent stimulation. The ANTHEM-HFpEF study demonstrates that autonomic regulation therapy, through cervical VNS, is safe and improves symptoms, exercise tolerance, autonomic function, and cardiac electrical stability in patients with heart failure with preserved or mildly reduced ejection fraction without changing mechanical cardiac functions.

Low-intensity Pulsed Ultrasound (Flowchart 4)

The LIPUS improves myocardial calcium-related protein processing by stimulating the eNOS-NO-cGMP-PKG signaling pathway, which in turn modulates myocardial diastolic function and facilitates HFpEF treatment and recovery.

Transcatheter Interatrial Shunt Device (Fig. 1)

One of the key hemodynamic features of HFpEF is elevated left atrial and pulmonary venous pressure at rest or on exertion, resulting in dyspnea and reduced exercise capacity. A transcatheter-implanted interatrial shunt device has been developed with the aim of opening an 8 mm large left-to-right atrial shunt and unloading left atrium.

The REDUCE LAP-HF I trial, a phase II clinical trial, demonstrated a greater reduction of exercise pulmonary capillary wedge pressure in patients on active treatment compared with patients treated with a sham procedure.

Another trial REDUCE LAP-HF II, was then conducted to test if the results could translate into CV death, nonfatal ischemic stroke and HF events reduction, or change in QoL measured by the Kansas City Cardiomyopathy Questionnaire overall summary score. The overall population results were neutral.

The RELIEVE-HF trial is a prospective, multicenter, randomized, double-blind, and sham-controlled trial.

Flowchart 3: Vagal nerve stimulation.

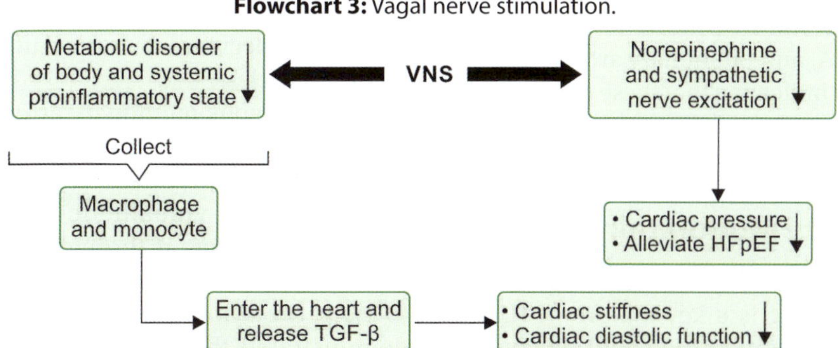

(HFpEF: heart failure with preserved ejection fraction; TGF-β: transforming growth factor beta; VNS: vagal nerve stimulation)

Flowchart 4: Low-intensity pulsed ultrasound (LIPUS).

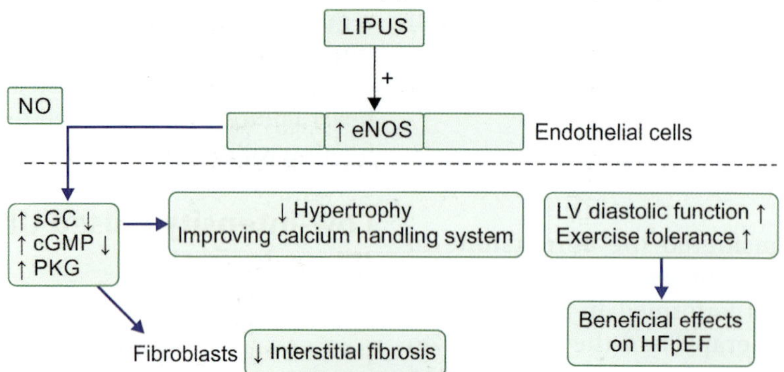

(cGMP: cyclic guanosine 3', 5'-monophosphate; HFpEF: heart failure with preserved ejection fraction; LV: left ventricular; PKG: protein Kinase G; sGC: soluble guanylate cyclase)

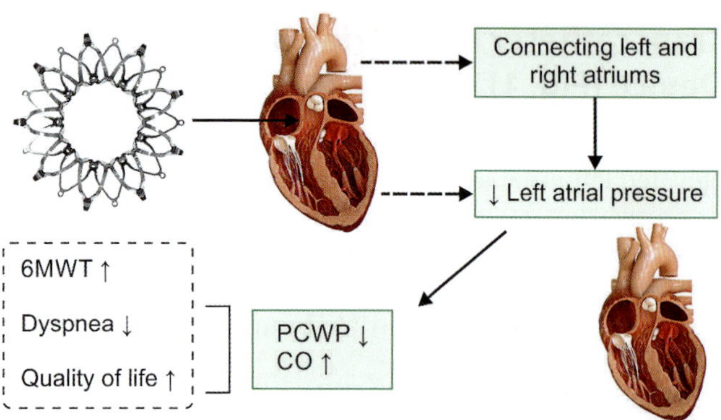

Fig. 1: Transcatheter interatrial shunt device. (CO: cardiac output; 6MWT: 6-minute walk test; PCWP: pulmonary capillary wedge pressure)

Patients with symptomatic HF with any LVEF were randomized 1:1 to transcatheter shunt implantation versus a placebo procedure, stratified by reduced (≤40%) versus preserved (>40%) LVEF. Transcatheter interatrial shunt implantation was safe but did not improve outcomes in patients with HF. However, the results from a prespecified exploratory analysis in stratified randomized groups suggest that shunt implantation is beneficial in patients with reduced LVEF and harmful in patients with preserved LVEF. The RELIEVE HF roll-in cohorts for HFpEF had poorer TAPSE, higher RA, and pulmonary artery pressure, and lower cardiac index indicating that these patients have more severe hemodynamic impairments which might explain why the IAS could be harmful in this subgroup.

Cardiac Contractility Modulation

Abnormal myocardial contractility, and pathological atrial and ventricular remodeling is a key feature of HFpEF. Nowadays, a new therapeutic option could be counted in this contest, cardiac contractility modulation (CCM). CCM is a new device acting through myocytes stimulation during the absolute refractory period of the action potential, leading to an increase in peak calcium concentration and inducing positive inotropism.

Renal Denervation and Pulmonary Artery Denervation

Renal denervation (RDN) is a technique that:

- Blocks the signaling between the central sympathetic nervous system and the kidney,
- Inhibits the activity of the RAAS,
- Suppresses the overactivation of the systemic sympathetic nervous system, and
- Reduces sympathetic activity by radiofrequency ablation of sympathetic fibers distributed in the vascular wall of the renal artery through a skin catheter.

Patients with HFpEF predominantly exhibit arterial stiffness, reduced aortic distensibility, increased pulse pressure, and increased pulse wave velocity. These are mediated either through elevated sympathetic nerve activity. So, reduction of sympathetic activity, improving vascular stiffness, and improving LV function are promising strategies to treat HFpEF. RDN reduces the sympathetic activity and regulates the RAAS system resulting in decrease in aortic stiffness and normalization of the ventricles.

Percutaneous pulmonary artery denervation (PADN) is a new technique that improves arterial pressure and promotes the function of the vascular system by damaging the sympathetic nerve of the pulmonary artery and altering it through radiofrequency ablation, ultrasound catheter denervation, and open-heart surgery to strip the sympathetic nerve. It has been clinically demonstrated that elevated circulatory catecholamine levels and impaired heart rate variability in patients with

HF with PAH are associated with excessive neurohumoral activation, suggesting that precapillary and postcapillary pulmonary hypertension may be treated with local denervation. Additionally, in the study, it was found that treatment with PADN significantly increased the 6-minute walk test. The precise mechanisms by which PADN exerts its therapeutic effects in the context of HFpEF remain to be fully elucidated.

Pericardial Resection

In HFpEF, diverse etiologies contribute to a spectrum of pathophysiological changes. These changes include myocardial hypertrophy, pulmonary hypertension, and diastolic dysfunction. Pericardial resection, by alleviating ventricular compression, may reduce elevated end-diastolic ventricular filling pressures. Such a reduction has the potential to mitigate the consequences of these pressures, such as pulmonary venous congestion, which can lead to symptoms like dyspnea, as well as complications including atrial fibrillation and compromised right ventricular function.

CONCLUSION

Several pharmacologic therapies and diagnostic devices are currently being tested in large trials in patients with HFpEF. More trials examining novel treatments such as antifibrotic, anti-inflammatory, and antioxidant agents, as well as cell therapies, are underway.

REFERENCES

1. Harikrishnan S, Sanjay G, Anees T, et al.; Trivandrum Heart Failure Registry. Clinical presentation, management, in-hospital and 90-day outcomes of heart failure patients in Trivandrum, Kerala, India: the Trivandrum Heart Failure Registry. Eur J Heart Fail. 2015;17(8):794-800.
2. Uijl A, Savarese G, Vaartjes I, et al. Identification of distinct phenotypic clusters in heart failure with preserved ejection fraction. Eur J Heart Fail. 2021;23(6):973-82.
3. Burkert Pieske, Carsten Tschöpe, Rudolf A de Boer, et al. How to diagnose heart failure with preserved ejection fraction: the HFA–PEFF diagnostic algorithm: a consensus recommendation from the Heart Failure Association (HFA) of the European Society of Cardiology (ESC). Eur Heart J. 2019;40(40):3297-317.
4. Mentz RJ, Anstrom KJ, Eisenstein EL, et al. Effect of Torsemide vs Furosemide After Discharge on All-Cause Mortality in Patients Hospitalized With Heart Failure: The TRANSFORM-HF Randomized Clinical Trial. JAMA. 2023;329(3):214-23.
5. Anker SD, Butler J, Filippatos G, et al.; EMPEROR-Preserved Trial Investigators. Empagliflozin in Heart Failure with a Preserved Ejection Fraction. N Engl J Med. 2021;385(16):1451-61.
6. Solomon SD, McMurray JJV, Claggett B, et al.; DELIVER Trial Committees and Investigators. Dapagliflozin in Heart Failure with Mildly Reduced or Preserved Ejection Fraction. N Engl J Med. 2022;387(12):1089-98.
7. Bhatt DL, Szarek M, Steg PG, et al.; SOLOIST-WHF Trial Investigators. Sotagliflozin in Patients with Diabetes and Recent Worsening Heart Failure. N Engl J Med. 2021;384(2):117-28.
8. Kosiborod MN, Abildstrøm SZ, Borlaug BA, et al.; STEP-HFpEF Trial Committees and Investigators. Semaglutide in Patients with Heart Failure with Preserved Ejection Fraction and Obesity. N Engl J Med. 2023;389(12):1069-84.
9. Packer M, Zile MR, Kramer CM, et al.; SUMMIT Trial Study Group. Tirzepatide for Heart Failure with Preserved Ejection Fraction and Obesity. N Engl J Med. 2024.
10. Yusuf S, Pfeffer MA, Swedberg K, et al.; CHARM Investigators and Committees. Effects of candesartan in patients with chronic heart failure and preserved left-ventricular ejection fraction: the CHARM-Preserved Trial. Lancet. 2003;362(9386):777-81.
11. Massie BM, Carson PE, McMurray JJ, et al.; I-PRESERVE Investigators. Irbesartan in patients with heart failure and preserved ejection fraction. N Engl J Med. 2008;359(23):2456-67.
12. Cleland JG, Tendera M, Adamus J, et al.; PEP-CHF Investigators. The perindopril in elderly people with chronic heart failure (PEP-CHF) study. Eur Heart J. 2006;27(19):2338-45.
13. Solomon SD, McMurray JJV, Anand IS, et al.; PARAGON-HF Investigators and Committees. Angiotensin-Neprilysin Inhibition in Heart Failure with Preserved Ejection Fraction. N Engl J Med. 2019;381(17):1609-20.
14. Mentz RJ, Ward JH, Hernandez AF, et al. Rationale, Design and Baseline Characteristics of the PARAGLIDE-HF Trial: Sacubitril/Valsartan vs Valsartan in HFmrEF and HFpEF With a Worsening Heart Failure Event. J Card Fail. 2023;29(6):922-30.
15. Pitt B, Pfeffer MA, Assmann SF, et al.; TOPCAT Investigators. Spironolactone for heart failure with preserved ejection fraction. N Engl J Med. 2014;370(15):1383-92.
16. Solomon SD, McMurray JJV, Vaduganathan M, et al.; FINEARTS-HF Committees and Investigators. Finerenone in Heart Failure with Mildly Reduced or Preserved Ejection Fraction. N Engl J Med. 2024;391(16):1475-85.
17. Tang F, Han H, Fu S, et al. Nonpharmacological approaches to managing heart failure with preserved ejection fraction. Circ Heart Fail. 2024;17(8):e011269.

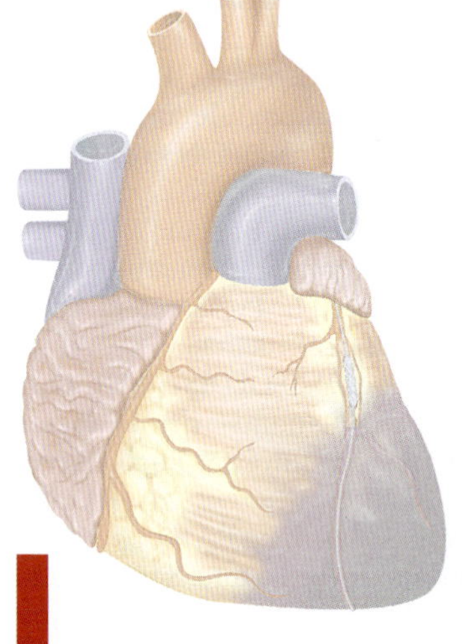

HFpEF Management: Recent Strategies

PC Manoria

INTRODUCTION

Heart failure with preserved ejection fraction (HFpEF) is a complex condition in which, besides LV diastolic dysfunction, comorbidities play a vital role in its outcome. If structural heart disease, heart failure (HF) symptoms, and evidence of diastolic dysfunction on echocardiography at rest or on a diastolic stress test are present, HFpEF is diagnosed. Biomarkers are less elevated in HFpEF than in heart failure with reduced ejection fraction (HFrEF). Besides diuretics, sodium-glucose cotransporter-2 (SGLT2) inhibitors now also have class-I recommendations. Glucagon-like peptide-1 receptor agonists (GLP-1 RA) semaglutide, recently in two trials, has shown benefit in the obese phenotype of HFpEF. Nonsteroidal mineralocorticoid receptor antagonist (MRA) finerenone has shown positive results in the FINE ARTS trial. Device therapy is still in the process of evolution.

Heart failure with preserved ejection fraction is a complex condition characterized by symptoms and signs of HF despite a normal or near-normal left ventricular ejection fraction (LVEF) of 50% or higher.[1] HFpEF is increasingly recognized as a multiorgan, systemic syndrome rather than just a result of left ventricular diastolic dysfunction. This produces elevated left atrial (LA) and ventricular filling pressures, leading to exertional dyspnea and other symptoms.

DIAGNOSIS OF HEART FAILURE WITH PRESERVED EJECTION FRACTION

The diagnosis of HFpEF is made by:

- *Presence of structural heart disease:* Left ventricular hypertrophy (LVH), left atrial enlargement (LAE).
- *Signs and symptoms of heart failure:* Systemic or pulmonary congestion.
- *Elevated serum markers:* A BNP level of >35 pg/mL in patients with sinus rhythm (SR), >100 in patients with acute heart failure (AHF) or >105 in patients with atrial fibrillation (AF). NT-proBNP levels >125 pg/mL in patients with SR, >300 in patients with AHF, and >365 in patients with AF.
- Documentation of diastolic dysfunction on the Echo Doppler at rest or on exercise if the resting parameter is equivocal. The following parameters are utilized to diagnose diastolic dysfunction, as shown in **Flowchart 1**.

Currently, the LA strain has also been used for assessment of LV diastolic function.[2] The current algorithm for diastolic dysfunction is outlined in **Flowchart 2**.

The comprehensive diagnosis of HFpEF by echocardiography is outlined in **Figure 1**.

TREATMENT OF HEART FAILURE WITH PRESERVED EJECTION FRACTION

The treatment of HFpEF revolves around drugs, treatment of etiology, and comorbidities. Device therapy is also being

Flowchart 1: Parameters for assessing diastolic dysfunction.

Diagnosis of Diastolic dysfunction in patients with normal systolic function

1. Average E/e′ >14
2. Septal e′ velocity <7 cm/s or Lateral e′ velocity <10 cm/s
3. TR velocity >2.8 m/s
4. LA volume index >34 mL/m²

0 or 1 positive → Normal diastolic function

2 positive → Indeterminate

3 or 4 positive → Diastolic dysfunction

Flowchart 2: Current algorithm for diastolic dysfunction.

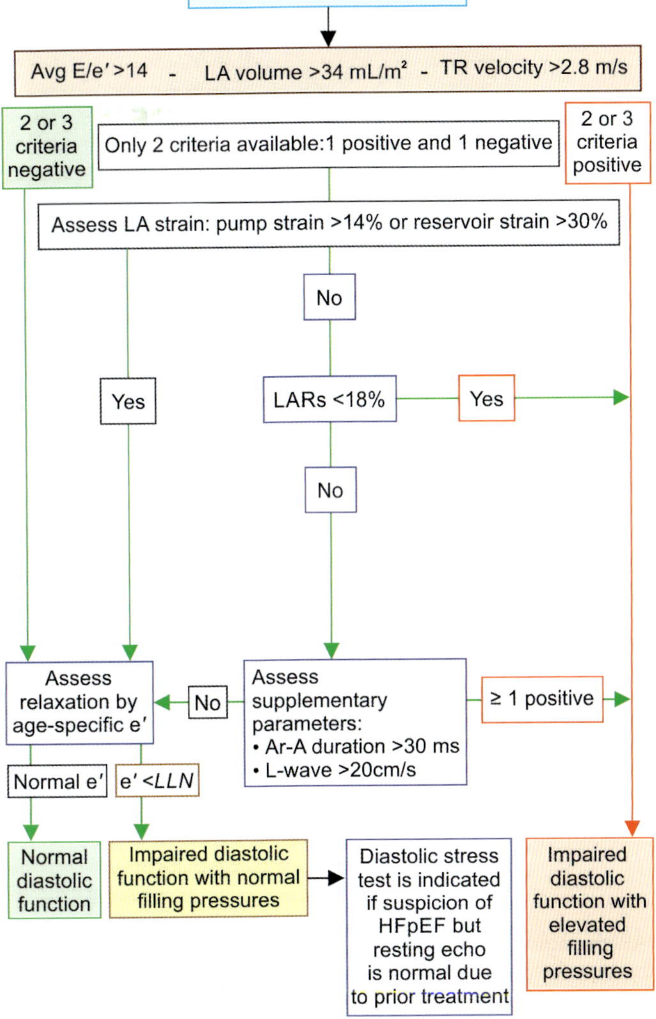

(HFpEF: Heart failure with preserved ejection fraction; LARs: left atrial reservoir strain LA: left atrial; LV: left ventricular; TR: tricuspid regurgitation)

evaluated for the treatment of HFpEF. The drug treatment for HFpEF is outlined in **Table 1**.

Diuretics are a class 1A recommendation for decreasing fluid retention and providing symptomatic relief. SGLT2 inhibitors, dapagliflozin, and empagliflozin, are also class 1 recommendations. Empagliflozin was approved after the positive EMPA preserved trial (2021)[3] and DAPA was approved after the DELIVER trial[4] (2022). Both of these trials have shown a statistically significant reduction in the primary endpoint of a composite of hospitalization for HF and cardiovascular (CV) death. CV death was not decreased in either of the trials. Angiotensin receptor-neprilysin inhibitor (ARNI), after the PARAGON[5] trial, has been approved for the treatment of HFpEF with a weak class IIb recommendation and is beneficial near the normal limit of ejection fraction. MRAs are also given a weak IIB recommendation. Injectable semaglutide has shown positive results in two HFpEF trials[6-7] in the obese phenotype of HFpEF and is likely to be approved in the future for this particular subset. Finerenone has also shown positive results in the FINEARTS-HF trial[8] and will also be approved in the future for the treatment of HFpEF and will replace steroidal MRA. The current recommendations for drug treatment and comorbidities for HFpEF are outlined in **Flowchart 3**.

Comorbidities are common in HFpEF, and they must be specifically looked for and treated (Class I recommendation). The common comorbidities associated with HFpEF are outlined in **Box 1**.

DEVICE THERAPY

Device therapy has emerged as an alternative approach to address certain structural and neurohormonal abnormalities in patients with HFpEF that are not amenable to pharmacologic interventions.

Current device therapies being investigated for HFpEF include LA unloading (e.g., left-to-right atrial shunts), cardiac contractility modulation, autonomic modulation, and respiratory modulation such as phrenic nerve stimulation.

Elevated LA pressure is a common physiological perturbation in symptomatic HFpEF. Several interatrial septal devices (IASD) have been studied to reduce LA pressure at rest and during exertion to improve symptoms. Although preliminary studies showed promising hemodynamic results and improvements in functional capacity, recent sham-controlled, randomized REDUCE LAP-HF II[9] (Reducing Elevated Left Atrial Pressure in Patients With Heart Failure II) and the Corvia Atrial Shunt in HF with preserved or mildly reduced ejection fraction have not shown favorable results.

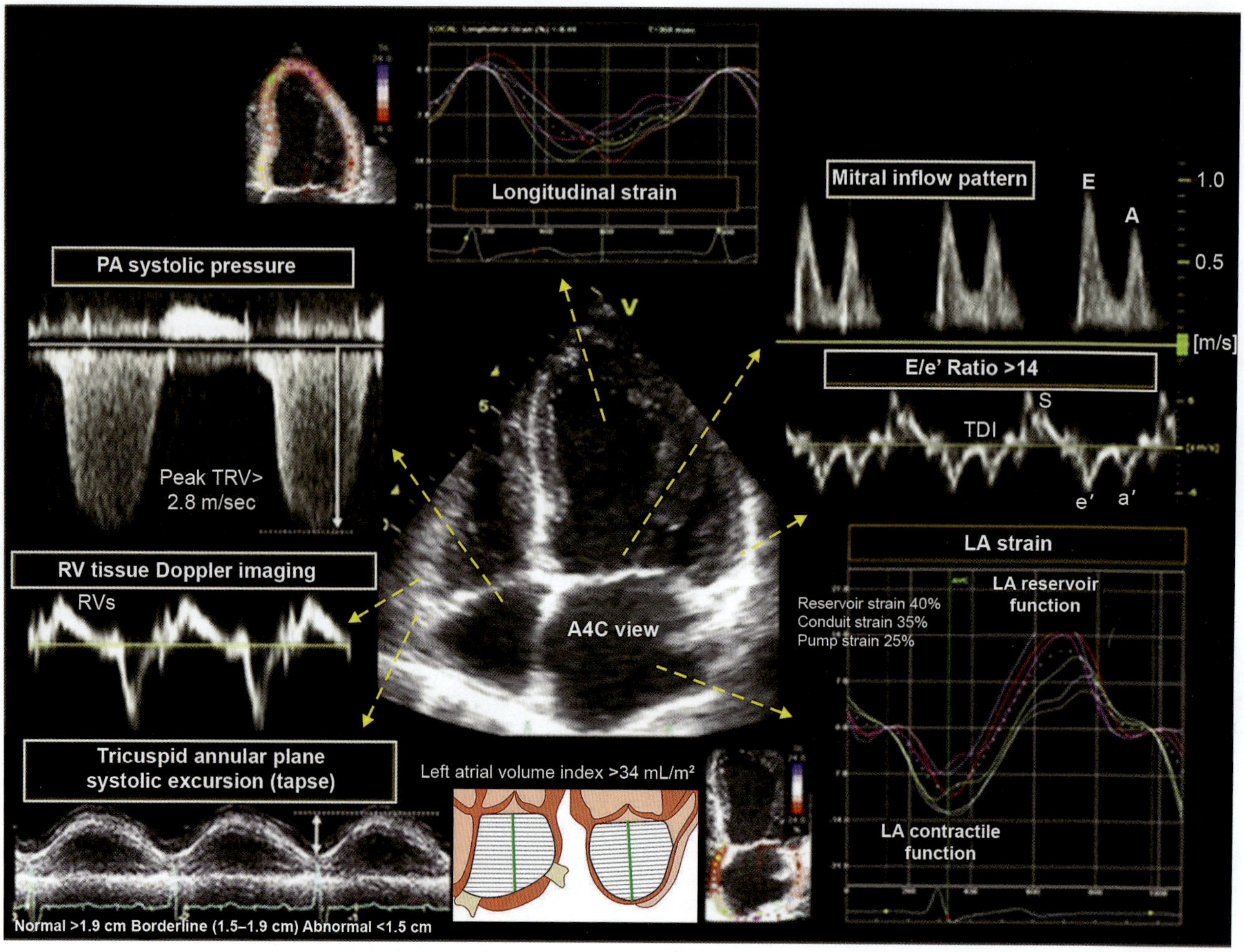

Fig. 1: Comprehensive echocardiographic evaluation of heart failure with preserved ejection fraction. (LA: left atrial; PA: pulmonary artery; RV: right ventricular)

TABLE 1: Drug treatment for heart failure.

S. No.	Drug	Level of recommendation
1	Diuretics	Class I
2	SGLT2 inhibitors	
	Empagliflozin	Class I
	Dapagliflozin	Class I
3	ARNI	Class IIb
4	MRAs	Class IIb
5	Nonsteroidal MRAs	Waiting for approval by Guidelines
6	Semaglutide	Waiting for approval by Guidelines

(ARNI: angiotensin receptor neprilysin inhibitor; MRA: mineralocorticoid receptor antagonist; SGLT2: sodium-glucose cotransporter-2)

Flowchart 3: Current recommendations for drug treatment and comorbidities for heart failure with preserved ejection fraction.

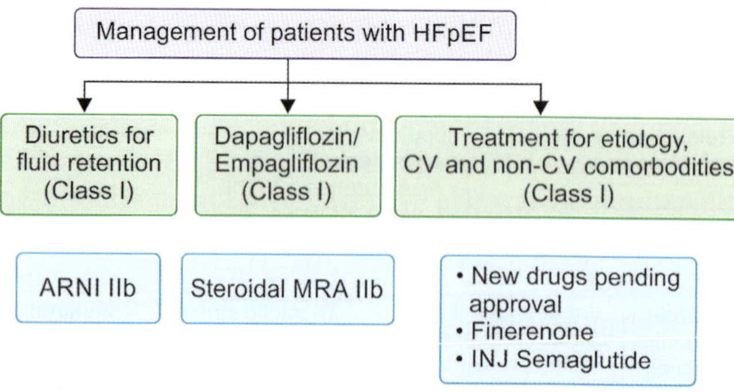

(ARNI: angiotensin receptor neprilysin inhibitor; HFpEF: Heart failure with preserved ejection fraction; MRA: mineralocorticoid receptor antagonist; SGLT2: sodium-glucose cotransporter-2)

The REDUCE LAP-HF II trial compared 309 patients with shunts and 312 patients in the sham control group. The primary endpoint, a composite of cardiovascular death, nonfatal ischemic/embolic stroke, total HF events, and change in health status, failed to show any statistically significant benefit, including its individual components. Major adverse cardiac events were more common in

BOX 1: Comorbidities in heart failure with preserved ejection fraction.

- Obesity
- Metabolic syndrome
- Type 2 diabetes
- Salt-sensitive hypertension
- Atrial fibrillation
- Chronic obstructive pulmonary disease
- Anemia
- Renal failure

patients assigned to shunt compared with the sham control group (6.9% vs. 2.7%; $p = 0.018$).

However, atrial shunt therapy showed potential efficacy in responders, i.e., no latent pulmonary vascular disease and no cardiac rhythm management device. Despite the challenges, IASD as a therapeutic strategy remains promising, and several ongoing studies will evaluate if certain patient phenotypes may benefit from this therapy.

The potential clinical benefit identified in the responder group after 1 and 2 years of follow-up is currently being evaluated in the RESPONDER-HF (Reevaluation of the Corvia Atrial Shunt Device in a Precision Medicine Trial to Determine Efficacy in Mildly Reduced or Preserved Ejection Fraction Heart Failure) trial and REDUCE LAP-HF II (Reducing Elevated Left Atrial Pressure in Patients With Heart Failure II).

CONCLUSION

Prior of SGLT2 inhibitors, HFpEF was considered an orphan disease, and all trials failed to show improvement in outcomes. SGLT2 inhibitors have been the first agents to show improved outcomes in HFpEF. New trials with injectable semaglutide in the obese phenotype of HFpEF and nonsteroidal MRA finerenone in HFpEF have shown positive results, and both drugs are likely to be approved in the future. However, the limitation of pharmacotherapy is that no trial as yet has shown a decrease in mortality. Device therapy is awaiting a proper phenotype for its benefit.

REFERENCES

1. Nagueh SF. Left ventricular diastolic function: understanding pathophysiology, diagnosis, and prognosis with echocardiography. JACC Cardiovasc Imaging. 2020;13:228-44.
2. Negishi K. Incremental diagnostic value of left atrial strain over left atrial volume. J Am Coll Cardiol Img. 2018;11(10):1416-8.
3. Anker S, Butler J, Filippatos G, et al. Empagliflozin in Heart Failure with a Preserved Ejection Fraction. N Engl J Med. 2021;385(16):1451-61.
4. Solomon SD, McMurray JJV, Claggett B, et al. Dapagliflozin in Heart Failure with Mildly Reduced or Preserved Ejection Fraction. N Engl J Med. 2022;387:1089-98.
5. Solomon SD, McMurray JJV, Anand Inder S, et al. Angiotensin–Neprilysin Inhibition in Heart Failure with Preserved Ejection Fraction. N Engl J Med. 2019;381:1609-20.
6. Kosiborod MN, Abildstrøm SZ, Borlaug BA, et al. Semaglutide in Patients with Heart Failure with Preserved Ejection Fraction and Obesity. N Engl J Med. 2023;389:1069-84.
7. Kosiborod MN, Petrie MC, Borlaug BA, et al. Semaglutide in Patients with Obesity-Related Heart Failure and Type 2 Diabetes. N Engl J Med. 2024;390:1394-407.
8. Solomon SD, McMurray JJV, Vaduganathan M, et al. Finerenone in Heart Failure with Mildly Reduced or Preserved Ejection Fraction. N Engl J Med. 2024;391:1475-85.
9. Patel Ravi B, Silvestry Frank E, Komtebedde Jan, et al. Atrial Shunt Device Effects on Cardiac Structure and Function in Heart Failure With Preserved Ejection Fraction: The REDUCE LAP-HF II Randomized Clinical Trial. JAMA Cardiol. 2024;9(6):507-22.

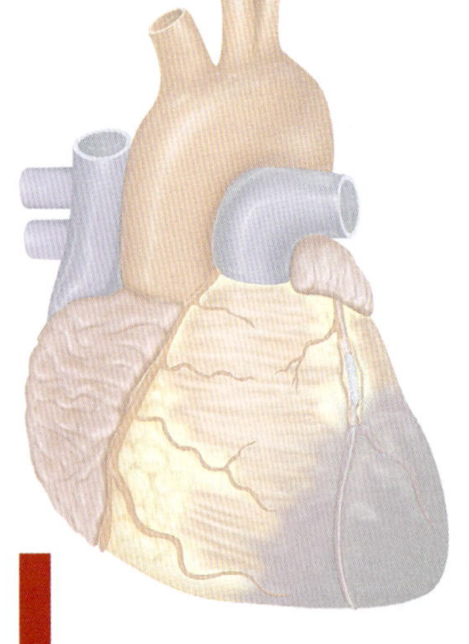

Recent Advances in Management of HFpEF

CK Ponde, HK Chopra

INTRODUCTION

Heart failure with preserved ejection fraction (HFpEF) is a complex clinical syndrome that affects up to 32 million people globally. It is primarily characterized by diastolic dysfunction (DD) and elevated left ventricular (LV) filling pressures, with a left ventricular ejection fraction (LVEF) of ≥50%. Despite a steadily rising prevalence, both in absolute terms and relative to the broader heart failure (HF) population, diagnosing HFpEF remains challenging. Two diagnostic tools, the H_2FPEF (Heavy, Hypertensive, atrial Fibrillation, Pulmonary hypertension, Elder, Filling pressure) score introduced in 2018 and the HFA-PEFF (Heart Failure Association Pretest assessment, Echocardiography, Functional testing, Final diagnosis) algorithm developed in 2020, have improved recognition of this syndrome; however, many cases still fall into an "uncertainty area" that complicates definitive diagnosis.[1] Even with therapeutic advances, HF remains a leading cause of morbidity and mortality worldwide, with a lifetime risk at age 40 estimated to be approximately 20%.[2]

ETIOLOGY AND PATHOPHYSIOLOGY OF HFpEF

The etiology of HFpEF is multifaceted, involving diverse cardiovascular (CV) and systemic conditions such as coronary artery disease (CAD), hypertension, valvular heart disease, cardiomyopathy, and infiltrative disorders like amyloidosis. Diabetes mellitus (DM), congenital heart anomalies, pericardial diseases, atrial fibrillation (AF), and exposure to cardiac toxins further contribute. These factors lead to structural and functional cardiac changes, particularly DD and drive ventricular and vascular stiffening, which are hallmarks of HFpEF.

At its core, HFpEF is characterized by DD, with impaired LV relaxation and increased stiffness, resulting in elevated diastolic pressures that transmit to the left atrium and pulmonary circulation, causing breathlessness and reduced lung compliance. Left atrial remodeling exacerbates atrial dysfunction, often culminating in AF, which worsens outcomes. Systemic factors like aging, hypertension, diabetes, and kidney disease increase arterial stiffness, compounding DD. Systemic inflammation and microvascular endothelial dysfunction, particularly in obesity and COPD, promote oxidative stress and myocardial remodeling, reinforcing the HFpEF pathophysiological cycle.[3]

SCORE-BASED DIAGNOSTIC ALGORITHMS FOR HFpEF

Two diagnostic tools, the H_2FPEF score and the HFA-PEFF algorithm have been developed to support the diagnosis of HFpEF, particularly in cases with inconclusive initial findings. The European Society of Cardiology (ESC) recommends using HFA-PEFF where expertise allows, while the American Heart Association (AHA)/American College of Cardiology (ACC)/Heart Failure Society of America (HFSA) does not favor one over the other. Both scores estimate the likelihood of HFpEF, though diagnostic uncertainty often persists, requiring further tests such as diastolic stress testing. Notably, discrepancies between the scores exist, and studies evaluating their accuracy have yielded mixed results.

CHALLENGES IN DIAGNOSING HFpEF

Diagnosing HFpEF presents significant challenges due to its complexity and nuanced criteria.[2,3] Unlike heart failure with reduced ejection fraction (HFrEF), HFpEF requires symptoms and/or signs of HF with structural or functional cardiac abnormalities, along with elevated natriuretic peptides or evidence of cardiogenic congestion.[2] Defining the ejection fraction (EF) threshold adds to the difficulty; HFpEF is classified as HF with LVEF ≥50%, while EFs between 40% and 50% are categorized as HF with mid-range EF (HFmrEF). This distinction helps identify stable HFpEF cases but is complicated by variability in EF measurement across imaging modalities.[2]

Heart failure with preserved ejection fraction is not synonymous with DD, as diastolic abnormalities alone are insufficient for diagnosis. Moreover, the absence of a single definitive test for HFpEF necessitates a clinical approach that accounts for noncardiac comorbidities and overlapping cardiac conditions, which often mimic HFpEF. Misdiagnosis is common, and active case-finding strategies in high-risk groups remain essential to improve diagnostic accuracy and guide effective treatment.[2,3]

LATEST PHARMACOLOGICAL THERAPIES FOR HFpEF

Heart failure with preserved ejection fraction presents unique therapeutic challenges due to its heterogeneous etiology and lack of definitive evidence-based targets. Traditional management of HFpEF has largely centered on symptomatic relief through decongestion and addressing underlying comorbidities such as diabetes, hypertension, obesity, ischemic heart disease, and arrhythmias. Additionally, treatment strategies have focused on identifying and managing specific pathologies like hypertrophic cardiomyopathy, amyloid cardiomyopathy, high-output heart failure, primary pulmonary hypertension, constrictive pericarditis, and cardiac sarcoidosis. Adjunctive therapies such as revascularization, exercise training, and physical rehabilitation have shown promise in improving functional outcomes and quality of life (QoL), particularly in frail patients recovering from HF hospitalization.

The overarching goals of therapy in HFpEF are to alleviate symptoms, enhance functional capacity, and reduce the risk of hospital admissions. A multifaceted approach is employed, involving risk stratification and comprehensive management of comorbid conditions like hypertension, DM, AF, CAD, chronic kidney disease (CKD), and obstructive sleep apnea. Nonpharmacological interventions, such as structured exercise programs, weight loss, and the use of implantable pulmonary artery monitors, play a significant role in symptom management. Pharmacological options include loop diuretics for congestion relief and disease-modifying agents like sodium-glucose cotransporter 2 (SGLT2) inhibitors mineralocorticoid receptor antagonists (MRAs), angiotensin receptor–neprilysin inhibitors (ARNIs), and angiotensin receptor blockers (ARBs).[2]

Historically, many trials investigating pharmacological therapies in HFpEF, including those assessing perindopril, irbesartan, beta-blockers, nitrates, digoxin, ivabradine, sildenafil, and serelaxin, have been disappointing, showing little to no benefit. However, recent advancements in guideline-directed medical therapy (GDMT) have demonstrated significant improvements in symptoms, functional capacity, and outcomes for HFpEF patients. Initiation of GDMT is recommended in both acute and chronic settings, as it is safe and effective in mitigating the morbidity and mortality associated with HFpEF **(Flowchart 1 and Table 1)**.[2]

Diuretics: Cornerstone of Symptomatic Relief

The use of diuretics for managing fluid retention in HFpEF is well-established. Loop diuretics, such as furosemide,

Flowchart 1: Treatment algorithm for guideline-directed medical therapy in HFpEF.[2]

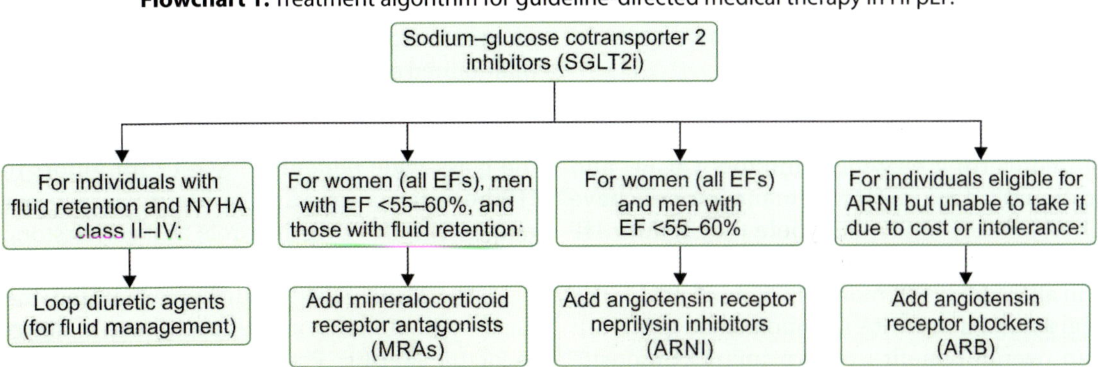

TABLE 1: Recommended starting and target doses for GDMT for HFpEF.

Drug class	*Starting dose*	*Target dose*
SGLT2is		
Dapagliflozin	10 mg daily	10 mg daily
Empagliflozin	10 mg daily	10 mg daily
Aldosterone antagonists		
Spironolactone	25 mg daily	50 mg daily
ARNIs		
Sacubitril/valsartan	24 mg/26 mg twice daily	97 mg/103 mg twice daily
ARBs		
Candesartan	4–8 mg daily	32 mg daily

(ARB: angiotensin receptor blocker; ARNI: angiotensin receptor–neprilysin inhibitor; GDMT: guideline-directed medical therapy; HFpEF: heart failure with preserved ejection fraction; SGLT2: sodium–glucose cotransporter-2)

are the first-line agents, with the lowest effective dose recommended initially. However, evidence does not support a prognostic benefit and there is some suggestion that diuretics may stimulate the sympathetic nervous system and renin–angiotensin–aldosterone system (RAAS).[4] For cases of diuretic resistance, sequential nephron blockade with thiazide or thiazide-like diuretics, such as metolazone, can be considered. Monitoring renal function and electrolytes is essential due to the risk of complications.[4,6]

The JCS/JHFS guideline recommends azosemide over furosemide due to its lower neurohormonal impact. Adjunctive therapies like tolvaptan and acetazolamide have also been explored. While tolvaptan has shown symptomatic improvements, it has not demonstrated reductions in mortality or rehospitalization. Recent evidence suggests acetazolamide may improve decongestion outcomes across the LVEF spectrum, but its use requires further validation.[4]

Angiotensin-Converting Enzyme Inhibitors, Angiotensin II Receptor Blockers, and Mineralocorticoid Receptor Antagonists

Angiotensin-converting enzyme inhibitors (ACEi) and ARBs, traditionally key in HFrEF management, have shown limited efficacy in HFpEF. While they reduce HF hospitalizations, they have not demonstrated significant reductions in all-cause or CV mortality (Kataria et al.). The TOPCAT trial assessed the MRA spironolactone in HFpEF, revealing no overall benefit in the primary composite outcome of all-cause mortality and HF hospitalizations. However, subgroup analysis indicated a reduction in HF hospitalizations among patients in the Americas, suggesting a regional benefit.

Angiotensin Receptor-Neprilysin Inhibitors

Sacubitril–valsartan, an ARNI, was compared to valsartan in patients with HF and LVEF ≥45%. Although it did not significantly reduce the composite endpoint of CV death and total HF hospitalizations, it demonstrated a notable reduction in HF hospitalizations. Subgroup analyses suggested greater benefit in patients with LVEF <57% and women. Ongoing trials are evaluating the efficacy of sacubitril–valsartan in acute HFpEF settings, focusing on biomarkers and clinical outcomes.[7] Sacubitril–valsartan got the US FDA approval for use in HFpEF in February 2021.

Sodium–Glucose Cotransporters 1 and 2 Inhibitors: Breakthrough Disease-modifying Therapies

The SGLT2 inhibitors represent a breakthrough in HFpEF treatment, marking the advent of disease-modifying therapies for this challenging condition. The EMPEROR-Preserved trial demonstrated that empagliflozin reduced the composite endpoint of HF hospitalization or CV death by 21%, with benefits evident within 18 days of initiation. This effect was consistent across patients with or without diabetes and was accompanied by improvements in kidney function and QoL.[6] However, the benefits of empagliflozin were less pronounced in patients with LVEF >65%.[4,6,7]

Dapagliflozin has shown similar promise. The PRESERVED-HF trial highlighted its ability to improve symptoms, physical function, and exercise capacity in HFpEF patients, regardless of diabetes status.[6] The DELIVER trial further reinforced dapagliflozin's efficacy, demonstrating an 18% reduction in the combined risk of worsening HF or CV death in patients with mildly reduced or preserved LVEF. Unlike empagliflozin, dapagliflozin maintained efficacy across the full LVEF spectrum, making it a robust option for a broader patient base.[4,6]

Meta-analyses of pooled trial data have confirmed the class-wide benefits of SGLT2 inhibitors in reducing HF hospitalizations and mortality across varying LVEF ranges, emphasizing their role as a cornerstone of HFpEF therapy.[4,6]

The EMPULSE trial further expanded the evidence base by demonstrating empagliflozin's clinical benefits in acute HFpEF. Patients treated with empagliflozin experienced significant improvements in composite endpoints, including mortality, HF events, and symptom scores, reinforcing its versatility in both chronic and acute settings.[6,7]

In addition to selective SGLT2 inhibitors, combined SGLT2 and SGLT1 inhibition has been explored. The SOLOIST-WHF trial evaluated sotagliflozin in patients with worsening HFpEF and T2DM, showing significant reductions in HF events despite early trial termination due to the COVID-19 pandemic. These findings have prompted recommendations for sotagliflozin use in select populations by ESC and AHA/ACC/HFSA guidelines. However, its broader application is tempered by higher incidences of adverse events, including diarrhea, genital infections, and diabetic ketoacidosis (Mahmood et al.). Ongoing trials, such as SOTA-P-CARDIA, aim to further delineate sotagliflozin's role, including its potential benefits in HFpEF patients without T2DM.[4]

The advent of SGLT2 inhibitors, with additional exploration of combined SGLT2/SGLT1 inhibition, has significantly expanded therapeutic options for HFpEF, providing both symptomatic relief and meaningful reductions in HF-related hospitalizations and mortality.

Glucagon-like peptide-1 Receptor Agonists: Emerging Therapeutics

Glucagon-like peptide-1 (GLP-1) receptor agonists have shown potential in improving HFpEF outcomes. The STEP-HFpEF and STEP-HFpEF DM trials demonstrated that semaglutide improved symptoms, exercise capacity, and weight loss in HFpEF patients, irrespective of baseline characteristics (Mahmood et al.). However, these trials primarily investigated secondary endpoints, such as HF hospitalization or mortality. The SUMMIT trial is currently exploring the efficacy of tirzepatide, a combined glucose-dependent insulinotropic polypeptide, and GLP-1 receptor agonist, on HF outcomes, offering potential insights into the role of these agents in HFpEF.[4]

Finerenone

Finerenone is a nonsteroidal MRA that is more selective for the mineralocorticoid receptor than spironolactone or eplerenone. It targets adverse hemodynamics (e.g., sodium retention and albuminuria) and nonhemodynamic (e.g. fibrotic and inflammatory) pathways related to mineralocorticoid receptor overactivation in heart, kidneys, and blood vessels. Finerenone has been shown to have more pronounced anti-inflammatory/antifibrotic effects, as well as a more balanced distribution in heart and kidney tissue, compared with spironolactone and eplerenone, which preferentially concentrate in the kidneys.

The FINEARTS-HF (Finerenone Trial to Investigate Efficacy and Safety Superior to Placebo in Patients with Heart Failure) trial was designed to test the hypothesis that finerenone, in addition to usual therapy, would reduce the rate of total worsening HF events and death from CV causes among patients with HF and mildly reduced or preserved ejection.

In the FINEARTS-HF study, finerenone demonstrated statistically significant *16% relative risk reduction* in the composite CV outcome (HF events and CV death) in patients with HF and LVEF ≥40%, compared to placebo.

This included *significant reductions in hospitalization* or urgent visits due to HF versus placebo. The effects of finerenone on the composite CV outcome were *consistent across a broad population*, regardless of baseline use of SGLT-2 inhibitors, LVEF, renal function, comorbidities or prior hospitalization status. Finerenone was *well tolerated*, with a comparable include of treatment-emergent SAEs to placebo.

TREATING UNDERLYING COMORBIDITIES

Managing comorbidities and modifiable HF risk factors has historically been the cornerstone of HFpEF management, with a focus on treating hypertension, AF, CAD, DM, CKD, hyperlipidemia, obesity, anemia, and sleep apnea. These conditions often coexist with HFpEF, though no HFpEF-specific therapies are available for their management.[6]

Hypertension

Hypertension, the leading cause of HFpEF (prevalence 60–89%), necessitates effective blood pressure (BP) control to prevent HF progression. ARBs, ACEi, and calcium channel blockers have shown greater efficacy in regressing left ventricular hypertrophy (LVH) compared to beta-blockers or diuretics. BP targets for HFpEF align with general population guidelines but may require adjustment based on comorbidities or symptoms of HF decompensation. Monitoring for exaggerated hypotensive responses to vasodilators is essential when titrating medications in HFpEF patients.[6]

Diabetes

The SGLT2 inhibitors are integral to HFpEF therapy, especially in diabetic patients, but these should be prioritized for individuals at high CV risk or when metformin is contraindicated. Adjustments to insulin or sulfonylurea doses are necessary to mitigate hypoglycemia risk. SGLT2 inhibitors are contraindicated in type 1 DM, those with a history of diabetic ketoacidosis (DKA), and patients with eGFR <15–20 mL/min/1.73 m^2.[6]

CHRONIC KIDNEY DISEASE

Evidence-based therapies like RAAS inhibitors and SGLT2 inhibitors slow CKD progression and improve outcomes in patients with HFpEF. Trials, such as DAPA-CKD, demonstrated reduced risks of eGFR decline, end-stage renal disease, and CV death with dapagliflozin, even in nondiabetic CKD patients. Short-term eGFR declines on SGLT2 inhibitor initiation are offset by long-term benefits.[6]

Chronic Coronary Syndrome

Coronary artery disease, prevalent in 35–60% of HFpEF patients, requires individualized evaluation and management. Diagnostic tools like CT coronary angiography and invasive coronary angiography are utilized based on CAD probability. While no prospective trials support revascularization in HFpEF, medical therapy with agents like beta-blockers, nitrates, calcium channel blockers, and ivabradine is recommended for angina relief.[6]

Atrial Fibrillation

In HFpEF with AF, adequate rate control is prioritized, commonly using beta-blockers or nondihydropyridine calcium channel blockers. Digoxin has demonstrated comparable QoL outcomes with fewer side effects than beta-blockers in elderly HFpEF patients (RATE-AF trial). While rhythm control strategies lack clear advantage, ablation may offer superior outcomes compared to antiarrhythmic drugs. In refractory cases, AV-node ablation with permanent pacemaker placement is an option.[6]

Renin–Angiotensin–Aldosterone System Inhibitors and Beta Blockers

The RAAS inhibitors, MRAs, and beta-blockers, though extrapolated from HFrEF guidelines, are considered in HFpEF management for select patients. Subgroup analyses suggest potential benefits, particularly in those with LVEF closer to 50%, though evidence remains inconclusive. Nonsteroidal MRAs like finerenone have shown promise in reducing HF hospitalizations in T2DM and CKD patients and are under investigation for broader HFpEF applicability.[6]

RECENT ADVANCES IN DEVICE-BASED ADJUNCT THERAPIES

Device-based therapies have emerged as promising adjuncts to pharmacological treatment in HFpEF, particularly for patients with specific phenotypes. These therapies aim to improve symptoms, enhance QoL, and reduce HF-related hospitalizations by addressing underlying physiological mechanisms.

Established Devices

The following are the established devices:

- *Inter-atrial shunt devices (IASDs):* Designed to reduce left atrial pressure by creating a shunt from the left to the right atrium, IASDs target the elevated left atrial pressures seen in HFpEF. The IASD received CE Mark approval in 2016, becoming the first transcatheter device for HFpEF treatment. While early studies showed symptom improvement in select subgroups, phase III trials yielded neutral primary endpoints, necessitating further investigation.[8,9]
- *Implantable pulmonary artery pressure (PAP) monitors:* Devices like CardioMEMS detect early rises in PAP, enabling proactive decongestion management. Clinical trials have demonstrated reduced HF hospitalizations, and CardioMEMS has earned a class IIb recommendation in guidelines for select HF patients.[8,9]
- *Baroreflex activation therapy:* The Barostim Neo system, approved by the FDA, helps restore autonomic balance in HF patients, showing promise in improving symptoms and reducing hospitalizations.

Emerging and Experimental Therapies

The emerging and experimental therapies are as follows:

- *Greater splanchnic nerve ablation:* Aimed at reducing LV filling pressure, this technique shows potential for symptom relief in HFpEF.
- *Left atrial pacing:* Used to correct interatrial dyssynchrony, this intervention may enhance cardiac function in specific HFpEF phenotypes.
- *Cardiac contractility modulation (CCM):* By improving calcium handling in the heart, CCM devices may enhance cardiac performance in HFpEF patients.
- *Renal denervation, vagus nerve stimulation, and baroreflex activation therapy:* These therapies aim to correct autonomic imbalance, a common issue in HFpEF.

While device-based therapies hold significant promise, many require further validation in larger studies to establish their efficacy and define their role in HFpEF management. Current clinical evidence supports the use of IASDs, PAP monitors, and baroreflex activation therapy for select patient groups, offering hope for tailored treatment strategies.[8,9]

CONCLUSION AND FUTURE PERSPECTIVES

Heart failure with preserved ejection fraction, once primarily attributed to LV DD, is now increasingly recognized as a complex, multiorgan syndrome. Its pathophysiology involves systemic changes linked to various comorbid conditions, which drive myocardial dysfunction in diverse ways. HFpEF remains difficult to diagnose, though recent guidelines have proposed a simplified three-step diagnostic pathway for most cases. For patients with inconclusive results, referral to specialized centers for additional testing is recommended. Regardless of LVEF, a diagnosis of HF has profound negative effects on quality and quantity of life.

Heart failure with preserved ejection fraction now represents approximately 50% of all HF cases and is considered one of the greatest unmet needs in cardiology. As the global population ages and comorbidities become more prevalent, the incidence of HFpEF is on the rise. Current outcomes in HFpEF are comparable to those in HFrEF, highlighting the importance of early intervention to prevent poor outcomes, including mortality, morbidity, and adverse patient-reported experiences. HFpEF is often accompanied by multimorbidity, with many patients managing five or more significant comorbidities, making its management particularly challenging.

Historically, treatment has centered on diuretics and managing comorbid conditions, with limited clinical trial data to guide decisions. However, recent breakthrough randomized controlled trials (RCTs) investigating the use of SGLT2 inhibitors (such as EMPEROR-Preserved and DELIVER) have demonstrated improved patient-reported outcomes, reductions in HF hospitalizations, and decreased CV death. This class of drugs has now earned a class IIa recommendation in the 2022 AHA guidelines for HFpEF, and further updates are expected in European and NICE clinical guidelines.

Despite recent advances in understanding the disease's pathophysiology, HFpEF continues to be under-recognized in clinical practice. This under-recognition remains a concern, especially given the advent of highly effective pharmacologic and lifestyle treatments that can significantly reduce morbidity and mortality. The ongoing identification of HFpEF "masqueraders"—conditions that mimic HFpEF but require different management approaches—further complicates recognition and treatment.

Looking ahead, ongoing large-scale studies into HFpEF pathobiology, as well as an increasing number of translational studies bridging the gap between laboratory research and clinical application offer hope for better management strategies. The growing body of clinical trials exploring novel therapeutics for HFpEF presents a promising future with the potential to reduce its prevalence, morbidity, and mortality. These advancements hold the promise of improving outcomes for a large segment of the population affected by this debilitating condition.

In conclusion, while HFpEF once lacked effective pharmacologic treatments, recent progress with drugs like ARNI, SGLT2 inhibitors, and finerenone has significantly improved the treatment landscape. Alongside continued research and the use of diuretics, these therapies have the potential to redefine outcomes for HFpEF patients, providing a clearer path toward better quantity and QoL.

REFERENCES

1. Balestrieri G, Limonta R, Ponti E, et al. The therapy and management of heart failure with preserved ejection fraction: New Insights on Treatment. Cardiac Fail Rev. 2024;10:e05.
2. Kittleson MM, Panjrath GS, Amancherla K, et al. 2023 ACC Expert Consensus Decision Pathway on Management of Heart Failure with Preserved Ejection Fraction: A report of the American College of Cardiology Solution Set Oversight Committee. J Am Coll Cardiol. 2023;81(18):1835-78.
3. Toth PP, Gauthier D. Heart failure with preserved ejection fraction: strategies for disease management and emerging therapeutic approaches. Postgrad Med. 2021; 133(2):125-39.
4. Mahmood A, Dhall E, Primus CP, et al. Heart failure with preserved ejection fraction management: a systematic review of clinical practice guidelines and recommendations. Eur Heart J Qual Care Clin Outcomes. 2024;10(7):571-89.
5. Devadoss R, Dhillon G, Sharma P, et al. Heartfelt Breakthroughs: Elevating Quality of Life with Cutting-Edge Advances in Heart Failure Treatment. J Cardiovasc Dev Dis. 2024;11(1):15.
6. Jasinska-Piadlo A, Campbell P. Management of patients with heart failure and preserved ejection fraction. Heart. 2023;109(11):874-83.
7. Kataria R, van Spall HG.; American College of Cardiology. 2022. Pharmacologic treatment for HFpEF: Role of drug therapies at the higher end of LVEF spectrum. [online] Available from https://www.acc.org/Latest-in-Cardiology/Articles/2022/03/08/18/51/Pharmacologic-Treatment-For-HFpEF [Last accessed January, 2025].
8. Wu Y, Song M, Wu M, et al. Advances in device-based treatment of heart failure with preserved ejection fraction: Evidence from clinical trials. ESC Heart Failure. 2024; 11(1):13-27.
9. Jeffries A. Heart failure with preserved ejection fraction: Advances in management. Medicine Today. 2023;24(10): 21-7.

CHAPTER 32

Impaired Pressure Natriuresis and Its Clinical Implications: From Uncontrolled Hypertension to Heart Failure

Anil Pareek, Franz H Messerli, C Venkata S Ram, HK Chopra, Mohsin Wali

INTRODUCTION

This chapter emphasizes the serious consequences of impaired natriuresis, especially in the Indian population, where the high prevalence of visceral adiposity has led to an epidemic of cardiovascular-kidney-metabolic (CKM) syndrome encompassing type 2 diabetes (T2D), cardiovascular disease (CVD), metabolic-associated fatty liver disease (MAFLD), and chronic kidney disease (CKD). Evidence supports a strong association between salt sensitivity, insulin resistance (IR), and an elevated risk of metabolic syndrome and CVD. Impaired natriuresis significantly contributes to a spectrum of health conditions, ranging from uncontrolled or resistant hypertension to heart failure (HF). Managing this complex condition requires a multifaceted approach, with dietary modifications and lifestyle changes being essential to reduce CV risks. Pharmacological interventions, including diuretics, calcium channel blockers (CCBs), and newer natriuretic agents, are effective for managing impaired natriuresis and helping patients achieve optimal blood pressure control. Notably, three of the four core treatment agents for HF [angiotensin receptor-neprilysin inhibitors (ARNis), sodium-glucose cotransporter-2 inhibitors (SGLT2is), and mineralocorticoid receptor antagonists (MRAs)] also enhance natriuresis, addressing both hypertension and fluid balance issues. These findings highlight the importance of integrated strategies in tackling CKM syndrome and its associated complications.

The relationship between renal perfusion and sodium excretion is fundamental to blood pressure (BP) regulation. The concept of pressure natriuresis (PN), originally proposed by Guyton,[1] describes a feedback mechanism that controls arterial pressure over the long term. This mechanism operates by decreasing sodium reabsorption and increasing sodium excretion in response to elevated renal perfusion pressure. This implies that, in hypertensive individuals, a higher systolic BP (SBP) becomes necessary for sodium excretion. When renal arterial pressure rises, the kidneys respond by increasing sodium excretion and reducing extracellular fluid volume, thereby maintaining the sodium balance and stabilizing BP. The equilibrium point for BP is reached when a balance between PN and extracellular fluid volume is achieved. Impaired PN, thus, reflects an atypical sodium excretion response at a given BP level and can lead to uncontrolled hypertension. Under these conditions, hypertension emerges as a kidney-related disease.[2]

High salt intake may lead to abnormalities in PN, hindering the regulation of the sodium balance and causing elevated BP and a heightened risk of hypertension.[3] Modern processed foods contain much higher amounts of sodium than natural foods, and high salt intake is a key contributor to the widespread prevalence of hypertension. Reducing salt intake can significantly lower average BP levels in humans. Notably, a one-third reduction in salt intake has been linked to a >10-mm Hg decline in average systolic and diastolic BP (DBP) levels. One study reported that the current salt intake of the population is five times higher than the physiological intake.[4] Additionally, the SCRIPT study found that Indian patients with hypertension and dyslipidemia consume significantly higher amounts of salt than recommended, with northern India reporting the highest daily intake of salt (14.13 g) in the country.[5]

In this context, the World Health Organization has established a global target to reduce sodium intake by 30% by 2025 as part of its strategy to prevent and control noncommunicable diseases.[6]

PATHOPHYSIOLOGY OF ELEVATED BLOOD PRESSURE AND HYPERTENSION—KIDNEYS ARE THE HEART OF THE MATTER

Blood pressure regulation is a complex physiological process that relies on the coordinated actions of several systems and involves CV, renal, neural, endocrine, and local tissue control mechanisms. Long-term BP control through renal-body fluid feedback is primarily driven by the balance between salt and water intake and excretion of these substances by the kidneys, which determines the extracellular fluid volume. PN and diuresis, which are critical for maintaining this balance, help stabilize both BP and body fluid volume under most conditions.[7]

The 2024 European Society of Cardiology (ESC) guidelines for the management of hypertension were the first to address the concept of impaired PN in the context of the renal pathophysiology of elevated BP.[8] The two key physiological components of BP, namely its static and pulsatile components, are regulated through multiple physiological mechanisms, with renal mechanisms playing an especially significant role. The dysregulation of these renal pathways can lead to BP elevations and adverse CV outcomes.

Therefore, the kidneys are essential for BP regulation, and their effects are primarily mediated by the PN mechanism and the renin-angiotensin-aldosterone system (RAAS). PN mechanisms allow the kidneys to adjust sodium excretion and thereby maintain normal BP in response to changes in dietary sodium intake. Low sodium intake activates the RAAS to enhance sodium reabsorption, conserving the intravascular volume and BP. Meanwhile, high sodium intake suppresses RAAS, thereby promoting natriuresis. However, chronic RAAS activation increases the BP required for effective sodium excretion.

MECHANISM OF PRESSURE NATRIURESIS

Increased renal perfusion pressure triggers the release of nitric oxide (NO), prostaglandin E2, and kinins. NO, in particular, increases medullary blood flow by decreasing vascular resistance specifically in the renal medulla rather than in the cortex. This selective vasodilation increases blood flow into the medulla, causing elevations in renal interstitial hydrostatic pressure (RIHP) without any significant changes in the total renal blood flow. Higher RIHP levels enhance natriuresis by increasing the concentration of sodium in the medullary interstitial space. This enables the kidneys to increase sodium excretion efficiently under elevated BP conditions, contributing to BP regulation.[2]

Elevated RIHP reduces the tubular reabsorption of sodium by influencing several processes in the proximal tubules. First, it alters tight junction permeability, facilitating higher sodium excretion, and redistributes the sodium transporters on tubule cells, inhibiting their sodium reabsorption capacity. Additionally, elevated RIHP stimulates the release of intrarenal prostaglandin E2, which further inhibits sodium reabsorption. In the absence of these responses, the kidneys may retain excess sodium, leading to fluid retention and higher BP. Together, these mechanisms enhance natriuresis to enable BP regulation under conditions of elevated renal perfusion pressure.[2]

MODULATION OF THE PRESSURE–NATRIURESIS RELATIONSHIP

Renin–Angiotensin–Aldosterone System

Renin–angiotensin–aldosterone system plays a crucial role in regulating long-term BP and sodium balance through its impact on PN. Preclinical studies show that normal renin–angiotensin system (RAS) function supports effective sodium balance with minimal BP changes, even when sodium intake varies. When angiotensin II (Ang II) levels remain high despite increased sodium intake, BP must rise significantly to maintain sodium balance, causing impaired PN. Conversely, blocking Ang II with angiotensin-converting enzyme inhibitors (ACEis) increases renal excretion at lower BP levels. This demonstrates that RAAS dysfunctions contribute to impaired PN and consequently hypertension.[9]

Atrial Natriuretic Peptide

Atrial natriuretic peptide (ANP) factor is another important factor that influences PN and renal excretion. Studies show that ANP promotes acute sodium excretion and has long-term effects on the kidneys, enhancing their excretory function at physiological levels. Infusing ANP directly into the kidneys has been shown to reduce BP, suggesting that ANP plays a role in modulating renal function independent of its systemic effects. Additionally, evidence shows that ANP may also interact with the RAAS by inhibiting renin secretion and counteracting the effects of Ang II. Although the precise mechanisms remain unclear, the ANP-mediated modulation of PN highlights its potential in managing body fluid volumes and BP over time.[9]

Other Factors

Genetics, dietary factors, and the sympathetic nervous system (SNS) all play significant roles in regulating PN. Although various studies have identified multiple genes that influence PN, the precise mechanisms via which these genetic factors affect BP regulation and salt sensitivity remain unclear. In addition, dietary influences are also crucial, since low potassium intake is linked to increased sodium reabsorption and elevated BP, while high fructose consumption combined with high sodium intake can exacerbate salt-sensitive hypertension. Additionally, SNS activation by Ang II promotes renal sodium reabsorption and raises BP, and norepinephrine is also believed to play a potential role in this process. Finally, other factors such as inflammation and reactive oxygen species (ROS) levels may also modulate PN.[2]

IMPAIRED NATRIURESIS AND ITS CLINICAL CONSEQUENCES

In chronic hypertension, PN mechanisms are impaired, as sodium excretion remains comparable to that in normotensive individuals despite higher BP levels.[9] Impaired PN refers to a condition where sodium excretion fails to increase in response to elevated BP, indicating a disruption of the renal mechanisms that regulate sodium homeostasis under hypertensive conditions. Factors such as transient BP spikes, oxidative stress, inflammation, and localized vasoconstriction can further disrupt the PN response, leading to PN disorders.[2]

Pressure natriuresis impairments can occur under various conditions, including CKD, in which the kidneys struggle to effectively excrete sodium; excessive salt intake, which overwhelms the renal handling capacity; renal nerve activation, which enhances sympathetic activity and promotes sodium retention; and conditions characterized by a deficiency of renal NO, a key vasodilator that facilitates sodium excretion. Additionally, certain medications can adversely affect kidney function, and the ineffective use of diuretics may also contribute to the development of impaired PN, further complicating the regulation of sodium and BP.[2]

A rightward shift in the pressure–natriuresis curve, as shown in **Figure 1**, signifies hypertension due to reduced sodium excretion at higher BP levels.[10]

Pressure natriuresis is a major determinant of systemic hemodynamics; when this process is impaired, hypertension occurs. Thus, understanding these mechanisms is vital for addressing hypertension and related disorders.

IMPAIRED NATRIURESIS: SALT SENSITIVITY

Salt sensitivity is characterized by an individual's susceptibility to changes in BP in response to dietary salt intake. In salt-sensitive individuals, the slope of the PN relationship is less steep and is shifted to the right, as depicted in **Figure 2**. This shift implies that higher BP levels are required to maintain sodium balance in these individuals, and that the physiological mechanisms of PN are impaired, preventing the kidneys from adequately excreting sodium under conditions of high sodium intake. This dysfunction can result in increased BP, contributing to the development of hypertension.[2]

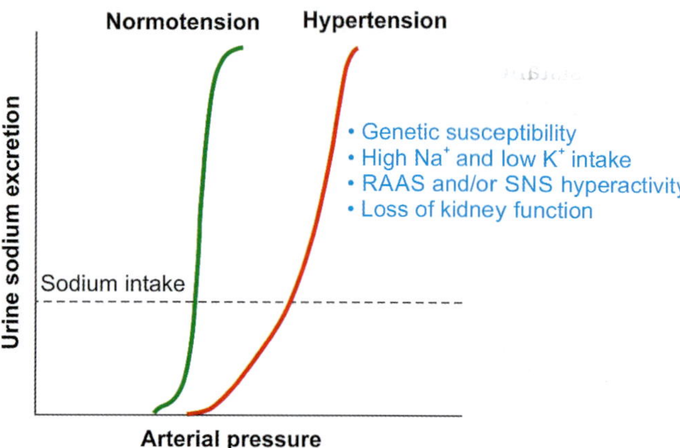

Fig. 1: Pressure–natriuresis curves in normotensive and hypertensive individuals.[10] (RAAS: renin–angiotensin–aldosterone system; SNS: sympathetic nervous system)

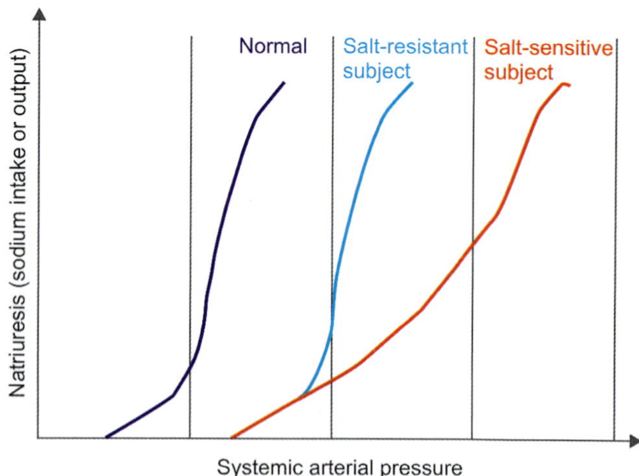

Fig. 2: Pressure–natriuresis curves in individuals with salt-resistant and salt-sensitive hypertension.[2]

The population can be broadly classified into salt-sensitive and salt-resistant individuals, with estimates suggesting that approximately 50–60% of people with hypertension exhibit salt sensitivity.[11] Several factors contribute to salt sensitivity, including aging, female sex, certain lifestyle factors, low-renin status, sympathetic overactivity, and comorbidities such as IR and CKD. Salt-sensitive hypertension is clinically significant due to its association with higher CV and renal risks.[12]

Guyton's classic concept illustrates that high salt intake leads to increased water retention, resulting in an expanded circulating blood volume, elevated cardiac output, and higher kidney perfusion pressure. This increase in kidney perfusion pressure subsequently enhances PN mechanisms, promoting sodium excretion to help restore fluid balance in the body. However, when this mechanism is impaired, hypertension may develop. Additionally, excessive sodium intake can increase systemic peripheral resistance due to the remodeling of small resistance arteries, further heightening the risk of hypertension. High salt consumption has also been linked to endothelial dysfunction, characterized by the reduced production of NO. Moreover, excessive sodium intake can lead to increased vascular stiffness and heightened sympathetic drive. Collectively, these factors contribute to elevated BP and various CV complications that can occur independently of BP. Therefore, understanding salt sensitivity is essential for developing targeted interventions to control BP and reduce CV risks.[11] Various mechanisms linking the high salt intake to hypertension are summarized in **Figure 3**.

Aging is another factor associated with changes in sodium homeostasis and kidney function, leading to salt retention and salt-sensitive hypertension. Older individuals often exhibit reduced sodium excretion, potentially due to altered renal function, increased sympathetic activity, decreased levels of natriuretic peptides, and heightened intrarenal RAAS activity, which collectively impair natriuresis.

Studies indicate that aging in both animals and humans is associated with blunted natriuretic responses, despite normal renal function, which may contribute to increased BP. PN is a crucial mechanism for regulating extracellular volume and ultimately affects BP. Therefore, the age-related rightward shift of pressure–natriuresis curves may be a primary cause of increased rates of salt-sensitive hypertension in the older population.

In a study involving 4,859 participants with normal kidney function (KoGES) and 235 individuals with nondiabetic CKD (ESPECIAL), older adults displayed lower estimated glomerular filtration rates (eGFRs), higher levels of albuminuria, and diminished PN responses. While olmesartan effectively lowered BP in both age groups, a low-salt diet (LSD) further reduced SBP only in older participants. Younger participants demonstrated a stronger correlation between BP and urine sodium levels than older participants under both experimental conditions, suggesting that aging diminishes the PN response, regardless of CKD status.

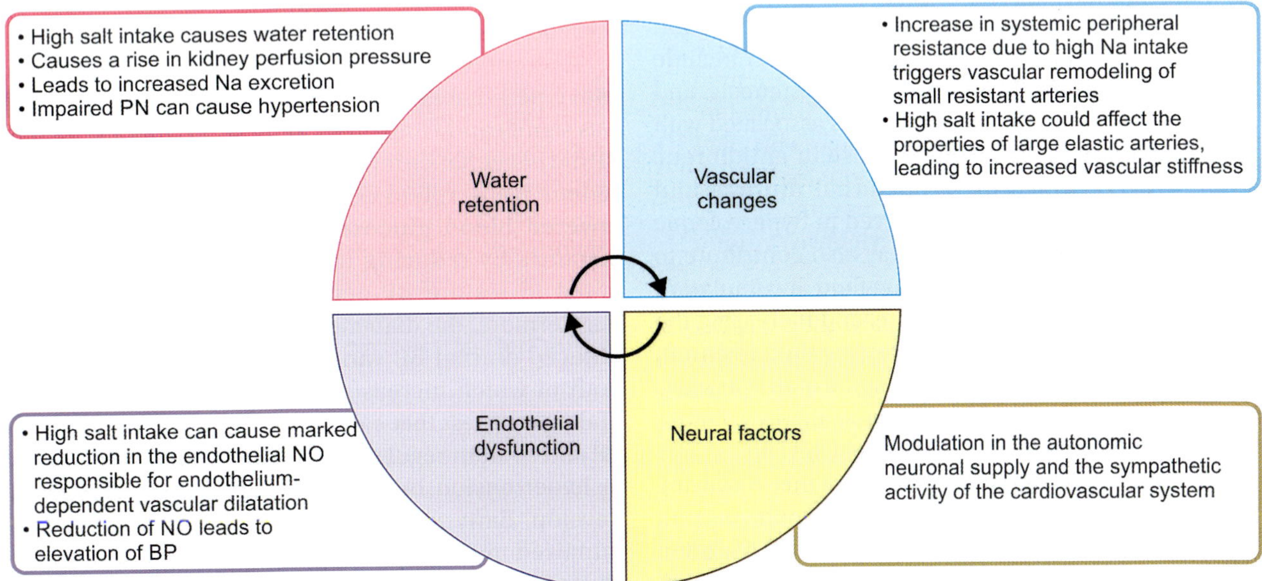

Fig. 3: Mechanisms linking high salt intake with hypertension.[11] (BP: blood pressure; NO: nitric oxide; PN: pressure natriuresis)

IMPAIRED NATRIURESIS: UNCONTROLLED OR RESISTANT HYPERTENSION

The kidneys are crucial for the long-term regulation of BP. Impaired PN, leading to increased extracellular fluid volume, is a key pathogenic factor in resistant hypertension. Higher BP thresholds for sodium excretion can result in sodium retention, particularly in individuals with reduced kidney function, leading to impaired extracellular fluid volume and resistant hypertension. This sodium retention is often accompanied by a decreased glomerular filtration rate and increased tubular sodium reabsorption. As a result, the kidneys fail to adequately excrete sodium despite elevated BP.[13]

In populations where primary hypertension is predominantly driven by excess fluid volume, patients with uncontrolled SBP exhibit a weakened correlation between ANP levels and signs of volume overload. Additionally, these individuals demonstrate a reduced vascular response to ANP. This diminished response to ANP can contribute to the persistence of elevated BP under conditions of volume-dependent hypertension.[14] This aligns with clinical and genetic studies, suggesting that hypertension in such individuals may represent a relative deficiency of ANP, resulting in impaired natriuresis.[15] High sodium intake exacerbates this issue, increasing the risk of treatment-resistant hypertension in these patients.[16]

Secondary Causes of Resistant Hypertension

In addition to volume-dependent mechanisms, common secondary contributors to resistant hypertension include obstructive sleep apnea (OSA), renal artery stenosis, and hyperaldosteronism.[17] In particular, OSA is associated with nocturnal increase in ANP and decrease in antidiuretic hormone (ADH), which drive nocturnal diuresis and natriuresis. The fluid retention observed in hypervolemic patients with high sodium intake may also contribute to the development of OSA by promoting fluid accumulation in the neck, increasing tissue pressure, and increasing the risk of upper airway narrowing. Addressing fluid retention and hypervolemia may help alleviate some of the pressure on the upper airway, reducing nocturnal airway collapse and subsequently lowering the burden of OSA.[18,19]

Renal artery stenosis, characterized by the narrowing of the renal arteries, can significantly impair sodium excretion and increase BP by activating the RAAS, often causing resistant hypertension. Reduced kidney perfusion due to this stenosis triggers renin release, leading to elevated levels of Ang II and aldosterone, which induce both vasoconstriction and sodium retention. In cases of bilateral renal artery stenosis, severe salt retention can result in episodic fluid overload and flash pulmonary edema.[13]

IMPAIRED NATRIURESIS: HYPERINSULINEMIA AND INSULIN RESISTANCE

In salt-sensitive individuals, high salt intake can exacerbate IR, which may further heighten the BP response to sodium. Several mechanisms link IR, salt sensitivity, and hypertension through renal, vascular, and immune pathways. IR selectively affects different tissues; while the expression of insulin receptor substrates (IRS1 and IRS2) decreases in tissues such as skeletal muscle, IRS2 expression in the kidneys remains high. This increased expression intensifies sodium retention due to compensatory hyperinsulinemia aimed at maintaining glucose levels, which may contribute to the development of hypertension.[20]

Insulin resistance partly contributes to hypertension via vascular dysfunction. Normally, insulin promotes vasodilation in skeletal muscle by increasing blood flow through NO production via the phosphatidylinositol 3-kinase (PI3K) pathway. However, in insulin-resistant states, this pathway becomes impaired, reducing NO synthesis. However, the mitogen-activated protein kinase (MAPK) pathway continues to produce the vasoconstrictor endothelin-1, tilting the balance toward vasoconstriction and hypertension. Notably, this vascular dysfunction precedes metabolic IR and worsens with high salt intake.[20]

A recent experimental study demonstrated that in rats with type 1 diabetes mellitus (T1DM), the PN mechanism was significantly impaired. In these T1DM rats, increased BP did not enhance renal medullary blood flow or decrease sodium reabsorption in the kidneys. While insulin therapy lowered blood glucose and restored the natriuretic response by reducing tubular sodium reabsorption, it failed to restore BP-dependent medullary perfusion. Furthermore, the diabetic rats exhibited higher DBP and reduced diurnal BP variation (nondipping BP pattern), both of which increased the long-term CV risk. These findings suggest that early T1DM leads to impairments in BP and sodium regulation, creating conditions conducive to hypertension before more advanced complications develop. Early interventions aimed at addressing this impaired natriuretic response, in conjunction with glycemic control, may help mitigate the CV risks associated with T1DM.[21]

IMPAIRED NATRIURESIS: VISCERAL OBESITY AND RENIN–ANGIOTENSIN–ALDOSTERONE SYSTEM ACTIVATION

The recognition of the pathophysiological relationships among metabolic risk factors, including obesity, diabetes, CKD, and CVD, has facilitated the development of the CKM syndrome concept. CKM syndrome often originates from excess or dysfunctional adipose tissue, which contributes to IR and hyperglycemia. Key processes such as inflammation, oxidative stress, and vascular dysfunction drive the progression of metabolic risk factors, promote kidney disease, and intensify heart–kidney interactions, ultimately leading to CVD. Additionally, metabolic risk factors and CKD further elevate the risk of CVD through various direct and indirect mechanisms.[22]

The ICMR-INDIAB-17 study reported a high prevalence of metabolic conditions across India. Notably, in this study, 39.5% of the population studied was found to have abdominal obesity (95% CI 37.7–41.4; 40,121 of 108,665 individuals).[23] Obesity-related hypertension is increasingly recognized as a unique phenotype of elevated BP that demands a tailored approach for both diagnosis and management. Many intricate and interrelated pathways connect obesity with hypertension.[24] Moreover, obese individuals require higher BP levels to maintain sodium balance, reflecting the impairment in renal PN. In these individuals, BP regulation via diuresis and natriuresis tends to promote hypertension, and obesity itself can heighten the risk of kidney impairment. In the early stages of obesity, enhanced tubular sodium reabsorption promotes sodium retention, which is a key trigger of the BP elevations associated with weight gain. Although renal vasodilation attempts to compensate by increasing glomerular filtration, this response is often inadequate, resulting in an expansion of extracellular volume and an upward recalibration of the PN mechanism. Additionally, obesity promotes renal sodium reabsorption through neural, hormonal, and renovascular pathways, shifting the pressure–natriuresis curve to the right. As a consequence, higher arterial pressure is needed to maintain sodium balance, contributing to the salt sensitivity associated with obesity-related hypertension.[25,26] Excess body weight and obesity are closely linked to adipose tissue dysfunction, which drives chronic vascular inflammation and oxidative stress, along with RAAS and SNS activation. Together, these factors contribute to the onset of hypertension in individuals with obesity.[24]

A schematic overview of the mechanisms linking obesity to hypertension is provided in **Flowchart 1**.[24]

Adipose Tissue Dysfunction

Obesity-related adipose tissue dysfunction plays a central role in the development of hypertension. As fat cells become dysfunctional, they undergo hypertrophy and exhibit macrophage infiltration. Dysfunctional adipose tissue can secrete elevated levels of various adipokines, including leptin, tumor necrosis factor-alpha (TNF-α), interleukin-6 (IL-6), and resistin, along with decreased adiponectin levels. This imbalance contributes to IR, vascular inflammation, and impaired endothelial function, disrupting NO production, increasing vascular tone, and promoting hypertension.[24]

Inflammation and Oxidative Stress

The increase in visceral adipose tissue promotes systemic inflammation and oxidative stress, primarily through proinflammatory cytokines such as IL-6 and TNF-α, as well as through the activity of adipose tissue macrophages, which release ROS. These factors impair endothelial function, promote vascular inflammation, and contribute to arterial stiffness and hypertension. Inflammation and oxidative stress are intricately linked to adipose tissue dysfunction, creating a vicious cycle. Specifically, adipocyte hypertrophy attracts macrophages, leading to the release of free fatty acids and TNF-α, which further amplify ROS production and suppress protective adiponectin, fueling chronic inflammation and hypertension in individuals with obesity.[24]

Flowchart 1: Schematic overview of the mechanisms linking obesity to hypertension.

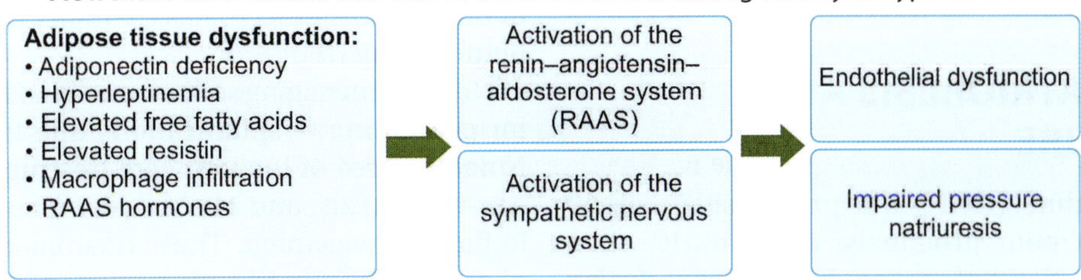

Activation of the Renin–Angiotensin–Aldosterone System

The activation of the RAAS is a key factor in the development of obesity-related hypertension. Ang II acts as a potent vasoconstrictor, leading to increased renal sodium retention and vascular hypertrophy. It also promotes aldosterone secretion, causing further sodium retention. Adipose tissue itself contributes to RAAS activity by producing components that regulate local adipocyte growth and differentiation while also potentially enhancing systemic RAAS activity. These tissues contain mineralocorticoid-stimulating factors that can increase aldosterone secretion, thereby promoting hypertension and IR. Elevated aldosterone levels, in turn, drive increase in sodium retention, inflammation, and oxidative stress, exacerbating hypertension.[24]

Activation of the Sympathetic Nervous System

Long-term activation of the SNS is another critical pathway linking obesity to hypertension. Obesity induces SNS activation, leading to peripheral vasoconstriction, increased heart rate, and impaired cardiac output, all of which elevate BP. Increased SNS outflow also stimulates renin release, amplifying RAAS activity and contributing to hypertension. Among the various key mediators, leptin triggers sympathetic activation in the hypothalamus, and insulin and Ang II have also been implicated in SNS activation. Although adiponectin is generally considered anti-inflammatory, its levels are reduced in obesity, which may indirectly contribute to sympathoactivation. Collectively, these mechanisms emphasize the role of SNS activation in the progression of obesity-related hypertension.[24]

Given the complex interplay of these factors, addressing obesity-related hypertension requires a nuanced approach that targets the metabolic and vascular abnormalities associated with excess weight. Comprehensive management strategies focusing on weight loss, improved metabolic health, and specific antihypertensive therapies are essential for mitigating the distinct effects of obesity on BP regulation.

IMPAIRED NATRIURESIS AND HEART FAILURE

Chronic heart failure (CHF) is a progressive clinical syndrome with a poor prognosis, particularly when accompanied by kidney dysfunction. Renal hypoperfusion is frequently observed in the early stages of HF, even when cardiac function is only mildly compromised. Traditionally, the kidneys have been viewed as a "victim" of chronic hypoperfusion and maladaptive responses to compensatory neurohormonal activation during HF progression. However, emerging evidence suggests that renal impairment may actually precede and contribute to the development of HF. Therefore, it is reasonable to speculate that the kidneys are not merely a victim but also a contributor to the onset, decompensation, and progression of HF.[27]

Chronic hypoperfusion and low renal perfusion pressure in the early stages of HF may impair PN, leading to sodium retention. This sodium retention is a significant contributor to the development of HF. It is widely accepted that sodium retention, volume overload, and congestion, along with renal dysfunction, are hallmarks of HF decompensation. Recent evidence even suggests that intrinsic renal derangements may impair natriuresis early in the course of the disease, even before clinical congestion or neurohumoral activation is evident.[28]

There is a substantial overlap between HF and renal dysfunction, with nearly half of all HF patients experiencing some level of renal impairment.[29] When renal dysfunction is present, the kidneys often struggle to produce effective PN.[28] This issue is particularly evident in cases of heart failure with preserved ejection fraction (HFpEF). Individuals diagnosed with HFpEF typically have a greater burden of comorbidities than those with heart failure with reduced ejection fraction (HFrEF).[30] A notably higher prevalence of renal impairment (approximately 49%) is also observed among individuals with HFpEF.[31]

Emerging insights into HFpEF reveal its complex relationship with kidney dysfunction. Renal insufficiency can propagate systemic inflammation and oxidative stress, both of which are known modifiers of PN. Salt and fluid retention, which are common features of CKD, may trigger the pathogenesis of HFpEF. Evidence suggests that abnormalities in renal sodium and fluid balance regulation often precede the onset of HFpEF. Prospective registry data indicate that even minor alterations in renal function can precede the development of HFpEF, distinguishing it from HFrEF. This syndrome of volume overload, regardless of the presence of detectable ventricular or vascular stiffness or other CVDs, exacerbates CV injury and risk, potentially perpetuating HFpEF.[32,33]

In CHF, managing sodium and fluid balance is essential for preventing hospitalizations due to fluid overload.[28] Notably, three of the four core treatment pillars for HF—ARNis, SGLT2is, and MRAs—promote natriuresis, aiding in fluid management. These treatments are components of the multifaceted approach for enhancing sodium excretion, improving fluid balance, and potentially reducing the need for hospitalizations in individuals with HF. This represents a paradigm shift in our understanding of HF pathophysiology, as it suggests that renal dysfunction leading to impaired PN is a critical contributor to disease progression. Recognizing the interplay between renal dysfunction and CHF, particularly in HFpEF, may provide insights into novel therapeutic strategies targeting the kidneys in order to improve patient outcomes.

THERAPEUTIC APPROACHES TO MANAGE IMPAIRED NATRIURESIS

In the absence of established guidelines, the consensus among experts emphasizes the importance of reducing salt intake in conjunction with conventional antihypertensive therapy as a foundational approach. A network meta-analysis has indicated that combining thiazide diuretics with CCBs is among the most effective pharmacological approaches for reducing BP in hypertensive populations.[34]

Diuretics

For patients with low plasma renin activity or salt-sensitive hypertension, particularly older adults, African Americans, and those with resistant hypertension or comorbidities such as metabolic syndrome, obesity, diabetes, or CKD, diuretics such as chlorthalidone, hydrochlorothiazide (HCTZ), and indapamide are effective BP-lowering options. Diuretics are especially beneficial for these patients due to their ability to counteract sodium retention, which is a key factor in salt-sensitive and low-renin hypertension.[35]

Multiple guidelines recommend chlorthalidone as the preferred diuretic due to its proven CV risk reduction benefits. These guidelines suggest replacing HCTZ with chlorthalidone or indapamide for patients with resistant hypertension. The landmark ALLHAT study demonstrated that chlorthalidone was more effective in preventing HF than amlodipine and lisinopril, achieving a reduction of >50% in HF incidence during the first year. After 5 years, HF rates were 38% higher with amlodipine and 19% higher with lisinopril compared to chlorthalidone. The advantage of chlorthalidone could be attributed to its effectiveness in enhancing sodium excretion, which is crucial for managing the fluid retention seen in CHF.[36]

The American Diabetes Association also recommends thiazide-like diuretics, specifically chlorthalidone and indapamide, for hypertensive patients with diabetes. These diuretics are favored due to their longer duration of action and their demonstrated impact on reducing CV events.[35]

In the context of CHF, loop diuretics are commonly used to manage fluid overload; however, their effectiveness can vary widely among different patients. Increasing loop diuretic doses often leads to diminishing returns, and high doses can cause side effects without providing additional benefits. To address these issues, a personalized approach that combines different types of diuretics or incorporates newer treatments, such as SGLT2is, may be more effective.[28]

The recent PUSH-AHF trial demonstrated the benefits of natriuresis-guided diuretic therapy in patients with acute heart failure (AHF). This approach significantly enhanced natriuresis and diuresis within 48 hours without affecting all-cause mortality or HF hospitalizations at 180 days. Most patients in the natriuresis-guided group received higher doses of loop diuretics; however, renal and electrolyte issues remained minimal despite the increased diuretic doses.[37]

Calcium Channel Blockers

Calcium channel blockers enhance natriuresis by dilating the afferent arterioles of the kidneys, which increase glomerular filtration pressure and subsequently promote sodium excretion. This natriuretic effect makes CCBs valuable in managing fluid balance and BP, particularly when used in combination with other medications, such as diuretics. This combined approach is particularly beneficial in conditions where impaired natriuresis contributes to hypertension or fluid overload, as it provides a more robust management of sodium and fluid levels.[34,38]

Sodium–Glucose Cotransporter-2 Inhibitors

Sodium-glucose cotransporter-2 inhibitors represent a breakthrough class of antidiabetic drugs with effects that extend beyond glucose control. By blocking the SGLT2 and partially inhibiting sodium–hydrogen exchanger 3 (NHE3) in the early proximal renal tubule, SGLT2is promote natriuresis and diuresis through enhanced sodium and glucose excretion. However, these effects are moderated by compensatory reabsorption mechanisms in downstream nephron segments. The enhanced delivery of sodium to the distal tubules activates tubuloglomerular feedback, which lowers glomerular pressure and helps preserve renal function.[2,39,40]

Beyond glycemic control, SGLT2is provide a wide range of metabolic, CV, and renal benefits. Clinical studies have demonstrated improved CV and renal outcomes after SGLT2is administration, even in nondiabetic populations. These benefits are attributed to mechanisms such as natriuresis and reduced BP, which improve the pressure–natriuresis curve.[2,12,39]

In patients with HFpEF, who have limited treatment options, SGLT2is have become the first drug to reduce hospitalizations for HF and decrease the risk of CV mortality. By inhibiting excessive sodium influx into atrial cardiomyocytes during atrial remodeling, SGLT2is provide potential antiarrhythmic benefits.[41] Moreover, SGLT2is block NHE1 activity in both the heart and vasculature, thereby reducing cardiac hypertrophy and fibrosis.[39]

Given their broad therapeutic benefits, SGLT2is have been dubbed the "statins of the 21st century," marking a major advancement in risk-based primary prevention for HF and other cardiorenal conditions.[42]

Mineralocorticoid Receptor Antagonists

Spironolactone, a well-established MRA, has demonstrated safety and efficacy in individuals with AHF who are at high risk for cardiorenal syndrome because it promotes natriuresis. This diuretic effect also makes spironolactone useful for treating resistant hypertension and CHF, enabling the management of fluid overload through enhanced sodium excretion.[43]

The nonsteroidal MRA finerenone has demonstrated CV benefits in the FIDELIO-DKD trial, with positive outcomes for CV end points observed early in treatment. These benefits are likely due to the natriuretic action of finerenone, which counters sodium and volume retention. This mechanism reduces fluid overload and contributes to improved CV and renal outcomes, particularly in patients with CKD and diabetes.[44]

Angiotensin Receptor-Neprilysin Inhibitors

Angiotensin receptor-neprilysin inhibitors are a novel class of drugs that simultaneously target two critical systems involved in regulating CV function: the RAS and natriuretic peptide system. By blocking neprilysin and angiotensin receptors concurrently, ARNIs enhance vasodilation, promote natriuresis, and reduce the activity of the endothelin, vasopressin, sympathetic, and RAS pathways, resulting in multiple CV benefits. The primary BP-lowering effect of ARNIs is achieved through enhanced natriuresis.[2] In a study by Wang et al., the effects of ARNI treatment were assessed in salt-sensitive hypertensive patients. The results demonstrated that ARNI therapy significantly increased cumulative sodium excretion over both 6 and 24 hours, leading to reduction in BP while promoting natriuresis and diuresis. This natriuretic effect could shift the pressure–natriuresis curve, potentially reducing salt sensitivity in affected individuals. The study concluded that the sacubitril/valsartan combination, when compared to valsartan alone, induced short-term increase in natriuresis and diuresis, providing superior office and ambulatory BP control and significantly reducing N-terminal pro-B-type natriuretic peptide levels in Asian patients with salt-sensitive hypertension.[45] Although ARNIs were initially approved for the treatment of HF, they also exert effects on BP and natriuresis, which could influence PN in conditions such as hypertension, CKD, and resistant hypertension.[2]

Newer Drugs

Recent early clinical trials involving new aldosterone synthase inhibitors have indicated the potential for lowering BP in patients with treatment-resistant and uncontrolled hypertension. These inhibitors function by reducing aldosterone production, which can help manage fluid retention and BP. However, further research is required to fully elucidate their benefits and determine their role in modulating the PN relationship.[12,46]

Renal Denervation

Increased SNS activity is a significant contributor to hypertension, particularly in conditions such as obesity, OSA, and CKD. SNS signals to the kidneys stimulate renin release, decrease renal blood flow and GFR, and increase sodium reabsorption in the renal tubules, resulting in a rightward shift of the pressure–natriuresis curve. Renal denervation (RDN) has been shown to decrease sympathetic activity both systemically and within the kidneys, which may positively attenuate PN impairments.[45]

PROGNOSTIC IMPLICATIONS OF IMPAIRED NATRIURESIS

Blood pressure is a recognized surrogate for CV and cerebrovascular risk. However, the real-world link between salt sensitivity/resistance and individual BP levels remains unclear. Salt sensitivity likely provides important insights into CV risk, though its direct impact on health outcomes is poorly understood at present.[47]

In a Japanese study, the salt sensitivity of hypertensive patients was assessed after a medication washout. The patients were alternated between low (1–3 g/day) and high (12–15 g/day) salt diets, and the BP was measured during each phase. In this study, salt sensitivity was defined as a >10% BP increase. After 7 years, the salt-sensitive patients were found to have a twofold higher rate of CV events than the salt-resistant patients, though neither group experienced kidney failure.[48]

A study from the United States assessed salt sensitivity by measuring BP changes after saline infusion and subsequent sodium depletion with furosemide. Here, salt sensitivity was defined based on a ≥10 mm Hg BP difference after saline infusion, and salt resistance based on a shift of <5 mm Hg. Over 25 years, salt-sensitive hypertensive subjects showed higher mortality, particularly due to CV causes. Notably, salt-sensitive normotensive individuals exhibited survival rates similar to hypertensive individuals, while salt-resistant normotensive participants experienced the best survival outcomes.[49]

Collectively, these findings indicate that impaired PN associated with salt-sensitive hypertension culminates in adverse CV outcomes.

FUTURE DIRECTIONS

Future research on impaired PN should focus on unraveling the mechanisms underlying RIHP, effects of reactive oxygen and nitrogen species, and role of prostaglandin E2 in regulating sodium balance. Understanding how oxidative stress affects these pathways could yield crucial insights into the pathophysiology of hypertension. The age-related decline in the PN response warrants further exploration, especially for developing potential interventions against salt-sensitive hypertension in older adults. Additionally, the genetic underpinnings of salt sensitivity must be identified. Recent evidence suggests that sodium may be stored nonosmotically in the skin and endothelial layers, highlighting the need for studies on extrarenal sodium buffering capacity. Targeting endothelial dysfunction and developing therapies that modulate nonrenal sodium storage could provide new approaches for managing salt-sensitive hypertension.

The discovery of novel mechanisms underlying salt-sensitive hypertension has highlighted the complexity of this condition. Beyond traditional kidney-centered pathways, evidence now suggests that vasoconstrictive mechanisms are crucial contributors to this phenotype, highlighting the role of these mechanisms in managing this condition. Future studies should explore the roles of emerging players, including the gut microbiome, endothelial function, nonosmotic sodium storage in the skin, and the influence of the mononuclear phagocytic and immune systems. These insights could enable the development of more effective, targeted treatments for salt-sensitive hypertension.

CONCLUSION

The interrelationships of salt sensitivity, IR, and the increased risk of metabolic syndrome and CVD highlight the importance of addressing impaired natriuresis. Impaired natriuresis in hypertension, often escalating to resistant hypertension and HF, is particularly concerning given the high rates of visceral adiposity and CKM syndrome in the Indian population. Diuretics, CCBs, and newer natriuretic agents have proven effective in managing impaired natriuresis and supporting better BP control. Additionally, three of the four core treatments for HF—ARNi, SGLT2i, and MRA—also promote natriuresis. In the future, research should focus on elucidating the mechanisms underlying impaired natriuresis to develop innovative treatment strategies for salt-sensitive hypertension, which may help enhance CVD mortality and morbidity benefits.

REFERENCES

1. Guyton AC. Blood pressure control—special role of the kidneys and body fluids. Science. 1991;252(5014):1813-6.
2. Baek EJ, Kim S. Current understanding of pressure natriuresis. Electrolyte Blood Press. 2021;19(2):38-45.
3. Grillo A, Salvi L, Coruzzi P, et al. Sodium intake and hypertension. Nutrients. 2019;11(9):1970.
4. Karppanen H, Mervaala E. Sodium intake and hypertension. Prog Cardiovasc Dis. 2006;49(2):59-75.
5. Kumbla D, Dharmalingam M, Dalvi K, et al. A study of salt and fat consumption pattern in regional Indian diet among hypertensive and dyslipidemic PaTients—SCRIPT study. J Assoc Physicians India. 2016;64(12):47-54.
6. Trieu K, Huang L, Aminde LN, et al. Estimated health benefits, costs, and cost-effectiveness of implementing WHO's sodium benchmarks for packaged foods in India: a modelling study. Lancet Public Health. 2024;9(11):e852-60.
7. Chopra S, Baby C, Jacob JJ. Neuro-endocrine regulation of blood pressure. Indian J Endocrinol Metab. 2011;15 Suppl 4(Supp l4):S281-8.
8. McEvoy JW, McCarthy CP, Bruno RM, et al. 2024 ESC guidelines for the management of elevated blood pressure and hypertension. Eur Heart J. 2024;45(38):3912-4018.
9. Hall JE, Mizelle HL, Hildebrandt DA, et al. Abnormal pressure natriuresis. A cause or a consequence of hypertension? Hypertension. 1990;15(6 Pt 1):547-59.
10. Kim GH. Primary role of the kidney in pathogenesis of hypertension. Life (Basel). 2024;14(1):119.
11. Youssef GS. Salt and hypertension: current views. Eur Soc Cardiol. 2022;22(3):1-10.
12. Vogt L, Marques FZ, Fujita T, et al. Novel mechanisms of salt-sensitive hypertension. Kidney Int. 2023;104(4):690-7.
13. Khawaja Z, Wilcox CS. Role of the kidneys in resistant hypertension. Int J Hypertens. 2011;2011:143471.
14. Yusuf SM, Norton GR, Peterson VR, et al. Attenuated relationships between indexes of volume overload and atrial natriuretic peptide in uncontrolled, sustained volume-dependent primary hypertension. Hypertension. 2023;80(1):147-59.
15. Macheret F, Heublein D, Costello-Boerrigter LC, et al. Human hypertension is characterized by a lack of activation of the antihypertensive cardiac hormones ANP and BNP. J Am Coll Cardiol. 2012;60(16):1558-65.
16. Shimosawa T. Salt, the renin-angiotensin-aldosterone system and resistant hypertension. Hypertens Res. 2013; 36(8):657-60.

17. Nagarajan N, Jalal D. Resistant hypertension: diagnosis and management. Adv Chronic Kidney Dis. 2019;26(2):99-109.
18. Ichioka M, Hirata Y, Inase N, et al. Changes of circulating atrial natriuretic peptide and antidiuretic hormone in obstructive sleep apnea syndrome. Respiration. 1992;59(3):164-8.
19. Giatti S, Santos RB, Aielo AN, et al. Association of sodium with obstructive sleep apnea. The ELSA-Brasil study. Ann Am Thorac Soc. 2021;18(3):502-10.
20. Ertuglu LA, Elijovich F, Laffer CL, et al. Salt-sensitivity of blood pressure and insulin resistance. Front Physiol. 2021;12:793924.
21. Culshaw GJ, Costello HM, Binnie D, et al. Impaired pressure natriuresis and non-dipping blood pressure in rats with early type 1 diabetes mellitus. J Physiol. 2019;597(3):767-80.
22. Ndumele CE, Neeland IJ, Tuttle KR, et al. A synopsis of the evidence for the science and clinical management of cardiovascular-kidney-metabolic (CKM) syndrome: a scientific statement from the American Heart Association. Circulation. 2023;148(20):1636-64.
23. Anjana RM, Unnikrishnan R, Deepa M, et al. Metabolic non-communicable disease health report of India: the ICMR-INDIAB national cross-sectional study (ICMR-INDIAB-17). Lancet Diabetes Endocrinol. 2023; 11(7):474-89.
24. Dorresteijn JA, Visseren FL, Spiering W. Mechanisms linking obesity to hypertension. Obes Rev. 2012;13(1):17-26.
25. Leggio M, Lombardi M, Caldarone E, et al. The relationship between obesity and hypertension: an updated comprehensive overview on vicious twins. Hypertens Res. 2017;40(12):947-63.
26. Hall JE, do Carmo JM, da Silva AA, et al. Obesity-induced hypertension: interaction of neurohumoral and renal mechanisms. Circ Res. 2015;116(6):991-1006.
27. Honetschlägerová Z, Sadowski J, Kompanowska-Jezierska E, et al. Impaired renal autoregulation and pressure-natriuresis: any role in the development of heart failure in normotensive and angiotensin II-dependent hypertensive rats? Hypertens Res. 2023;46(10):2340-55.
28. Verbrugge FH, Dupont M, Steels P, et al. The kidney in congestive heart failure: 'are natriuresis, sodium, and diuretics really the good, the bad and the ugly?'. Eur J Heart Fail. 2014;16(2):133-42.
29. Smith GL, Lichtman JH, Bracken MB, et al. Renal impairment and outcomes in heart failure: systematic review and meta-analysis. J Am Coll Cardiol. 2006; 47(10):1987-96.
30. Szlagor M, Dybiec J, Młynarska E, et al. Chronic kidney disease as a comorbidity in heart failure. Int J Mol Sci. 2023;24(3):2988.
31. Patel RN, Sharma A, Prasad A, et al. Heart failure with preserved ejection fraction with CKD: a narrative review of a multispecialty disorder. Kidney Med. 2023;5(12):100705.
32. Shah KS, Fang JC. Is heart failure with preserved ejection fraction a kidney disorder? Curr Hypertens Rep. 2019;21(11):86.
33. Fang JC. Heart failure with preserved ejection fraction: a kidney disorder? Circulation. 2016;134(6):435-7.
34. Qi H, Liu Z, Cao H, et al. Comparative efficacy of anti-hypertensive agents in salt-sensitive hypertensive patients: a network meta-analysis. Am J Hypertens. 2018;31(7): 835-46.
35. Burnier M, Bakris G, Williams B. Redefining diuretics use in hypertension: why select a thiazide-like diuretic? J Hypertens. 2019;37(8):1574-86.
36. ALLHAT Officers and Coordinators for the ALLHAT Collaborative Research Group. The Antihypertensive and Lipid-Lowering Treatment to Prevent Heart Attack Trial. Major outcomes in high-risk hypertensive patients randomized to angiotensin-converting enzyme inhibitor or calcium channel blocker vs diuretic: The Antihypertensive and Lipid-Lowering Treatment to Prevent Heart Attack Trial (ALLHAT). JAMA. 2002;288(23):2981-97.
37. Ter Maaten JM, Beldhuis IE, van der Meer P, et al. Natriuresis-guided diuretic therapy in acute heart failure: a pragmatic randomized trial. Nat Med. 2023;29(10):2625-32.
38. Elliott WJ, Ram CV. Calcium channel blockers. J Clin Hypertens (Greenwich). 2011;13(9):687-9.
39. Packer M, Wilcox CS, Testani JM. Critical analysis of the effects of SGLT2 inhibitors on renal tubular sodium, water and chloride homeostasis and their role in influencing heart failure outcomes. Circulation. 2023;148(4):354-72.
40. Zelniker TA, Braunwald E. Mechanisms of cardiorenal effects of sodium-glucose cotransporter 2 inhibitors: JACC state-of-the-art review. J Am Coll Cardiol. 2020; 75(4):422-34.
41. Trum M, Riechel J, Schollmeier E, et al. Empagliflozin inhibits increased Na influx in atrial cardiomyocytes of patients with HFpEF. Cardiovasc Res. 2024;120(9):999-1010.
42. Braunwald E. SGLT2 inhibitors: the statins of the 21st century. Eur Heart J. 2022;43(11):1029-30.
43. Verbrugge FH, Martens P, Ameloot K, et al. Spironolactone to increase natriuresis in congestive heart failure with cardiorenal syndrome. Acta Cardiol. 2019;74(2):100-7.
44. Filippatos G, Anker SD, Agarwal R, et al. Finerenone and cardiovascular outcomes in patients with chronic kidney disease and type 2 diabetes. Circulation. 2021;143(6):540-52.
45. Wang TD, Tan RS, Lee HY, et al. Effects of sacubitril/valsartan (LCZ696) on natriuresis, diuresis, blood pressures, and NT-proBNP in salt-sensitive hypertension. Hypertension. 2017;69(1):32-41.
46. Verma S, Pandey A, Pandey AK, et al. Aldosterone and aldosterone synthase inhibitors in cardiorenal disease. Am J Physiol Heart Circ Physiol. 2024;326(3):H670-88.
47. Bailey MA, Dhaun N. Salt sensitivity: causes, consequences, and recent advances. Hypertension. 2024;81(3):476-89.
48. Morimoto A, Uzu T, Fujii T, et al. Sodium sensitivity and cardiovascular events in patients with essential hypertension. Lancet. 1997;350(9093):1734-7.
49. Weinberger MH, Fineberg NS, Fineberg SE, et al. Salt sensitivity, pulse pressure, and death in normal and hypertensive humans. Hypertension. 2001;37(2 Pt 2):429-32.

CHAPTER

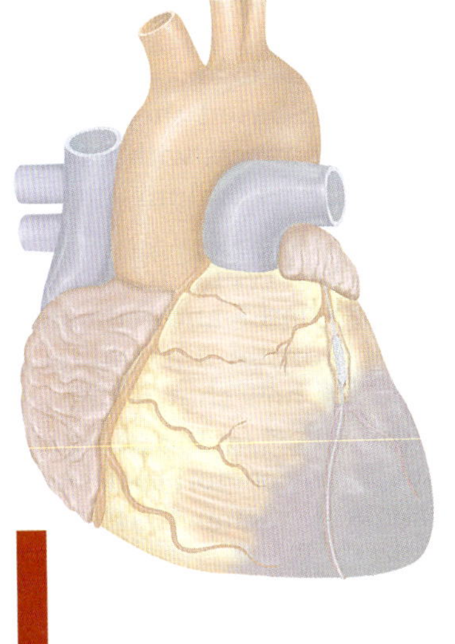

Exercise-induced Left Atrial Hypertension in HFpEF

Jayagopal PB

INTRODUCTION

The prevalence of heart failure with preserved ejection fraction (HFpEF) has continued to increase significantly during recent years. The incidence of HFpEF accounts for about 40–50% of overall heart failure (HF) cases worldwide and is associated with significant morbidity and mortality.[1] However, in India, this entity is seen only in one-third of patients with acute HF.[2] Earlier, the emphasis was on ejection fraction, but now the entity of HF with near-normal ejection fraction is recognized. This was earlier classified as diastolic HF. These patients have high filling pressures without a pronounced increase in ventricular chamber size. HFpEF is characterized by decreased stroke volume and cardiac output (CO).[3] This impaired left ventricular (LV) diastolic relaxation leads to elevated left atrial (LA) pressure during physical activity in HFpEF.[4] Exercise-induced left atrial hypertension (EILAH) is more prevalent in patients with HFmrEF and HFpEF.[5] Many patients with HFpEF have normal hemodynamics at rest, and abnormal values may arise during physiologically stressed conditions such as exercise.[6]

During exercise, the cardiovascular system undergoes several adaptive changes to meet the increased metabolic demands of the body. These include increased heart rate, stroke volume, CO, etc. During this time, the heart faces intermittent pressure and volume overload stress.[7] In a healthy heart, these changes lead to a moderate increase in LA pressure, which an efficient LV can easily accommodate. However, in HFpEF, the LV is stiff and nonefficient, which cannot accommodate increased volume and leads to elevated LA pressure.[8] The elevated LA pressure during exercise is transmitted backward to the pulmonary circulation, resulting in elevated pulmonary capillary wedge pressure (PCWP). This rise in PCWP is a key determinant factor of HFpEF.[9]

Exercise-induced left atrial hypertension patients are less likely to have comorbid conditions such as diabetes, hypertension, and chronic kidney diseases. Increased LA pressure during exertion is linked to HFpEF. Almost one-third of HFpEF patients have normal LA pressure at rest. EILAH patients demonstrate signs of an earlier or less severe stage of HF based on less cardiac remodeling and dysfunction, lack of atrial fibrillation, lack of loop diuretic therapy, lower systolic blood pressure, better 6-minute walk distance, and lower levels of natriuretic peptide. There was no difference in LV volume, LV mass, LVEF, or RA pressure during exercise and rest, but lower LA volume and lower pulmonary artery (PA) systolic pressure were observed during exercise in EILAH patients.[4]

Exercise-induced left atrial hypertension is predominately seen in patients who have HFpEF. Some patients have normal LA pressure at rest and elevated LA pressure during exercise.

DIAGNOSIS

In patients with EILAH with normal LV filling pressures at rest, diagnosis can be particularly difficult because the physical findings associated with congestion are frequently absent.[6] Invasive hemodynamic exercise testing is considered as a gold standard test for the diagnosis of HFpEF.[10] Diagnosis of EILAH can be difficult without exercise hemodynamic assessment. Exercise stress echocardiogram (ESE), cardiopulmonary exercise test (CPET), and right heart catheterization (RHC) during exercise were some diagnostic tools used for the detection of EILAH.

The gold standard for a different diagnosis of HFpEF is exercise testing and hemodynamic level. This would mean a PCWP ≥15 mm Hg at rest and a supine exercise PCWP >25 mm Hg at the end of the expiration and in upright exercise, PCWP ≥20 mm Hg is diagnostic. EILAH has been shown to predict long-term mortality. Age and LV mass were other predictors of increasing mortality.[9]

Pulmonary capillary wedge pressure relative to CO is considered as an indicator of dynamic left-sided filling pressure during increased exercise. An abnormal steep PCWP/CO slope >2.0 mm Hg/L/min is a key indicator for proper diagnosis. Three types of HFpEF have been described as per EILAH[9] **(Table 1)**.

Exercise PA systolic pressure >45 mm Hg is also associated with HFpEF.[6]

TABLE 1: Types of HFpEF.

Type	*Feature*
Type I HFpEF: Exercise-induced LA hypertension	Resting PCWP <15 mm Hg Peak exercise PCWP ≥25 mm Hg
Type II HFpEF: Resting LA hypertension	Resting PCWP ≥15 mm Hg, with no features of PVD, right ventricular (RV) dysfunction/failure, or tricuspid regurgitation (TR)
Type III HFpEF	Resting PCWP ≥15 mm Hg, with features of PVD, RV dysfunction/failure, or moderate TR

(HFpEF: heart failure and preserved ejection fraction; LA: left atrial; PCWP: pulmonary capillary wedge pressure; PVD: peripheral vascular disease)

MANAGEMENT

Management of EILAH is complex due to lack of specific therapies. Currently, no guideline-based therapeutic strategies are available for EILAH patients with HFpEF. The impact of approved drugs such as sodium–glucose cotransporter 2 inhibitors must be studied further. The EMPEROR-Preserved[11] and DELIVER[12] trials have shown excellent improvement in HFpEF and reduction in hospitalization. The newer nonsteroidal mineral receptor antagonist finerenone has now shown efficacy in this subset. What all these can reflect on the reduction in EILAH needs to be assessed. Many comorbidities and polypharmacy can further complicate therapy and lead to nonadherence.

Thus, a device therapy to unload the left atrium and divert blood to the right atrium and systemic veins to reduce LA pressure is appealing. Evidence suggests that atrial shunt therapy can dynamically unload LA and reduce LA pressure at rest and during exercise, which is beneficial for patients with EILAH with HFpEF than other categories.[10]

The initial trials in 44 patients showed reduced LA pressure with exercise. However, a larger randomized trial in 626 patients showed no difference in outcome at 1 year.[10] Some respondents in this group have been identified as all the same. Calculating exercise-induced increase in LA pressure and PA/RA pressure gradient on exercise is a bad sign. The presence of RV dysfunction and RHF are poor prognostic markers. It is, thus, essential to classify the HFpEF into three types as shown in **Flowchart 1**.

Thus, RV dysfunction and an increase in PA pressure and RA pressure during exercise would be a contraindication. If the PVR does not go beyond 1.75–1.8, it identifies a responder group.[10] CPET is a new method to identify responders. Impaired CO_2 augmentation during exercise showed a poor responder group. An increase in

Flowchart 1: HFpEF diagnosis.

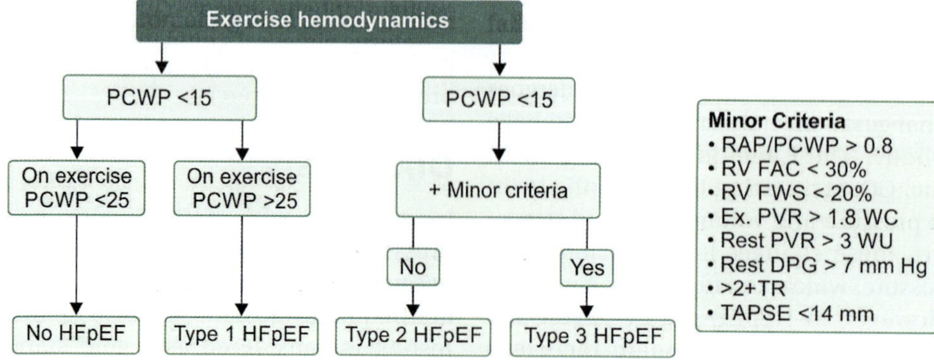

CO_2 during exercise probably explains the rise in PVR.[13] Newer therapies to reduce PVR and combine it with atrial shunting may be the future.

Wireless implantable PA pressure monitoring devices such as CardioMEMS[14] showed a 50% reduction in HF hospitalization, but the therapy, apart from the cost, needs support from the patients, doctors, and stakeholders.

Cardiac magnetic resonance imaging is useful for examining exercise-induced LV and RV volume changes. However, the availability of this modality is a severe limitation.

CONCLUSION

Exercise-induced left atrial hypertension present in HFpEF patients is a serious issue. It has been shown to predict long-term mortality.[4] Age and LV mass were other predictors of mortality. This will eventually worsen the severity of the disease. Early diagnosis of this entity can identify a group of patients who would be approached differently. The newer developments in medical and device therapy appear promising.

REFERENCES

1. Pfeffer MA, Shah AM, Borlaug BA, et al. Heart failure with preserved ejection fraction in perspective. Circ Res. 2019;124(11):1598-617.
2. Jayagopal PB, Sastry SL, Nanjappa V, et al. Clinical characteristics and 30-day outcomes in patients with acute decompensated heart failure: results from Indian College of Cardiology National Heart Failure Registry (ICCNHFR). Int J Cardiol. 2022;356:73-8.
3. Zile MR, Baicu CF, Gaasch WH. Diastolic heart failure–abnormalities in active relaxation and passive stiffness of the left ventricle. N Engl J Med. 2004;350:1953-9.
4. Dorfs S, Zeh W, Hochholzer W, et al. Pulmonary capillary wedge pressure during exercise and long-term mortality in patients with suspected heart failure with preserved ejection fraction. Eur Heart J. 2014;35(44):3103-12.
5. Litwin SE, Komtebedde J, Hu M, et al. Exercise-induced left atrial hypertension in heart failure with preserved ejection fraction. JACC Heart Fail. 2023;11(8):1103-17.
6. Borlaug BA, Nishimura RA, Sorajja P, et al. Exercise hemodynamics enhance diagnosis of early heart failure with preserved ejection fraction. Circ Heart Fail. 2010; 3(5):588-95.
7. Nystoriak MA, Bhatnagar A. Cardiovascular effects and benefits of exercise. Front Cardiovasc Med. 2018;5:135.
8. Omote K, Verbrugge FH, Borlaug BA, et al. Heart failure with preserved ejection fraction: mechanisms and treatment strategies. Annu Rev Med. 2022;73:321-37.
9. Eisman AS, Shah RV, Dhakal BP, et al. Pulmonary capillary wedge pressure patterns during exercise predict exercise capacity and incident heart failure. Circ Heart Fail. 2018;11(5):e004750.
10. Jagadeesan V, Gray WA, Shah SJ, et al. Atrial shunt therapy for heart failure: an update. J Soc Cardiovasc Angiogr Interv. 2023;2(6):101203.
11. Anker SD, Butler J, Filippatos G, et al. Empagliflozin in heart failure with a preserved ejection fraction. N Engl J Med. 2021;385:1451-61.
12. Solomon SD, McMurray JJV, Claggett B, et al. Dapagliflozin in heart failure with mildly reduced or preserved ejection fraction. N Engl J Med. 2022;387:1089-98.
13. Caravita S, Baratto C, Filippo A, et al. Shedding light on latent pulmonary vascular disease in heart failure with preserved ejection fraction. JACC Heart Fail. 2023;11(10): 1427-38.
14. Adamson PB, Abraham WT, Bourge RC, et al. Wireless pulmonary artery pressure monitoring guides management to reduce decompensation in heart failure with preserved ejection fraction. Circ Heart Fail. 2014;7(6): 935-44.

34

CHAPTER

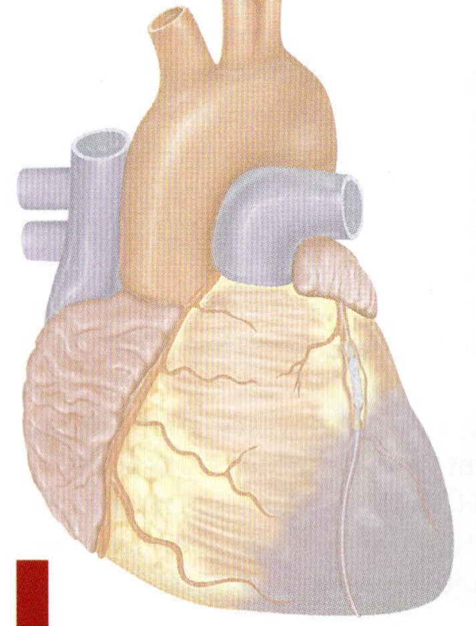

HFpEF and Left Atrial Cardiomyopathy: Advanced Therapeutic Navigation

HK Chopra, Viveka Kumar, CK Ponde, Aafreen Naik

INTRODUCTION

Heart failure with preserved ejection fraction (HFpEF) represents nearly half of all heart failure (HF) cases. Characterized by a left ventricular ejection fraction (LVEF) ≥50%, impaired diastolic function, and elevated natriuretic peptide levels, HFpEF is defined within the context of typical HF signs and symptoms.[1] The prevalence and incidence of HFpEF are rapidly growing, largely due to the aging population and increasing prevalence of predisposing conditions such as hypertension, obesity, metabolic syndrome, and diabetes.[2] Over the past two decades, the diagnostic approach to HFpEF has significantly evolved in parallel with our expanding scientific understanding of this complex syndrome.[3] HFpEF is associated with substantial morbidity and mortality, including a 35% 2-year hospitalization rate and a 14% 2-year mortality rate. HFpEF continues to increase by 10% relative to HF, with reduced ejection fraction (HFrEF) over the past decade.[2]

The HFpEF has long been considered primarily a disorder of the left ventricle (LV), characterized by increased stiffness in the LV and vasculature. However, recent insights reveal that HFpEF involves complex global myocardial and systemic abnormalities. Notably, the left atrium (LA) plays a critical role in HFpEF pathophysiology and disease progression. LA dysfunction in HFpEF is associated with a distinct phenotype featuring severe disease and poor outcomes.[4] The focus is now shifting from the LV to the LA, recognizing the latter's significant role in HFpEF. Historical debates about the definition and characterization of HFpEF have largely centered on LV, but emerging research emphasizes the importance of understanding LA remodeling and dysfunction.[5] Understanding and addressing LA dysfunction is crucial for improving HFpEF management and patient outcomes. Enhanced therapeutic strategies targeting the LA could pave the way for more effective treatments and better disease prognosis.[6]

Earlier studies have also highlighted the diagnostic and prognostic significance of LA size and pressure in HFpEF. Recent advancements, particularly echocardiographic speckle tracking strain, now allow for noninvasive assessment of LA function, including reservoir, conduit, and contractile strains. Among these, the LA reservoir strain has demonstrated robust prognostic value in HFpEF, surpassing both LV and right ventricular longitudinal strain.[6]

This chapter discusses the pathophysiological role of LA dysfunction in HFpEF and as a potential target in managing HFpEF.

HFpEF AS CLINICAL IMPLICATION OF LEFT ATRIUM DYSFUNCTION

The LA is a highly expandable, thin-walled structure essential for LV filling and optimizing cardiac output through its interactions with the LV and pulmonary veins throughout the cardiac cycle. The LA fulfills three primary functions, mechanical, endocrine, and regulatory. These functions are intricately connected and interdependent.[7] LA function has a distinct triphasic pattern, such as reservoir, conduit, and booster pump phases. During ventricular systole, the LA acts as a reservoir, collecting blood from the pulmonary veins. This phase is influenced by LA compliance and relaxation, as well as LV characteristics like the descent of the LV base during systole. In early diastole, the conduit phase occurs, where blood passively flows from the LA to the LV due to the pressure gradient. Finally, in late diastole, the booster pump phase involves active LA contraction, further enhancing LV filling and stroke volume.[8]

LEFT ATRIAL ATRIOPATHY AND LEFT ATRIAL DYSFUNCTION

The LA atriopathy includes a range of structural, functional, and electrical abnormalities. Structural abnormalities include left atrial enlargement and fibrosis, while the functional abnormalities include reduced contractility and decreased compliance. Electrical abnormalities associated with LA include atrial fibrillation (AF) and atrial flutter. Left atrial dysfunction is a specific subset of LA atriopathy, focusing on the impaired mechanical and electrical function of the LA.[8]

The LA dysfunction is critical in HF due to its impact on LV filling and cardiac output. LA stiffness impairs reservoir function, and LV longitudinal dysfunction worsens this by reducing passive LA stretch.[8] LA conduit dysfunction results from LV diastolic dysfunction, with early hypertensive heart disease temporarily enhancing LA pump function. In HFpEF, this compensation is absent due to high LV filling pressures.[8] LA dilatation initially compensates for early LV diastolic dysfunction by enhancing stroke volume but eventually leads to mechanical failure, causing pulmonary congestion and structural changes such as myocyte hypertrophy, fibrosis, and AF. LA dilatation also contributes to mitral regurgitation and worsens HF symptoms.[9] LA strain is a functional marker indicating LA stiffness and indirectly estimating LV end-diastolic pressure, but it should be interpreted cautiously due to its correlation with LV global longitudinal strain (GLS).[9]

Fibrosis is a key remodeling component in HFpEF. Clinical risk factors for HFpEF, such as obesity, hypertension, and diabetes, contribute to LA fibrosis through inflammation and oxidative stress.[6] LA remodeling and dysfunction, driven by elevated LV filling pressures, are prevalent and correlate with severe symptoms and adverse outcomes. Abnormal LA strain (<23%) and enlarged LA size predict worse NYHA class, higher hospitalization risk, and mortality.[10] The PROMIS-HFpEF study identified a distinct HFpEF subset with disproportionate left atrial myopathy, marked by significant LA dysfunction despite preserved LV function.[11]

ATRIAL FIBRILLATION IN HFpEF

The AF is a common comorbidity in HFpEF, leading to LA dysfunction and remodeling. HFpEF patients with AF exhibit reduced exercise capacity, severe right ventricular dysfunction, and higher mortality risk.[12] Increasing AF burden in HFpEF leads to a progressive decline in LA compliance and mechanics, leading to a distinct HFpEF phenotype with enhanced ventricular interaction, right HF, and worsening pulmonary vascular disease. Permanent AF in HFpEF is associated with severe biventricular dysfunction, high filling pressures, reduced LA function, and increased stiffness, necessitating distinct therapeutic approaches.[13] The close link between AF and HFpEF might be explained by intrinsic LA myopathy underlying both HFpEF and AF.[7]

DIAGNOSTIC AND PROGNOSTIC ROLE OF LEFT ATRIUM DYSFUNCTION IN HFpEF

The LA dilatation, indicating chronically elevated LA pressure, predicts hospitalization and mortality in HFpEF, especially with increased pulmonary pressure.[9] LA triphasic functions are sensitive markers for HFpEF severity.[14] LA dysfunction, measured by LA ejection fraction (LAEF), is linked to HF mortality and B-type natriuretic peptide (BNP) levels. It precedes HF in asymptomatic individuals, with LA reservoir strain being an independent predictor of HF and AF. Impaired LA reservoir strain (<18%) significantly increases mortality and HF risk.[8] Increased LA stiffness is a strong predictor of exercise intolerance and poor quality of life, particularly in older, obese patients. The LA stiffness index (LAS_r) correlates with adverse events, including HF hospitalization and mortality, highlighting its prognostic importance. High LA stiffness exacerbates exercise intolerance and dyspnea, suggesting that reducing LA stiffness could be a therapeutic target in HFpEF.[15] Monitoring LA dimensional changes may reflect treatment effects on LA pressure and function, benefiting atrial myocytes and the extracellular matrix, highlighting LA dysfunction as a potential therapeutic target in HFpEF.[16] Overall, LA dysfunction, particularly measured through LA strain and stiffness, holds significant diagnostic and prognostic value in HFpEF. Therapeutic strategies focusing on LA unloading and function augmentation may benefit HFpEF patients, potentially improving prognosis and quality of life.

DIAGNOSIS OF LEFT ATRIUM DYSFUNCTION

Evaluating LA function offers better prognostic value than measuring LA size in HF patients. Volumetric analysis, which measures maximum, minimum, and preatrial contraction volumes, is commonly used for this purpose.[9] Currently, there is no single gold-standard test for diagnosing LA dysfunction. The choice of diagnostic method varies with the clinical scenario, and a combination of multiple diagnostic approaches is recommended for the most sensitive detection of LA dysfunction.[17]

Role of Imaging Modalities

Noninvasive imaging techniques such as transthoracic echocardiography (TTE) and cardiac magnetic resonance (CMR) are vital for assessing LA deformation in cardiac diseases. Strain and strain rate imaging allows early detection of preclinical conditions by measuring myocardial deformation and its rate over time. LA strain (LAS) and LA strain rate (LASR) are less affected by loading conditions than LA volume, offering reliable atrial function indicators.[8] Both TTE and CMR can measure LAS and LASR during the LA reservoir, conduit, and contraction phases.[10] Using postprocessing software, TTE, and CMR analyze LAS and LASR from standard cine images, enhancing understanding of LA function in HFpEF and other atriopathies, supporting diagnosis and treatment.[8]

2D-Speckle Tracking Echocardiography

Speckle tracking echocardiography (STE) is a cutting-edge imaging technique crucial for assessing LA size, volume, and function. Unlike traditional tissue Doppler imaging (TDI), STE provides accurate myocardial deformation analysis without angle dependency using frame-by-frame tracking of the speckles pattern generated by the interactions between ultrasound and myocardial tissue.[9] STE can accurately quantify LA reservoir, conduit, and booster functions, detecting early dysfunction before visible changes occur.[4] STE generates strain and strain rate curves by tracing the LA endocardium. Nonforeshortened views and using ventricular end-diastole as the reference frame for zero strain are recommended, although image quality can be challenging in some patients.[8] STE provides comprehensive cardiac function data, crucial for detecting subtle myocardial damage. It also offers significant diagnostic and prognostic value in HF.[17] Overall, STE is a valuable tool in managing HFpEF and LA atriopathy, offering detailed myocardial insights, early dysfunction detection, and robust diagnostic and prognostic capabilities.

Feature Tracking Cardiac Magnetic Resonance

Feature tracking (FT) in CMR imaging assesses myocardial strain using standard cine images processed with specialized software. CMR offers better spatial resolution, signal, and contrast ratios compared to TTE, enhancing tracking accuracy.[8] ESC guidelines recommend measuring LA volumes and LV mass in suspected HFpEF. CMR is the gold standard for cardiac volumes, mass, and ejection fractions, especially with suboptimal echocardiographic images, and is key for assessing myocardial fibrosis.[10] The accuracy of echocardiography relies on a clear definition of the LA endocardial border, while CMR provides superior reproducibility for LA volumetric analysis.[18] The ability of CMR to scan any plane with excellent spatial resolution and contrast makes it the preferred imaging modality. Despite three-dimensional echocardiography (3DE) correlating well with CMR or cardiac computed tomography (CCT) volumes, CMR remains the gold standard for left atrial volume (LAV) measurement due to its precise endocardial definition and detection of myocardial pathologies.[9]

Biomarkers of Left Atrial Dysfunction

The HFpEF involves a distinct pathophysiological condition characterized by specific biomarker alterations. The RELAX trial has highlighted the elevation of biomarkers related to neurohormonal activation and myocardial necrosis in patients with HFpEF. Elevated NT-proBNP levels over time are indicative of continuous congestion in HFpEF, closely linked with diminished LA function.[19] The presence of elevated neurohormonal and myocardial necrosis biomarkers independently correlates with impaired LA mechanics, forming a unique profile in HFpEF patients. Lower LA reservoir strain is also associated with persistent NT-proBNP elevation, suggesting that impaired LA function contributes significantly to ongoing congestion and adverse clinical outcomes in HFpEF.[19]

LEFT ATRIUM DYSFUNCTION AS TARGET FOR TREATMENT OF HFpEF

In patients with HFpEF, the primary therapeutic goals are symptom relief, functional status improvement, and reduced hospital admissions. Diuretics, particularly loop diuretics, are the cornerstone of HFpEF management, tailored based on the degree of volume overload.[20] Current HFpEF guidelines emphasize managing underlying conditions such as hypertension and AF rather than HFpEF-specific therapies.[10] Unlike HFrEF, HFpEF lacks definitive therapies that improve outcomes.[9] Also, there is a lack of large-scale randomized controlled trials to establish specific therapies for HFpEF with AF.[20]

Advanced imaging techniques improved the evaluation of LA function, offering potential therapeutic targets in HFpEF. The concept of LA reverse remodeling, which involves improving LA function by reducing LA pressure and volume overload, is gaining more attention.

Notably, improvements in LA function often correlate with enhanced LVEF and reduced LA volume.[9] In response to the growing understanding of the critical role of LA in the pathophysiology of HFpEF, new devices to unload and/or decompress the LA are increasingly being evaluated.[21] These devices have the potential to address specific aspects of HFpEF that pharmacological treatments alone may not fully address.[6] Current device therapies for managing HFpEF are designed to mitigate LA pressure or pulmonary capillary wedge pressure (PCWP) through various means, which can effectively improve symptoms and quality of life while reducing the risk of readmission for HF. However, these device-based therapies for HFpEF are still in their early stages, and more research is required to identify which HFpEF phenotypes benefit most from these interventions.[22]

ATRIAL SHUNT DEVICES

Atrial shunt devices are designed to overcome the limitations of conventional treatments for patients with HFpEF. The rationale behind these devices is to create a controlled shunt between the atria, which helps to lower LA pressure, alleviate symptoms, and improve hemodynamic stability.[21] Several atrial shunt devices are under investigation, each with distinct designs and features. **Table 1** summarizes clinical trials evaluating different atrial shunt devices.

Interatrial Shunt Device

The interatrial shunt device (IASD) features a self-expanding nitinol frame that creates an 8 mm shunt between the atria.[31] This design facilitates a continuous left-to-right shunt, which helps in reducing LA pressure.[32] The concept of IASD is inspired by the observation that, in Lutembacher's syndrome, patients with mitral stenosis and a congenital atrial septal defect experience fewer symptoms due to the reduction in LA pressure.[32] The IASD received approval in 2016 as the first transcatheter device for HFpEF.[22]

Clinical trials, including the series of REDUCE LAP-HF studies, have shown that the IASD effectively lowers LA pressure and improves symptoms, with favorable safety outcomes and maintained device patency over 12 months.[22] Open-label REDUCE LAP-HF study showed

TABLE 1: Clinical trials evaluating atrial shunt devices and left atrial pacing therapy in heart failure with preserved ejection fraction.

Trial name	*Device/therapy*	*Study design*	*Patients*	*Follow-up*	*Primary outcomes*
REDUCE LAP-HF[23]	IASD	Phase 1, open-label, single-arm trial	*n* = 64 Symptomatic HFpEF (LVEF ≥40%) and elevated PCWP (>15 mm Hg) at rest and (*n* = >25 mm Hg during exercise)	6 months	Significant improvements in exercise hemodynamics, 6MWD, and MLWHFQ score; the device was well-tolerated
REDUCE LAP-HF I[24]	IASD	Phase 2, randomized, parallel-group, blinded, sham-multicenter trial	*n* = 44 NYHA III or ambulatory IV HF, LVEF ≥40%, exercise PCWP ≥25 mm Hg, and PCWP-right atrial pressure gradient ≥5 mm Hg	1 month	Reduction in PCWP during exercise compared to sham control
REDUCE LAP-HF II[25]	IASD	Phase 3, randomized, multicenter, blinded, sham-controlled trial	*n* = 326 Symptomatic HF patients with LVEF ≥40% and elevated resting or exercise PCWP	12 months	No reduction in cardiovascular death, nonfatal ischemic stroke, first and recurrent HF events, and no improvement in health status
First-in-human study (V-wave)[26]	V-wave device	Single-arm, open-label	*n* = 38 (HFrEF: *n* = 30; HFpEF: *n* = 8) NYHA class III HF	12 months	Significant improvement in NYHA functional class, QOL, and 6MWD; high incidence shunt stenosis or occlusion
RELIEVE-HF[27]	V-wave device	Prospective, randomized, double-blinded study	*n* = 97 Symptomatic HF patients, LVEF ≥40% in 50% of patients, NYHA class III	12 months	Favorable clinical effects improved KCCQ; safety endpoints achieved

Contd...

Contd...

Trial name	Device/ therapy	Study design	Patients	Follow-up	Primary outcomes
PRELIEVE[28]	Atrial flow regulator	Single-arm, open-label, prospective, nonrandomized, study	NYHA class III HF, LVEF ≥ 40%, elevated PCWP	12 months	AFR implantation was feasible and safe; improvements were observed in NYHA class, 6MWD, KCCQ, PCWP, and NT-proBNP in some individuals
myPACE[29]	Left atrial pacing therapy	Prospective, blinded, parallel-group, randomized trial	Stage B and C HFpEF	12 months	Improved MLHFQ scores, NT-proBNP, physical activity, and atrial fibrillation
RAPID-HF[30]	Left atrial pacing therapy	Single-center, double-blind, randomized, crossover trial	Symptomatic HFpEF and chronotropic incompetence	16 weeks	No significant improvement in cardiac output, exercise capacity, QOL score, and serum NT-proBNP levels with atrial pacing; increase in adverse events.

(6MWD: 6-min walk distance; AFR: atrial flow regulator; IASD: Interatrial Shunt Device; HFpEF: heart failure with preserved ejection fraction; KCCQ: Kansas City Cardiomyopathy Questionnaire; LVEF: left ventricular ejection fraction; MLHFQ: Minnesota Living With Heart Failure Questionnaire; NT-proBNP: N-terminal pro-B-type natriuretic peptide; PCWP: pulmonary capillary wedge pressure; QOL: quality of life)

that IASD is feasible and might be associated with improvements in exercise hemodynamics, functional capacity, and quality of life.[23] Subsequently, the sham-controlled REDUCE LAP-HF I trial confirmed these findings, showing long-term patency and a favorable safety profile for the IASD.[24] However, the small sample size of these two studies limited their ability to detect significant differences in hospitalization rates and quality of life measures.[33] REDUCE LAP-HF II, a phase 3, randomized, is underway. However, results from the 12-month follow-up indicate that the atrial shunt device did not reduce HF events or improve health status in this patient population.[25]

V-wave Device

The V-wave system is an hourglass-shaped, self-expanding prosthesis made of a nitinol frame, with a polytetrafluoroethylene (PTFE) skirt on both sides of the septum and a porcine trileaflet valve on the right atrial side to prevent right-to-left flow.[31,32] The first-in-human study assessing the V-wave system in patients with HFrEF and HFpEF demonstrated a 100% initial implant success rate. However, within 12 months, half of the devices became occluded or stenotic. Despite this, patients with preserved shunt patency showed improved hemodynamics.[26] The observations of this study prompted the creation of a second-generation device, which preserved the hourglass shape but eliminated the valve component; instead, a 5.1-mm central opening was created.[34] RELIEVE-HF trial is an ongoing randomized, sham-controlled trial evaluating the safety and efficacy of the second-generation V-wave shunt in advanced cases of both HFrEF and HFpEF. The primary outcomes of this trial are recently published. The study found that the V-wave system is safe and produces favorable clinical effects in patients with HF, regardless of LVEF, supporting the potential of this shunt device as a treatment for HF.[27]

Atrial Flow Regulator

The atrial flow regulator (AFR) is a self-expandable double-disc wired mesh device with a central penetration that facilitates IASD. This device is made from nitinol and is available in various fenestration (6, 8, and 10 mm) and total device diameters (18, 24, and 30 mm). It is implanted through a femoral vein using a 10- to 12-Fr sheath, and postimplantation antiplatelet therapy is typically administered.[22,31] ARF is designed to allow interatrial bidirectional flow.[34] The PRELIEVE study investigated AFR implantation in both HFpEF and HFrEF patients over a follow-up period of up to 1 year. The study found that AFR implantation was feasible and safe, with improvements observed in assessed parameters in some but not all patients.[28] Currently, several studies are ongoing to further assess the AFR. The ongoing PROLONGER study is aimed to identify invasive and noninvasive parameters predictive of a favorable response to AFR therapy in HF patients.[35]

Challenges and Future Directions

The long-term outcomes of atrial shunt devices, including their impact on mortality and hospitalization rates, are still uncertain. The durability of these devices and the potential for adverse effects need further investigation. Additionally, the optimal criteria for patient selection and the timing of device implantation are not yet fully defined.[21,22]

LEFT ATRIAL PACING THERAPY

Echocardiographic studies have identified interatrial dyssynchrony as a common issue in HFpEF, associated with reduced LA function and exacerbated clinical symptoms. This suggests that targeting interatrial dyssynchrony might be an effective treatment strategy.[22] LA pacing, which involves stimulating the LA via specially designed coronary sinus leads, is now being explored for atrial resynchronization in HFpEF patients.[36] **Table 1** summarizes clinical trials evaluating left atrial pacing therapy in HFpEF.

The myPACE trial, which focused on patients with HFpEF and preexisting pacemakers, demonstrated that personalized, moderately accelerated pacing improved quality of life, reduced NT-proBNP levels, increased physical activity, and positively impacted AF compared to conventional pacing settings.[29] This indicates that adjusting pacemaker settings to align with individual patients' heart rates could enhance clinical outcomes. While the outcomes of the RAPID-HF trial suggested that the benefits of pacing may be variable and potentially associated with risks.[30] Ongoing research includes the PACE HFpEF trial, which is evaluating the effects of continuously accelerated pacing in patients without standard pacing indications in HFpEF patients.[37]

CONCLUSION AND FUTURE PERSPECTIVES

The increasing prevalence of HFpEF calls for better diagnostic and therapeutic strategies. This chapter highlighted the role of LA dysfunction in HFpEF, emphasizing its impact on disease severity, prognosis, and symptom management. Advancements in imaging techniques, particularly echocardiographic speckle tracking and cardiac magnetic resonance, have improved our ability to assess LA function and predict disease progression. The emerging focus on LA as a therapeutic target has led to novel interventions, including atrial shunt devices and pacing strategies aimed at alleviating LA pressure and improving patient outcomes.

Future research should focus on large-scale randomized trials to validate the benefits and safety of atrial shunt therapy and explore its combination with other treatments. Innovations in imaging and device design will be crucial for improving patient outcomes and refining management strategies for HFpEF. A proactive approach to device therapy could enhance treatment efficacy beyond current standards.

REFERENCES

1. Harper AR, Patel HC, Lyon AR. Heart failure with preserved ejection fraction. Clin Med (Lond). 2018;18(Suppl 2):s24-9.
2. Roh J, Hill JA, Singh A, et al. Heart failure with preserved ejection fraction: heterogeneous syndrome, diverse preclinical models. Circ Res. 2022;130(12):1906-25.
3. Borlaug BA, Sharma K, Shah SJ, et al. Heart failure with preserved ejection fraction: JACC scientific statement. J Am Coll Cardiol. 2023;81(18):1810-34.
4. Omote K, Borlaug BA. Left atrial myopathy in heart failure with preserved ejection fraction. Circ J. 2023;87(8): 1039-46.
5. Khan MS, Memon MM, Murad MH, et al. Left atrial function in heart failure with preserved ejection fraction: a systematic review and meta-analysis. Eur J Heart Fail. 2020;22(3):472-85.
6. Freed BH, Shah SJ. Stepping out of the left ventricle's shadow: time to focus on the left atrium in heart failure with preserved ejection fraction. Circ Cardiovasc Imaging. 2017;10(4):e006267.
7. Jin X, Nauta JF, Hung CL, et al. Left atrial structure and function in heart failure with reduced (HFrEF) versus preserved ejection fraction (HFpEF): systematic review and meta-analysis. Heart Fail Rev. 2022;27(5):1933-55.
8. Alfuhied A, Kanagala P, McCann GP, et al. Multi-modality assessment and role of left atrial function as an imaging biomarker in cardiovascular disease. Int J Cardiovasc Imaging. 2021;37(11):3355-69.
9. Carpenito M, Fanti D, Mega S, et al. The central role of left atrium in heart failure. Front Cardiovasc Med. 2021;8:704762.
10. Dzhioeva O, Belyavskiy E. Diagnosis and management of patients with heart failure with preserved ejection fraction (HFpEF): current perspectives and recommendations. Ther Clin Risk Manag. 2020;16:769-85.
11. Patel RB, Lam CSP, Svedlund S, et al. Disproportionate left atrial myopathy in heart failure with preserved ejection fraction among participants of the PROMIS-HFpEF study. Sci Rep. 2021;11(1):4885.
12. Zheng R, Kusunose K. Linkage of left atrial function to heart failure with preserved ejection fraction. Int Heart J. 2023;64(1):4-9.
13. Reddy YNV, Obokata M, Verbrugge FH, et al. Atrial dysfunction in patients with heart failure with preserved ejection fraction and atrial fibrillation. J Am Coll Cardiol. 2020;76(9):1051-64.
14. Liu L, Sun M. Can left atrial function be used as a marker for evaluating the severity of heart failure with preserved ejection fraction? Int J Integr Cardiol. 2021;3(2):125.
15. Singleton MJ, Nelson MB, Samuel TJ, et al. Left atrial stiffness index independently predicts exercise intolerance and quality of life in older, obese patients with heart

failure with preserved ejection fraction. J Card Failure. 2022;28(4):567-75.
16. Inciardi RM, Pagnesi M, Lombardi CM, et al. Clinical implications of left atrial changes after optimization of medical therapy in patients with heart failure. Eur J Heart Fail. 2022;24(11):2131-9.
17. Peigh G, Shah SJ, Patel RB. Left atrial myopathy in atrial fibrillation and heart failure: clinical implications, mechanisms, and therapeutic targets. Curr Heart Fail Rep. 2021;18(3):85-98.
18. Kanagala P, Arnold JR, Cheng ASH, et al. Left atrial ejection fraction and outcomes in heart failure with preserved ejection fraction. Int J Cardiovasc Imaging. 2020;36(1):101-10.
19. Patel RB, Alenezi F, Sun JL, et al. Biomarker profile of left atrial myopathy in heart failure with preserved ejection fraction: Insights from the RELAX Trial. J Card Fail. 2020;26(3):270-5.
20. Jasinska-Piadlo A, Campbell P. Management of patients with heart failure and preserved ejection fraction. Heart. 2023;109(11):874-83.
21. Jagadeesan V, Gray WA, Shah SJ. Atrial shunt therapy for heart failure: an update. journal of the society for cardiovascular angiography and interventions. 2023;2(6):101203.
22. Wu Y, Song M, Wu M, et al. Advances in device-based treatment of heart failure with preserved ejection fraction: evidence from clinical trials. ESC Heart Fail. 2024;11(1):13-27.
23. Hasenfuß G, Hayward C, Burkhoff D, et al. A transcatheter intracardiac shunt device for heart failure with preserved ejection fraction (REDUCE LAP-HF): a multicentre, open-label, single-arm, phase 1 trial. Lancet. 2016;387(10025):1298-304.
24. Feldman T, Mauri L, Kahwash R, et al. Transcatheter Interatrial Shunt Device for the Treatment of Heart Failure With Preserved Ejection Fraction [REDUCE LAP-HF I (Reduce Elevated Left Atrial Pressure in Patients With Heart Failure)]: A Phase 2, Randomized, Sham-Controlled Trial. Circulation. 2018;137(4):364-75.
25. Shah SJ, Borlaug BA, Chung ES, et al. Atrial shunt device for heart failure with preserved and mildly reduced ejection fraction (REDUCE LAP-HF II): a randomised, multicentre, blinded, sham-controlled trial. The Lancet. 2022;399(10330):1130-40.
26. Rodés-Cabau J, Bernier M, Amat-Santos IJ, et al. Interatrial shunting for heart failure: early and late results from the first-in-human experience with the v-wave system. JACC Cardiovasc Interv. 2018;11(22):2300-10.
27. Rodés-Cabau J, Lindenfeld J, Abraham WT, et al. Interatrial shunt therapy in advanced heart failure: outcomes from the open-label cohort of the RELIEVE-HF trial. Eur J Heart Failure. 2024;26(4):1078-89.
28. Paitazoglou C, Özdemir R, Pfister R, et al. The AFR-PRELIEVE trial: a prospective, non-randomised, pilot study to assess the Atrial Flow Regulator (AFR) in heart failure patients with either preserved or reduced ejection fraction. EuroIntervention. 2019;15(5):403-10.
29. Infeld M, Wahlberg K, Cicero J, et al. Effect of personalized accelerated pacing on quality of life, physical activity, and atrial fibrillation in patients with preclinical and overt heart failure with preserved ejection fraction: The myPACE Randomized Clinical Trial. JAMA Cardiology. 2023;8(3):213-21.
30. Reddy YNV, Koepp KE, Carter R, et al. Rate-adaptive atrial pacing for heart failure with preserved ejection fraction. JAMA. 2023;329(10):801-9.
31. Miyagi C, Miyamoto T, Karimov JH, et al. Device-based treatment options for heart failure with preserved ejection fraction. Heart Fail Rev. 2021;26(4):749-62.
32. Kaye DM, Nanayakkara S. Interatrial shunt device for heart failure with preserved ejection fraction. Front Cardiovasc Med. 2019;6:143.
33. Maryniak A, Maisuradze N, Ahmed R, et al. Heart failure with preserved ejection fraction update: a review of clinical trials and new therapeutic considerations. Cardiol J. 2022;29(4):670-9.
34. Riccardi M, Tomasoni D, Vizzardi E, et al. Device-based percutaneous treatments to decompress the left atrium in heart failure with preserved ejection fraction. Heart Fail Rev. 2023;28(2):315-30.
35. Lewicki Ł, Kosmalska K, Liedtke S, et al. Pomeranian atRial flOw reguLatOr iN conGestive hEart failuRe (PROLONGER): Study protocol. Cardiol J. 2020;27(6):879-83.
36. Shear FE. Novel paradigms in the therapeutic management of heart failure with preserved ejection fraction: clinical perspectives. Am J Cardiovasc Dis. 2019;9(5):91-108.
37. Habel N, Infeld M, Bernknopf J, et al. Rationale and design of the PACE HFpEF trial: physiologic accelerated pacing as a holistic treatment of heart failure with preserved ejection fraction. Heart Rhythm O2. 2024;5(1):41-9.

Hypertrophic Cardiomyopathy: As a Mimicker of HFpEF in Consideration of ACC 2023 Expert Consensus Decision Pathway for HFpEF

S Shanmugasundaram, Ilayaraja Uthirapthi, Samuel Jebavaram, Vinodkumar BG

INTRODUCTION

Hypertrophic cardiomyopathy (HCM) is an inherited condition, transmitted in an autosomal dominant pattern with variable penetrance and expressivity. It is common globally, affecting one in 200–500 individuals in the population.[1] Heterogeneity is the hallmark of this condition in terms of causative genes, degree and distribution of hypertrophy, the presence and level of obstruction, severity of diastolic function impairment, clinical presentation, and arrhythmic potential including sudden cardiac arrest and outcomes. Though many have no or minimal symptoms, considerable number of individuals have limiting symptoms. In the HCM Registry of National Heart Lung and Blood Institute (NHLBI),[2] two-thirds of the enrolled 2,762 patients were asymptomatic. Class II dyspnea occurred in 26.2% and class III–IV in 7.2%. The other symptoms with which HCM may present include chest pain, palpitation, and syncope. Since the most common symptom is dyspnea, there is every likelihood that it may be misdiagnosed as heart failure with preserved ejection fraction (HFpEF). Diagnosis of HCM is straightforward if the characteristic clinical and echo features of dynamic obstruction are present or when hypertrophy is segmental and nonuniform with abrupt transition to the adjacent normal segments and when it occurs exclusively in unusual locations such as basal anterolateral wall, apex or inferior wall. But if LV hypertrophy is apparently uniform and mild-to-moderate in severity without features of dynamic obstruction, differentiating HCM from the syndrome of HFpEF is difficult. HFpEF is equally a heterogeneous disorder of different causes, phenotypes, and clinical presentation. Diagnosis of HFpEF is unambiguous when patients present with features of pulmonary or systemic congestion and echocardiography documents normal EF and rules out valvular, pericardial, and pulmonary vascular diseases. But a considerable number of individuals with HFpEF present with effort dyspnea without signs of congestion, the so-called ambulant HFpEF, in whom diagnosis may be difficult. Presence of left ventricular hypertrophy (LVH) and left atrial enlargement, occurrence of atrial fibrillation (AF) and elevation of natriuretic peptides (NP) are features that can occur in both the conditions. Despite such overlaps, differentiating HCM from HFpEF is mandatory as the prognosis and treatment options are different. This article addresses the important issues of how HCM could masquerade as HFpEF and why HCM should be viewed as an HFpEF mimic rather than one of the causes of it.

HYPERTROPHIC CARDIOMYOPATHY—A CAUSE OR MIMIC OF HEART FAILURE WITH PRESERVED EJECTION FRACTION

The HF and sudden cardiac death are important causes of cardiac death among HCM patients. In a cohort study of 4,893 patients with HCM recruited at 7 European referral centers followed up for a median period of 6.2 years, 2.8% died of HF and 1.7% required cardiac transplant. In this cohort, SCD occurred in 2.8% and aborted SCD in 0.6%.[3] Though the current consensus is to view HCM as a HF mimic, few authors have preferred to consider it as one of the causes of HFpEF. For example, in the single

Flowchart 1

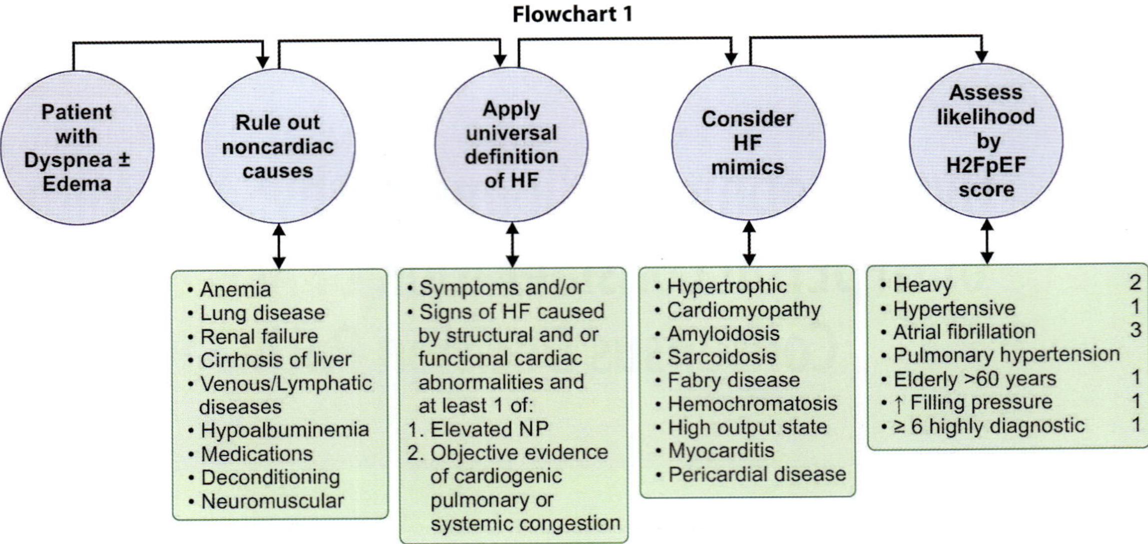

center study of Liu et al., 43.5% of 1,178 patients with HCM were diagnosed to have HFpEF based on 2017 AHA criteria (symptoms and signs of HF, EF >50% and elevated NT-proBNP >800 pg/mL). Those with the diagnosis of HFpEF were more often females and had greater LV wall thickness, higher left ventricular outflow gradient, and higher proportion of AF. The incidence of all cause death and cardiovascular death (CV death) was higher in the HFpEF group, 1.92 and 1.51 per 100 patient years respectively versus 0.96 and 0.70 in the non HF group. The incidence of SCD was similar, 0.53 versus 0.47 per 100 patient years. In the multivariate analysis, the presence of HF was an independent cause of all cause death and CV death with a HR of 2.0 and 1.82, respectively.[4] Contrary to this approach, the recently published ACC Expert Consensus decision pathway on management of HFpEF, has included HCM as one of the mimics rather than the cause of HFpEF.[5] The document recommends that the diagnostic pathway in an individual presenting with dyspnea and/or edema, should proceed stepwise, starting from exclusion of noncardiac causes of dyspnea or edema, application of Universal definition of HF, consideration of HF mimics, and finally using a valid scoring system like H2FpEF score to assess the probability of HFpEF **(Flowchart 1)**.

CLINICAL DIAGNOSIS OF HEART FAILURE

The first step in the algorithm is to identify the symptoms and signs of heart failure. Though not systematically used by clinicians, Framingham criteria provide a framework of assessing the symptoms/signs of heart failure.[6] Clinical diagnosis of HF requires the simultaneous presence of at least 2 major criteria or 1 major criterion in conjunction with 2 minor criteria. Major criteria include, paroxysmal nocturnal dyspnea, neck vein distension, rales, radiographic cardiomegaly (increasing heart size on chest radiography), acute pulmonary edema, S3 gallop, increased central venous pressure (>16 cm H_2O at right atrium), hepatojugular reflux, circulation time of >25 seconds, and weight loss >4.5 kg in 5 days in response to treatment. Minor criteria are bilateral ankle edema, nocturnal cough, dyspnea on ordinary exertion, hepatomegaly, pleural effusion, decrease in vital capacity by one-third from maximum recorded, and tachycardia (heart rate >120 beats/min). Minor criteria are acceptable only if they cannot be attributed to another medical condition such as pulmonary hypertension, chronic lung disease, cirrhosis, ascites, or the nephrotic syndrome. Noncardiac causes of dyspnea include anemia, obesity, lung and pleural diseases, upper airway obstruction, musculoskeletal disorders like polymyositis, muscular dystrophies or amyotrophic lateral sclerosis, kyphoscoliosis, restriction of diaphragmatic movement as in phrenic nerve palsy, ascites or intra-abdominal mass, chronic renal disease, thyroid disorders, anxiety, physical deconditioning, abnormal hemoglobins, etc. Noncardiac causes of edema include, hypoalbuminemia caused by malnutrition or malabsorption, chronic liver or renal diseases, obstructive sleep apnea, hypothyroidism, portal hypertension, venous disorders of legs like deep vein thrombosis (usually unilateral), varicose veins, May-Thurner syndrome (left leg edema), chronic venous insufficiency, post-thrombotic/phlebitis syndrome, pregnancy, medications like calcium blockers, pioglitazone, steroids, etc., inferior vena cava obstruction, and lymphatic disorders like filarial lymphangitis, Turner and Noonan syndrome, etc. Lipedema, a condition that mimics edema presents with limb swelling that starts from hip, progresses toward lower leg, and spares feet. It is nonpitting and lumpy with uneven surface. It may be painful and tender and skin may show bruises. By interfering with lymph drainage, secondary lymphedema may superimpose.

UNIVERSAL DEFINITION OF HEART FAILURE

Once such noncardiac causes are ruled out, the diagnosis of heart failure may be considered when the criteria of Universal definition of heart failure are present.[7]

It requires the presence of symptoms/signs of heart failure, caused by structural/functional cardiac abnormalities and at least one of the following: (1) elevated NP or (2) objective evidence of cardiogenic pulmonary or systemic congestion. Based on LV ejection fraction (EF), HF is classified into HF with reduced EF (<40%), HF with mildly reduced EF (41–50%) and HF with preserved EF (>50%). HFpEF is defined as a condition with a clinical diagnosis of HF and LVEF ≥50%, not attributable to an underlying cause such as an infiltrative cardiomyopathy, HCM, valvular disease, pericardial disease, or high-output HF.

HEART FAILURE WITH PRESERVED EJECTION FRACTION MIMICS

The HFpEF mimics are defined as those conditions that manifest the classical symptoms and signs of HF with an EF of ≥50% but with a primary noncardiac cause (kidney or liver disease) or a cardiac cause (infiltrative cardiomyopathy, HCM, valvular disease, pericardial disease, or high-output HF).[8] HFpEF is a systemic disease characterized by the presence of multiple metabolic/comorbid conditions with a common hemodynamic expression namely elevated filling pressures at rest or on exercise. The HFpEF mimics may also have the same hemodynamic feature that leads to effort intolerance and a congested state. But the underlying cause is unique as in infiltrative diseases such as amyloidosis, hemochromatosis, Fabry's disease, or as in genetically mediated condition like HCM. Most of the mimics, particularly the infiltrative diseases may have noncardiac systemic manifestations, but the cause remains singular. For example, in amyloidosis, the causative factor is extracellular deposition of a misfolded protein, amyloid in heart and other organs leading to protean manifestations. HCM is one of the mimics in which cardiac involvement is the only feature and noncardiac manifestations are absent. Since these conditions have a specific cause, the treatment and prognosis are different for each.

SIMILARITIES AND DISSIMILARITIES OF HYPERTROPHIC CARDIOMYOPATHY AND HEART FAILURE WITH PRESERVED EJECTION FRACTION

The clinical and imaging features of HCM may apparently fit in with the definition of HFpEF; effort dyspnea is the most common presenting symptom, EF is normal or supranormal, unless it progresses to dilated hypokinetic phenotype (burn out disease), structural abnormalities such as LVH and left atrial enlargement are universally present, filling pressures are elevated at rest or on effort and NP levels may be elevated. However, symptomatic HCM patients differ from conventional HFpEF in many ways. HFpEF is a systemic disease characterized by the presence of (1) systemic inflammation caused by the typical comorbid conditions such as obesity, hypertension, coronary artery disease (CAD), AF, chronic kidney disease (CKD), diabetes or metabolic syndrome (MS), chronic obstructive pulmonary disease (COPD), obstructive sleep apnea, etc. (2) structural and functional abnormalities of heart in the form of LVH, impairment of relaxation ± increased stiffness of myocardium caused by diseased myocytes or interstitium, left atrial enlargement or dysfunction, abnormal ventriculo-arterial coupling, chronotropic incompetence, subtle abnormalities of systolic function, and impaired contractile reserve, and (3) microvascular inflammation, and endothelial activation. But the pathophysiology of symptoms in HCM are limited to the heart.

In all the three phenotypes of HF, volume overload is common presenting with pulmonary edema/pedal edema, diastolic dysfunction of grade II–III occurs in the majority, functional MR, pulmonary hypertension and RV dysfunction are frequent, renal impairment and comorbid conditions are usually present, repeated hospitalizations for worsening of HF are common, and annual mortality is around 10%. On the contrary, signs of right heart failure such as elevation of jugular venous pressure, edema, and hepatomegaly are extremely rare in HCM, unless it progresses to the end stage or "burn out" phase. End-stage HCM often mimics HFrEF in terms of clinical presentation and echo findings. However, some degree of residual LVH is often present and LV dilatation is only mild-to-moderate. Documentation of classical features of HCM prior to the onset of this terminal phase might also help in establishing the diagnosis. Nearly two-thirds of the patients with HCM may present with obstruction either at rest or on provocation. In obstructive HCM (HOCM), HF symptoms such as dyspnea and fatigue are caused by low fixed cardiac output due to dynamic intracavitary obstruction and the secondary MR due to systolic anterior motion (SAM) of mitral valve. The symptoms may show day-to-day variability becoming pronounced postprandially or after alcohol ingestion and in states of dehydration. In HOCM, volume overload does not occur, comorbid conditions are rare because of younger age, EF is normal or supranormal, diastolic dysfunction is frequent, RV dysfunction is unusual, MR is classically due to SAM, hospitalization for HF almost never occurs, and annual mortality is very low (0.5%). In those with nonobstructive HCM, impairment of ventricular filling is responsible for symptoms of heart failure. Symptoms are often mild (NYHA class I–II) and the diastolic function impairment is often grade I–II. A small percentage of patients with nonobstructive HCM, may have advanced diastolic dysfunction with features of restrictive ventricular filling (grade III) in echo. Such patients are often called as restrictive phenotypes if HCM.[9,10] Volume overload features such as elevated JVP, hepatomegaly, and edema may be present. But the younger age of presentation, absence of comorbid conditions, presence of severe LVH, marked biatrial enlargement and a smaller LV cavity in echo and distribution of scarring in cardiac magnetic resonance (CMR) imaging may be helpful in differentiating this form of HCM from the garden variety of HFpEF. Moreover, if someone with suspected HCM presents with florid signs of HF namely PND, orthopnea, elevated JVP, edema, etc., phenocopies such as Fabry's disease, Danon disease, and amyloidosis should be seriously considered. In the later conditions which are also HFpEF mimics, and classical findings in systemic examination are suggestive enough to suspect the diagnosis.

Atrial fibrillation may occur both in HFpEF and in HCM. AF seems to be more prevalent in HFpEF than in HFrEF. In the long-term HF registry of European Society of Cardiology comprising of 14,964 patients, the prevalence of AF was 27% in HFrEF, 29% in HFmrEF and 39% in HFpEF. After adjusting for variables, the hazard ratio of AF for HF hospitalizations was: 1.036 in HFrEF, 1.430 in HFmrEF and 1.487 in HFpEF. For the combined all-cause death or HF hospitalizations the hazard ratios were: 0.957, 1.302, and 1.365.[11] Of 41,446 HF patients enrolled in Swedish Heart Failure Registry, 23% had HFpEF, 22% had HFmrEF, and 55% had HFrEF. The prevalence of AF was 65%, 60%, and 53% in HFpEF, HFmrEF, and HFrEF, respectively. The hazard ratio for death was 1.11, 1.22, and 1.17, for HF hospitalization or death, 1.17, 1.29, and, 1.15 and for stroke/TIA or death 1.15, 1.23, and 1.19 in HFpEF, HFmrEF, and HFrEF, respectively.[12] The reported prevalence of AF in HCM varies from 12.5–24% with an annual incidence of 2%. Subclinical AF has been reported in 24% of HCM patients implanted with ICD. Stroke risk is higher in HCM patients when compared to general population, even in the absence of documented AF in them. Increasing age and the presence of HF appeared to predict occurrence of ischemic stroke in HCM without AF with a HR of 1.75 for HF and 2.74 for age >65. Stroke risk in HCM with manifest AF is much higher—3.75% per year.[13] Because of the high risk of stroke/systemic embolism, oral anticoagulation is indicated in HCM with AF irrespective of CHADS2VASc score. The stroke rate in patients with HF (either HFrEF or HFpEF) and AF is 1.77 per 100 patient years.[14] Decision regarding oral anticoagulation is determined by CHADS2VASc score in HF patients having AF.

Effective drug treatments that improve survival are available for HFrEF and additionally biventricular pacing (BiVP) is found to be beneficial in improving symptoms and survival along with reverse remodeling of LV in those with left bundle branch block (LBBB).[15] Until recently, therapeutic options are limited for HFpEF, except for optimal management of comorbid conditions. Now we have evidence for sodium-glucose linked transporter protein 2 (SGLT2) inhibitors being useful in HFpEF, that too in terms of reducing HF hospitalizations but not mortality. Angiotensin receptor neprilysin inhibitors (ARNI) and mineralocorticoid receptor antagonists (MRA) have a limited role in reducing HF hospitalizations, particularly in those with an EF in the lower limit of normal range, i.e., <55–60%. Women with HFpEF seemed to derive greater benefit from ARNI with a higher cutoff for LVEF, i.e., <65–70%.[16-20]

In HCM, drug therapy options are limited but have a useful role in reducing symptoms and improving exercise capacity. β blockers, nonhydro pyridine calcium blockers, disopyramide, and mavacamten are being used for symptomatic patients. Mortality benefit of these drugs remains to be determined because of lack of evidence. Septal reduction therapies such as alcohol septal ablation or surgical myectomy are reserved for those with class II or more symptoms despite optimal drug therapy. Surgical myectomy appears to prolong survival in observational studies. If HCM is viewed as a cause of HFpEF rather than a mimic, there is a possibility that such nonpharmacological options might not be optimally used. Another area where HCM differs from HFpEF is the benefit of implantable cardioverter defibrillator (ICD) in effective prevention of sudden death in high risk individuals. In HFpEF, ICDs are indicated only for secondary prevention—resuscitated sudden cardiac arrest or documented ventricular tachycardia.

CONCLUSION

The HCM is ideally viewed as a HFpEF mimic rather than the cause of it because of different mechanisms of HF symptoms based on the phenotype of HCM, rare occurrence of clinically manifest congestion, younger age of presentation, lesser comorbid conditions, requirement of specific drugs and procedures to relieve the obstruction when present, higher occurrence of stroke even in the absence of AF with a need for oral anticoagulation irrespective of CHADS2VASc score in those with AF, need for risk stratification for sudden cardiac death, and different prognostic implications.

REFERENCES

1. Semsarian C, GradDipGenCouns JI, Maron MS, et al. New perspectives on the prevalence of Hypertrophic Cardiomyopathy. J Am Coll Cardiol. 2015;65(12): 1249-64.
2. Neubauer S, Kolm P, Ho CY, et al. Distinct subgroups in Hypertrophic Cardiomyopathy in the NHLBI Registry. J Am Coll Cardiol. 2019;74(19):2333-45.
3. Lorenzini M, Anastasiou Z, O'Mahony C, et al. Hypertrophic Cardiomyopathy Outcomes investigators. Mortality among referral patients with hypertrophic cardiomyopathy vs the general European population. JAMA Cardiol. 2020;5(1):73-80.
4. Liu J, Wang D, Ruan J, et al. Identification of heart failure with preserved ejection fraction helps risk stratification for hypertrophic cardiomyopathy. BMC Medicine. 2022; 20(1):21.
5. Kittleson MM, Panirat GS, Amancherla A, et al. 2023 ACC Expert Consensus Decision Pathway on Management of Heart Failure With Preserved Ejection Fraction: A Report of the American College of Cardiology Solution Set Oversight Committee. JACC. 2023;81(18): 1835.
6. McKee PA, Castelli WP, McNamara PM, et al. The Natural history of congestive heart failure: the Framingham study. New Engl J Med. 1971;285(26):1441-6.
7. Bozkurt B, Coats AJS, Tsutsui H, et al. Universal Definition and Classification of Heart Failure: A Report of the Heart Failure Society of America, Heart Failure Association of the European Society of Cardiology, Japanese Heart Failure Society and Writing Committee of the Universal Definition of Heart Failure. J Card Failure. 2021;27: 387-413.
8. Campbell P, Rutten FH, Lee MMY, et al. Heart failure with preserved ejection fraction: everything the clinician needs to know. Lancet. 2024;403(10431):1083-92.
9. Olivotto I, Cecchi F, Poggesi C, et al. Patterns of Disease Progression in Hypertrophic Cardiomyopathy: An Individualized Approach to Clinical Staging. Circ Heart Fail. 2012;5(4):535-46.
10. Rowin EJ, Maron BJ, Kiernan MS, et al. Advanced Heart Failure With Preserved Systolic Function in Nonobstructive Hypertrophic Cardiomyopathy: Under-Recognized Subset of Candidates for Heart Transplant. Circ Heart Fail. 2014; 7(6):967-75.
11. Zafrir B, Lund LH, Laroche C, et al. Prognostic implications of atrial fibrillation in heart failure with reduced, mid-range, and preserved ejection fraction: a report from 14,964 patients in the European Society of Cardiology Heart Failure Long-Term Registry. Eur Heart J. 2018;39:4277-84.
12. Sartipy U, Dahlström U, Fu M, et al. Atrial fibrillation in heart failure with preserved, mid-range, and reduced ejection fraction. JACC Heart Fail. 2017;5(8):565-74.
13. Dragasis S, Vlachos K, Kariki O, et al. Atrial fibrillation in hypertrophic cardiomyopathy - a contemporary mini review. Hellenic J Cardiol. 2022;67:66-72.
14. Inciardi RM, Giugliano RP, Park JG, et al. Risks of heart failure, stroke, and bleeding in atrial fibrillation according to heart failure phenotypes. JACC Clin Electrophysiol. 2023;9(4):569-80.
15. Heidenreich PA, Bozkurt B, Aguilar D, et al. 2022 AHA/ACC/HFSA Guideline for the Management of Heart Failure: A Report of the American College of Cardiology/American Heart Association Joint Committee on Clinical Practice Guidelines. Circulation. 2022;145:e895-e1032.
16. Anker SD, Butler J, Filippatos G, et al. Empagliflozin in heart failure with a preserved ejection fraction. N Engl J Med. 2021;385(16):1451-61.
17. Solomon SD, McMurray JJV, Claggett B, et al. Dapagliflozin in heart failure with mildly reduced or preserved ejection fraction. N Engl J Med. 2022;387(12):1089-98.
18. Kosiborod MN, Abildstrøm SZ, Borlaug BA, et al. Semaglutide in patients with heart failure with preserved ejection fraction and obesity. N Engl J Med. 2023;389(12): 1069-84.
19. Solomon SD, Vaduganathan M, Claggett B L, et al. Sacubitril/Valsartan across the Spectrum of Ejection Fraction in Heart Failure. Circulation. 2020;352-61.
20. Solomon SD, Claggett B, Lewis EF, et al. Influence of ejection fraction on outcomes and efficacy of spironolactone in patients with heart failure with preserved ejection fraction. Eur Heart J. 2016;37(5):455-62.

CHAPTER

Management of HFpEF: Normalizing the Apparently Normal Heart

Sarita Rao, Roshan Rao, Vaibhav Shukla, Abhishek Rathore, Achukatla Kumar

INTRODUCTION

The rapid global increase in heart failure (HF) cases has reached critical levels, and is recognized as a HF pandemic. Current estimates indicate that >60 million people are affected by HF worldwide, projected to rise further in the coming years.[1] This increase is driven by aging populations and the growing prevalence of risk factors such as hypertension, diabetes, obesity, and sedentary lifestyles. This escalating incidence underscores the urgent need for more effective prevention and management strategies for HF across diverse populations.

Traditionally, HF has been classified into two primary categories: heart failure with reduced ejection fraction (HFrEF) and heart failure with preserved ejection fraction (HFpEF), based on left ventricular ejection fraction (LVEF). While the exact LVEF thresholds defining these categories may vary, HFrEF is typically associated with an LVEF below 40%, and HFpEF is characterized by an LVEF of 50% or higher. Recently, an intermediate category, heart failure with mildly reduced ejection fraction (HFmrEF), has been identified, encompassing patients with an LVEF between 41 and 49%. Furthermore, a new classification, heart failure with improved ejection fraction (HFimpEF), has been introduced. This category includes individuals whose baseline LVEF was 40% or lower but who subsequently experienced a significant improvement of at least 10 percentage points, with a follow-up LVEF exceeding 40%. This recognizes the evolving nature of HF and the increasing prevalence of cases where EF significantly improves due to effective treatment.[2]

The HFpEF is characterized by myocardial dysfunction that leads to a disproportionate rise in left-sided filling pressures in order to sustain cardiac output. This condition is commonly associated with both cardiovascular (CV) and noncardiovascular comorbidities, which substantially contribute to the high rates of morbidity and mortality observed in HFpEF patients.[3] Although the exact pathophysiological mechanisms behind HF progression in HFpEF are not fully understood, prevailing models emphasize the role of various comorbidities such as obesity, hypertension, diabetes, chronic obstructive pulmonary disease, and chronic kidney disease in creating a systemic proinflammatory state. This inflammatory environment contributes to endothelial dysfunction, and subsequently, to the progression of HF.[4]

These comorbidities are not only prevalent among patients with HFpEF but are also accelerate disease progression and exacerbate functional limitations.[5] Given the significant impact of comorbidities on disease course and patient outcomes, a thorough and systematic approach to evaluating and managing these associated conditions should be central to HFpEF treatment strategies. Addressing these factors holistically may help mitigate disease progression and improve quality of life and functional capacity for HFpEF patients.

MANAGEMENT OF HEART FAILURE WITH PRESERVED EJECTION FRACTION

The management of HFpEF remains a substantial challenge due to the diverse clinical presentations and complex pathophysiology associated with this condition. Unlike HFrEF, where treatment approaches such as ACE inhibitors, β-blockers, and mineralocorticoid receptor antagonists (MRAs) have established efficacy, HFpEF has proven more resistant to traditional HF therapies.[6] HFpEF is frequently linked to multiple comorbidities, all of which contribute to its pathogenesis and progression. Recent advances in understanding the mechanisms underlying HFpEF have led to the exploration of new therapeutic strategies aimed at addressing both cardiac and systemic contributors. After diagnosing HFpEF and ruling out alternative conditions, a comprehensive treatment approach should be initiated. This includes addressing associated comorbidities alongside implementing both pharmacologic and nonpharmacologic therapeutic strategies.

Hypertension

Hypertension is a prevalent comorbidity in patients with HFpEF, and most patients with HFpEF have a history of elevated blood pressure.[7]

A meta-analysis of randomized trials suggests that lowering SBP below 130 mm Hg may reduce the likelihood of HF hospitalizations, though this may come at the cost of worsening renal function.[8] Optimal blood pressure targets in HFpEF remain unclear, as observational data suggest a possible J-shaped curve, where SBP below 120 mm Hg is associated with increased risk of hospitalizations and mortality.[9] Current consensus guidelines recommend aiming for a blood pressure target of <130/80 mm Hg in HFpEF patients, though this goal may vary based on individual patient characteristics.[10]

Diabetes

Diabetes and dysglycemia are highly prevalent in patients with HFpEF, with observational studies indicating that up to 30–40% have diabetes, and a further one-third may have prediabetes. Consequently, nearly three-quarters of HFpEF patients show some degree of insulin resistance or dysglycemia.[11-14] HFpEF patients with prediabetes or diabetes face higher HF hospitalization rates, while those with overt diabetes have an increased risk of all-cause and CV mortality. Notably, a "lean type 2 diabetes" phenotype, especially common among Asian patients, underscores the risk that extends beyond body mass index alone.[15,16]

Obesity

Obesity is prevalent in over 80% of patients with HFpEF, and these patients often experience worse outcomes compared to nonobese individuals. Obese HFpEF patients exhibit more right ventricular dysfunction, higher filling pressures, increased congestion, greater renal vulnerability, and more significant exercise intolerance, all of which contribute to a diminished quality of life.[17,18] Weight loss achieved through dietary intervention or bariatric surgery has demonstrated favorable hemodynamic outcomes, including reductions in blood pressure, heart rate, and cardiac filling pressures, both at rest and during exercise. However, systematic studies on weight loss specifically in HFpEF are limited.[19]

One key study is a 2 × 2 factorial randomized trial exploring caloric restriction and aerobic exercise in obese older adults with HFpEF, which showed that both interventions improved peak oxygen consumption over 20 weeks, though there was no significant improvement in overall quality of life. A recent randomized trial evaluating a multidomain physical therapy intervention in older patients (median BMI approximately 33 kg/m^2) hospitalized with HF demonstrated enhanced functional capacity and quality of life. Notably, the findings suggest that patients with HFpEF may derive even greater benefits from this intervention compared to those with HFrEF.[20]

Small studies of bariatric surgery in HFpEF have reported diastolic remodeling, diastolic function, and symptom relief; however, long-term clinical outcome data from large, randomized trials are still lacking.[21]

Chronic Kidney Disease

Chronic kidney disease (CKD) is a strong risk factor for developing HFpEF and may contribute directly to adverse cardiac remodeling, such as left ventricular hypertrophy, inflammation, myocardial fibrosis, and fluid retention, all of which drive HF pathogenesis.[22] Patients with CKD and HFpEF experience more severe symptoms and present with worse cardiac function, notably poorer right ventricular function and higher levels of cardiac biomarkers associated with wall stress, fibrosis, and neurohumoral and oxidative stress.[23] Lower estimated glomerular filtration rate and higher urinary albumin levels are both linked to increased risk of HFpEF and to worse outcomes, including higher rates of CV death and HF hospitalization.[24]

Coronary Artery Disease

Coronary artery disease (CAD) is prevalent in over 50% of patients with HFpEF, often worsening symptoms, limiting function, and heightening CV event risk.[25] Even when epicardial coronary blockages are absent, coronary microvascular dysfunction frequently occurs, marked by reduced coronary flow reserve, and is associated with increased HF hospitalization and CV mortality.[26] Observational data indicate that managing CV risk factors, including the use of statins, may benefit HFpEF patients with CAD.[27]

Several key trials have explored the impact of blood pressure management and related interventions in HFpEF patients, with outcomes regarding optimal treatment targets and strategies **(Table 1)**.

TABLE 1: Clinical trials of various comorbidity management in heart failure with preserved ejection fraction patients.

Disease	*Trial*	*N*	*Intervention*	*Key inclusion criteria*	*Primary composite Endpoint*	*Median follow-up (months)*	*Treatment effect (primary endpoint)*	*Overall efficacy and other notes*
Hypertension	SPRINT[28]	9,361	Intensive blood pressure (BP) control [systolic BP (SBP) <120] vs. standard (SBP <140)	Hypertensive patients without HF	Cardiovascular (CV) events and all-cause mortality	36	*Heart rate (HR):* 0.75 (0.64–0.89); $p < 0.001$	Reduced CV events and mortality but increased renal events in elderly
Hypertension	PARAMOUNT[29]	301	Sacubitril/valsartan vs. valsartan	Hypertensive HFpEF patients	Change in NT-proBNP, left atrial size	12	NT-proBNP ↓; Improved LA size	Suggested benefit in HF progression; more trials needed for long-term effects
Hypertension	TOPCAT[30]	3,445	Spironolactone vs. placebo	HFpEF with history of HF hospitalizations or BNP criteria	CV death and HF hospitalization	36	No effect on primary endpoint; ↓ in HF hospitalizations	Beneficial for HF-related hospitalization in Americas; mixed global efficacy
Hypertension	PRESERVE[31]	4,128	Valsartan vs. placebo	HFpEF patients	HF hospitalization and mortality	36	No significant reduction in HF hospitalizations or mortality	Good for BP control but limited impact on HF progression
Diabetes	DAPA-HF[32]	4,744	Dapagliflozin vs. placebo	HFrEF patients with/without T2D	CV death or HF hospitalization	18.2	HR: 0.74 (0.65-0.85); $p < 0.001$	Reduced HF hospitalizations, leading to trials in HFpEF
Diabetes	EMPEROR-Preserved[33]	5,988	Empagliflozin vs. placebo	HFpEF patients (LVEF >40%)	CV death or HF hospitalization	26	*HR:* 0.79 (0.69–0.90); $p < 0.001$	Significant benefit in reducing CV death and HF hospitalization
Diabetes	DELIVER[34]	6,263	Dapagliflozin vs. placebo	HFpEF (LVEF >40%)	CV death or HF hospitalizations	24	*HR:* 0.79 (0.69–0.91); $p < 0.001$	Reaffirmed benefits across HFpEF, regardless of diabetes status
Diabetes	CANVAS[35]	10,142	Canagliflozin vs. placebo	Type 2 diabetes (T2D) at high CV risk	CV events, including heart failure (HF) hospitalization	36	*HR:* 0.67 (0.52–0.87); $p < 0.001$	Reduced HF hospitalization by 33%, supporting HF prevention in diabetes
Diabetes	SCORED[36]	10,584	Sotagliflozin vs. placebo	T2D with chronic kidney disease (CKD)	CV death, HF hospitalization	16	*HR:* 0.74 (0.63–0.88); $p < 0.001$	Significant reduction in CV death and HF hospitalization in high-risk T2D

Contd...

Contd…

Disease	*Trial*	*N*	*Intervention*	*Key inclusion criteria*	*Primary composite Endpoint*	*Median follow-up (months)*	*Treatment effect (primary endpoint)*	*Overall efficacy and other notes*
Obesity	STEP-HFpEF[37]	400	Semaglutide vs. placebo	HFpEF patients with obesity	Weight loss and HF symptom improvement	Ongoing	–	Aiming to assess weight management's impact on HFpEF
Obesity	SUMMIT[38]	4,500	Tirzepatide vs. placebo	HFpEF with obesity	CV death and HF hospitalization	Ongoing	–	Exploring dual GIP/GLP-1 for HF outcomes
Chronic kidney disease	DAPA-CKD[39]	4,304	Dapagliflozin vs. placebo	CKD with albuminuria	CKD progression and HF hospitalization	24	*HR:* 0.61 (0.51–0.72); $p < 0.001$	Reduced CKD progression and HF hospitalization
Chronic kidney disease	CREDENCE[40]	4,401	Canagliflozin vs. placebo	CKD with T2D	CV death, HF hospitalization, and renal outcomes	34.4	*HR:* 0.70 (0.59–0.82); $p < 0.001$	Marked benefit in CKD and HF prevention in T2D
Chronic kidney disease	EMPA-KIDNEY[41]	6,609	Empagliflozin vs. placebo	CKD with/ without diabetes	CKD progression, renal or CV death	20	HR: 0.72 (0.64–0.82); $p < 0.001$	Significant CKD progression reduction, favorable for CV events
Chronic kidney disease	FIDELIO-DKD[42]	5,734	Finerenone vs. placebo	T2D with CKD and albuminuria	Kidney failure and CV events	30	*HR:* 0.82 (0.73–0.93); $p = 0.001$	Reduced kidney failure and CV events, supports use in diabetic CKD
Chronic kidney disease	FIGARO-DKD[43]	7,437	Finerenone vs. placebo	T2D with CKD	CV death and HF hospitalization	36	HR: 0.87 (0.76-0.98); $p = 0.03$	Lowered CV mortality, promotes finerenone in diabetic CKD
Coronary artery disease	NEAT-HFpEF[44]	110	Nitrates vs. placebo	HFpEF with coronaryartery disease (CAD)	Daily activity levels, quality of life (QoL), exercise tolerance	6	No benefit; reduced activity levels	Contradicts nitrate use in HFpEF; no QoL or exercise improvements

PHARMACOLOGICAL MANAGEMENT

Pharmacological therapies such as sodium-glucose cotransporter 2 (SGLT2) inhibitors, angiotensin receptor-neprilysin inhibitors (ARNIs), and MRAs have demonstrated varying degrees of efficacy in addressing the unique challenges of HFpEF.

Sodium–Glucose Cotransporter 2 Inhibitors

The SGLT2 inhibitors have emerged as a groundbreaking pharmacologic class in the management of HFpEF. Recent clinical trials have demonstrated the significant benefits of SGLT2 inhibitors in improving clinical outcomes for HFpEF patients. This class of drugs, initially developed for the treatment of type 2 diabetes, has shown promise in reducing HF hospitalizations, CV death, and improving overall quality of life in patients with HFpEF, regardless of diabetes status.

Recent data from large-scale trials, including the EMPEROR-Preserved[33] and DELIVER[34] studies, have provided compelling evidence supporting the use of SGLT2 inhibitors as first-line therapy for HFpEF. The EMPEROR-Preserved trial demonstrated that empagliflozin reduced the composite endpoint of first heart failure hospitalization (HHF) and CV death by 21% compared to placebo in patients with an LVEF >40%. Notably, the benefit of empagliflozin extended across the entire LVEF spectrum, including those with LVEF >50%, and it also slowed the decline in estimated glomerular filtration rate, while improving health-related quality of life (HRQoL). Similarly, the DELIVER trial, which included 6,263 patients with chronic or worsening HFpEF, showed that dapagliflozin significantly reduced the risk of first HHF and CV death, further improving HRQoL. Notably, the benefits of dapagliflozin were consistent across the LVEF range, with no attenuation of efficacy in patients with different LVEF subgroups. A subsequent meta-analysis of both the EMPEROR-Preserved and DELIVER trials reinforced these findings, confirming that SGLT2 inhibitors consistently reduce the risk of CV death and HHF, establishing them as a cornerstone of therapy for HFpEF.

Adverse effects of SGLT2 inhibitors, such as urinary/genital infections and rare cases of euglycemic ketoacidosis, are infrequent but should be considered during patient selection. Current guidelines strongly recommend SGLT2 inhibitors for HFpEF patients without contraindications.[45]

Angiotensin Receptor-Neprilysin Inhibitors

The ARNIs, particularly sacubitril/valsartan, have emerged as a promising treatment for HFpEF. The PARAGON-HF (Prospective Comparison of ARNI with ARB Global Outcomes in HFpEF) trial enrolled 4,822 patients with an LVEF ≥45% and compared sacubitril/valsartan with valsartan alone.[46] Although the primary composite endpoint of total HHF and CV death narrowly missed statistical significance (p = 0.06), subgroup analyses indicated potential benefits in patients with LVEF below the median (≤57%), particularly women. Sacubitril/valsartan significantly reduced the incidence of HHF in these subgroups.

Recent meta-analyses combining PARAGON-HF[46] and PARADIGM-HF[47] data suggest that ARNIs provide a consistent benefit across the HF spectrum, reinforcing their role in HFpEF. Current guidelines, including the 2021 European Society of Cardiology (ESC) guidelines, recommend ARNIs in patients with HFpEF who have elevated natriuretic peptides and recent hospitalization for HF to reduce HHF.

Mineralocorticoid Receptor Antagonists

Mineralocorticoid receptor antagonists, including spironolactone and eplerenone, have been explored as potential therapies for HFpEF. These drugs work by blocking the effects of aldosterone, a hormone that promotes sodium and water retention, contributing to fluid overload and worsening HF symptoms. MRAs have shown promise in other forms of HF, particularly in HFrEF, but their role in HFpEF remains less clear.

Clinical trials, such as the TOPCAT study, have provided mixed evidence for the efficacy of MRAs in HFpEF. While spironolactone did not significantly reduce the primary endpoint of CV death, aborted cardiac arrest, or HHFs, it did show a reduction in HHFs, suggesting a potential benefit in symptom management. However, the overall impact on long-term outcomes in HFpEF patients remains uncertain, with posthoc analyses suggesting regional variations in efficacy, particularly between the Americas and Russia/Georgia.[48]

Despite these mixed results, MRAs are still considered as a treatment option in certain HFpEF patients, particularly when symptoms of fluid overload are prominent. However, the risk of hyperkalemia and the need for careful monitoring make their use a balancing act, and further research from ongoing trials is needed to clarify their role in the broader HFpEF population. As of now, the current guidelines recommend considering MRAs after weighing the potential benefits against the risks.

Ongoing trials, including the SPIRIT-HF (Spironolactone in the Treatment of Heart Failure) and SPIRRIT (Spironolactone Initiation Registry Randomized Interventional Trial in Heart Failure With Preserved Ejection Fraction) studies, are actively investigating the role of MRAs in the management of HFpEF. The SPIRIT-HF trial is evaluating the impact of spironolactone on clinical outcomes in HFpEF patients, including its potential effects on symptom control and quality of life. Meanwhile, the SPIRRIT trial is examining real-world data regarding the initiation and long-term use of spironolactone in HFpEF patients, providing insights into its safety and effectiveness across diverse clinical settings. Both studies are critical as they seek to address the mixed results from previous trials, such as the TOPCAT study, where spironolactone demonstrated limited efficacy in reducing primary composite endpoints but showed benefits in specific regions.

CONCLUSION

The increasing global burden of heart failure, particularly HFpEF, highlights the urgent need for innovative and holistic management approaches. HFpEF is distinguished by its complex interplay of comorbidities, including hypertension, diabetes, obesity, chronic kidney disease, and CAD, which exacerbate disease progression and worsen patient outcomes. Despite significant advances in understanding HFpEF pathophysiology, effective therapies remain limited compared to HFrEF.

Recent clinical trials have underscored the potential benefits of targeted pharmacological therapies such as SGLT2 inhibitors, ARNIs, and MRAs in reducing hospitalizations and CV mortality in HFpEF patients. These findings mark a significant stride in addressing the unique challenges of HFpEF and offer a promising foundation for refining treatment strategies. Additionally, nonpharmacologic interventions, including weight management and exercise, have demonstrated modest improvements in functional capacity and quality of life, further emphasizing the importance of a comprehensive and individualized approach to care.

Future research should aim to address gaps in knowledge regarding optimal treatment thresholds, the long-term impact of emerging therapies, and strategies for effectively managing the multifaceted comorbidities associated with HFpEF. By advancing these objectives, it may be possible to transform the therapeutic landscape for HFpEF, ultimately improving outcomes and quality of life for this growing patient population.

REFERENCES

1. Shahim B, Kapelios CJ, Savarese G, et al. Global Public Health Burden of Heart Failure: An Updated Review. Card Fail Rev. 2023;9:e11.
2. Savarese G, Vedin O, D'Amario D, et al. Prevalence and prognostic implications of longitudinal ejection fraction change in heart failure. JACC Heart Fail. 2019;7:306-17.
3. ElGuindy A, Yacoub MH. Heart failure with preserved ejection fraction. Glob Cardiol Sci Pract. 2012;2012(1):10.
4. Stoicescu L, Crişan D, Morgovan C, et al. Heart Failure with Preserved Ejection Fraction: The Pathophysiological Mechanisms behind the Clinical Phenotypes and the Therapeutic Approach. Int J Mol Sci. 2024;25(2):794.
5. Pop C, Ştefan MG, Muntean DM, et al. Protective Effects of a Discontinuous Treatment with Alpha-Lipoic Acid in Obesity-Related Heart Failure with Preserved Ejection Fraction, in Rats. Antioxidants. 2020;9:1073.
6. Heinzel FR, Shah SJ. The future of heart failure with preserved ejection fraction: Deep phenotyping for targeted therapeutics. Herz. 2022;47:308-23.
7. Dunlay SM, Roger VL, Redfield MM. Epidemiology of heart failure with preserved ejection fraction. Nat Rev Cardiol. 2017;14:591-602.
8. Kawano H, Fuiwara A, Kai H, et al. Effects of blood pressure lowering in patients with heart failure with preserved ejection fraction: a systematic review and meta-analysis. Hypertens Res. 2019;42:504-13.
9. Tsimploulis A, Lam PH, Arundel C, et al. Systolic blood pressure and outcomes in patients with heart failure with preserved ejection fraction. JAMA Cardiol. 2018;3:288-97.
10. Heidenreich P, Bozkurt B, Aguilar D, et al. 2022 AHA/ACC/HFSA guideline for the management of heart failure: a report of the American College of Cardiology/American Heart Association Joint Committee on Clinical Practice Guidelines. J Am Coll Cardiol. 2022;79:e263-e421.
11. Owan TE, Hodge DO, Herges RM, et al. Trends in prevalence and outcome of heart failure with preserved ejection fraction. N Engl J Med. 2006;55:251-9.
12. Bhatia RS, Tu JV, Lee DS, et al. Outcome of heart failure with preserved ejection fraction in a population-based study. N Engl J Med. 2006;355:260-9.
13. Jackson AM, Rorth R, Liu R, et al. Diabetes and pre-diabetes in patients with heart failure and preserved ejection fraction. Eur J Heart Fail. 2022;24:497-509.
14. Inzucchi SE, Claggett BL, Vaduganathan M, et al. Efficacy and safety of dapagliflozin in patients with heart failure with mildly reduced or preserved ejection fraction by baseline glycemic status in DELIVER: subgroup analysis from a multi-centre randomised double blind placebo controlled trial. Lancet Diab Endocrinol. 2022; 10(12):869-81.
15. Tromp J, Tay WT, Ouwekerk W, et al. Multimorbidity in patients with heart failure from 11 Asian regions: a prospective cohort study using the ASIAN-HF registry. PLoS Med. 2018;15:31002541.
16. Chanrdamouli C, Teng TK, Tay WT, et al. Impact of diabetes and sex in heart failure with reduced ejection fraction patients from the ASIAN-HF registry. Eur J Heart Fail. 2019;31:297-307.
17. Obokata M, Reddy YN, Pislaru S, et al. Evidence supporting the existence of a distinct obese phenotype of heart failure with preserved ejection fraction. Circulation. 2010;3:202-6.
18. Reddy YNV, Lewis GD, Shah SJ, et al. Characterization of the obese phenotype of heart failure with preserved

ejection fraction: a RELAX trial ancillary study. Mayo Clin Proc. 2019;94:1199-209.

19. Reddy YNV, Anantha-Narayanan M, Obokata M, et al. Hemodynamic effects of weight loss in obesity: a systematic review and meta-analysis. J Am Coll Cardiol. 2019;8:678-87.
20. Kitzman DW, Whellan DJ, Duncan P, et al. Physical rehabilitation for older patients hospitalized for heart failure. N Engl J Med. 2021;385:203-16.
21. Mikhalkova D, Holman SR, Jiang H, et al. Bariatric surgery-induced cardiac and lipidomic changes in obesity-related heart failure with preserved ejection fraction. Obesity (Silver Spring). 2018;26:284-920.
22. Brouwers FP, de Boer RA, van der Harst P, et al. Incidence and epidemiology of new onset heart failure with preserved vs. reduced ejection fraction in a community-based cohort: 11-year follow up of PREVEND. Eur Heart J. 2013;34:1424-31.
23. Patel RB, Mehat R, Redfield MM, et al. Renal dysfunction in heart failure with preserved ejection fraction: insights from the RELAX trial. J Card Fail. 2020;26:233-42.
24. Lofman I, Szummer K, Dahlstrom U, et al. Associations with and prognostic impact of chronic kidney disease in heart failure with preserved, mid-range, and reduced ejection fraction. Eur J Heart Fail. 2017;19:1606-14.
25. Hwang SJ, Melenovsky V, Borlaug BA. Implications of coronary artery disease in heart failure with preserved ejection fraction. J Am Coll Cardiol. 2014;63:2817-27.
26. Taqueti VR, Solomon SD, Shah AM, et al. Coronary micro-vascular dysfunction and future risk of heart failure with preserved ejection fraction. Eur Heart J. 2018;39(10): 840-9.
27. Alehagen U, Benson L, Edner M, et al. Association between use of statins and mortality in patients with heart failure and ejection fraction ≥50. Circ Heart Fail. 2015;8: 862-70.
28. SPRINT Research Group; Wright JT Jr, Williamson JD, Whelton PK, et al. A Randomized Trial of Intensive versus Standard Blood-Pressure Control. N Engl J Med. 2017; 377(25):2506.
29. Solomon SD, Zile M, Pieske B, et al.; Prospective comparison of ARNI with ARB on Management Of heart failure with preserved ejection fraction (PARAMOUNT) Investigators. The angiotensin receptor neprilysin inhibitor LCZ696 in heart failure with preserved ejection fraction: a phase 2 double-blind randomised controlled trial. Lancet. 2012;380(9851):1387-95.
30. Selvaraj S, Claggett B, Shah SJ, et al. Systolic blood pressure and cardiovascular outcomes in heart failure with preserved ejection fraction: an analysis of the TOPCAT trial. Eur J Heart Fail. 2018;20(3):483-90.
31. Kasiakogias A, Rosei EA, Camafort M, et al. Hypertension and heart failure with preserved ejection fraction: position paper by the European Society of Hypertension. J Hypertens. 2021;39(8):1522-45.
32. Kaplinsky E. DAPA-HF trial: dapagliflozin evolves from a glucose-lowering agent to a therapy for heart failure. Drugs Context. 2020;9:2019-11-3.
33. Anker SD, Butler J, Filippatos G, et al.; EMPEROR-Preserved Trial Investigators. Empagliflozin in Heart Failure with a Preserved Ejection Fraction. N Engl J Med. 2021;385(16):1451-61.
34. Solomon SD, McMurray JJV, Claggett B, et al.; DELIVER Trial Committees and Investigators. Dapagliflozin in Heart Failure with Mildly Reduced or Preserved Ejection Fraction. N Engl J Med. 2022;387(12):1089-98.
35. Rådholm K, Figtree G, Perkovic V, et al. Canagliflozin and Heart Failure in Type 2 Diabetes Mellitus: Results From the CANVAS Program. Circulation. 2018;138(5):458-68.
36. Bhatt DL, Szarek M, Pitt B, et al., on behalf of the SCORED Investigators. Sotagliflozin in Patients with Diabetes and Chronic Kidney Disease. N Engl J Med. 2021;384:129-39.
37. Verma S, Petrie MC, Borlaug BA, et al.; STEP-HFpEF Trial Committees and Investigators. Inflammation in Obesity-Related HFpEF: The STEP-HFpEF Program. J Am Coll Cardiol. 2024;84(17):1646-62.
38. Packer M, Zile MR, Kramer CM, et al.; for the SUMMIT Trial Study Group. Tirzepatide for Heart Failure With Preserved Ejection Fraction and Obesity. N Engl J Med. 2024.
39. McMurray JJV, Wheeler DC, Stefánsson BV, et al.; DAPA-CKD Trial Committees and Investigators. Effects of Dapagliflozin in Patients With Kidney Disease, With and Without Heart Failure. JACC Heart Fail. 2022;10(6):446-7.
40. Sarraju A, Li J, Cannon CP, et al. Effects of canagliflozin on cardiovascular, renal, and safety outcomes in participants with type 2 diabetes and chronic kidney disease according to history of heart failure: Results from the CREDENCE trial. Am Heart J. 2021;233:141-8.
41. The EMPA-KIDNEY Collaborative Group. Empagliflozin in Patients With Chronic Kidney Disease. N Engl J Med. 2022;388:117-27.
42. Filippatos G, Pitt B, Agarwal R, et al.; FIDELIO-DKD Investigators. Finerenone in patients with chronic kidney disease and type 2 diabetes with and without heart failure: a prespecified subgroup analysis of the FIDELIO-DKD trial. Eur J Heart Fail. 2022;24(6):996-1005.
43. Filippatos G, Anker SD, Agarwal R, et al.; FIGARO-DKD Investigators. Finerenone reduces risk of incident heart failure in patients with chronic kidney disease and type 2 diabetes: analyses from the FIGARO-DKD trial. Circulation. 2022;145(6):437-47.
44. Wagdy K, Hassan M. NEAT HFpEF: Organic nitrates fail to deliver. Glob Cardiol Sci Pract. 2016;2016(1):e201601.
45. Cunningham JW, Vaduganathan M, Claggett BL, et al. Dapagliflozin in patients recently hospitalized with heart failure and mildly reduced or preserved ejection fraction. J Am Coll Cardiol. 2022;80(14):1302-10.
46. Solomon SD, McMurray JJV, Anand IS, et al. Angiotensin-neprilysin inhibition in heart failure with preserved ejection fraction. N Engl J Med. 2019;381(17):1609.
47. Chen CH. Critical Questions about PARADIGM-HF and the Future. Acta Cardiol Sin. 2016;32(4):387-96.
48. Cleland JGF, Bunting KV, Flather MD, et al. Beta-blockers for heart failure with reduced, mid-range, and preserved ejection fraction: an individual patient-level analysis of double-blind randomized trials. Eur Heart J. 2018;39(1):26-35.

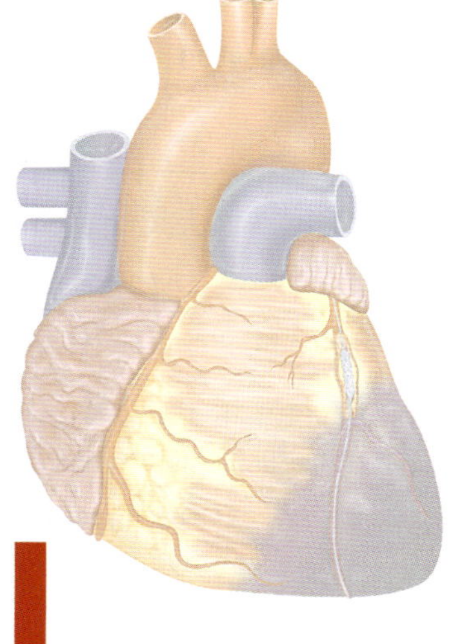

HFpEF: Definition, Pathology and Newer Management Strategies

Vinod Sharma

INTRODUCTION

Heart failure with preserved ejection fraction (HFpEF) is a clinical syndrome in which patients have signs and symptoms of HF as the result of high left ventricular (LV) filling pressure despite normal or near normal LV ejection fraction (LVEF ≥50%).

- HFpEF accounts for 50% of HF cases and its prevalence relative to HFrEF continues to rise.
- Most patients with HFpEF also display normal LV volumes and an abnormal diastolic filling pattern (i.e., diastolic dysfunction).
- Patients without signs and symptoms of HF but who have evidence of diastolic dysfunction on echocardiography do not meet criteria for HFpEF.

PATHOLOGY OF HEART FAILURE WITH PRESERVED EJECTION FRACTION

In last three decades, HFrEF has evolved to a distinct therapeutic entity, because large outcome trials demonstrated the efficacy of neurohormonal inhibition. While neurohormonal inhibition in HFpEF has failed to show any positive primary outcome either individually or in meta-analysis, this has led to consider HFpEF as a distinct HF phenotype, having different systemic and myocardial signaling **(Fig. 1)** as compared to HFrEF.

Heart failure with preserved ejection fraction patients are mostly of advanced age and predominantly female. They tend to have multiple comorbidities such as obesity/overweight (84%), systemic hypertension (60–80%), type 2 diabetes mellitus (T2DM) (20–45%), renal insufficiency, and obstructive sleep apnea.

All these comorbidities may initiate chronic systemic inflammation as evident from biomarkers levels in the patients with HFpEF, where plasma levels of soluble interleukin-1 receptor-like 1, C-reactive protein, and growth differentiation factor 15 were found to be elevated significantly.

This systemic inflammation may affect myocardial remodeling and dysfunction in HFpEF through a signaling cascade that begins with coronary microvascular endothelial dysfunction. This is followed by myocardial infiltration by activated macrophages, which includes reactive interstitial fibrosis and altered paracrine communication between endothelial cells and surrounding cardiomyocytes. These altered paracrine communications lead to deprivation of nitric oxide (NO) and cyclic guanosine monophosphate (CGMA) in cardiomyocytes, which render them hypertrophic and stiff.

The extracardiac morbidities are given in **Flowchart 1**.

High cardiomyocyte stiffness is caused by reduced distensibility of the giant cytoskeletal protein titin. The elastic property of titin is dynamically modulated by isoform shifts, phosphorylation, and oxidation.

The extramyocardial origin of HFpEF differs from the intramyocardial origin of HFrEF, where cardiac remodeling is driven by cardiomyocyte cell death due to myocardial ischemia, necrosis, infection, or toxicity.

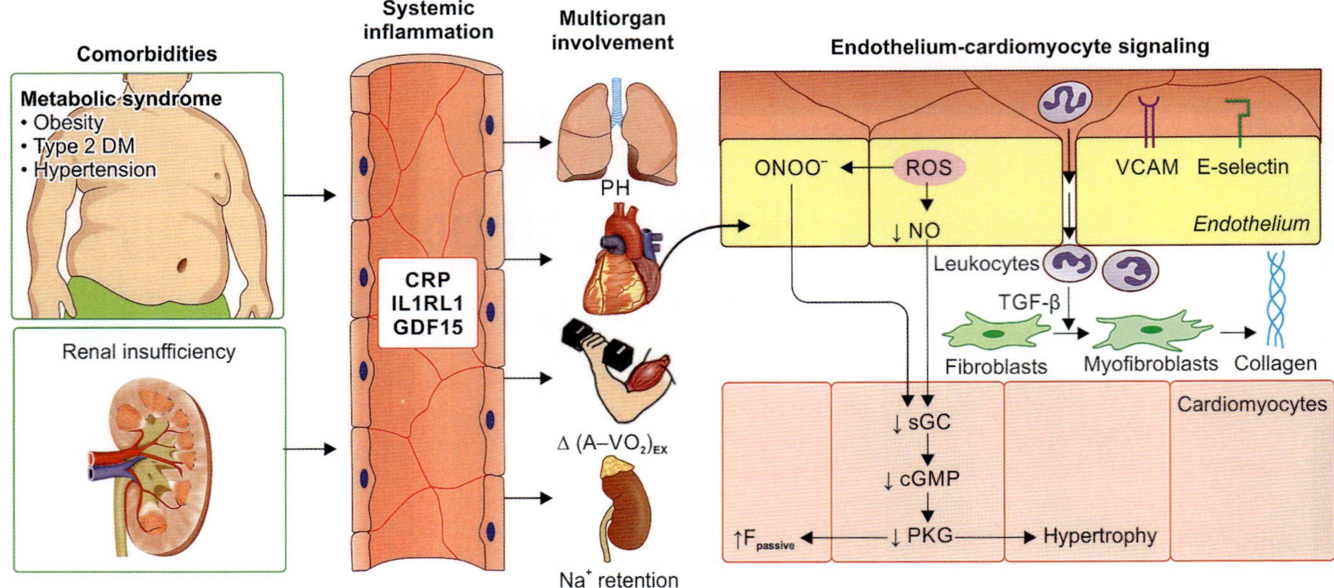

Fig. 1: Systemic and myocardial signaling in HFpEF.
Source: Shah et al. (2016).

Flowchart 1: Extracardiac morbidities.

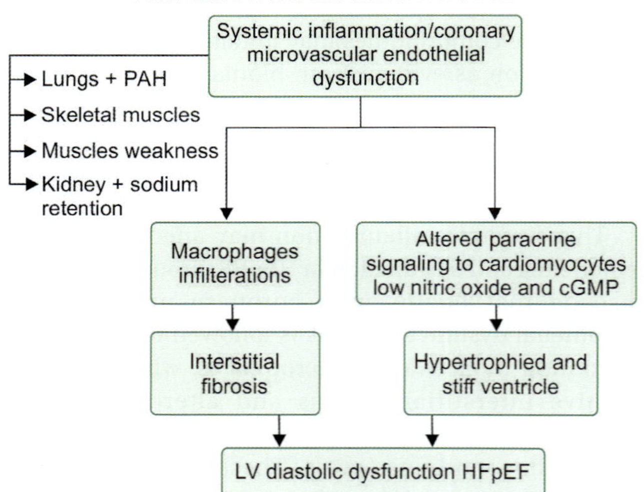

The distinct origins of HFpEF and HFrEF are evident by:
- Unequal LV structural and ultrastructural remodeling
- Lower markers of myocardial injury (high sensitive troponin T), due to less cardiomyocyte damage and myocardial stress (NT-proBNP) because of concentric LV remodeling/hypertrophy in HFpEF in contrast to eccentric LV remodeling in HFrEF, and also by visceral distribution of adipose tissue in mostly overweight or obsess patients of HFpEF, in whom there is decreased production and increased clearance of natriuretic peptides (NPs)

Chronic inflammation in HFpEF affects not only myocardium, but also other organs like skeletal muscles, lungs, and kidneys. Limited effort tolerance and dyspnea in patients with HFpEF are attributed to inflammation of skeletal muscles, rapid and brisk rise in LV filling pressure, and inappropriate pulmonary vasoconstriction as evident from pulmonary hypertension in majority of patients of HFpEF.

There is also inadequate peripheral skeletal muscle vasodilatation, perfusion, and oxygen use evident from absent widening of arteriovenous oxygen difference.

Systemic inflammation also affects the renal microvasculature and the ability of kidneys to excrete sodium. Inability to excrete a sodium load contributes to progressive volume expansion, eventually leading to transition from chronic compensated to decompensated stage in natural history of HFpEF. This altered pathophysiology also explains the efficacy of diuretics in HFpEF, as they restore the pressure–natriuresis relationship.

*The three most common HFpEF phenotypes observed in different studies of HFpEF are **(Fig. 2)**:*

1. The most common phenotype is "older, vascular aging", which comprises group of elderly patients with arterial stiffness leading to hypertension and chronic kidney disease. These patients typically have concentric use on echocardiogram, a higher association with chronic kidney disease, and elevated levels of inflammatory molecules in the blood. This group overlaps with "metabolic obese group". Inflammation is responsible for remodeling of left atrial (LA) muscle and conduction tissue leading to LA myopathy in these patients. This LA myopathy leads to increase in pulmonary artery

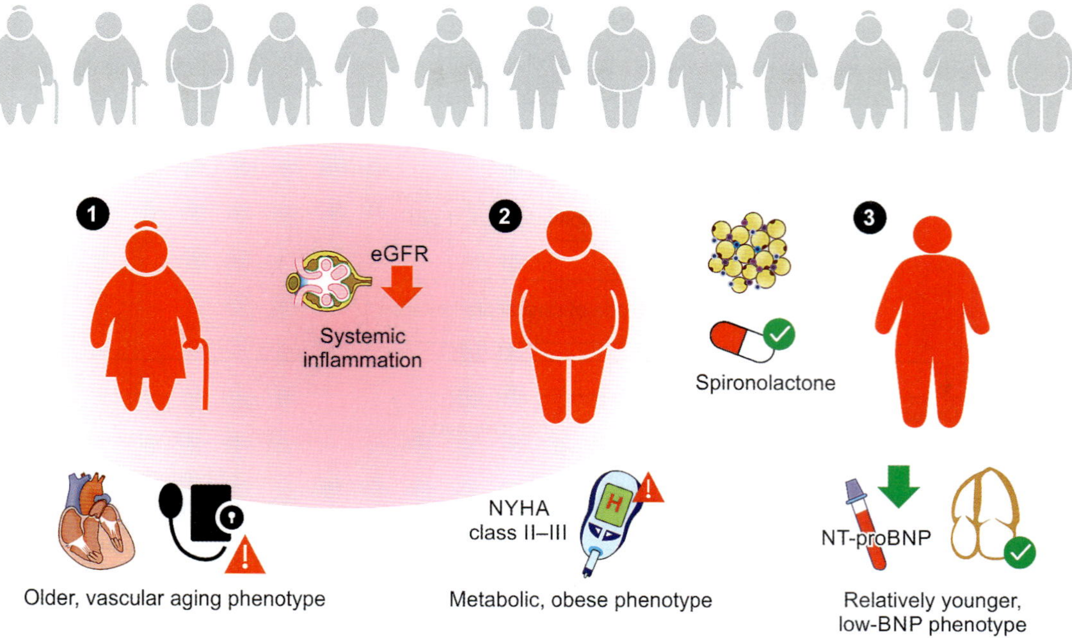

Fig. 2: Three heart failure with preserved ejection fraction phenotypes.
Source: Coats A. (2024). Cardiac failure review, Volume 10. [online] Available from https://www.cfrjournal.com/editions/cfr-volume-10-2024 [Last accessed January, 2025].

pressure and right ventricular (RV) dysfunction. In this subset of patients, blood pressure control with drugs targeting RAAS plays a central role.

2. Second common phenotype of HFpEF is "metabolic, obese" typified by patients with high body weight and T2DM, having different atherosclerotic vascular diseases, particularly affecting renal vessels, which accounts for high prevalence of chronic kidney disease in this subset of patients. Obesity results in increased renin–angiotensin activity and aldosterone levels. This group of patients showed better responsiveness to spironolactone in the TOPCAT trial.
3. Third phenotype of HFpEF consists of younger patients with lower levels of stress biomarkers such as B-type natriuretic peptide (BNP)/N-terminal fraction of pro-BNP (NT-ProBNP) and soluble ST2.

In these patients, resting echocardiogram and peptide biomarker assay may not help in diagnosis. They may require additional testing including diastolic stress testing and invasive and noninvasive assessment of pulmonary artery pressure during exercise.

This phenotype also overlaps with "metabolic, obese" type, and in post hoc analysis of TOPCAT trial, they were found to benefit from spironolactone therapy.

HFpEF is characterized by different phenotypes driven by different cardiac and noncardiac comorbidities; underlying assumption behind this phenotypic classification is that HFpEF is not a single disease but a group of different disease processes that shares heart failure symptoms and signs as clinical manifestation.

CLASSIFICATION OF HFpEF BASED ON CLINICAL PRESENTATION

The classification of HFpEF based on clinical presentation is given in **Flowchart 2**.

TREATMENT OF HEART FAILURE WITH PRESERVED EJECTION FRACTION

Recently, there has been newer understanding in differentiating and defining distinct phenotype of HFpEF. Progressive decrease of LV relaxation and LA compliance in HFpEF causes higher LA pressure resulting in high pulmonary capillary wedge pressure (PCWP), especially during exercise. Exercise intolerance is an important clinical component of HFpEF. It has been found that a large LA correlates with a higher risk of incidence of hospitalization in patients with HFpEF, and also it has been found that LA size is independently associated with morbidity and mortality in patients with HFpEF. In one of the comparative analyses by Reddy et al., in 285 patients of HFpEF with and without atrial fibrillation, it was shown that progression to permanent atrial fibrillation was strongly correlated with their baseline LA myopathy and compliance. Atrial fibrillation is associated with adverse

Flowchart 2: Classification of HFpEF based on clinical presentation.

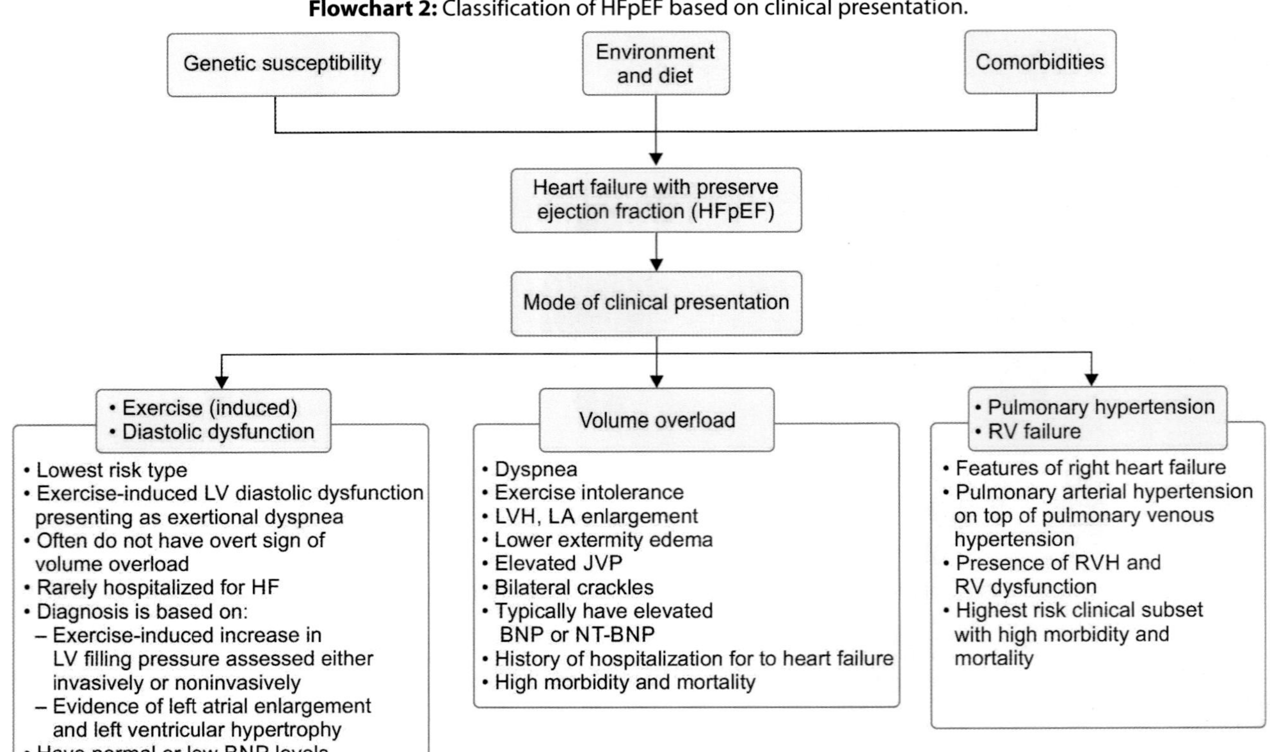

outcomes in HFpEF patients, especially when it becomes permanent. As a result of all these observations, the LA size and function have been a potential therapeutic target to reduce morbidity and mortality in HFpEF. Despite broader understanding of the features of HFpEF, the pharmacological treatment modality is still not as effective as in HFrEF. In meta-analysis of seven prospective studies comprising 2,554 patients evaluating the effect of angiotensin-converting enzyme inhibitors for HFpEF patients, there was no significant reduction in mortality or rehospitalization due to heart failure. On similar note, angiotensin-receptor blocker irbesartan was evaluated in randomized study of 4,128 patients and there was no significant improvement in outcomes in patients with HFpEF. In meta-analysis relating to the use of beta-blockers in HFpEF and their role in terms of affecting mortality and hospitalization comprising 12 clinical studies involving 21,216 patients of HFpEF, it was found that there was only lower risk of all-cause mortality but no association with HF-related mortality or hospitalization. Another meta-analysis by Bonsu et al. tried to evaluate the impact of several pharmacological interventions, including mineral corticoid antagonists, beta-blockers, angiotensin-converting enzyme inhibitors, and angiotensin-receptor blockers. In this study, they examined 15 randomized controlled trials with 5,930 HFpEF patients, but no drug treatment showed any significant difference between treatment for mortality and hospitalization (except that spironolactone and eplerenone, which showed a tendency to reduce mortality and hospitalization compared with other interventions). New therapeutic agent, angiotensin receptor–neprilysin inhibitor (ARNI), sacubitril–valsartan had shown a lower mortality and hospitalization rate in HFrEF patients, and its efficacy was superior to that of enalapril. However, a randomized, double-blind trial PARAGON-HF (prospective comparison of angiotensin receptor neprilysin inhibitor (ARNI) with angiotensin-receptor blockers Global Outcome in HFpEF) (was conducted to assess the efficacy of sacubitril–valsartan on HFpEF patients in comparison to valsartan in 4,796 patients. The sacubitril–valsartan did not result in significant benefit in total hospitalizations for heart failure nor mortality due to cardiovascular causes in patients with HFpEF. Another therapeutic agent, the sodium–glucose cotransporter type-2 (SGLT2) inhibitors were found to have effect in lowering the rate of cardiovascular death or hospitalization in heart failure patients. Tanaka et al. analyzed the data of prospective multicenter studies from Japan in which the effect of SGLT2 inhibitor on LV diastolic function and parameters of T2DM patients with stable heart failure were investigated. They reported that within 53 T2DM patients with stable heart failure, HFpEF patients

(n = 37) showed more significant improvement in global longitudinal strain (17.0 ± 1.9% to 18.8 ± 2.0%, *p < 0.001)* at 6 months after administration of dapagliflozin, compared to HFmrEF and HFrEF patients. The Semaglutide in patients with Heart Failure with Preserved Ejection Fraction and obesity (STEP-HFpEF) trial has come out with conclusion that weight loss with a glucose-like peptide-1 agonist in obese HFpEF patients provides benefits in terms of quality of life (QoL) measured by the Kansas City cardiomyopathy questionnaire clinical summary score and 6-minute-walk distance (6MWD). However, long-term sustainability of clinical improvement outcomes is yet to be seen.

Because of phenotypic diversity in HFpEF, personalized therapeutic strategies are proposed, which are configured in a matrix with HFpEF presentation in the abscissa and HFpEF predispositions in the ordinate.

Pathophysiological-specific interventions in HFpEF are given in **Table 1**.

The HFpEF clinical presentation phenotypes are listed in **Table 2**.

Diuretics

- Lowering LV filling pressures with diuretics is of paramount importance for HFpEF patients to achieve symptomatic benefit, reduce pulmonary artery pressures, and improve RV loading.
- Administration of diuretics can be guided by the use of implantable hemodynamic monitors that either directly and continuously measure diastolic LV pressures or provide surrogates of pressure.

Other Drugs

Besides diuretics to reduce congestion, the following three classes of drugs have shown remarkable benefits in HFpEF.

1. *Antialdosterone drugs* have shown immense clinical benefit in the TOPCAT trial.
2. *SGLT2 inhibitors:* This class of drugs appears to be fundamental drugs in patients with and without diabetes, as they have shown a reduction in cardiovascular mortality and hospitalization for heart failure

TABLE 1: Pathophysiological-specific interventions In HFpEF.

• Metabolic risk	• Calorie restriction
• Systemic inflammation	• Statins
• Pulmonary hypertension	• PDE inhibitors
• Sodium retention	• Diuretics
• Myocardial cGMP	• Neprilysin
• Myocardial fibrosis	• Spironolactone

TABLE 2: HFpEF clinical presentation phenotypes.

HFpEF predisposition phenotypes	*Lung congestion*	*+Chronotropic incompetence*	*+Pulmonary hypertension (CpcPH)*	*+Skeletal muscle weakness*	*+Atrial fibrillation*
Overweight/ obesity/ metabolic syndrome/ type 2 DM	• Diuretics (loop diuretic in DM) • Caloric restriction • Statins • Inorganic nitrite/ nitrate • Sacubitril • Spironolactone	+Rate adaptive atrial pacing	+Pulmonary vasodilators (e.g., PDE5I)	+Exercise training program	+Cardioversion +Rate Control +Anticoagulation
+Arterial hypertension	+ACEI/ARB	• +ACEI/ARB • +Rate adaptive atrial pacing	• +ACEI/ARB • +Pulmonary vasodilators (e.g., POE5I)	• +ACEI/ARB • +Exercise training program	• +ACEI/ARB • + Cardioversion • +Rate control • +Anticoagulation
+Renal dysfunction	+Ultrafiltration if needed	• +Ultrafiltration if needed • +Rate adaptive atrial pacing	• +Ultrafiltration if needed • Pulmonary vasodilators (e.g., POE5I)	• +Ultrafiltration if needed • +Exercise training program	• +Ultrafiltration if needed • +Cardioversion • +Rate control • +Anticoagulation
+CAD	• +ACEI • +Revasculari-zation	• +ACEI • +Revasculari-zation • +Rate adaptive atrial pacing	• +ACEI • +Revasculari-zation • +Pulmonary vasodilators (e.g., POE5I)	• +ACEI • +Revasculari-zation • +Exercise training program	• +ACEI • +Revascularization • +Cardioversion • +Rate control • +Anticoagulation

Source: Shah et al. (2016).

in EMPEROR-PRESERVED and DELIVER Trials. DECLARE-TIMI-58 Trial reported that diabetic patients without atrial fibrillation may benefit by use of SGLT2 inhibitors because they have preventive effect on this arrhythmia.

3. *ARNI:* Obesity is a common comorbidity in many patients of HFpEF. Excess visceral adipose tissue promotes the hyperactivation of neurohormonal system, which along with reduced neprilysin activity, typical of obese HFpEF, makes the proinflammatory and fibrotic effect of aldosterone unopposed, leading to diastolic dysfunction and progressive rise of LV filling pressure.

The RAASI, particularly ARNI, plays central role along with SGLT2 in the management of HFpEF. Another promising agent in management of obese patients of HFpEF is semaglutide. STEP-HFpEF trial recently has demonstrated that in comparison to placebo, semaglutide administration led to significant reduction in body weight, improvement in symptoms, physical limitation, and exercise function with a positive impact on QoL, inflammatory status, and survival in patients with HFpEF.

Caloric Restriction

- Because increased body adiposity promotes inflammation and impairs cardiac, arterial, renal, and skeletal muscle function, weight loss should be considered as a treatment strategy for the majority of HFpEF patients.
- The QoL improvement was significantly greater with diet than with exercise.

Statins

- The presence of systemic inflammation supports the use of statins in HFpEF. Statins improve endothelial redox balance and restore NO bioavailability, independently of low-density lipoprotein lowering.
- In an observational study, statin-treated HFpEF patients were also less prone to develop atrial fibrillation.

Inorganic Nitrite/Nitrate

- In the HFpEF signaling cascade, cardiomyocytes are deprived of NO and cGMP because of altered paracrine communication between inflamed microvascular endothelial cells and cardiomyocytes **(Fig. 1)**.
- Organic NO donors were therefore suggested to be potentially useful in HFpEF because they could restore myocardial NO content and concomitantly correct the elevated arterial load.
- Organic nitrates may produce greater than expected hypotensive effects in people with HFpEF or potentially impair cardiac output because of excessive preload reduction.
- Organic nitrates typically increase local NO levels and require bioactivation in the tissues.
- In contrast to organic nitrates, the inorganic nitrate–nitrite pathway represents an important alternative route to restore NO signaling in HFpEF.
- Nitrite is now known to function as an important *in vivo* NO reservoir. Importantly, nitrite is preferentially reduced to NO in the presence of hypoxia and acidosis, which occurs during physical exercise, thus delivering NO in time and locations (i.e., skeletal and cardiac muscles) of greatest need.
- Nitrate–nitrite preparations have been shown to improve conduit artery stiffness in healthy volunteers and improve systemic vasodilation during exercise in patients with HFpEF.

Arterial Hypertension

Arterial hypertension is found in ≥80% of HFpEF patients. Treatment of arterial hypertension in older people without heart failure reduces incidence of heart failure.

Coronary Artery Disease

The presence of coronary artery disease also identifies a distinct HFpEF group with a larger LV systolic functional deficit, poor prognosis, and a high incidence of sudden death. Use of ACEIs is recommended for prevention of new cardiovascular events. In HFpEF patients with coronary artery disease, observational data suggest that complete revascularization is associated with better preservation of LV systolic function and an improved prognosis, although prospective trial data are still lacking.

Chronotropic Incompetence

- Many patients with HFpEF display marked impairments in cardiac output reserve during exercise, despite normal resting values. Impaired cardiac output reserve in HFpEF is related not only to decreased stroke volume augmentation, but also to chronotropic incompetence. This observation was supported by the worsened exercise capacity when heart rate was slowed by the ivabradine.
- Because there is a direct relationship between heart rate response to activity and aerobic capacity, a clinical trial is currently testing whether rate-adaptive atrial pacing can improve exercise capacity in patients with HFpEF.

Pulmonary Hypertension

- Recent evidence stressed the importance in HFpEF of pathophysiologic targets beyond the heart **(Fig. 1)**. Pulmonary hypertension is frequently present at rest and patients can also develop an exaggerated pulmonary hypertensive response to exercise. In HFpEF, pulmonary pressures can be augmented by increased LA pressure and by pulmonary vasoconstriction. When both mechanisms prevail, combined precapillary and postcapillary pulmonary hypertension is present. Because of pulmonary hypertension and shared predisposing mechanisms, RV dysfunction is common in HFpEF and is associated with increased morbidity and mortality. The right ventricle in HFpEF displays heightened afterload sensitivity, suggesting favorable potential for benefit from reduction in pulmonary pressures. A number of trials have or are currently testing the effects of pulmonary vasodilators targeting cGMP, endothelin, and NO (NCT02713126; NCT02262078) in patients with HFpEF.
- Impairments in pulmonary function predict incident development of HFpEF independent of cardiac function. HFpEF patients with increased interstitial pulmonary edema display greater pulmonary vascular abnormalities and RV dysfunction, supporting aggressive therapies to reduce left heart filling pressures chronically in patients with HFpEF.

Atrial Fibrillation

- Prevalent atrial fibrillation in HFpEF goes along with a more advanced stage of cardiac remodeling evident from a larger left atrium and uniformly carries a worse prognosis.
- Incident atrial fibrillation in HFpEF also accompanies worse LV diastolic dysfunction and was inversely related to statin use.
- Atrial fibrillation to beget HFpEF and vice versa and efforts to restore sinus rhythm could be included in a HFpEF treatment strategy. Similar to HFpEF, atrial fibrillation reacts favorably to exercise training and weight loss. To restore sinus rhythm, only cardioversion is recommended because catheter ablation of atrial fibrillation had limited long-term success in HFpEF with single- and multiple-procedure drug-free success rates of 27% and 45%, respectively. If cardioversion is unsuccessful, rate control and permanent anticoagulation become mandatory.

DEVICES IN MANAGEMENT OF HEART FAILURE WITH PRESERVED EJECTION FRACTION

With the limitation of the pharmacological treatment in patients with heart failure, other avenues have been probed in, and some of the newer treatment modalities in form of device treatments or getting more attention. The various devices that are being used or under trial in these patients with HFpEF are:

- Interatrial shunt device
- Left ventricle expander
- Electrical therapy
- Left ventricular assist device (LVAD)
- Mechanical circulatory support devices (which are under development)

Transcatheter Interatrial Shunt Device

In patients with HFpEF, higher pressure and larger LA size are important targets for treatment since they are strongly related to symptom, hospitalization, and the devices which are intended to reduce LA pressure for device therapy in HFpEF. The use of interatrial device is based on a concept derived from the Lutembacher syndrome (a patient with mitral stenosis and interatrial septal defect who manifests fewer symptom than a patient with mitral stenosis only) to reduce LA pressure. There are three interatrial shunt devices **(Figs. 3A to C)**.

1. Interatrial shunt device
2. V-wave
3. Atrial flow regulator

All these devices can be inserted percutaneously via femoral access under the guidance of transesophageal echocardiography, and these devices can be implanted through transseptal puncture performed in the middle of interatrial septum. The main objective of using these devices is to relieve symptoms temporarily by reducing LA pressure.

V-wave Device

The V-wave interatrial shunt (V-wave Caesarea, Israel) **(Fig. 3B)** is an hourglass-shaped nitinol self-expanding prosthesis covered with a polytetrafluoroethylene polymer on the left side and a trileaflet porcine pericardium valve on the right side to prevent right-to-left flow, paradoxical embolism, and early closure. After implantation, the patient receives anticoagulation with warfarin for 3 months, and aspirin (81–100 mg/day) is administered indefinitely.

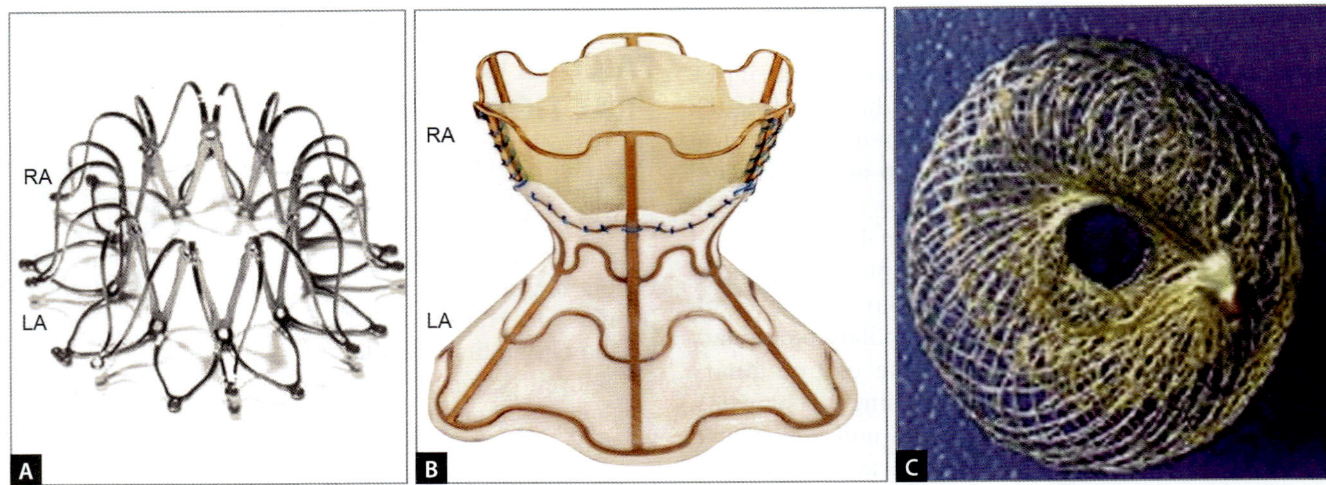

Figs. 3A to C: Devices for interatrial shunting. (A) Interatrial shunt device; (B) V-wave; (C) Atrial flow regulator. (LA left atrial; RA right atrial)

This device underwent a prospective multicenter single-arm open-label trial and clarified its safety and feasible outcomes for heart failure patients, the targets of which were HFpEF and HFrEF patients. 8 HFpEF patients and 30 HFrEF patients were enrolled in the trial and implanted with a V-wave shunt device. One patient (2.6%) had a cardiac tamponade within the hours following the procedure, but there were no other major adverse cardiovascular or neurological events. At 12 months from the device insertion, two patients died due to noncardiac causes, not related to the device or to study procedures. The major adverse event rate was 7.9%. 5 of 36 case patients (14%) had total occlusions and 13 (36%) had shunt restenosis due to pannus formation 1 year after device insertion.

The V-wave-implanted patients' New York Heart Association class improved in 78% of the patients at 3 months and 60% at 12 months, along with an increase of QoL and 6-minute-walk tests after 1 year. Importantly, the HFrEF patients who maintained patent shunts ($n = 14$) exhibited a significant improvement in PCWP at 12 months (from 23.3 ± 5.4 mm Hg at baseline to 18.0 ± 4.0 mm Hg at 12 months, $p = 0.011$) and a rise in LVEF (from 23 ± 7 to 26 ± 8%, $p = 0.007$), even though their baseline features, including older age, more severe underlying cardiac disease and comorbidities, reduced exercise capacity, poorer systolic function, and worse hemodynamic status, were generally consistent with a poorer prognosis.

Atrial Flow Regulator

The atrial flow regulator (AFR) (Occlutech, Istanbul, Turkey) is a nitinol self-expandable double-disk wired mesh with a central penetration that enables interatrial bidirectional flow **(Fig. 3C)**. It is available in 6-, 8-, and 10-mm fenestration diameters and 18-, 24-, and 30-mm total device diameters, derived via 10- or 12-Fr sheath from the femoral vein.[28,43] Antiplatelets were usually given to the patients after implantation of an AFR.

There are two reports on the AFR: A case report of 54-year-old woman with severe and irreversible pulmonary artery hypertension (PAH) and a nonrandomized pilot study reported by Kumar et al., including 12 patients with severe irreversible PAH. All procedures were successful without any major complications, and all patients had relief of syncope, improved 6MWD, and improved cardiac index. Inferior vena cava congestion and pericardium effusions were reduced, even though right ventricular function did not show significant changes. Also, the device was patent in all patients at a median follow-up of 189 days.

Even though the AFR has been used for the treatment of PAH, an international nonrandomized clinical trial (PRELIEVE, NCT03030274) is currently recruiting up to 30 patients with symptomatic HF (including HFpEF and HFrEF), based on the success of the other interatrial shunt devices.

Left Ventricle Expander

The basic pathophysiology of HFpEF is diastolic stiffness, and therefore the concept of expanding the LV from inside or outside has been under experiment and it can be a radical considering the anatomical feature of HFpEF. Currently, two devices are being tested; however, their safety, efficacy, and influence on cardiac function or need for an anticoagulant are still not defined. There is also a concern that LV expander might be temporary if further hypertrophic changes occur in LV chamber. Currently, there are two devices:

1. *CORolla Assist Device:* The CORolla (Co-Assist INC. HAIFA, Israel) is an elastic cell expanding device, which is attached to the endocardium and enhances LV diastolic expansion, improves LV filling, and lowers LV and LA pressures. The trial for percutaneous transapical insertion of the devices is ongoing. In PILOT study, it was found that following implant of this device, there was significant improvement in LV mass, LA index volume, and consistent LV remodeling at 6 months. It seems that this device may be of certain efficacy and safety.
2. *Im-Cardia:* The Im-Cardia (Co-Assist INC. HAIFA, Israel) in an elastic cell expanding device attached to the epicardial surface of LV. These devices in certain surgically by median astronomy as procedure during the surgery for aortic valve disease. In initial study with patients with severe optic stenosis who underwent a surgical treatment with Im-cardia insertion, there was significant LV mass decrease (–126 ± 33 gm) and decrease in LA area (–2.29 ± 3.09 cm^2), which were observed at 1 year of cardiac contractility modulation (CCM).

Cardiac Contractility Modulation

Cardiac contractility modulation is a type of pacemaker used for patients with heart failure. It involves applying high-voltage, long-duration, biphasic electric signals to the RV septum during the absolute myocardial refractory period. CCM delivers nonexcitatory electrical signal and improves the contraction of heart. This concept of CCM was originally developed for symptomatic HFrEF, i.e., HFrEF patients with slightly prolong who were not eligible for cardiac resynchronization therapy (CRT). The benefit of CCM in terms of quality of exercise tolerance has been demonstrated in patients with HFrEF in different studies (FIX-HF-4, FIX-HF-5, and FIX-HF-5C). These trials have been conducted in different areas in Europe and United States. In particular, subgroup analysis of FIX-HF-5 revealed that CCM has more been efficient in patients with baseline ejection fraction between 35% and 45%. Based on encouraging results of this therapy in patients with HFrEF, Tschöpe et al. prospectively investigated the effect of CCM in a few patients who had dyspnea and exercise intolerance was the primary symptom. These patients had shown early improvements in diastolic function with CCM with an increase in EF reserved for 3 months. They performed frequent endomyocardial biopsies and found an early in continues increase in pressure now key contractile proteins. Chronically, there was improvement in collision composition. Moreover, there was an increase in the cardiac protein pressure, both near the CCM probe and remotely, which indicates that the CCM leads to a global beneficial effect in cardiac reverse remodeling of HFpEF patients as was observed in patient with HFrEF patients.

There is ongoing study that is evaluating safety efficacy of CCM therapy in patients of HFpEF who were symptomatic despite appropriate guideline-directed medical treatment.

Left Atrial Permanent Pacing

The basic pathophysiological mechanism of HFpEF is LA electrical desynchrony following reduced LV function. This has been a new target of treatment in patients of HFpEF. There has been an independent correlation between the severity of the intra-atrial desynchrony and reduced LA function in patients with HFpEF. The prolonged intra-atrial desynchrony has been linked to deteriorating clinical symptoms in patients with HFpEF. This observation led to the concept of using LA pacing for HFpEF patients.

Physiological Accelerated Pacing

In HFpEF, it has been found that heart rate lowering results in adverse outcomes, and has been suggested that the opposite may be beneficial. The shortening of diastolic filling time with a higher heart rate might normalize the elevated filling pressure that is the *sine qua non* of HFpEF. The initial clinical studies assess the effect of accelerated heart rates in pacemakers, and patients with preclinical and overt HFpEF provide support for this hypothesis and have shown improvement in QoL, BNP level, and activity level at atrial fibrillation. The PACE HFpEF (physiologic accelerated pacing as treatment for Heart Failure preserved Ejection Fraction) trial is an prospective patient-blinded multiple crossover pilot study to assess the impact of accelerated pacing on QoL, physical activity, N-terminal Pro-BNP, and echocardiographic measures of cardiac structure and function. In this study, 20 patients were enrolled in dual chamber pacemaker implantation under the US Food Drug Administration. Investigation device exemption with both atrial and ventricular physiologic lead placement targeting the Bachmann Bundle and the His Bundle. The enrollment for this study has been completed. All study participants underwent successful dual chamber pacemaker implantation and completed outcome.

Baroreceptor Activation Therapy

Arterial baroreceptors are located at carotid sinuses and arterial baroreflex induced by these baroreceptors are strong regulators of intravascular stressed blood volume, which provides regulation of blood pressure in heart rate. The reduced baroreceptor heart rate reflects sensitivity that has been shown to be an independent predictor of outcomes in heart failure, and therefore baroreceptor activation therapy (BAT) is being tested as a device for treating autonomic dysregulation in patients of HFpEF.

Baroreceptor activation therapy is an electrical technology that stimulates the carotid sinuses with an implanted pacemaker-like device. BAT was initially developed for resistant hypertension. In patients with HFpEF, there is an ongoing prospective registry (BAROSTIM THERAPY in Heart Failure with Preserved Ejection Fraction), the results for which will be available soon.

Left Ventricular Assist Device for HFpEF and Diastolic Dysfunction

The left ventricular assist device (LVAD) is a standard and essential option for the patients with end-stage HFrEF with dilated or ischemic cardiomyopathy. LVAD has demonstrated improved morbidity and mortality in this subset of patients. However, there are limited reports of LVAD being implanted in HFpEF patients because of their typical feature of relatively small left ventricle.

Left Atrial Assist Device

A left atrial assist device (LAAD) **(Figs. 4A and B)** has been under development that can be implanted in mitral position so that the blood from left atrium will fill the left ventricle. This is a mixed-flow pump with a diameter and height of approximately 30–40 mm.

This will be able to pump up to 10 liter/minute and up to 180 mm Hg. In the INVETRO study, LAAD has been found to increase cardiac output and decrease LA pressure under diastolic heart failure conditions whereas the atrial pulsatility and full function of aortic valves are maintained. The concept of LAAD is that the entire flow is from left ventricle through the aortic valve and LV remodeling may be expected by dilatation of the LV cavity and an increase in LV compliance. LAAD may provide a bridge-to-recovery therapy for HFpEF patients. There is less risk of suction event with this device because the typical left atrium of HFpEF patients is dilated and LA pressure is significantly elevated. However, when HFpEF patients improve, careful maintenance of pump speed or consideration of pump explant is needed because the smaller or normal size of LA could be risk for LA suction events. One major limitation of LAAD support is the possible impact of elevated LV end-diastolic pressure because it may hamper coronary blood flow and affect right ventricular function.

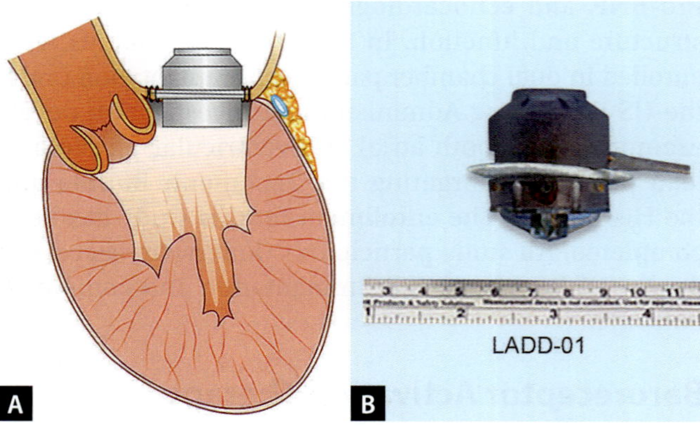

Figs. 4A and B: *Left atrial assist device (LAAD):* (A) Implanted at the mitral position; (B) Dimension of the LAAD.

CONCLUSION

- HFpEF is a condition with vast pathophysiological complexity and clinical heterogeneity; as a result of this, any specific pharmacological treatment appears to be a distant possibility.
- The identification of specific clinical subtypes has helped in choosing specific strategies to handle specific pathophysiological alterations and comorbidities with aim to improve QoL and mortality.
- Currently, aldosterone antagonist and more importantly, SGLT2 inhibitors have been shown to have beneficial role in HFpEF due to their spectrum of action affecting multiple common pathophysiological aspects of different phenotypes of HFpEF.

REFERENCES

1. Shah SJ, Kitzman DW, Borlaug BA, et al. Phenotype-specific treatment of heart failure with preserved ejection fraction: a multiorgan roadmap: Circulation. 2016;134(1):73-90.
2. Shah SJ, Katz DH, Deo RC. Phenotypic spectrum of heart failure with preserved ejection fraction. Heart Fail Clin. 2014;10(3):407-18.
3. Haass M, Kitzman DW, Anand IS, et al. Body mass index and adverse cardiovascular outcomes in heart failure patients with preserved ejection fraction: result from the Ibesartan in Heart Failure with Preserved Ejection Fraction (I-PRESERVE) trial. Circ Heart Fail. 2011;4(3): 324-31.
4. D'Elia E, Vaduganathan M, Gori M, et al. Role of biomarkers in cardiac structure phenotyping in heart failure with preserved ejection fraction: critical appraisal and practical use. Eur J Heart Fail. 2015;17(12):1231-9.
5. Franssen C, Chen S, Unger A, et al. Myocardial micro-vascular inflammatory endothelial activation in heart

failure with preserved ejection fraction. JACC Heart Fail. 2016;4(4):312-4.
6. Westermann D, Lindner D, Kasner M, et al. Cardiac inflammation contributes to changes in the extracellular matrix in patients with heart failure and normal ejection fraction. Circ Heart Fail. 2011;4(1):44-52.
7. Bishu K, Deswal A, Chen HH, et al. Biomarkers in acutely decompensated heart failure with preserved or reduced ejection fraction. Am Heart J. 2012;164(5):763-70.e3.
8. Neeland IJ, Winders BR, Ayers CR, et al. Higher natriuretic peptide levels associate with a favorable adipose tissue distribution profile. J Am Coll Cardiol. 2013;62(8):752-60.
9. Paulus WJ. Culprit mechanism(s) for exercise intolerance in heart failure with normal ejection fraction. J Am Coll Cardiol. 2010;56:864-6.
10. van Empel VP, Mariani J, Borlaug BA, et al. Impaired myocardial oxygen availability contributes to abnormal exercise hemodynamics in heart failure with preserved ejection fraction. J Am Heart Assoc. 2014;3(6):e001293.
11. Senni M, Paulus WJ, Gavazzi A., et al. New strategies for heart failure with preserved ejection fraction: The importance of targeted therapies for heart failure phenotypes. Eur Heart J. 2014;35(40):2797-815.
12. Sharma K, Kass DA. Heart failure with preserved ejection fraction: mechanisms, clinical features, and therapies. Circ Res. 2014;115(1):79-96.
13. Wohlfahrt P, Redfield MM, Lopez-Jimenez F, et al. Impact of general and central adiposity on ventricular-arterial aging in women and men. JACC Heart Fail. 2014;2(5):489-99.
14. Borlaug BA. The pathophysiology of heart failure with preserved ejection fraction. Nat Rev Cardiol. 2014;11(9):507-15.
15. Abraham WT, Stevenson LW, Bourge RC, et al; CHAMPION Trial Study Group. Sustained efficacy of pulmonary artery pressure to guide adjustment of chronic heart failure therapy: Complete follow-up results from the CHAMPION randomised trial. Lancet. 2016;387(10017):453-61.
16. Kitzman DW, Brubaker P, Morgan T, et al. Effect of caloric restriction or aerobic exercise training on peak oxygen consumption and quality of life in obese older patients with heart failure with preserved ejection fraction: A randomized clinical trial. JAMA. 2016;315(1):36-46.
17. Ramasubbu K, Estep J, White DL, et al. Experimental and clinical basis for the use of statins in patients with ischemic and non-ischemic cardiomyopathy. J Am Coll Cardiol. 2008;51(4):415-26.
18. Antoniades C, Bakogiannis C, Leeson P, et al. Rapid, direct effects of statin treatment on arterial redox state and nitric oxide bioavailability in human atherosclerosis via tetrahydrobiopterin-mediated endothelial nitric oxide synthase coupling. Circulation. 2011;124:335-45.
19. Zakeri R, Chamberlain AM, Roger VL, et al. Temporal relationship and prognostic significance of atrial fibrillation in heart failure patients with preserved ejection fraction: a community-based study. Circulation. 2013;128:1085-93.
20. Fukuta H, Sane DC, Brucks S, et al. Statin therapy may be associated with lower mortality in patients with diastolic heart failure: a preliminary report. Circulation. 2005;112:357-63.
21. Gomberg-Maitland M, Shah SJ, Guazzi M. Inflammation in heart failure with preserved ejection fraction: Time to put out the fire. JACC Heart Fail. 2016;4:325-8.
22. Redfield MM, Anstrom KJ, Levine JA, et al; NHLBI Heart Failure Clinical Research Network. Isosorbide mononitrate in heart failure with preserved ejection fraction. N Engl J Med. 2015;373(24):2314-24.
23. Schwartzenberg S, Redfield MM, From AM, et al. Effects of vasodilation in heart failure with preserved or reduced ejection fraction implications of distinct pathophysiologies on response to therapy. J Am Coll Cardiol. 2012;59(5):442-51.
24. Thomas GR, DiFabio JM, Gori T, et al. Once daily therapy with isosorbide-5-mononitrate causes endothelial dysfunction in humans: Evidence of a free-radical-mediated mechanism. J Am Coll Cardiol. 2007;49(12): 1289-95.
25. Vanderpool R, Gladwin MT. Harnessing the nitrate-nitrite-nitric oxide pathway for therapy of heart failure with preserved ejection fraction. Circulation. 2015;131(4):334-6.
26. Omar SA, Fok H, Tilgner KD, et al. Paradoxical normoxia-dependent selective actions of inorganic nitrite in human muscular conduit arteries and related selective actions on central blood pressures. Circulation. 2015;131(4):381-9; discussion 389.
27. Borlaug BA, Koepp KE, Melenovsky V. Sodium nitrite improves exercise hemodynamics and ventricular performance in heart failure with preserved ejection fraction. J Am Coll Cardiol. 2015;66(15):1672-82.
28. Eggebeen J, Kim-Shapiro DB, Haykowsky M, et al. One week of daily dosing with beetroot juice improves submaximal endurance and blood pressure in older patients with heart failure and preserved ejection fraction. JACC Heart Fail. 2016;4(6):428-37.
29. Lee DI, Zhu G, Sasaki T, et al. Phosphodiesterase 9A controls nitric-oxide-independent cGMP and hypertrophic heart disease. Nature. 2015;519(7544):472-6.
30. Takimoto E, Champion HC, Li M, et al. Chronic inhibition of cyclic GMP phosphodiesterase 5A prevents and reverses cardiac hypertrophy. Nat Med. 2005;11(2):214-22.
31. Lee DI, Kass DA. Phosphodiesterases and cyclic GMP regulation in heart muscle. Physiology (Bethesda). 2012;27:248-58.
32. Gheorghiade M, Greene SJ, Filippatos G, et al; COMPOSE Investigators and Coordinators. Cinaciguat, a soluble guanylate cyclase activator: Results from the randomized, controlled, phase IIb COMPOSE programme in acute heart failure syndromes. Eur J Heart Fail. 2012;14(9):1056-66.
33. Ghofrani HA, Galiè N, Grimminger F, et al; PATENT-1 Study Group. Riociguat for the treatment of pulmonary arterial hypertension. N Engl J Med. 2013;369(4):330-40.
34. Solomon SD, Zile M, Pieske B, et al; Prospective comparison of ARNI with ARB on Management Of heart failure with preserved ejection fraction (PARAMOUNT) Investigators. The angiotensin receptor neprilysin inhibitor LCZ696

in heart failure with preserved ejection fraction: a phase 2 double-blind randomised controlled trial. Lancet. 2012;380:1387-95.
35. Hoendermis ES, Liu LC, Hummel YM, et al. Effects of sildenafil on invasive haemodynamics and exercise capacity in heart failure patients with preserved ejection fraction and pulmonary hypertension: a randomized controlled trial. Eur Heart J. 2015;36:2565-73.
36. Pitt B, Pfeffer MA, Assmann SF, et al; TOPCAT Investigators. Spironolactone for heart failure with preserved ejection fraction. N Engl J Med. 2014;370:1383-92.
37. Pfeffer MA, Claggett B, Assmann SF, et al. Regional variation in patients and outcomes in the Treatment of Preserved Cardiac Function Heart Failure With an Aldosterone Antagonist (TOPCAT) trial. Circulation. 2015;131:34-42.
38. Zile MR, Jhund PS, Baicu CF, et al; Prospective Comparison of ARNI With ARB on Management of Heart Failure With Preserved Ejection Fraction (PARAMOUNT) Investigators. Plasma biomarkers reflecting profibrotic processes in heart failure with a preserved ejection fraction: data from the Prospective Comparison of ARNI With ARB on Management of Heart Failure With Preserved Ejection Fraction Study. Circ Heart Fail. 2016;9(1): e002551.
39. Hummel SL, Seymour EM, Brook RD, et al. Low-sodium DASH diet improves diastolic function and ventricular-arterial coupling in hypertensive heart failure with preserved ejection fraction. Circ Heart Fail. 2013;6(6): 1165-71.
40. Ter Maaten JM, Damman K, Verhaar MC, et al. Connecting heart failure with preserved ejection fraction and renal dysfunction: the role of endothelial dysfunction and inflammation. Eur J Heart Fail. 2016;18(6):588-98.
41. Gori M, Senni M, Gupta DK, et al; PARAMOUNT Investigators. Association between renal function and cardiovascular structure and function in heart failure with preserved ejection fraction. Eur Heart J. 2014;35(48): 3442-51.
42. Hwang SJ, Melenovsky V, Borlaug BA. Implications of coronary artery disease in heart failure with preserved ejection fraction. J Am Coll Cardiol. 2014;63(25 pt A): 2817-27.
43. Borlaug BA, Melenovsky V, Russell SD, et al. Impaired chronotropic and vasodilator reserves limit exercise capacity in patients with heart failure and a preserved ejection fraction. Circulation. 2006;114(20):2138-47.
44. Brubaker PH, Joo KC, Stewart KP, et al. Chronotropic incompetence and its contribution to exercise intolerance in older heart failure patients. J Cardiopulm Rehabil. 2006;26(2):86-9.
45. Melenovsky V, Hwang SJ, Lin G, et al. Right heart dysfunction in heart failure with preserved ejection fraction. Eur Heart J. 2014;35(48):3452-62.
46. Edelmann F, Gelbrich G, Düngen HD, et al. Exercise training improves exercise capacity and diastolic function in patients with heart failure with preserved ejection fraction: Results of the Ex-DHF (Exercise training in Diastolic Heart Failure) pilot study. J Am Coll Cardiol. 2011;58:1780-91.
47. Melenovsky V, Hwang SJ, Redfield MM, et al. Left atrial remodeling and function in advanced heart failure with preserved or reduced ejection fraction. Circ Heart Fail. 2015;8:295-303.
48. Machino-Ohtsuka T, Seo Y, Ishizu T, et al. Efficacy, safety, and outcomes of catheter ablation of atrial fibrillation in patients with heart failure with preserved ejection fraction. J Am Coll Cardiol. 2013;62:1857-65.
49. Paulus WJ, Tschöpe C. A novel paradigm for heart failure with preserved ejection fraction: comorbidities drive myocardial dysfunction and remodeling through coronary microvascular endothelial inflammation. J Am Coll Cardiol. 2013;624(4):263-71.
50. Ha JW, Oh JK, Pellikka PA, et al. Diastolic stress echocardiography: a novel noninvasive diagnostic test for diastolic dysfunction using spine bicycle exercise Doppler echocardiography. J Am Soc Echocardiogr. 2005;18(1):63-8.

CHAPTER

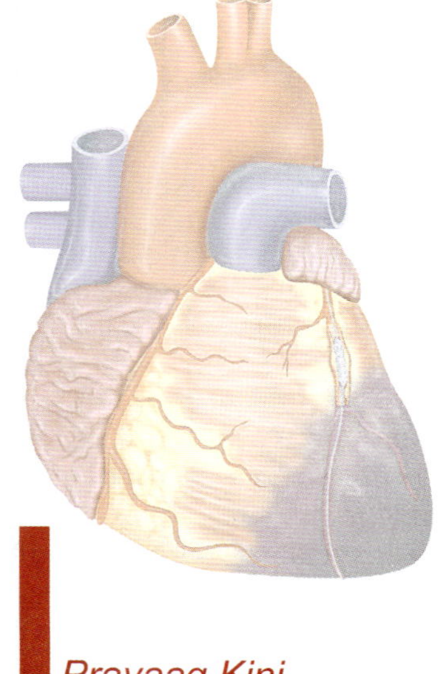

Advances in Management of HFpEF: Chasing the Elusive "Jigsaw"

Prayaag Kini

INTRODUCTION

Heart failure with preserved ejection fraction (HFpEF) is a complex clinical syndrome affecting approximately up to 32 million people worldwide.[1] HFpEF is mainly characterized by the presence of diastolic dysfunction (DD) and elevated left ventricular (LV) filling pressure in the setting of a LV ejection fraction (LVEF) ≥50%.[2] Despite epidemiological evidence of a steadily increasing prevalence now recognized worldwide, both in absolute and relative terms, its diagnosis and management can still pose a challenge. Today, HFpEF is understood as being characterized by different phenotypes driven by varying profiles of cardiac and noncardiac comorbidities. Patients with HFpEF are hospitalized approximately more than once within 1 year after diagnosis and have a mortality rate of approximately 15% per year.[1] Two scores have been created to better recognize this syndrome: (1) The H2FPEF score in 2018 and (2) the HFA-PEFF algorithm in 2020.[3-5] A head-to-head comparison has shown differences in sensitivity and specificities and even ethnic polarizations. Heterogeneity in HFpEF etiologies could be one reason why several HFpEF clinical trials did not reach strong outcomes to recommend a single therapy for this syndrome, as against HF with reduced ejection fraction (HFrEF), where four pillars have been elected as optimal medical therapy from international guidelines.[6,7]

With clarity coming in from various quarters, HFpEF treatment paradigm has changed for the better in recent times with the advent of the sodium-glucose cotransporter-2 inhibitors (SGLT2i), which beneficially act through the whole spectrum of LVEF.[8] Implantable devices like interatrial shunt-based devices and the CardioMEMS and use of cardiac contractility modulation, vagal and tragal stimulation, and renal denervation (RDN) have opened up newer vistas for monitoring and guiding therapy adding yet another layer of solace. Although all of these represent a remarkable leap forward in management of HFpEF, there are still areas of uncertainty and lack of clarity.

In this chapter, we focus on the HFpEF phenotypes according to the latest evidence, the role of the new drugs, and the potential role of new devices to treat this complex syndrome.

BACKGROUND

Understanding HFpEF Phenotypes: HFrEF versus HFpEF Pathophysiology

The term "preserved ejection fraction" was first coined in the CHARM program to split the enrolled population into two subgroups on the basis of the most validated and readily available tool to define LV contractile abilities, which was LVEF that was ubiquitously measured by simple outpatient echocardiography and primarily studied subgroup of patients who could benefit from therapies targeting neurohormonal activation.[9] HFpEF, however, turned out to be a "different animal" and it was easily recognized that the mainstays of the *reduced "LVEF paradigm",* which consisted of a single organ involved with recognizable dysfunction and lesser need to deeply investigate the underlying etiology (most likely Ischemic with its relevant treatment), did not fit in the HFpEF setting

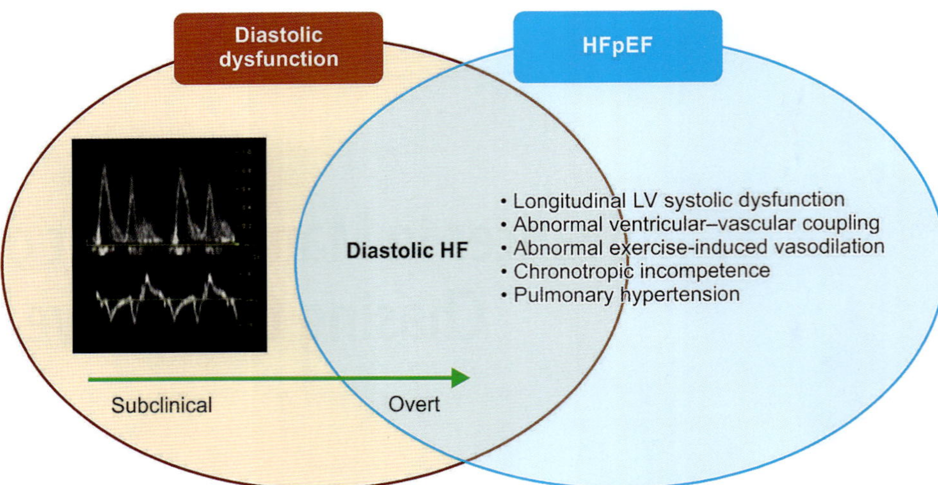

Fig. 1: Diastolic dysfunction and evolution towards diastolic HF.

where multiple organs and systems are involved, with the heart playing an important, but not exclusive, role. A variety of morphological and functional abnormalities of uncertain significance coexisted; however, rest echocardiography still plays a pivotal role as a primary diagnostic role. Further trial evidence led us to consider the importance of phenotype in HFpEF and to address a tailored therapy rather than "one size fits all" paradigm in HFrEF.

The DD and evolution towards diastolic HF are given in **Figure 1**.

From a hemodynamic perspective, a hallmark of HFpEF is a pulmonary capillary wedge pressure of ≥15 mm Hg (at rest) or ≥25 mm Hg (after exercise), or LV end-diastolic pressure ≥16 mm Hg (at rest).[3,4] Right heart catheterization at rest and during exercise is indeed the diagnostic gold standard for an accurate HFpEF diagnosis.[5] However, direct hemodynamic measurement during exercise is an invasive procedure and should be reserved for selected cases only.

Phenotyping for Tailored Therapy

Complexity and multimorbidity are the hallmarks of HFpEF. The underlying understanding is that HFpEF is not a single disease, but rather a group of different disease processes that share HF symptoms and signs as clinical manifestations. According to a HFpEF model,[10] patients with HFpEF could fall into one or another part of the circle and they could develop the syndrome on the basis of a single mechanism or as the result of multiple concurrent injuries. Addressing the single components of the picture seems to be the way to tailored treatment.[11,12] The studies supporting this view divide HFpEF cohorts into mutually exclusive subgroups, the so-called phenotypes, on the basis of the clinical and epidemiological characteristics of patients.[13-20] The cluster of comorbidities characterizing a specific phenotype is the result of a specific pathological pathway that could be hopefully targeted by specific treatments.

HFpEF Phenotypic Clustering: Pieces of the Jigsaw

The physiopathological complexity of HFpEF has prompted cardiologists to use artificial intelligence and machine learning techniques to analyze the complex relationships within this diverse population and identify specific subgroups that could be treated homogeneously to an extent. Following pioneering studies by Shah et al.[11], Uijl et al. proposed a model consisting of five clusters obtained from HFpEF patients recorded in the Swedish Heart Failure Registry and validated it externally with the Chronic Heart Failure European Society of Cardiology guideline-based Cardiology Practice Quality project registry **(Fig. 2)**.[18]

The first cluster is that of young patients, with an average age <60 years and a reduced burden of comorbidities, including arterial hypertension and obesity. This group also includes those with HF with improved ejection fraction (EF). Weight loss and blood pressure control using renin–angiotensin–aldosterone system (RAAS) inhibitors (RAASi) are central to these patients.

The second cluster is the most prevalent of the four clusters of HFpEF population and consists of patients with an average age of 77 years who have AF, in the absence of diabetes. These patients predominantly benefit from a less stringent heart rate control to avoid further reducing their already compromised chronotropic reserve.

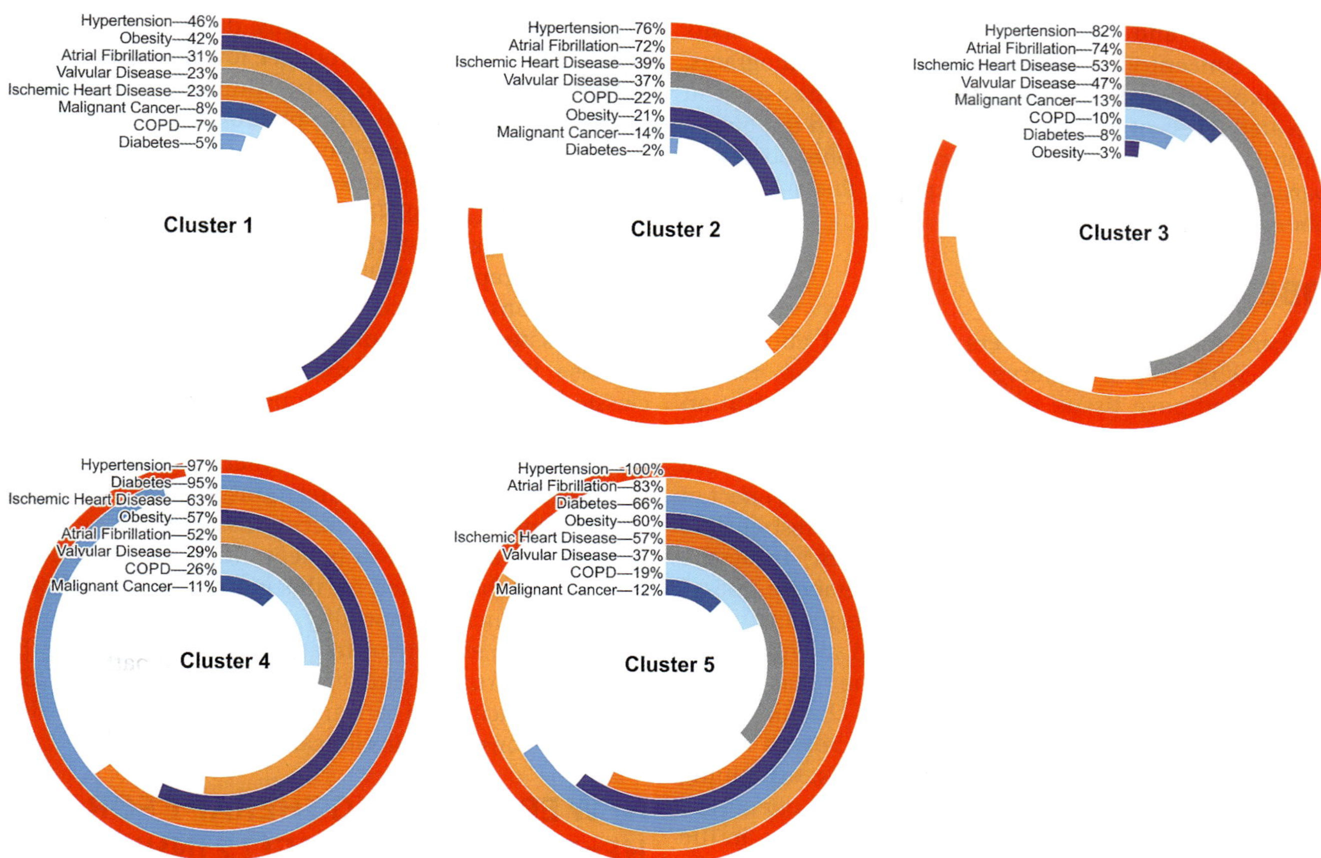

Fig. 2: Identification of distinct phenotypic clusters in heart failure with preserved ejection fraction.
Source: Uijl et al. (2021).

The third cluster is the second most represented and consists of the oldest patients, with an average age of 88 years, the highest burden of comorbidities, and the highest concentration of natriuretic peptides. These patients derive the highest prognostic benefit from the intensive treatment of all comorbidities. They present with clinically overt HF with frank congestion, which must be treated with diuretics, including antialdosterone agents, which have shown remarkable clinical benefit in clinical trials such as the TOPCAT trial.[21]

The fourth cluster consists of patients with an average age of 71 years, AF, and diabetes. In this group of patients, in addition to glycemic control, the introduction of an SGLT2i appears to be fundamental, as the EMPEROR-Preserved and DELIVER trials have shown a reduction in cardiovascular (CV) mortality and hospitalization for HF.

Finally, the fifth cluster is the fusion of the second and fourth clusters as it includes elderly patients with an average age of 82 years, diabetes, and AF. The DECLARE-TIMI 58 trial found that diabetes patients without AF may benefit from the use of SGLT2i because they have a preventive effect on this arrhythmia.[22-24]

Thus, these four clusters broadly include a population that is, on average, older (aged between 60 and 90 years), with a higher burden of comorbidities, including arterial hypertension.

CURRENT PROGRESS IN "PHENOMAPPING": DOES IT SHOW THE WAY AHEAD?

Recently, a review conducted by Peters et al. identified the three most recurrent HFpEF phenotypes in studies that focused on specific characteristics through statistical analysis of large datasets, known as "phenomapping".[25] These three phenotypes were also observed in studies where researchers did not employ this static strategy, demonstrating some robustness in the results **(Fig. 1)**.[26]

The first two analyzed phenotypes closely reflect everyday clinical practice, as they represent two patient groups commonly encountered in outpatient settings. The most prevalent phenotype is "older, vascular aging", which conforms with the findings of Shah et al., describing a group of elderly patients with arterial stiffness leading to hypertension and chronic kidney disease.[11] These patients exhibit concentric LV hypertrophy on echocardiograms, a higher incidence of chronic kidney disease, and elevated levels of inflammatory molecules in the blood, contributing to the pathophysiology of this phenotype and partially justifying its partial overlap with the "metabolic, obese" group.

OBESITY AND HFpEF

Beyond the different clusters mentioned above, the obese with HFpEF deserve special mention. Excess visceral adipose tissue promotes the hyperactivation of neurohormonal systems that, together with the reduced plasma activity of neprilysin typical of these patients, make the proinflammatory and fibrotic effect of aldosterone unopposed, favoring DD that is responsible for the progressive increase in filling pressures.[27] In fact the second most frequent phenotype is the "metabolic, obese", represented by patients with high body weight and type 2 diabetes, predisposing them to widespread atherosclerotic vascular disease, particularly affecting the renal vessels, which accounts for the high prevalence of chronic kidney disease in this group. Obesity leads to increased renin-angiotensin activity and aldosterone levels, explaining why patients with characteristics related to this phenotype showed better responsiveness to spironolactone in the TOPCAT trial.[28] Likewise, the STEP-HFpEF trial has recently demonstrated in obese HFpEF patients that take semaglutide versus placebo significantly reduced body weight, improving symptoms, physical limitations and exercise function, with a positive impact on quality of life (QoL), inflammatory status, and survival.[29] Considering the typical pathophysiological changes of the obese phenotype, RAASi, particularly aldosterone antagonists and neprilysin inhibitors (ARNI), play a central role, in addition to the use of SGLT2i.

It is also understood that inflammation is responsible for remodeling the left atrial muscle and conduction tissue, promoting in sense a "left atrial myopathy", associated with increased pulmonary pressures and RV dysfunction (**Fig. 2** ensemble). Arterial stiffness and kidney disease mandate more stringent blood pressure control with drugs targeting the RAAS and will continue to play a central role. These elderly hypertensive patients are at a higher risk of AF, which is deleterious in HFpEF patients by loss of the "atrial kick" (**Fig. 3**).

AGING AND HFpEF: SEMINAL CONSIDERATIONS

There is a gradient of age, inflammation, diagnostic tools, and poor prognosis, which is highest in the "older, vascular aging" phenotype and gradually decreases from the "metabolic, obese" to the "younger, low BNP" phenotype. While the patients in the first phenotype are older, those belonging to the third phenotype are "relatively younger", with lower levels of stress biomarkers, such as B-type natriuretic peptide (BNP)/N-terminal fraction of pro-BNP (NT-proBNP) and soluble ST2. Identifying these patients solely through peptide assays and resting echocardiography is challenging; thus, prompt additional investigations are necessary, including noninvasive or invasive assessment of pulmonary artery pressures during exercise. While older HFpEF patients often experience classic symptoms, such as dyspnea and fatigue, younger patients with low BNP levels may present with other symptoms, such as exercise intolerance, unexplained dyspnea on exertion or other nonspecific complaints. Medications, lifestyle modifications, and interventions that have been shown to benefit older HFpEF patients may need to be tailored for this group. Traditional hard endpoints, such as mortality, may not be suitable for assessing the efficacy of treatments in younger HFpEF patients. Alternative outcome measures, including QoL, exercise capacity, and early markers of HFpEF progression should be considered in clinical trials.

NEW ERA OF DRUG THERAPY FOR HFpEF: ADVENT OF SGLT2 INHIBITORS

In recent years, cardiologists have added SGLT2i to their pharmacological arsenal.[6,7] Initially, these molecules were shown to reduce the incidence of CV events, including HF, in patients with type 2 diabetes who were at high or very high CV risk.[24,30-32]

The introduction of SGLT2i has opened up a new avenue for HF treatment beyond neurohormonal activation control. The mechanism of action of this drug class is complex and not yet fully understood. However, it is known that inhibiting SGLT2 at the proximal convoluted tubule level causes glucose and sodium to be excreted in the urine, which, due to osmotic effects, promotes diuresis.[33] This diuresis, however, is different from that caused by loop diuretics, as it appears to have a selective effect on interstitial volume, with minimal impact on vascular volume. This leads to a reduction in preload and, albeit modestly, blood pressure without triggering compensatory activation of the RAAS (**Fig. 4**).[34]

Two randomized controlled clinical trials, DAPA-HF and EMPEROR-Reduced, were conducted with patients of HFrEF.[35,36] In these trials, dapagliflozin and empagliflozin, respectively, significantly reduced the incidence of fatal CV events and hospitalization for HF, leading to their inclusion as the "fourth pillar" of HFrEF pharmacological therapy. The efficacy of these molecules was also studied

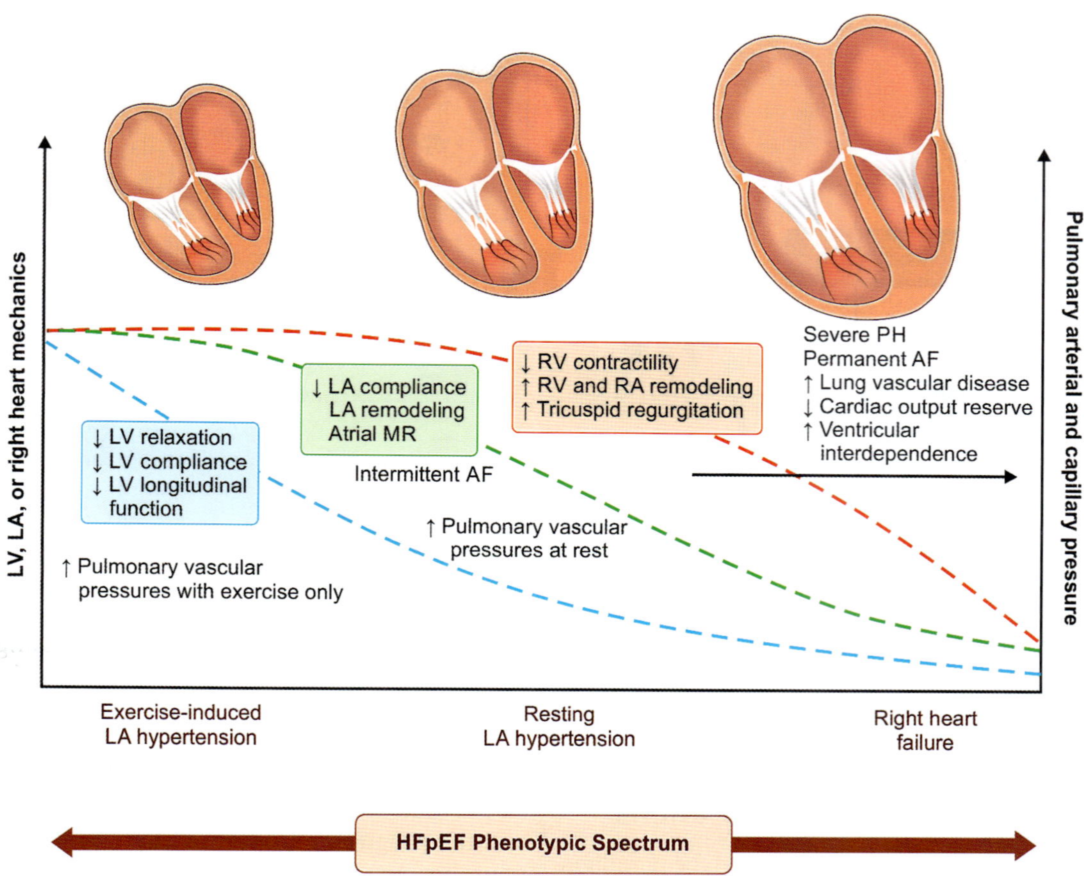

Fig. 3: Hemodynamics of HFpEF.
Source: Borlaug BA, Sharma K, Shah SJ, et al. Heart failure with preserved ejection fraction: JACC scientific statement. J Am Coll Cardiol. 2023;81(18):1810-34.

in HFpEF and heart failure with moderately reduced EF (HFmrEF) in the EMPEROR-Preserved and DELIVER clinical trials.[22,23] Both trials had positive results, with a significant reduction in the primary outcome (a composite of CV death and hospitalization for HF) **(Flowchart 1)**.

The magnitude of the effect was similar in EMPEROR-Preserved (HR 0.79, 95% CI 0.69–0.90, p <0.001) and in DELIVER (HR 0.82, 95% CI 0.73–0.92, p <0.001). The positive result was driven by a lower risk of hospitalization for HF and worsening HF events. The effect on CV deaths was almost significant in both trials (HR 0.88, 95% CI 0.74–1.05 in DELIVER; HR 0.91, 95% CI 0.76–1.09 in EMPEROR-Preserved). Given the large number of patients needed to reach a significant result, a prespecified meta-analysis of DELIVER and EMPEROR-Preserved was planned, and it proved a significant reduction in CV mortality (HR 0.88, 95% CI 0.77–1.00).[37] SGLT2i also improved health status and QoL, as measured by the Kansas City Cardiomyopathy Questionnaire.[38,39] In summary, empagliflozin and dapagliflozin significantly reduced the incidence of CV events and worsening HF in HFpEF, demonstrating that SGLT2i improved the prognosis of HF patients across the entire LVEF spectrum.

Additionally, we also understand that the increase in sodium concentration in the ultrafiltrate promotes the restoration of a normal tubuloglomerular feedback, which, through the macula densa, induces vasoconstriction of the afferent arteriole. This leads to a reduction in intraglomerular pressure, which, due to hemodynamic effects, reduces the extent and rate of the glomerular filtration and proteinuria reduction.[40-42] The beneficial effect on the kidneys is purely hemodynamic and visible from the beginning of drug administration. Simultaneously, a transient mild reduction in the glomerular filtration rate and, equally slightly, an increase in creatinine levels can be observed. SGLT2i reduce insulin resistance and contribute to weight loss, both for their diuretic effect and, over time, for the loss of calories in the urine, which induces a fasting-like state promoting lipolysis and ketogenesis.[43,44]

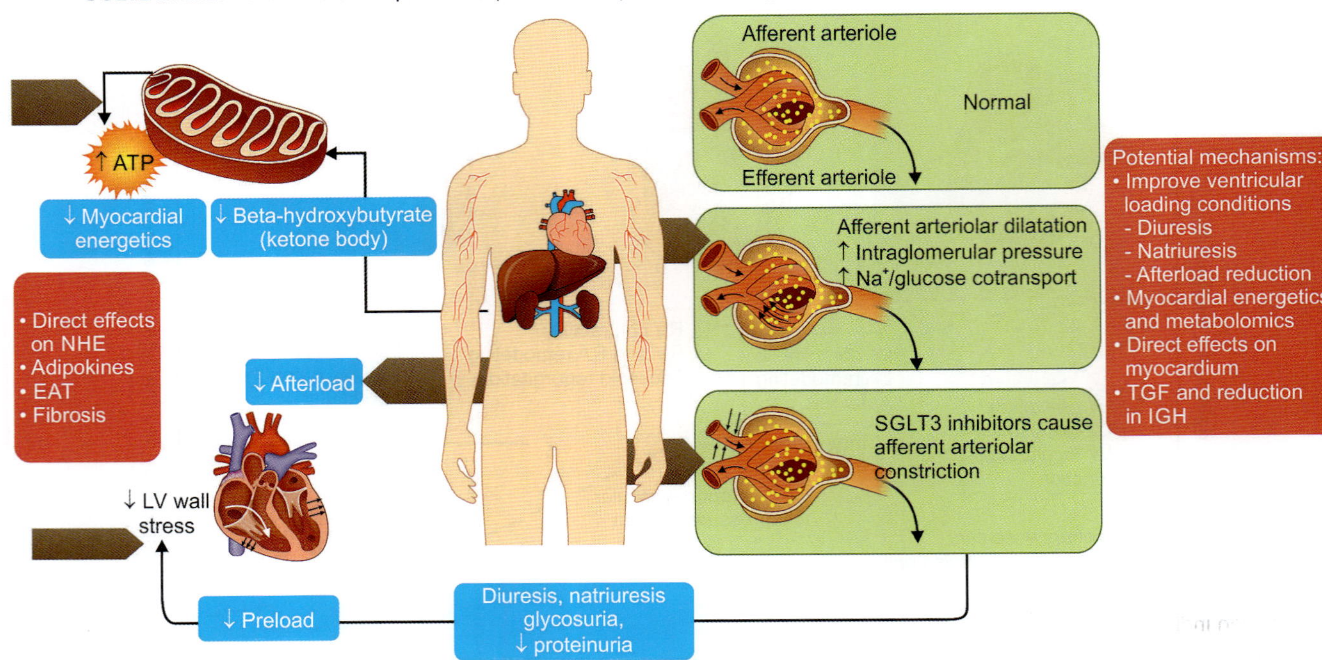

Fig. 4: Proposed mechanism of cardiovascular benefits of SGLT2i in HF.

SGLT2 Inhibitors: Practical Implications

The introduction of SGLT2i has transformed the paradigm of HFpEF treatment.[45-47] Rather than solely targeting neurohormonal activation, this class of drugs addresses comorbidities, which are a peculiar feature of HFpEF, and offers a valuable opportunity for cross-sectional intervention on the cardio-renal-metabolic continuum, which is profoundly altered in these patients.

According to new evidence, SGLT2i should be introduced during hospitalization for acute HF.[48] Clinical studies have shown that their use is safe, well-tolerated, and effective in achieving faster decongestion. Furthermore, their use in combination with ARNI and mineralocorticoid receptor antagonists (MRA) has an additive effect, facilitating faster titration of the latter due to improved potassium control.[49,50]

The multidimensional composite benefits of SGLT2i are given in **Figure 5**.

NEUROHORMONAL ANTAGONISM AND RAAS BLOCKADE IN HFpEF

Patterns of neurohormonal activation are different in HF cohorts according to LVEF.[51,52] Sympathetic and RAAS activation, resulting in elevated levels of plasma renin activity, aldosterone, catecholamines, and NT-proBNP, is a key feature of HFrEF. Just a small proportion of HFpEF patients display the same cascade of activation, and the prognostic impact of elevated plasma levels of neurohormones (well established in HFrEF patients) is uncertain in the HFpEF subgroup.[53] The heterogeneity of the HFpEF population is at least in part responsible for the puzzling results of the several neutral trials that tried to replicate the success achieved in the HFrEF trials **(Fig. 6)**.[54,55]

ANGIOTENSIN-CONVERTING ENZYME INHIBITORS AND ANGIOTENSIN RECEPTOR BLOCKERS

Three large-scale randomized clinical trials tested the safety and efficacy of angiotensin-converting enzyme inhibitors in HFpEF.[56-58] Two of them, the CHARM-Preserved and the I-PRESERVE used an angiotensin receptor blocker (ARB), and the PEP-CHF trial used an angiotensin-converting enzyme inhibitor.[56-58] CHARM-Preserved inclusion criteria were: LVEF >40%, New York Heart Association (NYHA) class II–IV, and previous hospital admission for HF. The primary outcome of composite CV death and HF admission was not met (HR 0.89, 95% CI 0.77–1.03, $p = 0.118$). The echocardiographic CHARM substudy proved that only half of patients enrolled had a moderate or severe DD, given that a worse DD was a strong prognostic predictor.[59] Based on these observations, the clinical trials

Flowchart 1: SGLT2i in HFpEF—proposed mechanism of usage.

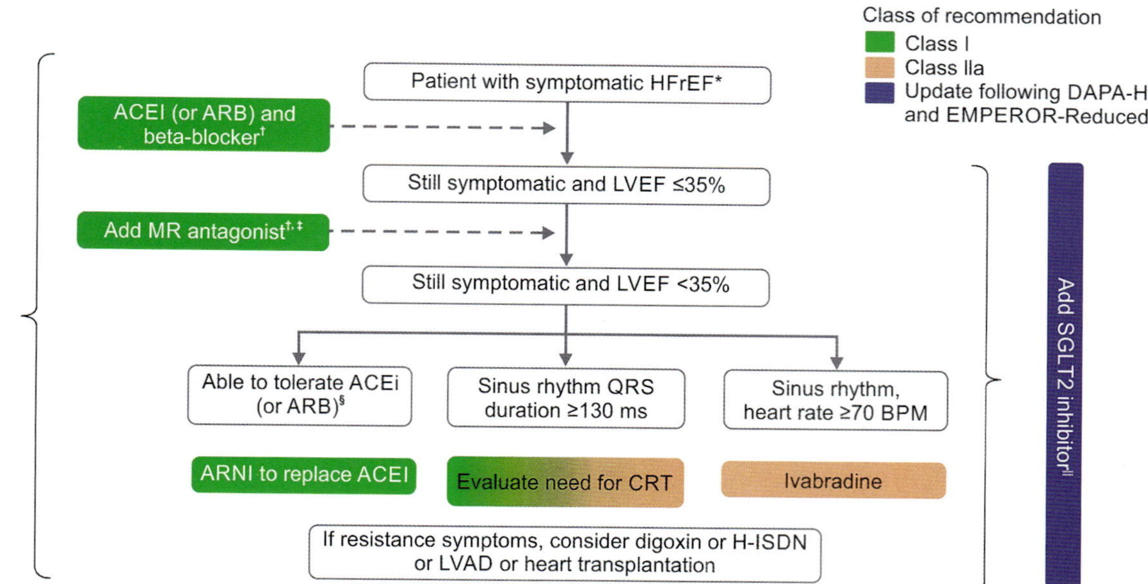

Note: Green indicates a class I recommendation; orange indicates a class IIa recommendation; blue indicates the suggested revision to the algorithm based on recent DAPA-HF trial results.

*NYHA class II–IV, LVEF <40%; †Uptitrate to maximum tolerated evidence-based dose; ‡With a hospital admission for HF within the last 6 months or with elevated natriuretic peptides (BNP >250 pg/mL or NT-proBNP >500 pg/mL in men and 750 pg/mL in women); §With an elevated plasma natriuretic peptide level (BNP ≥150 pg/mL or plasma NT-ProBNP ≥600 pg/mL, or if hospitalization within 12 months plasma BNP ≥100 pg/mL or plasma NT-proBNP ≥400 pg/mL); ||Dapagliflozin is the only SGLT2 inhibitor that has demonstrated significant and clinically meaningful reductions in both the CV deaths and worsening HF components of the primary composite endpoint in patients with HFrEF, both with and without T2D.

(ACEI: angiotensin-converting enzyme inhibitor; ARB: angiotensin-receptor blocker; ARNI: angiotensin receptor–neprilysin inhibitor; BNP: B-type natriuretic peptide; CRT: cardiac resynchronization therapy; H-ISDN: hydralazine and isosorbide dinitrate; HF: heart failure; HFrEF: heart failure with reduced ejection fraction; LVAD: left ventricular assist device; LVEF: left ventricular ejection fraction: MR: mineralocorticoid receptor, NT-ProBNP: N-terminal pro-B-type natriuretic peptide; NYHA: New York Heart Association: SGLT2: sodium–glucose cotransporter 2)

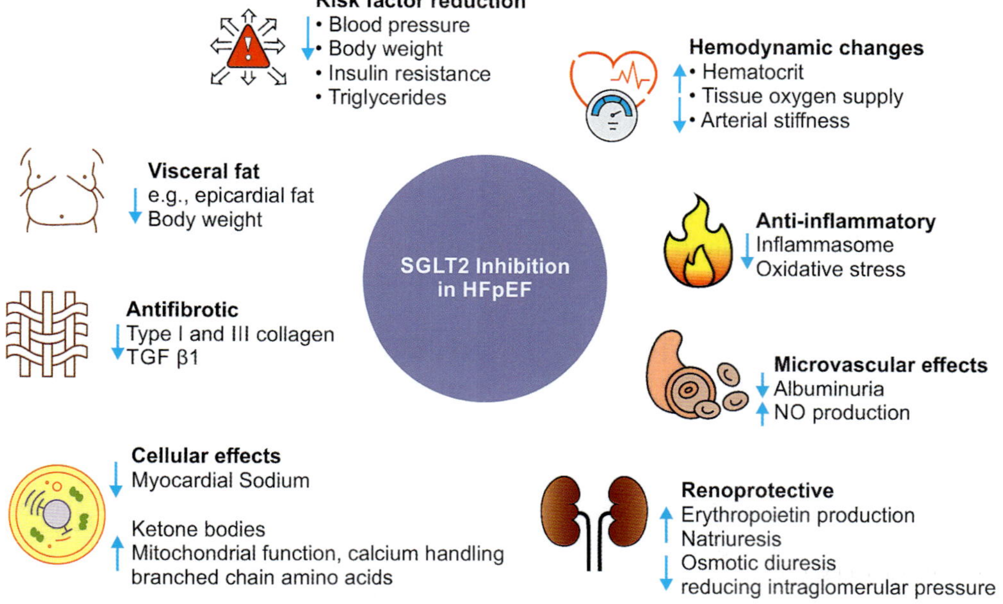

Fig. 5: Multidimensional composite benefits of SGLT2i.

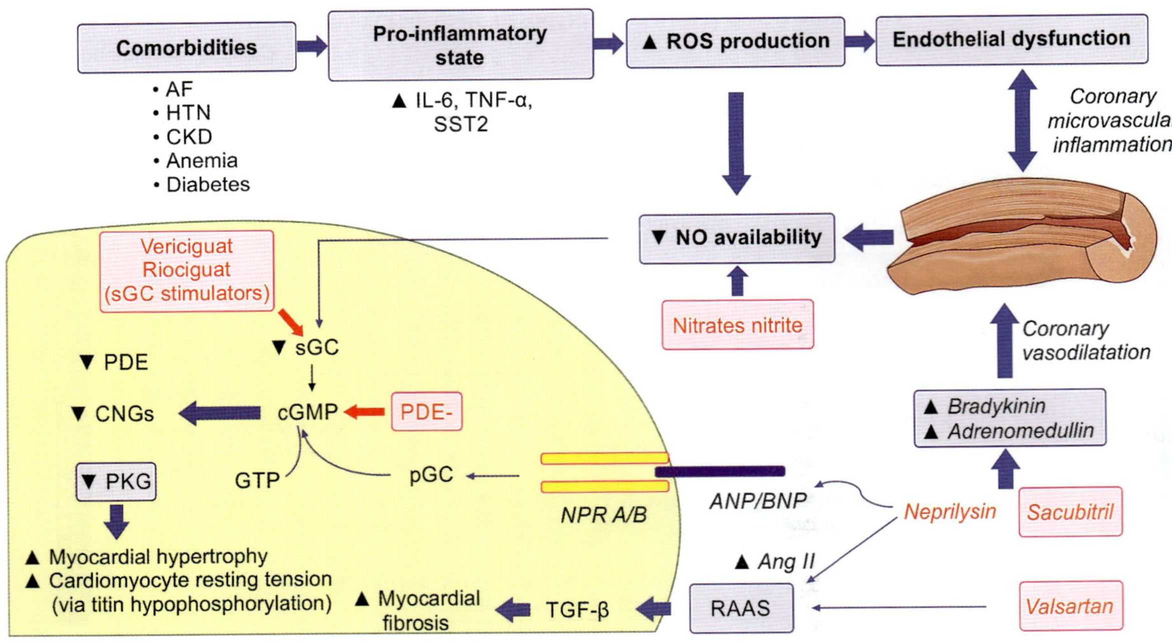

Fig. 6: NP, c-GMP, and RAAS blockade in HF with potential therapeutic targets.

that followed tried to target a more selected cohort, adding in the inclusion criteria both echocardiographic evidence of DD and congestion. All trials had similar results confirming no effects on mortality and some effect on HF hospitalization.

A large metanalysis that included the aforementioned clinical trials and other smaller-size studies concluded that both ARB and angiotensin-converting enzyme inhibitors have no effect on all-cause mortality (HR 1.01, 95% CI 0.92–1.11), CV death (HR 1.02, 95% CI 0.90–1.14), and HF hospitalization (HR 0.92, 95% CI 0.83–1.02).[60] A subanalysis of the CHARM study examined LVEF as a continuous variable and found a significant effect on HF hospitalization for values <50%.[21,61] Based on this evidence, the 2022 American Heart Association/American College of Cardiology/Heart Failure Society of America guidelines give a class 2b recommendation for ARB use with the aim of reducing HF hospitalization, especially in the lower end of the LVEF.[7]

MINERALOCORTICOID RECEPTOR ANTAGONISTS IN HFpEF

The TOPCAT trial shaped much of our knowledge around the use of MRA in HFpEF, being the only large-scale clinical trial on clinically relevant outcomes. It enrolled patients aged >50 years with at least one sign or symptom of HF, VEF >45%, and history of HF hospitalization in the previous 12 months or elevated natriuretic peptide (NP) level.[21] The overall result on the primary outcome of a composite CV death and HF hospitalization was neutral (HR 0.89, 95% CI 0.77–1.04, $p = 0.14$), as only HF hospitalizations were significantly reduced in the treatment arm (HR 0.83, 95% CI 0.69–0.99, $p = 0.04$). Patients enrolled with the HF hospitalization criterion recorded a far lower rate of events than those enrolled with the NP criterion.[62] Smaller studies found beneficial effects of MRA on surrogate outcomes (mainly, echocardiographically assessed DD parameters, reverse remodeling, and NP decrease), but not on QoL, symptoms, and exercise capacity.[63,64] New trials such as the SPIRRIT-HFpEF and FINEARTS-HF (NCT04435626) are ongoing to better define the role of MRA in HFpEF.[65]

The 2022 American Heart Association/American College of Cardiology/Heart Failure Society of America guidelines give a class 2b recommendation for MRA use, with the aim of reducing HF hospitalization, especially in the lower LVEF range.[7] However, the European guidelines do not mention MRA for HFpEF.[6]

ANTAGONIST RECEPTOR–NEPRILYSIN INHIBITORS FOR HFpEF

The PARAGON-HF trial randomized 4,822 patients with NYHA class II–IV, EF >45%, elevated NP, and structural heart disease to valsartan alone or sacubitril/valsartan.[66] The primary endpoint was narrowly missed but a split of components of the outcomes demonstrated a truly neutral effect on CV mortality (HR 0.95, 95% CI 0.79–1.16) yet a modest positive effect on HF hospitalizations. NYHA class improvement, change in QoL assessed by the Kansas City Cardiomyopathy Questionnaire, and renal function preservation showed benefit from ARNI treatment compared with valsartan.

Prespecified subgroups analysis highlighted a different response to treatment in women (who benefitted most) compared with men and, as seen in the CHARM Preserved and TOPCAT trials, in the lower end of the EF spectrum, with an efficacy of the treatment up to an EF of 57%.[67]

Recently, the PARAGLIDE study randomized 466 patients with LVEF >40% and a recent event of worsening HF to sacubitril/valsartan versus valsartan, showed that the primary endpoint of N-terminal fraction of pro-BNP reduction was greater in the sacubitril/valsartan group ($p = 0.0049$) and was associated with clinical benefit as reduced worsening renal failure compared with valsartan alone was reported, despite a more symptomatic hypotension.[68]

A recent pool analysis of PARAGLIDE and PARAGON showed that in a population of 5,262 patients, sacubitril/valsartan versus valsartan alone significantly reduced CV death and total worsening heart failure events ($p = 0.027$). These data encourage the use of ARNI in HF with mildly reduced or preserved LVEF, particularly in those with a LVEF below normal.[69]

BETA-BLOCKER THERAPY IN HFpEF

Beta-blockers have been studied less intensively and in smaller clinical trials compared with the RAASi agents. The SENIORS trial enrolled HF patients across the entire spectrum of the LVEF and randomized them to nebivolol or a placebo.[70] The subgroup analysis of 752 patients with LVEF >35% is the largest cohort randomized to a placebo we have till date. A smaller study, the J-DHF, tested carvedilol compared with a placebo in a smaller cohort of patients; several meta-analyses put together data from randomized clinical trials and observational cohorts with or without propensity score analysis, but the overall quality of the data was low, were the results are inconsistent throughout the studies.

Nonetheless, meta-analyses suggest that beta-blockers could reduce CV mortality or all-cause mortality without significant effect on HF hospitalization.[71-74] The heterogeneity of the HFpEF population, the various underlying mechanisms, and etiologies make the design of clinical trials even more difficult than with other agents. In all these clinical trials, beta-blocker withdrawal was high due to drug intolerance. Chronotropic incompetence related to beta-blockers is a well-recognized contributor to exercise intolerance commonly observed in HFpEF.[75] One study reported significant improvement in functional capacity measured by peak oxygen consumption after beta-blocker withdrawal in patients with HFpEF and chronotropic incompetence.[76]

ADDRESSING CONCOMITANT CARDIAC COMORBIDITIES

The HFpEF is a multidimensional syndrome characterized by noncardiac and cardiac comorbidities, conditioning phenotypes and affecting prognosis. Addressing underlying potential therapeutic options individually is needed to improve symptoms, QoL, and outcomes **(Flowchart 2)**.[77]

ISCHEMIC HEART DISEASE: GENERAL TERM FOR SEVERAL CONDITIONS RELATED TO HFpEF

Ischemic heart disease and HF are strongly and tightly connected conditions.[78-82] Ischemic heart disease is a common cardiac comorbidity in HFpEF, even though prevalence varies across studies, also depending on the imaging modalities used to ascertain it, and on the general arterial involvement. Ischemic heart disease includes microvascular dysfunction (MVD), coronary artery disease, or previous "silent" MI.[83,84] The most important mechanisms leading to MVD in HFpEF consist of microvascular inflammation, capillary rarefaction, and cardiac fibrosis.[85-88] MVD contributes to the proinflammatory state, exacerbated by the multiple comorbidities present in HFpEF, promotes oxidative stress, and endothelial dysfunction. SGLT2s have shown beneficial effects of cardiac microvascular endothelial cells on cardiomyocyte function and demonstrated an improvement in myocardial flow reserve in a single-center prospective randomized clinical trial.[89] Ranolazine inhibits the late sodium current, reduces intracellular calcium in cardiomyocytes, and promotes ventricular relaxation by decreasing diastolic tone and microcirculatory resistance, thus improving coronary blood flow. It also acts on cardiac fibrosis; thus, it could improve the most important physiological mechanisms of MVD in this syndrome.[90] New studies on antidiabetic agents, glucagon-like peptide-1 agonists, are ongoing in the obese HFpEF phenotype, and they could also have a role in chronic inflammation and MVD.

ATRIAL FIBRILLATION

Atrial fibrillation is a highly prevalent cardiac comorbidity in HFpEF, ranging from 32 to 65% in epidemiological studies.[91,92] Despite this difference in absolute prevalence, AF is consistently reported to be more common in HFpEF than in HFrEF, and to be associated with older age.

Flowchart 2: Addressing concomitant comorbidities in HFpEF.

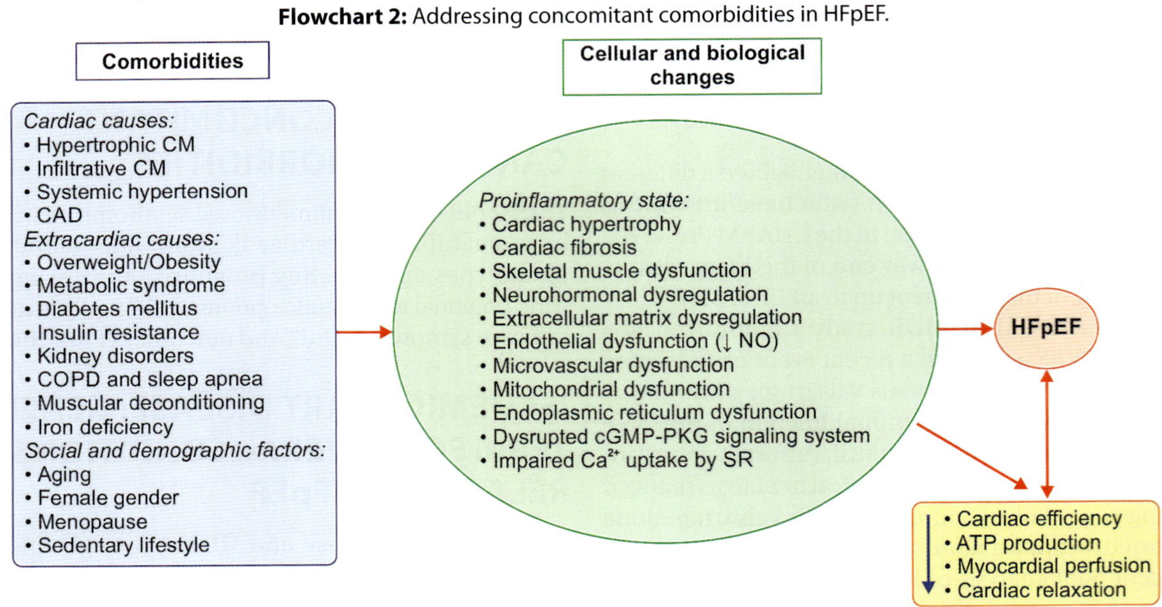

An interesting analysis of the HF Long-Term Registry of the European Society of Cardiology, evaluating both ambulatory and hospitalized HF patients, showed that after multivariable adjustment, AF significantly increased long-term mortality and hospitalization just in the HFpEF and HFmrEF population, but not in the HFrEF population.[93] Patients with AF and HFpEF should be anticoagulated according to guidelines, keeping in mind the high incremental thromboembolic risk added by HF.[94] Based on the available evidence, no firm recommendation can be drawn on rhythm versus rate control strategy preference.

Rate control is still more popular choice among clinicians with convincing evidence to support a routine rhythm control strategy still missing. The two major trials on this subject and subsequent meta-analysis suggest no benefit of one strategy over the other.[95] Three drug classes are valuable options for rate control in HFpE: (1) β-blockers, (2) nondihydropyridine calcium channel blockers, and (3) digoxin. Few studies have directly compared these drugs. The RATE-AF trial compared low-dose digoxin and bisoprolol in HF patients with permanent AF.[96,97] The vast majority of the trial cohort (81%) had HFpEF. The primary endpoint (QoL at 6 months from randomization) was not different in the two groups, and fewer adverse events were recorded in the digoxin group ($p < 0.001$).

DIABETES AND METABOLISM DISORDERS

Diabetes, excess weight, and obesity, typical features of HFpEF patients, as already documented in the previously mentioned phenotypes, cause inactivity and deconditioning, justifying the high prevalence of dyspnea and exercise intolerance in this population. Weight loss, through caloric restriction or increased physical activity, and glycemic control have a positive effect on prognosis and CV events. Notably, visceral and pericardial adipose tissues play a negative, proinflammatory role compared to subcutaneous adipose tissue, emphasizing that "not all fat is equal". Metabolically active fat, responsible for releasing inflammatory adipokines into circulation, exerts a detrimental impact on the heart and other organs, particularly the kidneys, where fibrotic degeneration leads to diastolic dysfunction and chronic kidney disease. Additionally, obesity is associated with obstructive sleep apnea, contributing to increased right ventricular afterload, promoting functional deterioration, and eventually its failure.

From the therapeutic perspective, glucagon-like peptide-1 agonists may represent a future therapeutic target for patients with HFpEF, acting on several pathways involved in the pathophysiology of HFpEF, including diabetes and obesity. It has been demonstrated that the use of liraglutide is associated with reduced body weight and improved metabolic control. The LEADER study demonstrated that the rate of the first occurrence of death from CV causes, nonfatal MI, or nonfatal stroke among patients with type 2 diabetes was lower with liraglutide than with a placebo.[98,99] Moreover, in the STEP-HFpEF trial, semaglutide significantly reduced body weight, improving symptoms with a positive impact on QoL in obese HFpEF patients.

DEVICES IN HFpEF: CURRENT ROLE AND LOOKING AHEAD

Drug therapy options for HFpEF are currently limited, and the associated high risk of cardiovascular mortality and HF rehospitalization significantly impact patients' QoL and longevity while imposing a substantial economic burden on society. Recent research indicates that certain device-based therapies may serve as valuable adjuncts to drug therapy in patients with specific phenotypes of HFpEF, effectively improving symptoms and QoL while reducing the risk of readmission for HF.[100,101] These include interatrial shunt and greater splanchnic nerve ablation to reduce left ventricular filling pressure, implantable heart failure monitor to guide diuresis, left atrial pacing to correct interatrial dyssynchrony, cardiac contractility modulation to enhance cardiac calcium handling, as well as renal denervation, baroreflex activation therapy (BAT), and vagus nerve stimulation to restore the autonomic imbalance. A basic overview of the mechanisms and clinical evidence pertaining to these devices with the aim of enhancing therapeutic strategies for HFpEF is presented in **Table 1**.[102]

Interatrial Shunt-based Devices

Despite heterogeneity in the etiology and pathophysiology of HFpEF, left atrial pressure (LAP) overload has been identified as a common cause of HFpEF-related exercise intolerance. Therefore, establishing an artificial interatrial shunt that relies on a pressure gradient to drain blood from the left heart to the right heart can effectively reduce LAP both at rest and during exercise. This approach has shown promising results in relieving symptoms and improving clinical outcomes for patients with HFpEF, making it a potential therapeutic option.

To date, several atrial shunt devices, including the interatrial shunt device (IASD) (Corvia Medical Inc.), the V-wave shunt (V-Wave Ltd), and the atrial flow regulator (Occlutech), have been developed to reduce LAP by artificially constructing access from the left atrium to the right atrium **(Fig. 7)**.

Consisting of a nitinol frame and an 8 mm central channel, the IASD is currently the most extensively researched interatrial shunt in HFpEF/HFmEF patients. The REDUCE LAP-HF (REDUCe Elevated Left Atrial Pressure in Patients with Heart Failure) was the first

TABLE 1: Summary of devices for HFPEF that are currently available.

	IASD	*V-Wave shunts*	*AFR*	*Transcatheter atrial shunt system*	*NoYA system*
Site	LA to RA	LA to RA	LA to RA	LA to CS	LA to RA
Access (French)	Femoral vein (16-F)	Femoral vein (14-F)	Femoral vein (10/12-F)	Right Internal jugular vein (24-F)	Femoral vein (14F)
Shunt diameter	8 mm	5.1 mm	8–10 mm	10 mm	4–12 mm
Patency at 12 months	100%	• 50% (either stenosis or closure) with 1° generation device • 100% with 2° generation device	100%	100%	70% (at 6 months) for 2 closure and one missing data
Therapy postimplantation	Aspirin (75–325 mg daily) indefinitely + clopidogrel or anticoagulant therapy for 6 months. Anticoagulant therapy indefinitely if AF or other indication	Aspirin (7–325 mg) indefinitely + clopidogrel for 3 months or warfarin/ DOACs indefinitely (in patients with prior anticoagulant indication)	• Aspirin (75–325 mg daily) indefinitely + P2YI2 inhibitor or anticoagulant therapy for 6 months • Anticoagulant therapy indefinitely if AF or other indication	Aspirin + clopidogrel or oral anticoagulant + clopidogrel monotherapy (in those with prior indications for anti-coagulation)	Aspirin 100 mg for 1 month

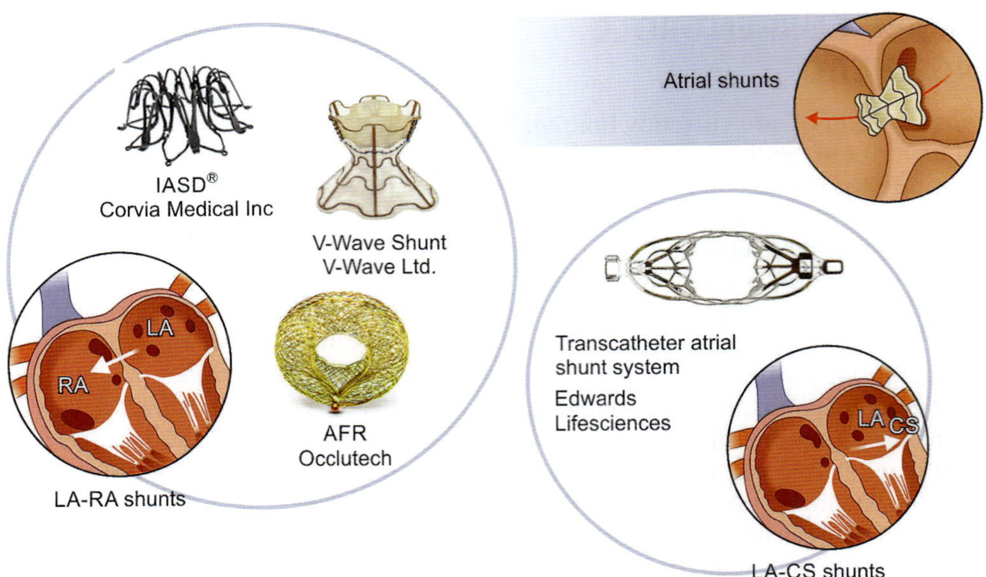

Fig. 7: Interatrial shunt-based devices for HFPEF.

open-label, single-arm, phase 1 trial designed to investigate the effect of IASD in 64 patients with symptomatic HFpEF (LVEF ≥40%) and elevated PCWP (>15 mm Hg at rest and >25 mm Hg during exercise). Results showed that the device was well tolerated, with significant improvements in exercise hemodynamics, 6-minute-walk distance (6MWD), and Minnesota Living with Heart Failure Questionnaire (MLWHFQ) score at 6 months. These observations were corroborated by the randomized, sham-controlled, phase 2 REDUCE LAP-HF I trial, which demonstrated a favorable mechanistic impact of IASD on exercise PCWP. At 1 year, the IASD remained patent in all patients, with no significant differences in major adverse cardiac, cerebrovascular, and renal events. Moreover, patients with the IASD placement showed a trend for improved NYHA functional class and reduced HF hospitalization. However, the phase 3 REDUCE LAP-HF II trial involving 626 symptomatic HF patients with LVEF ≥40% and elevated resting or exercise PCWP failed to confirm better outcomes for IASD in cardiovascular death, nonfatal ischemic stroke, first and recurrent HF events, and health status compared with a sham procedure.

The V-wave shunt is a self-expanding nitinol frame covered with porcine pericardial tissue, shaped like an hourglass. In a single-arm, open-label study involving 38 patients with HFrEF and HFpEF, the implantation of the first-generation V-Wave system was deemed both safe and feasible, resulting in significant improvements in NYHA functional class, QOL, and 6MWD. However, after 12 months, a high incidence of shunt stenosis or occlusion resulted in loss of efficacy. The ongoing RELIEVE-HF trial (NCT03499236) aims to enroll 500 patients to evaluate the safety and efficacy of the second-generation V-wave shunt in advanced HF, irrespective of LVEF.

The atrial flow regulator (AFR) is a self-expandable double-disc wired mesh with a central penetration that enables interatrial shunting. PRELIEVE was an open-label, prospective, nonrandomized, first-in-man study investigating the feasibility of AFR implantation up to 1-year follow-up in patients with HFrEF or HFpEF. Findings indicated that the AFR device in patients with HF was both feasible and safe and was associated with improved NYHA class, 6MWD, Kansas City Cardiomyopathy Questionnaire (KCCQ), PCWP, and NT- proBNP in some but not all patients. The Pomeranian atRial flOw reguLatOr iN conGestive hEart failuRe (PROLONGER) study was designed to establish invasive and noninvasive parameters capable of predicting a favorable response to AFR therapy in patients with HF.

Implantable Heart Failure Monitor

Volume overload remains a primary contributor to the exacerbation of HFpEF. Continuous monitoring of intracardiac pressures reveals that elevated LV filling pressure occurs 1–2 weeks before the onset of dyspnea and signs of edema in patients with HF, providing a more sensitive indicator of volume overload and predicting HF deterioration. In recent years, there has been growing evidence that pulmonary artery (PA) pressure-guided management of HF by the CardioMEMS HF system, where PA pressure is remotely monitored by a wireless PA sensor implanted in the left inferior PA to guide diuresis, further reduces the hospitalization for HF compared with conventional treatment strategy. The CHAMPION (CardioMEMS Heart Sensor Allows Monitoring of Pressure to Improve Outcomes in New York Heart Association Class III Heart Failure Patients) trial, which enrolled 550 individuals with NYHA functional class III HF, irrespective of the LVEF, and a history of HF hospitalization 1 year ago, showed that HF events in the experiment group were reduced by 28% compared with those in the control group (HR 0.72, 95% CI 0·60– 0·85, p = 0·0002), and 99% patients had no device or system-related complications. Notably, the reduction in hospitalization for HF was more pronounced in patients with LVEF ≥50%, reaching 70% (HR, 030, 95% CI 0.18–0.48; p < 0.0001).

The implantable heart failure monitors for HF monitoring are given in **Figures 8A to C**.

Based on the CHAMPION results, the Food and Drug Administration (FDA) approved CardioMEMS for the treatment of patients with HFpEF and HFrEF in 2014. After approval of CardioMEMS, a real-world study involving 1,200 patients with NYHA functional class III HF (46.8% with preserved EF) and a prior HF hospitalization within 12 months showed that hemodynamically-guided management significantly reduced HF hospitalization by 57% and all-cause hospitalization by 27% compared to 1 year before procedure. The benefit was consistent across baseline LVEF, and >99% of patients were free of device-related complications or sensor failure. The GUIDE-HF (hemodynamic-GUIDEed management of Heart Failure) trial extended the indication for CardioMEMS implantation to earlier HF populations where it was shown that though at 12 months of follow-up, the primary outcomes of all-cause mortality and readmission for HF were not reduced in the experiment group compared with the control group, a prespecified pre-COVID-19 analysis showed that hemodynamically-guided HF management strategies significantly reduced the composite endpoint of HF events and all-cause mortality by 19% (p = 0.049) and the risk for HF hospitalization by 28% (p = 0.007). A retrospective analysis of 29 patients with HFpEF (LVEF ≥45%) showed that CardioMEMS improved not only pulmonary artery diastolic pressures but also metabolic markers including body weight, body mass index, systolic blood pressure, high-density lipoprotein, and triglycerides 6 months after implantation.

For clinical use, the latest HF guidelines gave a class IIb recommendation for CardioMEMS implantation in selected HF patients to reduce the risk of HF hospitalization. Future trials are warranted to investigate the potential of CardioMEMS implantation in HF in the post-COVID-19 era, particularly in reducing cardiovascular mortality.

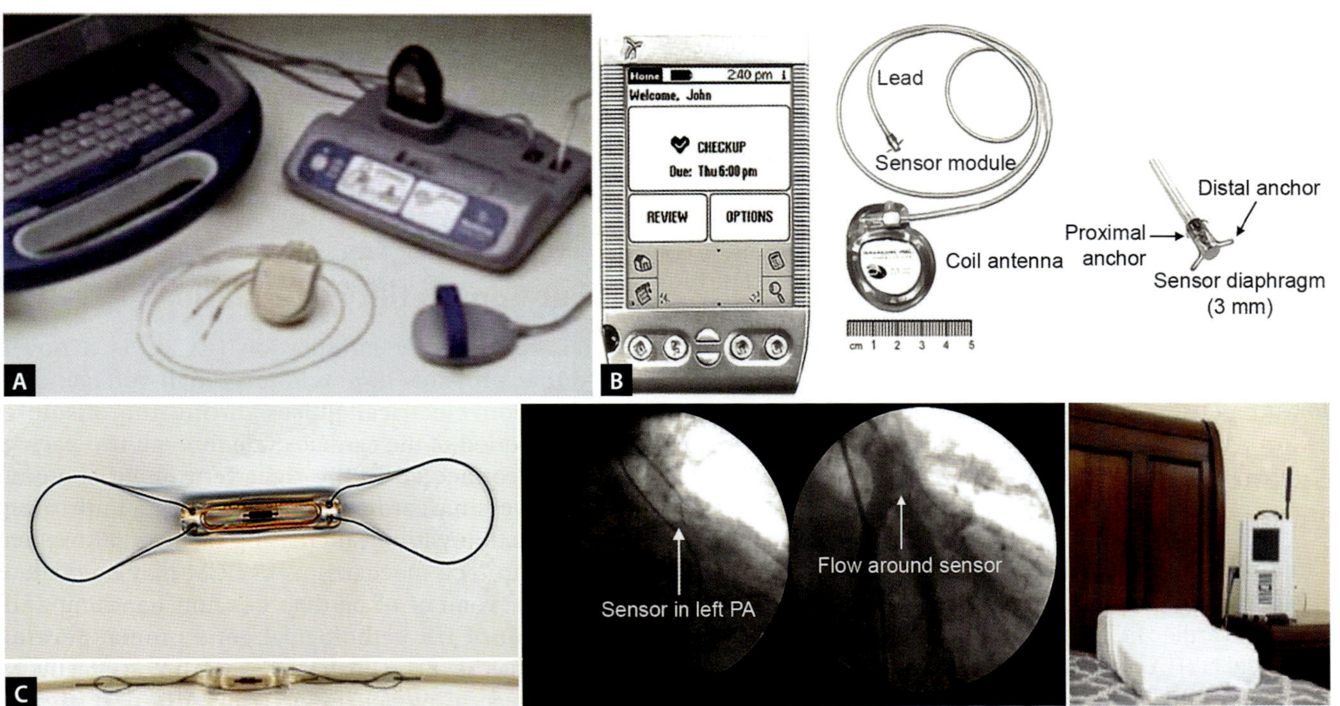

Figs. 8A to C: Implantable heart failure monitors for HF monitoring.

Left Atrial Pacing

Echocardiographic studies have shown that interatrial dyssynchrony is common in patients with HFpEF and is associated with decreased left atrial function and worsening clinical symptoms, suggesting that amelioration of interatrial dyssynchrony may be a potential treatment target for HFpEF. Left atrial pacing is performed using specially designed coronary sinus that stimulates the middle and distal coronary sinus region, initially for atrial tachyarrhythmias and more recently for atrial resynchronization in HFpEF patients. In 2013, a pilot study conducted by Laurent et al. enrolling six patients with severe HFpEF with interatrial conduction delay showed that left atrial pacing significantly improved the 6MWD, mitral A-wave duration, and E/A and E/e′ ratio after 3 months of active pacing. Importantly, after 1 week of pacing inactivation, a significant decrease in 6MWD happened with an on/off response. In addition, recent studies have found that left atrial pacing at about 125 beats per minute could lead to beneficial cardiac remodeling and reduced left ventricular end-diastolic volume and filling pressure in anesthetized patients with hypertensive heart disease-associated HFpEF and in pigs with concentric LV hypertrophy and fibrosis. It is believed that these benefits from left atrial permanent pacing open a new avenue for the treatment of HFpEF. More recently, the myPACE (Personalized Pacing: A New Paradigm for Patients with Diastolic Dysfunction or Heart Failure With Preserved Ejection Fraction) trial showed that, among patients with stage B and C HFpEF and pacemakers, moderately accelerated, personalized pacing was well tolerated and improved QoL, NT-proBNP, physical activity, and atrial fibrillation compared to conventional care at 1-year follow-up. However, the RAPID-HF (Efficacy Study of Pacemakers to Treat Slow Heart Rate in Patients with Heart Failure) trial, a randomized, double-blind, cross-over study conducted in 29 patients with HFpEF/HFmEF and chronotropic incompetence, indicates that atrial pacing did not significantly improve parameters calling upon larger RCTs with extended follow-up periods to warrant use of this modality for HFpEF.

Splanchnic Ablation for Volume Management

The first-in-human study of the right GSN blockade by thoracoscopic surgery in 10 HFpEF patients showed reduced cardiac filling pressure during exercise, improved QoL, and NYHA class at 12 months of follow-up. However, adverse events associated with the procedure itself have prompted the development of a less invasive, endovascular, transvenous procedure known as splanchnic ablation for volume management (SAVM) **(Fig. 9)**. The first-in-human study of SAVM using the Axon ablation system in 11 HFpEF patients showed that the procedure was safe and resulted in sustained improvements in NT-proBNP, health status, and 6MWD over a 12-month follow-up period.

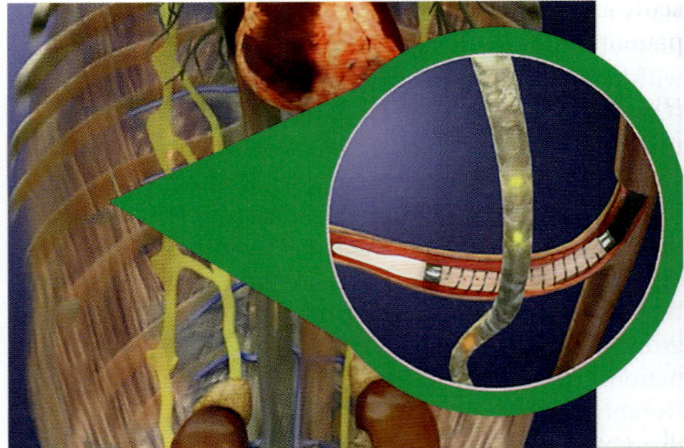

Fig. 9: Splanchnic ablation for HFpEF.

The ongoing randomized, sham-controlled, phase 2 clinical trial REBALANCE-HF (Endovascular Ablation of the Right Greater Splanchnic Nerve in Subjects Having HFpEF) was designed to enroll 80 patients for transvenous SAVM at 20 centers. Inclusion criteria included ejection fraction ≥50% and elevated PCWP ≥25 mm Hg during exercise. Early findings from the initial 18 patients indicate that after 1 month following SAVM intervention, there was a significant reduction of 7.5 mm Hg (p <0.01) in mean PCWP during exercise at 20 W, with an improvement of at least one NYHA class observed in 33% of patients, thus verifying that the modulation of splanchnic bed capacitance via GSN ablation offers a potential treatment strategy for HFpEF.

Cardiac Contractility Modulation

Cardiac contractility modulation (CCM) is a novel device that provides nonexcitatory, high-voltage, and long-duration electrical pulses during the absolute refractory period of the cardiac cycle through two pacing electrodes connected to the right ventricular septum, thereby reversing cardiac remodeling and improving cardiac function without increasing myocardial oxygen consumption. The mechanisms of CCM may be related to the improvement of cardiac calcium handling and modification of HF pathological gene profile. Several clinical studies have shown that CCM safely and effectively improved physical tolerance as determined by peak oxygen uptake (VO_2) and QoL as determined by the MLWHFQ score and reduced cardiac death and HF hospitalization in patients with HFrEF.

However, unlike the clear evidence for CCM use in HFrEF, there is little clinical evidence for CCM use in HFpEF. Subgroup analysis of the FIX-HF-5 (Evaluate Safety and Efficacy of the OPTIMIZER System in Subjects with Moderate-to-Severe Heart Failure) trial suggested that HF patients with LVEF 35–45% had more significant improvement in peak VO_2 and MLWHFQ score compared with those with LVEF 25–34% at 6 months after CCM implantation. The CCM-REG prospective registry study also showed that patients with baseline LVEF of 35–45% had a better 3-year survival benefit than those with LVEF of 25–34% after the CCM procedure. The greater benefit of CCM in patients with a higher LVEF range suggests that CCM may be suitable for HFpEF. In 2016, Tschöpe C et al. first reported an overall symptomatic, functional, and histological improvement in two female HFpEF patients (LVEF of 50% and 47%, respectively) treated with CCM for 3 months. The CCM-HFpEF (CCM in Heart Failure With Preserved Ejection Fraction, NCT03240237) trial, a prospective, multicenter, single-arm, pilot study assessing the efficacy and safety of CCM therapy in HFpEF patients with NYHA class II or III, showed that CCM significantly improved patients' health status as determined by the increase of KCCQ overall score by 18.0 points ($p <0.001$), also being generally safe, with 93.6% of patients experiencing no device-related complications. The randomized, quadruple-blind, sham-controlled, 1,500-patient AIM HIGHer (Assessment of CCM in HF With Higher Ejection Fraction) trial is underway to validate the potential impacts of CCM on cardiovascular death and HF hospitalization in HFpEF patients.

OTHER THERAPIES FOR HFpEF

Renal Denervation

Although RDN has been proven effective in treating refractory hypertension, its efficacy in HF, particularly HFpEF, remains uncertain due to insufficient evidence.[103-133] Current literature suggests that sympathetic nerve activation is present in patients with HFpEF, similar to those with HFrEF. This phenomenon is often associated with the pathological process of common comorbidities of HFpEF, such as hypertension, atrial fibrillation, metabolic syndrome, chronic kidney disease, and pulmonary hypertension.[61] RDN can enhance the function of remote organs, including the heart, skeletal muscle, vasculature, and lungs by reducing renal afferent and efferent sympathetic tone.

The first randomized, open-controlled trial to evaluate the effectiveness of RDN in HFpEF patients was terminated early due to recruitment difficulties (only 25 HFpEF patients were randomized 2:1 to receive RDN or medication). The trial was inadequate in its ability to detect whether RDN improved QoL (MLWHFQ score), exercise function, BNP, and cardiac remodeling at 12 months, although RDN improved VO_2 peak and E/e' at 3 months.[134] Kresoja et al. retrospectively analyzed cardiac magnetic resonance imaging and echocardiogram data from 164 hypertensive patients undergoing RDN procedure, of whom 99 were HFpEF patients. After RDN treatment, LV diastolic stiffness and LV filling pressures as well as NT-proBNP were improved in patients with HFpEF, suggesting RDN might be a promising therapy for patients with HFpEF and uncontrolled arterial hypertension.[63] Whether the efficacy of RDN for HFpEF depends on its effect on lowering blood pressure and heart rate remains controversial as per other studies The ongoing UNLOAD-HFpEF (Renal Denervation to Treat Heart Failure With Preserved Ejection Fraction) trial is the first randomized, sham-controlled, double-blind pilot trial that will further address the role of RDN in HFpEF.

Baroreflex Activation Therapy

Baroreceptor dysfunction is a prevalent pathophysiological feature in most cases of HF and closely links to LV impairment regardless of LVEF. BAT chronically stimulates carotid baroreceptors to reduce centrally mediated sympathetic outflow and increase parasympathetic activity, thereby counteracting sympathetic overactivation and parasympathetic withdrawal associated with HF. Notably, the improvement in LV mass was weakened when renal SNA suppression was blocked during BAT, suggesting that BAT primarily enhances cardiac structure and function by inhibiting renal SNA.

Results from feasibility studies in 21 subjects with normal LVEF showed that after 12 months, BAT delivered by the first-generation Rheos System reduced blood pressure and improved 6MWD and LV mass in patients with refractory hypertension and symptomatic HFpEF. Clemmer et al. utilized HumMod, a comprehensive physiological model, to simulate HFpEF and predict the dynamic changes in blood pressure, cardiac structure, and sympathetic nerve activity (SNA) during baroreflex activation. The results showed that simulating baroreflex activation for a period of 6 months led to reduced LV mass, lowered blood pressure, decreased cardiac SNA, and restoration of β1-adrenergic activity.

The HOPE4HF (Hope Heart Failure Study) and BeAT-HF (Baroreflex Activation for Heart Failure) trials showed that, compared with GDMT alone, BAT with the Barostim Neo system plus GDMT significantly improved the 6MWD, MLWHFQ-rated QoL, NYHA functional class, and NT-proBNP in patients of HFrEF (LVEF ≤35%) with NYHA functional class III, and were associated with a trend of reduced hospital days for HF. The safety of BAT was also demonstrated, with over 94% of patients having no major neurologic, cardiovascular, or procedure-related events. Based on these results, the BAT with the second-generation Barostim Neo system is approved by the FDA for symptomatic HF patients with NYHA functional class III, LVEF ≤35%, NT-proBNP <1,600 pg/mL, and no indication for cardiac resynchronization therapy.[69] A patient-level meta-analysis suggested that BAT improved exercise capacity, NYHA class, and QoL in GDMT-treated patients with NYHA class II/III HFrEF. The BAROSTIM THERAPY in HFpEF (NCT02876042) is an ongoing registry to evaluate the feasibility and effectiveness of BAT in patients with HFpEF combined with refractory hypertension.

Vagus Nerve and Tragus Stimulation

Schwartz et al. first reported the feasibility of long-term VNS in eight patients with HFrEF, showing improvements in functional status, QoL, and LV volume after implantation of a vagus stimulator. However, three larger clinical trials, including ANTHEM-HF (Autonomic Neural Regulation Therapy to Enhance Myocardial Function in Heart Failure), INOVATE-HF (INcrease Of VAgal TonE in CHF), and NECTAR-HF (Neural Cardiac Therapy for Heart Failure), have failed to consistently validate the prognosis-improving effects of VNS in patients with HFrEF.

The recently published ANTHEM-HFpEF (Autonomic Regulation Therapy to Enhance Myocardial Function in Heart Failure with Preserved Ejection Fraction) trial first investigated the safety and feasibility of chronic VNS in 52 patients with HFpEF/HFmrEF. At the 1-year follow-up, VNS showed good tolerance and was associated with significant improvements in NYHA class, 6MWD, QoL, autonomic tone, and cardiac electrical stability, although it did not alter cardiac mechanical function.

Low-level tragus stimulation (LLTS) is a noninvasive method of percutaneous VNS that has been demonstrated to reduce cardiac inflammation and fibrosis and improve LV diastolic function in a rat model of HFpEF. Tran et al. showed for the first time that LLTS can acutely

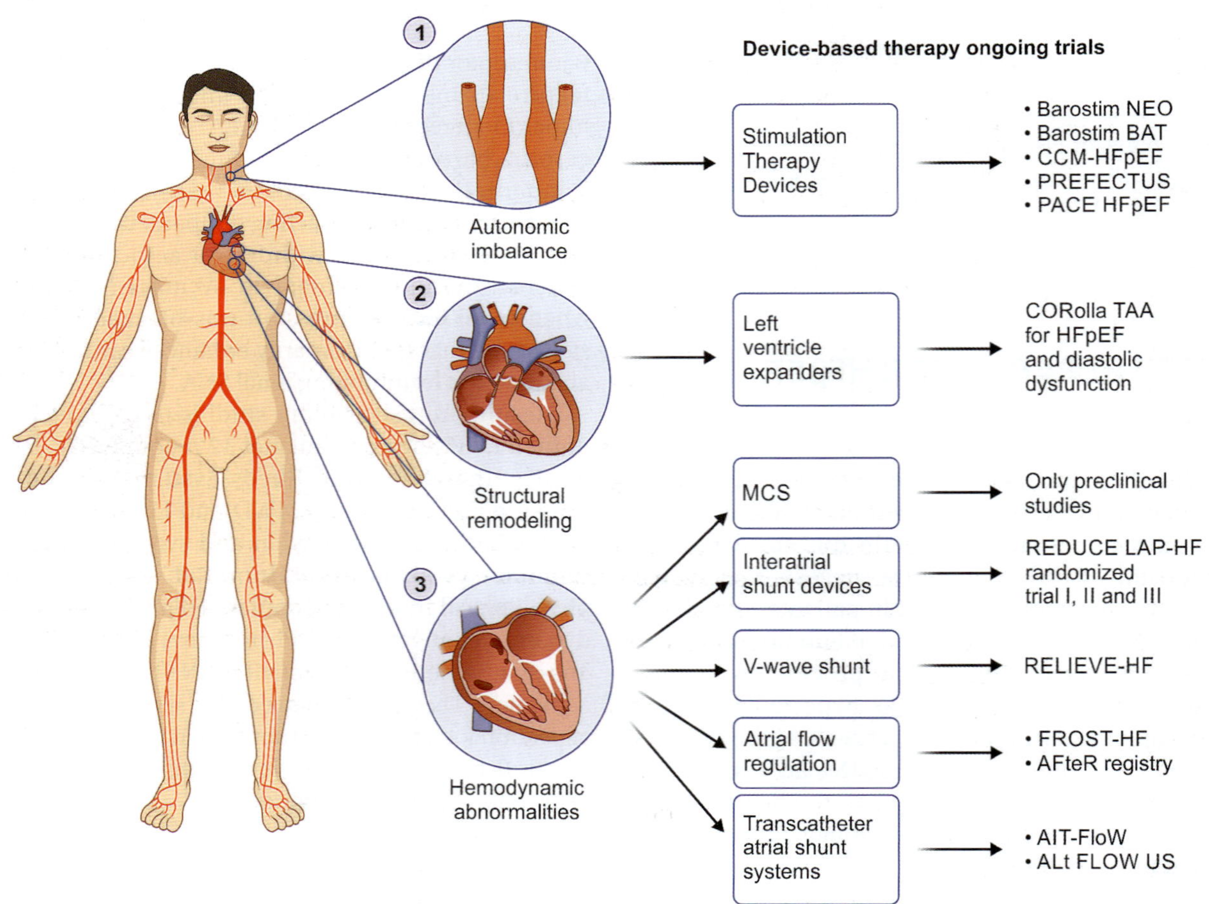

Fig. 10: Device-based therapies in HF—a summary.

improve the global longitudinal strain of LV in HFpEF patients by regulating autonomic tone. Subsequently, a pilot, sham-control, double-blind, randomized clinical trial evaluating the effects of chronic LLTS on cardiac function, exercise capacity, and inflammation in HFpEF patients with a predominantly inflammatory-metabolic phenotype showed that the LV global longitudinal strain, tumor necrosis factor-α level, and QoL were significantly improved after treatment with LLTS for 3 months. Of note, the decreases in tumor necrosis factor-α were associated with improvements in the LV global longitudinal strain, suggesting that patients with a proinflammatory state may benefit more from LLTS. Future studies are warranted to elucidate the effectiveness of VNS on distinct phenotypes of HFPEF.

A summary of device-based therapies in HF is given in **Figure 10**.

CONCLUSION AND FUTURE PERSPECTIVES

The HFpEF encompasses nearly half of HF worldwide and still remains a poor prognostic indicator. Due to the heterogeneity of HFpEF as a disease process, targeted pharmacotherapy has become increasingly difficult. Although there is data supporting beta-blockers, MRAs, angiotensin-converting enzyme inhibitor, revascularization, cardiac rehabilitation, and more recently SGLT2i as therapeutic targets to reduce hospitalizations, no therapeutic category has found a mortality benefit. We are continuing to learn more about HFpEF as a complex interplay of not only neurohormonal but also myocardial interstitial disturbances driven by comorbid and systemic inflammatory conditions. Future targeted therapies need to focus on treatment of HFpEF as a systemic disease process.

Device-based therapies for HFpEF are an exciting and emerging field of research. The IASD gained CE Mark approval in 2016, becoming the world's first transcatheter device for the treatment of HFpEF, and the CardioMEMS and Barostim Neo systems have also been approved by the FDA for use in selected HF patients. The fact that CardioMEMS has received a IIb recommendation in current guidelines for selected HF patients, with the aim of reducing HF hospitalizations, is also encouraging. Overall, the clinical evidence of phase-3 RCTs is less, the follow-up period is short, and the endpoints are mostly NYHA class, 6MWD, QOL, and biomarkers of HF, rather than cardiovascular death or HF hospitalization. Therefore, the effectiveness of these devices in concert with other emerging therapies like ARNI and SGLT2i still needs to be further studied.

REFERENCES

1. Redfield MM, Borlaug BA. Heart failure with preserved ejection fraction: A review. JAMA. 2023;329(10):827-38.
2. Gori M, D'Elia E, Zambelli G, et al. Heart failure with preserved ejection fraction: An update on diagnosis and treatment. G Ital Cardiol (Rome). 2020;21(2):119-27.
3. Reddy YNV, Carter RE, Obokata M, et al. A simple, evidence-based approach to help guide diagnosis of heart failure with preserved ejection fraction. Circulation. 2018;138(9):861-70.
4. Pieske B, Tschöpe C, de Boer RA, et al. How to diagnose heart failure with preserved ejection fraction: The HFA-PEFF diagnostic algorithm: A consensus recommendation from the Heart Failure Association (HFA) of the European Society of Cardiology (ESC). Eur Heart J. 2019;40:3297-317.
5. Kittleson MM, Panjrath GS, Amancherla K, et al. 2023 ACC expert consensus decision pathway on management of heart failure with preserved ejection fraction: A report of the American College of Cardiology Solution Set Oversight Committee. J Am Coll Cardiol. 2023;81(18):1835-78.
6. McDonagh TA, Metra M, Adamo M, et al. 2021 ESC guidelines for the diagnosis and treatment of acute and chronic heart failure. Eur Heart J. 2021;42(36):3599-726
7. Heidenreich PA, Bozkurt B, Aguilar D, et al. 2022 AHA/ACC/HFSA guideline for the management of heart failure: A report of the American College of Cardiology/American Heart Association joint committee on clinical practice guidelines. Circulation. 2022;145(18):e895-1032.
8. Talha KM, Butler J, Greene SJ, et al. Potential global impact of sodium glucose cotransporter-2 inhibitors in heart failure. Eur J Heart Fail. 2023;25(7):999-1009.
9. Swedberg K, Pfeffer M, Granger C, et al. Candesartan in heart failure—assessment of reduction in mortality and morbidity (CHARM): Rationale and design. Charm-Programme Investigators. J Card Fail. 1999;5(3):276-82.
10. Obokata M, Reddy YNV, Borlaug BA. Diastolic dysfunction and heart failure with preserved ejection fraction: Understanding mechanisms by using noninvasive methods. JACC Cardiovasc Imaging. 2020;13(1 Pt 2): 245-57.
11. Shah SJ, Katz DH, Selvaraj S, et al. Phenomapping for novel classification of heart failure with preserved ejection fraction. Circulation. 2015;131(3):269-79.
12. Kao DP, Lewsey JD, Anand IS, et al. Characterization of subgroups of heart failure patients with preserved ejection fraction with possible implications for prognosis and treatment response. Eur J Heart Fail. 2015;17(9):925-35.
13. Senni M, Paulus WJ, Gavazzi A, et al. New strategies for heart failure with preserved ejection fraction: The importance of targeted therapies for heart failure phenotypes. Eur Heart J. 2014;35(40):2797-815.
14. Jones E, Randall EB, Hummel SL, et al. Phenotyping heart failure using model-based analysis and physiology-informed machine learning. J Physiol. 2021;599(22): 4991-5013.
15. Gu J, Pan JA, Lin H, et al. Characteristics, prognosis and treatment response in distinct phenogroups of heart

failure with preserved ejection fraction. Int J Cardiol. 2021;323:148-54.

16. Casebeer A, Horter L, Hayden J, et al. Phenotypic clustering of heart failure with preserved ejection fraction reveals different rates of hospitalization. J Cardiovasc Med (Hagerstown). 2021;22(1):45-52.
17. Hedman ÅK, Hage C, Sharma A, et al. Identification of novel pheno-groups in heart failure with preserved ejection fraction using machine learning. Heart 2020;106(5):342-9.
18. Uijl A, Savarese G, Vaartjes I, et al. Identification of distinct phenotypic clusters in heart failure with preserved ejection fraction. Eur J Heart Fail. 2021;23(6):973-82.
19. Nguyen NT, Tran DT, Le An P, et al. Clinical phenotypes and age-related differences in presentation, treatment, and outcome of heart failure with preserved ejection fraction: a Vietnamese multicenter research. Cardiol Res Pract. 2021;2021:4587678.
20. Gevaert AB, Tibebu S, Mamas MA, et al. Clinical phenogroups are more effective than left ventricular ejection fraction categories in stratifying heart failure outcomes. ESC Heart Fail. 2021;8(4):2741-54.
21. Pitt B, Pfeffer MA, Assmann SF, et al. Spironolactone for heart failure with preserved ejection fraction. N Engl J Med. 2014;370(15):1383-92.
22. Anker SD, Butler J, Filippatos G, et al.; EMPEROR-Preserved Trial Investigators. Empagliflozin and cardiovascular outcomes in heart failure with a preserved ejection fraction. N Engl J Med. 2021;385(16):1451-61.
23. Solomon SD, McMurray JJV, Claggett B, et al.; DELIVER Trial Committees and Investigators. Dapagliflozin in heart failure with mildly reduced or preserved ejection fraction. N Engl J Med. 2022;387(12):1089-98.
24. Wiviott SD, Raz I, Bonaca MP, et al.; DECLARE–TIMI 58 Investigators. Dapagliflozin and cardiovascular outcomes in type 2 diabetes. N Engl J Med. 2019;380(4):347-57.
25. Peters AE, Tromp J, Shah SJ, et al. Phenomapping in heart failure with preserved ejection fraction: Insights, limitations, and future directions. Cardiovasc Res. 2023;118(18):3403-415.
26. Segar MW, Patel KV, Ayers C, et al. Phenomapping of patients with heart failure with preserved ejection fraction using machine learning-based unsupervised cluster analysis. Eur J Heart Fail. 2020;22(1):148-58.
27. Lin CY, Sung HY, Chen YJ, et al. Personalized management for heart failure with preserved ejection fraction. J Pers Med. 2023;13(5):746.
28. Anand IS, Claggett B, Liu J, et al. Interaction between spironolactone and natriuretic peptides in patients with heart failure and preserved ejection fraction. JACC Heart Fail. 2017;5(4):241-52.
29. Kosiborod MN, Abildstrøm SZ, Bourlag BA, et al.; STEP-HFpEF Trial Committees and Investigators. Semaglutide in patients with heart failure with preserved ejection fraction and obesity. N Engl J Med. 2023;389(12):1069-84.
30. Zinman B, Wanner C, Lachin JM, et al.; EMPA-REG OUTCOME Investigators. Empagliflozin, cardiovascular outcomes, and mortality in type 2 diabetes. N Engl J Med. 2015;373(22):2117-28.
31. Neal B, Perkovic V, Mahaffey KW, et al. Canagliflozin and cardiovascular and renal events in type 2 diabetes. N Engl J Med 2017;377(7):644–57.
32. Bhatia K, Jain V, Gupta K, et al. Prevention of heart failure events with sodium-glucose co-transporter 2 inhibitors across a spectrum of cardio-renal-metabolic risk. Eur J Heart Fail. 2021;23(6):1002-8.
33. Lopaschuk GD, Verma S. Mechanisms of cardiovascular benefits of sodium glucose co-transporter 2 (SGLT2) inhibitors: A state-of-the-art review. JACC Basic Transl Sci. 2020;5(6):632-44.
34. Packer M. Molecular, cellular and clinical evidence that sodium-glucose cotransporter 2 inhibitors act as neurohormonal antagonists when used for the treatment of chronic heart failure. J Am Heart Assoc. 2020;9(16): e016270.
35. McMurray JJV, Solomon SD, Inzucchi SE, et al. Dapagliflozin in patients with heart failure and reduced ejection fraction. N Engl J Med. 2019;381(21):1995-2008.
36. Packer M, Anker SD, Butler J, et al.; EMPEROR-Reduced Trial Investigators. Cardiovascular and renal outcomes with empagliflozin in heart failure. N Engl J Med. 2020; 383(15):1413-24.
37. Vaduganathan M, Docherty KF, Claggett BL, et al. SGLT-2 inhibitors in patients with heart failure: A comprehensive meta-analysis of five randomised controlled trials. Lancet. 2022;400(10345):757-67.
38. Butler J, Filippatos G, Siddiqi TJ, et al. Empagliflozin, health status, and quality of life in patients with heart failure and preserved ejection fraction: The EMPEROR-Preserved trial. Circulation. 2022;145(3):184-93.
39. Kosiborod MN, Bhatt AS, Claggett BL, et al. Effect of dapagliflozin on health status in patients with preserved or mildly reduced ejection fraction. J Am Coll Cardiol. 2023;81(5):460-73.
40. Gronda E, Jessup M, Iacoviello M, et al. Glucose metabolism in the kidney: Neurohormonal activation and heart failure development. J Am Heart Assoc. 2020;9(23):e018889.
41. Yale JF, Bakris G, Cariou B, et al. Efficacy and safety of canagliflozin over 52 weeks in patients with type 2 diabetes mellitus and chronic kidney disease. Diabetes Obes Metab. 2014;16:1016-27.
42. Perkovic V, Jardine M, Vijapurkar U, et al. Renal effects of canagliflozin in type 2 diabetes mellitus. Curr Med Res Opin. 2015;31(12):2219-31.
43. Vallon V, Gerasimova M, Rose MA, et al. SGLT2 inhibitor empagliflozin reduces renal growth and albuminuria in proportion to hyperglycemia and prevents glomerular hyperfiltration in diabetic Akita mice. Am J Physiol Ren Physiol. 2014;306(2):F194–204.
44. Packer M, Zannad F, Butler J, et al. Influence of endpoint definitions on the effect of empagliflozin on major renal outcomes in the EMPEROR-Preserved trial. Eur J Heart Fail. 2021;23(10):1798-9.

45. Scholtes RA, Muskiet MHA, van Baar MJB, et al. Natriuretic effect of two weeks of dapagliflozin treatment in patients with type 2 diabetes and preserved kidney function during standardized sodium intake: Results of the DAPASALT trial. Diabetes Care. 2021;44(2):440-7.
46. Sciatti E, Gori M, D'Elia E, et al. Empagliflozin in heart failure with preserved ejection fraction: First success in mission impossible. Eur Heart J Suppl. 2022;24(Suppl I): I153-9.
47. Gori M, D'Elia E, Sciatti E, et al. Sodium-glucose cotransporter 2 inhibitors in heart failure with preserved ejection fraction: Rationale for and practical use of a successful therapy. Card Fail Rev. 2022;8:e26.
48. Biegus J, Voors AA, Collins SP, et al. Impact of empagliflozin on decongestion in acute heart failure: the EMPULSE trial. Eur Heart J. 2023;44(1):41-50.
49. Butler J, Usman MS, Filippatos G, et al. Safety and efficacy of empagliflozin and diuretic use in patients with heart failure and preserved ejection fraction: A post hoc analysis of the EMPEROR-Preserved trial. JAMA Cardiol. 2023;8(7):640-9.
50. Ferreira JP, Zannad F, Pocock SJ, et al. Interplay of mineralocorticoid receptor antagonists and empagliflozin in heart failure: EMPEROR-Reduced. J Am Coll Cardiol. 2021;77(11):1397-407.
51. Vergaro G, Aimo A, Prontera C, et al. Sympathetic and renin-angiotensin-aldosterone system activation in heart failure with preserved, mid-range and reduced ejection fraction. Int J Cardiol. 2019;296:91-7.
52. Jimenez-Marrero S, Moliner P, Rodríguez-Costoya I, et al. Sympathetic activation and outcomes in chronic heart failure: Does the neurohormonal hypothesis apply to mid-range and preserved ejection fraction patients? Eur J Intern Med. 2020;81:60-6.
53. Gronda E, Dusi V, D'Elia E, et al. Sympathetic activation in heart failure. Eur Heart J Suppl. 2022;24(Suppl E):E4-11.
54. Gori M, Marini M, Gonzini L, et al. Combined neuro-humoral modulation and outcome in patients with chronic heart failure and mildly reduced or preserved ejection fraction. J Clin Med. 2022;11(22):6627.
55. Gori M, D'Elia E, Iorio A, et al. Clinical application of personalized medicine: Heart failure with preserved left ventricular fraction. Eur Heart J Suppl. 2020;22 (Suppl L):L124-8.
56. Yusuf S, Pfeffer MA, Swedberg K, et al. Effects of candesartan in patients with chronic heart failure and preserved left-ventricular ejection fraction: The CHARM-Preserved Trial. Lancet. 2003;362(9386):777-81.
57. Massie BM, Carson PE, McMurray JJ, et al.; I-PRESERVE Investigators. Irbesartan in patients with heart failure and preserved ejection fraction. N Engl J Med. 2008;359(23): 2456-67.
58. Cleland JG, Tendera M, Adamus J, et al. The perindopril in elderly people with chronic heart failure (PEP-CHF) study. Eur Heart J. 2006;27(19):2338-45.
59. Persson H, Lonn E, Edner M, et al. Diastolic dysfunction in heart failure with preserved systolic function: Need for objective evidence: Results from the CHARM Echocardiographic substudy–CHARMES. J Am Coll Cardiol. 2007;49(6):687-94.
60. Martin N, Manoharan K, Davies C, et al. Beta-blockers and inhibitors of the renin-angiotensin aldosterone system for chronic heart failure with preserved ejection fraction. Cochrane Database Syst Rev. 2021;5:CD012721.
61. Lund LH, Claggett B, Liu J, et al. Heart failure with mid-range ejection fraction in CHARM: Characteristics, outcomes and effect of candesartan across the entire ejection fraction spectrum. Eur J Heart Fail. 2018;20(8):1230–9.
62. McMurray JJ, O'Connor C. Lessons from the TOPCAT trial. N Engl J Med. 2014;370(15):1453-4.
63. Edelmann F, Wachter R, Schmidt AG, et al. Effect of spironolactone on diastolic function and exercise capacity in patients with heart failure with preserved ejection fraction: The Aldo-DHF randomized controlled trial. JAMA. 2013;309(8):781-91.
64. Boccanelli A, Mureddu GF, Cacciatore G, et al. Anti-remodelling effect of canrenone in patients with mild chronic heart failure (AREA IN-CHF study): Final results. Eur J Heart Fail. 2009;11(1):68-76.
65. Lund LH, Oldgren J, James S. Registry-based pragmatic trials in heart failure: Current experience and future directions. Curr Heart Fail Rep. 2017;14(2):59-70.
66. Solomon SD, McMurray JJV, Anand IS, et al. Angiotensin-neprilysin inhibition in heart failure with preserved ejection fraction. N Engl J Med. 2019;381(17):1609-20.
67. McMurray JJV, Jackson AM, Lam CSP, et al. Effects of sacubitril-valsartan versus valsartan in women compared with men with heart failure and preserved ejection fraction: Insights from PARAGON-HF. Circulation. 2020;141(5):338-51.
68. Mentz RJ, Ward JH, Hernandez AF, et al.; PARAGLIDE-HF Investigators. Angiotensin-neprilysin inhibition in patients with mildly reduced or preserved ejection fraction and worsening heart failure. J Am Coll Cardiol. 2023;82(1): 1-12.
69. Vaduganathan M, Mentz RJ, Claggett BN, et al. Sacubitril/valsartan in mildly reduced or preserved ejection fraction: a pre-specified participant-level pooled analysis of PARAGLIDE-HF and PARAGON-HF. Eur Heart J. 2023; 44(31):2982-93.
70. van Veldhuisen DJ, Cohen-Solal A, Böhm M, et al. Beta-blockade with nebivolol in elderly heart failure patients with impaired and preserved left ventricular ejection fraction: data from SENIORS (Study of Effects of Nebivolol Intervention on Outcomes and Rehospitalization in Seniors with Heart Failure). J Am Coll Cardiol. 2009; 53(23):2150-8.
71. Yamamoto K, Origasa H, Hori M; J-DHF Investigators. Effects of carvedilol on heart failure with preserved ejection fraction: The Japanese Diastolic Heart Failure study (J-DHF). Eur J Heart Fail. 2013;15(1):110-8.
72. Liu F, Chen Y, Feng X, et al. Effects of beta-blockers on heart failure with preserved ejection fraction: A meta-analysis. PLoS One. 2014;9(3):e90555.

73. Bavishi C, Chatterjee S, Ather S, et al. Beta-blockers in heart failure with preserved ejection fraction: A meta-analysis. Heart Fail Rev. 2015;20(2):193-201.
74. Fukuta H, Goto T, Wakami K, et al. The effect of beta-blockers on mortality in heart failure with preserved ejection fraction: A meta-analysis of observational cohort and randomized controlled studies. Int J Cardiol. 2017;228:4-10.
75. Zweerink A, van der Lingen ACJ, Handoko ML, et al. Chronotropic incompetence in chronic heart failure. Circ Heart Fail. 2018;11(8):e004969.
76. Palau P, Seller J, Domínguez E, et al. Effect of β-blocker withdrawal on functional capacity in heart failure and preserved ejection fraction. J Am Coll Cardiol. 2021;78(21): 2042-56.
77. D'Elia E, Vaduganathan M, Gori M, et al. Role of biomarkers in cardiac structure phenotyping in heart failure with preserved ejection fraction: Critical appraisal and practical use. Eur J Heart Fail. 2015;17(12):1231-9.
78. Rush CJ, Berry C, Oldroyd KG, et al. Prevalence of coronary artery disease and coronary microvascular dysfunction in patients with heart failure with preserved ejection fraction. JAMA Cardiol. 2021;6(10):1130-43.
79. Trevisan L, Cautela J, Resseguier N, et al. Prevalence and characteristics of coronary artery disease in heart failure with preserved and mid-range ejection fractions: a systematic angiography approach. Arch Cardiovasc Dis. 2018;111(2):109-18.
80. Hwang SJ, Melenovsky V, Borlaug BA. Implications of coronary artery disease in heart failure with preserved ejection fraction. J Am Coll Cardiol. 2014;63(25 Pt A): 2817-27.
81. Lopes RD, Alexander KP, Stevens SR, et al. Initial invasive versus conservative management of stable ischemic heart disease in patients with a history of heart failure or left ventricular dysfunction: Insights from the ISCHEMIA trial. Circulation. 2020;142(18):1725-35.
82. Bilak JM, Alam U, Miller CA, et al. Microvascular dysfunction in heart failure with preserved ejection fraction: Pathophysiology, assessment, prevalence and prognosis. Card Fail Rev. 2022;8:e24.
83. Del Buono MG, Montone RA, Camilli M, et al. Coronary microvascular dysfunction across the spectrum of cardiovascular disease: JACC state-of-the-art review. J Am Coll Cardiol. 2021;78(13):1352-71.
84. Berry C, Skyles R. Microvascular dysfunction in heart failure with preserved ejection fraction: A modifiable therapeutic target? JACC Cardiovasc Imaging. 2022;15(6):1012-4.
85. Mohammed SF, Hussein S, Mirzoyev SA, et al. Coronary microvascular rarefraction and myocardial fibrosis in heart failure with preserved ejection fraction. Circulation. 2015;131(6):550-9.
86. Leccisotti L, Cinti F, Sorici GP, et al. Dapagliflozin improves myocardial flow reserve in patients with type 2 diabetes: The DAPAHEART Trial: A preliminary report. Cardiovasc Diabetol. 2022;21(1):173.
87. Ren L, Chen X, Nie B, et al. Ranolazine inhibits pyroptosis via regulation of miR-135b in the treatment of diabetic cardiac fibrosis. Front Mol Biosci. 2022;9:806966.
88. Sartipy U, Dahlström U, Fu M, et al. Atrial fibrillation in heart failure with preserved, mid-range, and reduced ejection fraction. JACC Heart Fail. 2017;5(8):565-74.
89. Eapen ZJ, Greiner MA, Fonarow GC, et al. Associations between atrial fibrillation and early outcomes of patients with heart failure and reduced or preserved ejection fraction. Am Heart J. 2014;167(3):369-75.e2.
90. Zafrir B, Lund LH, Laroche C, et al. Prognostic implications of atrial fibrillation in heart failure with reduced, mid-range, and preserved ejection fraction: A report from 14,964 patients in the European Society of Cardiology Heart Failure Long-Term Registry. Eur Heart J. 2018;39(48):4277-84.
91. Hindricks G, Potpara T, Dagres N, et al. 2020 ESC guidelines for the diagnosis and management of atrial fibrillation developed in collaboration with the European Association for Cardio-Thoracic Surgery (EACTS): The Task Force for the diagnosis and management of atrial fibrillation of the European Society of Cardiology (ESC) developed with the special contribution of the European Heart Rhythm Association (EHRA) of the ESC. Eur Heart J. 2021;42(5):373-498.
92. Wyse DG, Waldo AL, DiMarco JP, et al. A comparison of rate control and rhythm control in patients with atrial fibrillation. N Engl J Med. 2002;347(23):1825-33.
93. Van Gelder IC, Hagens VE, Bosker HA, et al.; Rate Control versus Electrical Cardioversion for Persistent Atrial Fibrillation Study Group. A comparison of rate control and rhythm control in patients with recurrent persistent atrial fibrillation. N Engl J Med. 2002;347(23):1834-40.
94. Miyagi C, Miyamoto T, Karimov JH, et al. Device-based treatment options for heart failure with preserved ejection fraction. Heart Fail Rev. 2021;26(4):749-62.
95. Freed BH, Shah SJ. Stepping out of the left ventricle's shadow: Time to focus on the left atrium in heart failure with preserved ejection fraction. Circ Cardiovasc Imaging. 2017;10(4):0062678.
96. Hasenfuß G, Hayward C, Burkhoff D, et al. A transcatheter intracardiac shunt device for heart failure with preserved ejection fraction (REDUCE LAP-HF): A multicentre, open-label, single-arm, phase 1 trial. Lancet. 2016;387(10025):1298-304.
97. De Rosa R, Piscione F, Schranz D, et al. Transcatheter implantable devices to monitoring of elevated left atrial pressures in patients with chronic heart failure. Transl Med IniSa. 2017;17:19-21.
98. Rosalia L, Ozturk C, Shoar S, et al. Device-based solutions to improve cardiac physiology and hemodynamics in heart failure with preserved ejection fraction. JACC Basictransl Sci. 2021;6(9-10):772-95.
99. Shah SJ, Borlaug BA, Chung ES, et al.; REDUCE LAP-HF II investigators. Atrial shunt device for heart failure with preserved and mildly reduced ejection fraction (REDUCE

LAP-HF II): A randomised, multicentre, blinded, sham-controlled trial. Lancet. 2022;399(10330):1130-40.
100. Feldman T, Mauri L, Kahwash R, et al. Transcatheter interatrial shunt device for the treatment of heart failure with preserved ejection fraction (REDUCE LAP-HF I [Reduce Elevated Left Atrial Pressure in Patients With Heart Failure]): A phase 2, randomized, sham-controlled trial. Circulation. 2018;137(4):364-75.
101. Shah SJ, Feldman T, Ricciardi MJ, et al. One-year safety and clinical outcomes of a transcatheter interatrial shunt device for the treatment of heart failure with preserved ejection fraction in the reduce elevated left atrial pressure in patients with heart failure (REDUCE LAP-HF I) trial: A randomized clinical trial. JAMA Cardiol. 2018;3:968-77.
102. Wu Y, Song M, Wu M, et al. Advances in device-based treatment of heart failure with preserved ejection fraction: Evidence from clinical trials. ESC Heart Fail. 2024;11(1): 13-27.
103. Shah SJ, Borlaug BA, Chung ES, et al. Atrial shunt device for heart failure with preserved and mildly reduced ejection fraction (REDUCE LAP-HF II): a randomised, multicentre, blinded, sham-controlled trial. Lancet. 2022 Mar 19;399(10330):1130-40.
104. Borlaug BA, Blair J, Bergmann MW, et al.; REDUCE LAP-HF-II Investigators. Latent pulmonary vascular disease may alter the response to therapeutic atrial shunt device in heart failure. Circulation. 2022;145(21):1592-604.
105. Rodés-Cabau J, Bernier M, Amat-Santos IJ, et al. Interatrial shunting for heart failure: Early and late results from the first-in-human experience with the V-wave system. JACC Cardiovasc Interv. 2018;11(22):2300-10.
106. Paitazoglou C, Özdemir R, Pfister R, et al. The AFR-PRELIEVE trial: A prospective, non-randomised, pilot study to assess the atrial flow regulator (AFR) in heart failure patients with either preserved or reduced ejection fraction. EuroIntervention. 2019;15:403-10.
107. Lewicki Ł, Kosmalska K, Liedtke S, et al. Pomeranian atrial flow regulator in congestive heart failure (prolonger): Study protocol. Cardiol J. 2020;27:879-83.
108. Volpe M, Liuzzo G. Unloading left heart with a shunt device shows no benefits in heart failure with preserved ejection fraction but supports the importance of phenotyping patients in clinical trials. Eur Heart J. 2022;43:1700-1.
109. Burlacu A, Simion P, Nistor I, et al. Novel percutaneous interventional therapies in heart failure with preserved ejection fraction: An integrative review. Heart Fail Rev. 2019;24:793-803.
110. Griffin JM, Borlaug BA, Komtebedde J, et al. Impact of interatrial shunts on invasive hemodynamics and exercise tolerance in patients with heart failure. J Am Heart Assoc. 2020;9(17):e016760.
111. Brugts JJ, Radhoe SP, Aydin D, et al. Clinical update of the latest evidence for CardioMEMS pulmonary artery pressure monitoring in patients with chronic heart failure: A promising system for remote heart failure care. Sensors (Basel). 2021;21(7):2335.
112. Abraham WT, Adamson PB, Bourge RC, et al.; CHAMPION Trial Study Group Wireless pulmonary artery haemodynamic monitoring in chronic heart failure: A randomised controlled trial. Lancet. 2011;377:658-66.
113. Adamson PB, Abraham WT, Bourge RC, et al. Wireless pulmonary artery pressure monitoring guides management to reduce decompensation in heart failure with preserved ejection fraction. Circ Heart Fail. 2014;7(6):935-44.
114. Shavelle DM, Desai AS, Abraham WT, et al. Lower rates of heart failure and all-cause hospitalizations during pulmonary artery pressure-guided therapy for ambulatory heart failure: One-year outcomes from the Cardio-MEMS Post-approval study. Circ Heart Fail. 2020;13(8):e006863.
115. Lindenfeld J, Zile MR, Desai AS, et al. Haemodynamic-guided management of heart failure (GUIDE-HF): A randomised controlled trial. Lancet. 2021;398(10304): 991-1001.
116. Abbott. (2022). Abbott's CardioMEMS HF system receives FDA approval to support patients battling earlier-stage heart failure. [online] Available from https://abbott.mediaroom.com/2022-02-21-Abbotts-CardioMEMS-TM-HF-System-Receives-FDA-Approval-to-Support-Patients-Battling-Earlier-Stage-Heart-Failure [Last accessed January, 2025].
117. Eicher JC, Laurent G, Mathé A, et al. Atrial dyssynchrony syndrome: An overlooked phenomenon and a potential cause of 'diastolic' heart failure. Eur J Heart Fail. 2012;14(3): 248-58.
118. Maass AH, van Gelder IC. Atrial resynchronization therapy: A new concept for treatment of heart failure with preserved ejection fraction and prevention of atrial fibrillation? Eur J Heart Fail. 2012;14(3):227–29.
119. Laurent G, Eicher JC, Mathe A, et al. Permanent left atrial pacing therapy may improve symptoms in heart failure patients with preserved ejection fraction and atrial dyssynchrony: A pilot study prior to a national clinical research programme. Eur J Heart Fail. 2013;15(1): 85-93.
120. Silverman DN, Rambod M, Lustgarten DL, et al. Heart rate-induced myocardial Ca^{2+} retention and left ventricular volume loss in patients with heart failure with preserved ejection fraction. J Am Heart Assoc. 2020;9(17):e017215.
121. Klein FJ, Bell S, Runte KE, et al. Heartrate-induced modifications of concentric left ventricular hypertrophy: Exploration of a novel therapeutic concept. Am J Physiol Heart Circ Physiol. 2016;311(4):H1031-39.
122. Infeld M, Wahlberg K, Cicero J, et al. Effect of personalized accelerated pacing on quality of life, physical activity, and atrial fibrillation in patients with preclinical and overt heart failure with preserved ejection fraction: The myPACE randomized clinical trial. JAMA Cardiol. 2023;8(3): 213-21.
123. Reddy YNV, Koepp KE, Carter R, et al. Rate-adaptive atrial pacing for heart failure with preserved ejection fraction: The RAPID-HF randomized clinical trial. JAMA. 2023;329:801-9.

124. Fudim M, Hernandez AF, Felker GM. Role of volume redistribution in the congestion of heart failure. J Am Heart Assoc. 2017;6(8):e006817.
125. Fudim M, Ponikowski PP, Burkhoff D, et al. Splanchnic nerve modulation in heart failure: mechanistic overview, initial clinical experience, and safety considerations. Eur J Heart Fail. 2021;23(7):1076-84.
126. Bapna A, Adin C, Engelman ZJ, et al. Increasing blood pressure by greater splanchnic nerve stimulation: A feasibility study. J Cardiovasc Transl Res. 2020;13(4):509-18.
127. Fudim M, Khan MS, Paracha AA, et al. Targeting preload in heart failure: Splanchnic nerve blockade and beyond. Circ Heart Fail. 2022;15(3):e009340.
128. Reddy V, Sievert H, Zirakashvili T, et al. TCT-432 greater splanchnic nerve ablation in chronic heart failure: Preserved versus reduced left ventricular ejection fraction. J Am Coll Cardiol. 2021;78:B177-8.
129. Málek F, Gajewski P, Zymliński R, et al. Surgical ablation of the right greater splanchnic nerve for the treatment of heart failure with preserved ejection fraction: First-in-human clinical trial. Eur J Heart Fail. 2021;23:1134-43.
130. Fudim M, Zirakashvili T, Shaburishvili N, et al. Transvenous right greater splanchnic nerve ablation in heart failure and preserved ejection fraction: First-in-human study. JACC Heart failure. 2022;10(10):744-52.
131. Fudim M, Fail PS, Litwin SE, et al. Endovascular ablation of the right greater splanchnic nerve in heart failure with preserved ejection fraction: Early results of the REBALANCE-HF trial roll-in cohort. Eur J Heart Fail 2022;24:1410-4.
132. Patel RB, Shah SJ. The splanchnic reservoir: An oasis for blood volume in heart failure with preserved ejection fraction? Eur J Heart Fail. 2021;23(7):1144-6.
133. Cappannoli L, Scacciavillani R, Rocco E, et al. Cardiac contractility modulation for patient with refractory heart failure: An updated evidence-based review. Heart Fail Rev. 2021;26:227-35.
134. De Denus S, O'Meara E, Desai AS, et al. Spironolactone metabolites in TOPCAT–new insights into regional variation. N Engl J Med. 2017;376(17):1690-2.

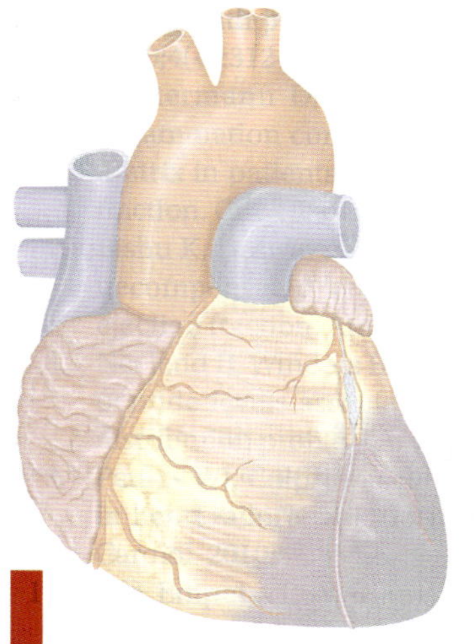

HFpEF: As Multimorbidities Disease—Advances in Management

Prabhakar Dorairaj, Samuel Jebavaram

INTRODUCTION

Heart failure (HF) is a growing pandemic with dramatic improvements in clinical and survival outcomes in HFrEF. However, HFpEF has lagged in creating such improvements but currently there is a surge in the evidence supporting its management. The present chapter will focus on the advances in the management strategies of HFpEF.

DIAGNOSIS OF HEART FAILURE WITH PRESERVED EJECTION FRACTION

The definition of HF is "clinical syndrome with current or prior symptoms and signs of a structural and/or functional cardiac abnormality that is corroborated with either elevated natriuretic peptides or objective evidence of cardiogenic pulmonary or systemic congestion".[1] HF with an ejection fraction of >50% is defined as HFpEF.

MANAGEMENT OF HEART FAILURE WITH PRESERVED EJECTION FRACTION

The cornerstone of acute HFpEF management is decongestion with a diuretic that takes a class 1 indication. Interestingly, most of the studies on HFpEF have included HFmrEF as a part of cohort of patients who do not have HFrEF.

It is important to understand that HFpEF is not like HFrEF where the four-pillar management has become the norm. HFpEF is a multimorbidity disease involving cardiovascular, pulmonary, renal, metabolic, and geriatric conditions. Management of HFpEF involves management of all these comorbidities.[2]

SODIUM–GLUCOSE COTRANSPORTER-2 INHIBITORS

The EMPEROR preserved trial with empagliflozin and DELIVER trial with dapagliflozin had significant reduction in hospitalization due to heart failure (HHF) by 27% and 23%, respectively. However, both studies did not show a significant reduction in cardiovascular death. The efficacy was noted irrespective of the presence of diabetes mellitus, age, sex, previous use of RAAS inhibitors, NTpro BNP levels, or previous HHF.[3,4] With two successful trials on two different molecules, sodium–glucose cotransporter-2 inhibitors (SGLT2i) are now class I indication in the management of HFpEF. SGLT2i should be avoided when eGFR is <20 mL/min/1.73m^2.

Mineralocorticoid Receptor Antagonist

The TOPCAT trial tested spironolactone and reported a negative trial with the primary endpoint (composite CV death, HHF, or aborted cardiac arrest). But there was a significant reduction in first HHF. A post-hoc analysis showed that the study was significant in the America and not beneficial in Eastern Europe where there were pointers toward poor compliance.[5] This controversy will be addressed by future trials on spironolactone—SPIRIT-HF and SPIRRIT.

Finerenone is a nonsteroidal mineralocorticoid receptor antagonist (MRA) that reduced the worsening HF events significantly by 18%, and an insignificant trend toward reduction in deaths due to cardiovascular causes (7%) was reported in the FINEARTS-HF trial.[6]

Angiotensin Receptor Blocker and Neprilysin Inhibitor

Two trials with angiotensin receptor blocker and neprilysin inhibitor (ARNI) in HFpEF, PARAGON and PARAGLIDE separately did not achieve statistical significance. However, In the pooled analysis among patients who were recently hospitalized for HF, ARNI significantly reduced cardiovascular death and HHF by 22%. The benefits were higher when the LVEF was ≤60%.[7]

Beta-blockers

Chronotropic incompetence contributes to exercise intolerance in HFpEF. Beta-blockers can blunt the heart rate response to exercise and have been subject to a lot of scrutiny in HFpEF. ELANDD study (Effects of Long-term Administration of Nebivolol on the clinical symptoms, exercise capacity, and left ventricular function of patients with Diastolic Dysfunction), CIBIS-ELD, and SWEDIC (Swedish Doppler Echocardiographic) study showed that beta-blocker use was associated with higher natriuretic peptide levels.

Compared to resting heart rate, atrial pacing at 120 beats/minute reduced the LVEDP from 17 to 8 mm Hg. There was also a reduction in LV end-systolic, end-diastolic, and stroke volumes. Prolonged diastolic period will increase the filling period, which will increase the volumes and pressures.[8]

In the PRESERVE HR trial for HFpEF patients with chronotropic incompetence, withdrawal of carvedilol improved maximal functional capacity.[9]

With available evidence, it will be prudent to have a more lenient approach toward heart rate lowering agents in HFpEF patients already on these agents and to avoid these agents in the absence of a clear indication if they are not already on heart rate lowering agents.

Glucagon-like Peptide-1 Receptor Agonists

In the STEP-HFpEF trial, in patients with HFpEF and BMI ≥30 kg/m², once weekly semaglutide significantly produced the weight loss by 10% points, improved the six-minute-walk test by 20 meters, and reduced CRP levels.[10] In the SELECT trial, which included ASCVD patients with a BMI ≥27 kg/m², weekly semaglutide reduced the composite cardiovascular outcomes and MACE in patients with or without HF irrespective of the type of HF.[11]

Exercise

Exercise training has been shown to produce beneficial adaptations in arterial and skeletal muscle function. The results of exercise on the systolic and diastolic functions of the heart have been inconsistent. However, the overall benefit of exercise in improving cardiorespiratory fitness is emphasized in HFpEF.[2]

Salt and Water Restriction

A major meta-analysis of salt and water restriction in HF advised 3.75–10 grams of salt every day—same as ESC guidance in chronic HF. Fluid intake is guided by thirst and environmental conditions. In acute HF, there is no evidence of extreme sodium intake (<1 gm Na/day) or fluid restriction. A fluid intake that is less than urine output is advised.[12]

An average Indian consumes more than 10 grams of salt per day and a salt restriction is prudent.

Device-based Therapies in HFpEF

The elevated left atrial pressure or pulmonary capillary wedge pressure is the basic physiology of HFpEF and reduction of the same is the basis of device-based therapies in HFpEF.[13] The various device-based therapies are discussed in **Table1**.

TABLE 1: Device-based therapies in HFpEF.

Treatment	*Comment*
Interatrial shunt for left atrial decompression into the right atrium: Interatrial shunt device (IASD), V-wave shunt, and atrial flow regulator (Occlutech)	Variable response to devices—correct hemodynamic responders have to be identified. Concern about anticoagulation and right-sided volume overload
Implantable monitoring of PCWP to guide diuretic therapy: CardioMEMS PA sensor system, remotely monitors LPA pressure	• CHAMPION study in NYHA Class III showed 70% reduction in HF in HFpEF, while it was 50% in overall HF. GUIDE HF trial expanded modest improvement in previous HF • Future studies for mortality reduction are needed

Contd...

Contd...

Treatment	*Comment*
Left atrial pacing: Ameliorates atrial dyssynchrony, p-wave duration >120 mseconds is paced	• Improvement in 6-minute-walk test in initial trials • myPACE and RAPID-HF showed conflicting results • Further large-scale studies are required
• *Splanchnic ablation:* It leads to favorable redistribution of fluid • Right greater splanchnic nerve stimulation increases the right heart volumes and pressures • Ablation leads to reverse	• SAVM showed the safety of ablation, improvement in NTproBNP and 6-minute-walk distance • *Ongoing REBALANCE:* HF early results showed 7.5 mm Hg reduction in PCWP and improved quality of life • Long-term safety and efficacy results awaited
• *Cardiac contractility modulation* improves calcium handling • Nonexcitatory, high-voltage, long-duration electrical pulse of the RV septum during the absolute refractory period • This reverses cardiac remodeling and improves cardiac function	• Optimizer smart device—FIX HF-5. CCF-HFpEF—showed better outcomes when LVEF is 35–45% • Sham-controlled AIM-HIGHer trial in HFpEF is underway
Renal denervation, whether the BP reduction or changes in LVH are responsible for improvements in HFpEF is unclear	• Initial results are not conclusive due to smaller number of patients. • Improvement in diastolic filling pressures and NT pro-BNP have been noted • Safety, long-term results, and mechanisms are unclear • UNLOAD-HFpEF is a sham-controlled ongoing trial
Baroreflex activation therapy (BAT): Baroreceptor dysfunction noted in HF	• HOPE4HF and BeAT-HF improved exercise capacity in HFrEF • In HumMod model, BAT was effective by inhibiting renal sympathetic nerve activity. BAROSTIM in HFpEF is an ongoing registry and results are awaited
• *Vagus nerve stimulation (VNS)* relieves proinflammatory state and improves cardiac remodeling • Low-level tragus stimulation (LLTS) is a percutaneous method of VNS	• ANTHEM-HFpEF improvement in functional capacity was noted. • LLTS has been acutely shown to improve longitudinal strain of LV in HFpEF • Further studies are needed to identify the duration, frequency, and intensity of LLTS

CONCLUSION

The HFpEF is a multimorbidity disease. Three pillars in the management of HFpEF are SGLT2i, ARNI, and MRAs, especially finerenone. In a congested state, the diuretics are most useful. Beta-blockers are reserved for definite indications and a lenient use of beta-blockers in HFpEF is prudent. The future of device-based therapies is evolving and is likely the future in this complex disease.

REFERENCES

1. Bozkurt B, Coats AJS, Tsutsui H, et al. Universal definition and classification of heart failure: a report of the Heart Failure Society of America, Heart Failure Association of the European Society of Cardiology, Japanese Heart Failure Society and Writing Committee of the Universal Definition of Heart Failure: Endorsed by the Canadian Heart Failure Society, Heart Failure Association of India, Cardiac Society of Australia and New Zealand, and Chinese Heart Failure Association. Eur J Heart Fail. 2021;23(3):352-80.
2. Anker SD, Usman MS, Anker MS, et al. Patient phenotype profiling in heart failure with preserved ejection fraction to guide therapeutic decision making. A scientific statement of the Heart Failure Association, the European Heart Rhythm Association of the European Society of Cardiology, and the European Society of Hypertension. Eur J Heart Fail. 2023;25(7):936-55.
3. Anker SD, Butler J, Filippatos G, et al.; EMPEROR-Preserved Trial Investigators. Empagliflozin in heart failure with a preserved ejection fraction. N Eng J Med. 2021;385(16):1451-61.
4. Solomon SD, McMurray JJV, Claggett B, et al. DELIVER Trial Committees and Investigators. Dapagliflozin in heart failure with mildly reduced or preserved ejection fraction. N Eng J Med. 2022;387(12):1089-98.
5. Pfeffer MA, Claggett B, Assmann SF, et al. Regional variation in patients and outcomes in the Treatment of Preserved Cardiac Function Heart Failure With an Aldosterone Antagonist (TOPCAT) trial. Circulation. 2015;131(1):34-42.
6. Solomon SD, McMurray JJV, Vaduganathan M, et al.; FINEARTS-HF Committees and Investigators. Finerenone in heart failure with mildly reduced or preserved ejection fraction. N Eng J Med. 2024;391(16):1475-85.

7. Vaduganathan M, Mentz RJ, Claggett BL, et al. Sacubitril/valsartan in heart failure with mildly reduced or preserved ejection fraction: A pre-specified participant-level pooled analysis of PARAGLIDE-HF and PARAGON-HF. Eur Heart J. 2023;44(31):2982-93.
8. Meyer M, LeWinter MM. Heart rate and heart failure with preserved ejection fraction: Time to Slow β-Blocker Use? Circ Heart Fail. 2019;12(8):e006213.
9. Palau P, Seller J, Domínguez E, et al. Effect of β-blocker withdrawal on functional capacity in heart failure and preserved ejection fraction. J Am Coll Cardiol. 2021;78(21): 2042-56.
10. Kosiborod MN, Abildstrøm SZ, Borlaug BA, et al. Semaglutide in patients with heart failure with preserved ejection fraction and obesity. N Eng J Med. 2023;389(12): 1069-84.
11. Deanfield J, Verma S, Scirica BM, et al. Semaglutide and cardiovascular outcomes in patients with obesity and prevalent heart failure: A prespecified analysis of the SELECT trial. Lancet. 2024;404(10454):773-86.
12. Mullens W, Damman K, Dhont S, et al. Dietary sodium and fluid intake in heart failure. A clinical consensus statement of the Heart Failure Association of the ESC. Eur J Heart Fail. 2024;26(4):730-41.
13. Wu Y, Song M, Wu M, et al. Advances in device-based treatment of heart failure with preserved ejection fraction: Evidence from clinical trials. ESC Heart Fail. 2024;11(1): 13-27.

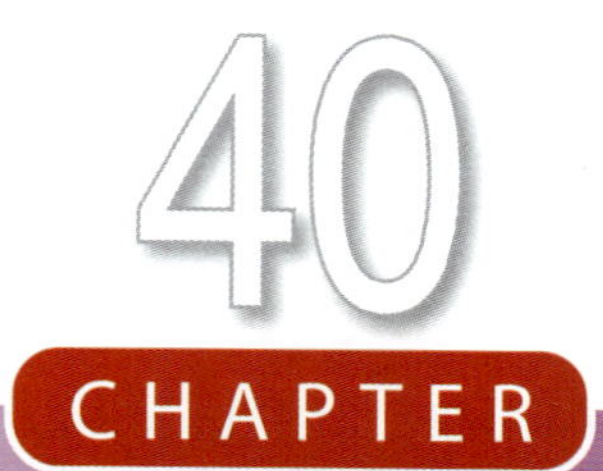

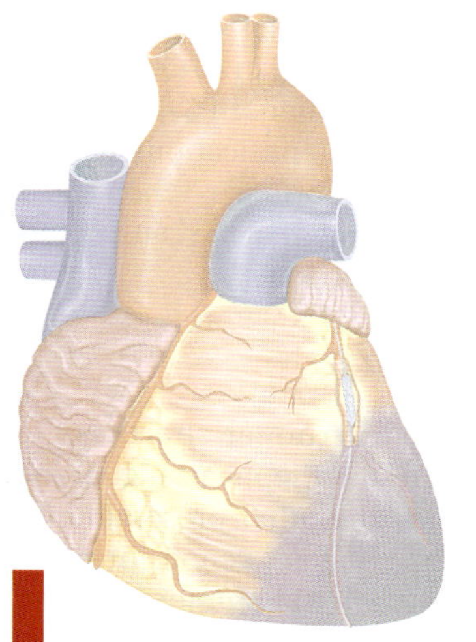

HFpEF to Acute Heart Failure: What is It? Management Strategies

Tapan Ghose, Sutapa Chaudhuri

INTRODUCTION

Heart failure (HF) is a clinical syndrome with current or prior symptoms and or signs caused by a structural and/or functional cardiac abnormality as determined by an EF <50%, abnormal cardiac chamber enlargement, E/E' of >15, moderate-to-severe ventricular hypertrophy or moderate/severe valvular obstructive or regurgitant lesion and corroborated by at least—one of the following (1) elevated natriuretic peptide levels (2) objective evidence of cardiogenic pulmonary or systemic congestion by diagnostic modalities, such as imaging (e.g., chest X-ray or elevated filling pressures by echocardiography) or hemodynamic assessment (e.g., right heart study) at rest—or with provocation (e.g., exercise). Heart failure with preserved EF (HFpEF) is HF with EF >50%. HFpEF encompasses a disease group of patient of varied etiologies.[1]

PHENOTYPES OF HEART FAILURE WITH PRESERVED EJECTION FRACTION

Four clinical phenotypes were identified initially (1) aging, (2) coronary artery disease (CAD), (3) obesity, and (4) pulmonary hypertension (PH).[2] Currently 14 phenotypes are under consideration, they are age, sex, type 2 diabetes mellitus, obesity, sleep apnea, hypertension, hypotension, COPD, iron deficiency, CAD, atrial fibrillation, high heart rate, and chronotropic.[3]

Acute heart failure (AHF) is defined as new or worsening of symptoms and signs of HF. This is the most frequent cause of unplanned hospitalization in age group of >65 years of age. De novo HF denotes symptoms of HF without a previous history of HF. Acute decompensated heart failure (ADHF) denotes worsening signs or symptoms in a previously diagnosed patient of HF.[3,4]

EPIDEMIOLOGY

No global data on the HFrEF versus HFpEF is available on the prevalence of HF. Global burden of disease (GBD) collaborations reported 37.7 million cause of HF prevalence worldwide.[4] Annual hospitalization in USA and Europe exceed 1 million per year. INTER-CHF study, reported on 5,823 patients of HF from 108 countries in six geographical regions. The overall 1 year mortality was 16.5%. Country wise mortality were (Africa 34%), India (23%), South America (9%), Middle East (9%), and China (7%).[5]

RISK FACTORS

Ischemic heart disease (IHD) is the most common (>50%) risk factors in high income regions, eastern and central Europe. In Asia pacific high income regions and Latin America IHD contributed to 30–40% cases. In Africa, it contributed to <10% cases. Hypertension contributed to 17% cases globally. Rheumatic disease contributed to 34% cases in East Asia and 14% cases in Sub-Saharan Africa. Since the obesity epidemic affects women more, hypertensive heart disease leading to AF is more common in women.[5,6]

MORBIDITY AND MORTALITY

Globally, AHF in hospital mortality is 4%. 60–90 days mortality is 10%. 1 year mortality is 25–30%. Highest 1 year mortality is reported from India and African countries. Unless treated properly 5-year mortality in HF is similar irrespective of EF.[5]

PATHOPHYSIOLOGICAL MECHANISM OF TRANSITIONS OF HEART FAILURE WITH PRESERVED EJECTION FRACTION TO ACUTE HEART FAILURE

The substrate is either a functional or structural disorder. They may be acute of chronic. Examples are hypertension, diabetes, IHD, cardiomyopathies, etc. These changes lead to response of the body which is initially adaptive and later on becomes maladaptive. This may be punctuated by acute events such as arrhythmias, infection, anemia, stress, etc. Initial response of LV in diastolic dysfunction. Increased LV filling pressure leads to pulmonary congestion. Relaxation of LV is active process which require removal of cytoplasmic calcium by the sarcoplasmic reticulum Ca^{++} ATPase (SERCA) pump and in part via extraction from plasma membrane. Reduction in ATP generation due to ischemia impairs the relaxation function. LV filling is impaired due to hypertrophy and or fibrosis in hypertension, diabetes, CKD, aortic stenosis, and aging. In mitral stenosis there is diastolic dysfunction not due to structural abnormality but due to chronic underfilling. ADHF is triggered by sudden development of atrial fibrillation in mitral stenosis, aortic stenosis, and hypertrophic cardiomyopathy.

Increased extracellular fluid and/or change in venous compliance leads to increased filling pressure in ventricles which triggers AHF. Only 50% of the patient has weight gain >0.9% kg proceeding hospitalization of ADHF which indicates the enormous role of venous compliance. In normal individual increased sodium in the body is retained by intestinal glycosaminoglycans network which prevents edema formation. In HF this network is dysfunctional. Fluid redistribution also plays an important role. Normally, one-fourth of the blood volume is in venous system. Sympathetic stimulation diverts fluid from splanchnic and peripheral venous systemic to pulmonary bed leading to congestion.[7]

PRECIPITATING FACTORS

Acute coronary syndrome, arrhythmias (atrial fibrillation is particular) infection (particularly lower respiratory tract), hypertension, noncompliance with activity restrictions, dietary sodium restriction, fluid restrictions, and drug regimen are the precipitating causes in most cases. Psychological stress is also a precipitating cause. In 40–50% causes no precipitating cause can be identified. In 5–20% cases multiple causes may be present. Identifications of precipitation cause has prognostic importance. Whenever a cause is identified, proper management of the cause alters the natural history in a positive direction.[8,9]

CLINICAL PRESENTATION

Most common symptoms in exertional shortness of breath. Shortness of breath at rest, orthopnea, fatigue, and reduced exercise tolerance are the other presentations. Signs include peripheral edema, jugular venous pressure elevation, S3 gallop, and bilateral basal pulmonary rates. Liver is soft, enlarged, and tender. Cold clammy skin, altered mentation, and oliguria suggest cardiogenic shock.

Criteria for ICU admission are (1) hemodynamic instability (HF <40 bpm or >130 bpm, SBP <90, or hypoperfusion), (2) respiratory distress (respiratory rate >25/min, O_2 saturation <90% despite O_2 supplementation), use of accessory muscles of respiration or exhaustion by patient which dictates needs for mechanical ventilation.[10,11]

DIAGNOSIS

Measurement of plasma natriuretic peptides is indicated in either brain natriuretic peptide (BNP) or N-terminal pro-BNP (NT pro BNP) or mid regional proatrial natriuretic peptide (MR pro ANP). Very high value is suggestive of AHF. Elevation from a euvolemic BNP level to higher level also indicates ADHF. Several new biomarkers are available. However, their role in routine practice is not clear. Chest X-ray, echocardiography, ECG, troponin, and blood workup are other diagnostic modalities.

A recently proposed protocol is helpful in evaluation and personalization of the management. The elements are (1) phenotype (2) pathophysiology (3) precipitating cause (4) pathology (5) polymorbidity (6) iatrogenic element (7) patient preference **(Box 1)**.[12] The initial protocol was 7P protocol which has been modified by authors to 9P protocol. HFpEF should be considered in a patient with dyspnea with any one of the following: (1) Age >60 years (2) atrial fibrillation, (3) CKD, (4) CAD, (5) diabetes, (6) hypertension, (7) overweight. H2FPEF[11] and HFA-PEFF[12] are other diagnostic algorithms. Lung ultrasonography is emerging as a great diagnostic modality in AHF.[13,14] ECG, vitals monitoring, and oxygen saturation are the standardized practices. Holter monitoring, extended loop recorder (ELR), are important in selected cases. C-reactive protein (CRP) and procalcitonin help to identify inflammation. Basic assessment of kidney, liver, and blood panel is important.[15-17]

BOX 1: 9P protocol in acute heart failure.

1. *Phenotype:* Clinically access good peripheral perfusion (warm) was low perfusion (cold) and congestion (no congestion—dry; presence of congestion—wet). Most common acute heart failure (AHF) patient is warm-wet
2. *Pathophysiology:* Initial need for intravenous (IV) diuretic for congestion, inotropic support, and use of vasodilators should be promptly addressed and executed
3. *Precipitating cause:* Identify a cause and treat the cause. This alters the natural history quickly
4. *Pathology:* Identify the pathology and tailor the management.
5. *Polymorbidity:* Renal, hepatic, pregnancy status, bleeding disorder, allergies, drug intolerance, and past history of toxicity should be assessed
6. *Potential iatrogenic contribution:* The relative benefit of procedures such as diagnostic angiography, endoscopic procedures, and bronchoscopic procedures should be assessed. Use of nonsteroidal anti-inflammatory drugs (NSAIDs) as analgesics is a classical example which should be avoided
7. *Preference:* Patient preferences, patient directives, living will, family preferences, and ethical issues should be addressed early. Discussion with the patient and or relatives should be done very early as AHF patient may deteriorate very fast
8. *Planning:* Plan the step down care trial, from IV to oral therapy, shifting from intensive care unit (ICU) to ward to discharge. Plan a rehabilitation and exercise program. Assess the social and home condition and need for support of social system and paramedics. In advanced heart failure the need for devices and transplant listing should be planned
9. *Prognostication:* Estimate, document, and communicate the prognosis by using algorithms such as Stevenson's classification, ADHERE risk Tree, GWTG-HF score, and MEESSI–AHF score

Source: Modified after Arrigo1 M, Jessup M, Mullens W, et al. Acute heart failure. Nat Rev Dis Primers. 2020;6(1):16.

MANAGEMENT

Current management of AHF is based on the expert opinion, experience, and trial evidence involving short-term outcomes. Prehospital management include back rest of 45°, supplemental nasal oxygen. Prehospital management should not delay the hospital admission. The principles of management are reduced congestion, increased oxygenation, reduced preload, reduced afterload, increased myocardial contractility, reduced negative troponin factors, and to institute drugs which reduce mortality in the long run.

Oxygen saturation should be restored by either supplemental oxygen, noninvasive ventilation, or invasive ventilation. Decongestive therapy principle is similar in HFpEF and HFrEF. Intravenous diuretic in the form of 3 or 4 doses or intravenous infusion continuously can be administered with equal success. Urinary volume and spot urine sodium after 1 hour of administration of IV diuretic can be used as a response to diuretic. Hourly urine 100–150 mL/hour in first of 6 hours and/or spot urinary sodium of >50–70 mmol 2 hours postloop diuretic injection is an adequate response. Reassessment is indicated early in the course. Doubling of the dose to attain a "ceiling dose" is indicated. When a "ceiling dose" is achieved, a second diuretic with separate site of action (sequential nephron blockade) should be considered. Renal replacement therapy should be considered next. Decongestive therapy should be switched to oral form once euvolemia is reached.[18-20]

ETIOLOGICAL TREATMENT

Treatment of the underlying cardiac cause and precipitating cause should be considered next. Treatment myocardial ischemia, infection, specific therapies for amyloidosis, surgical or interventional therapy for valvular heart disease should be considered.[20]

SODIUM GLUCOSE COTRANSPORTER 2 INHIBITOR

Sodium glucose cotransporter 2 inhibitor (SGLT2) class of drugs have shown to alter the natural history of the disease by reducing mortality.

The empagliflozin heart failure with preserved ejection fraction (EMPEROR-PRESERVED)[21] demonstrated reduced mortality, risk of rehospitalization, kidney function detection with improved quality of life in 5,988 patients with HF and EF >40%. There was 21% reduction in composite of death and HF hospitalization. Dapagliflozin evaluation to improve the lives of patient with preserved EF heart failure (DELIVER)[22] demonstrated decreased risk of worsening HF or cardiovascular death (n = 6,263). A meta-analysis of these two trials confirmed the benefits. SGLT2 should be administered in all patients of HFpEF once clinical stabilization is achieved irrespective of diabetes status. The drug should be avoided in active urinary tract infection, euglycemic ketosis, or eGFR <20 mL/min 1.73 m^2 or patient with risk factors of foot amputation.[23]

Steroidal and Nonsteroidal Mineralocorticoid Receptor Antagonist

The spironolactone with the treatment of preserved cardiac function heart failure with an aldosterone antagonist (TOPCAT), trial involving 3,445 patient with HFpEF showed reduced hospitalization. There was no reduction in either total or cardiovascular mortality. Higher the EF and BNP greater was the benefit. Either spironolactone 25 mg or eplerenone 25–100 mg/day may be titrated based on the response, tolerance electrolyte disturbances, and renal output.[24]

Nonsteroidal MRA finerenone has been studied in two large trials of diabetic CKD without HF. Finerenone reduced the kidney disease progression and HF hospitalization. In the Finerenone Trial to Investigate Efficacy and Safety superior to placebo in Patients with Heart Failure (FINEARTS-HF). 6,001 patients with HFpEF ≥40 years were randomized to placebo or 20 mg finerenone (maximum dose 40 mg). The primary outcome was composite of worsening HF or CV death. 1,083 primary outcome events occurred in 624 of 3,003 patients in the finerenone arm and 1,283 events occurred in 719 of 2,998 patients in the placebo arm (Rate ratio 0.84; 95% CI 0.74–0.95; *p* 0.007). Each component of primary outcome was lower in the drug arm. The benefit were in addition to SGLT2 inhibitor usage. Among secondary outcome measures KCCQ score improved, NYHA class remained unchanged, kidney composite outcome and all-cause death, were not different. The incidence of hyperkalemia was 14.3% as compared to 6.9% in placebo arm. Based on the results of TOPCAT and FINEARTS-HF trial finerenone should be added next to SGLT2 in HFpEF.[25]

Angiotensin Receptor Neprilysin Inhibitor

Subgroup analysis of patient from prospective comparison of ARNI with ARB global outcomes in HFpEF (PARAGON HF) demonstrated that angiotensin receptor neprilysin inhibitor (ARNI) reduced the risk of rehospitalization and reduced the BNP level as compared to valsartan alone. ARNI may be used and uptitrated based on the clinical response if hemodynamics allow the usage. The presence of hypertension supports the use of ARNI.[26]

Miscellaneous Drugs

IV NTG in accelerated hypertension with AHF reduces preload and helps stabilization quickly. β-blocker or non DHF calcium blocker should be used for rate control in AFib with HFpEF. Digitals is preferred in patient with hypotension. Atrial fibrillation in HFpEF and hypertrophic cardiomyopathy, cardiac amyloidosis, rheumatic mitral stenosis, or mechanical heart valve require anticoagulation regardless of CHA2DS2-VASC score.

In patient with HFpEF and suspected sleep apnea, polysomnography is indicated and either CPAP or BiPAP should be used, as indicated. In HFpEF patient with obesity (BMI ≥30), 2–4 mg weekly subcutaneous injection of glucagen-like peptide (GLP-1) receptor agonist semaglutide reduced the risk of hospitalization, improved quality of life irrespective of diabetic status. The mean change of body weight is 13.3% with semaglutide 2.6% with placebo. Recently published SUMMIT trial was presented at AHA in November 2024. Tirzepatide, a long acting agonist of glucose dependent insulinotropic polypeptide (GIP) and GLP-1 receptor was administered subcutaneous every week (up to 15 mg) in 731 patient with HFpEF, obesity (BMI ≥30). 364 patient were in active arm and 367 in placebo arm. At 104 weeks, combined death and HF hospitalization occurred in 9.9% patient in the drug arm compared to 15.3% patient's in placebo arm (HR 0.62, CI 0.41–0.95, $p = 0.026$). The study concluded that tirzepatide caused lower risk of death and hospitalized due to HF and improved quality of life. Thiazolidinediones and dipeptidyl peptidase-4 (DPP-4) inhibitors such as sitagliptin and saxagliptin are contraindicated in acute HFpEF.[27]

PREDISCHARGE MANAGEMENT PLAN

One who survives an episode of AHF has a subsequent risk of rehospitalization. Goals include prevention of rehospitalization and improve survival. Congestion is the most common cause of rehospitalization. Persistent congestion and renal dysfunction are considered poor postdischarge prognostic markers. Clinical markers (weight gain and fluid loss), biochemical markers (BNP), renal function, oxygenation, etc., should be optimized predischarge. Benefit of achieving specific lower target values for biomarkers has not been documented. Biomarkers of myocardial fibrosis, soluble ST-2 receptor has been corelated with disease severity and poor long-term prognosis. Clinicians, patient, caregivers, and ancillary services must collaborate for titration of drugs, fluid volume, treat coexisting condition, and discuss about the discharge, life style changes, and possible readmission protocol.[28,29]

POSTDISCHARGE MANAGEMENT

Efforts should be made to delay disease progression, improve symptom, and quality of life (QOL). ACC foundation—AHA guideline recommend first telephonic contact at day 3 and a follow-up visit 7–14 days after discharge. Clinicians should identify patient at risk of readmission.

Quality of Life

Dyspnea, fatigue, dry mouth, orthopnea, disturbed sleep duration and quality, and concentration difficulty are markers of poor QOL. Major depression is present in 20% patient of HF. Women has worse QOL scores.[30,31]

PROGNOSIS

Short-term mortality of acute decompensated HFpEF is similar to HFpEF with decongestion. Presence of multiple comorbidities or biomarker elevation adversely effort the mortality in long term. Poor prognostic markers are (1) older age, (2) male gender, (3) NYHA class, (4) lower EF, (5) CAD, (6) diabetes, (7) renal impairment, (8) PH, (9) RV dysfunction, (10) atrial fibrillation, and (10) increased red cell distribution width.

CONCLUSION

Many therapies have been tested in HF management. Inotropic agents (levosimendan and omecamtiv mecarbil), vasodilators (nesiritide, ularitide, and serelaxin), and diuretic (tolvaptan) have been studied with neutral outcome. Slides suggest that tested HF drugs should be administered during first 48 hours of hospital contact. Several new medications are under study in AHF. Some drugs act by modulating the adrenomedullin pathway and some act by modulating intracellular enzymes like DPP-3. A multimarker strategy based on serial biomarker evaluation (BNP HS, CRP, HS troponin, ST-2, growth differentiation factors 15, cystatin-c, and galactin 3) may improve prognosis which remains to be proved. QOL studies in HFpEF patient, translational research on the progression of HFpEF to AHF is the need of the hour.[32-36]

REFERENCES

1. Bozkurt B, Coats AJ, Tsutsui H, et al. Universal Definition and Classification of Heart Failure: A Report of the Heart Failure Society of America, Heart Failure Association of the European Society of Cardiology, Japanese Heart Failure Society and Writing Committee of the Universal Definition of Heart Failure. J Card Fail. 2021:S1071-9164(21)00050-6.
2. Samson R, Jaiswal A, Ennezat PV, et al. Clinical phenotypes in heart failure with preserved ejection fraction. J Am Heart Assoc. 2016;5:e002477.
3. Anker SD, Usman MS, Anker MS, et al. Patient phenotype profiling in heart failure with preserved ejection fraction to guide therapeutic decision making. A scientific statement of the Heart Failure Association, the European Heart Rhythm Association of the European Society of Cardiology, and the European Society of Hypertension. Eur J Heart Fail. 2023;25(7):936-55.
4. Ambrosy AP, Fonarow GC, Butler J, et al. The global health and economic burden of hospitalizations for heart failure: lessons learned from hospitalized heart failure registries. J Am Coll Cardiol. 2014;63(12):1123-33.
5. Dokainish H, Teo K, Zhu J, et al. Global mortality variations in patients with heart failure: results from the International Congestive Heart Failure (INTER-CHF) prospective cohort study. Lancet Glob Health. 2017;5(7):e6650-72.
6. Khatibzadeh S, Farzadfar F, Oliver J, et al. Worldwide risk factors for heart failure: a systematic review and pooled analysis. Int J Cardiol. 2013;168(2):1186-94.
7. Arrigo M, Parissis JT, Akiyama E, et al. Understanding acute heart failure: pathophysiology and diagnosis. Eur Heart J Suppl. 2016;18:G11-8.
8. Fonarow GC, Abraham WT, Albert NM, et al. Factors identified as precipitating hospital admissions for heart failure and clinical outcomes: findings from OPTIMIZE-HF. Arch Intern Med. 2008;168(8):847-54.
9. Arrigo M, Gayat E, Parenica J, et al. Precipitating factors and 90-day outcome of acute heart failure: a report from the intercontinental GREAT registry. Eur J Heart Fail. 2017;19(2):201-8.
10. Van Aelst LNL, Arrigo M, Placido R, et al. Acutely decompensated heart failure with preserved and reduced ejection fraction present with comparable haemodynamic congestion. Eur J Heart Fail. 2018;20(4):738-47.
11. Mebazaa A, Yilmaz MB, Levy P, et al. Recommendations on pre-hospital & early hospital management of acute heart failure: a consensus paper from the Heart Failure Association of the European Society of Cardiology, the European Society of Emergency Medicine and the Society of Academic Emergency Medicine. Eur J Heart Fail. 2015; 17(6):544-58.
12. Arrigol M, Jessup M, Mullens W, et al. Acute heart failure. Nat Rev Dis Primers. 2020;6(1):16.
13. Reddy YNV, Carter RE, Obokata M, et al A simple evidence based approach to help guide diagnosis of heart failure with preserved ejection fraction. Circulation. 2018;138(9):861-70.
14. Pieske B, Tschope C, de Boer RA, et al. How to diagnose heart failure with preserved ejection fraction. The HFA-PEEF diagnostic algorithm: a consensus recommendation from the heart failure association of European society of Cardiology (ESC). Europe Heart J. 2019;40(40):3297-317.
15. Fonarow GC, Adams Jr KR, Abraham WT, et al. Risk stratification for in-hospital mortality in acutely decompensated heart failure: classification and regression tree analysis. JAMA. 2005;293(5):572-80.
16. Platz E, Lewis EF, Uno H, et al. Detection and prognostic value of pulmonary congestion by lung ultrasound in ambulatory heart failure patients. Eur. Heart J. 2016; 37(15):1244-51.
17. Aras MA, Teerlink JR. Lung ultrasound: a 'B-line' to the prediction of decompensated heart failure. Eur. Heart J. 2016;37(15):1252-4.
18. Matsue Y, Damman K, Voors AA, et al. Time-to-furosemide treatment and mortality in patients hospitalized with acute heart failure. J Am Coll Cardiol. 2017;69(25):3042-51.
19. ter Maaten, JM, Valente MA, Damman K, et al. Diuretic response in acute heart failure–pathophysiology, evaluation and therapy. Nat Rev Cardiol. 2015;12:184-92.

20. Yancy CW, Jessup M, Bozkurt B, et al. 2017 ACC/AHA/HFSA focused update of the 2013 ACCF/AHA guideline for the management of heart failure: a report of the American College of Cardiology/American Heart Association Task Force on Clinical Practice Guidelines and the Heart Failure Society of America. Circulation. 2017;136: e137-e161.
21. Anker SF, Butler J, Gerasimos F, et al.; for the EMPEROR-Preserved Trial Investigators. Empagliflozin in Heart Failure with a Preserved Ejection Fraction. N Engl J Med. 2021;385:1451-61.
22. Solomon SD, McMurray JV, Claggett B, et al.; for the DELIVER Trial Committees and Investigators. Dapagliflozin in Heart Failure with Mildly Reduced or Preserved Ejection Fraction. N Engl J Med. 2022;387: 1089-98.
23. Vaduganathan M, Docherty F, Claggett BL, et al. SGLT2 inhibitors in patients with heart failure: a comprehensive meta-analysis of five randomised controlled trials. Lancet. 2022;400(10354):757-67.
24. Pitt B, Pfeffer MA, Assmann S, et al.; for the TOPCAT Investigators. Spironolactone for heart failure with preserved ejection fraction. N Engl J Med. 2014;370:1383-92.
25. Solomon SD, McMurray JJV, Vaduganathan M, et al.; for the FINEARTS-HF Committees and Investigators. Finerenone in Heart Failure with Mildly Reduced or Preserved Ejection Fraction. N Engl J Med. 2024;391: 1475-85.
26. Solomon SD, McMurray JJV, Anand IS, et al.; the PARAGON-HF Investigators and Committees. Angiotensin-neprilysin inhibition in heart failure with preserved ejection fraction. N Engl J Med. 2019;381:1609-20.
27. Zile R, Kramer CM, Baum SJ, et al.; the SUMMIT Trial Study Group. Tirzepatide for Heart Failure with Preserved Ejection Fraction and Packer. New Engl J Med. 2024.
28. Gayat E, Arrogo M, Littnerova S, et al. Heart failure oral therapies at discharge are associated with better outcome in acute heart failure: a propensity-score matched study. Eur. J. Heart Fail. 2018;20(2):345-54.
29. Demissei BG, Cotter G, Prescott MF, et al. A multimarker multi-time point-based risk stratification strategy in acute heart failure: results from the RELAX-AHF trial. Eur. J. Heart Fail. 2017;19(8):1001-10.
30. Freedland KE, Rich MW, Skala JA, et al. Prevalence of depression in hospitalized patients with congestive heart failure. Psychosom Med. 2003;65(1):119-28.
31. Warraich HJ, Kitzman DW, Whellan DJ, et al. Physical function, frailty, cognition, depression, and quality of life in hospitalized adults ≥60 years with acute decompensated heart failure with preserved versus reduced ejection fraction: insights from the REHAB-HF trial. Circ. Heart Fail. 2018;11(11):e005254.
32. Mebazaa A, Nieminen MS, Packer M, et al. Levosimendan vs dobutamine for patients with acute decompensated heart failure: the SURVIVE randomized trial. JAMA. 2007; 297(17):1883-91.
33. Teerlink JR, Felker GM, McMurray JJV, et al. Acute treatment with omecamtiv mecarbil to increase contractility in acute heart failure. J Am Coll Cardiol. 2016;67(12): 1444-55.
34. Packer M, O'Connor C, McMurray JJV, et al. Effect of ularitide on cardiovascular mortality in acute heart failure. N Engl J Med. 2017;376:1956-64.
35. Voors AA, Kremer D, Geven C, et al. Adrenomedullin in heart failure: pathophysiology and therapeutic application. Eur J Heart Fail. 2019;21(2):163-71.
36. Takagi K, Blet A, Levy B, et al. Circulating dipeptidyl peptidase 3 and alteration in haemodynamics in cardiogenic shock: results from the OptimaCC trial. Eur J Heart Fail. 2020;22(2):279-86.

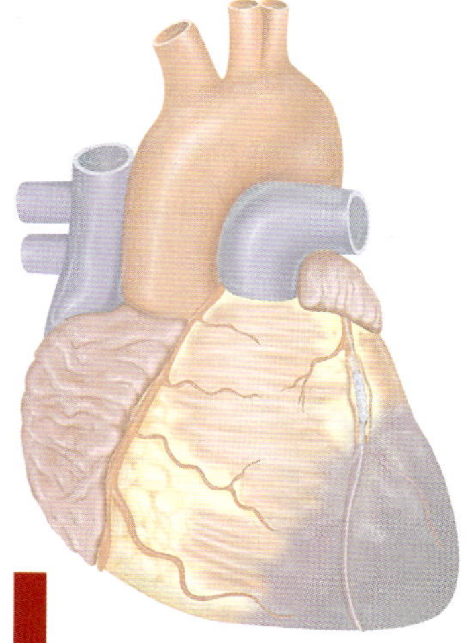

Advances and New Dimensions in HFpEF Management

Ranabrata Sen, Debabrata Roy

INTRODUCTION

Patients with heart failure with preserved ejection fraction (HFpEF) account for nearly 50% of all patients with heart failure (HF). The proportion of HFpEF in India is approximately 19–25% as per the registry data such as the Trivandrum Heart Failure Registry[1] and ASIAN-HF.[2] The mean age of presentation of patients from India is around 58–68 years, which is about 10 years younger than the data reported from the West. Still, the evidence-based treatment options for HFpEF have historically been limited. Treatment guidelines have accordingly emphasized symptomatic management through relief of congestion and treatment of comorbidities.[3,4] However, recent data from prospective, randomized trials have now provided newer directions toward pharmacologic approaches to modify disease progression in selected patients with HFpEF.

Significant questions remain:

- How to approach a person with shortness of breath?
- How to overcome diagnostic dilemma and identify a need for further testing?
- How to rule out mimics to avoid missed diagnosis?
- How to manage comorbidities and address complexities in care?
- How to initiate and optimize GDMTs?

GENERAL APPROACH TO MANAGEMENT

Three steps to be followed are:

1. Establish the diagnosis of HF and exclude potentially treatable alternatives
2. Manage congestion and address comorbidities
3. Evidence-based medical therapy

Establish the Diagnosis of Heart Failure

The diagnosis of HFpEF begins with recognizing the clinical syndrome of HF based on the identification of cardinal symptoms and signs from bedside evaluation or initial diagnostic assessment **(Flowchart 1)**.

In HFpEF, cardiac output is maintained at the cost of abnormally elevated filling pressure, which is responsible for the symptoms and signs. Neurohumoral activation (sympathetic and renin–angiotensin–aldosterone system activation) is present only in a proportion of HFpEF patients unlike in all patients with heart failure with reduced ejection fraction (HFrEF).[5] Thus, the cornerstone of diagnosing HFpEF is rest and exercise noninvasive or invasive hemodynamics assessment. Exercise testing is critical as such patients may have normal filling pressures at rest but a brisk rise in pressures during exercise.[6] Multiparameter risk scores such as the H_2FPEF or Heart Failure Association (HFA)-PEFF algorithms may help to estimate the likelihood of HFpEF and identify those in whom additional exercise hemodynamic evaluation or diastolic stress testing may be helpful **(Flowchart 2)**.

The gold standard for confirming the diagnosis of HFpEF is right heart catheterization, which is cumbersome and not easily available. An invasively measured pulmonary capillary wedge pressure of ≥15 mm Hg (at rest) or left ventricular end-diastolic pressure ≥16 mm Hg (at rest) is generally considered diagnostic in the presence of clinical features. If resting echocardiographic findings

Flowchart 1: Suggested algorithm for establishing the diagnosis of HFpEF.

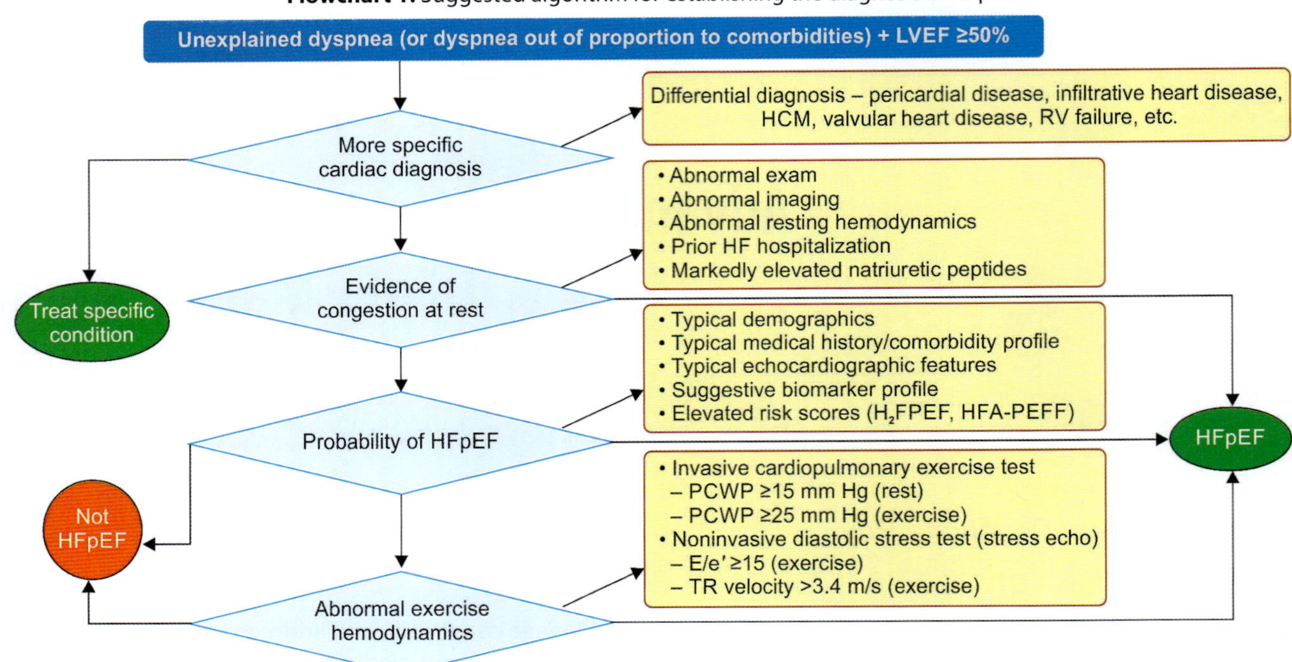

(HCM: hypertrophic cardiomyopathy; HF: heart failure; HFA: Heart Failure Association; HFpEF: heart failure with preserved ejection fraction; LVEF: left ventricular ejection fraction; PCWP: pulmonary capillary wedge pressure; RV: right ventricular; TR: tricuspid regurgitation)

and laboratory parameters are equivocal, a diastolic stress (exercise) test is recommended.

EXCLUSION OF MIMICKERS

Patients with HF symptoms and normal or near-normal LVEF comprise a heterogeneous group. Many cardiac conditions commonly coexist with HFpEF such as coronary artery disease, atrial fibrillation, functional mitral or tricuspid regurgitation, postcapillary pulmonary hypertension, and chronotropic incompetence. This makes diagnosis even more challenging, and treating these conditions is also an initial target for the management of HFpEF **(Flowchart 3)**.

MANAGE CONGESTION

Although not all patients with HFpEF are congested at rest, signs and symptoms of volume overload are frequently present in HFpEF and are correlated with functional status as well as the risk for HF hospitalization and death.[7] Data from implantable hemodynamic monitoring studies highlight that intracardiac filling pressures steadily rise weeks in advance of HF hospitalization in both patients with HFrEF and HFpEF. This can be identified as an opportunity to prevent HF decompensation with early management of congestion.[8] Loop diuretic agents have been the mainstay of decongestion in patients with HF. They are used in >80–90% of patients enrolled in clinical trials. Though there are concerns that these agents may worsen neurohormonal activation, electrolyte derangements, and renal dysfunction, particularly at higher doses.[9] The results of the TRANSFORM-HF (ToRsemide compArisoN With furoSemide FOR Management of Heart Failure) trial did not suggest a difference between furosemide and torsemide with regard to all-cause mortality or all-cause hospitalization among HFpEF patients.[10]

Data from trials of angiotensin receptor blockers (ARBs), angiotensin receptor-neprilysin inhibitors (ARNIs), and sodium-glucose cotransporter-2 (SGLT2) inhibitors in HFrEF suggest that loop diuretic requirement may reduce with the use of these agents. But in patients with HFpEF, this effect of ARNI may be attenuated.[11-13] Accordingly, in less urgent scenarios, consideration may be given to initiating agents such as SGLT2 inhibitors or ARNIs before adding/increasing loop diuretics, particularly in those with a lower end of preserved ejection fraction.

Hemodynamic congestion in HFpEF may also be exacerbated by the redistribution of stressed blood volume from the splanchnic compartment. So, alternate

Flowchart 2: Application of multiparameter scores to facilitate the diagnosis of HFpEF.

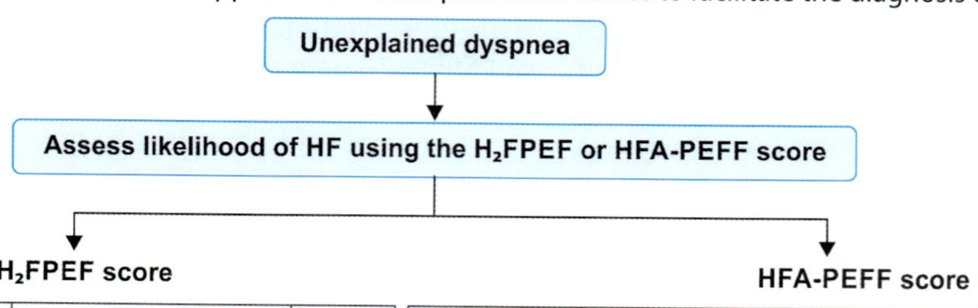

H_2FPEF score

	Parameter	Definition	Points
H_2	Heavy	BMI >30 kg/m²	2
	Hypertensive	≥2 antihypertensive medications	1
F	Atrial fibrillation	Persistent or paroxysmal	3
P	Pulmonary hypertension	PASP >35 mm Hg by Doppler	1
E	Elderly	Age >60 years	1
F	Elevated filling pressure	E/e′ ratio by Doppler	1

HFA-PEFF score

	Major criteria (2 points)	Minor criteria (1 point)
Functional	• Septal e' <7 cm/s • Laterial e' <10 cm/s • Average E/e' ratio ≥15 • TR velocity >2.8 m/s (est. PASP >35 mm Hg)	• Average E/e' ratio 9–14 • GLS <16%
Morphological	• LAVI 35 mL/m² • LVMI ≥149/122 g/m² (m/f) and RWT > 0.42	• LAVI 29–34 mL/m² • LVMI 155/95 g/m² (m/f) • RWT >0.42 • LV wall thickness ≥12 mm
Biomarker		
Ainus rhythm	• NT proBNP >220 pg/mL • BNP >80 pg/mL	• NT proBNP 125–220 pg/mL • BNP 35–80 pg/mL
Atrial fibrillation	• NT proBNP >660 pg/mL • BNP >240 pg/mL	• NT proBNP 365–660 pg/mL • BNP 105–240 pg/mL

HFpEF unlikely (Low probability) (HFpEF 0–1, HFA-PEFF 0–1)

HFpEF possible (Intermediate probability) (H_2FPEF 2–5, HFA-PEFF 2–4)

HFpEF likely (High probability) (H_2FPEF ≥6, HFA-PEFF ≥5)

HFpEF likely (High probability) (H_2FPEF ≥6, HFA-PEFF ≥5)

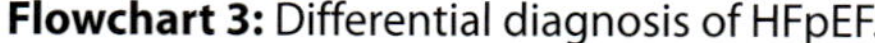

Flowchart 3: Differential diagnosis of HFpEF.

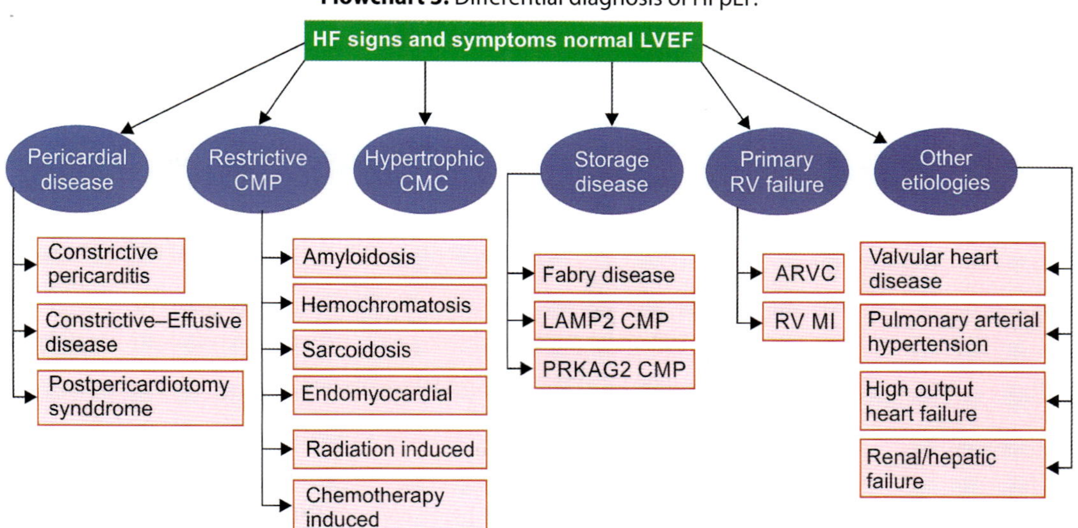

(ARVC: arrhythmogenic right ventricular cardiomyopathy; CMP: cardiomyopathy)

decongestive strategies, including splanchnic nerve ablation, are also under study for the management of HFpEF [e.g., REBALANCE-HF (Endovascular Ablation of the Right Greater Splanchnic Nerve in Subjects Having HFpEF); NCT04592445]. Other strategies to enhance loop diuretic efficiency (e.g., acetazolamide) in HF (including HFpEF) are also the focus of ongoing investigation.[14]

ADDRESS COMORBIDITIES

Both cardiovascular and noncardiovascular comorbidities are highly prevalent in patients with HFpEF and have a significant role in the burden of morbidity and mortality in this population.[15-20] The precise pathophysiologic mechanisms leading to HF progression in HFpEF remain poorly understood. But current models highlight the contribution of comorbidities, including obesity, hypertension, diabetes, chronic obstructive pulmonary disease, and chronic kidney disease (CKD), to a systemic proinflammatory state that may promote endothelial dysfunction and HF progression **(Table 1)**.[21,22]

EVIDENCE-BASED MANAGEMENT

Exercise

Exercise intolerance is a key symptom of HFpEF, and improvement in functional capacity is an important goal. Increased physical activity, preferably aerobic physical activity (e.g., brisk walking) for 150 min/week (30 min/day on most days of the week), is recommended for initial weight loss.[23] The ongoing REHAB-HFpEF (Physical Rehabilitation for Older Patients With Acute Heart Failure With Preserved Ejection Fraction) trial is likely to provide specific guidance regarding optimal exercise prescription in patients with HFpEF.

Pharmacologic Therapy

Early randomized trials of pharmacologic therapy in HFpEF aimed to apply the success of treatment with neurohormonal antagonists, including angiotensin-converting enzyme (ACE) inhibitors (PEP-CHF), ARBs (CHARM-Preserved, I-PRESERVE), and mineralocorticoid receptor antagonists (MRAs) (TOPCAT), from patients with HFrEF to those with higher ejection fractions but were mostly unsuccessful.[24-27] HFpEF treatment guidelines have historically emphasized decongestion for relief of symptoms and aggressive management of comorbidities. With the publication of recent randomized trials of ARNI and SGLT2 inhibitors, specific pharmacologic interventions are now appropriate to consider in many patients with HFpEF.

Sodium–Glucose Cotransporter-2 Inhibitors

Trial evidence: In the EMPEROR-Preserved trial, empagliflozin group experienced a 21% reduction in rates of the primary composite outcome of cardiovascular death or HF [HR: 0.79 (95% CI: 0.69–0.90); $p < 0.001$], primarily directed by a 29% reduction in the risk of HF hospitalization [HR: 0.71 (95% CI: 0.60–0.83)].[28]

In the DELIVER trial, compared to those assigned to placebo, patients assigned to dapagliflozin experienced

TABLE 1: Management of key noncardiac and cardiac comorbidities in patients with HFpEF.

Conditions	*Recommended strategies*
Diabetes/dysglycemia	Management of BP to guideline-recommended targets, typically <130/80 mm Hg
Obesity	• Priority SGLT2 inhibitors (as in all patients) • ACE inhibitor/ARB for CKD/proteinuria • Finerenone for ongoing proteinuria despite ACE inhibitor/ARB
Chronic kidney disease	• ACE inhibitor/ARB for proteinuria • SGLT2 inhibitors • Finerenone (if diabetes and ongoing proteinuria despite ACE inhibitor/ARB)
Coronary artery disease/coronary microvascular dysfunction	• Antiplatelet therapy • Moderate–high-intensity statin therapy for those with elevated LDL • Revascularization for patients with angina or ischemia on provocative testing
Atrial fibrillation	• Anticoagulation for stroke prophylaxis • Consider a trial of rhythm control
Chronotropic incompetence	• Avoid routine use of beta-blockers • Compelling indication

(ACE: angiotensin-converting enzyme; ARB: angiotensin receptor blocker; BP: blood pressure; CKD: chronic kidney disease; GLP: glucagon-like peptide; LDL: low-density lipoprotein; SGLT2: sodium–glucose cotransporter-2)

an 18% reduction in the primary composite outcome [HR: 0.82 (95% CI: 0.73–0.92)], with a significant reduction of 21% in worsening HF events [HR: 0.79 (95% CI: 0.69–0.91)] and numerical (nonsignificant) reduction in cardiovascular death [HR: 0.88 (95% CI: 0.74–1.05)].[29]

The SOLOIST-WHF trial of sotagliflozin, a composite SGLT1/2 inhibitor, suggests that initiation of SGLT inhibitor treatment during HF hospitalization or early after hospital discharge results in robust benefits in higher-risk HFpEF patients, supporting the rationale for predischarge initiation of these agents in eligible patients.[30]

What do guidelines say?
The 2022 American College of Cardiology/American Heart Association (ACC/AHA) guidelines now suggest that the use of SGLT2 inhibitors to treat patients with HF and LVEF ≥ 50% is reasonable [class of recommendation (COR) IIa].[1]

The 2023 focused update of the 2021 ESC guidelines recommend SGLT2 inhibitor (dapagliflozin or empagliflozin) in patients with HFpEF to reduce the risk of HF hospitalization or CV death (COR I).[31]

Angiotensin Receptor-Neprilysin Inhibitors

Trial evidence: The PARAGON-HF trial suggests that the use of ARNI may be a superior approach to ARB monotherapy for selected patients with HFpEF.[20]

What do guidelines say?
The 2022 ACC/AHA treatment guidelines suggest that the use of ARNI may be considered to reduce HF hospitalization in patients with HFpEF, emphasizing the likely greater benefit in those patients closer to the lower LVEF boundary of the universal definition [COR: 2b, level of evidence (LOE): B–R].

Angiotensin-converting Enzyme Inhibitors and Angiotensin Receptor Blockers

Trial evidence: In the PEP-CHF trial of elderly patients with symptomatic HF, LVEF >40%, and evidence of diastolic dysfunction, treatment with the ACE inhibitor such as perindopril did not reduce rates of all-cause death or HF hospitalization [HR: 0.92 (95% CI: 0.7–1.21)] despite improvements in the NYHA functional class and 6-minute walk distance compared with placebo.[19]

In the CHARM-Preserved trial, a possible signal of reduction in HF hospitalizations with the ARB such as candesartan was seen in patients with symptomatic HF and ejection fraction >40% [HR: 0.84 (95% CI: 0.70–1.00)]. On the contrary, the I-PRESERVE trial showed no impact of irbesartan on the primary composite of cardiovascular death or cardiovascular hospitalization.[32,33]

What do guidelines say?
The 2022 ACC/AHA guidelines continue to support the consideration of ARB in patients with HFpEF to reduce hospitalizations (COR IIb). Based on data from the PARAGON-HF trial, these agents may be most appropriate as a second-line alternative for those who cannot tolerate or afford ARNIs.

ACE inhibitors are not considered as a reasonable alternative.

Mineralocorticoid Receptor Antagonists

Activation of the mineralocorticoid receptor by aldosterone is a potent stimulus for myocardial fibrosis, left ventricular hypertrophy, and endothelial dysfunction that may contribute to pathophysiologic remodeling, myocardial stiffening, and diastolic dysfunction in patients with HF.

Trial evidence: In the TOPCAT trial done in patients with symptomatic HF, LVEF ≥45% did not show any discernible treatment benefit with spironolactone with regard to the primary composite outcome of cardiovascular death, aborted cardiac arrest, or hospitalization for HF [HR: 0.89 (95% CI: 0.77–1.04)] despite lower rates of HF hospitalization observed in the spironolactone group [HR: 0.83 (95% CI: 0.69–0.99)]. In a post hoc secondary analysis of the TOPCAT trial, there were concerns regarding patient selection, treatment adherence, and study conduct in the Russian/Georgian sites. It has been argued that the favorable treatment effect observed in subgroup of patients enrolled in the America [HR for primary composite: 0.82 (95% CI: 0.69–0.98)] may be a better summary of the effect of spironolactone in a "true" HFpEF population.

Two ongoing trials will provide greater clarity concerning potential benefit of MRAs in HFpEF (SPIRIT-HF and SPIRRIT). The nonsteroidal MRA such as finerenone will reduce morbidity and mortality in patients with HF, and mildly reduced or preserved LVEF is the subject of the ongoing FINEARTS-HF trial.

What do guidelines say?
The ACC/AHA 2022 guidelines indicate that spironolactone can be considered to reduce HF hospitalization in appropriately selected HFpEF patients matching the eligibility criteria of the TOPCAT trials, emphasizing greater benefit in those with LVEF closer to 50% (COR IIb).

Device-based Therapy for Heart Failure with Preserved Ejection Fraction

Traditional approaches to monitoring congestion such as surveillance of daily weights, symptom burden, and natriuretic peptides may be particularly limited in patients with HFpEF due to confounding by obesity and comorbid medical illness.

Trial evidence: Data from the CHAMPION and GUIDE-HF trials of wireless hemodynamic monitoring using an implantable pulmonary artery pressure sensor suggest that hemodynamic-guided HF management may be an effective strategy to reduce HF hospitalizations in HFpEF.[34,35]

What do guidelines say?

The ACC/AHA 2022 guidelines have indicated that implantable hemodynamic monitoring may be considered for patients with symptomatic HFpEF and either elevated natriuretic peptides or prior HF hospitalization to reduce HF hospitalizations (COR IIb).

CONCLUSION

Following confirmation of the diagnosis and exclusion of mimickers, treatment should focus on decongestion and optimal management of cardiac and noncardiac comorbidities. Based on the cumulative evidence of efficacy, all patients with symptomatic HFpEF should be treated with SGLT2 inhibitors in the absence of contraindications or previous intolerance. For those who remain symptomatic despite SGLT2 inhibition, particularly those with hypertension, LVEF below normal, elevated natriuretic peptides, or recent HF hospitalization, addition of ARNI or substitution of ARB/ACE inhibitor with ARNI is recommended. For those without advanced CKD (eGFR <45 mL/min/1.73 m^2), a three-drug regimen with further addition of MRA may also be appropriate. Consideration should be given to withdrawal of beta-blockers in patients without a compelling indication, with substitution by ARNI and MRA for the management of hypertension. Given the potential volume sensitivity of patients with HFpEF, consideration may be given to dose reduction in loop diuretic agents following the introduction of SGLT2 inhibitors, ARNIs, and MRAs to prevent excessive dehydration, hypotension, or worsening renal function. Optimization of loop diuretic therapy may be further guided by the use of ambulatory hemodynamic monitoring in selected patients with recurrent HF hospitalization and ongoing HF symptoms despite optimization of pharmacologic therapy.

REFERENCES

1. Harikrishnan S, Sanjay G, Anees T, et al. Clinical presentation, management, in-hospital and 90-day outcomes of heart failure patients in Trivandrum, Kerala, India: the Trivandrum Heart Failure Registry. Eur J Heart Fail. 2015; 17(8):794-800.
2. Tromp J, Teng TH, Tay WT, et al. Heart failure with preserved ejection fraction in Asia. Eur J Heart Fail. 2019;21(1):23-36.
3. Heidenreich P, Bozkurt B, Aguilar D, et al. 2022 AHA/ACC/HFSA guideline for the management of heart failure. J Am Coll Cardiol. 2022;79:e263-421.
4. McDonagh TA, Metra M, Adamo M, et al. 2021 ESC guidelines for the diagnosis and treatment of acute and chronic heart failure. Eur Heart J. 2021;42(36):3599-726.
5. Vergaro G, Aimo A, Prontera C, et al. Sympathetic and renin-angiotensin-aldosterone system activation in heart failure with preserved, mid-range and reduced ejection fraction. Int J Cardiol. 2019;296:91-7.
6. Anjan VY, Loftus TM, Burke MA, et al. Prevalence, clinical phenotype, and outcomes associated with normal B-type natriuretic peptide levels in heart failure with preserved ejection fraction. Am J Cardiol. 2012;110:870-6.
7. Jering K, Claggett B, Redfield MM, et al. Burden of heart failure signs and symptoms, prognosis, and response to therapy: the PARAGON-HF trial. J Am Coll Cardiol. 2021; 9(5):386-97.
8. Zile MR, Bennett TD, Sutton M, et al. Transition from chronic compensated to acute decompensated heart failure: pathophysiological insights obtained from continuous monitoring of intracardiac pressures. Circulation. 2008;118(14):1433-41.
9. Solomon SD, Rizkala AR, Lefkowitz MP, et al. Baseline characteristics of patients with heart failure and preserved ejection fraction in the PARAGON-HF trial. Circ Heart Fail. 2018;11(7):e004962.
10. Mentz RJ, Anstrom KJ, Eisenstein EL, et al. Effect of torsemide vs furosemide after discharge on all-cause mortality in patients hospitalized with heart failure: the TRANSFORM-HF randomized clinical trial. JAMA. 2023; 329(3):214-23.
11. Vardeny O, Claggett B, Kachadourian J, et al. Reduced loop diuretic use in patients taking sacubitril/valsartan compared with enalapril: the PARADIGM-HF trial. Eur J Heart Fail. 2019;21(3):337-41.
12. Jackson AM, Dewan P, Anand IS, et al. Dapagliflozin and diuretic use in patients with heart failure and reduced ejection fraction in DAPA-HF. Circulation. 2020;142(11): 1040-54.
13. Chatur S, Claggett BL, Vardeny O, et al. Sacubitril/valsartan and loop diuretic requirement in heart failure with preserved ejection fraction in the PARAGON-HF trial. Eur J Heart Fail. 2023;25(1):87-94.
14. Mullens W, Dauw J, Martens P, et al. Acetazolamide in acute decompensated heart failure with volume overload. N Engl J Med. 2022;387(13):1185-95.
15. Ather S, Chan W, Bozkurt B, et al. Impact of noncardiac comorbidities on morbidity and mortality in a predominantly male population with heart failure and preserved versus reduced ejection fraction. J Am Coll Cardiol. 2012; 59:998-1005.
16. Mentz RJ, Kelly JP, von Lueder TG, et al. Noncardiac comorbidities in heart failure with reduced versus preserved ejection fraction. J Am Coll Cardiol. 2014;64: 2281-93.

17. Bhatt AS, Ambrosy AP, Dunning A, et al. The burden of non-cardiac comorbidities and association with clinical outcomes in an acute heart failure trial—insights from ASCEND-HF. Eur J Heart Fail. 2020;22:1022-31.
18. Vaduganathan M, Patel RB, Michel A, et al. Mode of death in heart failure with preserved ejection fraction. J Am Coll Cardiol. 2017;69(5):556-69.
19. Solomon SD, Wang D, Finn P, et al. Effect of candesartan on cause-specific mortality in heart failure patients: the Candesartan in Heart failure Assessment of Reduction in Mortality and morbidity (CHARM) program. Circulation. 2004;110(15):2180-3.
20. Desai AS, Vaduganathan M, Cleland JG, et al. Mode of death in patients with heart failure and preserved ejection fraction: insights from PARAGON-HF trial. Circ Heart Fail. 2021;14(12):e008597.
21. Paulus WJ, Tschope C. A novel paradigm for heart failure with preserved ejection fraction: comorbidities drive myocardial dysfunction and remodeling through coronary microvascular endothelial inflammation. J Am Coll Cardiol. 2013;62:263-71.
22. Borlaug B. The pathophysiology of heart failure with preserved ejection fraction. Nat Rev Cardiol. 2014;11: 507-15.
23. Arnett DK, Blumenthal RS, Albert MA, et al. 2019 ACC/AHA guideline on the primary prevention of cardiovascular disease: a report of the American College of Cardiology/ American Heart Association Task Force on clinical practice guidelines. J Am Coll Cardiol. 2019;74:e177-232.
24. Cleland JG, Tendera M, Adamus J, et al. The perindopril in elderly people with chronic heart failure (PEP-CHF) study. Eur Heart J. 2006;27:2338-45.
25. Yusuf S, Pfeffer MA, Swedberg K, et al. Effects of candesartan in patients with chronic heart failure and preserved left-ventricular ejection fraction: the CHARM-Preserved trial. Lancet. 2003;362:777-81.
26. Massie BM, Carson PE, McMurray JJ, et al. Irbesartan in patients with heart failure and preserved ejection fraction. N Engl J Med. 2008;359:2456-67.
27. Pitt B, Pfeffer MA, Assmann SF, et al. Spironolactone for heart failure with preserved ejection fraction. N Engl J Med. 2014;370:1383-92.
28. Anker SD, Filippatos BG, Ferreira JP, et al. Empagliflozin in heart failure with a preserved ejection fraction. N Engl J Med. 2021;385:1451-61.
29. Solomon SD, McMurray JJV, Claggett B, et al. Dapagliflozin in heart failure with mildly reduced or preserved ejection fraction. N Engl J Med. 2022;387(12):1089-98.
30. Bhatt DL, Szarek M, Steg PG, et al. Sotagliflozin in patients with diabetes and recent worsening heart failure. N Engl J Med. 2021;384(2):117-28.
31. McDonagh TA, Metra M, Adamo M, et al. 2023 focused update of the 2021 ESC guidelines for the diagnosis and treatment of acute and chronic heart failure. Eur Heart J. 2023;44:3627-39.
32. McMurray JJ, Carson PE, Komajda M, et al. Heart failure with preserved ejection fraction: clinical characteristics of 4,133 patients enrolled in the I-PRESERVE trial. Eur J Heart Fail. 2008;10(2):149-56.
33. Shah SJ, Heitner JF, Sweitzer NK, et al. Baseline characteristics of patients in the treatment of preserved cardiac function heart failure with an aldosterone antagonist trial. Circ Heart Fail. 2013;6(2):184-92.
34. Adamson PB, Abraham WT, Bourge RC, et al. Wireless pulmonary artery pressure monitoring guides management to reduce decompensation in heart failure with preserved ejection fraction. Circ Heart Fail. 2014;7(6): 935-44.
35. Lindenfeld J, Zile MR, Desai AS, et al. Haemodynamic-guided management of heart failure (GUIDE-HF): a randomised controlled trial. Lancet. 2021;398(10304): 991-1001.

SECTION 2

HFpEF and Diagnostic Biomarkers

42. NT-proBNP: Diagnostic, Prognostic, and Therapeutic Implications
43. Multiple Plasma Biomarkers for Risk Stratification in Patients with HFpEF in Emergency
44. Use of Color Scalograms in the Diagnosis of HFpEF

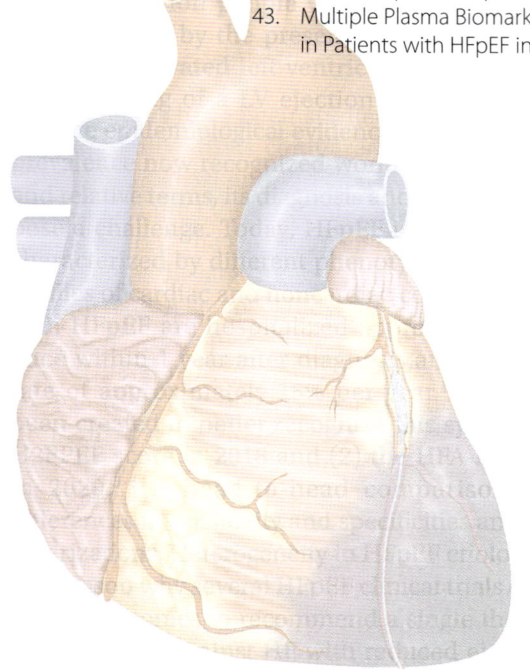

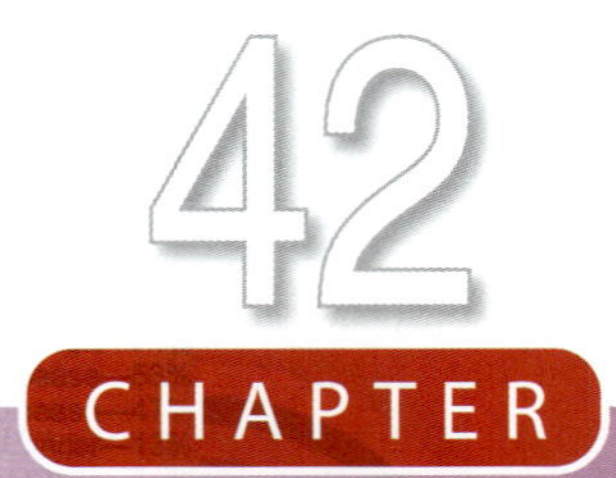

CHAPTER

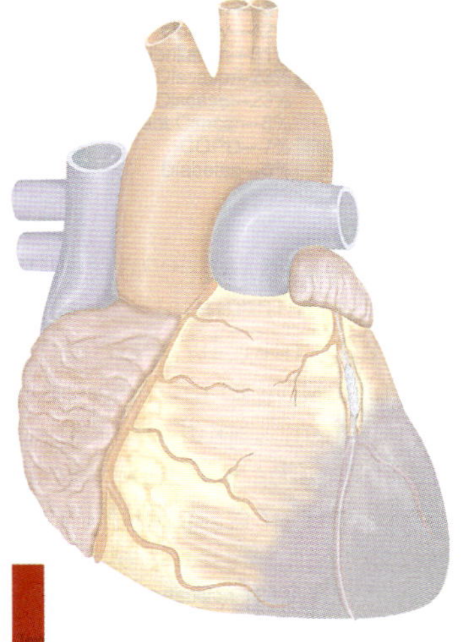

NT-proBNP: Diagnostic, Prognostic, and Therapeutic Implications

Srikanta Sharma, Aayushi Gupta, Soumit Sharma, HK Chopra

INTRODUCTION

The N-terminal fragment of proBNP (NT-proBNP) is a peptide released by the heart's ventricles in response to myocardial stretching and increased wall tension. It is a precursor to brain natriuretic peptide (BNP) and has become an essential biomarker for diagnosing, risk stratification, therapeutic decision-making, and prognosis in cardiovascular diseases. Over the past decade, several novel biomarkers, such as galectin-3 and soluble ST2, have shown potential, but most have yet to be implemented in clinical practice. NT-proBNP and BNP, however, remain the most reliable and routinely used biomarkers in cardiovascular care as NT-proBNP levels reflect not only heart failure (HF) but also myocardial damage, stress, systemic inflammation, and fibrosis, and their routine measurement helps assess the presence of structural heart disease. European guidelines recommend age-specific diagnostic thresholds due to differences in BNP and NT-proBNP levels, with an observed 10 pg/mL difference in BNP and a 100% difference in NT-proBNP between men and women.[1,2] The reasons for these variations are usually hormonal influences on gene expression, gender differences in body composition, and potential extracardiac sources of natriuretic peptides, particularly in the female reproductive system.[3,4]

CLINICAL APPLICATIONS

Heart Failure

Heart failure with preserved ejection fraction (HFpEF) accounts for nearly half of all patients diagnosed with HF. Despite having the same poor prognosis as heart failure with reduced ejection fraction (HFrEF), HFpEF can be challenging to diagnose. NT-proBNP is a critical tool in diagnosing HF, helping to rule out HF quickly and guide treatment and prognosis. Natriuretic peptides are the most frequently used biomarkers for diagnosing HF patients, with elevated levels serving as a diagnostic criterion regardless of LVEF.[5] NT-proBNP levels have a high negative predictive value (0.94–0.98), meaning they are particularly useful for ruling out HF, though their positive predictive value remains lower (0.64–0.67). Age-specific NT-proBNP thresholds are recommended, for diagnosis of HF, with values >450 pg/mL for patients younger than 50 years, >900 pg/mL for those between 50 and 75 years, and >1,800 pg/mL for those older than 75.[1,6-8] However, the diagnosis of HFpEF can be underestimated in patients with obesity due to the effect of body mass on natriuretic peptide secretion.

Guideline	Recommendation	Class of evidence
2024 American Heart Institute of America/ Heart failure society of America	Confirm the diagnosis of HF	1A
	Assess the severity of HF	1A
	Assess the prognosis of HF	1A

Risk Stratification

NT-proBNP is also valuable in identifying individuals at risk of developing HF, allowing for targeted preventative strategies. Two major trials, PONTIAC[9] and STOP-HF,[10] demonstrated that measuring NT-proBNP in at-risk populations, such as those with diabetes, facilitates the early identification of patients who could benefit from more aggressive prevention strategies, thereby reducing the incidence of HF.[11] NT-proBNP can also predict HF onset in at-risk populations, helping clinicians develop targeted intervention plans.

Clinical use in heart failure: In acute HF, NT-proBNP has both diagnostic and prognostic value. Elevated NT-proBNP levels offer additional diagnostic accuracy, particularly when the etiology of dyspnea is unclear. Natriuretic peptides help confirm or exclude acute HF in patients with ambiguous clinical presentations as well it helps in diagnosis of chronic HF, HFpEF, and HFrEF.[12,13] However, NT-proBNP levels in HFpEF patients can sometimes be misleading. Up to 20–25% of HFpEF patients may exhibit low BNP/NT-proBNP levels, despite evidence of increased pulmonary wedge pressures. This is thought to be due to genetic factors, obesity, or other confounding variables.[2,14] Nevertheless, NT-proBNP is a valuable tool in ruling out HF in emergency settings due to its high negative predictive value and ability to reduce decision-making time.

Therapeutic Value

NT-proBNP correlates with left ventricular filling pressure and is used to monitor responses to intravenous therapy, assess hemodynamic congestion, and guide discharge decisions in patients hospitalized for HF. Studies have shown that therapies targeting a reduction in NT-proBNP levels correspond to improved patient outcomes.[15-17] The measurement of NT-proBNP before hospital discharge, once the patient reaches an optimal fluid balance; and can inform decisions on frequency, and intensity of follow-up care. Lower NT-proBNP levels at discharge, or a significant reduction in levels post-therapy, are associated with improved outcomes.[18-20]

Prognostic Value

NT-proBNP is a well-established prognostic marker in both chronic and acute HF, regardless of LVEF. Higher NT-proBNP levels are associated with increased mortality and poorer outcomes in HF patients.[14,21-23] For instance, in patients with exertional dyspnea and preserved left ventricular ejection fraction, NT-proBNP levels at rest were strongly correlated with elevated wedge pressures during peak exercise.[24,25] In the STRONG-HF study, intensified therapy guided by NT-proBNP levels resulted in better outcomes for patients, with those showing a greater reduction in NT-proBNP levels after acute HF treatment faring better than those with persistently high levels.[18,19] Failure to reduce NT-proBNP by 30% posttreatment is associated with significantly increased mortality. For chronic HF patients, long-term outcomes are also correlated with NT-proBNP levels, with elevated levels being predictive of recurrent hospitalizations.[26,27]

Hypertrophic Obstructive Cardiomyopathy

In patients with hypertrophic obstructive cardiomyopathy (HOCM), NT-proBNP levels help differentiate HOCM from other causes of left ventricular hypertrophy. Elevated NT-proBNP levels are indicative of increased left ventricular outflow tract obstruction, septal thickness, and adverse clinical outcomes, including sudden cardiac death and HF.[28] Serial measurements of NT-proBNP can be used to track disease progression and assess treatment response, with decreases in NT-proBNP indicating effective management.

Acute Coronary Syndrome

NT-proBNP is increasingly recognized for its role in the diagnosis, treatment, and prognosis of coronary artery disease (CAD). In acute coronary syndrome (ACS), NT-proBNP levels reflect left ventricular dysfunction caused by myocardial ischemia and increased wall stress.[15,16] Elevated NT-proBNP levels after myocardial infarction predict a higher risk of mortality and adverse cardiovascular events. Additionally, NT-proBNP is valuable in assessing coronary wall stress during procedures such as balloon inflation during coronary intervention.[29]

Stable Coronary Artery Disease

NT-proBNP levels are elevated in patients with significant coronary stenosis, even in the absence of acute ischemic events. In stable CAD, NT-proBNP correlates with disease extent and provides valuable prognostic information.[30]

Valvular Heart Diseases

Valvular heart diseases, which cause either volume or pressure overload of the left ventricle, lead to elevated NT-proBNP levels. NT-proBNP is correlated with left atrial enlargement and left ventricular dysfunction, and higher levels indicate the severity of valvular disease.[31,32] In patients undergoing valve repair or replacement, NT-proBNP levels can inform surgical timing and predict postoperative outcomes.[33,34]

LIMITATIONS OF NT-proBNP

NT-proBNP levels are influenced by several factors, including age, gender, obesity, renal function, and ethnicity. In elderly patients and women, NT-proBNP levels tend to be higher, while levels are lower in obese patients, potentially leading to underdiagnosis.[33] Comorbidities such as chronic obstructive pulmonary disease (COPD), pulmonary embolism, and sepsis can also elevate NT-proBNP levels. Additionally, medications such as beta-blockers, diuretics, and angiotensin-converting enzyme (ACE) inhibitors affect NT-proBNP concentrations, complicating its interpretation.[31,35] To improve diagnostic and prognostic accuracy, NT-proBNP should be used in conjunction with other clinical assessments, serial measurements, and consideration of patient-specific characteristics. Future advancements in assay development may help overcome some of these limitations.

CONCLUSION

NT-proBNP has proven to be a robust biomarker for a variety of cardiovascular diseases. It reflects hemodynamic myocardial stress independent of the underlying pathology, making it a valuable tool for diagnosing and managing HF, coronary artery disease, hypertrophic cardiomyopathy, and valvular heart diseases. While NT-proBNP is not specific to a single condition, its greatest strength lies in ruling out HF in patients presenting with dyspnea. Additionally, NT-proBNP provides significant prognostic information across various cardiovascular conditions, including chronic and acute heart HF, stable coronary artery disease, acute coronary syndromes, hypertrophic cardiomyopathy, and valvular heart diseases.

REFERENCES

1. McDonagh TA, Metra M, Adamo M, et al. 2023 Focused Update of the 2021 ESC Guidelines for the diagnosis and treatment of acute and chronic heart failure: Developed by the task force for the diagnosis and treatment of acute and chronic heart failure of the European Society of Cardiology (ESC) with the special contribution of the Heart Failure Association (HFA) of the ESC. Eur J Heart Fail. 2024;26:5-17.
2. Bansal M, Marwick TH. Natriuretic peptides and filling pressure at rest and stress. Heart Fail Clin. 2008;4:71-86.
3. Welsh P, Campbell RT, Mooney L, et al. Reference ranges for NTproBNP (N-Terminal Pro-B-Type Natriuretic Peptide) and risk factors for higher NT-proBNP concentrations in a large general population cohort. Circ Heart Fail. Oct;15(10):e009427.
4. Cediel G, Codina P, Spitaleri G, et al. Gender-related differences in heart failure biomarkers. Front Cardiovasc Med. 2020;7:617705.
5. Ponikowski P, Voors AA, Anker SD, et al. 2016 ESC Guidelines for the diagnosis and treatment of acute and hronic heart failure: The Task Force for the diagnosis and treatment of acute and chronic heart failure of the European Society of Cardiology (ESC). Developed with the special contribution of the Heart Failure Association (HFA) of the ESC. Eur J Heart Fail. 2016;18:891-975.
6. Bozkurt B, Coats AJS, Tsutsui H, et al. Universal definition and classification of heart failure: a report of the Heart Failure Society of America, Heart Failure Association of the European Society of Cardiology, Japanese Heart Failure Society and Writing Committee of the Universal Definition of Heart Failure: Endorsed by the Canadian Heart Failure Society, Heart Failure Association of India, Cardiac Society of Australia and New Zealand, and Chinese Heart Failure Association. Eur J Heart Fail. 2021;23:352-80.
7. Siddiqui MH, Dixit R, Agarwal S, et al. Determining the role of NT-proBNP levels in diabetic patients with heart failure: a study from North India. J Educ Health Promot. 2024;13:20.
8. Maisel A, Mueller C, Adams K Jr, et al. State of the art: using natriuretic peptide levels in clinical practice. Eur J Heart Fail. 2008;10(9):824-39.
9. Huelsmann M, Neuhold S, Resl M, et al. PONTIAC (NT-proBNP Selected PreventiOn of cardiac events in a population of dIabetic patients without a history of Cardiac disease): a prospective randomized controlled trial. J Am Coll Cardiol. 2013;62:1365-72.
10. Ledwidge M, Gallagher J, Conlon C, et al. Natriuretic peptide-based screening and collaborative care for heart failure: the STOP-HF randomized trial. JAMA. 2013; 310:66-74.
11. Wang TJ, Larson MG, Levy D, et al. Plasma natriuretic peptide levels and the risk of cardiovascular events and death. N Engl J Med. 2004;350:655-63.
12. Bachmann KN, Gupta DK, Xu M, et al. Unexpectedly low natriuretic peptide levels in patients with heart failure. JACC Heart Fail. 2021;9:192-200.
13. Sakane K, Kanzaki Y, Tsuda K, et al. Disproportionately low BNP levels in patients of acute heart failure with preserved vs. reduced ejection fraction. Int J Cardiol 2021;327: 105-10.
14. Myhre PL, Vaduganathan M, Claggett B, et al. B-type natriuretic peptide during treatment with sacubitril/ valsartan: The PAR-ADIGM-HF trial. J Am Coll Cardiol. 2019;73:1264-72.
15. Butt JH, Adamson C, Docherty KF, et al. Efficacy and safety of dapagliflozin in heart failure with reduced ejection fraction according to N-terminal pro-B-type natriuretic peptide: Insights from the DAPA-HF trial. Circ Heart Fail. 2021;14:e008837.
16. Ordu S, Yildiz BS, Alihanoglu YI, et al. Effects of ivabradine therapy on heart failure biomarkers. Cardiol J. 2015;22: 501-9.
17. Fragopoulou E, Panagiotakos DB, Pitsavos C, et al. N-terminal ProBNP distribution and correlations with biological characteristics in apparently healthy Greek population: ATTICA study. Angiology. 2010;61:397-404.
18. Kociol RD, Horton JR, Fonarow GC, et al. Admission, discharge, or change in B-type natriuretic peptide and

long-term outcomes: data from Organized Program to Initiate Lifesaving Treatment in Hospitalized Patients with Heart Failure (OPTIMIZE-HF) linked to Medicare claims. Circ Heart Fail. 2011;4:628-36.

19. Maisel A, Januzzi J, Xue Y, et al. Post-acute care: the role of natriuretic peptides. Congest Heart Fail. 2012;18: S14-6.
20. Salah K, Kok WE, Eurlings LW, et al. A novel discharge risk model for patients hospitalised for acute decompensated heart failure incorporating N-terminal pro-B-type natriuretic peptide levels: a European collaboration on Acute decompensated Heart Failure: ELAN-HF Score. Heart. 2014;100:115-25.
21. Anand IS, Fisher LD, Chiang YT, et al. Changes in brain natriuretic peptide and norepinephrine over time and mortality and morbidity in the Valsartan Heart Failure Trial (Val-HeFT). Circulation. 2003;107:1278-83.
22. van Veldhuisen DJ, Linssen GC, Jaarsma T, et al. B-type natriuretic peptide and prognosis in heart failure patients with preserved and reduced ejection fraction. J Am Coll Cardiol. 2013;61:1498-506.
23. Letsas KP, Filippatos GS, Pappas LK, et al. Determinants of plasma NT-pro-BNP levels in patients with atrial fibrillation and preserved left ventricular ejection fraction. Clin Res Cardiol. 2009;98:101-6.
24. Saito Y, Omae Y, Harada T, et al. Exercise stress echocardiography-based phenotyping of heart failure with preserved ejection fraction. J Am Soc. Echocardiogr. 2024; 37(8): 759-68.
25. Backhaus SJ, Lange T, George EF, et al. Exercise stress real-time cardiac magnetic resonance imaging for noninvasive characterization of heart failure with preserved ejection fraction: The HFpEF-Stress Trial. Circulation. 2021;143: 1484-98.
26. Gaggin HK, Truong QA, Rehman SU, et al. Characterization and prediction of natriuretic peptide "nonresponse" during heart failure management: results from the ProBNP Outpatient Tailored Chronic Heart Failure (PROTECT) and the NT-proBNP-Assisted Treatment to Lessen Serial Cardiac Readmissions and Death (BATTLESCARRED) study. Congest Heart Fail. 2013;19:135-42.
27. Masson S, Latini R, Anand IS, et al.; the Val-HeFT Investigators. Prognostic value of changes in N-terminal pro-brain natriuretic peptide in Val-HeFT (Valsartan Heart Failure Trial) J Am Coll Cardiol. 2008;52:997-1003.
28. Gębka A, Rajtar-Salwa R, Dziewierz A, et al. Serum N-terminal pro-B-type natriuretic peptide levels are associated with left atrial dilation, resting left ventricular outflow tract gradient, and pulmonary hypertension in patients with hypertrophic cardiomyopathy. Postepy Kardiol Interwencyjnej. 2020;16(1):97-101.
29. Heeschen C, Hamm CW, Mitrovic V, et al. N-terminal pro-B-type natriuretic peptide levels for dynamic risk stratification of patients with acute coronary syndromes. Circulation. 2004;110(20):3206-12.
30. Dokainish H. Left ventricular diastolic function and dysfunction: central role of echocardiography. Glob Cardiol Sci Pract. 2021;2021:3.
31. Suda A, Takahashi J, Schwidder M, et al.; Coronary Vasomotor Disorders International Study COVADIS Group. Prognostic association of plasma NT-proBNP levels in patients with microvascular angina: a report from the international cohort study by COVADIS. Int J Cardiol Heart Vasc. 2022;43:101139.
32. Parajuli P, Ahmed AA. Left Atrial Enlargement. [Updated 2023 Jul 24]. In: StatPearls [Internet]. Treasure Island (FL): StatPearls Publishing; 2023.
33. Seewöster T, Büttner P, Nedios S, et al. Association Between Cardiovascular Magnetic Resonance-Derived Left Atrial Dimensions, Electroanatomical Substrate and NT-proANP Levels in Atrial Fibrillation. J Am. Heart Assoc. 2018;7:e009427.
34. Dokainish H. Left ventricular diastolic function and dysfunction: central role of echocardiography. Glob Cardiol Sci Pract. 2021;2021:3.
35. Parajuli P, Ahmed AA. Left Atrial Enlargement. [Updated 2023 Jul 24]. In: StatPearls [Internet]. Treasure Island (FL): StatPearls Publishing; 2023.

CHAPTER

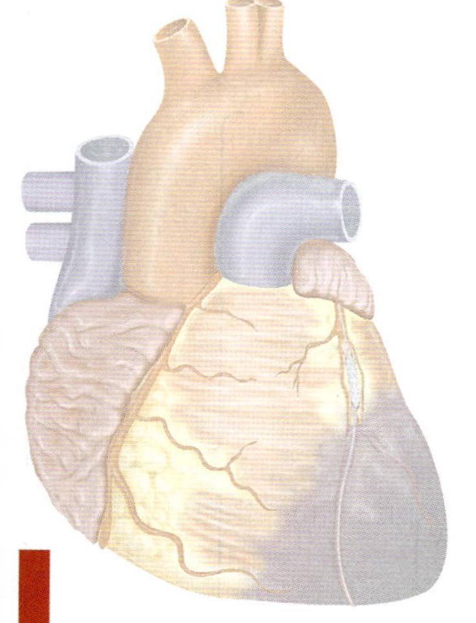

Multiple Plasma Biomarkers for Risk Stratification in Patients with HFpEF in Emergency

Nitish Kumar Parmar, Sheikh Ubair Nabi

INTRODUCTION

Heart failure with preserved ejection fraction (HFpEF) is a complex clinical syndrome characterized by signs and symptoms of heart failure (HF) despite a normal or near-normal left ventricular ejection fraction (LVEF ≥50%).[1] It accounts for approximately half of all HF cases and the prevalence is continuously increasing.[2] Unlike heart failure with reduced ejection fraction (HFrEF), HFpEF lacks a well-defined treatment strategy, and its diagnosis and management, especially in acute settings like the emergency department.

Biomarkers have emerged as essential tools in understanding the pathophysiology, improving diagnosis, and assessing prognosis in HFpEF.[2] The cornerstone biomarkers of HF are B-type natriuretic peptide (BNP) and N-terminal pro-B-type natriuretic peptide (NT-proBNP).[3] However, in HFpEF, natriuretic peptide levels tend to be lower than in heart failure with reduced ejection fraction (HFrEF), and their interpretation can be complicated by factors such as atrial fibrillation, obesity, and renal impairment.[4] Also, HFpEF pathophysiology involves multiple mechanisms that are not captured by natriuretic peptides alone. Therefore, combining natriuretic peptides with other biomarkers has the possibility of offering a more holistic view of the disease. This chapter explores the possibility of using multiple plasma biomarkers for risk stratification in patients with HFpEF.

PATHOPHYSIOLOGICAL DOMAINS OF HEART FAILURE WITH PRESERVED EJECTION FRACTION AND ASSOCIATED BIOMARKERS

The pathophysiology of HFpEF is different from that of HFrEF. The key underlying mechanism in the pathophysiology of HFrEF is cardiomyocyte damage resulting in the development of systolic dysfunction. Whereas in HFpEF inflammation, fibrosis, myocardial stress, vascular dysfunction, and neurohormonal activation are keystones in the pathophysiology.[5] Several biomarkers have been reported for HFpEF, each corresponding to specific underlying processes. The various pathophysiological mechanisms associated with the development of HFpEF and corresponding biomarkers are shown in **Table 1**. The novel biomarkers that have been evaluated most extensively in HFpEF are soluble suppression of tumorigenicity (sST2) protein, galectin-3 (Gal-3), and growth differentiation factor 15 (GDF-15).

Inflammation and Fibrosis

Galectin-3 and sST2 are well-established markers associated with inflammation and fibrosis, which are central to the development of myocardial stiffness and diastolic dysfunction in HFpEF. Serum levels of Gal-3 are

TABLE 1: The Pathophysiologic mechanism of heart failure with preserved ejection fraction and associated biomarkers.

Myocardial stretch and injury	• BNP/NT-ProBNP • Soluble neprilysin • hs-cTnI/T
Cardiac remodeling	• sST2 • Galectin 3
Inflammation and oxidative stress	• CRP • GDF 15 • TNF-alpha • Interleukins
Vascular derangements	• Adrenomedullin • Endothelin
Obesity	• FABP4 • Leptin • Adiponectin
Kidney dysfunction	• NGAL • Cystatin C • KIM-1
Senescence	IGFBP7
Anemia	• Hb • Ferritin • TSAT

(BNP: brain natriuretic peptide; CRP: C-reactive protein; FABP-4: fatty acid-binding protein 4; GDF-15: growth differentiation factor-15; Hb: hemoglobin; hs-cTnI/T: high sensitive cardiac troponin I and T; IGFBP7: insulin-like growth factor binding protein 7; KIM 1: kidney injury molecule-1; NGAL: neutrophil gelatinase-associated lipocalin; NT-proBNP: N-terminal pro-B-type natriuretic peptide; sST2: soluble suppression of tumorigenicity-2 protein; TNF: tumor necrosis factor; TSAT: transferrin saturation)

elevated in both acute and chronic HFpEF, and they have been related to 1-year and 5-year all-cause mortality.[6] Elevated plasma levels of sST2 have been reported to be an independent predictor of mortality and disease progression in both acute and chronic HFpEF.[7,8] GDF-15 is another emerging biomarker associated with adverse outcomes in HFpEF. GDF-15 is a stress-responsive cytokine that plays a role in regulating inflammation, apoptosis, and tissue repair. Several studies reported that GDF-15 was an independent predictor for long-term death and the composite outcome of death or HF rehospitalization in patients with HFpEF.[9,10]

Myocardial Stress

The NT-proBNP is a widely used biomarker for HF, reflecting myocardial stress and ventricular wall tension. It is elevated in HFpEF due to the increased filling pressures in the stiffened left ventricle. While NT-proBNP is highly sensitive for detecting HF, its levels may be confounded by other factors such as obesity (which suppresses NT-proBNP) or chronic kidney disease (which elevates it).[4] In addition to NT-proBNP, high-sensitivity troponins have been explored as markers of subclinical myocardial injury. It has been shown that elevated levels of troponins are associated with poor outcomes in patients with HFpEF.[11,12]

Endothelial Dysfunction and Vascular Health

Biomarkers such as adrenomedullin and endothelin-1 have been investigated for their roles in reflecting vascular dysfunction in HFpEF.[13,14] Studies show that increased endothelin-1 levels correlate with poor cardiovascular outcomes, suggesting that vascular health plays a pivotal role in the progression of HFpEF.[13]

Neurohormonal Activation

Aldosterone and renin levels indicate the activation of the renin-angiotensin-aldosterone system (RAAS), a pathway critical to fluid retention, vascular stiffening, and cardiac remodeling. High plasma renin levels is an independent predictor of mortality in patients with HFpEF.[15]

Overall, HFpEF is a heterogeneous syndrome involving complex interactions between the heart, vasculature, and systemic factors. These diverse mechanisms explain the variability in clinical presentation and the challenges in treating this condition, highlighting the need for individualized approaches in its management.[16] In clinical practice, most patients with HFpEF show a combination of these phenotypes, where several pathophysiological procedures overlap and cause differing expressions of circulating biomarkers and cardiac imaging results.[17]

Multibiomarker Strategy

Due to the heterogeneous nature of HFpEF it might not be possible to capture the full spectrum of the pathophysiologic changes using a single biomarker. A multibiomarker approach has the potential to increase diagnostic certainty by providing a comprehensive view of myocardial stretch, injury, fibrosis, and inflammation. Also combining multiple biomarkers, such as natriuretic peptides, ST2, and Gal-3, can lead to improved risk stratification, and the development of more personalized therapeutic strategies.

In a recent study on multiple biomarker-based risk stratification in patients with acute HF, the authors performed a subanalysis on patients included in the REDINSCOR II study.[18] They included multiple biomarkers

[NT-proBNP, Cystatin-C, GDF-15, Gal-3, and high sensitive C reactive protein (hs-CRP)] for analysis both at admission and discharge. The primary outcome was 12-month mortality. The authors observed that a model including NT-proBNP, hs-CRP, and GDF-15 had a higher mortality prediction than most currently used scores.

In another study on patients with acute decompensated HF, the authors evaluated NT-proBNP, high-sensitivity cardiac troponin T (hs-TNT), and sST2 for mortality prediction.[19] Raised levels of each biomarker were associated with a higher risk of death. In patients where all three biomarkers were below the cutoff levels the death rate was 0% as compared to 53% in patients where levels of all three biomarkers were above the cutoff. Other studies using multi-marker strategies involving novel biomarkers of prognosis in acute HF have also been published.[20-23] However, most of the studies included patients with acute HF or undifferentiated dyspnea. There is a paucity of studies exclusively on patients with HFpEF.

The EMPEROR-Preserved trial examined the effects of empagliflozin in patients with chronic HF and a LVEF of over 40%.[24] Using the data from this trial Pocock and colleagues developed a multi-biomarker risk tool aimed at predicting 2-year survival and the combined risk of cardiovascular death or HF hospitalization in HFpEF patients.[24] 35 potential variables were evaluated and the final model included NT-proBNP, hs-cTnT, and several chronic conditions such as chronic obstructive pulmonary disease, insulin-treated diabetes, and anemia (hemoglobin <12 g/dL).[25] The authors observed that there was a positive association (Pearson correlation of $r = 0.34$) between the biomarker combination of NT-proBNP and hs-CTnT. The patients with the highest combination of both biomarkers had 8.7 times mortality as compared to those with the lowest combination of both biomarkers. Subsequent external validation of the two multivariable models in the PARAGON-HF trial showed similar performance.[12]

Wu et al. studied the relationship between the novel biomarkers and the development of cardiac fibrosis in patients with HFpEF.[26] The authors developed a scoring system using the presence of diabetes mellitus and the median levels of Matrix metalloproteinase-2 (MMP-2), Gal-3, and endothelin-1 to detect the presence of cardiac fibrosis. The combined score had an area under the curve (AUC) of 0.838 for the prediction of cardiac fibrosis. The authors also observed that TIMP2 and NT-proBNP were significantly associated with the aggravation of HF symptoms.

The use of machine learning algorithms to integrate multiple biomarkers and clinical data is an emerging area of research. It is possible to process large data sets and identify complex patterns and interactions between biomarkers, clinical features, and patient outcomes using machine learning models. This allows for far more precise risk stratification, overcoming the limitations of traditional statistical methods.

In a study conducted by Chirinos and colleagues, the investigators evaluated 49 plasma biomarkers in 379 patients with chronic HFpEF and assessed the prognostic utility of a supervised machine-learning model. The authors identified biomarkers that predicted the combined endpoint of all-cause death and HF-related hospitalization using advanced statistical modeling to develop a multi-marker predictive model. They identified two closely related biomarker clusters dominated by markers of fibrosis, tissue remodeling, inflammation, renal injury, and dysfunction. Several biomarkers were found to predict both death and HF hospitalizations. The machine-learning model combining these biomarkers significantly enhanced risk prediction for death and HF hospitalization when added to the MAGGIC (Meta-Analysis Global Group in Chronic HF) risk score. Validation in the HFpEF subset of the Penn Heart Failure Study yielded similar findings. The study highlighted the potential of biomarker analysis to detect critical biological signals, that can reflect both clinical and subclinical pathophysiology potentially aiding in early diagnosis and treatment strategies.[27]

A recent study by Yan Gao and colleagues examined 18 biomarkers from key pathophysiological domains of HF in 380 patients hospitalized with HFpEF. Using a supervised machine (SVM) learning approach, the researchers developed a model to predict 2-year all-cause and cardiovascular mortality based on a combination of the 18 biomarkers and clinical factors. Several biomarkers independently predicted 2-year mortality risk, including NT-proBNP, hs-TnT, GDF-15, tumor necrosis factor-α (TNFα), endoglin, and three biomarkers of extracellular matrix turnover (TIMP-1, MMP-2, and MMP-9). The SVM model successfully predicted the 2-year risk of all-cause mortality in both the training and validation sets, significantly improving patient classification when compared to the reference model.[28]

Woolley and colleagues conducted an unsupervised cluster analysis using 363 biomarkers from a cohort of 429 HFpEF patients.[29] The differences in biomarker expression between the identified clusters were analyzed and used for pathway over-representation analyses. Four distinct patient subgroups emerged based on their biomarker profiles. During a 21-month follow-up, clusters with activation of inflammatory pathways had the highest percentage of death (62.1% and 62.8%) whereas the cluster associated with pathways related to cell proliferation and survival had the lowest mortality.

CONCLUSION

The use of multiple biomarkers to help stratify patients of HFpEF holds great promise in future. Also with the development of machine learning models, it is possible to further improve the predictive power of multi-biomarker panels. However, despite recent advances this strategy faces multiple challenges. There is a marked paucity of data regarding the use of multiple biomarker strategies in patients with HFpEF. The cutoff values of various novel biomarkers are not well established. Also, variability in assay methods and the cost-effectiveness of routine multi-biomarker testing are significant barriers. Future studies are necessary to evaluate the role of multi-biomarker strategies in HFpEF.

REFERENCES

1. Harper AR, Patel HC Lyon AR. Heart failure with preserved ejection fraction. Clin Med. 2018;18(2):s24-9.
2. Borlaug BA, Sharma K, Shah SJ, et al. Heart failure with preserved ejection fraction: JACC Scientific Statement. J Am Coll Cardiol. 2023;81(18):1810-34.
3. Ponikowski P, Voors AA, Anker SD, et al. 2016 ESC Guidelines for the diagnosis and treatment of acute and chronic heart failure: the task force for the diagnosis and treatment of acute and chronic heart failure of the European Society of Cardiology (ESC). Developed with the special contribution of the Heart Failure Association (HFA) of the ESC. Eur J Heart Fail. 2016;18(8):891-975.
4. Remmelzwaal S, van Ballegooijen AJ, Schoonmade LJ, et al. Natriuretic peptides for the detection of diastolic dysfunction and heart failure with preserved ejection fraction—a systematic review and meta-analysis. BMC Med. 2020;18(1):290.
5. Gevaert AB, Boen JRA, Segers VF, et al. Heart failure with preserved ejection fraction: a review of cardiac and noncardiac pathophysiology. Front Physiol. 2019; 10:638.
6. Sanchez FJC, Bodas OA, Bautista PS, et al. Predictive value of serum galectin-3 levels in patients with acute heart failure with preserved ejection fraction. Int J Cardiol. 2013;169(3):177-82.
7. Manzano-Fernández S, Mueller T, Pascual-Figal D, et al. Usefulness of soluble concentrations of interleukin family member ST2 as predictor of mortality in patients with acutely decompensated heart failure relative to left ventricular ejection fraction. Am J Cardiol. 2015;107(2):259-67.
8. Zile MR, Jhund PS, Baicu CF, et al. Plasma biomarkers reflecting profibrotic processes in heart failure with a preserved ejection fraction: Data from the prospective comparison of ARNI with ARB on management of heart failure with preserved ejection fraction study. Circ Heart Fail. 2016;9(1):e002551.
9. Mendez Fernandez AB, Ferrero-Gregori A, Garcia-Osuna A, et al. Growth differentiation factor 15 as a mortality predictor in heart failure patients with non-reduced ejection fraction. ESC Heart Fail. 2020;7(5):2223-9.
10. Chan MMY, Santhakrishnan R, Chong JPC, et al. Growth differentiation factor 15 in heart failure with preserved vs. reduced ejection fraction. Eur J Heart Fail. 2016;18(1):81-8.
11. Hu H, Li J, Wei X, et al. Elevated level of high-sensitivity cardiac troponin I as a predictor of adverse cardiovascular events in patients with heart failure with preserved ejection fraction. Chin Med J (Engl). 2023;136(18):2195-202.
12. Gori M, Senni M, Claggett B, et al. Integrating High-Sensitivity Troponin T and Sacubitril/Valsartan Treatment in HFpEF: The PARAGON-HF Trial. JACC Heart Fail. 2021;9(9):627-35.
13. Chowdhury MA, Moukarbel GV, Gupta R, et al. Endothelin 1 is associated with heart failure hospitalization and long-term mortality in patients with heart failure with preserved ejection fraction and pulmonary hypertension. Cardiology. 2019;143(3–4):124-33.
14. Obokata M, Kane GC, Reddy YNV, et al. The neuro-hormonal basis of pulmonary hypertension in heart failure with preserved ejection fraction. Eur Heart J. 2019;40(45):3707-17.
15. Binder C, Poglitsch M, Duca F, et al. Renin feedback is an independent predictor of outcome in HFpEF. J Pers Med. 2021;11(5):370.
16. Omote K, Verbrugge FH, Borlaug BA, et al. Heart failure with preserved ejection fraction: mechanisms and treatment strategies. Annu Rev Med. 2022;73:321-37.
17. Verweft J, Soens L, Wynants J, et al. Heart failure with preserved ejection fraction: relevance of a dedicated dyspnoea clinic. Eur Heart J. 2023;44(17):1544-56.
18. Álvarez-García J, García-Osuna Á, Vives-Borras M, et al. A 3-Biomarker 2-Point-based risk stratification strategy in acute heart failure. Front Physiol. 2021;12:708890.
19. Pascual-Figal DA, Manzano-Fernández S, Boronat M, et al. Soluble ST2, high-sensitivity troponin T- and N-terminal pro-B-type natriuretic peptide: complementary role for risk stratification in acutely decompensated heart failure. Eur J Heart Fail. 2011;13(7):718-25.
20. Chen Y, Zhao X, Liang L, et al. sST2 and Big ET-1 as alternatives of multi-biomarkers strategies for prognosis evaluation in patients hospitalized with heart failure. Int J Gen Med. 2023;16:5003-16.
21. Januzzi JL, Peacock WF, Maisel AS, et al. Measurement of the interleukin family member st2 in patients with acute dyspnea: results from the PRIDE (Pro-Brain Natriuretic Peptide Investigation of Dyspnea in the Emergency Department) Study. J Am Coll Cardiol. 2007;50(7): 607-13.
22. Rehman SU, Martinez RA, Mueller T, et al. Independent and incremental prognostic value of multimarker testing in acute dyspnea: Results from the ProBNP Investigation of Dyspnea in the Emergency Department (PRIDE) study. Clin Chim Acta. 2008;392(1):41-5.

23. Van Kimmenade RR, Januzzi JL, Ellinor PT, et al. Utility of amino-terminal pro-brain natriuretic peptide, galectin-3, and apelin for the evaluation of patients with acute heart failure. J Am Coll Cardiol. 2006;48(6):1217-24.
24. Anker SD, Butler J, Filippatos G, et al. Empagliflozin in heart failure with a preserved ejection fraction. N Engl J Med. 2021;385(16):1451-61.
25. Pocock SJ, Ferreira JP, Packer M, et al. Biomarker-driven prognostic models in chronic heart failure with preserved ejection fraction: the EMPEROR-Preserved trial. Eur J Heart Fail. 2022;24(10):1869-78.
26. Wu CK, Su MYM, Wu YF, et al. Combination of plasma biomarkers and clinical data for the detection of myocardial fibrosis or aggravation of heart failure symptoms in heart failure with preserved ejection fraction patients. J Clin Med. 2018;7(11):427.
27. Chirinos JA, Orlenko A, Zhao L, et al. Multiple plasma biomarkers for risk stratification in patients with heart failure and preserved ejection fraction. J Am Coll Cardiol. 2020;75(11):1281-95.
28. Gao Y, Bai X, Lu J, et al. Prognostic value of multiple circulating biomarkers for 2-year death in acute heart failure with preserved ejection fraction. Front Cardiovasc Med. 2021;8:779282.
29. Woolley RJ, Ceelen D, Ouwerkerk W, et al. Machine learning based on biomarker profiles identifies distinct subgroups of heart failure with preserved ejection fraction. Eur J Heart Fail. 2021;23(6):983-91.

CHAPTER

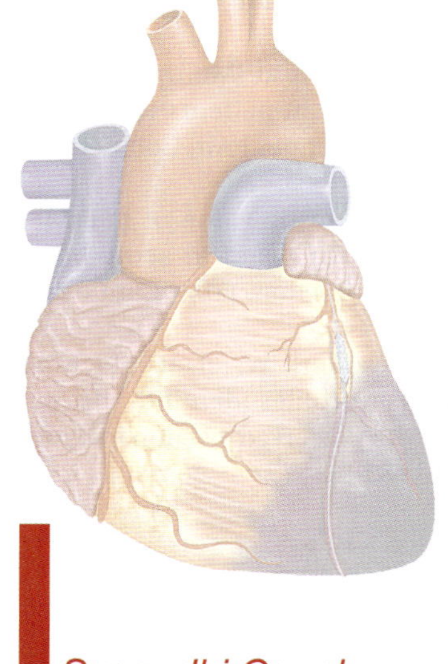

Use of Color Scalograms in the Diagnosis of HFpEF

Sugandhi Gopal

INTRODUCTION

Until recently, patients presenting with dyspnea on exertion were often misjudged regarding the cause of their symptoms. If clinical evaluations and echocardiograms revealed no other discernible findings, lack of physical fitness or mental state were considered. The *Universal Definition and Classification of Heart Failure* by the American College of Cardiology describes heart failure as a clinical syndrome with symptoms and/or signs caused by a structural and/or functional cardiac abnormality. This definition is corroborated by elevated natriuretic peptide levels and/or objective evidence of pulmonary or systemic congestion.

DISCUSSION

Diagnosing heart failure with preserved ejection fraction (HFpEF) is relatively straightforward when patients are decompensated. However, as our understanding has advanced, it has become clear that diastolic dysfunction leads to HFpEF and that the above universal definition is not always adequate. We must identify the subset of patients who were wrongly labelled as "normal."

Clinically differentiating between "lack of physical fitness" and a cardiac-related diagnosis like diastolic dysfunction is challenging. Currently, the gold standard is by invasive methods involving catheters and measurement of pulmonary capillary wedge pressure (PCWP) and right-sided pressures at rest and stress (with bicycle ergometry) in the Cath Lab. HFpEF is often a diagnosis of elimination. An additional complicating factor in diagnosis is that diastolic dysfunction may initially be asymptomatic (up to stage 2 dysfunction). Identifying this is important because it is more amenable to treatment, before progressing to symptomatic HFpEF (stages C and D). Early HFpEF may be present for many years before manifesting as overt heart failure.

It is clear that a low-cost screening method for diastolic dysfunction would be clinically valuable and is the aim of this chapter. Beyond all this, the importance of diagnostic methods lies in the availability of treatments—a compelling reason for mass screening, noninvasively.

Among noninvasive strategies, echocardiograms are currently the standard tests for diagnosing diastolic dysfunction. While ECGs are universally available, they have not traditionally been used for functional assessment of the heart. Echocardiograms provide two critical sets of data:

1. Ensuring that the ejection fraction is normal—a requirement for diagnosing HFpEF.
2. Identifying severe diastolic dysfunction through mitral flows and tissue Doppler imaging.

However, this strategy is 5–8 times more expensive than the more widely available ECG.

Until recently, mechanical events in the heart were not identifiable through electrical monitoring, which is why ECGs were not used to comment on systolic or diastolic functions. The development of algorithms to detect changes in contraction and relaxation now allows for the early identification of at-risk patients and timely intervention. This process is now well established.

Further discussions focus on the use of real data versus a virtual "black box." AI-rendered diagnosis and accuracy levels, especially for grading diastolic dysfunction.

TABLE 1: Changing scenario for color scalogram.

The HFpEF tool box	*What makes the difference in advanced ECGs*
• *The physical exam:* Be thorough! from heart sounds to sign of heart failure • *Biomarkers:* Brain natriuretic peptide • *Advanced ECG: Will replace recommendations after GDMT review* • *Echocardiography:* Always include exercise from leg raising to bicycle ergometry • *Coronary evaluation:* If the etiology is not identified • Cardiac MRI if myocardial inflammatory or infiltrative disease is suspected • Cardiopulmonary exercise testing • Invasive exercise hemodynamics • Follow-up repeat of above parameters with intervention	• Digital acquisition and storage • Cloud storage • Large and complicated computations • Matlab and Python • Python Libraries • Data science and displays • Machine learning and AI • Automation • Reporting formats • Massive cloud registries • Near real time transfer of data and Bandwidth

(GDMT: guideline-directed medical therapy; MRI: magnetic resonance imaging)

Flowchart 1: The step wise electrocardiogram (ECG) diagnosis of diastolic dysfunction.

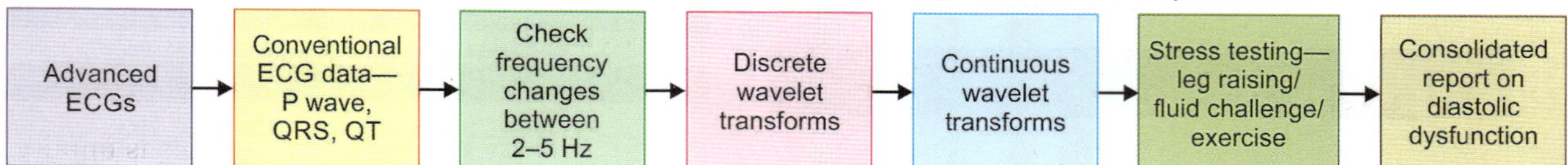

An additional factor is the use of parameters generated by conventional ECGs, combined with newer data science methods. These include waveform amplitudes, axes, and durations, as well as measures derived from three-dimensional vector cardiography (VCG) and waveform complexity via singular value decomposition. Note that parts of A-ECG analysis can also be performed on digitized ECG data recordings stored by any modern ECG vendor.

Noninvasive diagnosis of diastolic dysfunction, including data collection under stress provocation, has the potential to alter the progression toward HFpEF. Early, remote, repeated, and definitive diagnoses can significantly enhance patient care and preventive measures **(Table 1)**.

We hypothesize that combined measures of A-ECG derived data from the standard resting 12-lead ECG could be used to accurately identify the presence of diastolic dysfunction. This new paradigm shift for approach to diastolic dysfunction and HFpEF is with machine learning and AI techniques.

By implementing a stepwise diagnostic approach for HFpEF, incorporating parameters from conventional ECGs such as QRS width, P morphology, and QT intervals and combining them with frequency analysis, and color scalograms, and leveraging machine learning (and eventually AI)/We can achieve a medically acceptable level of accuracy exceeding >95%. Here is a presentation of the work in these cutting-edge technologies and developments. Such advancements are poised to significantly impact the current heart failure statistics **(Flowchart 1)**.

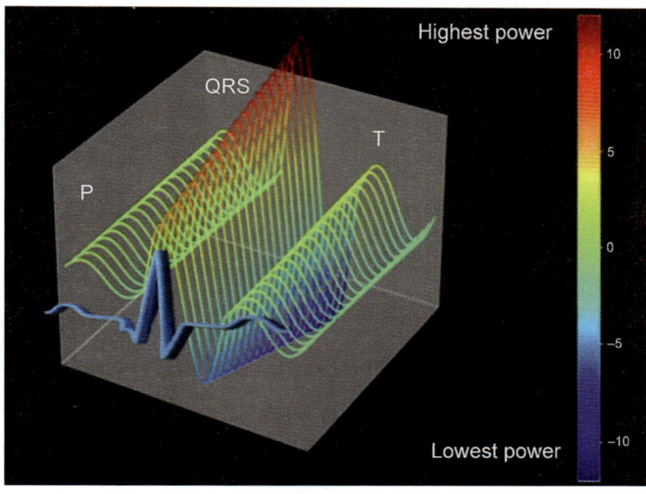

Fig. 1: Color scalogram representation of electrocardiogram (ECG).

Color scalograms represent a cutting-edge, noninvasive machine learning method for analyzing ECGs from a single digital ECG sampling. A scalogram visualizes the amplitude of different frequencies over time by plotting the absolute values of continuous wavelet transform (CWT) or discrete wavelet transform (DWT) coefficients of a signal. This visual representation of the heart's electrical activity can help identify patterns associated with diastolic dysfunction, such as abnormalities in the T wave frequencies that represent diastole and repolarization **(Fig. 1)**.

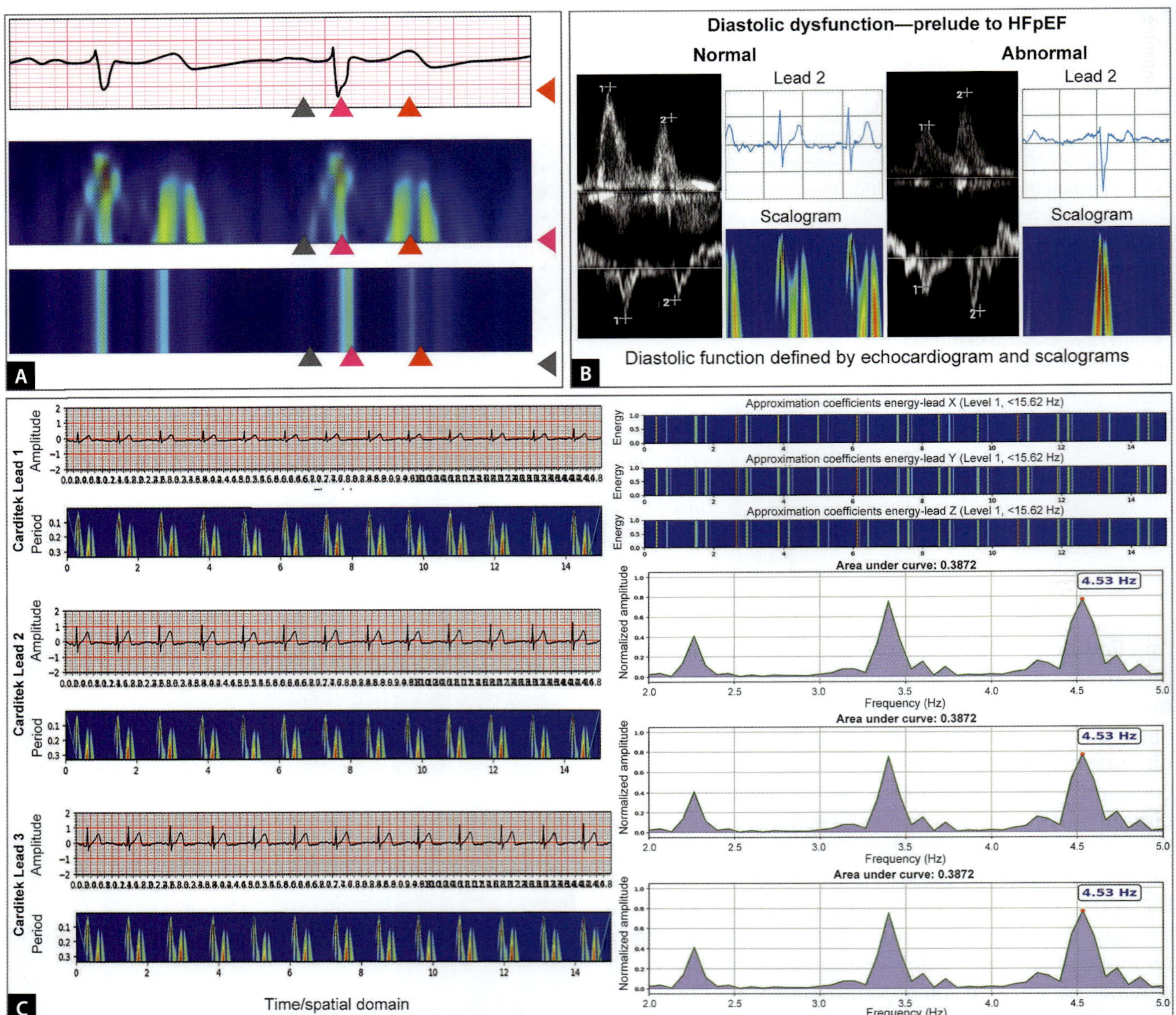

Figs. 2A to C: (A) Basics of color scalograms—PQRS are shown in color scalogram, highest power in red progressing through oranges, green, and blue based on energy. DWT shows a line corresponding to T, and color coded as above. Normal diastolic function shows T intensities in reds and oranges while dysfunction is more represented by blues; (B) The correlation between echocardiogram findings and color scalograms—distinct pattern are seen—normal on the left and dysfunction on the right, where T wave has lost intensity; and (C) Different components of ECG waveform (P, QRS, and T wave) have very distinct frequency characteristics which can be visualized through time frequency analysis technique by color scalogram. The input is a calculated analysis, condensing 12 lead ECG to a modified 3 leads (Carditek algorithm) from which a CWT and DWT are generated as above. The changes may also be corroborated with frequency analysis of the T wave itself to look for a left ward shift in dysfunction.

These patterns are generated by passing a chosen mother wavelet through the ECG wave at the optimal morphological transform. Research indicates that traditional 12-lead ECG wave analysis using mother wavelets is often inadequate. Consequently, many companies have developed proprietary algorithms for modifying input ECGs, eliminating noise, focusing on specific frequencies, and selecting mother wavelets. These algorithms, along with advanced display transformations, enhance the analysis of ECG waves.

This innovative approach holds significant potential for mass screening and heart failure prevention, offering a more detailed and accurate assessment of cardiac health.

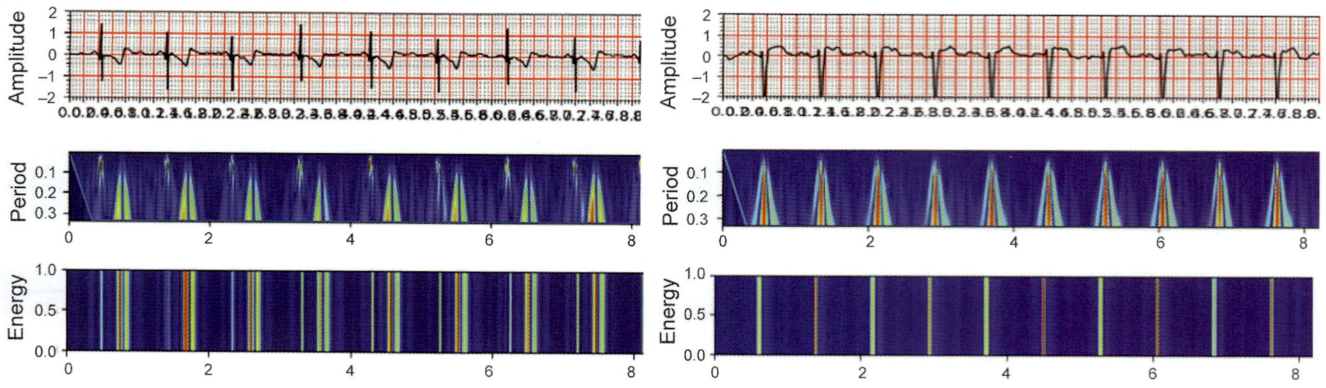

Fig. 3: Normal and abnormal—hypertension/diabetes/lifestyle changes, high heart rates—all lead to diastolic dysfunction.

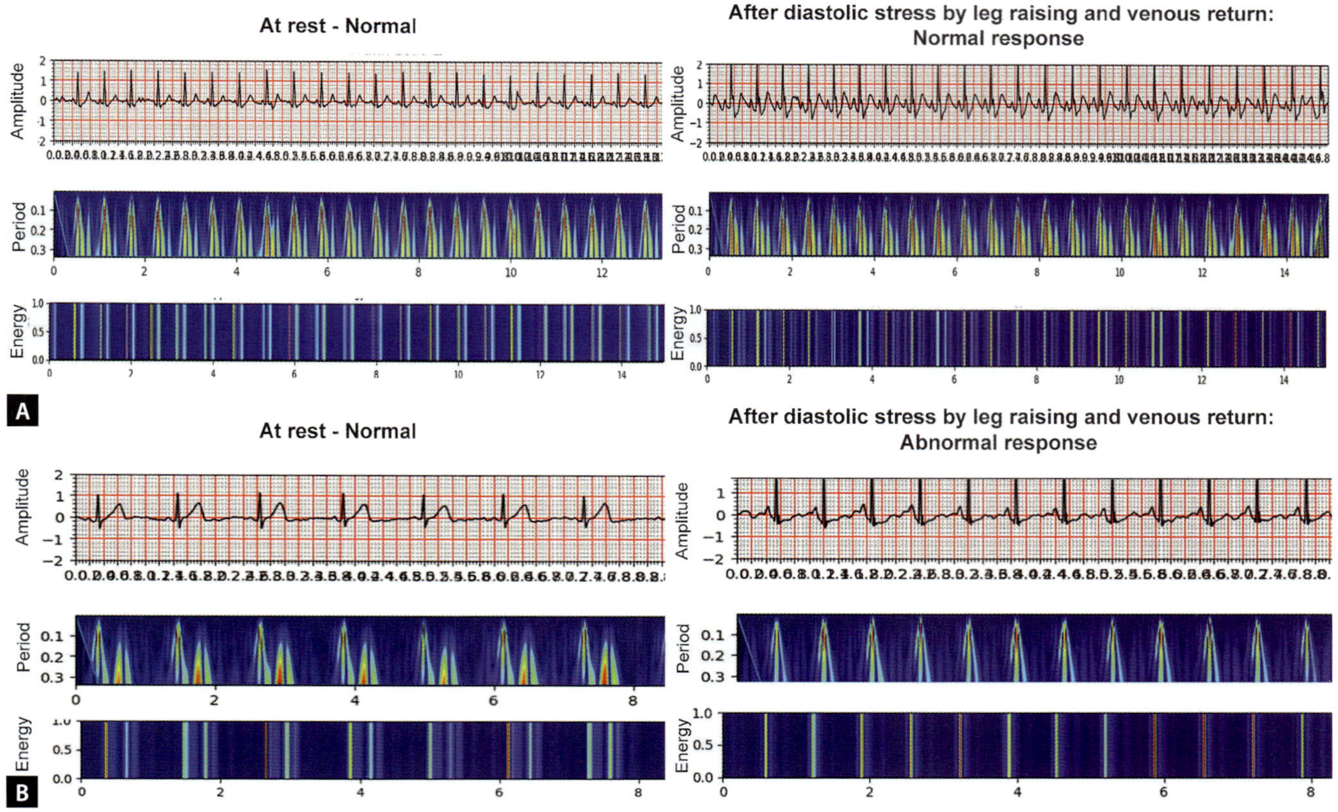

At rest - Normal

After diastolic stress by leg raising and venous return: Normal response

A

At rest - Normal

After diastolic stress by leg raising and venous return: Abnormal response

B

Figs. 4A and B: (A) Scalogram with response to diastolic stress (normal response); (B) Scalogram with response to diastolic stress (abnormal response).

ECGs are complex waves—they are filled with wavelets of different frequencies, with different energy levels and varying in the time domain. Wavelets can produce scalograms, which are visual representations of how the frequency content of a signal changes over time. The choice of a particular mother function will depend a lot on the signal to be treated, we can even create our own wavelet function. Common mother wavelets used are as follows: "Haar," "Daubechies," "Symlets," "Coiflets," "Biorthogonal," "Reverse biorthogonal," "Discrete Meyer (FIR Approximation)," "Gaussian," "Mexican hat wavelet," "Morlet wavelet," "Complex Gaussian wavelets," "Shannon wavelets," "Frequency B-Spline wavelets," "Complex Morlet wavelets."

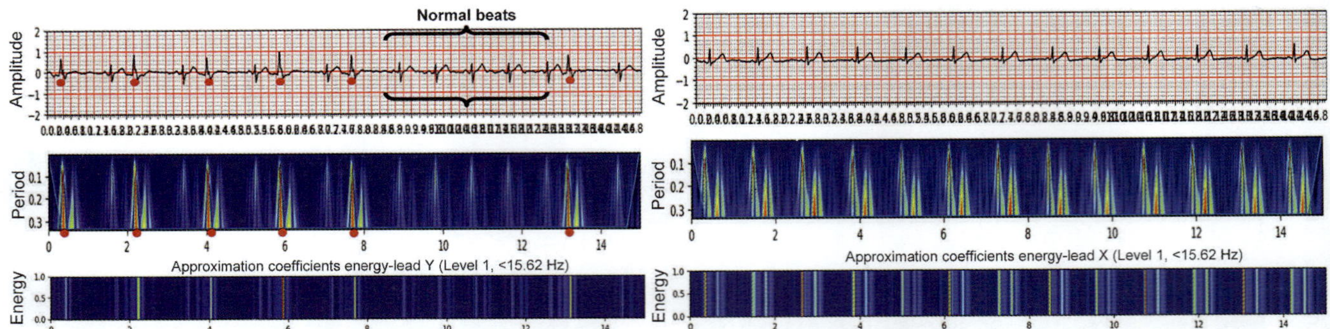

Fig. 5: Scalogram with response to treatment of myocardial disease.

CONCLUSION

Analyzing wavelets is complex maths. It needs the power of the cloud, algorithms and a good database function with the software suitable for millions of simultaneous ECG recordings. Given all this power, CWT and DWT analysis are nevertheless done in seconds in the cloud **(Figs. 2A to C)**.

Diastolic stress testing: Leg raising for 1 minute or IV fluid loading of 300 mL in <10 minutes. A bicycle ergometry, or less desirably a treadmill stress test may be used **(Figs. 4A and B)**.

The above patient with arrhythmia associated cardiomyopathy recovered after control with medications. Even the normal beats in **Figure 5** had diastolic dysfunction. There was a surprising and complete recovery after medical management—this would not be visible without color scalogram, and may reflect recovery of inflammation.

REFERENCES

1. Carditek.com. Clinical Studies with Sydantek from Carditek Medical Devices. [onlone] Available from sydantek@carditek.com [Last accessed January 2025].
2. Bozkurt B, Coats AJ, Tsutsui H, et al. Universal Definition and Classification of Heart Failure: A Report of the Heart Failure Society of America, Heart Failure Association of the European Society of Cardiology, Japanese Heart Failure Society and Writing Committee of the Universal Definition of Heart Failure. J Card Fail. 2021:S1071-9164(21) 00050-6.
3. McColl H, Chowdhury S, Schlegel TT, et al. Diagnosing diastolic dysfunction using explainable advanced electrocardiography. medRxiv. 2023;04(19):23288666.
4. Peterson A, Krubsack D, Sengupta P. (2023). Electrocardiogram-based assessment of diastolic function. [online] Available from https://patents.google.com/patent/EP4252651A2/en [Last accessed January 2025].

SECTION 3

HFpEF, Echo and Imaging

45. Role of Three-dimensional Echocardiography in the Assessment of HFpEF
46. Effect of ARNI on Left Atrial and Left Ventricular Strain by Speckle Tracking Echocardiography in Heart Failure
47. Echocardiographic Evaluation of Atrial Function in HFpEF
48. 3D Echocardiography and BNP Screening in HFpEF
49. Echocardiographic Evaluation of Atrial Fibrillation with Atriopathy and Thromboembolism
50. Echocardiographic Remodeling Reversal with SGLT2i and ARNI in HFpEF
51. Echocardiographic-guided Therapy in HFpEF
52. Echocardiographic Evaluation of Diastolic Functions Beyond Guideline
53. Echocardiography Evaluation of the Left Atrial Strain on Patients with SGLT2i and ARNI with HFpEF
54. Echocardiographic Evaluation of Left Atrium and Mitral Annulus in HFpEF Patients on ARNI and SGLT2i Therapy
55. Atrial Strain: A Piece of the HFpEF Puzzle Found, but is It Yet in Place
56. Echocardiographic Evaluation of HFpEF in Emergency
57. Echocardiographic Diagnostic, Prognostic, and Therapeutic Indications of E/e' and LAVI in HFpEF
58. Effect of E/e' in HFpEF Management on SGL2i, ARNI, and Beta-blocker Therapy
59. Echocardiographic Variables on Cardiac Atrial and Ventricular Remodeling Reversal by ARNI and SGLT2i in HFpEF
60. Effect of SGLT2 Inhibitors and ARNI on Increased Left Atrial Stiffness Index in HFpEF
61. Atrial Dysfunction: Echocardiographic Evaluation in Patients with HFpEF and AF
62. Deciphering the Dilemma: Anticoagulation for HFpEF with AF
63. The Evolving Role of Nonimplant Interatrial Shunts in Managing HFpEF
64. Deterioration in RV Structure and Function in HFpEF Echocardiographic Evaluation
65. Echocardiographic Evaluation of HFpEF in Oncology
66. Echocardiographic Evaluation of Left Atrial Stiffness Index and Right Ventricular and Right Atrial Strain in HFpEF
67. HFpEF and Left Atrial Atriopathy: Advanced Therapeutic Navigation
68. Computed Tomography Angiography in HFpEF
69. CMR Evaluation on Cardiac Remodeling Reversal after ARNI in HF
70. Cardiac Magnetic Resonance to Enhance Phenotypic Characterization of HFpEF
71. Focal and Diffuse Fibrosis in HFpEF: Cardiac Magnetic Resonance Evaluation and Outcomes
72. Role of CT Evaluation for Transcatheter Aortic Valve Implantation in HFpEF

Role of Three-dimensional Echocardiography in the Assessment of HFpEF

Vijayadithyan Jaganathan, Vaidehi Mendpara, Kousalya Rajendran, Shruti Hegde, Navin C Nanda, HK Chopra

INTRODUCTION

Heart failure with preserved ejection fraction (HFpEF) is as clinically significant as heart failure with reduced ejection fraction (HFrEF), since nearly half of all HF patients are diagnosed with HFpEF in recent years.[1] Traditionally, two-dimensional transthoracic echocardiography (2DTTE) has been utilized for assessing HFpEF. However, three-dimensional (3D) TTE is potentially superior to 2DTTE due to the addition of the third dimension. This chapter will focus on the comparison of 3DTTE with 2DTTE in relation to cardiac magnetic resonance (CMR) in the assessment of left ventricular (LV) EF which is an essential parameter in the diagnosis of HFpEF.

COMPARISON OF LEFT VENTRICULAR VOLUMES AND EJECTION FRACTION BY 2DTTE AND 3DTTE IN VALIDATION WITH CMR

The LVEF by 2DTTE forms the basis to differentiate the three common types of HF in clinical practice. These are HFpEF with LVEF 50% or more, HFrEF with LVEF 40% or less, and HF with mildly reduced (mr)EF with LVEF in the range of 41–49%.[2] 2DTTE is widely available in major hospitals across the world, does not use radiation, is cost effective, and many cardiologists consider it an essential component of a thorough patient work up. Incomplete LV endocardial border definition in subjects with small acoustic windows such as those with thick chest walls and pulmonary disease has been circumvented with the use of intravenous contrast echocardiography, which fully delineates LV cavity. Many studies in literature show acceptable correlation of LVEF with other techniques and reasonable intra- and interobserver variability. However, 2DTTE assessment of LVEF suffers from several limitations. Errors occur due to LV apex foreshortening, especially in sick patients who are unable to be repositioned or are on ventilators. In addition, when calculating LV volumes and LVEF using the traditional modified Simpson biplane method of discs, 2DTTE assumes a bullet-shaped LV morphology, which may not be applicable to all patients.[3] This is because each 2D image represents only a thin slice of LV, making it challenging to fully assess its correct shape resulting in errors in LVEF estimation. 3DTTE overcomes these limitations of 2DTTE.

A major advantage of 3DTTE over 2DTTE is the ability to encompass the whole LV in the 3D dataset in most patients. Thus, no assumption is made regarding the shape of LV and cropping the dataset can eliminate or markedly reduce LV foreshortening. Thus, 3DTTE has the potential to improve accuracy compared to 2D TTE in the assessment of LV function. However, 3DTTE is not without drawbacks. 3DTTE images are based on 2DTTE images, hence there is no improvement in image quality compared to 2DTTE. As a matter of fact, image quality tends to decrease because of lower frame rate and lower temporal resolution when acquiring 3D datasets. The following section offers an in-depth overview of studies comparing 3DTTE with 2DTTE and CMR for assessing LV volumes and EF.

A meta-analysis published in 2012 by Dorosz et al.[3] reviewed studies from 1990 to 2011, comparing LV volumes and EF measured by 3DTTE and CMR imaging. The analysis included 23 studies with 1,638 echocardiograms. Most were adult males averaging around 65 years of age. Most studies used equipment from a single vendor for imaging, but employed different techniques such as automated border detection, mesh, and slice methods. In a subgroup, the meta-analysis also compared 3DTTE with standard 2DTTE and CMR imaging, assessing overall bias and limits of agreement for LV volumes and EF. The results indicated that 3DTTE often underestimated LV volumes as compared to CMR but had a narrower 95% confidence interval compared to 2DTTE. For LVEF measurements, there was no significant bias between 3DTTE and 2DTTE and the variance difference was modest (4.7%). However, a notable advantage of 3DTTE was its lower intraobserver and interobserver variability, which is crucial in clinical practice where consistent and reliable measurements are needed, especially for serial examinations to monitor clinical changes.[3]

In a study conducted in 2013 in which our group was involved, the aim was to evaluate and compare the accuracy and reproducibility of LV volumes and EF measurements obtained from various echocardiographic methods against CMR. Data was reviewed from 18 studies (2 multicenter and 16 single-center), each included at least 30 patients, total 1,299 patients, and focusing on both normal and abnormal LV function. In contrast to the Dorosz et al. study, which did not include contrast echocardiography, this study compared both noncontrast and contrast 2DTTE as well as noncontrast and contrast 3DTTE with CMR. The findings revealed that LVEF measurements were fairly consistent between CMR and both contrast 2DTTE and noncontrast 3DTTE. Among the echocardiographic methods, contrast 2DTTE showed better reproducibility and alignment with CMR measurements of LVEF compared to noncontrast 2DTTE. Likewise, 3DTTE demonstrated greater accuracy compared to 2DTTE in terms of agreement with CMR. However, the study did not conclusively determine the relative efficacy of contrast 2DTTE versus contrast 3DTTE. In terms of LV volume measurements, echocardiographic methods generally reported smaller and more variable volumes compared to CMR. Hence, it was concluded that while contrast 2DTTE and noncontrast 3DTTE provide reliable LVEF measurements, volume measurements from these methods are less accurate.[4]

Another study focused specifically on comparing the intra- and interobserver variability between 2DTTE and 3DTTE for assessing LV function in a general population. The study included 150 participants, where two observers evaluated LV volumes and LVEF, using both 2DTTE and 3DTTE. The findings revealed that 3DTTE consistently outperformed 2DTTE, showing lower mean differences, narrower limits of agreement, as well as higher correlation coefficients (r) and intraclass correlation coefficients (ICC). Overall, 3DTTE demonstrated greater robustness and reproducibility compared to 2DTTE, establishing 3DTTE as the preferred method for evaluating LV function.[5]

A more recent systematic review and meta-analysis published in 2019 included a larger number of studies with a higher number of patients. As many as 38 studies with 1,881 adult subjects from 2011 to 2018, were assessed for correlation of LVEF and volumes by 3DTTE and CMR. Unlike the previously mentioned meta-analysis, this study included a substantial number of patients with fully automated 3D echocardiography software, reflecting contemporary practices in the field. Because semiautomated software requires manual initialization of LV contours before automatic detection, there are chances of introduction of errors. On the other hand, fully automated software generates LV casts and analyzes volume curves without manual input, which would potentially increase accuracy. This meta-analysis concluded that while 3DTTE still underestimated LV volumes compared to CMR, LVEF measurements were similar to CMR values for both types of software. Furthermore, fully automated software showed less biases and variability in LV volume measurements compared to semiautomated software. Thus, adoption of fully automated software during 3DTTE enhanced measurement accuracy with reduction in observer variability.[6]

Another study published in 2019 evaluated the impact of image quality and echocardiography contrast enhancement (CE) to improve LV endocardial border definition for LV volume measurements using 2DTTE and 3DTTE, compared to CMR. The study, which included 32 postmyocardial infarction patients, revealed that 2DTTE had the largest negative bias in LV volume measurements when compared to CMR. In contrast, using CE with 2DTTE and 3DTTE reduced this bias, with CE 3DTTE showing the smallest bias. The correlation of LVEF with CMR was also stronger with 3DTTE as compared to 2DTTE. CE improved accuracy and reduced variability for both 2DTTE and 3DTTE, with better image quality further enhancing agreement with CMR. Overall, in patients with both poor and optimal quality images, 3DTTE proved to be more accurate than 2DTTE in estimating LV volumes and EF and with less inter- and intraobserver variability in EF estimation.[7] CMR imaging offers a greater ability to exclude papillary muscles and trabeculations, resulting in potentially more accurate LV volume estimates compared to echocardiography, where trabeculations often overlaid on the endocardium blur the distinction between the two structures resulting in smaller LV cavity size and smaller LV volume calculations.

In summary, studies reviewed suggest that 3DTTE offers superior performance compared to 2DTTE in the evaluation of LV volumes and EF, especially when we use software to track LV endocardium automatically during 3DTTE. Enough data is currently not available to assess the role of CE during 3DTTE in comparison with CMR. However, as previously mentioned 3DTTE has its limitations and has not yet replaced 2DTTE in assessing LV function. Instead, it can serve as a valuable supplement to 2DTTE, especially when more accurate information is needed for a definitive diagnosis of HFpEF. CMR which has been used as a comparison method ("gold standard") for 3D and 2DTTE assessment of LV function has its own limitations. It is generally more expensive and less accessible and available only at certain centers. Also, patients may face issues such as claustrophobia or interference from implanted devices. Other technical challenges include motion artifacts, longer scan times, and the need for extensive postprocessing, which add complexities to the workflow. Additionally, gadolinium-based contrast agents can pose risks for patients with severe renal impairment. So far, there are no studies to date specifically comparing 2DTTE with 3DTTE in patients with HFpEF.

LEFT ATRIUM

In HFpEF, the left atrium (LA) enlarges gradually due to elevated LV filling pressure and diastolic dysfunction, making it an important prognostic marker.[8] However, LA volume is affected significantly due to foreshortening of the atrium when captured by 2DTTE. This issue can be addressed by using 3DTTE that captures the entire atrium within the pyramidal beam.[9] A study published in 2016 found that 3DTTE provides more accurate and larger LA volume measurements compared to 2DTTE, with better correlation with CMR. Thus, 3DTTE assessment of LA volume could provide more accurate assessment of prognosis as compared to 2DTTE.[10]

RIGHT VENTRICLE

Pulmonary hypertension associated with HFpEF may lead to right ventricular (RV) dysfunction, which is also an important prognostic marker in HFpEF.[11] Due to the complex shape of RV, 3DTTE has demonstrated greater accuracy in assessing RV volumes and RV EF, potentially offering improved prognostic capabilities in HFpEF compared to 2DTTE.[12]

SPECKLE TRACKING ECHOCARDIOGRAPHY

In 2D TTE, there is a high chance of specific speckles moving out of the examining plane because of thin slice like 2D images resulting in incorrect results. In contrast, the likelihood of this occurring is much less with 3DTTE because of the larger pyramidal dataset. Thus, evaluating LV global longitudinal strain with 3DTTE may provide superior prognostic value compared to 2DTTE in HFpEF.[13]

CONCLUSION

The 3D TTE can offer incremental value over 2D TTE, particularly when accuracy in assessing LVEF is paramount in the assessment of HFpEF. This is especially important for the precise categorization and differentiation of HFpEF from other types of heart failure. In the future, the application of 3DTTE is expected to increase as more echocardiography laboratories implement software for the automatic assessment of LV function. This advancement will not only enhance accuracy but also save considerable time compared to 2DTTE. The anticipated advancements in strain analysis includes complete automation using 3D software with improved tracking and automatic border detection, less variability among vendors, and the capacity to simultaneously quantify strain in all four chambers of the heart.[14] The recent advent of artificial intelligence in noninvasive cardiac imaging is expected to further enhance the rapidity and accuracy of echocardiography in evaluating LV function.[15-17]

REFERENCES

1. Shah SJ, Borlaug BA, Kitzman DW, et al. Research priorities for heart failure with preserved ejection fraction: National Heart, Lung, and Blood Institute Working Group summary. Circulation. 2020;141(12):1001-26.
2. Writing Committee Members; ACC/AHA Joint Committee Members. 2022 AHA/ACC/HFSA guideline for the management of heart failure. J Card Fail. 2022;28(5): e1-e167.
3. Dorosz JL, Lezotte DC, Weitzenkamp DA, et al. Performance of 3-dimensional echocardiography in measuring left ventricular volumes and ejection fraction: a systematic review and meta-analysis. J Am Coll Cardiol. 2012;59(20):1799-808.
4. Wood PW, Choy JB, Nanda NC, et al. Left ventricular ejection fraction and volumes: it depends on the imaging method. Echocardiography. 2014;31(1):87-100.
5. Lyng Lindgren F, Tayal B, Bundgaard Ringgren K, et al. The variability of 2D and 3D transthoracic echocardiography applied in a general population: intermodality, inter- and intraobserver variability. Int J Cardiovasc Imaging. 2022;38(10):2177-90.
6. Kitano T, Nabeshima Y, Otsuji Y, et al. Accuracy of left ventricular volumes and ejection fraction measurements by contemporary three-dimensional echocardiography with semi- and fully automated software: systematic review

and meta-analysis of 1,881 subjects. J Am Soc Echocardiogr. 2019;32(9):1105-15.e5.

7. Jenner J, Sörensson P, Pernow J, et al. Contrast enhancement and image quality influence two- and three-dimensional echocardiographic determination of left ventricular volumes: comparison with magnetic resonance imaging. Clin Med Insights Cardiol. 2019;13:1179546819831980.
8. Backhaus SJ, Nasopoulou A, Lange T, et al. Left atrial roof enlargement is a distinct feature of heart failure with preserved ejection fraction. Circ Cardiovasc Imaging. 2024;17(7):e016424.
9. Hung J, Lang R, Flachskampf F, et al. 3D echocardiography: a review of the current status and future directions. J Am Soc Echocardiogr. 2007;20(3):213-33.
10. Badano LP, Miglioranza MH, Mihăilă S, et al. Left atrial volumes and function by three-dimensional echocardiography: reference values, accuracy, reproducibility, and comparison with two-dimensional echocardiographic measurements. Circ Cardiovasc Imaging. 2016;9(7):e004229.
11. Barilli M, Tavera MC, Valente S, et al. Structural and hemodynamic changes of the right ventricle in PH-HFpEF. Int J Mol Sci. 2022;23(9):4554.
12. Ahmad A, Li H, Zhang Y, et al. Three-dimensional echocardiography assessment of right ventricular volumes and function: technological perspective and clinical application. Diagnostics (Basel). 2022;12(4):806.
13. Medvedofsky D, Maffessanti F, Weinert L, et al. 2D and 3D echocardiography-derived indices of left ventricular function and shape: relationship with mortality. JACC Cardiovasc Imaging. 2018;11(11):1569-79.
14. Collier P, Phelan D, Klein A. A test in context: myocardial strain measured by speckle-tracking echocardiography. J Am Coll Cardiol. 2017;69(8):1043-56.
15. Pandey A, Kagiyama N, Yanamala N, et al. Deep-learning models for the echocardiographic assessment of diastolic dysfunction. JACC Cardiovasc Imaging. 2021;14(10):1887-900.
16. Lau ES, Di Achille P, Kopparapu K, et al. Deep learning-enabled assessment of left heart structure and function predicts cardiovascular outcomes. J Am Coll Cardiol. 2023;82(20):1936-48.
17. Akerman AP, Porumb M, Scott CG, et al. Automated echocardiographic detection of heart failure with preserved ejection fraction using artificial intelligence. JACC: Advances. 2023;2:100452.

CHAPTER

Effect of ARNI on Left Atrial and Left Ventricular Strain by Speckle Tracking Echocardiography in Heart Failure

Vijayadithyan Jaganathan, Vaidehi Mendpara, Kousalya Rajendran, Navin C Nanda, HK Chopra

INTRODUCTION

Heart failure is a complex clinical syndrome which is classified based on left ventricular ejection fraction (LVEF) measured by two-dimensional echocardiography: heart failure with reduced ejection fraction (HFrEF), defined as LVEF of 40% or less; heart failure with mildly reduced ejection fraction (HFmrEF), with LVEF between 41 and 49%; and heart failure with preserved ejection fraction (HFpEF), characterized by LVEF of 50% or more.[1] Sacubitril/valsartan, an angiotensin receptor-neprilysin inhibitor (ARNI), has been shown to not only lower the risk of cardiovascular death and heart failure hospitalizations in HFrEF, but also improve symptoms as well as echocardiographic parameters and serum biomarkers. This chapter will explore the effects of ARNI therapy on left atrial (LA) and LV strain by speckle tracking echocardiography (STE) in heart failure.[2,3]

Myocardial strain, evaluated through STE, offers a reliable method for assessing systolic and diastolic function. This technique allows for the objective measurement of myocardial deformation, providing insights into cardiac performance that supplement conventional parameters such as LVEF evaluation by echocardiography.[4]

The LV global longitudinal strain (GLS) by STE measures LV longitudinal shortening as the base moves toward the apex in systole, unlike LVEF, which measures inward motion of LV cavity during systole. LV GLS has been shown to detect subtle reduction in LV function before any decrease is noted in LVEF and is therefore a valuable parameter in the evaluation of LV function. Similar to LV GLS, LA strain is also a measure of longitudinal deformation of the left atrium. LA reservoir strain that also represents peak LA longitudinal strain (PALS) has been shown in some studies to detect increased left sided filling pressures earlier than standard LV diastolic parameters. It is therefore a more sensitive marker of symptom severity related to LA congestion. **Table 1** summarizes key studies in the literature that investigated the effect of ARNI therapy on LV and LA strain parameters, highlighting their findings and clinical significance.[5-18]

Most studies indicate a significant improvement in LV GLS and LA strain parameters following sacubitril/valsartan therapy. These are accompanied by improvements in other echocardiographic indices of LV systolic and diastolic function such as LVEF as well as salutary changes in serum biomarkers. One study also demonstrated reduction in cardiovascular and total mortality as well as rehospitalization in HFrEF patients. The majority employed a single-arm design as prospective cohorts using ARNI, except for four studies that compared ARNI against renin angiotensin system (RAS) inhibitors and one that contrasted it with traditional heart failure therapy. However, studies with long-term follow up on ARNI therapy are not many.

Among all the studies, three are particularly noteworthy. One study (#3 in **Table 1**) identified clinical, biohumoral, and echocardiographic predictors of LV reverse remodeling (LVRR) associated with sacubitril/valsartan therapy. It found LV GLS greater than –9.3% predicted LVRR after 6 months of therapy, and PALS correlated with reduction in symptoms and congestion parameters, such as New York Heart Association functional class status. Another study (#8 in **Table 1**) assessed the persistence of implantable cardioverter-defibrillator (ICD) indications after 6 months of sacubitril/valsartan therapy in patients who did not have a baseline ICD but met implantation criteria according to European Society of Cardiology (ESC) guidelines.

TABLE 1: Effect of angiotensin receptor-neprilysin inhibitor (ARNI) on left ventricular (LV) and left atrial (LA) strain parameters in heart failure.

Study	*Study design*	*Objective/Primary endpoint*	*Strain parameters*	*Echocardiographic (echo) and other parameters*
1. Kalanatari et al. (2024) Number of patients (*n*) g = 40	• Sacubitril/Valsartan (S/V) in single arm with optimal medical therapy (OMT) • Heart failure with reduced ejection fraction (HFrEF) (Follow-up: 6 months)	Echo parameters, left ventricular (LV) global longitudinal strain (LV GLS) and LV reverse remodeling (RR)	• LV GLS improved from −12.8% ± 2.8% to −15.4% ± 3.4% • Right ventricular (RV) GLS improved (from −14.9% ± 3.4% to −19.3% ± 4.3%	• Reduction in LV end diastolic volume (EDV) and LV end systolic volume (ESV) • LVEF improved from 32% ± 7% to 44% ± 9% • Reduction in RV EDV • Decrease in NT-proBNP • 6MWT distance improved from 428 ± 105 m to 486 ± 124 m
2. Setouhi et al. (2024) (n = 200)	• S/V in single arm with OMT • HFrEF (Follow-up: 6 months)	LV ejection fraction (EF), LVGLS, mitral E/e′ ratio	• 41% patients showed improved LVEF and LVGLS • 37% showed improved LV GLS but none in LVEF	Improved LVESV and mitral E/è ratio
3. Mandoli et al. (2023) (*n* = 341)	• S/V in single arm with OMT • HFrEF (Follow-up: 6 months)	LVEF, LV GLS, left atrial (LA) strain	Improvement in LV GLS and peak LA longitudinal strain (PALS)	• 40% pts. showed LVRR. Of those with LVRR, 24% showed LVEF ≥35% (early complete responders, Group 1) and 16% still had LVEF <35% (early incomplete responders, Group 2). The remaining 60% of patients did not show any LVRR (nonearly responders, Group 3) • Group 1 demonstrated significant improvements in all parameters, while Group 2 exhibited some improvements. In contrast, Group 3 showed no improvement • LV GLS > −9.3% predicted LV RR • Global PALS predicted improved symptoms and congestion parameters (NYHA class and NT-proBNP at baseline) • Reduction in NT-pro BNP levels by 42%
4. Correale et al. (2023) (*n* = 47)	• S/ V in single arm with OMT • HFrEF (Follow-up: 6 months)	LA Strain	• Improved LA strain (both PALS and LA conduit) • LVGLS not studied	• 40% showed LARR. Reduction in indexed LVEDVi and LVESVi • Increase in LVEF, LAEF at follow-up compared to baseline • Reduction in LA volume • Reduction in mitral E/e′ ratio • Improvement in NYHA class and NT-proBNP levels

Contd…

Contd...

Study	*Study design*	*Objective/Primary endpoint*	*Strain parameters*	*Echocardiographic (ECHO) and other parameters*
5. Bras et al. (2023) (*n* = 65)	• S/V in single arm with OMT • HFrEF (Follow-up: 6 months)	LA strain and LV GLS	• LV GLS improved from –10.2% to -13.9% • Improvement in LA peak/ reservoir, LA conduit, and LA contractile strains and strain rate	• Reduction in LV dimensions and LA volumes • Increase in LVEF
6. Moon et al. (2022) (n = 409)	• S/V in single arm with OMT • HFrEF (Follow-up: 27 months)	• LA reservoir strain (RS) and LVGLS • To analyze composite cardiovascular (CV) death and HF hospitalization in relation to LVRR and LARR	LVGLS increased from –10.2% to –13.9% and LARS increased from 11.4% to 15.9%	• 39.6% achieved complete LVRR and LARR, 28.1% showed partial and 32.3% no LVRR and LARR • 101 patients (24.7%) experienced composite events (17 deaths from CV causes; 95 from HF hospitalizations), depicting lower event rate observed with ARNI therapy attributed to LVRR and LARR
7. Elshafey et al. (2021) (*n* = 73)	• S/V compared with traditional treatment • HFrEF (Follow up: 6-11 months)	LVEF and torsion dynamics in HFrEF	Increase in GLS (also increase in LV untwist and twist parameters)	Improvement in diastolic parameters and increase in LV EF
8. Pastore et al. (2021) (*n* = 113)	• S/V in single arm with OMT • HFrEF (Follow-up: 6 months)	• Percentage of ICD indication persistence • Clinical, bio-humoral and echocardiographic parameters including LV GLS. Predictors of persistence of ICD indications	Increase in LVGLS	• LV GLS cut off of –8.3% predicted persistence of ICD indications. LA volume indexed ≥42 mL/m^2 was another predictor • Nearly 60% of patients no longer met ICD indications, while 40% still did • Improvement in NYHA class, with none classified as NYHA class IV
9. Mazzetti et al. (2020) (*n*=30)	• S/V compared with ACEI (enalapril, ramipril, captopril) and ARBs (candesartan) • HFrEF (Follow-up: 3–6 months)	• LV GLS • Myocardial mechanics in HFrEF	Improvement in LV GLS	Nonlinear trend in reduction of NT-proBNP values
10. Castrichini et al; (2020) (*n* = 77)	• S/V single arm, • HFrEF (Follow-up: 3–18 months)	• Rates of LV and LARR by echo • PALS.	Improvements in LV GLS, total LA emptying fraction, and PALS	• Increase in LVEF • Decrease in LVEDVi

Contd...

Contd…

Study	*Study design*	*Objective/Primary endpoint*	*Strain parameters*	*Echocardiographic (ECHO) and other parameters*
11. De Vecchis et al. (2020) (*n* = 40)	S/V compared with RASi (Follow-up: 12 months)	LA strain (PALS)	Improvement in PALS	Lower risk of atrial fibrillation recurrences
12. Goncalves et al. (2020) (*n* = 42)	• S/V single arm • HFrEF (Follow-up: 6 months)	LV GLS	Improvement in LV GLS	• Increase in LVEF • Reduction in LA volume and Pulmonary artery systolic pressure
13. Desai et al. (2019) (*n* = 464)	• S/V compared with enalapril • HFrEF (12 weeks)	• LV GLS • Aortic characteristic impedance, measure of central aortic stiffness	No significant change in LV GLS.	No significant change in aortic characteristic impedance but significant changes in LA volume, LV volumes indices, and mitral E/e′ ratio
14. Chung et al. (2023) (*n* = 1,075)	• S/V compared with RASi • HFmrEF (LVEF: 40–50%) (Follow-up: 1–1.8 years)	• Prognostic value of LV GLS • All-cause death, composite CV death and HF hospitalizations	Improvement in LV GLS.	• Also, improvement in LVEF, but LV GLS independently linked to clinical outcomes after adjusting for LVEF • Lower all-cause and CV deaths. Lower HF hospitalizations

All reductions and improvements shown in the Table were statistically significant.
(6MWT: 6-minute walk test; ACEI: angiotensin converting enzyme inhibitor; ARBs: angiotensin receptor blockers; HFmrEF: heart failure with mildly reduced LV ejection fraction; ICD: implantable cardiac defibrillator; NT ProBNP: N Terminal pro brain natriuretic peptide; NYHA: New York Heart Association; RASi: renin angiotensin system inhibitor)

This study concluded that LV GLS, with a cutoff point of –8.3%, was the primary predictor of ICD indication persistence after 6 months of ARNI treatment.

One other study by Desai et al (#13 in **Table 1**), was a double-blind clinical trial involving 464 participants with (HFrEF) randomized to receive either sacubitril-valsartan or enalapril for 3 months. Measurement of central aortic stiffness, LVEF and LVGLS showed no significant difference between the two groups but sacubitril-valsartan demonstrated greater reductions in LA volume index, LV volumes indices and mitral E/e′ ratio. However, the study is older compared to all others and was of short duration, which could be a significant limitation.

All studies dealt with HFrEF patients except one that involved a small number of subjects with HFmrEF. This study (#14 in **Table 1**) compared sacubitril/valsartan therapy with RAS inhibitors in HFmrEF and found that ARNI therapy compared with RAS inhibitors improved both LV GLS and LVEF, but LV GLS was independently linked to clinical outcomes after adjusting for LVEF.

CONCLUSION

In conclusion, many studies in the literature indicate significant improvements in LV GLS and LA strain parameters following sacubitril/valsartan therapy. Concomitantly, improvements were observed in symptom relief, the 6-minute walk test, and other echocardiographic parameters, including LVEF, LV end-systolic, and end-diastolic volumes, as well as diastolic markers like mitral E/e′ ratios.

REFERENCES

1. Ponikowski P, Voors AA, Anker SD, et al. 2016 ESC Guidelines for the diagnosis and treatment of acute and chronic heart failure: the task force for the diagnosis and treatment of acute and chronic heart failure of the European Society of Cardiology (ESC). Developed with the special contribution of the Heart Failure Association (HFA) of the ESC. Eur J Heart Fail. 2016;18(8):891-975.
2. Pascual-Figal D, Bayés-Genis A, Beltrán-Troncoso P, et al. Sacubitril-Valsartan, clinical benefits and related mechanisms of action in heart failure with reduced ejection fraction: a review. Front Cardiovasc Med. 2021;8:754499.
3. McMurray JJ, Packer M, Desai AS, et al. Angiotensin-neprilysin inhibition versus enalapril in heart failure. N Engl J Med. 2014;371(11):993-1004.
4. Teske AJ, De Boeck BW, Melman PG, et al. Echocardiographic quantification of myocardial function using tissue deformation imaging: a guide to image acquisition and analysis using tissue Doppler and speckle tracking. Cardiovasc Ultrasound. 2007;5:27.
5. Kalanatari S, Oren D, Medvedofsky D, et al. Reverse remodeling effects of sacubitril-valsartan: structural and functional optimization in stage C heart failure. Am J Cardiol. 2024;210:249-55.
6. Setouhi A, Mohamed ON, Farrag HMA, et al. Does speckle tracking transthoracic echocardiography indicate subtle changes in left ventricular function in heart failure patients with reduced ejection fraction treated by sacubitril-valsartan? J Cardiovasc Echogr. 2024;34(1):19-24.
7. Mandoli GE, Pastore MC, Giannoni A, et al. Deformation imaging by strain in chronic heart failure over sacubitril-valsartan: a multicenter echocardiographic registry. ESC Heart Fail. 2023;10(2):846-57.
8. Correale M, Magnesa M, Mazzeo P, et al. Left atrial functional remodeling in patients with chronic heart failure treated with sacubitril/valsartan. J Clin Med. 2023; 12(3):1086.
9. Brás PG, Gonçalves AV, Branco LM, et al. Sacubitril/valsartan improves left atrial and ventricular strain and strain rate in patients with heart failure with reduced ejection fraction. Life. 2023;13(4):995.
10. Moon MG, Hwang IC, Lee HJ, et al. Reverse remodeling assessed by left atrial and ventricular strain reflects treatment response to sacubitril/valsartan. JACC Cardiovasc Imaging. 2022;15(9):1525-41.
11. Elshafey WEH, Al Khoufi EA, Elmelegy EK. Effects of sacubitril/valsartan treatment on left ventricular myocardial torsion mechanics in patients with heart failure reduced ejection fraction: 2D speckle tracking echocardiography. J Cardiovasc Echogr. 2021;31(2):59-67.
12. Pastore MC, Mandoli GE, Giannoni A, et al. Sacubitril/valsartan reduces indications for arrhythmic primary prevention in heart failure with reduced ejection fraction: insights from DISCOVER-ARNI, a multicenter Italian register. Eur Heart J Open. 2021;2(1):oeab046.
13. Mazzetti S, Scifo C, Abete R, et al. Short-term echocardiographic evaluation by global longitudinal strain in patients with heart failure treated with sacubitril/valsartan. ESC Heart Fail. 2020;7(3):964-72.
14. Castrichini M, Manca P, Nuzzi V, et al. Sacubitril/valsartan induces global cardiac reverse remodeling in long-lasting heart failure with reduced ejection fraction: standard and advanced echocardiographic evidences. J Clin Med. 2020;9(4):906.
15. De Vecchis R, Paccone A, Di Maio M. Favorable effects of sacubitril/valsartan on the peak atrial longitudinal strain in patients with chronic heart failure and a history of one or more episodes of atrial fibrillation: a retrospective cohort study. J Clin Med Res. 2020;12(2):100-7.
16. Valentim Gonçalves A, Galrinho A, Pereira-da-Silva T, et al. Myocardial work improvement after sacubitril-valsartan therapy: a new echocardiographic parameter for a new treatment. J Cardiovasc Med (Hagerstown). 2020;21(3):223-30.
17. Desai AS, Solomon SD, Shah AM, et al. Effect of sacubitril-valsartan vs enalapril on aortic stiffness in patients with heart failure and reduced ejection fraction: a randomized clinical trial. JAMA. 2019;322(11):1077-84.
18. Chung FP, Chao TF, Lee AS, et al. Discriminative ability of left ventricular strain in mildly reduced ejection fraction heart failure. JACC Adv. 2023;2(9):100654.

CHAPTER

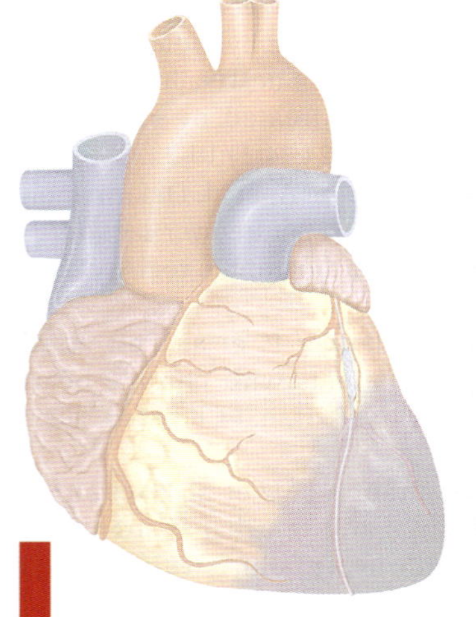

Echocardiographic Evaluation of Atrial Function in HFpEF

Mark Hellerman, Smadar Kort

INTRODUCTION

Heart failure with preserved ejection fraction (HFpEF) is a complex clinical syndrome for which diagnosis and management is guided by echocardiography. While earlier studies focused primarily on echocardiographic signals of delayed ventricular relaxation or abnormal systolic function, recent insights reveal that HFpEF is also significantly affected by structural and functional abnormalities in the atria. Current phenotyping techniques, which consider atrial myopathy, promise more precise insights into pathophysiology which can guide personalized interventions that target core mechanisms of the disease.

CONTENTS AND DESCRIPTION

Chronic elevation of left ventricular (LV) filling pressures, a consequence of LV diastolic dysfunction, can lead to both structural and functional changes in the left atria (LA). Structural changes include LA enlargement, which has long been associated with HFpEF and remains an important marker for disease progression. LA enlargement, however, is not present in all individuals with HFpEF, as functional abnormalities may manifest prior to structural changes. LA function is coordinated between three integrated phases which include the reservoir, conduit, and booster-pump phase **(Fig. 1)**. During the reservoir phase, the LA expands to facilitate storage of blood from pulmonary venous return during LV systole. Next, during the conduit phase the LA passively transfers the stored blood into the LV during ventricular diastole. Finally, during the booster phase, active contraction of the LA during the final part of diastole contributes 15–30% of the LV stroke volume, boosting the ejection force and stroke volume.[1]

Strain analysis during each phase of the LA cycle can provide prognostic and diagnostic value for patients with HFpEF. Reduced LA strain is associated with adverse outcomes in HFpEF, including increased risk of cardiovascular hospitalization and death.[2-4] In particular, LA reservoir strain is a strong predictor of adverse events and is independently associated with worse clinical outcomes.[2,3] And while LA strain garners predictive value alone, risk stratification can be further enhanced when it is combined with diastolic transmitral inflow and annular diastolic velocities.[5] In a study of over 300 patients with HFpEF, LA stiffness index—defined as the ratio of E/e' divided by peak atrial longitudinal strain (LS)—found that elevated LA stiffness was associated with a considerably higher incidence of multiple HF hospitalizations, even after adjusting for relevant clinical and echocardiographic variables.[5] LA strain can also provide significant diagnostic value in distinguishing HFpEF from noncardiac causes of dyspnea—especially in patients with paroxysmal atrial fibrillation (AF).[6] Moreover, LA strain can aid in earlier diagnosis of HFpEF, as reduced strain is associated with markers of diastolic dysfunction and increased LV filling pressures.[7] Lower LA strain is also linked to a higher incidence of AF in HFpEF patients and has been demonstrated to provide incremental predictive information about the risk of developing AF, beyond traditional clinical and echocardiographic parameters.[8,9]

Importantly, measuring LA compliance during exercise using speckle-tracking echocardiography has

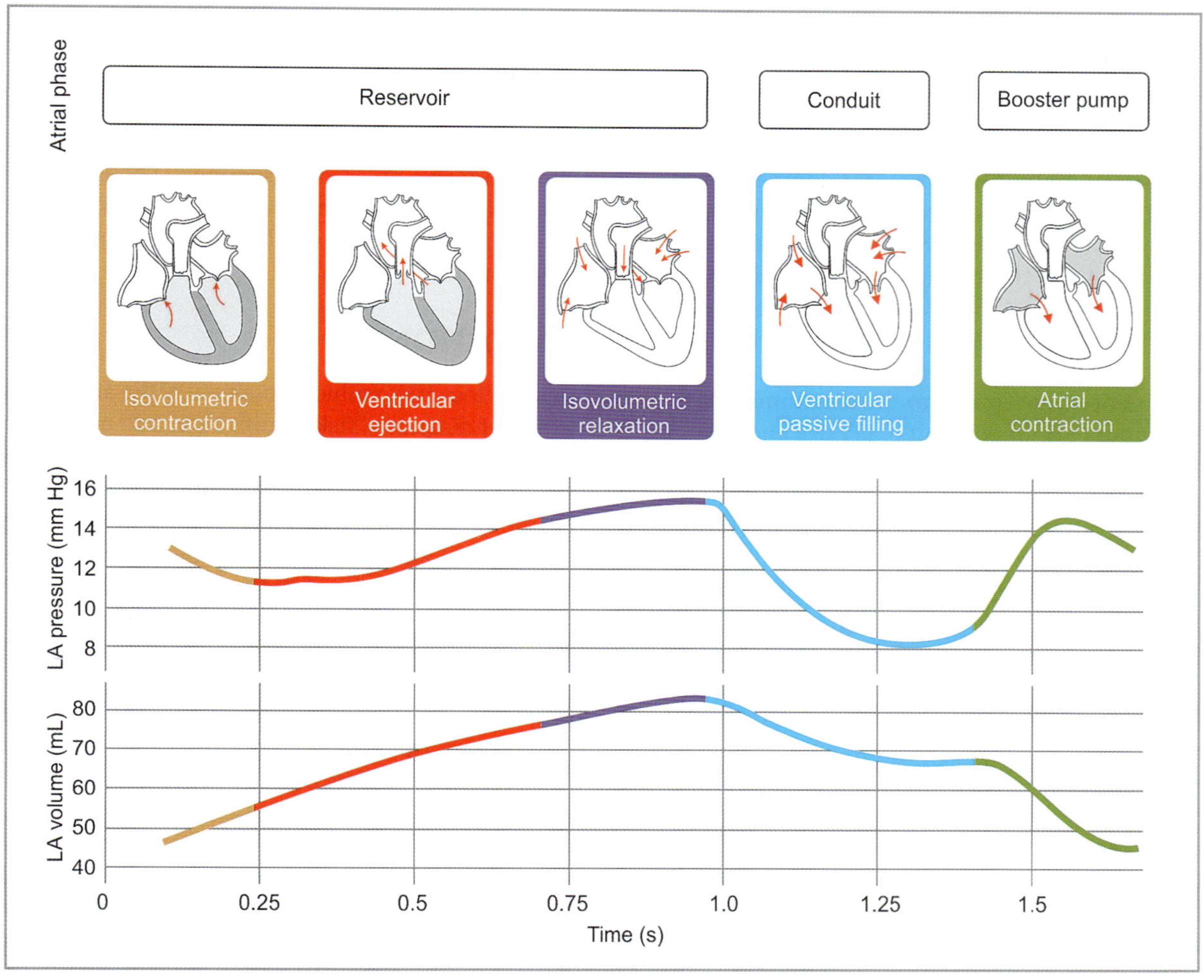

Fig. 1: Atrial phases with corresponding left atrial (LA) pressure and volume waveforms.
Source: Wikipedia Commons. Phases of cardiac cycle. [online] Available from https://commons.wikimedia.org/wiki/File:Phases_of_the_cardiac_cycle.svg) [Last accessed January, 2025]

been demonstrated to significantly enhance the diagnosis of HFpEF in patients with dyspnea.[10] Impaired LA strain response during exercise is associated with right ventricular-to-pulmonary circulation uncoupling and ventilation inefficiency, highlighting its role in exercise intolerance in HFpEF.[11]

Atrial-secondary mitral regurgitation (MR)—a clinical entity characterized by isolated annular dilation and LA dysfunction—has also been increasingly recognized in patients with HFpEF, especially those with comorbid AF. It holds significant prognostic importance as it is associated with worse clinical outcomes, including increased morbidity and mortality.[12,13] Atrial-secondary MR is primarily caused by LA dilation, which leads to mitral annular enlargement and reduced leaflet coaptation, even in the absence of LV dilation. This mechanism is well-documented using three-dimensional transesophageal echocardiography.[13-16]

Patients with secondary MR exhibit worse LA function during exercise compared to those with primary MR. This includes lower LA strain and strain rate, leading to reduced exercise performance and higher event rates such as mortality and hospitalization for heart failure.[17] Handgrip exercise during echocardiography can unmask atrial MR in patients who appear to have nonsevere atrial MR at rest. This method improves risk stratification and can influence clinical decision-making regarding the need for mitral valve interventions.[18] In a cohort of 80 patients with atrial-secondary MR, the addition of handgrip exercise testing to echocardiographic assessment at rest improved the global chi-square (from 21.2–30.2) and the Harrell's c-index (from 0.69–0.78) for prediction of mitral valve surgery/interventions during follow-up.[18]

Echocardiographic assessment of the right atrium (RA) has also been the subject of recent study in patients with HFpEF, especially in the presence of pulmonary hypertension (PH). Patients with HFpEF and pulmonary hypertension (HFpEF-PH) exhibit significantly increased RA stiffness and higher RA pressures compared to those with HFpEF without PH and those with pulmonary arterial hypertension (PAH).[19] HFpEF-PH patients demonstrate worse RA function, characterized by reduced total right atrial emptying fraction (RAEF) and slightly reduced active RAEF, indicating impaired RA performance.[19] Patients with PAH have significantly impaired RA reservoir and passive conduit functions compared to those without PAH—and this impairment is independent of RA size and pressure.[20]

Importantly, impaired RA LS has been associated with RV enlargement, RV dysfunction and higher NT-proBNP levels, independent of RA size and pressure—implicating RA LS as a sensitive marking of RV dysfunction in patients with HFpEF-PH.[20] The findings of RA LS using echocardiography parallel those observed using cardiac magnetic resonance (CMR) imaging, which have also identified impaired RA reservoir function as an independent predictor of death in individuals with HFpEF.[21]

Moreover, RA size has been found to have prognostic value in patients with HFpEF—associated with a more than two-fold increased risk adverse clinical outcomes including all-cause mortality and HF hospitalizations.[22] Notably, among patients with HFpEF, those who have findings of both LA and RA myopathy (biatrial myopathy) appear to be at higher risk for adverse outcomes than those with isolated LA myopathy.[23] In a recent study of 476 patients with HFpEF who underwent invasive hemodynamic exercise testing and comprehensive echocardiography imaging it was found that those with biatrial myopathy had an 84% higher risk of HF hospitalization or death compared to those with isolated LA myopathy.[23]

Secondary tricuspid regurgitation (STR) is a common condition in patients with HFpEF and can be classified into two distinct phenotypes: atrial secondary tricuspid regurgitation (A-STR), and ventricular secondary tricuspid regurgitation (V-STR).[24] A-STR is characterized by predominant dilation of the RA and tricuspid annulus (TA), with preservation of right ventricular function, whereas V-STR is primarily driven by RV dysfunction and is often caused by left-sided heart diseases, PH, and LV systolic dysfunction.[25] As these conditions progress, however, the distinctions of these phenotypes often blur. Identification of STR is important, as recent studies have identified RA dysfunction as an independent predictive marker in patients with HFpEF. Patients with severe STR and HFpEF exhibit higher right atrial pressure both at rest and during exercise compared to those with mild or no STR. This increased pressure is associated with impaired stroke volume (SV) and cardiac output (CO), leading to pulmonary vascular derecruitment and relative left heart underfilling.[24,26] For accurate diagnosis of STR, comprehensive assessments using 3D echocardiography or transesophageal echocardiography is advised and can help guide potential surgical or transcatheter interventions.[25]

LIMITATIONS

While echocardiographic assessment of the atria can be very useful for diagnosis, risk stratification and management of patients with HFpEF, several technical limitations must be considered. First, there remains significant variability in reported reference ranges for left atrial strain. Reference ranges for LA strain vary significantly across studies due to differences in sample sizes, heart rates, and body surface areas, leading to heterogeneity in the data.[27,28] There also exist limitations with respect to the prognostic value of LA strain. Although LA strain provides incremental prognostic information, robust clinical outcome data from large prospective trials are still needed to confirm its predictive ability before it can be widely accepted in clinical practice.[29] Similar limitations exist for the evaluation of the right atria in patients with HFpEF. Specifically, there remains variability across software vendors, image quality, lack of standardized reference values, and uncertain prognostic value. Different echocardiography software vendors produce varying RAS measurements, leading to inconsistencies. For example, EchoPAC measurements are significantly less negative compared to TomTec and VVI, which can affect clinical interpretations.[30] Just as there is a lack of universally accepted normal reference values for LA strain, there remains a lack of universally accepted normal reference values for RAS which complicates the clinical application of these measurements. Different studies have reported varying normal ranges, influenced by factors such as age, gender, and the specific echocardiographic technique used.[31,32] Despite growing acknowledgment that LA strain is a crucial tool for early diagnosis and risk stratification in HFpEF, routine evaluation is yet common practice, and further research is needed to fully integrate LA strain into routine clinical practice and explore its potential as a therapeutic target.

CONCLUSION

Ultimately, echocardiographic assessment of atrial function is increasingly recognized as a crucial component of managing patients with HFpEF. Both the LA and RA play vital roles in cardiac function, and atrial myopathy can significantly impact clinical outcomes. LA strain analysis, particularly during the reservoir phase, provides valuable prognostic and diagnostic information, helping to predict adverse events and distinguish HFpEF from other causes of dyspnea. Moreover, the assessment of LA compliance during exercise enhances the diagnosis of HFpEF, especially in patients with paroxysmal AF. Similarly, RA assessment, especially in the context of PH, reveals important insights into disease severity and prognosis. Notably, the presence of biatrial myopathy, characterized by dysfunction in both the LA and RA, is associated with a significantly higher risk of adverse outcomes compared to isolated LA myopathy. Therefore, integrating a comprehensive evaluation of atrial function into routine clinical practice is essential for early diagnosis, risk stratification, and the development of personalized treatment strategies that target the core mechanisms of HFpEF.

REFERENCES

1. Freed BH, Daruwalla V, Cheng JY, et al. Prognostic Utility and Clinical Significance of Cardiac Mechanics in Heart Failure With Preserved Ejection Fraction. Circ Cardiovasc Imaging. 2016;9:e003754.
2. Santos ABS, Roca GQ, Claggett B, et al. Prognostic Relevance of Left Atrial Dysfunction in Heart Failure With Preserved Ejection Fraction. Circ: Hear. Fail. 2016;9:e002763.
3. Katahira M, Kiko T, Endo K, et al. Abstract 13033: Usefulness of MR-Derived Left Ventricular Global Longitudinal Strain and Left Atrial Strain to Predict Cardiovascular Events in Patients With HFpEF. Circulation. 2023;148:A13033.
4. Mehrzad R, Rajab M, Spodick D. The Three Integrated Phases of Left Atrial Macrophysiology and Their Interactions. Int. J. Mol. Sci. 2014;15:15146-60.
5. Reddy YNV, Obokata M, Egbe A, et al. Left atrial strain and compliance in the diagnostic evaluation of heart failure with preserved ejection fraction. Eur J Heart Fail. 2019;21:891-900.
6. Katbeh A, Potter TD, Geelen P, et al. Heart failure with preserved ejection fraction or non-cardiac dyspnea in paroxysmal atrial fibrillation: The role of left atrial strain. Int J Cardiol. 2021;323:161-7.
7. Buggey J, Hoit BD. Left atrial strain. Curr Opin Cardiol. 2019;33:479-85.
8. Jasic-Szpak E, Marwick TH, Kosmala Przewlocka M, et al. P325Incremental value of left atrial strain in predicting atrial fibrillation in heart failure with preserved ejection fraction. Eur Hear J. 2019;40:ehz747.0160.
9. Hristova K, Tselov N, Tsonev SV, et al. S-29-5: Early changes in left atrial strain and global ventricular function in hypertensive patients with heart failure with preserved EF. J Hypertens. 2023;41:e70.
10. Harada T, Kagami K, Shina T, et al. Diagnostic value of reduced left atrial compliance during ergometry exercise in heart failure with preserved ejection fraction. Eur J Heart Fail. 2023;25(8):1293-303.
11. Sugimoto T, Bandera F, Generati G, et al. Left Atrial Function Dynamics During Exercise in Heart Failure Pathophysiological Implications on the Right Heart and Exercise Ventilation Inefficiency. JACC: Cardiovasc. Imaging. 2017;10(10 Pt B):1253-64.
12. Lupasteanu I, Vijan I, Delcea C, et al. P1087Prevalence and significance of mitral regurgitation in atrial fibrillation coexisting with HFpEF and HFmEF. EP Eur. 2020;22:euaa162.292.
13. Deferm S, Dauw J, Vandervoort PM, et al. Atrial Functional Mitral and Tricuspid Regurgitation. Curr Treat Options Cardiovasc Med. 2020;22:30.
14. Ring L, Dutka DP, Wells FC, et al. Mechanisms of atrial mitral regurgitation: insights using 3D transoesophageal echo. Eur Heart J Cardiovasc. Imaging. 2014;15(5):500-8.
15. Deferm S, Bertrand PB, Verbrugge FH, et al. Atrial Functional Mitral Regurgitation JACC Review Topic of the Week. J Am Coll Cardiol. 2019;73:2465-76.
16. Schutter SD, Damme EV, Hout GV, et al. Atrial functional mitral regurgitation during exercise is associated with impaired longitudinal left ventricular systolic function and annular dilation: an exercise echocardiographic study. Eur. Hear. J. 2022;43:ehac544.141.
17. Sugimoto T, Bandera F, Generati G, et al. Left Atrial Dynamics During Exercise in Mitral Regurgitation of Primary and Secondary Origin Pathophysiological Insights by Exercise Echocardiography Combined With Gas Exchange Analysis. JACC: Cardiovasc. Imaging. 2020;13(1 Pt 1):25-40.
18. Spieker M, Sidabras J, Lagarden H, et al. Handgrip echocardiography improves risk stratification in patients with atrial functional mitral regurgitation. Eur Heart J. 2023;44:ehad655.1742.
19. van Wezenbeek J, van der Bovenkamp A, Wessels JN, et al. Abstract 15161: Increased Right Atrial Stiffness in Patients With Heart Failure With Preserved Ejection Fraction and Pulmonary Hypertension. Circulation. 2020;142(3):15161.
20. Querejeta Roca G, Campbell P, Claggett B, et al. Right Atrial Function in Pulmonary Arterial Hypertension. Circ Cardiovasc Imaging. 2015;8(11):e003521; discussion e003521.
21. Jain S, Kuriakose D, Edelstein I, et al. Right Atrial Phasic Function in Heart Failure With Preserved and Reduced Ejection Fraction. JACC: Cardiovasc Imaging. 2019;12(8 Pt 1):1460-70.
22. Ikoma T, Obokata M, Okada K, et al. Impact of Right Atrial Remodeling in Heart Failure With Preserved Ejection Fraction. J Card Fail. 2021;27(5):577-84.
23. Omote K, Sorimachi H, Obokata M, et al. Biatrial myopathy in heart failure with preserved ejection fraction. Eur J Heart Fail. 2024;26(2):288-98.
24. Harada T, Obokata M, Omote K, et al. Functional Tricuspid Regurgitation and Right Atrial Remodeling in Heart Failure With Preserved Ejection Fraction. Am J Cardiol. 2022;162:129-35.

25. Muraru D, Badano LP, Hahn RT, et al. Atrial secondary tricuspid regurgitation: pathophysiology, definition, diagnosis, and treatment. Eur Hear J. 2024;45(11):895-911.
26. Baratto C, Caravita S, Corbetta G, et al. Impact of severe secondary tricuspid regurgitation on rest and exercise hemodynamics of patients with heart failure and a preserved left ventricular ejection fraction. Front Cardiovasc Med. 2023;10:1061118.
27. Nielsen AB, Skaarup KG, Hauser R, et al. Normal values and reference ranges for left atrial strain by speckle-tracking echocardiography: the Copenhagen City Heart Study. Eur Hear J. Cardiovasc Imaging. 2021;23(1):42-51.
28. Pathan F, D'Elia N, Nolan MT, et al. Normal Ranges of Left Atrial Strain by Speckle-Tracking Echocardiography: A Systematic Review and Meta-Analysis. J Am Soc Echocardiogr. 2017;30:59-70.e8.
29. Hoit BD. Assessment of Left Atrial Function by Echocardiography: Novel Insights. Curr Cardiol Rep. 2018; 20(10):96.
30. Agrawal A, Dahdah JE, Arockiam AD, et al. Abstract 17044: Normal Ranges of Right Atrial Strain by Contemporary Echocardiography Software: A Prospective Comparative Cohort Study. Circulation. 2023;148:A17044.
31. Nemes A, Kormányos Á, Domsik P, et al. Normal reference values of right atrial strain parameters using three-dimensional speckle-tracking echocardiography (results from the MAGYAR-Healthy Study). Int J Cardiovasc Imaging. 2019;35(11):2009-18.
32. Muraru D, Onciul S, Peluso D, et al. Sex- and Method-Specific Reference Values for Right Ventricular Strain by 2-Dimensional Speckle-Tracking Echocardiography. Circ Cardiovasc Imaging. 2016;9(2):e003866.

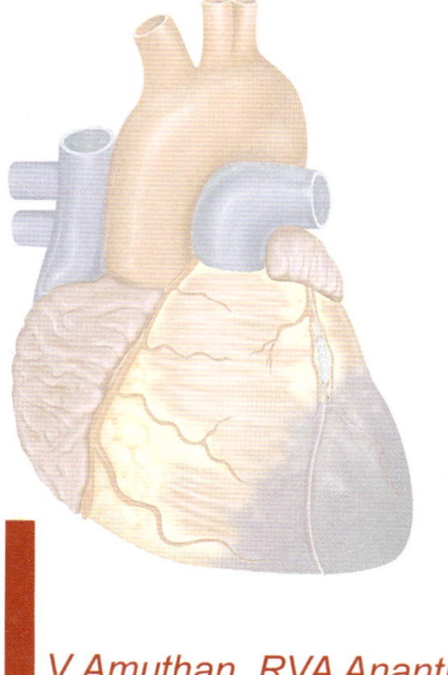

3D Echocardiography and BNP Screening in HFpEF

V Amuthan, RVA Ananth

INTRODUCTION

Echocardiography has been the marvel of 20th century. This ultrasound technique since its inception from the days of elder, has revolutionized the diagnosis and treatment in the management of cardiac patients. From the days of single crystal probe to M Mode, 2D, Color flow mapping, the advancement has reached the stage of three-dimensional echocardiogram with added fourth dimension of time [4D echocardiography—the real-time three-dimensional (3D) echocardiography]. The newer 3D matrix array transducers have a more uniform atomic structure, larger band, and have efficient electromechanical coupling. They have >2,500 crystals arranged as 50 rows and 50 columns.[1-5] The performance of the 3D echocardiogram has the same methodology as standard two dimensional echocardiography.[6-8] The image data set is essentially acquired from the same parasternal and apical windows.[9-13] The acquisition of optimized two dimensional images along with routine ECG connection is the most important prerequisite.

EXAMINATION OF LEFT VENTRICLE AND LEFT VENTRICLE FUNCTION ASSESSMENT

The LV ejection fraction (EF): The cornerstone of the prognostication and treatment schedule for echocardiographic evaluation starts with evaluation of left ventricular ejection fraction (LVEF). Despite its limitations, EF has become part of the lingua franca of cardiology.[13] The evidence base for modern cardiology is so heavily based on this simple measurement that it is unlikely to disappear. The advantages and problems in calculating EF as the ratio between stroke volume and end-diastolic volume and their solutions are enumerated in **Table 1**. 3D imaging is available with echocardiography, MRI, and CT. The main attraction and advantage of 3D imaging is to avoid geometric assumptions when calculations of LV volumes are being obtained, and to avoid errors created by cutting a 3D structure in two dimensions.[14,15] The current software for 3D evaluation of LVEF is much easier and can be performed within minutes in the setting of the emergency room. LVEF is important in classification of HFpEF where the LVEF is >50% and heart failure with reduced ejection fraction (HFrEF) when it is <40% and midrange when it is 40–50%. This classification is important because of differing prognosis, response to treatment, and major clinical trials selecting patients based on their LVEF **(Table 1)**. However, this concept is flawed as a patient with HFpEF can progress to HFrEF **(Table 2)**. Similarly, a patient with HFrEF, the EF can be improved and then it is called heart failure with improved ejection fraction.

HEART FAILURE WITH PRESERVED EJECTION FRACTION

The diagnosis of heart failure with preserved ejection fraction (HFpEF) can be easily made in a patient with overt heart failure and echocardiographic evidence of normal EF.[16] However, in patients with subtle symptoms and symptoms occurring after stress it becomes immensely difficult to diagnose. We have two important scoring strategies to aid us: H2FPEF and HFA-PEFF algorithms **(Table 3)**.

TABLE 1: Clinical applications of 3D echocardiography for left ventricular (LV) function.

Clinical application	*Images*
LV function The main advantage of 3D LV function is that: • It avoids geometric assumptions of LV volumes calculated from 2D; • It avoids errors created by cutting a 3D structure in two dimensions; • The current software for 3D evaluation of LVEF is much easier and can be performed within minutes in the setting of the emergency room. On the right is the technique of calculation of LVEF from heart model.	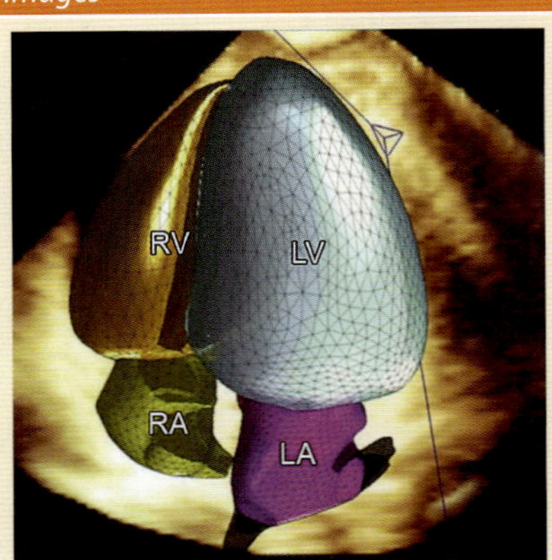

(LA: left atrium; LVEF: left ventricular ejection fraction; RV: right ventricular; RA: right atrium)

TABLE 2: Demonstration of progression of heart failure with preserved ejection fraction (HFpEF) to heart failure with reduced ejection fraction (HFrEF).

Clinical application	*Images*
A 40-year-old patient with secondary hypertension due to polycystic kidney disease was admitted with heart failure in March 2022. He had a normal left ventricular (LV) ejection fraction of 50%, global longitudinal strain (GLS)—10.3% and territorial longitudinal strain (TLS) abnormality involving anterior septum. E' was 4 cm/sec and E/e' 23.79. The left atrial reservoir strain (LASr) was 23%, LA Vmax 32 mL. The coronary angiogram was done which was normal.	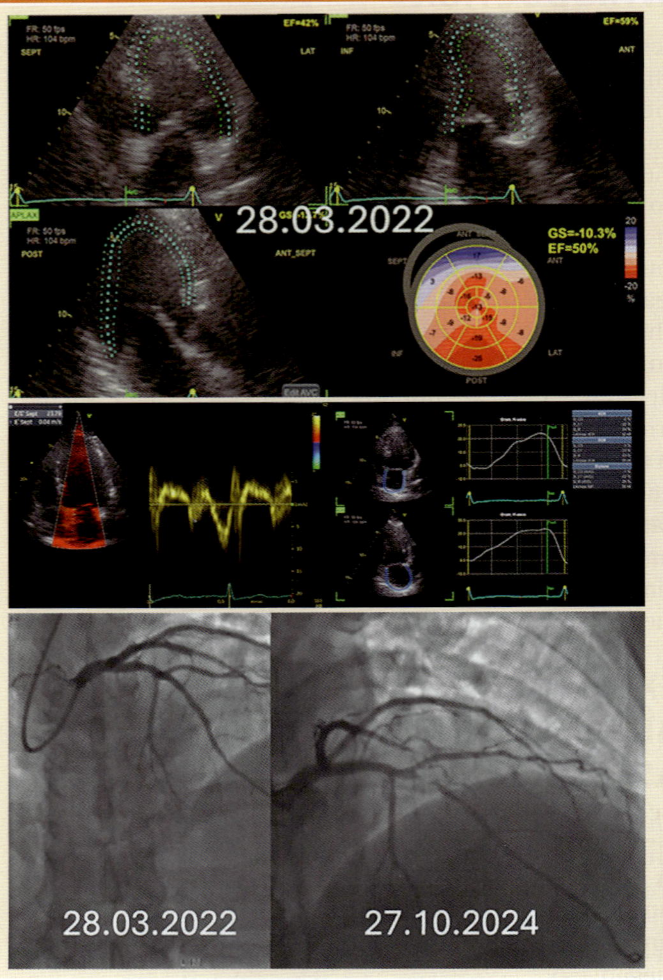

Contd...

Contd...

Clinical application	*Images*
He was readmitted in October 2024 with CCF. His LVEF 25%, GLS—4% e′ 3, and E/e′ 25, LASr 17%, and LA Vmax 32 mL. He had 90% narrowing of mid LAD. This case proves the fact that the HFpEF can progress to HFrEF for obvious reasons.	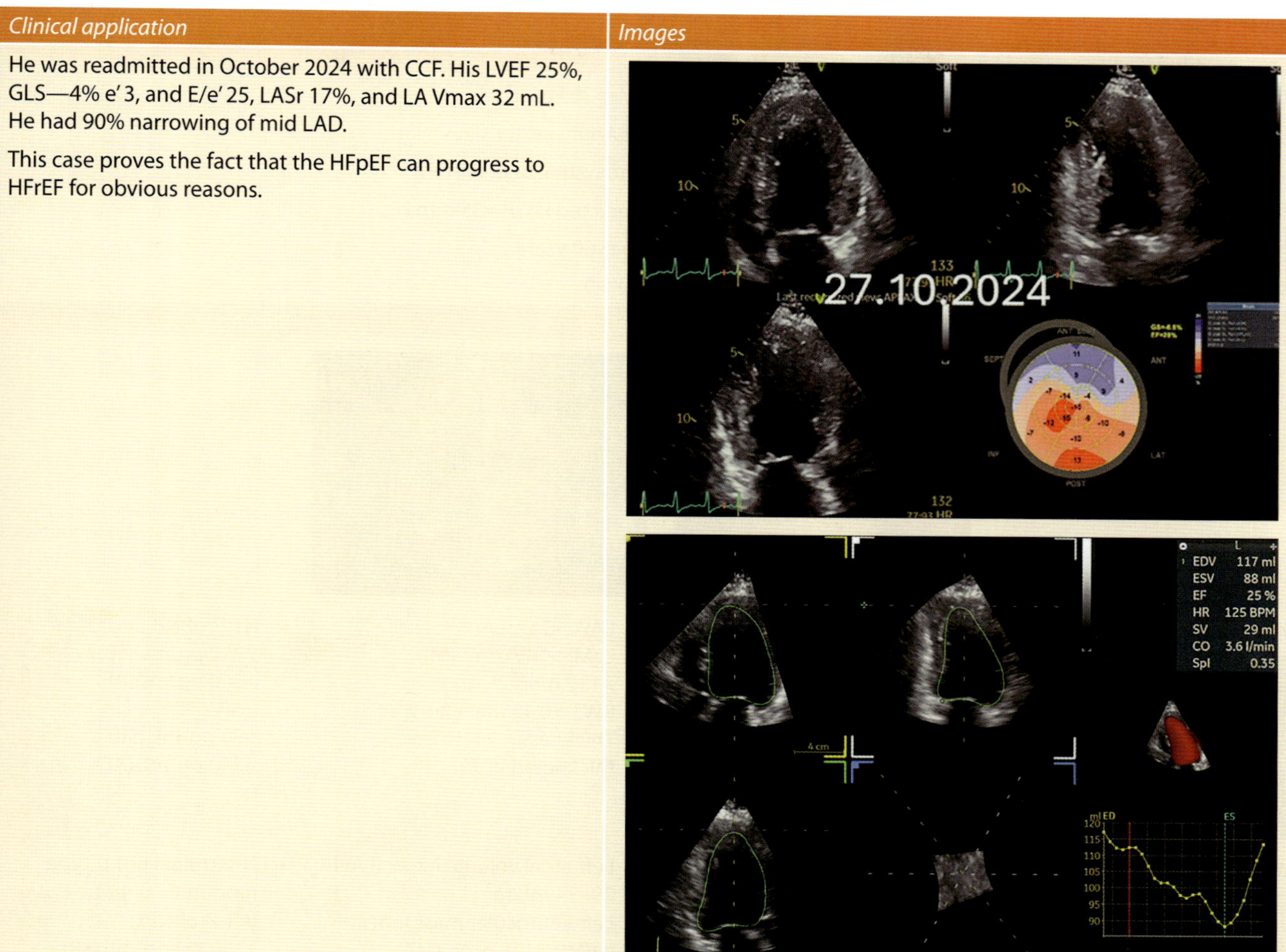

In the H2FPEF algorithm, weightage is given for *H*eavy (BMI >30 kg/m^2), *H*ypertensive (Use of >2 antihypertensive drugs) with atrial *F*ibrillation (paroxysmal or persistent), *P*ulmonary hypertension (Doppler predicted PA pressure >35 mm Hg), *E*lderly patient (age >60) and elevated *F*illing pressures (Doppler E/e′ >9). It is considered to be significant if the score is ≥6 and is considered to be ruled out if the score is 0–1. HFA-PEFF algorithm has been proposed by *H*eart *F*ailure *A*ssociation of European Society of Cardiology *P*retest assessment *E*chocardiographic and natriuretic peptide major and minor criteria and a score *F1* Functional testing in case of uncertainty and *F2* final etiology. A score of ≥5 is considered significant.[17-19] A high H2FPEF score (6–9) has a high specificity (97%) and positive predictive accuracy for diagnosing HFpEF and a low score (0–1) has a high sensitivity (97%) and negative predictive accuracy for ruling out HFpEF. HFA-PEFF high score has 84% specificity in diagnosing HFpEF and a low score, sensitivity of 99% in ruling out HFpEF.[20] However, in presence of atrial fibrillation, the sensitivity and specificity are reduced.[21-27] Case examples are shown in **Table 4**.

4D Left Ventricular Strain

Shortening and lengthening, which are the basic functions of the myocardial fibers result in a systolic twist followed by a diastolic untwisting of the left ventricle due to helical orientation of fibers. In systole, the LV apex undergoes a counterclockwise rotation about its longitudinal axis as viewed from the apex, preceded by a brief clockwise rotation due to the earlier shortening of the subendocardial fibers during isovolumic contraction. Rotation of the LV base in systole is opposite in direction compared to apical rotation, with a brief counterclockwise rotation during isovolumic contraction followed by a

TABLE 3: Clinical applications of 3D echocardiography for heart failure with preserved ejection fraction (HFpEF): H2FPEF score versus HFA-PEFF score.

H2FPEF score	*Clinical variables*	*Values*	*Points*
H2	Heavy	BMI >30 kg/m^2	2
	Hypertensive	≥2 Antihypertensives	1
F	Atrial fibrillation	Paroxysmal or persistent	3
P	Pulmonary hypertension	Predicted PASP >35 mm Hg	1
E	Elder	Age>60 years	1
F	Filling pressure	E/e' >9	1
HFA-PEFF score	*Functional*	*Morphological*	*Biomarker*
Major	• Septal e' <7 cm/sec or Lateral e' <10 cm/sec • Average E/e' >15 • Tricuspid regurgitation (TR) velocity >2.8 m/sec Pulmonary arterial systolic pressure (PASP) >35 mm Hg	• LAVI ≥34 mL/m^2 • LVMI >149 g/m^2 (M) >122 g/m^2 (F) and RWT >0.42 (Relative Wall Thickness = 2 × LVPW thickness/LVIDd)	• NT-ProBNP >220 pg/mL (SR) >660 pg/mL (AF) • BNP >80 pg/mL (SR) >240 pg/mL (AF)
Minor	• Average E/e' 9-14 • Global longitudinal strain (GLS) <-16	• Left atrial volume index (LAVI) 29–34 mL/m^2 • Left ventricular mass index (LVMI) >115 g/m^2 (M) >95 g/m^2 (F) • Relative wall thickness (RWT) >0.42 • LV wall thickness >1.2 cm	• N-terminal pro b-type natriuretic peptide (NT-ProBNP) 125–220 pg/mL (SR) 325–660 pg/mL (AF) • Brain natriuretic peptide (BNP) 35–80 pg/mL (SR) 105–240 pg/mL (AF)
Major criteria 2 points	>5 points HFpEF		
Minor criteria 1 point	2–4 points	Diastolic stress test or	Invasive hemodynamics

clockwise rotation during LV ejection. This motion has been compared with that used to squeeze water out of a wet towel.[28] The main determinant of the LV twist is the apical rotation **(Table 5)**. A recent study by Muhammad Ashraf et al., to compute left ventricular (LV) twist from 3D echocardiography concluded LV twist and torsion can be computed accurately.[29,30] 3D speckle tracking has improved the accuracy of LV deformation imaging and torsion dynamics. To date, no prognostic information exists on the role of rotational parameters of LV function. The areas most likely to benefit are HFpEF and cardiac dyssynchrony resynchronization therapy.[31-33.]

Global longitudinal strain has evolved as one of the most robust parameters, and this has been shown to identify subclinical LV dysfunction. GLS is calculated using a variety of proprietary software (EchoPac, GE Medical Systems, Milwaukee, Wisconsin, USA; Syngo velocity vector imaging, Siemens, Mountain View, California, USA; LV analysis, Tomtec GmbH, Unterschlessheim, Germany). GLS is well validated as a marker for the measurement of LV longitudinal deformation, which has emerged as a sensitive and specific marker to detect early and subtle myocardial dysfunction. In one of the recent meta-analysis, Kalam et al., have shown the independent prognostic

TABLE 4: Clinical application of HFA-PEFF scoring: Case examples.

Case examples: Clinical application of HFA-PEFF scoring	*Images*
Case 1: This 59-year-old gentleman with nonobstructive hypertrophic cardiomyopathy with heart failure had e' septal 4 cm/sec e' lateral 6 cm/sec E/e' 15 TRP 3.27 m/sec, PASP 42 mm Hg	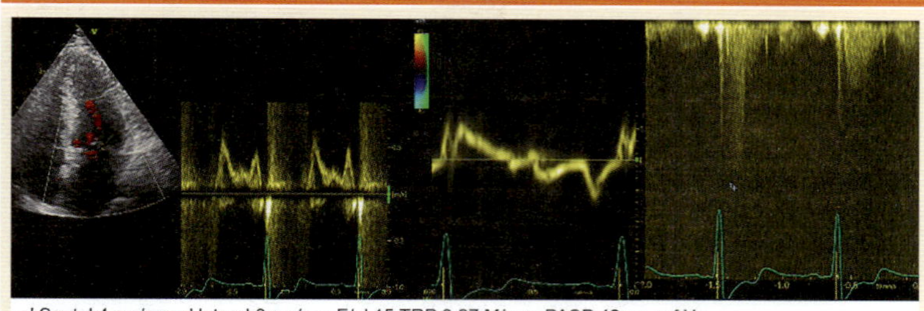 e' Septal 4 cm/sec e' lateral 6 cm/sec E/e' 15 TRP 3.27 M/sec, PASP 42 mm of Hg
• He had a left atrial volume index (LAVI) 45 mL/m^2 • Left ventricular mass index (LVMI) of 172 g/m^2 • Relative wall thickness (RWT) 0.42 • Left ventricular (LV) wall thickness of 1.2 cm	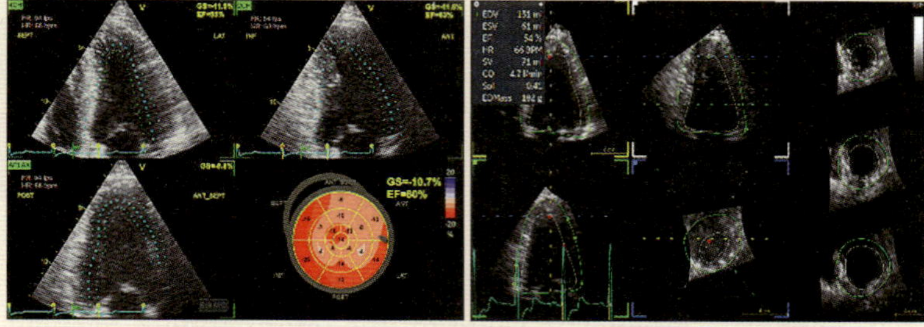
Thus, he has fulfilled the criteria for HFA-HEFF score.	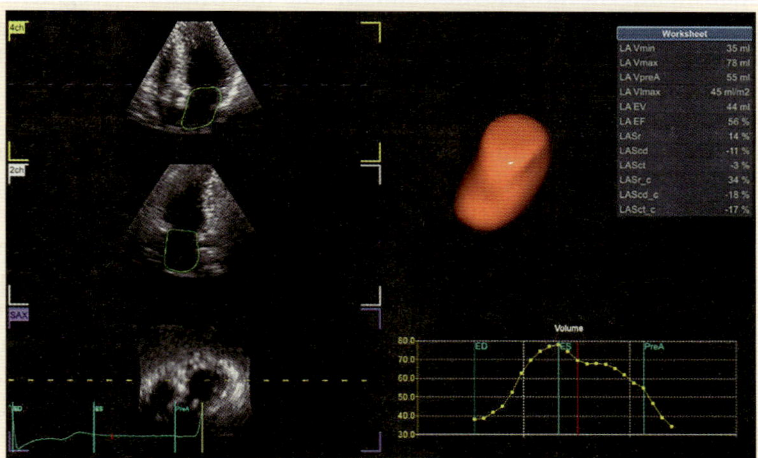
Case 2: This 69-year-old hyperthyroid lady with heart failure had an LVEF of 56% Septal e' of 3 cm/s Lateral e' of 8 cm/sec and average E/e' of 25 The TR jet velocity of 2.8 m/sec	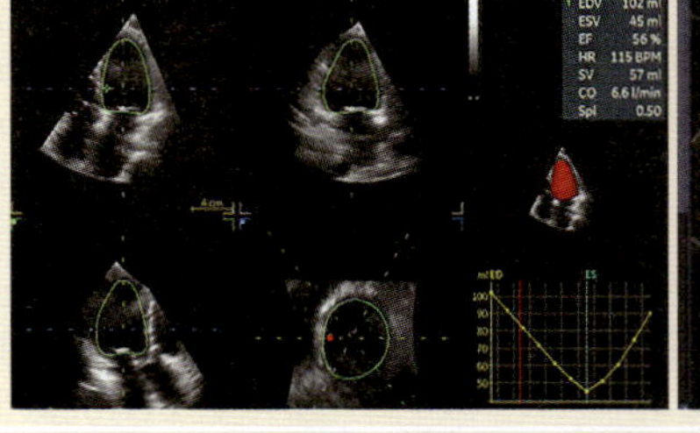 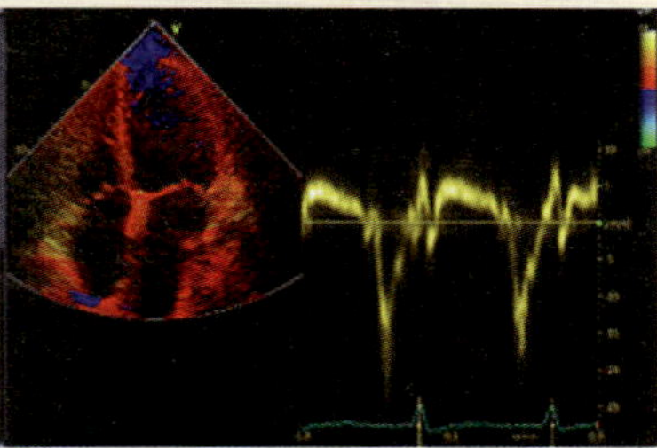
However, she had an LV GLS of 15% LA Vmax of 74 mL/m^2 LVMI of 137 g/m^2	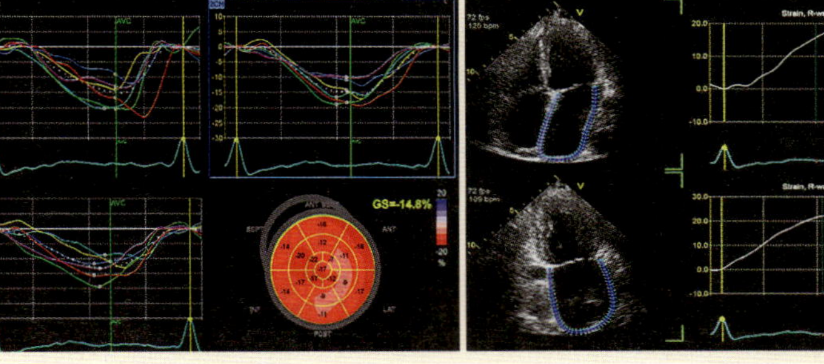

TABLE 5: Clinical applications of 4D LV strain.

Clinical applications	*Images*
4D left ventricular (LV) strain *The advantages of 4D strain are:* • Out of plane speckle motion is avoided • The Bull's eye map is dynamic • The global strain calculation is simultaneous in all segments • Area strain and left ventricular (LV) twist can be calculated with ease • At present their use is limited to patients with heart failure with preserved ejection fraction (HFpEF) and selection of patients for cardiac resynchronization therapy (CRT)	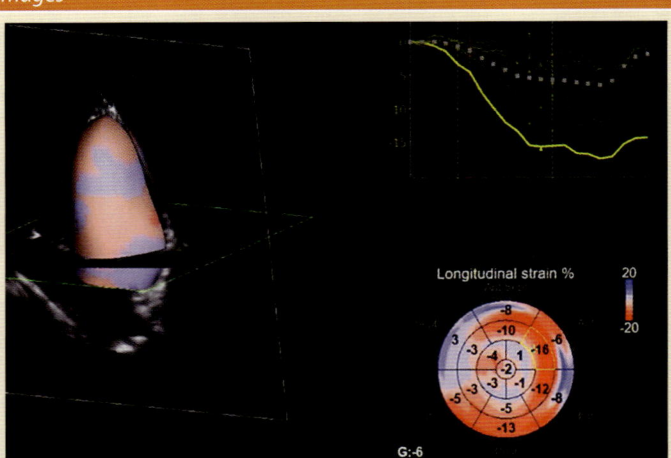

significance of GLS in patients with mild LV global impairment. The prognostic value of this information seems likely to be superior to that provided by LVEF.[34] LV GLS before discharge after ST-segment-elevation myocardial infarction is independently associated with LV dilatation at follow-up.[35] In another study of 576 patients who underwent echocardiography ≤24 hours after primary percutaneous coronary intervention for STEMI, GLS, and wall motion score index (WMSI) were comparable and both superior for early risk assessment compared with volume-based left ventricular function indicators such as LVEF and ESVI. Compared with WMSI, the advantage of GLS is the provision of a semiautomated quantitative measure.[36]

3D Evaluation of Left Ventricular Regional Function

The American Society of Echocardiography has recently recommended a 17-segment model for this.[37,38] In a 17-segment model, beginning at the anterior junction of the interventricular septum and the RV free wall and continuing counterclockwise, basal and mid ventricular segments should be labeled as anteroseptal, inferoseptal, inferior, inferolateral, anterolateral, and anterior. The apex is divided into five segments, including septal, inferior, lateral, and anterior segments, as well as the "apical cap," which is defined as the myocardium beyond the end of the LV cavity. A Bulls-eye plot can be constructed where the outer ring represents the basal segments, the middle ring represents the segments at mid-papillary muscle level, and the inner ring represents the distal level. The fact is that some manufacturers and many echocardiography laboratories never adopted these guidelines.[39] The severity of contractile dysfunction is scored visually in each segment as 1 for normal contraction or hyperkinesia, 2 for hypokinesia, 3 for akinesia, and 4 for dyskinesia. The global wall motion score is there after calculated by averaging the readings in all the segments. A score of 5 for aneurysmal segments has been deleted from the recent guidelines statement from American Society of Echocardiography.[38] A normal LV has a WMSI of 1, and the index increases as wall motion abnormalities increase in severity. A WMSI of 1.1–1.9 can predict a small infarct size, and an index ≥2.0 can predict a larger infarct size. However, this approach is subjective and operator dependent, demands complete visualization of the endocardium, and is subject to the vicissitudes of cardiac loading and heart rate. The ability of 3D echocardiography in providing tomographic slicing of Left ventricle to nine short axis tomographic slices with simultaneous display of left ventricle in apical two chamber, three chamber, and four chamber views greatly enhances diagnostic accuracy. 4D strain analysis would help in this in depicting the bull's eye plot or the automated functional imaging of the longitudinal, circumferential, area and radial strain on a scale of -20–+20 instead of the four grade regional wall motion score analysis. Further myocardial deformation analysis by speckle-tracking echocardiography has been shown to accurately predict viability in patients with chronic ischemic left ventricular dysfunction.[40] **Table 6** illustrates a case study emphasizing the use of speckle-tracking echocardiography in the importance of territorial longitudinal strain analysis.

3D Evaluation of Right Ventricular Function

Echocardiographic assessment of the right ventricle is difficult because of its complex shape. Right ventricular (RV)

TABLE 6: Left ventricular (LV) regional function and stress echo.

LV regional function and stress echo
3D echocardiography has the advantage of acquiring triplane images from LV apex, before and after treadmill Exercise from single beat acquisition. From these triplane images, the automated function imaging (AFI) bull's eye plot can be plotted easily. In this, 75-year-old diabetic patient treadmill exercise electrocardiogram (ECG) was normal. However, the postexercise bull's eye plot clearly demonstrates the new strain abnormality in the anterior septum, poststress. The coronary angiogram revealed a 99% tight mid LAD lesion.

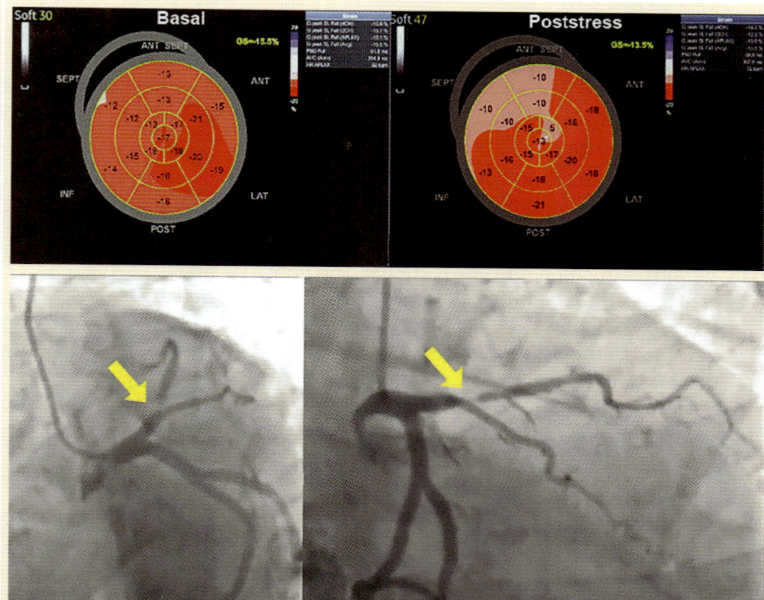

performance is known to be a major determinant of clinical status and long-term outcomes in patients with pulmonary hypertension, cardiomyopathies, and congenital heart disease. Apical acquisition of volumes is recommended in the adult population. The modified RV apical four-chamber view is used. One way (the medial approach) is to move the transducer medially to get the RV modified apical four-chamber view and then tilt the transducer cranially and anteriorly—and even rotate—to include the pulmonary valve in the guidance images. Because of the complicated structure and geometry of the right ventricle, conventional two-dimensional echocardiography is unable to correctly estimate RV volume using reasonable geometric assumptions. From the echocardiographer's perspective, the right ventricle is divided into four segments: (1) the infundibulum (or outflow tract), (2) anterior free wall, (3) lateral wall, and (4) inferior wall.[41-43] The dual blood supply (RCA and LAD) of the infundibulum and the anterior wall makes these segments the most resistant to ischemia, while the inferior wall is the most susceptible and the lateral wall has an intermediate level of susceptibility to ischemia. Steps involved in 3D evaluation of RV are shown in **Table 7**.

3D Evaluation of Left Atrium

Although 2D assessment remains the current standard for left atrial volume assessment in clinical practice, the visualization of the left atrium in 3D shape, independent of geometric assumptions, favors its use, and it may be the preferred method for LA volume assessment.[44-46] The 3D LA quantification software has the advantage in that it can be used for calculation of left atrial volume as well as left atrial strain as shown in **Table 8**. For assessing the 3D LA function, LA focused apical four chamber view is acquired and the image is optimized for alignment and temporal resolution. The mitral valve coaptation center point is land marked and the LV end diastolic, end systolic, and preatrial contraction phases are set. The results of 3D LA function analysis is displayed as LA volumetric data (LA Vmax, LA EF), LA strain values [LA Reservoir Strain (LASr), LA Conduit Strain (LAScd), and LA contraction Strain (LASct)]. LA volume and index are important factors in stress test but however they do not form part of stress echocardiography.[47-50] The advantages of LAVI stress echo are enumerated in the following text.[51-52]

- A normal LAVI (<28 mL/m^2) is a strong predictor of low cardiac risk.
- LA size predicts myocardial ischemia during stress test.
- LA dilatation during stress echo predicts abnormal contractile reserve.
- In patients with hypertrophic cardiomyopathy, LAVI predicts increased risk of arrhythmias and major cardiac events.[53]

LAVI stress echocardiography case studies are shown in **Tables 9 and 10**.

TABLE 7: Clinical applications of 3D echocardiography for right ventricular (RV) function in heart failure preserved ejection fraction (HFpEF).

Clinical application	*Images*
RV function: 3D echocardiographic RV functional analysis correlates with cardiovascular magnetic resonance (CMR) because of inclusion of RV inlet, trabecular body and outlet. *Case 1:* On the right the RV function analysis in a patient with Brugada syndrome is shown. The right ventricular ejection fraction (RVEF) of 59% correlated with CMR derived RVEF.	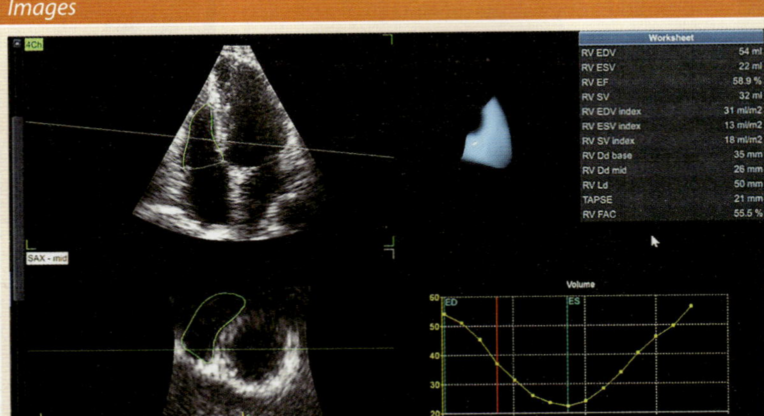
Case 2: The figures from a known case of systemic lupus erythematosus with severe pulmonary hypertension are shown. **Figures 1A, D, and E** show the dilated and hypertrophic RV. She had grade III tricuspid regurgitation and trivial pulmonary regurgitation. The predicted pulmonary artery pressure was 104/35 mm of mercury.	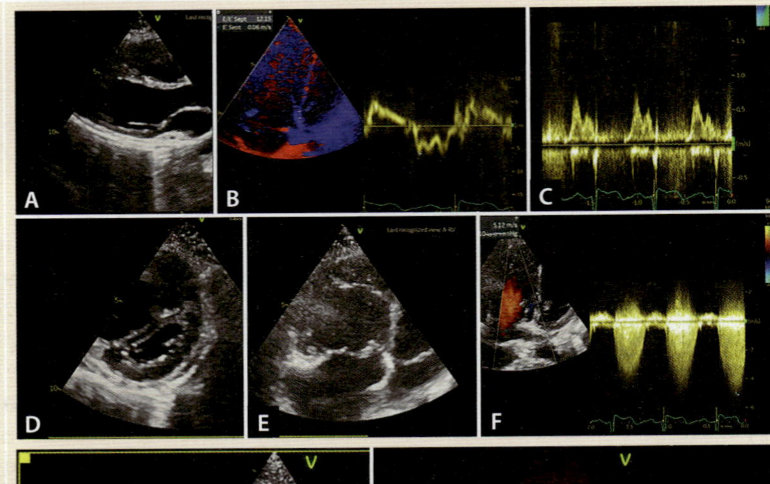
Figs. 2A and B: Interatrial septum bulges into left atrium with opening of flap valve and minimal right-to-left shunt.	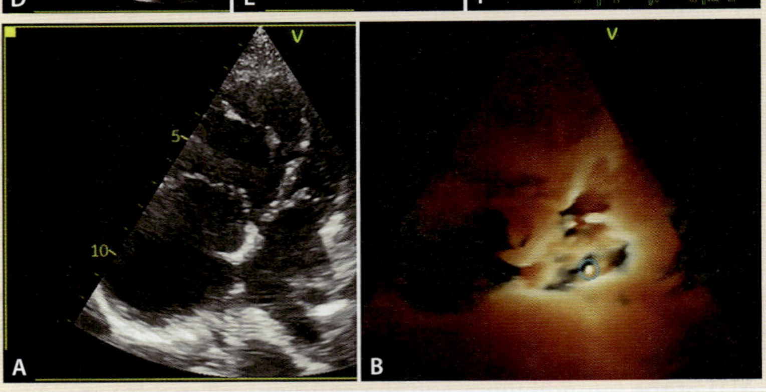
Fig. 3: There was right ventricular dysfunction with right ventricular (RV) ejection fraction of 35%, RV free wall strain of -18% and TAPSE 17 mm. She had a normal left ventricular ejection fraction (LVEF) of 59%. The LV GLS was—20% and she had normal left ventricular pressure strain loop.	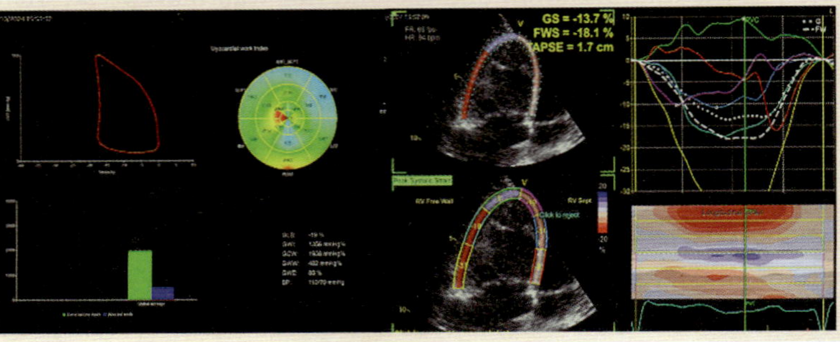

Contd...

Contd...

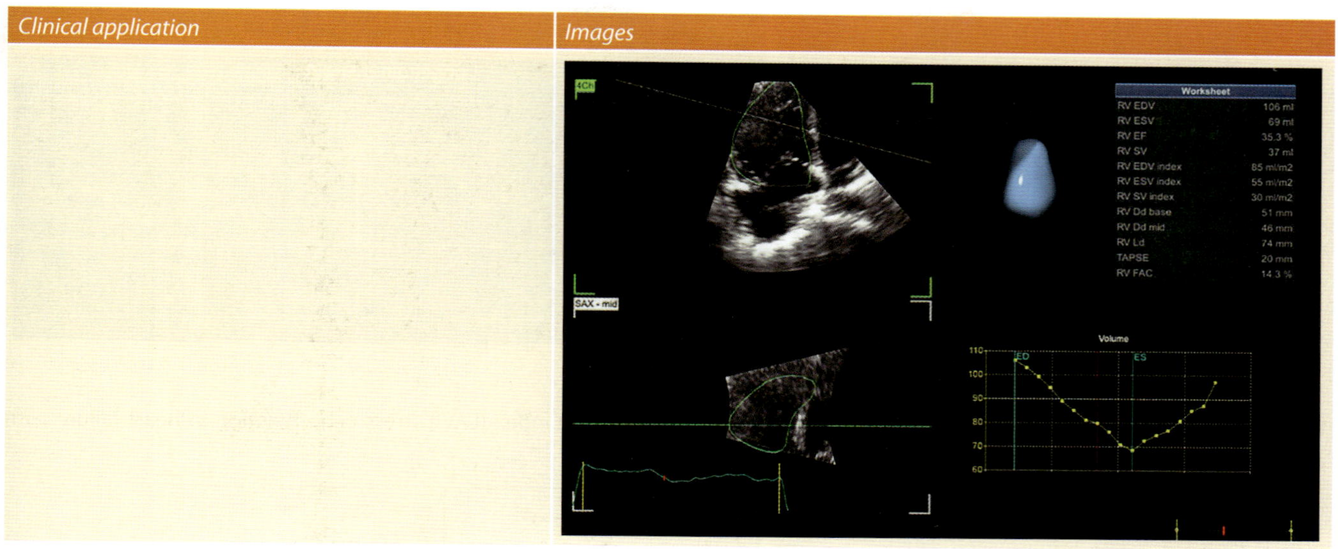

TABLE 8: Clinical application of 3D echocardiography for left atrium (LA) function.

Clinical application	*Images*
LA function A. For assessing the 3D LA function, LA focused apical four chamber view is acquired and the image is optimized for alignment and temporal resolution. The mitral valve coaptation center point is land marked and the LV end diastolic, end systolic and preatrial contraction phases are set. The results of 3D LA function analysis is displayed as LA volumetric data (LA Vmax, LAEF), LA strain values [LA reservoir strain (LASr), LA conduit strain LAScd, and LA contraction strain LASct].	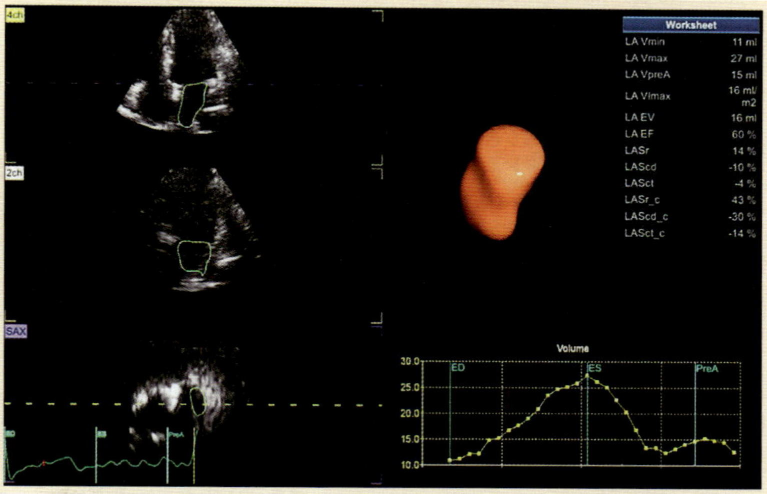
B. Normal LA strain curve is displayed (The normal LA reservoir strain is around 40%).	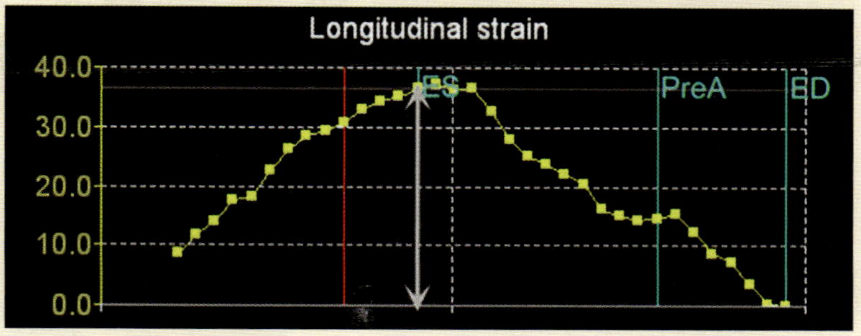

Contd...

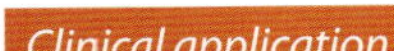

Contd...

Clinical application	*Images*
C. LA strain curve in the patient with Brugada syndrome referred above: Showing abnormally reduced LASr to 14%.	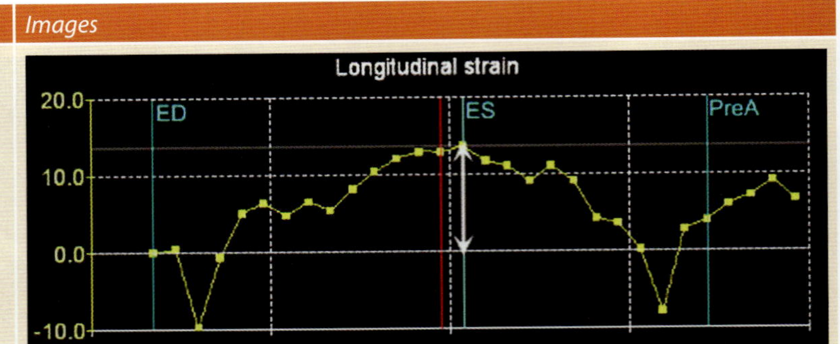

TABLE 9: Clinical application of 3D echocardiography for left atrial volume index (LAVI) stress echo function in heart failure with preserved ejection fraction (HFpEF).

Figs. 1A and B: For performing the 3D LAVI stress echocardiography, standard treadmill exercise electrocardiogram can be combined with acquisition of triplane left atrial focused four chamber view at basal and peak exercise or poststress. **Figure 1A** depicts left ventricular (LV) focused apical four chamber view and **Figure 1B** depicts left atrium (LA) focused apical four chamber view. Global and territorial longitudinal strain analysis of left ventricle are performed initially at the basal and poststress.	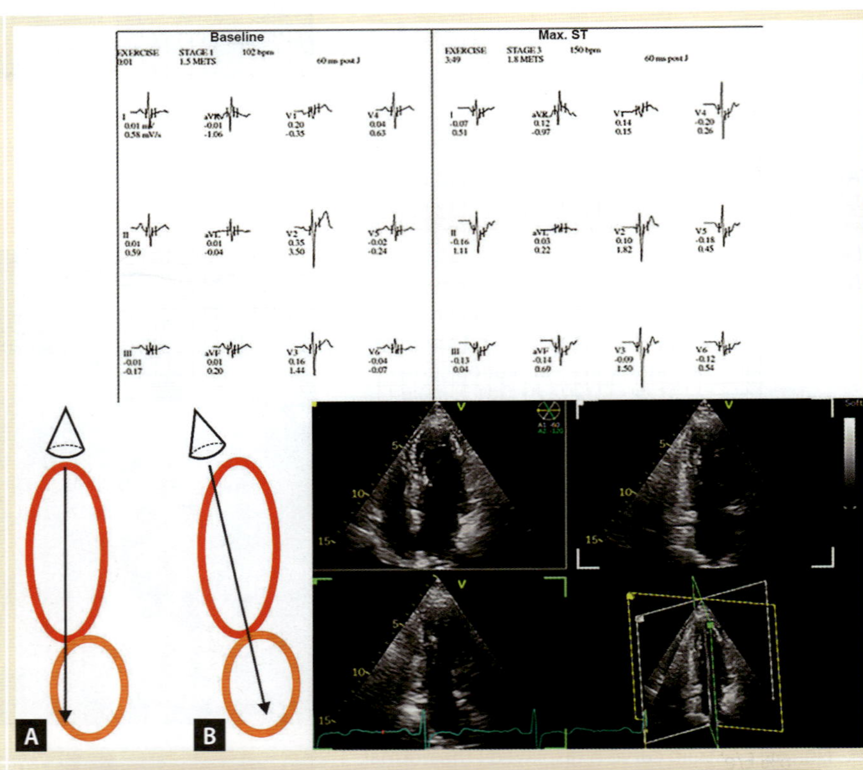
Fig. 2: In a 59-year-old diabetic patient, with unstable angina and markedly positive Bruce protocol treadmill exercise ECG shown above, LAVI stress echocardiogram was done. The basal left ventricular ejection fraction (LVEF) 57%, global longitudinal strain (GLS)—18.7%, LAVI 25 mL/m^2 LASr 37%.	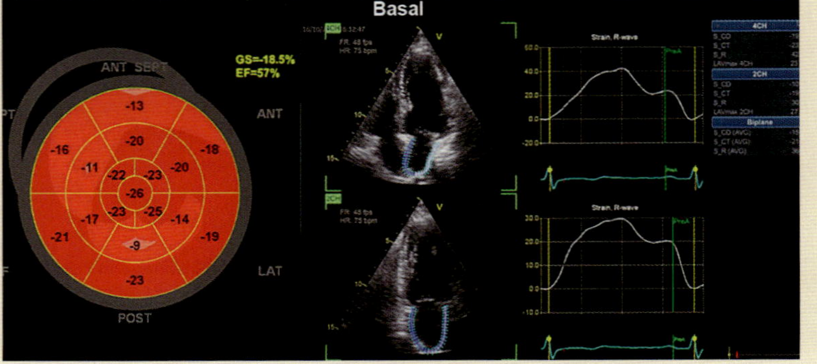

Contd...

Contd...

The poststress LVEF 68%, GLS—18% with stress, there was new territorial longitudinal strain abnormality in anterior septum and anterolateral wall. LAVI 21 mL/m^2 LASr 31%. This hemodynamic profile is suggestive of LAVI reduction or nondilation with stress. The predictors of LAVI reduction and nondilation with stress are E/e' <14, LVEF >50% and rest LAVI <35 mL/m^2 LAVI dilation is three times more common with heart failure with reduced ejection fraction (HFrEF).	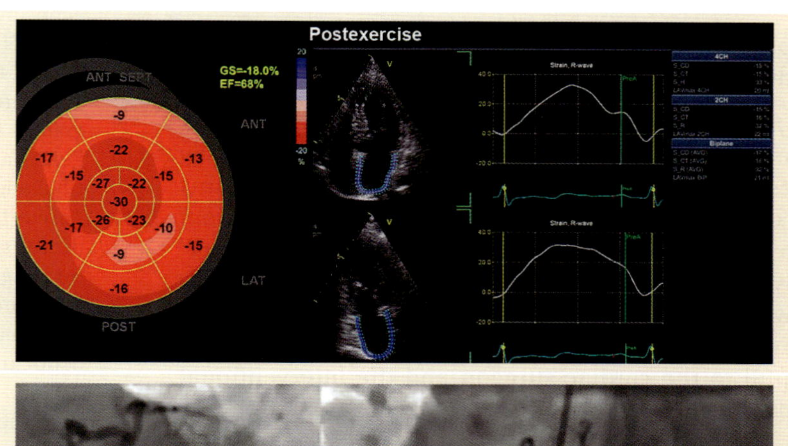
The angiogram in this patient revealed 90% lesion of the main OM, for which he underwent stenting.	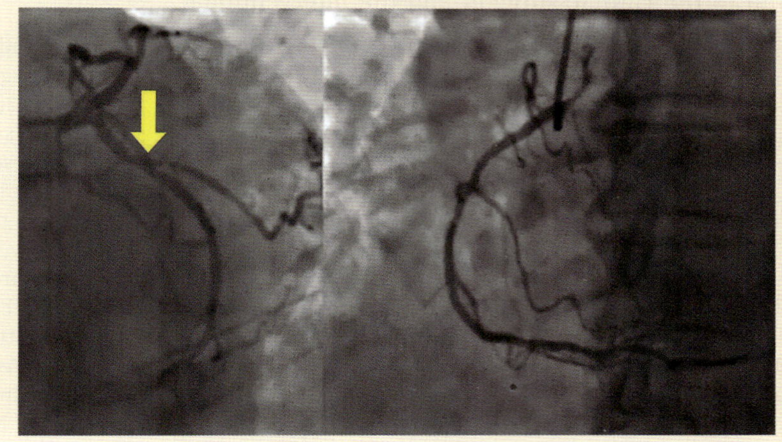

TABLE 10: Clinical application of 3D echocardiography for left atrial volume index (LAVI) stress echo function in heart failure with reduced ejection fraction (HFrEF).

Clinical application	*Images*
This 62-year-old diabetic patient with history of chronic alcoholism, (200 mL of whisky/day for 20 years) performed treadmill exercise electrocardiogram (ECG). His basal left ventricular ejection fraction (LVEF) was 26%, global longitudinal strain (GLS)—6% E/e' 25. He performed only 3 Mets of Ex with LVEF 33%, GLS—8%, and E/e' 25.	Basal GS=-5.7% EF=26% Poststress GS=-8.3% EF=33%
LAVI basal 70 mL left atrial reservoir strain (LASr)—2% Poststress 81 mL LASr 12%.	Basal Poststress

CONCLUSION

At present the following are the areas where 3D echocardiography has demonstrated the usefulness:[54]

LV function assessment: By eliminating the need for geometric modeling and avoiding errors caused by foreshortened views, 3D echocardiography remains the choice of methods for determination of LV function. Its results are comparable to cardiac MRI and are economically cheaper. By the current photo realistic *enFace* views of cardiac valves, congenital abnormalities and their supporting structures, 3D imaging is particularly helpful to the cardiac surgeon and the interventional cardiologist.

RV volume assessment: 3D echocardiography is the only economically viable alternative to cardiac MRI in evaluation of RV function. Permits evaluation of regional LV function and objective detection of wall motion abnormalities. Regional wall motion abnormality and LV systolic dyssynchrony assessment by 3D echocardiography serve as an additional referral criterion for cardiac resynchronization therapy. 3D derived LA volume and index along with LA strain are important factors in stress echocardiography though may not be part of routine stress echocardiography.

REFERENCES

1. Savarese G, Becher PM, Lund LH, et al. "Global burden of heart failure: a comprehensive and updated review of epidemiology." Cardiovasc Res. 2023;118(17):3272-87.
2. Heidenreich PA, Albert NM, Allen LA, et al. "Forecasting the impact of heart failure in the United States: a policy statement from the American Heart Association." Circ Heart Fail. 2013;6(3):606-19.
3. Kittleson MM, Panjrath GS, Amancherla K, et al. 2023 ACC expert consensus decision pathway on management of heart failure with preserved ejection fraction: a report of the American College of Cardiology Solution Set Oversight Committee. J Am Coll Cardiol. 2023;81(18):1835-78.
4. Handke M, Heinrichs G, Moser U, et al. Transesophageal real-time three-dimensional Echocardiography. Methods and initial in vitro and human in vivo studies. J Am Coll Cardiol. 2006;48(10):2070-6.
5. Sugeng L, Shernan SK, Salgo IS, et al. Live 3-dimensional transesophageal echocardiography initial experience using the fully-sampled matrix array probe. Am Coll Cardiol. 2008;52(6):446-9.
6. Mor-Avi V, Sugeng L, Lang RM. Real-time 3-dimensional echocardiography. An integral component of the routine echocardiographic examination in adult patients? Circulation. 2009;119(2):314-29.
7. Bhan A, Kapetanakis S, Monaghan MJ. Three-dimensional echocardiography. Heart. 2010;96(2):153-63.
8. Johri AM, Passeri JJ, Picard MH. Three dimensional echocardiography: approaches and clinical utility. Heart. 2010;96(5):390-7.
9. Faletra FF, Ho SY, Auricchio PA. Anatomy of right atrial structures by real-time 3D transesophageal echocardiography. JACC Cardiovasc imaging. 2010;3(3):966-75.
10. Pearlman AS. Echocardiography 2020: Opportunities and Challenges. JASE. 2010;23(8):P898-900.
11. Latcu DG, Rinaldi JP, Saoudi N. Real-time three-dimensional transoesophageal echocardiography for diagnosis of left atrial appendage thrombus. Eur J Echocardiogr. 2009;10(5):711-2.
12. Szmigielski C, Rajpoot K, Grau V, et al. Real-time 3D fusion echocardiography. J Am Coll Cardiol Img. 2010;3(7):682-90.
13. Hilberath JN, Oakes DA, Shernan SK, et al. Safety of transesophageal echocardiography. J Am Soc Echocardiogr. 2010; 23(11):1115-27.
14. Rulands FA, Breithardt D, Brehmer OA, et al. Transthoracic high-resolution real-time three-dimensional echocardiography for the analysis of regional left-ventricular wall motion patterns in patients with cardiac resynchronization therapy. Eur Heart J. 2003;24:396.
15. Heidenreich PA, Bozkurt B, Aguilar D, et al. 2022 AHA/ACC/HFSA Guideline for the Management of Heart Failure: A Report of the American College of Cardiology/American Heart Association Joint Committee on Clinical Practice Guidelines. J Am Coll Cardiol. 2022;79(17):e263-e421.
16. Pfeffer MA, Shah AM, Borlaug BA. Heart failure with preserved ejection fraction in perspective. Circ Res. 2019; 124(11):1598-617.
17. Reddy YNV, Kaye DM, Handoko ML, et al. Diagnosis of heart failure with preserved ejection fraction among patients with unexplained dyspnea. JAMA Cardiol. 2022; 7(9):891-9.
18. McDonagh TA, Metra M, Adamo M, et al. 2021 ESC Guidelines for the diagnosis and treatment of acute and chronic heart failure Developed by the Task Force for the diagnosis and treatment of acute and chronic heart failure of the European Society of Cardiology (ESC). With the special contribution of the Heart Failure Association (HFA) of the ESC. Eur Heart J. 2021;42(36):3599-726.
19. Pieske B, Tschöpe C, de Boer RA, et al. How to diagnose heart failure with preserved ejection fraction: the HFA-PEFF diagnostic algorithm: a consensus recommendation from the Heart Failure Association (HFA) of the European Society of Cardiology (ESC). Eur Heart J. 2021;42(13):1274.
20. Tada A, Nagai T, Omote K, et al. Performance of the H_2FPEF and the HFA-PEFF scores for the diagnosis of heart failure with preserved ejection fraction in Japanese patients: A report from the Japanese multicenter registry. Int J Cardiol. 2021;342:43-8.
21. Bonelli A, Degiovanni A, Beretta D, et al. H2FPEF and HFA-PEFF scores performance and the additional value of cardiac structure and function in patients with atrial fibrillation. Int J Cardiol. 2024;413:132385.

22. Mert GÖ, Özlek B, Özlek E, et al. Comparing the Diagnostic Performance of HFA-PEFF and H2FPEF Scoring Systems in Heart Failure with Preserved Ejection Fraction Patients: Insights from the APOLLON Registry. Anatol J Cardiol. 2023;27(9):539-48.
23. Ariyaratnam J, Mishima R, Kadhim K, et al. Utility and validity of the HFA-PEFF and H2FPEF scores in patients with symptomatic atrial fibrillation. J Am Coll Cardiol. 2024;12(6):1015-25.
24. Golla MSG, Shams P. Heart Failure With Preserved Ejection Fraction (HFpEF). In: Stat Pearls [Internet]. Treasure Island (FL): Stat Pearls Publishing; 2024.
25. Forsyth F, Brimicombe J, Cheriyan J, et al.; OPTIMISE HFPEF investigators and collaborator. Diagnosis of patients with heart failure with preserved ejection fraction in primary care: cohort study. ESC Heart Fail. 2021;8:4562-71.
26. Arques S. Clinical Relevance of the Spectral Tissue Doppler E/e' Ratio in the Management of Patients with Atrial Fibrillation: a Comprehensive Review of the Literature. J Atr Fibrillation. 2018;11(2):2038.
27. Tsang W, Salgo IS, Medvedofsky D, et al. Transthoracic 3D echocardiographic left heart chamber quantification using an automated adaptive analytics algorithm. J Am Coll Cardiol Img. 2016;9(7):769-82.
28. Beladan CC, Călin A, Roşca M, et al. Left ventricular twist dynamics: principles and applications. Heart. 2014;100: 731-40.
29. Helle-Valle T, Crosby J, Edvardsen T, et al. New noninvasive method for assessment of left ventricular rotation: speckle tracking echocardiography. Circulation. 2005;112: 3149-56.
30. Ashraf M, Myronenko A, Nguyen T, et al. Defining left ventricular apex-to-base twist mechanics computed from high-resolution 3D echocardiography: validation against sonomicrometry. JACC Cardiovasc Imaging. 2010;3: 227-34.
31. Marwick TH. Methods used for the assessment of LV systolic function: common currency or tower of Babel? Heart. 2013;99:1078-86.
32. Mannaerts HF, van der Heide JA, Kamp O, et al. Early identification of left ventricular remodelling after myocardial infarction, assessed by transthoracic 3D echocardiography. Eur Heart J. 2004;25:680-7.
33. Mollema SA, Nucifora G, Bax JJ. Prognostic value of echocardiography after acute myocardial infarction. Heart. 2009;95:1732-45.
34. Kalam K, Otahal P, Marwick TH. Prognostic implications of global LV dysfunction: a systematic review and meta-analysis of global longitudinal strain and ejection fraction. Heart. 2014;100:1673-80.
35. Joyce E, Hoogslag GE, Leong DP, et al. Association between left ventricular global longitudinal strain and adverse left ventricular dilatation after ST-segment–elevation myocardial infarction. Circulation: Cardiovasc Imaging. 2014;7(1):74-81.
36. Munk K, Andersen NH, Terkelsen CJ, et al. Global left ventricular longitudinal systolic strain for early risk assessment in patients with acute myocardial infarction treated with primary percutaneous intervention. J Am Soc Echocardiogr. 2012;25(6):644-51.
37. Schiller NB, Shah PM, Crawford M, et al. Recommendations for quantitation of the left ventricle by two-dimensional echocardiography. American Society of Echocardiography Committee on Standards, Subcommittee on Quantitation of Two-Dimensional Echocardiograms. J Am Soc Echocardiogr. 1989;2(5):358-67.
38. Lang RM, Badano LP, Mor-Avi V, et al. Recommendations for Cardiac Chamber Quantification by Echocardiography in Adults: An Update from the American Society of Echocardiography and the European Association of Cardiovascular Imaging. J Am Soc Echocardiogr. 2015; 28(1):1-39.
39. Feigenbaum H. Echocardiographic chamber quantification in the era of multimodality imaging: beware of unintended consequences. J Am Soc Echocardiogr. 2015; 28(7):847-50.
40. Altiok E, Tiemann S, Becker M, et al. Myocardial Deformation Imaging by Two-Dimensional Speckle-Tracking Echocardiography for Prediction of Global and Segmental Functional Changes after Acute Myocardial Infarction: A Comparison with Late Gadolinium Enhancement Cardiac Magnetic Resonance. J Am Soc Echocardiogr. 2014;27(3):249-57.
41. Rudski LG, Lai WW, Afilalo J, et al. Guidelines for the echocardiographic assessment of the right heart in adults: a report from the American Society of Echocardiography endorsed by the European Association of Echocardiography, a registered branch of the European Society of Cardiology, and the Canadian Society of Echocardiography. J Am Soc Echocardiogr. 2010;23(7):685-713.
42. Rallidis LS, Makavos G, Nihoyannopoulos P. Right ventricular involvement in coronary artery disease: role of echocardiography for diagnosis and prognosis. J Am Soc Echocardiogr. 2014;27(3):223-9.
43. Ostenfeld E, Flachskampf FA. Assessment of right ventricular volumes and ejection fraction by echocardiography: from geometric approximations to realistic shapes. Echo Res Pract. 2015;2(1):R1-R11.
44. Miyasaka Y, Tsujimoto S, Maeba H, et al. Left atrial volume by real-time three-dimensional echocardiography: validation by 64-slice multidetector computed tomography. J Am Soc Echocardiogr. 2011;24(6):680-6.
45. Marsan NA, Tops LF, Holman ER, et al. Comparison of left atrial volumes and function by real-time three dimensional echocardiography in patients having catheter ablation for atrial fibrillation with persistence of sinus rhythm versus recurrent atrial fibrillation three months later. Am J Cardiol. 2008;102:847-53.
46. Delgado V, Vidal B, Sitges M, et al. Fate of left atrial function as determined by real-time three-dimensional echocardiography study after radiofrequency catheter

ablation for the treatment of atrial fibrillation. Am J Cardiol. 2008;101:1285-90.
47. Nagueh SF, Smiseth OA, Appleton CP, et al. Recommendations for the Evaluation of Left Ventricular Diastolic Function by Echocardiography: An Update from the American Society of Echocardiography and the European Association of Cardiovascular Imaging. Eur Heart J Cardiovasc Imaging. 2016;17(12):1321-60.
48. Poulsen MK, Dahl JS, Henriksen JE, et al. Left atrial volume index: relation to long-term clinical outcome in type 2 diabetes. J Am Coll Cardiol. 2013;62(25):2416-21.
49. Abhayaratna WP, Seward JB, Appleton CP, et al. Left atrial size: physiologic determinants and clinical applications. J Am Coll Cardiol. 2006;47(12):2357-63.
50. Prota C, Cortigiani L, Campagnano E, et al. Left atrium stress echocardiography: correlation between left atrial volume, function, and B-lines at rest and during stress. Explor Cardiol. 2024;2:19-30.
51. Alsaileek AA, Osranek M, Fatema K, et al. Predictive value of normal left atrial volume in stress echocardiography. J Am Coll Cardiol. 2006;47(5):P1024-8.
52. Badano LP, Kolias TJ, Muraru D, et al. Industry representatives, Reviewers: This document was reviewed by members of the 2016–2018 EACVI Scientific Documents Committee. Standardization of left atrial, right ventricular, and right atrial deformation imaging using two-dimensional speckle tracking echocardiography: a consensus document of the EACVI/ASE/Industry Task Force to standardize deformation imaging. Eur Heart J Cardiovasc Imaging. 2018;19(6):591-600.
53. Wierzbowska-Drabik K, Kasprzak JD, Haberka M, et al. Left atrial volume changes during exercise stress echocardiography in heart failure and hypertrophic cardiomyopathy. Hellenic J Cardiol. 2022;67:9-18.
54. Mor Avi V, Lang RM. Three dimensional echocardiography. UpToDate. 2024;1-43.

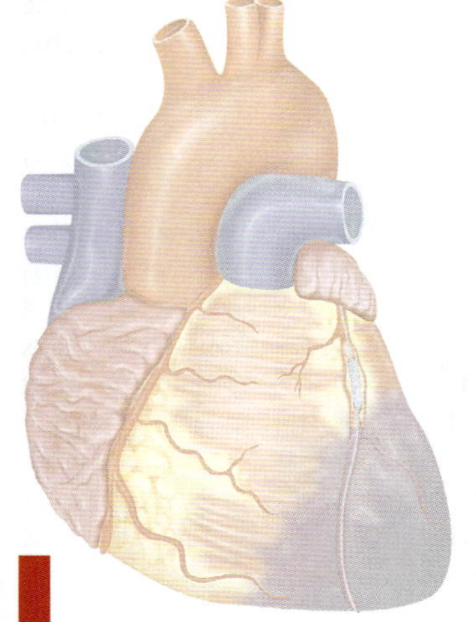

Echocardiographic Evaluation of Atrial Fibrillation with Atriopathy and Thromboembolism

Manish Bansal, Ravi R Kasliwal, HK Chopra

INTRODUCTION

Atrial fibrillation (AF) is the most common arrhythmia encountered in clinical practice. The estimated global prevalence of AF was 50 million in 2020.[1,2] The overall lifetime risk of AF is about 15–40% in different ethnic groups with the highest risk in the White individuals.[3] Aging is one of the most important risk factors for AF, with every 5-year increase in the age associated with a hazard ratio of 1.43–1.66 for AF.[4,5]

Systemic thromboembolism, especially stroke, is the most dreadful complication of AF. Overall, there is a 2.4-fold increase in the risk of stroke in patients with AF.[6] The risk increases with the increasing number of predisposing risk factors accompanying AF. The CHA_2DS_2-VASc score, which incorporates many of these risk factors, is a clinically useful tool to predict the risk of stroke in AF and for guiding management.

Left atrial (LA) dilatation, fibrosis, and dysfunction are the primary pathophysiological substrates for AF. Once AF sets in, it propagates these abnormalities, initiating a vicious cycle. The same pathophysiological abnormalities also lead to the formation of thrombi in the left atrium and LA appendage (LAA), creating a source of systemic embolism. Given the intrinsic role of LA dilatation and dysfunction in the initiation and propagation of AF as well as the occurrence of systemic embolism, a thorough evaluation of the left atrium is essential in all patients who present with an embolic event due to AF. Echocardiography is the best modality for this purpose.

ECHOCARDIOGRAPHIC ASSESSMENT OF LEFT ATRIUM IN ATRIAL FIBRILLATION WITH SYSTEMIC EMBOLISM

The LA abnormalities in AF can arise from several different mechanisms. Increased left ventricular (LV) filling pressure is one of the most common reasons. The raised LV filling pressure is transmitted back to the left atrium, causing its dilatation and subsequent dysfunction. There are many conditions that cause AF through this mechanism, including heart failure (HF) with reduced ejection fraction, HF with preserved ejection fraction, severe aortic stenosis, restrictive cardiomyopathy, etc.

Atrial fibrillation can also occur in the absence of elevated LV filling pressure. Significant mitral stenosis or regurgitation increases LA load and can lead to AF. Numerous other cardiac conditions that cause myopericardial inflammation such as rheumatic heart disease, pericarditis, and acute myocarditis can also trigger AF. Lastly, AF can also occur as a primary event without any hemodynamic abnormalities affecting the left atrium and without any identifiable cause. The cardiac diseases that affect the right atrium may also lead to the development of AF.

Regardless of the mechanism, AF is associated with LA dilatation and dysfunction, both of which can be reliably assessed with echocardiography. In addition, echocardiography also helps to rule out any LA/LAA clot and allows assessment of the LAA structure and function.

ECHOCARDIOGRAPHIC ASSESSMENT OF LEFT ATRIAL SIZE

Left atrial size has a direct relationship with the risk of AF. Larger the left atrium, greater the risk of AF and its recurrence after successful restoration of sinus rhythm, either through pharmacological or electrical cardioversion or catheter ablation.

Traditionally, the LA anteroposterior diameter obtained from the parasternal long-axis view has been the primary measurement used for assessing the LA size. However, being a unidimensional measurement, it often underestimates the LA enlargement; therefore, the current guidelines do not recommend LA diameter as a preferred measure of the LA size.[7]

Left atrial volume (LAV) is the current gold standard for quantifying the LA size.[7] Two echocardiographic methods are used most commonly for estimating the LAV—the area-length method and biplane Simpson's method. Of the two, the latter is currently preferred because of the ease of the measurement. More recently, the three-dimensional echocardiography-based LAV estimation has also become feasible.

The basic principles for LAV estimation using the biplane Simpson's method are the same as for the left ventricle. First, the LA-focused apical four- and two-chamber views that avoid LA foreshortening are acquired. Subsequently, the LA endocardial border is traced in both these views in the end-systolic frame (ventricular end-systole). The tracing extends from one end of the mitral annulus to the other, while excluding the pulmonary vein openings and LAA. The inbuilt software available on the echocardiography machine then calculates the LAV automatically **(Fig. 1)**. LAV is then indexed to the body surface area to yield the LAV index (LAVI), which is the recommended volumetric measure of the LA size. The upper limit of normal for LAVI is 34 mL/m^2 for both genders.[7]

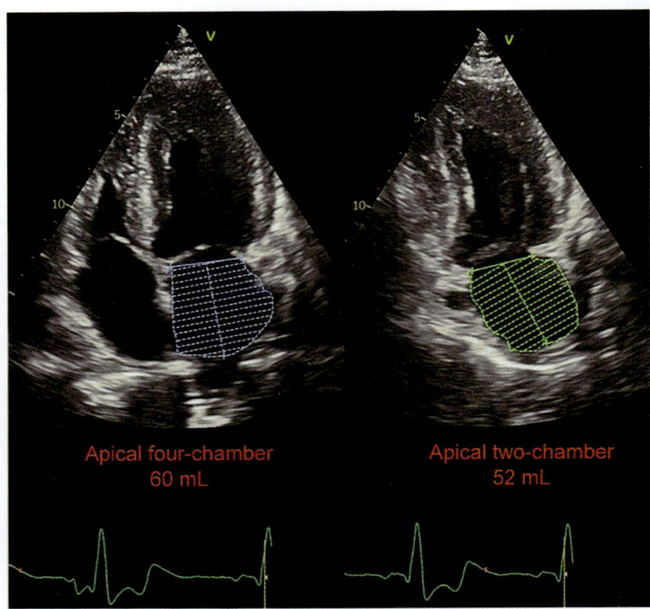

Fig. 1: Measurement of left atrial volume using the biplane Simpson's method. The average left atrial volume in this patient was 56 mL.

Utility of Left Atrial Volume for Predicting Atrial Fibrillation and Systemic Embolism

Left atrial size (LA diameter in older studies and LAV or LAVI in the recent studies) is a strong predictor of adverse cardiovascular outcomes. It is associated with increased risk of AF, HF hospitalizations, stroke, and cardiovascular as well as all-cause mortality.[8-18] A meta-analysis of several studies showed that each 10 mL/m^2 increase in the baseline LAVI was associated with a 22% increased adjusted hazard for all-cause mortality.[19]

Several studies have shown that increased LAVI is a strong predictor of new-onset AF or AF recurrence after interventions. A meta-analysis was performed, which included 31 studies with 2,725 patients with a mean follow-up period of 6.5 months. Each unit increase in the LAVI was associated with a 6% increase in the risk of AF recurrence after electrical cardioversion.[20] Another meta-analysis showed similar findings in patients undergoing radiofrequency ablation.[21] Larger LAV/LAVI significantly increased the odds of having AF recurrence after ablation. LAVI has also been shown to predict AF recurrence after other modes of ablation such as cryoablation.[22,23]

Left atrial volume is also a strong predictor of stroke risk with or without preexisting AF. In a study, including 1,554 elderly subjects with no prior AF, LAV was independently predictive of the first ischemic stroke and death.[15] Among patients presenting with cryptogenic stroke, increased LAVI is associated with greater likelihood of cardioembolic stroke, stroke recurrence, and the new-onset AF.[24,25] LAV is also associated with the presence of LAA thrombus.[26,27]

LEFT ATRIAL STRAIN

Although LAVI has good prognostic value, it is limited by the fact that it only reflects the chronic changes in the LA loading conditions. For this reason, it is also known as the glycosylated hemoglobin of the LV diastolic dysfunction. The LA strain offers unique advantages in this context. Most importantly, it is more sensitive than LAVI to subtle and short-term changes in LA hemodynamics. It is also easier to measure than LAVI.

Speckle tracking echocardiography (STE) is the modality used for measuring LA strain. It is a grayscale-based technique, and the same LA-focused apical four-chamber image as used for the LAV assessment can be used for LA strain measurement also. A good quality electrocardiogram with well visible P waves is essential for STE. The image sector should be narrowed to improve the lateral resolution. Artifacts should be minimized. Once a proper image is acquired, it is analyzed using the STE software. The LA endocardial border is traced in the same manner as for LAV estimation. Once the endocardial border is traced, the software generates a region of interest, which is usually 3 mm thick. After verifying that the region of interest follows the LA contour, covers the LA myocardium properly, and does not extend into the pericardium, the software is allowed to process the image and generates the LA strain curve.

The default analysis method uses QRS as the reference, and the LA strain curve thus generated is depicted in **Figure 2**. The strain value at the beginning is zero, and as the left atrium stretches during systole, the LA strain increases and reaches a peak just before the opening of the mitral valve. This peak represents the LA reservoir strain (LARS) or peak atrial longitudinal strain (PALS), which is the primary LA strain measure used for clinical purposes. Once the mitral valve opens, the LA size decreases, resulting in a reduction in the LA strain, which reaches a plateau during diastasis. The difference between the earlier peak and this plateau represents the LA conduit strain. Subsequently, as the left atrium contracts during the late diastole, there is further reduction in the LA strain, which eventually reaches the baseline. This last phase represents the LA contraction strain.

A meta-analysis of 40 studies showed that the normal value of LARS is 39% (95% confidence interval 38–41%).[28] However, a value of approximately 22–23% is considered the lower limit of the normal.[29]

Clinical Utility of Left Atrial Strain in Atrial Fibrillation and Systemic Embolism

Left atrial strain has emerged as a useful measure of the cumulative LA overload and is a sensitive measure of LA dysfunction and remodeling. It correlates well with the invasively measured LV filling pressure as well as the extent of the LA myocardial fibrosis.[30-32] The incorporation of

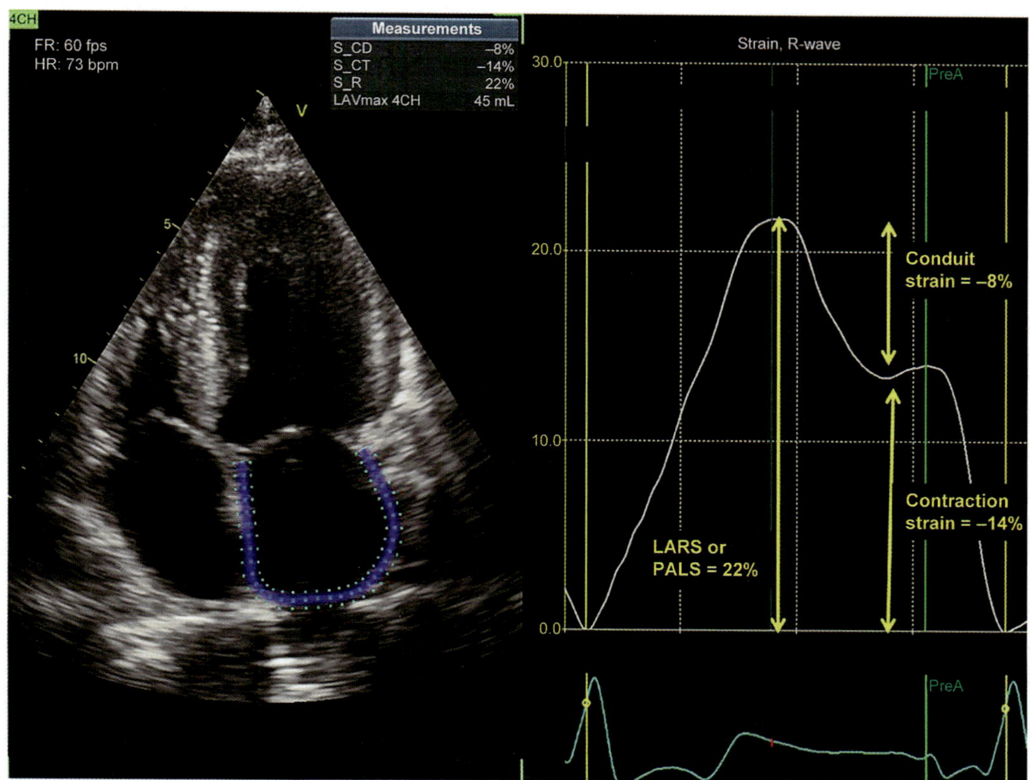

Fig. 2: Left atrial strain measurement using QRS as the reference point (please see the text for more details). (LARS: left atrial reservoir strain; PALS: peak atrial longitudinal strain)

LARS in the echocardiographic algorithms recommended for LV diastolic function assessment has been shown to improve their diagnostic accuracy. Furthermore, LARS performs better than LAVI for this purpose.[31,33-36]

Left atrial strain is also a good predictor of AF in patients who are at risk for developing it.[33,37-43] In a recent study, which followed up 4,312 consecutive patients admitted with acute HF, the incidence of new-onset AF among 2,461 patients in sinus rhythm at baseline was assessed. Reduced LARS (<18%) was a significant predictor of AF risk over a follow-up of 5 years. The authors also developed a risk score (HAS-BAP), which included LARS and had good accuracy for predicting AF.[37]

Left atrial strain also predicts AF recurrence after cardioversion or catheter ablation.[44-47] In a study involving 256 patients with paroxysmal or persistent AF undergoing catheter ablation, reduced LA strain (<23.2%) was associated with a higher risk of AF recurrence after ablation.[45] Similar findings have also been shown in patients undergoing electrical cardioversion.[44]

Left atrial strain is also a good predictor of LAA thrombosis and the stroke risk in AF.[44,48,49] A study followed up 190 patients with persistent AF for a mean duration of 29 months during which 15 strokes occurred. LA strain was one of the independent predictors of the stroke risk and enhanced the prognostic value of CHA_2DS_2-VASc score for this purpose.[48] Another study found LA strain to have a stronger association than CHA_2DS_2-VASc score with the embolic risk in 286 patients with AF, 82 of which had presented with acute embolism. LA strain also predicted mortality risk in these patients with embolism over a median follow-up period of 425 days.[49]

LEFT ATRIAL APPENDAGE ASSESSMENT

The LAA is the most common site for thrombus formation and subsequent embolism in AF. Approximately, 90% of intracardiac thrombi in nonrheumatic AF and 60% in patients with rheumatic mitral valve disease form within the LAA **(Fig. 3)**.[50] Hence, exclusion of LAA thrombus is mandatory prior to cardioversion or catheter ablation of AF.

The LAA is a small, pyramidal structure situated on the lateral aspect of the left atrium, abutting the main pulmonary artery and left superior pulmonary vein. It has a very variable and complex anatomy with multiple lobes,[51] and hence, a comprehensive assessment is needed to reliably rule out LAA thrombus **(Fig. 4)**.[52] Transesophageal echocardiography (TEE) is highly accurate for this purpose with sensitivity and specificity

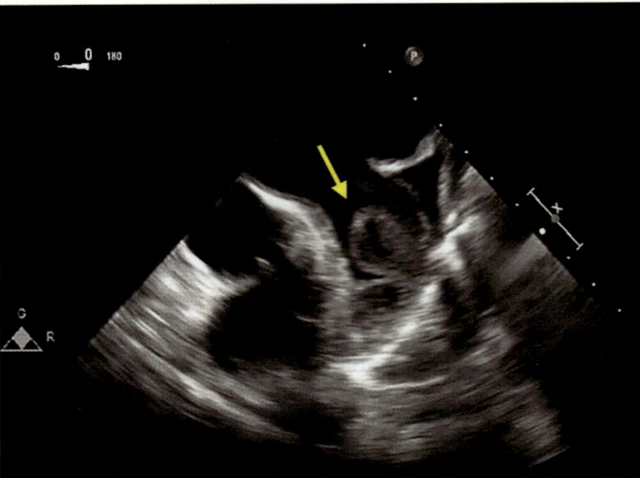

Fig. 3: A large left atrial thrombus in a patient with atrial fibrillation.

reported to be as high as 100 and 99%, respectively.[53] The presence of spontaneous echo contrast is also a predictor of thromboembolism, even if no thrombus is found at the time of examination.[54,55]

Apart from the LAA thrombus, LAA function can also be assessed during echocardiography and can provide useful information.[56] The LAA velocities are measured by placing the pulsed-wave sample volume in the proximal one-third segment of the LAA (toward the LAA mouth). In patients with sinus rhythm, especially when the heart rate is slow, a typical quadriphasic flow pattern can be seen as depicted in **Figures 5A to C**. The late diastolic emptying velocity (also known as LAA contraction velocity), which occurs immediately after the P wave on the electrocardiogram, is the most important wave since it reflects the LAA contractile function. It is also a significant predictor of thromboembolic risk.[57] The average LAA contraction velocity is 50–60 cm/s.[58-60]

The LAA flow pattern and velocities are quite variable during AF. Usually, saw-tooth waves of varying amplitude and regularity are seen.[61,62] The peak and/or mean LAA velocities may be measured, though there is no consensus regarding this.

Numerous studies have shown the prognostic value of LAA dysfunction for systemic thromboembolism. The presence of LAA dysfunction implies an increased stroke risk even if no clot is found at the time of initial examination.[59,63-65] The patients with reduced LAA contraction velocity (≤20 cm/s) have been shown to have a higher prevalence of LAA thrombi, spontaneous echo contrast, and the risk of ischemic stroke.[63] The LAA dysfunction may also occur during sinus rhythm in conditions such as mitral stenosis, severe LV systolic dysfunction, and hypertrophic cardiomyopathy and is a marker of thromboembolism risk in these patients.[66-70] Lastly, the LAA contraction velocity is also a good predictor of conversion to and maintenance of sinus rhythm after cardioversion.[71-74] In a multicenter study involving 408 patients undergoing cardioversion of AF, the mean LAA velocity >31 cm/s was one of the few independent predictors of the success of cardioversion.[74]

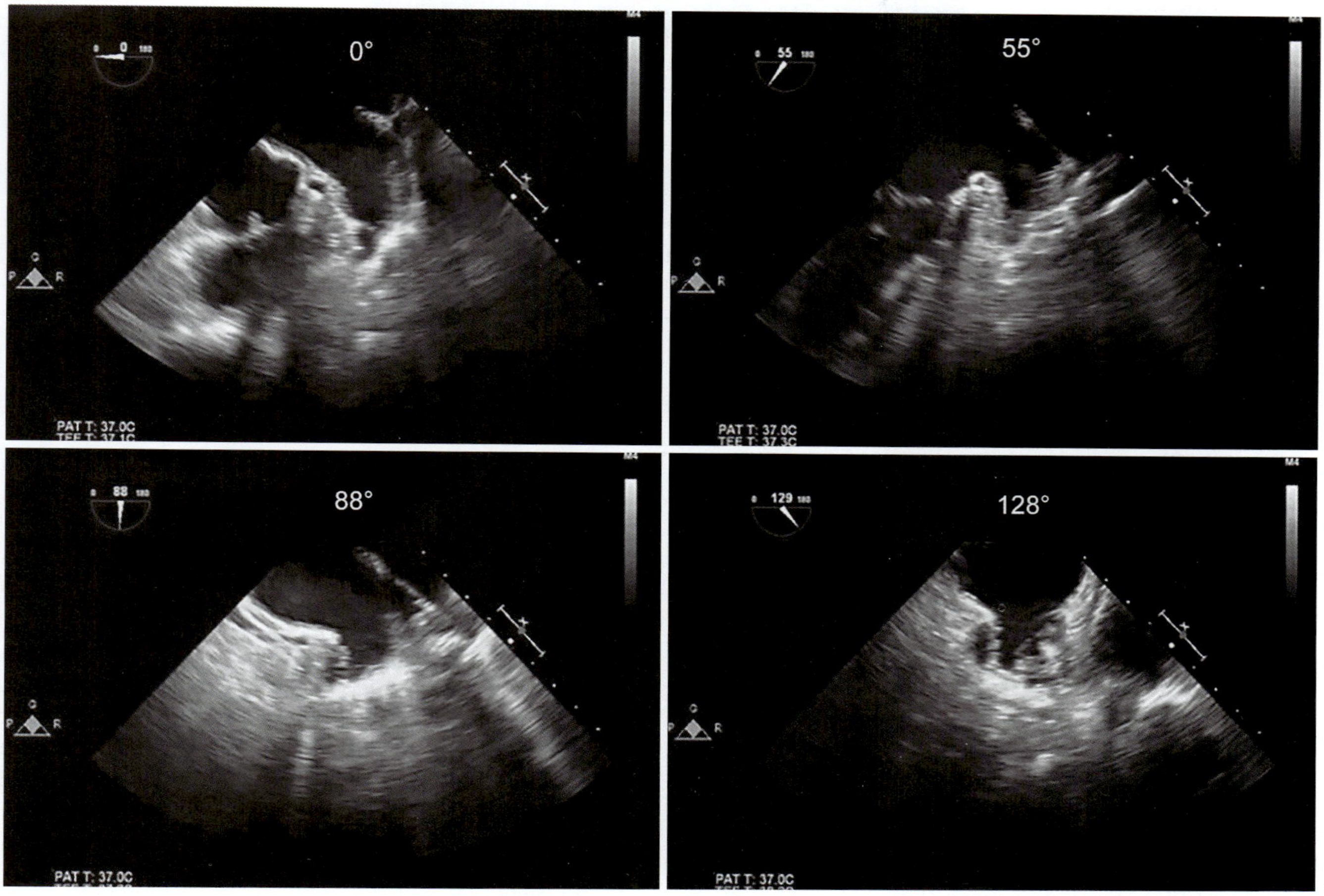

Fig. 4: Scanning of the left atrial appendage in multiple imaging planes during transesophageal echocardiography.

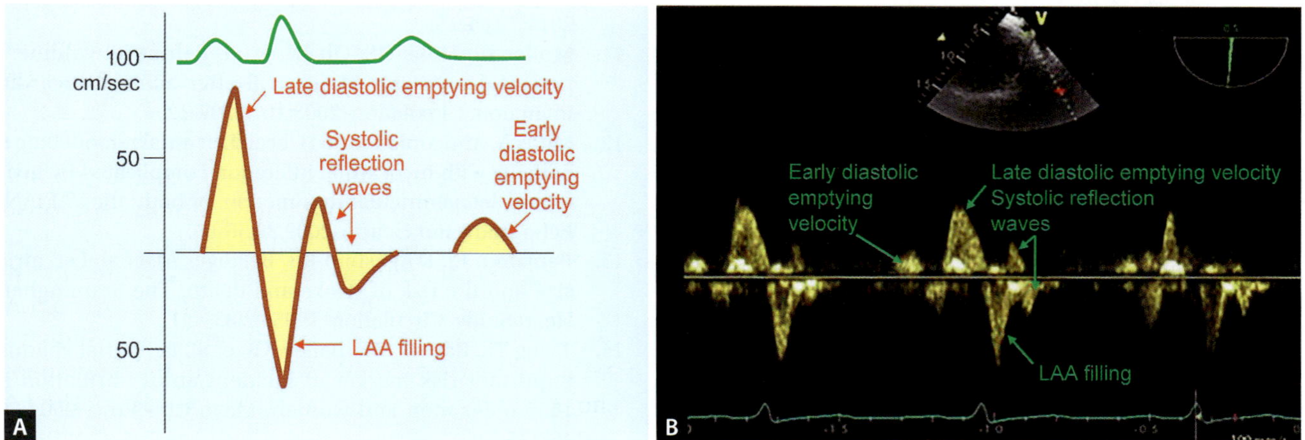

Figs. 5A and B

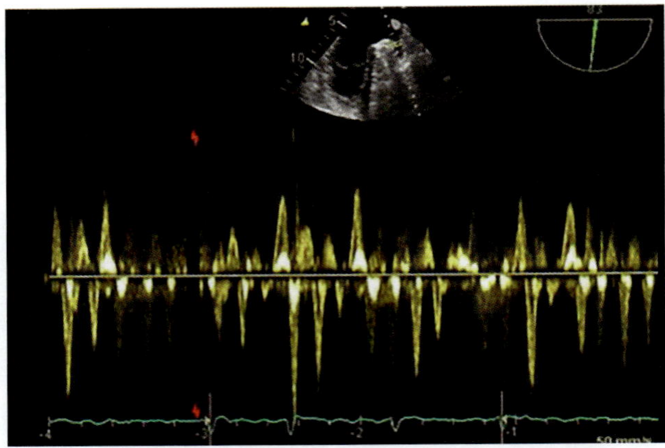

Fig. 5C

Figs. 5A to C: Left atrial appendage (LAA) flow pattern. (A) A schematic diagram showing the different flow waves during sinus rhythm; (B) Pulsed-wave Doppler tracing of the LAA flow in sinus rhythm; and (C) Pulsed-wave Doppler tracing of the LAA flow in atrial fibrillation. *Source:* Reproduced with permission from Bansal and Kasliwal.[56]

CONCLUSION

Atrial fibrillation is the most common arrhythmia encountered in clinical practice. Systemic thromboembolism is a serious complication of AF. In patients presenting with AF, with or without an embolic event, a thorough assessment of the LA size and function is essential. LAVI is the preferred measure of LA size, whereas LARS has emerged as the preferred measure of LA function. In addition, a detailed assessment of the LAA to rule out any preexisting clot and for quantifying its contractile function is also required for the complete evaluation of these patients.

REFERENCES

1. Tsao CW, Aday AW, Almarzooq ZI, et al. Heart Disease and Stroke Statistics-2023 update: a report from the American Heart Association. Circulation. 2023;147:e93-621.
2. Chugh SS, Havmoeller R, Narayanan K, et al. Worldwide epidemiology of atrial fibrillation: a Global Burden of Disease 2010 Study. Circulation. 2014;129:837-47.
3. Joglar JA, Chung MK, Armbruster AL, et al. 2023 ACC/AHA/ACCP/HRS guideline for the diagnosis and management of atrial fibrillation: a report of the American College of Cardiology/American Heart Association Joint Committee on Clinical Practice Guidelines. J Am Coll Cardiol. 2024;83:109-279.
4. Allan V, Honarbakhsh S, Casas JP, et al. Are cardiovascular risk factors also associated with the incidence of atrial fibrillation? A systematic review and field synopsis of 23 factors in 32 population-based cohorts of 20 million participants. Thromb Haemost. 2017;117:837-50.
5. Alonso A, Krijthe BP, Aspelund T, et al. Simple risk model predicts incidence of atrial fibrillation in a racially and geographically diverse population: the CHARGE-AF consortium. J Am Heart Assoc. 2013;2:e000102.
6. Odutayo A, Wong CX, Hsiao AJ, et al. Atrial fibrillation and risks of cardiovascular disease, renal disease, and death: systematic review and meta-analysis. BMJ. 2016;354:i4482.
7. Lang RM, Badano LP, Mor-Avi V, et al. Recommendations for cardiac chamber quantification by echocardiography in adults: an update from the American Society of Echocardiography and the European Association of Cardiovascular Imaging. J Am Soc Echocardiogr. 2015;28:1-39.e14.
8. Surkova E, Badano LP, Genovese D, et al. Clinical and prognostic implications of methods and partition values used to assess left atrial volume by two-dimensional echocardiography. J Am Soc Echocardiogr. 2017;30:1119-29.
9. Zile MR, Gottdiener JS, Hetzel SJ, et al. Prevalence and significance of alterations in cardiac structure and function in patients with heart failure and a preserved ejection fraction. Circulation. 2011;124:2491-501.
10. Shah AM, Shah SJ, Anand IS, et al. Cardiac structure and function in heart failure with preserved ejection fraction: baseline findings from the echocardiographic study of the treatment of preserved cardiac function heart failure with an aldosterone antagonist trial. Circ Heart Fail. 2014;7:104-15.
11. Moller JE, Hillis GS, Oh JK, et al. Left atrial volume: a powerful predictor of survival after acute myocardial infarction. Circulation. 2003;107:2207-12.
12. Meris A, Amigoni M, Uno H, et al. Left atrial remodelling in patients with myocardial infarction complicated by heart failure, left ventricular dysfunction, or both: the VALIANT Echo study. Eur Heart J. 2009;30:56-65.
13. Benjamin EJ, D'Agostino RB, Belanger AJ, et al. Left atrial size and the risk of stroke and death. The Framingham Heart Study. Circulation. 1995;92:835-41.
14. Tsang TS, Barnes ME, Bailey KR, et al. Left atrial volume: important risk marker of incident atrial fibrillation in 1655 older men and women. Mayo Clin Proc. 2001;76:467-75.
15. Barnes ME, Miyasaka Y, Seward JB, et al. Left atrial volume in the prediction of first ischemic stroke in an

elderly cohort without atrial fibrillation. Mayo Clin Proc. 2004;79:1008-14.

16. Flaker GC, Fletcher KA, Rothbart RM, et al. Clinical and echocardiographic features of intermittent atrial fibrillation that predict recurrent atrial fibrillation. Am J Cardiol. 1995;76:355-8.
17. Katsiki N, Mikhailidis DP, Papanas N. Left atrial volume: an independent predictor of cardiovascular outcomes. Int J Cardiol. 2018;265:234-5.
18. Taniguchi N, Miyasaka Y, Suwa Y, et al. Usefulness of left atrial volume as an independent predictor of development of heart failure in patients with atrial fibrillation. Am J Cardiol. 2019;124:1430-35.
19. Ramu B, Elwan AM, Coleman CI, et al. The association between baseline left atrial volume index and all-cause mortality in patients with heart failure: a meta-analysis. Conn Med. 2015;79:469-75.
20. Raniga D, Goda M, Hattingh L, et al. Left atrial volume index: a predictor of atrial fibrillation recurrence following direct current cardioversion: a systematic review and meta-analysis. Int J Cardiol Heart Vasc. 2024;51:101364.
21. Njoku A, Kannabhiran M, Arora R, et al. Left atrial volume predicts atrial fibrillation recurrence after radiofrequency ablation: a meta-analysis. Europace. 2018;20:33-42.
22. Celik AI, Kanadasi M, Demir M, et al. Predictors of the paroxysmal atrial fibrillation recurrence following cryoballoon-based pulmonary vein isolation: assessment of left atrial volume, left atrial volume index, galectin-3 level and neutrophil-to-lymphocyte ratio. Indian Pacing Electrophysiol J. 2019;19:9-14.
23. Albano AJ, Bush J, Parker JL, et al. Left atrial volume index predicts arrhythmia-free survival in patients with persistent atrial fibrillation undergoing cryoballoon ablation. J Atr Fibrillation. 2019;12:2192.
24. Jordan K, Yaghi S, Poppas A, et al. Left atrial volume index is associated with cardioembolic stroke and atrial fibrillation detection after embolic stroke of undetermined source. Stroke. 2019;50:1997-2001.
25. Tan BYQ, Ho JSY, Sia CH, et al. Left atrial volume index predicts new-onset atrial fibrillation and stroke recurrence in patients with embolic stroke of undetermined source. Cerebrovasc Dis. 2020;49:285-91.
26. Osawa K, Nakanishi R, Ceponiene I, et al. Predicting left atrial appendage thrombus from left atrial volume and confirmation by computed tomography with delayed enhancement. Tex Heart Inst J. 2020;47:78-85.
27. Shiraki H, Tsunamoto H, Onishi T, et al. Left atrial volume index as a predictor for left atrial appendage thrombus in patients with non-valvular atrial fibrillation receiving appropriate oral anticoagulation therapy: a prospective multi-center study. Echocardiography. 2024;41:e15735.
28. Pathan F, D'Elia N, Nolan MT, et al. Normal ranges of left atrial strain by speckle-tracking echocardiography: a systematic review and meta-analysis. J Am Soc Echocardiogr. 2017;30:59-70.e8.
29. Singh A, Singulane CC, Miyoshi T, et al. Normal values of left atrial size and function and the impact of age: results of the World Alliance Societies of Echocardiography Study. J Am Soc Echocardiogr. 2022;35:154-64.e3.
30. Cameli M, Sparla S, Losito M, et al. Correlation of left atrial strain and doppler measurements with invasive measurement of left ventricular end-diastolic pressure in patients stratified for different values of ejection fraction. Echocardiography. 2016;33:398-405.
31. Ye Z, Miranda WR, Yeung DF, et al. Left atrial strain in evaluation of heart failure with preserved ejection fraction. J Am Soc Echocardiogr. 2020;33:1490-9.
32. Habibi M, Lima JA, Khurram IM, et al. Association of left atrial function and left atrial enhancement in patients with atrial fibrillation: cardiac magnetic resonance study. Circ Cardiovasc Imaging. 2015;8:e002769.
33. Morris DA, Belyavskiy E, Aravind-Kumar R, et al. Potential usefulness and clinical relevance of adding left atrial strain to left atrial volume index in the detection of left ventricular diastolic dysfunction. JACC Cardiovasc Imaging. 2018;11:1405-15.
34. Singh A, Addetia K, Maffessanti F, et al. LA strain for categorization of LV diastolic dysfunction. JACC Cardiovasc Imaging. 2017;10:735-43.
35. Frydas A, Morris DA, Belyavskiy E, et al. Left atrial strain as sensitive marker of left ventricular diastolic dysfunction in heart failure. ESC Heart Fail. 2020;7:1956-65.
36. Hwang IC, Cho GY, Choi HM, et al. H2FPEF score reflects the left atrial strain and predicts prognosis in patients with heart failure with preserved ejection fraction. J Card Fail. 2021;27:198-207.
37. Park JJ, Park JH, Hwang IC, et al. Left atrial strain as a predictor of new-onset atrial fibrillation in patients with heart failure. JACC Cardiovasc Imaging. 2020;13:2071-81.
38. Jasic-Szpak E, Marwick TH, Donal E, et al. Prediction of AF in heart failure with preserved ejection fraction: incremental value of left atrial strain. JACC Cardiovasc Imaging. 2021;14:131-44.
39. Reddy YNV, Obokata M, Verbrugge FH, et al. Atrial dysfunction in patients with heart failure with preserved ejection fraction and atrial fibrillation. J Am Coll Cardiol. 2020;76:1051-64.
40. Pourafkari L, Ghaffari S, Bancroft GR, et al. Factors associated with atrial fibrillation in rheumatic mitral stenosis. Asian Cardiovasc Thorac Ann. 2015;23:17-23.
41. Gabrielli L, Corbalan R, Cordova S, et al. Left atrial dysfunction is a predictor of postcoronary artery bypass atrial fibrillation: association of left atrial strain and strain rate assessed by speckle tracking. Echocardiography. 2011;28:1104-8.
42. Her AY, Kim JY, Kim YH, et al. Left atrial strain assessed by speckle tracking imaging is related to new-onset atrial fibrillation after coronary artery bypass grafting. Can J Cardiol. 2013;29:377-83.
43. Cameli M, Lisi M, Reccia R, et al. Pre-operative left atrial strain predicts post-operative atrial fibrillation in patients undergoing aortic valve replacement for aortic stenosis. Int J Cardiovasc Imaging. 2014;30:279-86.
44. Costa C, Gonzalez-Alujas T, Valente F, et al. Left atrial strain: a new predictor of thrombotic risk and successful electrical cardioversion. Echo Res Pract. 2016;3:45-52.
45. Motoki H, Negishi K, Kusunose K, et al. Global left atrial strain in the prediction of sinus rhythm maintenance

after catheter ablation for atrial fibrillation. J Am Soc Echocardiogr. 2014;27:1184-92.
46. Yasuda R, Murata M, Roberts R, et al. Left atrial strain is a powerful predictor of atrial fibrillation recurrence after catheter ablation: study of a heterogeneous population with sinus rhythm or atrial fibrillation. Eur Heart J Cardiovasc Imaging. 2015;16:1008-14.
47. Sarvari SI, Haugaa KH, Stokke TM, et al. Strain echocardiographic assessment of left atrial function predicts recurrence of atrial fibrillation. Eur Heart J Cardiovasc Imaging. 2016;17:660-7.
48. Hsu PC, Lee WH, Chu CY, et al. Prognostic role of left atrial strain and its combination index with transmitral E-wave velocity in patients with atrial fibrillation. Sci Rep. 2016;6:17318.
49. Obokata M, Negishi K, Kurosawa K, et al. Left atrial strain provides incremental value for embolism risk stratification over CHA_2DS_2-VASc score and indicates prognostic impact in patients with atrial fibrillation. J Am Soc Echocardiogr. 2014;27:709-16.e4.
50. Odell JA, Blackshear JL, Davies E, et al. Thoracoscopic obliteration of the left atrial appendage: potential for stroke reduction? Ann Thorac Surg. 1996;61:565-9.
51. Veinot JP, Harrity PJ, Gentile F, et al. Anatomy of the normal left atrial appendage: a quantitative study of age-related changes in 500 autopsy hearts: implications for echocardiographic examination. Circulation. 1997;96:3112-5.
52. Burkule N, Govind SC, Sola S, et al. The Indian Academy of Echocardiography practice guideline for the performance of transesophageal echocardiographic evaluation of a patient with cerebrovascular stroke. J Indian Acad Echocardiogr Cardiovasc Imaging. 2018;2:1-18.
53. Manning WJ, Silverman DI, Gordon SP, et al. Cardioversion from atrial fibrillation without prolonged anticoagulation with use of transesophageal echocardiography to exclude the presence of atrial thrombi. N Engl J Med. 1993;328:750-5.
54. Black IW, Hopkins AP, Lee LC, et al. Left atrial spontaneous echo contrast: a clinical and echocardiographic analysis. J Am Coll Cardiol. 1991;18:398-404.
55. Kasliwal RR, Mittal S, Kanojia A, et al. A study of spontaneous echo contrast in patients with rheumatic mitral stenosis and normal sinus rhythm: an Indian perspective. Br Heart J. 1995;74:296-9.
56. Bansal M, Kasliwal RR. Echocardiography for left atrial appendage structure and function. Indian Heart J. 2012;64:469-75.
57. Agmon Y, Khandheria BK, Meissner I, et al. Left atrial appendage flow velocities in subjects with normal left ventricular function. Am J Cardiol. 2000;86:769-73.
58. Tabata T, Oki T, Fukuda N, et al. Influence of aging on left atrial appendage flow velocity patterns in normal subjects. J Am Soc Echocardiogr. 1996;9:274-80.
59. Mugge A, Kuhn H, Nikutta P, et al. Assessment of left atrial appendage function by biplane transesophageal echocardiography in patients with nonrheumatic atrial fibrillation: identification of a subgroup of patients at increased embolic risk. J Am Coll Cardiol. 1994;23:599-607.
60. Mikael Kortz RA, Delemarre BJ, van Dantzig JM, et al. Left atrial appendage blood flow determined by transesophageal echocardiography in healthy subjects. Am J Cardiol. 1993;71:976-81.
61. Li YH, Lai LP, Shyu KG, et al. Clinical implications of left atrial appendage function: its influence on thrombus formation. Int J Cardiol. 1994;43:61-6.
62. Jue J, Winslow T, Fazio G, et al. Pulsed Doppler characterization of left atrial appendage flow. J Am Soc Echocardiogr. 1993;6:237-44.
63. Transesophageal echocardiographic correlates of thromboembolism in high-risk patients with non-valvular atrial fibrillation. Ann Intern Med. 1998;128:639-47.
64. Li YH, Lai LP, Shyu KG, et al. Clinical implications of left atrial appendage flow patterns in nonrheumatic atrial fibrillation. Chest. 1994;105:748-52.
65. Li YH, Hwang JJ, Lin JL, et al. Importance of left atrial appendage function as a risk factor for systemic thromboembolism in patients with rheumatic mitral valve disease. Am J Cardiol. 1996;78:844-7.
66. Hwang JJ, Li YH, Lin JM, et al. Left atrial appendage function determined by transesophageal echocardiography in patients with rheumatic mitral valve disease. Cardiology. 1994;85:121-8.
67. Golbasi Z, Cicek D, Canbay A, et al. Left atrial appendage function in patients with mitral stenosis in sinus rhythm. Eur J Echocardiogr. 2002;3:39-43.
68. Saygi S, Turk UO, Alioglu E, et al. Left atrial appendage function in mitral stenosis: is it determined by cardiac rhythm? J Heart Valve Dis. 2011;20:417-24.
69. Ito T, Suwa M, Kobashi A, et al. Influence of altered loading conditions on left atrial appendage function in vivo. Am J Cardiol. 1998;81:1056-9.
70. Yakar Tuluce S, Kayikcioglu M, Tuluce K, et al. Assessment of left atrial appendage function during sinus rhythm in patients with hypertrophic cardiomyopathy: transesophageal echocardiography and tissue Doppler study. J Am Soc Echocardiogr. 2010;23:1207-16.
71. Tanabe K, Yoshitomi H, Asanuma T, et al. Prediction of outcome of electrical cardioversion by left atrial appendage flow velocities in atrial fibrillation. Jpn Circ J. 1997;61:19-24.
72. Perez Y, Duval AM, Carville C, et al. Is left atrial appendage flow a predictor for outcome of cardioversion of nonvalvular atrial fibrillation? A transthroacic and transesophageal echocardiographic study. Am Heart J. 1997;134:745-51.
73. Verhorst PM, Kamp O, Welling RC, et al. Transesophageal echocardiographic predictors for maintenance of sinus rhythm after electrical cardioversion of atrial fibrillation. Am J Cardiol. 1997;79:1355-9.
74. Palinkas A, Antonielli E, Picano E, et al. Clinical value of left atrial appendage flow velocity for predicting of cardioversion success in patients with non-valvular atrial fibrillation. Eur Heart J. 2001;22:2201-8.

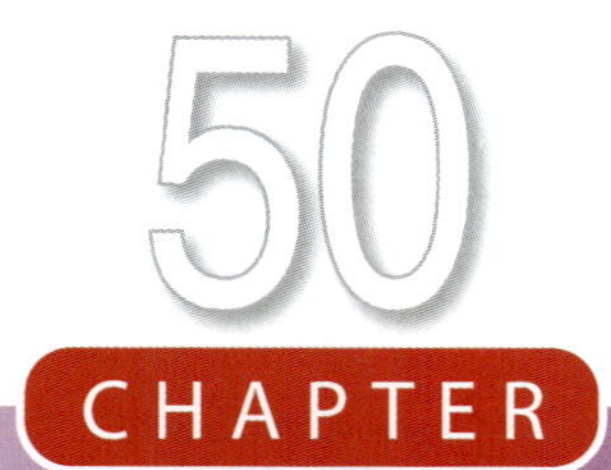

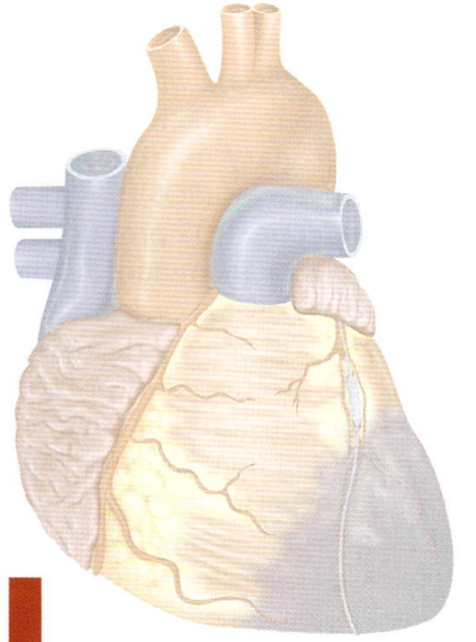

Echocardiographic Remodeling Reversal with SGLT2i and ARNI in HFpEF

Abdirahman Wardhere, Wissam I Khalife, Masood Ahmad

INTRODUCTION

Heart failure with preserved ejection fraction (HFpEF) is increasingly recognized as a significant public health concern, constituting about 50% of all heart failure (HF) cases with a female-to-male ratio of 2:1[1] and contributing to considerable morbidity and mortality.[2] HFpEF is characterized by abnormalities in the structure and diastolic function of the left ventricle (LV) despite preserved left ventricular ejection fraction (LVEF). Due to the heterogeneity of HFpEF, there is a limited understanding of its mechanistic underpinnings.[3] Consequently, there are few effective therapeutic options for HFpEF, with only a limited number of trials providing evidence of their efficacy.[4] The sodium-glucose cotransporter 2 inhibitors (SGLT2i) and mineralocorticoid receptor antagonists (MRA) have the most substantial evidence supporting their use in HFpEF. Furthermore, there are promising indications for using angiotensin receptor-neprilysin inhibitors (ARNI) or angiotensin receptor blockers (ARB) in specific subsets of the HFpEF population.

MECHANISM OF CARDIAC REMODELING

Cardiac remodeling refers to a series of maladaptive molecular, cellular, and interstitial alterations that present clinically as changes in the heart's size, mass, geometry, and function, often leading to poor prognosis **(Fig. 1)**.[5,6] HFpEF involves neurohormonal activation, including the renin-angiotensin-aldosterone and sympathetic nervous systems. However, this activation is generally less pronounced than heart failure with reduced ejection fraction (HFrEF).[7] In the context of HFpEF, cardiac remodeling is typically seen as LV hypertrophy coupled with abnormal diastolic function.[8,9] Impairments of LV global longitudinal strain, left atrial strain, and right ventricular (RV) strain are observed in patients with HFpEF **(Figs. 2A to D)**.[10] Reverse remodeling is the process by which these pathological changes are reversed in response to therapy and is associated with improved clinical outcomes, serving as a biomarker for therapeutic success.[4] The developments in noninvasive imaging techniques over the past decade, especially in transthoracic echocardiography (TTE) and cardiac magnetic resonance imaging (CMRI), have significantly enhanced the assessment of reverse remodeling. This chapter will focus on the echocardiographic findings of reverse remodeling with SGLT2i and ARNI in HFpEF patients.

ANGIOTENSIN RECEPTOR-NEPRILYSIN INHIBITORS

Angiotensin receptor-neprilysin inhibitor therapy (sacubitril/valsartan) targets maladaptive neurohormonal pathways while promoting adaptive natriuretic peptide expression. This treatment has demonstrated life-prolonging effects in patients with mild-to-moderate HFrEF symptoms compared with ACE inhibitors.[11] These findings led to the design of the landmark trial, PARAGON-HF (Prospective Comparison of ARNI with ARB Global Outcomes in HF with Preserved Ejection Fraction) study, which found that sacubitril/valsartan did not significantly reduce total HF hospitalizations and

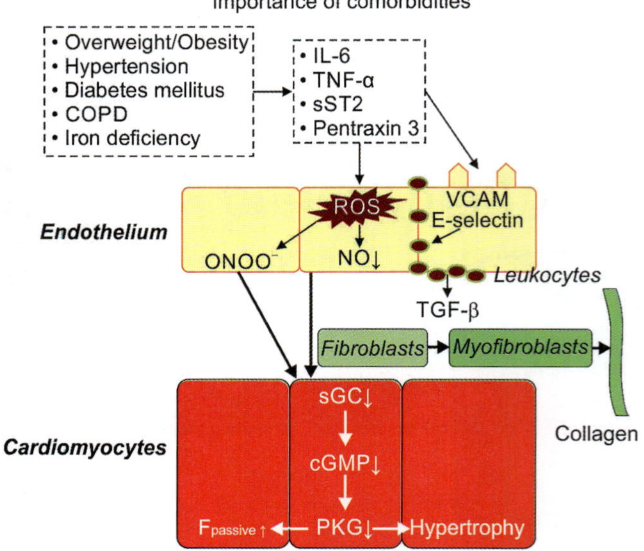

Fig. 1: Comorbidities induce a proinflammatory state with elevated plasma levels of interleukin (IL)-6, tumor necrosis factor (TNF)-α, soluble ST2 (sST2), and pentraxin 3. Coronary microvascular endothelial cells produce reactive oxygen species (ROS), vascular cell adhesion molecule (VCAM), and E-selectin. ROS production leads to the formation of peroxynitrite ($ONOO^-$) and reduced nitric oxide (NO) bioavailability, lowering soluble guanylate cyclase (sGC) activity in adjacent cardiomyocytes. Lower sGC activity decreases cyclic guanosine monophosphate concentration and protein kinase G (PKG) activity, increases resting tension (Fpassive) of cardiomyocytes due to hypophosphorylation of titin, and promotes prohypertrophic stimuli for cardiomyocyte hypertrophy. VCAM and E-selectin expression in endothelial cells favors migration into the subendothelium of monocytes with release of transforming growth factor-β (TGF-β). These changes facilitate the conversion of fibroblasts to myofibroblasts, which deposit collagen in the interstitial space. (COPD: chronic obstructive pulmonary disease; HFpEF: heart failure with preserved ejection fraction)

Source: With permission from Paulus and Tschöpe.[6]

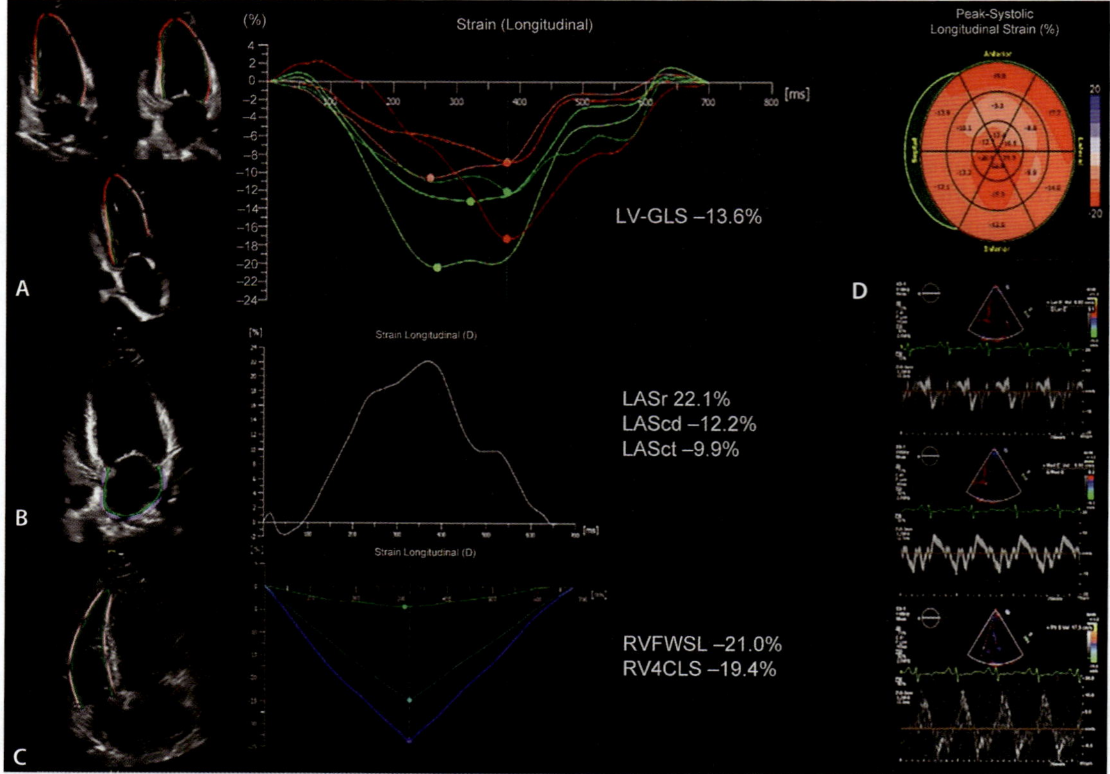

Figs. 2A to D: Parameters of myocardial mechanics in HFpEF. (A) Impaired LV global longitudinal strain and mechanical dispersion are common HFpEF mechanical changes. (B) Reductions in left atrial reservoir, conduit, and contractile function are commonly seen in symptomatic HFpEF. (C) HFpEF-associated impairment of right ventricular free wall and four-chamber deformation. (D) Despite normal or near-normal tissue Doppler-derived parameters of diastolic function, significant deteriorations of mechanical deformation may exist. (LAScd: left atrial strain during conduit phase; LASct: left atrial strain during contraction phase; LASr: left atrial strain during reservoir phase; LV-GLS: left ventricular global longitudinal strain; RV4CLS: right ventricular four-chamber longitudinal strain; RVFWLS: right ventricular free-wall longitudinal strain)

Source: Reproduced with permission from Seetharam et al.[10]

cardiovascular death compared with valsartan in patients with LVEF ≥45.[12] However, subanalyses indicated benefits for patients with mildly reduced and borderline LVEF (45–57%) and in women regardless of LVEF. A post hoc analysis showed more pronounced benefits when treatment began soon after an HF hospitalization, highlighting a group at high risk for short-term morbidity.[13] The PARAGON-HF echocardiographic substudy showed that cardiac structure and function measures were generally consistent with those reported in the I-PRESERVE (Irbesartan in Heart Failure with Preserved Ejection Fraction) trial, particularly regarding LV mass, LVH prevalence, LA area, E/e′ ratio, and estimated PASP.[14,15]

The PARAMOUNT trial,[16] a phase 2 randomized controlled trial, involved 301 patients, with 149 receiving LCZ696 (ARNI) and 152 receiving valsartan. NT-proBNP levels decreased more with LCZ696 than with valsartan [ratio of change, 0.77 (0.64–0.92), $p = 0.005$] at 12 weeks, but this difference was not significant at 36 weeks [ratio of change, 0.88 (0.65–1.09), $p = 0.20$]. Left atrial volume was significantly reduced with a mean change of −4.6 mL in the ARNI group compared with valsartan group with a mean change of +0.37 mL after 36 weeks of treatment ($p = 0.003$). Other echocardiographic measurements, including LVEF, ventricular volumes, or diastolic function parameters, did not differ significantly at 9 months. ARNI also improves RV performance and pulmonary hypertension in HFrEF; however, the mechanism is not entirely dependent on reverse remodeling.[17] In a post hoc analysis of the PARAMOUNT trial, sacubitril/valsartan improved global circumferential strain but not global longitudinal strain when compared with valsartan for 36 weeks.[18]

SODIUM–GLUCOSE COTRANSPORTER 2 INHIBITORS

Sodium–glucose cotransporter 2 inhibitors have demonstrated significant benefits in reducing hospitalizations due to HF and cardiovascular mortality in patients with HFpEF, as evidenced by the results from the DELIVER and EMPEROR-Preserved trials. The SGLT2i do this by inducing a state of nutrient deprivation and hypoxia-like conditions, which promote increased ketosis, erythropoiesis, autophagy, and modified iron homeostasis, thereby boosting cardiac energy and function.[19] The EMPEROR-Preserved trial showed that empagliflozin notably lowered the combined risk of cardiovascular death or HF hospitalization in patients with chronic HFpEF.[20] Similarly, the DELIVER trial showed that dapagliflozin resulted in prompt and sustained reductions in clinical events among HFpEF patients.[21] Although HF hospitalizations were the main outcomes in these trials, pooled analyses have shown reductions in cardiovascular deaths and HF hospitalizations across different HF patient populations, regardless of ejection fraction or care settings.

A prospective study conducted by Sakai and Miura indicated that 12 weeks of SGLT2i treatment led to improvements in diastolic function parameters in HFpEF patients, with noted significant reductions in E/A ratio (meanΔ ± SD, −0.06 ± 0.007; $p = 0.048$), septal E/e (−6.73 ± 0.009; $p = 0.003$), and lateral E/e′ (−8.35 ± 0.008, $p = 0.044$).[22] Changes in E/e′ were correlated with vascular and metabolic markers, including the cardio-ankle vascular index, flow-mediated dilation, and homeostatic model assessment of insulin resistance. In a pig model of HFpEF, dapagliflozin alleviated heart concentric remodeling **(Figs. 3A to E)**.[23] These results support the concept of HFpEF as a systemic condition influenced by multiple metabolic factors.

LIMITATIONS

This chapter includes reliance on early data. Longer-term follow-up is needed to better understand the effects of ARNI and SGLT2i in reverse remodeling. The chapter also underscores the ongoing evolution of imaging techniques for evaluating novel therapeutic effects and the need for further validation of these techniques.

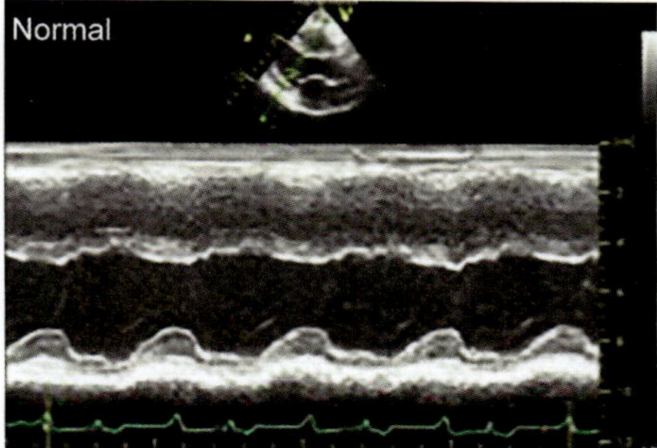

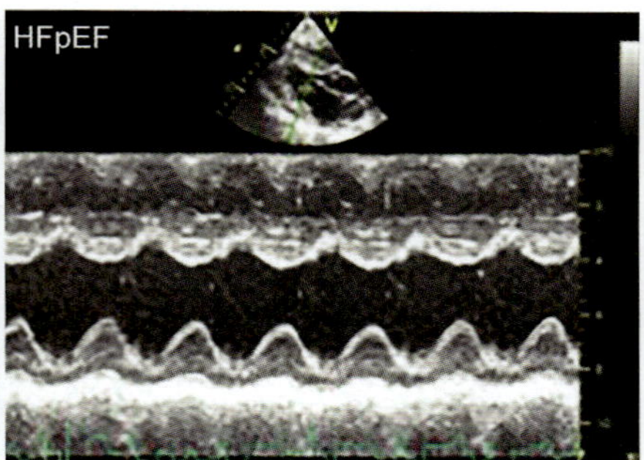

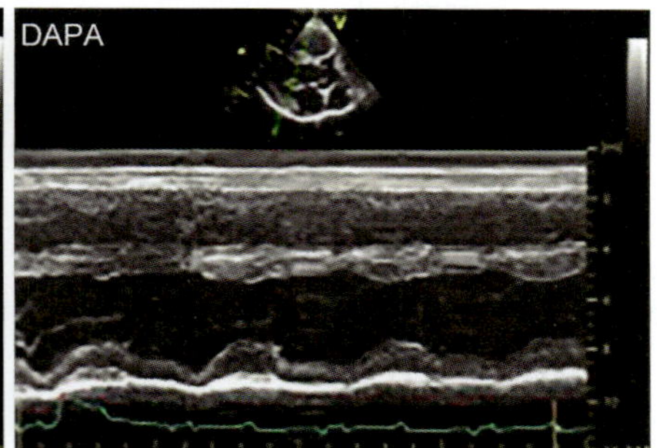

Fig. 3A

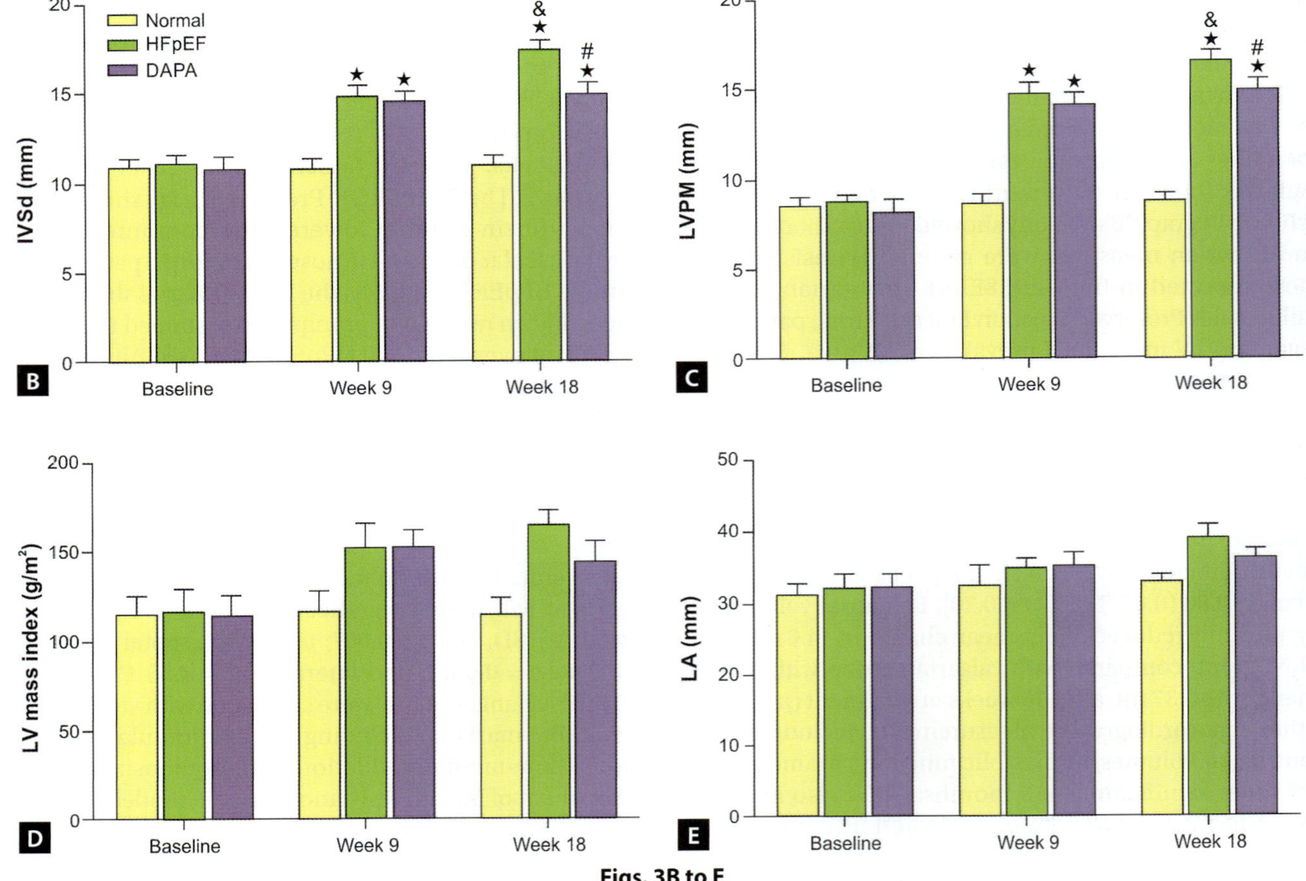

Figs. 3B to E

Figs. 3A to E: Dapagliflozin alleviated heart concentric remodeling in HFpEF pigs. Structural changes in the heart are measured by echocardiography. Representative images of the following are shown. (A) Echocardiographic M-mode Doppler imaging. (B) Interventricular septum thickness at end-diastole (IVSd). (C) Left ventricular posterior wall (LVPW). (D) LV mass index. (E) Left atrium (LA). The data are presented as the mean ± SD. $n = 10$ pigs per group. Two-way repeated-measures ANOVA was performed. ★$p < 0.05$ versus the normal group, $^{\#}p < 0.05$ versus the HFpEF group, and $p < 0.05$ versus the 9th week of the same group.
Source: With permission from Zhang et al.[23]

TABLE 1: The effect of SGLT2i and ARNI on echocardiographic reverse remodeling parameters in HFpEF.

Reverse remodeling in heart failure with preserved ejection fraction				
	Drug	*Follow-up time*	*Parameter assessed*	*Effects on reverse remodeling*
Solomon et al.[16]	Valsartan–sacubitril	12 weeks	LA size	Improvement in LAV and LA dimensions
Biering-Sørensen et al.[18]	Valsartan–sacubitril	36 weeks	LV GLS, GCS	Improvement of LV GCS but not GLS
Sakai and Miura[22]	Empagliflozin, luseogliflozin, and tofogliflozin	12 weeks	Mitral peak E and A velocity, mitral annular e′ velocity	Improvement in assessed diastolic parameters

(ARNI: angiotensin receptor-neprilysin inhibitors; GCS: global circumferential strain; GLS: global longitudinal strain; HFpEF: heart failure with preserved ejection fraction; LA: left atrial; LAV: left atrial volume; LV: left ventricle; SGLT2i: sodium–glucose cotransporter 2 inhibitors)

SUMMARY

Pertinent studies summarizing the roles of ARNI and SGLT2i medication groups in cardiac reverse remodeling in HFpEF patients are listed in **Table 1**. ARNI medications result in significant reductions in LA size and improvement in global circumferential strain, while SGLT2i medications improve diastology parameters.

Further studies with longer-term follow-up are needed to confirm these results.

CONCLUSION

Reverse remodeling has become an innovative method for objectively evaluating the therapeutic effects of HF. It demonstrates correlations between biochemical markers and clinical outcomes. Significant improvements in reverse remodeling echocardiographic parameters were observed with ARNI and SGLT2i medication groups. Advanced imaging techniques have emphasized the potential of reverse remodeling as a biomarker for assessing therapeutic response. However, further validation of these techniques and their prognostic significance is essential to support their incorporation into standard clinical practice.

REFERENCES

1. Duca F, Zotter-Tufaro C, Kammerlander AA, et al. Gender-related differences in heart failure with preserved ejection fraction. Sci Rep. 2018;8(1):1080.
2. Zile M, Gottdiener JS, Hetzel SJ, et al. Prevalence and significance of alterations in cardiac structure and function in patients with heart failure and a preserved ejection fraction. Circulation. 2011;124(23):2491-501.
3. Heidenreich P, Bozkurt B, Aguilar D, et al. 2022 AHA/ACC/HFSA guideline for the management of heart failure: a report of the American College of Cardiology/American Heart Association Joint Committee on clinical practice guidelines. Circulation. 2022;145(18):e895-1032.
4. Kodsi M, Makarious D, Gan GCH, et al. Cardiac reverse remodeling by imaging parameters with recent changes to guideline medical therapy in heart failure. ESC Heart Fail. 2023;10(6):3258-75.
5. Azevedo P, Polegato B, Minicucci MF, et al. Cardiac remodeling: concepts, clinical impact, pathophysiological mechanisms and pharmacologic treatment. Arq Bras Cardiol. 2016;106(1):62-9.
6. Paulus WJ, Tschöpe C. A novel paradigm for heart failure with preserved ejection fraction: comorbidities drive myocardial dysfunction and remodeling through coronary microvascular endothelial inflammation. J Am Coll Cardiol. 2013;62(4):263-71.
7. Castiglione V, Gentile F, Ghionzoli N, et al. Pathophysiological rationale and clinical evidence for neurohormonal modulation in heart failure with preserved ejection fraction. Card Fail Rev. 2023:9:e09.
8. Douglas PS, Morrow R, Ioli A, et al. Left ventricular shape, afterload and survival in idiopathic dilated cardiomyopathy. J Am Coll Cardiol. 1989;13:311-5.
9. Konstam MA, Rousseau MF, Kronenberg MW, et al. Effects of the angiotensin converting enzyme inhibitor enalapril on the long-term progression of left ventricular dysfunction in patients with heart failure. Circulation. 1992;86(2):431-8.
10. Seetharam K, Sengupta PP, Bianco CM. Cardiac mechanics in heart failure with preserved ejection fraction. Echocardiography. 2020;37(11):1936-43.
11. McMurray JJV, Packer M, Desai AS, et al. Angiotensin-neprilysin inhibition versus enalapril in heart failure. N Engl J Med. 2014;371:993-1004.
12. Solomon SD, McMurray JJV, Anand IS, et al. Angiotensin-neprilysin inhibition in heart failure with preserved ejection fraction. N Engl J Med. 2019;381:1609-20.
13. Ventura HO, Lavie CJ, Mehra MR. Heart failure with preserved ejection fraction: separating the wheat from the chaff. J Am Coll Cardiol. 2020;75:255-7.
14. Massie BM, Carson PE, McMurray JJ, et al. Irbesartan in patients with heart failure and preserved ejection fraction. N Engl J Med. 2008;359:2456-67.
15. Shah AM, Cikes M, Prasad N, et al. Echocardiographic features of patients with heart failure and preserved left ventricular ejection fraction. J Am Coll Cardiol. 2019;74:2858-73.
16. Solomon SD, Zile M, Pieske B, et al. The angiotensin receptor neprilysin inhibitor LCZ696 in heart failure with preserved ejection fraction: a phase 2 double-blind randomized controlled trial. Lancet. 2012;380(9851):1387-95.
17. Zhang J, Du L, Qin X, et al. Effect of sacubitril/valsartan on the right ventricular function and pulmonary hypertension in patients with heart failure with reduced ejection fraction: a systematic review and meta-analysis of observational studies. J Am Heart Assoc. 2022;11(9):e024449.
18. Biering-Sørensen T, Lassen MCH, Shah A, et al. The effect of sacubitril/valsartan on left ventricular myocardial deformation in heart failure with preserved ejection fraction (PARAMOUNT trial). J Card Fail. 2023;29(6):968-73.
19. Pandey A, Bhatt B, Pandey A, et al. Mechanisms of benefits of sodium-glucose cotransporter 2 inhibitors in heart failure with preserved ejection fraction. Eur Heart J. 2023;44(37):3640-51.
20. Anker SD, Butler J, Filippatos G, et al. Empagliflozin in heart failure with a preserved ejection fraction. N Engl J Med. 2021;385:1451-61.
21. Solomon SD, McMurray JJV, Claggett B, et al. Dapagliflozin in heart failure with mildly reduced or preserved ejection fraction. N Engl J Med. 2022;387:1089-98.
22. Sakai T, Miura S. Effects of sodium-glucose cotransporter 2 inhibitor on vascular endothelial and diastolic function in heart failure with preserved ejection fraction: novel prospective cohort study. Circ Rep. 2019;1:286-95.
23. Zhang N, Feng B, Ma X, et al. Dapagliflozin improves left ventricular remodeling and aorta sympathetic tone in a pig model of heart failure with preserved ejection fraction. Cardiovasc Diabetol. 2019;18(1):107.

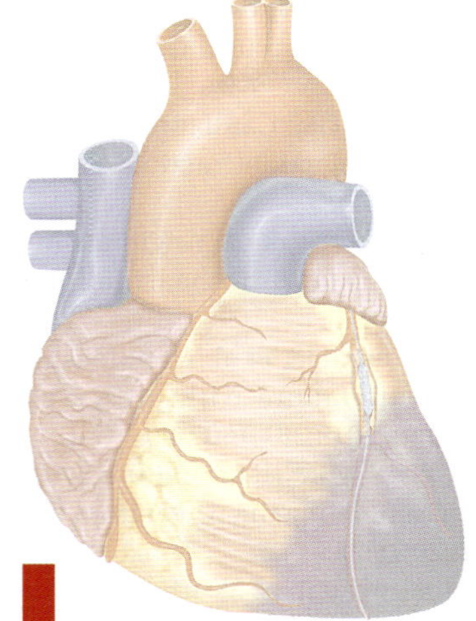

Echocardiographic-guided Therapy in HFpEF

Iniya Rajendran, Dennis Fong, Rajesh Janardhanan

INTRODUCTION

Echocardiography is vital in diagnosing, phenotyping, and managing heart failure with preserved ejection fraction (HFpEF). It provides information on cardiac structure, function, and hemodynamics. Unlike heart failure with reduced ejection fraction (HFrEF), patients with HFpEF have normal or near-normal left ventricular ejection fraction (LVEF) yet exhibit debilitating symptoms of heart failure, which often go undiagnosed for years. The underlying pathology in HFpEF is primarily related to impaired diastolic filling, ventricular stiffness, and increased filling pressures.[1] Echocardiography has allowed for a more nuanced understanding of HFpEF's pathophysiology, enabling more precise targeting of interventions.

ECHOCARDIOGRAPHIC ASSESSMENT OF DIASTOLOGY AND ITS ROLE IN HFpEF

The overarching contributor to HFpEF is diastolic dysfunction, which exists in a majority of patients with clinical heart failure syndrome and normal ejection fraction. Echocardiography provides a comprehensive assessment of diastolic dysfunction. Patients exhibit symptoms of heart failure when there is an elevation of left ventricular end-diastolic filling pressures, which is central to the pathophysiology of diastolic dysfunction. In population-based studies, diastolic dysfunction was classified as normal, abnormal left ventricular (LV) relaxation (grade I), pseudonormal (grade II), or restrictive (grade III).[1] The intracardiac hemodynamics during diastole can be measured using echocardiographic Doppler parameters to determine the level of diastolic function as recommended by the American Society of Echocardiography (ASE) and European Association of Cardiovascular Imaging (EACVI). The simplified and validated flowchart algorithm uses a combination of transmitral Doppler flow, mitral annular tissue Doppler, left atrial volume index (LAVI), and TR velocity.[2]

Transmitral flow velocity is typically obtained in the apical four-chamber view by placing a continuous Doppler on the mitral valve tips. The resultant Doppler signal consists of an early diastolic E wave immediately at the initiation of diastole. The E wave consists of an upgoing acceleration slope followed by a deceleration slope. The time interval from the peak of the E until it drops to its baseline constitutes the deceleration time, which signifies the duration of pressure equalization between the two chambers. The E wave is followed by an atrial systolic A wave toward the end of diastole.

In normal physiological conditions and preserved LV myocardial relaxation, the E wave is higher than the A wave due to a rapid decrease in LV pressure during early diastole, causing filling from the atrium to the ventricle. The deceleration time is in the normal range between 150 and 240 milliseconds. Subsequently, the A wave is small due to only a small remainder of blood in the atrium producing an E/A ratio >1, signifying normal diastolic function. The E wave is blunted in grade-I diastolic dysfunction, where there is an impairment in LV relaxation alone with a resultant increase in early diastolic pressure. Filling of the ventricle now depends on atrial contraction

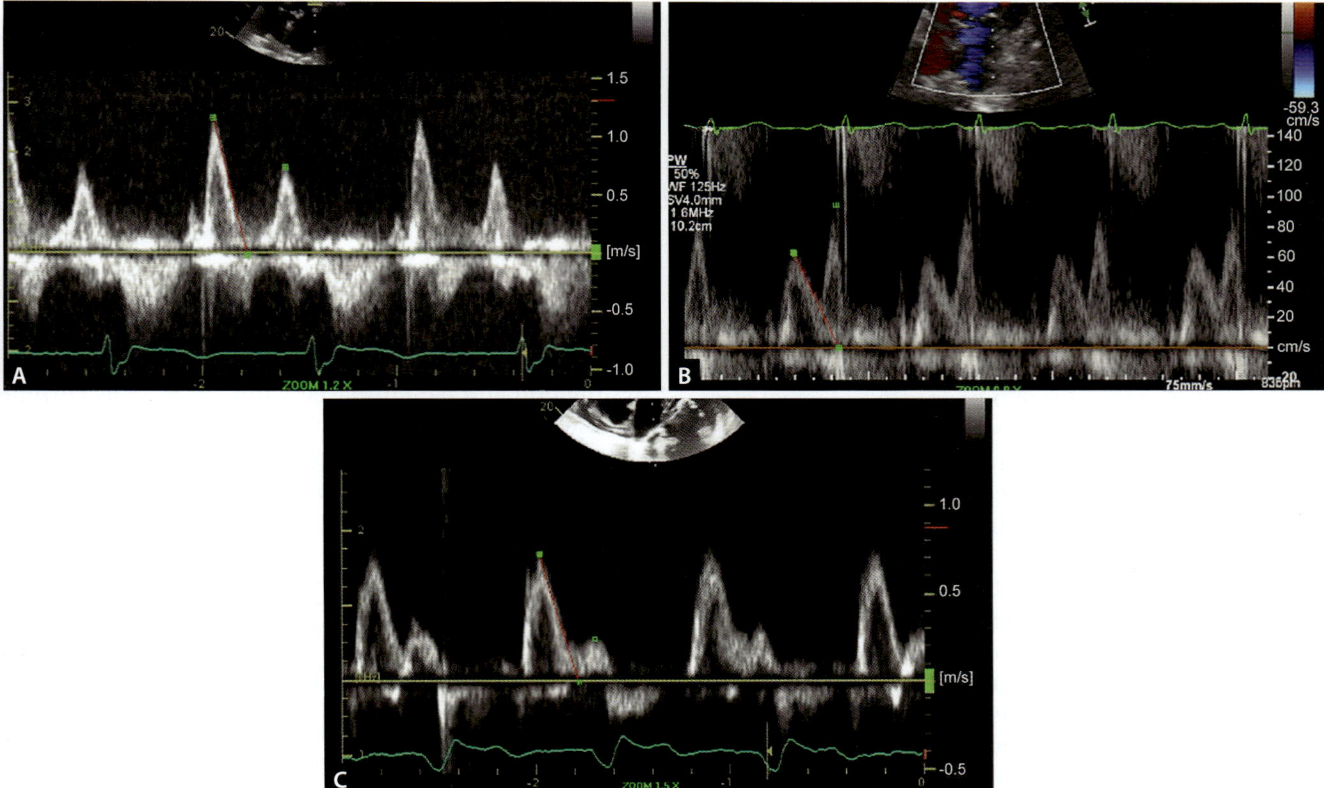

Figs. 1A to C: (A) Normal mitral inflow pattern consistent with normal diastolic function; (B) Reversal of E and A waveforms indicating impaired relaxation with normal left atrial pressures; (C) Markedly elevated E/A ratio consistent with elevated left atrial pressures and impaired relaxation.

alone, generating a larger A wave producing an E/A ratio >1. In grade-II diastolic function, in addition to impaired relaxation, there is an increase in left atrial pressure in response to persistent elevation in filling pressures. This phenomenon returns the E/A to a normal ratio, but individually, both parameters remain abnormal, hence, the term pseudonormal pattern. In grade-III diastolic dysfunction with restrictive filling, the E wave is severely elevated due to elevated left atrial pressures where the E/A ratio is >2.[2] Normal, impaired relaxation and pseudonormal transmitral Doppler waveforms are shown in **Figures 1A to C**.

Like continuous wave Doppler, tissue Doppler imaging of the lateral and medial mitral excursion in diastole creates an e' and a' wave during the E and A wave in the opposite direction. An E/e' ratio >14 should raise suspicion of diastolic dysfunction, prompting the echocardiographer to search for other parameters that may confirm or negate the presence of diastolic dysfunction. The ASE guidelines also utilize a TR velocity value >2.8 m/s and LAVI >34 mL/m^2 as surrogates to pulmonary pressures and left atrial pressures, respectively, to determine the diastolic dysfunction grade.[2] Other echocardiographic parameters, such as pulmonary vein flow velocities, M-mode assessment of B bump, and Tei index, among others, aid in supplementing the assessment of diastology and elevated filling pressures.

Although these parameters and algorithms can identify patients with diastolic dysfunction with excellent specificity, these tests have poor sensitivity.[3] The addition of other nonechocardiographic parameters overcomes this limitation. The two most validated scores, the H_2FPEF and HFA-PEFF scores, have been shown to improve the diagnostic performance of HFpEF. The H_2FPEF score includes four clinical variables (age, body mass index, hypertension, and presence of atrial fibrillation) and two echocardiographic variables(E/e' and estimated pulmonary pressure).[4] The HFA-PEFF score is multistep process and uses symptoms, EKG, and brain natriuretic peptide along with functional echo features, including tissue Doppler or E/e' ratio or TR velocity, and morphological markers, including LA volume index or left ventricular mass index or relative wall thickness.[5]

On a clinical level, something as basic as adequate hypertension management can lead to improvements in diastolic function. A randomized control trial of

384 patients with hypertension, dividing between control versus valsartan, showed improvement in diastolic function based on echo-measured diastolic relaxation velocity.[6]

USE OF STRESS ECHOCARDIOGRAPHY IN THE DIAGNOSIS OF HFpEF

Despite the use of a systematic approach to HFpEF diagnosis as described earlier, a proportion of patients remain undiagnosed with normal preliminary tests but have ongoing HFpEF symptoms on exertion. It is well known that in normal individuals, physiological stress, such as exercise, augments myocardial relaxation to overcome elevated filling pressures. In the presence of impaired LV relaxation, this compensatory mechanism is blunted, lending itself to using stress echocardiography to diagnose occult HFpEF and subclinical diastolic dysfunction.[2] ASE and EACVI guidelines recommend the use of diastolic stress echo in the presence of symptoms and evidence of grade-I diastolic dysfunction to diagnose HFpEF. Its use is limited in a completely structurally normal heart or clearly abnormal diastology parameters. It is best performed with exercise rather than pharmacological stress agents such as dobutamine to stimulate patients' day-to-day activities. An abnormal test is indicated by E/e' >14 or septal E/e' ratio >15 and peak TR velocity >2.8 m/sec with exercise, although there is no universal consensus on this diagnostic criteria.[2] Some limitations of diastolic stress echo are difficulties with accurate image acquisition during tachycardia and fusion of inflow and annular velocities during peak exercise, especially when treadmill testing is used instead of a supine bicycle test. Further, Doppler signals could be contaminated if diastolic stress data is needed during an ischemic stress test, usually done with an ultrasound-enhancing agent (echo contrast). Given these limitations, the need for additional equipment, the lack of consensus on universal diagnostic criteria, and approach to equivocal test results, the real-world uptake of diastolic stress echocardiography remains low.[7]

MONITORING THERAPY IN HFpEF

The strength of echocardiography lies in its ability to diagnose diastolic abnormalities and estimate filling pressures. The role of echocardiography in monitoring therapy using sodium-glucose cotransporter-2 inhibitors and mineralocorticoid receptor antagonists in classic HFpEF patients is less clear. In patients with progressive worsening of diastolic dysfunction over time, we know that patient prognosis worsens. Specific echo parameters that could be targeted for future studies include a reduction in TR velocity, improvement in the mitral inflow velocity pattern, improvement in the E/e' ratio and e' velocities, and a reduction in LA and IVC size. Although no large-scale studies exist to offer guidance for using these parameters over time in patient treatment, on a practical basis, guideline-directed treatment of HFpEF should improve some of these parameters. An interesting future direction includes a better assessment of the left atrial size and function, especially regarding atrial fibrillation and HFpEF. This could be a target to guide such patients' rhythm management decisions. Other limitations to utilizing echo to guide therapy monitoring include the inherently variable nature of the diagnosis of diastolic dysfunction and patient-based variables such as current volume status and heart rate. As machine learning and AI technologies evolve, large-scale data mining can utilize specific echo parameters to identify correlations with patient outcomes.

ROLE OF ECHOCARDIOLOGY IN ASSESSMENT AND MANAGEMENT OF HFpEF MASQUERADERS

With HFpEF being such a heterogeneous disease process, echocardiography becomes critical as a first-line tool to identify potential "masqueraders". Specifically, the clinician should be mindful of screening patients with suspected HFpEF for other cardiac conditions, including hypertrophic cardiomyopathy (HCM), constrictive pericarditis, restrictive cardiomyopathy, and infiltrative disorders. In HCM, classic echo findings include disproportionate LV hypertrophy and LV outflow obstruction. In pericardial disease states, thickening of the pericardium along with interventricular dependence and respiratory variation of the mitral inflow pattern are clues to suggest constriction. Infiltrative disorders often present on echo with LV wall thickening and/or abnormal diastolic dysfunction. Cardiac sarcoidosis can have abnormal septal motion and asymmetric thickening. Hemochromatosis commonly has diastolic dysfunction, and cardiac MRI is typically a more sensitive test. High output heart failure, as seen in disease states such as anemia, cirrhosis, and large AV fistulas, typically has findings on echocardiogram of four chamber enlargement and increased LV outflow velocity-time integral (VTI).[8] The role of echocardiography in HCM, constrictive cardiomyopathy, and amyloid cardiomyopathy will be described as follows.

Diagnosis and Therapy Monitoring in Hypertrophic Cardiomyopathy

Patients with HCM develop heart failure symptoms and inability to exert themselves due to dynamic obstruction

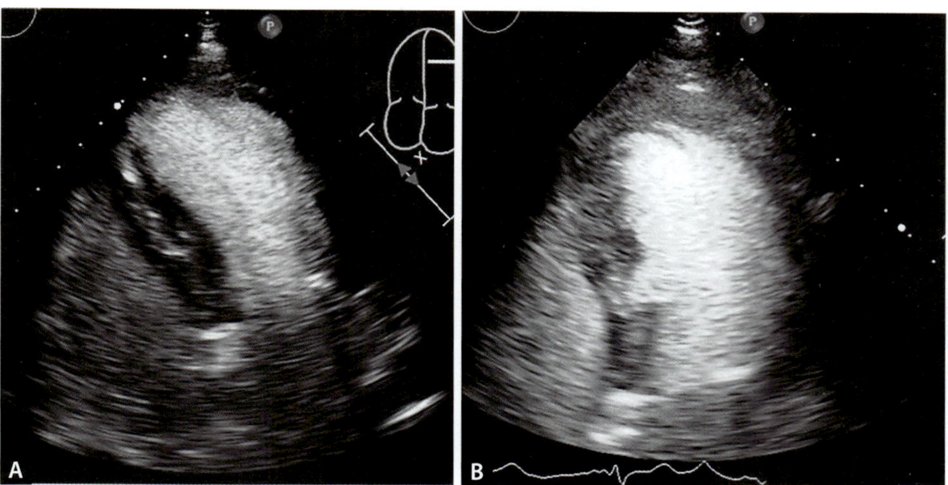

Figs. 2A and B: A patient with severe hypertrophic obstructive cardiomyopathy who underwent septal alcohol ablation. (A) Thickened septum causing outflow obstruction; (B) Infarcted and thinned out portion of the septum after alcohol ablation of a septal perforator causing lowering of the gradient.

to the left ventricular outflow tract (LVOT), hyperdynamic contraction, and impaired relaxation. This obstruction can be due to subaortic obstruction caused by abnormal septal anterior motion (SAM) of the mitral valve, other abnormalities of the mitral valve apparatus, and increased septal thickness.[9] Most patients with HCM have preserved ejection fraction. Reduction in ejection fraction typically occurs in the end stage of the disease. Echo is essential for assessing the LVOT gradient and initiating therapy, as it provides information on the maximum gradient and the precise location where the gradient is created. A significant LVOT gradient is defined as a peak gradient of 30 mm Hg, and therapies are reserved for a gradient of 50 mm Hg. Provocation maneuvers such as Valsalva and standing may be performed if a gradient is not present at rest. In severely symptomatic individuals who do not have a gradient at rest, an exercise stress echocardiogram may be used to determine eligibility for therapies.

Septal myectomy is the gold standard treatment for HCM with obstruction (HOCM), but alcohol septal ablation is equally effective and is reserved for nonsurgical candidates. Alcohol septal ablation uses concurrent fluoroscopy and transthoracic or transesophageal echo to identify the septal perforator supplying the hypertrophied septum. Intracoronary ultrasound-enhancing agent injection is used to localize the vessel to be ablated and to monitor the LVOT gradient during the procedure. Intraprocedural echo guidance has been shown to improve procedural success and decrease intervention time and is currently routinely used.[9] Patients who have undergone either surgery or alcohol septal ablation will need to be monitored with echocardiography either for routine surveillance or at onset of recurrent symptoms. **Figures 2A and B** depict a septal infarct induced by alcohol septal ablation.

Medical management of HOCM includes using beta-blockers, calcium channel blockers, and the subsequent use of echo to assess changes in the LVOT gradient as a response to therapy. Mavacamten is a novel cardiac myosin inhibitor that reduces actin-myosin bridging, resulting in decreased contractility, LVOT gradient, and SAM.[10] It is approved for use in patients with a gradient >50 mg Hg and New York Heart Association (NYHA) class II and III symptoms. Echo features observed after 30 weeks of Mavacamten therapy include resolution of SAM, reduction in LVOT gradient, and improvement in LAVI, and E/e'.[10] Echo monitoring is essential for dose titration.[11] Therapy should only be initiated if the ejection fraction is >55%. At 4 and 8 weeks of treatment, echo is used to reassess the LVOT gradient. A dose reduction is done if the gradient drops to <20 mm Hg. If the gradient remains >20 mm Hg, then the higher dose is maintained. This is to subject the patient to the lowest possible therapeutic dose to minimize the toxic effects of the drug. At 12 weeks of maintenance therapy, if the gradient remains <30 mm Hg, the same dose is continued, and the dose is uptitrated for a gradient >30 mm Hg. At any point during the monitoring period, if LVEF reduces to below 50%, treatment should be terminated.[11]

Diagnosis and Therapy Monitoring in Constrictive Cardiomyopathy

Constrictive physiology as a cause of HFpEF symptoms can be identified by transmitral Doppler flow echocardiography. In constrictive cardiomyopathy, the parietal

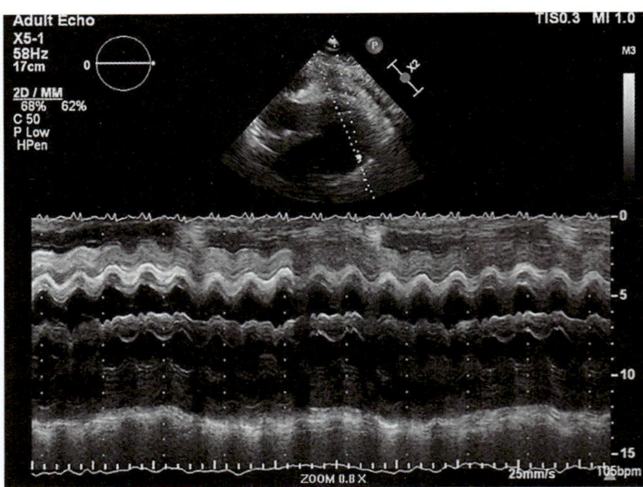

Fig. 3: M-mode in a subcostal window through the interventricular septum shows a septal shift toward the left ventricle in diastole that varies with inspiration versus expiration.

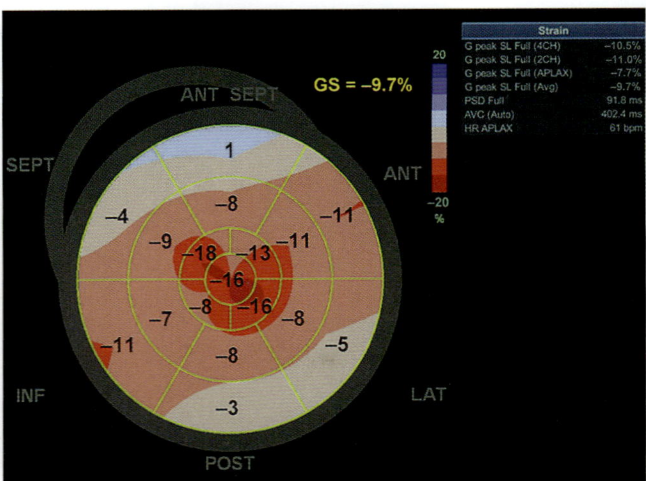

Fig. 4: Strain imaging of a patient with amyloidosis showing the characteristic "cherry-on-top" pattern.

and visceral layers of the pericardium become fused and fibrotic, often due to prior cardiac surgery, thoracic radiation, pericarditis, or idiopathic causes.[12] Two hallmark features of constrictive physiology include the dissociation between intrathoracic and intracardiac pressure changes and ventricular interdependence resulting from a rigid pericardium.[13] These physiological features are evident in Doppler echocardiography. The mitral inflow pattern, observed during inspiration and expiration provides diagnostic clues. Other echocardiographic findings may include pericardial thickening and a characteristic "septal bounce" where the septum abruptly shifts towards the left ventricle in early diastole, as shown in **Figure 3**. For the management of pericarditis and prevention of its recurrence, which can progress to constriction, colchicine is considered the drug of choice.[14] However, definitive treatment for constrictive cardiomyopathy in patients with NYHA class III or IV symptoms involves surgical pericardiectomy to remove the abnormal pericardium and alleviate the restriction on the heart chambers. Doppler echocardiography is also employed to monitor the resolution of constrictive physiology post-surgery, with about 60% of patients showing improvement in Doppler parameters following pericardiectomy.[15]

Diagnosis and Therapy Monitoring in Amyloid Cardiomyopathy

Unlike constrictive cardiomyopathy, where a rigid pericardium impairs ventricular filling, restrictive cardiomyopathy is characterized by a stiff myocardium, leading to increased diastolic ventricular pressure, and decreased ventricular filling. This results in signs and symptoms of heart failure. Notably, the respiratory variation in transmitral Doppler flow seen in constriction is absent in restriction.[16] The etiologies of restrictive cardiomyopathy are diverse and include infiltrative diseases, storage disorders, and conditions that cause myocardial fibrosis. General management focuses on guideline-directed HFpEF therapy and addressing the underlying cause. Among the various conditions associated with restrictive cardiomyopathy, echocardiography plays a particularly crucial role in the diagnosis and treatment monitoring of amyloidosis, where abnormal, misfolded proteins called amyloid fibrils deposit in the extracellular space in the myocardium. There is either an overproduction of light chains in AL amyloidosis or a misfolding of liver-derived transthyretin in ATTR amyloidosis.[17] Key echocardiographic features that raise suspicion for amyloidosis include left ventricular wall thickness greater than 12 mm (in the absence of hypertension), increased myocardial echogenicity, biatrial enlargement, valve thickening, and a decreased global longitudinal strain (GLS) with the characteristic "cherry on top" sign observed on speckle tracking as shown in **Figure 4**. Diastolic dysfunction is universal in amyloidosis with very low septal and lateral tissue Doppler velocities and the presence of any grade of diastolic dysfunction—I, II, or III.[18] These findings should prompt further diagnostic evaluation for amyloidosis. A recently validated score called the ATTR-CM score comprises three clinical parameters (age, sex, and hypertension) and three echocardiographic parameters (ejection fraction, posterior wall thickness, and relative wall thickness) to identify high-risk ATTR amyloid patients who should undergo further diagnostic evaluation.[19] Although echocardiography cannot reliably differentiate between the different types of amyloid cardiomyopathy, it is essential in therapeutic monitoring with either chemotherapy or protein stabilizer/reducer therapies. Expert consensus suggests serial measurements when monitoring response to therapy, including diastology assessments, GLS, and stroke volume.[20]

LEFT ATRIAL STRAIN IMAGING

There has been increasing awareness of the importance of the left atrium in relation to LV function and relaxation. The three phases of left atrial function are serving as a reservoir during LV systole, serving as a conduit for passive LV filling, and booster pump to provide active LV filling. While the size of the left atrium is a critical part of assessing diastolic function, there has been limited clinical data to correlate left atrial function to diastolic function. Strain imaging of the left atrium is a relatively niche topic in echocardiography that has yet to gain widespread adoption but serves as a potential target to better characterize and standardize left atrial function. A prospective multicenter study of 706 patients was carried out in 2015 to characterize normal strain rates in healthy adults compared to a validation group with diastolic dysfunction. Healthy patients had a strain percent of 45.5 ± 11.5%, with a strain rate of –2.11 ± 0.61 , which serve to characterize LA reservoir function and pump function, respectively.[21] Additionally, use of strain imaging detected LA dysfunction in patients with normal left atrial size, and strain parameters were inversely related to NYHA class severity.[21] LA strain imaging may serve as a target for future research in identifying patients earlier who are at risk for developing significant diastolic dysfunction.

CONCLUSION

Echocardiography remains a cornerstone in the evaluation and management of HFpEF. It provides essential insights into diastolic dysfunction, ventricular geometry, and filling pressures, helping to tailor treatment strategies and monitor disease progression. While HFpEF can be challenging to manage due to its complex nature, echocardiography offers a noninvasive, widely available, and highly informative method to assess and manage these patients effectively.

REFERENCES

1. Redfield MM, Jacobsen SJ, Burnett JC Jr, et al. Burden of systolic and diastolic ventricular dysfunction in the community: Appreciating the scope of the heart failure epidemic. JAMA. 2003;289(2):194-202.
2. Nagueh SF, Smiseth OA, Appleton CP, et al. Recommendations for the evaluation of left ventricular diastolic function by echocardiography: An update from the American Society of Echocardiography and the European Association of Cardiovascular Imaging. J Am Soc Echocardiogr. 2016;29(4):277-314.
3. Harada T, Kagami K, Kato T, et al. Echocardiography in the diagnostic evaluation and phenotyping of heart failure with preserved ejection fraction. J Cardiol. 2022;79(6):679-90.
4. Reddy YNV, Carter RE, Obokata M, et al. A simple, evidence-based approach to help guide diagnosis of heart failure with preserved ejection fraction. Circulation. 2018;138(9):861-70.
5. Pieske B, Tschöpe C, de Boer RA, et al. How to diagnose heart failure with preserved ejection fraction: the HFA–PEFF diagnostic algorithm: a consensus recommendation from the Heart Failure Association (HFA) of the European Society of Cardiology (ESC). Eur Heart J. Eur Heart J. 2019;40(40):3297-317.
6. Solomon SD, Janardhanan R, Verma A, et al. Effect of angiotensin receptor blockade and antihypertensive drugs on diastolic function in patients with hypertension and diastolic dysfunction: A randomised trial. Lancet. 2007;369(9579):2079-87.
7. Tani Y, Reddy YNV, Verbrugge FH, et al. Variability in approach to exercise stress echocardiography for diagnosis of heart failure with preserved ejection fraction: An international survey on real-world practice. Eur Heart J Imaging Methods Pract. 2024;2(1):qyae059.
8. Kittleson MM, Panjrath GS, Amancherla K, et al. 2023 ACC Expert Consensus Decision Pathway on Management of Heart Failure with Preserved Ejection Fraction: A Report of the American College of Cardiology Solution Set Oversight Committee. J Am Coll Cardiol. 2023;81(18):1835-78.
9. Ommen SR, Mital S, Burke MA, et al. 2020 AHA/ACC Guideline for the Diagnosis and Treatment of Patients with Hypertrophic Cardiomyopathy: A Report of the American College of Cardiology/American Heart Association Joint Committee on Clinical Practice Guidelines. Circulation. 2020;142(25):e558-631.
10. Hegde SM, Lester SJ, Solomon SD, et al. Effect of mavacamten on echocardiographic features in symptomatic patients with obstructive hypertrophic cardiomyopathy. J Am Coll Cardiol. 2021;78(25):2518-32.
11. Olivotto I, Oreziak A, Barriales-Villa R, et al. Mavacamten for treatment of symptomatic obstructive hypertrophic cardiomyopathy (EXPLORER-HCM): a randomised, double-blind, placebo-controlled, phase 3 trial. Lancet. 2020;396(10253):759-69.
12. Dal-Bianco JP, Sengupta PP, Mookadam F, et al. Role of Echocardiography in the diagnosis of constrictive pericarditis. J Am Soc Echocardiogr. 2009;22(1):24-33.
13. Oh JK. Echocardiography in heart failure: Beyond diagnosis. Eur J Echocardiogr. 2007;8(1):4-14.
14. Chiabrando JG, Bonaventura A, Vecchié A, et al. Management of acute and recurrent pericarditis. J Am Coll Cardiol. 2020;75:76-92.

15. Adler Y, Charron P, Imazio M, et al. 2015 ESC Guidelines for the Diagnosis and Management of Pericardial Diseases: The Task Force for the Diagnosis and Management of Pericardial Diseases of the European Society of Cardiology (ESC) Endorsed by: The European Association for Cardio-Thoracic Surgery (EACTS). Eur Heart J. 2015;36(42):2921-64.
16. Wood MJ, Picard MH. Utility of echocardiography in the evaluation of individuals with cardiomyopathy. Heart. 2004;90(6):707-12.
17. Donnelly JP, Hanna M. Cardiac amyloidosis: An update on diagnosis and treatment. Cleve Clin J Med. 2017; 84(12 suppl 3):12-26.
18. Garcia-Pavia P, Bengel F, Brito D, et al. Expert consensus on the monitoring of transthyretin amyloid cardiomyopathy. Eur J Heart Fail. 2021;23(6):895-905.
19. Davies DR, Redfield MM, Scott CG, et al. A simple score to identify increased risk of transthyretin amyloid cardiomyopathy in heart failure with preserved ejection fraction. JAMA Cardiol. 2022;7(10):1036-44.
20. Dorbala S, Ando Y, Bokhari S, et al. ASNC/AHA/ASE/EANM/HFSA/ISA/SCMR/SNMMI expert consensus recommendations for multimodality imaging in cardiac amyloidosis: Part 1 of 2—evidence base and standardized methods of imaging. J Nucl Cardiol. 2019;26(6):2065-123.
21. Morris DA, Takeuchi M, Krisper M, et al. Normal values and clinical relevance of left atrial myocardial function analysed by speckle-tracking echocardiography: multicentre study. Eur Heart J Cardiovasc Imaging. 2015;16(4):364-72.

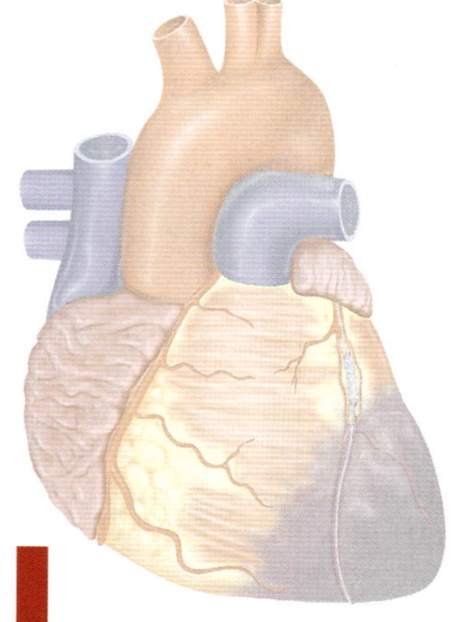

CHAPTER 52

Echocardiographic Evaluation of Diastolic Functions Beyond Guideline

Rohit Tandon, SK Parashar

INTRODUCTION

Evaluation of left ventricular (LV) diastolic function is routinely employed while performing a standard echocardiographic examination. Various echocardiographic parameters [both two-dimensional (2D) and Doppler] can give robust information regarding LV relaxation and compliance properties, a prerequisite for estimating LV filling pressure (LVFP). Echocardiographic estimation of LVFP proves useful in evaluating patients with dyspnea of unknown etiology and also those with symptoms and signs of heart failure with preserved ejection fraction (HFpEF). In this chapter, we discuss the pathophysiology of diastolic dysfunction, and a comprehensive review of techniques used in echocardiographic examination, beyond earlier ASE guidelines of 2016.

Diagnosis of HFpEF is based on (1) presence of clinical syndrome of heart failure, (2) absence of cardiomegaly: with LVEDVI <97 mL/m^2 and LVESV <49 mL/m^2, (3) presence of signs of increased LVFP, (4) other helpful signs including left ventricular hypertrophy (LVH) and/or left atrial enlargement with normal LV ejection fraction >50%, and (5) presence of comorbidities, namely hypertension, diabetes mellitus, CAD, infiltrative disorders (amyloidosis), obesity with/without sleep apnea syndrome, renal dysfunction, constrictive pericarditis, etc.

ECHOCARDIOGRAPHIC METHODS TO ASSESS DIASTOLIC DYSFUNCTION

The ASE 2016 guidelines streamlined the algorithms by restricting the number of variables used to assess LV diastolic function to four key parameters (shown in **Flowcharts 1 and 2**), which are well documented in the literature.

Flowchart 1: Algorithm for the assessment of diastolic dysfunction in patients with normal LVEF.

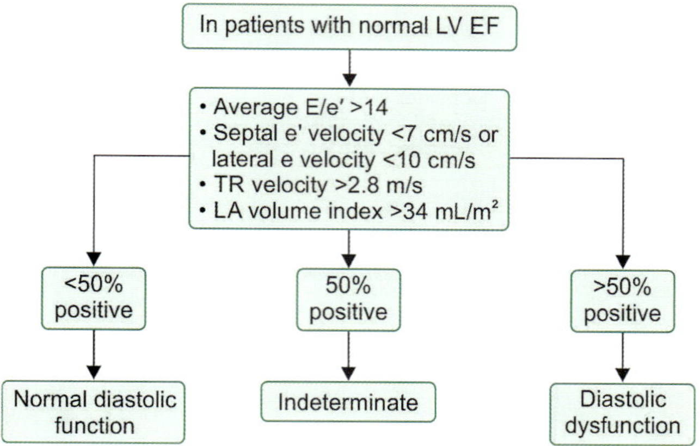

(LVEF: left ventricular ejection fraction)

However, to reduce the frequency of indeterminate cases and to assess the functions at bed side, some more methods have been devised. Before discussing them, two additional parameters such as principle of Valsalva technique and mitral "L" wave are briefly mentioned in the following text.

Valsalva Procedure (Figs. 1 and 2)

Valsalva procedure is a valuable technique in classifying grades of diastolic dysfunction. The patient is first familiarized about how to perform a routine Valsalva and assess if the patient is able to do it. Alternatively, the patient

Flowchart 2: Algorithm for estimation of LV filling pressures and grading LV diastolic function in patients with depressed LVEFs and patients with myocardial disease and normal LVEF.

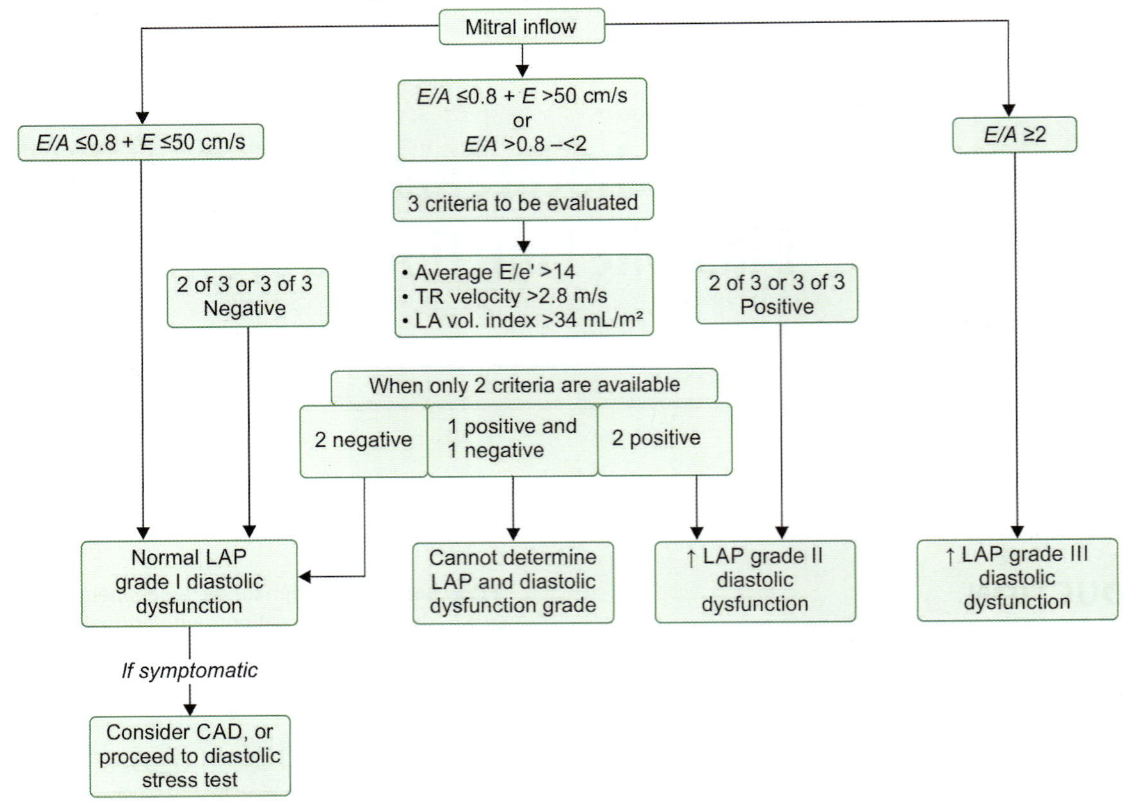

(LVEF: left ventricular ejection fraction)

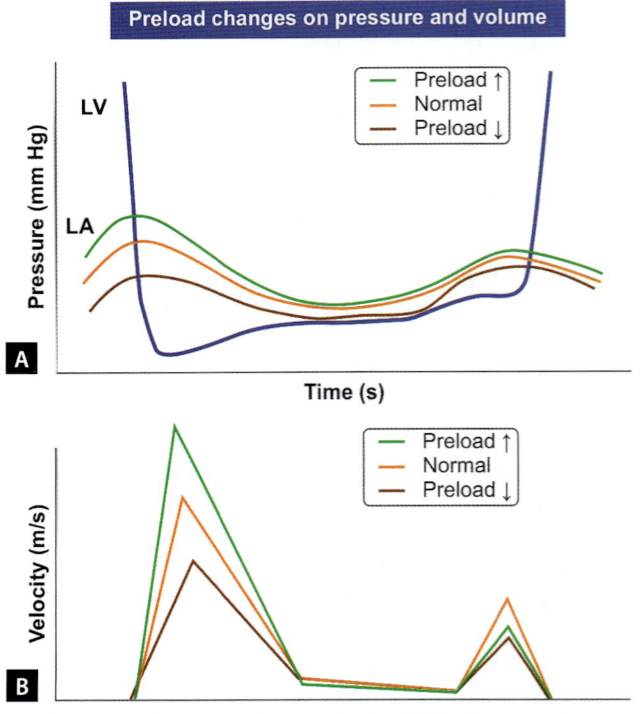

Figs. 1A and B: Hemodynamic basis of Valsalva technique.

is asked to forcefully blow into a sphygmomanometer tube to raise a pressure up to 40 mm of Hg and hold it for 10 seconds. These procedures result in reduction in LV preload, thereby reducing LV end-diastolic pressure. In normal individuals, there is reduction of mitral *E* and *A* velocities (>20 cm/s in *E* wave) along with lengthening of deceleration time with no significant change in *E/A* ratio.

In case of pseudonormal filling, during Valsalva technique, the mean LA pressure is decreased resulting in >50% reduction in *E/A* ratio, with conversion to grade I dysfunction, thereby unmasking a higher grade of diastolic dysfunction. Similarly, in grade III diastolic dysfunction with restrictive physiology, it helps in determining whether the dysfunction is reversible or irreversible which is of significant prognostic value.

Mitral "L" Wave

Mitral "L" wave is an abnormal mid-diastolic positive wave, seen like a "hump", in mitral Doppler, of about 20–30 cm/s velocity, associated with an increased *E/e'* ratio **(Fig. 3)**. L waves are best seen when E and A waves are well separated, as in slow heart rate, or A waves are absent as in atrial fibrillation. It is due to strikingly prolonged LV

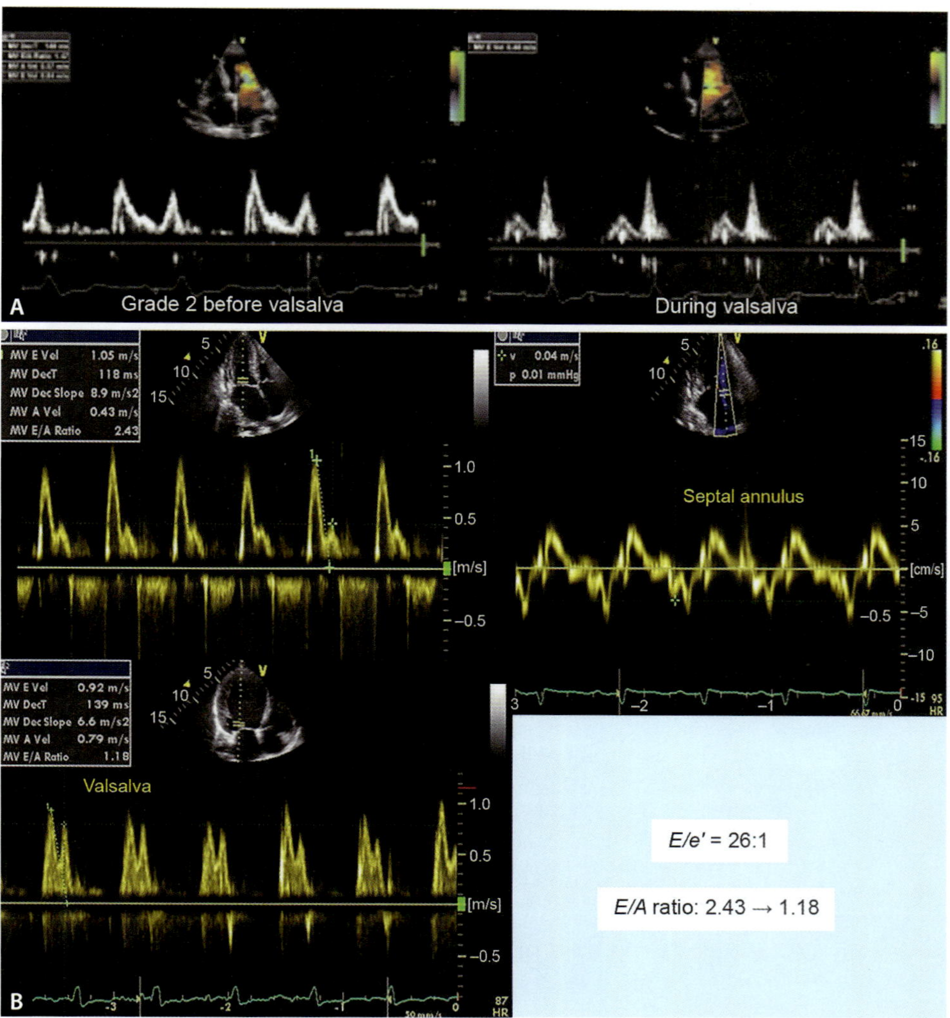

Figs. 2A and B: (A) A pseudonormal pattern being converted to grade I diastolic function during Valsalva; (B) A case of grade III diastolic dysfunction with an *E/e′* ratio of 26:1 and mitral *E/A* ratio of 2.43 which, following Valsalva, is reduced to 1.18 indicative of reversible physiology.

relaxation during transmitral Doppler imaging, associated with increased LVFP. As such, following preload reduction, it tends to regress or disappear because of a decrease in mean LAP **(Fig. 4)**. Occasionally, it can also be seen in TDI recordings **(Fig. 5)**.

DIASTOLIC MITRAL REGURGITATION

During transmitral PW recordings, diastolic mitral regurgitation (MR) may be seen which is highly suggestive of elevated LVEDP. When operational compliance is considerably reduced during late diastole, blood pumping into LV during atrial systole will increase the LV pressure more than the left atrium causing some amount of blood to regurgitate called diastolic MR. This can be identified on transmitral PW recordings.

SIMPLIFICATION IN THE DIAGNOSIS OF DIASTOLIC DYSFUNCTION USING CLINICAL ALGORITHMS

- In the last few years, there have been attempts to (1) simplify the diagnosis, (2) make it more clinically and bedside oriented, (3) reduce indeterminates, and (4) avoid sophisticated tests including invasive hemodynamic exercise monitoring. One such method is the heart failure scoring system—*H_2FPEF scoring system*. Reddy et al. proposed a simple, rapid bedside scoring system utilizing six simple and universally available clinical and echocardiographic variables and gave a point to each variable to create a composite score ranging from 0 to 9 **(Table 1)**.

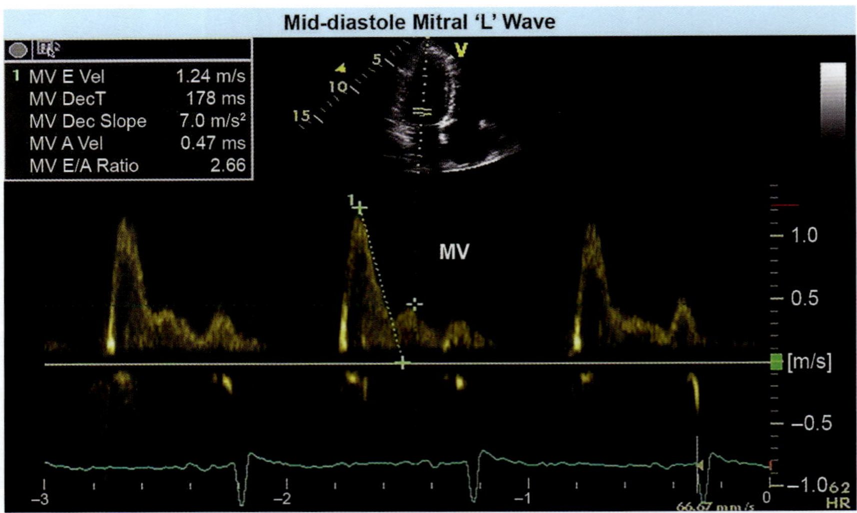

Fig. 3: "L" wave in mitral inflow seen as a "hump" in mid-diastole.

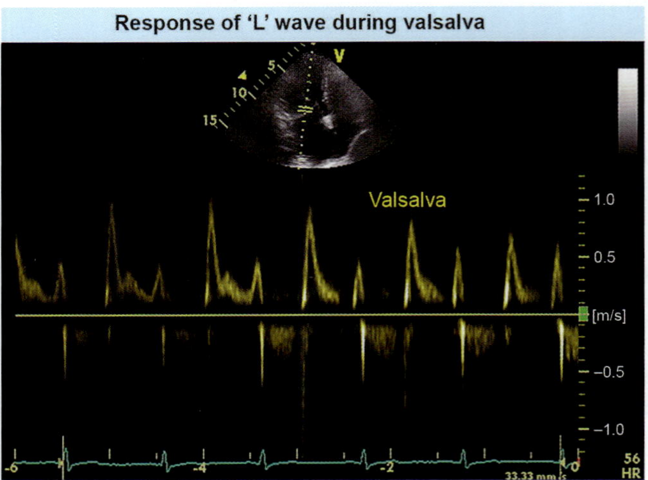

Fig. 4: During Valsalva, there is significant regression of L wave.

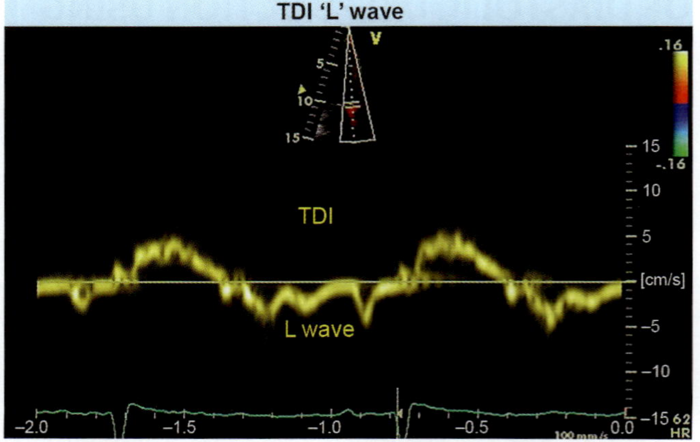

Fig. 5: Mid-diastolic L wave seen in TDI recording.

TABLE 1: Six variables and point given for each variable.

Variable	*Values*	*Points*
(H_2)	Body mass index >30 kg/m^2	2
	Hypertension with two or more antihypertensive medications	1
(F)	Atrial fibrillation—paroxysmal or persistent	3
(P)	Pulmonary hypertension >35 mm Hg	1
(E)	Elderly with age >60 years	1
(F)	Filling pressure: Doppler derived *E/e'* >9	1
H_2FPEF score		9

It can be observed that the presence of two comorbidities, namely obesity and atrial fibrillation, independently increase the probability for HFpEF. By establishing the probability of disease, the H_2FPEF score may be used to effectively rule out disease among patients with low scores (0 or 1), to establish the diagnosis with reasonably high confidence at higher scores (6–9), and to identify patients for whom additional testing is needed with intermediate scores (2–5).

- *Updated recommendations of Heart Failure Association (HFA) of the European Society of Cardiology (ESC)*

A diagnostic algorithm comprising steps for evaluating HFpEF is shown in **Flowchart 3**. *Step 1 (P = Pretest assessment)* is typically performed in the ambulatory setting and includes assessment for HF symptoms and signs, typical clinical demographics and diagnostic laboratory tests, electrocardiogram, and basic echocardiography. In the absence of overt noncardiac causes of breathlessness,

Flowchart 3: Recommended steps in evaluating HFpEF.

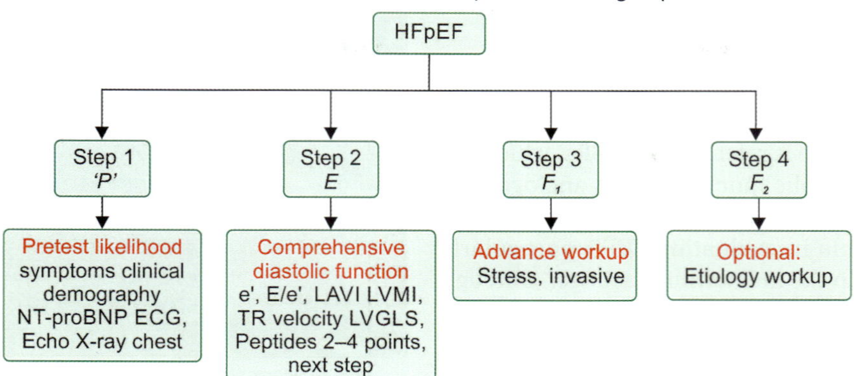

TABLE 2: Diagnostic criteria of points allotted (see the text for details).

Point system: >5 points: HFpEF 2–4 points: Diastolic stress/Invasive: Values corrected for atrial fibrillation		
	Major	*Minor*
E' velocity	Septal (5–7 cm/s) Lateral (7–10 cm/s)	
Average *E/e'*	>15	9–14
PASP	>35 mm Hg	
GLS	>–16%	LV mass index
LAVI	>34 mL/m^2 (SR) >40 mL/m^2 (AF)	Peptides
	>149/122 g/m^2	>115/95
	NT-proBNP > 220 pg/mL (SR) or BNP >80 pg/mL (SR) AF: 3 times the above values	125–220 pg/mL 35–80 3 times the values

HFpEF could be suspected if there is a normal LV ejection fraction, no significant heart valve disease or cardiac ischemia, and at least one typical risk factor. Elevated natriuretic peptides support but normal levels do not exclude a diagnosis of HFpEF. *Step 2 (E = Echocardiography and Natriuretic Peptide Score)* requires comprehensive echocardiography assessing measures which include mitral annular early diastolic velocity (*e'*), LVFP estimated by using *E/e'* ratio, left atrial volume index, LV mass index, LV relative wall thickness, tricuspid regurgitation velocity, LV global longitudinal systolic strain, and serum natriuretic peptide levels. From these measures **(Table 2)**, major (2 points) and minor (1 point) criteria were defined. A score ≥5 points implies definite HFpEF; ≤1 point makes HFpEF unlikely. An intermediate score (2–4 points) implies diagnostic uncertainty, in which case one proceeds to Step 3. *Step 3 (F_1 = Functional testing)* was recommended with echocardiographic noninvasive or invasive hemodynamic exercise stress tests. *Step 4 (F_2 = Final etiology)* was recommended to establish a possible specific cause of HFpEF or alternative explanations. In summary, if step *P* is positive, then second step *E* should be done, which includes a comprehensive echocardiography and brain natriuretic peptide/*N*-terminal natriuretic peptide levels, if not already done in Step *P*. Step F_1 should be done, if step *E* is inconclusive. Step F_2 is optional in confirmed cases, to define underlying etiology.

- *Newer diagnostic parameters:* Recently, some novel diagnostic parameters have been employed for diastolic function assessment, although they were present earlier also and utilized for other clinical conditions:
  - *3D echo/CMR:* As compared to 2D echo, they are more helpful in evaluation of LA and LV volumes and hence LVEF. They are more informative in better tissue characterization, ventricular mass, and hypertrophy. They help in unmasking alternative pathologies.
  - *Diastolic ventricular strain, strain rate, twist:*
- In systolic dysfunction, radial, circumferential and longitudinal strains are affected. Involvement of twist is also observed.
- Radial and longitudinal strains are mainly involved in diastolic dysfunction, whereas circumferential strain and twist are preserved.
- Delayed relaxation is observed by speckle tracking echocardiography to recognize ischemic myocardium while evaluating diastolic function. This is the basis of diastolic strain where even after recovery from transient myocardial ischemia, delayed relaxation persists for a considerable period of time and can be detected by measurement of strain during diastole.

MYOCARDIAL DEFORMATION MEASUREMENTS

Myocardial deformation measurement of strain rate during IVRT is called strain rate during isovolumic relaxation (SR_{IVR}) and during E wave is referred to as (SR_E) which are useful in assessing diastolic function. SR_{IVR}, analogous to *e*′, is inversely related to Tau, similar to *E/e*′. The ratio of E/SR_{IVR} is also suitable in evaluating LVFP, particularly where *E/e*′ ratio falls in the indeterminate range. Although SR_E also represents LV relaxation, the relationship of E/SR_E with LVFP is not as accurate as that of E/SR_{IVR}. These parameters can be performed in mitral valve disease and mitral annular calcification (MAC) where annular velocities are altered. SR_{IVR} is measured at the isovolumic relaxation period. Hence, a transmitral pressure gradient will not be a problem here and also not affected by any changes in preload.

Left Ventricular Twist and Untwisting

Another important cardiac function of the left ventricle is twisting and untwisting. When one looks from the apex of LV during systole, the LV apex normally twists counterclockwise but the base twists clockwise and potential energy is stored by this process. Immediately after, systole LV untwists and the intraventricular pressure gradient is created by untwisting. LV torsion is the sum of both apical and basal twist. Twisting stores potential energy which is released during untwisting at early diastole. The requisite is to obtain good-quality basal and apical LV and basal LV short-axis images. Since it is mainly a research-oriented technique, details are not discussed.

Limitations of the above techniques: Some of the limitations which preclude routine use are (1) technical quality of imaging, (2) multiple artifacts, (3) lack of standardization and reproducibility, (4) lack of consensus on normal and abnormal values, (5) need for more training to achieve satisfactory acquisition and analysis, and (6) lower accuracy with tachycardia.

Left Atrial Function and Strain (Fig. 6)

Left atrial strain has generated a lot of interest recently. It is a promising, simple, noninvasive technique with a diagnostic accuracy of up to 95%, if performed correctly. It is more sensitive than the conventional parameters of atrial function.

Moreover, abnormalities in LA play an important role in pathophysiology and disease progression of HFpEF. LA modulates LV filling by three functions: (1) Reservoir function which occurs during ventricular systole when LA is relaxing and stores pulmonary venous blood (2) conduit. This phase occurs during ventricular diastole when LA transfers blood passively in LV (3) booster. This occurs in the final phase of diastole when LA actively contracts and contributes between 15% and 30% of LV stroke volume. The normal values, average, and range are shown in **Table 3**.

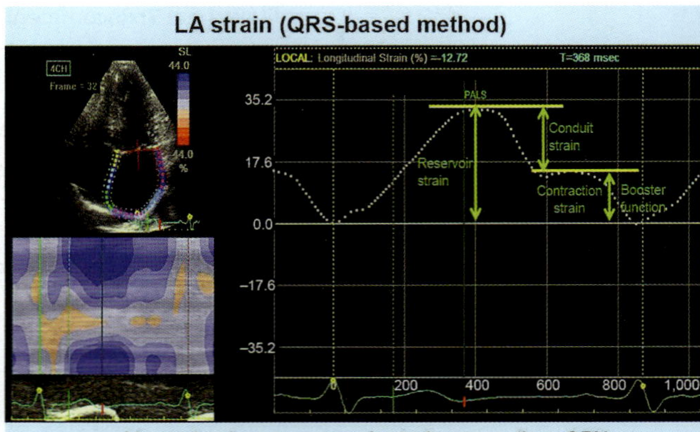

Fig. 6: Left atrial strain showing various functional waves.

TABLE 3: Normal values of LA strain components.

Strain component	Mean	95% CI
Reservoir	39.4	38–40.8
Conduit	23	20.7–25.2
Contractile	17.4	16–19

Atrial fibrosis is responsible for the pathogenesis of LV diastolic dysfunction. Advanced LV diastolic dysfunction may also cause atrial fibrosis due to chronic afterload mismatch. Atrial scarring is ultimately responsible for the reduced LA reservoir, booster pump, and conduit function seen with LV diastolic dysfunction which may be evaluated by LA deformation imaging. In a normal person, pressure elevated during left atrial filling is dampened by increased compliance due to atrial relaxation and mitral annular descent. But at some stage, the atrium becomes stiff at the onset of fibrotic scarring and fills at higher pressures. As a result, reservoir strain or peak LA strain is reduced which is found to correlate well with LVFP. LA strain is calculated as the global strain averaged in six segments utilizing four- and two-chamber views to calculate reservoir, conduit, and booster strain, though reservoir function is more correlated with adverse LV and LA remodeling and is an independent prognostic marker. It may be particularly more useful in situations where annular motion is altered, such as pacing, bundle branch block, and MAC. It is measured by maximal strain during LV systole. It is independent of LAVI.

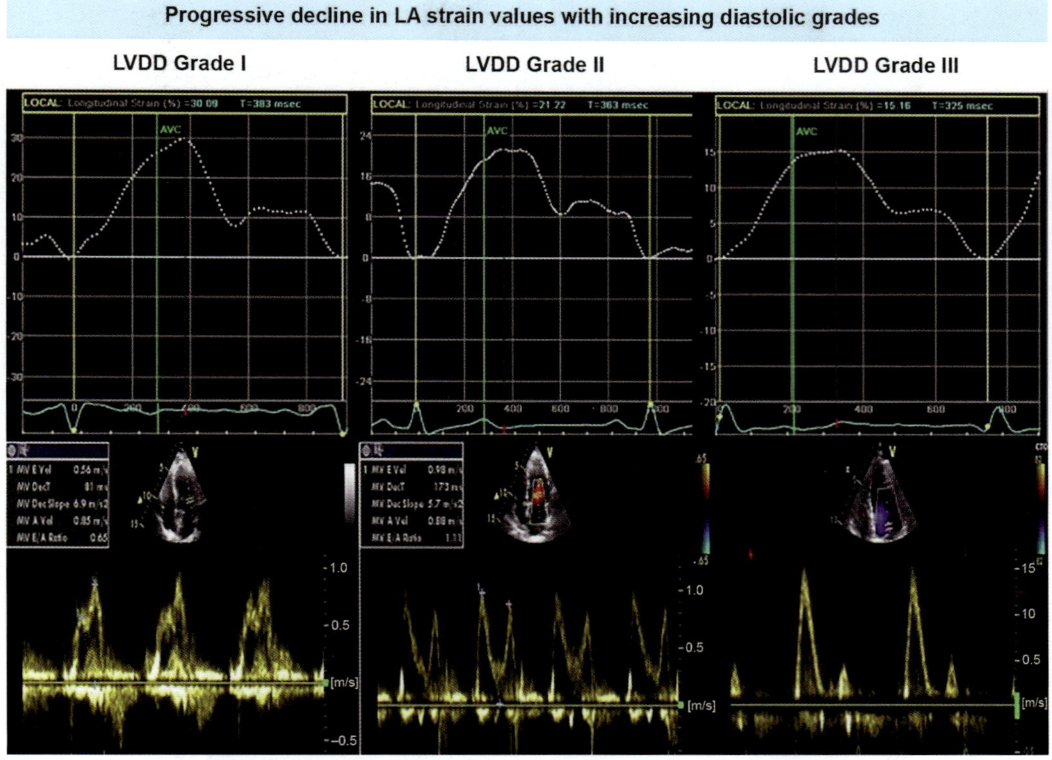

Fig. 7: LA strain showing progressive decline in LA strain from 30% to 22% to 15%.
Courtesy: Nitin Burkule.

There is a significant inverse relationship between values of reservoir strain and LVEDP **(Fig. 7)**. The normal average peak LA strain is 30–40%. A value below 18% is considered significant to predict increased LA filling pressure. One should avoid LA dropouts. It can also track the grade of diastolic function severity, especially between grades I and II in which LA volume may not be able to distinguish.

Limitations: Some of the limitations of LA strain imaging include AF, MAC, MV disease, hypertension, obesity, and LA dropouts.

Left Atrial Stiffness Index

{(E/e')/LARs} incorporates echocardiographic estimates of LAP (E/e') and LA reservoir functions (LARs) to describe left atrial compliance in the setting of impaired diastolic function. In those with diastolic impairment and raised LVFP, elevated LAP causes increased LA wall stress, decreasing LA compliance and leading to reduced LA filling. An index of >0.26 identifies patients who are at a greater risk of heart failure hospitalization or death at 5 years in those with HFpEF (LVEF ≥50%) and LVEDP >16 mm Hg **(Figs. 8A to C)**.

Left Atrial Filling Index

(E wave/LA strain ratio) is a measurement that combines LA and LV diastolic measurements to estimate LVFP **(Flowchart 4; Figs. 8A to C)**.

Left atrial filling index is calculated by dividing the mitral early diastolic inflow peak velocity (E) by the LA reservoir strain (LASr). LA filling index can be a useful tool for estimating LVFP in patients with cardiovascular risk factors and preserved LV ejection fraction. Elevated values (>3.2) are associated with worse functional capacity, heart failure hospitalization at 2 years, and symptomatic status (sensitivity of 83% and specificity of 79%).

ASSESSMENT OF DIASTOLIC DYSFUNCTION IN FEW COMMON CLINICAL CONDITIONS

Atrial Fibrillation

In patients with AF, Doppler assessment of LV diastolic function is limited by the variability in cycle length due to the absence of organized atrial activity and the frequent occurrence of LA enlargement regardless of filling pressure.

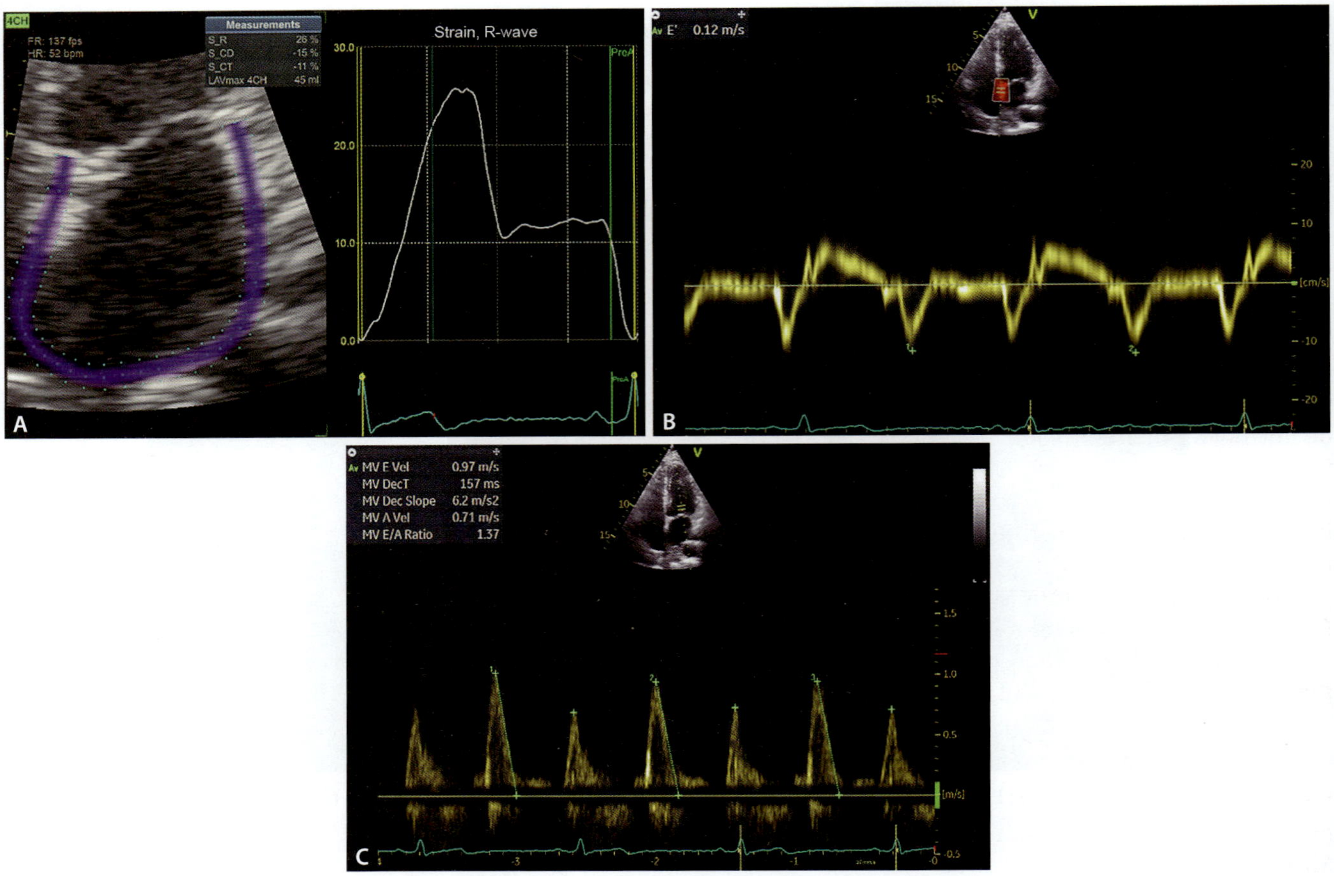

Figs. 8A to C: Calculation of both left atrial stiffness index (0.34) and left atrial filling index (3.3) from left atrial reservoir strain and mitral annular tissue Doppler and inflow velocities.

Flowchart 4: Algorithm of LA filling index explaining the reason for low reservoir strain.

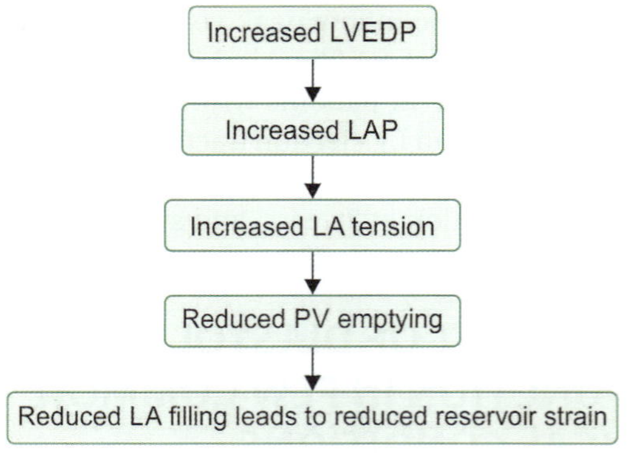

E/septal *e*′ >11 suggests that mean LAP is increased in patients with AF. Because of RR variability, at least 5–10 values should be averaged. Alternatively, three nonconsecutive *E* and *e*′ velocities may be averaged as long as they are within 10–20% of the mean heart rate. An additional clue to the presence of elevated mean LAP is lack of variability in peak E-wave velocity despite varying RR intervals. In summary, the following findings are suggestive of increased LVFPs:

- Mitral "E" peak acceleration rate >1,900 cm/s
- Mitral deceleration time <160 ms in patients with depressed EF
- IVRT <65 ms; "L" wave if present
- Septal *E*/*e*′ >11 indicating filling pressure >15 mm Hg with a sensitivity of 75% and specificity of 93%
- Pulmonary vein diastolic wave DT <220 ms

Atrioventricular Block and Pacing

Abnormalities of cardiac conduction system due to disease, aging, drugs, or pacing can adversely affect atrioventricular (AV) synchrony as well as synchronous LV contraction and relaxation.

Advanced AV Blocks

A first-degree AV block of 200–280 ms is usually well tolerated only if LVEF and heart rate are normal. However, in patients with shortened diastolic filling periods due to markedly impaired LV relaxation, faster heart rates, bundle branch block or ventricular pacing, a first-degree AV block of >280 ms usually results in "fusion" of *E* and *A* velocities. Hence, AV synchrony becomes "unphysiological" as filling occurs only with atrial contraction (uniphasic A wave) and diastolic MR. In this case, only TR velocity can be used as a possible indicator of LVFPs in the absence of any pulmonary disease.

Bundle Branch Blocks

No study has established diastolic LV function impairment with isolated right bundle branch, left anterior hemiblock, or left posterior hemiblock. Left bundle branch block is frequently associated with organic heart disease and impaired LV diastolic function. With normal LAP, an impaired LV relaxation filling pattern is seen, while pseudonormal and restrictive patterns occur with progressive increases in LV stiffness and increased LAP. As long as no fusion of mitral *E* and *A* velocities occurs, the variables used to evaluate diastolic function and filling pressures should remain valid.

Mitral Annular Calcification

Left ventricular diastolic parameters are altered in the presence of MAC. This could be due to direct effects of MAC or might reflect truly reduced diastolic function. Interpretation of diastolic parameters in patients with MAC should be performed with caution. This is because these patients have lower annular velocities and higher transmitral flow velocities. In patients having mild mitral annular calcification, the *E/A* ratio gives modest correlation with LVFPs ($r = 0.66$). *E/A* ratios <0.8 or >1.8 are classified as having normal or elevated LVFP. In the intermediate group (MV ratio 0.8–1.8), measuring IVRT is suggested as a short IVRT (<80 ms) indicates elevated LVFP **(Flowchart 5)**.

Flowchart 5: Algorithm showing evaluation of LV filling pressure in MAC.

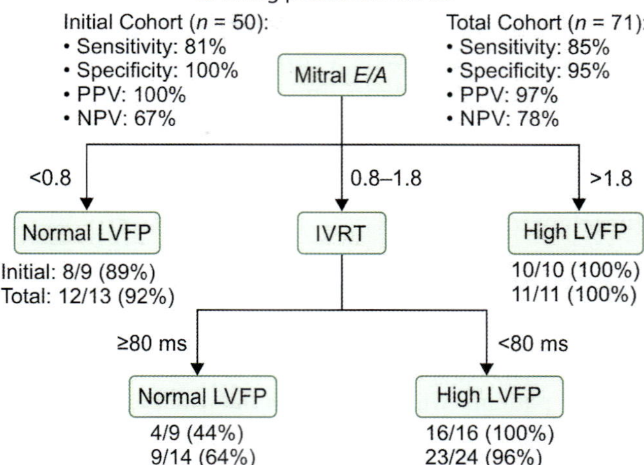

Courtesy: With permission from W Zoghbi.

CAVEATS IN THE DIAGNOSIS OF HEART FAILURE WITH PRESERVED EJECTION FRACTION

- The availability of an objective parameter is essential for the diagnosis of HF because it is a highly subjective condition. Indeed, it has been shown that a majority of HF cases (almost 90%) were actually misdiagnosed. This illustrates the poor diagnostic reliability of the common signs and symptoms of HF.
- Almost >30% may have normal diastolic function, which could also be related to fortuitous LV unloading because of prior administration of diuretics.
- BNP and NT-proBNP, in general, are elevated in patients with acute heart failure, rather than chronic heart failure. They can also be normal in stable, symptomatic HFpEF. Hence, normal NP levels do not exclude HFpEF.
- Many individuals have abnormal diastolic functions with a normal EF, and this combination, per se, does not mean that they have HF.
- Noninvasive diagnosis of HFpEF remains challenging in euvolemic patients where resting LVFPs may be normal. Hence, objective documentation of elevated LVFP may be difficult. Conversely, LV diastolic pressure may be increased in the setting of normal LV diastolic properties if total body water is inappropriately increased.
- Assessment of various global diastolic strain studies needs more experience in routine practice.

CONCLUSION

Diastolic dysfunction (HFpEF) is an intriguing disease which is either over- or underdiagnosed. However, assessment should be done in all vulnerable patients for heart failure and those presenting with unexplained dyspnea, either at rest or on exertion. A clinical correlation, including age and comorbidities and good 2D echo, is always the starting point. Some simple bedside techniques have been described to assess a rapid evaluation of HFpEF. Deformation imaging like LA strain has emerged as an important step in evaluation. Hence, it is imperative to have a step-wise approach. It should always be mentioned in the final report if filling pressure is normal, increased, or indeterminate and should be compared in every follow-up following therapy. Increased PA systolic pressure, in the absence of COPD, is an indirect and good criterion for diastolic dysfunction. It is imperative to integrate several echo variables to arrive at a correct diastolic assessment. Various diagnostic algorithms have been proposed to simplify the diagnosis. Newer and novel indices and artificial intelligence have the potential to advance in this field to fill up the gaps in knowledge and may play an important role in future.

SUGGESTED READING

1. Abudiab MM, Chebrolu LH, Schutt RC, et al. Doppler echocardiography for the estimation of LV filling pressure in patients with mitral annular calcification. JACC Cardiovasc Imaging. 2017;10(12):1411-20.
2. Bianco CM, Sengupta PP, Farjo PD, et al. Myocardial mechanics in patients with normal LVEF and diastolic dysfunction. JACC Cardiovasc Imaging. 2020;13:258-71.
3. Braunauer K, Düngen HD, Belyavskiy E, et al. Potential usefulness and clinical relevance of a novel left atrial filling index to estimate left ventricular filling pressures in patients with preserved left ventricular ejection fraction. Eur Heart J. 2020;21(3):260-9.
4. Kim D, Seo JH, Choi KH, et al. Prognostic implications of left atrial stiffness index in heart failure patients with preserved ejection fraction. JACC Cardiovasc Imaging. 2023;16(4):435-45.
5. Nagueh SF, Smiseth OA, Appleton CP, et al. Recommendations for the evaluation of left ventricular diastolic function by echocardiography: an update from the American Society of Echocardiography and the European Association of Cardiovascular Imaging. J Am SocEchocardiogr. 2016;29:277-314.
6. Nagueh SN. Left ventricular diastolic function: Understanding pathophysiology, diagnosis, and prognosis with echocardiography. JACC Cardiovasc Imaging. 2020; 13:228-44.
7. Oh JK, Miranda WR, Bird JG, et al. The 2016 diastolic function guideline: Is it already time to revisit or revise them? JACC Cardiovasc Imaging. 2020;13(1 Part 2):327-35.
8. Pieske B, Tschöpe C, de Boer RA, et al. How to diagnose heart failure with preserved ejection fraction: the HFA–PEFF diagnostic algorithm: a consensus recommendation from the Heart Failure Association (HFA) of the European Society of Cardiology (ESC). Eur Heart J. 2019;40:3297-317.
9. Reddy YNV, Obokata M, Egbe A, et al. Left atrial strain and compliance in the diagnostic evaluation of heart failure with preserved ejection fraction. Eur J Heart Fail. 2019;21(7):891-900.
10. Silbiger JJ. Pathophysiology and echocardiographic diagnosis of left ventricular diastolic dysfunction. J Am Soc Echocardiogr. 2019;32(2):216-32.
11. Singh A, Addetia K, Lang RM. LA strain for categorization of LV diastolic dysfunction. JACC Cardiovasc Imaging. 2017;10(7):735-43.
12. Sorrentino R, Espusito R, Santoro C, et al. Practical Impact of new diastolic recommendations on noninvasive estimation of left ventricular diastolic function and filling pressures. J Am Soc Echocardiogr. 2020;33(2):161-71.
13. Yogesh NV, Reddy Rickey E, Margaret M, et al. A simple, evidence-based approach to help guide diagnosis of heart failure with preserved ejection fraction. Circulation. 2018;138:861-70.

CHAPTER 53

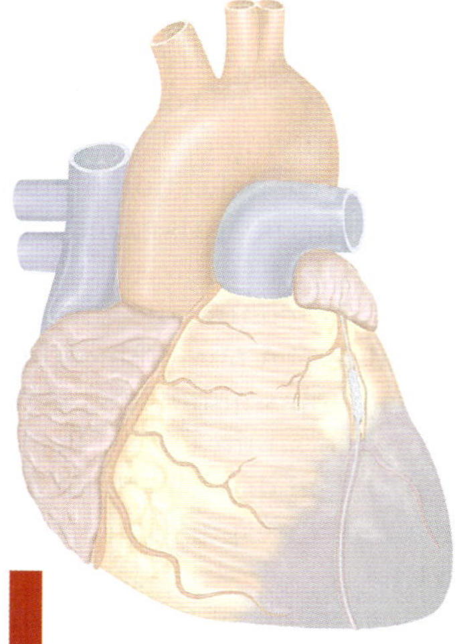

Echocardiography Evaluation of the Left Atrial Strain on Patients with SGLT2i and ARNI with HFpEF

Amrish Agrawal, Vishal Agrawal, Thair Al Jumaily

INTRODUCTION

The left atrium (LA) has an important role in mastering left ventricular (LV) filling during the whole diastole. It modulates LV filling by providing LA boost toward the end of ventricular diastole. Its dysfunction is a powerful predictor of heart failure (HF), myocardial infarction, atrial fibrillation (AF), and cardiovascular death.

The time-dependent adaptive response of atrial myocytes to mechanical and metabolic stressors gives rise to LA remodeling, which at the tissue level is due to the alterations leading to myocyte hypertrophy, necrosis, and changes in the composition of the extracellular matrix.

Over the years, varied echocardiography parameters were looked into, ranging from volumetric to Doppler approaches, as a prognostic indicator for adverse cardiovascular outcomes. Though LA size and volume assessment are commonly used and well established, increasingly LA function assessment by strain imaging has an important role in many conditions, especially for the impact of therapy for HF.

EVOLUTION OF ECHOCARDIOGRAPHY FOR LEFT ATRIAL FUNCTION ASSESSMENT

With the evolution of the technology of echocardiography, there have been incremental advances and refinement about parameters used to define LA function.[1] With the advent of tissue Doppler imaging (TDI), which is less dependent on load, A velocity was utilized as a measure of LA contractile function, and it demonstrated a good correlation with traditional Doppler and LA volumetric measurements. Assessment of A velocity mandates the presence of sinus rhythm, and LA function index (LAFI) was derived to evaluate LA function even in AF.[2] Another common assessment is the use of LA volume index (LAVI), which shows reduction with HF improvement but lacks sensitivity as a marker of improvement of diastolic dysfunction.[3]

Two-dimensional speckle-tracking echocardiography (2D-STE) analysis provides an assessment of myocardial deformation and is based on tracking change of speckle position in an echocardiographic image, during the movement of the heart wall over the course of a heart cycle. Assessment of left atrial strain (LAS) by 2D-STE provides an angle-free assessment of the atrial deformation,[4] and many of the limitations and shortcomings of previous methods can be bypassed.[3] As we will discuss in the next section, strain evaluates myocardial deformation, while strain rate examines the rate of change in the strain. Both strain and strain rate can be measured throughout the cardiac cycle, thereby enabling the evaluation of LA function in all three phases of LA contraction, which include the reservoir, conduit, and contractile phases. This improves the sensitivity for early detection as well as the prognosis of diastolic dysfunction.

METHODOLOGY AND PITFALLS IN OBTAINING LEFT ATRIAL STRAIN

Assessment of LAS by 2D-STE has come to the fore in the current decade, mirroring its rise for the assessment of

LV global longitudinal strain (GLS), and it is much more superior to TDI and velocity vector imaging (VVI).[5]

The EACVI/ASE/Industry Taskforce consensus document[4] (2018) recommends standardized LAS analysis using apical four-chamber nonforeshortened views with a higher frame rate (50–70 frames/min). Subdivision of the LA wall into segments is not recommended, as orifices of pulmonary veins and LA appendage are anyway extrapolated for tracking purposes. Biplane assessment can be done, but it is optional. LA longitudinal strain is referred to as the global longitudinal strain of the entire wall. Methodological challenges for LAS include contouring the LA endocardial surface due to the thin LA wall, far-field localization of LA on echo and mobile interatrial septum, as well as aneurysms.

The LA function is divided into three distinct phases: (1) Reservoir, (2) conduit, and (3) contraction, each associated with pressure and volumetric portions of the respective LV cardiac cycle.[4] In the reservoir phase, when the mitral valve is closed and as the pulmonary veins fill the LA with blood, the LA stretches. Expansion of LA in the longitudinal axis gives rise to an atrial strain that is positive and reaches its peak at the end of LA filling before the opening of the mitral valve. The peak strain, referred to as peak atrial longitudinal strain (PALS), is considered the most important due to its prognostic value in cardiovascular diseases.[6]

Subsequently, with the opening of the mitral valve, passive LA emptying ensues into the LV (corresponding to the E wave), which is modulated by atrial compliance, LV relaxation, and compliance. Emptying of LA results in decreased atrial strain with negative deflection of the strain curve up to a plateau period. This phase is called the conduit phase.[6]

The last phase is labeled as the contractile phase. It represents the atrial systole and the LA pump function. It corresponds to the A wave (late transmitral flow) and causes a second deflection on the strain curve. Peak atrial contraction strain (PACS), or late-diastolic strain, is measured following the P wave and corresponds to active atrial contraction **(Figs. 1A to C)**.

Commonly, strain processing begins at the nadir of LAS, which coincides with the mitral valve closure and is situated at the onset of QRS. This is the zero reference, and hence PALS corresponds to atrial reservoir function, strain during early diastole reflects atrial conduit function, and strain during late diastole (PACS) corresponds to atrial contractile function.

Left atrial strains are dependent on image quality and influenced with acoustic window, which influences delineation of chamber endocardial borders. LAS is also dependent on electrocardiogram gating, and R-to-R gating is preferred to avoid influence of atrial arrhythmias

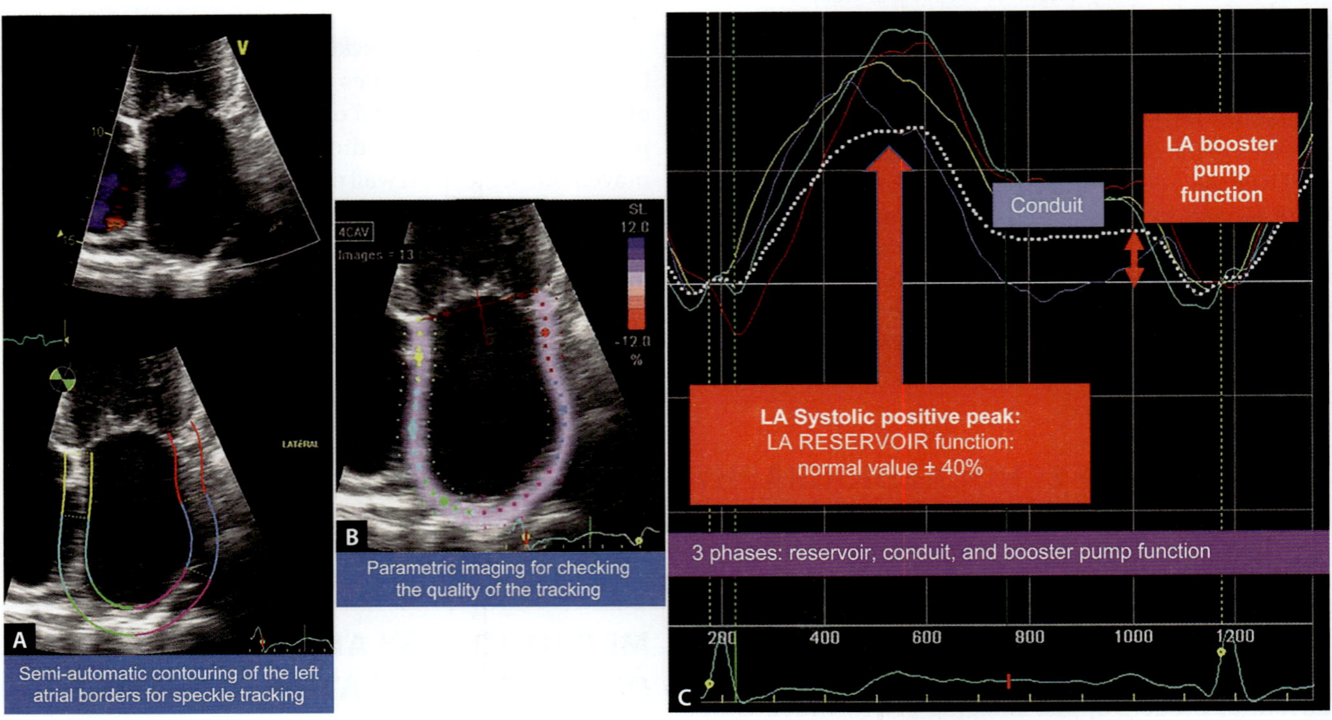

Figs. 1A to C: Example of how to get left atrial strain for quantifying left atrial function.
Source: Adapted from Donal et al.[7]

TABLE 1: Normal values of LA reservoir, conduit, and booster strain.[8]

Phasic left atrial strain	Mean with 95% CI
Left atrial reservoir strain (PALS)	39.4% (38–40.8)
Left atrial conduit strain (LAS-cd)	23% (20.7–25.2)
Left atrial booster or contractile strain (LAS-ct)	17.4% (16–19)

influencing atrial contraction. The normal values of LAS from each phase are listed in **Table 1**.[8]

SUPERIORITY OF LEFT ATRIAL STRAIN IN HEART FAILURE

Heart failure is an important condition that requires careful and detailed evaluation of the function of left ventricle and LA. Currently, European and American guidelines[9] describe phenotypes [HFrEF, heart failure with preserved ejection fraction (HFpEF), and heart failure with mildly reduced ejection fraction (HFmrEF)] based on the cutoffs of ejection fraction (EF), and preserved ejection fraction (pEF) is defined as those with EF >50%. Though LA function is impaired in all subtypes of HF, assessment of diastolic dysfunction is very important in HFpEF as well as in HFmrEF, as it is its main pathophysiological mechanism.

The echo assessment algorithm for diastolic function is complex and multiparametric, using transmitral flow, tissue velocity, the maximum LAVI, and estimated pulmonary artery pressure.[8] Both LAVI and E/e′ ratios can lose their diagnostic value at more severe grades of diastolic dysfunction. LA function deteriorates progressively with increasing LV filling pressure and dilatation of the LA chamber.[5] Serial LAS assessment by showing gradual progression can represent a sensitive diagnostic tool to differentiate between stages of advanced diastolic dysfunction.[10] During the early stages of HFpEF, an increase in LV pressure conducts to LA and causes decrease in LA relaxation and PALS. As the severity increases, LAVI also increases, which is used as one of the components to diagnose diastolic dysfunction.[10]

Singh et al.[11] found that an LAS cutoff of 19% separates grade III diastolic dysfunction with >90% accuracy, and an LAS threshold of >24% differentiates grade I from grade II or grade III diastolic dysfunction. Multiple studies suggest that PALS correlated well with escalating patient symptomatology, with lower values associated with a higher NYHA class.[12] It has also demonstrated utility in HFpEF patients as it is decreased in the early stages of the disease, being able to predict admissions, cardiovascular mortality, and sudden death.[13]

Atrial fibrillation is common in all categories of HF due to atrial overload, dilatation, and fibrosis. Atrial arrhythmias are common in patients with setting of HFpEF and restrictive cardiomyopathy, particularly in cardiac amyloidosis related to amyloid deposition. In a large cohort of patients with cardiac amyloidosis, Bandera et al.[14] found increased atrial stiffness and reduced LA reservoir and contraction function, which was independently associated with reduced clinical outcomes.

THERAPEUTIC RECOMMENDATION FOR TREATMENT OF PATIENTS WITH HFpEF

Guideline-directed medical therapy (GDMT) has improved medical outcomes for patients with HFrEF.[9] Class I recommendation medications include a beta blocker, angiotensin receptor–neprilysin inhibitors (ARNI, if not possible then, ACEi or ARB), a mineralocorticoid-receptor antagonist, and sodium–glucose cotransporter-2 inhibitors (SGLT2i). All the above drugs have been tested in the setting of HFpEF.

Currently, ARNI is a class IIb recommendation for HFpEF. By inhibiting the renin–angiotensin–aldosterone system, ARNI/ACEi/ARB therapy was shown to have a major effect on collagen synthesis, reducing interstitial fibrosis, and inflammation. In 2021 ESC guidelines for HF,[9] SGLT2 inhibitors were a class IIa recommendation in HFmrEF and HFpEF; however, in their 2023-focused update of HF, these have been upgraded to class IA recommendation and as the first specific therapeutic agents to be used in both types of HF, irrespective of the diabetic state.

IMPACT OF ANGIOTENSIN RECEPTOR–NEPRILYSIN INHIBITORS ON LEFT ATRIAL STRAIN IN HFpEF

Currently, ARNIs carry a class IIb indication in the setting of HFpEF. The putative mechanism for improvement in LA function in the setting of HFpEF includes sustained improvement in cardiac hemodynamics and filling pressure, and reduction in the burden of myocardial fibrosis.[15] With ARNI, the amount of LV remodeling is decreased or reversed with improved cardiac efficiency. Therefore, patients with less fibrosis and at an early stage of atrial disease may respond more quickly with a decrease in overall chamber compliance and a resultant decrease in LA dimension.[16] On the other hand, LA assessment may be less sensitive to capture the effect of HF treatment in patients with advanced atrial disease, as those with a history of AF.

The relationship between treatments with ARNI and the treatment effects on LV GLS and LAS has been studied, providing valuable information for clinical practice. A multicenter study in Italy looked at LV GLS and PALS as predictors of reverse LV remodeling after 6 months and found that an increase in PALS was associated with decreased NT-proBNP and NYHA class, once again demonstrating its utility for congestive states.[17] Similar to other studies, ARNIs were associated with improved LV GLS and LAS for a minimum of 3–6 months in patients with optimal GDMT.[16] Increased LV GLS and LAS also demonstrated an associated decrease in hospitalizations and cardiovascular death.[18]

The PARAMOUNT (Prospective Comparison of ARNI with ARB on Management of Heart Failure with Preserved Ejection Fraction) trial studied the effect of ARNI versus ARB on NT-proBNP, finding lower values in the group treated with ARNI.[16] LA dimensions and left atrial volume (LAV) were significantly reduced in the ARNI group after 36 weeks of treatment ($p = 0.003$ and $p = 0.034$), respectively. Other echocardiographic measurements, including LVEF, ventricular volumes, or diastolic function parameters, did not differ significantly at 9 months. A substudy compared the two pharmacological approaches to assess the impact on LV GLS though its impact on LAS was not studied. The PARAGON-HF trial studied the comparison of ARNI with ARBs in the treatment of HFpEF, demonstrating lower cardiovascular deaths and hospitalization in the ARNI group; however, this just missed statistical significance when compared to the ARB group.

IMPACT OF TREATMENT WITH SODIUM–GLUCOSE COTRANSPORTER-2 INHIBITORS ON LEFT ATRIAL STRAIN IN HFpEF

Over the last few years, the role of SGLT2 inhibitors has been well established across the full spectrum of HF,[19] and their use has resulted in significant benefits in patients with HF, irrespective of LVEF.

The reasons for these benefits are multiple, but one of the mechanisms is SGLT2 inhibition in HF promotes reverse cardiac remodeling. Cardiac remodeling is a pivotal mechanism in HF progression and is associated with poor clinical outcomes. Congestive treatment unloads the LA, resulting in an improvement in reservoir function. Studies looking into this matter of ACR have small numbers and need to be clubbed to get relevant supporting information.[20]

In a systematic review and meta-analysis published in 2022,[21] where 32 studies with 2,351 patients were included, the use of SGLT2 inhibitors was associated with an improvement in markers of cardiac function. SGLT2 inhibitors are able to decrease LA afterload mismatch, which improves LA booster pump function in the failing heart. There is also improvement in operative atrial distensibility in congestive HF.

In another paper published in 2022, the authors[20] studied the effect of empagliflozin on LAS in patients with type 2 diabetes (T2D) and ACS in 44 participants in an Australian hospital. The baseline LAS was similar between the groups. LA reservoir, conduit, and contractile strain increased in the empagliflozin group but remained unchanged in the comparison group. The difference in change between the groups was significant for the LA reservoir ($p = 0.003$) and contractile strain ($p = 0.005$).

In a subanalysis of the EMPA hemodynamic study,[22] which was a prospective, randomized placebo-controlled exploratory trial, the authors examined the effect of SGLT2 inhibitor empagliflozin on LAS in patients with diabetes. Output variables were analyzed at baseline, day 1, day 3, and 3 months. The study was well conducted, with low-interobserver variability of 0.97 and intraobserver variability of 0.98 for LAS reservoir. There was no effect of empagliflozin on hemodynamic parameters or EF, whereas diastolic filling pressure as measured by E/e′ was significantly improved after 1 day of treatment and sustained until the end of the study. In addition, LAS analysis showed empagliflozin significantly improved LA function after 3 months of treatment, as assessed by an increase in the LAS reservoir and LAS contraction phase values compared with placebo.

In a research thesis submitted in March 2023, Strohhofer[22] looked at echocardiographic loops of 219 patients after AMI, within the framework of the EMMY trial, at three points in time (weeks 0, 6 ± 2, and 26 ± 2) regarding LA structure and function. Mean GLS was 22.2 (95% CI 20.6–23.8). The measured echocardiographic LA structural and functional parameters did not significantly differ between the intervention and placebo groups at any time. Over time, both groups demonstrated a significant increase in LA GLS and LAVI.

Tanaka et al.[23] studied the impact of adding dapagliflozin in diabetic patients with different types of chronic stable HF. They found significant improvement of LVEF%, LAVI, and E/e′, together with the improvement of LV GLS after administration of dapagliflozin for all HF patients. This improvement was superior in patients with

HFpEF, which were 69% of all patients, compared to non-HFpEF patients.

Thiele et al.[24] enrolled 44 diabetic patients to receive empagliflozin 10 mg for 3 months. Even though there was no effect on hemodynamic parameters, there was a significant improvement in the E/e′ ratio, which was detected from the first day of treatment and maintained till the end of study. In addition, empagliflozin significantly improved LAS parameters after 3 months of treatment with LA reservoir and LA contraction phase values changed from 26.4 ± 8.0 to 29.0 ± 7.4%; $p = 0.011$ and from 10.9 ± 5.7 to 12.5 ± 6.0%; $p = 0.008$, respectively compared with placebo.

In a study published in 2023, El-Saied et al.[25] looked at the impact of SGLT2i on LA functions in 70 patients with T2D and HFmrEF. LA volumes and deformation analysis were conducted using 2D-STE. Three LAS parameters were obtained (LA reservoir strain, contractile strain, and conduit strain). After 6 months of SGLT2i treatment, there was better control of HbA1c and improvement of diastolic functions (E/e′ ratio and LAVI significantly decreased, $p < 0.001$). LA reservoir increased from 17.3 ± 2.0 to 23.8 ± 3.6, LA conduit from 11.0 ± 2.2 to 13.7 ± 2.8, and LA contractile from 6.5 ± 1.4 to 10.5 ± 2.6, $p < 0.001$ for all. Changes in LAS values were significantly associated with the changes in LV GLS, LAEF%, E/e′ ratio, and LAVI. The authors concluded that adding SGLT2i to the existing GDMT in patients with T2DM and HFmrEF is associated with favorable clinical outcomes and significant improvement of LA volume and functions, with further improvement of LV diastolic and longitudinal functions.

CONCLUSION

The LA by virtue of the chamber being proximal to the left ventricle influences and is also influenced by changes occurring in hemodynamic stress of HF. There is the emergence of LAS, a novel marker of LA function to reliably predict the diastolic dysfunction and outperforms conventional parameters. Both ARNI and SGLT2 inhibitors improve HF outcomes in the setting of pEF and can play a substantial role in reversing adverse cardiac remodeling, including improving LV systolic and diastolic functions, LV mass, and volume. All these translate to an improvement of LA function as assessed by LAS. Reversed cardiac remodeling may partially explain the favorable effects of SGLT2i on LA function.

REFERENCES

1. Hoit BD. Left atrial size and function: role in prognosis. J Am Coll Cardiol. 2014;63(6):493-505.
2. Gan GCH, Ferkh A, Boyd A, et al. Left atrial function: evaluation by strain analysis. Cardiovasc Diagn Ther. 2018;8(1):29-46.
3. Morris DA, Belyavskiy E, Aravind-Kumar R, et al. Potential usefulness and clinical relevance of adding left atrial strain to left atrial volume index in the detection of left ventricular diastolic dysfunction. JACC Cardiovasc Imaging. 2018;11(10):1405-15.
4. Badano LP, Kolias TJ, Muraru D, et al. Standardization of left atrial, right ventricular, and right atrial deformation imaging using two-dimensional speckle tracking echocardiography: a consensus document of the EACVI/ASE/Industry Task Force to standardize deformation imaging. Eur Heart J Cardiovasc Imaging. 2018;19(6):591-600.
5. Molnár AÁ, Merkely B. The added value of atrial strain assessment in clinical practice. Diagnostics (Basel). 2022;12(4):982.
6. Thomas L, Muraru D, Popescu BA, et al. Evaluation of left atrial size and function: relevance for clinical practice. J Am Soc Echocardiogr. 2020;33(8):934-52.
7. Donal E, Galli E, Schnell F. Left atrial strain: a must or a plus for routine clinical practice? Circ Cardiovasc Imaging. 2017;10(10):e007023.
8. Pathan F, D'Elia N, Nolan MT, et al. Normal ranges of left atrial strain by speckle-tracking echocardiography: a systematic review and meta-analysis. J Am Soc Echocardiogr. 2017;30(1):59-70.e8.
9. McDonagh TA, Metra M, Adamo M, et al. 2021 ESC guidelines for the diagnosis and treatment of acute and chronic heart failure. Eur Heart J. 2021;42(36):3599-726.
10. Nagueh SF, Smiseth OA, Appleton CP, et al. Recommendations for the evaluation of left ventricular diastolic function by echocardiography: an update from the American Society of Echocardiography and the European Association of Cardiovascular Imaging. J Am Soc Echocardiogr. 2016;29(4):277-314.
11. Singh A, Medvedofsky D, Mediratta A, et al. Peak left atrial strain as a single measure for the non-invasive assessment of left ventricular filling pressures. Int J Cardiovasc Imaging. 2019;35(1):23-32.
12. Singh A, Addetia K, Maffessanti F, et al. LA strain for categorization of LV diastolic dysfunction. JACC Cardiovasc Imaging. 2017;10(7):735-43.
13. Fan JL, Su B, Zhao X, et al. Correlation of left atrial strain with left ventricular end-diastolic pressure in patients with normal left ventricular ejection fraction. Int J Cardiovasc Imaging. 2020;36(9):1659-66.
14. Bandera F, Martone R, Chacko L, et al. Clinical importance of left atrial infiltration in cardiac transthyretin amyloidosis. JACC Cardiovasc Imaging. 2022;15(1):17-29.
15. Kim GH, Uriel N, Burkhoff D. Reverse remodelling and myocardial recovery in heart failure. Nat Rev Cardiol. 2018;15(2):83-96.
16. Zile MR, Jhund PS, Baicu CF, et al. Plasma biomarkers reflecting profibrotic processes in heart failure with a

preserved ejection fraction: data from the prospective comparison of ARNI with ARB on management of heart failure with preserved ejection fraction study. Circ Heart Fail. 2016;9(1):e002551.

17. Mandoli GE, Pastore MC, Giannoni A, et al. Deformation imaging by strain in chronic heart failure over sacubitril-valsartan: a multicenter echocardiographic registry. ESC Heart Fail. 2023;10(2):846-57.
18. Deferm S, Martens P, Verbrugge FH, et al. LA mechanics in decompensated heart failure: insights from strain echocardiography with invasive hemodynamics. JACC Cardiovasc Imaging. 2020;13(5):1107-15.
19. Talha KM, Anker SD, Butler J. SGLT-2 inhibitors in heart failure: a review of current evidence. Int J Heart Fail. 2023;5(2):82-90.
20. Sehly A, He A, Ihdayhid AR, et al. Early SGLT2 inhibitor use is associated with improved left atrial strain following acute coronary syndrome. Acta Cardiol. 2024;79(2): 224-34.
21. Theofilis P, Antonopoulos AS, Katsimichas T, et al. The impact of SGLT2 inhibition on imaging markers of cardiac function: a systematic review and meta-analysis. Pharmacol Res. 2022;180:106243.
22. Strohhofer C. (2023). The impact of the SGLT inhibitor empagliflozin on the left atrial function after acute myocardial infarction - the EMMY-trial. [online] Available from https://online.medunigraz.at/mug_online/wbAbs.getDocument?pThesisNr=71399&pAutorNr=&pOrgNr=1. [Last accessed January, 2025].
23. Tanaka H, Soga F, Tatsumi K, et al. Positive effect of dapagliflozin on left ventricular longitudinal function for type 2 diabetic mellitus patients with chronic heart failure. Cardiovasc Diabetol. 2020;19(1):6.
24. Thiele K, Rau M, Grebe J, et al. Empagliflozin improves left atrial strain in patients with type 2 diabetes: data from a randomized, placebo-controlled study. Circ Cardiovasc Imaging. 2023;16(4):e015176.
25. El-Saied SB, El-Sherbeny WS, El-Sharkawy SI. Impact of sodium glucose co-transporter-2 inhibitors on left atrial functions in patients with type-2 diabetes and heart failure with mildly reduced ejection fraction. Int J Cardiol Heart Vasc. 2023;50:101329.

CHAPTER 54

Echocardiographic Evaluation of Left Atrium and Mitral Annulus in HFpEF Patients on ARNI and SGLT2i Therapy

Satish C Govind

INTRODUCTION

Heart failure with preserved left ventricular (LV) ejection fraction (HFpEF) accounts for nearly half of all heart failure cases and is associated with significant morbidity and mortality.[1] Unlike heart failure with reduced LV ejection fraction—termed HFrEF—, HFpEF is characterized by preserved LV ejection fraction (LVEF), impaired LV diastolic function, elevated LV filling pressures, left atrial (LA) enlargement, and dysfunction.[2] Assessing LA size, function, pressure, and presence of pulmonary hypertension, usually by tricuspid regurgitation peak velocity, is essential in establishing the diagnosis and understanding of disease progression and therapeutic response in HFpEF.

Two novel drugs—angiotensin receptor-neprilysin (ARN) inhibitors and sodium-glucose cotransporter-2 (SGLT2) inhibitors—have emerged as effective therapies in HFpEF management.[3] Studies have shown that these drugs can improve LV diastolic function, reduce LA pressure, and potentially prevent adverse cardiac events. This article focuses on the echocardiographic assessment of the LA and mitral annulus in HFpEF patients undergoing ARN inhibitor and SGLT2 inhibitor therapy.

LEFT ATRIAL EVALUATION

Left Atrial Size or Diameter

Echocardiography can assess LA size by measuring its diameter (anterior-posterior dimension) in the parasternal long-axis view.[4] However, this method is somewhat limited because it needs to account for LA shape variations that can also happen mediolaterally and superoinferiorly. Measurements are typically taken at the end of ventricular systole. Dilated LA often indicates chronic pressure and volume overload, commonly seen in conditions such as hypertension, heart failure, and atrial fibrillation (AF). A dilated LA is associated with higher cardiovascular risk, reflecting prolonged and chronic exposure to elevated LV filling pressures.

Left Atrial Volume

Two-dimensional Left Atrial Volume

The LA volume index (LAVi) is an essential marker of chronic LV diastolic dysfunction in HFpEF. Increased LAVi (>34 mL/m^2) suggests chronic elevation of LV filling pressures and correlates with disease severity and burden.[5] Echocardiographic measurement of LAVi is performed in the apical four-chamber view and indexed to body surface area (BSA) to account for patient size. LAVi is usually measured using the biplane area-length method in the apical four-chamber and two-chamber views. This approach is superior to LA diameter sizing because it provides a more comprehensive assessment of LA shape and size. LAVi is calculated by indexing the volume to the BSA, helping adjust for patient size **(Fig. 1)**.

Three-dimensional Left Atrial Volume

Three-dimensional (3D) echocardiography captures the entire LA chamber in a single volumetric dataset, allowing for more precise quantification of LA size and volume without relying on geometric assumptions, as required in two-dimensional (2D) echocardiography. Images are typically acquired from an apical four-chamber view, capturing the complete LA structure. The volumetric data is then processed to measure maximum and minimum LA volumes in one cardiac cycle. The 3D application calculates the LA volume, producing accurate maximum, minimum, and preatrial contraction LA volumes **(Fig. 1)**.

By capturing the full LA chamber in a single volume, 3D echocardiography minimizes interobserver and intraobserver variability, which is higher in 2D methods due to image foreshortening and geometrical assumptions. 3D imaging allows for comprehensive assessment across the cardiac cycle, including maximum and minimum LA volumes and volumes at various phases of diastole and systole.

A larger LAVi is associated with adverse outcomes, including an increased risk of AF, stroke, and heart failure hospitalization. LAVi is particularly useful for tracking disease progression and the impact of therapeutic interventions over time.

ARN inhibitor and SGLT2 inhibitor therapies have been associated with reductions in LAVi, reflecting improved hemodynamic status and decreased LA pressure. Regular monitoring of LAVi can provide valuable insights into disease progression and response to therapy in HFpEF patients.

Left Atrial Emptying Fraction

Left atrial emptying fraction (LAEF) is calculated as the difference between the maximum and minimum LA volumes during the cardiac cycle, expressed as a percentage of the maximum LA volume:

- LA maximum volume at end-systole minus LA minimum volume at end-diastole divided by LA maximum volume

Left atrial emptying fraction reflects the LA's reservoir function, i.e., its ability to store blood during LV systole and release it during early diastole. A reduced LAEF indicates impaired LA function, often in conditions associated with elevated LV filling pressures. A lower LAEF is associated with worse cardiovascular outcomes, especially in HFpEF and AF.

Left Atrial Strain

Left atrial strain, especially the reservoir strain, is increasingly recognized as a sensitive marker of LA function. It provides insight into LA compliance and the ability of the LA to accommodate LV filling pressures.[6] Reduced LA reservoir strain (<23%) indicates impaired LA function, commonly observed in HFpEF due to increased LV stiffness.

Left atrial strain is measured using speckle-tracking echocardiography (STE) to evaluate LA deformation throughout the cardiac cycle. There are three phases of LA strain:

1. *Reservoir strain* (positive strain during ventricular systole): This measures LA stretching and reflects LA compliance. Normal reservoir strain is typically >23–25%.
2. *Conduit strain* (negative strain during early diastole): This represents passive emptying from the LA to the LV.
3. *Contractile strain* (during late diastole, atrial contraction): This reflects the active contractile function of the LA, which is particularly relevant in patients with sinus rhythm.

Both conduit and contractile strains are not used as routine measures and are awaiting validation.

Left atrial strain is a sensitive indicator of LA function, particularly useful in detecting subclinical dysfunction even before LA dilatation or enlargement is visible. Reduced LA reservoir strain suggests impaired LA compliance and is often seen in LV diastolic dysfunction, heart failure, and AF. LA strain can predict cardiovascular outcomes and provide insights into disease severity and therapeutic response.

Speckle tracking echocardiography LA strain allows clinicians to detect sensitive and subtle changes in LA function. It is a promising parameter for better understanding of LA changes compared to the existing echocardiographic parameters of LA assessment. ARN inhibitor and SGLT2 inhibitor therapies may improve LA strain, positively impacting LA compliance and reducing LV filling pressures **(Table 1)**.

MITRAL ANNULUS EVALUATION

Tissue Doppler Imaging

Mitral annular relaxation velocities (e′ and a′) are measured using tissue Doppler imaging (TDI) to assess LV diastolic function. A reduced e′ velocity, <7 cm/s, indicates impaired LV relaxation, a characteristic feature of HFpEF **(Fig. 2)**.

Left Atrial Pressure

Estimating LA pressure is crucial in evaluating HFpEF. Direct measurement of LA pressure is not feasible with routine echocardiography, but indirect markers such as the E/e′ ratio can be used.[7]

The E/e′ ratio is an echocardiographic parameter used to estimate LV filling pressures, particularly in patients

TABLE 1: Left atrial echocardiographic parameters.

Parameter	*Measurement method*	*Normal values*	*Clinical significance*
LA size	Diameter in parasternal long-axis view	Varies with age/sex	Enlargement indicates chronic volume/pressure overload
LA volume index (LAVI)	Biplane area-length method in apical views	<34 mL/m²	High LAVI reflects diastolic dysfunction, elevated filling pressures, and adverse outcomes
LA emptying fraction (LAEF)	Difference between maximum and minimum LA volumes	>45%	Low LAEF indicates impaired LA reservoir function and is linked to adverse outcomes
LA strain	Speckle-tracking echocardiography	>23%	Low LA reservoir strain reflects poor LA compliance and predicts cardiovascular risk in diastolic dysfunction

(LA: left atrium)

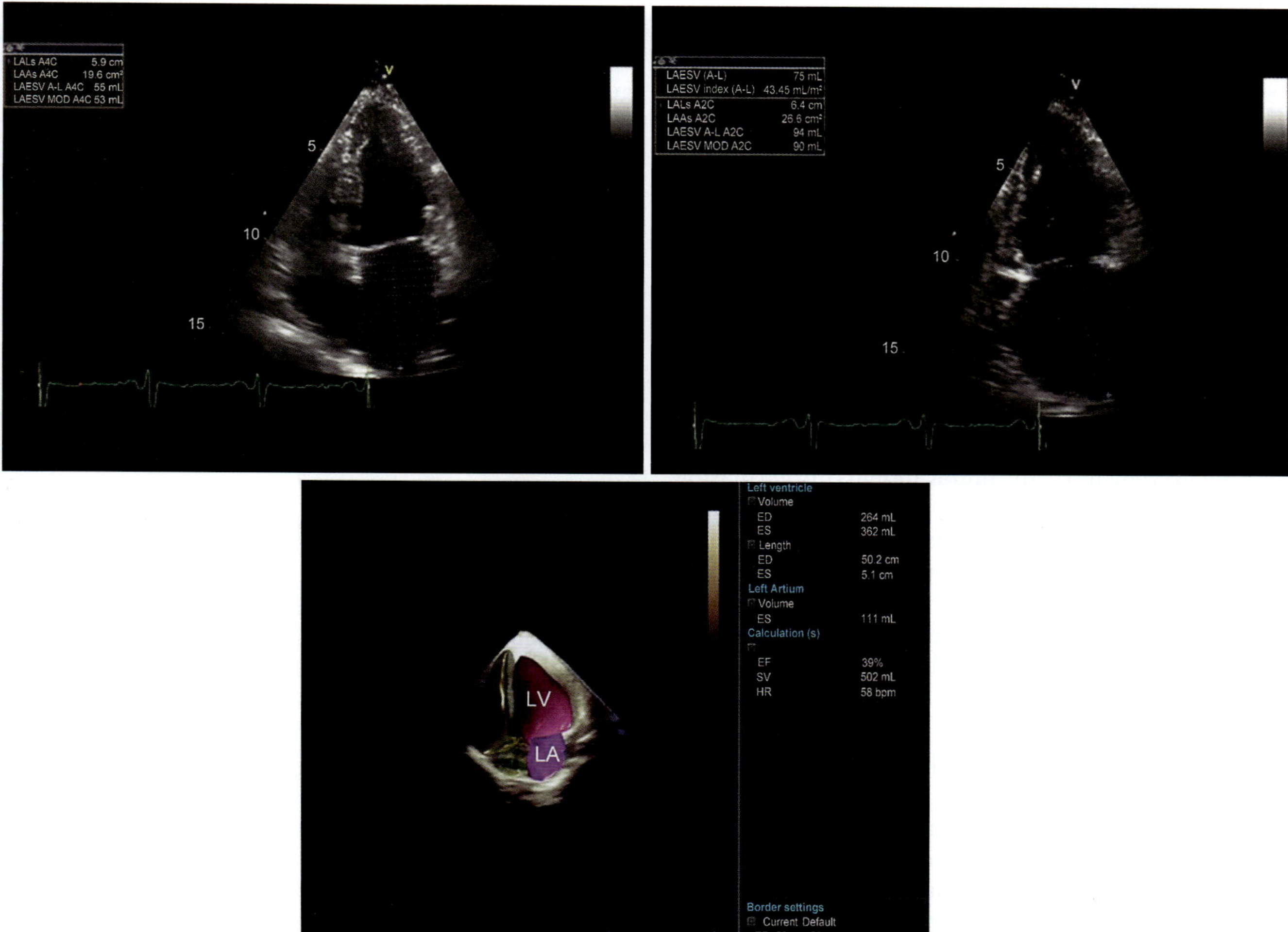

Fig. 1: Left atrial volume by 2D and 3D echocardiography.

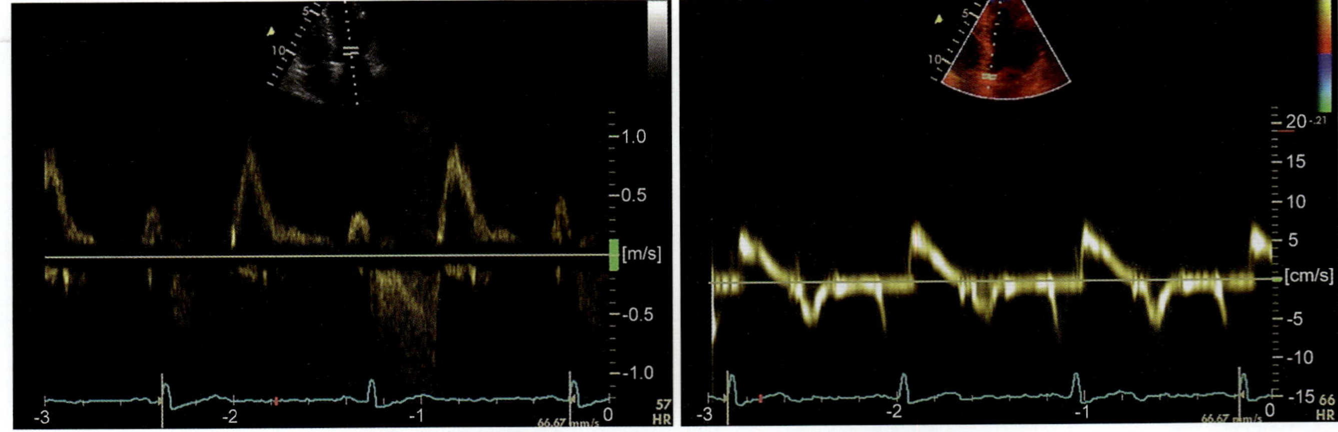

Fig. 2: E transmitral E velocity and e′ by tissue Doppler imaging.

with LV diastolic dysfunction and HFpEF. The E/e′ ratio, combining TDI e′ and transmitral inflow E velocity, provides a reliable estimate of LV filling pressures.

Transmitral Doppler Imaging: E Velocity

The E velocity represents the early diastolic filling phase due to passive relaxation.

It is measured by placing the Doppler sample volume at the tips of the mitral leaflets in the apical four-chamber view and recording the peak velocity of the E wave.

Tissue Doppler Imaging: e′ Velocity

The e′ wave is measured using TDI, which assesses the movement (velocity) of the mitral annulus during diastole. This reflects the relaxation capacity of the LV myocardium. The TDI sample is placed at the lateral or septal mitral annulus, preferably both in the apical four-chamber view. The early diastolic velocity (e′) is recorded at both sample sites. Lower e′ velocities indicate impaired LV relaxation, which is common in patients with diastolic dysfunction.

Calculating E/e′ Ratio

The E/e′ ratio is calculated by dividing the peak E wave velocity by the e′ velocity.

Separate values are reported for the septal and lateral e′ measurements, but an average of septal and lateral e′ values is often used for a more comprehensive assessment. The E/e′ ratio, which compares early mitral inflow velocity (E) to mitral annular early diastolic velocity (e′), is also a surrogate for LA pressure. An elevated E/e′ ratio (>14), averaged to septal and lateral mitral annulus, suggests elevated LV filling pressures in sinus rhythm, which is common in HFpEF. In the presence of AF, >11 indicates raised LV filling pressure. An E/e′ ratio >15 generally correlates with a mean pulmonary capillary wedge pressure (PCWP) >15 mm Hg, indicating elevated LV filling pressures.

An ARN inhibitor therapy, particularly sacubitril/valsartan, has been shown to enhance myocardial relaxation, increasing e′ velocity over time. Similarly, SGLT2 inhibitors, such as empagliflozin and dapagliflozin, may improve diastolic function, decreasing E/e′ ratio, indicating reduced LV filling pressures. ARN inhibitor and SGLT2 inhibitor therapies can reduce E/e′ ratio over time, indicating improved LV compliance and reduced LA pressure. Tracking the E/e′ ratio can thus help monitor treatment response in HFpEF patients.

Mitral Annular Plane Systolic Excursion

Mitral annular plane systolic excursion (MAPSE) is an index of longitudinal LV function and is measured as the total distance of mitral annular motion during systole. Sample points at five mitral annular points are placed (septal, lateral, inferior, anterior, and posterior annulus), and M-mode is applied. The normal range is from 10–12 mm, with <10 mm being associated with impaired LV systolic function; it provides indirect information about longitudinal LV systolic function. This technique has its limitations and cannot be used when there is significant mitral annular calcification or when there is a mitral prosthesis.

Mitral annular plane systolic excursion may be reduced in HFpEF due to global LV impairment. Improvement in MAPSE following ARN inhibitor and SGLT2 inhibitor therapy may suggest a favorable remodeling response in HFpEF patients.

IMPACT OF ARN INHIBITOR AND SGLT2 INHIBITOR THERAPY ON ECHOCARDIOGRAPHIC PARAMETERS

Both ARN inhibitor and SGLT2 inhibitor therapies have shown beneficial effects on LA and mitral annular function in HFpEF patients:[8]

- *ARN inhibitor (Sacubitril/Valsartan):* Studies have shown that ARNI can lead to reverse remodeling of the LA, reducing LA size, LAVi and LA pressure reflected by E/e′ LV filling pressure. Improvements in LA strain and mitral annular velocities indicate enhanced myocardial relaxation, a key therapeutic objective in HFpEF.[9]
- *SGLT2 inhibitor (Empagliflozin, Dapagliflozin):* SGLT2 inhibitors are also associated with LA size and LAVi reductions, possibly due to their diuretic and anti-inflammatory effects. They may also improve LA strain and lower the E/e′ ratio, reflecting a decrease in LV filling pressures.[10]

Regular echocardiographic monitoring allows clinicians to assess the efficacy of these therapies and adjust treatment as necessary to achieve optimal outcomes in HFpEF patients.[11]

CONCLUSION

Echocardiography remains a vital tool in assessing and managing HFpEF, particularly in evaluating the effects of ARN inhibitor and SGLT2 inhibitor therapies on LA and mitral annular function. Monitoring parameters such as LAVi, LA strain, mitral annular velocities, and E/e′ ratio provides valuable insights into LV diastolic function and cardiac mechanics. By tracking changes in these measurements, clinicians can assess treatment response and tailor therapy for improved patient outcomes in HFpEF. ARN inhibitor and SGLT2 inhibitor therapies have been associated with reductions in the above-mentioned echocardiographic parameters, reflecting improved hemodynamic status and decreased LA pressure.

REFERENCES

1. McDonagh TA, Metra M, Adamo M, et al.; ESC Scientific Document Group. 2021 ESC Guidelines for the diagnosis and treatment of acute and chronic heart failure. Eur Heart J. 2021;42(36):3599-726. Erratum in: Eur Heart J. 2021;42(48):4901.
2. Borlaug BA, Paulus WJ. Heart failure with preserved ejection fraction: pathophysiology, diagnosis, and treatment. Eur Heart J. 2011;32(6):670-9.
3. Solomon SD, McMurray JJV, Anand IS, et al.; PARAGON-HF Investigators and Committees. Angiotensin-neprilysin inhibition in heart failure with preserved ejection fraction. N Engl J Med. 2019;381(17):1609-20.
4. Lang RM, Badano LP, Mor-Avi V, et al. Recommendations for cardiac chamber quantification by echocardiography in adults: an update from the American Society of Echocardiography and the European Association of Cardiovascular Imaging. J Am Soc Echocardiogr. 2015;28(1):1-39.e14.
5. Thomas L, Muraru D, Popescu BA, et al. Evaluation of Left Atrial Size and Function: Relevance for Clinical Practice. J Am Soc Echocardiogr. 2020;33(8):934-952.
6. Nagueh SF, Smiseth OA, Appleton CP, et al. Recommendations for the Evaluation of Left Ventricular Diastolic Function by Echocardiography: An Update from the American Society of Echocardiography and the European Association of Cardiovascular Imaging. J Am Soc Echocardiogr. 2016;29(4):277-314.
7. Singh A, Carvalho Singulane C, Miyoshi T, et al.; WASE Investigators. Normal values of left atrial size and function and the impact of age: Results of the World Alliance Societies of Echocardiography study. J Am Soc Echocardiogr. 2022;35(2):154-64.e3.
8. Anker SD, Butler J, Filippatos G, et al.; EMPEROR-Preserved Trial Investigators. Empagliflozin in Heart Failure with a Preserved Ejection Fraction. N Engl J Med. 2021;385(16):1451-61.
9. Aziri B, Begic E, Jankovic S, et al. Systematic review of sodium-glucose cotransporter 2 inhibitors: a hopeful prospect in tackling heart failure-related events. ESC Heart Fail. 2023;10(3):1499-530.
10. Verma S, McMurray JJV. The serendipitous story of SGLT2 inhibitors in heart failure. Circulation. 2019;139(22):2537-41.
11. Simes BC, MacGregor GG. Sodium-glucose cotransporter-2 (SGLT2) inhibitors: a Clinician's guide. Diabetes Metab Syndr Obes. 2019;12:2125-36.

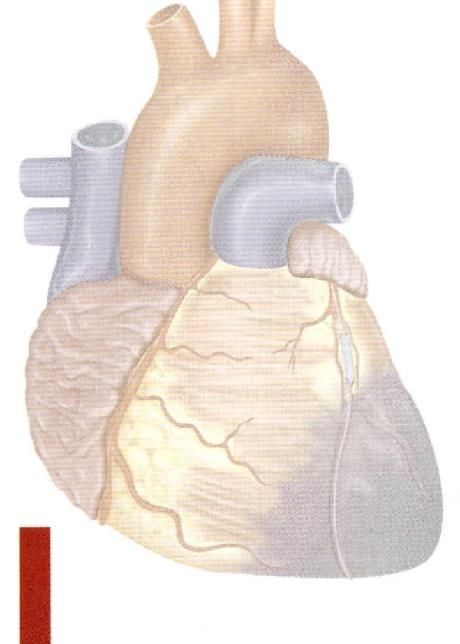

Atrial Strain: A Piece of the HFpEF Puzzle Found, but is It Yet in Place

Aniruddha De

INTRODUCTION

Heart failure with preserved ejection fraction (HFpEF) is a common and complex form of heart failure (HF) characterized by a preserved left ventricular ejection fraction (LVEF) but with symptoms of HF due to impaired diastolic function. This condition poses a significant diagnostic challenge, as traditional measures of cardiac function, such as LVEF, are often normal.[1] Therefore, additional diagnostic tools are needed to better identify and manage HFpEF. This chapter explores the key mechanisms of one such emerging tool, the assessment of atrial strain, which has shown promise in enhancing the diagnosis and understanding of HFpEF.[2]

Also, HFpEF has traditionally been thought of as a disorder of the left ventricle. However, recent studies have shown that abnormalities in the left atrium play an important role in the pathophysiology and disease progression of HFpEF.[1-13] Speckle-tracking strain has emerged as a valuable tool to assess left atrial (LA) function by allowing measurement of LA performance at various phases of the cardiac cycle in a single beat.[1]

Multiple echocardiographic indices have been applied for diagnosis of HFpEF, including LA volume, left ventricular (LV) hypertrophy (LVH), e velocity, E/e′ ratio, and tricuspid regurgitation velocity.[1-3] LA reservoir strain quantifies the deformation of the left atrium during atrial filling, where less deformation (lower strain) has been associated with adverse LA remodeling and increased fibrosis.[14] This is thought to reflect the cumulative impact of adverse LV and LA remodeling over time from high filling pressures, mediated through atrioventricular uncoupling and systemic inflammation.[3] LA reservoir strain may also offer technical advantages compared to other indices, particularly in patients where annular motion is altered, such as with pacing, bundle branch block, and mitral annular calcification.

Because abnormal LA function and left atrial strain (LAS) have been consistently identified in HFpEF and are associated with greater disease severity, according to their hypotheses, measurement of LAS might be useful in its diagnostic evaluation. To test this hypothesis, they evaluated the ability of LAS to discriminate patients with HFpEF from individuals with etiologies of noncardiac dyspnea (NCD) as defined invasively using gold standard methods, and then compared LAS with other echocardiographic indices commonly used in this evaluation. According to the 2022 AHA/ACC/HFSA guideline for the management of HF, the criteria for diagnosing HFpEF include: A normal or near-normal LVEF ≥50%, evidence of cardiac dysfunction by echocardiography (e.g., abnormal LV filling and elevated filling pressures), and elevated natriuretic peptides.[3]

The sensitivity, however, varies substantially for this approach, ranging from 25 to 80%.[3-5] In addition, patients at the early stage of the disease may be assessed as normal or indeterminant.[4]

Given the complexity of HFpEF, various parameters, including clinical (patient's history and physical examination), biochemical [serum B-type natriuretic peptide (BNP) level], hemodynamic, and radiographic data, are all utilized to reach a diagnosis.[4,5] Scoring criteria, including H2FPEF and HFA-PEFF scores, can assist in diagnosis but are not entirely validated; therefore, it is recommended to explore further. Moving on, we should understand different types of atrial strain.[4]

UNDERSTANDING HFpEF

Heart failure with preserved ejection fraction, previously known as diastolic HF, represents a heterogeneous group of disorders where the heart muscle can contract normally but has difficulty relaxing and filling with blood.[5] This leads to elevated pressures in the heart and lungs, causing symptoms such as shortness of breath, fatigue, and fluid retention. HFpEF is often associated with various comorbidities, including hypertension, obesity, diabetes, and chronic kidney disease. The pathophysiology of HFpEF involves complex interactions between myocardial stiffness, impaired relaxation, and altered atrial function. Despite the normal EF, patients with HFpEF can exhibit significant symptoms and a reduced quality of life, making accurate diagnosis and management crucial.[6]

DIAGNOSTIC CHALLENGES IN HFpEF

Diagnosing HFpEF is challenging due to the overlap of symptoms with other conditions and the lack of specific biomarkers or imaging techniques that definitively diagnose the disease. Traditional diagnostic tools, including echocardiography, cardiac MRI, and blood biomarkers, are often used but may not always provide a clear diagnosis in cases of HFpEF.[5,6]

- *Echocardiography:* While echocardiography is a cornerstone in evaluating heart function, standard parameters such as LVEF, LV dimensions, and diastolic function indices can be normal in HFpEF. This necessitates the use of more advanced echocardiographic techniques to enhance diagnostic accuracy.[6]
- *Cardiac MRI:* It can offer detailed images of myocardial structure and function, but it is not always readily available and may be costly. Furthermore, while it provides valuable information about myocardial fibrosis and structural abnormalities, it may not always capture subtle functional changes.[6,7]
- *Biomarkers:* Although biomarkers like BNP can indicate HF, they are not specific to HFpEF and can be influenced by other conditions.[7]

These limitations highlight the need for novel diagnostic approaches to improve the accuracy of HFpEF diagnosis and management.

ATRIAL STRAIN: A NOVEL DIAGNOSTIC TOOL

Atrial strain imaging, particularly using speckle-tracking echocardiography (STE), has emerged as a promising tool for evaluating atrial function and providing additional diagnostic insight into HFpEF.[7] Atrial strain measures the deformation of atrial myocardium during the cardiac cycle and provides information about atrial contractility and relaxation.

Atrial Strain Measurement

Speckle-tracking echocardiography assesses atrial strain by tracking the movement of speckles in the myocardium throughout the cardiac cycle. This technique provides detailed information about the extent and direction of myocardial deformation.[7-17]

Understanding Atrial Strain

Atrial strain is a measure of myocardial deformation within the atria, obtained using STE. It quantifies how the atrial myocardium stretches and contracts during the cardiac cycle, providing insights into atrial function beyond conventional parameters such as EF and diastolic filling pressures. Atrial strain can be categorized into:[8-17]

- *Longitudinal strain:* It measures deformation along the length of the atrium. Reduced longitudinal strain often indicates impaired atrial contraction.
- *Radial strain:* It measures deformation perpendicular to the atrial long axis. Changes in radial strain can reflect alterations in atrial stiffness and filling pressures.

These measurements offer a more nuanced view of atrial performance, which is crucial for patients with HFpEF, where traditional markers often appear normal despite symptomatic HF **(Figs. 1A and B)**.

Components of Left Atrial Strain

The LA function operates in three distinct phases during each cardiac cycle: (1) The "reservoir" phase (PALS) during ventricular systole, (2) the "conduit" phase (FnC) during early diastole, and (3) the "booster pump" phase (PACS) in late diastole **(Fig. 2)**.[11,12]

Despite the straightforward nature of measuring LA two-dimensional (2D) strain by STE, methodological differences initially led to some variation in average values. However, this has been improved through recent systematization and standardization proposed by various international societies and the industry. These entities have defined longitudinal strain, which is the strain in the direction tangential to the endocardial atrial border in an apical view, as the recommended method. The guidance advises against a segmental study;[12] therefore, it recommends only the overall value obtained in the analyzed view. Combining measures obtained by the four- and two-chamber views to calculate global longitudinal

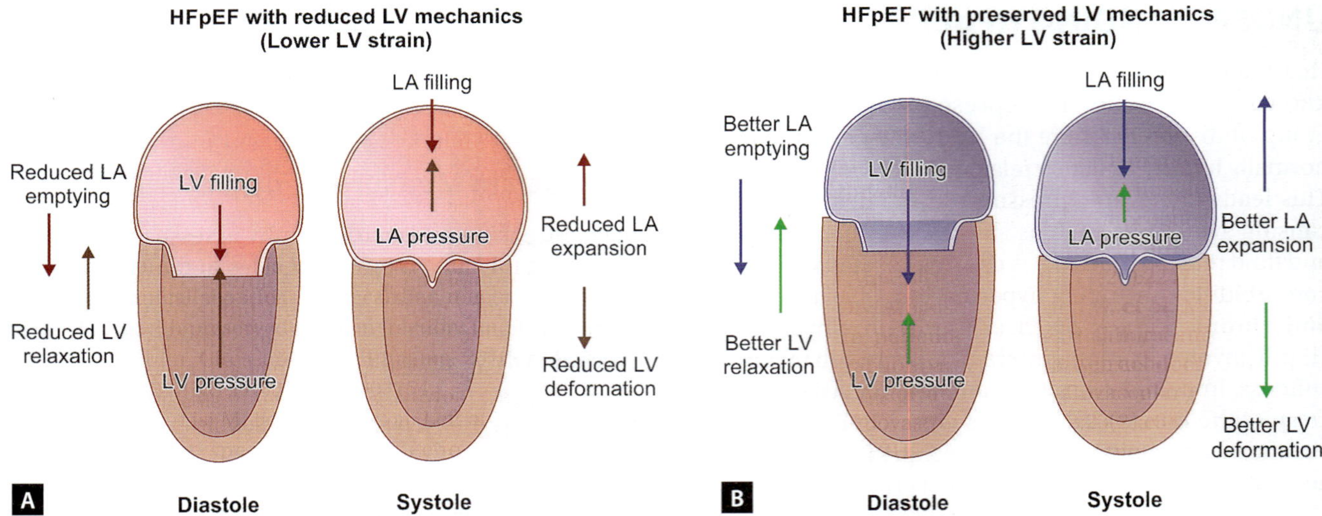

Figs. 1A and B: Impact of different degrees of LV strain on LA mechanics in HFpEF. LV mechanics and effects on LA mechanics: Summary of mechanism that explains the relationship between LV and LA mechanics in HFpEF and its role in the development of symptoms. Examples of LA strain–time curve from HFpEF with lower LV strain.[11] (HFpEF: heart failure with preserved ejection fraction; LA: left atrial; LV: left ventricular)

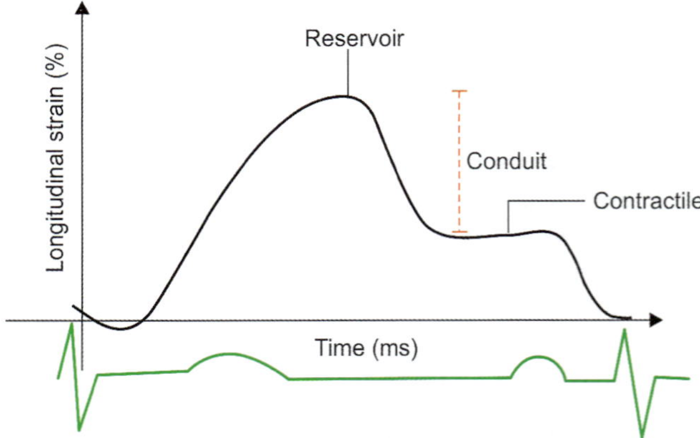

Fig. 2: Components of left atrial strain.

LAS is possible, and this was previously recommended. However, conducting the study using a single view, precisely the four-chamber view, is acceptable due to its practicality **(Figs. 3A to D)**.[12]

Strain versus Ejection Fraction

Ejection fraction and global strain are relative (unitless) parameters describing LV global function. EF describes a relative volume change, considering both the length change of the ventricle (longitudinal deformation) and its diameter change (mainly circumferential but also radial deformation). Global strain, usually global longitudinal strain (GLS), considers only one of these deformation components. Strain imaging has been shown to be more sensitive for the detection of subtle systolic dysfunction than LVEF,[16] likely due to the compensation of early-longitudinal dysfunction by the augmentation of other strain components, which allows the LV to maintain an EF within the normal range.[11-13] Some authors suggest that the (semi) automated image processing contributes to a higher reproducibility of strain measurements compared with EF, which directly impacts the sensitivity to detect small changes.[7,12,16]

Factors affecting Strain Values

Assessment of myocardial function is one of the most frequent indications for echocardiography and also frequently reported by other cardiac imaging modalities. In research, the concept of "contractility," which describes the intrinsic ability of the muscle to shorten with a certain velocity against a certain load, is used as a load-independent measure of myocardial function. However, imaging-related parameters, such as EF or strain, consider only myocardial deformation and neglect the pre- and afterload under which the fibers have to shorten and are, therefore, only load-dependent surrogate parameters. The afterload to the myofibers is determined by cavity pressure, but its translation into the relevant parameter of "wall stress" (force per cross-sectional area) depends on chamber geometry [e.g., diameter (wall curvature) and wall thickness], as described by LaPlace's law or more sophisticated models.[15] Furthermore, regional or temporal inhomogeneity of myocardial function or changes in passive properties of the myocardium may interact **(Fig. 4)**.

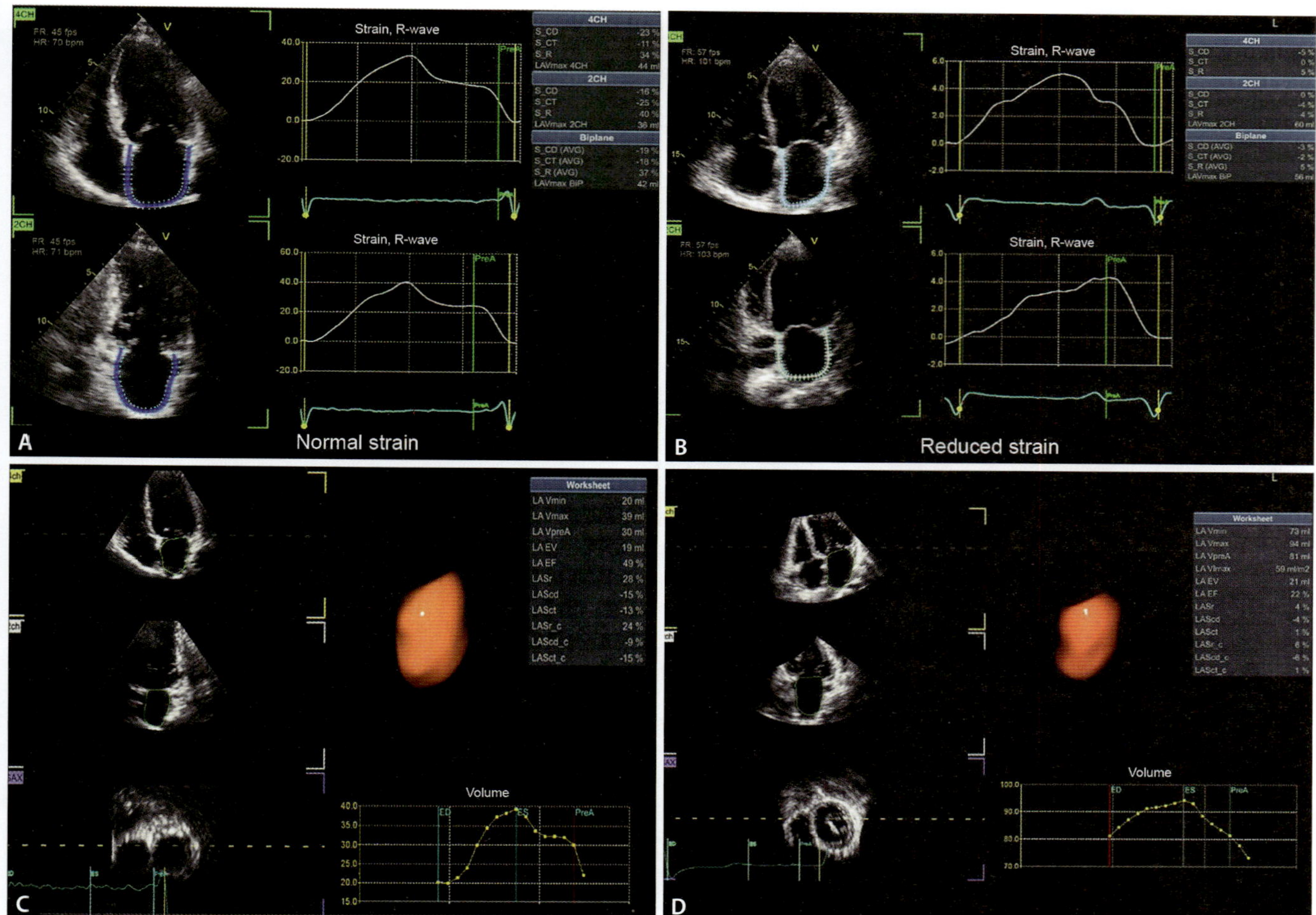

Figs. 3A to D: 2D and 3D speckle tracking can determine measures of left atrial strain, including peak reservoir strains, for the four- and two-chamber echocardiographic views. Automatic results can be obtained for the reservoir, conduit, and contraction measures in the four- and two-chamber views, with overall results (mean values) calculated for the two views.

To foster the conceptual understanding of how a load-dependent parameter like strain should be interpreted, the following clinical review is organized, according to the main factors that lead to changes in measured strain values rather than pathology.[14]

Elevated left ventricular filling pressure (LVFP) during exercise is a significant marker of heart dysfunction, particularly in patients with HF or other cardiovascular diseases. LVFP refers to the pressure within the left ventricle of the heart during the filling phase, also known as diastole. When this pressure is elevated it suggests that the left ventricle is not properly relaxing or filling with blood, which can impair cardiac function and lead to symptoms such as shortness of breath, fatigue, and exercise intolerance.[13]

Patients with HFpEF can experience elevated LVFPs during exercise, even when their resting LVFP appears normal. This phenomenon is a crucial challenge in diagnosing and managing HFpEF, especially in individuals presenting with exertional dyspnea. A study by Ye et al. assessed the diagnostic value of LAS in detecting elevated LVFP during exercise in 669 patients undergoing stress echocardiography. The findings indicated that peak atrial longitudinal strain (PALS) and conduit function (FnC) were significantly lower in patients with elevated LVFP during exercise, regardless of their diastolic function at rest.[14,15]

Additionally, Telles et al. demonstrated that PALS and peak atrial contraction strain (PACS) correlated with invasive measurements of pulmonary capillary pressure during exercise. They remained independent predictors of HFpEF in multivariate analyses. In their study, a PALS value of ≤33% was shown to predict HFpEF with a sensitivity of 88% and specificity of 77%, based on invasively verified diagnoses. This highlights the clinical value of PALS as a noninvasive tool for detecting exercise-induced

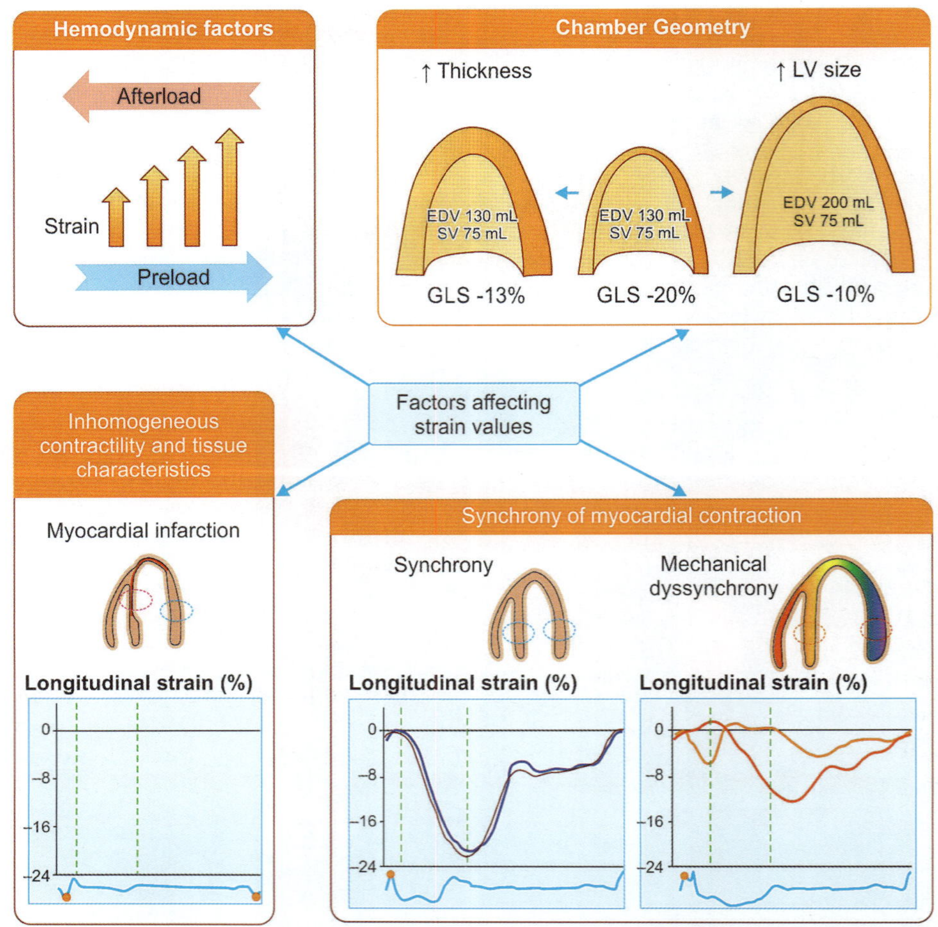

Fig. 4: Central illustration for factors affecting strain values. Left atrial strain in a subset of patients with elevated left ventricular filling pressure occurring only after exercise but remaining normal at rest.

Source: Voigt JU, Cvijic M. 2- and 3-dimensional myocardial strain in cardiac health and disease. JACC Cardiovasc Imaging. 2019;12(9): 1849-63.

LVFP elevation, providing significant insights into LV diastolic dysfunction, which plays a central role in HFpEF pathophysiology.[16,17]

Initially, the left atrium compensates for increased filling pressure by enhancing its pump function. However, as diastolic dysfunction worsens, LA compliance decreases, leading to impaired function and LA enlargement. LAS reflects the cumulative impact of LV diastolic dysfunction on the left atrium and provides essential information regarding the heart's ability to manage increased pressures during exercise.[17,18]

The clinical utility of resting LAS in predicting LVFP elevations during exercise remains an area of interest. Current studies suggest that the inclusion of LAS in the diagnostic workup for HFpEF could improve the detection of patients who may require exercise testing.[18,19]

ROLE OF DIASTOLIC EXERCISE ECHOCARDIOGRAPHY IN HFpEF

Diastolic exercise echocardiography plays a pivotal role in diagnosing and managing HFpEF, a condition characterized by normal LVEF but impaired diastolic function.[19,20] Unlike systolic HF, patients with HFpEF exhibit normal ventricular contraction but have difficulty filling the left ventricle during diastole. This leads to increased filling pressures, particularly during exertion, resulting in symptoms such as shortness of breath and exercise intolerance. The challenge in HFpEF diagnosis is that many patients exhibit normal hemodynamics at rest, making exercise stress testing essential for uncovering abnormal heart function under stress.

Diastolic exercise echocardiography involves evaluating the heart's response to stress by measuring parameters such as LVFPs, LAS, and pulmonary pressures during and after exercise. The test is particularly useful for detecting elevated LVFP, which is often hidden at rest but becomes evident during exertion. By comparing echocardiographic indices such as E/e′ ratio (a measure of LVFP) at rest and during exercise, clinicians can identify patients with exercise-induced diastolic dysfunction, a hallmark of HFpEF.

In a case study by Reddy et al., a 62-year-old woman presented with dyspnea and fatigue despite having a normal EF and no significant coronary artery disease. Resting echocardiography showed normal diastolic function and LVFP. However, during diastolic exercise echocardiography, her E/e′ ratio significantly increased, indicating elevated LVFP during exertion. This finding led to a diagnosis of HFpEF, which was missed during resting evaluation. The patient was subsequently managed with tailored therapies, including diuretics and lifestyle changes, aimed at reducing diastolic pressures during physical activity.[20,21]

This case highlights the critical importance of diastolic exercise echocardiography in identifying HFpEF, particularly in patients whose symptoms are exacerbated by exercise but who appear normal at rest.

ROLE OF ATRIAL STRAIN IN PREDICTING ATRIAL FIBRILLATION

Atrial strain, particularly LAS, has emerged as an important tool for predicting the onset of atrial fibrillation (AF). A common arrhythmia, AF is often associated with structural and functional changes in the left atrium. LAS, measured through echocardiography, provides insights into the atrium's mechanical function by assessing its deformation during the cardiac cycle.

Several studies have demonstrated the predictive value of atrial strain for AF. In particular, a study by Morris et al. found that reduced LAS was strongly associated with an increased risk of developing AF, even in patients with no previous history of the condition. The study highlighted that impaired atrial strain was linked to LA dysfunction, a known precursor to AF. Similarly, Cameli et al. showed that LAS could predict the recurrence of AF after cardioversion, supporting its role as a reliable marker for long-term outcomes in AF management.

Atrial strain offers clinicians a noninvasive method to detect subclinical atrial dysfunction before the onset of AF. Its predictive power makes it a valuable tool in identifying high-risk patients and guiding early interventions to prevent or manage AF more effectively.[22,23]

ROLE OF ATRIAL STRAIN TO DISTINGUISH LEFT ATRIAL MYOPATHY FROM HFpEF

Atrial strain, mainly LAS, has emerged as a valuable tool for distinguishing LA myopathy from HFpEF. Both conditions share overlapping clinical features, such as diastolic dysfunction and elevated LA pressures, making them challenging to differentiate those using conventional diagnostics. LAS provides detailed insight into atrial mechanics by assessing the deformation of the left atrium during the cardiac cycle. This allows for a more nuanced evaluation of atrial function.[24]

A study by Santos et al. demonstrated that reduced LAS was significantly associated with atrial myopathy, independent of LV diastolic function. In contrast, patients with HFpEF often exhibit preserved LAS until the advanced stages of the disease. This distinction is crucial as LAS helps in identifying subclinical atrial dysfunction before the onset of overt structural changes or symptoms.

Further research, such as that by Singh et al., emphasized the prognostic value of LAS in patients with LA myopathy, where reduced atrial strain correlated with a higher risk of adverse cardiovascular outcomes, including AF and stroke. Incorporating LAS into routine assessments enables clinicians to better differentiate between HFpEF and LA myopathy, guiding more tailored therapeutic interventions.[25,26]

CLINICAL EVIDENCE SUPPORTING ATRIAL STRAIN

Several studies provide clinical evidence supporting the role of atrial strain in the diagnosis and management of HFpEF:

- *Nagueh et al.:*[1]
    - *Study overview:* Nagueh et al. investigated the relationship between atrial strain and diastolic function in HFpEF patients. The study used STE to measure atrial strain and compared it with traditional diastolic function indices.
    - *Findings:* The study found that patients with HFpEF had reduced atrial strain compared to healthy controls. The results indicated that atrial strain abnormalities correlated with diastolic dysfunction parameters, suggesting that atrial strain can enhance the diagnostic assessment of HFpEF.
- *Sanna et al.:*[2]
    - *Study overview:* Sanna et al. explored the prognostic value of atrial strain in HFpEF patients. The study aimed to determine whether atrial strain measurements could predict adverse clinical outcomes.

- *Findings:* The research demonstrated that reduced atrial strain was associated with worse clinical outcomes, including increased hospitalization rates and mortality. The study highlighted the potential of atrial strain as a prognostic tool in HFpEF management.

- *Reddy et al.:*[3]
  - *Study overview:* Reddy et al. examined the incremental value of atrial strain measurements in diagnosing HFpEF. The study compared atrial strain with traditional echocardiographic parameters to assess its added diagnostic value.
  - *Findings:* The study found that incorporating atrial strain measurements improved diagnostic accuracy and risk stratification in HFpEF. The research emphasized the value of atrial strain in providing additional information that complements conventional diagnostic methods.

CLINICAL IMPLICATIONS OF ATRIAL STRAIN IN HFpEF

Heart failure with preserved ejection fraction is characterized by normal LVEF but impaired diastolic function, which traditional echocardiographic parameters may not fully capture. Atrial strain adds value to the diagnostic process in several ways:[27]

- *Enhanced sensitivity and specificity:* Atrial strain can detect subtle atrial dysfunction that may precede or accompany diastolic abnormalities. Studies have shown that atrial strain abnormalities are prevalent in HFpEF patients even when standard echocardiographic measures are normal. For instance, reduced longitudinal atrial strain has been associated with impaired LV filling and increased LA pressures.[28]
- *Early detection of atrial dysfunction:* Abnormal atrial strain can indicate early atrial dysfunction, which may be an early marker of HFpEF. Identifying these changes early allows for prompt intervention and management, potentially before more severe symptoms develop.[12]
- *Complementary to existing tests:* Atrial strain provides additional diagnostic information that complements other echocardiographic findings. For example, in cases where diastolic dysfunction indices are borderline or ambiguous, atrial strain can clarify the presence of HFpEF by highlighting atrial abnormalities that support the diagnosis.[27,28]

Prognostic Significance of Atrial Strain

Atrial strain has significant prognostic implications for patients with HFpEF. Several studies have demonstrated that atrial strain measurements correlate with clinical outcomes and can be used to predict adverse events:[29-31]

- *Risk stratification:* Reduced atrial strain is associated with worse outcomes in HFpEF. For example, lower longitudinal strain has been linked to increased hospitalizations and mortality. This correlation helps stratify patients based on their risk of adverse events, guiding more personalized treatment strategies.
- *Disease progression:* Serial assessment of atrial strain can monitor disease progression. Deterioration in atrial strain over time may indicate worsening HF or increased atrial pressure, necessitating adjustments in treatment or closer monitoring.
- *Predictive value:* Atrial strain can predict outcomes such as HF, hospitalization, and all-cause mortality. Studies have shown that patients with significantly impaired atrial strain are more likely to experience these events, emphasizing the need for ongoing evaluation and management.

Guiding Treatment and Management

Incorporating atrial strain into clinical practice can guide treatment and management decisions for HFpEF patients:[31-34]

- *Tailored therapy:* Understanding a patient's atrial strain profile can influence therapeutic choices. For instance, patients with significant atrial dysfunction may benefit from treatments aimed at reducing atrial pressures and improving atrial compliance, such as aggressive hypertension management or diuretics.
- *Treatment monitoring:* Atrial strain can be used to monitor the efficacy of treatments. Improvements in atrial strain following therapy may indicate a positive response to treatment, while persistent abnormalities might suggest the need for alternative strategies.
- *Personalized management plans:* By integrating atrial strain data, clinicians can develop more personalized management plans. This approach allows for targeted interventions that address specific aspects of atrial dysfunction, potentially improving patient outcomes and quality of life.

CURRENT GUIDELINES BY EUROPEAN ASSOCIATION OF CARDIOVASCULAR IMAGING

The 2022 European Association of Cardiovascular Imaging (EACVI) guidelines have introduced updated algorithms for assessing diastolic dysfunction. They aim to provide a more precise and systematic approach to diagnosing HFpEF and related diastolic abnormalities. These guidelines emphasize the integration of multiple imaging modalities to enhance diagnostic accuracy **(Flowchart 1)**.[35]

Simplified Diagnostic Algorithm

The revised algorithm refines the assessment of diastolic dysfunction by focusing on key accessible parameters. Historically, evaluating diastolic dysfunction involved complex metrics such as the E/A ratio (early-to-late ventricular filling velocities), E/e′ ratio (the ratio of mitral inflow velocity to mitral annular velocity), and LA volume index (LAVI). The EACVI 2022 guidelines streamline this process by concentrating on more practical measurements and adjusting thresholds to improve diagnostic reliability **(Flowchart 2)**.[35]

The guidelines recommend an initial screening based on the patient's clinical presentation and an echocardiographic evaluation. This includes integrating tissue Doppler imaging, 2D echocardiography, and potentially advanced techniques like strain imaging for cases with inconclusive results.

Key Updates in the Guidelines[36]

Role of Left Atrial Strain

The new guidelines acknowledge the "grey zone" challenges where diastolic dysfunction is difficult to quantify. They highlight LAS as a valuable parameter due to its high specificity and sensitivity. LAS, which is straightforward to measure, correlates with LVFP both at rest and during exercise. This makes LAS a promising tool for diagnosing HFpEF, providing a more accurate assessment of diastolic dysfunction and enhancing overall diagnostic precision.[35]

LIMITATIONS AND FUTURE DIRECTIONS

While atrial strain is a promising tool, there are limitations to its current application:[32-34]

- *Technical limitations:* The accuracy of atrial strain measurements can be affected by factors such as image quality and operator expertise. Standardization of measurement techniques and equipment calibration are essential for reliable results.
- *Need for validation:* Further validation in larger, diverse patient populations is needed to confirm the utility of atrial strain in routine clinical practice and to establish reference values for different patient groups.
- *Integration with other tools:* Atrial strain should be used in conjunction with other diagnostic tools and clinical assessments to provide a comprehensive evaluation of HFpEF.

Flowchart 1: Algorithm for the diagnosis of HFpEF in patients presenting with suspected symptoms and/or signs of heart failure.[35]

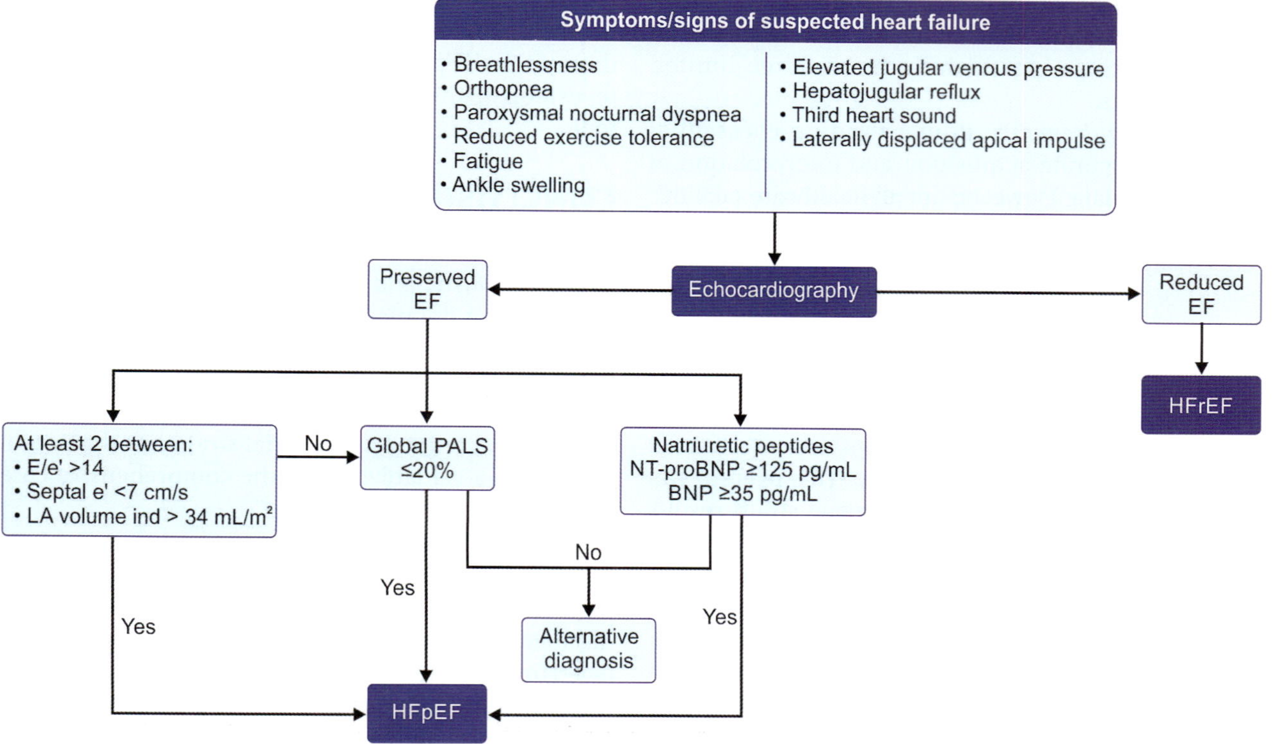

Flowchart 2: Current EACVI algorithm.

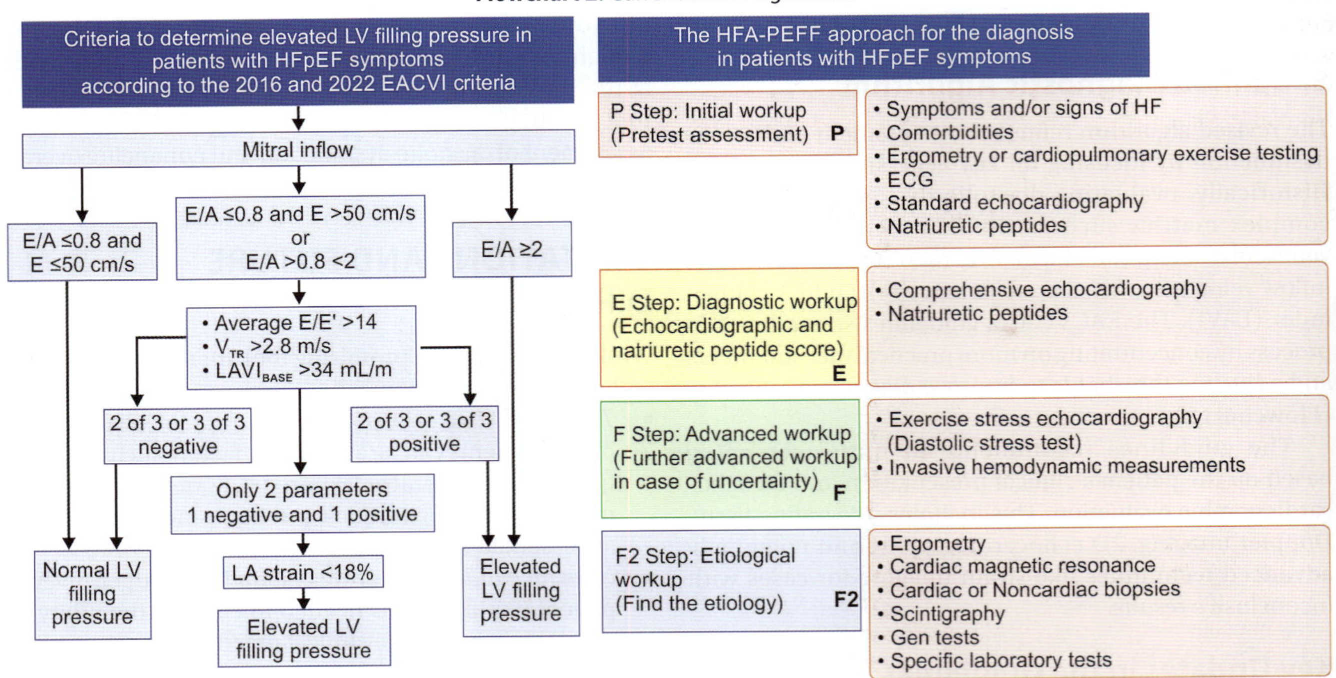

Limited Availability and Access

- *Specialized equipment:* STE, the technique used to measure atrial strain, requires specialized equipment and software, which may not be available in all clinical settings, particularly in resource-limited environments.
- *Training requirements:* Proper training is essential to ensure accurate acquisition and interpretation of atrial strain data. However, not all healthcare facilities have the necessary resources to train their personnel effectively.

Interpretation Challenges

- *Overlap with other conditions:* Reduced atrial strain is not specific to HFpEF and can be observed in other cardiac conditions such as AF, valvular heart disease, and hypertrophic cardiomyopathy. This overlap can complicate the interpretation of atrial strain results and reduce specificity for diagnosing HFpEF.
- *Prognostic uncertainty:* While atrial strain has shown prognostic value in some studies, its role in predicting long-term outcomes in HFpEF patients remains under investigation. More research is needed to establish how atrial strain measurements can be integrated into risk stratification models and treatment planning.

Longitudinal Data and Prognostic Value

Insufficient longitudinal data: There is limited longitudinal data on how changes in atrial strain over time correlate with disease progression or response to therapy in HFpEF patients. More studies are needed to establish the role of atrial strain as a monitoring tool.

CONCLUSION

Atrial strain imaging represents a promising advancement in the diagnostic and management landscape of HFpEF. By providing detailed insights into atrial function and identifying early changes, atrial strain can enhance the accuracy of HFpEF diagnosis, aid in risk stratification, and guide treatment decisions. As research continues to validate and refine its use, atrial strain has the potential to become a valuable tool in the comprehensive care of patients with HFpEF.

Heart failure with preserved ejection fraction represents a unique and challenging subset of HF with distinct underlying mechanisms.[21] The interplay of diastolic dysfunction, endothelial dysfunction, myocardial hypertrophy, and systemic inflammation contributes to the pathophysiology of HFpEF and distinguishes it from other forms of HF.[22] Understanding these mechanisms is crucial for developing targeted therapies and improving outcomes for patients with HFpEF. The author concludes with Brage Høyem Amundsen's editorial comment about the atrial strain: "A Piece of the HFpEF Puzzle Found, But Not Yet in Place."[36]

REFERENCES

1. Nagueh SF, et al. Atrial strain and its relationship to diastolic function in patients with heart failure with preserved ejection fraction. J Am Coll Cardiol. 2016;68(16):1680-8.
2. Sanna G, et al. Prognostic value of atrial strain in heart failure with preserved ejection fraction. Circ Heart Fail. 2018;11(4):e004239.
3. Reddy YNV, et al. Incremental value of atrial strain measurements for the diagnosis of heart failure with preserved ejection fraction. J Am Soc Echocardiography. 2019;32(7):855-63.
4. Murphy TM, Waterhouse DF, James SA, et al. Comparison of HFrEF vs HFpEF's clinical workload and cost in the first year following hospitalization and enrollment in a disease management program. Int J Cardiol. 2017;232:330-5.
5. Morris DA, Belyavskiy E, Aravind-Kumar R, et al. Potential usefulness and clinical relevance of adding left atrial strain to left atrial volume index in the detection of left ventricular diastolic dysfunction. JACC Cardiovasc Imaging. 2018;11(10):1405-15.
6. Blume GG, McLeod CJ, Barnes ME, et al. Left atrial function: physiology, assessment, and clinical implications. Eur J Echocardiogr. 2011;12(6):421-30.
7. Katbeh A, De Potter T, Geelen P, et al. Heart failure with preserved ejection fraction or non-cardiac dyspnea in paroxysmal atrial fibrillation: the role of left atrial strain. Int J Cardiol. 2021;323:161-7.
8. Cameli M, Mandoli GE, Loiacono F. Left atrial strain: a useful index in atrial fibrillation. Int J Cardiol. 2016;220: 208-13.
9. Cameli M, Pastore MC, Mandoli GE, et al. Prognosis and risk stratification of patients with advanced heart failure (from PROBE). Am J Cardiol. 2019;124(1):55-62.
10. Morris DA, et al. Left atrial function as assessed by speckle tracking echocardiography in heart failure with preserved ejection fraction: a systematic review and meta-analysis. Euro J Heart Fail. 2017;19(9):1132-49.
11. Singh A, et al. Left atrial strain: a new prognostic marker in heart failure with preserved ejection fraction. J Am Coll Cardiol Cardiovasc Imaging. 2019;12(8):1389-92.
12. Santos AB, et al. Diastolic dysfunction diagnostic algorithms in HFpEF: importance of left atrial function. Eur Heart J Cardiovasc Imaging. 2015;16(2):234-42.
13. Kurt M, et al. Left atrial strain as a predictor of exercise capacity in patients with heart failure and preserved ejection fraction. J Am Soc Echocardiogr. 2015;28(6): 636-44.
14. Telles F, Nanayakkara S, Evans S, et al. Impaired left atrial strain predicts abnormal exercise haemodynamics in heart failure with preserved ejection fraction. Eur J Heart Fail. 2019;21(4):495-505.
15. Pieske B, Tschöpe C, de Boer RA, et al. How to diagnose heart failure with preserved ejection fraction: the HFA–PEFF diagnostic algorithm: a consensus recommendation from the Heart Failure Association (HFA) of the European Society of Cardiology (ESC). Eur Heart J. 2019;40(40): 3297-317.
16. Heidenreich PA, Bozkurt B, Aguilar D, et al. 2022 AHA/ACC/HFSA guideline for the management of heart failure: a report of the American College of Cardiology/American Heart Association Joint Committee on Clinical Practice Guidelines. Circulation. 2022;145(18):e895-1032.
17. Almeida ALC, de Melo MDT, de Souza Le Bihan DC, et al. Posicionamento do Departamento de Imagem Cardiovascular da Sociedade Brasileira de Cardiologia sobre o Uso do Strain Miocárdico na Rotina do Cardiologista – 2023. Arq Bras Cardiol. 2023;120(12):e20230646.
18. Loizou CP, Pattichis CS, D'hooge J (Eds). Handbook of Speckle Filtering and Tracking in Cardiovascular Ultrasound Imaging and Video. Cyprus: The Institution of Engineering and Technology; 2017.
19. de Sousa RD, Regis CDM, Silva IDS, et al. Software for post-processing analysis of strain curves: the D-station. Arq Bras Cardiol. 2020;114(3):496-506.
20. Badano LP, Kolias TJ, Muraru D, et al. Standardization of left atrial, right ventricular, and right atrial deformation imaging using two-dimensional speckle tracking echocardiography: a consensus document of the EACVI/ASE/industry task force to standardize deformation imaging. Eur Heart J Cardiovasc Imaging. 2018;19(6):591-600.
21. Sirbu C, Herbots L, D'hooge J, et al. Feasibility of strain and strain rate imaging for the assessment of regional left atrial deformation: a study in normal subjects. Eur J Echocardiogr. 2006;7(3):199-208.
22. Morris DA, Gailani M, Vaz Pérez A, et al. Left atrial systolic and diastolic dysfunction in heart failure with normal left ventricular ejection fraction. J Am Soc Echocardiogr. 2011;24(6):651-62.
23. Ye Z, Miranda WR, Yeung DF, et al. Left atrial strain in evaluation of heart failure with preserved ejection fraction. J Am Soc Echocardiogr. 2020;33(12):1490-9.
24. Appleton CP, Hatle LK. The natural history of left ventricular filling abnormalities: assessment by two-dimensional and doppler echocardiography. Echocardiography. 1992; 9(4):437-57.
25. Fauchier L, Bisson A, Bodin A. Heart failure with preserved ejection fraction and atrial fibrillation: recent advances and open questions. BMC Med. 2023;21(1):54.
26. Shah S, Segar MW, Kondamudi N, et al. Supranormal left ventricular ejection fraction, stroke volume, and cardiovascular risk: findings from population-based cohort studies. JACC Heart Fail. 2022;10(8):583-94.
27. Gorter TM, et al. Left atrial dysfunction as a feature of HFpEF: influence of left ventricular filling pressure and left atrial volume. Eur J Heart Fail. 2016;18(11):1369-76.

28. Hummel YM, et al. Prognostic value of left atrial strain in heart failure with preserved ejection fraction. Eur J Heart Fail. 2018;20(8):1113-22.
29. Thomas L, et al. Impact of left atrial function on the prognosis of patients with heart failure with preserved ejection fraction: implications for assessment of diastolic function. J Am Coll Cardiol Cardiovasc Imaging. 2014; 7(4):376-84.
30. Freed BH, Daruwalla V, Cheng JY, et al. Prognostic utility and clinical significance of cardiac mechanics in heart failure with preserved ejection fraction: importance of left atrial strain. Circ Cardiovasc Imaging. 2016;9(3):10.1161/CIRCIMAGING.115.003754 e003754.
31. Cameli M, Lisi M, Focardi M, et al. Left atrial deformation analysis by speckle tracking echocardiography for prediction of cardiovascular outcomes. Am J Cardiol. 2012;110(2):264-9.
32. Mitter SS, Shah SJ, Thomas JD. A test in context: E/A and E/e′ to assess diastolic dysfunction and LV filling pressure. J Am Coll Cardiol. 2017;69(11):1451-64.
33. Morris DA, et al. The left atrial strain in heart failure with preserved ejection fraction: prognostic relevance and the impact of right ventricular function. J Am Soc Echocardiogr. 2018;31(9):1203-12.
34. Andersen OS, et al. Diagnostic and prognostic utility of left atrial function in heart failure with preserved ejection fraction. J Am Coll Cardiol. 2018;71(20):2247-57.
35. Smiseth OA, Morris DA, Cardim N, et al. Multimodality imaging in patients with heart failure and preserved ejection fraction: an expert consensus document of the European Association of Cardiovascular Imaging. Eur Heart J Cardiovasc Imaging. 2022;23(2):e34-61.
36. Amundsen BH. Atrial strain: a piece of the HFpEF puzzle found, but not yet in place. J Am Coll Cardiol. 2021;78(3):258-9.

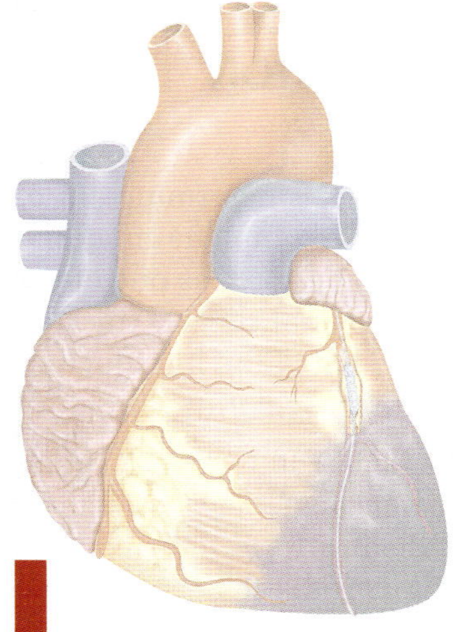

Echocardiographic Evaluation of HFpEF in Emergency

Rekha Mishra, Manisha Sharma

INTRODUCTION

Heart failure with preserved ejection fraction (HFpEF) is a common clinical syndrome that is increasing in prevalence coupled with the growing population burden of aging and comorbidities. It can be described as a clinical syndrome of heart failure (HF) manifesting its signs and symptoms (such as dyspnea, fatigue, ankle edema, neck vein distension, pulmonary edema, etc.) due to structural or functional cardiac abnormality coupled with left ventricular ejection fraction (LVEF) ≥50% along with elevated left ventricular filling pressures (LVFPs).[1-4]

EPIDEMIOLOGY

Presently, HF irrespective of LVEF has a prevalence of >64 million people globally which is approximately 1–3% of total world population.[5] Community-based epidemiological studies and registries with LVEF assessments report that the percentage of HFpEF is somewhere between 19 and 55% of all HF cases.[6] Large number of people participated in the Framingham Heart Study over three decades, which showed an increasing trend in the percentage of HF constituting HFpEF (LVEF ≥50%), from 41% in 1985–1994 to 56% in 2005–2014.[7] HFpEF is rather unusual in younger patients, but its importance grows in the aging population and the rate is comparatively higher in females than male, moreover there is an associated history of hypertension.[8]

The Olmsted County cohort, one of the largest and most comprehensive epidemiological assessment of cardiac structure and function in HFpEF, showed an occurrence of left ventricle (LV) hypertrophy of 42% among 244 HFpEF cases.[9] In a study of all incident HF cases in Olmsted County, MN, in 1991, 43% of cases with LVEF evaluated had an LVEF ≥50%.[1] Echocardiography was found to be the most commonly used imaging modality in epidemiological, registry, and clinical trial studies of HFpEF.

ROLE OF ECHOCARDIOGRAPHY IN CLASSIFICATION OF HEART FAILURE

In 2022, the American College of Cardiology (ACC), American Heart Association (AHA), and Heart Failure Society of America (HFSA) recommended guidelines[10] for prognostication and management of HF incorporating the classification of HF based on LVEF:

- *Heart failure with reduced ejection fraction (HFrEF):* Patients with an LVEF ≤40%.
- *Heart failure with improved ejection fraction (HFimpEF):* Patients with a previous LVEF ≤40% and a subsequent measurement of LVEF >40%.
- *Heart failure with mildly reduced ejection fraction (HFmrEF):* Patients with an LVEF 41–49% with evidence of spontaneous or provokable increased LVFPs, characterized by elevated natriuretic peptides or hemodynamic measurements. HFmrEF is sometimes referred to as HF with midrange ejection fraction in the literature.
- *Heart failure with preserved ejection fraction:* Patients with an LVEF ≥50% with evidence of spontaneous or provokable increased LVFPs, characterized by elevated natriuretic peptides or hemodynamic measurements.

PATHOPHYSIOLOGY OF HEART FAILURE WITH PRESERVED EJECTION FRACTION

The new paradigm suggests that myocardial remodeling and dysfunction in HFpEF are consequent of the following intracellular changes:

- *Comorbidities particularly obesity:* These induce a systemic proinflammatory state.
- *Proinflammatory state:* Leads to the production of reactive oxygen species (ROS) by coronary microvascular endothelial cells, limiting nitric oxide (NO) bioavailability to the adjacent cardiomyocytes.
- *Limited NO bioavailability:* Declines protein kinase G (PKG) activity in cardiomyocytes.
- *Low PKG activity:* Accelerates the cardiomyocyte hypertrophy, leading to concentric LV remodeling and stiffening of cardiomyocytes due to hypophosphorylation of giant cytoskeletal protein titin.
- *Stiff cardiomyocytes and collagen deposition* by myofibroblasts results in diastolic LV dysfunction, the prime cardiac functional deficit in HFpEF.[11-16]

EVALUATION OF A PATIENT WITH DYSPNEA IN EMERGENCY

Exertional/resting dyspnea is a common clinical complaint. It is reasonable to suspect HFpEF as a possible diagnosis in any patient with exertional/resting dyspnea with one of the following clinical parameters not otherwise explained by an alternative diagnosis:

- Age 60 or older
- Atrial fibrillation
- Chronic kidney disease
- Coronary artery disease
- Diabetes
- Hypertension
- Overweight/obesity

Echocardiography is the most helpful tool in diagnosing HFpEF in a patient with dyspnea in emergency and is strongly recommended. It provides not only essential information on cardiac structure and function but also hemodynamics and is performed in all patients where there is clinical suspicion for HFpEF.[17] It is crucial in identifying HFpEF among patients with dyspnea, especially when overt congestion is absent. Echocardiography also provides valuable insight into the pathophysiology and underlying phenotypes of HFpEF, treatment, and risk stratification.[18,19]

ECHOCARDIOGRAPHY TO DETERMINE LEFT VENTRICULAR EJECTION FRACTION

The first step in identifying HFpEF is determination of LVEF, which should be measured by biplane modified Simpson's method.[20] LVEF should be ≥50% as one of the criteria to define HFpEF. The advent of speckle tracking echocardiography (STE) has facilitated the introduction into clinical practice of strain based imaging as an alternative assessment of myocardial systolic contractility. Its value is maximal among patients with preserved or mild LV dysfunction. LV diameters and volumes should be recorded and the assessment for the presence of concentric remodeling or LV hypertrophy and nondilated LV and left atrial (LA) enlargement **(Figs. 1A to D)**.

ECHOCARDIOGRAPHY TO IDENTIFY ELEVATED FILLING PRESSURE IN PRESENCE OF NORMAL LEFT VENTRICULAR EJECTION FRACTION

The HFpEF by definition requires the presence of elevated filling pressures either at rest or with exertion without which systemic perfusion cannot be maintained.[21] Although diastolic dysfunction is a central feature in HFpEF, the pathophysiology is complex with variable contributions from diastolic dysfunction, impaired contractile reserve, impaired atrial function, relative pericardial restraint, and abnormal ventricular vascular coupling which all contribute to the elevation in pulmonary venous and left sided filling pressures.[22-24] Echocardiography with Doppler readily helps in assessing not only LV diastolic function but also in assessment of severity/grading, identification of etiology, important differential diagnosis, and management of acute HF.[25]

The assessment of diastolic dysfunction is complex, and multiple factors must be assessed and no one parameter can be used in isolation. Therefore, different parameters are used to evaluate the performance of LV as well as RV. The following parameters are more frequently used: the peak acceleration rate of mitral E velocity, mitral filling velocity ratio (E/A), ratio between rapid ventricular filling velocity, and ventricular myocardial relaxation velocity (E/e'), isovelocity relaxation time (IVRT), peak tricuspid regurgitation(TR) velocity, RV fractional area change (FAC), and tricuspid annular plane systolic excursion (TAPSE).[20] According to the latest guidelines (2016) from American society of Echocardiography and European Association of Cardiovascular imaging mainly

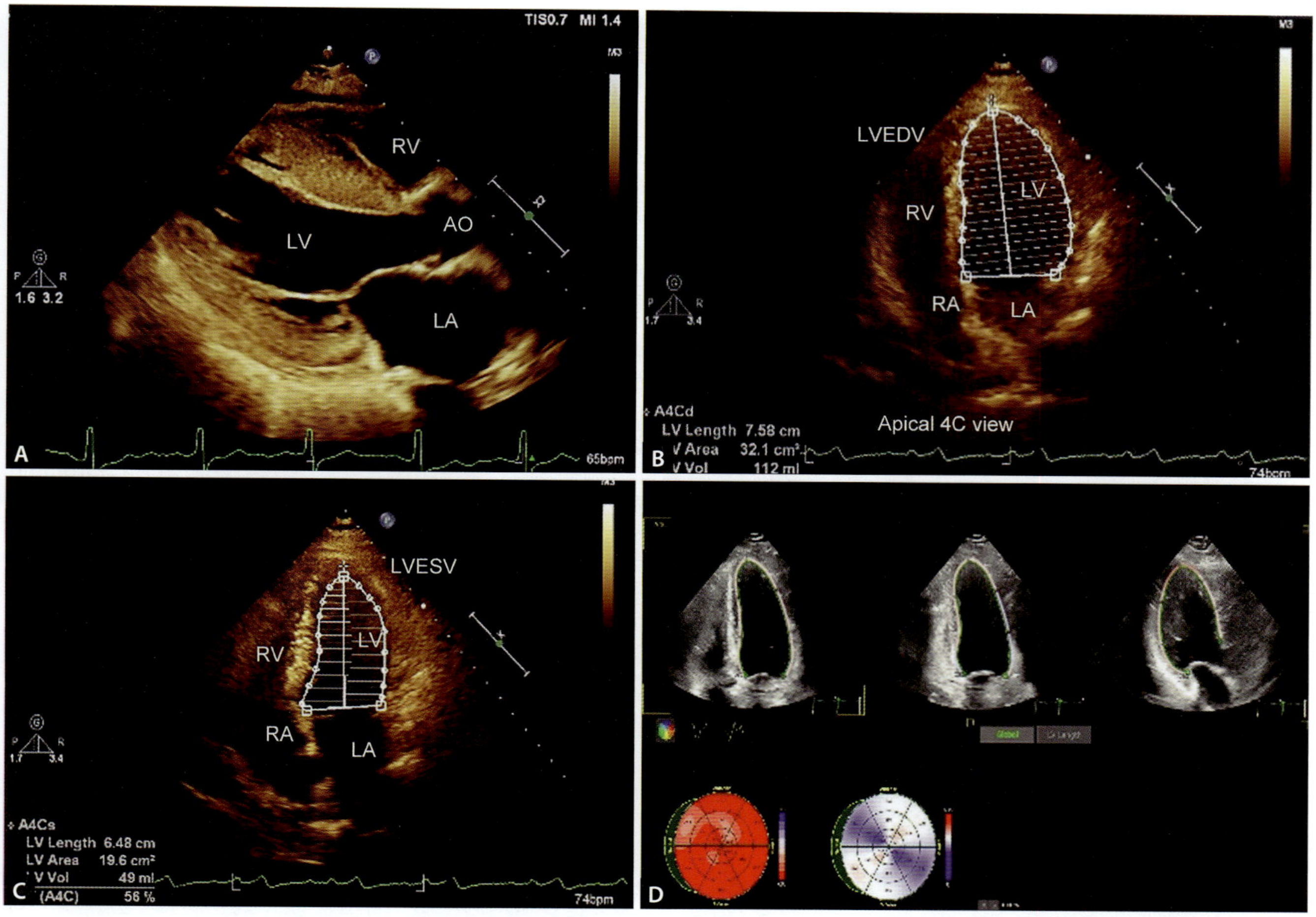

Figs. 1A to D: (A) Parasternal long axis view showing end diastolic frame with left ventricular concentric hypertrophy and dilatation of left atrium; (B and C) Two orthogonal views, apical four chamber (B) and apical two chamber (C) views to calculate volume and left ventricular ejection fraction; (D) Speckle tracking echocardiography of LV with apical four chamber, two chamber, and apical long-axis views with bull's-eye longitudinal strain imaging of left ventricle (LV). (RA: right atrial; RV: right ventricle; LV: left ventricle; LA: left atrial; LVEDV: left ventricle end-diastolic volume; LVESV: left ventricular end-systolic volume; AO: aorta)

four variables need to be evaluated in determining the diastolic function if LV systolic function is preserved[17] **(Flowchart 1)**.

These four variables and their abnormal variables are **(Figs. 2A to F)**:

1. Annular e' velocity (septal e' velocity <7.0 cm/sec, lateral e' <10 cm/sec)
2. An average E/e' ratio of >14
3. LA maximum volume index of 34 mL/m^2
4. Peak TR velocity of >2.8 m/sec

At times only the medial or lateral e' velocity is available and, in these circumstances, medial E/e' ratio >15 cm/sec or a lateral E/e' >13 cm/sec is considered abnormal.

The LA volume is a surrogate marker of the severity and chronicity of LV diastolic dysfunction.[26] LA maximum volume index (Biplane LA volume) is currently recommended and not LA anteroposterior diameter by M-mode, as LA enlargement can occur in the medial-lateral and superior-inferior directions only, resulting in an increased LA volume while the LA anteroposterior diameter is still within the normal range.[20]

Flowchart 1: Algorithm for determining if left ventricle (LV) diastolic dysfunction is present in patients with normal LVEFs and no evidence of myocardial disease.[17]

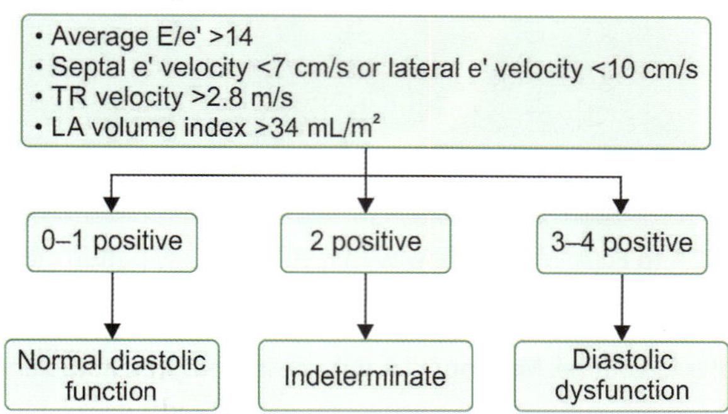

(LA: left atrial; TR: tricuspid regurgitation)

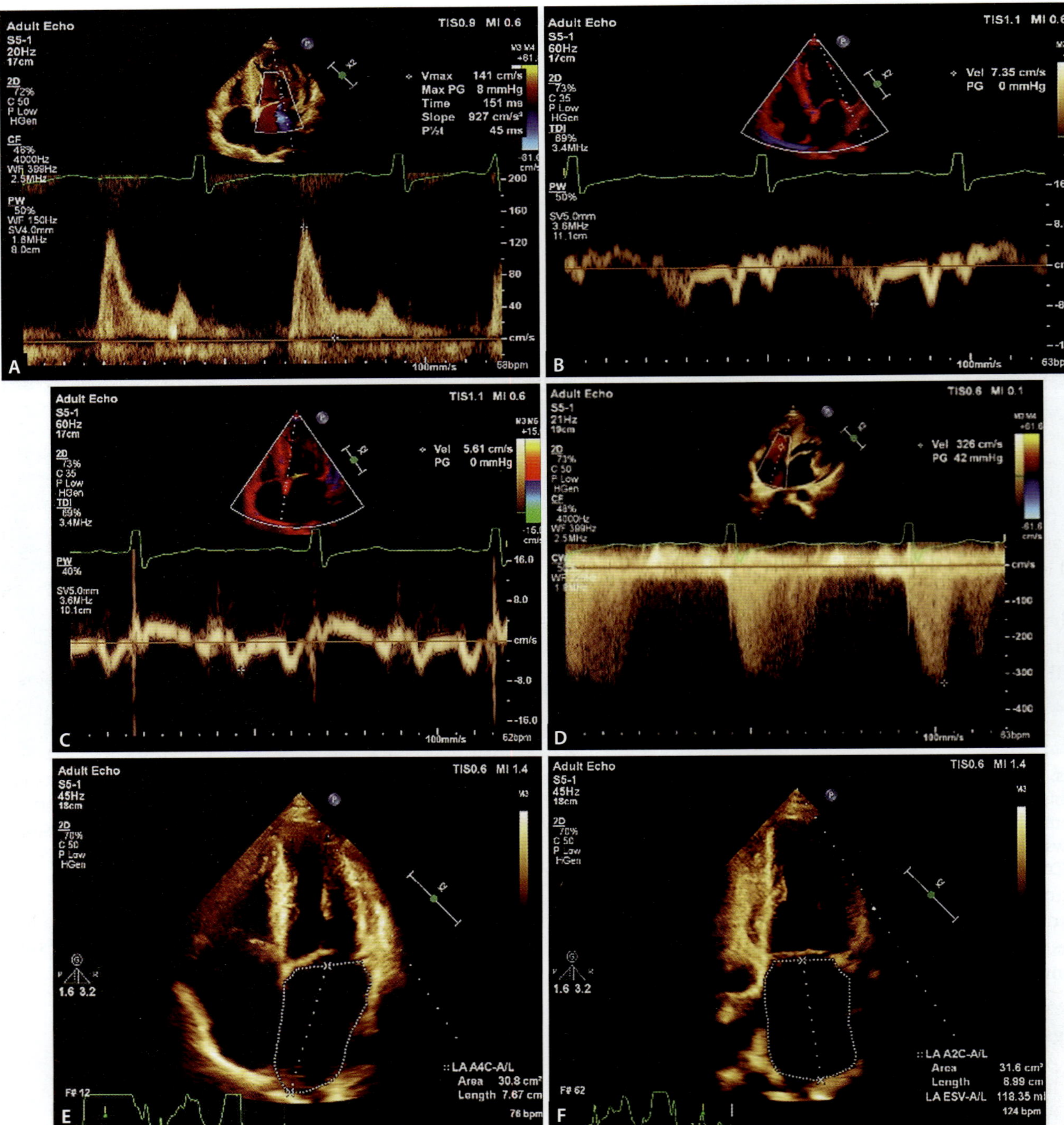

Figs. 2A to F: (A) Mitral inflow with restrictive flow pattern; (B and C) Tissue Doppler velocity recording from the lateral and septal mitral annulus respectively. E/e'(Av)–21.8 is consistent with elevated left ventricle (LV) filling pressures; (D) Tricuspid regurgitation velocity with peak flow velocity of 3.2 m/s; (E and F) Apical four and two chamber views demonstrating biplane Simpson's method for calculating left atrial (LA) volume. Maximum LA volume is measured at the end systole.

LV diastolic function is normal if more than half of the available variables do not meet the cutoff values for identifying abnormal function. LV diastolic dysfunction is present if more than half of the available parameters meet these cutoff values. The study is inconclusive if half of the parameters do not meet the cutoff values.

ECHOCARDIOGRAPHY FOR EVALUATION OF LEFT ATRIAL FUNCTION

Echocardiography is also used to determine LA remodeling and atrial dysfunction. LA enlargement and/or dysfunction are increasingly recognized as biomarkers for adverse cardiovascular events. LA function is important and may demonstrate alterations prior to changes in LA volume.[27] LA strain has emerged as a superior method for LA function quantification compared with measures based on volume changes, such as LAEF.[28] Two dimensional STE is currently the preferred technique for the routine measurement of LA strain, as it is semiautomated, less angle-dependent, and less affected by artifacts than tissue Doppler imaging. The only recommended strain parameter of LA function is the global longitudinal strain.[29] Peak LA longitudinal strain represents atrial reservoir function and is reduced in HFpEF[30] **(Fig. 3)**.

DIAGNOSTIC SCORES IN HEART FAILURE WITH PRESERVED EJECTION FRACTION

The diagnosis of HFpEF at times can be challenging and diagnostic scores have been proposed to aid in the diagnosis. Therefore, two scores have been validated for the diagnosis of HFpEF, namely H_2FPEF and HFA-PEFF. The H_2FPEF score relies mostly on comorbidities

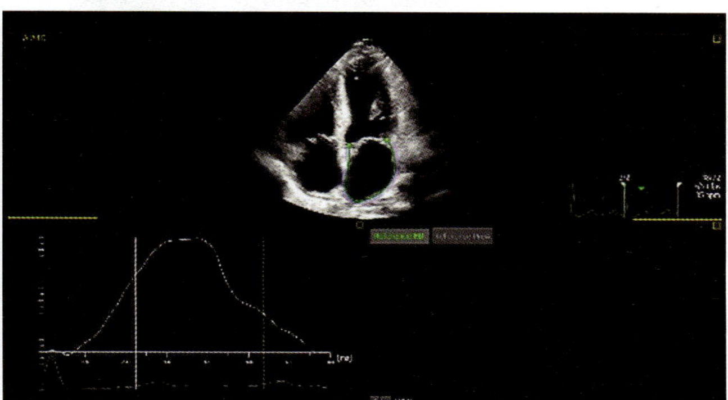

Fig. 3: Apical four chamber view—measurement of left atrial strain by 2D speckle tracking echocardiography analysis: Analysis of conduit, pump, and reservoir function of left atrium.

and includes clinical-obesity, hypertension, atrial fibrillation, age and echocardiographic data—pulmonary hypertension and E/e' ratio. The HFA-PEFF uses multiple echocardiographic parameters on structural and functional cardiac abnormalities and includes natriuretic peptide blood levels. A high rating in either of the two scores has a high positive predictive value, and the scores are most useful when HFpEF is clinically suspected, but the diagnosis is uncertain.

H_2FPEF Score

The H_2FPEF score was developed by at the Mayo Clinic,[31] Rochester, USA. They defined HFpEF as elevated pulmonary capillary wedge pressure (PCWP) at rest (≥15 mm Hg) or during exercise (≥25 mm Hg). They built a score using six parameters and each parameter is given a score according to the presence of the respective criteria **(Table 1)**. The final H_2FPEF score is calculated by the sum of points, indicating low probability (<2 points), intermediate probability (2–5 points) or high probability (>5 points) of HFpEF.

HFA-PEFF Score

A consensus recommendation from the Heart Failure Association (HFA) of the European Society of Cardiology (ESC) proposed a four-step diagnostic algorithm for HFpEF: Step 1 (P)—pretest assessment; Step 2 (E)—echocardiographic and natriuretic peptide HFpEF score; Step 3 (F1)—Functional testing; and Step 4 (F2)—Final etiology. On Step 2 (E), the authors proposed the HFA-PEFF score, which was based on echocardiographic and

TABLE 1: The H_2FPEF score.

Clinical variable		*Values*	*Points*
H_2	*Heavy*	Body mass index >30 kg/m^2	2
	Hypertension	2 or more antihypertensive medicines	1
F	*Atrial Fibrillation*	Paroxysmal or persistent	3
P	*Pulmonary Hypertension*	Doppler echocardiographic estimated right ventricular systolic pressure >35 mm Hg	1
E	*Elderly*	Age >60 years	1
F	*Filling pressures*	Doppler echocardiographic E/e' >9	1
H_2FPEF Score sum (0–9)			
Interpretation: 0–1: Low probability (unlikely HFpEF) 2–5: Intermediate probability 6–9: High probability (likely HFpEF)			

TABLE 2: HFA-PEFF score.[32]

	Functional	*Morphological*	*Biomarker (SR)*	*Biomarker (AF)*
Major	Septal e′ <7 cm/s or Lateral e′ <10 cm/s or Average E/e′ ≥15 or TR velocity >2.8 m/s PASP >35 mm Hg	LAVI > 34 mL/m² or LVMI ≥149/122 g/m² (m/w) and RWT >0.42	NT-proBNP >220 pg/mL or BNP >80 pg/mL	NT-proBNP >660 pg/mL or BNP >240 pg/mL
Minor	Average E/e′ 9–14 or GLS <16%	LAVI 29–34 mL/m² or LVMI ≥115/95 g/m² (m/w) and RWT >0.42 or LV wall thickness ≥12 mm	NT-proBNP 125–220 pg/mL or BNP 35–80 pg/mL	NT-proBNP 365–660 pg/mL or BNP 105–240 pg/mL
Major criteria: 2 points		*≥5 points; High probability (diagnosis HFpEF)* *2–4 points: Intermediate probability (Diastolic Stress Test or Invasive Hemodynamic Measurement)*		
Minor points: 1 point		*0–1 point: Low probability (unlikey HFpEF)*		

(BNP: B-type natriuretic peptide; GLS: global longitudinal strain; HFpEF: heart failure with preserved ejection fraction; LAVI: left atrial volume index; LVMI: left ventricular mass index; LVWT: left ventricular wall thickness; m: men; NT-proBNP: N-terminal B-type natriuretic peptide; PASP: Pulmonary artery systolic pressure; RWT: relative wall thickness; TR: Tricuspid regurgitation; w: women)

natriuretic peptide measurements. The HFA-PEFF score has three domains: Functional, morphological, and biomarker **(Table 2)**.

ECHOCARDIOGRAPHY TO IDENTIFY HEART FAILURE WITH PRESERVED EJECTION FRACTION PHENOTYPES

Echocardiography provides valuable insight into the pathophysiology and underlying phenotypes in HFpEF as it has been recognized that HFpEF is a heterogeneous syndrome.

- *Left atrial dysfunction phenotype*—LA remodeling and dysfunction secondary to increased LVFPs are associated with worse symptoms of dyspnea, more pulmonary vascular disease, greater RV dysfunction, depressed exercise capacity and adverse outcomes in HFpEF.[33,34] LA myopathy may be mediated by atrial fibrillation (AF), mitral regurgitation (MR), coronary microvascular dysfunction, and inflammation.[35,36] Multiple studies have shown the use of LA reservoir strain assessed by STE to identify LA dysfunction, help diagnosis, and predict outcomes in HFpEF.[37,38]
- *Pulmonary hypertension (PH) and pulmonary vascular phenotype*—PH is common in patients with HFpEF, and is associated with worse exercise capacity and clinical outcomes.[39-41] While PH is predominantly associated with LA hypertension, but a number of patients develop pulmonary vascular disease, manifest by elevation in pulmonary vascular resistance and reduction in pulmonary arterial compliance.[42] Echocardiography helps in identifying the presence of pulmonary vascular disease from mid systolic notching in the RV outflow Doppler profile, along with a short acceleration time caused by increased pulmonary arterial resistance with enhanced early wave reflection.[43,44] **(Fig. 4)**. A recent study reported that RV and pulmonary vascular coupling (RV-PA coupling) assessed by TAPSE to RVSP (<0.36 mm/mm Hg) predicts the pulmonary vascular disease in HFpEF.[45]

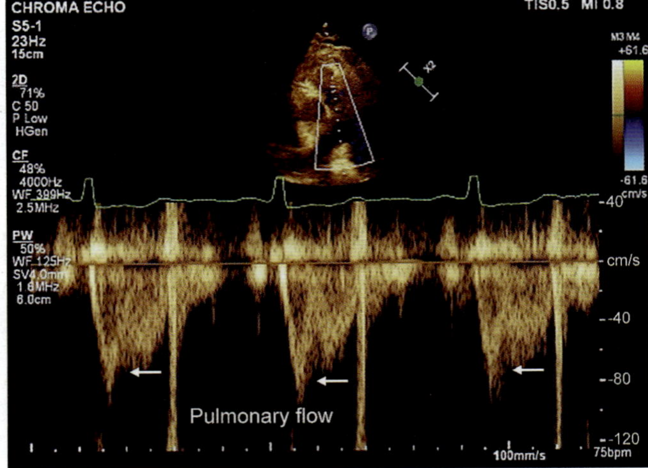

Fig. 4: Pulse wave Doppler of pulmonary flow with short acceleration time and a notch (arrow) in the deceleration time consistent with high resistant flow seen in pulmonary vascular disease.

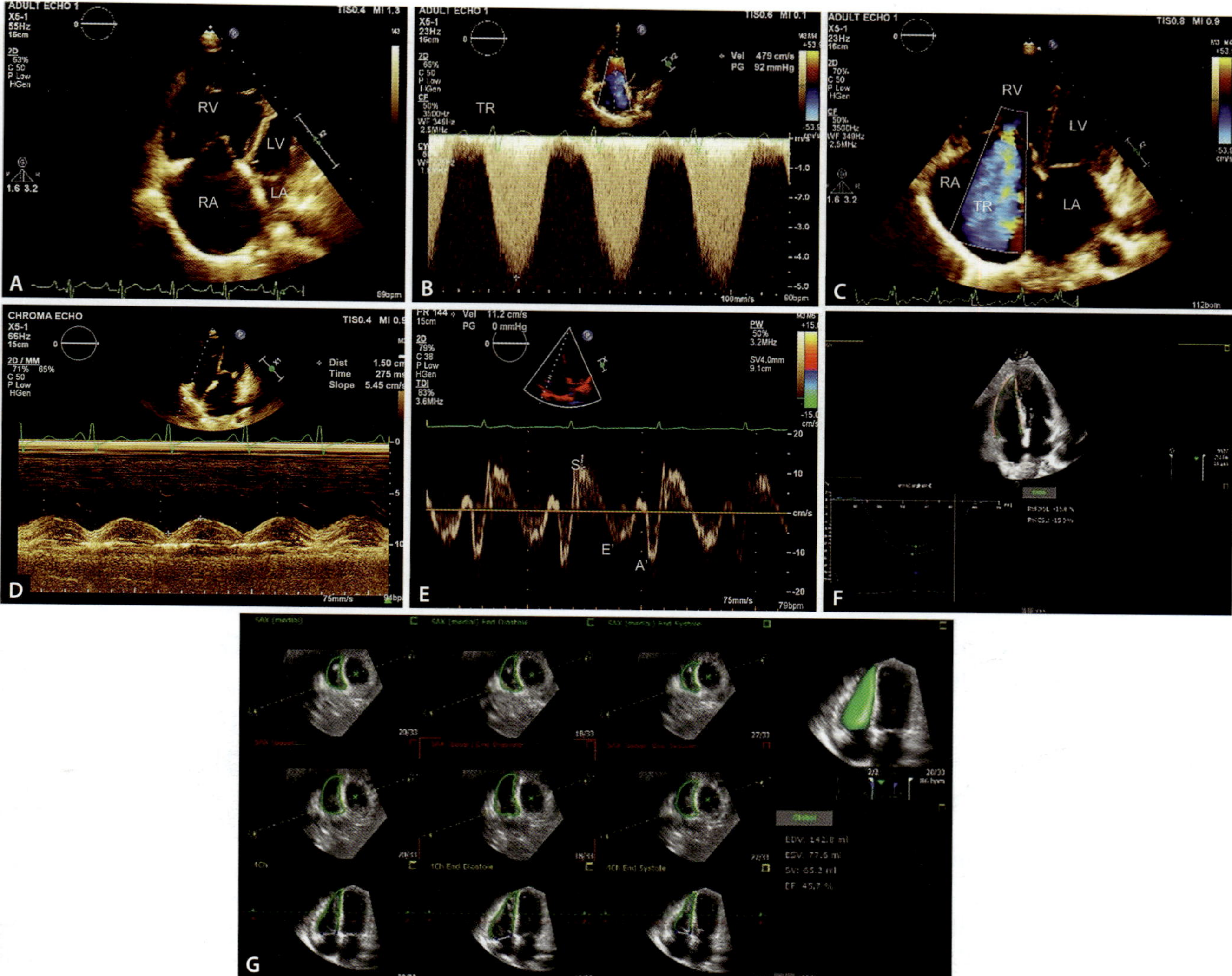

Figs. 5A to G: (A) Apical four chamber view in a patient with advanced pulmonary hypertension, demonstrating marked right ventricle (RV) and right atrial (RA) enlargement, interventricular, and interatrial septum shifted to the left, small left ventricle (LV) and left atrial (LA); (B) Spectral continuous wave Doppler signal of the tricuspid regurgitation in apical four chamber view showing peak pressure gradient of 92 mm Hg; (C) Apical four chamber view demonstrating enlargement of RV and RA with evidence of severe tricuspid regurgitation by color Doppler; (D) Measurement of tricuspid annular plane systolic excursion (TAPSE) of the tricuspid lateral annulus in apical four-chamber view; (E) Tissue Doppler of the Tricuspid lateral annulus in apical four chamber view; S' is used in the assessment of RV systolic function; (F) Longitudinal systolic strain of the RV in the apical four chamber view, showing marked reduction of global as well as RV free wall longitudinal strain; (G) 3D echocardiography for assessment of RV function with calculation of RV end diastolic and end systolic volumes, RV stroke volume, and RV ejection fraction.

- *Right ventricular dysfunction phenotype*—the presence of PH causes RV systolic dysfunction in HFpEF. Echocardiography helps in measuring the various indices of RV systolic dysfunction, namely, TAPSE, RV FAC, free wall strain, tricuspid annular s' velocity, and RV index of myocardial performance.[46,47]

The RV dysfunction is associated with RV remodeling. Echocardiography helps in assessment of RV dilatation (RV basal, mid and longitudinal dimensions, and areas), RV hypertrophy as well as right atrial (RA) dilatation. RA and RV dilatation leads to tricuspid annular dilatation and resultant secondary TR. The progression of PH and TR adversely affects RA structure and function by increasing both afterload and preload.[48-50] RA enlargement and subsequent annular dilatation may further worsen TR, forming a vicious cycle **(Figs. 5A to G)**.

- *Obesity phenotype*—obesity is now recognized as an important phenotype of HFpEF,[51] patients with the

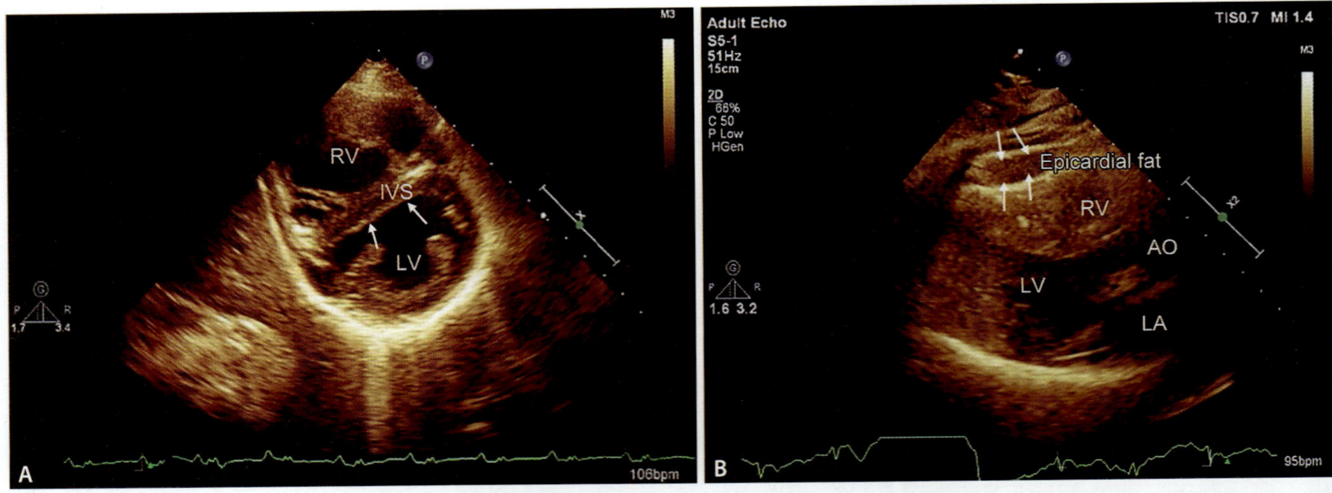

Figs. 6A and B: (A) Short axis view demonstrating flattening of interventricular septum (IVS) (arrow) with D-shaped left ventricle (LV) cavity and enlarged right ventricle symptoms of (s/o) pulmonary hypertension; (B) Parasternal long axis view at end-systole in an obese heart failure with preserved ejection fraction (HFpEF) patient. Increased epicardial fat thickness identified between the right ventricular free wall and the pericardium (arrow).

obese phenotype display a number of key differences such as greater relationships between body weight and cardiac filling pressures, greater plasma volume expansion, more ventricular remodeling, more adverse hemodynamics, altered right ventricular-pulmonary artery coupling, worse exercise capacity, and enhanced pericardial restraint.[51]

Echocardiography helps in detecting the adverse effects of obesity like the degree of pericardial restraint is recognized as a D-shaped LV cavity in the short axis view which can be quantified by assessment of eccentricity index.[51] Abdominal obesity is associated with epicardial fat and has recently been found to be associated with increased mortality in HFpEF.[52] Measurement of epicardial fat thickness can be estimated by echocardiography in parasternal long axis view **(Figs. 6A and B)**.

- *Ishemia/microvascular dysfunction phenotype*—the presence of coronary artery disease (CAD) in patients with HFpEF have a greater risk of deterioration of LV function related to ischemic mechanisms, which implies a poorer prognosis compared to patients with HFpEF without CAD. Subendocardial ischemia may also develop in the absence of epicardial CAD in HFpEF, caused by the combination of coronary microvascular dysfunction and hemodynamic derangements that compromise subendocardial perfusion.[53]

ROLE OF ECHOCARDIOGRAPHY IN HEART FAILURE WITH PRESERVED EJECTION FRACTION MIMICS TO IDENTIFY SPECIFIC ETIOLOGY

As the final step in the HFpEF diagnostic process, care should be taken to exclude other differential diagnosis that mimic HFpEF **(Table 3)**. Echocardiography is very helpful in ruling out the less common causes of HFpEF including hypertrophic cardiomyopathy, constrictive pericarditis (CP), and restrictive cardiomyopathies which include infiltrative cardiomyopathies such as amyloidosis, storage disorders, radiation-induced heart disease, and endomyocardial fibrosis. Although, these diseases account for a small minority of cases of HFpEF, the clinical presentation in older persons with HFpEF may be identical. The main use of echocardiography in acute cardiac care of patients affected by these cardiomyopathies relates to the diagnosis and management of acute HF.

Current ESC guidelines include increased LV mass index as one of the criteria for the diagnosis of HFpEF.[25] Whenever significant LV hypertrophy is identified, the diagnosis of amyloidosis must be considered, particularly in the presence of a pericardial effusion or apical sparing pattern of LV strain.[54] Pericardial disease, particularly CP should be considered when HF and normal EF coexist. Pericardial thickening is a hallmark of constriction but is a relatively insensitive finding. The distinction between

TABLE 3: Differential diagnoses of HFpEF and their echocardiographic clues.[55]

Differential diagnosis	*Echocardiographic clues*
1. Hypertrophic cardiomyopathy	Asymmetric hypertrophy, ↑↑LV wall thickness, LVOT obstruction, SAM
2. Restrictive cardiomyopathy	Small LV cavity, ↑LV wall thickness, sparkling myocardium, apical sparing in GLS, severely reduced tissue Doppler, PE
3. Pulmonary arterial hypertension	↑RVSP with no sign of elevated LV filling pressure, Isolated right heart dilation, PA dilatation, RVOT Doppler midsystolic notch
4. Constrictive pericarditis	Pericardial thickening, Septal bounce, annulus paradoxus and annulus reversus, ↑Respiratory variation in mitral/tricuspid flow, absence of IVC collapse
5. Valvular heart disease	Morphological valvular abnormalities, Color Doppler
6. Coronary artery disease	Regional wall motion abnormality and thinning
7. Chronic thromboembolic pulmonary hypertension	↑RVSP with no sign of elevated LV filling pressure, Isolated right heart dilation, PA dilatation, RVOT Doppler midsystolic notch
8. High output heart failure	↑Doppler-derived cardiac output
9. Fabry disease	LVH, valvular dysfunction, preferential ↓ GLS in inferolateral segments

(GLS: global longitudinal strain; IVC: inferior vena cava; LV: left ventricle; LVH: left ventricular hypertrophy; LVOT: left ventricular outflow tract; PA: pulmonary arterial; RVOT: right ventricular outflow tract; RVSP: right ventricular systolic pressure; SAM: systolic anterior motion)

CP and other causes of diastolic HF is essential since the treatment is totally different. Findings that suggest CP include a normal or high e′ velocity (medial annulus velocity > lateral annulus velocity), which is unusual in other causes of restrictive fillings **(Figs. 7A and B)**.

ROLE OF ECHOCARDIOGRAPHY IN RISK STRATIFICATION

Finally, echocardiographic parameters provide prognostic information reflecting specific pathophysiologic abnormalities in HFpEF **(Box 1)**.

TRIGGERS FOR ACUTE DECOMPENSATION IN HEART FAILURE WITH PRESERVED EJECTION FRACTION SEEN IN EMERGENCY

Patients with HFpEF are indeed at risk for acute decompensation due to various cardiovascular and

BOX 1: Prognostic information in heart failure with preserved ejection fraction (HFpEF).

- Left ventricular (LV) hypertrophy (↑LV mass index)
- Impaired LV systolic performance (↓GLS)
- High filling pressure (↑E/e′, restrictive filling pattern)
- Left atrial (LA) dysfunction (↓LA reservoir strain)
- Pulmonary hypertension (↑RVSP)
- Right ventricular (RV) dysfunction (↓TAPSE, ↓FAC, ↓RVEF, ↓TAPSE/RVSP)

(FAC: fractional area change GLS: global longitudinal strain; RVSP: right ventricular systolic pressure; RVEF: right ventricular ejection fraction; TAPSE: tricuspid annular plane systolic excursion)

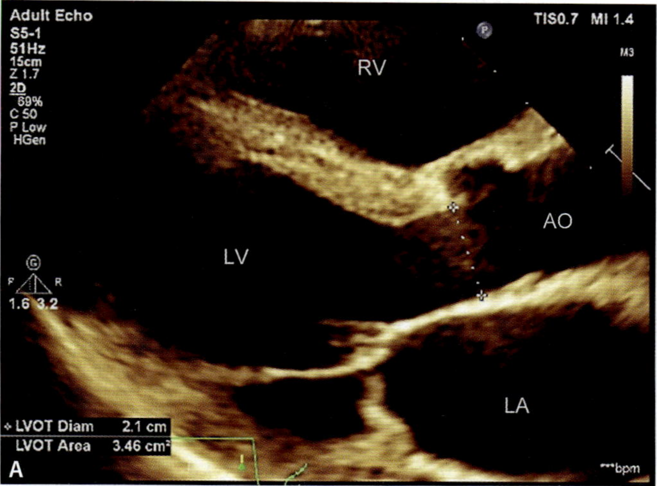

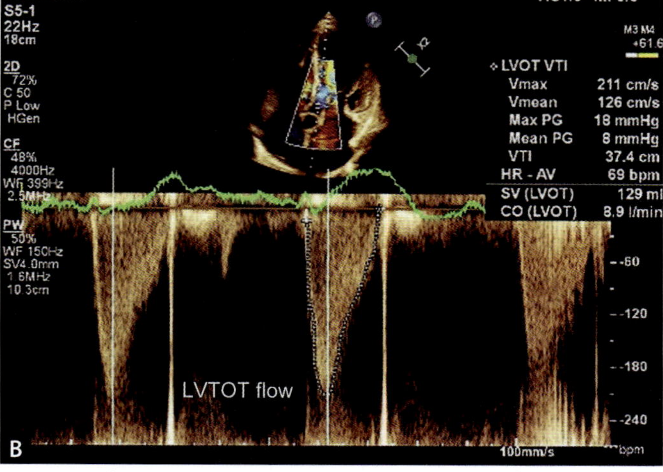

Figs. 7A and B: High output heart failure in a patient with liver cirrhosis. (A) Parasternal long axis view in end systole to calculate diameter of left ventricle outflow tract (LVOT), diameter is converted into area using the formula, LVOT = $\pi r^2 = D^2 \times 0.785$; (B) Pulse wave sample volume of LVOT in apical four chamber view; Stroke volume calculated was 129 mL and cardiac output was 8.9 L/min.

BOX 2: Common triggers for acute decompensation of heart failure with preserved ejection fraction (HFpEF).

- Poorly controlled or uncontrolled hypertension
- Acute kidney injury or worsening chronic kidney disease
- Anemia
- Chronic pulmonary disease or its exacerbation
- Dysrhythmia, particularly tachyarrhythmia, especially new-onset atrial fibrillation
- Infection
- Ischemia
- Increased salt intake or water retention
- Medication noncompliance, including antihypertensives or diuretics

noncardiovascular conditions. These conditions can lead to increased cardiac output demands that the failing heart cannot meet, resulting in acute pulmonary and systemic venous congestion[56] **(Box 2)**.

CONCLUSION

The HFpEF has become a very common condition, in tandem with the aging of the population and the increasing burden of metabolic comorbidities and is associated with high morbidity and mortality. Echocardiography is indispensable tool in the evaluation, management as well as prognostic stratification of HFpEF. It provides valuable insight into the pathophysiology and underlying phenotypes in HFpEF.

REFERENCES

1. Senni M, Tribouilloy CM, Rodeheffer RJ, et al. Congestive heart failure in the community: a study of all incident cases in Olmsted County, Minnesota, in 1991. Circulation. 1998;98:2282-9.
2. Owan TE, Hodge DO, Herges RM, et al. Trends in prevalence and outcome of heart failure with preserved ejection fraction. N Engl J Med. 2006;355:251-9.
3. Bhatia RS, Tu JV, Lee DS, et al. Outcome of heart failure with preserved ejection fraction in a population-based study. N Engl J Med. 2006;355:260-9.
4. Lam CS, Lyass A, Kraigher-Krainer E, et al. Hemodynamics, dyspnea, and pulmonary reserve in heart failure with preserved ejection fraction. Eur Heart J. 2018;39:2810-21.
5. GBD 2017 Disease and Injury Incidence and Prevalence Collaborators. Global, regional, and national incidence, prevalence, and years lived with disability for 354 diseases and injuries for 195 countries and territories, 1990–2017: a systematic analysis for the Global Burden of Disease Study 2017. Lancet. 2017;392:P1789-858.
6. Devereux RB, Roman MJ, Liu JE, et al. Congestive heart failure despite normal left ventricular systolic function in a population-based sample: the Strong Heart study. Am J Cardiol. 2000;86:1090-6.
7. Vasan RS, Xanthakis V, Lyass A, et al. Epidemiology of left ventricular systolic dysfunction and heart failure in the Framingham study: an echocardiographic study over 3 decades. JACC Cardiovasc Imaging. 2018;11:1-11.
8. Smith GL, Masoudi FA, Vaccarino V, et al. Outcomes in heart failure patients with preserved ejection fraction: mortality, readmission, and functional decline. J Am Coll Cardiol. 2003;41:1510-8.
9. Lam CS, Roger VL, Rodeheffer RJ, et al. Cardiac structure and ventricular-vascular function in persons with heart failure and preserved ejection fraction from Olmsted County, Minnesota. Circulation. 2007;115:1982-90.
10. Douglas PS, DeCara JM, Devereux RB, et al. American Society of Echocardiography Standards; American College of Cardiology Foundation. Echocardiographic imaging in clinical trials: American Society of Echocardiography Standards for echocardiography core laboratories: endorsed by the American College of Cardiology Foundation. J Am Soc Echocardiogr. 2009;22:755-65.
11. Borbély A, van der Velden J, Papp Z, et al. Cardiomyocyte stiffness in diastolic heart failure. Circulation. 2005;111:774-81.
12. Heidenreich PA, Bozkurt B, Aguilar D, et al. 2022 AHA/ACC/HFSA Guideline for the Management of Heart Failure: A Report of the American College of Cardiology/American Heart Association Joint Committee on Clinical Practice Guidelines. J Am Coll Cardiol. 2022;79(17):e263-e421.
13. Van Heerebeek L, Hamdani N, Falcão-Pires I, et al. Low myocardial protein kinase G activity in heart failure with preserved ejection fraction. Circulation. 2012;126:830-9.
14. Westermann D, Lindner D, Kasner M, et al. Cardiac inflammation contributes to changes in the extracellular matrix in patients with heart failure and normal ejection fraction. Circ Heart Fail. 2011;4:44-52.
15. Kasner M, Westermann D, Lopez B, et al. Diastolic tissue Doppler indexes correlate with the degree of collagen expression and cross linking in heart failure and normal ejection fraction. J Am Coll Car diol. 2011;57:977-85.
16. Zile MR, Gottdiener JS, Hetzel SJ, et al. Prevalence and significance of alterations in cardiac structure and function in patients with heart failure and a preserved ejection fraction. Circulation. 2011;124:2491-501.
17. Nagueh SF, Smiseth OA, Appleton CP, et al. Recommendations for the evaluation of left ventricular diastolic function by echocardiography: An update from the American society of echocardiography and the European association of cardiovascular imaging. J Am Soc Echocardiogr. 2016;29:277-314.
18. Obokata M, Olson TP, Reddy YN, et al. Hemodynamics, dyspnea, and pulmonary reserve in heart failure with preserved ejection fraction. Eur Heart J. 2018;39:2810-21.
19. Shah SJ, Borlaug BA, Kitzman DW, et al. Research priorities for heart failure with preserved ejection fraction. Circulation. 2020;141:1001-26.
20. Lang RM, Badano LP, Mor-Avi V, et al. Recommendations for cardiac chamber quantification by echocardiography

in adults: an update from the American Society of Echocardiography and the European Association of Cardiovascular Imaging. J Am Soc Echocardiogr. 2015; 16:233-71.
21. Abudiab MM, Redfield MM, Melenovsky V, et al. Cardiac output response to exercise in relation to metabolic demand in heart failure with preserved ejection fraction. Eur J Heart Fail. 2013;15:776-85.
22. Borlaug BA. The pathophysiology of heart failure with preserved ejection fraction. Nat Rev Cardiol. 2014;11:507-15.
23. Borlaug BA, Kane GC, Melenovsky V, et al. Abnormal right ventricular-pulmonary artery coupling with exercise in heart failure with preserved ejection fraction. Eur Heart J. 2016;37:3293-302.
24. Borlaug BA, Olson TP, Lam CS, et al. Global cardiovascular reserve dysfunction in heart failure with preserved ejection fraction. J Am Coll Cardiol. 2010;56:845-54.
25. Ponikowski P, Voors AA, Anker SD, et al. 2016 ESC guidelines for the diagnosis and treatment of acute and chronic heart failure: the TASK Force for the diagnosis and treatment of acute and chronic heart failure of the European society of cardiology (ESC). Developed with the special contribution of the heart failure association (HFA) of the ESC. Eur Heart J. 2016;37:2129-200.
26. Thomas L, Hoy M, Byth K, et al. The left atrial function index: a rhythm independent marker of atrial function. Eur J Echocardiogr. 2008;9:356-62.
27. Thomas L, Muraru D, Popescu BA, et al. Evaluation of left atrial size and function: relevance for clinical practice. J Am Soc Echocardiogr. 2020;33(8):934-52.
28. Cameli M, Lisi M, Focardi M, et al. Left atrial deformation analysis by speckle tracking echocardiography for prediction of cardiovascular outcomes. Am J Cardiol. 2012;110(2):264-9.
29. Badano LP, Kolias TJ, Muraru D, et al. Standardization of left atrial, right ventricular, and right atrial deformation imaging using two-dimensional speckle tracking echocardiography: a consensus document of the EACVI/ASE/Industry Task Force to standardize deformation imaging. Eur Heart J Cardiovasc Imaging. 2018;19(6):591-600.
30. Obokata M, Negishi K, Kurosawa K, et al. Incremental diagnostic value of la strain with leg lifts in heart failure with preserved ejection fraction. JACC Cardiovasc Imaging. 2013;6(7):749-58.
31. Reddy YNV, Carter RE, Obokata M, et al. A simple, evidence-based approach to help guide diagnosis of heart failure with preserved ejection fraction. Circulation. 2018; 138(9):861-70.
32. Pieske B, Tschöpe C, de Boer RA, et al. How to Diagnose Heart Failure with Preserved Ejection Fraction: The HFA-PEFF Diagnostic Algorithm: A Consensus Recommendation from the Heart Failure Association (HFA) of the European Society of Cardiology (ESC). Eur Heart J. 2019;40(40):3297-317.
33. Melenovsky V, Borlaug BA, Rosen B, et al. Cardiovascular features of heart failure with preserved ejection fraction versus nonfailing hypertensive left ventricular hypertrophy in the urban baltimore community: The role of atrial remodeling/dysfunction. J Am Coll Cardiol. 2007; 49(2):198-207
34. Santos AB, Kraigher-Krainer E, Gupta DK, et al. Impaired left atrial function in heart failure with preserved ejection fraction. Eur J Heart Fail. 2014;16(10):1096-103.
35. Patel RB, Lam CSP, Svedlund S, et al. Disproportionate left atrial myopathy in heart failure with preserved ejection fraction among participants of the PROMIS HFpEF study. Sci Rep. 2021;18(3):1-11.
36. Tamargo M, Obokata M, Reddy YNV, et al. Functional mitral regurgitation and left atrial myopathy in heart failure with preserved ejection fraction. Eur J Heart Fail. 2020;22(3):489-98.
37. Santos AB, Roca GQ, Claggett B, et al. Prognostic relevance of left atrial dysfunction in heart failure with preserved ejection fraction. Circ Heart Fail. 2016;9(4):e002763.
38. Freed BH, Daruwalla V, Cheng JY, et al. Prognostic utility and clinical significance of cardiac mechanics in heart failure with preserved ejection fraction: Importance of left atrial strain. Circ Cardiovasc Imag. 2016;9(3):10.1161.
39. Lam CS, Roger VL, Rodeheffer RJ, et al. Pulmonary hypertension in heart failure with preserved ejection fraction: A community-based study. J Am Coll Cardiol. 2009;53(13):1119-26.
40. Melenovsky V, Hwang SJ, Lin G, et al. Right heart dysfunction in heart failure with preserved ejection fraction. Eur Heart J. 2014;35(48):3452-62.
41. Mohammed SF, Hussain I, Abou Ezzeddine OF, et al. Right ventricular function in heart failure with preserved ejection fraction: A community-based study. Circulation. 2014;130(25):2310-20.
42. Gorter TM, Obokata M, Reddy YN, et al. Exercise unmasks distinct pathophysiologic features in heart failure with preserved ejection fraction and pulmonary vascular disease. Eur Heart J. 2018;39(30):2825-35.
43. Arkles JS, Opotowsky AR, Ojeda J, et al. Shape of the right ventricular Doppler envelope predicts hemodynamics and right heart function in pulmonary hypertension. Am J Respir Crit Care Med. 2011;183(2):268-76.
44. Takahama H, McCully RB, Frantz RP, et al. Unraveling the RV ejection Doppler envelope: Insight into pulmonary artery hemodynamics and disease severity. JACC Cardiovasc Imaging. 2017;10(10 Pt. B):1268-77.
45. Gorter TM, van Veldhuisen DJ, Voors AA, et al. Right ventricular-vascular coupling in heart failure with preserved ejection fraction and pre- vs. Post-capillary pulmonary hypertension. Eur Heart J Cardiovasc Imaging. 2018;19(4):425-32.
46. Guazzi M, Bandera F, Pelissero G, et al. Tricuspid annular plane systolic excursion and pulmonary arterial systolic pressure relationship in heart failure: An index of right ventricular contractile function and prognosis. Am J Physiol Heart Circ Physiol. 2013;305(9):H1373-81.

47. Rudski LG, Lai WW, Afilalo J, et al. Schiller NB. Guidelines for the echocardiographic assessment of the right heart in adults: A report from the American society of echocardiography endorsed by the European association of echocardiography, a registered branch of the European society of cardiology, and the Canadian society of echocardiography. J Am Soc Echocardiogr. 2010;23(7):685-713.
48. Obokata M, Reddy YNV, Melenovsky V, et al. Deterioration in right ventricular structure and function over time in patients with heart failure and preserved ejection fraction. Eur Heart J. 2019;40(8):689-98.
49. Ikoma T, Obokata M, Okada K, et al. Impact of right atrial remodeling in heart failure with preserved ejection fraction. J Card Fail. 2021;27(5):577-84.
50. Gorter TM, van Melle JP, Rienstra M, et al. Right heart dysfunction in heart failure with preserved ejection fraction: the impact of atrial fibrillation. J Card Fail. 2018;24(3):177-85.
51. Obokata M, Reddy YN, Pislaru SV, et al. Evidence supporting the existence of a distinct obese phenotype of heart failure with preserved ejection fraction. Circulation. 2017;136(1):6-19.
52. Tsujimoto T, Kajio H. Abdominal obesity is associated with an increased risk of all-cause mortality in patients with HFpEF. J Am Coll Cardiol. 2017;70(22):2739-49.
53. Obokata M, Reddy YNV, Melenovsky V, et al. Myocardial injury and cardiac reserve in patients with heart failure and preserved ejection fraction. J Am Coll Cardiol. 2018;72(1):29-40.
54. Phelan D, Collier P, Thavendiranathan P, et al. Relative apical sparing of longitudinal strain using two-dimensional speckle-tracking echocardiography is both sensitive and specific for the diagnosis of cardiac amyloidosis. Heart. 2012;98(19):1442-8.
55. Obokata M, Reddy YNV, Borlaug BA. The Role of Echocardiography in Heart Failure with Preserved Ejection Fraction: What Do We Want from Imaging? Heart Fail Clin. 2019;15(2):241-56.
56. Yancy CW, Lopatin M, Stevenson LW, et al. ADHERE Scientific Advisory Committee and Investigators. Clinical presentation, management, and in-hospital outcomes of patients admitted with acute decompensated heart failure with preserved systolic function: a report from the Acute Decompensated Heart Failure National Registry (ADHERE) Database. J Am Coll Cardiol. 2006;47(1):76-84.

CHAPTER

Echocardiographic Diagnostic, Prognostic, and Therapeutic Indications of E/e' and LAVI in HFpEF

Naveen Garg, KK Kapur

INTRODUCTION

Heart failure (HF) has been classified into two broad categories based on left ventricular ejection fraction (LVEF) viz.—heart failure with preserved ejection fraction (HFpEF; LVEF >50%) and heart failure with reduced ejection fraction (HFrEF; LVEF <40%). More than 50% of HF patients are considered to have preserved EF (HFpEF).

Heart failure with preserved ejection fraction is a clinical syndrome which is characterized by evidence of:

- Symptoms and signs of HF.
- An LVEF ≥50%.
- Objective evidence of cardiac structural and/or functional abnormalities consistent with the presence of LV diastolic dysfunction/raised LV end diastolic pressures (LVEDP).

Symptoms and signs of HFpEF are generally non-specific; impaired exercise tolerance is the usual complaint in patients with HFpEF. These patients are generally obese, elderly, and majority of them are females. They are also likely to have comorbidities such as hypertension, diabetes, atrial fibrillation (AF), COPD, anemia, sleep apnea, or renal disease.

The assessment of LV filling pressures (LVEDP) is performed noninvasively using the echocardiographic Doppler technique. This procedure is cost effective, accurate, and reproducible.[1-7]

PATHOPHYSIOLOGY OF HFPEF

The etiopathogenesis of HFpEF involves an abnormal diastolic relaxation process of the left ventricle (diastolic dysfunction DD). This syndrome is due to increased ventricular stiffness. This intern leads to increased stress on the left atrium leading to left atrial dilatation, elevated left atrial volumes (LAV) as well as left atrial pressures (LAP). Increased stress on LA fibers leads to elevated natriuretic peptides (BNP or NT-pro-BNP). Thus, the functional and structural changes in the left atrium results in elevated left atrial volume index (LAVi) as well as BNP/NT-pro-BNP.[8-14]

Assessment of LV filling pressures involves a combined use of transmitral blood flow velocities (E, A and E/A) as well as tissue Doppler velocities (e' a'). The ratio of E/e' is positively correlated with severity of diastolic dysfunction and is almost proportional to the degree of elevation of LV filling pressures **(Fig. 1)**.[15-17]

In comparison with HFrEF (LVEF <40%), HFpEF has complex etiopathogenesis, as well as controversial management plan; given the limited number of drug trials. However, certain indices for the definitive diagnosis of this condition have now been established. The diagnostic echocardiographic criteria in patients with reduced exercise tolerance with or without signs of HF are as follows:

- Elevated LAVi >34 mL/m^2.
- Elevated transmitral E/A ratios >2.
- Septal e' <7 cm/s and lateral e' <10 cm/s.
- Elevated E/e' >15 (combination of transmitral and tissue Doppler and annular peak velocities).
- Elevated PA systolic pressure (TR jet peak velocity >2.8 m/s).

If three or more of above criteria are present, the diagnosis of elevated LV filling pressures is established. Additional use of natriuretic biomarkers (BNP >80 pg/mL

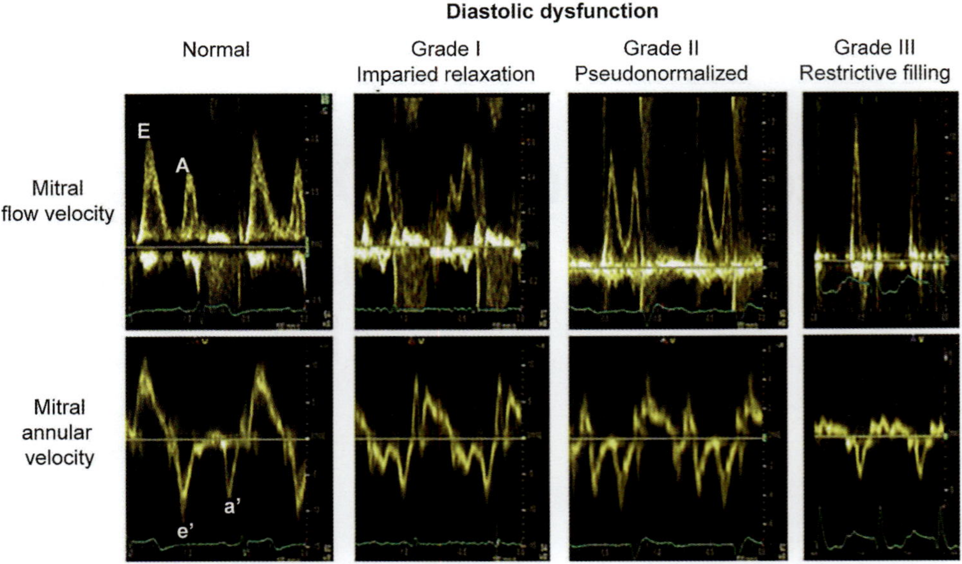

Fig. 1: Transmitral inflow Doppler as well as mitral annular tissue Doppler in different grades of diastolic dysfunction.

Flowchart 1: Algorithm for stress analysis.

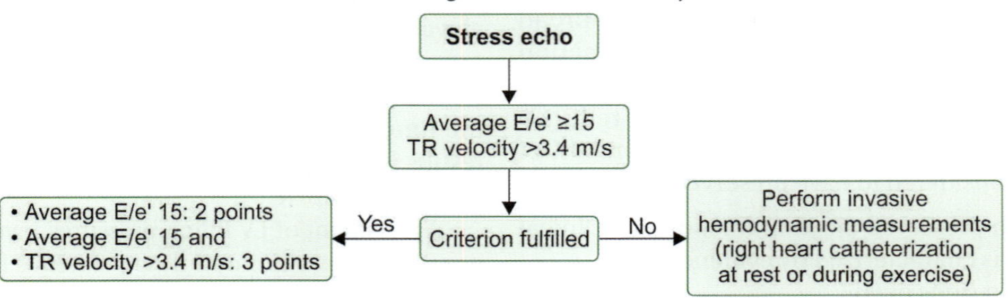

(TR: tricuspid regurgitation)

or NT-pro-BNP >220 pg/mL) as well as use of global left ventricular strain (GLS <16) as well as relatively more recent addition of LA strain parameters, adds to the diagnostic assessment.[18-24]

These indices show greater inter as well as intra-observer reproducibility in patients with sinus rhythm, but accuracy and reproducibility is inversely affected in patients with nonsinus rhythms (especially AF, ventricular ectopics, SVT, or VT). In patients with AF the LAVi criteria has increased from 34 to 40 mL/m^2 so have the natriuretic biomarkers (BNP 80–240 pg/mL and NT-pro-BNP 220–660 pg/mL) (**Flowchart 1; Tables 1 and 2**).

The well-established formula for estimating LV filling pressures from E/e′ ratios is the one given Stephen Nagueh as under:

$$\text{Nagueh formula - LVEDP/PCWP} = (1.24 \times E/e') + 1.9$$

Left atrial volume is calculated by multiplying the atrial area in two-chamber and four-chamber views (using the biplane area-length method) by 0.85 and then dividing it by the shortest length of the atrium.

$$\text{Biplane A/L method: Uses the formula (LAV)} = 0.85\,(A1 \times A2)/L$$

It is recommended to index LAV with body surface area (BSA) for standard calculations.

$$\text{LAVi} = \text{LAV/BSA}\ (\text{BSA} = \sqrt{(\text{weight} \times \text{height}/3{,}600)})$$

DIAGNOSTIC, PROGNOSTIC, AND THERAPEUTIC IMPLICATIONS

The sensitivity and specificity of an *E*/*e*′ ratio >9 were found to be 78% and 59%, respectively; while it is 46% and 86% for *E*/*e*′ >13. Both the sensitivity and specificity of LA volume index >30 mL/m^2 were about 70%. Measurements of LV mass had low sensitivity (26%) for HFpEF but high specificity (86%) if LVH was present. Tricuspid regurgitation (TR)

TABLE 1: Major and minor criteria for diagnosing HFpEF by echocardiography. Points >5 are diagnostic whereas patients with <5 points are subjected to stress test for analysis as shown in **Flowchart 1**.

	Functional	*Morphological*	*Biomarker (SR)*	*Biomarker (AF)*
Major	septal e' <7 cm/s or lateral e' <10 cm/s or Average E/e* ≥15 or TR velocity >2.8 m/s (PASP >35 mm Hg)	LAVI >34 mL/m^2 or LVMI ≥ 149/122 g/m^2 (m/w) and RWT >0.42	NT-pro-BNP >220 pg/mL or BNP >80 pg/mL	NT-pro-BNP >660 pg/mL or BNP >240 pg/mL
Minor	Average E/e' 9–14 or GLS <16%	LAVI 29–34 mL/m^2 or LVMI >115/95 g/m^2 (m/w) or RWT >0.42 or LV wall thickness ≥12 mm	NT-pro-BNP 125–220 pg/mL or BNP 35–80 pg/mL	NT-pro-BNP 365, 660 pg/mL or BNP 105–240 pg/mL
Major criteria: 2 points 5 points: HFpEF				
Minor criteria: 1 point 2–4 points: Diastolic stress test or invasive hemodynamic measurements.				

(GLS: global longitudinal strain; HFpEF: heart failure with preserved ejection fraction; LAVI: left ventricular mass index; LV: left ventricular; LVMI: left ventricular mass index; NT-pro-BNP: N-terminal pro b-type natriuretic peptide; PASP: pulmonary artery systolic pressure; RWT: relative wall thickness; TR: tricuspid regurgitation)

TABLE 2

Indices	*Criteria*	*SR*	*AF*
LAVI	Major	>34 mL/m^2	>40 mL/m^2
	Minor	29–34 mL/m^2	34–40 mL/m^2
NT-pro-BNP	Major	>220 pg/mL	>660 pg/mL
	Minor	125–220 pg/mL	375–660 pg/mL
BNP	Major	>80 pg/mL	>240 pg/mL
	Minor	35–80 pg/mL	105–240 pg/mL

(LAVI: left atrial volume index; NT-pro-BNP: N-terminal pro b-type natriuretic peptide)

velocity derived PASP >35 mm Hg has sensitivity and specificity of 46% and 86%, respectively for HFpEF, which also makes it an important diagnostic criterion. The utility of GLS <16% was moderate (sensitivity 62% and specificity 56%) and is considered as minor criterion.[11,25-30]

For NT-pro-BNP the sensitivity and specificity is 59% and 77% at values of >275 pg/mL; while sensitivity decreases to 46% and specificity increased to 85% if the cutoff proposes to >450 pg/mL. At recommended cutoff of 125 pg/mL (minor criterion, if the patient is in sinus rhythm), the sensitivity reported is 77% and specificity is 53%. There is a great limitation of NT-pro-BNP while diagnosing HFpEF; near about in 20% of invasively proven HFpEF patients has NT-pro-BNP in normal range, particularly in obese patients. Combining the results of echocardiography indices (E/e') and NT-pro-BNP can increase the predictive value of HFpEF.[14,30-38]

The LA mass as well as LA size was independently associated with high risk of mortality in I-PRESERVED substudy among LVEF >50%. In TOPCAT study, E/e′ and TR peak velocities were predictive of outcomes.

A proposed algorithm consisting LAVI ≥34 mL/m^2 and septal (or lateral) E/e′ >8 could determine diastolic dysfunction with a 95.6% sensitivity and 54.5% specificity. Septal E/e′ (≥15) and LAVI (≥34 mL/m^2) were the better predictors of the increased LVEDP than the other echocardiographic parameters. There were statistically significant moderate positive correlations of LVEDP with septal E/e′ and LAVI. Similar results were observed in CEAL-HFpEF study; where lateral E/e′ >12 and LAVI 34 mL/m^2, have the greatest diagnostic value for diagnosing diastolic dysfunction in HFpEF patients and have good correlation with invasively measured LVEDP.

Blanco et al. found that >50% reduction in admission E/e′ was correlated with better outcomes. Therefore, patients with worse prognosis have a constantly higher E/e′ ratio. Also, the KaRen study found that E/e′ ratio has been an important prognostic marker, and in the mean follow-up of 28 months of this cohort, E/e′ ratio was the only echocardiographic predictor associated with adverse outcome. E/e′ ratio >13 had worse prognosis compared with ≤13 **(Table 3)**.[39-43]

There are no standard treatment guidelines for HFpEF, due to its multifaceted etiopathology. However, preload reduction (pressure reduction in LA) remains the mainstay of treatment strategies. Achieving a ratio of E/A <1 or E/e′ <15 is considered as a good therapeutic as well as prognostic success. Diuresis is thus remains the foremost treatment pathway for HFpEF. Since HFpEF is more prevalent in patients with obesity; the antidiabetic drug SGPL2i and GLP-1 appears as promising agents as they help in weight reduction as well as have diuretic effect too. Other drugs such as angiotensin-receptor neprilysin inhibitor (ARNI), ARBs, and β-blockers are used in HFpEF with reasonably good efficacy in patients with comorbidities such as AF, diabetes, hypertension, etc., **(Flowchart 2)**.

In the TOPCAT trial (Patients and Outcomes in the Treatment of Preserved Cardiac Function Heart Failure with an Aldosterone Antagonist), which studied patients, who were metabolic obese and had high prevalence of CKD; had showed better responsiveness (BNP and hospitalization) to spironolactone. Since obesity tends to increase the levels of aldosterone [renin angiotensin aldosterone system (RAAS)]. TOPCAT trial echocardiographic substudy showed that spironolactone (MRAs) reduced the E/A ratio, which was associated with reduced cardiovascular death and HF hospitalizations.

EMPEROR-Preserved and DELIVER and DECLARE-TIMI trials had shown diabetes patients without AF may benefit from the use of SGLT2i because they have a preventive effect on this arrhythmia. Based on these studies the 2022 American College of Cardiology (ACC)/

TABLE 3: Diagnostic and prognostic value of E/e′ in different studies.

Study	*LVEF criteria*	*E/e′*
TOPCAT	>45%	Prognostic
CEAL-HFpEF	>50%	Diagnostic
R Blanco et al.	>50%	Prognostic
KaRen	>45%	Prognostic

(LVEF: left ventricular ejection fraction; HFpEF: heart failure with preserved ejection fraction)

Flowchart 2: Etiopatholgy and therapeutic intervention in heart failure with preserved ejection fraction (HFpEF).[44]

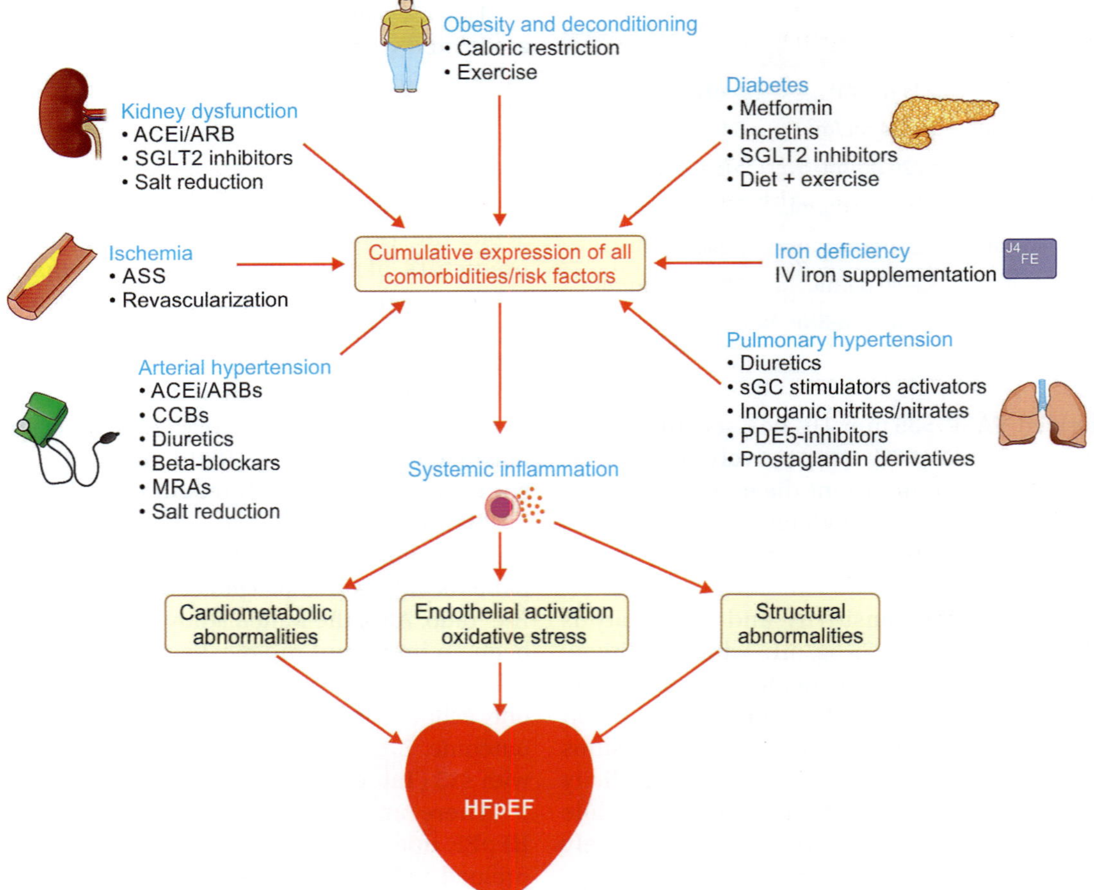

(ARB: angiotensin receptor blockers; ARNi: angiotensin-receptor neprilysin inhibitor LVEF: left ventricular ejection fraction; HF: heart failure; HFpEF: heart failure with preserved ejection fraction; MRA: Mineralocorticoid receptor antagonists; SGLT2i: Sodium-glucose cotransporter 2 inhibitors)

American Heart Association (AHA) recommend SGPL2i to treat patients with HF and LVEF >50%. (Class of Recommendation IIa). Meta-analysis of 12,251 patients of HFpEF in the EMPEROR-Preserved and DELIVER trials suggested that treatment with SGLT2 inhibitors reduced both cardiovascular death [HR: 0.88/(95% CI: 0.77–1.00)] and hospitalization for HF [HR: 0.74 (95% CI: 0.67–0.83)] with consistent effects across all examined subgroups. Patients with type-1 diabetes, end-stage CKD on dialysis, or eGFR <20 mL/min/1.73 m^2 are not candidates for SGLT2 inhibitors.

As yet, the use of GLP-1 agonists are not recommended in HFpEF. The recent trials STEP-HFpEF and STEP-HFpEF DM had concluded that semaglutide treatment result in improved exercise function and increased weight loss compared with placebo.

The clinical trials on role of RAAS inhibitors (ACEi/ARBs) in HFpEF had shown that though these agents show improvements in NYHA functional class and 6-minute walk distance compared with placebo; but fail to reduce all-cause death or HF hospitalization (PEP-CHF trial). The possible significant results of ARBs in HFpEF shown in CHARM trial were not validated in I-PRESERVE trial.

The PARAGON-HF trial suggests that use of ARNI may be a superior approach to ARB monotherapy for selected patients with HFpEF. This study depicted the significant benefit of ARNI in hospitalizations and cardiovascular death in HF patients with LVEF >45%. Although no improvement on submaximal exercise capacity was observed in similar PARALLAX Trail. Though the precise cutoff LVEF not clear for the use of ARNI in HF but results of many studies appeared to have extended benefits to many patients with LVEF >50%, especially the women population. However, in 2024 it was finally concluded that ARNI has no role in reducing the adverse events among patients with HFpEF **(Table 4)**.

The current guidelines suggest diuretics as class-1 (strongly beneficial) and SGLT2i are class-2a (moderately beneficial); whereas ARNI, MRA, and ARBs are considered weakly beneficial in patients with *LVEF near to 50%*. This statement was given due to varying LVEF (>40%, >45%, or >50%) in different study groups while defining HFpEF **(Fig. 2)**.[44-54]

TABLE 4: Depicting various drug trials using different criteria for LVEF in HFpEF patients.

Study	LVEF	Drug	Conclusion
TOPCAT	>45%	Spirolactone	Not superior to placebo
EMPEROR-P	>40%	Empagliflozin	May be indicated
DELIVER	>40%	Dapagliflozin	May be indicated
DECLARE-TIMI	>40%	Dapagliflozin	May be indicated
STEP-HFpEF-DM	>45%	Semaglutide	More studies needed
PEP-CHF	40–50%	Perindopril	Not superior to placebo
I-PRESERVE	>45%	Irbesartan	Not superior to placebo
PARAGON-HF	>45%	ARNI	Failed to reduced adverse effects
PARALLAX	>40%	ARNI	Not superior to placebo

(ARNI: angiotensin-receptor neprilysin inhibitor; LVEF: left ventricular ejection fraction; HFpEF: heart failure with preserved ejection fraction)

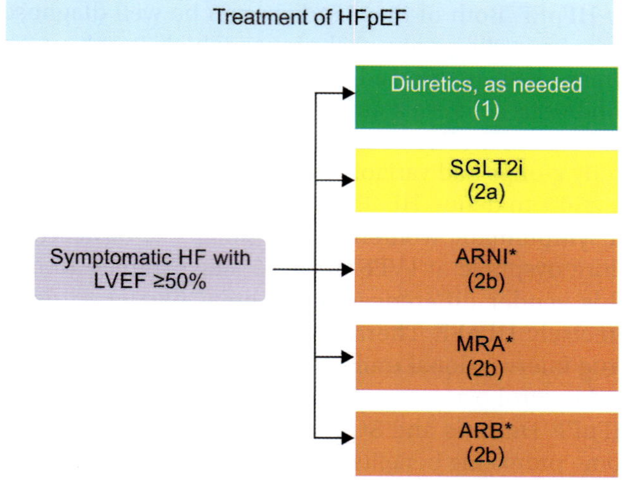

Fig. 2: 2022 AHA/ACC/HFSA Guideline for the Management of Heart Failure: A Report of the American College of Cardiology/American Heart Association Joint Committee on Clinical Practice Guidelines. (ARB: angiotensin receptor blockers; ARNi: angiotensin-receptor neprilysin inhibitor LVEF: left ventricular ejection fraction; HF: heart failure; HFpEF: heart failure with preserved ejection fraction; MRA: Mineralocorticoid receptor antagonists; SGLT2i: Sodium-glucose cotransporter 2 inhibitors)
*Greater benefit in patients with LVEF closer to 50%.

NOVEL INDICATORS IN DIAGNOSIS OF HEART FAILURE WITH PRESERVED EJECTION FRACTION

Many novel echocardiographic diagnostic indicators has been proposed for the diagnosis of HFpEF. Since increased LVEDP or LV filling pressures affect the physiology of LA and there is notable remodeling of LA during diastolic failure of LV. This conclusions had proposed that LA strain may be a good diagnostic as well as prognostic indicator of HFpEF.

Another similar physiological indicator in pipeline is (E + LAVi)/2. This marker had demonstrated the highest discriminatory power, with a threshold of 40.1, yielding high sensitivity (97%), and relatively low specificity (30%) in predicting LVEDP >20 (ECHO-PREDICT study).[56]

Other upcoming novel diagnostic approaches include; 3D evaluations of chambers; detecting HFpEF with artificial intelligence (AI incorporation with echocardiography).

CONCLUSION

Heart failure with preserved ejection fraction is the most common subtype of HF. Many diagnostic tools has been designed to evaluate its severity but none has shown its sturdiness. E/e′ though is found to be a good diagnostic as well as prognostic indicator; but it also has several limitations. Since, *sine qua non* of HFpEF is increased preloading conditions in the presence of normal afterloads. This happens because of diastolic or relaxation pathology. This diastolic failure leads to remodeling of LA which can be appreciated by increased LA volumes or disturbed LA strain patterns. Many studies has concluded that LA volume index along with E/e′; both carry high degree of accuracy in diagnosing HFpEF. These both indices show functional and structural aspect of changes lead by HFpEF. Both of these indices can be well diagnosed by echocardiography techniques which is robust and cheap. E/e′ is affected by the changes in preloading conditions so it is a sound marker of therapeutic success and also an indictors of prognosis of disease. Different study groups had variably classified LVEF as >40%, >45%, or ≥50% to define HFpEF. It is also true that particularly in symptomatic women due to small size of heart; are more dyspneic at LVEF of 50–55% as compare to men. This gender differences poses great barrier to define precisely HFpEF. Therapeutically, there are not many drug interventional trails. Reduction in weight, exercise, and control over comorbidities are known remedies for HFpEF. Diuresis and SGLT2i are only medications with some promising benefits. The limitations of all the above trials is that E/e′ and LAVi were utilized only in minority of studies for diagnosis, therapeutics, and prognosis.

REFERENCES

1. Upadhya B, Kitzman DW. Heart failure with preserved ejection fraction: New approaches to diagnosis and management. Clin Cardiol. 2020;43(2):145-55.
2. Redfield MM, Borlaug BA. Heart failure with preserved ejection fraction: A review. JAMA. 2023;329(10): 827-38.
3. Garg N. Diagnostic Prognostic and Therapeutic Implications of E/e′ in Heart Failure. In: Chopra HK, Nanda NC, Narula J, (Eds). Advances and Innovations in Heart Failure (AIHF): A Textbook of Cardiology; 2023.
4. Harper AR, Patel HC, Lyon AR. Heart failure with preserved ejection fraction. Clin Med (Lond). 2018;18(Suppl 2): s24-s29.
5. Dunlay SM, Roger VL, Redfield MM. Epidemiology of heart failure with preserved ejection fraction. Nat Rev Cardiol. 2017;14(10):591-602.
6. Borlaug BA, Sharma K, Shah SJ, et al. Heart failure with preserved ejection fraction: JACC Scientific Statement. Am Coll Cardiol. 2023;81(18):1810-34.
7. Paulus WJ, Tscope C. A Novel paradigm for heart failure with preserved ejection fraction. J Am Coll Cardiol. 2013;62(4):263-71.
8. Teramoto K, Tay WT, Tromp J, et al. Longitudinal NT-proBNP: Associations with echocardiographic changes and outcomes in heart failure. 2024;13(9):032254.
9. Robinson S, Ring L, Oxborough D, et al. The assessment of left ventricular diastolic function: guidance and recommendations from the British Society of Echocardiography. Echo Res Pract. 2024;11(1):16.
10. van de Bovenkamp AA, Enait V, de Man FS, et al.; Validation of the 2016 ASE/EACVI Guideline for Diastolic Dysfunction in Patients With Unexplained Dyspnea and a Preserved Left Ventricular Ejection Fraction. J Am Heart Assoc. 2021;10(18):e021165
11. Sharifov OF, Schiros CG, Aban I, et al. Diagnostic Accuracy of Tissue Doppler Index E/e for Evaluating Left Ventricular Filling Pressure and Diastolic Dysfunction/ Heart Failure With Preserved Ejection Fraction: A Systematic Review and Meta Analysis. J Am Heart Assoc. 2016;5(1):e002530.
12. Tangen J, Nguyen TN, Melichova D, et al. Left atrial volume assessed by echocardiography identifies patients with high risk of adverse outcome after acute myocardial infarction. Echo Res Pract. 2024;11(1):24.
13. Oh JK, Miranda WR, Kane GC. Diagnosis of Heart Failure With Preserved Ejection Fraction Relies on Detection of Increased Diastolic Filling Pressure, But How. J Am Heart Assoc. 2023;12(6):e028867.
14. Chrysohoou C, Konstantinou K, Tsioufis K. The Role of NT-proBNP Levels in the Diagnosis and Treatment of Heart Failure with Preserved Ejection Fraction—It Is Not Always a Hide-and-Seek Game. J Cardiovasc Dev Dis. 2024;11(7):225.
15. Geske JB, Sorajja P, Nishimura RA, et al. Evaluation of left ventricular filling pressures by Doppler echocardiography in patients with hypertrophic cardiomyopathy. Circulation. 2007;116(23):2702-8.
16. Pieske B, Tschope C, Boer R, et al. How to diagnose heart failure with preserved ejection fraction: the HFA–PEFF diagnostic algorithm: a consensus recommendation from the Heart Failure Association (HFA) of the European Society of Cardiology (ESC). Eur Heart J. 2019;40(40):3297-317.
17. Mitter SS, Shah SJ, Thomas JD. A Test in Context E/A and E/e′ to Assess Diastolic Dysfunction and LV Filling Pressure. J Am Coll Cardiol. 2017;69(11):1451-64.
18. Morris DA, Belyavskiy E, Aravind-Kumar R, et al. Potential usefulness and clinical relevance of adding left atrial

strain to left atrial volume index in the detection of left ventricular diastolic dysfunction. J Am Coll Cardiol Cardiovasc Img. 2018;11(10):1405-15.
19. Fernandes SL, Carvalho RR, Santos LG, et al. Pathophysiology and treatment of heart failure with preserved ejection fraction: state of the art and prospects for the future. Arq Bras Cardiol. 2020;114(1):120-9.
20. Berry NC, Manyoo A, Oldham WM, et al. Protocol for exercise hemodynamic assessment: performing an invasive cardiopulmonary exercise test in clinical practice. Pulm Circ. 2015;5(4):610-8.
21. Nagueh SF, Smiseth OA, Appleton CP, et al. Recommendations for the Evaluation of Left Ventricular Diastolic Function by Echocardiography: An Update from the American Society of Echocardiography and the European Association of Cardiovascular Imaging. J Am Soc Echocardiogr. 2016;29(4):277-314.
22. Sharma AK, Kumar H, Razi MM, et al. To determine the correlation between echocardiographic diastolic parameters and invasively measured left ventricular end diastolic pressure in patients with heart failure with preserved ejection fraction- an observational, descriptive study. (CEAL-HFpEF study). Indian Heart J. 2021;73(4):470e475.
23. Jong-Won Ha, Andersen OS, Smiseth OA. Diastolic Stress Test Invasive and Noninvasive Testing. J Am Coll Cardiol Cardiovasc Img. 2020;13:272-82.
24. Fauchier L, Bisson A, Bodin A. Heart failure with preserved ejection fraction and atrial fibrillation: recent advances and open questions. BMC Med. 2023;21(1): 54.
25. Ozer N, Okutucu S, Kepez A, et al. Diagnostic accuracy and clinical utility of echocardiographic indices for detecting left ventricular diastolic dysfunction in patients with coronary artery disease and normal ejection fraction. Anadolu Kardiyol Derg. 2011;11(8):666-73.
26. Obokata M, Borlaug BA. The strengths and limitations of E/e′ in heart failure with preserved ejection fraction. Eur J Heart Fail. 2018;20(9):1312-4.
27. Zamfirescu MB, Ghilencea LN, Popescu MR, et al. The E/e′ ratio—role in risk stratification of acute heart failure with preserved ejection fraction. Medicina (Kaunas). 2021;57(4):375.
28. Harada T, Obokata M, Kagami K, et al. Utility of E/e′ ratio during low-level exercise to diagnose heart failure with preserved ejection Fraction. JACC Cardiovasc Imaging. 2023;16(2):145-55.
29. Ibrahim IM, Hafez H, Al-Shair MHA, et al. Echocardiographic parameters differentiating heart failure with preserved ejection fraction from asymptomatic left ventricular diastolic dysfunction. Echocardiography. 2020; 37(2):247-52.
30. Obokata M, Reddy YNV, Borlaug BA, et al. Diastolic dysfunction and heart failure with preserved ejection fraction: understanding mechanisms by using noninvasive methods. JACC Cardiovasc Imaging. 2020;13(1 Pt 2): 245-57.
31. Chen S, Zhou Y, Wu X, et al. The value of echocardiography combined with NT-pro BNP level in assessment and prognosis of diastolic heart failure. Comput Math Methods Med. 2022;2022:2102496.
32. Verbrugge FH, Omote K, Reddy YNV, et al. Heart failure with preserved ejection fraction In patients with normal natriuretic peptide Levels is associated with increased morbidity and mortality. Eur Heart J. 2022;43(20):1941-51.
33. Salah K, Stienen S, Pinto YM, et al. Prognosis and NT-proBNP in heart failure patients with preserved versus reduced ejection fraction. Heart. 2019;105(15):1182-9.
34. Sakamoto D, Sotomi Y, Mutsuoka Y, et al. Prognostic Utility and Cutoff Differences in NT-proBNP Levels Across Subgroups in Heart Failure With Preserved Ejection Fraction: Insights From the PURSUIT-HFpEF Registry. J Card Fail. 2024:S1071-9164(24)00925.
35. Birrell H, Isles C, Fersia O, et al. Assessment of the diagnostic value of NT-proBNP in heart failure with preserved ejection fraction. Br J Cardiol. 2024;31(1):17-22.
36. Eriksson B, Wändell P, Dahlström U, et al. Limited value of NT-proBNP as a prognostic marker of all-cause mortality in patients with heart failure with preserved and mid-range ejection fraction in primary care: A report from the swedish heart failure register. Scand J Prim Health Care. 2019;37(4):434-43.
37. Kristensen SL, Mogensen UM, Jhund PS, et al. N-Terminal Pro-B-Type Natriuretic Peptide Levels for Risk Prediction in Patients With Heart Failure and Preserved Ejection Fraction According to Atrial Fibrillation Status. Circ Heart Fail. 2019;12(3):e005766.
38. Tanaka A, Node K. So-far overlooked HFpEF patients with normal natriuretic peptide level need more evidence. ESC Heart Fail. 2022;9(5):3659-60.
39. Kumbhani D. Treatment of preserved cardiac function heart failure with an aldosterone antagonist - TOPCAT. JACC Heart Fail. 2021;9:803-6.
40. Blanco R, Ambrosio G, Belziti C, et al. Prognostic value of NT-proBNP, and echocardiographic indices of diastolic function, in hospitalized patients with acute heart failure and preserved left ventricular ejection fraction. Int J Cardiol. 2020;317:111-20.
41. Shahim A, Hourqueig M, Donal E, et al. Predictors of long-term outcome in heart failure with preserved ejection fraction: a follow-up from the KaRen study. ESC Heart Fail. 2021;8(5):4243-54.
42. Gehlken C, Screever EM, Suthahar N, et al. Left atrial volume and left ventricular mass indices in heart failure with preserved and reduced ejection fraction. ESC Heart Fail. 2021;8(4):2458-66.
43. McDonagh TA, Metra M, Adamo M, et al. 2023 Focused Update of the 2021 ESC Guidelines for the diagnosis and treatment of acute and chronic heart failure. Eur Heart J. 2023;44(37):3627-39.
44. Wintrich J, Kindermann I, Ukena C, et al. Therapeutic approaches in heart failure with preserved ejection fraction: past, present, and future. Clin Res Cardiol. 2020; 109(9):1079-98.

45. Balestrieri G, Limonta R, Ponti E, et al. The therapy and management of heart failure with preserved ejection fraction: new insights on treatment. Card Fail Rev. 2024;10:e05.
46. Shear FE. Novel paradigms in the therapeutic management of heart failure with preserved ejection fraction: clinical perspectives. Am J Cardiovasc Dis. 2019;9(5):91-108.
47. Kommu S, Berg RL. The efficacy and safety of sacubitril/valsartan compared to valsartan in patients with heart failure and mildly reduced and preserved ejection fractions: a systematic review and meta-analysis of randomized controlled trials. J Clin Med. 2024;13(6):1572.
48. Meyer M, LeWinter MM, Zile MR. A targeted treatment opportunity for HFpEF taking advantage of diastolic tone. Circulation. 2021;144(16):1269-71.
49. Desai AS, Lam CSP, McMurray JJV, et al. How to manage heart failure with preserved ejection fraction practical guidance for clinicians. JACC Heart Fail. 2023;11(6):619-36.
50. Zhao Z, Jiang C, He L, et al. Impact of sodium-glucose cotransporter 2 inhibitor on E/e′ in patients with heart failure. Advances and Revolutions in Heart Failure (ARHF): A Textbook of Cardiology. J Am Heart Assoc. 2023;12(24):e031269.
51. Garg N. Effect of E/e′ in Heart Failure Patients on Angiotensin Receptor-Neprilysin Inhibitor Therapy. In: Chopra HK, Nanda NC, Narula J, (Eds). Advances & Revolutions in Heart Failure (ARHF): A Textbook of Cardiology; 2023.
52. Heidenreich P, Bozkurt B, Aguilar D, et al. 2022 AHA/ACC/HFSA Guideline for the Management of Heart Failure: A Report of the American College of Cardiology/American Heart Association Joint Committee on Clinical Practice Guidelines. Circulation. 2022;145(18).
53. Cunningham J. Prospective Comparison of ARNI With ARB Global Outcomes in HF With Preserved Ejection Fraction - PARAGON-HF. Am Coll Cardiol. 2024.
54. Suleman M, Saqib M, Mumtaz H, et al. Novel echocardiographic markers for left ventricular filling pressure prediction in heart failure with preserved ejection fraction (ECHO-PREDICT): a prospective cross-sectional study. Ann Med Surg (Lond). 2023;85(11):5384-95.

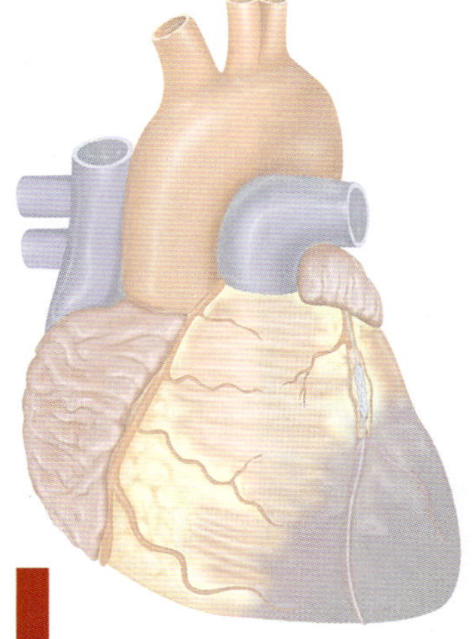

Effect of E/e′ in HFpEF Management on SGL2i, ARNI, and Beta-blocker Therapy

Simmi Manocha, Naveen Garg, Naveen Sharma

INTRODUCTION

Heart failure (HF) is a global epidemic affecting at least 26 million people worldwide. It is expected that its prevalence will increase by more than 45% by 2030.[1,2] As the prognosis of HF remains poor, early intervention and treatment of causative factors are the only tools to control its progression. The most important causes of HF include lifestyle diseases such as hypertension, diabetes, or obesity, whereas other causes include coronary artery disease, rheumatic heart diseases, arrhythmias, etc.

PATHOPHYSIOLOGY

Heart failure is a complex clinical syndrome with symptoms and signs that result from any structural or functional impairment of ventricular filling or ejection of blood.

Heart failure was considered to be equivalent to a "pump failure", where the pumping capacity or the ejection fraction of the left ventricle is reduced to meet the demands of the resting body. However, with advancement of medical science, it had been observed that relaxation of the left ventricle (diastole) is also an active process similar to muscular contraction in systole. The diastole (especially the isovolumic relaxation phase) is an ATP intake process. The dysfunction during diastole thus leads to abnormal ventricle filling (also known as left ventricular filling pressures), atrial congestion, and later pulmonary congestion. Thus, during the process of left ventricular diastolic dysfunction (LVDD), the ejection fraction of left ventricle (LVEF) remains normal or preserved.[3-6]

The functional capacity of the left ventricle, i.e., ejection fraction (LVEF), is assessed noninvasively with echocardiography. HF is now being classified into subtypes on the basis of ejection fractions as HFrEF (heart failure with reduced ejection fraction) when LVEF <40% and HFpEF (heart failure with preserved ejection fraction) when LVEF >50%. The gray area of LVEF between 40% and 49% is labeled as HFmrEF (heart failure with mildly reduced EF).

HFpEF is an entity of HF where a symptomatic patient presents with normal LVEF. However, it must also be noted that an asymptomatic patient can also depict the signs of HFpEF, especially when they undergo stress testing (pre-HF stage).[7-10]

ECHOCARDIOGRAPHY

Normally, in a cardiac cycle, during the early phase of ventricle filling, most of blood enters the ventricle and atrial kick contributes later to filling phase. This whole process can be evaluated via pulse Doppler study at the mitral level. Normally, the early filling wave (E-wave of Doppler study) is slightly bigger than the late filling wave (A-wave). However, during LVDD, due to restrictive filling in the later phase, A-wave is increased in altitude depicting more force being exerted by left atria to fill in the left ventricle. This reflects increased left ventricular end diastolic pressures (LVEDP). As this dysfunction progresses, the atrial pressures also rise which in turn lead to increased pulmonary venous congestion and later increased pulmonary capillary wedge pressure (PCWP) and hence pulmonary artery hypertension (PAH). Thus, noninvasive measurement of LVEDP becomes the biomarker for the invasively measured PCWP. The ratio of E/A waves reflects LVEDP. With the advent of tissue Doppler technique, the *e′*

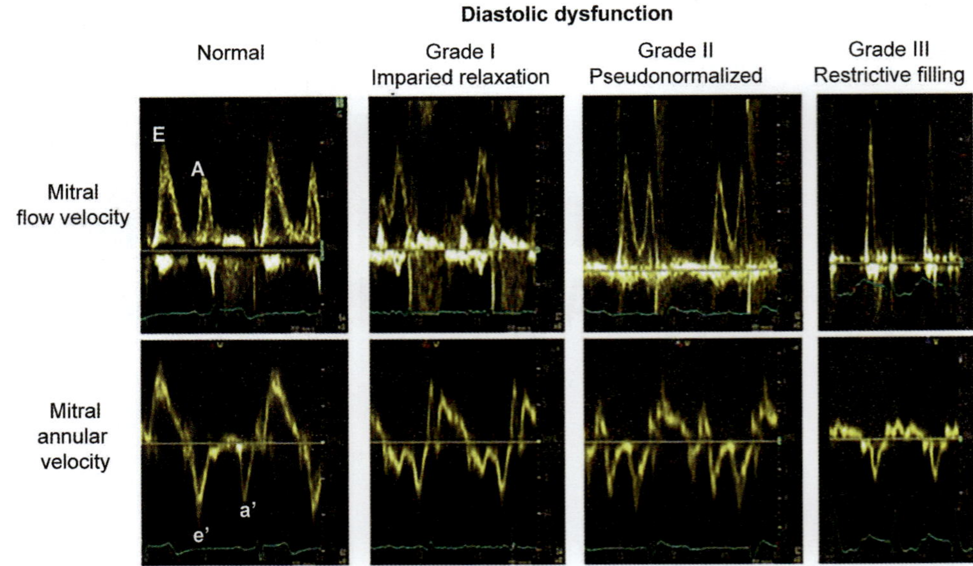

Fig. 1: Mitral inflow Doppler as well as mitral annular tissue Doppler in different grades of diastolic dysfunction.

velocity is measured as the mean of lateral or septal edge tissue *e'* waves of mitral orifice.[7,11-18] The ratio of *E/e'* is considered as the most accurate correlation with LVEDP (or PCWP) and hence forms the basis for diagnosing LVDD (**Fig. 1**).

DIAGNOSIS AND PROGNOSIS

Diagnosis of HFpEF is challenging and is made mostly via echocardiography as well as Doppler studies. The blood biomarker "NT-proBNP" is also an excellent indicator of atrial congestion. Increased levels of this peptide almost rule in HF. This peptide contributes to defining patients with HFpEF when other clinical or diagnostic criteria do not match properly. NT-proBNP is also used as a prognostic indicator. Higher values have been linked to an increased risk of cardiovascular events and mortality in patients.

Thus, keeping all of the above in view, the latest universal definition of HF is a condition with symptoms and/or signs caused by a structural and/or functional cardiac abnormality and corroborated by elevated natriuretic peptide levels and/or objective evidence of pulmonary or systemic congestion.[19-22]

THERAPEUTICS

In consideration of all the above-mentioned pathophysiology, it becomes imperative to find a therapy which could help in:

- Reducing LV muscular stiffness so that filling pressures or LVEDP may get reduced
- Reducing pulmonary venous hypertension

However, the therapy of HFpEF is very tricky as well as challenging. Many medications have been assessed to fulfil the above criteria, but none provides satisfying results.

BETA BLOCKERS

In a patient with HFpEF, prevention of tachycardia or controlling the heart rate allows to maximize the diastolic filling period. In addition to it, beta blockers have proven benefits in reducing blood pressure and myocardial ischemia, promoting regression of left ventricular hypertrophy, and antagonizing the excessive adrenergic stimulation during HF.

Experimental studies have shown that beta blockers increase survival rates and halt the progression of diastolic dysfunction by attenuation of inflammatory changes, oxidative stress, and preventing myocardial fibrosis when used in high doses.

The SWEDIC study has shown benefits of carvedilol in patients with HFpEF which were mostly attributed to heart rate reduction. However, the study has its own limitations: Small in sample size, heart rate of 70 beats/min is not high, and Doppler indices of LVDD were not easy to obtain in all cases.

In another study, J-DHF study, which was a prospective, randomized, open, blinded-endpoint design, the results suggested that there was no significant difference in the outcomes (all-cause death) between the control group and the treated group. However, this study also favored the fact that standard dose prescription of carvedilol is effective in HFpEF (less hospitalization rate).

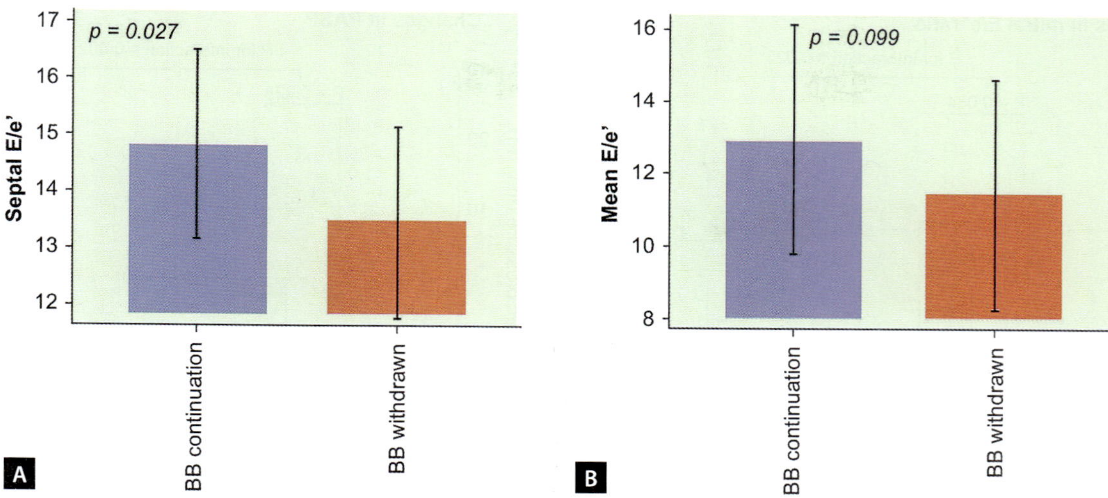

Figs. 2A and B: No significant changes were found in the mean *E/e'* ratio, but septal *E/e'* ratio decreased significantly when beta-blockers were withdrawn.
Source: Palau P, et al.[29]

Although the OPTIMIZE-HF study demonstrated the effect of beta blockers in patients with HF with reduced LVEF, patients with preserved systolic function had poor outcomes, and beta blockers did not significantly influence the mortality and rehospitalization risks for these patients. Although it was emphasized that HFpEF patients in this study had received low-dose beta blockers, the ongoing study analysis over the next few years concluded that the dose of beta blocker does not affect the clinical outcome in HFpEF patients.

Interestingly, another study, which was a meta-analysis of the previous studies, indicated that the benefits of beta blockers emerged at follow-up for 3 years but not for 1 year in patients with HF. Thus, the dose as well as the duration of beta-blocker therapy may influence the effects of clinical events in HFpEF patients.

Many other studies also suggested similar conflicting data for the use of beta blockers in patients with HFpEF. On one hand, beta blockers have benefits as they prevent the progression of disease and associated complications such as atrial fibrillation whereas on the other hand, they do not offer any survival benefit and also reduce the quality of life by interfering with exercise tolerance. Their use have failed to improve the *E/e'* ratio, walk distance, and NT-proBNP levels in patients with HFpEF, whereas discontinuation of beta-blockers had shown some beneficial effects **(Figs. 2A and B)**.

Thus, it was ultimately concluded that beta blockers are the first-line treatment for rate control in permanent AF as well as in uncontrolled hypertensive patients.[23-29]

SODIUM–GLUCOSE COTRANSPORTER 2 INHIBITORS

Sodium–glucose cotransporter 2 (SGLT2) is the major cotransporter involved in glucose reabsorption in the kidney, and the inhibition of SGLT2 has been established as a novel therapeutic measure for diabetic control. The EMPA-REG OUTCOME trial has demonstrated robust benefits of SGLT2 inhibitor in terms of the prevention of HF and reduction in cardiovascular mortality, which was the first evidence for prevention of major cardiovascular events by antidiabetic medications. Later, DELIVER and EMPEROR-Preserved trials demonstrated large cardiovascular benefits of the SGLT2 inhibitor, especially in patients with HFpEF irrespective of their diabetic status.

A recent trial, CAMEO-DAPA trial, demonstrated that treatment with dapagliflozin (a SGLT2 inhibitor) reduces resting and exercise PCWP, along with favorable effects on plasma volume and body weight. These findings provide new insight into the hemodynamic mechanisms of benefit with sodium–glucose cotransporter-2 inhibitors in HFpEF.

Thus, this antidiabetic molecule, SGLT2 inhibitor, has become an important agent in the management of all types of HF.

Many mechanisms are conceptualized for its protective action on heart:

- SGLT2 inhibitors have been shown to induce nutrient deprivation and increased ketotic state, which may contribute to improved cardiac energetics and function.

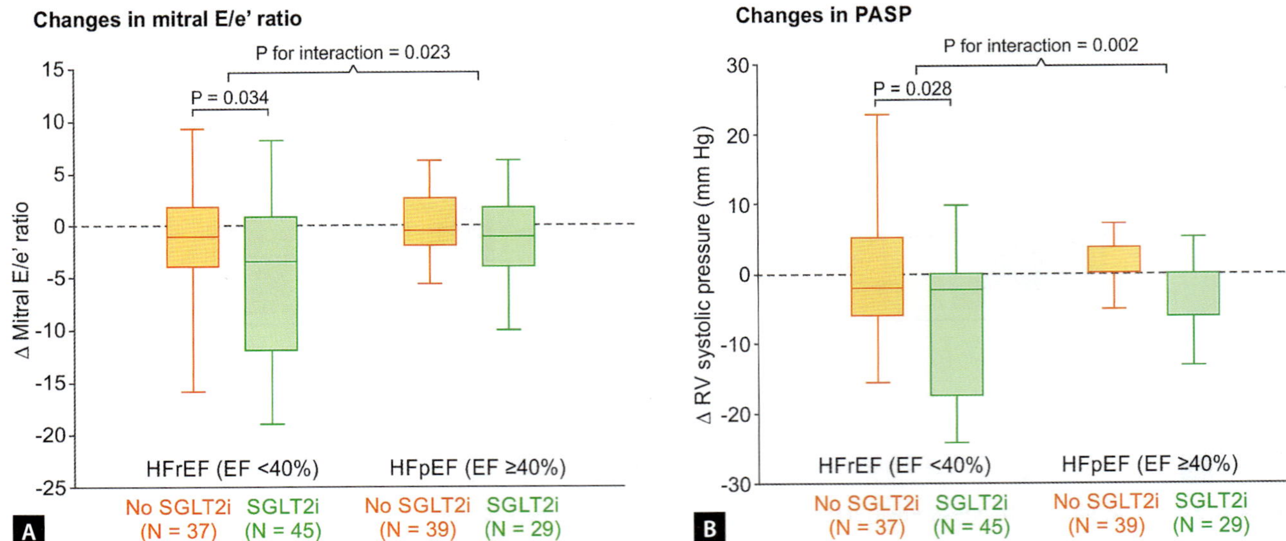

Figs. 3A and B: Significant change has been observed in patients with HFrEF with SGLT2 inhibitor than HFpEF with SGLT2 inhibitor when compared with the corresponding control group.
Source: Hwang et al.[39]

- These agents also reduce epicardial adipose tissue and alter adipokine signaling, which may reduce oxidative stress and inflammation.
- SGLT2 inhibitors have been shown to reduce myofilament stiffness as well as extracellular matrix remodeling/fibrosis in the heart, hence improving diastolic function.

All these methods lead to reductions in plasma volume, cardiac preload and afterload, alterations in cardiac metabolism, reduced arterial stiffness, and interaction with the Na^+/H^+ exchanger.

The principal effect of SGLT2 inhibitor (dapagliflozin) on LV diastolic function has been shown in the IDDA trial. It has demonstrated a significant improvement in LV diastolic function as well as a significant decrease in estimated LV filling pressure during exercise compared to the placebo group. This is the first randomized clinical trial to provide the beneficial effect of dapagliflozin on LV diastolic dysfunction in patients with type 2 diabetes.

A meta-analysis by Theofilis et al. had shown significant improvement in *E/e′* as well as an increase in the global strain of LV in patients. Similar findings were observed by Wee et al. in their meta-analysis. However, both these analyses were oriented to HFrEF rather than HFpEF. The study conducted by Hwang et al. depicts that benefits of the SGLT2 inhibitor are more prominent in HFrEF than in HFpEF **(Figs. 3A and B)**.

A significant effect of SGLT2 inhibitor in patients with HFpEF was observed by Soga et al. In their prospective multicenter trial, they followed diabetic patients for

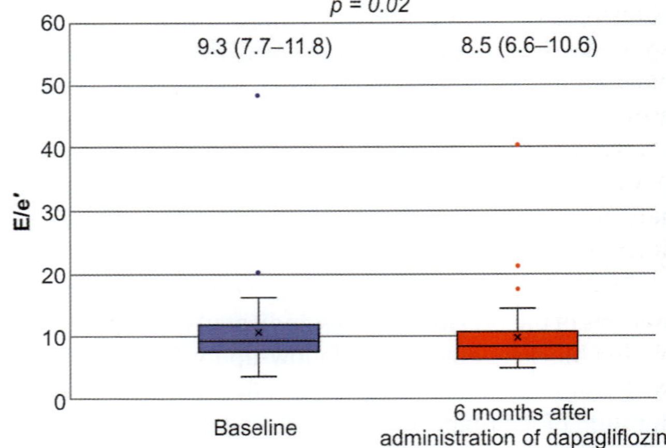

Fig. 4: Result for primary end point, showing a significant decrease in *E/e′* 6 months after administration of dapagliflozin.
Source: Soga et al.[40]

6 months and showed a significant decrease in *E/e′* from 9.3 to 8.5 cm/s ($p = 0.020$) **(Fig. 4)**.[30-40]

Although trends to use SGLT2 inhibitor in patients with HFpEF without diabetes are rising, it is still recommended for patients with type 2 diabetes.

ANGIOTENSIN RECEPTOR/NEPRILYSIN INHIBITOR

In the past few decades, many pathophysiologic studies were conducted to understand the maladaptive response

Flowchart 1: ARNI pathway in heart failure (HF).

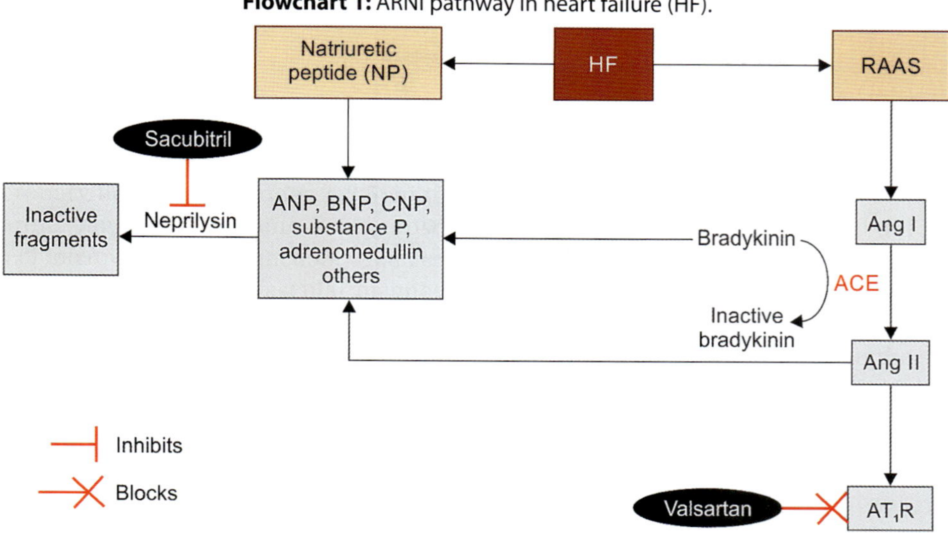

during HF on activation of the renin–angiotensin–aldosterone system (RAAS). Activation of RAAS leads to vasoconstriction, hypertension, increased aldosterone levels, increased sympathetic tone, and eventually cardiac remodeling, all of which are detrimental to the progression of the disease. Compensatory mechanism to RAAS is called the natriuretic peptide system, which leads to increased levels of BNP or NT-pro-BNP, resulting in vasodilation, natriuresis, and diuresis. Natriuretic peptides are broken down by an enzyme called neprilysin.

Thus, it was agreed that ACE inhibitors or ARBs in combination with natriuretic peptides may give better results in patients with HF. However, of many such combinations, only one combination, sacubitril–valsartan, is not yet approved. Sacubitril is a prodrug that, upon activation, acts as a neprilysin inhibitor and valsartan is an ARB **(Flowchart 1)**.

The first study on the role of ARNI in HF was the PARAMOUNT trial (Prospective comparison of ARNI with ARB on Management of heart failure with preserved ejection fraction). In this trial, although the early decrease in NT-proBNP after 4 weeks of treatment with ARNI was not significant compared with the valsartan group ($p = 0.063$), it decreased significantly after week 12 ($p = 0.005$). However, the difference at week 36 became insignificant ($p = 0.20$).

The PARAMOUNT study, after 36 weeks of treatment, had shown a significant reduction in the left atrial volume and left atrial width with ARNI compared with before treatment ($p = 0.003$ and 0.03, respectively), indicating reverse left atrial remodeling. However, other echocardiographic measures at week 36, including LVEF, and diastolic functional indicators namely *E/e′*, measures did not differ between groups.

The PARAGON-HF (Prospective Comparison of ARNI with ARB Global Outcomes in HF With Preserved Ejection Fraction) study had narrowly missed the significance of ARNI in its primary endpoint and concluded that the sacubitril–valsartan combination, compared with valsartan alone, did not result in a significantly lower rate of total HF hospitalizations or death from cardiovascular events among patients with HF and an EF of 45% or higher. But the study group did note a benefit (improved NYHA class and renal function) in a particular group of patients comprising women having HF with LVEF 45–60%. This landmark study noted that there is some significant role of ARNI in HFmrEF and HFpEF.

Similarly, the PARALLEX (the Prospective Comparison of ARNI vs. Comorbidity Associated Conventional Therapy on Quality of Life and Exercise Capacity) study noted that at 12 weeks, NT-proBNP levels were significantly reduced in the sacubitril/valsartan group versus the comparator group but did not significantly improve 6-minute walk distance at 24 weeks.

However, in an experimental model on rats, it was found that ARNI had shown significant improvement among rats with HFpEF over the valsartan group. HFpEF was induced by feeding rats with a high dose of saline. Later, these rats were divided into two groups to be treated with ARNI and valsartan. After a certain period, the ARNI group had shown strong improvement than valsartan alone[22,23,41-47] **(Figs. 5A and B)**.

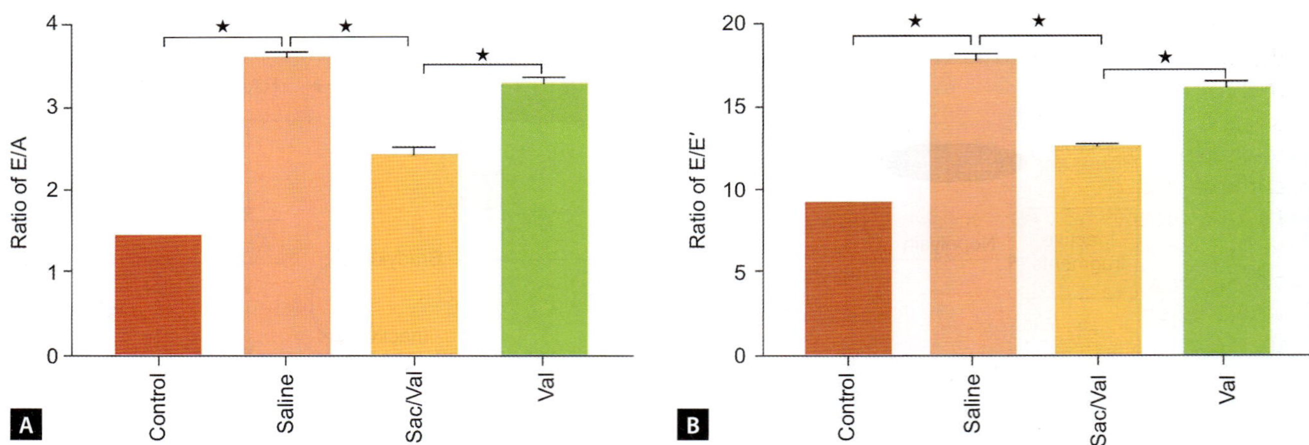

Figs. 5A and B: Change in *E/A* as well as *E/e'* among rats treated with sacubitril/valsartan (Sac/Val) combination and valsartan alone. *Source:* Zhang et al.[46]

Flowchart 2: Green color identifies a Class 1 therapy from clinical practice guidelines, yellow color indicates a Class 2a therapy, and orange color denotes a Class 2b therapy. However, recent trials had indicated a better place of SGLT2 inhibitor in the algorithm in future.

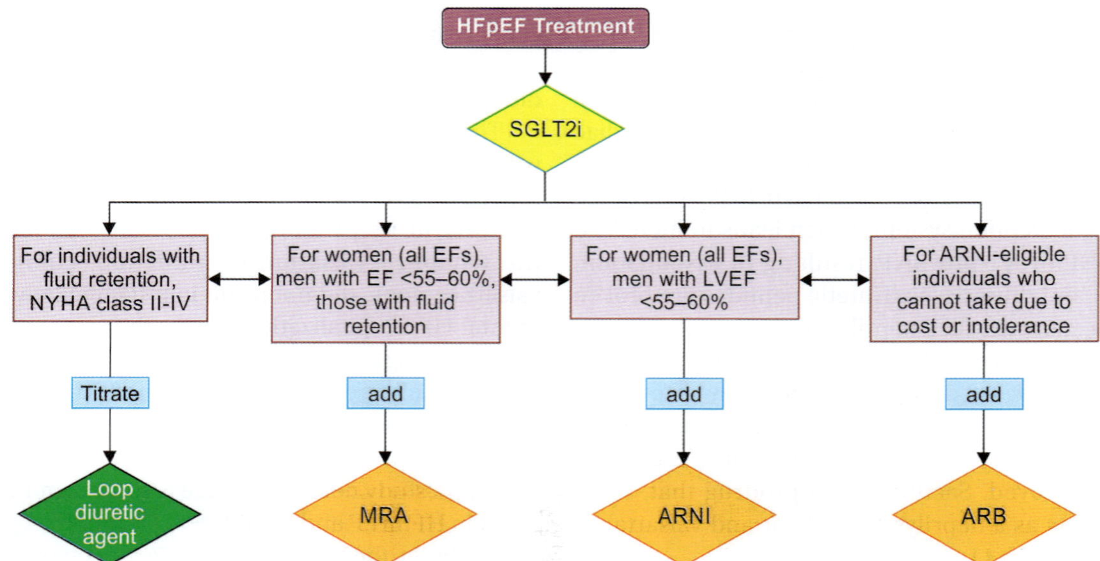

Sources: Solomon et al.[48]; Anker et al.[49]

CONCLUSION

- HFpEF is an advancing age problem—a true geriatric syndrome. It is estimated that after the age of 90 years, almost everyone is suffering from HFpEF.
- The diagnosis of HFpEF is also challenging. It involves echocardiographic, Doppler, and chemical indicators to diagnose.
- Apart from those given earlier, the treatment or management strategies to cure HFpEF are also limited. Most of them are restricted to lifestyle management or control of risk factors such as hypertension, diabetes, or obesity.
- Unlike in HFrEF, among the available medications, such as beta blockers, SGLT2 inhibitors, ACE/ARBs, ARNI, or other medications such as diuretics, nitrates, or aldosterone antagonists, none is found to be comprehensively effective for HFpEF.
- A number of studies had shown that the effect of medications stays only for short periods rather for long time intervals, which also indicates that short-period benefits are may be due to control of risk factors rather than the disease as such.
- The algorithm recommended for treatment of HFpEF is shown in **Flowchart 2**.

- The role of beta blockers in HFpEF is individualized that they may be used in who have specific indications, including prior myocardial infarction (for up to 3 years), angina, or AF. The major side effect of exercise tolerance should be monitored due to the potential for chronotropic incompetence.
- Last but not least to mention that women response to treatment therapies for HFpEF is better than men; especially with ARNI or SGLT2 inhibitor. The reason why women may respond more favorably to these therapies at a relatively higher LVEF may be because women tend to have smaller LV chamber size and are thus more prone to demonstrate higher LVEFs when compared with men.[48,49]

REFERENCES

1. Savarese G, Lund LH. Global public health burden of heart failure. Card Fail Rev. 2017;3(1):7-11.
2. Roger VL. Epidemiology of heart failure: A contemporary perspective. Circ Res. 2021;128(10):1421-34.
3. Satpathy C, Mishra TK, Satpathy R, et al. Diagnosis and management of diastolic dysfunction and heart failure. Am Fam Physician. 2006;73:841-6.
4. Golla MSG, Shams P. Heart failure with preserved ejection fraction (HFpEF). Treasure Island (FL): StatPearls Publishing; 2025 Jan. [online] Available from https://www.ncbi.nlm.nih.gov/books/NBK599960/ [Last accessed January, 2025].
5. Gevaert AB, Boen JRA, Segers VF. Heart failure with preserved ejection fraction: A review of cardiac and noncardiac pathophysiology. Front Physiol. 2019;10:638.
6. Borlaug BA. The pathophysiology of heart failure with preserved ejection fraction. Nature Rev Cardiol. 2014;11:507-15.
7. Pfeffer MA, Shah AM, Borlaug BA. Heart failure with preserved ejection fraction in perspective. Circ Res. 2019;124(11):1598-617.
8. Gazewood JD, Turner PL. Heart failure with preserved ejection fraction: Diagnosis and management. Am Fam Physician. 2017;96(9):582-8.
9. Campbell P, Rutten FH, Lee MM, et al. Heart failure with preserved ejection fraction: everything the clinician needs to know. Lancet. 2024;403(10431):1083-92.
10. Mol EE, Hartmann C, Moura LAZ, et al. HFrEF, HFmrEF, and HFpEF: Are They a Continuum or Different Faces of a Syndrome? DOI: 10.36660/ijcs.20240048.
11. Formiga F, Nuñez J, Moraga MJC, et al. Diagnosis of heart failure with preserved ejection fraction: a systematic narrative review of the evidence. Heart Fail Rev. 2024;29: 179-89.
12. Garg N, Kapur KK. Advances in LA strain evaluation by echocardiography in hypertension. In: Nanda NC, Chopra HK, Narula J (Eds). Advances in Clinical Cardiovascular Imaging, Echocardiography & Interventions: A Textbook of Cardiology. New Delhi: Jaypee Brothers Medical Publishers; 2019. pp. 49-57.
13. Karnik A, Jankowski M, Narang A. Unmasking HFpEF with artificial intelligence: A disruptive opportunity for disease detection. J Cardiac Fail. 2024;30(11):1533-4.
14. Istratoaie S, Gargani L, Popescu BA, et al. How to diagnose heart failure with preserved ejection fraction. Eur Heart J. 2024;25(11):1505-16.
15. Reddy YNV, Olson TP, Obokata M, et al. Hemodynamic Correlates and Diagnostic Role of Cardiopulmonary Exercise Testing in Heart Failure With Preserved Ejection Fraction. JACC Heart Fail. 2018;6(8):665-75.
16. Borlaug BA, Olson TP, Lam CSP, et al. Global cardiovascular reserve dysfunction in heart failure with preserved ejection fraction. J Am Coll Cardiol. 2010;56(11):845-54.
17. Pieske B, Tschöpe C, de Boer RA, et al. How to diagnose heart failure with preserved ejection fraction: the HFA-PEFF diagnostic algorithm: a consensus recommendation from the Heart Failure Association (HFA) of the European Society of Cardiology (ESC). Eur Heart J. 2019;40:3297-317.
18. Reddy YNV, Carter RE, Obokata M, et al. A simple, evidence-based approach to help guide diagnosis of heart failure with preserved ejection fraction. Circulation. 2018;138:861-70.
19. McDowell K, Kondo T, Talebi A, et al. Prognostic Models for Mortality and Morbidity in Heart Failure With Preserved Ejection Fraction. JAMA Cardiol. 2024;9(5):457-65.
20. Balestrieri G, Limonta R, Ponti E, et al. The Therapy and Management of Heart Failure with Preserved Ejection Fraction: New Insights on Treatment. Cardiac Fail Rev. 2024;10:e05.
21. Abdin A, Böhm M, Shahim B, et al. Heart failure with preserved ejection fraction epidemiology, pathophysiology, diagnosis and treatment strategies. Int J Cardiol. 2024;412:132304.
22. Böhm M, Perez AC, Jhund PS, et al. Relationship between heart rate and mortality and morbidity in the irbesartan patients with heart failure and preserved systolic function trial (I-Preserve). Eur J Heart Fail. 2014;16:778-87.
23. Takada T, Sakata Y, Miyata S, et al. Impact of elevated heart rate on clinical outcomes in patients with heart failure with reduced and preserved ejection fraction: a report from the CHART-2 Study. Eur J Heart Fail. 2014;16:309-16.
24. Bergström A, Andersson B, Edner M, et al. Effect of carvedilol on diastolic function in patients with diastolic heart failure and preserved systolic function. Results of the Swedish Doppler-echocardiographic study (SWEDIC). Eur J Heart Fail. 2004;6:453-61.
25. Hernandez AF, Hammill BG, O'Connor CM, et al. Clinical effectiveness of beta-blockers in heart failure: findings from the OPTIMIZE-HF (Organized Program to Initiate Lifesaving Treatment in Hospitalized Patients with Heart Failure) registry. J Am Coll Cardiol. 2009;53:18492.
26. Lam PH, Gupta N, Dooley DJ, et al. Role of high-dose beta-blockers in patients with heart failure with preserved ejection fraction and elevated heart rate. Am J Med. 2018; 131:1473-81.

27. Wernhart S, Papathanasiou M, Rassaf T, et al. The controversial role of beta-blockers in heart failure with preserved ejection fraction. Pharmacol Ther. 2023;243:108356.
28. Jun G, Fan YQ, Bian L, et al. Long-term prescription of beta-blocker delays the progression of heart failure with preserved ejection fraction in patients with hypertension: A retrospective observational cohort study. Eur J Prevent Cardiol. 2016;23(13):1421-8.
29. Palau P, Seller J, Domínguez E, et al. Effect of β-blocker withdrawal on functional capacity in heart failure and preserved ejection fraction. JACC. 2021;78(21):2042-56.
30. Peikert A, Chandra A, Kosiborod MN, et al. Association of dapagliflozin vs placebo with individual Kansas City Cardiomyopathy Questionnaire components in patients with heart failure with mildly reduced or preserved ejection fraction: a secondary analysis of the DELIVER trial. JAMA Cardiol. 2023;8:684-90.
31. Wagdy K, Nagy S. EMPEROR-Preserved: SGLT2 inhibitors breakthrough in the management of heart failure with preserved ejection fraction. Glob Cardiol Sci Pract. 2021;2021:e202117.
32. Wee CF, Teo YH, Teo YN, et al. Effects of Sodium/Glucose Cotransporter 2 (SGLT2) Inhibitors on Cardiac Imaging Parameters: A Systematic Review and Meta-analysis of Randomized Controlled trails. J Cardiovasc Imaging. 2022;30(3):153-68.
33. Theofilis P, Antonopoulos AS, Katsimichas T, et al. The impact of SGLT2 inhibition on imaging markers of cardiac function: A systematic review and meta-analysis. Pharmacol Res. 2022;180:106243.
34. Rau M, Thiele K, Hartmann NUK, et al. Empagliflozin does not change cardiac index nor systemic vascular resistance but rapidly improves left ventricular filling pressure in patients with type 2 diabetes: A randomized controlled study. Cardiovasc Diabetol. 2021;20:6.
35. Shim CY, Seo J, Cho I, et al. Randomized, Controlled Trial to Evaluate the Effect of Dapagliflozin on Left Ventricular Diastolic Function in Patients with Type 2 Diabetes Mellitus: The IDDIA Trial. Circulation. 2021;143:510-2.
36. Marketou M, Kontaraki J, Maragkoudakis S, et al. Effects of Sodium-Glucose Cotransporter-2 Inhibitors on Cardiac Structural and Electrical Remodeling: From Myocardial Cytology to Cardiodiabetology. Curr Vasc Pharmacol. 2022;20:178-88.
37. Scheffer M, Driessen-Waaijer A, Hamdani N, et al. Stratified Treatment of Heart Failure with preserved Ejection Fraction: Rationale and design of the STADIA-HFpEF trial. ESC Heart Fail. 2020;7:4478-87.
38. Malhotra Kapoor P. Impact of sodium-glucose cotransporter 2 inhibitor on E/e' in patients with heart failure. In: Nanda NC, Chopra HK, Narula J (Eds). Advances & Revolutions in Heart Failure (ARHF): A Textbook of Cardiology. New Delhi: Jaypee Brothers Medical Publishers; 2024. pp. 770-8.
39. Hwang IC, Cho GY, Yoon YE, et al. Different effects of SGLT2 inhibitors according to the presence and types of heart failure in type 2 diabetic patients. Cardiovasc Diabetol. 2020;19:69.
40. Soga F, Tanaka H, Tatsumi K, et al. Impact of dapagliflozin on left ventricular diastolic function of patients with type 2 diabetic mellitus with chronic heart failure. Cardiovasc Diabetol. 2018;17:132.
41. Solomon SD, Zile M, Pieske B, et al. The angiotensin receptor neprilysin inhibitor LCZ696 in heart failure with preserved ejection fraction: a phase 2 double-blind randomised controlled trial. Lancet. 2012;380: 1387-95.
42. Morrow DA, Velazquez EJ, DeVore AD, et al. Clinical outcomes in patients with acute decompensated heart failure randomly assigned to Sacubitril/Valsartan or enalapril in the Pioneer-HF trial. Circulation. 2019;139:2285-8.
43. Solomon SD, McMurray JJV, Anand IS, et al. Angiotensin-neprilysin inhibition in heart failure with preserved ejection fraction. N Engl J Med. 2019;381:160920.
44. Jackson AM, Jhund PS, Anand IS, et al. Sacubitril–valsartan as a treatment for apparent resistant hypertension in patients with heart failure and preserved ejection fraction. Eur Heart J. 2021;42:374152.
45. Suzuki K, Claggett B, Minamisawa M, et al. Pulse pressure, prognosis, and influence of sacubitril/valsartan in heart failure with preserved ejection fraction. Hypertension. 2021;77(2):546-56.
46. Zhang W, Liu J, Fu Y, et al. Sacubitril/valsartan reduces fibrosis and alleviates high-salt diet-induced HFpEF in rats. Front Pharmacol. 2021;11:600953.
47. Wachter R, Shah SJ, Cowie MR, et al. Angiotensin receptor neprilysin inhibition versus individualized RAAS blockade: design and rationale of the PARALLAX trial. ESC Heart Fail. 2020;7(3):856-64.
48. Solomon SD, McMurray JJV, Claggett B, et al. Dapagliflozin in heart failure with mildly reduced or preserved ejection fraction. N Engl J Med. 2022;387:1089-98.
49. Anker SD, Butler J, Filippatos G, et al. Empagliflozin in heart failure with a preserved ejection fraction. N Engl J Med. 2021;385:1451-61.

Echocardiographic Variables on Cardiac Atrial and Ventricular Remodeling Reversal by ARNI and SGLT2i in HFpEF

Ankush Sachdeva, Sanil Omar, AK Omar

INTRODUCTION

Heart failure with preserved ejection fraction (HFpEF) is now recognized as a difficult-to-treat subset in cardiology in comparison with heart failure with reduced ejection fraction (HFrEF) and has become a more diagnosed form of heart failure (HF) with its incidence increasing by 1% annually.[1] There is no gold standard in diagnosing HFpEF, and it is not as simple when compared to HFrEF as the ejection fraction (EF) remains normal as seen in patients with noncardiac causes. The 2022 AHA/ACC/HFSA guideline for the HF management has published the criteria for diagnosing HFpEF, which includes a normal or near-normal left ventricular ejection fraction (LVEF ≥50%), raised left ventricular filling pressures by echocardiography, and increased natriuretic peptide (NP) levels.[2] The sensitivity for this approach ranges from 25–80%.[3-5] The patients in their initial stage of the disease may be diagnosed as normal or indeterminate.[6]

Parameters including clinical (patient history, physical examination), biochemical (serum BNP level), hemodynamic, and radiographic data are all used to reach a diagnosis.[7,8] Scoring criteria including the H2FPEF score and HFA-PEFF scores can help in diagnosis but are not completely validated.

HISTORY TAKING AND CLINICAL EXAMINATION

General physical examination is done in patients with impending HF along with history taking to search for risk factors and comorbidities linked to HFpEF.[2] HFpEF symptoms may be similar to HFrEF such as breathlessness on exertion, orthopnea, fatigue, and paroxysmal nocturnal dyspnea. Signs of HF such as elevated jugular venous pressure, pulmonary rhonchi, and lower extremity edema might be present.[9] Presence of obesity, atrial fibrillation (AF), and diabetes increases the chances of HFpEF.[10] Patients with HFpEF might complain of chest discomfort resembling angina. Patients with HFpEF can also present with tachycardia, sweating, narrow pulse pressure, and vasoconstriction in advanced stages. Dizziness and orthostatic hypotension suggest the possibility of cardiac amyloidosis.[11] Framingham criteria base the diagnosis on the presence of major symptoms such as nocturnal dyspnea and orthopnea as well as minor symptoms such as edema of the extremities and exertional dyspnea.[12] Framingham's clinical criteria have good sensitivity to exclude the diagnosis of HF but has poor specificity to confirm its diagnosis. Some patients with HF may not have symptoms as only 50% of patients even with left ventricular dysfunction on an echocardiogram are symptomatic. Symptoms and signs of HF are nonspecific, which makes the clinical diagnosis of HF challenging with <25% of accuracy.[13]

Echocardiography

Echocardiography for HFpEF gives information to estimate raised LV filling pressure, which includes Doppler (E/e′) ratio, LVEF estimation, and pulmonary artery systolic pressure (PASP).[14] Features that increase the chances of HFpEF are left atrial enlargement, decreased left atrial strain, impaired LV early diastolic tissue velocity (e′), decreased global longitudinal strain (GLS), and right ventricular (RV) dilatation/dysfunction.[14] These abovementioned echocardiography criteria are specific but have low sensitivity.[15] In patients who are euvolemic, mildly hypervolemic, or are in early disease stage, diastolic function may be normal or indeterminate. Diastolic dysfunction might not be seen at rest in one-third of patients with HFpEF by echocardiography **(Figs. 1A to H)**.

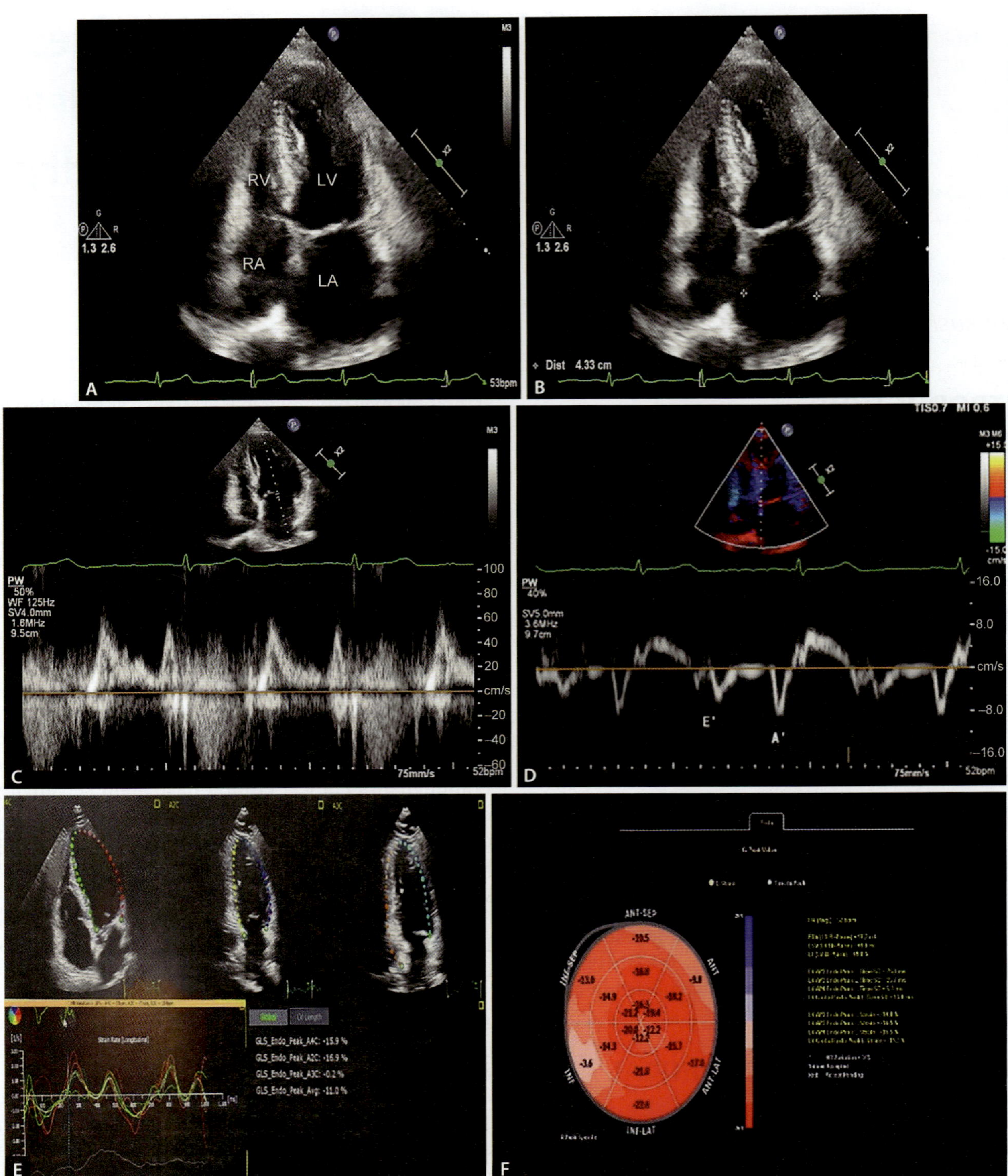

Figs. 1A to F

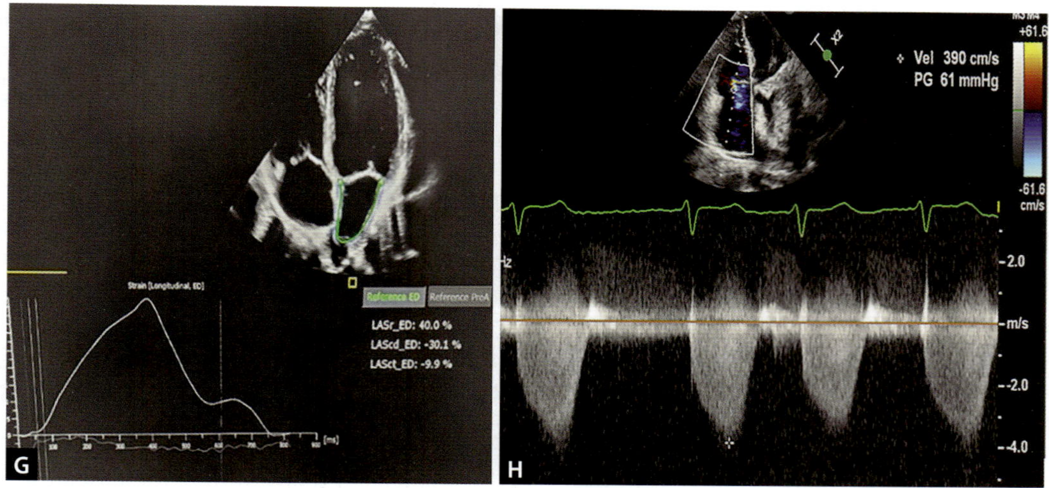

Figs. 1G and H

Figs. 1A to H: Spectrum of parameters used in echocardiography to diagnose HFpEF.

Natriuretic Peptides

Natriuretic peptides such as BNP/N-terminal pro-B-type natriuretic peptide (NT-proBNP) measurement are helpful in supporting HFpEF diagnosis when the cause of dyspnea is unclear. Plasma NP levels increase in response to cardiac wall stress, which is related to chamber dimension and distending pressure, according to the law of Laplace. Patients with HFpEF and raised NP levels have an increased risk of HF. NP level has been recommended in international guidelines, but one-third of patients with HFpEF have normal NP levels; therefore, their value must be interpreted in the clinical context. The diagnostic gold standard is cardiac catheterization for showing increased LV filling pressures.[16]

Stress Test and Invasive Testing

Invasive stress methods to evaluate HFpEF, where cardiac filling pressures are elevated during hemodynamic exercise testing, involve right heart catheterization for the direct measurement of central hemodynamics at rest and then during graded increases in exercise workload to volitional fatigue, ideally with simultaneous expired gas analysis to evaluate aerobic capacity (peak oxygen consumption).[17-20] Diagnosis of HFpEF is defined as elevated PCWP at rest (≥15 mm Hg) or during exercise (≥25 mm Hg). Invasive exercise testing directly assesses the parameters that define HFpEF, which serves as the gold standard test to prove that HFpEF is the cause of symptoms.[14] It is more expensive, requires operator expertise, and is invasive. Exercise echocardiography has increasingly been used as an alternative to invasive stress testing.[18] Some studies have shown correlations of variables measured using exercise echocardiography with invasively obtained data, but other studies have not shown favorable results.[21]

TABLE 1: H2FPEF score chart.

	Clinical variable	*Values*	*Points*
H_2	*Heavy*	Body mass index >30 kg/m^2	2
	Hypertensive	Two or more antihypertensive medicine	1
F	*Atrial fibrillation*	Paroxysmal or persistent	3
P	*Pulmonary hypertension*	Pulmonary artery systolic pressure >35 mm Hg on echocardiography	1
E	*Elder*	Age >60 years	1
F	*Filling pressure*	E/e' >9	1
	H2FPEF score		Sum (0–9)

DIAGNOSTIC METHODOLOGIES

The clinical score H2FPEF[14] can be used for risk stratification, which combines risk factors such as obesity, AF, and age >60 years, into a weighted score. A score <2 has a low chance of having HFpEF, while those patients with a score >6 have a greater possibility. Patients in the midrange of the score need more workup **(Table 1)**.

More definitive tests are required for in-between probability of such disease. The H2FPEF score calculation is simple, which involves clinical and echocardiographic data that are readily available. A further scoring algorithm, the HFA-PEFF score, was given by the ESC/HFA for diagnostic evaluation of HFpEF in 2019.[19] This diagnostic algorithm was not evidence-based like the H2FPEF score but is very similar in methodology.

MANAGEMENT OF HEART FAILURE WITH PRESERVED EJECTION FRACTION

Other than risk factor modification and physical exercise, aldosterone-blocking agents, and sodium-glucose cotransporter-2 inhibitor (SGLT2i), targeted therapies have come up for specific HFpEF causes such as hypertrophic cardiomyopathy or cardiac amyloidosis **(Table 2)**.

González-López et al., in the year 2015, studied consecutive patients aged 60 years or older with newly diagnosed HFpEF with a septal thickness of 12 mm on echocardiography using 99mTc-3,3-diphosphono-1,2-propanodicarboxylic acid (DPD) scintigraphy, which found a rate of 13% of wild-type transthyretin cardiac amyloidosis,[22] showing that umbrella of HFpEF is distinct and treatable diseases may hide, which can be identified by correct cardiac imaging **(Table 2)**. A large proportion of HFpEF patients has no specific underlying cause except for hypertension, obesity, diabetes mellitus, presence of AF, etc. Modification of risk factors and lifestyle changes such as regular exercise have shown benefit in HFpEF.[23] Medical therapy of such classical HFpEF patients without specific etiology has shown modest benefits.

ROLE OF VARIOUS MEDICATIONS IN HFpEF

Medical therapy in HFpEF patients without specific etiology has shown some benefits.

Mineralocorticoid Antagonist Drugs

Mineralocorticoid antagonist drugs treat myocardial fibrosis, which is beneficial in HFrEF but show mixed results in HFpEF. The TOPCAT trial[24] of spironolactone did not show clinical benefits, but delayed analysis by geographic area shows significant regional variation in patient characteristics, and also in patients from America, they had a positive effect on hospitalization for HF and cardiovascular mortality.[25]

Guanylate Cyclase Stimulator, Angiotensin Receptor-neprilysin Inhibitor, and Sodium–Glucose Cotransporter-2 Inhibitor

The guanylate cyclase stimulator vericiguat did not fulfill expectations of clinical improvement in HFpEF in a published large trial.[26] Drugs primarily given for HFrEF, such as angiotensin receptor blockers, mineralocorticoid antagonists, and angiotensin receptor-neprilysin inhibitors (ARNIs) can be considered in HF with EF near the lower limit or at the borderline of normal EF. SGLT2 inhibitors such as empagliflozin and dapagliflozin improved symptoms and modestly reduced hospitalizations due to HF, but not death, in HFpEF trials.[27-30]

There are several mimics or "phenocopies" of HFpEF that are amenable to specific therapies and need to be identified, where imaging plays a central diagnostic role in the differential diagnosis.[31,32] In HFpEF, the role of epicardial CAD is not much clear. It is generally accepted that microvascular coronary dysfunction may contribute to HFpEF and diastolic dysfunction. In a study of patients with reduced coronary flow reserve by positron emission tomography (PET) and no flow-limiting epicardial coronary stenosis, diastolic left ventricular

TABLE 2: Umbrella concept of HFpEF.

HFpEF	*Final diagnosis informed by imaging*	*Main current therapeutic options*
• Symptoms/signs of HF • EF ≥50% • Structural/functional abnormality	• Classical HFpEF • CAD/coronary microvascular dysfunction • HCM • Cardiac amyloidosis • Anderson–Fabry disease • Cardiac hemochromatosis • Cardiac sarcoidosis • Constrictive pericarditis • Right-sided heart disease	• Risk factor modification • Aldosterone antagonists • SGLT2 inhibitors • Anti-ischemic drugs, statins, and revascularization • Beta-blockers, calcium antagonists, mavacamten, and aficamten • Chemotherapy—AL amyloidosis, tafamidis—ATTR amyloidosis • Enzyme replacement therapy • Chaperone therapy • Iron chelation therapy • Immunosuppressive therapy, ICD • Pericardiectomy • Medical or interventional/surgical therapy

(CAD: coronary artery disease; HC: hypertrophic cardiomyopathy; ICD: implantable cardioverter defibrillator)

function was impaired and the risk of hospitalization for HFpEF substantially increased.[33] Microvascular coronary dysfunction cannot be easily visualized by invasive or noninvasive coronary angiography, though postprocessing of angiography images might allow identification of increased microvascular resistance.[34,35] A reduction of coronary flow reserve under 2–2.5, in the absence of epicardial flow-limiting stenoses, is mostly accepted as a sign of microvascular dysfunction, which can be demonstrated by PET, stress cardiovascular magnetic resonance,[36] or sophisticated invasive measurements. The underlying mechanism of microvascular dysfunction includes endothelial dysfunction/inflammation, which is partly treatable by modification of cardiovascular risk factors, angiotensin-converting enzyme inhibitors, and statins.

DISCUSSION

Angiotensin receptor-neprilysin inhibitor, sacubitril/valsartan, which inhibits maladaptive neurohormonal pathways while upregulating adaptive NP expression, has shown to prolong life in patients with mild-to-moderate symptoms of HFrEF when it was used in place of ACE inhibitors.[37,38] These findings led to the PARAGON-HF (Prospective Comparison of ARNI with ARB Global Outcomes in HF with Preserved Ejection Fraction) study in HFpEF, which narrowly missed significance in primary endpoint and concluded that the sacubitril/valsartan combination, compared with the ARB valsartan, did not result in a significantly lower the rate of total HF hospitalizations (HFHs) and death from cardiovascular causes among patients with HF and in an EF of 45% or higher.[39,40] Suggestion of benefit was noted in those patients with an EF in the lower range (45–57%) studied, as well as in women, who represent a high proportion of patients with HFpEF. On the basis of these data, the US Food and Drug Administration expanded approval of sacubitril/valsartan to this narrower group of patients with HFpEF (<60%), the first such approval. A post hoc analysis of PARAGON-HF concluded that benefits of sacubitril/valsartan became evident when treatment was initiated closer to an episode of HFH, comprising a vulnerable group of patients with a higher risk of short-term morbidity.[41]

The PARAGLIDE-HF study enrolled 466 patients, and it was prospectively powered to detect a relative 23% greater reduction in the primary endpoint of time-averaged reduction in NT-proBNP from baseline to the average of the 4- and 8-week measurements in the sacubitril/valsartan group compared with the valsartan group. The study formally met its primary endpoint, thus demonstrating a nominally significant 15% greater reduction in the sacubitril/valsartan arm (95% CI: 0–27%; $p = 0.049$). Although the study was not powered to examine clinical outcomes, a hierarchical secondary endpoint was prespecified for analysis using a win ratio, which included cardiovascular death, number and timing of worsening HF events, and meaningful change in time-averaged NT-proBNP (either reduction 1.33 as loss). The win ratio analysis (1.19; 95% CI: 0.93–1.52) did not suggest benefit in these patients. Notably, data to analyze the primary endpoint were not available for a substantial number of patients because of higher numbers of missing biomarker values and patient withdrawals in the sacubitril/valsartan group. Safety analyses noted a 50% higher (24 vs. 16%) rate of symptomatic hypotension in sacubitril/valsartan arm compared with valsartan-treated patients.

CONCLUSION

Although the trial nominally achieved significance on its primary endpoint, the margin of benefit was less than anticipated on the basis of the prospective power calculation. The finding that clinically meaningful outcomes on cardiac events did not show a difference suggests that the magnitude of reduction in the NP levels may not have been sufficient to reach threshold for clinical benefit. Mentz et al.[42] did not report baseline or longitudinal use of diuretic agent dosing among the two groups, which if different between groups could have contributed to the differential reduction in NT-proBNP levels and also to the observed rates of symptomatic hypotension. The use of SGLT2is was low in both groups, and with the known benefits of this drug class on reducing HFH rates in HFpEF, one is left wondering whether the putative benefits of sacubitril/valsartan would be positively or negatively affected in a scenario of greater proportional use of these agents, especially with respect to tolerability, including symptomatic hypotension.[43] Overall, these data echo the results of PARAGON-HF and suggest that the evidence for treatment benefit of ARNI in unselected patients with HFpEF appears limited. However, in the subgroup of patients with an EF lower than normal (<60%) had a greater relative reduction in NT-proBNP levels and a strong trend to clinical benefit (win ratio: 1.46; 95% CI: 1.09–1.95). This analytic methodology also ignores ties, and given that ties occurred in more than one-third of the comparisons in PARAGLIDE-HF, the win ratio calculation, which is restricted only within the category of winners and losers, likely overestimates treatment effect.[44] Furthermore, NT-proBNP as a final tiebreaker was responsible for the majority of "wins" for sacubitril/valsartan. The number of clinical events alone may have been small, and the duration of observation might be short to demonstrate benefit in meaningful outcomes. Thus, although the study suggests some evidence of a beneficial trend of sacubitril/valsartan in HFpEF and a recent episode of worsening HF, the data are still far from reaching a conclusion.

REFERENCES

1. Stringer B, Hyder S, Nozadze N, et al. Analysis of clinical, biochemical and echocardiographic criteria for heart failure with preserved ejection fraction. J Card Fail. 2022;28(5):S107.
2. Heidenreich PA, Bozkurt B, Aguilar D, et al. 2022 American College of Cardiology/American Heart Association/Heart Failure Society of America guideline for the management of heart failure: executive summary. J Card Fail. 2022; 28(5):810-30.
3. Penicka M, Bartunek J, Trakalova H, et al. Heart failure with preserved ejection fraction in outpatients with unexplained dyspnea: a pressure-volume loop analysis. J Am Coll Cardiol. 2010;55(16):1701-10.
4. Lam CS, Roger VL, Rodeheffer RJ, et al. Pulmonary hypertension in heart failure with preserved ejection fraction: a community-based study. J Am Coll Cardiol. 2009;53(13):1119-26.
5. Obokata M, Reddy YN, Borlaug BA. Diastolic dysfunction and heart failure with preserved ejection fraction: understanding mechanisms by using noninvasive methods. JACC Cardiovasc Imaging. 2020;13(1 Part 2):245-57.
6. Mitter SS, Shah SJ, Thomas JD. A test in context: E/A and E/e′ to assess diastolic dysfunction and LV filling pressure. J Am Coll Cardiol. 2017;69(11):1451-64.
7. Snipelisky D, Kelly J, Levine JA, et al. Accelerometer-measured daily activity in heart failure with preserved ejection fraction: clinical correlates and association with standard heart failure severity indices. Circ Heart Fail. 2017;10(6):e003878.
8. Huis In 't Veld AE, de Man FS, van Rossum AC, et al. How to diagnose heart failure with preserved ejection fraction: the value of invasive stress testing. Neth Heart J. 2016;24(4):244-51.
9. Solomon SD, Rizkala AR, Lefkowitz MP, et al. Baseline characteristics of patients with heart failure and preserved ejection fraction in the PARAGON-HF trial. Circ Heart Fail. 2018;11(7):e004962.
10. Packer M, Metra M. Guideline-directed medical therapy for heart failure does not exist: a non-judgmental framework for describing the level of adherence to evidence-based drug treatments for patients with a reduced ejection fraction. Eur J Heart Fail. 2020;22(10):1759-67.
11. Borlaug BA. Evaluation and management of heart failure with preserved ejection fraction. Nat Rev Cardiol. 2020;17(9):559-73.
12. Löfström U, Hage C, Savarese G, et al. Prognostic impact of Framingham heart failure criteria in heart failure with preserved ejection fraction. ESC Heart Fail. 2019;6(4): 830-9.
13. Golla MSG, Hajouli S, Ludhwani D. Heart failure and ejection fraction. In: StatPearls. Treasure Island: StatPearls Publishing; 2024. [online] Available from https://www.ncbi.nlm.nih.gov/books/NBK553115/. [Last accessed January, 2025].
14. Reddy YNV, Carter RE, Obokata M, et al. A simple, evidence-based approach to help guide diagnosis of heart failure with preserved ejection fraction. Circulation. 2018;138(9):861-70.
15. Nakamura T, Iwanaga Y, Miyaji Y, et al. Cardiovascular efficacy of sitagliptin in patients with diabetes at high risk of cardiovascular disease: a 12-month follow-up. Cardiovasc Diabetol. 2016;15:54.
16. De Keulenaer GW, Brutsaert DL. Systolic and diastolic heart failure are overlapping phenotypes within the heart failure spectrum. Circulation. 2011;123(18):1996-2004.
17. Borlaug BA, Nishimura RA, Sorajja P, et al. Exercise hemodynamics enhance diagnosis of early heart failure with preserved ejection fraction. Circ Heart Fail. 2010; 3(5):588-95.
18. Obokata M, Reddy YNV, Pislaru SV, et al. Evidence supporting the existence of a distinct obese phenotype of heart failure with preserved ejection fraction. Circulation. 2017;136(1):6-19.
19. Pieske B, Tschöpe C, de Boer RA, et al. How to diagnose heart failure with preserved ejection fraction: the HFA-PEFF diagnostic algorithm: a consensus recommendation from the heart failure association (HFA) of the European society of cardiology (ESC). Eur Heart J. 2019;40(40):3297-317.
20. Mueller C, McDonald K, de Boer RA, et al. Heart failure association of the European society of cardiology practical guidance on the use of natriuretic peptide concentrations. Eur J Heart Fail. 2019;21(6):715-31.
21. Maeder MT, Thompson BR, Brunner-La Rocca HP, et al. Hemodynamic basis of exercise limitation in patients with heart failure and normal ejection fraction. J Am Coll Cardiol. 2010;56(11):855-63.
22. González-López E, Gallego-Delgado M, Guzzo-Merello G, et al. Wild-type transthyretin amyloidosis as a cause of heart failure with preserved ejection fraction. Eur Heart J 2015;36(38):2585-94.
23. Edelmann F, Gelbrich G, Düngen HD, et al. Exercise training improves exercise capacity and diastolic function in patients with heart failure with preserved ejection fraction: results of the ex-DHF (exercise training in diastolic heart failure) pilot study. J Am Coll Cardiol. 2011;58(17):1780-91.
24. Pitt B, Pfeffer MA, Assmann SF, et al. Spironolactone for heart failure with preserved ejection fraction. N Engl J Med. 2014;370(15):1383-92.
25. Pfeffer MA, Claggett B, Assmann SF, et al. Regional variation in patients and outcomes in the treatment of preserved cardiac function heart failure with an aldosterone antagonist (TOPCAT) trial. Circulation. 2015;131(1):34-42.
26. Armstrong PW, Lam CSP, Anstrom KJ, et al. Effect of vericiguat vs placebo on quality of life in patients with heart failure and preserved ejection fraction: the VITALITY-HFpEF randomized clinical trial. JAMA. 2020; 324(15):1512-21.

27. Anker SD, Butler J, Filippatos G, et al. Empagliflozin in heart failure with a preserved ejection fraction. N Engl J Med. 2021;385(16):1451-61.
28. Solomon SD, McMurray JJV, Claggett B, et al. Dapagliflozin in heart failure with mildly reduced or preserved ejection fraction. N Engl J Med. 2022;387(12):1089-98.
29. McDonagh TA, Metra M, Adamo M, et al. 2021 ESC guidelines for the diagnosis and treatment of acute and chronic heart failure. Eur Heart J. 2021;42(36):3599-726.
30. Heidenreich PA, Bozkurt B, Aguilar D, et al. 2022 AHA/ACC/HFSA guideline for the management of heart failure: a report of the American college of cardiology/American heart association joint committee on clinical practice guidelines. Circulation. 2022;145(18):e895-1032.
31. Kittleson MM, Panjrath GS, Amancherla K. 2023 ACC expert consensus decision path way on management of heart failure with preserved ejection fraction: a report of the American College of Cardiology solution set oversight committee. J Am Coll Cardiol. 2023;81(18):1835-78.
32. Borlaug BA, Sharma K, Shah SJ, et al. Heart failure with preserved ejection fraction: JACC scientific statement. J Am Coll Cardiol. 2023;81(18):1810-34.
33. Taqueti VR, Solomon SD, Shah AM, et al. Coronary microvascular dysfunction and future risk of heart failure with preserved ejection fraction. Eur Heart J. 2018;39(10):840-9.
34. Mejia-Renteria H, Lee JM, Choi KH, et al. Coronary microcirculation assessment using functional angiography: development of a wire-free method applicable to conventional coronary angiograms. Catheter Cardiovasc Interv. 2021;98(6):1027-37.
35. Milzi A, Dettori R, Lubberich RK, et al. Coronary microvascular dysfunction as assessed by angiography-derived index of microvascular resistance co-localizes with and may explain the presence of ischemia in stress-cardiac magnetic resonance imaging in the absence of coronary artery disease. Front Cardiovasc Med. 2022;9:1060764.
36. Indorkar R, Kwong RY, Romano S, et al. Global coronary flow reserve measured during stress cardiac magnetic resonance imaging is an independent predictor of adverse cardiovascular events. JACC Cardiovasc Imaging. 2019; 12(8 Pt 2):1686-95.
37. Cohn JN, Johnson G. Heart failure with normal ejection fraction. The V-HeFT study. Veterans administration cooperative study group. Circulation. 1990;81(2 Suppl.): III48-53.
38. Shah KS, Xu H, Matsouaka RA, et al. Heart failure with preserved, borderline, and reduced ejection fraction: 5-year outcomes. J Am Coll Cardiol. 2017;70(20):2476-86.
39. McMurray JJV, Packer M, Desai AS, et al. Angiotensin-neprilysin inhibition versus enalapril in heart failure. N Engl J Med. 2014;371(11):993-1004.
40. Solomon SD, McMurray JJV, Anand IS, et al. Angiotensin-neprilysin inhibition in heart failure with preserved ejection fraction. N Engl J Med. 2019;381(17):1609-20.
41. Ventura HO, Lavie CJ, Mehra MR. Heart failure with preserved ejection fraction: separating the wheat from the chaff. J Am Coll Cardiol. 2020;75(3):255-7.
42. Mentz RJ, Ward JH, Hernandez AF, et al. Angiotensin-neprilysin inhibition in patients with mildly reduced or preserved ejection fraction and worsening heart failure. J Am Coll Cardiol. 2023;82(1):1-12.
43. Heidenreich PA, Bozkurt B, Aguilar D, et al. 2022 AHA/ACC/HFSA guideline for the management of heart failure: a report of the American College of Cardiology/American Heart Association Joint Committee on Clinical Practice Guidelines. J Am Coll Cardiol. 2022;79(17):e263-421.
44. Ajufo E, Nayak A, Mehra MR. Fallacies of using the win ratio in cardiovascular trials: challenges and solutions. JACC Basic Transl Sci. 2023;8(6):720-7.

CHAPTER

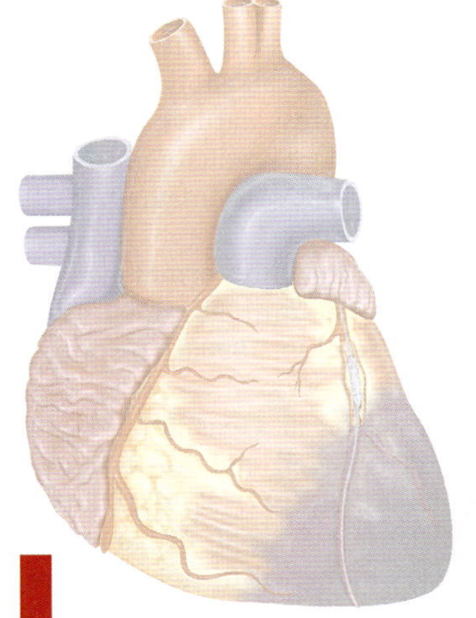

Effect of SGLT2 Inhibitors and ARNI on Increased Left Atrial Stiffness Index in HFpEF

Rahul Mehrotra, Mohit M Bhagwati, Anamika Roy

INTRODUCTION

Heart failure with preserved ejection fraction (HFpEF) represents nearly half of all heart failure cases, characterized by normal left ventricular ejection fraction (LVEF ≥50%) and impaired diastolic function. Left atrial (LA) dysfunction, including increased LA stiffness, is a critical component in the pathophysiology of HFpEF. Elevated LA stiffness index is linked to adverse outcomes such as atrial fibrillation, stroke, and worsening heart failure. Recent pharmacologic advancements, particularly sodium-glucose cotransporter 2 inhibitors (SGLT2i) and angiotensin receptor-neprilysin inhibitors (ARNI), have shown promise in managing HFpEF. This chapter explores the impact of SGLT2i and ARNI on LA stiffness index in HFpEF patients.

PATHOPHYSIOLOGY OF LEFT ATRIAL STIFFNESS IN HEART FAILURE WITH PRESERVED EJECTION FRACTION

The left atrium plays a pivotal role in modulating left ventricular filling and maintaining cardiac output. In HFpEF, elevated filling pressures and diastolic dysfunction lead to LA remodeling and fibrosis, which increase LA stiffness. This pathological alteration contributes to impaired reservoir and conduit function of the LA, promoting atrial fibrillation and further exacerbating heart failure symptoms.

The pathophysiological process underlying increased LA stiffness in HFpEF involves multiple interrelated factors:

- *Elevated left ventricular filling pressures:* Diastolic dysfunction in HFpEF leads to elevated left ventricular filling pressures, which are transmitted backward to the left atrium, causing LA dilation and increased wall stress.
- *LA remodeling:* Chronic pressure overload results in structural remodeling of the LA, characterized by myocyte hypertrophy, interstitial fibrosis, and changes in the extracellular matrix. These changes contribute to increased LA stiffness and impaired LA compliance.
- *Atrial fibrosis:* Fibrosis is a hallmark of atrial remodeling in HFpEF. It disrupts the normal architecture of the atrial myocardium, leading to increased stiffness and reduced contractile function.
- *Inflammation:* Inflammatory processes play a significant role in the development of atrial fibrosis and stiffness. Elevated levels of proinflammatory cytokines and markers of systemic inflammation have been observed in HFpEF patients, correlating with LA dysfunction.
- *Neurohormonal activation:* Activation of the renin-angiotensin-aldosterone system (RAAS) and sympathetic nervous system contributes to LA remodeling and increased stiffness through promoting fibrosis and hypertrophy.

LEFT ATRIAL STIFFNESS INDEX: A KEY INDICATOR IN CARDIOVASCULAR ASSESSMENT

The left atrial stiffness index (LASI) is an emerging parameter in cardiovascular medicine, particularly in the evaluation of atrial function and its impact on various cardiovascular conditions. LASI is calculated by the ratio of left ventricular end-diastolic pressure (LVEDP) to LA strain during the reservoir phase. This index provides insight into the mechanical properties of the left atrium, specifically, its compliance and distensibility, and has gained attention as a prognostic tool in different cardiac pathologies, particularly HFpEF.[1]

The left atrium plays a critical role in modulating left ventricular filling pressures by serving as a reservoir, conduit, and booster pump. In conditions like hypertension, HFpEF, atrial fibrillation (AF), and valvular heart diseases, the left atrium often undergoes remodeling, leading to increased stiffness. This remodeling is characterized by fibrosis, which reduces atrial compliance and impairs its function. LASI, by quantifying this stiffness, reflects the extent of atrial remodeling and provides valuable information about the hemodynamic burden placed on the left atrium.

Clinical relevance of LASI is seen in the following conditions.

- *Heart failure with preserved ejection fraction:* HFpEF is frequently associated with increased LA stiffness. Patients with HFpEF often present with elevated LASI, which correlates with worse outcomes. Studies suggest that LASI can be used to differentiate HFpEF from other forms of heart failure, as well as to predict adverse events such as hospitalizations and mortality in these patients.
- *Atrial fibrillation:* In patients with AF, increased LASI is indicative of atrial remodeling and fibrosis, both of which are critical in the pathogenesis and perpetuation of AF. Higher LASI values have been associated with a greater likelihood of AF recurrence after ablation procedures, making it a potential marker for procedural success, and long-term rhythm outcomes.
- *Valvular heart disease:* In conditions like mitral valve disease, LASI is elevated due to the increased pressure load on the left atrium. This index not only reflects the severity of the disease but also has prognostic implications, as higher LASI values have been linked to poorer postoperative outcomes in patients undergoing valve surgery.
- *Hypertension:* LASI has been shown to be elevated in hypertensive patients even in the absence of overt heart failure or AF. This suggests that LASI could be an early marker of subclinical cardiac dysfunction in hypertensive individuals, potentially guiding early intervention strategies.

MECHANISMS OF ACTION OF SODIUM-GLUCOSE COTRANSPORTER 2 INHIBITORS

The SGLT2 inhibitors, initially developed for glucose control in diabetes mellitus, have shown cardiovascular benefits beyond glycemic control. These benefits are believed to stem from multiple mechanisms, including:

- *Diuresis and natriuresis:* SGLT2i induce diuresis and natriuresis, reducing preload and afterload, which can decrease LA pressure and stiffness. The reduction in intravascular volume and blood pressure helps alleviate the hemodynamic burden on the LA.[2]
- *Reduction in inflammation and fibrosis:* SGLT2i have been shown to reduce myocardial fibrosis and inflammation, which can mitigate LA stiffness. This effect is mediated through mechanisms such as inhibition of the RAAS, reduction in oxidative stress, and modulation of inflammatory pathways.[3]
- *Improved myocardial energetics:* By shifting substrate utilization from glucose to ketones, SGLT2i may enhance myocardial energetics, improving overall cardiac function. This metabolic shift is associated with reduced myocardial oxygen demand and improved efficiency of cardiac muscle cells.[4]

MECHANISMS OF ACTION OF ANGIOTENSIN RECEPTOR-NEPRILYSIN INHIBITORS

The ARNI, combining an angiotensin receptor blocker (valsartan) with a neprilysin inhibitor (sacubitril), addresses neuro hormonal activation in heart failure. The therapeutic effects on LA stiffness include:

- *Neurohormonal modulation:* ARNI reduces the detrimental effects of angiotensin II and increases beneficial natriuretic peptides, leading to vasodilation and reduced cardiac remodeling. By blocking angiotensin II receptors and inhibiting neprilysin, ARNI lowers blood pressure, reduces cardiac afterload, and mitigates RAAS-mediated fibrosis.[5]
- *Reduction of myocardial fibrosis:* By inhibiting neprilysin, ARNI increases the levels of natriuretic peptides, which have antifibrotic properties, thereby reducing LA fibrosis and stiffness. Natriuretic peptides promote vasodilation, natriuresis, and inhibition of myocardial fibrosis, contributing to improved diastolic function and reduced LA stiffness.[6]
- *Enhanced diastolic function*: ARNI improves diastolic function by reducing ventricular stiffness and improving ventricular relaxation. This, in turn, reduces the backward pressure transmission to the LA, alleviating LA stiffness.

CLINICAL EVIDENCE ON SODIUM-GLUCOSE COTRANSPORTER 2 INHIBITORS IN HEART FAILURE WITH PRESERVED EJECTION FRACTION

Several clinical trials and studies have assessed the impact of SGLT2i on HFpEF, focusing on LA function and stiffness **(Table 1)**:

- *EMPEROR-preserved trial:* This pivotal trial demonstrated that empagliflozin significantly reduced the composite outcome of cardiovascular death or hospitalization for heart failure in HFpEF patients. The trial also noted improvements in LA function, suggesting a potential reduction in LA stiffness.[7] In a subanalysis, empagliflozin was shown to decrease LA volume index and improve LA strain, indicating reduced LA stiffness.
- *DAPA-HF and DELIVER trials:* Studies with dapagliflozin showed similar benefits, including improved diastolic function and potential reductions in LA stiffness. In the DELIVER trial, dapagliflozin significantly reduced the risk of cardiovascular death and worsening heart failure in patients with HFpEF, with secondary analyses suggesting improvements in LA function and stiffness.[8,9]
- *Mechanistic studies:* Mechanistic studies have provided insights into how SGLT2i improve LA function. These studies suggest that SGLT2i reduce LA stiffness through a combination of hemodynamic effects, reduction in myocardial fibrosis, and improved myocardial energetics.[3]

CLINICAL EVIDENCE ON ANGIOTENSIN RECEPTOR-NEPRILYSIN INHIBITORS IN HEART FAILURE WITH PRESERVED EJECTION FRACTION

Clinical trials evaluating ARNI in HFpEF have also highlighted its beneficial effects on LA stiffness and overall cardiac function **(Table 2)**:

- *PARAGON-HF trial:* This trial compared sacubitril/valsartan with valsartan alone in HFpEF patients. Although it did not meet its primary endpoint, secondary analyses indicated improvements in LA size and function, suggesting a reduction in LA stiffness. The trial demonstrated that ARNI reduced NT-proBNP levels, improved quality of life, and decreased LA volume index, indicative of reduced LA stiffness.[9]
- *PARAMOUNT trial:* This earlier phase II trial demonstrated that ARNI significantly reduced NT-proBNP levels and LA volumes, markers associated with decreased LA stiffness. The PARAMOUNT trial provided the initial evidence supporting the beneficial effects of ARNI on LA remodeling and function in HFpEF.[6]
- *Real-world evidence:* Real-world studies have corroborated the findings from clinical trials, showing that ARNI improves diastolic function, reduces LA volume, and over all cardiac remodeling in HF patients. These studies suggest that ARNI can be effectively used in routine clinical practice to manage LA stiffness in HFpEF.[10]

TABLE 1: Summary of key clinical trials on sodium-glucose cotransporter 2 inhibitors in heart failure with preserved ejection fraction.

Trial	*Drug*	*Primary endpoint*	*Results*	*Secondary outcomes related to left atrial (LA) stiffness*
EMPEROR-Preserved	Empagliflozin	Cardiovascular (CV) death or heart failure (HF) hospitalization	Reduced by 21%	Improvement in LA function, decreased LA volume index
DELIVER	Dapagliflozin	CV death or HF hospitalization	Reduced by 18%	Improved diastolic function, potential reduction in LA stiffness

TABLE 2: Summary of key clinical trials on angiotensin receptor-neprilysin inhibitors (ARNI) in heart failure with preserved ejection fraction.

Trial	*Drug*	*Primary endpoint*	*Results*	*Secondary outcomes related to left atrial (LA) stiffness*
PARAGON-HF	Sacubitril/valsartan	Total heart failure (HF) hospitalizations and cardiovascular (CV) death	Did not meet primary endpoint	Reduction in LA volume index, improved LA function
PARAMOUNT	Sacubitril/valsartan	Change in N-terminal-prohormone B-type natriuretic peptide (NT-proBNP) levels	Significant reduction	Decreased LA volumes, indicative of reduced LA stiffness

COMBINATION THERAPY: SODIUM-GLUCOSE COTRANSPORTER 2 INHIBITORS AND ANGIOTENSIN RECEPTOR-NEPRILYSIN INHIBITORS

The combination of SGLT2i and ARNI may offer synergistic benefits in reducing LA stiffness in HFpEF:

- *Complementary mechanisms:* SGLT2i and ARNI target different pathophysiological pathways, potentially providing additive effects in reducing LA stiffness and improving diastolic function. SGLT2i primarily exert their effects through diuresis, natriuresis, and metabolic modulation, while ARNI acts through neurohormonal modulation and antifibrotic effects.
- *Improved outcomes:* Preliminary data suggest that combined therapy can lead to better clinical outcomes, including reduced hospitalization rates and improved quality of life in HFpEF patients. The combination therapy may enhance LA function, reduce LA stiffness, and improve overall cardiac performance.[11]
- *Enhanced diastolic function:* The combination of SGLT2i and ARNI may synergistically improve diastolic function by reducing ventricular stiffness, improving ventricular relaxation and alleviating LA stiffness. This multifaceted approach addresses the complex pathophysiology of HFpEF more comprehensively than monotherapy.

POTENTIAL MECHANISTIC INSIGHTS FROM PRECLINICAL STUDIES

Preclinical studies offer valuable insights into how SGLT2i and ARNI may synergistically reduce LA stiffness **(Table 3)**:

- *Animal models:* Studies in animal models of HFpEF have shown that SGLT2i and ARNI can reduce LA fibrosis and improve diastolic function. These preclinical models provide a mechanistic basis for the observed clinical benefits of SGLT2i and ARNI on LA stiffness.[12]
- *Molecular pathways:* Research indicates that these agents modulate key molecular pathways involved in inflammation, fibrosis, and oxidative stress, contributing to reduced LA stiffness. For instance, SGLT2i have been shown to inhibit the TGF-β signaling pathway, which is a key mediator of fibrosis, while ARNI increases levels of natriuretic peptides, which have antifibrotic properties.[13]

TABLE 3: Mechanisms of action of sodium-glucose cotransporter 2 inhibitors (SGLT2i) and angiotensin receptor-neprilysin inhibitors (ARNI) on LA stiffness.

Mechanism	*SGLT2i*	*ARNI*
Diuresis and natriuresis	✓	✓
Reduction in inflammation and fibrosis	✓	✓
Improved myocardial energetics	✓	×
Neurohormonal modulation	×	✓
Reduction of myocardial fibrosis	✓	✓
Enhanced diastolic function	✓	✓

PRACTICAL CONSIDERATIONS IN CLINICAL MANAGEMENT

Implementing SGLT2i and ARNI in the management of HFpEF requires careful consideration:

- *Patient selection:* Identifying patients with significant LA stiffness who are likely to benefit from these therapies is crucial. Echocardiographic assessment and biomarkers can aid in this process. Parameters such as LA volume index, LA strain, and NT-proBNP levels can help identify patients with elevated LA stiffness who may benefit from SGLT2i and ARNI therapy.
- *Dosing and monitoring:* Optimal dosing and monitoring for potential side effects, such as hypotension and renal dysfunction, are essential to maximize benefits and minimize risks. Regular monitoring of renal function, electrolytes, and blood pressure is necessary to ensure patient safety. Adjustments in medication doses may be required based on individual patient responses and tolerability.[8]
- *Combination therapy:* When considering combination therapy with SGLT2i and ARNI, it is important to start with low doses and titrate gradually to avoid adverse effects. Coordination between cardiologists and primary care providers is crucial to ensure appropriate monitoring and follow-up.
- *Patient education:* Educating patients about the benefits and potential side effects of SGLT2i and ARNI is important for adherence and successful management. Patients should be informed about the signs and symptoms of hypotension, electrolyte imbalances, and renal dysfunction, and encouraged to report any adverse effects promptly.
- *Lifestyle modifications:* In addition to pharmacologic therapy, lifestyle modifications such as dietary changes, weight management, and regular physical activity should be encouraged to optimize cardiovascular health and reduce LA stiffness. These nonpharmacologic interventions can complement the effects of SGLT2i and ARNI and improve overall outcomes in HFpEF patients.

FUTURE DIRECTIONS

Ongoing research and future studies will continue to elucidate the role of SGLT2i and ARNI in managing LA stiffness in HFpEF:

- *Large-scale trials:* Further large-scale randomized trials are needed to confirm the long-term benefits and safety of combined therapy in HFpEF patients. These trials should include diverse populations to ensure generalizability of the findings.
- *Biomarker development:* Developing and validating biomarkers for LA stiffness can enhance patient stratification and treatment monitoring. Biomarkers such as LA strain, fibrosis markers, and circulating natriuretic peptides can help identify patients who are most likely to benefit from SGLT2i and ARNI therapy and monitor their response to treatment.
- *Mechanistic studies:* Mechanistic studies exploring the molecular and cellular pathways modulated by SGLT2i and ARNI can provide deeper insights into their effects on LA stiffness. Understanding the precise mechanisms of action can guide the development of more targeted therapies and optimize treatment strategies.
- *Combination therapy trials:* Clinical trials specifically designed to evaluate the combination of SGLT2i and ARNI in HFpEF are needed to determine the optimal dosing, safety, and efficacy of this approach. These trials should assess clinical outcomes, LA function, and patient-reported outcomes to provide a comprehensive evaluation of combination therapy.
- *Real-world evidence:* Real-world studies and registries can provide valuable information on the effectiveness and safety of SGLT2i and ARNI in routine clinical practice. These studies can complement randomized trials and provide insights into the long-term impact of these therapies on LA stiffness and HFpEF outcomes.

CONCLUSION

The LA stiffness index is a valuable, noninvasive marker that provides critical information about the mechanical properties of the left atrium. It holds significant prognostic value across a spectrum of cardiovascular diseases, particularly in conditions characterized by atrial remodeling and fibrosis. As research continues to evolve, LASI may become an integral part of routine cardiovascular assessment, aiding in the diagnosis, risk stratification, and management of patients with heart disease.

The management of increased LA stiffness in HFpEF remains a clinical challenge. Emerging evidence suggests that SGLT2i and ARNI can positively impact LA stiffness and improve clinical outcomes in HFpEF patients. The combination of these therapies offers a promising strategy, leveraging their complementary mechanisms to address the multifaceted pathophysiology of HFpEF. Ongoing research will further clarify their roles and optimize treatment paradigms for this complex condition.

REFERENCES

1. Kim D, Seo JH, Choi KH, et al. Prognostic Implications of Left Atrial Stiffness Index in Heart Failure Patients With Preserved Ejection Fraction. JACC Cardiovasc Imaging. 2023;16(4):435-45.
2. Verma S, McMurray JJV. SGLT2 inhibitors and mechanisms of cardiovascular benefit: a state-of-the-art review. Diabetologia. 2018;61(10):2108-17.
3. Kolijn D, Pabel S, Tian Y, et al. Empagliflozin improves endothelial and cardiomyocyte function in human heart failure with preserved ejection fraction via reduced pro-inflammatory-oxidative pathways and protein kinase Gα oxidation. Cardiovasc Res. 2021;117(2):495-507.
4. Ferrannini E, Mark M, Mayoux E. CV Protection in the EMPA-REG OUTCOME Trial: A "Thrifty Substrate" Hypothesis. Diabetes Care. 2016;39(7):1108-14.
5. Solomon SD, McMurray JJV, Anand IS, et al. Angiotensin-Neprilysin Inhibition in Heart Failure with Preserved Ejection Fraction. N Engl J Med. 2019;381(17):1609-20.
6. Solomon SD, Zile M, Pieske B, et al. Prospective comparison of ARNI with ARB on Management Of heart failure with preserved ejection fraction (PARAMOUNT) Investigators. The angiotensin receptor neprilysin inhibitor LCZ696 in heart failure with preserved ejection fraction: a phase 2 double-blind randomised controlled trial. Lancet. 2012; 380(9851):1387-95.
7. Anker SD, Butler J, Filippatos G, et al. Empagliflozin in Heart Failure with a Preserved Ejection Fraction. N Engl J Med. 2021;385(16):1451-61.
8. McMurray JJV, Solomon SD, Inzucchi SE, et al. Dapagliflozin in Patients with Heart Failure and Reduced Ejection Fraction. N Engl J Med. 2019;381(21):1995-2008.
9. Solomon SD, Vaduganathan M, L Claggett B, et al. Sacubitril/Valsartan Across the Spectrum of Ejection Fraction in Heart Failure. Circulation. 2020;141(5):352-61.
10. Paolini C, Mugnai G, Dalla Valle C, et al. Effects and clinical implications of sacubitril/valsartan on left ventricular reverse remodeling in patients affected by chronic heart failure: A 24-month follow-up. Int J Cardiol Heart Vasc. 2021;35:100821.
11. Docherty KF, Jhund PS, Inzucchi SE, et al. Effects of dapagliflozin in DAPA-HF according to background heart failure therapy. Eur Heart J. 2020;41(25):2379-92.
12. Chin KL, Ofori-Asenso R, Hopper I, et al. Potential mechanisms underlying the cardiovascular benefits of sodium glucose cotransporter 2 inhibitors: a systematic review of data from preclinical studies. Cardiovasc Res. 2019;115(2):266-76.
13. Lam CS, Roger VL, Rodeheffer RJ, et al. Pulmonary hypertension in heart failure with preserved ejection fraction: a community-based study. J Am Coll Cardiol. 2009;53(13):1119-26.

CHAPTER 61

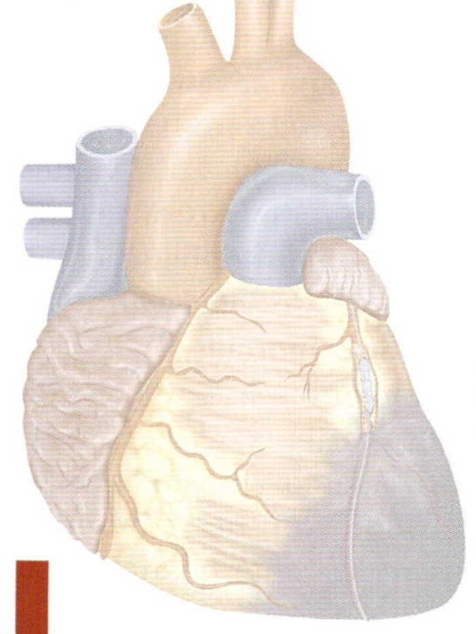

Atrial Dysfunction: Echocardiographic Evaluation in Patients with HFpEF and AF

Hansa Gupta, Madhu Mary, Ranjan Kumar

INTRODUCTION

With spurt in cardiometabolic diseases, there is a rise in cases of heart failure with preserved ejection fraction (HEpEF). It is an entity wherein person is in clinical heart failure with LVEF ≥50% due to intermittent or sustained elevation in left ventricular filling pressure (LVFP).

Left atrial (LA) dysfunction due to remodeling of LA is the result of raised LVFP.

Hence, there is a resurgence of interest toward assessment of LA size and function with various emerging softwares in the echocardiography machine so as to detect the impact of raised LVFP on LA dysfunction relatively quickly, noninvasively in an affordable way. Echocardiography can help the clinicians in establishing their diagnosis of HFpEF over and above the clinical examination.

Several noninvasive indices have been studied over a period of time which shall be discussed subsequently.

STANDARD ECHOCARDIOGRAPHIC PARAMETERS

Left Atrial Size

Left atrial size is an indicator of severity and chronicity of LA pressure elevation and LV diastolic dysfunction in absence of mitral valve disease, AF, conduction defects, etc.[1] **(Figs. 1A to C)**.

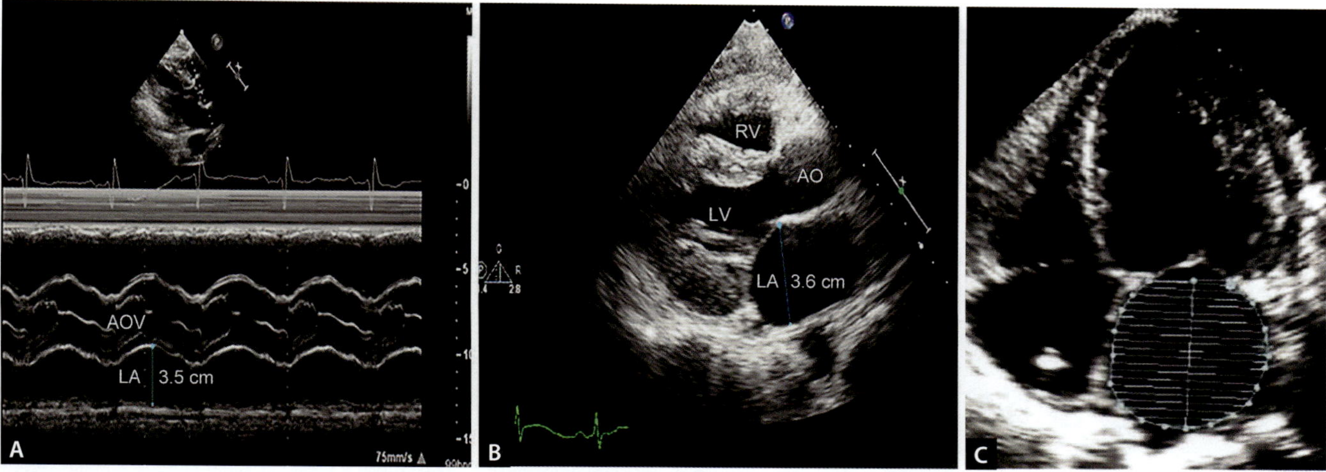

Figs. 1A to C: (A) LA size in M-mode; (B) 2D-PLAX; (C) LA area in 4C.

Left atrial size is best measured from M-mode and 2-dimensional echocardiography (2DE). The LA size is measured at its maximum diameter in PLAX view (anterior-posterior diameter) perpendicular to the aortic root long axis and at the level of the aortic sinuses by using the leading edge to leading edge convention at the end of ventricular systole (end of T-wave on ECG). Normal reference values are 27–38 mm in women and 30–40 mm in men.[2]

But because of the asymmetrical geometry, insertion of pulmonary veins and the presence of LA appendage, the exact dimension estimation is not very reliable.

Left Atrial Volume

Left atrial volume (LAV) is considered the current gold standard for quantifying LA size, which is considered as the glycosylated hemoglobin of LA dysfunction.

The current guidelines recommend the biplane Simpson's method for estimating LAV instead of biplane area length method which was cumbersome.

Left atrial volume is measured by obtaining the endocardial tracings of the blood–tissue interface on apical 4C and 2C chamber views (excluding LA appendage and pulmonary veins) at the end systole when LA is at its maximum size. At the mitral valve level, the tracing is closed by connecting the two opposite ends of the mitral annulus with a straight line. LA volume then calculated and divided by body surface area to obtain the LAV index (normal LAVi <34 mL/m^2).

Left atrial volume can be calculated using the disk summation technique by adding the volume of a stack of cylinders of height "h" and area calculated by orthogonal minor and major transverse axes (D1 and D2) assuming an oval shape: $\frac{\pi}{4h\Sigma}(D1)(D2)$

The 3D method is a promising robust method of LAV measurement as no geometric assumptions are made. The data sets can be obtained from the apical views using a multibeat full-volume acquisition **(Figs. 2A to C)**.

It shows excellent correlation with the LAVI values derived from CT and CMR.[3] A meta-analysis of several studies including patients with HF showed that each 10 mL/m^2 increase in baseline LAVI was associated with a 22% increased adjusted hazard of all-cause mortality.[4]

LAVI can also be used to monitor disease progression in HFpEF. In a study of 409 patients with HFpEF, improvement in LAVI was associated with lower rate of HF-hospitalization over a follow-up of 22 months, as compared to the patients with stable or increased LAVI.[5]

Increase LAVI is a strong predictor of new-onset AF or AF recurrence after radiofrequency ablation.

Limitations

Although LAVI has been an important measure of LA remodeling, it has several limitations. The use of improper views and incorrect endocardial border tracing can lead to measurement variability. In addition, the time and effort required to perform LAVI estimation discourages its routine measurement. Several different techniques such as the use of three-dimensional echocardiography and automated image recognition and analysis are being developed to overcome these challenges.[6-8]

Another limitation of LAVI is that it is not sensitive to detect milder forms of LV diastolic dysfunction. It is also not responsive to dynamic changes in the LVFP. In addition due to the complex nature of HFpEF, the relationship between LAVI and LVFP is not perfect. A significant scatter has been found between LAVI and LVFP in patients with HFpEF.[9] This has been also reflected in a

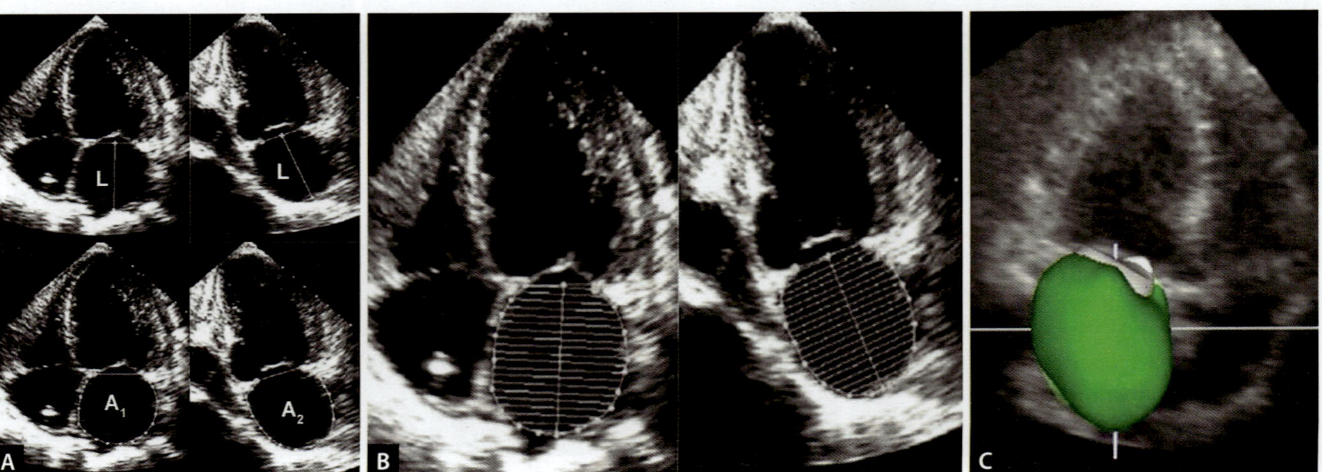

Figs. 2A to C: (A) Area length technique; (B) Biplane method of discs; (C) 3D data sets.

relatively inconsistent correlation between LAVI and other echocardiographic parameters in HFpEF.[10]

Left Atrial Function

Volumetric Methods

These methods can be used to assess LA reservoir, conduit, and booster pump functions by obtaining LA volume at their maximum, V_{max} (just before mitral valve opening, at end-systole) and minimum, V_{min} (when the mitral valve closes, at end-diastole), and immediately before atrial systole, V_p (before the P-wave on ECG). From these volumes, total, passive, and active ejection (or emptying) fractions can be calculated. LA active volumes are:

LA reservoir volume or LA filling volume (LAFV) $= V_{max} - V_{min}$;

LA conduit volume or LA passive emptying volume $= V_{max} - V_p$

LA contractile volume $= V_p - V_{min}$[11]

The difference between maximum and minimum LA volume divided by the minimum LA volume is used as index of atrial compliance.[12]

Doppler Method: Transmitral Flow and Pulmonary Flow

The pattern of mitral inflow exhibits a "E wave," which reveals passive ventricular filling in early diastole and "A wave," which reveals the late active filling phase during atrial contraction and depends on LA systolic function, LV compliance, and AV conduction[13] **(Figs. 3A to C)**.

We place the sample volume at the tips of the mitral leaflets in 4C view.

In early LV diastolic dysfunction, LV filling decreases during early diastole, and LA contracts extra to maintain an adequate LV output. As LV dysfunction progresses, LA pressure increases, and the contribution due to LA contraction decreases. LV filling during early diastole begins earlier and lasts for a short time. Later, LA pump function reduces because it has to work against high LV late diastolic pressure; hence, peak A wave velocity is reduced. Also, some blood flows back in the pulmonary veins from LA at this stage.

To measure pulmonary venous flow, the sample volume is placed into any pulmonary veins in 4C view **(Figs. 4A and B)**. We can measure peak systolic (S) velocity, peak anterograde diastolic (D) velocity, and peak atrial reversal (Ar) velocity.

- An increase in mean LA pressure will reverse the normal pattern of S/D >1, to S/D ratio <1 with a diastolic filling predominance.
- Ar velocity, exceeding 35 cm/s implies elevated filling pressures.

Tissue Doppler Imaging and 2D Speckle Tracking Echocardiography to Measure LA Myocardial Deformation (Fig. 5)

Strain and strain rate measure the extent and the rate of myocardial deformation, respectively by TDI or 2-D speckle-tracking echocardiography.

It is used to evaluate global and regional LA function.[14]

The sample volume is placed at mitral annulus in 4C and 2C apical views to obtain systolic (S), early diastolic (E′), and late diastolic (A′) velocities. Peak velocity in late diastole secondary to atrial contraction (A′) is shown to be marker of atrial function[15] is reduced in diseased states associated with LA dysfunction.

The technical challenges of TDI-based strain rate imaging is that it is sensitive to both translational motion and the interrogating angle.[16]

Speckle tracking echocardiography (STE) is the latest imaging technique that has been used to quantify and prognosticate cardiac functions. LA strain (LAS) is used to assess LA phasic physiology in which 2D tracking of speckles, or acoustic markers of myocardium, is performed via automated software. The software

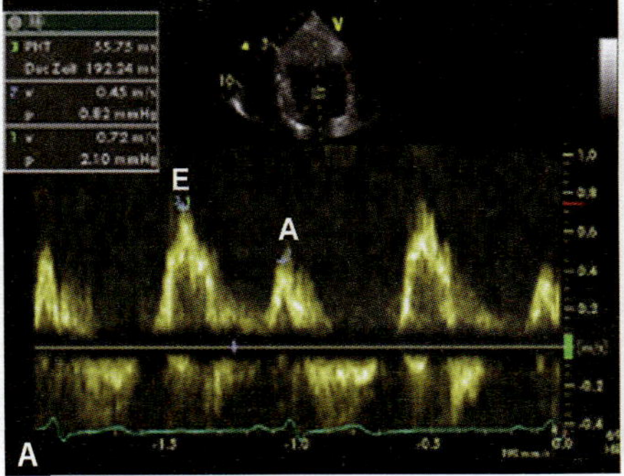

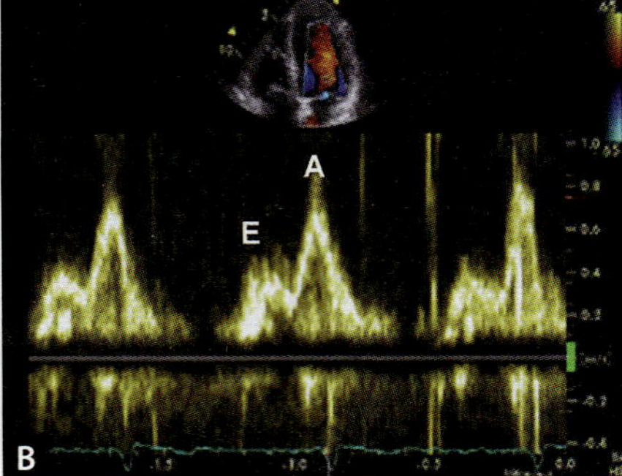

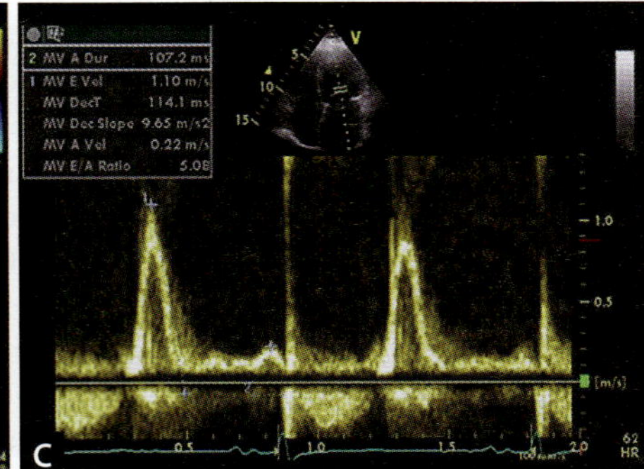

Figs. 3A to C: Mitral inflow pattern.

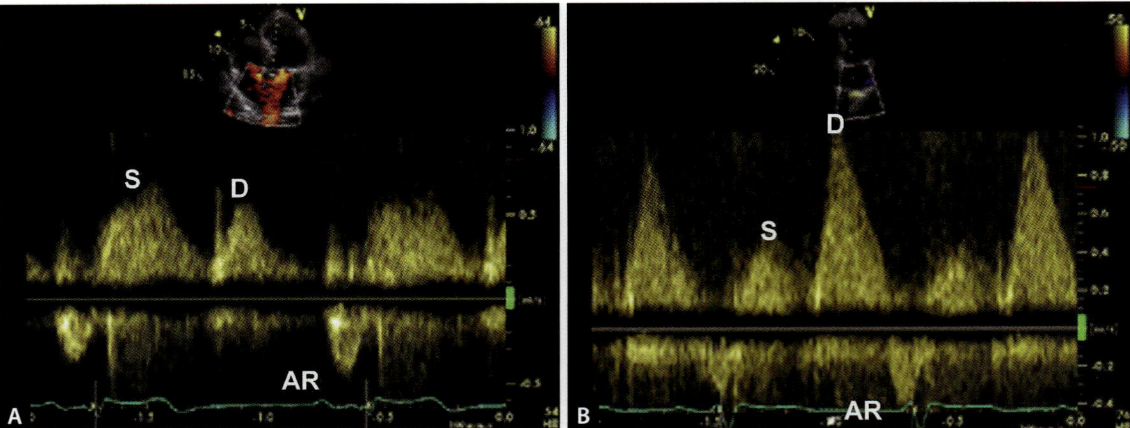

Figs. 4A and B: Pulmonary venous flow.

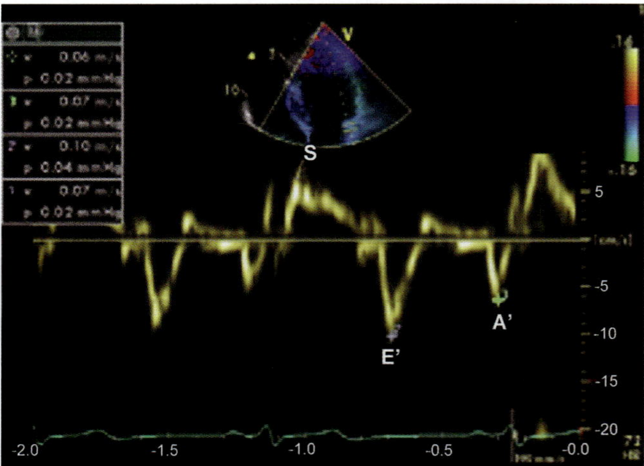

Fig. 5: Tissue Doppler.

constructs a longitudinal strain and strain rate curve for each segment and denotes the integral functionality and interdependence of the LA and LV.

To assess LA strain an apical, a non-foreshortened 4C view is obtained **(Fig. 6)**. The reference time point would be the LV end-diastole (strain = zero) as determined by the mitral valve inflow. The automated software requires users to define the atrial wall/endocardial border to perform calculations. LA deformation may be assessed by means of two peaks: maximum deformation also known as reservoir stain which is the peak strain before the opening of the mitral valve during the LV systole; booster strain or contractile strain is the strain at the ventricular end-diastole minus the strain at the onset of atrial contraction. Conduit strain is defined as the difference between booster and reservoir strain.[17] STE is not as load or angle dependent as tissue Doppler imaging.[18]

Normal values currently accepted are the following:[19]

- Reservoir strain 39% (95% confidence interval: 38–41%)
- Conduit strain 23% (95% confidence interval: 21–25%)
- Contractile strain 17% (95% confidence interval: 16–19%)

Addition of LA reservoir strain (LARS) increases the sensitivity to detect LV diastolic dysfunction compared to conventional parameters.[20] Reduced LARS (<23%) is significantly associated with worst functional class even when LAVI was normal. LA strain impairment occurs earlier than the increase in LA size and is more responsive to changes in LVFP.

Atrial Function in Heart Failure with Preserved EF and Atrial Fibrillation

Left atrial reservoir function contributes majorly to cardiac output. In LV dysfunction, the LA reservoir function gets affected due to reduced LV longitudinal systolic shortening. To compensate, the LA pump function becomes more active to help the diseased LV to accommodate more blood and maintain adequate cardiac output (by Frank Starling mechanism)[21] In AF, this compensation does not occur; hence, there is increased incidence of heart failure.[22]

Left atrial reservoir strain is another complimentary parameter to assess high filling pressure. A value <18% corresponded to an increased LVFP.[23]

In HFpEF, patients who develop AF, LAS is reduced. Moreover, peak atrial contractile strain (PACS), peak atrial longitudinal strain (PALS), and LAVi show a high predictive value for occurrence of AF in HFpEF.[24]

In 2021, Jasic-Szpak et al. demonstrated that LAS indices, mainly LA booster strain and LARS, can help to predict the development of AF in patients with HFpEF.[24]

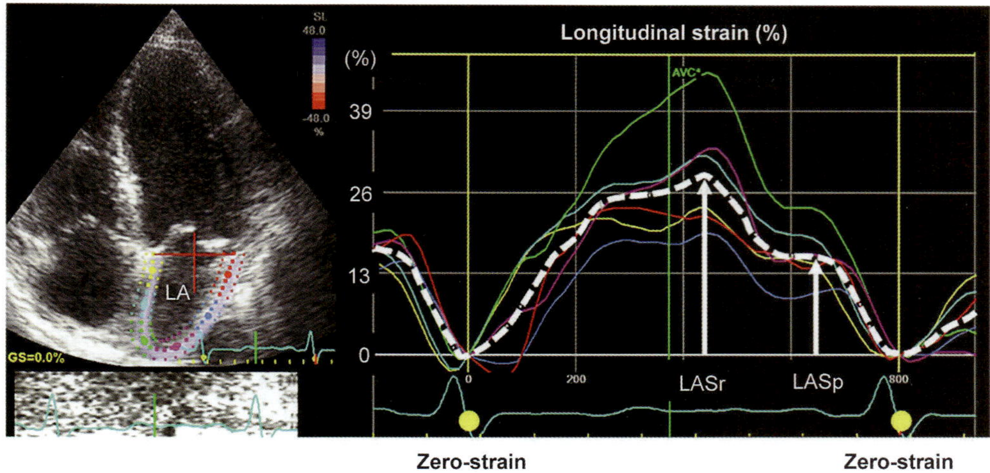

Fig. 6: Longitudinal strain.

SUMMARY

Echo indices s/o elevated LVFP and moderately severe LV dysfunction:

- Mitral E/A ratio is >2
- Average E/e' >14
- Peak TR velocity >2.8 ms
- Ar velocity –>35 cm/sec
- Ar duration exceeds transmitral "A" wave duration by >30 ms
- LAVi >34 mL/m ^{2}
- LA reservoir strain <18%

CONCLUSION

Left atrial enlargement is virtually diagnostic of advanced LV diastolic dysfunction. LA size (LA diameter in older studies and LAVI in recent studies) is a strong predictor of cardiovascular outcomes. It is associated with increased risk of HF, AF, hospitalizations, stroke, and all-cause mortality. LAVI can be used to monitor disease progression in HFpEF. LA strain, in addition, significantly enhances the sensitivity to detect LV diastolic dysfunction and occurrence of AF.

Timely assessment of LA dysfunction can help in risk stratification and early preventive and therapeutic intervention to reduce morbidity and mortality related to heart failure.

REFERENCES

1. Tsang TSM, Barnes ME, Gersh BJ, et al. Left atrial volume as a morphophysiologic expression of left ventricular diastolic dysfunction and relation to cardiovascular risk burden. Am J Cardiol. 2002;90(12):1284-9.
2. Vyas H, Jackson K, Chenzbraun A. Switching to volumetric left atrial measurements: Impact on routine echocardiographic practice. Eur J Echocardiogr. 2011; 12:107-11.
3. Rohner A, Brinkert M, Kawel N, et al. Functional assessment of the left atrium by real-time three-dimensional echocardiography using a novel dedicated analysis tool: Initial validation studies in comparison with computed tomography. Eur J Echocardiogr. 2011;12(7):497-505.
4. Ramu B, Elwan AM, Coleman CI, et al. The association between baseline left atrial volume index and all cause mortality in patients with heart failure: Meta-analysis. Conn Med. 2015;79:469-75.
5. Hao Z, Xu G, Yuan M, et al. The predictive value of changes in left atrial volume index for rehospitalization in heart failure with preserved ejection fraction. Clin Cardiol. 2023;46:151-8.
6. Canciello G, de Simone G, Izzo R, et al. Validation of left atrial volume estimation by left atrial diameter form the parasternal long axis view. J Am Soc Echocardiogr. 2017;30:262-9.
7. HU J, Olaisen SH, Smistad E, et al. Automated 2-D and 3-D left atrial volume measurements using deep learning. Ultrasound Med Biol. 2024;50:47-56.
8. Takeuchi M, Nabeshima Y, Kitano T, et al. Prognostic value of the left ventricular - left atrial volume ration assessed using three-dimensional echocardiography with fully automated analytical software. J Cardiol. 2021;78: 406-12.
9. Hoshida S, Watanabe T, Shinoda Y, et al. Considerable scatter in the relationship between left atrial volume and pressure in heart failure with preserved left ventricular ejection fraction. Sci Rep. 2020;10:90.
10. Gehlken C, Screever EM, Suthahar N, et al. Left atrial volume and left ventricular mass indices in heart failure with preserved and reduced ejection fraction. ESC Heart Fail. 2021;8:2458-66.

11. Lang RM, Bierig M, Devereux RB, et al. Recommendations for chamber quantification: a report from the American Society of Echocardiography's Guidelines and Standards Committee and the Chamber Quantification Writing Group, developed in conjunction with the European Association of Echocardiography, a branch of the European Society of Cardiology. J Am Soc Echocardiogr. 2005;18(12):1440-63.
12. Salvo GD, Caso P, Piccolo RL, et al. Atrial myocardial deformation properties predict maintenance of sinus rhythm after external cardioversion of recent-onset lone atrial fibrillation: a color Doppler myocardial imaging and transthoracic and transesophageal echocardiographic study. Circulation. 2005;112(3):387-95.
13. Choong CY, Herrmann HC, Weyman AE, et al. Preload dependence of Doppler-derived indexes of left ventricular diastolic function in humans. J Am Coll Cardiol. 1987;10(4):800-8.
14. Zhang Q, Yip GWK, Yu CM. Approaching regional left atrial function by tissue Doppler velocity and strain imaging. Europace. 2008;10 Suppl 3:iii62-9.
15. Hesse B, Schuele SU, Thamilasaran M, et al. A rapid method to quantify left atrial contractile function: Doppler tissue imaging of the mitral annulus during atrial systole. Eur J Echocardiogr. 2004;5(1):86-92.
16. Hoit BD. Left atrial size and function: Role in prognosis. J Am Coll Cardiol. 2014;63:493-505.
17. Badano LP, Badano LP, Kolias TJ, et al. Standardization of left atrial, right ventricular, and right atrial deformation imaging using two-dimensional speckle tracking echocardiography: a consensus document of the EACVI/ASE/industry task force to standardize deformation imaging. Eur Heart J Cardiovasc Imaging. 2018;19(6):591-600.
18. Molnár A, Merkely B. The added value of atrial strain assessment in clinical practice. Diagnostics. 2022;12: 982.
19. Pathan F, D'Elia N, Nolan MT, et al. Normal ranges of left atrial strain by speckle-tracking echocardiography: A systematic review and meta-analysis. J Am Soc Echocardiogr. 2017;30(1):59-70.e8.
20. Morris DA, Belyavskiy E, Aravind-Kumar R, et al. Potential usefulness and clinical relevance of adding left atrial strain to left atrial volume index in detection of left ventricular diastolic dysfunction. JACC Cardivasc imaging. 2018;11:1405-15.
21. Suga H. Importance of atrial compliance in cardiac performance. Circ Res. 1974;35(1):39-43.
22. Benjamin EJ, Levy D, Vaziri SM, et al. Independent risk factors for atrial fibrillation in a population-based cohort. The Framingham Heart Study. JAMA. 1994;271(11):840-4.
23. Smiseth OA, Morris DA, Cardim N, et al. Multimodality imaging in patients with heart failure and preserved ejection fraction: An expert consensus document of the European Association of Cardiovascular Imaging. Eur Heart J Cardiovasc Imaging. 2022;23(2):e34-e61.
24. Jasic-Szpak E, Jasic-Szpak E, Marwick TH, et al. Prediction of AF in heart failure with preserved ejection fraction: Incremental value of left atrial strain. JACC Cardiovasc Imaging. 2021;14(1):131-44.

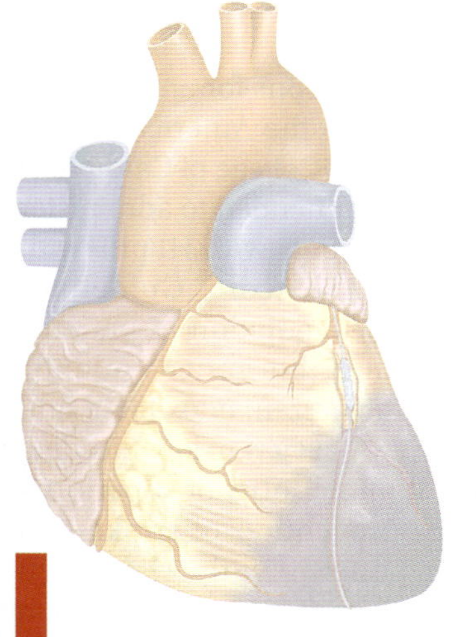

Deciphering the Dilemma: Anticoagulation for HFpEF with AF

Jabir Abdullakutty, Vijin Joseph

INTRODUCTION

This chapter discusses about the need for anticoagulation in the management of heart failure with preserved ejection fraction (HFpEF) in patients with atrial fibrillation (AF). There is a lot of dilemma about whether to give anticoagulation to all patients who suffer from HFpEF and AF. They are associated with old age, hypertension, and diastolic dysfunction, which increases in prevalence and usually coexist. The combination of these two can increase the risk of stroke and heart failure (HF) hospitalization. It is very difficult to differentiate whether HFpEF or AF comes first.[1] So the therapeutic strategy is based on risk classification and individualized therapy choices. This review emphasizes the need for the best use of anticoagulation in HFpEF with AF so that it successfully helps manage thromboembolic risk and reduce bleeding consequences in these patients. Finally, this will improve the prognosis and quality of life for patients who suffer from this difficult and mysterious ailment.[2]

DESCRIPTION

Heart failure can be classified into three types: (1) Heart failure with reduced ejection fraction (HFrEF ≤40%), (2) heart failure with mildly reduced ejection fraction (HFmrEF 41–49%), and (3) HFpEF ≥50%. Here we mainly describe the incidence and prevalence of HFpEF with AF and vice versa. There are few studies that describe the incidence and prevalence of HFpEF with AF. One such study is the PREVEND (Prevention of Renal and Vascular End-stage Disease) study, where the incidence of HFpEF per 1,000 person-years was 4.90 for those with AF versus 0.85 for those without AF.[3] Other studies and registries show that the prevalence of HFpEF with AF varies between 8 and 24%. In the Framingham Heart Study, AF was identified as a major risk factor for new-onset HFpEF. This study also shows that HFpEF has a higher incidence in women compared with men.[3]

Similarly, the incidence and prevalence of AF with HFpEF in the Framingham Heart Study were six times higher. In HFpEF, the prevalence of AF varies between 15 and 41%. In four major trials such as AFFIRM, REALISE-AF, EORP-AF Pilot, and RACE II trial, the prevalence of HFpEF in AF was 8, 18, 17, and 24%, respectively.[1] In seven major trials such as OPTIMIZE-HF, ADHERE, EuroHF Survey, New York HF Registry, MISCHF, I-PRESERVE, and CHARM-Preserved, the prevalence of AF in HFpEF was 33, 21, 25, 23, 29, 29, and 29%, respectively. A recent study showed that patients with HFpEF were more likely to have prevalent AF compared to patients with HFrEF.[4]

Shared Mechanism for Heart Failure with Preserved Ejection Fraction and Atrial Fibrillation

There are certain risk factors that predispose to both; they are advanced age, hypertension, obesity, and sleep apnea.

The main mechanism by which HFpEF gives rise to AF is via structural and functional remodeling of the left atrium (LA). In HFpEF, there is larger LA volume, reduced emptying fractions, and contractile reserve. LA enlargement in HFpEF is associated with atrial fibrosis, which contributes to electrical remodeling, increased atrial refractoriness, and the development of AF.[1]

The mechanism by which AF gives rise to HFpEF is by causing LA dilation, impaired atrial function, and atrial fibrosis. AF can also be associated with LV myocardial fibrosis, which results in diastolic dysfunction and HFpEF. Furthermore, atrioventricular annular remodeling with progressive mitral and tricuspid regurgitation and depletion of ANP, which leads to more vasoconstriction and congestion, can lead to HFpEF.[1]

In a meta-analysis of 10 studies, all-cause mortality was significantly higher in patients with HFrEF and AF than in those with HFpEF and AF, whereas HF hospitalization and incidence of stroke were similar, regardless of ejection fraction.

LIMITATIONS

As HFpEF is a multifaceted and diverse condition, there is a scarcity of clinical trials in this subgroup. The majority of clinical trials in HF are primarily focused on reduced ejection fraction. Although no trial has specifically randomized AF patients with HFpEF to anticoagulation, subgroup data from the nonvitamin K antagonist (VKA) oral anticoagulant (NOAC) trials suggest similar efficacy in patients with and without HF.

MANAGEMENT

In the treatment of patients with HFpEF and AF, manage HF with diuretics and SGLT2 inhibitors and treat the underlying etiology. Anticoagulation in HFpEF with AF patients is required when they have clinical risk factors for stroke or thromboembolism, and current guidelines highlight the risk associated with both HFrEF and HFpEF on the basis of growing evidence that stroke rates are increased in AF patients with either type of HF.[1] Both AF and HFpEF are characterized by endothelial dysfunction, leading to an imbalance of vasoactive substances and the promotion of a prothrombotic state. Endothelial dysfunction plays a significant role in promoting platelet activation and adhesion, thereby heightening the likelihood of thrombosis. So anticoagulation is very important in patients with HFpEF with AF to prevent stroke.[2,5] The primary prevention of stroke in these patients is by the use of oral anticoagulation, which can be achieved with either direct oral anticoagulants (DOACs) or VKAs. Although HFpEF is an independent risk factor for stroke and thromboembolism, the need for anticoagulation is decided based on the CHA2DS2-VASc score, because of the potential risk for bleeding in the elderly population with multiple comorbidities. AF patients with HFpEF derive similar protection against thrombotic events with no significant difference in major bleeding or all-bleeding events while on NOACs when compared to VKA.[6]

GUIDELINES

Current guidelines and recommendations for anticoagulation in HFpEF with AF are based on the American Heart Association (AHA) and the American College of Cardiology (ACC) guidelines in 2017. It is recommended to administer oral anticoagulants (OACs) for patients with HFpEF with AF based on their CHA2DS2-VASc score. Guidelines do not recommend starting anticoagulation in patients with HFpEF without AF. Among the anticoagulants, NOACs (including apixaban, dabigatran, edoxaban, and rivaroxaban) are preferred over VKA in view of low-bleeding risk, and they have exhibited noninferiority or superiority compared to warfarin in the prevention of stroke and systemic embolism among patients with AF.[2] When making a decision between warfarin (VKA) and NOACs, it is important to take into account various factors, including renal function, drug interactions, and patient's preference.[2]

CONCLUSION

The management of anticoagulation in patients with HFpEF with AF presents a therapeutic challenge due to the intricate nature of the condition and diverse characteristics of the patient population. However, implementing a multidimensional approach can help healthcare providers in selecting the best anticoagulation therapy, thereby decreasing the risk of bleeding manifestations and preventing stroke and systemic embolism. We need to have well-designed clinical trials that are specific to HFpEF with AF and the outcomes with anticoagulation therapy.[2]

REFERENCES

1. Kotecha D, Lam CSP, Van Veldhuisen DJ, et al. Heart failure with preserved ejection fraction and atrial fibrillation: vicious twins. J Am Coll Cardiol. 2016;68(20):2217-28.
2. Jyotsna Fnu, Mahfooz K, Sohail H, et al. Deciphering the dilemma: anticoagulation for heart failure with preserved ejection fraction (HFpEF). Cureus. 2023;15(8):e43279.
3. Vermond RA, Geelhoed B, Verweij N, et al. Incidence of atrial fibrillation and relationship with cardiovascular events, heart failure, and mortality: a community-based study from the Netherlands. J Am Coll Cardiol. 2015;66(9):1000-7.
4. Santhanakrishnan R, Wang N, Larson MG, et al. Atrial fibrillation begets heart failure and vice versa: temporal associations and differences in preserved versus reduced ejection fraction. Circulation. 2016;133(5):484-92.
5. Xian Y, O'Brien EC, Liang L, et al. Association of preceding antithrombotic treatment with acute ischemic stroke severity and in-hospital outcomes among patients with atrial fibrillation. JAMA. 2017;317(10):1057-67.
6. Xiong Q, Lau YC, Senoo K, et al. Non-vitamin K antagonist oral anticoagulants (NOACs) in patients with concomitant atrial fibrillation and heart failure: a systemic review and meta-analysis of randomized trials. Eur J Heart Fail. 2015;17(11):1192-200.

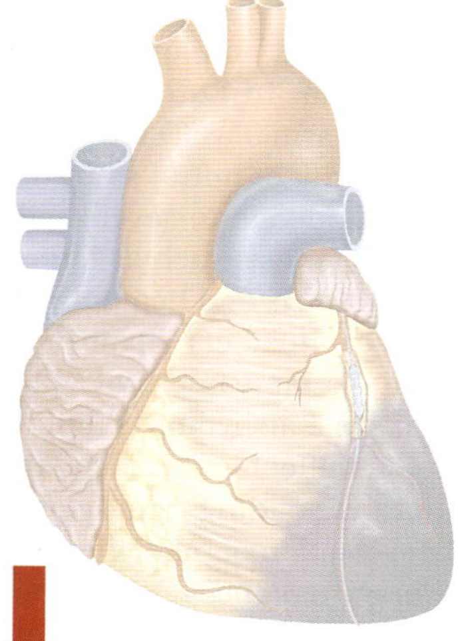

The Evolving Role of Nonimplant Interatrial Shunts in Managing HFpEF

S Shanmugasundaram, Ilayaraja Uthirapthi, Samuel Jebavaram, Vinodkumar BG

INTRODUCTION

Heart failure (HF) is a frequent disease affecting 1–2% of the population. Its prevalence increases with age with 7.0% of the subjects aged 70–79 years and 10.1% of those ≥80 years suffering from this condition.[1] Despite progress in the management of HF, in terms of drugs, devices, and surgery, considerable number of patients with HF continue to face the risk of dying and suffering from disease exacerbation and progression. This is particularly true in heart failure with preserved ejection fraction (HFpEF) for which the proven therapies are limited. Thus far, sodium-glucose linked transporter protein 2 (SGLT2) inhibitors are the only proven drug therapy for HFpEF, that too in terms of reducing HF hospitalizations but not mortality.[2-4] Angiotensin receptor neprilysin inhibitors (ARNI) and mineralocorticoid receptor antagonists (MRA) have also been found to be useful in reducing HF hospitalizations, particularly in those with an ejection fraction (EF) in the lower limit of normal range, i.e., <55–60%.[5,6] Women with HFpEF seemed to derive greater benefit from ARNI with a higher cutoff for LVEF, i.e., <65–70%. Moreover, medical therapy has its own limitations that include pill burden because of polypharmacy (≥5 drugs) and hyperpolypharmacy (≥10 drugs), adverse effects, interactions, and noncompliance. In such a scenario, device therapies appear to be alternate attractive options for improving symptoms, exercise capacity, and quality of life (QOL). The device therapies available for managing HF patients of entire spectrum of EF include those which detect pulmonary congestion early (Pacemakers/ICDs which can measure intrathoracic impedance and give alerts, CardioMEMS, an implantable pulmonary artery pressure monitoring system, noninvasive detection of lung fluid by ReDS which uses remote dielectric sensing with radar sensors in a wearable vest), cardiac resynchronization therapy (CRT) in eligible patients and transcatheter edge-to-edge repair (TEER) for secondary mitral regurgitation (MR). Creation of interatrial shunts (IASh) with or without implanted devices is a novel method to decompress left atrium (LA) the pressure of which is elevated at rest or on exercise. With reduction of LA pressure, pulmonary congestion and the resultant symptoms are expected to improve and HF admissions might decrease. By reducing the resting and exercise induced elevations of LA pressure, IASh appear to be promising therapy to improve the outlook of patients with HF particularly HFpEF.[7]

PATHOPHYSIOLOGY OF HEART FAILURE WITH PRESERVED EJECTION FRACTION

The HFpEF is diagnosed in the presence of (1) symptoms and/or signs of HF with an EF of ≥50%, and (2) evidence of structural and/or functional cardiac abnormalities (LVH or increased LA volume) corroborated by (3) documentation of systemic/pulmonary congestion either clinically or by imaging (chest X-ray or lung ultrasound revealing interstitial and alveolar pulmonary edema or hydrothorax or Doppler echo revealing an elevated E/e' ratio of >15 or TR velocity exceeding 2.8 m/s in the presence of left heart disease) or elevation of natriuretic peptide levels. It is a systemic disease characterized by the presence of

(1) systemic inflammation caused by the typical comorbid conditions such as obesity, hypertension, coronary artery disease (CAD), atrial fibrillation (AF), chronic kidney disease (CKD), diabetes or metabolic syndrome (MS), chronic obstructive pulmonary disease (COPD), obstructive sleep apnea, etc. (2) structural and functional abnormalities of heart in the form of left ventricular hypertrophy (LVH), impairment of relaxation ± increased stiffness of myocardium caused by diseased myocytes or interstitium, left atrial enlargement or dysfunction, abnormal ventriculo-arterial coupling, chronotropic incompetence, subtle abnormalities of systolic function, and impaired contractile reserve, and (3) microvascular inflammation and endothelial activation.

HFpEF is a heterogeneous disorder with multiple etiologies, phenotypes, and clinical presentation. However, the core hemodynamic abnormality in all these subtypes is similar in the form of elevation of LV filling pressure [LV end diastolic pressure (LVEDP) or pulmonary artery wedge pressure (PAWP)] at rest (≥ 15 mm Hg) or on exercise (≥25 mm Hg). Based on the resting and exercise hemodynamics, HFpEF may be classified into three subtypes: *Type I*—resting PAWP <15 mm Hg but the peak exercise PAWP is ≥25 mm Hg. *Type II*—resting PAWP ≥15 mm Hg ± clinical evidence of pulmonary and/or systemic congestion but without pulmonary hypertension (PH) or right ventricular dysfunction (RVD) or tricuspid regurgitation (TR) of at least moderate severity. *Type III*—Resting PAWP ≥15 mm Hg with features of PH and/or RVD and/or TR.[7] Drugs have a limited value in patients with normal resting LA pressure and exercise induced LA hypertension (EILAH) who experience episodic, unpredictable increase in LA pressure with exercise or stress. IASh devices have a particular value in this category by promptly decompressing LA whenever LA pressures increase episodically.

EVOLUTION OF THE CONCEPT

The concept of creating an iatrogenic atrial septal defect (ASD) originated from clinical observations of patients with Lutembacher syndrome and elderly patients who develop acute left HF after ASD closure. In patients with Lutembacher syndrome, left-to-right shunt through ASD could effectively decompress LA in such a way that LA pressure and PAWP are near normal despite the presence of moderate-to-severe mitral stenosis. On the other hand, some vulnerable older adults develop pulmonary edema after device closure of ASD, because of abrupt rise of LA pressure which was all along decompressed by the left-to-right shunt across the defect. The preexisting raised LV filling pressure due to the common comorbid conditions such as hypertension, CAD, etc., is masked by ASD and once the defect is closed, LV filling pressures are transmitted to LA (unmasking) and pulmonary vein leading to acute pulmonary edema. In Lutembacher syndrome, the potential benefit or harm of ASD in mitral stenosis is determined by the severity of mitral stenosis and the size of the defect. If MS is moderate-to-severe and ASD is large, symptoms of mitral stenosis such as effort dyspnea, paroxysmal nocturnal dyspnea, and hemoptysis cease to manifest but augmented overload of right atrium (RA) and right ventricle (RV) due to increased flow may lead to PH, RV dysfunction, and atrial arrhythmias. But if the defect is small to medium, net effect is beneficial in terms of unloading LA without overloading right heart. This principle applies well to the creation of IASh, the size of which should be optimal enough to reduce LA pressure but at the same time not resulting in large left-to-right shunt.

Increased LV filling pressures and LA pressure either at rest or while exercising is the hemodynamic hallmark of HFpEF. Elevation of LA pressure is passively transmitted into pulmonary veins, capillaries, and arteries resulting in pulmonary venous and arterial hypertension (isolated postcapillary PH). Increased pulmonary capillary pressure causes dyspnea and at times acute pulmonary edema when the pressures increase markedly and suddenly. This initial phase is followed by vasoconstriction and structural alterations in pulmonary arterioles and small pulmonary arteries leading to further elevation of PA pressures (combined postcapillary PH). This will eventually lead to RV dysfunction and right HF. Chronic elevation of LA pressure (LA hypertension) may induce structural remodeling of LA which may predispose the individual to AF. AF begets AF by worsening HF and by promoting electrical and structural remodeling of LA. Reducing the LA pressure by creating an interatrial communication, is expected to lower LA pressure which may reduce symptoms and improve QoL and exercise capacity, reduce or prevent HF hospitalizations, and possibly the occurrence of AF.

It all started with balloon/blade atrial septostomy done in four children with myocarditis who were on extracorporeal membrane oxygenator (ECMO) with evidence of elevated pressures in LV and LA.[8] Subsequently, atrial septostomy was performed in adults with acute on chronic HF with cardiogenic shock on ECMO, who manifested refractory pulmonary edema or upper body hypoxemia. These initial efforts paved the way for the subsequent attempts in designing ideal devices for achieving optimal hemodynamics and keeping the defect open at long term. Then came in the idea of creating a defect in the atrial septum with no implants—the concept of "leaving nothing behind." This manuscript attempts to review the indications, technical aspects, and clinical outcomes of the no-implant interatrial shunt procedures.

Different types of atrial shunt therapies have been (and are being) tried out in open label studies and randomized studies after adequate bench testing, animal experiments and feasibility studies in human beings.[7,9] However, evidence of benefit is only slowly evolving because of heterogeneity of HF phenotypes included in the studies, varied trial designs, and lack of power of studies due to small number of subjects enrolled. Atrial shunting procedures with implant devices include, Corvia IASD system II, a nitinol based double disc device with the shunt size of 8 mm; V-wave system, Ventura, a nitinol hour-glass shaped device covered with polytetrafluoroethylene with a shunt size of 5.1 mm; Occlutech atrial flow regulator, a dual-disk nitinol device available in 6, 8, and 10 mm shunt sizes, and Apture shunt from Edwards, a tubular nitinol device with retention arms for creating a communication between coronary sinus and LA. These devices have been tested in clinical trials with documented benefit at least at short term which is beyond of the scope of this article.

The ideal candidates for the shunt procedure include those HF patients with an EF of >40% in Class II–IVa (ambulatory) functional status on optimal drug therapy for the HF and comorbid conditions and have a resting PAWP ≥15 mm Hg or peak exercise PAWP ≥25 mm Hg measured at end expiration or exercise induced increase of PAWP by ≥10 mm Hg from the resting value and the gradient between LA (PAWP) and RA of ≥5 mm Hg . The studies on interatrial shunt devices for HFpEF mostly have included the following inclusion criteria: (1) Diagnosed to have HFpEF by valid criteria, (2) Class II–IVa symptoms despite guideline directed therapy, (3) Recent or recurrent hospitalizations for worsening of HF or need for intravenous diuretics to relieve symptoms, (4) LVEF >40%, (5) echocardiographic evidence of elevated filling pressures in the form of reduced tissue Doppler velocities (lateral e' <10 cm/s; septal e' <8 cm/s) and increased E/e' ratio of >15 or left atrial enlargement (LA anteroposterior dimension >40 mm or LA volume index >28 mL/m^2), (6) age >40 years, (7) resting PAWP of ≥15 mm Hg or end expiratory PAWP during supine ergometer exercise ≥25 mm Hg with a gradient between PAWP to RA pressure ≥5 mm Hg or increase of PAWP by ≥10 mm Hg at peak exercise when compared to resting value with a gradient between PAWP to RA pressure ≥5 mm Hg , and (8) life expectancy >1 year. The benefit if the procedure appears to be more when exercise pulmonary vascular resistance (PVR) is <1.75 Wood units. Those with the following conditions are excluded from atrial shunting therapies: (1) Advanced HF—on inotropes or mechanical circulatory support either at present or in recent times, cardiac index <2.0 L.min/m^2, heart transplant listing, (2) PH with PA systolic pressure of ≥70 mm Hg or PVR of >4 Wood units, (3) RV dysfunction (TAPSE <14 mm or RV fractional area shortening ≤30%), (4) Elevated RA pressure >14 mm Hg, (5) moderate-to-severe valve disease, (6) infiltrative or hypertrophic cardiomyopathy, (7) significant coronary or carotid atherosclerotic disease, (8) CKD with an eGFR <25 mL/min/1.73 m^2, (9) recent stroke or transient ischemic attack, (10) deep vein thrombosis/pulmonary embolism, (11) prior surgical or device closure of ASD, and (12) unsuitable anatomy.

NONIMPLANT INTERATRIAL COMMUNICATION

The advantages of nonimplant atrial shunting methods include lower risk of infection, thromboembolism, and device embolization, provision for future transseptal access for left sided interventions, and easier closure of the shunt at times of need. However, the potential for anatomic or functional reduction in shunt orifice size due to tissue ingrowth or partial collapse of the opening during phases of cardiac cycle remains a disadvantage of this method.

One such nonimplant method is using a novel transcatheter device (Alleviant Medical)[10] that can create a durable interatrial shunt by using a short pulse of radiofrequency energy to excise a precise segment of the interatrial septum **(Table 1; Figs. 1 and 2)**. The system is a 16F catheter intended for transfemoral approach. After transseptal puncture, the device is advanced over a guidewire into the LA. The tip of the device is opened in the LA and slowly retracted under image guidance until the electrode is in contact with the right side of atrial septum in RA. The tip of the device is closed, securing the septal tissue to be removed within the device. A short pulse of radiofrequency energy is applied to cut the tissue. The guidewire and device (with excised septal tissue contained within) are withdrawn, leaving a durable passageway to permit LA-to-RA shunt flow. It creates a 7 mm shunt. The clinical studies, Evaluation of the Safety and Feasibility of a Percutaneously Created Interatrial Shunt to Alleviate Heart Failure Symptoms in Patients With Chronic Heart Failure and Preserved or Mid-Range Left Ventricular Ejection Fraction, ALLEVIATE-HF-1 (single center) and ALLEVIATE-HF-2 (multicentric) were the prospective, open-label, uncontrolled, nonrandomized studies. From August 2020 to March 2022, a total of 28 patients were enrolled and the mean age was 68 ± 9 years, majority (68%) being female. LVEF was 60.8% ± 8.4%, and body mass index was 36.1 ± 7.5 kg/m^2. 20 were in class III and 8 in class II. Mean 6 minute walk test distance (6MWT) was 252 ± 67 meters. Baseline resting and peak exercise PAWP were 19 ± 7 mm Hg and 40 ± 11 mm Hg, respectively. Mean baseline N-terminal pro-B-type natriuretic

TABLE 1: Interatrial shunt therapies currently under investigation in humans.

Device/procedure	*Corvia*	*V-Wave*	*Occlutech*	*Edwards*	*Alleviant*	*NoYA*	*InterShunt*
Type	Implant	Implant	Implant	Implant	Procedure	Procedure	Procedure
Description	Nitinol stent	Nitinol/PTFE hourglass	Nitinol braid with central orifice	Tubular nitinol device with retention arms	Coring catheter	RF catheter	Cutting catheter
Shunt flow	LA → RA	LA → RA	LA → RA	LA → CS	LA → RA	LA → RA	LA → RA
Shunt size	8 mm	5.1 mm	4, 6, 8, 10 mm	7 mm	6 mm	4–12 mm	6 mm
Development stage	Pivotal RCT complete, follow-up confirmatory RCT in responder subgroup ongoing	Pivotal RCT enrollment complete, follow-up ongoing	Pivotal RCT enrollment ongoing	Phase 2 feasibility/ mechanistic RCT ongoing	Pivotal RCT enrollment ongoing	Open-label trial ongoing	Small pilot studies in humans

(CS: coronary sinus; LA: left atrium; PTFE: polytetrafluoroethylene; RA: right atrium; RCT: randomized clinical trial).
Source: Jagadeesan V, Gray WA, Shah SJ. Atrial shunt therapy for heart failure: An update. J Soc Cardiovasc Angiogr Interv. 2023;2(6Part B):101203.

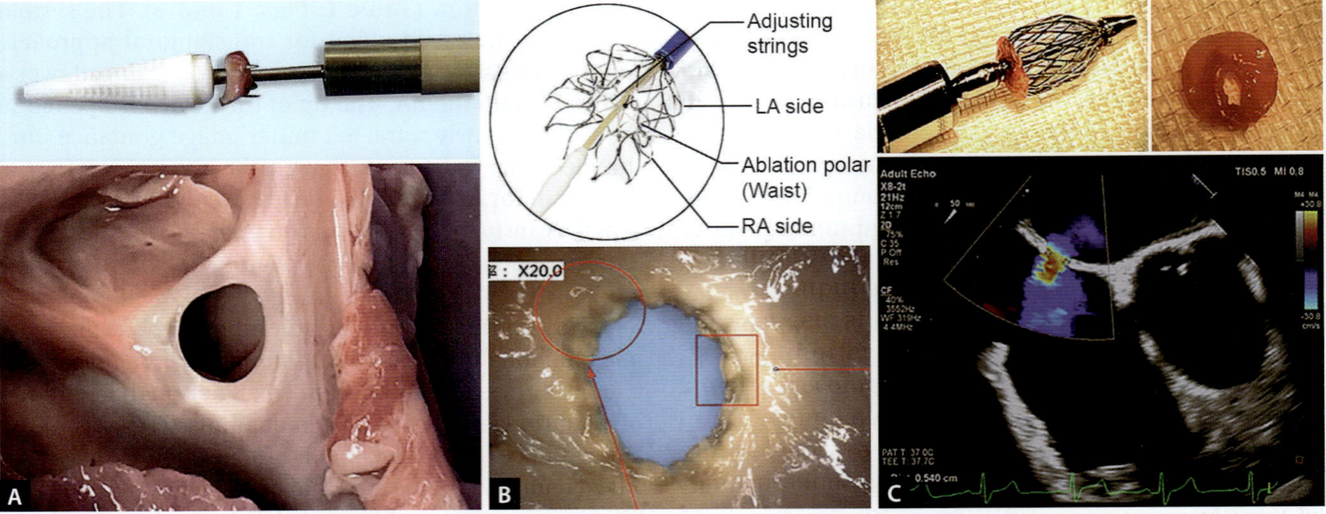

Figs. 1A to C: No-implant atrial shunts: (A) Implant-free Alleviant Medical septal cutting device; (B) Implant-free NoYa radiofrequency system (NoYA MedTech); (C) InterShunt (InterShunt Technologies).
Source: Rabecca TH, Lindenfield J, Lim SD, et al. Structural cardiac interventions in patients with heart failure – JACC Scientific statement. J Am Coll Cardiol. 2024;84(9):832-47.

peptide (NT-proBNP) level was 1,151 ± 993 pg/mL. All the 28 procedures were technically successful with a shunt diameter as assessed by postprocedure echo was 7.1 ± 0.9 mm. Peak exercise PAWP reduced by 5.4 ± 9.6 mm Hg ($p = 0.011$). Mean PAWP with passive leg raise and during intermediate-stage activity (20 W) decreased by 4.1 ± 5.8 mm Hg ($p = 0.005$) and 5.3 ± 10.6 mm Hg ($p = 0.014$), respectively. Mean right atrial pressure at rest and during peak exercise increased by 1.0 ± 4.2 mm Hg and 1.2 ± 6.6 mm Hg (p = NS). During the clinical follow-up

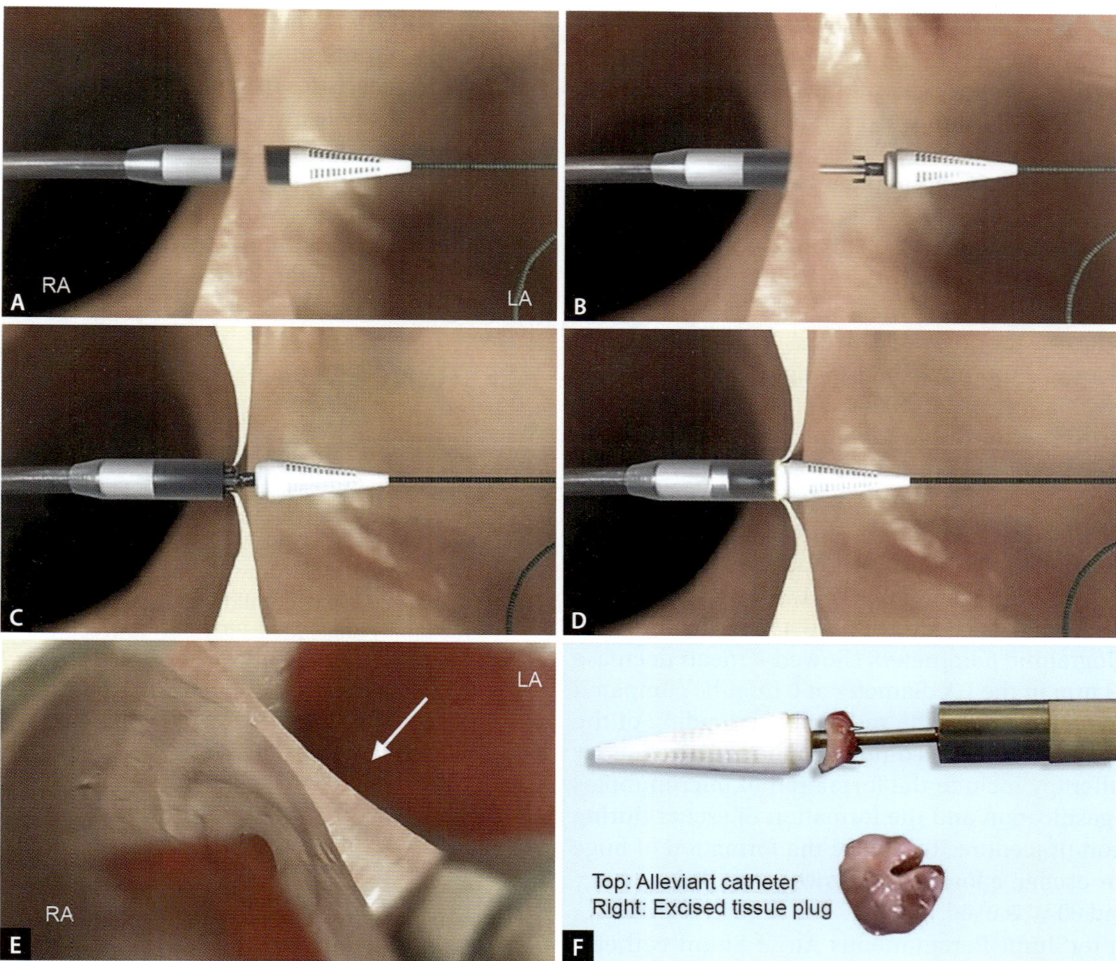

Figs. 2A to F: Creation of a no-implant interatrial shunt using the Alleviant system. (A) After transseptal puncture, the device is advanced over a guidewire into the left atrium (LA); (B) The tip of the device is opened in the LA and slowly retracted under image guidance until the electrode resides in the right atrium (RA); (C) The tip of the device is closed, securing the septal tissue to be removed within the device; (D) A short pulse of radiofrequency energy is applied to cut the tissue; (E) The guidewire and device (with excised septal tissue contained within) are withdrawn, leaving a durable passageway to permit LA-to-RA shunt flow (arrow); (F) Alleviant Medical Catheter with excised septal tissue after the procedure.

Source: Udelson JE, Barker CM, Wilkins G, et al. No-implant interatrial shunt for HPpEF: 6-month outcomes from multicentre pilot feasibility studies. JACC Heart Failure. 2023;11(8):1121.

at 6 months, 14 patients improved by 1 NYHA functional class, and 4 patients improved by 2 classes. Mean 6MWT distance increased by 101 ± 71 m (p <0.001), and the Kansas City Cardiomyopathy Questionnaire (KCCQ) overall summary score increased by 26 ± 19 points (p < 0.001) and the mean NT-proBNP level decreased by 372 ± 857 pg/mL. All 28 patients demonstrated shunt patency measured by echo, at the 6-month follow-up visit, with a mean shunt diameter of 7.0 ± 0.9 mm. The ratio of pulmonary to systemic flow indicating left-to-right shunt (Qp/Qs) was 1.3 ± 0.1. EF did not change and there was nonsignificant decrease in LAVI of 1.6 ± 8.9 mL/m^2 and the mean LA diameter decreased significantly by 0.2 ± 0.5 cm. There was a small, nonsignificant increase in the right atrial volume index of 0.6 ± 11.2 mL/m^2. The results of this study match with the results of implantable shunts. The authors had extended its application to patients with HFrEF in a study that included five patients in whom the clinical benefit was documented.[11] NT-ProBNP was reduced by 558 ± 139 pg/mL, walking distance in 6MWT improved by 151 ± 76 meters and the KCCQ-overall summary score improved by 19 ± 5. Enrollment for the randomized sham-controlled pivotal study (ALLAY-HF, FDA IDE approved) is currently underway.

Another radiofrequency ablation-based interatrial shunt (RAIAS)' named the NoYA system (NoYA MedTech,

Hangzhou, China), consists of a self-expanded flowerlike nitinol stent connected to the radiofrequency generator. The flowerlike stent was configured with a diameter adjustable from 4–12 mm waist in the middle, on which the electric poles are located. Under the radial force of the stent and the power of radiofrequency energy, an interatrial communication was made. After ablation, the device was removed from the body. This novel approach was evaluated first in 11 domestic pigs and then in nine HFpEF patients and one with HFmrEF with NYHA functional classes.[12] RAIAS therapy was successful in all patients, and an evidence interatrial left-to-right shunt flow was detected with a mean Qp:Qs of 1.3 ± 0.3. No major safety event occurred. But, there was a progressive reduction in diameter of the defect from 5.0 mm postprocedure to 3.0 at 6 months, and two patients showed complete closure of the defect. Patients showed improvements of NYHA functional class at 6 months, a reduction of median NT-proBNP from 3,533 to 1,347 pg/mL and an improvement in 6MWD from 349 to 440 m. In addition, echocardiographic parameters showed a mean decrease of 3.1 ± 3.9 mm in the LA diameter at 6 months compared with baseline, reflecting the reduced overloading of the LA after RAIAS. The shortcomings of the radiofrequency ablation therapy include the formation of microbubbles by tissue gasification and the formation of eschar during the ablation procedure. To reduce the formation of huge bubbles or eschar, a lower total power of radiofrequency with 45 and 60 W is used.

The InterShunt Percutaneous Atrial Shunt catheter system (InterShunt Technologies, Inc)[13] is another device-less atrial shunt procedure that excises a 6-mm circular portion of the tissue of atrial septum **(Table 1)** had been tested eight patients with class II–IVa HFpEF patients. The procedure was successful and there were no device-related harm. At the 1-month follow-up, all shunts were patent with left-to-right flow. The mean peak exercise pulmonary capillary wedge pressure decreased by 6 ± 2.2 mm Hg, and the mean NT-proBNP decreased by 405.6 ± 277 pg/mL. LVEF improved to 66.3% ± 7.4%.

CONCLUSION

Although further validation is needed, these results show promise toward novel minimally invasive methods to treat patients with HFpEF or HFmrEF with limiting symptoms and an appropriate hemodynamic profile. But we need to wait for randomized trials with a larger number of HFpEF patients included for a meaningful conclusion and widespread clinical application. Meanwhile, there are lot of questions that remain to be answered regarding this therapy; the role of exercise PASP or PVR in identifying potential responders, relationship between the PAWP-RAP gradient and the benefit, need for individualizing the size of the shunt rather than using a fixed size, the clinical characteristics or imaging parameters of cardiac remodeling or subtle myocardial dysfunction in identifying the potential responders, the influence of AF or atrial myopathy in determining the efficacy of these devices, the reason for the patients with pacemakers faring worse with shunt therapies, application of the treatment in those with HFrEF or valvular heart diseases, long-term safety, and efficacy are some of them.

REFERENCES

1. Roger VL. Epidemiology of heart failure: a contemporary perspective. Circ Res. 2021;128(10):1421-34.
2. Anker SD, Butler J, Filippatos G, et al. Empagliflozin in heart failure with a preserved ejection fraction. N Engl J Med. 2021;385(16):1451-61.
3. Solomon SD, McMurray JJV, Claggett B, et al. Dapagliflozin in heart failure with mildly reduced or preserved ejection fraction. N Engl J Med. 2022;387(12):1089-98.
4. Kosiborod MN, Abildstrøm SZ, Borlaug BA, et al. Semaglutide in patients with heart failure with preserved ejection fraction and obesity. N Engl J Med. 2023;389(12):1069-84.
5. Solomon SD, Vaduganathan M, Claggett B L, et al. Sacubitril/Valsartan across the spectrum of ejection fraction in heart failure. Circulation. 2020;141(5):352-61.
6. Solomon SD, Claggett B, Lewis EF, et al. Influence of ejection fraction on outcomes and efficacy of spironolactone in patients with heart failure with preserved ejection fraction. Eur Heart J. 2016;37(5):455-62.
7. Jagadeesan V, Gray WA, Shah SJ. Atrial shunt therapy for heart failure: An update. J Soc Cardiovasc Angiogr Interv. 2023;2(6Part B):101203.
8. Koenig PR, Ralston MA, Kimball TR, et al. Balloon atrial septostomy for left ventricular decompression in patients receiving extracorporeal membrane oxygenation for myocardial failure. J Pediatr. 1993;122(6):S95-9.
9. Rabecca TH, Lindenfield J, Lim SD, et al. Structural cardiac interventions in patients with heart failure – JACC Scientific statement. J Am Coll Cardiol. 2024;84(9):832-47.
10. Udelson JE, Barker CM, Wilkins G, et al. No-implant interatrial shunt for HPpEF: 6-month outcomes from multicentre pilot feasibility studies. JACC Heart Failure. 2023;11(8):1121.
11. Fudim M, Barker C, Wilkins G, et al. Multi-center Clinical Outcomes Of A No-implant Interatrial Shunt For Heart Failure With Preserved And Reduced Ejection Fraction: Update From Early Feasibility Program. J Card Failure. 2024;30(1):124.
12. Sun W, Zou H, Yong Y, et al. The RAISE Trial: a novel device and first-in-man trial. Circ Heart Fail. 2022;15(4):e008362
13. Vardi G, Shaburishvili T, Fudim M, et al. Evaluation of an implant free interatrial shunt to improve heart failure: EASE HF. Presented at TVT 2022. J Am Coll Cardiol. 2022;80(12_Supplement):B139.

CHAPTER 64

Deterioration in RV Structure and Function in HFpEF Echocardiographic Evaluation

Sunil S Bohra, Akash Jain, Prashuka Jain

INTRODUCTION

Heart failure with preserved ejection fraction (HFpEF) is a clinical syndrome characterized by symptoms and signs of heart failure despite a preserved left ventricular ejection fraction (LVEF ≥50%). Unlike heart failure with reduced ejection fraction (HFrEF), where systolic dysfunction of the left ventricle (LV) is the primary abnormality, HFpEF involves complex pathophysiological mechanisms affecting multiple cardiac structures, including the right ventricle (RV). In recent years, it has become evident that RV structure and function play a significant role in HFpEF pathophysiology and prognosis. RV dysfunction (RVD) in HFpEF is increasingly recognized as a significant determinant of morbidity and mortality. The deterioration of RV function in HFpEF is an under-recognized but a critical aspect of the disease.

This chapter aims to provide a comprehensive overview of RV structure and function deterioration in HFpEF, with a focus on echocardiographic evaluation, which remains the cornerstone imaging modality for assessing both RV and LV function. The chapter will cover the importance of RV function in HFpEF, the mechanisms contributing to RV deterioration, and echocardiographic techniques used for evaluation.

PREVALENCE OF RIGHT VENTRICULAR FUNCTION IN HEART FAILURE WITH PRESERVED EJECTION FRACTION

Reporting exact prevalence data for RVD is challenging, because HFpEF severity across different studies has varied, as well as the echocardiographic methods, criteria and cutoff values employed for the assessment of RVD.[1,2,3-5] Some of these cutoff values for RVD are less well established or have also changed over time.[6-8]

A study by Puwanant et al.[9] reported prevalence of RV systolic dysfunction in HFpEF of 33%, 40%, and 50%, as categorized by reduced RV fractional area change (FAC), tricuspid annular plane systolic excursion (TAPSE), and tricuspid annular systolic velocity (RV S′), respectively. Aschauer et al.[4] reported RVD in 19% of the patients using cardiac magnetic resonance (CMR) imaging. In a meta-analysis, the prevalence of RVD was 18%, 28%, and 21% using RV FAC, TAPSE, and RV S′, respectively.[10]

There is growing evidence that RVD is also a major predictor of the clinical course of HFpEF.[10] A 2.2-fold increased risk for all-cause mortality per 7% decrease in FAC after adjustment for pulmonary pressures was reported in a study by Melenovsky et al.[1] In another prospective study, 55% of patients with HFpEF died with clinical signs of right heart failure. Pooled data from individual studies recently showed that the risk of mortality increases by ~26% per 5 mm decrease in TAPSE and by ~16% per 5% decrease in FAC.[10]

Staging of right heart dysfunction and failure in HFpEF as per Heart Failure Association of the European Society of Cardiology (2018):

- *Stage 1:* At risk for right heart failure without RVD and without signs/symptoms of right heart failure.
- *Stage 2:* RVD without signs/symptoms of right heart failure.
- *Stage 3:* RVD with prior or current signs/symptoms of right heart failure.

- *Stage 4:* RVD with refractory signs/symptoms of right heart failure at rest (requiring specialized interventions).

MECHANISMS OF RIGHT VENTRICULAR DETERIORATION IN HEART FAILURE WITH PRESERVED EJECTION FRACTION

Several studies have demonstrated that RVD is a critical prognostic marker in HFpEF. The development of RVD, often secondary to pulmonary hypertension (PH), significantly worsens outcomes in HFpEF patients.[11]

The deterioration of RV structure and function in HFpEF results from several pathophysiological processes:

- *Pulmonary vascular remodeling and pulmonary hypertension:* In HFpEF, LV diastolic dysfunction leads to elevated left atrial pressure, which is transmitted to the pulmonary circulation, increasing the afterload on the RV.[12] This increased afterload strains the RV, leading to hypertrophy, dilation, and eventual failure.
- *Ventricular interdependence:* RV function is linked to LV function through ventricular interdependence, where the two ventricles share the interventricular septum and pericardium.[2] The close anatomical and functional relationship between the LV and RV means that any dysfunction of the LV affects the RV. In HFpEF, LV diastolic dysfunction, increased LA pressure, and the presence of concentric LV hypertrophy alter the septal motion and thus impair RV filling and contraction.
- *RV-PA coupling:* "RV-pulmonary artery (PA) coupling" is an assessment of the RV contractile capacity with consideration of the afterload. The gold standard for measuring RV-PA coupling is the "Ees/Ea" ratio, originally obtained invasively using a conductance catheter. The Ees/Ea ratio is a measure of how well the RV's contractility adjusts to afterload. It is calculated by dividing the RV end-systolic elastance (Ees) by the pulmonary arterial elastance (Ea). A normal Ees/Ea ratio is between 1.5 and 2.0 which indicates that RV contractility works effectively under the afterload exerted on the RV and generates an appropriate stroke volume. Conversely, a decreased Ees/Ea ratio signifies "uncoupling", where RV contractility diminishes under the existing afterload conditions and is unable to supply the necessary stroke volume to pulmonary circulation. Although RV is tolerant to changes in preload, its function can be easily impaired by a slight increase in afterload;[13] thus, emphasizing that afterload is crucial when evaluating RV function. In HFpEF, this coupling is often impaired due to increased pulmonary vascular resistance (PVR), leading to RVD even in the absence of overt RV dilation.
- *Systemic inflammation and fibrosis:* HFpEF is often associated with systemic inflammation, which can lead to myocardial fibrosis. Fibrosis in the RV myocardium contributes to stiffening and impaired contractility. Additionally, the chronic inflammatory state often seen in HFpEF can exacerbate endothelial dysfunction and pulmonary vascular remodeling, further worsening RV function.
- *Neurohormonal activation:* Neurohormonal systems, particularly the renin-angiotensin-aldosterone system (RAAS) and the sympathetic nervous system, are activated in HFpEF and contribute to RVD. Elevated levels of circulating catecholamines and angiotensin II promote RV hypertrophy, fibrosis, and eventual failure.

ECHOCARDIOGRAPHIC EVALUATION OF RIGHT VENTRICULAR STRUCTURE AND FUNCTION

The tricuspid valve has a crucial role in the normal function of the RV. Evaluation of the morphological features of the RV requires the following projections:[11]

- Parasternal long axis plane (to evaluate the RV outflow tract and moderator band).
- RV inflow tract views (evaluation of the anterior and inferior RV wall and the Eustachian valve).
- RV outflow tract views (to evaluate the RV outflow tract curving over the LV, the pulmonary valve, the pulmonary trunk and its bifurcation into the left and right arteries).
- Short axis planes (to display the crescentic shape of the RV and to display the RV outflow).
- RV focused apical four-chamber plane (this is optimal for morphological assessment of the tricuspid valve and measurement of RV dimensions).
- Subcostal projection (to evaluate the diaphragmatic wall of the RV).

Echocardiography is the primary imaging modality used for evaluating RV structure and function in HFpEF due to its accessibility, noninvasive nature, and ability to provide real-time assessment of RV size, shape, and contractility. Several echocardiographic parameters are commonly used to assess RV function:

- *RV size and shape:* The measurement of the following dimensions is recommended for right heart assessment:
  - *RV basal-apical:* In the four-chamber view, the RV is measured at the base with an upper reference limit of 41 mm, at mid-diameter at the level of the LV papillary muscles with a maximum dimension

of 35 mm, and in the longitudinal dimension with an upper reference limit of 86 mm.
    - *RV wall thickness:* It is evaluated in subcostal long axis view at end-diastole with measurements >5 mm considered abnormal. The trabeculations and papillary muscle must be excluded for this measurement.
    - *RV area:* It is best evaluated in RV focused four-chamber view at end-diastole, with an upper reference limit at end-diastole of 24 cm^2 in men and 20 cm^2 in women excluding trabeculations and the moderator band).
    - *RV outflow tract (RVOT):* RVOT is located between the supraventricular crest and pulmonary valve. Measurement is done of the proximal diameter of the RVOT at the subvalvular level (parasternal long axis, maximum limit is 33 mm), and the distal diameter of the RVOT at the pulmonary valve level (parasternal short axis, upper reference limit 27 mm).
    - *Inferior vena cava (IVC) dimension:* The dilatation of the IVC with diameter >21 mm in the case of chronic heart failure suggests hemodynamic congestion. The RA pressure is calculated by measuring the diameter and the degree of inspiratory collapse of the IVC (IVC diameter ≤2.1 cm with a collapse >50% during sniff indicates normal RA pressure; IVC diameter ≥2.1 cm with a collapse <50% during sniff indicates high RA pressure). When the parameters of IVC diameter and collapse do not fall within these limits, an intermediate value of RA pressure may be used, or other secondary markers of elevated RA pressure could be involved.[14-17]
- *TAPSE:* TAPSE is a simple measure of longitudinal RV systolic function. It is obtained by placing an M-mode cursor over the lateral tricuspid annulus and measuring the excursion during systole. A TAPSE value <17 mm is indicative of RV systolic dysfunction.
The width of excursion correlates with RVEF (5 mm = 20% RVEF, 10 mm = 30% RVEF, 15 mm = 40% RVEF, 20 mm = 50% RVEF). RV systolic function as evaluated with TAPSE can be used to assess the risk of cardiovascular death in many cardiovascular diseases.[16,18-20]

  Mohammed and colleagues' finding of a 33% incidence of abnormal TAPSE is consistent with previous reports in HFpEF populations. Lower TAPSE did not predict all-cause mortality in fully adjusted models but was independently associated with cardiovascular mortality and HF hospitalizations.
- *RV FAC:* FAC is another parameter used to assess RV systolic function. It is calculated by measuring the difference between the RV end-diastolic area and the RV end-systolic area, divided by the end-diastolic area. FAC <35% suggests RVD.
- *Tissue Doppler imaging (TDI) of the tricuspid annulus:* TDI is used to measure the velocity of the tricuspid annulus during systole (S′ wave). This parameter reflects RV longitudinal contraction, with values <9.5 cm/s indicating RV systolic dysfunction.
- *RV strain:* Speckle-tracking echocardiography allows for the assessment of RV global longitudinal strain (GLS), a sensitive marker of RV systolic function. Strain imaging can detect subclinical RVD before overt changes in RV size or TAPSE occur. GLS values more negative than –20% are considered normal, while values closer to zero indicate impaired RV function.
- *Pulmonary artery pressure (PAP):* Echocardiographic estimates of PAP can be made by measuring the velocity of tricuspid regurgitation (TR) jet using continuous-wave Doppler and applying the simplified Bernoulli equation. Elevated PAP is often present in HFpEF and contributes to RV deterioration.
- *Right atrium volume:* Increased RA pressure is an indication of RVD as increased RA dimensions can be an indication of volume and pressure overload. Measurement of RA volume requires evaluation from the four-chamber view. Normal values are 21 ± 6 mL/m^2 for men and 25 ± 7 mL/m^2 for women.[18]
- *Right ventricular diastolic function:* RV diastolic dysfunction increases atrial pressures and decreases collapsibility of the IVC. RV diastolic dysfunction can be a result of pressure and volume overload mechanisms. The evaluation of the following parameters is recommended for the assessment of RV diastolic function: 2D morphological assessment of the RV, size of the IVC with inspiratory collapse as explained in previous sections, Doppler velocities of the trans-tricuspid flow (E, A, E/A) (susceptible to preload and afterload), tissue Doppler velocities of the tricuspid annulus (E′, A′, E/A′), deceleration time, and isovolumetric relaxation time.[16]
- Pulsed-wave Doppler of hepatic vein flow assessment includes systolic wave (S), systolic reversal wave (SR), diastolic wave (D), and the atrial reversal wave (AR). Increased RA pressure is indicated by S/D <1, hepatic vein systolic filling fraction <55%, and by a prominent systolic and atrial reversal wave.
- *RV dP/dt:* The rate of pressure rise in the ventricles (dP/dt) is an invasive measurement developed and validated as an index of ventricular contractility or systolic function. RV dP/dt is load dependent. Because of neglect of the inertial component of the Bernoulli equation and the rise in RA pressure, RV dP/dt will be

less accurate in severe TR. RV dP/dt <approximately 400 mm Hg/s is likely abnormal. RV dP/dt cannot be recommended for routine uses because of the lack of data in normal subjects although it can be considered in follow-up of subjects with suspected RVD.

- *Myocardial performance index (MPI):* The MPI also known as the RIMP or Tei index, is a global estimate of both systolic and diastolic function of the RV. The MPI is defined as the ratio of isovolumic time divided by ET, or [(IVRT + IVCT)/ET].
- *The right-sided MPI can be obtained by two methods:* The pulsed Doppler method and the tissue Doppler method. In the pulsed Doppler method, the ET is measured with pulsed Doppler of RV outflow (time from the onset to the cessation of flow), and the tricuspid valve closure-opening time is measured with either pulsed Doppler of the tricuspid inflow (time from the end of the transtricuspid A wave to the beginning of the transtricuspid E wave) or continuous Doppler of the TR jet (time from the onset to the cessation of the jet). In the tissue Doppler method, all time intervals are measured from a single beat by pulsing the tricuspid annulus. Correlation between both methods is modest and that normal values differ based on the method chosen. The upper reference limit for the right-sided MPI is 0.40 using the pulsed Doppler method and 0.55 using the tissue Doppler method. The MPI may be used for initial and serial measurements as an estimate of RV function to complement with other methods of measurements. It should not be used as the sole quantitative method for RV functional evaluation and in patients with irregular heart rates.
- *Myocardial acceleration during isovolumic contraction:* Myocardial acceleration during isovolumic contraction is defined as the peak isovolumic myocardial velocity divided by time to peak velocity. It is typically measured for the RV by Doppler tissue imaging at the lateral tricuspid annulus. RV IVA is not recommended as a screening parameter for RV systolic function in the general echocardiography laboratory population.

There are limited normative data available, and RV IVA is an angle-dependent Doppler measurement that appears to vary with age and heart rate. Because of the broad confidence interval around its lower reference limit in various studies, no reference value can be recommended.

- *3D echocardiography:* Three-dimensional (3D) echocardiography provides a more accurate assessment of RV volumes and ejection fraction than traditional two-dimensional (2D) imaging. RV ejection fraction (RVEF) obtained from 3D echocardiography is a robust indicator of RV systolic function.

ECHOCARDIOGRAPHIC ASSESSMENT OF RV-PA COUPLING

TAPSE:PASP ratio—This ratio was first proposed and evaluated as a surrogate of RV-PA coupling in a series of patients with HF and showed a prognostic role independent of the severity of LV dysfunction.[21-23] The ratio of TAPSE to systolic PAP (i.e., TAPSE/SPAP) enhances the prognostic risk stratification in patients with heart failure and a ratio <0.36 mm/mmHg indicates a higher probability of mortality in patients with heart failure.[21] *TAPSE:PASP ratio* has also been tested in precapillary PH where it correlated with hemodynamics and was an independent predictor of survival.[24-26] *TAPSE:*PASP has been validated with invasive RV pressure-volume (P-V) analysis in a small group of patients with severe PAH.[27] Consequently, TAPSE:PASP ratio has been incorporated into the risk assessment algorithm of the 2022 ESC/ERS PH Guidelines and has a potential role in suspected PH in patients with systemic sclerosis.[28] Its limitations relate to incomplete/inaccurate estimation of PASP from TR jet velocity and IVC profile.

RVFWLS:PASP ratio—A recent study has highlighted an independent prognostic role for the baseline RV free wall longitudinal strain *RVFWLS:PASP ratio* in treatment-naive patients with precapillary PH.[29] A preliminary analysis by an independent group has offered some retrospective validation for this parameter in a small cohort using invasive P-V loop analysis.[30]

PROGNOSTIC IMPLICATIONS OF RIGHT VENTRICULAR DYSFUNCTION IN HEART FAILURE WITH PRESERVED EJECTION FRACTION (TABLE 1)

The RVD is a powerful prognostic marker in HFpEF. Patients with evidence of RV systolic dysfunction, particularly those with concomitant PH, have worse clinical outcomes, including higher mortality rates and increased hospitalizations. Several studies have demonstrated the association between reduced TAPSE, FAC, RV strain, and adverse prognosis in HFpEF. In the treatment of preserved cardiac function heart failure with an aldosterone antagonist trial (TOPCAT) echocardiographic substudy, TR velocity was measurable in 450 subjects (48% of substudy patients) and was abnormal (>2.9 m/s) in 162 (36%).

In a community-based study of HFpEF, Mohammed et al. described that RV enlargement and a higher grade of TR were prominent.[2] Parrinello et al. also showed in an observational study of a small number of patients (n = 135) that RVD could be a distinctive prognostic factor

TABLE 1: Summary of key trials evaluating right ventricular dysfunction in heart failure with preserved ejection fraction.

Trial/study	*Objective*	*Intervention/ focus*	*Key findings*	*Implications for RV dysfunction*	*Reference*
PARAMOUNT	Compare effects of ARNI (sacubitril/ valsartan) vs. ARB in HFpEF	Sacubitril/ valsartan	Reduced NT-proBNP levels, improved LA function, indirect benefit on RV function	No significant direct effect on RV dysfunction; reduced pulmonary congestion benefits RV	Solomon, et al. (2012) Lancet
RELAX	Evaluate PDE-5 inhibition (sildenafil) in HFpEF	Sildenafil	No improvement in exercise capacity, symptoms, or RV function	Targeting PH did not improve RV function in HFpEF	Redfield, et al. (2013) JAMA
SILK	Assess sildenafil in HFpEF with PH	Sildenafil	No change in RV function or clinical outcomes	Similar to RELAX; sildenafil ineffective in improving RV function	Bonderman, et al. (2013) EHJ
DIAST-CHF	Study RV dysfunction in HFpEF patients with PH and CTEPH	RV dysfunction and PH in CTEPH	PH worsened RV function, leading to poorer outcomes	Strong association between PH and RV dysfunction; worsens HFpEF outcomes	Hoeper, et al. (2016) Circulation
TOPCAT	Evaluate spirono-lactone in HFpEF	Spironolactone	No significant reduction in death/hospitalization, potential benefit on RV fibrosis	Indirect benefit on RV via reduced fibrosis and improved cardiac structure	Pitt, et al. (2014) NEJM
HEPHF	Explore hemodynamic responses to PDE-5 inhibition	Sildenafil	No significant improvement in RV function or hemodynamics	Reinforced findings that targeting PH alone does not improve RV function	Hoendermis, et al. (2015) EJHF
PRESERVE (Phase 2)	Study macitentan in HFpEF and PH	Macitentan (Endothelin receptor antagonist)	Early data suggest potential benefit in reducing RV afterload and pulmonary pressures	Ongoing trial; promising for reducing RV stress in PH-HFpEF	NCT02070991 (ClinicalTrials.gov)

(ARB: angiotensin receptor blocker; ARNI: Angiotensin receptor-neprilysin inhibitor; CTEPH: Chronic thromboembolic pulmonary hypertension; EJHF: European Journal of Heart Failure; EHJ: European Heart Journal; LA: Left atrium; PH: Pulmonary hypertension; PDE-5: Phosphodiesterase-5; NEJM: New England Journal of Medicine)

for patients with HFpEF but not for those with HFrEF.[31] Obokata et al. reported that RV structure and function deteriorate over time in HFpEF patients, compared with changes seen in the LV among them.[32] Regarding the pathogenic processes underlying RVD in HFpEF, RV dilatation, and contractile impairment occur secondary to the failure to compensate for the pressure overload caused by the decline in pulmonary arterial compliance and the increase in vascular resistance.[4,13,33] RV enlargement and remodeling are observed in an advanced stage of RVD even in HFpEF. Additional deterioration could promote further pulmonary remodeling and create a vicious cycle that leads to a worse prognosis.[34]

The presence of RVD also influences therapeutic decision-making. For example, patients with significant RV failure may be less responsive to conventional heart failure therapies, such as diuretics and vasodilators, and may require more specialized interventions targeting the pulmonary circulation and RV afterload.

THERAPEUTIC CONSIDERATIONS

The treatment of RVD in HFpEF is challenging due to the complex interplay between RV function, pulmonary pressures, and LV diastolic dysfunction. Management strategies focus on reducing RV afterload, optimizing RV preload, and preventing further deterioration of RV function.

Pharmacological

Since RVD in HFpEF is often secondary to elevated LV filling pressures, optimizing LV diastolic function is crucial.

- SGLT2 inhibitors should be initiated in all HFpEF patients without contraindications, ideally once stable during hospitalization for index event. MRA may be beneficial in some HFpEF subsets with LVEF <55–60% or elevated B-type natriuretic peptide with close monitoring of potassium and renal function.

ARNIs have been proven to be beneficial in HFpEF patients with EF <60% and particularly in women. ARBs can be used when ARNI is cost prohibitive.
- β-blockers should be considered in patients with a history of myocardial infarction or AF for rate control.
- PAP monitoring with CardioMEMS reduces risk for HFpEF hospitalizations. It may be most useful for individuals with recurrent hospitalizations and those who experience lability in volume status.
- Target for glycosylated hemoglobin HbA_{1c} is <7–7.5% for individuals with lower comorbidity burden or less severe HF and HbA_{1c} target is <8–8.5% for more severe HF, higher comorbidity burden, and the elderly.
- SGLT2 inhibitors should be first line for diabetic HFpEF. Metformin may be considered if estimated glomerular filtration rate (eGFR) is >30.
- Glucagon-like peptide-1 (GLP-1) agonists or GIP antagonist may be considered for obese individuals with diabetes mellitus and HFpEF.
- Dipeptidyl peptidase-4 (DPP4) inhibitors saxagliptin and alogliptin and thiazolidinediones are contra-indicated in HF.

Nonpharmacological

Vagus nerve stimulation, low-intensity pulsed ultrasound (LIPUS), transcatheter insertion of an atrial shunt, personalized accelerated pacemaker, cardiac contractility modulator (CCM), renal denervation (RDN), percutaneous pulmonary artery denervation, and pericardial resection are newer modalities, majority being in investigational phase for treatment of HFpEF. In severe cases of RV failure, advanced therapies such as extracorporeal membrane oxygenation (ECMO), right ventricular assist devices (RVAD), and mechanical circulatory support or lung transplantation may be required.

CONCLUSION

The deterioration of RV structure and function is a critical aspect of HFpEF pathophysiology, with significant implications for prognosis and treatment. Echocardiography provides invaluable insight into the assessment of RV function, allowing for early detection of dysfunction and guiding clinical management. As our understanding of the role of RVD in HFpEF evolves, it is likely that RV-targeted therapies will play an increasingly important role in improving outcomes for these patients. The recognition of RVD in HFpEF underscores the need for a more holistic approach to heart failure management, one that considers both ventricles and the intricate relationships between the pulmonary circulation and the heart.

REFERENCES

1. Melenovsky V, Hwang SJ, Lin G, et al. Right heart dysfunction in heart failure with preserved ejection fraction. Eur Heart J. 2014;35(48):3452-62.
2. Mohammed SF, Hussain I, Abou Ezzeddine OF, et al. Right ventricular function in heart failure with preserved ejection fraction: a community-based study. Circulation. 2014;130(25):2310-20.
3. Morris DA, Gailani M, Vaz Perez A, et al. Right ventricular myocardial systolic and diastolic dysfunction inheart failure with normal left ventricular ejection fraction. J Am Soc Echocardiogr. 2011;24(8):886-97.
4. Aschauer S, Kammerlander AA, Zotter-Tufaro C, et al. The right heart in heart failure with preserved ejection fraction: insights from cardiac magnetic resonance imaging and invasive haemodynamics. Eur J Heart Fail. 2016;18(1):71-80.
5. Ghio S, Guazzi M, Scardovi AB, et al.; all investigators. Different correlates but similar prognostic implications for right ventricular dysfunction in heart failure patients with reduced or preserved ejection fraction. Eur J Heart Fail. 2017;19(7):873-9.
6. Lang RM, Bierig M, Devereux RB, et al.; Chamber Quantification Writing Group; American Society of Echocardiography's Guidelines and Standards Committee; European Association of Echocardiography. Recommendations for chamber quantification: are port from the American Society of Echocardiography's Guidelines and Standards Committee and the Chamber Quantification Writing Group, developed in conjunction with the European Association of Echocardiography, a branch of the European Society of Cardiology. J Am Soc Echocardiogr. 2005;18(12):1440-63.
7. Lang RM, Badano LP, Mor-Avi V, et al. Recommendations for cardiac chamber quantification by echocardiography in adults: an update from the American Society of Echocardiography and the European Association of Cardiovascular Imaging. J Am Soc Echocardiogr. 2015;28: 1-39.e14.
8. Lang RM, Badano LP, Mor-Avi V, et al. Recommendations for cardiac chamber quantification by echocardiography in adults: an update from the American Society of Echocardiography and the European Association of Cardiovascular Imaging. Eur Heart J Cardiovasc Imaging. 2015;16:233-70.
9. Puwanant S, Priester TC, Mookadam F, et al. Right ventricular function in patients with preserved and reduced ejection fraction heart failure. Eur J Echocardiogr. 2009;10(6):733-7.
10. Gorter TM, Hoendermis ES, van Veldhuisen DJ, et al. Right ventricular dysfunction in heart failure withpreserved ejection fraction: a systematic review and meta-analysis. Eur J Heart Fail. 2016;18(12):1472-87.
11. Hoeper MM, Lam CSP, Vachiery JL, et al. Pulmonary Hypertension in Chronic Heart Failure with Preserved

Ejection Fraction: A Systematic Analysis of Heart and Lung Interactions. Circulation. 2016;134(5):365-73.

12. Obokata M, Reddy YNV, Borlaug BA. Diastolic Dysfunction and HFpEF: Mechanisms and Noninvasive Methods. JACC: Cardiovasc Imaging. 2017;10(5):525-37.
13. Vonk Noordegraaf A, Westerhof BE, Westerhof N. The relationship between the right ventricle and its load in pulmonary hypertension. J Am Coll Cardiol. 2017; 69(2):236-43.
14. Schneider M, Binder T. Echocardiographic evaluation of the right heart. Wien Klin Wochenschr. 2018;130:413-20.
15. Choudhary G, Malik AA, Stapleton D, et al. Assessment of right ventricle by echocardiogram. In: Lakshmanadoss U (Ed). Echocardiography in Heart Failure and Cardiac Electrophysiology. IntechOpen; 2016.
16. Rudski LG, Lai WW, Afilalo J, et al. Guidelines for the echocardiographic assessment of the right heart in adults: a report from the American Society of -Echocardiography. J Am Soc Echocardiogr. 2010;23:685-713.
17. Jones N, Burns AT, Prior DL. Echocardiographic assessment of the right ventricle: state of the art. Heart Lung Circ. 2019;28(9):1339-50.
18. De Vecchis R, Baldi C, Giandomenico G, et al. Estimating right atrial pressure using ultrasounds: an old issue revisited with new methods. J Clin Med Res. 2016;8(8): 569-74.
19. Bleeker GB, Steendijk P, Holman ER, et al. Assessing right ventricular function: the role of echocardiography and complementary technologies. Heart. 2006;92(Suppl 1): i19-26.
20. Modin D, Møgelvang R, Andersen DM, et al. Right ventricular function evaluated by tricuspid annular plane systolic excursion predicts cardiovascular death in the general population. J Am Heart Assoc. 2019;8:e012197.
21. Guazzi M, Bandera F, Pelissero G, et al. Tricuspid annular plane systolic excursion and pulmonary arterial systolic pressure relationship in heart failure: an index of right ventricular contractile function and prognosis. Am J Physiol Heart Circ Physiol. 2013;305(9):H1373-81.
22. Guazzi M, Dixon D, Labate V, et al. RV contractile function and its coupling to pulmonary circulation in heart failure with preserved ejection fraction: stratification of clinical phenotypes and outcomes. JACC Cardiovasc Imaging. 2017;10(10):1211-21.
23. Gorter TM, van Veldhuisen DJ, Voors AA, et al. Right ventricular-vascular coupling in heart failure with preserved ejection fraction and pre- vs. post-capillary pulmonary hypertension. Eur Heart J Cardiovasc Imaging. 2018;19(4):425-32.
24. Tello K, Wan J, Dalmer A, et al. Validation of the Tricuspid Annular Plane Systolic Excursion/Systolic Pulmonary Artery Pressure Ratio for the Assessment of Right Ventricular-Arterial Coupling in Severe Pulmonary Hypertension. Circ Cardiovasc Imaging. 2019;12(9): e009047.
25. Tello K, Axmann J, Ghofrani AJ, et al. Relevance of the TAPSE/PASP ratio in pulmonary arterial hypertension. Int J Cardiol. 2018;1(266):229-35.
26. Hameed A, Condliffe R, Swift AJ, et al. Assessment of right ventricular function—a state of the art. Curr Heart Fail Rep. 2023;20(3):194-207.
27. Richter MJ, Peters D, Ghofrani HA, et al. Evaluation and prognostic relevance of right ventricular-arterial coupling in pulmonary hypertension. Am J Respir Crit Care Med. 2020;201(1):116-9.
28. Colalillo A, Grimaldi MC, Vaiarello V, et al. In systemic sclerosis, the TAPSE/sPAP ratio can be used in addition to the DETECT algorithm for pulmonary arterial hypertension diagnosis. Rheumatology. 2022;61(6):2450-6.
29. Ünlü S, Bézy S, Cvijic M, et al. Right ventricular strain related to pulmonary artery pressure predicts clinical outcome in patients with pulmonary arterial hypertension. Eur Heart J Cardiovasc Imaging. 2023;24(5): 635-42.
30. Richter MJ, Rako ZA, Tello K. Ratio between right ventricular strain and systolic pulmonary artery pressure as a surrogate for right ventricular to pulmonary arterial coupling: validation against the gold standard. Eur Heart J Cardiovasc Imaging. 2023;24(3):e50-e52.
31. Parrinello G, Torres D, Buscemi S, et al. Right ventricular diameter predicts all-cause mortality in heart failure with preserved ejection fraction. Intern Emerg Med. 2019;14(7):1091-100.
32. Obokata M, Reddy YNV, Melenovsky V, et al. Borlaug Deterioration in right ventricular structure and function over time in patients with heart failure and preserved ejection fraction. Eur Heart J. 2019;40:689-97.
33. Kammerlander AA, Marzluf BA, Graf A, et al. Right ventricular dysfunction, but not tricuspid regurgitation, is associated with outcome late after left heart valve procedure J Am Coll Cardiol. 2014;64(24):2633-42.
34. Gorter TM, van Veldhuisen DJ, Voors AA, et al. Rapid right-sided deterioration in heart failure with preserved ejection fraction. Eur Heart J. 2019;40(8):699-702.

CHAPTER

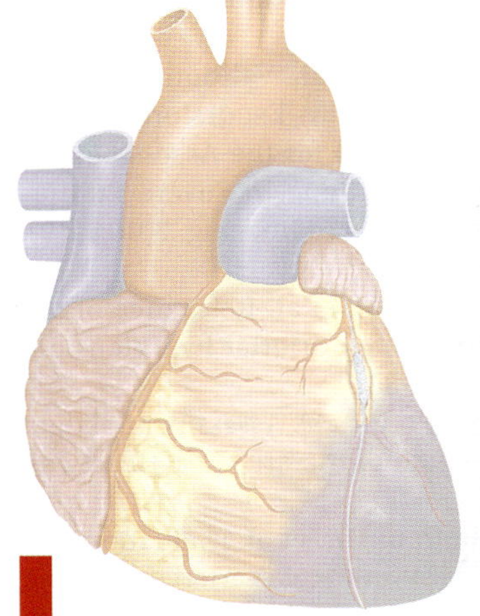

Echocardiographic Evaluation of HFpEF in Oncology

Manish Bansal, Ravi R Kasliwal, HK Chopra

INTRODUCTION

The advances in cancer diagnostics and therapeutics have significantly improved the survival of patients treated for various cancers.[1] However, the improved survival of these patients has presented another challenge as they are now living long enough to experience the long-term adverse effects of their cancer therapies. Cardiac complications are among the most common long-term consequences of various cancer therapies and are a significant source of morbidity and mortality among cancer survivors.[2,3]

Left ventricular (LV) myocardial dysfunction presenting as heart failure with reduced ejection fraction (HFrEF) is the most important cardiac complication observed among cancer survivors. It is termed cancer therapy-related cardiac dysfunction (CTRCD) and has attracted the most attention.[4] Numerous studies have been performed to understand the incidence of CTRCD, its mechanisms, prognostic implications, and the methods to predict, prevent, and treat it. However, left ventricular diastolic dysfunction (LVDD) is also known to occur in these patients and may even be more common than LV systolic dysfunction. When advanced, LVDD may manifest as heart failure with preserved ejection fraction (HFpEF).[5,6] Unfortunately, the exact incidence of HFpEF in cancer patients and its prognostic implications remain inadequately understood.

WHAT IS HEART FAILURE WITH PRESERVED EJECTION FRACTION?

Heart failure with preserved ejection fraction is an entity characterized by the presence of:

- Symptoms and/or signs of heart failure (HF)
- Left ventricular ejection fraction (LVEF) ≥50%
- Objective evidence of cardiac structural and/or functional abnormalities consistent with LVDD or raised LV filling pressure[7,8]

Left ventricular diastolic dysfunction is, thus, an integral component of HFpEF. However, nearly half of all patients with HFpEF are also known to have either overt (i.e., low normal LVEF) or subclinical [reduced LV global longitudinal strain (LV-GLS) with normal LVEF] LV systolic dysfunction.[9] For this reason, HFpEF is no longer considered to be pure diastolic HF.

ROLE OF ECHOCARDIOGRAPHY IN DIAGNOSING HFpEF

Echocardiography is among the most important diagnostic modalities in the evaluation of HFpEF **(Figs. 1A to E)**. Many different diagnostic algorithms, which include several different echocardiographic parameters, have been proposed for diagnosing HFpEF.[10,11]

In a patient with clinical features suggestive of HF, LVEF estimation using echocardiography is the first step in categorizing the patients into HFrEF, HFpEF,

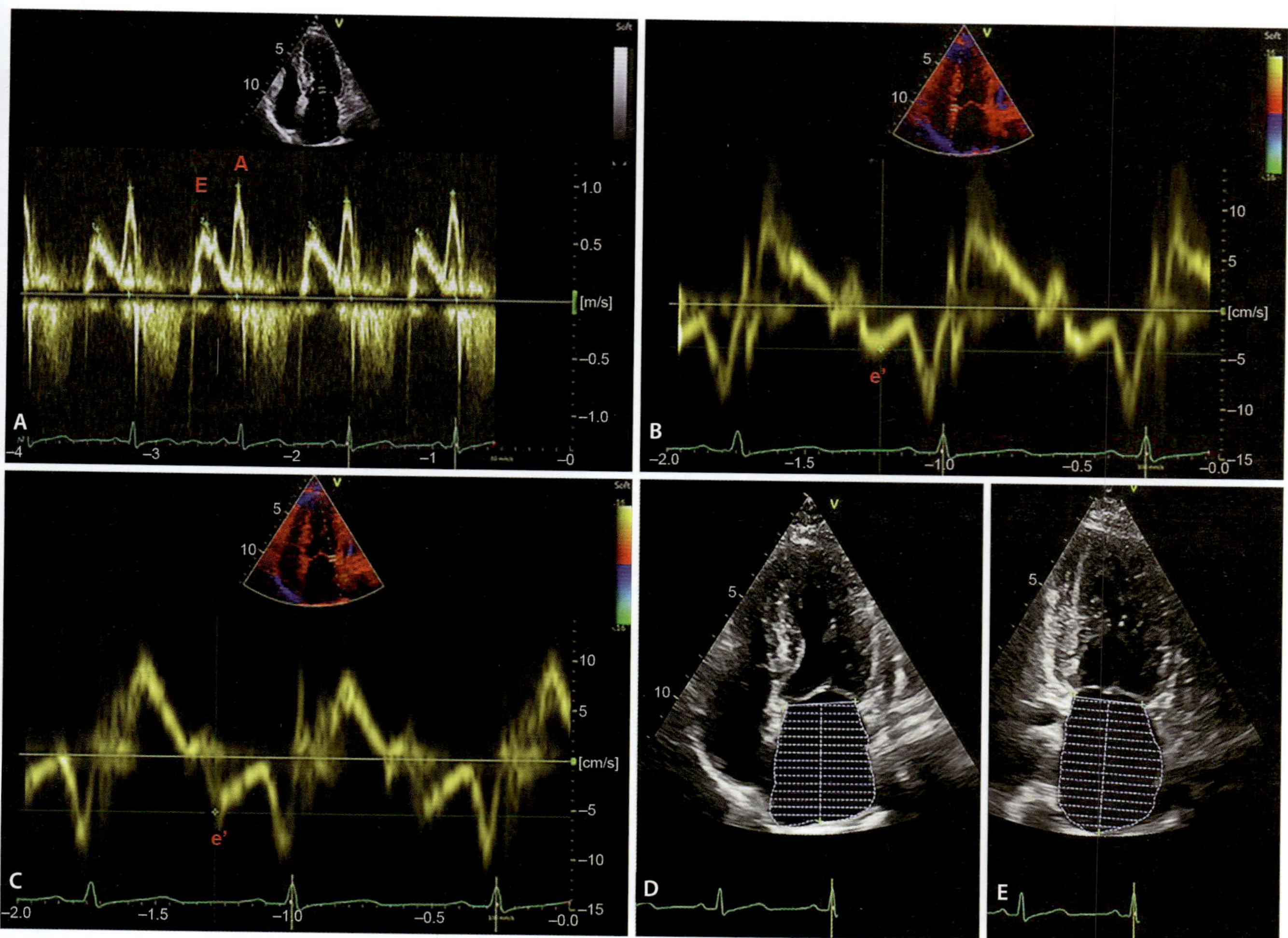

Figs. 1A to E: Left ventricular diastolic dysfunction in a 62-year-old lady receiving trastuzumab for breast cancer. (A) The early diastolic mitral inflow velocity (E) is reduced (59 cm/s), whereas the late diastolic velocity (A) is increased (92 cm/s), resulting in an abnormal mitral E/A ratio. The deceleration time of E is also prolonged (256 ms); (B and C) The septal and lateral early diastolic mitral annular velocities are also significantly reduced (4 and 6 cm/s, respectively); and (D and E) The left atrial volume is increased (36 mL/m^2).

or HF with mildly reduced EF (HFmrEF). If HFpEF is suspected, echocardiography helps in identifying the cardiac structural and functional abnormalities that could explain the clinical phenotype. LV hypertrophy and left atrial enlargement are the two most relevant structural abnormalities consistent with a diagnosis of HFpEF, whereas the abnormalities of LV diastolic function, reduced LV-GLS, and reduced LA strain are the most important functional abnormalities.[11] The 2016 American Society of Echocardiography guidelines provide detailed guidance on using echocardiography for the assessment of LVDD.[12] Lastly, echocardiography is also helpful in excluding other potential conditions that could mimic HFpEF, such as hypertrophic cardiomyopathy, severe aortic stenosis, infiltrative heart disease like amyloidosis, and pericardial diseases.

LEFT VENTRICULAR DIASTOLIC DYSFUNCTION AND HFpEF IN ONCOLOGY

Several studies have evaluated LV diastolic function in cancer patients, but most of these studies did not specify whether LVDD was associated with the clinical syndrome of HFpEF. Hence, the following discussion focuses primarily on LVDD in oncology patients.

Incidence of Left Ventricular Diastolic Dysfunction in Cancer Patients

The overall incidence of LVDD in cancer patients remains uncertain because of the differences in the patient profiles, cancer treatment received by the patients, criteria used for diagnosing LVDD, and the timing of assessment in relation to the cancer therapy.[13-18] Anthracyclines have been studied the most as they are the most likely chemotherapeutic agents to cause myocardial dysfunction. Radiation therapy (RT) is another potential source of LVDD.

In a recent study, Palmer et al. studied 3,342 adult survivors of childhood cancers who had received anthracyclines with or without RT. Two echocardiographic examinations were performed 6 years apart. The overall prevalence of LVDD was 15.2% at the baseline and 15.7% at the time of follow-up assessment. The prevalence of LVDD was 86.3 and 91.8%, respectively, in patients with reduced LVEF, 9.2 and 9.0%, respectively, in patients with normal LVEF but reduced LV-GLS, and 2.2 and 3.7%, respectively, in patients with normal LVEF and LV-GLS.[13]

In another study, Upshaw et al. studied 362 breast cancer participants treated with doxorubicin, doxorubicin followed by trastuzumab, or trastuzumab alone.[17] The patients were followed for a median duration of 2.1 years. Those treated with doxorubicin with or without subsequent trastuzumab showed a persistent worsening in LV diastolic function. The ratio of early diastolic to late diastolic mitral inflow velocity (E/A), lateral and septal mitral annular diastolic velocities (e′), and the ratio of mitral E to e′ (E/e′) decreased with time. Similar changes were not seen in patients who received only trastuzumab. Overall, 60, 70, and 80% of patients had abnormal LVDD at 1, 2, and 3 years, respectively. However, only 5% of patients developed an E/e′ >5, even though the reduction in mitral e′ to below normal values (<7 cm/s for septal e′ and <10 cm/s for lateral e′) was quite common. Thus, this study showed a very high prevalence of LVDD.[17] A few previous studies had also reported similar findings.[14-16]

In the above study, RT had a negative association with the occurrence of LVDD.[17] However, most other studies have shown opposite findings. A high incidence of LVDD has been reported in patients with Hodgkin's lymphoma receiving at least 35 Gy of mediastinal irradiation.[19,20] Other studies have shown an association between RT and the development of LVDD or even HFpEF in breast cancer patients.[21-23]

Mechanism of Left Ventricular Diastolic Dysfunction

Numerous different mechanisms have been proposed to explain the development of LVDD secondary to cancer therapies. Oxidative stress, inflammation, endothelial dysfunction, mitochondrial dysfunction, abnormal intracellular Ca^{2+} handling, coronary microvascular dysfunction, and cell apoptosis with subsequent myocardial fibrosis have all been implicated in LVDD caused by anthracyclines. Similar mechanisms may also operate with other chemotherapeutic agents and RT.[24] It has been estimated that the inflection point for the development of LVDD with anthracyclines occurs at a cumulative dose 150 mg/m^2 with a 5% incidence at a dose of 190 mg/m^2.[25] These dose levels are much lower than those responsible for causing overt LV systolic dysfunction (inflection point at 250–300 mg/m^2 and 5% risk at 400–425 mg/m^2).[26]

Apart from the cancer therapy-related risk factors, many conventional cardiovascular risk factors associated with LVDD such as hypertension and diabetes are also common in adult patients currently or previously treated for cancers. These risk factors may contribute to the LVDD caused by cancer therapies.[6] A "multi-hit" hypothesis has been proposed, which suggests that the initial cancer treatment serves as the "first hit," which makes the LV myocardium vulnerable to the adverse effects of various cardiovascular risk factors developing later in life. These traditional cardiovascular risk factors then serve as the "second hit" and unmask the LVDD.[24,27] However, in such cases, it is often difficult to determine the exact role of previous cancer-related treatment in causing LVDD. Indeed, in a study of 1,807 childhood cancer survivors (median age, 32 years), the development of cardiovascular risk factors such as hypertension, insulin resistance, and obesity contributed equally or even more than the cancer treatment-related factors to the development of LV systolic and diastolic dysfunction.[28]

Prognostic Significance of Left Ventricular Diastolic Dysfunction in Cancer Patients

Much like the incidence of LVDD in cancer patients, its prognostic significance also remains unclear.

In the study by Upshaw et al., abnormal LV diastolic function was associated with a subsequent decrease in LVEF and LV-GLS, whereas changes in E/e′ were associated with worsening LV-GLS alone.[17] Several other studies have shown that LVDD predicts subsequent LV systolic dysfunction, whereas many others have shown opposite results.[14-16,22,29-32] These studies have used several different echocardiographic parameters, either in isolation or in combination, to diagnose LVDD. These include mitral E velocity, E/A ratio, e′, E/e′, isovolumic relaxation time, myocardial performance index, etc.

Nagiub et al. performed a meta-analysis of the studies that evaluated the ability of nonstrain diastolic parameters to predict doxorubicin-induced cardiotoxicity. Four studies met the inclusion criteria. Only mitral E,

E/A ratio, lateral e′, and lateral mitral annular systolic velocity could predict subsequent CTRCD.[33]

GUIDELINE RECOMMENDATIONS

The current societal guidelines recommend comprehensive echocardiographic examination at baseline in most patients undergoing cancer treatment, especially those receiving potentially cardiotoxic therapies or those with risk factors for developing cardiac complications.[4] The timing and frequency of subsequent echocardiographic examination after a baseline study vary according to the patient's underlying cardiac risk and the type of cancer therapy being used. However, the main aim of these studies is to recognize LV systolic dysfunction occurring during the treatment. Although an assessment of LVDD is also an integral part of every echocardiographic examination, the guidelines do not specify the implications of LVDD in these patients. The protocol for repeat evaluation is also not defined. The lack of any guidance on these issues reflects the current knowledge gap in our overall understanding of the importance of LVDD in the setting of cardio-oncology.

CONCLUSION

Cardiac complications are among the most important causes of morbidity and mortality in patients successfully treated for various cancers. LV systolic dysfunction resulting in HFrEF is the most important cardiac complication in these patients. However, LVDD may also occur and is even more common than LV systolic dysfunction. Unfortunately, the overall incidence of LVDD and its prognostic implications in cancer patients are unclear, which has precluded wider attention to LVDD in this setting.

REFERENCES

1. Siegel RL, Miller KD, Wagle NS, et al. Cancer statistics, 2023. CA Cancer J Clin. 2023;73(1):17-48.
2. Abdel-Qadir H, Austin PC, Lee DS, et al. A population-based study of cardiovascular mortality following early-stage breast cancer. JAMA Cardiol. 2017;2(1):88-93.
3. Armenian SH, Xu L, Ky B, et al. Cardiovascular disease among survivors of adult-onset cancer: a community-based retrospective cohort study. J Clin Oncol. 2016;34(10):1122-30.
4. Plana JC, Galderisi M, Barac A, et al. Expert consensus for multimodality imaging evaluation of adult patients during and after cancer therapy: a report from the American Society of Echocardiography and the European Association of Cardiovascular Imaging. J Am Soc Echocardiogr. 2014;27(9):911-39.
5. Kwan ML, Cheng RK, Iribarren C, et al. Risk of heart failure with preserved versus reduced ejection fraction in women with breast cancer. Breast Cancer Res Treat. 2022;193(3):669-75.
6. Reding KW, Cheng RK, Vasbinder A, et al. Lifestyle and cardiovascular risk factors associated with heart failure subtypes in postmenopausal breast cancer survivors. JACC CardioOncol. 2022;4(1):53-65.
7. McDonagh TA, Metra M, Adamo M, et al. 2021 ESC guidelines for the diagnosis and treatment of acute and chronic heart failure. Eur Heart J. 2021;42(36):3599-726.
8. Kittleson MM, Panjrath GS, Amancherla K, et al. 2023 ACC expert consensus decision pathway on management of heart failure with preserved ejection fraction: a report of the American College of Cardiology Solution Set Oversight Committee. J Am Coll Cardiol. 2023;81(18):1835-78.
9. Shah AM, Claggett B, Sweitzer NK, et al. Prognostic importance of impaired systolic function in heart failure with preserved ejection fraction and the impact of spironolactone. Circulation. 2015;132(5):402-14.
10. Reddy YNV, Carter RE, Obokata M, et al. A simple, evidence-based approach to help guide diagnosis of heart failure with preserved ejection fraction. Circulation. 2018;138(9):861-70.
11. Pieske B, Tschöpe C, de Boer RA, et al. How to diagnose heart failure with preserved ejection fraction: the HFA-PEFF diagnostic algorithm: a consensus recommendation from the Heart Failure Association (HFA) of the European Society of Cardiology (ESC). Eur Heart J. 2019;40(40):3297-317.
12. Nagueh SF, Smiseth OA, Appleton CP, et al. Recommendations for the evaluation of left ventricular diastolic function by echocardiography: an update from the American Society of Echocardiography and the European Association of Cardiovascular Imaging. J Am Soc Echocardiogr. 2016;29(4):277-314.
13. Palmer C, Mazur W, Truong VT, et al. Prevalence of diastolic dysfunction in adult survivors of childhood cancer: a report from SJLIFE cohort. JACC CardioOncol. 2023;5(3):377-88.
14. Reuvekamp EJ, Bulten BF, Nieuwenhuis AA, et al. Does diastolic dysfunction precede systolic dysfunction in trastuzumab-induced cardiotoxicity? Assessment with multigated radionuclide angiography (MUGA). J Nucl Cardiol. 2016;23(4):824-32.
15. Serrano JM, González I, Del Castillo S, et al. Diastolic dysfunction following anthracycline-based chemotherapy in breast cancer patients: incidence and predictors. Oncologist. 2015;20(8):864-72.
16. Klein R, Nadouri D, Osler E, et al. Diastolic dysfunction can precede systolic dysfunction on MUGA in cancer patients receiving trastuzumab-based therapy. Nucl Med Commun. 2019;40(1):22-9.
17. Upshaw JN, Finkelman B, Hubbard RA, et al. Comprehensive assessment of changes in left ventricular diastolic function with contemporary breast cancer therapy. JACC Cardiovasc Imaging. 2020;13(1 Pt 2):198-210.

18. Appel JM, Sogaard P, Mortensen CE, et al. Tissue-Doppler assessment of cardiac left ventricular function during short-term adjuvant epirubicin therapy for breast cancer. J Am Soc Echocardiogr. 2011;24(2):200-6.
19. Heidenreich PA, Hancock SL, Vagelos RH, et al. Diastolic dysfunction after mediastinal irradiation. Am Heart J. 2005;150(5):977-82.
20. Adams MJ, Lipsitz SR, Colan SD, et al. Cardiovascular status in long-term survivors of Hodgkin's disease treated with chest radiotherapy. J Clin Oncol. 2004;22(15): 3139-48.
21. Saiki H, Petersen IA, Scott CG, et al. Risk of heart failure with preserved ejection fraction in older women after contemporary radiotherapy for breast cancer. Circulation. 2017;135(15):1388-96.
22. Cao L, Cai G, Chang C, et al. Diastolic dysfunction occurs early in HER2-positive breast cancer patients treated concurrently with radiation therapy and trastuzumab. Oncologist. 2015;20(6):605-14.
23. Saiki H, Moulay G, Guenzel AJ, et al. Experimental cardiac radiation exposure induces ventricular diastolic dysfunction with preserved ejection fraction. Am J Physiol Heart Circ Physiol. 2017;313(2):H392-407.
24. Camilli M, Ferdinandy P, Salvatorelli E, et al. Anthracyclines, diastolic dysfunction and the road to heart failure in cancer survivors: an untold story. Prog Cardiovasc Dis. 2024;86:38-47.
25. Minotti G, Salvatorelli E, Reggiardo G, et al. Cardiac anthracycline accumulation and B-type natriuretic peptide to define risk and predictors of cancer treatment-related early diastolic dysfunction. J Pharmacol Exp Ther. 2022;381(3):266-73.
26. Swain SM, Whaley FS, Ewer MS. Congestive heart failure in patients treated with doxorubicin: a retrospective analysis of three trials. Cancer. 2003;97(11):2869-79.
27. Thavendiranathan P, Calvillo-Argüelles O. Breast cancer treatment and diastolic dysfunction: should we worry about relaxing in cardio-oncology? JACC Cardiovasc Imaging. 2020;13(1 Pt 2):211-14.
28. Nolan MT, Marwick TH, Plana JC, et al. Effect of traditional heart failure risk factors on myocardial dysfunction in adult survivors of childhood cancer. JACC Cardiovasc Imaging. 2018;11(8):1202-3.
29. Rohde LE, Baldi A, Weber C, et al. Tei index in adult patients submitted to adriamycin chemotherapy: failure to predict early systolic dysfunction. Diagnosis of adriamycin cardiotoxicity. Int J Cardiovasc Imaging. 2007;23(2):185-91.
30. Honda K, Takeshita K, Murotani K, et al. Assessment of left ventricular diastolic function during trastuzumab treatment in patients with HER2-positive breast cancer. Breast Cancer. 2017;24(2):312-8.
31. Dorup I, Levitt G, Sullivan I, et al. Prospective longitudinal assessment of late anthracycline cardiotoxicity after childhood cancer: the role of diastolic function. Heart. 2004;90(10):1214-6.
32. Eidem BW, Sapp BG, Suarez CR, et al. Usefulness of the myocardial performance index for early detection of anthracycline-induced cardiotoxicity in children. Am J Cardiol. 2001;87(9):1120-2, A9.
33. Nagiub M, Nixon JV, Kontos MC. Ability of nonstrain diastolic parameters to predict doxorubicin-induced cardiomyopathy: a systematic review with meta-analysis. Cardiol Rev. 2018;26(1):29-34.

CHAPTER

Echocardiographic Evaluation of Left Atrial Stiffness Index and Right Ventricular and Right Atrial Strain in HFpEF

Nilufar Fatema

INTRODUCTION

More than half of the heart failure (HF) patients belong to heart failure with preserve ejection fraction (HFpEF) group. But still, it is a challenge for cardiologists to diagnose HFpEF group. According to ESC HF guidelines of 2021, the diagnostic criteria of HFpEF were: (1) Symptoms and signs of HF, (2) LVEF ≥50%, and (3) objective evidence of cardiac structural and/or functional abnormalities consistent with the presence of LV diastolic dysfunction (LVDD)/raised LV filling pressure, including raised natriuretic peptides.[1]

ASSESSMENT OF LEFT ATRIAL FUNCTION, LEFT ATRIAL STRAIN, AND LEFT ATRIAL STIFFNESS INDEX

There are three phases of left atrial (LA) function that are reservoir, conduit, and contractile.[2] In reservoir phase, the filling of the left atrium via pulmonary veins occurs after closure of the mitral valve. The LA conduit phase occurs during early diastole when the mitral valve opens while the passive LV filling occurs which corresponds to the E wave that is early transmitral flow in Doppler. The LA contractile phase correlates with the A wave that is late transmitral flow due to left atrial contraction.[3,4] LA function is affected by abnormal loading conditions and heart rate in all three phases. LA reservoir strain (LASr) has prognostic value in a variety of cardiovascular diseases.[5] It also predicts morbidity and mortality in the humans.[6] Due to volume or pressure overload, the anatomy of LA is changed as LA has thin walls, which are susceptible to atrial remodeling. That is why arrhythmic focus is generated in LA wall. During reservoir phase, LA filling leads to stretching of the atrial wall, so the disease conditions that cause a reduction in LA compliance have a direct effect on LA reservoir phasic function.[7] The degree of LA interstitial fibrosis correlates to LA reservoir function, and this can be evaluated by LA strain imaging.[7] LA stiffness index for identifying HFpEF from diastolic dysfunction is the most accurate way that correlates well with pulmonary artery systolic pressure. LA stiffness can be assessed by the ratio of change of LA pressure to volume during passive filling of LA. LA stiffness is calculated as E/e'/LA reservoir strain. LA stiffness has prognostic value in case of HFpEF, is an early marker for target organ damage in case of hypertension, predicts exercise capacity, and improves quality of life in older age and obesity-induced HFpEF. It is also association between LA stiffness index and can predict the recurrence of atrial fibrillation (AF) and the cardiac death events.

Left atrial contractile strain (LASct) and LA conduit strain (LAScd) have some clinical utility, but these are more used for research purposes. LASct correlates to the active contraction of the atria. LA contractile function is reduced if there are elevated LV filling pressures. In case of AF, LASct is lower, which has predictive value for the development of new AF in future.[8] Walek P et al. showed maintenance of sinus rhythm in post-DCR who had preserved LASct.[9] LASct may predict recurrence of AF in postcatheter ablation in normal-sized LA.[10] LASct has demonstrated prognostic value in specific populations such as patients with congenital aortic stenosis and patients with ESRF.[11,12]

The LAScd is an indirect marker of LV relaxation as it results from the pressure gradient between LA and LV when mitral valve opens. LAScd is reduced in case of HFpEF and diastolic dysfunction.[13,14] Further researches are required to find out the wider application of LASct and LAScd **(Figs. 1 and 2)**.

TECHNICAL ASPECTS OF LEFT ATRIAL STRAIN MEASUREMENT

The EACVI/ASE/Industry Taskforce has released a consensus statement to standardize LA strain assessment to reduce intervendor variability.[3] LA strain should be assessed by an optimized apical four-chamber cine view with high frame rate of 50–70 frames/minute. Evidence supports the use of global rather than regional LA strain and sample over the LA wall probably, as it provides less opportunity for sampling error than a single view. We use apical four- and two-chamber views for automated tracking.[3] Manual correction to endocardial tracking is often needed due to the thin LA and mobile interatrial septum in case of atrial septal aneurysm.[4] The recent development of a specific LA-strain software (e.g., Auto strain LA and LA Automated Function Imaging) has further consolidated a uniform approach to LA-strain measurement. Nonexpert operators can also do these measurements easily.[15]

Two temporal reference points may be used for tracking the LA border (QRS-guided or P-wave-guided). Current LA-strain software automatically detects the upslope of the R-wave as the marker for end-diastole and endocardial tracing is generated. In MASCOT-HIT study took place in 26 expert centers showed that both reference points for LA-strain assessment were reproducible and demonstrated that QRS-guided LA-strain was more feasible and needed shorter analysis time.[15]

Normal values for LASr have been assessed in two meta-analyses.[16,17] Variation in the "normal value" of LASr was influenced by different ECG gating, sample size, and vendor, as well as age, gender, and race. LA reservoir and conduit function were deteriorating with increasing age and in women.[18,19] The normal value for LASr is ≈ – 38% **(Table 1)**; however, studies have shown that a LASr cutoff of ≈ ≥22% identifies risk of adverse outcomes.[20,21]

TABLE 1: Normal values for LA strain.

LA reservoir strain	*Normal value*
LASr	–38%

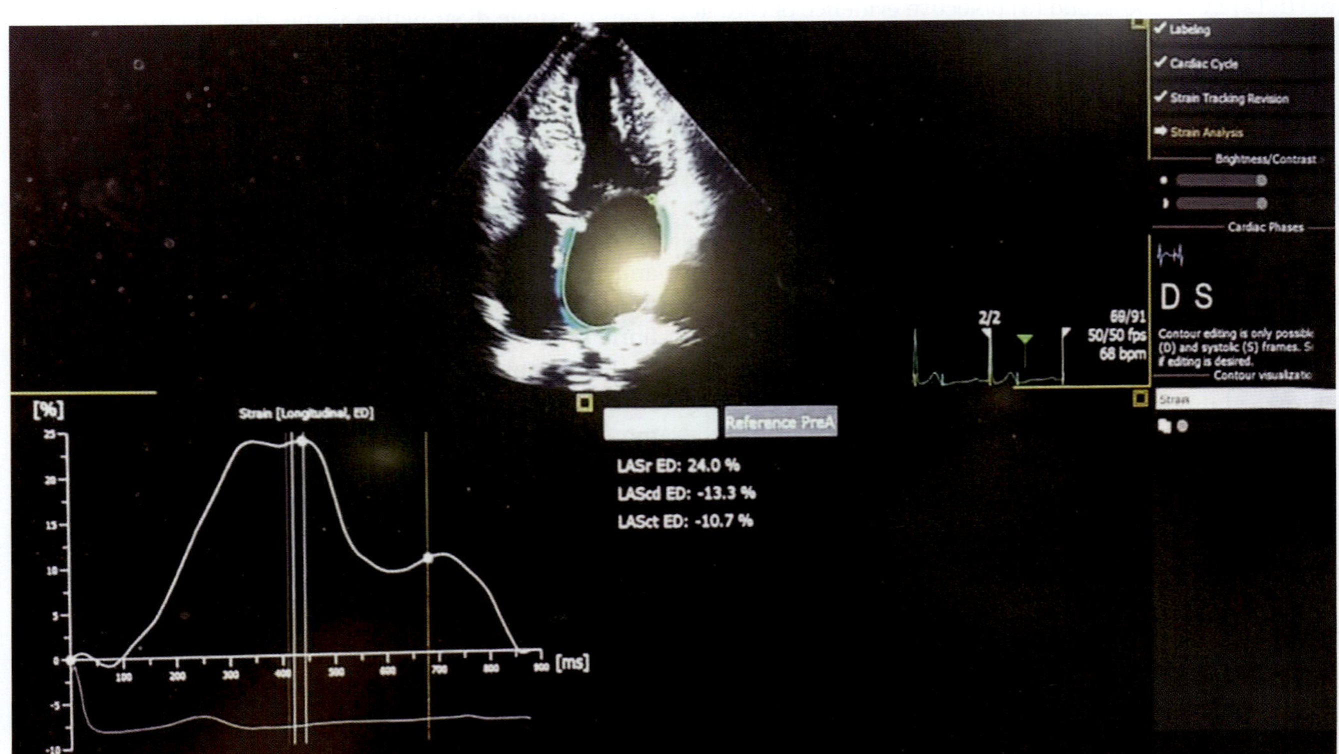

Fig. 1: Strain curve demonstrating LA strain with tracing of LA border in hypertensive patient A with dilated LA size.

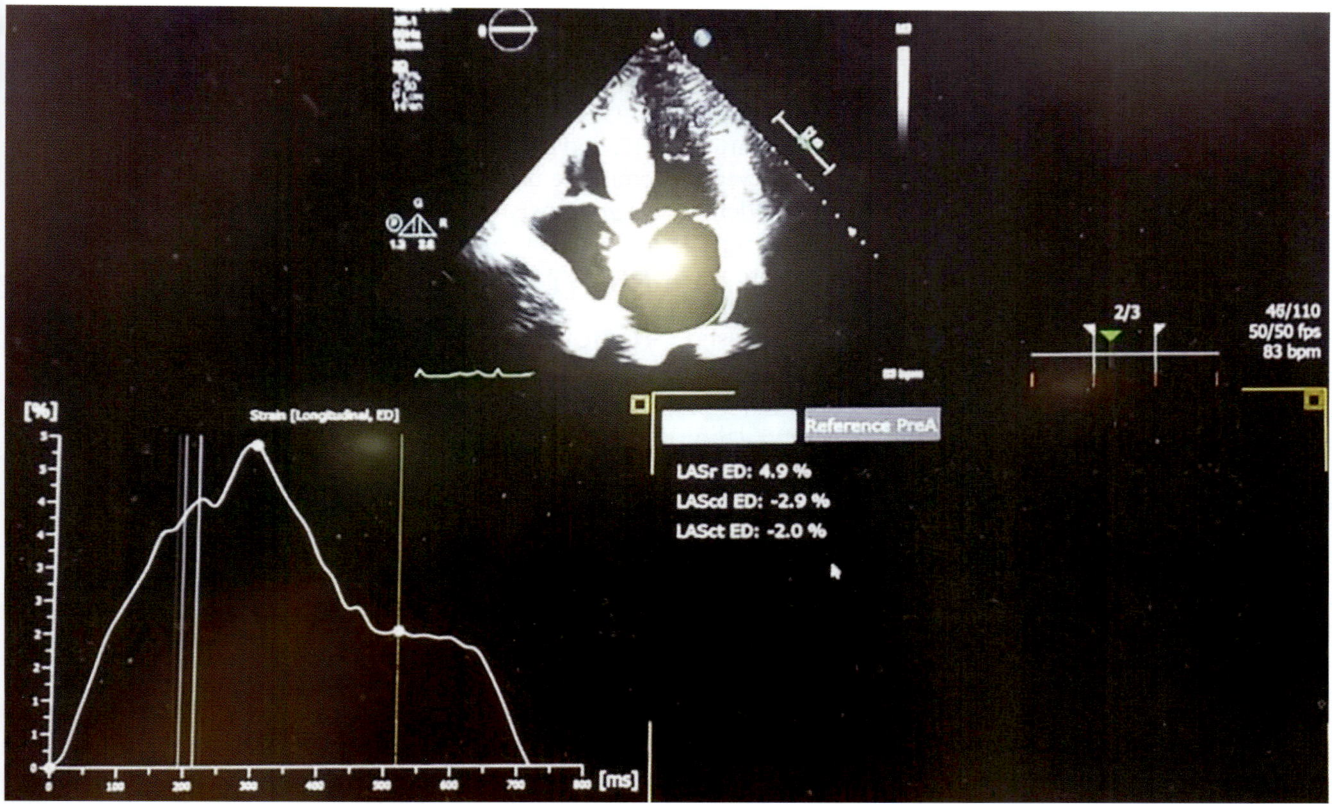

Fig. 2: Strain curve demonstrating LA strain with tracing of LA border in hypertensive patient B with dilated LA.

CLINICAL IMPLICATIONS OF LEFT ATRIAL STRAIN

Clinical applications of LA strain are more in case of AF, HFpEF, and valvular heart disease.[22] To asses LA function, LA strain has capability to predict AF in different disease conditions.[23-36] In the Copenhagen City Heart Study,[23] LA strains were done in 4,466 healthy participants and they were followed for 5.3 years for incident development of new AF. About 4.3% of participants developed AF. Results showed a LA strain of <23% was associated with increased risk of AF in 6.8% compared to those with LA strain ≥23%. Abnormal LASr and LASct were independent predictors of AF. Abnormal LASr (≤19%) is also a useful predictor of AF occurrence in patients with hypertension.[37] In case of cryptogenic stroke, abnormal LA strain is predictive of new-onset AF in future. Atriopathy was reclassified after demonstrating a potential clinical benefit.[26-28] In a meta-analysis, 1,025 post radiofrequency ablation AF patients were studied, and reported that LASr was significantly lower preablation in patients with recurrent AF compared with patients with sinus rhythm (15.7 ± 5.7% vs. 23.0 ± 7.0%, $p = 0.016$). Lower LASr was associated with AF recurrence,[34] and it reflects arteriopathy and fibrosis in AF patients. LA strain is an independent predictor in AF patients without dilated LA.[29,33] This ability of strain to risk-stratify the recurrence of AF may aid in determining the patients who will be benefited from longer-term anticoagulation and monitoring.[28]

More than 50% of HF is due to HFpEF.[38] LA strain can give information that is useful for the diagnosis of HFpEF. In 517 HFpEF patients with elevated filling pressures have reduced LASr (<23%) and increased left atrial volume index (LAVi) (62.4 and 33.6%, $p < 0.01$).[39] Sub-analyses of the large HFpEF management trials such as TOPCAT (Treatment Of Preserved Cardiac Function Heart Failure With an Aldosterone Antagonist Trial) showed that LASr of <26% was detected in 52% of HFpEF patients whereas in PARAMOUNT (Prospective comparison of ARNI with ARB on Management Of heart failUre with preserved ejectioN fracTion) trial, LASr was consistently shown to be impaired in patients with HFpEF in comparison with controls (48.4 ± 1.2% vs. controls 58.4 ± 2.1%, $p < 0.001$).[40,41]

The diagnosis of HFpEF is based on multiple clinical and echocardiographic variables. The LA strain may facilitate this diagnosis. Traditional echocardiographic assessment of HFpEF includes pulmonary artery pressure, transmitral flow with tissue velocity imaging, and LAVi.[38,42] Reddy et al. proposed the "H2PEFF" score to simplify the diagnostic process of HFpEF, which includes echocardiographic and clinical parameters (such as E/e′ ratio >9, pulmonary artery systolic pressure >35 mm Hg, obesity, AF, age >60 years, and ≥2 antihypertensive agents).[43] These variables derive a composite score from 0 to 9 where the odds of HFpEF doubled for each 1-unit score increase. This score was found useful to differentiate unexplained dyspnea due to HFpEF from noncardiac dyspnea. However, an invasive hemodynamic exercise testing is the gold standard for the diagnosis of HFpEF. Another diagnostic algorithm is the ESC Heart Failure Association algorithm "HFA-PEFF":[44] Pretest assessment (P), diagnostic workup with echocardiogram and natriuretic peptide (E), functional testing in case of uncertainty (F), and final etiological workup (F). In this diagnostic approach, a score of ≥5 is diagnostic of HFpEF whilst a score of ≤1 is unlikely to be HFpEF, and scores 2–4 are indeterminate and require further testing. Both these scores have evolved to estimate the likelihood of HFpEF. But still, there is variability that has been shown when both the algorithms were applied to the same population with suspected 41% HFpEF patients and they were classified differently by either score.[45]

The importance of LA filling pressure is not restricted to HFpEF whereas the current diagnostic algorithm for diastolic dysfunction is also dependent on measurement of LAVi and E/e′. But the diagnosis is not clear cut when it provides equivocal findings.[46] The raised LA filling pressures lead to LA dilatation and remodeling due to stretching of atrial cardiomyocytes.[47] This process is nonspecific as it is also caused by AF where delayed reverse remodeling occurs. Assessment of LA function by LA strain has been shown to be a sensitive tool in its ability to differentiate between all stages of diastolic dysfunction.[46] LASr improves the feasibility and diagnostic accuracy of the 2016 ASE/EACVI diastolic algorithm in patients with HFpEF.[48] LA strain measurements allow for accurate classification of diastolic dysfunction with a LASr of >35% correlating to patients with normal diastolic function with an accuracy of 72%.[49] Abnormal LASr of ≤19% identified patients with grade-3 diastolic dysfunction with an accuracy of 95%.[49]

LA strain is impaired in valvular heart disease and has prognostic importance. Mitral regurgitation (MR) due to any cause is associated with reduced both reservoirs and contractile LA strain.[50] Sugimoto et al. found significantly impaired LA strain profile in both primary and secondary MR. In the same study, LASr >16% at peak exercise was associated with 3-year event-free survival.[50,51] In asymptomatic patients with moderate MR, a reduced LASr was associated with the development of subsequent cardiovascular events.[51] Preoperative mitral valve surgery patients with severe primary MR demonstrated reductions in LASr (<21%) as an independent predictor of mortality, HF, and functional capacity.[52] Future applications of LASr could be used to find out the accurate timing of mitral valve surgery to improve postoperative outcomes.

RIGHT VENTRICULAR STRAIN

Rationale for Assessment of Right Ventricular Function

The assessment of right ventricular (RV) function is essential for the diagnosis of pulmonary hypertension, HF, and valvular abnormalities. The assessment of the RV by echocardiography is challenging due to its retrosternal position, crescent-shaped geometry, and volume dependency.[53] RV function occurs by three mechanisms: (1) Longitudinal shortening with movement of tricuspid annulus toward the apex, (2) radial motion with movement of free wall inward producing a bellows effect, and (3) anteroposterior shortening from free wall movement over the septum.[54] The current gold standard for assessment of RV function is RV volumetric analysis and RV ejection fraction (RVEF) using CMR. The accessibility to CMR remains restricted till date in some places due to limitations such as being costly, lack of skilled people, and contraindications in patients with noncompatible devices.

The quantitative echocardiographic markers, which are tricuspid annular plane systolic excursion (TAPSE) and RV fractional area change (FAC), are subject to translational motion. These parameters have limited prognostic and diagnostic significance.[55] The TAPSE can be overestimated with translational motion and is partially representative as it evaluates just one segment of the RV. RV FAC has some limitations in its image quality and depends on the correct identification of the endocardial delineation.[56] At this point, the RV strain and three-dimensional echocardiography (3DE) are emerging as promising additions to earlier parameters.

The RV strain is not angle-dependent and it can measure longitudinal function in RV free wall. The RV strain can detect the subclinical RV dysfunction where the conventional method of RV function shows normal, which is same as LV.[55] RV longitudinal strain is a highly sensitive marker of RV dysfunction, is reproducible,[57] and is useful in cardiomyopathies, cardiac amyloidosis, and cancer.[58] 3DE is helpful to detect the complex structure of the RV and overcomes limitations of foreshortened images in 2D echocardiography.[59] CMR is gold standard for accuracy and reproducibility in assessing RV.[60] The standard 2D echocardiography has some prognostic value.[61]

Right ventricular–pulmonary artery (RV–PA) coupling represents how RV contractility matches RV afterload. The more RV afterload the more RV contractility due to the "RV–PA coupling" and adverse outcome is associated with RV–PA "uncoupling". The gold standard assessment of RV–PA coupling is invasive multibeat RV pressure-volume evaluation of arterial and ventricular elastance. It can be measured noninvasively using the ratio of TAPSE to PASP with a cutoff value of TAPSE/PASP = 0.31 mm/mm Hg and it helps to know the prognosis.[62] Determination of RVEF/PASP ratio by 3DE can be used as a novel marker of RV–PA coupling.[63,64] Indexing strain assessment of RV function against PASP (via RV-GLS/PASP and RV-FWS/PASP) can provide a representation of RV–PA coupling and demonstrates an increased risk of mortality.[65]

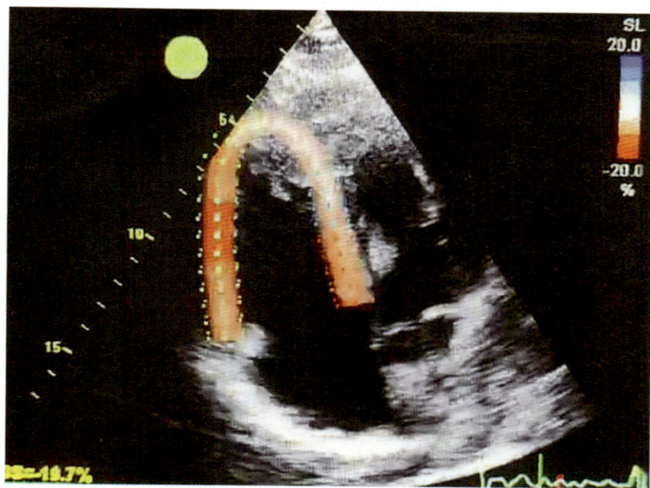

Fig. 3: RV strain in patient C.

Technical Aspects of Right Ventricular Strain Measurement

Right ventricular (RV) strain should be assessed in RV-focused apical four-chamber view. The RV should be completely visualized with optimization of the RV-free wall as standard apical four-chamber view will give a smaller strain value.[55,66] The RV strain can be assessed in two ways, (1) RV-GLS (six-segment model involving the interventricular septum (IVS) and free-wall) or (2) RV free-wall strain (RV-FWS), which is a three-segment model.[66] The measurement of either RV-GLS or RV-FWS will be dependent on the situations. The diseases that are involved with the right-sided circulation such as pulmonary hypertension are best assessed by RV-FWS while RV function assessment is needed, for example, tricuspid regurgitation or RV infarction might need to include the septum. The EACVI/ASE/Industry Task Force supports measurement of RV-FWS.[3,66,67]

A recent meta-analysis of normal values for RV strain reviewed 788 articles, which included 4,439 healthy subjects. The analysis defined normal reference values with a pooled mean and lower limit of normal with 95% confidence interval for RV-FWS of –26.9% (–28.0%, –25.9%) and RV-GLS of –23.4% (–24.2, –22.6%), respectively.[68]

A new software has been introduced for dedicated RV strain, which may overcome some of the technical challenges of using the LV strain software package to assess the RV. A study using CMR as the gold standard found that traditional parameters for RV function (TAPSE, FAC, and RV S') and contemporary RV strain all provided good correlation with RVEF. However, RV-FWS provided the strongest diagnostic accuracy to predict an impaired RVEF (<45%) with a high specificity and sensitivity.[69] The limitations of 2D strain are the transition of speckles to outside the imaging plane during systole and introducing artefact. The 3D strain can partially overcome this problem **(Fig. 3)**.

Clinical Implications of Right Ventricular Strain

Right ventricular strain assessment is important in pulmonary arterial hypertension (PAH), cardiomyopathies, and valvular heart disease.

In PAH, the status of the RV has the major role to determine the outcome. RV strain may be impaired whilst conventional parameters for RV function are still normal. This situation is described as subclinical RV dysfunction.[70] Abnormal RV-FWS in PAH has been shown as a powerful predictor of future cardiovascular events in a study with 4-year follow-up of these patients.[71] RV FWS was an independent predictor for all-cause mortality in patients with PAH.[72]

In case of left heart failure (LHF), RV strain plays important role in prognostic value. RV strain may deteriorate early in LHF if LA pressure is increased, but it is more commonly impaired in late-stage disease.[73] In a study of 98 HF patients who are candidates for heart transplantation, a low RV FWS was the strongest predictor of the combined outcome of HF hospitalization, cardiovascular (CV) death, insertion of intra-aortic balloon pump or ventricular assist device, and need for heart transplant.[74] Multiple studies have shown that RV FWS strain was an independent predictor of overall and CV mortality in patients with HFrEF and superior to TAPSE, FAC, and RV S' in this regard.[75-77] The sensitivity of RV strain by RV FWS to predict poor outcomes in HFrEF is the most precise functional measure that correlates with the degree of myocardial fibrosis.[78]

Tricuspid regurgitation (TR) is most commonly secondary to pulmonary hypertension and annular dilatation in the setting of RV volume/pressure overload due to left heart disease.[79] "Primary" TR is due to valve disease being uncommon. Accurate assessment of RV function is necessary for decision-making regarding TR. In case of primary TR, delayed intervention on the tricuspid valve may lead to permanent RV dysfunction.[80-82] Reduced RV FWS in patients with functional TR is more sensitive for detecting RV impairment and is associated with worse outcomes when compared to conventional measurements of RV function.[83] In this population, a significant proportion of patients had abnormal RV FWS but preserved FAC and TAPSE suggesting that subclinical myocardial dysfunction occurs prior to the reduction of RVEF.[83] RV strain is a highly sensitive and prognostic tool in TR patients. Future clinical applications to utilize strain to determine the proper timing of tricuspid valve intervention are promising.[84]

RIGHT ATRIAL STRAIN

Rationale for the Assessment of Right Atrial Function

The right atrium is neglected and undervalued for its contribution to overall cardiac function. For this reason, the assessment of right atrial (RA) function is done in a few disease conditions. The RA has phasic functions like LA, which can be evaluated by echocardiography and CMR.[85]

The evaluation of size and function of RA is important in the outcomes of disease conditions such as pulmonary hypertension, HF, atrial arrhythmias, and RV infarction. 1,085 pulmonary hypertension patients were evaluated in a meta-analysis of 12 studies, those with an enlarged RA area had poor prognosis.[86] Another study showed an impairment of RA reservoir, conduit functions, and RA strain in patients with pulmonary hypertension, it is also correlated with worse functional class.[87] In HFpEF, impaired CMR-derived RA conduit and reservoir function were independent predictors of mortality.[85] Atrial arrhythmias are more common with RA dilatation in both 2D and 3D echocardiography.[88] The ability of the RA to reverse remodeling can be assessed by RA volume detection in post-radiofrequency ablation for AF.[89] In post-RV infarction patients, RA function as assessed by reservoir and conduit RA strain has a role in prognosis.[90]

Technical Aspects of Right Atrial Strain Measurement

The accurate assessment of RA function continues to be a challenge due to the impact of volume overloading and off-axis imaging with echocardiography.[91] Traditional 2D echocardiographic assessment of RA area by planimetry is susceptible to errors arising from geometric assumptions and off-axis of RA. RA volume assessment is not routine or supported by current guidelines due to the lack of standardized RA volume data.[92] RA strain may be assessed via both CMR and standard transthoracic echo (STE). The CMR feature tracking assessment of RA strain has strong inter- and intraobserver reliability, which has consistency with STE RA strain. The limitations of CMR revolve around access and cost.[93] That is why STE RA strain aims to add to the assessment of RA function given the promising outcomes. A review article by Khan et al.

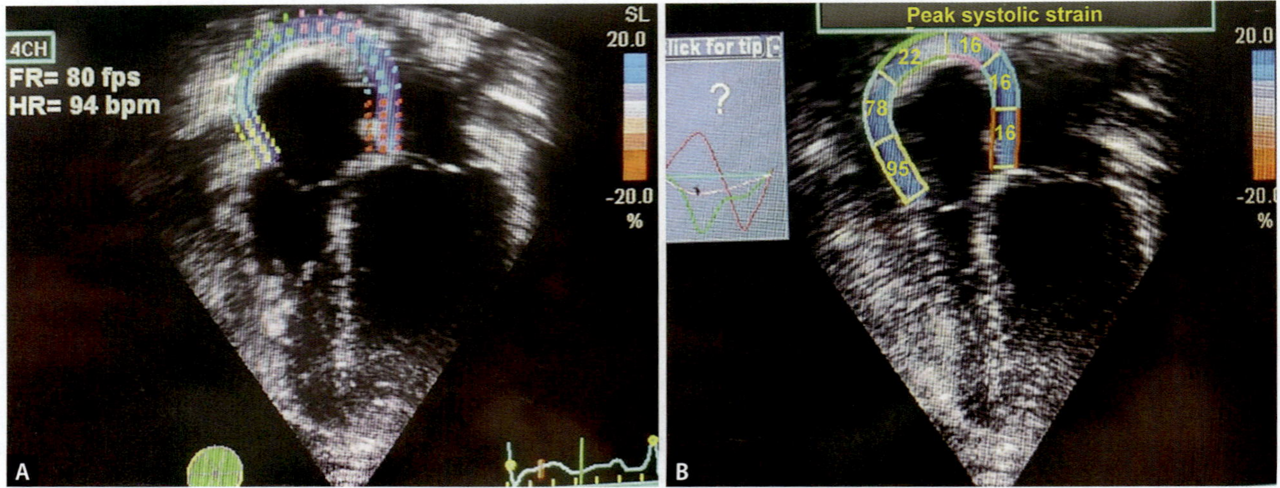

Figs. 4A and B: RA strain in patient D and patient E.

in 2018 showed that only 59 studies were found on STE RA strain. About 80% of these studies were retrospective. A single study highlighted the need for future prospective and randomized controlled trials to strengthen the clinical utility of STE RA strain **(Figs. 4A and B)**.[94]

Clinical Implications of Right Atrial Strain

The clinical utility of RA strain remains limited due to the lack of established normal values.[95] A meta-analysis of RA strain which included 4,111 normal adults concluded that there is limited clinical utility of RA strain due to the extensive variability in currently reported normal values of RA strain.[96] Until technical capabilities improve, RA strain may be used as a research tool.

CONCLUSION

The diagnostic utility and clinical applications of strain have been improved in last decade. The chamber-specific strain software and taskforce consensus statements have helped overcome the previous limitations of reproducibility and intervendor variability like LV GLS. The usefulness of RV and LA strains is more evident. Clinical outcomes will improve in the future if strain-directed therapy can be provided.

REFERENCES

1. McDonagh TA, Metra M, Adamo M, et al.; ESC Scientific Document Group. 2021 ESC Guidelines for the diagnosis and treatment of acute and chronic heart failure. Eur Heart J. 2021;42(36):3599-726.
2. Matsuda Y, Toma Y, Ogawa H, et al. Importance of left atrial function in patients with myocardial infarction. Circulation. 1983;67(3):566-71.
3. Badano LP, Kolias TJ, Muraru D, et al. Standardization of left atrial, right ventricular, and right atrial deformation imaging using two-dimensional speckle tracking echocardiography: a consensus document of the EACVI/ASE/Industry Task Force to standardize deformation imaging. Eur Heart J Cardiovasc Imaging. 2018;19(6):591-600.
4. Voigt JU, Mălăescu GG, Haugaa K, et al. How to do LA strain. Eur Heart J Cardiovasc Imaging. 2020;21(7): 715-7.
5. Thomas L, Muraru D, Popescu BA, et al. Evaluation of left atrial size and function: relevance for clinical practice. J Am Soc Echocardiogr. 2020;33(8):934-52.
6. Modin D, Biering-Sørensen SR, Mogelvang R, et al. Prognostic value of left atrial strain in predicting cardiovascular morbidity and mortality in the general population. Eur Heart J Cardiovasc Imaging. 2019;20(7): 804-15.
7. Cameli M, Lisi M, Righini FM, et al. Usefulness of atrial deformation analysis to predict left atrial fibrosis and endocardial thickness in patients undergoing mitral valve operations for severe mitral regurgitation secondary to mitral valve prolapse. Am J Cardiol. 2013;111(4):595-601.
8. Hirose T, Kawasaki M, Tanaka R, et al. Left atrial function assessed by speckle tracking echocardiography as a predictor of new-onset non-valvular atrial fibrillation: Results from a prospective study in 580 adults. Eur Heart J Cardiovasc Imaging. 2012;13(3):243-50.
9. Walek P, Grabowska U, Cieśla E, et al. Left atrial longitudinal strain in the contractile phase as a predictor of sinus rhythm maintenance after electrical cardioversion performed due to persistent atrial fibrillation. Kardiol Pol. 2021;79(4):458-60.
10. Nielsen AB, Skaarup KG, Djernaes K, et al. Left atrial contractile strain predicts recurrence of atrial tachyarrhythmia after catheter ablation. Int J Cardiol. 2022;358:51-7.
11. Mutluer FO, Bowen DJ, van Grootel RWJ, et al. Prognostic value of left atrial strain in patients with congenital aortic stenosis. Eur Heart J Open. 2022;2(3):23.
12. Ayer A, Banerjee U, Mills C, et al. Left atrial strain is associated with adverse cardiovascular events in patients with end-stage renal disease: findings from the cardiac, endothelial function and arterial stiffness in ESRD (CERES) study. Hemodial Int. 2022;26(3):323-34.
13. Marino PN, Degiovanni A, Zanaboni J. Complex interaction between the atrium and the ventricular filling process: the role of conduit. Open Heart. 2019;6(2):e001042.
14. Savelev A, Solovev O, Baturova M, et al. Reduction of left atrial strain and strain rate during conduit phase as the earliest marker of left ventricular diastolic disfunction. Eur Heart J Cardiovasc Imaging. 2021;22:31.
15. Cameli M, Miglioranza MH, Magne J, et al. Multicentric atrial strain comparison between two different modalities: MASCOT HIT study. Diagnostics (Basel). 2020;10(11):946.
16. Pathan F, D'Elia N, Nolan MT, et al. Normal ranges of left atrial strain by speckle-tracking echocardiography: a systematic review and meta-analysis. J Am Soc Echocardiogr. 2017;30(1):59-70.
17. Mohseni-Badalabadi R, Mirjalili T, Jalali A, et al. A systematic review and meta-analysis of the normal reference value of the longitudinal left atrial strain by three dimensional speckle tracking echocardiography. Sci Rep. 2022;12(1):4395.
18. Sugimoto T, Robinet S, Dulgheru R, et al. Echocardiographic reference ranges for normal left atrial function parameters: Results from the EACVI NORRE study. Eur Heart J Cardiovasc Imaging. 2018;19(6):630-8.
19. Liao JN, Chao TF, Kuo JY, et al. Age, sex, and blood pressure-related influences on reference values of left atrial deformation and mechanics from a large-scale Asian population. Circ Cardiovasc Imaging. 2017;10(10):e006077.
20. Stassen J, van Wijngaarden AL, Butcher SC, et al. Prognostic value of left atrial reservoir function in patients

with severe primary mitral regurgitation undergoing mitral valve repair. Eur Heart J Cardiovasc Imaging. 2022;24(1): 142-51.

21. Maffeis C, Morris DA, Belyavskiy E, et al. Left atrial function and maximal exercise capacity in heart failure with preserved and mid-range ejection fraction. ESC Heart Fail. 2021;8(1):116-28.
22. Leung M, van Rosendael PJ, Abou R, et al. Left atrial function to identify patients with atrial fibrillation at high risk of stroke: new insights from a large registry. Eur Heart J. 2018;39(16):1416-25.
23. Hauser R, Nielsen AB, Skaarup KG, et al. Left atrial strain predicts incident atrial fibrillation in the general population: The Copenhagen City Heart Study. Eur Heart J-Cardiovasc Imaging. 2021;23(1):52-60.
24. Park JJ, Park JH, Hwang IC, et al. Left atrial strain as a predictor of new-onset atrial fibrillation in patients with heart failure. JACC Cardiovasc Imaging. 2020;13(10): 2071-81.
25. Raman B, Smillie RW, Mahmod M, et al. Incremental value of left atrial booster and reservoir strain in predicting atrial fibrillation in patients with hypertrophic cardiomyopathy: a cardiovascular magnetic resonance study. J Cardiovasc Magn Reson. 2021;23(1):109.
26. Ramkumar S, Pathan F, Kawakami H, et al. Impact of disease stage on the performance of strain markers in the prediction of atrial fibrillation. Int J Cardiol. 2021;324:233-41.
27. Rasmussen SMA, Olsen FJ, Jørgensen PG, et al. Utility of left atrial strain for predicting atrial fibrillation following ischemic stroke. Int J Cardiovasc Imaging. 2019;35(9): 1605-13.
28. Deferm S, Bertrand PB, Churchill TW, et al. Left atrial mechanics assessed early during hospitalization for cryptogenic stroke are associated with occult atrial fibrillation: a speckle-tracking strain echocardiography study. J Am Soc Echocardiogr. 2021;34(2):156-65.
29. Ble M, Benito B, Cuadrado-Godia E, et al. Left atrium assessment by speckle tracking echocardiography in cryptogenic stroke: seeking silent atrial fibrillation. J Clin Med. 2021;10(16):3501.
30. Kawakami H, Ramkumar S, Pathan F, et al. Use of echocardiography to stratify the risk of atrial fibrillation: comparison of left atrial and ventricular strain. Eur Heart J Cardiovasc Imaging. 2020;21:399-407.
31. Moreno-Ruiz LA, Madrid-Miller A, Martínez-Flores JE, et al. Left atrial longitudinal strain by speckle tracking as independent predictor of recurrence after electrical cardioversion in persistent and long standing persistent non-valvular atrial fibrillation. Int J Cardiovasc Imaging. 2019;35(9):1587-96.
32. Wałek P, Ciesla E, Gorczyca I, et al. Left atrial wall dyskinesia assessed during contractile phase as a predictor of atrial fibrillation recurrence after electrical cardioversion performed due to persistent atrial fibrillation. Medicine (Baltimore). 2020;99:e23333.
33. Motoc A, Luchian ML, Scheirlynck E, et al. Incremental value of left atrial strain to predict atrial fibrillation recurrence after cryoballoon ablation. PLoS One. 2021; 16(11):e0259999.
34. Nielsen AB, Skaarup KG, Lassen MCH, et al. Usefulness of left atrial speckle tracking echocardiography in predicting recurrence of atrial fibrillation after radiofrequency ablation: a systematic review and meta-analysis. Int J Cardiovasc Imaging. 2020;36(7):1293-309.
35. Ma XX, Boldt LH, Zhang YL, et al. Clinical relevance of left atrial strain to predict recurrence of atrial fibrillation after catheter ablation: A meta-analysis. Echocardiography. 2016;33(5):724-33.
36. Mouselimis D, Tsarouchas AS, Pagourelias ED, et al. Left atrial strain, intervendor variability, and atrial fibrillation recurrence after catheter ablation: a systematic review and meta-analysis. Hellenic J Cardiol. 2020;61(3):154-64.
37. Petre I, Onciul S, Iancovici S, et al. Left atrial strain for predicting atrial fibrillation onset in hypertensive patients. High Blood Press Cardiovasc Prev. 2019;26(4):331-7.
38. Koca H, Demirtas AO, Kaypakli O, et al. Decreased left atrial global longitudinal strain predicts the risk of atrial fibrillation recurrence after cryoablation in paroxysmal atrial fibrillation. J Interv Card Electrophysiol. 2020;58(1):51-9.
39. McDonagh TA, Metra M, Adamo M, et al.; Corrigendum to: 2021 ESC Guidelines for the diagnosis and treatment of acute and chronic heart failure. Eur Heart J. 2021;42(36):3599-726. Developed by the task force for the diagnosis and treatment of acute and chronic heart failure of the European Society of Cardiology (ESC) With the special contribution of the Heart Failure Association (HFA) of the ESC. Eur Heart J. 2021 Dec 21;42(48):4901.
40. Morris DA, Belyavskiy E, Aravind-Kumar R, et al. Potential usefulness and clinical relevance of adding left atrial strain to left atrial volume index in the detection of left ventricular diastolic dysfunction. JACC: Cardiovasc Imaging. 2018;11:1405-15.
41. Santos AB, Kraigher-Krainer E, Gupta DK, et al. Impaired left atrial function in heart failure with preserved ejection fraction. Eur J Heart Fail. 2014;16(10):1096-103.
42. Santos AB, Roca GQ, Claggett B, et al. Prognostic relevance of left atrial dysfunction in heart failure with preserved ejection fraction. Circ Heart Fail. 2016;9(4):e002763.
43. Nagueh SF, Smiseth OA, Appleton CP, et al. Recommendations for the evaluation of left ventricular diastolic function by echocardiography: An update from the American Society of Echocardiography and the European Association of Cardiovascular Imaging. J Am Soc Echocardiogr. 2016;29(4):277-314.
44. Reddy YNV, Carter RE, Obokata M, et al. A simple, evidence-based approach to help guide diagnosis of heart failure with preserved ejection fraction. Circulation. 2018; 138(9):861-70.
45. Pieske B, Tschöpe C, de Boer RA, et al. How to diagnose heart failure with preserved ejection fraction: the HFA-PEFF

diagnostic algorithm: A consensus recommendation from the Heart Failure Association (HFA) of the European Society of Cardiology (ESC). Eur Heart J. 2019;40(40): 3297-317.

46. Sanders-van Wijk S, Barandiarán Aizpurua A, Brunner-La Rocca HP, et al. The HFA-PEFF and H2FPEF scores largely disagree in classifying patients with suspected heart failure with preserved ejection fraction. Eur J Heart Fail. 2021; 23(5):838-40.
47. Singh A, Medvedofsky D, Mediratta A, et al. Peak left atrial strain as a single measure for the non-invasive assessment of left ventricular filling pressures. Int J Cardiovasc Imaging. 2019;35(1):23-32.
48. Cameli M, Mandoli GE, Mondillo S. Left atrium: the last bulwark before overt heart failure. Heart Fail Rev. 2017; 22(1):123-31.
49. Venkateshvaran A, Tureli HO, Faxén UL, et al. Left atrial reservoir strain improves diagnostic accuracy of the 2016 ASE/EACVI diastolic algorithm in patients with preserved left ventricular ejection fraction: insights from the KARUM haemodynamic database. Eur Heart J Cardiovasc Imaging. 2022;23(9):1157-68.
50. Singh A, Addetia K, Maffessanti F, et al. LA Strain for categorization of LV diastolic dysfunction. JACC Cardiovasc Imaging. 2017;10(7):735-43.
51. Sugimoto T, Bandera F, Generati G, et al. Left atrial dynamics during exercise in mitral regurgitation of primary and secondary origin. JACC Cardiovasc Imaging. 2020;13(1 Pt 1):25-40.
52. Cameli M, Pastore MC, Righini FM, et al. Prognostic value of left atrial strain in patients with moderate asymptomatic mitral regurgitation. Int J Cardiovasc Imaging. 2019;35(9): 1597-604.
53. Mandoli GE, Pastore MC, Benfari G, et al. Left atrial strain as a pre-operative prognostic marker for patients with severe primary mitral regurgitation. Int J Cardiol. 2021;324:139-45.
54. Tadic M. Multimodality evaluation of the right ventricle: an updated review. Clin Cardiol. 2015;38(12):770-6.
55. Haddad F, Hunt SA, Rosenthal DN, et al. Right ventricular function in cardiovascular disease. Part I: Anatomy, physiology, aging, and functional assessment of the right ventricle. Circulation. 2008;117(11):1436-48.
56. Tadic M, Nita N, Schneider L, et al. The predictive value of right ventricular longitudinal strain in pulmonary hypertension, heart failure, and valvular diseases. Front Cardiovasc Med. 2021;8:698158.
57. Dutta T, Aronow WS. Echocardiographic evaluation of the right ventricle: Clinical implications. Clin Cardiol. 2017; 40(8):542-8.
58. Stolfo D, Albani S, Biondi F, et al. Global right heart assessment with speckle-tracking imaging improves the risk prediction of a validated scoring system in pulmonary arterial hypertension. J Am Soc Echocardiogr. 2020;33(11):1334-44.e2.
59. Steen H, Giusca S, Montenbruck M, et al. Left and right ventricular strain using fast strain-encoded cardiovascular magnetic resonance for the diagnostic classification of patients with chronic non-ischemic heart failure due to dilated, hypertrophic cardiomyopathy or cardiac amyloidosis. J Cardiovasc Magn Reson. 2021;23(1):45.
60. Lang RM, Badano LP, Mor-Avi V, et al. Recommendations for cardiac chamber quantification by echocardiography in adults: An update from the American Society of Echocardiography and the European Association of Cardiovascular Imaging. J Am Soc Echocardiogr. 2015; 28(1):1-39.e14.
61. Park JB, Lee SP, Lee JH, et al. Quantification of right ventricular volume and function using single-beat three-dimensional echocardiography: a validation study with cardiac magnetic resonance. J Am Soc Echocardiogr. 2016; 29(5):392-401.
62. Nagata Y, Wu VC, Kado Y, et al. Prognostic value of right ventricular ejection fraction assessed by transthoracic 3D echocardiography. Circ Cardiovasc Imaging. 2017;10(2): e005384.
63. Tello K, Wan J, Dalmer A, et al. Validation of the tricuspid annular plane systolic excursion/systolic pulmonary artery pressure ratio for the assessment of right ventricular-arterial coupling in severe pulmonary hypertension. Circ Cardiovasc Imaging. 2019;12(9):e009047.
64. van de Veerdonk MC, Kind T, Marcus JT, et al. Progressive right ventricular dysfunction in patients with pulmonary arterial hypertension responding to therapy. J Am Coll Cardiol. 2011;58(24):2511-9.
65. Kubba S, Davila CD, Forfia PR. Methods for evaluating right ventricular function and ventricular-arterial coupling. Prog Cardiovasc Dis. 2016;59(1):42-51.
66. Iacoviello M, Monitillo F, Citarelli G, et al. Right ventriculo-arterial coupling assessed by two-dimensional strain: a new parameter of right ventricular function independently associated with prognosis in chronic heart failure patients. Int J Cardiol. 2017;241:318-21.
67. Badano LP, Muraru D, Parati G, et al. How to do right ventricular strain. Eur Heart J Cardiovasc Imaging. 2020; 21(8):825-7.
68. Muraru D, Onciul S, Peluso D, et al. Sex- and method-specific reference values for right ventricular strain by 2-dimensional speckle-tracking echocardiography. Circ Cardiovasc Imaging. 2016;9(2):e003866.
69. Wang TKM, Grimm RA, Rodriguez LL et al. Defining the reference range for right ventricular systolic strain by echocardiography in healthy subjects: a meta-analysis. PLoS One. 2021;16(8):e0256547.
70. Focardi M, Cameli M, Carbone SF, et al. Traditional and innovative echocardiographic parameters for the analysis of right ventricular performance in comparison with cardiac magnetic resonance. Eur Heart J Cardiovasc Imaging. 2015;16(1):47-52.
71. van Kessel M, Seaton D, Chan J, et al. Prognostic value of right ventricular free wall strain in pulmonary hypertension patients with pseudo-normalized tricuspid annular plane systolic excursion values. Int J Cardiovasc Imaging. 2016;32(6):905-12.

72. Motoji Y, Tanaka H, Fukuda Y, et al. Efficacy of right ventricular free-wall longitudinal speckle-tracking strain for predicting long-term outcome in patients with pulmonary hypertension. Circ J. 2013;77(3):756-63.
73. Haeck ML, Scherptong RW, Marsan NA, et al. Prognostic value of right ventricular longitudinal peak systolic strain in patients with pulmonary hypertension. Circ Cardiovasc Imaging. 2012;5(5):628-36.
74. Shah AM, Cikes M, Prasad N, et al. Echocardiographic features of patients with heart failure and preserved left ventricular ejection fraction. J Am Coll Cardiol. 2019; 74(23):2858-73.
75. Cameli M, Righini FM, Lisi M, et al. Comparison of right versus left ventricular strain analysis as a predictor of outcome in patients with systolic heart failure referred for heart transplantation. Am J Cardiol. 2013;112(11):1778-84.
76. Houard L, Benaets MB, de Meester de Ravenstein C, et al. Additional prognostic value of 2D right ventricular speckle-tracking strain for prediction of survival in heart failure and reduced ejection fraction: a comparative study with cardiac magnetic resonance. JACC Cardiovasc Imaging. 2019;12(12):2373-85.
77. Vizzardi E, D'Aloia A, Caretta G, et al. Long-term prognostic value of longitudinal strain of right ventricle in patients with moderate heart failure. Hellenic J Cardiol. 2014;55(2):150-5.
78. Carluccio E, Biagioli P, Alunni G, et al. Prognostic value of right ventricular dysfunction in heart failure with reduced ejection fraction: superiority of longitudinal strain over tricuspid annular plane systolic excursion. Circ Cardiovasc Imaging. 2018;11(1):e006894.
79. Lisi M, Cameli M, Righini FM, et al. RV Longitudinal deformation correlates with myocardial fibrosis in patients with end-stage heart failure. JACC Cardiovasc Imaging. 2015;8(5):514-22.
80. Furlani AC, Garcia MJ. Right ventricular strain. Circ Cardiovasc Imaging. 2019;12(3):e008862.
81. Kadri AN, Menon V, Sammour YM, et al. Outcomes of patients with severe tricuspid regurgitation and congestive heart failure. Heart. 2019;105(23):1813-7.
82. Kilic A, Saha-Chaudhuri P, Rankin JS, et al. Trends and outcomes of tricuspid valve surgery in North America: An analysis of more than 50,000 patients from the Society of Thoracic Surgeons database. Ann Thorac Surg. 2013;96(5):1546-52; discussion 1552.
83. Dreyfus J, Ghalem N, Garbarz E, et al. Timing of referral of patients with severe isolated tricuspid valve regurgitation to surgeons (from a French nationwide database). Am J Cardiol. 2018;122(2):323-6.
84. Prihadi EA, van der Bijl P, Dietz M, et al. Prognostic implications of right ventricular free wall longitudinal strain in patients with significant functional tricuspid regurgitation. Circ Cardiovasc Imaging. 2019;12(3): e008666.
85. Aalen JM, Smiseth OA. Strain identifies pseudo-normalized right ventricular function in tricuspid regurgitation. Eur Heart J Cardiovasc Imaging. 2021;22(8):876-7.
86. Jain S, Kuriakose D, Edelstein I, et al. Right atrial phasic function in heart failure with preserved and reduced ejection fraction. JACC Cardiovasc Imaging. 2019;12(8 Pt 1): 1460-70.
87. Liu K, Zhang C, Chen B et al. Association between right atrial area measured by echocardiography and prognosis among pulmonary arterial hypertension: a systematic review and meta-analysis. BMJ Open. 2020;10(9):e031316.
88. Meng X, Li Y, Li H, et al. Right atrial function in patients with pulmonary hypertension: a study with two-dimensional speckle-tracking echocardiography. Int J Cardiol. 2018;255:200-5.
89. Müller H, Burri H, Lerch R. Evaluation of right atrial size in patients with atrial arrhythmias: comparison of 2D versus real time 3D echocardiography. Echocardiography. 2008;25(6):617-23.
90. Müller H, Noble S, Keller PF, et al. Biatrial anatomical reverse remodelling after radiofrequency catheter ablation for atrial fibrillation: evidence from real-time three-dimensional echocardiography. Europace. 2008; 10(9):1073-8.
91. Nourian S, Hosseinsabet A, Jalali A, et al. Evaluation of right atrial function by two-dimensional speckle-tracking echocardiography in patients with right ventricular myocardial infarction. Int J Cardiovasc Imaging. 2017; 33(1):47-56.
92. Li J, Lu C, Wang W, et al. Assessment of right atrium dysfunction in patients with obstructive sleep apnea syndrome using velocity vector imaging. Cardiovasc Ultrasound. 2018;16(1):32.
93. Rudski LG, Lai WW, Afilalo J, et al. Guidelines for the echocardiographic assessment of the right heart in adults: A report from the American Society of Echocardiography: Endorsed by the European Association of Echocardiography, a registered branch of the European Society of Cardiology, and the Canadian Society of Echocardiography. J Am Soc Echocardiogr. 2010;23:685-713.
94. Truong VT, Palmer C, Young M, et al. Right atrial deformation using cardiovascular magnetic resonance myocardial feature tracking compared with two-dimensional speckle tracking echocardiography in healthy volunteers. Sci Rep. 2020;10(1):5237.
95. Khan S, Alenezi F, Bloomfield G. Right atrial speckle tracking strain echocardiography in heart failure. J Cardiac Fail. 2018;24(8):S38.
96. Hosseinsabet A, Mahmoudian R, Jalali A, et al. Normal ranges of right atrial strain and strain rate by two-dimensional speckle-tracking echocardiography: a systematic review and meta-analysis. Front Cardiovasc Med. 2021;8:771647.

CHAPTER

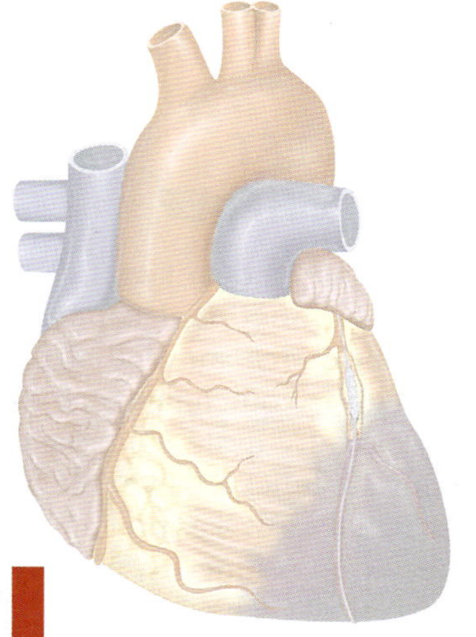

HFpEF and Left Atrial Atriopathy: Advanced Therapeutic Navigation

HK Chopra, Viveka Kumar, Anil Pareek, Anu Grover, Ruhani Bali

INTRODUCTION

Heart failure with preserved ejection fraction (HFpEF) is a condition of global concern, currently accounting for approximately half of all heart failure (HF) cases.[1] HFpEF is notably prevalent in the outpatient setting, particularly among elderly, female, and hypertensive patients, and is frequently associated with atrial fibrillation (AF). This condition is challenging to diagnose due to its complex and diverse pathophysiology. It also contributes significantly to hospitalizations for decompensated HF and is associated with high morbidity and all-cause mortality.

Diagnosing HFpEF typically involves identifying signs or symptoms of HF, confirming preserved ejection fraction (EF), and detecting elevated biomarkers and/or increased filling pressure. Traditionally, HFpEF was attributed to abnormal left ventricular (LV) diastolic function, including abnormalities in active relaxation and passive stiffness.[2] A hallmark of HF is the reduction in left ventricular ejection fraction (LVEF). However, left atrium (LA) enlargement is considered as a surrogate marker for diastolic dysfunction of the LV and is independently associated with increased morbidity and mortality.

Recent insights suggest that functional impairment in the LA significantly contributes to the pathogenesis of HFpEF.[3] Although increased LA size is present in the majority of HFpEF patients, approximately one-third do not exhibit LA enlargement. The role of all three phases of LA function in HFpEF patients is less well understood, especially in those without a history of AF and with normal LA size.

HFpEF, once considered primarily a disorder of the LV, is now understood involve multiple cardiac, vascular, and noncardiac abnormalities. Among these, LA dysfunction plays a critical role in the pathophysiology and progression of HFpEF.[4] Despite these advancements in understanding, a major challenge in managing HFpEF remains the lack of definitive therapies that improve outcomes. This underscores the necessity for ongoing research to elucidate the heterogeneous mechanisms underlying HFpEF and to develop targeted, effective treatments.

CENTRAL ROLE OF THE LEFT ATRIUM IN HEART FAILURE: MYTH OR REALITY?

Overlooked Role of the Left Atrium in Heart Failure

The HF is typically classified based on LV function, often overlooking the critical role of the LA. Traditionally seen merely as a conduit for blood from the pulmonary veins to the LV, the LA's function has received less attention. However, in HFpEF, where LV function is relatively preserved, the importance of the LA is increasingly recognized. Assessing LA function can provide valuable insights into HFpEF's pathophysiology, with some phenotypes suggesting that LA dysfunction may occur early and drive HF symptoms. This underscores the need to consider LA function in HF evaluation and management. Understanding LA's role in HFpEF may lead to new treatment strategies targeting LA dysfunction to improve patient outcomes.[3]

Historically, LV was viewed as the primary indicator and determinant of cardiac health. Recent advancements in cardiovascular (CV) imaging have enhanced our understanding of the LA, revealing its significant contribution to various CV diseases. The LA's mechanical and neurohormonal properties impact symptoms and prognosis in HF patients, making it a potential therapeutic and prognostic target.[2]

ANATOMY AND PHYSIOLOGY OF THE LEFT ATRIUM IN HFpEF

Understanding the anatomy and physiology of LA provides insights into its dynamic nature. The LA performs three primary mechanical functions; reservoir, conduit, and booster pump. As a reservoir, it restores oxygenated blood from the pulmonary veins. During early diastole, the LV relaxes and expands to fill with blood, impacting LA function.[2] The conduit function ensures the efficient transfer of blood from pulmonary veins and the LV, with compliance of both atrial and ventricular chambers affecting this process. Better compliance facilitates smoother blood movement, enhancing the LA's reservoir function.[2]

The booster pump function refers to the LA's ability to contract and actively contribute to ventricular filling. This function depends on intrinsic LA contractility, venous return, and LV end-diastolic pressures.[2] Additionally, the LA helps maintain mitral valve competence, particularly in early or mild HFpEF stages, compensating for LV diastolic dysfunction. Over time, this compensation can lead to LA dilation and dysfunction, known as left atrial atriopathy **(Fig. 1)**. This increases the risk of AF, pulmonary hypertension (PH), and atrial functional mitral regurgitation (MR).[4]

PATHOPHYSIOLOGY OF LEFT ATRIAL DYSFUNCTION IN HFpEF

The LA dysfunction in HFpEF can lead to significant complications, resulting in poor functional capacity and worsening HF symptoms. Evidence shows that LA dysfunction is associated with adverse outcomes such as severe pulmonary vascular disease, RV dysfunction, and increased mortality.[4,5] Assessing LA function, in addition to size, provides valuable therapeutic as well as prognostic information in HF. This is because LA function directly indicates heart's efficiency and overall CV health.[2]

LA cardiomyocytes can be affected by hypertension systemic inflammation, metabolic abnormalities like diabetes, and valvular heart diseases. These factors can alter LA structure, contractility, and electrical activity, leading to atrial cardiomyopathy. This condition can disrupt normal electrical signals, causing atrial arrhythmias and impairing the LA's ability to pump blood into the ventricles, which can result in symptoms like exercise intolerance. Atrial cardiomyopathy can also cause LA enlargement and thickening, further compromising its function.[3]

Recognizing and addressing LA atriopathy is crucial for effectively diagnosing and treating HFpEF. While ventricular cardiomyopathy's definition and understanding are clearer, atriopathy's role in conditions such as AF and HF is increasingly acknowledged. By focusing on LA function, clinicians can better manage and treat heart conditions involving the LA.[3]

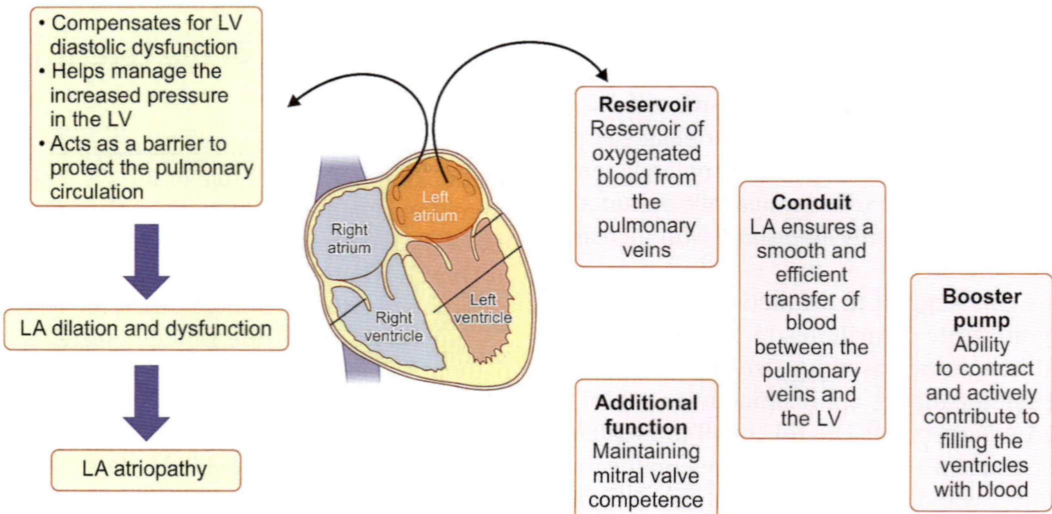

Fig. 1: Normal functions and compensatory mechanisms of the left atrium in heart failure. (LA: left atrium; LV: left ventricular)

DIAGNOSTIC APPROACHES FOR ASSESSING LEFT ATRIAL ATRIOPATHY IN HFpEF

Assessing LA atriopathy in HFpEF involves multiple diagnostic methods to capture structural and functional changes. Tools such as electrocardiography (ECG), echocardiography, cardiac magnetic resonance imaging (MRI), computed tomography (CT) have been explored to diagnose atriopathy.[6] These tools vary in their predictive value and applicability across different HF conditions, highlighting the need for a comprehensive assessment approach.

Echocardiography is a primary tool for evaluating LA function, offering several key measurements. **Table 1** summarizes each of these echocardiographic measurements with their specific uses and limitations, requiring a nuanced interpretation to accurately assess LA function in HFpEF.

Additional parameters such as LA ejection fraction or percentage of blood the LA pumps out with each contraction; LA coupling index; and LA function index are suggested for assessing LA function in cases of either type of heart failure.[3]

TABLE 1: Echocardiographic measurements with their specific uses and limitations.

Left atrium diameter (LAD)[3]	• Aims to provide measurement of anteroposterior LA linear dimension by M-mode • LAD does not provide an accurate size of the LA due to the complex and irregular shape of the LA
LA volume[3]	• LA volume reflects the chronic effect of left ventricular (LV) filling pressures over time, and is an important marker of diastolic dysfunction and LA structural remodeling
Maximum left atrial volume (LAV)	• Assessed at end-systole and is a strong predictor of cardiovascular (CV) outcomes • It has been recommended for the measurement of LA size
Minimum LAV	• Assessed at end-diastole, represents atrial afterload, and is more closely related to left ventricular end-diastolic pressure (LVEDP) and LV filling pressures
Left atrial strain[7]	• It is a marker of LA deformation which indicates various changes in the length of the atrial myocardium (both shortening and lengthening) • A valuable parameter that offers understanding of the pathophysiology and prognosis • Its multifaceted role focuses on its correlation with LV filling pressures, major adverse CV events (MACE), and the risk of atrial fibrillation along with heart failure with preserved ejection fraction (HFpEF)
Peak atrial longitudinal strain (PALS)[3]	Greater diagnostic importance versus LA geometry for documenting the presence and severity of diastolic dysfunction

CLINICAL IMPLICATIONS AND PROGNOSTIC SIGNIFICANCE OF LEFT ATRIAL ATRIOPATHY IN HFpEF

Clinical Implications of Left Atrium Atriopathy in HFpEF

In patients with HFpEF, elevated LA pressure, especially during exercise, is linked to symptoms and increased mortality. LA dysfunction, characterized by impaired LA strain, serves as a marker for reduced exercise tolerance or functional capacity.

A study using echocardiography and right heart catheterization assessed 71 subjects with exertional dyspnea. HFpEF patients exhibited impaired LA reservoir and booster strain along with increased stiffness. These LA abnormalities correlated with higher exercise pulmonary capillary wedge pressure (PCWP) and remained significant predictors after adjusting for other factors. LA stiffness was also strongly related to B-type natriuretic peptide (BNP) levels.[4,8]

Data from the multi-ethnic study of atherosclerosis, showed that lower LA reservoir strain and impaired LA functional reserve were associated with reduced submaximal exercise capacity, as reflected with shorter 6-minute walk distance (6MWD).[9]

Another study using cardiac MRI quantified LA reservoir strains and measured peak oxygen levels (VO_2max). Patients with HFpEF showed significantly lower LA reservoir and conduit strain compared to those without HFpEF. LA conduit strain strongly correlated with VO_2max, indicating a stronger predictor of exercise capacity and impaired early ventricular filling.[10] A similar study from the German HFpEF registry found that lower LA reservoir strain was independently associated with impaired peak VO_2 in HFpEF patients. Thus, reduced LA reservoir strain is a valuable marker for decreased exercise capacity in HFpEF patients.[11]

Prognostic Significance of Left Atrium Atriopathy in HFpEF

The LA dysfunction significantly increases the risk of HF hospitalization and death. A cohort of 308 HFpEF patients identified LA reservoir strain as the strongest correlate of adverse events, independently associated with CV hospitalization or death. Decreased LA reservoir strain was linked to increased pulmonary vascular resistance and decreased peak oxygen consumption.[4,12]

A 2015 Mayo clinic study compared the structure and function of the LA in HFpEF and HF with reduced ejection fraction (HFrEF). Both HF types showed abnormal LA size and function compared to controls. HFpEF group showed greater LA stiffening and pressure. This suggested a higher prevalence of AF with HFpEF. LA dysfunction was more strongly linked to mortality in HFpEF, indicating a worse prognosis in this group. These findings underscore the significance of addressing atriopathy in HFpEF.[13]

TARGETING LEFT ATRIUM DYSFUNCTION

Considering the association of LA dysfunction with poor prognosis, reduced functional capacity, and abnormal hemodynamics, interventions aimed at unloading the LA, improving its function, and restoring sinus rhythm could enhance outcomes in HFpEF patients with atriopathy. These findings highlight the importance of exploring targeted therapeutic approaches to address LA dysfunction in HFpEF.

Therapeutic Strategies and Management of Left Atrial Atriopathy in HFpEF

The management of HFpEF is challenging due to the complexity and diversity within the syndrome. Current treatments include pharmacological interventions, lifestyle modifications, and interventional therapies targeting common comorbidities. Among the unique presentations of HFpEF is LA atriopathy, which requires a tailored approach for effective management.[4]

Lifestyle and Nonpharmacological Interventions

Cardiac rehabilitation (CR) programs, combining exercise training, education, and counseling are crucial for improving physical and psychological outcomes in HFpEF patients.[14] For patients hospitalized for acute HFpEF exacerbation, these programs help enhance recovery, reduce hospital readmissions, and improve overall quality of life by gradually increasing physical activity under professional supervision.[15]

Weight management through moderate physical activity can also alleviate LA atriopathy, although excessive exercise could have the opposite effect.[4]

Pharmacological Interventions

Mineralocorticoid receptor antagonist: Mineralocorticoid receptor antagonist (MRAs) like spironolactone have shown promise in HFpEF management. In the TOPCAT trial, spironolactone significantly reduced the primary outcome of CV-related death, aborted cardiac arrest, and HF hospitalization among patients with elevated natriuretic peptide (NP) levels.[4]

Angiotensin receptor-neprilysin inhibitor: Neprilysin plays a significant role in the degradation of NPs. The PARAMOUNT trial showed a greater decrease in N-terminal pro BNP (NT-proBNP) levels, and LA volume with ARNI treatment compared to valsartan, at the 12-week follow-up. However, the larger PARAGON trial showed only a narrow miss in reducing the composite outcome of CV death and total HF hospitalizations.[4]

SGLT2 inhibitors: The SGLT2 inhibitors, such as empagliflozin and dapagliflozin, have shown positive effects in HF management. In the EMPEROR-Preserved trial, empagliflozin reduced the combined risk of CV death or HF hospitalization in patients with HFpEF. Notably, over half the patients in the EMPEROR-Preserved trial had a history of AF, and there was no difference in the efficacy of empagliflozin between patients with or without AF. Further support for SGLT2 inhibitors comes from a post hoc analysis of the DECLARE-TIMI58 trial, which showed reduced rates of new-onset AF with dapagliflozin.[4]

Novel pharmacologic approaches: New pharmacologic approaches are being explored for HF treatment. Relaxin, a vasodilator, activates the relaxin family peptide receptor RXFP1, which is expressed in atrial but not ventricular myocytes. In human atrial tissue, relaxin increases inotropy, suggesting its potential as an LA-targeted therapy. This specific targeting could provide new avenues for managing HF, especially in cases involving atrial dysfunction.[4]

Device-based therapies: Restoring sinus rhythm in patients with AF and HFpEF may improve clinical outcomes. Few trials advocate the benefits of catheter ablation in HFpEF patients. However, concerns exist regarding its adverse effects on LA hemodynamics in patients with increased LA stiffness. Clinical trials are necessary to assess the efficacy and safety of this procedure.

Devices like the interatrial shunt device (IASD) have shown promise in improving exercise hemodynamics, symptoms, and exercise capacity by reducing LA pressure in HFpEF patients. Other innovative approaches, such as percutaneous pericardial resection and novel assist devices, are also under investigation for their potential benefits in HFpEF.[4]

In summary, addressing LA atriopathy in HFpEF requires a multifaceted approach, combining lifestyle modifications, pharmacological treatments, and advanced interventional therapies. Targeted therapeutic strategies focusing on the LA's function and hemodynamics offer new opportunities for individualized HFpEF management and improving patient outcomes.

FUTURE DIRECTIONS FOR LEFT ATRIAL ATRIOPATHY IN HFpEF

As LA structure and function play a crucial role in both HFpEF and HFrEF, their assessment assumes increasing importance, particularly in HFpEF where evidence-based therapies are lacking.

Future research should focus on investigating the effects of current and future HF agents on LA atriopathy specifically in patients with HFpEF. Understanding how these therapies impact LA structure and function could lead to the development of new treatment options to improve outcomes in this patient population.[4] LAS has emerged as an important tool in the noninvasive diagnosis and stratification of HFpEF. Therefore, it should be integrated into the standard diagnostic workflow for HFpEF assessment. Future heart failure guidelines should include clear directives for the utilization of LAS in the evaluation of HFpEF, ensuring its consistent incorporation into clinical practice.[2,7]

Further studies are needed to validate the comprehensive contribution of atrial function indices in HFpEF assessment. Precise imaging of LA function is essential for accurately assessing the severity and progression of HFpEF, highlighting the importance of advancing imaging techniques.[3]

CONCLUSION

Left atrial dysfunction is a key determinant of prognosis and adverse outcomes in heart failure with preserved ejection fraction. Recognizing and addressing left atrial atriopathy is vital for improving outcomes in these patients. Abnormalities in the left atrium, such as reduced LA reservoir strain and increased stiffness, are strongly associated with cardiovascular hospitalization and mortality. Therefore, implementing targeted therapeutic strategies to alleviate left atrial burden and improving its function holds great promise for enhancing outcomes in HFpEF patients.

REFERENCES

1. Jasinska-Piadlo A, Campbell P. Management of patients with heart failure and preserved ejection fraction. Heart. 2023;109(11):874-83.
2. Carpenito M, Fanti D, Mega S, et al. The central role of left atrium in heart failure. Front Cardiovasc Med. 2021; 8:704762.
3. Zheng R, Kusunose K. Linkage of left atrial function to heart failure with preserved ejection fraction. Int Heart J. 2023;64(1):4-9.
4. Omote K, Borlaug BA. Left atrial myopathy in heart failure with preserved ejection fraction. Circ J. 2023; 87(8): 1039-46.
5. Obokata M, Borlaug BA. Left atrial dysfunction: the next key target in heart failure with preserved ejection fraction. Eur J Heart Fail. 2019;21(4):506-8.
6. Kreimer F, Gotzmann M. Left atrial cardiomyopathy—a challenging diagnosis. Front Cardiovasc Med. 2022;9: 942385.
7. Shinzato MH, Santos N, Nishida G, et al. Left ventricular and atrial myocardial strain in heart failure with preserved ejection fraction: the evidence so far and prospects for phenotyping strategy. Cardiovasc Ultrasound. 2024; 22(1):4.
8. Telles F, Nanayakkara S, Evans S, et al. Impaired left atrial strain predicts abnormal exercise haemodynamics in heart failure with preserved ejection fraction. Eur J Heart Fail. 2019;21(4):495-505.
9. Patel RB, Freed BH, Beussink-Nelson L, et al. Associations of Cardiac Mechanics With Exercise Capacity: The Multi-Ethnic Study of Atherosclerosis. J Am Coll Cardiol. 2021;78(3):245-57.
10. von Roeder M, Rommel KP, Kowallick JT, et al. Influence of left atrial function on exercise capacity and left ventricular function in patients with heart failure and preserved ejection fraction. Circ Cardiovasc Imaging. 2017;10(8):e006785.
11. Maffeis C, Morris DA, Belyavskiy E, et al. Left atrial function and maximal exercise capacity in heart failure with preserved and mid-range ejection fraction. ESC Heart Fail. 2021;8(1):116-28.
12. Freed BH, Daruwalla V, Cheng JY, et al. Prognostic Utility and Clinical Significance of Cardiac Mechanics in Heart Failure With Preserved Ejection Fraction: Importance of Left Atrial Strain. Circ Cardiovasc Imaging. 2016;9(3):e003754.
13. Melenovsky V, Hwang SJ, Redfield MM, et al. Left atrial remodeling and function in advanced heart failure with preserved or reduced ejection fraction. Circ Heart Fail. 2015;8(2):295-303.
14. Bozkurt B, Fonarow GC, Goldberg LR, et al. Cardiac rehabilitation for patients with heart failure: JACC expert panel. J Am Coll Cardiol. 2021;77(11):1454-69.
15. Sachdev V, Sharma K, Keteyian SJ, et al. Supervised Exercise Training for Chronic Heart Failure With Preserved Ejection Fraction: A Scientific Statement From the American Heart Association and American College of Cardiology. Circulation. 2023;147(16):e699-e715.

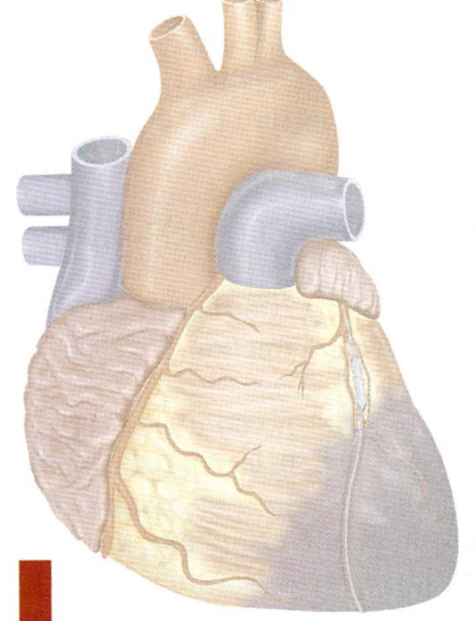

Computed Tomography Angiography in HFpEF

Priya Jagia, Sreelal Variar

INTRODUCTION

Heart failure (HF) is characterized by the heart's inability to pump blood effectively to meet the oxygenation and perfusion demands of the body. It leads to symptoms such as shortness of breath, fatigue, and fluid retention. Heart failure with preserved ejection fraction (HFpEF) is defined as heart failure with an ejection fraction (EF) of 50% or greater in the absence of other causes like hypertrophic cardiomyopathy, infiltrative diseases, or pericardial diseases.[1] It is increasingly recognized as a prevalent condition, particularly among older adults and those with comorbidities such as hypertension and diabetes.[2] The diagnosis and management of HFpEF pose unique challenges due to its heterogeneous nature and the absence of a single identifiable cause.[3] Traditional imaging modalities, particularly echocardiography, play a crucial role in the assessment of cardiac structure and function in patients with HFpEF. However, computed tomography angiography (CTA) has emerged as a valuable tool in the evaluation of this condition. This chapter explores the role of CTA in the assessment of HFpEF, discussing its applications, advantages, limitations, and prospects.

ROLE OF COMPUTED TOMOGRAPHY ANGIOGRAPHY

Cardiac Abnormalities

Cardiac computed tomography angiography (CCTA) is a noninvasive imaging modality that uses radiation to create detailed cross-sectional images of the heart and surrounding structures. CCTA has gained prominence in the evaluation of coronary artery disease (CAD) and other cardiac conditions due to its high spatial resolution and excellent sensitivity for the detection of CAD. It can also give insights into the morphology of the cardiac chambers and the pericardium.

Evaluation of Coronary Artery Disease

More than half of the patients with HFpEF have involvement of the epicardial coronary arteries.[4] Given the high prevalence of CAD in patients with HF, it is essential to rule out significant coronary lesions that may contribute to symptoms. Patients with CAD are more likely to have worsening of their EFs and have higher mortality rates. Complete revascularization in these patients provides symptomatic relief and improves mortality rates.[5] According to the 2021 European Society of Cardiology Guidelines, a CCTA is recommended in patients with chronic heart failure when they are having low-to-intermediate probability of CAD or when the initial functional evaluation is equivocal **(Figs. 1A to F)**.[6] The ACC 2023 guidelines on evaluation of chronic coronary disease recommends CCTA as an appropriate investigation in newly diagnosed HFpEF with no prior CAD evaluation[7] **(Table 1)**. Patients with nonobstructive CAD on CCTA have better outcomes compared with those having obstructive CAD.[8]

Evaluation of Diastolic Dysfunction

Left ventricular diastolic function can be calculated using the diastolic expansion index (DAI) measurement using CCTA.[9,10] The left atrium (LA) volume can be calculated

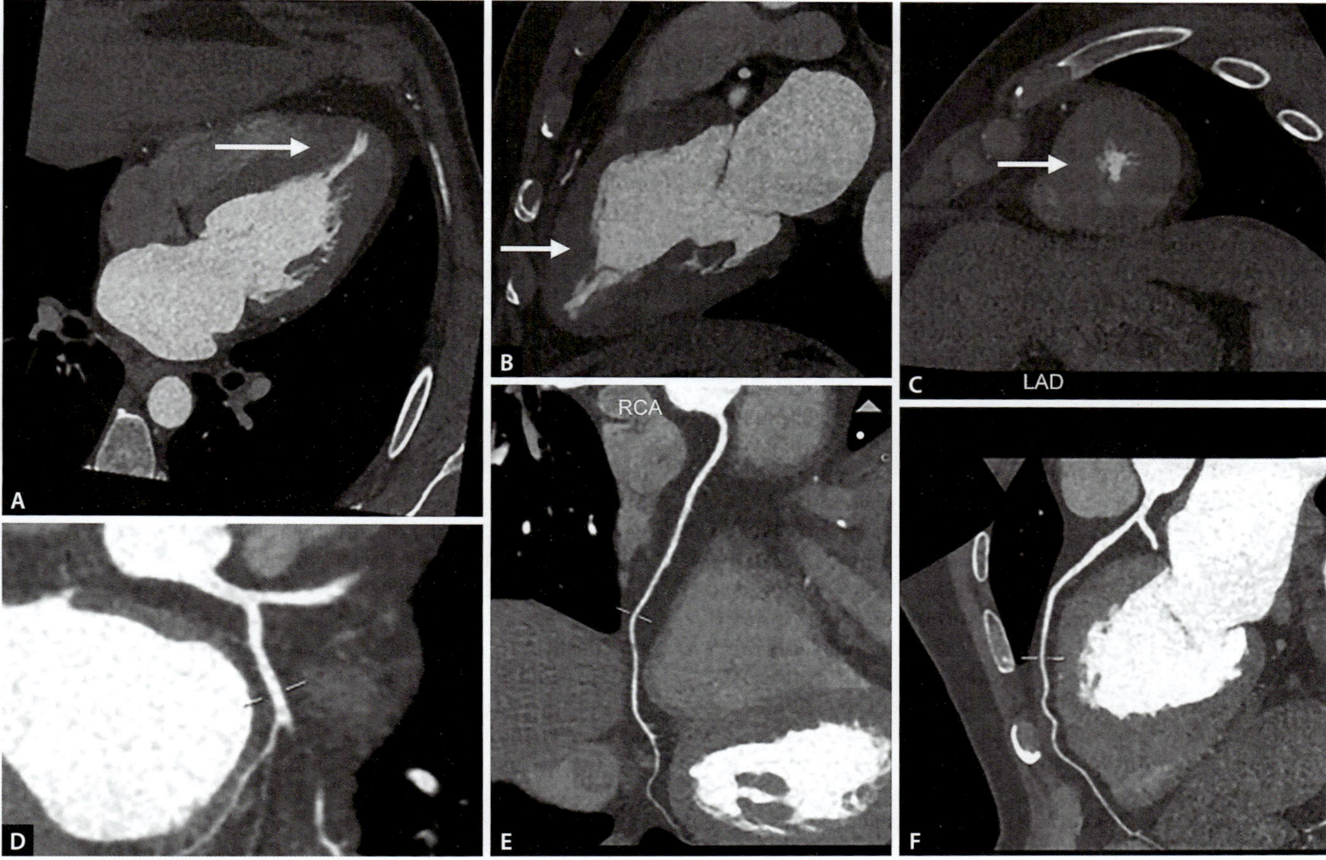

Figs. 1A to F: A 49-year-old gentleman with heart failure with preserved ejection fraction and low-to-intermediate pretest probability for CAD. The exercise ECG revealed equivocal results. A CCTA performed revealed presence of apical hypertrophic cardiomyopathy, demonstrated by white arrows in the (A) four-chamber, (B) two-chamber, and (C) short-axis views. The CCTA also showed (D) normal left coronary, (E) LAD, and (F) RCA.

TABLE 1: Indications for CT coronary angiography in HFpEF.

ESC Guidelines 2021	*ACC/AHA guidelines 2023*
Low-to-intermediate pretest probability for CAD	Newly diagnosed HFpEF with no prior evaluation for CAD
Equivocal functional tests for stress-induced CAD	

by drawing the contours for LA and extrapolating using the region growing tools available in most post processing software packages. LV volume is calculated through semiautomated detection of endocardial and epicardial contours by post processing algorithms, as shown in **Figures 2A and B**. The diastolic expansion index is calculated as the ratio of LV and LA volumes.

$$\text{DAI} = \text{LV volume} / \text{LA volume}$$

There is substantial agreement between CCTA and echocardiography for higher grades of diastolic dysfunction.[9]

Evaluation of Late Iodine Enhancement

Cardiac computed tomography angiography can also be utilized to assess myocardial tissue characteristics, using late iodine enhancement. The late iodine enhancement is assessed on scans done ~12 minutes after iodine injection using monochromatic low kilovolt peak acquisition in dual energy systems. Like late gadolinium enhancement on CMR, pathology-specific patterns of enhancement can be seen. In patients where CMR is contraindicated, this can be useful for evaluation of etiology in HFpEF.[11]

Assessment of Cardiac Anatomy and Function

Cardiac computed tomography angiography provides comprehensive anatomical information about the heart, including the size and morphology of the chambers, wall thickness, and volumes. Functional evaluation of the valves and ventricles can also be done when there is poor echocardiographic window and contraindication to CMR. In patients with HFpEF, CCTA can help identify:

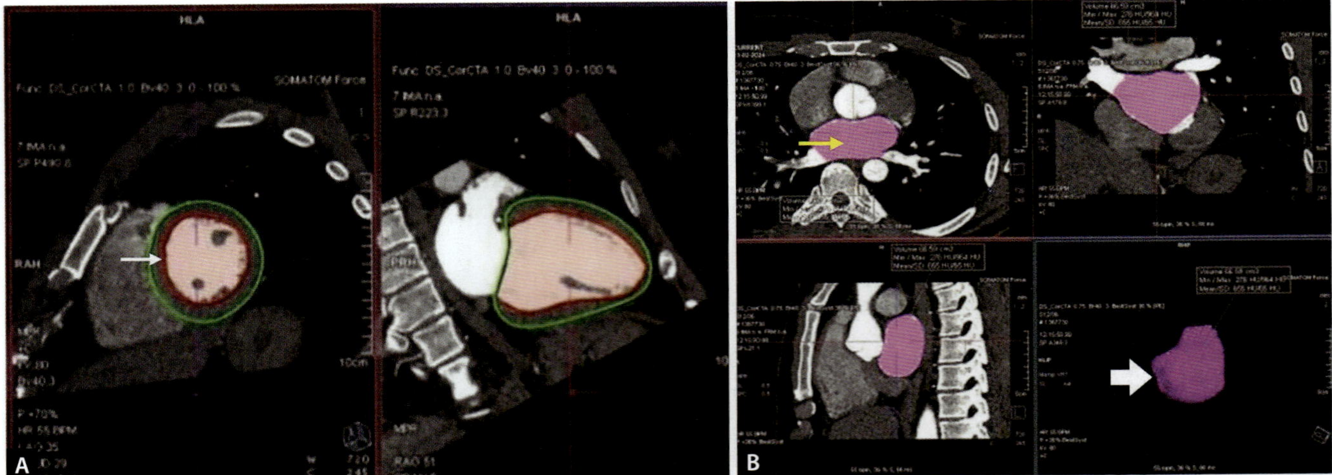

Figs. 2A and B: A 33-year-old female patient with HFpEF. CMR could not be performed due to claustrophobia. Diastolic function could not be accurately evaluated on echocardiography due to suboptimal windows. (A) Calculation of LV volume was done by semiautomated contour detection as shown by white arrows; (B) LA volumes were calculated using region growing (yellow arrow) at end systole, by excluding the appendage and pulmonary veins. Final volume used for calculation is shown by the white arrowhead.

TABLE 2: Morphological and functional changes of cardiac chambers on CCTA in conditions mimicking HFpEF.

HFpEF	*Restrictive cardiomyopathy*	*Hypertrophic cardiomyopathy*	*Constrictive pericarditis*
• Dilated LA • Concentric LVH • CAD • Normal indexed end diastolic volume (EDV) • RA–RV dilatation	• Dilated LA and RA • Concentric LVH • Pleural/pericardial effusion • Normal indexed EDV • Interatrial septal thickening	• Dilated LA • Asymmetrical LVH • Systolic anterior motion of mitral leaflet/LV outflow obstruction	• Dilated LA and RA • Pericardial thickening/ calcification • Pericardial effusion • Tubular ventricles and increased septal excursion

- *Left ventricular hypertrophy (LVH):* LVH is a common finding in HFpEF and is associated with increased myocardial stiffness and impaired diastolic function.
- *Left atrial (LA) enlargement:* Left atrial enlargement is often observed in HFpEF and is indicative of elevated filling pressures and diastolic dysfunction. Both LA diameters and LA volumes can be calculated.
- *Right atrial (RA) enlargement:* RA volume and maximum diameters can also be similarly calculated. RA dilatation occurs later in the disease and is a poor prognostic marker.
- *Right ventricle (RV):* Right ventricular dilatation and dysfunction is another poor prognostic marker in the disease spectrum. As calculation of RA and RV volumes are suboptimal in echocardiography due to window limitations, CCTA can be an alternative modality when CMR is contraindicated.

Table 2 lists morphological and functional changes of cardiac chambers on CCTA in conditions mimicking HFpEF.

EVALUATION OF EXTRACARDIAC STRUCTURES

The evaluation of extracardiac structures is done as follows:

- *Lung water quantification:* Pulmonary congestion is present in many patients with HFpEF. These changes may not be apparent on chest X ray/clinical examination, unlike HFrEF. However, they carry prognostic significance.[12,13] Patients with subclinical congestion can be detected using quantitative computed tomography.[14] The quantification is performed using measurement of lung density by artificial intelligence-enabled computation algorithms, as shown in **Figures 3A to E**. The increase in lung density due to increase in lung water is often missed on visual inspection alone, underlining the importance of quantitative methods. The left upper lobe is often chosen for measuring lung water density, with cutoff value of –825 indicating pulmonary edema.[15]

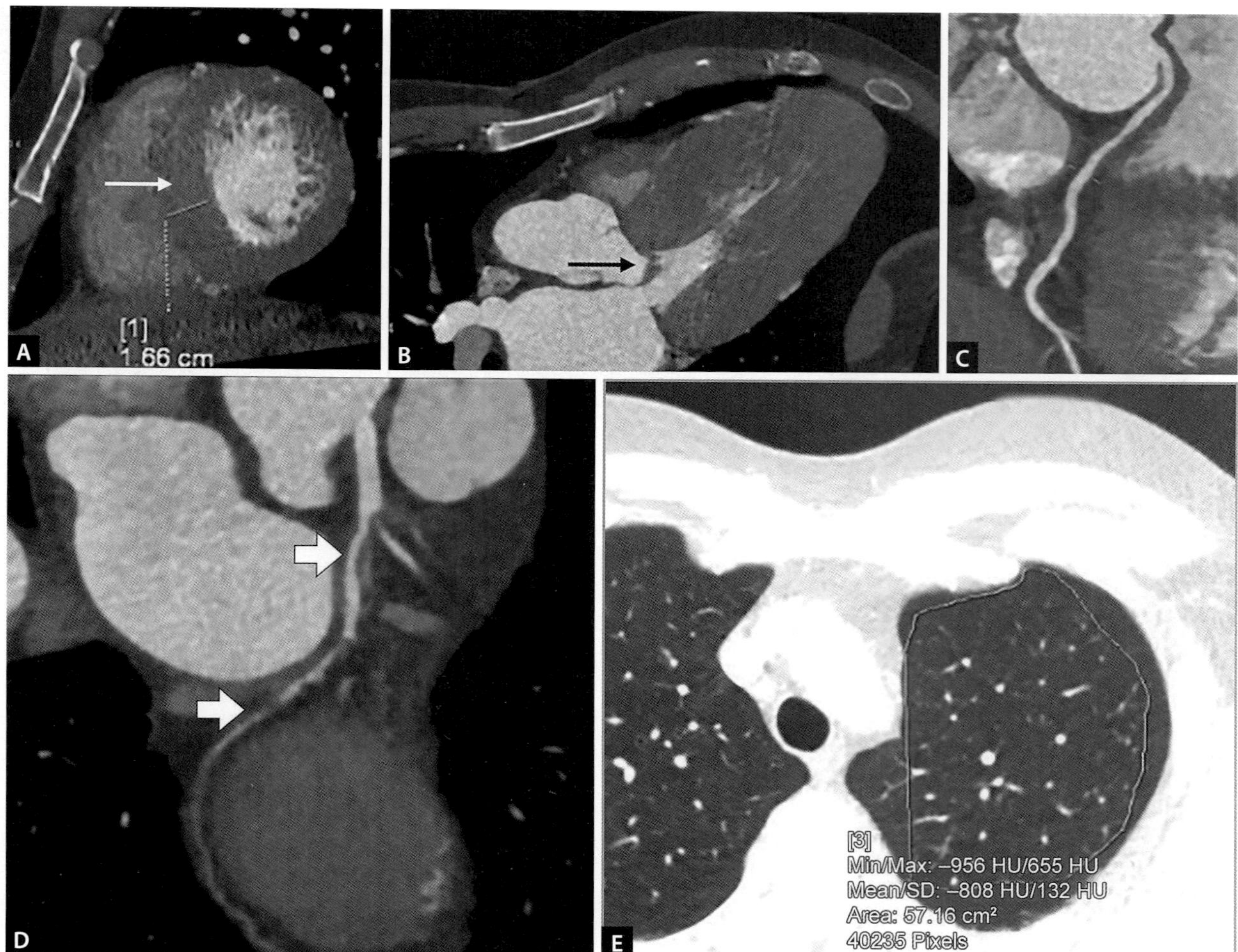

Figs. 3A to E: A 56-year-old man with HFpEF. Echocardiography revealed presence of hypertrophic obstructive cardiomyopathy. CCTA was advised for evaluation of coronary arteries. (A and B) Asymmetrical septal hypertrophy and systolic anterior motion of anterior mitral leaflet (black arrow in part B). Significant disease of the left anterior descending artery was seen (D) with eccentric non calcified plaques (white arrowheads). (E) Lung attenuation showed increased values (part of the volume shown in E) with mean attenuation of –760 HU, indicating increased lung water content.

- *Epicardial adipose tissue (EAT):* It is thought to play an important role in the pathogenesis of HFpEF. It has both metabolic and inflammatory effects on the heart.[16] Another potential mechanism is through the creation of a pericardial constraint, affecting myocardial relaxation and increasing filling pressures. Ventricular interdependence is also altered when EAT volumes are increased.[17] Using a contrast or noncontrast scan of the chest, epicardial volumes can be easily calculated using region growing tools, as shown in **Figures 4A to F**.[18,19] Calculation of EAT volume can be a potential prognostic marker in patients with HFpEF. Changes in EAT volume can be used to assess treatment response to agents like SGLT-2 inhibitors. The volume of EAT has been found to correlate with global longitudinal strain in patients with HFpEF.[20] As they can be assessed on low radiation noncontrast scans, follow-up for EAT volume can be done to evaluate response to treatment.
- Evaluation of the lung parenchyma and mediastinum also helps in ruling out other etiologies. Patients with connective tissue diseases may show signs, including ground glass opacities, nodules, or interlobular interstitial thickening. Mediastinal lymphadenopathy and parenchymal changes may also be seen in sarcoidosis **(Figs. 5A to D)**.
- *Pulmonary vasculature:* Patients often have associated dysplasia of pulmonary vasculature.[21] This leads to features of pulmonary hypertension. Dilated pulmonary arteries, pruning of segmental branches

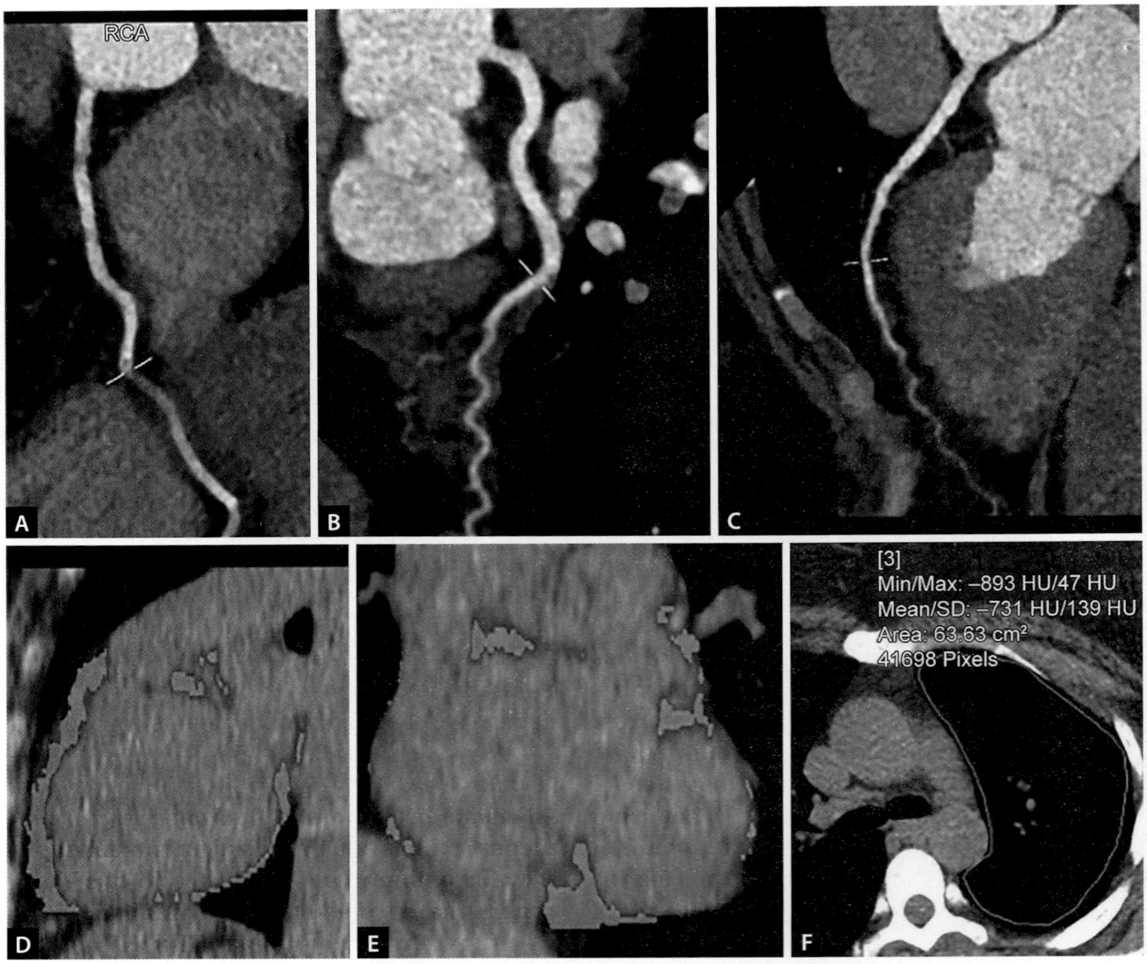

Figs. 4A to F: A 44-year-old obese man with HFpEF. The coronary evaluation showed normal (A) RCA, (B) LCx, and (C) LAD. (D and E) Region growing tools were used to isolate the epicardial adipose tissue volume (green areas) in the noncontrast phase of acquisition (done for calcium scoring). He also showed (F) increased lung attenuation, indicating lung congestion and increased lung water content.

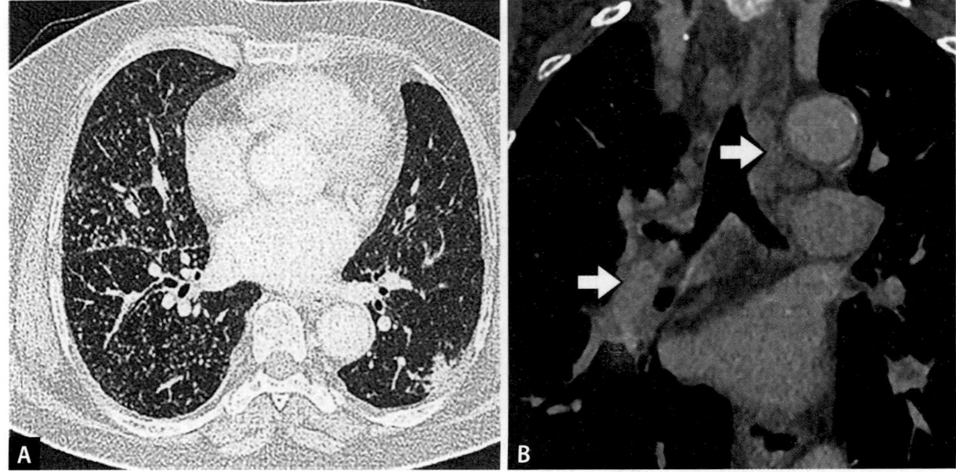

Figs. 5A and B

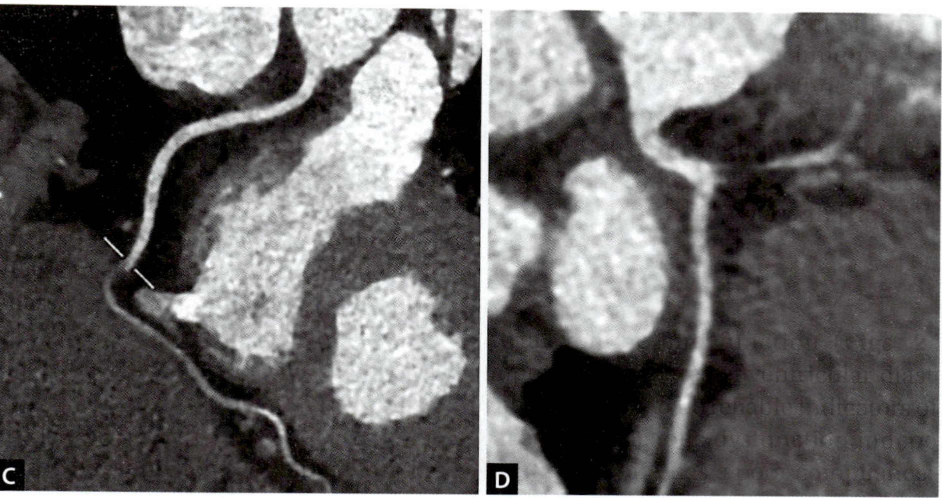

Figs. 5C and D

Figs. 5A to D: A 60-year-old female with HFpEF. CCTA advised for coronary artery evaluation showed (A) multiple interstitial nodules and patchy subpleural consolidations, with (B) enlarged mediastinal and bilateral hilar lymph nodes (B), suggesting sarcoidosis. (C and D) The CCTA showed normal coronary arteries. Sarcoidosis was confirmed histopathologically on endobronchial lymph node biopsy.

and ground glass opacities can be visualized. Perfusion abnormalities may be present, which can be visualized on dual energy CT.

LIMITATIONS

- *Radiation exposure:* CCTA involves exposure to ionizing radiation, which carries a small risk of radiation-induced cancer. Although advancements in technology have reduced radiation doses, the risk remains a consideration, particularly in younger patients or those requiring multiple imaging studies.
- *Contrast-induced nephropathy:* CCTA requires the use of iodinated contrast agents, which can pose risks for patients with preexisting kidney disease. Contrast-induced nephropathy is a potential complication, and clinicians must weigh the risks and benefits of contrast administration in this population.
- *Limited assessment of diastolic function:* While CCTA can provide valuable anatomical information, it is not as effective as echocardiography in assessing diastolic function. CCTA does not provide direct measurements of intracardiac pressures or flow dynamics, which are critical for diagnosing and managing HFpEF.

CONCLUSION

Cardiac computed tomography angiography plays a significant role in the evaluation of HFpEF. While it is not a first-line imaging modality, CCTA offers unique advantages in assessing coronary artery disease, cardiac anatomy, and myocardial characteristics. Its ability to provide comprehensive information in a noninvasive manner makes it a valuable tool in the diagnostic arsenal for HFpEF. However, clinicians must remain aware of the limitations and potential risks associated with CCTA, ensuring that its use is appropriate and guided by clinical context. As research and technology continue to advance, the role of CCTA in HFpEF evaluation is likely to expand, paving the way for improved diagnosis and management of this complex condition.

REFERENCES

1. Heidenreich PA, Bozkurt B, Aguilar D, et al. 2022 AHA/ACC/HFSA Guideline for the Management of Heart Failure: A Report of the American College of Cardiology/American Heart Association Joint Committee on Clinical Practice Guidelines. Circulation. 2022;145(18):e895-1032.
2. Ponikowski P, Voors AA, Anker SD, et al. 2016 ESC Guidelines for the diagnosis and treatment of acute and chronic heart failure: The Task Force for the diagnosis and treatment of acute and chronic heart failure of the European Society of Cardiology (ESC) Developed with the special contribution of the Heart Failure Association (HFA) of the ESC. Eur Heart J. 2016;37(27):2129-200.
3. Borlaug BA, Lam CS, Roger VL, et al. Contractility and ventricular systolic stiffening in hypertensive heart disease insights into the pathogenesis of heart failure with preserved ejection fraction. J Am Coll Cardiol. 2009;54(5):410-8.
4. Hwang SJ, Melenovsky V, Borlaug BA. Implications of coronary artery disease in heart failure with preserved

ejection fraction. J Am Coll Cardiol. 2014;63(25 Pt A): 2817-27.
5. Rush CJ, Berry C, Oldroyd KG, et al. Prevalence of coronary artery disease and coronary microvascular dysfunction in patients with heart failure with preserved ejection fraction. JAMA Cardiol. 2021;6(10):1130-43.
6. McDonagh TA, Metra M, Adamo M, et al. 2021 ESC Guidelines for the diagnosis and treatment of acute and chronic heart failure. Eur Heart J. 2021;42(36): 3599-726.
7. Multimodality Writing Group for Chronic Coronary Disease; Winchester DE, Maron DJ, Blankstein R, et al. ACC/AHA/ASE/ASNC/ASPC/HFSA/HRS/SCAI/SCCT/SCMR/STS 2023 Multimodality Appropriate Use Criteria for the Detection and Risk Assessment of Chronic Coronary Disease. J Am Coll Cardiol. 2023;81(25): 2445-67.
8. Yu MM, Zuo WX, Zhao X, et al. Prognostic value of coronary CT angiography in heart failure patients with preserved ejection fraction. Eur Radiol. 2023;33(5):3052-63.
9. van der Veen HA, Lessick J, Abadi S, et al. Accuracy of diastolic function by cardiac computed tomography relative to echo-doppler: additive clinical and prognostic value. J Comput Assist Tomogr. 2021;45(2):242-7.
10. Ghersin I, Ghersin E, Abadi S, et al. Assessment of diastolic function in hypertrophic cardiomyopathy by computed tomography-derived analysis of left ventricular filling. J Comput Assist Tomogr. 2017;41(3):339-43.
11. Im DJ, Youn JC, Lee HJ, et al. Role of cardiac computed tomography for etiology evaluation of newly diagnosed heart failure with reduced ejection fraction. J Clin Med. 2020;9(7):2270.
12. Anderson LW, Krathwohl DR, Airasian PW, et al. A taxonomy for learning, teaching and assessing: a revision of B taxonomy of educational objectives. In: Anderson LW, Krathwohl DR (Eds). New York: Longman; 2001.
13. Jain CC, Tschirren J, Reddy YNV, et al. Subclinical pulmonary congestion and abnormal hemodynamics in heart failure with preserved ejection fraction. JACC Cardiovasc Imaging. 2022;15(4):629-37.
14. Barile M, Hida T, Hammer M, et al. Simple quantitative chest CT for pulmonary edema. Eur J Radiol Open. 2020;7:100273.
15. Packer M. Epicardial adipose tissue may mediate deleterious effects of obesity and inflammation on the myocardium. J Am Coll Cardiol. 2018;71(20):2360-72.
16. van Woerden G, van Veldhuisen DJ, Manintveld OC, et al. Epicardial adipose tissue and outcome in heart failure with mid-range and preserved ejection fraction. Circ Heart Fail. 2022;15(3):e009238.
17. Marwan M, Koenig S, Schreiber K, et al. Quantification of epicardial adipose tissue by cardiac CT: Influence of acquisition parameters and contrast enhancement. Eur J Radiol. 2019;121:108732.
18. Yin L, Yan C, Yang C, et al. Measurement of epicardial adipose tissue using non-contrast routine chest-CT: A consideration of threshold adjustment for fatty attenuation. BMC Med Imaging. 2022;22(1):114.
19. Ishikawa H, Otsuka K, Kono Y, et al. Extent of coronary atherosclerosis is associated with deterioration of left ventricular global longitudinal strain in patients with preserved ejection fraction undergoing coronary computed tomography angiography. IJC Hear Vasc. 2023;44:101176.
20. Omote K, Sorimachi H, Obokata M, et al. Pulmonary vascular disease in pulmonary hypertension due to left heart disease: Pathophysiologic implications. Eur Heart J. 2022;43(36):3417-31.

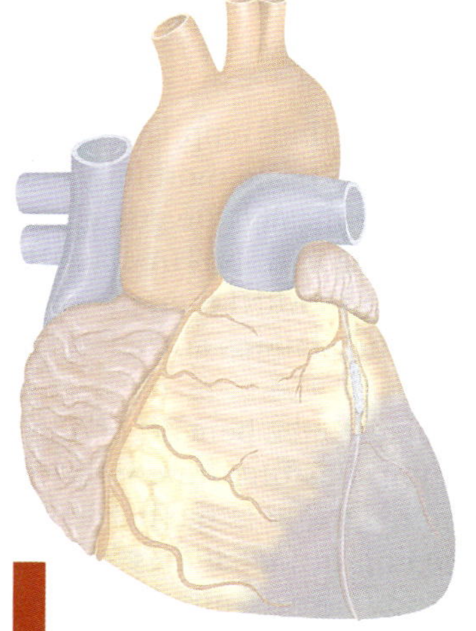

CMR Evaluation on Cardiac Remodeling Reversal after ARNI in HF

Mona Bhatia, Karthika Gopal D, Prasit Maity, Amit Garg, Sachin Raiya

INTRODUCTION

Cardiac remodeling is a pathological phenomenon characterized by persistent alterations in the shape and function of the heart, often triggered by various stressors such as myocardial injury and chronic volume overload.[1] In heart failure with reduced ejection fraction (HFrEF), adverse cardiac remodeling typically manifests as increased ventricular volumes and impaired cardiac function, further contributing to the disease's progression.

Conversely, reverse cardiac remodeling—the improvement of ventricular function and reduction of cardiac dimensions—represents a critical therapeutic goal in managing heart failure (HF). This transformation is primarily achieved through the application of guideline-directed medical therapy (GDMT), which includes a spectrum of pharmacological and nonpharmacological interventions designed to restore cardiac function.

Among them, angiotensin receptor-neprilysin inhibitors (ARNIs) have emerged as a cornerstone in HF management, demonstrating significant efficacy in promoting reverse remodeling.[2,3] The integration of ARNI therapy into clinical practice has been supported by robust clinical evidence indicating improved outcomes, including reductions in hospitalizations and mortality.

Cardiac magnetic resonance (CMR) imaging has become an invaluable tool in evaluating the effects of ARNI therapy on cardiac remodeling. CMR provides high-resolution images of cardiac structures and function, allowing for precise assessments of changes in ventricular size and mass over time.

ANGIOTENSIN RECEPTOR-NEPRILYSIN INHIBITOR

Angiotensin receptor-neprilysin inhibitors represent a significant advancement in the pharmacological management of HF, particularly HFrEF. At the heart of ARNI therapy is neprilysin, also known as neutral endopeptidase, an enzyme that plays a pivotal role in the degradation of various vasoactive peptides, including natriuretic peptides, adrenomedullin, bradykinin, and substance P. These peptides are crucial for cardiovascular regulation and contribute to the pathophysiology of HF.[4] Importantly, angiotensin II also serves as a substrate for neprilysin, which implies that neprilysin inhibition can result in elevated angiotensin II levels. This pharmacodynamic interaction necessitates the concurrent administration of angiotensin receptor blockers (ARBs) with neprilysin inhibitors to mitigate the consequences of increased angiotensin II.

It is essential to note the contraindication of combining neprilysin inhibitors with angiotensin-converting enzyme inhibitors (ACEIs).[5] This is due to the increased risk of angioedema, a potentially life-threatening side effect associated with elevated bradykinin levels when both classes of drugs are administered together. Thus, the strategic use of ARNI therapy allows for the synergistic effects of increased beneficial peptides alongside the regulation of the renin–angiotensin system, ultimately improving outcomes in HF management.

CARDIAC REMODELING REVERSAL AFTER ANGIOTENSIN RECEPTOR-NEPRILYSIN INHIBITOR IN HEART FAILURE

Cardiac remodeling is a crucial pathological process that accompanies HF, particularly in patients with HFrEF. The PARADIGM-HF (Prospective Comparison of ARNI with ACEI to Determine Impact on Global Mortality and Morbidity in HF) trial provides substantial evidence regarding the efficacy of sacubitril/valsartan in facilitating cardiac remodeling reversal in chronic HFrEF patients.[2,6]

In the PARADIGM-HF study, a total of 10,513 individuals were screened, with 2,079 excluded due to intolerance to target doses of either sacubitril/valsartan or enalapril, the comparator drug. The trial focused on patients with the New York Heart Association (NYHA) class II–IV symptoms and a baseline ejection fraction of ≤40%, later revised to ≤35% after 1 year. Eligible participants were required to be on stable doses of GDMT to ensure a uniform background treatment regimen. This rigorous selection process underlines the importance of identifying a patient population that could most benefit from ARNI therapy.

The results of the trial were striking, demonstrating a significant absolute reduction of 4.7% in the primary composite endpoint of cardiovascular death or hospitalization due to HF in patients treated with sacubitril/valsartan compared to those on enalapril. The hazard ratio of 0.80 and a 95% confidence interval of 0.73–0.87 confirmed the robustness of the findings, with a p-value <0.001 indicating statistical significance. Notably, the number needed to treat to prevent one primary endpoint event over 27 months was 21, showcasing the clinical utility of sacubitril/valsartan in managing HFrEF.

Furthermore, sacubitril/valsartan treatment resulted in a remarkable 20% reduction in instances of sudden cardiac death, an impactful observation for improving patient outcomes. It is noteworthy, however, that the incidence of symptomatic hypotension was higher in the ARNI group (14.0 vs. 9.2%; $p < 0.001$). Importantly, this hypotensive effect did not translate into a deterioration of renal function, a critical consideration given the renal implications frequently associated with HF therapies. Although there was a slight increase in cases of angioedema in the sacubitril/valsartan group, this variation did not reach statistical significance compared to enalapril.

The trial's outcomes highlight its potential to significantly reduce both cardiovascular mortality and hospitalizations, ultimately improving the quality of life for patients suffering from HFrEF. As such, the integration of ARNI into standard HF treatment protocols should be considered to enhance clinical outcomes in this patient population.

The 2016 update to the HF guidelines emphasized the need for ARNI, ACEIs, or ARBs to mitigate morbidity and mortality in affected patients. Specifically, the guidelines advocate for transitioning patients with NYHA class II–III symptoms from ACEIs or ARBs to ARNI therapy when feasible, based on class I recommendations and a level of evidence: B-R.

Recent studies have corroborated the benefits of ARNI therapy, notably in enhancing diastolic function, left ventricular (LV) function, and reduction in the burden of ventricular arrhythmias while improving patients' quality of life.[7,8] The PROVE-HF study stands out, revealing remarkable benefits after 12 months of treatment with sacubitril/valsartan. Participants exhibited a significant median increase in left ventricular ejection fraction (LVEF), from 28.2 to 37.8%, alongside marked reductions in both LV end-diastolic volume index and left ventricular end-systolic volume (LVESV) index. Additionally, reductions in indexed left atrial volume and the E/e′ ratio suggest substantial improvements in cardiac function. The PROVE-HF trial included patient demographics often excluded from previous studies, such as those with newly diagnosed HF and individuals with low baseline levels of N-terminal pro-B-type natriuretic peptide (NT-proBNP). These findings were further validated by the EVALUATE-HF trial, which documented early improvements in echocardiographic parameters as early as 12 weeks when comparing sacubitril/valsartan with enalapril, reinforcing the growing evidence supporting ARNI therapy.[9]

CARDIAC MAGNETIC RESONANCE EVALUATION OF CARDIAC REMODELING REVERSAL

Cardiac imaging has emerged as the definitive method for evaluating cardiac remodeling, with CMR imaging gaining prominence due to its superior capability in assessing both structural and functional alterations in the heart. Among the various echocardiographic measurements used to assess reverse remodeling, a reduction in LVESV is particularly noteworthy, as it encompasses both geometric and functional aspects of cardiac performance **(Fig. 1)**.

Research has demonstrated that patients exhibiting a lower LVEF or larger LV volumes typically face poorer prognoses. However, it is intriguing to note that patients with more compromised cardiac function or more dilated LV chambers often show a greater tendency toward reverse remodeling.[10] This phenomenon may be attributed to the

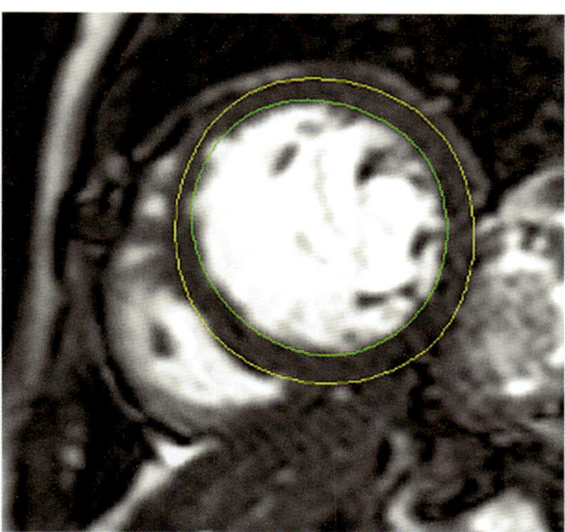

Fig. 1: Short-axis noncontrast cine sequence demonstrating ventricular volumetrics calculation on cardiac MRI as the gold standard.

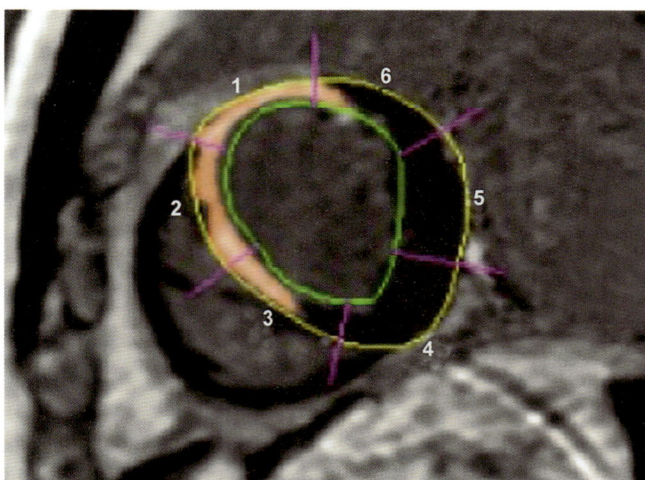

Fig. 3: Four-chamber noncontrast cine sequence demonstrating delayed subendocardial enhancement of the left ventricle at the septal, basal, midcavity, and apical regions.

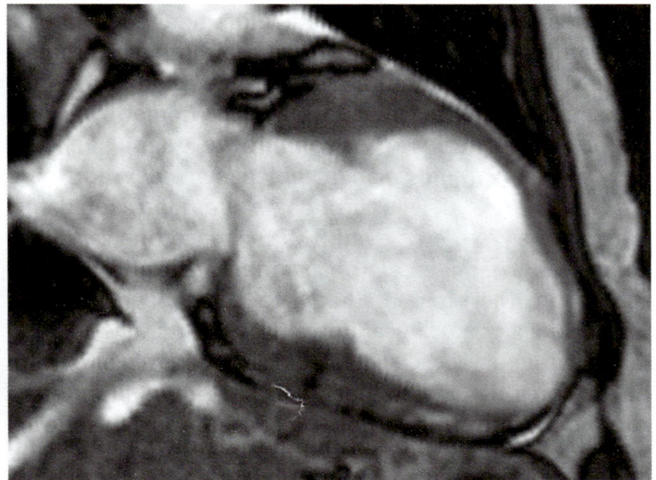

Fig. 2: Long-axis noncontrast cine sequence demonstrating a dilated left ventricle in a patient with low ejection fraction with thinning and bulging of the left ventricular anterior wall in the left anterior descending artery territory.

nature of reverse remodeling assessments, which typically involve examining proportional changes in LVEF and LV volumes from baseline values. Consequently, alterations in cardiac function may be more readily achievable when starting from a baseline characterized by significant dysfunction or dilation **(Fig. 2)**.

Strain imaging is another valuable technique that complements traditional measurements. By assessing the systolic deformation of the LV, strain imaging operates relatively independently of LV volume and geometry, providing a higher sensitivity for tracking systolic dysfunction.[11] This capability suggests that strain imaging may reveal subtle systolic abnormalities, further indicating a potential for significant reverse remodeling when compared to conventional measures such as LVEF.

When juxtaposed with echocardiography, CMR stands out due to its enhanced contrast resolution and reproducibility, as it is not influenced by factors such as acoustic windows. Additionally, CMR can provide insights into the presence and extent of myocardial fibrosis through late gadolinium enhancement (LGE).[12] The degree of LGE has been shown to correlate inversely with the likelihood of reverse remodeling;[13-15] specifically, in a study of 58 patients with idiopathic dilated cardiomyopathy, the absence of LGE was a strong predictor of improvements in LV size and function, independent of the severity of LV dilation and dysfunction.[16]

Moreover, research indicates that the absence of LGE is associated with a high degree of specificity and positive predictive value in forecasting reverse remodeling outcomes,[17] reinforcing its role as a reliable prognostic indicator across varying baseline LV volumes and LVEF. Such instances of reverse remodeling often correlate with a more favorable prognosis, underscoring the relevance of CMR in guiding clinical decision making **(Figs. 3 and 4)**.

Recent developments, such as T1 mapping, have further enhanced CMR's utility by quantifying extracellular volume and myocardial fibrosis, demonstrating potential for prognostic assessment in patients with HFrEF. But it is important to note that data regarding remodeling outcomes derived from this technique remain relatively limited, indicating an area for future research and exploration.

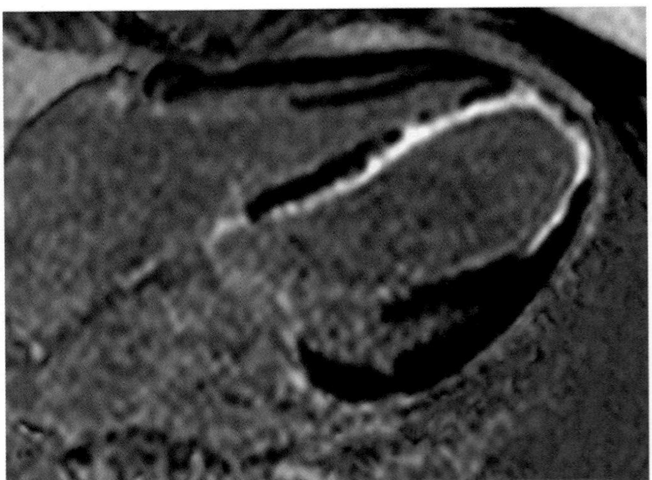

Fig. 4: Short-axis postcontrast sequence demonstrating measurement of scar volumetrics on delayed subendocardial enhancement of the left ventricle at the midcavity level.

In recent research led by Kieran et al., a pivotal prospective, multicenter, randomized, double-blind, active-comparator trial was conducted to evaluate the effects of sacubitril/valsartan compared to valsartan alone in patients post myocardial infarction. The study specifically targeted individuals who had experienced a myocardial infarction at least 3 months prior and presented with a LVEF of 40% or lower. Participants were already on treatment regimens that included a renin-angiotensin system inhibitor and a beta-blocker, unless contraindicated.

The primary endpoint of the study was to analyze changes in LVESV index over 52 weeks, employing CMR imaging as a measurement tool. Secondary objectives encompassed a range of factors, including additional magnetic resonance imaging parameters, levels of NT-proBNP, high-sensitivity cardiac troponin I, and a patient global assessment of change. Notably, the study excluded participants classified as the NYHA class ≥II or those exhibiting symptoms of HF, focusing instead on asymptomatic individuals.

The study's results revealed significant insights: sacubitril/valsartan did not significantly improve LV remodeling compared to valsartan alone in the studied population. Specifically, the potential advantages of neprilysin inhibition, a mechanism inherent to sacubitril/valsartan, were not demonstrated in patients who displayed asymptomatic LV systolic dysfunction late post myocardial infarction. The authors suggest that further investigation is warranted, particularly among subgroups with more severe systolic dysfunction or elevated natriuretic peptide levels.[18]

CONCLUSION

The interplay between ARNI therapy and cardiac remodeling underscores a transformative approach in the management of HFrEF. Future research will undoubtedly continue to elucidate the complex mechanisms underlying cardiac remodeling and potential for innovative treatments to further mitigate its adverse effects.

However, the existing methodologies for assessing myocardial status often rely upon a singular imaging test. This approach yields a binary categorization of the myocardium, which may fail to capture the multifaceted physiological dynamics that characterize various forms of HF. It may obscure the complex interplay of pathophysiological changes that occur during disease progression and treatment.

Consequently, there is a pressing need for future clinical trials to explore the clinical implications of employing modality-based strategies or integrating multiple imaging modalities. By adopting a more nuanced approach to imaging, healthcare providers may be better positioned to refine treatment decisions, ultimately enhancing patient outcomes. The integration of advanced imaging techniques could facilitate a deeper understanding of myocardial behavior and contribute to more personalized therapeutic regimens.

REFERENCES

1. Cohn JN, Ferrari R, Sharpe N. Cardiac remodeling—concepts and clinical implications: a consensus paper from an international forum on cardiac remodeling. J Am Coll Cardiol. 2000;35:569-82.
2. McMurray JJ, Packer M, Desai AS, et al. Angiotensin-neprilysin inhibition versus enalapril in heart failure. N Engl J Med. 2014;371(11):993-1004.
3. Velazquez EJ, Morrow DA, DeVore AD, et al. Angiotensin-neprilysin inhibition in acute decompensated heart failure. N Engl J Med. 2019;380:539-48.
4. Vardeny O, Miller R, Solomon SD. Combined neprilysin and renin-angiotensin system inhibition for the treatment of heart failure. J Am Coll Cardiol. 2014;2:663-70.
5. Packer M, Califf RM, Konstam MA, et al. Comparison of omapatrilat and enalapril in patients with chronic heart failure: the omapatrilat versus enalapril randomized trial of utility in reducing events (OVERTURE). Circulation. 2002;106:920-6.
6. SOLVD Investigators, Yusuf S, Pitt B, et al. Effect of enalapril on mortality and the development of heart failure in asymptomatic patients with reduced left ventricular ejection fractions. N Engl J Med. 1992;327:685-91.
7. Lewis EF, Claggett BL, McMurray JJV, et al. Health-related quality of life outcomes in PARADIGM-HF. Circ Heart Fail. 2017;10:e003430.

8. Martens P, Nuyens D, Rivero-Ayerza M, et al. Sacubitril/valsartan reduces ventricular arrhythmias in parallel with left ventricular reverse remodeling in heart failure with reduced ejection fraction. Clin Res Cardiol. 2019; 108:1074-82.
9. Desai AS, Solomon SD, Shah AM, et al. Effect of sacubitril-valsartan vs enalapril on aortic stiffness in patients with heart failure and reduced ejection fraction: a randomized clinical trial. JAMA. 2019;322:1-10.
10. Lupón J, Gaggin HK, de Antonio M, et al. Biomarker-assist score for reverse remodeling prediction in heart failure: the ST2-R2 score. Int J Cardiol. 2015;184: 337-43.
11. Park SM, Kim YH, Ahn CM, et al. Relationship between ultrasonic tissue characterization and myocardial deformation for prediction of left ventricular reverse remodeling in non-ischaemic dilated cardiomyopathy. Eur J Echocardiogr. 2011;12:887-94.
12. Barison A, Grigoratos C, Todiere G, et al. Myocardial interstitial remodeling in non-ischaemic dilated cardiomyopathy: insights from cardiovascular magnetic resonance. Heart Fail Rev. 2015;20:731-49.
13. Ishii S, Inomata T, Fujita T, et al. Clinical significance of endomyocardial biopsy in conjunction with cardiac magnetic resonance imaging to predict left ventricular reverse remodeling in idiopathic dilated cardiomyopathy. Heart Vessels. 2016;31:1960-68.
14. Chimura M, Onishi T, Tsukishiro Y, et al. Longitudinal strain combined with delayed-enhancement magnetic resonance improves risk stratification in patients with dilated cardiomyopathy. Heart. 2017;103:679-86.
15. Barison A, Aimo A, Ortalda A, et al. Late gadolinium enhancement as a predictor of functional recovery, need for defibrillator implantation and prognosis in non-ischemic dilated cardiomyopathy. Int J Cardiol. 2018;250:195-200.
16. Masci PG, Schuurman R, Andrea B, et al. Myocardial fibrosis as a key determinant of left ventricular remodeling in idiopathic dilated cardiomyopathy: a contrast-enhanced cardiovascular magnetic study. Circ Cardiovasc Imaging. 2013;6:790-9.
17. Kida K, Yoneyama K, Kobayashi Y, et al. Late gadolinium enhancement on cardiac magnetic resonance images predicts reverse remodeling in patients with nonischemic cardiomyopathy treated with carvedilol. Int J Cardiol. 2013;168:1588-9.
18. Docherty KF, Campbell RT, Brooksbank KJM, et al. Effect of neprilysin inhibition on left ventricular remodeling in patients with asymptomatic left ventricular systolic dysfunction late after myocardial infarction. Circulation. 2021;144(3):199-209.

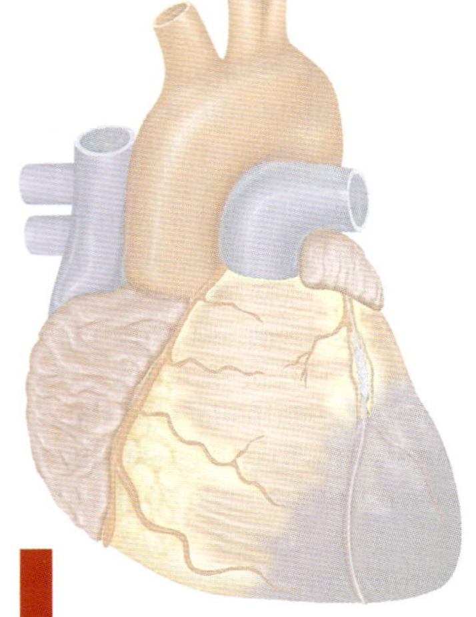

CHAPTER 70

Cardiac Magnetic Resonance to Enhance Phenotypic Characterization of HFpEF

Johann Christopher, Nilay S Nimbalkar, Richa Kothari

INTRODUCTION

Heart failure with preserved ejection fraction (HFpEF) is an important global health problem. It is commonly seen in elderly patients with hypertension and obesity and is associated with left ventricular hypertrophy (LVH). Patients with HFpEF usually present with symptomatic heart failure (HF) despite a normal left ventricle (LV) ejection fraction (LVEF) but have similar morbidity and mortality as patients with HF with reduced ejection fraction (HFrEF).[1]

Heart failure with preserved ejection fraction involves a complex interplay of pathophysiological changes involving diastolic dysfunction, remodeling of the LV, and left atrium (LA), and it is associated with a poor prognosis. Echocardiography is the first-line method for evaluation of diastolic dysfunction, the use of multimodality imaging is increasing, including nuclear imaging, CT, and MRI.[2-4]

According to the latest defining criteria for HfpEF, it is obviously impossible to predict LV dimensions and hemodynamics with sole clinical data. Need for further imaging modalities like Cardiac MRI (CMR) is inevitable.[1]

Cardiac MRI is the gold standard cardiovascular imaging modality for the atrial and ventricular volume assessment and ejection fraction quantification. It is also the best alternative imaging modality in patients with suboptimal echocardiographic image quality that does not only make morphological and functional evaluations but also gives information about perfusion, viability, and tissue characterization, which may provide a better understanding of the pathophysiological mechanism of the HFpEF.

It allows assessment of LA enlargement, LVH, permanent replacement fibrosis, and dynamic interstitial fibrosis using late gadolinium enhancement (LGE) and T1 mapping.

By providing tissue characterization with T1 and T2 mapping, CMR is the best imaging modality in the differential diagnosis of myocarditis, infiltrative disorders such as Fabry's disease, sarcoidosis, amyloidosis, noncompaction cardiomyopathy, arrhythmogenic RV cardiomyopathy, hypertrophic cardiomyopathy, or Chagas disease.[5-7]

Cardiac MRI has high reproducibility and good spatial and temporal resolution. It has reduced geometric assumptions for volume calculations, is less operator-dependent than other cardiovascular imaging modalities, and there is no fear of ionizing radiation. New methods such as feature tracking enable myocardial strain analysis as well.

Cardiac MRI plays a pivotal role, particularly, in patients with nondiagnostic echocardiographic examinations secondary to suboptimal image quality.

It has been shown that abnormal longitudinal strain despite preserved LVEF is a strong prognostic factor for worse outcomes in HFpEF patients. Myocardial strain and torsion can be acquired by CMR as well. Feature tracking analysis helps to detect anatomical features of interest in the LV subendocardium and subepicardium on segmented steady-state free precession (SSFP) cine images similar to echocardiographic speckle tracking. CMR feature tracking method provides LA strain and strain rate calculation. These measures have been demonstrated to be impaired and associated with exercise intolerance in HFpEF patients. It is the preferred imaging tool for volume and ejection fraction estimation in HF patients due to its 3D approach for nonsymmetrical ventricles and superior image quality, which is less user-dependent and has a higher reproducibility.[8-12] Volumes are measured from a cine stack of short-axis biventricular contiguous slices. Modern cine sequences use breath hold, electrocardiographic-gated, and segmented SSFP to produce images with high spatial/temporal resolution, which are superior to other cardiac imaging modalities. Myocardial mass is also measured from the same short axis slices and CMR is considered the ideal method for the assessment of LV mass.[1-3]

LEFT VENTRICLE DIASTOLIC FUNCTION BY CARDIAC MRI

Diastolic dysfunction is generally considered a key component for the diagnosis of HFpEF. Use of noninvasive techniques for the assessment of LV diastolic function is preferred over invasive techniques.[13] CMR may provide other various LV diastolic function parameters such as LA size and function, LV hypertrophy and mass, and myocardial deformation imaging with strain method **(Figs. 1A to E)**, which are the most useful parameters for the assessment of patients with HfpEF.[6,13,14]

Left Atrial Evaluation by Cardiac MRI

Atrial volume and function **(Figs. 2A to D)** are two important measures of ventricular diastolic performance and are shown to be reliable indicators of the duration and severity of diastolic dysfunction independent of loading conditions.[15] LA has a poor compliance; thus, LA dilation is an indicator of diastolic dysfunction with elevation of LV

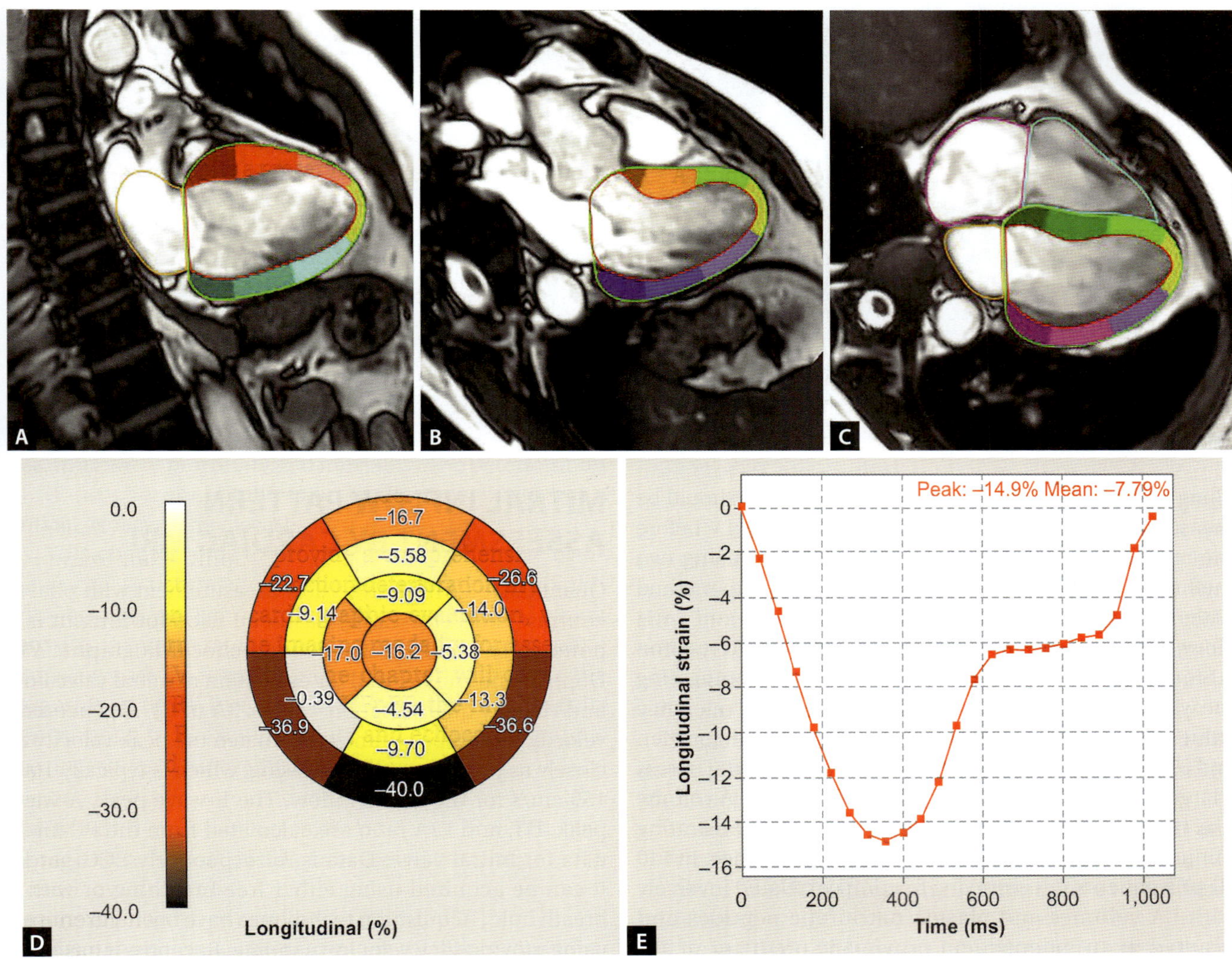

Figs. 1A to E: (A to C) Long-axis strain assessment by CMR; (D) Bull's eye pictorial in 17-segment model; and (E) GLS curve demonstrating the same.

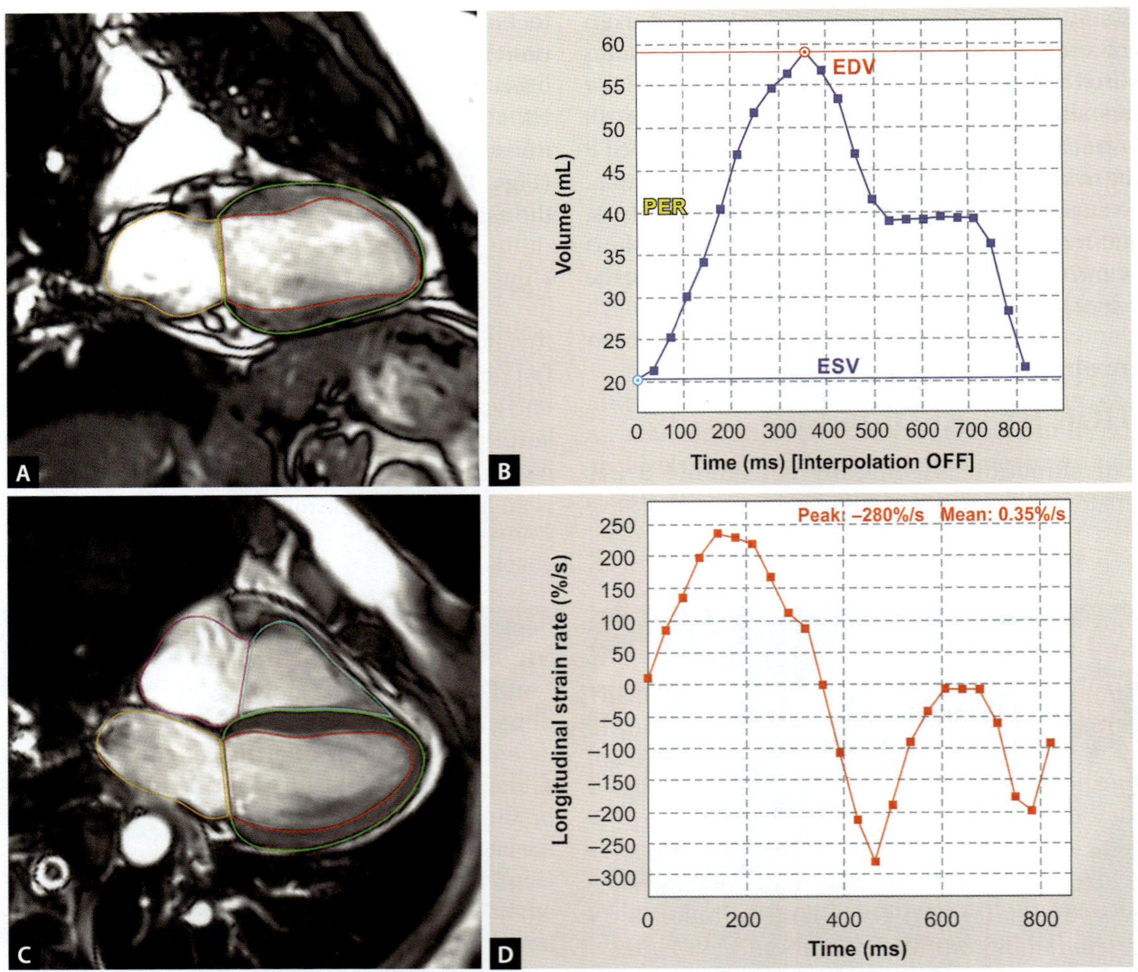

Figs. 2A to D: (A and C) Long-axis cine images demonstrating the LA assessment (orange curve). On the right, are seen (B) The LA function and (D) LA strain graphs as assessed by CMR.

filling pressure in the diastolic phase. LA volume should be measured at the end of the systolic phase of the LV before the mitral valve opening. It can be measured using two methods. First method is the bi-plane area-length method with manually drawn endocardial contours in 2- and 4-CH views with exclusion of pulmonary veins. Second method is Simpson's method on the short axis slices encompassing the whole left atrium. The study reported normal reference values in 108 healthy volunteers as 103 ± 30 mL for men and 89 ± 21 mL for women by area-length method. There is a large amount of data supporting the maximal LA volume use. However, there are also several studies demonstrating minimal LA volume to be of prognostic significance. In 140 HFpEF patients, LA emptying fraction correlated inversely with LA volumes and plasma natriuretic peptides and resulted in an independent prognostic predictor of all-cause death or hospitalization for HF.[16-18]

MITRAL INFLOW PATTERN ASSESSMENT BY CARDIAC MRI

Quantitative CMR-derived flow measurement with phase-contrast CMR (PC-CMR) has been used for long. It is a potentially useful alternative to echocardiographic-PW Doppler and can be used for evaluation of mitral valve flow and velocity quantification[19] **(Figs. 3A to C)**. An encoding velocity should be optimized to match the peak velocity as closely as possible without aliasing, which is typically 100–150 cm/s for the mitral inflow. The E-wave peak, A-wave peak, DT, and E/A ratio are calculated from the PC-CMR data for mitral valve. Data is retrospectively ECG-gated. It can be acquired using either free breathing or with a breath hold. Acquisition techniques have been introduced using moving slice velocity mapping. Recently, it has been demonstrated that three-directional 3D velocity-encoded

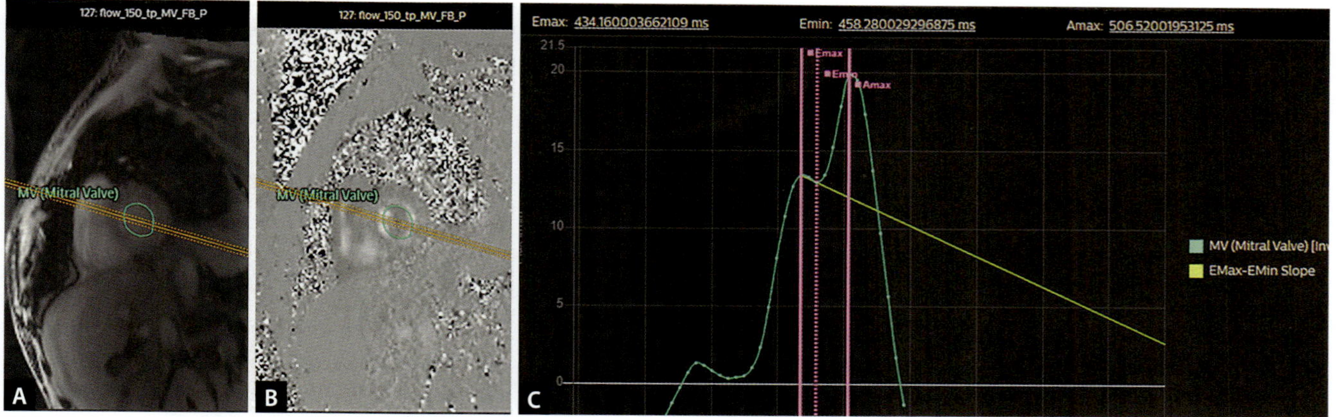

Figs. 3A to C: Mitral inflow pattern assessment by CMR. (A and B) Phase and magnitude images obtained at mitral valve level by CMR and (C) graph which calculates the E/A ratio.

MRI with retrospective valve tracking showed better agreement with echo-Doppler when differentiating a restrictive filling pattern from other patterns.[13,20-22] In line with echocardiography, CMR-derived E/Ea <8 has 100% positive predictive value for pulmonary capillary wedge pressure (PCWP) ≤15 mm Hg, and E/Ea ratio >15 has 100% positive predictive value for PCWP >15 mm Hg.[23]

PULMONARY VENOUS FLOW PATTERN BY CARDIAC MRI

Waveform analysis of pulmonary venous flow is a helpful way to assess LV diastolic dysfunction. Pulmonary vein velocity-encoded MRI is an alternative method of PW Doppler to investigate atrial filling patterns.[6] 2D one-directional velocity encoding at the pulmonary vein and 3D three-directional velocity-encoding approach of the intra-atrial blood flow field are two different ways of obtaining a pulmonary venous time–velocity curve. The pulmonary vein flow is sampled 1 cm into the pulmonary vein ostium similar to Doppler echocardiography. The use of pulmonary venous flow for the LV diastolic dysfunction assessment is limited in conditions such as sinus tachycardia, first-degree atrioventricular block, and AF.[19] Velocity-encoded MRI offers a useful alternative to PW Doppler for pulmonary venous flow assessment and several studies have shown good correlations when compared with Doppler echocardiography.[6,19]

TISSUE CHARACTERIZATION BY CARDIAC MRI

Several diseases that have similar clinical presentations may have the same clinical phenotype as HFpEF and should be considered mimics, which confuses the diagnostic process.[24] It is of utmost importance to recognize other alternative cardiac diseases, which should be considered in the differential diagnosis for HFpEF.[10] Those diseases are mainly restrictive cardiomyopathy, constrictive pericarditis, and severe tricuspid regurgitation. Specific findings with LGE include subendocardial LV, RV free wall, and septum hyperenhancement.[10] Amyloidosis **(Figs. 4A to D)**, cardiac sarcoidosis **(Figs. 5A to C)**, and hemochromatosis are the primary restrictive cardiomyopathies that are encountered in daily practice.[25] CMR is the only noninvasive technique for quantifying myocardial iron overload. Introduced in 1999, the T2* technique is a robust, fast, reproducible method that is the method of choice for cardiac iron quantification, which is transferable among different CMR scanners. Different online calculators or simple Excel sheet methods are available for myocardial iron quantification.

Tissue characterization plays a pivotal role in the context of HFpEF in identifying specific patterns of fibrosis and scarring in most of the cardiomyopathies that could be a differential diagnosis for HFpEF. The identification of mimics of HFpEF may allow an individualized approach to molecular targets and functional abnormalities, such as the use of some important drugs in senile amyloidosis, and beta-blockers, and/or calcium channel antagonists in patients with hypertrophic cardiomyopathy.[10,11,26]

Identification of myocardial scar and fibrosis can be done by following methods:

- *LGE:* CMR using LGE can detect myocardial scarring and fibrosis, which are common in ischemic cardiomyopathy and can also occur in nonischemic forms of HFrEF. Identifying these areas helps in understanding the underlying pathology and risk stratification.

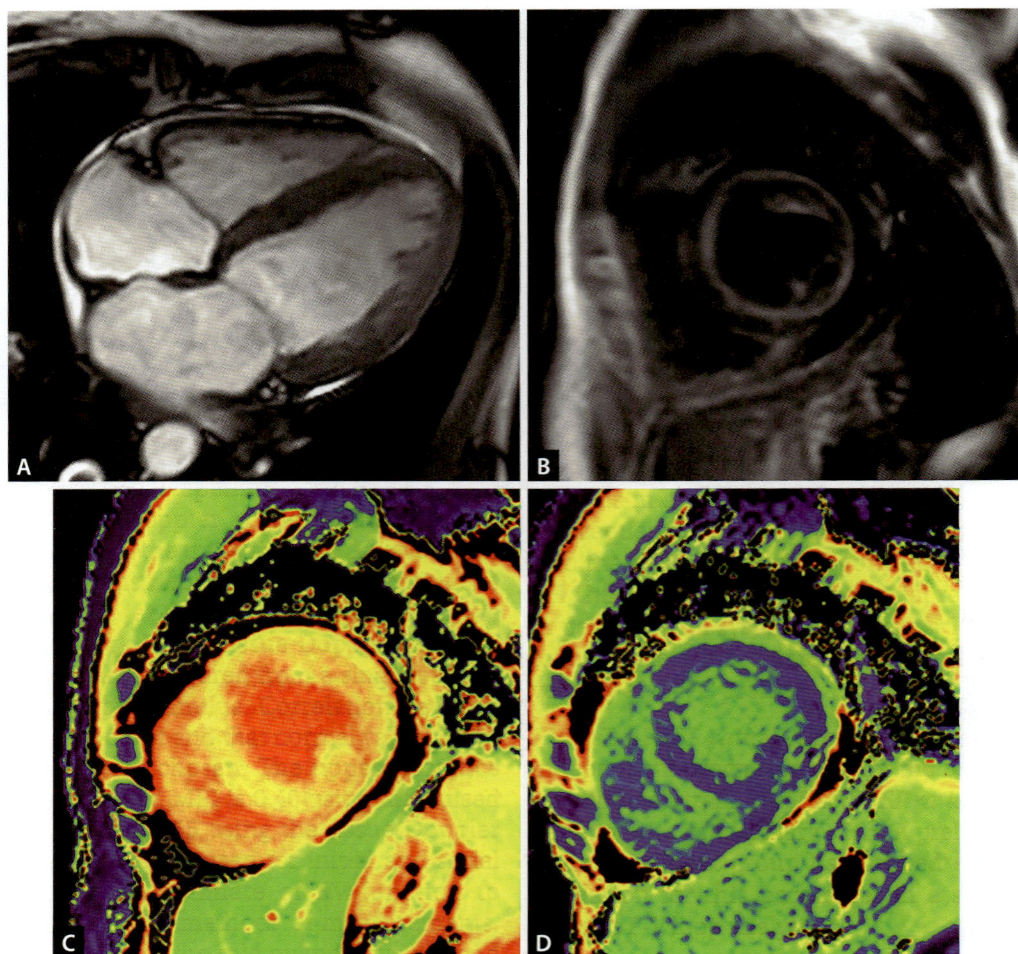

Figs. 4A to D: Four-chamber, LGE, T1 mapping, and ECV images of a patient with amyloidosis. LGE image shows diffuse smooth global subendocardial enhancement. T1 mapping and ECV show corresponding raised values.

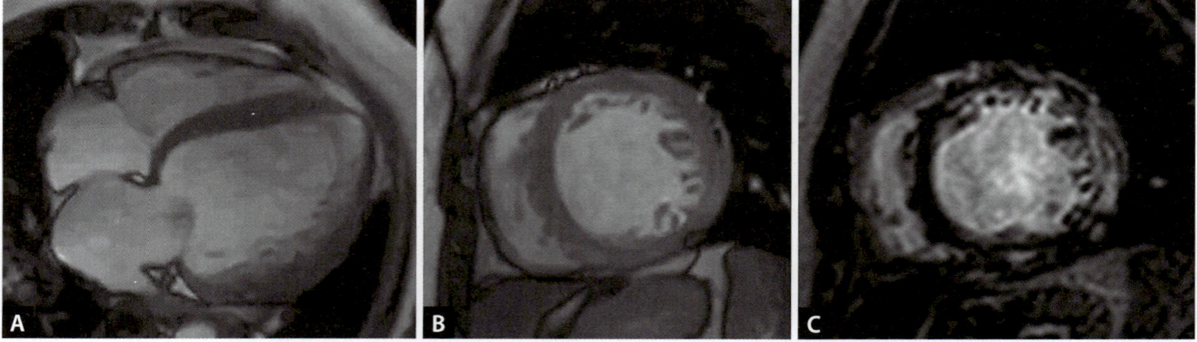

Figs. 5A to C: 4 chamber, short axis, LGE images in a patient with sarcoidosis. LGE image shows patchy areas of mid to epicardial enhancement, especially along the lateral wall.

- *T1 mapping and extracellular volume (ECV):* Advanced techniques like T1 mapping **(Figs. 6A to C)** can quantify diffuse myocardial fibrosis, providing additional insights into myocardial health and fibrosis that might not be detected with LGE alone.

CARDIAC MRI TECHNIQUES IN RESEARCH

Although it is well known that myocardial stiffness plays an important role in cardiac function and increased

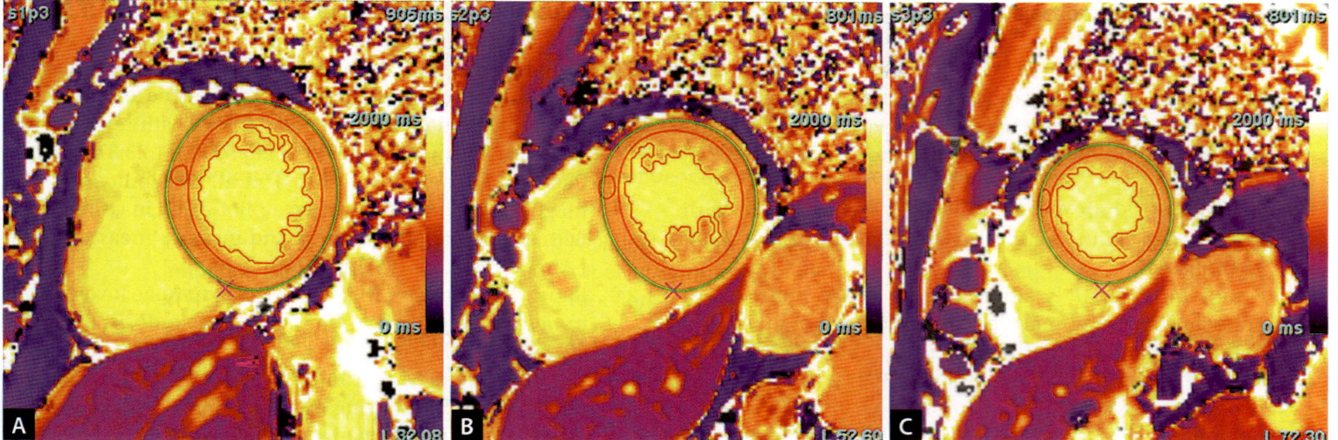

Figs. 6A to C: T1 mapping assessed by CMR software at basal, mid, and apical LV levels.

stiffness may cause restrictive diastolic filling, there is still no conventional imaging method to measure myocardial stiffness directly in vivo.[27,28] High-resolution magnetic resonance elastography is a novel technique based on a stiffness map produced by an external vibrating source that generates shear waves inside a tissue of interest. Arani et al. have demonstrated the feasibility of 3D high-frequency CMR elastography diagnostic imaging technique for quantitatively measuring myocardial stiffness in vivo, which does not require a contrast agent.[28]

Stress and exercise CMR have emerged as important tools in HFpEF diagnosis during the past few years. Considering that patients with HFpEF develop symptoms on exertion, an exercise test for the diagnosis becomes inevitable. Stress perfusion CMR may help identify HFpEF patients at higher cardiovascular risk with no known coronary artery disease.[29] Additional to that, in a study by Backhaus et al., real-time-CMR bicycle exercise stress testing showed high accuracy in the diagnosis of HFpEF, and LA longitudinal shortening during the exercise was demonstrated as the best independent predictor of HFpEF proven with an invasive method.[30]

Four-dimensional flow is another new method that can quantitively assess LV 3D blood flow over the cardiac cycle.[31] It is possible to identify and monitor diastolic dysfunction with 4D flow. Analysis of flow components and the kinetic energy and momentum will provide a precise assessment of the dynamic of ventricular filling and ejection.[5] It can differentiate restrictive diastolic filling and normal diastolic filling patterns, and can also evaluate kinetic energy, vorticity, or particle tracing-based metrics.[32,33] Machine learning and artificial intelligence (AI) are gaining importance in the medical imaging field and are expected to transform clinical practice. CMR can use machine learning to help guide diagnosis and therapy management as it relies on complex acquisition strategies. AI is associated with radiomics, which is a novel image analysis technique. Digital images are converted into numeric data, which can then be analyzed to obtain multiple numerical quantifiers of shape and tissue character, and it has been demonstrated that disease conditions or clinical outcomes may be identified with high accuracy with this new method.[34-36]

CONCLUSION

Cardiac MRI is a valuable tool in the management of HFpEF, offering insights into myocardial structure, function, and fibrosis, which are crucial for accurate diagnosis and effective treatment planning.

REFERENCES

1. McDonagh TA, Metra M, Adamo M, et al. 2021 ESC guidelines for the diagnosis and treatment of acute and chronic heart failure. Eur Heart J. 2021;42(36):3599-726.
2. Pieske B, Tschöpe C, De Boer RA, et al. How to diagnose heart failure with preserved ejection fraction: The HFA-PEFF diagnostic algorithm: a consensus recommendation from the Heart Failure Association (HFA) of the European Society of Cardiology (ESC). Eur Heart J. 2019;40:3297-317.
3. Smiseth OA, Morris DA, Cardim N, et al. Multimodality imaging in patients with heart failure and preserved ejection fraction: An expert consensus document of the European Association of Cardiovascular Imaging. Eur Heart J Cardiovasc Imaging. 2022;23(2):e34-61.
4. Sorrentino R, Esposito R, Santoro C, et al. Practical impact of new diastolic recommendations on noninvasive estimation of left ventricular diastolic function and filling pressures. J Am Soc Echocardiogr. 2020;33:171-81.
5. Webb J, Fovargue L, Tøndel K, et al. The emerging role of cardiac magnetic resonance imaging in the evaluation of patients with HFpEF. Curr Heart Fail Rep. 2018;15:1-9.
6. Barison A, Aimo A, Todiere G, et al. Cardiovascular magnetic resonance for the diagnosis and management of

heart failure with preserved ejection fraction. Heart Fail Rev. 2022;27:191-205.
7. Kanagala P, Cheng ASH, Singh A, et al. Diagnostic and prognostic utility of cardiovascular magnetic resonance imaging in heart failure with preserved ejection fraction–implications for clinical trials. J Cardiovasc Magn Reson. 2018;20:4.
8. Pfeffer MA, Shah AM, Borlaug BA. Heart failure with preserved ejection fraction in perspective. Circ Res. 2019; 124:1598-617.
9. Kinno M, Nagpal P, Horgan S, et al. Comparison of echocardiography, cardiac magnetic resonance, and computed tomographic imaging for the evaluation of left ventricular myocardial function: Part 2 (diastolic and regional assessment). Curr Cardiol Rep. 2017;19(1):6.
10. Nagueh SF, Chang SM, Nabi F, et al. Cardiac imaging in patients with heart failure and preserved ejection fraction. Circ Cardiovasc Imaging. 2017;10(9):e006547.
11. Nagueh SF, Bierig SM, Budoff MJ, et al. American Society of Echocardiography clinical recommendations for multimodality cardiovascular imaging of patients with hypertrophic cardiomyopathy: Endorsed by the American Society of Nuclear Cardiology, society for cardiovascular magnetic resonance, and Society of Cardiovascular Computed Tomography. J Am Soc Echocardiogr. 2011; 24(5):473-98.
12. Nagueh SF, Appleton CP, Gillebert TC et al. Recommendations for the evaluation of left ventricular diastolic function by echocardiography. Eur J Echocardiogr. 2009;10: 165-93.
13. Rathi VK, Doyle M, Yamrozik J, et al. Routine evaluation of left ventricular diastolic function by cardiovascular magnetic resonance: a practical approach. J Cardiovasc Magn Reson. 2008;10:36.
14. Bellenger NG, Burgess MI, Ray SG, et al. Comparison of left ventricular ejection fraction and volumes in heart failure by echocardiography, radionuclide ventriculography and cardiovascular magnetic resonance; are they interchangeable? Eur Heart J. 2000;21(16):1387-96.
15. Simek CL, Feldman MD, Haber HL, et al. Relationship between left ventricular wall thickness and left atrial size: comparison with other measures of diastolic function. J Am Soc Echocardiogr. 1995;8:37-47.
16. Hoit BD. Left atrial size and function: role in prognosis. J Am Coll Cardiol. 2014;63:493-505.
17. Hudsmith LE, Petersen SE, Francis JM, et al. Normal human left and right ventricular and left atrial dimensions using steady state free precession magnetic resonance imaging. J Cardiovasc Magn Reson. 2005;7:775-82.
18. Thomas L, Hoy M, Byth K, et al. The left atrial function index: a rhythm independent marker of atrial function. Eur J Echocardiogr. 2008;9:356-62.
19. Chamsi-Pasha MA, Zhan Y, Debs D, et al. CMR in the evaluation of diastolic dysfunction and phenotyping of HFpEF: current role and future perspectives. JACC Cardiovasc Imaging. 2020;13:283-96.
20. Pandey T, Jambhekar K. Evaluation of diastolic dysfunction using cardiac magnetic resonance imaging. Eur Cardiol. 2010;6:21-5.
21. Westenberg JJM. CMR for assessment of diastolic function. Curr Cardiovasc Imaging Rep. 2011;4:149-58.
22. Brandts A, Bertini M, Van Dijk EJ, et al. Left ventricular diastolic function assessment from three-dimensional three-directional velocity-encoded MRI with retrospective valve tracking. J Magn Reson Imaging. 2011;33:312-9.
23. Paelinck BP, de Roos A, Bax JJ, et al. Feasibility of tissue magnetic resonance imaging: a pilot study in comparison with tissue Doppler imaging and invasive measurement. J Am Coll Cardiol. 2005;45(7):1109-16.
24. Rapezzi C, Longhi S, Milandri A, et al. Cardiac involvement in hereditary-transthyretin related amyloidosis. Amyloid. 2012;19(Suppl 1):16-21.
25. Nojima Y, Ihara M, Kurimoto T, et al. Amyloid light-chain amyloidosis manifesting as heart failure with preserved ejection fraction in a patient with hyper-immunoglobulin E-emia. Am J Case Rep. 2016;17:235-40.
26. Mörner S, Hellman U, Suhr OB, et al. Amyloid heart disease mimicking hypertrophic cardiomyopathy. J Intern Med. 2005;258(3):225-30.
27. Zile MR, Baicu CF, Gaasch WH. Diastolic heart failure–abnormalities in active relaxation and passive stiffness of the left ventricle. N Engl J Med. 2004;350: 1953-9.
28. Arani A, Arunachalam SP, Chang ICY, et al. Cardiac MR elastography for quantitative assessment of elevated myocardial stiffness in cardiac amyloidosis. J Magn Reson Imaging. 2017;46(5):1361-7.
29. Pezel T, Hovasse T, Sanguineti F, et al. Long-term prognostic value of stress CMR in patients with heart failure and preserved ejection fraction. JACC Cardiovasc Imaging. 2021;14(12):2319-33.
30. Backhaus SJ, Lange T, George EF, et al. Exercise stress real-time cardiac magnetic resonance imaging for noninvasive characterization of heart failure with preserved ejection fraction: The HFpEF-Stress trial. Circulation. 2021;143: 1484-98.
31. Pica S, Piatti F, Milani P, et al. 4D flow CMR for diastolic function assessment in cardiac amyloidosis. Eur Heart J Cardiovasc Imaging. 2019;20(Supplement_2):408-9.
32. Ashkir Z, Myerson S, Neubauer S, et al. Four-dimensional flow cardiac magnetic resonance assessment of left ventricular diastolic function. Front Cardiovasc Med. 2022;9:866131.
33. Alattar Y, Soulat G, Gencer U, et al. Left ventricular diastolic early and late filling quantified from 4D flow magnetic resonance imaging. Diagn Interv Imaging. 2022;103:345-52.
34. Krittanawong C. The rise of artificial intelligence and the uncertain future for physicians. Eur J Intern Med. 2018;48:e13-4.
35. Leiner T, Rueckert D, Suinesiaputra A, et al. Machine learning in cardiovascular magnetic resonance: basic concepts and applications. J Cardiovasc Magn Reson. 2019;21(1):61.
36. Lambin P, Rios-Velazquez E, Leijenaar R, et al. Radiomics: extracting more information from medical images using advanced feature analysis. Eur J Cancer. 2012;48(4): 441-6.

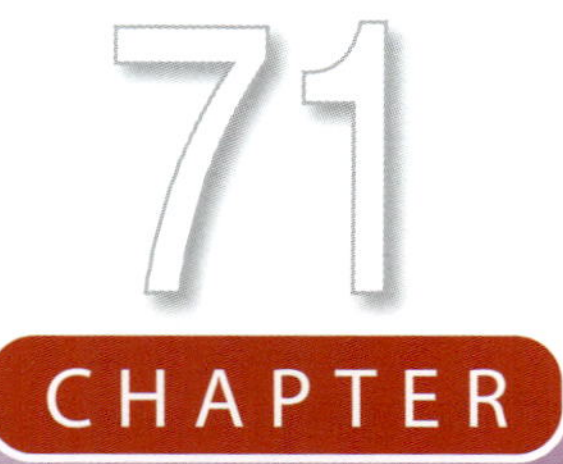

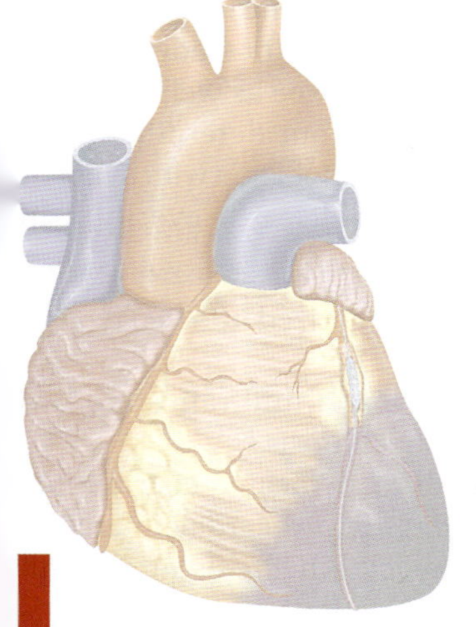

CHAPTER 71

Focal and Diffuse Fibrosis in HFpEF: Cardiac Magnetic Resonance Evaluation and Outcomes

Shoma Mukerjee Sharma, Harsh Mahajan

INTRODUCTION

Heart failure with preserved ejection fraction (HFpEF) is defined as a clinical syndrome with symptoms and signs of heart failure but preserved ejection fraction (EF ≥50%). The presence of diastolic dysfunction and elevated levels of natriuretic peptides (NPs) are also hallmarks of this condition.[1,2] HFpEF accounts for approximately half of all heart failure cases and is associated with significant morbidity and mortality.[3] The syndrome shows increased prevalence in the elderly and has been linked to comorbidities, such as hypertension, obesity, diabetes, and atrial fibrillation (AF).[4]

ABNORMALITIES IN CARDIOVASCULAR STRUCTURE AND FUNCTION IN HFpEF (FLOWCHART 1)

- *Diastolic dysfunction:* Poor relaxation and filling of the left ventricle (LV), especially during exercise resulting in increased left atrial (LA) and pulmonary venous pressures.[5]
- *LV remodeling:* Increased LV wall thickness and mass with little to no change in LV volume due to chronic pressure overload.[6]

Flowchart 1: Abnormalities in cardiovascular structure and function in HFpEF.

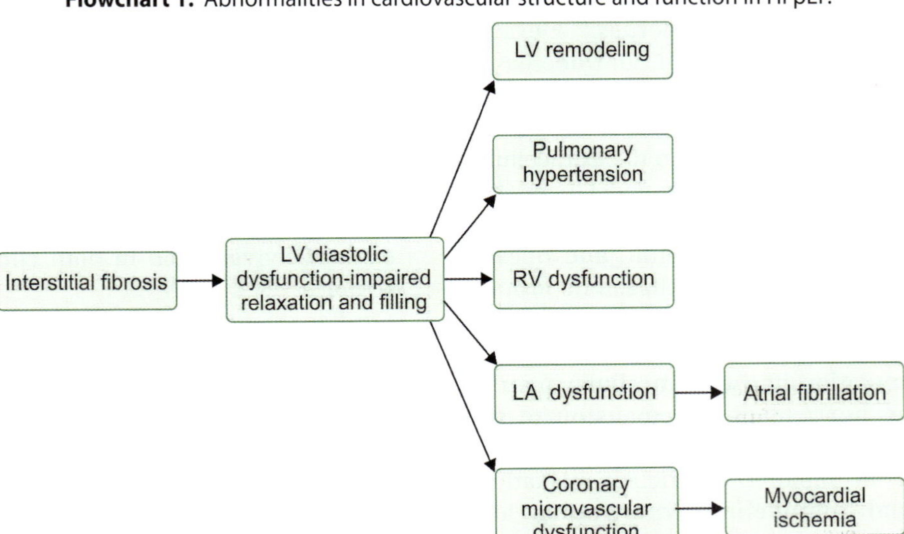

- *Pulmonary hypertension:* Increased LA and pulmonary venous pressures from diastolic dysfunction cause elevated pulmonary artery pressure.[7]
- *Right ventricular (RV) dysfunction:* Occurs in 20–35% of HFpEF patients, often in advanced stages, and is a predictor of morbidity and mortality, especially when associated with pulmonary hypertension and AF.[5]
- *Coronary microvascular dysfunction:* Seen in approximately 75% of HFpEF patients. This results in reduced blood flow to small coronary vessels and myocardial ischemia.[8]
- *LA myopathy and enlargement:* LA dysfunction is associated with worse outcomes, and is often independent of AF.[9]
- *AF:* Found in approximately two-thirds of patients. AF is linked to worse RV function, lower exercise capacity, and increased mortality. It is often seen independent of atrial myopathy being related to pulmonary hypertension.[9]
- *Pericardial constriction:* Epicardial fat deposition and obesity are associated with hemodynamic signs of pericardial constriction in patients, particularly women with HFpEF.[10]
- *Impaired exercise tolerance:* In HFpEF, mechanisms that balance cardiac input and output during exercise are compromised, leading to reduced LV distensibility and increased pulmonary pressure.[5]

PATHOPHYSIOLOGY OF MYOCARDIAL FIBROSIS IN HFpEF

Myocardial fibrosis causing increased passive myocardial stiffness is an essential element in the pathophysiology of HFpEF. Myocardial fibrosis is the end result of alterations in the cardiac extracellular matrix and to some extent changes in cardiomyocyte properties.[11] Elevated expression of collagen types I and III, and decreased levels of collagenase and metalloproteinase-1 are induced by myocardial injury or inflammation and have been found to promote collagen deposition in the extracellular matrix.[12] The comorbidity-inflammation model theory has emerged over the last decade and postulates that systemic inflammation in diabetes, hypertension, and obesity causes a chain reaction resulting in collagen deposition and myocardial fibrosis. This has been implicated in the onset and progression of HFpEF.[13]

Collagen accumulation in the extracellular matrix/interstitium of the heart leads to expansion of the extracellular space and increased myocardial stiffness. This in turn results in impaired ventricular relaxation, adverse ventricular remodeling/hypertrophy, and diastolic dysfunction; these constitute the hallmark features of HFpEF. Myocardial fibrosis precedes clinical symptoms and diagnosis. The presence as well as extent of cardiac fibrosis serve as important determinants of clinical outcomes with both being associated with a higher incidence of arrhythmias, higher disease severity, and mortality.[14]

Myocardial fibrosis is broadly categorized into two types:

1. Replacement fibrosis
2. Interstitial fibrosis (reactive and infiltrative are two further subtypes of interstitial fibrosis.[15]

Replacement fibrosis tends to be focal in distribution. It is typically seen in the settings of myocardial infarction where ischemia-induced myocyte necrosis and death are replaced by scar tissue.[16] Reactive interstitial fibrosis shows mostly a diffuse distribution pattern and has been associated with conditions such as aging, diabetes, and hypertension.[17] The infiltrative subtype type of fibrosis results from the accumulation of insoluble proteins such as seen in amyloidosis, glycosphingolipids, as seen in Anderson–Fabry disease, and other storage disorders within the interstitial space. Both forms of interstitial fibrosis can eventually progress to cardiomyocyte injury and replacement fibrosis.[18]

In HFpEF, the diffuse pattern of interstitial fibrosis is more commonly seen. The focal pattern of replacement fibrosis has also been observed and can represent both ischemic and nonischemic pathologies.[19]

EVALUATION OF DIASTOLIC DYSFUNCTION IN HFpEF

Comprehensive evaluation requires a combination of clinical and diagnostic tools: Physical examination, electrocardiogram (ECG), chest radiographs, laboratory tests, and multimodality imaging. Invasive measurements of LV diastolic properties and pressures are rarely used due to impracticality on a large scale.

Multimodality imaging relies primarily on the following:

- *Echocardiography:* This remains the first choice for assessing diastolic function in HFpEF. It has been extensively validated in both clinical and research settings.[20,21]
- *Cardiac magnetic resonance imaging (CMRI):* This has emerged as a valuable supporting tool for the diagnosis of HFpEF. The advantages of CMR are higher spatial resolution, superior accuracy in quantifying structural heart changes, and unmatched ability to characterize tissue properties. CMR disadvantages are its limited availability, higher cost, challenges for patients with

claustrophobia, difficulty in older or obese individuals due to breath-holding, and image degradation in patients with AF or cardiac devices.[22]

CARDIAC MAGNETIC RESONANCE IMAGING IN HFpEF

Overview

Cardiac magnetic resonance imaging (MRI) evaluation of indices of diastolic dysfunction in HFpEF includes the following:

- Biventricular volumetric measurements including ventricular volumes, mass, and function, along with detailed morphological information.
- LA size and function.
- Mitral inflow and pulmonary venous velocity profiles.
- Assessment of interstitial and focal myocardial fibrosis
- Myocardial strain imaging.

Protocol (Table 1)

Clinical CMR is performed on 1.5 T or 3 T, systems A cardiac imaging-specific surface coil with multiple coil elements (typically ≥8 elements) is recommended Parallel imaging techniques are employed that reduce scan and breath hold times. ECG-gating hardware and software are essential. The ECG-gating system should be capable of performing prospective gating, retrospective gating, as well as triggered gating techniques to ensure accurate synchronization with the cardiac cycle.[23]

ASSESSMENT OF FOCAL AND DIFFUSE FIBROSIS WITH CARDIAC MAGNETIC RESONANCE

Cardiac magnetic resonance is established as a preferred noninvasive imaging method for identifying and

TABLE 1: CMR protocol for HFpEF.

CMR sequence	*Purpose*	*Key parameters and sequences*
Cine MRI	Assess cardiac structure, LV, RV volumes, function, and mass	• Short-axis and long-axis views. Breath-hold and ECG gating • Sequence-bSSFP
T1 mapping (precontrast)	Detect diffuse myocardial fibrosis	• Parametric color maps • Sequence options: – MOLLI – ShMOLLI technique – SASHA
T2 mapping	Evaluate myocardial edema.	• Sequence options: – BSSFP acquisitions with varying T2 preparation times – Gradient and spin echo (GraSE)
Perfusion imaging (optional)	Assess coronary microvascular function, and detect inducible ischemia.	• First-pass perfusion, pharmacological stress (e.g., adenosine) • Sequence -GRE-EPI
Late gadolinium enhancement (LGE)	Identify focal fibrosis/scar tissue.	• Acquired 10–15 minutes postgadolinium contrast injection • Sequence options: – 2D segmented inversion recovery GRE – PSIR – 3D sequences free breathing option – Black blood options for subendocardial scar detection
T1 mapping (postcontrast)	Quantify extracellular volume (ECV) fraction, indirect assessment of diffuse fibrosis	• Acquired at least 15 minutes postcontrast • Software-generated ECV color maps
Myocardial strain imaging	Quantify strain patterns and indicators of diastolic dysfunction	Feature tracking or tagging techniques
Phase-contrast imaging (optional)	Assess blood flow patterns across the mitral valve, an indicator of diastolic dysfunction of LV	Through-plane velocity encoding, 2D phase-contrast • 4D flow options

(CMR: cardiac magnetic resonance; bSSFP: balanced steady-state free precession; GRE-EPI: gradient echo-echo planar imaging; PSIR: phase-sensitive inversion recovery; MOLLI: modified Look–Locker imaging; ShMOLLI: shortened MOLLI; SASHA: saturation recovery single-shot acquisition; MRI: magnetic resonance imaging)

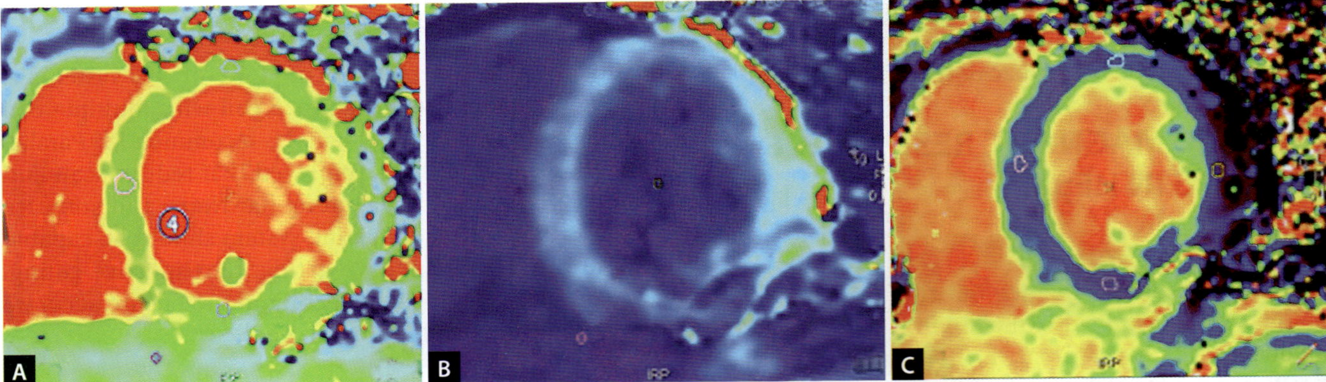

Figs. 1A to C: (A) Native T1 map, 3T MOLLI; (B) Postcontrast T1map; (C) ECV map derived from pre- and postcontrast T1maps. (ECV: extracellular volume; MOLLI: Modified Look-Locker Inversion-recovery)

quantifying myocardial fibrosis. The two key techniques that are currently in use are:

- LGE for detecting replacement fibrosis
- T1 mapping/extracellular volume (ECV) fraction for identifying interstitial fibrosis.[24]

Native T1 Mapping (Figs. 1A to C)

Principle: Native T1 mapping is a quantifiable marker of interstitial fibrosis and shows a strong correlation with histological measurements of fibrosis.

T1 mapping is based on the evaluation of longitudinal proton relaxation times following an electromagnetic pulse. The technique generates color-coded maps from multiple T1-weighted images, with each pixel representing a specific T1 value.[25] Native T1 values measured before the administration of contrast agents, are unique to different tissue types, with each having a defined normal range. Deviation from these ranges can indicate disease or physiological abnormalities.[26] The precontrast mean T1 value for normal myocardium is approximately 977 ± 63 milliseconds at 1.5 T and 1,100 ± 54 at 3 T.[27,28] Precontrast T1 values in fibrotic myocardium are significantly longer compared to normal myocardium (1,060 ± 61 milliseconds vs. 987±34 milliseconds), making T1 mapping an effective tool for differentiating both interstitial and replacement fibrosis from healthy tissue.[29]

Native T1 values are influenced by several factors such as the strength of the magnetic field, the specific region of interest, and the phase of the cardiac cycle.[30] *Therefore, it is crucial to standardize T1 mapping methodologies within institutions and establish normal T1 value ranges based on the specific parameters used in each institution's imaging protocols.*[31]

Techniques

- *Look-locker technique*: Acquires multiple image data segments, along the T1 recovery curve after application of an inversion pulse, each data segment having a defined inversion time (TI). The image acquisition is repeated after a period allowing complete magnetization recovery. There are two main variations of the technique:
  1. *Modified Look-Locker Sequence (MOLLI):* The most widely used clinical T1 mapping technique This captures images during diastole over 3–5 heartbeats and requires a total of 17 heartbeats. It is dependent on heart rate and image degradation can occur if full magnetization recovery is not achieved.
  2. *Shortened Modified Look-Locker Sequence (shMOLLI):* This is a faster sequence than MOLLI, reducing breath-hold time. It is suitable for patients with difficulty holding their breath.[32]
- *Saturation recovery-based t1 mapping techniques:* This employs a saturation radiofrequency (RF) pulse to null longitudinal magnetization, eliminating dependence on heart rate. This technique avoids biases from MOLLI-based techniques but has a lower signal-to-noise ratio than inversion recovery (IR) methods. The most commonly used sequence is SASHA (Saturation Recovery Single-Shot Acquisition).[33]
- *ECV mapping:* ECV serves as a valuable method for assessing both focal and diffuse myocardial fibrosis. Excessive collagen deposition causes an increase in ECV thereby making it a reliable indicator of myocardial fibrosis and a marker for myocardial tissue remodeling.

To estimate ECV, the myocardial and blood T1 values of the myocardium are measured before and after administration of contrast agents. The patient's hematocrit level is required for ECV calculation. The formula for calculating ECV is as follows:

ECV = (1 – hematocrit) × (1/postcontrast T1 myo – 1/native T1 myo)/(1/postcontrast T1 blood – 1/native T1 blood).

As compared to both native and post-contrast T1 values, ECV values demonstrate greater reproducibility across different magnetic field strengths, vendors, and acquisition techniques. Various postprocessing software can generate ECV maps using pixel-wise native and postcontrast T1 values.[34]

DELAYED GADOLINIUM IMAGING

Late gadolinium enhancement imaging is a key technique in CMR, widely used to distinguish viable from non-viable myocardium across various ischemic and nonischemic heart conditions. It has become the gold standard for identifying myocardial scarring. LGE images are usually obtained after cine imaging and other structural or tissue characterization techniques.[35]

Gadolinium-based contrast agents (GBCAs) are administered intravenously at doses ranging from 0.1 to 0.15 mmol/kg, at an injection rate of 4–7 mL/s. Group II GBCAs are preferred due to their favorable safety profile, with minimal risk of nephrogenic systemic fibrosis. Imaging is typically performed after an 8–10-minute delay following the contrast injection.[36]

In normal myocardium, GBCA exhibits rapid wash-in/wash-out kinetics, while in cardiomyopathies, the extravascular-extracellular space expands due to fibrosis, leading to altered GBCA kinetics. Differences in GBCA distribution between healthy and fibrotic tissue create varying relaxivity rates on T1-weighted images, making these differences more visible after several minutes when equilibrium between blood and myocardium is reached.

In normal myocardium, GBCAs are confined to the interstitial space, in acute myocardial injury; however, ruptured myocyte membranes allow GBCA to enter the intracellular space, increasing its distribution volume. In chronic injuries, the formation of scar tissue and collagen replacement of affected cells further expands the interstitial space and increases the distribution volume of GBCAs.[35]

The combination of slower GBCA kinetics and increased distribution volume in injured tissue results in delayed accumulation, appearing as delayed hyperenhancement on images, around 10 minutes postinjection.[37] LGE image acquisition timing is, therefore, crucial to maximizing the contrast between healthy (dark) and fibrotic (bright) myocardium. LGE's role in identifying and differentiating between various cardiomyopathies based on scar patterns and tissue characteristics is well validated.

Scar Patterns in Late Gadolinium Enhancement (Figs. 2A to E)

- Ischemic patterns. This is usually a subendocardial or transmural pattern and focal in distribution, following a vascular territory.
- Nonischemic patterns can be the following:
  - Patchy/midwall, seen in nonischemic cardiomyopathies.
  - Subepicardial, seen mostly associated with postinflammatory conditions, such as myocarditis.
  - Diffuse subendocardial as observed in amyloidosis or endomyocardial fibrosis

Standard Late Gadolinium Enhancement Sequences

- T1-weighted segmented, IR gradient echo pulse sequence. This is initiated with a 180° IR pulse, after which a delay or TI is required to enhance contrast between healthy and damaged myocardium.
- Look-Locker (TI scout). This is performed prior to LGE imaging to determine the optimal TI. The goal is to null normal myocardium (appear dark) while highlighting damaged areas (appear hyperenhanced).
- *Phase-sensitive inversion recovery (PSIR) sequence.* This is an alternative to the conventional IR sequence, it reduces sensitivity to the chosen TI, minimizing artifacts and potential misinterpretations by acquiring a reference image every two heartbeats.
- 3D LGE imaging is a free-breathing technique useful for patients unable to hold their breath. Multiplanar reformatting (MPR) is possible with this sequence.

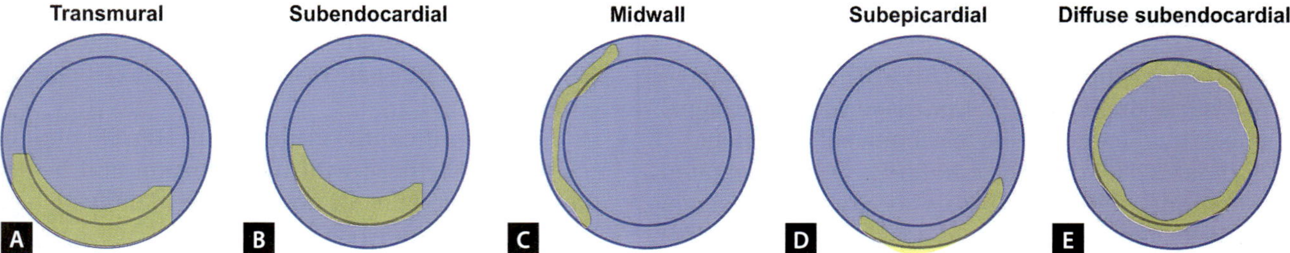

Figs. 2A to E: (A and B) Ischemic pattern of LGE and (C to E) Nonischemic patterns.

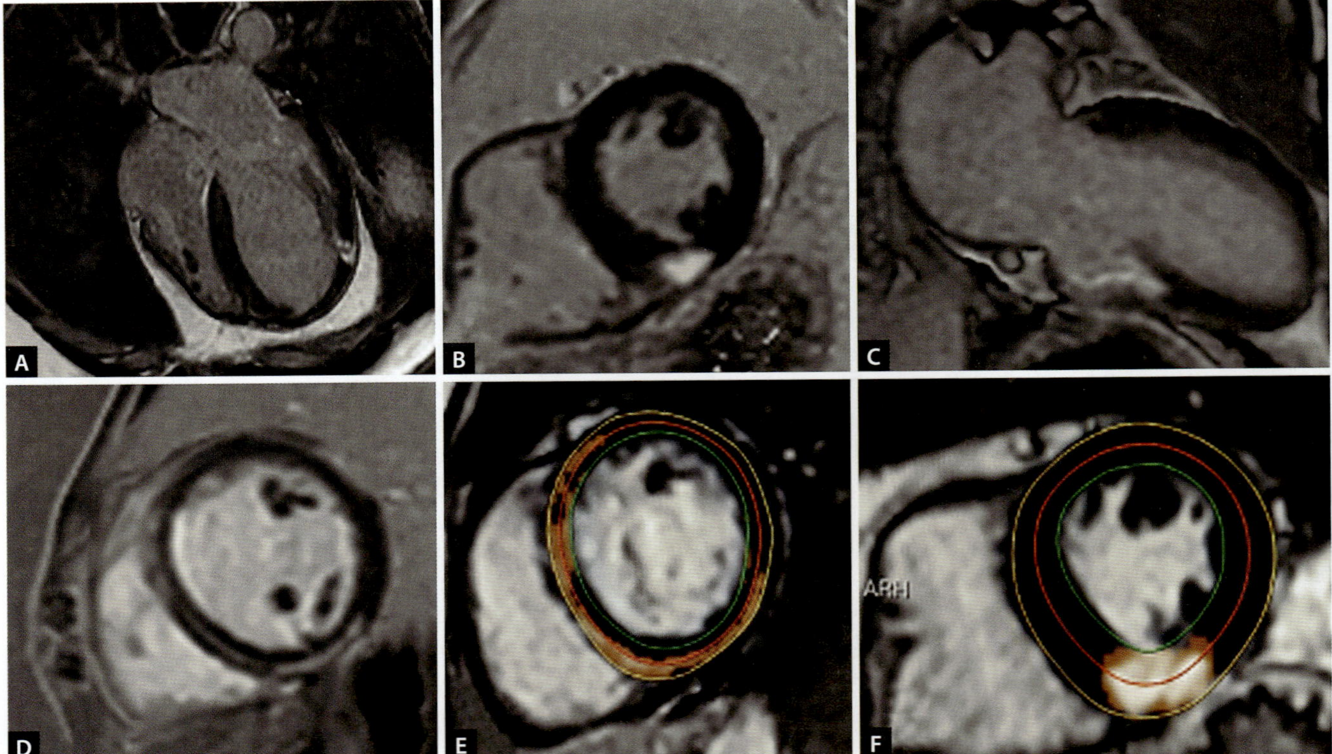

Figs. 3A to F: (A) PSIR HLA image showing focal LGE in the lateral wall; (B and C) PSIR SA and VLA view showing a transmural ischemic pattern of LGE in basal inferior wall, RCA territory infarction; (D) PSIR SA image showing diffuse midwall LGE suggestive of fibrosis; (E and F) Scar quantification using the FWHM technique. (FWHM: full width at half maximum; HLA: human leukocyte antigen; LGE: late gadolinium enhancement; RCA: right coronary artery; SA: short axis; VLA: vertical long axis)

- *Dark blood imaging:* LGE techniques that aim to improve scar visibility by increasing the contrast between blood and scar tissue. These use methods, such as T2 preparation, magnetization transfer, spin-locking, or multiple inversion pulses, to partially suppress (gray-blood) or completely null (black-blood) the blood pool signal.[38,39]

Scar Quantification (Figs. 3A to F)

The scar or fibrosis picked up by LGE imaging can be further quantified using various algorithms and expressed as a percentage of ventricular volume. Common methods of CMR scar quantification include:

- Manual contouring. The clinician manually traces the fibrotic region.
- *Full-width half maximum (FWHM):* An automated technique that identifies scar tissue where the signal intensity is 50% above the maximum enhancement.
- *Standard deviation thresholding:* Semiautomated technique, defining fibrosis as areas with signal intensity above 2–6 standard deviations from normal myocardium.
- Machine learning and AI emerging automated methods that use AI to segment and quantify LGE regions in real-time.
- These techniques vary in precision, automation, and operator dependence.

OUTCOMES OF CARDIAC MAGNETIC RESONANCE ASSESSMENT IN HFpEF (FLOWCHART 2)

Diffuse Myocardial Fibrosis and HFpEF

- Diffuse myocardial fibrosis, measured by native T1 mapping and ECV, is associated with diastolic dysfunction and increased left ventricular (LV) stiffness in HFpEF patients, but not in HFrEF or healthy controls.[40]
- ECV is significantly elevated in HFpEF patients compared to those with hypertension and healthy controls, suggesting its potential for identifying high-risk HFpEF phenotypes.[41]

Flowchart 2: Outcomes of cardiac magnetic resonance assessment in HFpEF.

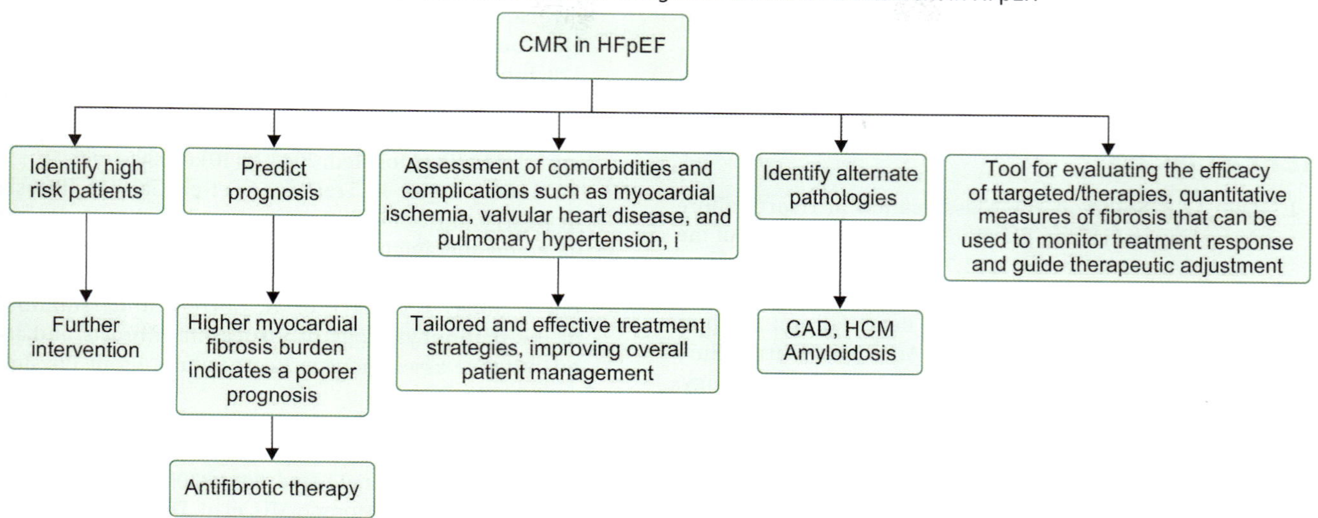

(CAD: coronary artery disease; CMR: cardiac magnetic resonance; HCM: hypertrophic cardiomyopathy; HFpEF: heart failure with preserved ejection fraction)

- Higher myocardial fibrosis burden, detected via CMR, is linked to poorer prognosis in HFpEF patients.[42]
- ECV and indexed ECV (iECV) may serve as markers for risk stratification and prognosis in HFpEF, with iECV emerging as a novel tool for assessing diffuse fibrosis. Diffuse fibrosis measured by iECV is an independent predictor of prognosis in HFpEF, associated with ventricular and LA remodeling, as well as renal dysfunction.[43]

Focal Fibrosis and Late Gadolinium Enhancement in HFpEF

- Increased LGE size is strongly linked to higher cardiovascular mortality and heart failure hospitalizations, making LGE quantification useful for risk stratification in HFpEF.[44]
- HFpEF patients exhibit greater focal fibrosis (ischemic and non-ischemic) compared to controls. Previously undetected small myocardial infarctions, consistent with preserved LVEF, were identified in HFpEF patients.[45]

Thus, assessment of myocardial fibrosis using cardiac MRI has significant implications for the management of HFpEF. Identifying the extent and type of fibrosis can inform prognosis, guide therapeutic decisions, and help monitor treatment response.[46]

Antifibrotic therapies targeting specific pathways involved in fibrosis are currently being investigated in clinical trials. Cardiac MRI can serve as a valuable tool for evaluating the efficacy of these therapies, providing quantitative measures of fibrosis that can be used to monitor treatment response and guide therapeutic adjustments.[47]

FUTURE DIRECTIONS

Myocardial stiffness plays a crucial role in various cardiac diseases.[48] Recent advancements in 2D and 3D high-frequency magnetic resonance elastography (MRE) techniques allow for the measurement of vibrational shear waves generated by an external source, using either ultrasound or CMR. The resulting wave-field images are transformed into stiffness maps. Studies have shown that myocardial stiffness is higher in end-systole compared to end-diastole and increases with aging. Another study using 3D high-frequency MRE found significantly higher myocardial stiffness in patients with cardiac amyloidosis compared to healthy controls.[49-53]

CONCLUSION

Cardiac MRI provides comprehensive insights into myocardial fibrosis in HFpEF, facilitating improved understanding, diagnosis, and management of this complex condition. The ability to accurately assess both focal and diffuse fibrosis using LGE and T1/ECV mapping techniques makes cardiac MRI an invaluable tool in the evaluation of HFpEF patients.

Continued advancements in imaging techniques and their integration into clinical practice will likely enhance the care of HFpEF patients, ultimately improving outcomes. Future research should focus on standardizing imaging protocols, exploring the potential of novel MRI techniques, and investigating the role of cardiac MRI in guiding personalized treatment strategies for HFpEF.

REFERENCES

1. Lam CSP, Solomon SD. Classification of Heart Failure According to Ejection Fraction: JACC Review Topic of the Week. J Am Coll Cardiol. 2021;77(25):3217-25.
2. Bozkurt B, Coats AJS, Tsutsui H, et al. Tsutsui Universal definition and classification of heart failure: a report of the Heart Failure Society of America, Heart Failure Association of the European Society of Cardiology, Japanese Heart Failure Society and Writing Committee of the Universal Definition of Heart Failure: Endorsed by the Canadian Heart Failure Society, Heart Failure Association of India, Cardiac Society of Australia and New Zealand, and Chinese Heart Failure Association. Eur J Heart Fail. 2021;23(3):352-80.
3. Brown S, Biswas D, Wu J, et al. Race- and ethnicity-related differences in heart failure with preserved ejection fraction using natural language processing. JACC Adv. 2024;3(8):101064.
4. Seferovic PM, Vardas P, Jankowska EA, et al. The heart failure association atlas: heart failure epidemiology and management statistics 2019. Eur J Heart Fail. 2021; 23(6):906-14.
5. Borlaug BA. The pathophysiology of heart failure with preserved ejection fraction. Nat Rev Cardiol. 2014;11(9): 507-15.
6. Aurigemma GP, Zile MR, Gaasch WH. Contractile behavior of the left ventricle in diastolic heart failure: with emphasis on regional systolic function. Circulation. 2006;113(2):296-304.
7. Ruocco G, Gavazzi A, Gonnelli S, et al. Pulmonary arterial hypertension and heart failure with preserved ejection fraction: are they so discordant? Cardiovasc Diagn Ther. 2020;10(3):534-45.
8. Taqueti VR, Solomon SD, Shah AM, et al. Coronary microvascular dysfunction and future risk of heart failure with preserved ejection fraction. Eur Heart J. 2018; 39(10):840-49.
9. Omote K, Borlaug BA. Left atrial myopathy in heart failure with preserved ejection fraction. Circ J. 2023; 87(8):1039-46.
10. Crum Y, Hoendermis ES, van Veldhuisen DJ, et al. Epicardial adipose tissue and pericardial constraint in heart failure with preserved ejection fraction. ESC Heart Fail. 2024;11(3):1698-706.
11. Borbély A, van der Velden J, Papp Z, et al Cardiomyocyte stiffness in diastolic heart failure. Circulation. 2005; 111(6):774-81.
12. Spinale FG. Matrix metalloproteinases: regulation and dysregulation in the failing heart. Circ Res. 2002; 90(5):520-30.
13. Paulus WJ, Zile MR. From systemic inflammation to myocardial fibrosis: the heart failure with preserved ejection fraction paradigm revisited. Circ Res. 2021; 128(10):1451-67.
14. Sweeney M, Corden B, Cook SA. Targeting cardiac fibrosis in heart failure with preserved ejection fraction: mirage or miracle? EMBO Mol Med. 2020;12(10):e10865.
15. Ravassa S, López B, Treibel TA, et al. Cardiac fibrosis in heart failure: focus on non-invasive diagnosis and emerging therapeutic strategies. Mol Aspects Med. 2023; 93:101194.
16. Liu T, Song D, Dong J, et al. Current understanding of the pathophysiology of myocardial fibrosis and its quantitative assessment in heart failure. Front Physiol. 2017;8:238.
17. Zile MR, Baicu CF, Gaasch WH. Diastolic heart failure—abnormalities in active relaxation and passive stiffness of the left ventricle. N Engl J Med. 2004;350(19):1953-59.
18. Lopez B, Ravassa S, Moreno MU, et al. Diffuse myocardial fibrosis: mechanisms, diagnosis and therapeutic approaches. Nat Rev Cardiol. 2021;18(7):479-98.
19. Lee DS, Gona P, Vasan RS, et al. Relation of disease pathogenesis and risk factors to heart failure with preserved or reduced ejection fraction: insights from the framingham heart study of the national heart, lung, and blood institute. Circulation. 2009;119(24):3070-7.
20. Smiseth OA. Evaluation of left ventricular diastolic function: state of the art after 35 years with Doppler assessment. J Echocardiogr. 2018;16(2):55-64.
21. Harada T, Kagami K, Kato T, et al. Echocardiography in the diagnostic evaluation and phenotyping of heart failure with preserved ejection fraction. J Cardiol. 2022;79(6):679-90.
22. Ambale-Venkatesh B, Lima JA. Cardiac MRI: a central prognostic tool in myocardial fibrosis. Nat. Rev. Cardiol. 2015;12(1):18-29.
23. Lau C, Elshibly MMM, Kanagala P, et al. The role of cardiac magnetic resonance imaging in the assessment of heart failure with preserved ejection fraction. Front Cardiovasc Med. 2022;9:922398.
24. Zhu L, Wang Y, Zhao S, et al. Detection of myocardial fibrosis: Where we stand. Front Cardiovasc Med. 2022; 9:926378.
25. Taylor AJ, Salerno M, Dharmakumar R, et al. T1 mapping: basic techniques and clinical applications. JACC Cardiovasc Imaging. 2016;9(1):67-81.
26. Triadyaksa P, Kuijpers D, Akinci D'Antonoli T, et al Early detection of heart function abnormality by native T1: a comparison of two T1 quantification methods. Eur Radiol. 2020;30(1):652-62.
27. Messroghli DR, Plein S, Higgins DM, et al. Human myocardium: single-breath-hold MR T1 mapping with high spatial resolution—reproducibility study. Radiology. 2006;238(3):1004-12.
28. Roy C, Slimani A, de Meester C, et al. Age and sex corrected normal reference values of T1, T2 T2* and ECV in healthy subjects at 3T CMR. J Cardiovasc Magn Reson. 2017;19(1):72.

29. Hamilton-Craig CR, Strudwick MW, Galloway GJ. T_1Mapping for Myocardial Fibrosis by Cardiac Magnetic Resonance Relaxometry-A Comprehensive Technical Review. Front Cardiovasc Med. 2017;3:49.
30. Tribuna L, Oliveira PB, Iruela A, et al. Reference Values of Native T1 at 3T Cardiac Magnetic Resonance-Standardization Considerations between Different Vendors. Diagnostics (Basel). 2021;11(12):2334.
31. Messroghli DR, Moon JC, Ferreira VM, et al. Clinical recommendations for cardiovascular magnetic resonance mapping of T1, T2, T2 and extracellular volume: A consensus statement by the Society for Cardiovascular Magnetic Resonance (SCMR) endorsed by the European Association for Cardiovascular Imagin. J Cardiovasc Magn Reson. 2017;19:1-24.
32. Messroghli DR, Radjenovic A, Kozerke S, et al. Modified Look-Locker inversion recovery (MOLLI) for high-resolution T1 mapping of the heart. Magn Reson Med. 2004;52(1):141-6.
33. Chow K, Flewitt JA, Green JD, et al. Saturation recovery single-shot acquisition (SASHA) for myocardial T(1) mapping. Magn Reson Med. 2014;71(6):2082-95.
34. Haaf P, Garg P, Messroghli DR, et al. Cardiac T1 Mapping and Extracellular Volume (ECV) in clinical practice: a comprehensive review. J Cardiovasc Magn Reson. 2016;18(1):89.
35. Jenista ER, Wendell DC, Azevedo CF, et al. Revisiting how we perform late gadolinium enhancement CMR: insights gleaned over 25 years of clinical practice. J Cardiovasc Magn Reson. 2023;25(1):18.
36. Nacif MS, Arai AE, Lima JA, et al. Gadolinium-enhanced cardiovascular magnetic resonance: administered dose in relationship to United States Food and Drug Administration (FDA) guidelines. J Cardiovasc Magn Reson. 2012;14(1):18.
37. Holtackers RJ, Emrich T, Botnar RM, et al. Late Gadolinium Enhancement Cardiac Magnetic Resonance Imaging: From Basic Concepts to Emerging Methods. Rofo. 2022;194(5):491-504.
38. Franco A, Javidi S, Ruehm SG. Delayed Myocardial Enhancement in Cardiac Magnetic Resonance Imaging. J Radiol Case Rep. 2015;9(6):6-18.
39. Holtackers RJ, Van De Heyning CM, Chiribiri A, et al. Dark-blood late gadolinium enhancement cardiovascular magnetic resonance for improved detection of subendocardial scar: a review of current techniques. J Cardiovasc Magn Reson. 2021;23(1):961.
40. Su MY, Lin LY, Tseng YH, et al. CMR-verified diffuse myocardial fibrosis is associated with diastolic dysfunction in HFpEF. JACC Cardiovasc Imaging. 2014;7(10):991-7.
41. Del Torto A, Guaricci AI, Pomarico et al. Advances in multimodality cardiovascular imaging in the diagnosis of heart failure with preserved ejection fraction. Front Cardiovasc Med. 2022;9:758975.
42. Roy C, Slimani A, De Meester C, et al. Associations and prognostic significance of diffuse myocardial fibrosis by cardiovascular magnetic resonance in heart failure with preserved ejection fraction. J Cardiovasc Magn Reson. 2018;20(1):1-12.
43. Kanagala P, Arnold JR, Singh A, et al. Characterizing heart failure with preserved and reduced ejection fraction: an imaging and plasma biomarker approach. PLoS One. 2020;15(4):e0232280.
44. Yang Z, Xu R, Wang JR, et al. Association of myocardial fibrosis detected by late gadolinium-enhanced MRI with clinical outcomes in patients with diabetes: a systematic review and meta-analysis. BMJ Open. 2022;12(1):e055374.
45. Kanagala P, Cheng ASH, Singh A, et al. Relationship Between Focal and Diffuse Fibrosis Assessed by CMR and Clinical Outcomes in Heart Failure With Preserved Ejection Fraction. JACC Cardiovasc Imaging. 2019;12(11 Pt 2):2291-301.
46. Zhang X, Yang S, Hao S, et al. Myocardial fibrosis and prognosis in heart failure with preserved ejection fraction: a pooled analysis of 12 cohort studies. Eur Radiol. 2024;34(3):1854-62.
47. Borlaug BA, Sharma K, Shah SJ, et al. Heart Failure With Preserved Ejection Fraction: JACC Scientific Statement. J Am Coll Cardiol. 2023;81(18):1810-34.
48. Xu J, Yang W, Zhao S, Lu M. State-of-the-art myocardial strain by CMR feature tracking: clinical applications and future perspectives. Eur Radiol. 2022;32(8):5424-35.
49. DeVore AD, McNulty S, Alenezi F, et al. Impaired left ventricular global longitudinal strain in patients with heart failure with preserved ejection fraction: insights from the RELAX trial. Eur J Heart Fail. 2017;19(7):893-900.
50. Pezeshki PS, Ghorashi SM, Houshmand G, et al. Feature tracking cardiac magnetic resonance imaging to assess cardiac manifestations of systemic diseases. Heart Fail Rev.2023;28(5):1189-99.
51. Kammerlander AA, Donà C, Nitsche C, et al. Feature tracking of global longitudinal strain by using cardio-vascular MRI improves risk stratification in heart failure with preserved ejection fraction. Radiology. 2020;296(2): 290-98.
52. Rajiah PS, Kalisz K, Broncano J, et al. Myocardial strain evaluation with cardiovascular MRI: Physics, principles, and clinical applications. Radiographics. 2022;42(4):968-90.
53. Chamsi-Pasha MA, Zhan Y, Debs D. CMR in the evaluation of diastolic dysfunction and phenotyping of HFpEF: current role and future perspectives. JACC Cardiovasc Imaging. 2020;13(1 Pt 2):283-96.

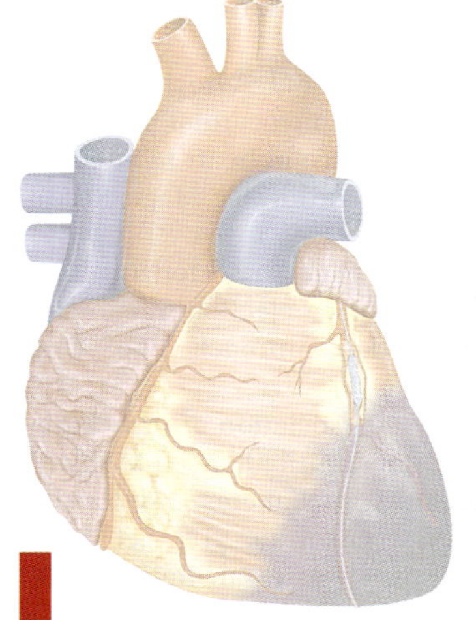

Role of CT Evaluation for Transcatheter Aortic Valve Implantation in HFpEF

Anshika Gulati, Parveen Gulati

INTRODUCTION

Heart failure with preserved ejection fraction (HFpEF) refers to diastolic heart failure (HF) presenting with symptoms and signs of HF, with evidence of structural and/or functional cardiac abnormalities and/or rising levels of biochemical markers (NT-proBNP) while maintaining LV ejection fraction (EF) *of 50% or greater.*[1,2]

Diastolic dysfunction (DD) is a key component in the diagnosis of HFpEF. This leads to elevated pressures in the heart and pulmonary circulation, contributing to symptoms of heart failure, such as dyspnea and fatigue.

Among various causes, aortic valve pathologies are significant contributor to HFpEF.

HEART FAILURE WITH PRESERVED EJECTION FRACTION AND AORTIC STENOSIS

The AS is a common condition, with its prevalence steadily increasing, especially among the elderly population. Increase in afterload caused by AS triggers adaptive hypertrophic remodeling of LV myocardium. Initially, cardiac compensatory mechanisms help maintain adequate wall stress, but over time, this causes structural damage reducing LV compliance leading to HFpEF.[3]

HEART FAILURE WITH PRESERVED EJECTION FRACTION AND AORTIC REGURGITATION

The AR causes a chronic volume and pressure overload on LV triggering LV eccentric remodeling, characterized by an increased diameter-to-volume ratio and mass in early stages. When LV remodeling is no longer able to compensate for the detrimental effects of the regurgitated blood volume caused by AR, end-diastolic pressure rises significantly, leading to the onset of HFpEF. AR has been found to significantly increase the risk of all-cause mortality in HFpEF patients owing to small LV cavity and increased LV wall stiffness, that even a small amount of AR can cause a disproportionately elevated end-diastolic pressure.[4]

TRANSCATHETER AORTIC VALVE IMPLANTATION IN HEART FAILURE WITH PRESERVED EJECTION FRACTION

Aortic valve replacement has been shown to potentially induce a process of reverse remodeling leading to structural and functional improvements in HFpEF patients.[5]

Traditional surgical aortic valve replacement was earlier considered as the only established method for providing a curative solution for HFpEF associated with aortic valve pathologies. TAVI emerged as the standard of care for patients who were at high surgical risk or deemed unfit for surgery. However, recent studies have demonstrated encouraging results with TAVI even among patients with lower surgical risk.[6]

These pioneering findings are a direct result of the advancements in device technology and the growing experience of interventionists. Nevertheless, directly visualizing the size of aortic valve is unfeasible during the TAVI procedure, in contrast to the surgical valve replacement method. Under sizing the valve can result in paravalvular aortic regurgitation or even valve embolization. Conversely, oversizing the valve can lead to complications such as rupture of the aortic root, coronary ostia occlusion, or aortic valve block.[7]

Therefore, precise sizing is mandatory prior to the procedure. CT has established itself as the benchmark for procedural planning in TAVI. Distinguishing it from conventional echocardiography, CT provides an operator-independent, all-encompassing, three-dimensional (3D), and even four-dimensional (4D) assessment that can be analyzed remotely in preparation for the procedure. Recent technological strides have led to swifter image acquisition and enhanced spatial and temporal resolution, along with a reduced requirement for contrast agents and diminished radiation exposure. Apart from precise sizing of THV, routine utilization of CT scans has enabled procedural planning by aiding in the selection of optimal access site.

AIMS AND OBJECTIVES

This chapter aims to offer a comprehensive review of the role of CT evaluation in preprocedural assessment for viability and strategic planning of TAVI in HFpEF patients and in assessment of post-TAVI complications in these patients.

TRANSCATHETER AORTIC VALVE IMPLANTATION PLANNING COMPUTED TOMOGRAPHY PROTOCOL

Essential technical requirements for TAVI CT include a scanner with at least 64 slices, ability to perform ECG-gated triggering for cardiac imaging, and detector elements smaller than 0.625 mm.

The patient is positioned supine with arms comfortably raised above the head. Tube potential of 100 kVp is recommended for patients weighing up to 100 kg and 120 kVp for heavier patients. ECG-gated dose modulation of tube current (mA) is employed. Scanning occurs during inspiration in the craniocaudal direction using a spiral acquisition mode with retrospective ECG gating. An ideal heart rate of around 60 bpm is needed to capture a stable aortic valve.[8]

For enhanced image quality, contrast agents with high iodine concentrations between 270 and 400 mg iodine/mL are recommended. Careful timing of the contrast is crucial with region of interest (ROI) places at ascending aorta. A test bolus of 10–20 mL of contrast media is initiated at a flow rate of 5–6 mL/s for accurate tracking. For the main contrast injection, administer 50–70 mL at a flow rate of 5–6 mL/s. Finally, ensure proper delivery by following up with a 50–80 mL saline chaser at a flow rate of 4–5 mL/s.

The scout scan extends from aortic arch to femoral arteries. For calcium scoring, noncontrast scanning is done first, focusing primarily on the valve area, followed by a complete assessment of the heart for TAVI preparation. Finally, an aortogram is conducted from aortic arch to femoral arteries, providing comprehensive visualization and helping to determine the access site.

The datasets are transmitted to a dedicated workstation for analysis, where images from both the systolic and diastolic phases are reconstructed. Postprocessing techniques, including 3D multiplanar reconstruction (MPR), curved MPR, maximum intensity projection, and volume rendering, are applied to the images.[8]

PREPROCEDURAL COMPUTED TOMOGRAPHY EVALUATION

Accurate Assessment of Aortic Anatomy

Quantification of Aortic Valve Calcification

Aortic valve calcification is assessed on NCCT using conventional coronary artery calcium scoring software. Calcified plaques are identified as areas of attenuation greater than 130 HU, with each area assigned a "calcium score" based on its density and size. These individual scores are then summed to obtain the total Agatston score. A score of 3,000 or higher in men and 1,600 or higher in women strongly suggests severe AS. Conversely, an Agatston score of <1,600 in men and <800 in women strongly suggests the absence of severe AS.[9]

Landing Zone Calcium

Aortic valve complex which includes the valve cusps, aortic annulus, and left ventricular outflow tract (LVOT) is the landing zone where the device makes contact. It is assessed in late-diastolic phase and graded according to the extent of calcification as none, mild, moderate, or severe, considering factors such as circumferential involvement, depth of extension into the lower LVOT, and the radial thickness of the calcification **(Fig. 1)**.

Paravalvular regurgitation (PVR) is a significant complication of TAVI and is associated with increased mortality rates. Aortic valve complex calcification is an important predictor of PVR development following TAVI.[9]

Aortic Annulus Measurements

Aortic annulus is defined as the virtual plane formed by connecting the basal hinge points or nadir of the three aortic valve leaflets. Once the annular plane is accurately identified, all measurements are taken during midsystole,

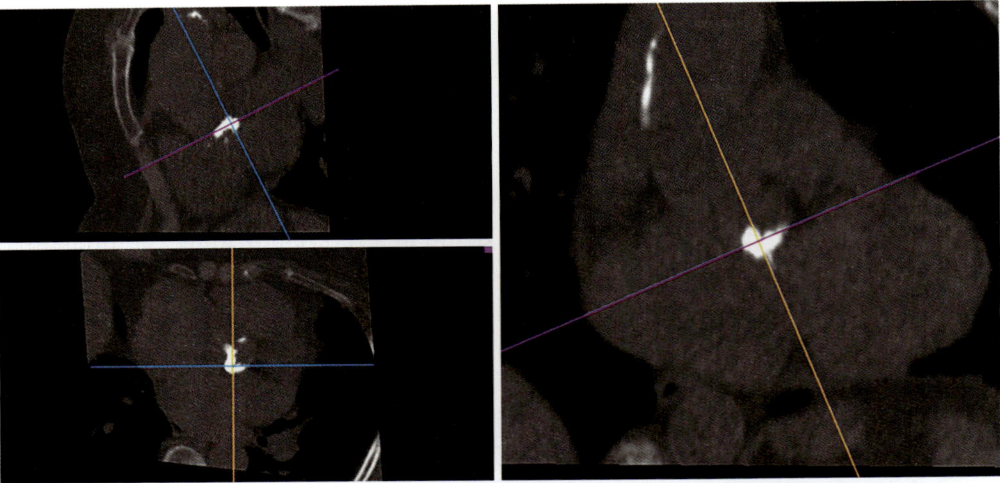

Fig. 1: Noncontrast computed tomography (CT) showing aortic root calcification.

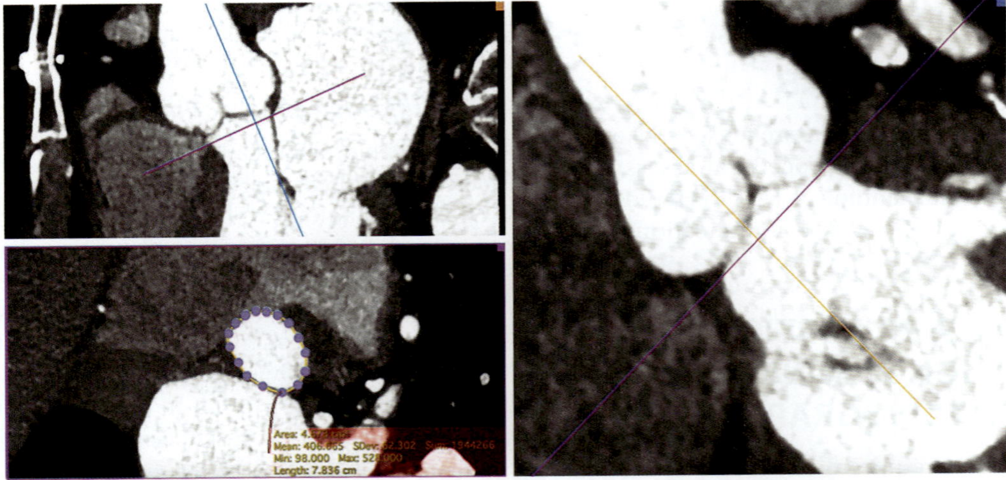

Fig. 2: Measurement of surface area and diameter of aortic annulus by three-dimensional multiplanar reconstruction of electrocardiographically (ECG)-gated cardiac computed tomography (CT) at the level of nadir of each cusp.

when valve opening is at its maximum. During this phase, the aortic annulus assumes a more oval shape, which has been shown to provide the most accurate measurements for transcatheter heart valve (THV) sizing. Aortic annulus experiences dynamic changes; on average, there is approximately a 10% reduction in area and about a 5% decrease in diameter and perimeter during diastolic phases.[8]

The key measurements for selecting appropriate valve size include annulus diameters, circumference, and area, all of which are measured in the short-axis plane. Longest diameter (LD) and shortest diameter (SD) of aortic annulus are recorded. Mean diameter (D), calculated by averaging LD and SD, is used to calculate nominal THV area using the formula π (D/2) 2 .

The planimetry tool on workstation is then used to manually trace the annular perimeter. Based on this tracing, the workstation software computes the area (A), circumference (C), and mean diameter (D) of the aortic annulus **(Fig. 2)**.

The CT area cover index, which indicates the degree of oversizing of THV relative to the measured annulus size, is calculated using the formula: [(Nominal THV area—measured area)/ nominal THV area] × 100%.[10]

Aortic Root Assessment

The aortic root extends from the aortic annulus up to the sinotubular junction (STJ). It consists of the sinuses of Valsalva, valve cusps, and fibrous interleaflet triangles. To ensure proper sizing of THV and to identify potential

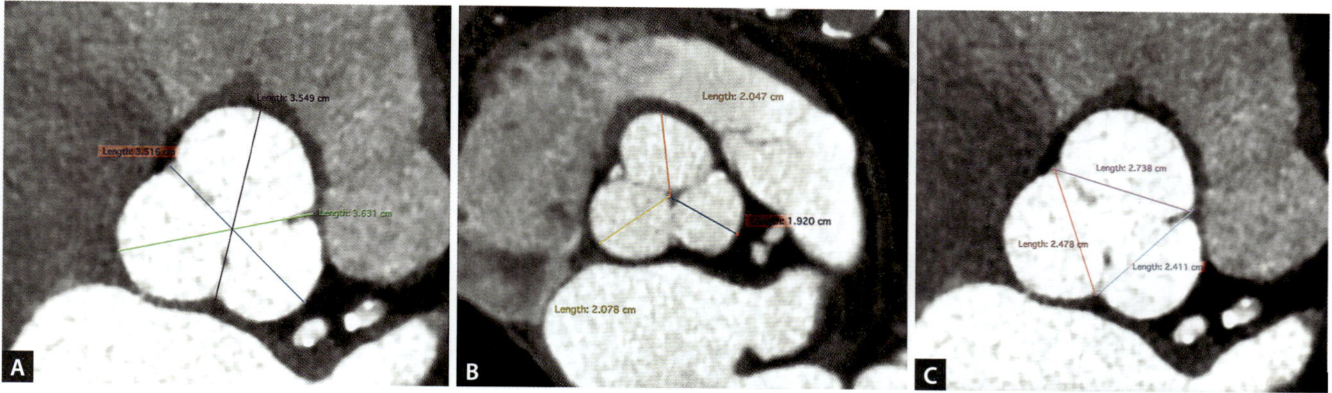

Figs. 3A to C: (A) Measurement of sinus of Valsalva width; (B) Measurement of leaflet length; (C) Measurement of intercommissural distance.

challenges during the TAVI procedure, it is crucial to precisely evaluate the structures of the aortic root.[11]

Sinuses of Valsalva Measurements

Sinuses of Valsalva are optimally assessed during the diastolic phase. After identifying the annulus in axial plane, images are scrolled toward the midportion of the aortic root. The sinus width for each cusp is measured from one commissure to the opposite cusp edge **(Fig. 3A)**. Length of each leaflet and intercommissural distance are measured in the axial plane, as shown in **Figures 3B and 3C**, respectively. Height of sinuses of Valsalva is determined by measuring the distance from the annulus to the STJ for each cusp in the coronal or sagittal plane. Sinus of Valsalva mean diameter <30 mm indicates an increased risk of coronary occlusion, particularly when the coronary ostia are low lying. Therefore, accurate measurement of sinuses of Valsalva is essential for pre-TAVI assessment.[12]

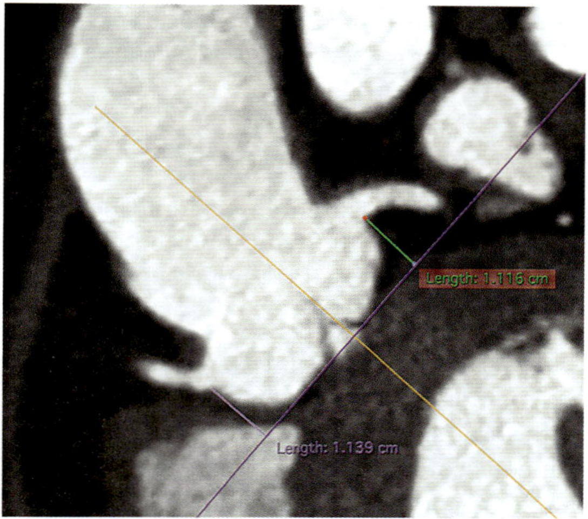

Fig. 4: Measurement of coronary ostia height from annular plane.

Coronary Ostia Measurements

Coronary occlusion is a significant complication of TAVI, though it occurs infrequently. However, it is associated with severe clinical outcomes, including a reported 30-day mortality rate as high as 40.9%. A notable risk factor for coronary occlusion is a low coronary ostial height (<10–12 mm) relative to the annulus. The coronary ostium height is assessed in a plane perpendicular to the annular plane by measuring the distance from the lower edge of the annulus to the left main (LM) ostium and the right coronary artery (RCA) ostium, respectively **(Fig. 4)**.[12]

Sinotubular Junction Measurements

It is critical to identify anatomies where there may be potential contact between the THV and STJ. This is especially important when using balloon-expandable devices in cases with low STJ height. STJ height is measured perpendicular to the annular plane and recorded in millimeters (mm).

Additionally, STJ diameter is determined using a caliper tool on an imaging plane that is properly aligned with the STJ. Comparing the STJ diameter to the anticipated THV size is essential, as an STJ diameter smaller than the THV increases the risk of STJ injury **(Fig. 5)**.

It is also important to assess the size and distribution of calcifications on STJ, particularly circumferential calcifications, as these can influence the sizing of balloon aortic valvuloplasty balloons.[13]

Left Ventricular Outflow Tract Width

After measuring the annulus plane, the transverse MPR plane is scrolled by 5 mm into the LVOT to achieve the LVOT short-axis view. LVOT diameters are mentioned in the report. This evaluation can aid in detecting any constriction or dilation of the LVOT.[11]

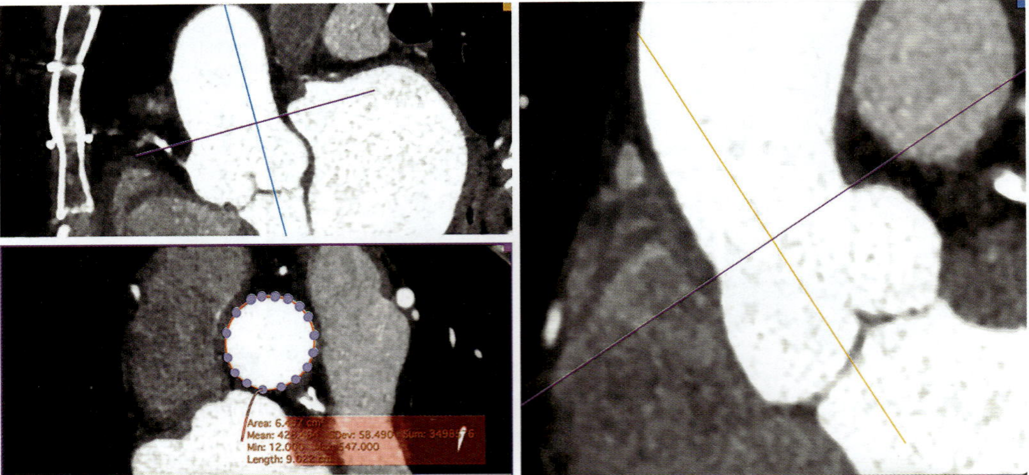

Fig. 5: Measurement of surface area and diameter of sinotubular junction by three-dimensional multiplanar reconstruction of electrocardiographically (ECG)-gated cardiac computed tomography (CT).

Assessment of Ascending Aorta

Ascending aortic measurements should be performed using double-oblique MPR and reported in millimeters. It is also crucial to assess for the presence of any other aortic pathologies.[13]

Detection of coronary artery disease (CAD): CT can identify CAD, a common comorbidity in HFpEF patients. Patients with both aortic stenosis and significant CAD benefit from simultaneous coronary artery bypass grafting (CABG) or percutaneous coronary intervention (PCI) during TAVI, leading to improved outcomes. CT coronary angiography can accurately detect CAD and grade its severity to determine the need for such concurrent procedures, enhancing overall treatment effectiveness. The evaluation of CAD can also influence the choice of transcatheter valve type and appropriate sizing of the THV, reducing complications like coronary obstruction.[14]

Evaluation of LV function: Apart from providing insights into the underlying pathophysiology of HFpEF, CT evaluation of LV function plays a critical role in TAVI planning, influencing both patient selection and risk stratification. Reduced LVEF (<50%) in patients with AS is associated with poorer outcomes following TAVI.[15]

Identifying LV remodeling: CT imaging allows for the evaluation of LV remodeling, including parameters such as LV mass and volume. Patients with significant LV hypertrophy or dilatation may experience worse outcomes post-TAVI. By assessing these parameters, clinicians can identify patients at higher risk of complications and tailor their management strategies accordingly.[16]

Identification of other cardiac abnormalities: CT can detect other cardiac abnormalities which may influence the decision-making process for TAVI.

- *Pericardial effusion:* CT can detect pericardial effusion, which can increase the risk of complications, including cardiac tamponade during the TAVI procedure.[17]
- *Left atrial (LA) enlargement:* Increased LV afterload resulting from severe AS leads to progressive cardiac remodeling in form of LV hypertrophy and LA enlargement which may affect clinical outcomes after valvular replacement therapy. LA enlargement secondary to AS was documented in a significant proportion of patients undergoing TAVI and was associated with a more than threefold increased risk of CVD at 1-year. CT can identify these structural changes thereby aiding in preprocedural planning and predicting prognosis in these patients.[18]

Procedural Planning

- *Access site selection:* In the early days of TAVI, vascular complications were a significant contributor to mortality, largely due to larger device profiles and case selection. To address this issue, multidetector CT (MDCT) has now replaced angiography as the standard of care for iliofemoral assessment in TAVI. CT imaging is used to assess the dimensions, curvature, and degree of calcification in the iliofemoral arteries to determine the suitability of the transfemoral approach.

  Use of large-diameter delivery sheaths in TAVI necessitates precise vascular access with a luminal diameter of at least 6 mm. However, many patients with severe aortic stenosis have unfavorable iliofemoral arteries, which may exhibit narrow luminal diameters,

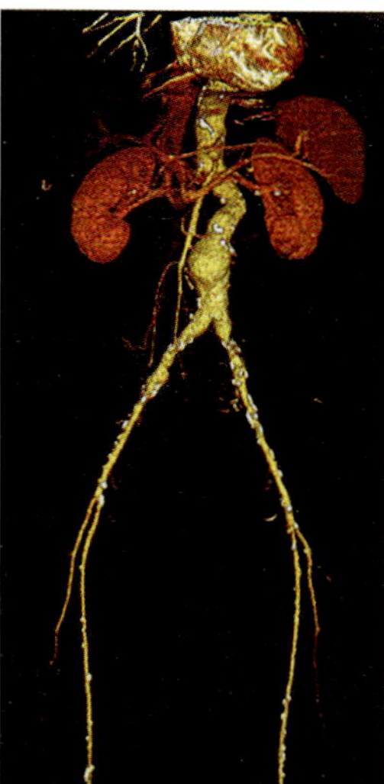

Fig. 6: Computed tomography (CT) evaluation of tortuosity and calcification of arterial access site.

dense circumferential or horseshoe-shaped calcifications, and significant tortuosity. These factors elevate the risk of access site complications and central embolization. In such instances, alternative access routes may be considered, including transapical, transaortic, transaxillary/subclavian, transcarotid, suprasternal transaortic/innominate, and transcaval approaches. CT imaging is essential for evaluating the safety and feasibility of these alternative access methods **(Fig. 6)**.[19]

Optimal Projection Curve

The TAVI procedures typically require fluoroscopic angulations to obtain a coplanar view of the aortic annulus with minimal parallax. Patient-specific, optimal C-arm angulations can be determined using CT scans. The ideal projection angles during TAVI include the three-cusp view, noncoronary cusp view (overlapping the LCC and RCC), left coronary cusp view (overlapping the NCC and RCC), and right coronary cusp view (overlapping the LCC and NCC).

Various techniques are used to determine the best implant projection for TAVI. One effective method is to first identify the annulus plane in the 3D MPR module and mark the lowest point of each cusp. Then, in the 3D volume rendering module, contrast is adjusted to highlight these three points. Using the "rotate around a focal point" tool, the projection is adjusted until the three points align in a single line. The optimal C-arm angulation is then displayed in the lower right corner.[20]

POSTPROCEDURE EVALUATION

Patients undergoing TAVI may develop implant leaflet thrombosis, referred to as hypoattenuating leaflet thrombosis/ thickening (HALT) which can restrict leaflet movement and lead to outflow tract obstruction, known as hypoattenuation affecting motion (HAM). This complication has been linked to transient ischemic attacks and can occur in both transcatheter and surgical bioprosthetic valves, typically resolving with anti-coagulation. Four-dimensional cardiac CT, which uses scan data collected throughout the cardiac cycle to create a cine loop of valve leaflet motion, can aid in identifying HAM and differentiating it from other causes of postprocedural valve gradients, such as pannus formation and prosthetic valve underexpansion that may occur in cases of densely calcified native valves.[21]

IMPROVED PROCEDURAL OUTCOMES

Under sizing the valve can result in paravalvular aortic regurgitation or even valve embolization. Conversely, oversizing the valve can lead to complications such as rupture of the aortic root, coronary ostia occlusion, or aortic valve block.[7]

Studies have shown that CT-guided TAVI can lead to better outcomes, including lower rates of complications and improved patient survival.

FURTHER ADVANCES

Recent studies have incorporated computational fluid dynamics (CFD) into preprocedural cardiac CT to enhance understanding of flow gradients following implantation and to offer personalized risk prediction models.[22]

In future, integrating artificial intelligence-driven computational predictive modeling into decision support tools may aid in predicting post-TAVI complications including annular rupture, paravalvular leak and HALT.[23]

CONCLUSION

By providing detailed information about the patient's anatomy and cardiac function, CT has emerged as a gold standard in preprocedural evaluation of patients undergoing TAVI, and helps to significantly reduce mortality and postprocedural complications in HFpEF patients. Abundance of evidence-based data and remarkable image quality offered by CT emphasize its indispensable role, rendering it a resource that should be fully harnessed in the lead-up to any TAVI procedure.

REFERENCES

1. Writing Committee Members; Yancy CW, Jessup M, Bozkurt B, et al. 2013 ACCF/AHA Guideline for the Management of Heart Failure A Report of the American College of Cardiology Foundation/American Heart Association Task Force on Practice Guidelines. J Am Coll Cardiol. 2013;62(16):E147-E239.
2. McDonagh TA, Metra M, Adamo M, et al. ESC Scientific Document Group, 2021 ESC Guidelines for the diagnosis and treatment of acute and chronic heart failure: Developed by the Task Force for the diagnosis and treatment of acute and chronic heart failure of the European Society of Cardiology (ESC) With the special contribution of the Heart Failure Association (HFA) of the ESC. Eur Heart J. 2021;ehab368.
3. Lindman BR, Dweck MR, Lancellotti P, et al. Management of asymptomatic severe aortic stenosis: evolving concepts in timing of valve replacement. JACC Cardiovasc Imaging. 2020;13:481-93.
4. Abdurashidova T, Monney P, Tzimas G, et al. Nonsevere aortic regurgitation increases short-term mortality in acute heart failure with preserved ejection fraction. ESC Heart Fail. 2020;7(6):3901-9.
5. Mehdipoor G, Chen S, Chatterjee S, et al. Cardiac structural changes after transcatheter aortic valve replacement: systematic review and meta-analysis of cardiovascular magnetic resonance studies. J Cardiovasc Magn Reson. 2020;22(1):41.
6. Rode's-Cabau J, Webb JG, Cheung A, et al. Transcatheter aortic valve implantation for the treatment of severe symptomatic aortic stenosis in patients at very high or prohibitive surgical risk: acute and late outcomes of the multicenter Canadian experience. J Am Coll Cardiol. 2010;55(11):1080-90
7. Piazza N, Kalesan B, van Mieghen N. A 3 center comparison of 1 year mortality outcomes between transcatheter aortic valve implantation and surgical aortic valve replacement on the basis of propensity score matching among intermediate risk patients. J Am Coll Cardiol Interv. 2013;6(5):443-51.
8. Schoenhagen P, Hausleiter J, Achenbach S, et al. Computed tomography in the evaluation for transcatheter aortic valve implantation. Cardiovasc Diagn Ther. 2011;1(1):446.
9. Baumgartner H, Falk V, Bax JJ, et al. 2017 ESC/EACTS guidelines for the management of valvular heart disease. Eur Heart J. 2017;38(36):2739-91.
10. Khalique OK, Hahn RT, Gada H, et al. Quantity and location of aortic valve complex calcification predicts severity and location of paravalvular regurgitation and frequency of post-dilation after balloon-expandable transcatheter aortic valve replacement. JACC Cardiovasc Interv. 2014;7(8):885-94.
11. Sattar Sakrana AA, Abuelatta RA, Fattah Ali SA, et al. Variables affecting the accuracy of MDCT in prediction of the proper prosthesis deployment projection for transcatheter aortic valve implantation. Egypt J Radiol Nucl Med. 2017;48(2):357-63.
12. Ribeiro HB, Nombela-Franco L, Urena M, et al. Coronary obstruction following transcatheter aortic valve implantation: a systematic review. J Am Coll Cardiol Interv. 2013;6(5):452-61.
13. Masson JB, Kovac J, Schuler G, et al. Transcatheter aortic valve implantation: review of the nature, management, and avoidance of procedural complications. J Am Coll Cardiovasc Interv. 2009;2(9):811-20.
14. Maeno Y et al. Efficacy and safety of percutaneous coronary intervention during transcatheter aortic valve replacement. Euro Intervention; 2014.
15. Goel S et al. Cardiac imaging for the assessment of left ventricular function in patients undergoing transcatheter aortic valve replacement. JACC: Cardiovascular Imaging; 2015.
16. Chen CH et al. Prognostic significance of left ventricular hypertrophy in patients with aortic stenosis undergoing transcatheter aortic valve replacement. Eur Heart J; 2018.
17. Boccuzzi G et al. Impact of preexisting pericardial effusion on TAVR outcomes. Eur Heart J; 2020.
18. Asami M, Dobner S, Stortecky S, et al. Cardiovascular outcomes in patients with left atrial enlargement undergoing transcatheter aortic valve implantation. Catheter Cardiovasc Interv. 2022;99(6):1908-17.
19. Okuyama K, Jilaihawi H, Mirocha J, et al. Alternative access for balloon-expandable transcatheter aortic valve replacement: comparison of the transaortic approach using right anterior thoracotomy to partial J-sternotomy. J Thorac Cardiovasc Surg. 2015;149(3):789-97.
20. Généreux P, Webb JG, Svensson LG, et al. Vascular complications after transcatheter aortic valve replacement: insights from the PARTNER (Placement of Aortic Transcatheter Valve) trial. J Am Coll Cardiol. 2012; 60(12):1043-52.
21. Hansson NC, Grove EL, Andersen HR, et al. Transcatheter Aortic ValveThrombosis: Incidence, Predisposing Factors, and Clinical Implications. J Am Coll Cardiol. 2016;68(19):2059-69.
22. Karabelas E, Longobardi S, Fuchsberger J, et al. Global Sensitivity Analysis of Four Chamber Heart Hemodynamics Using Surrogate Models. IEEE TransBiomed Eng. 2022;69(10):3216-23.
23. Hatoum H, Singh-Gryzbon S, Esmailie F, et al. Predictive Model for Throm-bus Formation After Transcatheter Valve Replacement. Cardiovasc Eng Tech-nol. 2021;12(6): 576-88.

SECTION 4

HFpEF and Coronary Artery Disease

73. Dapagliflozin after AMI: Cardiometabolic Benefits (With or Without HFpEF)
74. Treatment of STEMI with HFpEF: Focusing on Mortality Benefits
75. ARNI Postpercutaneous Coronary Intervention in STEMI to Prevent HFpEF
76. CABG in LV Dysfunction and Heart Failure

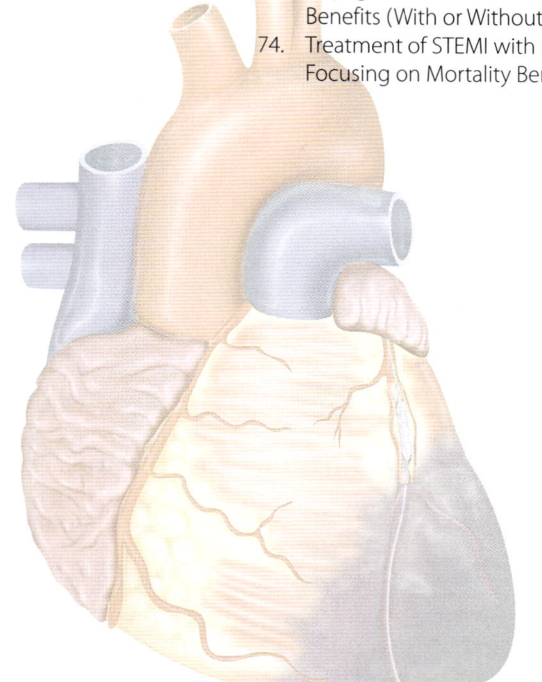

CHAPTER 73

Dapagliflozin after AMI: Cardiometabolic Benefits (With or Without HFpEF)

Jai Bharat Sharma, Kunal Mahajan, Surender Himral

INTRODUCTION

The extensive body of medical research accumulated over the years has significantly enhanced our understanding of acute myocardial infarction (AMI) and has dramatically improved patient prognosis. Despite advancements in early invasive management and adherence to standard guideline-directed medical therapy, there remains a pressing need to explore further improvements, as the incidence of adverse events continues to be alarmingly high. Sodium–glucose cotransporter 2 inhibitors (SGLT2i) present a promising avenue for such advancements. SGLT2i, initially known for their role in treating type-2 diabetes mellitus, have been recognized for their potential to enhance cardiovascular outcomes, even in patients without diabetes mellitus. These benefits are particularly significant in heart failure (HF), covering reduced and preserved ejection fractions and positioning SGLT2i as a transformative option in managing HF.[1-4] This ongoing pursuit to improve patient outcomes has garnered global interest among investigators, marking SGLT2i as a potential milestone in treating AMI. This chapter aims to explore the role of dapagliflozin post-AMI, with a focus on its cardiometabolic effects.

SCOPE IN ACUTE MYOCARDIAL INFARCTION

Patients experiencing an AMI are at heightened risk for a range of complications, such as recurrent myocardial infarction (MI), chronic HF, life-threatening arrhythmias, and cardiovascular death.[5,6] The risk begins with the onset of MI symptoms, escalates with extended ischemic time, and stays high over the medium and long term, particularly if complicated by left ventricular systolic dysfunction or HF.[7-9] Currently, a significant number of patients hospitalized due to acute decompensated heart failure (ADHF) post-MI are classified as having HF with preserved ejection fraction (HFpEF), followed by those with HF with mid-range ejection fraction (HFmrEF), and HF with reduced ejection fraction (HFrEF). This classification must be considered when managing patients with AMI. To mitigate the risks of adverse cardiac remodeling that might result in chronic HF, sudden cardiac death, or progression to end-stage heart disease, various evidence-based therapies are initiated shortly after AMI. Despite advancements in treatment, the rates of adverse cardiovascular outcomes remain concerningly high, highlighting the ongoing need to develop additional evidence-based strategies.[10,11] SGLT2i offers hope by addressing various pathophysiological mechanisms, as evidenced in myriad studies.

PATHOPHYSIOLOGY

Various potential mechanisms have been explored in previous research that may prevent ventricular remodeling, altering natural history, and progression to chronic HF and end-stage heart disease **(Box 1)**.[12] A metabolic hypothesis suggests that SGLT2i may enhance cardiovascular protection, cardiac efficiency, and contractility by promoting a shift in metabolic substrates from traditional fatty acids to ketone bodies.[13] Other hypotheses suggest several mechanisms by which

BOX 1: Potential mechanisms of action of SGLT2i.

- Metabolic hypothesis—substrate shift from conventional fatty acids to ketone bodies
- Restoration of tubuloglomerular feedback and attenuation of RAAS
- Osmotic diuresis
- Decrease in myocardial calcium overload
- Attenuating myocardial ischemia/reperfusion injury

SGLT2i may confer cardiovascular benefits. These include restoring tubuloglomerular feedback, which subsequently reduces activation of the renin–angiotensin–aldosterone system and sympathetic nervous system; inducing osmotic diuresis, thereby lowering ventricular overload; inhibiting the sodium–hydrogen exchanger pump, which decreases myocardial calcium overload; improving cardiac energy metabolism; and increasing hematocrit due to hemoconcentration or an increase in red cell mass with increased renal erythropoietin production.[14] The exact mechanism for myocardial protection against ischemia remains unclear, but animal studies prove that SGLT2i can mitigate ischemic injury. For example, an experimental study in mice demonstrated that empagliflozin reduced myocardial oxidative stress, interstitial fibrosis, and macrophage infiltration.[15] A recent animal study demonstrated that prolonged oral administration of canagliflozin significantly reduced myocardial infarct size by lessening myocardial ischemic/reperfusion injury.[16]

RECENT EVIDENCE

Recent cardiovascular trials of SGLT2i over the last few years have established the benefits of SGLT2i in lowering the risk of HF hospitalization and cardiovascular death in patients with HFrEF and high-risk groups, including those with type-2 diabetes mellitus or chronic kidney disease. The findings from key trials, such as EMPEROR-Preserved,[3,17] EMPEROR-Reduced,[18,19] and DAPA-HF,[19-21] support the broadening use of SGLT2i across a wide range of HF populations. This paved the way for various studies and trials to evaluate the role of SGLT2i in acute MI.

In one of the most extensive population-based cohort studies, Kwon et al. analyzed the association between early SGLT2i use (within the first 14 days) and recurrent cardiovascular events in patients with type-2 diabetes mellitus and AMI undergoing percutaneous intervention, with the primary endpoint of composite risk of HF hospitalization and all-cause death and the secondary endpoint of the incidence of major adverse cardiac events (MACE), i.e., composite of all-cause death, nonfatal MI, and ischemic stroke. The authors compared two groups matched by propensity score in a 1:2 ratio—those initiated on SGLT2i early (938) and those not started on SGLT2i (1,876). The patients initiated on SGLT2i early following MI showed a significantly lower risk of primary and secondary endpoints after a median follow-up of 2.1 years. The adjusted hazard ratio for the primary endpoint was 0.68 [95% confidence interval (CI) 0.54–0.87, $p = 0.002$] and for the secondary endpoint, it was 0.77 (95% CI 0.60–0.99, $p = 0.04$). However, the study also had essential limitations: Its retrospective nature and, therefore, inability to establish causality or rule out residual confounding. Ultimately, only a small number of patients with type-2 diabetes mellitus following early MI were treated with an SGLT2i (n = 938; 3.3%) compared with the rest of the eligible post-MI type-2 diabetes mellitus population studied (nearly 30,000 patients). Thus, there is a considerable risk of unmeasured bias in selecting these rare patients, and further efforts to mitigate this risk could have included factoring physician- and hospital-based characteristics into the modeling. Although the authors ardently concluded that the use of early SGLT2i following an AMI in patients with type-2 diabetes mellitus was associated with lower all-cause death and HF hospitalizations compared with those not receiving these therapies, it was more hypothesis-generating.[22,23] Further meta-analysis of multiple observational studies regarding the safety and efficacy of SGLT2i in the acute post-AMI setting suggested a promising therapeutic effect, and investigators looked up to RCTs for this, which include the EMMY (Empagliflozin in acute myocardial infarction), DAPA-MI (Dapagliflozin in Patients with Myocardial Infarction), and EMPACT-MI (Empagliflozin after Acute Myocardial Infarction) trials[24-28] **(Table 1)**.

EMMY Trial

The EMMY trial enrolled 476 AMI patients within 72 hours of percutaneous coronary intervention and randomized them to receive either empagliflozin (10 mg daily) or placebo. The primary outcome was the change in NT-proBNP levels over 26 weeks. Empagliflozin resulted in a 15% greater reduction in NT-proBNP than placebo (adjusted mean difference: –85% vs. –81.7%, $p < 0.05$), indicating significant efficacy in lowering this cardiac biomarker. The baseline median NT-proBNP level was 1,294 (757–2,246) pg/mL, with modest improvements observed in left ventricular ejection fraction (LVEF), a decrease in mean E/e' ratio, and reduced left ventricular end-systolic and end-diastolic volumes in the empagliflozin group. Hospitalization for HF occurred in three patients from the empagliflozin group compared to four patients in the placebo group, with no significant differences in serious adverse events reported.

TABLE 1: Key findings from the randomized controlled trials addressing the use of SGLT2i in acute myocardial infarction.

Trial	*EMMY 2022*	*DAPA-MI 2023*	*EMPACT-MI*
Design	RCT	RCT-Registry based	RCT
Number	476	4,017	6,522
Drug	Empagliflozin, 10 mg	Dapagliflozin, 10 mg	Empagliflozin, 10 mg
Primary endpoint	Changes in NT-pro-BNP at 6 months	Death, hospitalization for HF, nonfatal AMI, atrial fibrillation/flutter, type-2 diabetes mellitus, NYHA class, body weight decrease	All-cause mortality and time to first HF hospitalization
Result	Empagliflozin 10 mg is superior to placebo in reducing NT-proBNP levels at 26 weeks among patients with AMI	Improvement in cardiometabolic outcomes but no impact on the composite of cardiovascular death or hospitalization for HF compared with placebo	Empagliflozin reduced first and total HF hospitalizations across the range of LVEF with and without congestion

DAPA-MI Trial

The DAPA-MI trial included 4,017 AMI patients without preexisting diabetes mellitus or chronic HF, followed for 1 year. Patients were assigned to receive either dapagliflozin (10 mg once daily) or placebo. The primary composite endpoint included death from any cause, hospitalization for HF, nonfatal MI, atrial fibrillation/flutter, new-onset type-2 diabetes mellitus, functional classification according to NYHA at the final visit, and a minimum body weight reduction of 5% or greater at the final visit. The trial population comprised 72% STEMI, with a mean HbA1c of 5.7% and an average eGFR of 83.5 mL/min/1.73 m^2. Baseline LVEF was <30% in 6.5% and between 30–49% in 67% of participants. Although the study did not yield a statistically significant difference in predefined composite endpoints [hazard ratio (HR) 0.95; 95% CI 0.64–1.40], the win ratio analysis revealed significant advantages for dapagliflozin with a win ratio of 1.34 (95% CI 1.20–1.50; $p < 0.001$).

EMPACT-MI Trial

The EMPACT-MI trial enrolled 6,522 AMI patients aged 18 or older within 14 days post-event, with a median follow-up period of 17.9 months. Patients were randomly assigned to receive either empagliflozin (10 mg daily) or placebo, with the primary outcome being a composite endpoint of the first occurrence of hospitalization for HF or death from any cause. There was no statistically significant difference between groups for the primary endpoint: 8.2% in the empagliflozin group experienced hospitalization or death compared to 9.1% in the placebo group (HR 0.90, 95% CI 0.76–1.06, $p = 0.21$). However, HF hospitalization rates were significantly reduced by 21% (HR 0.79, 95% CI 0.60–0.98) in the empagliflozin group, while cardiovascular-related deaths showed no significant reduction (HR 0.96, 95% CI 0.78–1.19).

In conclusion, while the EMMY trial demonstrated that empagliflozin effectively improves cardiac biomarkers and function after AMI, it did not evaluate clinical outcomes directly. In contrast, the DAPA-MI and EMPACT-MI trials aimed to assess SGLT2i's impact on hospitalization and mortality rates among AMI patients, revealing mixed results that underscore the need for further research into their clinical efficacy in this population.

However, certain design limitations may have obscured the trials' full potential benefits. Early patient enrolment and a lower-than-expected primary event rate contributed to the lack of statistically significant effects on the primary endpoints. Additionally, the influence of the COVID-19 pandemic on hospitalization rates may have further masked potential benefits. Specifically, concerns regarding the EMPACT-MI trial's design arise from the absence of monitoring for outpatient HF symptoms and treatment adjustments, such as intravenous diuretics and medication modifications.

A compelling argument can be made for initiating SGLT2i therapy later in the AMI trajectory, potentially after myocardial stunning resolves or even during ischemia. While the trials incorporated effective standard-of-care treatments to mitigate left ventricular remodeling and reduce the need for additional interventions, it is conceivable that an isolated evaluation of SGLT2i in these settings—absent concomitant therapies—could yield more pronounced benefits akin to those observed in early angiotensin-converting enzyme (ACE) inhibitor trials in the 1990s. However, conducting such trials in the present era seems improbable.

In a recent meta-analysis by Idowu et al., which pooled data from 11,204 patients, SGLT2i use after AMI was significantly associated with a reduced risk of HF hospitalization [odds ratio (OR) 0.77, 95% CI 0.62–0.96, $p = 0.02$). However, it was not associated with a reduced risk of all-cause mortality (OR 1.05, 95% CI 0.77–1.43, $p = 0.75$), cardiac-related death (OR 1.04, 95% CI 0.83–1.30, $p = 0.76$), or MACE (OR 0.90, 95% CI 0.77–1.05, $p = 0.18$).[28] This analysis adds another dimension to the evidence supporting SGLT2i in patients with AMI; however, the population with preserved ejection fraction after MI remains underrepresented, highlighting the need for further evaluation in future studies.

CONCLUSION

Despite the lack of statistically significant benefits observed in DAPA-MI and EMPACT-MI trials, the potential of SGLT2i in AMI management remains promising. Future trials, meticulously designed to address the limitations mentioned previously, hold the key to unlocking the full potential of this class of medications. The ongoing exploration of novel therapeutic approaches underscores our commitment to finding effective strategies for AMI patients. Patients with complicated AMIs are a distinct population at high risk for both early and progressive HF or cardiac death. Despite current medical therapy, these patients have a clear unmet need for further risk reduction, particularly during the crucial early period following AMI, to prevent the onset of adverse cardiac remodeling, chronic HF, and cardiac death. The potential mechanistic effects of SGLT2i therapy may be particularly beneficial in patients with AMI.

REFERENCES

1. McMurray JJV, Solomon SD, Inzucchi SE, et al. Dapagliflozin in patients with heart failure and reduced ejection fraction. N Engl J Med. 2019;381(21):1995-2008.
2. Solomon SD, McMurray JJV, Clagget B, et al. Dapagliflozin in heart failure with mildly reduced or preserved ejection fraction. N Engl J Med. 2022;387(12):1089-98.
3. Anker SD, Butler J, Filippatos G, et al.; EMPEROR-Preserved Trial Investigators. Empagliflozin in heart failure with a preserved ejection fraction. N Engl J Med. 2021;385(16):1451-61.
4. Packer M, Anker SD, Butler J, et al. Cardiovascular and renal outcomes with empagliflozin in heart failure. N Engl J Med. 2020;383:1413-24.
5. Wellings J, Kostis JB, Sargsyan D, et al. Risk factors and trends in incidence of heart failure following acute myocardial infarction. Am J Cardiol. 2018;122(1):1-5.
6. Mercado-Lubo R, Yarzebski J, Lessard D, et al. Changing trends in the landscape of patients hospitalized with acute myocardial infarction (2001 to 2011). (from the Worcester Heart Attack Study). Am J Cardiol. 2020;125(5):673-677.
7. Solomon SD, Zelenkofske S, McMurray JJ, et al. Sudden death in patients with myocardial infarction and left ventricular dysfunction or heart failure. N Engl J Med. 2005;352(25):2581-8.
8. Giustino G, Redfors B, Brener SJ, et al. Correlates and prognostic impact of new-onset heart failure after ST-segment elevation myocardial infarction treated with primary percutaneous coronary intervention: Insights from the INFUSE-AMI trial. Eur Heart J Acute Cardiovasc Care. 2018;7:339-47.
9. Kamon D, Sugawara Y, Soeda T, et al. Predominant subtype of heart failure after acute myocardial infarction is heart failure with non-reduced ejection fraction. ESC Heart Fail. 2021;8(1):317-25.
10. Desai NR, Udell JA, Wang Y, et al. Trends in performance and opportunities for improvement on a composite measure of acute myocardial infarction care. Circ Cardiovasc Qual Outcomes. 2019;12(3):e004983.
11. Harrington JL, Jones WS, Udell JA, et al. Acute Decompensated Heart Failure in the Setting of Acute Coronary Syndrome. J Am Coll Cardiol Heart Fail. 2022;10(6):404-14.
12. Verma S, Anker SD, Butler J, et al. Early initiation of SGLT2 inhibitors is important irrespective of ejection fraction: SOLOIST-WHF in perspective. ESC Heart Fail. 2020;7:3261-7.
13. Ferrannini E, Mark M, Mayoux E. CV protection in the EMPA-REG OUTCOME trial: a "thrifty substrate" hypothesis. Diabetes Care. 2016;39:1108-14.
14. Furtado RHM, Bonaca MP, Raz I, et al. Dapagliflozin and cardiovascular outcomes in patients with type 2 diabetes mellitus and previous myocardial infarction. Circulation. 2019;139(22):2516-27.
15. Lin B, Koibuchi N, Hasegawa Y, et al. Glycemic control with empagliflozin ameliorates cardiovascular injury and cognitive dysfunction in obese type 2 diabetic mice. Cardiovasc Diabetol. 2014;13:148.
16. Lim VG, Bell RM, Arjun S, et al. SGLT2 inhibitor canagliflozin attenuates myocardial infarction in the diabetic and nondiabetic heart. JACC Basic Transl Sci. 2019;4(1):15-26.
17. Wagdy K, Nagy S. EMPEROR-Preserved: SGLT2 inhibitors breakthrough in the management of heart failure with preserved ejection fraction. Glob Cardiol Sci Pract. 2021;2021(3):e202117.
18. Zannad F, Ferreira JP, Pocock SJ, et al. SGLT2 inhibitors in patients with heart failure with reduced ejection fraction: A meta-analysis of the EMPEROR-Reduced and DAPA-HF trials. Lancet. 2020;396(10254):819-29.
19. Wagdy K. The EMPEROR-Reduced trial: SGLT2 inhibitors for heart failure get more support. Glob Cardiol Sci Pract. 2020;2020(3):e202031.
20. McMurray JJV, De Mets DL, Inzucchi SE, et al.; DAPA-HF Committees and Investigators. A trial to evaluate the effect of the sodium-glucose co-transporter 2 inhibitor dapagliflozin on morbidity and mortality in patients with

heart failure and reduced left ventricular ejection fraction (DAPA-HF). Eur J Heart Fail. 2019;21(5):665-75.

21. Wagdy K, Selwanos P. DAPA-HF trial signals the birth of "diabetic cardiology" and more. Global Cardiol Sci Pract. 2020;2020(2):e202022.
22. Kwon O, Myong JP, Lee Y, et al. Sodium-glucose cotransporter-2 inhibitors after acute myocardial infarction in type 2 diabetes patients: A population-based investigation. J Am Heart Assoc. 2023;12:e0027824.
23. Nunes JT, Udell JA. So much to say on the best of what's around regarding sodium-glucose cotransporter-2 inhibitors acute myocardial infarction. J Am Heart Assoc. 2023;12(14):e030495.
24. Sinha T, Khilji F, Laraib F, et al. The effectiveness sodium-glucose cotransporter-2 (SGLT2) inhibitors cardiovascular outcomes all-cause mortality patients acute coronary syndrome: Systematic Review Meta-Analysis. Cureus. 2024;16(4):e58019.
25. Von Lewinski DV, Kolesknic E, Tripolt NJ, et al. Empagliflozin in acute myocardial infarction: The EMMY trial. Eur Heart J. 2022;43(41):4421-32.
26. James S, Erlinge D, Storey RF, et al. Dapagliflozin in myocardial infarction without diabetes or heart failure. NEJM Evid. 2024;3(2):EVIDoa2300286.
27. Butler J, Jones WS, Udell JA, et al. Empagliflozin after acute myocardial infarction. N Engl J Med. 2024;390(16):1455-66.
28. Idowu A, Adebolu O, Wattanachayakul P, et al. Cardiovascular outcomes of sodium-glucose co-transporter 2 inhibitors use after myocardial infarction: A systematic review and meta-analysis of randomized controlled trials. Curr Probl Cardiol. 2024;49(8):102648.

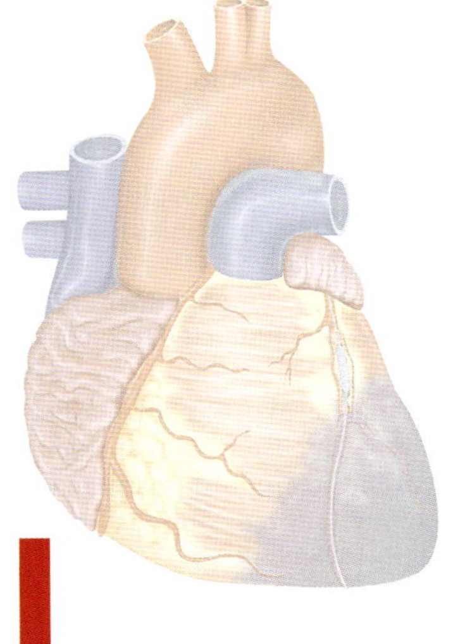

Treatment of STEMI with HFpEF: Focusing on Mortality Benefits

VK Shah, Simit V Shah

INTRODUCTION

ST-elevation myocardial infarction (STEMI) and heart failure with preserved ejection fraction (HFpEF) are significant health challenges that require specialized medical care. While both conditions have been extensively studied, their simultaneous occurrence in patients adds a layer of complexity. STEMI is a critical emergency marked by a complete blockage of a coronary artery[1] whereas HFpEF is a form of heart failure where the heart struggles to relax and fill properly, despite maintaining normal contraction.[2] The combination of these two conditions necessitates careful management strategies to achieve positive outcomes, particularly regarding mortality rates.

In recent decades, there have been significant advancements in treatment protocols for STEMI, leading to improved survival rates.[3] However, managing STEMI in patients with HFpEF remains an area that needs further research, as current guidelines primarily address STEMI treatment within the broader heart failure context, often overlooking the unique characteristics of HFpEF.[4] This manuscript examines the latest strategies and potential approaches to enhance survival outcomes for STEMI patients with HFpEF, emphasizing key interventions such as revascularization, medication therapy, and management of risk factors.

CONTENTS AND DESCRIPTION

Epidemiology and Pathophysiology

ST-elevation Myocardial Infarction

The STEMI accounts for a significant proportion of cardiovascular mortality worldwide. It is often triggered by the rupture of an atherosclerotic plaque, leading to an acute thrombotic occlusion of the coronary artery.[5] Rapid intervention, primarily through reperfusion therapies such as percutaneous coronary intervention (PCI) or thrombolysis, is crucial to minimize myocardial damage and reduce mortality rates.[6] Despite these advancements, mortality remains high, especially in patients with comorbidities such as heart failure.[7]

Heart Failure with Preserved Ejection Fraction

The HFpEF, on the other hand, represents nearly half of all heart failure cases, with its prevalence rising, particularly among older adults.[8] Unlike heart failure with reduced ejection fraction (HFrEF), HFpEF is characterized by normal or near-normal left ventricular ejection fraction but with impaired diastolic function.[9,10] This leads to elevated filling pressures, resulting in heart failure symptoms.[11] Patients with HFpEF typically present with a range of comorbidities, including hypertension, obesity, and diabetes, all of which contribute to the complexity of managing STEMI in this group.[12]

The coexistence of STEMI and HFpEF exacerbates the challenges in treatment, as the pathophysiology of HFpEF complicates postinfarct myocardial remodeling.[13] Patients with HFpEF are more prone to diastolic dysfunction, increased ventricular stiffness, and left atrial enlargement, all of which increase the risk of adverse cardiovascular events following STEMI.[14] Understanding these pathophysiological nuances is essential for developing targeted treatment strategies.

CHALLENGES IN ST-ELEVATION MYOCARDIAL INFARCTION MANAGEMENT WITH HEART FAILURE WITH PRESERVED EJECTION FRACTION

Pathophysiological Considerations

The unique myocardial alterations in HFpEF patients impact the traditional management of STEMI. Postinfarction, patients with HFpEF may experience more pronounced myocardial stiffness and reduced compliance, which can hinder the heart's ability to recover. As a result, the therapeutic strategies typically employed in STEMI, such as revascularization and pharmacological therapy, may not yield the same benefits as they do in patients without HFpEF.[15]

Moreover, the risk of left ventricular hypertrophy and myocardial fibrosis is higher in HFpEF patients, making it essential to adapt therapies that account for these structural changes.[4] Consequently, STEMI treatment in HFpEF must focus not only on restoring coronary perfusion but also on addressing the underlying diastolic dysfunction.[10]

Diagnostic Challenges

Distinguishing between acute coronary syndrome and acute decompensated heart failure can be particularly challenging in patients with HFpEF. The symptoms of STEMI, such as chest pain and shortness of breath, often overlap with those of heart failure exacerbation, which can lead to delays in diagnosis and treatment.[16] Early and accurate identification of STEMI in HFpEF patients is critical, as timely reperfusion has been shown to improve survival.[17]

Diagnostic imaging techniques, such as echocardiography and cardiac magnetic resonance (CMR), play an important role in differentiating STEMI from heart failure exacerbation.[18] These tools help in assessing left ventricular function, identifying wall motion abnormalities, and detecting the presence of infarction or ischemia.[4] Biomarkers such as troponins and natriuretic peptides also aid in the diagnostic process, although elevated levels of these markers may be seen in both STEMI and HFpEF exacerbation, necessitating careful clinical evaluation.

Treatment Response Variability

One of the significant challenges in managing STEMI in HFpEF patients is the variability in response to standard therapies. HFpEF patients often have altered pharmacokinetics and pharmacodynamics, which can affect the efficacy of medications such as antiplatelet agents, β-blockers, and anticoagulants.[19]

For example, while antiplatelet therapy is a cornerstone of STEMI treatment, HFpEF patients may have a heightened risk of bleeding complications, necessitating a careful balance between the benefits of antithrombotic therapy and the risks of adverse effects. Similarly, β-blockers, commonly used to reduce myocardial oxygen demand, may have less favorable outcomes in HFpEF patients due to their potential to exacerbate diastolic dysfunction.[20]

LIMITATIONS IN CURRENT MANAGEMENT

One of the primary limitations in the management of STEMI with HFpEF is the lack of robust randomized controlled trials (RCTs) that specifically address this patient population. Most clinical trials focus on STEMI patients with HFrEF or without heart failure, leaving a gap in evidence for those with preserved ejection fraction.[7]

Furthermore, the heterogeneity of HFpEF itself poses challenges in creating a one-size-fits-all treatment approach.

GUIDELINES AND ALGORITHM FOR ST-ELEVATION MYOCARDIAL INFARCTION MANAGEMENT IN HEART FAILURE WITH PRESERVED EJECTION FRACTION PATIENTS TO REDUCE MORTALITY

Based on current evidence and expert consensus, the following algorithm is proposed for the management of STEMI in patients with HFpEF (**Flowchart 1**):

Step 1: Rapid Diagnosis

The first step in managing STEMI in HFpEF patients is the rapid differentiation between STEMI and heart failure exacerbation. This requires a combination of clinical assessment, electrocardiography (ECG), and biomarker analysis to confirm the diagnosis and rule out other potential causes of chest pain and dyspnea.[16]

Step 2: Prompt Revascularization

Once STEMI is diagnosed, revascularization should be initiated as quickly as possible. PCI remains the preferred method of reperfusion, but in settings where PCI is not immediately available, fibrinolysis may be considered.[3]

Revascularization, either through PCI or fibrinolysis, remains the primary treatment for STEMI, significantly

Flowchart 1: Management of ST-elevation myocardial infarction (STEMI) in patients with heart failure with preserved ejection fraction (HFpEF).

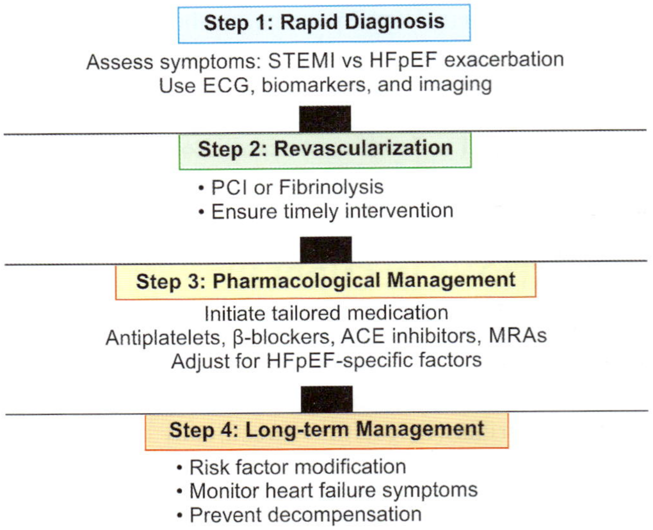

Step 1: Rapid Diagnosis

Assess symptoms: STEMI vs HFpEF exacerbation
Use ECG, biomarkers, and imaging

Step 2: Revascularization

- PCI or Fibrinolysis
- Ensure timely intervention

Step 3: Pharmacological Management

Initiate tailored medication
Antiplatelets, β-blockers, ACE inhibitors, MRAs
Adjust for HFpEF-specific factors

Step 4: Long-term Management

- Risk factor modification
- Monitor heart failure symptoms
- Prevent decompensation

(ACE: angiotensin-converting-enzyme inhibitors; ECG: electrocardiography; MRA: mineralocorticoid receptor antagonist; PCI: percutaneous coronary intervention)

reducing infarct size and improving survival rates.[7] In patients with HFpEF, early revascularization is equally crucial, although the diastolic dysfunction present in these patients may influence the extent of myocardial recovery postreperfusion.[15]

Studies have shown that prompt revascularization within guideline-recommended timelines leads to better long-term outcomes, even in high-risk populations like those with HFpEF.[17] However, the timing of revascularization must be coupled with careful monitoring for potential complications such as arrhythmias and heart failure exacerbation.[6]

Step 3: Optimization of Pharmacological Therapy

Pharmacological therapy for STEMI in HFpEF patients must address both ischemic injury and the underlying heart failure. This requires a tailored approach, as standard therapies may need to be modified to accommodate the specific needs of HFpEF patients.

- *Antiplatelet therapy:* Dual antiplatelet therapy (DAPT) with aspirin and a P2Y12 inhibitor is standard post-STEMI. In HFpEF patients, however, the increased bleeding risk warrants a more individualized approach to the duration and intensity of antiplatelet therapy.
- *β-blockers:* While β-blockers are beneficial in reducing myocardial oxygen demand, their use in HFpEF patients should be cautiously monitored, as they can lead to worsening diastolic dysfunction.[20]

Renin-angiotensin-aldosterone system (RAAS) inhibitors: RAAS inhibitors, including ACE inhibitors and angiotensin receptor blockers (ARBs), play a pivotal role in managing heart failure and preventing adverse remodeling post-MI. HFpEF patients may particularly benefit from these agents, although the evidence is less robust compared to HFrEF.[21]

Step 4: Long-term Risk Factor Management

Following acute management, long-term care should focus on reducing the risk of recurrent cardiovascular events through aggressive risk factor management. This includes strict control of blood pressure, glucose, and cholesterol levels, as well as lifestyle interventions aimed at weight reduction and increasing physical activity.[19]

Managing cardiovascular risk factors is essential in preventing recurrent ischemic events and improving long-term survival in STEMI patients with HFpEF. Aggressive control of hypertension, diabetes, and dyslipidemia has been shown to reduce the risk of subsequent myocardial infarctions and heart failure hospitalizations.[19]

In addition to pharmacotherapy, lifestyle modifications such as dietary changes, weight management, and physical activity are integral to reducing cardiovascular risk. These interventions are especially relevant for HFpEF patients, who often present with multiple comorbidities that exacerbate their condition.[18]

CONCLUSION

Managing STEMI in patients with HFpEF presents unique challenges, but with targeted interventions, there is potential to significantly improve mortality outcomes. Early revascularization is crucial as it reduces infarct size, preserves myocardial function, and mitigates the risk of heart failure progression, offering direct mortality benefits. Tailored pharmacological therapy, including the optimal use of β-blockers, ACE inhibitors, and MRAs, further contributes to survival by addressing the unique physiological considerations of HFpEF patients. Comprehensive risk factor management, such as controlling hypertension, diabetes, and lipid levels, reduces the likelihood of recurrent ischemic events, which in turn lowers long-term mortality risk. Despite these advances, future research, particularly large-scale RCTs, is necessary to provide clearer guidance on optimizing treatment strategies in this population. By addressing the specific pathophysiological and clinical challenges of this group, healthcare providers can better tailor treatments to not only enhance survival rates but also improve overall quality of life for HFpEF patients experiencing STEMI.

REFERENCES

1. O'Gara PT, Kushner FG, Ascheim DD, et al. 2013 ACCF/AHA guideline for the management of ST-elevation myocardial infarction. J Am College Cardiol. 2013;61(4): e78-e140.
2. Dunlay SM, Roger VL, Redfield MM. Epidemiology of heart failure with preserved ejection fraction. Nat Rev Cardiol. 2017;14(10):591-602.
3. Ibanez B, James S, Agewall S, et al. 2017 ESC Guidelines for the management of acute myocardial infarction in patients presenting with ST-segment elevation. Eur Heart J. 2018;39(2):119-77.
4. Shah SJ, Katz HD, Deo CR. Clinical phenotype of heart failure with preserved ejection fraction. Heart Fail Clin. 2014;10(3):377-86.
5. Windecker S, Kolh P, Alfonso F, et al. 2014 ESC/EACTS guidelines on myocardial revascularization. Eur Heart J. 2014;35(37):2541-619.
6. Niccoli G, Scalone G, Lerman A, et al. Coronary microvascular obstruction in acute myocardial infarction. Eur Heart J. 2016;37(13):1024-33.
7. Redfield MM, Chen HH, Borlaug BA, et al. Effect of phosphodiesterase-5 inhibition on exercise capacity and clinical status in heart failure with preserved ejection fraction. JAMA. 2013;309(12):1268-77.
8. Lam CSP, Donal E, Kraigher-Krainer E, et al. Epidemiology and clinical course of heart failure with preserved ejection fraction. Eur J Heart Failure. 2011;13(1): 18-28.
9. McMurray JJV, Packer M, Desai AS, et al. Angiotensin-neprilysin inhibition versus enalapril in heart failure. New Engl J Med. 2014;371(11):993-1004.
10. Shah AM, Pfeffer MA. The many faces of heart failure with preserved ejection fraction. Nat Review Cardiol. 2012;9(10):555-6.
11. Paulus WJ, Tschöpe C. A novel paradigm for heart failure with preserved ejection fraction: comorbidities drive myocardial dysfunction and remodeling through coronary microvascular endothelial inflammation. J Am Coll Cardiol. 2013;62(4):263-71.
12. Bhatia RS, Tu JV, Lee DS, et al. Outcome of heart failure with preserved ejection fraction in a population-based study. New Engl J Med. 2006;355(3):260-9.
13. Borlaug BA, Redfield MM. Diastolic and systolic heart failure are distinct phenotypes within the heart failure spectrum. Circulation. 2011;123(18):2006-13.
14. Gjesdal O, Bluemke DA, Lima JAC. Cardiac remodeling at the population level—risk factors, screening, and outcomes. Nat Rev Cardiol. 2011;8(12):673-85.
15. Steg PG, James SK, Atar D, et al. ESC Guidelines for the management of acute myocardial infarction in patients presenting with ST-segment elevation. Eur Heart J. 2012;33(20):2569-619.
16. Thygesen K, Alpert JS, Jaffe AS, et al. Fourth universal definition of myocardial infarction. J Am Coll Cardiol. 2019;72(18):2231-64.
17. Wiviott SD, Braunwald E, McCabe CH, et al. Prasugrel versus clopidogrel in patients with acute coronary syndromes. New Engl J Med. 2007;357(20):2001-15.
18. Piepoli MF, Hoes AW, Agewall S, et al. 2016 European Guidelines on cardiovascular disease prevention in clinical practice. Eur Heart J. 2016;37(29):2315-81.
19. Grundy SM, Stone NJ, Bailey AL, et al. 2018 AHA/ACC/AACVPR/AAPA/ABC/ACPM/ADA/AGS/APhA/ASPC/NLA/PCNA guideline on the management of blood cholesterol. J Am Coll Cardiol. 2019;73(24):e285-e350.
20. Yusuf S, Pfeffer MA, Swedberg K, et al. Effects of candesartan in patients with chronic heart failure and preserved left-ventricular ejection fraction: The CHARM-Preserved Trial. Lancet. 2003;362(9386):777-81.
21. Cleland JGF, Tendera M, Adamus J, et al. The perindopril in elderly people with chronic heart failure (PEP-CHF) study. Eur Heart J. 2006;27(19):2338-45.

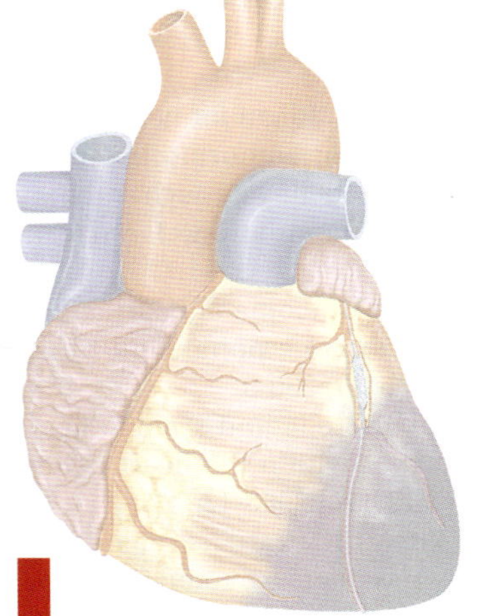

ARNI Postpercutaneous Coronary Intervention in STEMI to Prevent HFpEF

Sameer Gupta, Purshotam Lal

INTRODUCTION

Heart failure (HF) occurs when heart is unable to pump enough blood to fulfil the body's demands for oxygen and nutrients. Regardless of the underlying cause, HF is often a progressive medical condition, and advancement is linked to a lower chance of survival.[1,2] To emphasize these risks and the advancement of disease New York Heart Association (NYHA) classifies the HF as given in **Table 1**.

TABLE 1: Different classes of heart failure (HF) under New York Heart Association (NYHA) classification.

NYHA class	*Symptoms*
Class I	No limitation of physical activity. Normal physical activity does not cause undue fatigue, palpitation, or shortness of breath
Class II	Slight restriction on physical exercise. Comfortable at rest. Frequent physical exercise causes palpitations, exhaustion, dyspnea, or chest discomfort
Class III	Marked limitation in physical activities. Comfortable at rest. Excessive restlessness results in exhaustion, palpitations, dyspnea, or chest discomfort
Class IV	Heart failure symptoms when at rest. Any physical exertion exacerbates the pain

Source: Marvin HM. Diseases of the Heart and Blood Vessels: Nomenclature and Criteria for Diagnosis. Arch Intern Med. 1964; 113(6):906-7.

WHAT IS HEART FAILURE WITH PRESERVED EJECTION FRACTION?

Heart failure with preserved ejection fraction (HFpEF) is the situation where the heart pumps correctly but is too stiff to fill.

Together with aging and an increased risk of obesity, inactivity, and cardiometabolic diseases, there is an increasing chance of HFpEF. HFpEF is still not well understood in clinical practice, despite recent developments in our knowledge of its pathophysiological consequences on the heart, lungs, and extracardiac tissues as well as the advent of novel, simple diagnostic techniques.[3]

Patients with a left ventricular ejection fraction (LVEF) of ≥50% exhibiting either spontaneous or provokable elevated left ventricular filling pressures (LVFPs), as evidenced by natriuretic peptides and invasive hemodynamic parameters, are considered to have HFpEF.[1] HFpEF is a heterogeneous disease due to the fact that there exist few well-defined clinical phenotypes accountable for HF. On the contrary, disease arises in people with different risk factors that might or not be characterized by a particular HFpEF phenotype.[4] Some predisposing factors for the development of HFpEF include age, female sex, type II diabetes, hypertension, coronary artery disease (CAD), atrial fibrillation, and chronic obstructive pulmonary disease (COPD) but these are not entirely inclusive **(Fig. 1)**.

When epidemiological statistics revealed the prevalence of HFpEF in the public, especially among older persons, treatment aimed at these patients received more attention.[5]

ROLE OF ANGIOTENSIN RECEPTOR-NEPRILYSIN INHIBITOR

Angiotensin receptor-neprilysin inhibitor (ARNI) is one of the pharmacologic treatment that is rapidly gaining favor and excitement because of its capacity to lessen the unfavorable symptoms associated with HF diagnosis.[6]

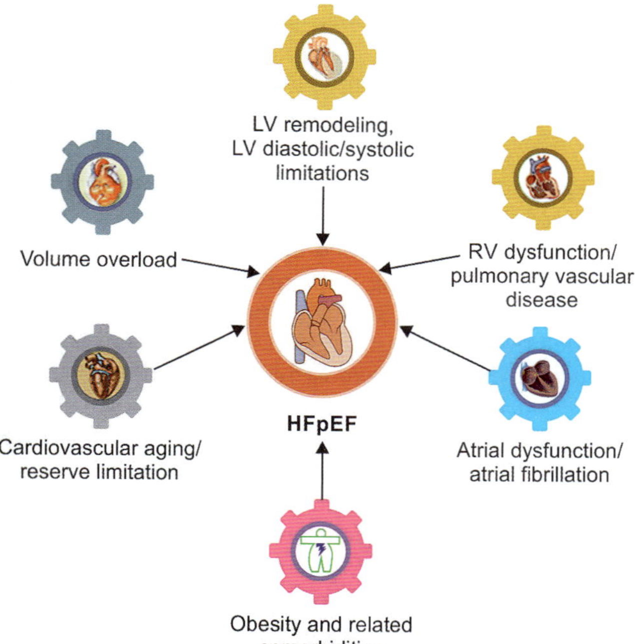

Fig. 1: Mechanisms in patients with heart failure with preserved ejection fraction (HFpEF). (LV: left ventricular; RV: right ventricular) *Source:* Ma C, Luo H, Fan L, et al. Heart failure with preserved ejection fraction: an update on pathophysiology, diagnosis, treatment, and prognosis. Braz J Med Biol Res. 2020;53(7):e9646.

CONTENTS AND DESCRIPTION

What is an Angiotensin Receptor-Neprilysin Inhibitor Drug?

The ARNI is a combination of two classes of drug, i.e., angiotensin II receptor blocker (ARB) and a neprilysin inhibitor. Sacubitril/valsartan is the only available ARNI currently and was approved by the Food and Drug Administration (FDA) in 2015.

What does Angiotensin Receptor-Neprilysin Inhibitor do?

The two active ingredients, valsartan and sacubitril, function differently. Through inhibiting the receptors that angiotensin II typically connects to, valsartan inhibits the function of angiotensin II. This action widens or dilates blood vessels and counteracts the detrimental effects of the hormone on the heart.

Sacubitril prevents the natriuretic peptides from being broken down. Water and salt are excreted in the urine as a result of natriuretic peptides. Blood pressure is lowered and the heart's workload decreases as a result. The two medications work together to lessen the load on the weakening heart **(Fig. 2)**.

ST-elevated Myocardial Infarction Patients Postpercutaneous Coronary Intervention

The PCI aims to alleviate occlusion or narrowing of the coronary artery and to improve blood flow to the ischemic region.[7] The ability of PCI to target chest pain, coronary artery stenosis, and associated clinical symptoms has demonstrated its usefulness in management of AMI.[8-10] However, it is important to remember that there is

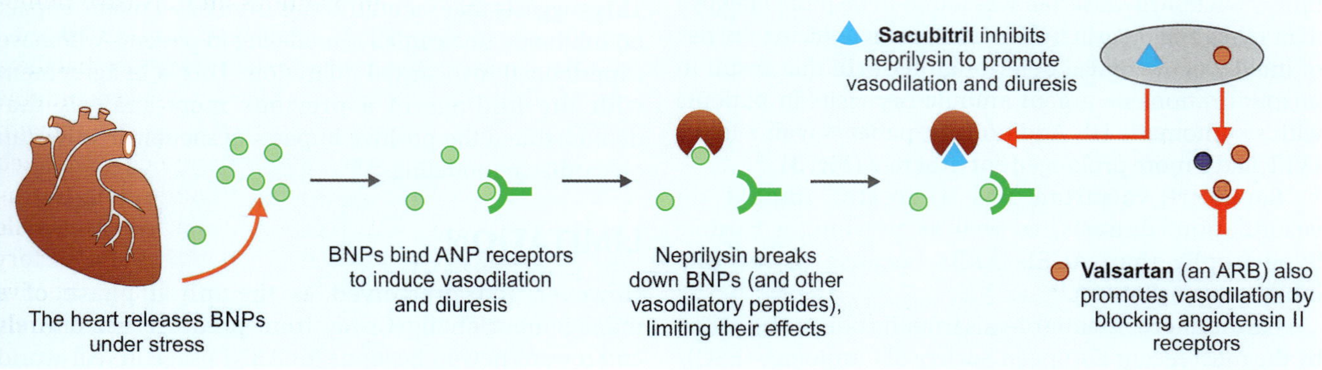

Fig. 2: Mechanism of action of sacubitril + valsartan.
Source: Dargad RR, Prajapati MR, Dargad RR, et al. Sacubitril/valsartan: A novel angiotensin receptor-neprilysin inhibitor. Indian Heart J. 2018;70(1):S102-10.

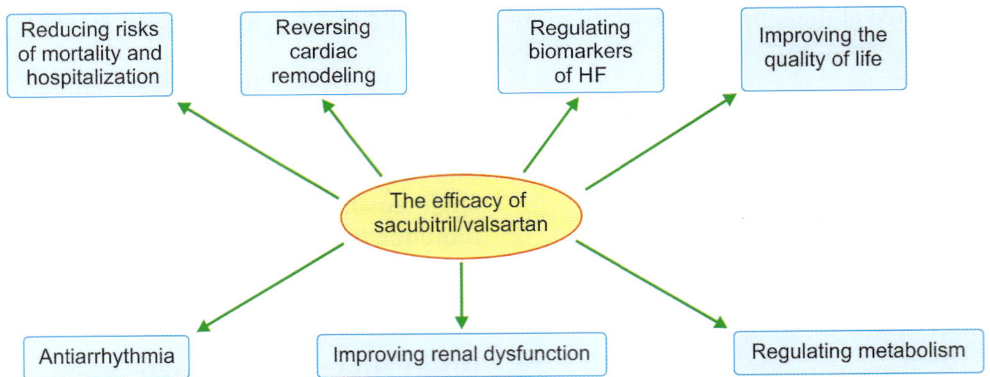

Fig. 3: Efficacy of sacubitril/valsartsan in heart failure (HF) patients.
Source: Zhang R, Sun X, Li Y, et al. The efficacy and Safety of Sacubitril/Valsartan in Heart Failure Patients: A Review. J Cardiovasc Pharmacol Therapeutics. 2022;27:1-12.

a high prevalence of postoperative complications, and these complications are linked to higher death rates. Such complications include stent thrombosis and the requirement for target lesion blood transport reconstruction. More importantly, irrespective of the patient demographic, left ventricular dysfunction is a major cause of hospitalized patient death, notably when first PCI revascularization fails.[11] Statistics show that left ventricular remodeling occurs in up to 30% of individuals having ST-elevated myocardial infarction (STEMI).[12] Yang et al., suggested in their study that compared to individuals with LVEF over 40%, those with LVEF below 40% had 7.54 times more risk of 30-day cardiovascular mortality and even had 6.54 times of higher cardiovascular mortality risk during a 1-year period.[13]

Current Role of ARNI to Treat HFpEF

Sacubitril-valsartan, an ARNI, is the first of its kind which prevents the degradation of various vasoactive peptides and blocks the renin-angiotensin system at the same time.[14] Sacubitril-valsartan was found to be more effective than renin-angiotensin inhibitors alone in reducing the risk of incidents of clinical deterioration of HF that result in hospitalizations or urgent ambulatory visits in patients with symptomatic HF. Additionally, patients with a lower LVEF had a more prolonged survival rate **(Fig. 3)**.[15]

Sacubitril-valsartan has a greater impact on vasodilation, diuresis, as well as preventing cardiac hypertrophy than ACEIs/ARBs because of its dual inhibitory mechanism.[16]

Furthermore, sacubitril-valsartan has been suggested by the most recent European Society of Cardiology (ESC)/American Heart Association (AHA) recommendations for HF over standard ACEI/ARB, with the objective of reducing morbidity and mortality.[1,17] Sacubitril-valsartan has been shown to reduce left ventricular remodeling in rat models of HFpEF; cardiac color Doppler ultrasonography has confirmed these findings.[18]

Rezq et al., study showed that, ARNI is more effective than ACEI at reducing unfavorable clinical outcomes that occur early-at 30 days-and enhancing reverse remodelling.[19]

Furthermore, in the most recent PARADISE-MI trial study,[20] the primary outcome determined by the clinical endpoint committee (CEC) demonstrated that ARNI significantly decreased the total number of primary endpoint events (first and recurrent) by 21% when compared to ramipril [rate ratio 0.79; 95% confidence interval (CI): 0.65–0.97; $p = 0.02$]. In line with this, PARAGON-HF trial also recommended ARNI use to treat HFpEF as in this study they compare the results of ARNI with ARB global outcomes in HF.[15,21]

According to some studies, after 6 months of treatment, the cardiac remodeling indexes left ventricle stroke volume, left ventricular diastolic volume, and left atrial volume (LVSV, LVDV, and LAV) respectively, were substantially improved in the sacubitril/valsartan group. This suggests that sacubitril/valsartan has a major impact on inhibiting myocardial remodeling in patients who have experienced myocardial infarction. This is in agreement with the findings of a previous meta-analysis that demonstrated the positive impacts of sacubitril/valsartan on cardiac remodeling.[22-24]

LIMITATION

However, it is perceived as the initial phase of a management change away from predetermined goals and toward new indications for ARNI usage in real-world HFpEF therapy. In order to validate that the activity of ARNI on a bigger sample can be responsible for the clinical improvement in patients, more studies with larger sample size needs to be done.

Moreover, there can be concerns regarding the accurateness of the HFpEF diagnosis because it's probable that the LVEF was initially lower than needed for the diagnosis 3 months before admission, which could have culminated in a misclassification.

CONCLUSION

Sacubitril/valsartan is safer to use in clinical settings and is equally effective as valsartan in avoiding HF and preventing ventricular remodeling in patients having acute myocardial infarction without raising the probability of side effects such as hyperkalemia, symptomatic hypotension, and renal failure following PCI.

The results provide evidence in favor of a novel strategy to outcome-improving treatment that is more effective than the current drugs used in patients with HFpEF.

REFERENCES

1. Heidenreich PA, Bozkurt B, Aguilar D, et al. 2022 AHA/ACC/HFSA Guideline for the Management of Heart Failure: A Report of the American College of Cardiology/American Heart Association Joint Committee on Clinical Practice Guidelines. J Am Coll Cardiol. 2022;79(17):e263-421.
2. Ammar KA, Jacobsen SJ, Mahoney DW, et al. Prevalence and prognostic significance of heart failure stages: application of the American College of Cardiology/American Heart Association heart failure staging criteria in the community. Circulation. 2007;115(12):1563-70.
3. Borlaug BA, Sharma K, Shah SJ, et al. Heart Failure With Preserved Ejection Fraction: JACC Scientific Statement. J Am Coll Cardiol. 2023;81(18):1810-34.
4. Anker SD, Usman MS, Anker MS, et al. Patient phenotype profiling in heart failure with preserved ejection fraction to guide therapeutic decision making. A scientific statement of the Heart Failure Association, the European Heart Rhythm Association of the European Society of Cardiology, and the European Society of Hypertension. Eur J Heart Fail. 2023;25(7):936-55.
5. Shah KS, Xu H, Matsouaka RA, et al. Heart Failure With Preserved, Borderline, and Reduced Ejection Fraction: 5-Year Outcomes. J Am Coll Cardiol. 2017 Nov 14;70(20):2476-86.
6. Mujadzic H, Prousi GS, Napier R, et al. Angiotensin Receptor-Neprilysin Inhibitors. The Impact of Angiotensin Receptor-Neprilysin Inhibitors on Arrhythmias in Patients with Heart Failure: A Systematic Review and Meta-analysis online) CC BY 4.0 license. J Innov Card Rhythm Manag. 2022;13(9):5164-75.
7. Ahmad M, Mehta P, Reddivari AKR, et al. Percutaneous Coronary Intervention. In: StatPearls. Treasure Island (FL): StatPearls Publishing; 2023.
8. Heyse A, Manhaeghe L, Mahieu E, et al. Sacubitril/valsartan in heart failure and end-stage renal insufficiency. ESC Hear Fail. 2019;6(6):1331-3.
9. Liu Y, Liu H, Hao Z, et al. Efficacy and safety of different doses of tirofiban combined with ticagrelor on diabetic patients with AMI receiving in emergency percutaneous coronary intervention (PCI). Int J Clin Exp Med. 2015; 8(7):11360.
10. Sauer AJ, Cole R, Jensen BC, et al. Practical guidance on the use of sacubitril/valsartan for heart failure. Heart Fail Rev. 2019;24(2):167-76.
11. Saia F, Grigioni F, Marzocchi A, et al. Management of acute left ventricular dysfunction after primary percutaneous coronary intervention for ST elevation acute myocardial infarction. Am Heart J. 2010;160(6):S16-21.
12. Bellis A, Mauro C, Barbato E, et al. The Rationale of Neprilysin Inhibition in Prevention of Myocardial Ischemia-Reperfusion Injury during ST-Elevation Myocardial Infarction. Cells. 2020;9(9):2134.
13. Yang M, Guo F, Yang YJ, et al. Prognostic Value of Preoperative Assessment of Left Ventricular Function in Patients Undergoing Percutaneous Coronary Intervention. Rev Cardiovasc Med. 2023;24(3):80.
14. Vardeny O, Miller R, Solomon SD. Combined neprilysin and renin-angiotensin system inhibition for the treatment of heart failure. JACC Heart Fail. 2014;2(6):663-70.
15. JJ M, M P, AS D, et al. Angiotensin-neprilysin inhibition versus enalapril in heart failure. N Engl J Med. 2014; 371(11):132-3.
16. Campbell DJ. Long-term neprilysin inhibition—implications for ARNIs. Nat Rev Cardiol. 2016;14(3):171-86.
17. McDonagh TA, Metra M, Adamo M, et al. 2023 Focused Update of the 2021 ESC Guidelines for the diagnosis and treatment of acute and chronic heart failure. Eur J Heart Fail. 2024;26(1):5-17.
18. Shi YJ, Yang CG, Qiao WB, et al. Sacubitril/valsartan attenuates myocardial inflammation, hypertrophy, and fibrosis in rats with heart failure with preserved ejection fraction. Eur J Pharmacol. 2023;961.
19. Rezq A, Saad M, El Nozahi M. Comparison of the Efficacy and Safety of Sacubitril/Valsartan versus Ramipril in Patients With ST-Segment Elevation Myocardial Infarction. Am J Cardiol. 2021;143:7-13.
20. Jering KS, Claggett B, Pfeffer MA, et al. Prospective ARNI vs. ACE inhibitor trial to DetermIne Superiority in reducing heart failure Events after Myocardial Infarction (PARADISE-MI): design and baseline characteristics. Eur J Heart Fail. 2021;23(6):1040-8.
21. Solomon SD, McMurray JJV, Anand IS, et al. Angiotensin-Neprilysin Inhibition in Heart Failure with Preserved Ejection Fraction. N Engl J Med. 2019;381(17):1609-20.
22. Zhao J, Zeng Y, Shen X. Efficacy and safety of early initiation of Sacubitril/Valsartan in patients after acute myocardial infarction: a meta-analysis. Clin Cardiol. 2021;44(10):1354-9.
23. Yandrapalli S, Aronow WS, Mondal P, et al. The evolution of natriuretic peptide augmentation in management of heart failure and the role of sacubitril/valsartan. Arch Med Sci. 2017;13(5):1207-16.
24. Wang Y, Zhou R, Lu C, et al. Effects of the angiotensin-receptor neprilysin inhibitor on cardiac reverse remodeling: Meta-analysis. J Am Heart Assoc. 2019;8(13):e012272.

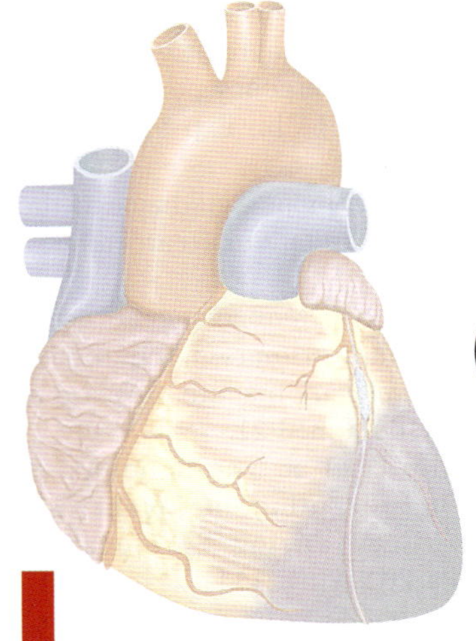

CABG in LV Dysfunction and Heart Failure

OP Yadava

INTRODUCTION

In India, coronary artery disease (CAD) is the most common etiology for heart failure (HF)[1] and left ventricular (LV) dysfunction may be present in up to 20% of CAD patients.[2] Even the resultant phenotype is very different from the western world. These patients present at a younger age, with more LV dysfunction and a heavier load of atherosclerosis, due to the higher prevalence of diabetes mellitus (DM) in India.[1] Velazquez and Bonow sum it succinctly, "This more aggressive course represents the convergence of ischemia, myocardial fibrosis, and endothelial dysfunction, which are superimposed on the inherent progressive nature of LV dysfunction, often with associated comorbidities, such as diabetes, which accelerate the adverse clinical trajectory."[3]

PREOPERATIVE EVALUATION AND DECISION MAKING

Heart Failure versus Ejection Fraction

Heart failure and LV dysfunction often coexist, and patients should be investigated for each individually, as they act independently. In a Swedish Nationwide Population-based Cohort Study, Dalen et al. showed that HF was an important risk factor for poor short-term and long-term outcomes after coronary artery bypass graft (CABG) surgery, regardless of preoperative reduced ejection fraction (EF). In fact, HF is more important than the EF. Though reduced EF more than doubled the risk of early death after CABG, it was HF which influenced long-term outcomes.[4]

Coronary Artery Disease Severity versus Ischemia

In the secondary analysis of International Study of Comparative Health Effectiveness with Medical and Invasive Approaches (ISCHEMIA) trial, it has been categorically shown that when the cohort of patients with moderate to severe ischemia were compared with those with no or minimal demonstrable ischemia, there was no difference in mortality between the invasive and the conservative arm. However, when the atherosclerotic burden on computed tomography (CT) angiography was examined, increasing CAD burden was shown to increase mortality as well as myocardial infarction (MI). Therefore, assessment of the anatomical extent of CAD was a better predictor of outcomes of CABG in patients with LV dysfunction in HF, compared to functional imaging. Patients with triple vessel CAD and those with extensive remodeling with LV systolic dysfunction receive maximum benefit from surgical myocardial revascularization.[5]

Role of Imaging

Imaging plays an important role in evaluating a patient of LV dysfunction. Advanced 2D and 3D echocardiography-based imaging technologies such as tissue Doppler imaging, speckle tracking, contrast echocardiography, and tricuspid annular plane systolic excursion (TAPSE) are key to accurate assessment of biventricular function, pulmonary hypertension, and structural heart disease.[6] Dobutamine stress echocardiography (DSE) and nuclear myocardial perfusion imaging are complemented by cardiac magnetic resonance (CMR) for assessing myocardial viability and transmurality of infarction (using delayed gadolinium enhancement), and for assessing the contractile reserves to prognosticate outcomes. This helps in predicting survival and all-cause mortality, independent of the LVEF.[7,8] Positron emission tomography (PET) and single photon emission computed tomography (SPECT) too may be helpful in assessing ischemia and myocardial viability.

Role of Viability Testing

There are four prerequisites for myocardium to be labelled viable, each affirmed by a different mode of investigation. It must have preserved cell membrane integrity (assessed by uptake of thallium 201 or 99-m technetium), preserved metabolism (uptake of 18 F-Fluorodeoxyglucose-FDG), contractile reserve during stimulation (DSE or stress CMR imaging), and absence of scar (late gadolinium enhancement on CMR). None of these modalities is fool proof, but nuclear tests have higher sensitivity and wall motion imaging has greater specificity. Therefore, more than one of these complementary technologies may be needed to demonstrate hibernating myocardium.[9]

Viability testing to detect hibernating myocardium has not been validated by randomized data, yet it is widely used based on observational studies. In a widely quoted landmark meta-analysis, myocardial revascularization was associated with a reduction in annual mortality from 16 to 3.2% ($p < 0.0001$) with medical treatment in patients with viability, as compared to no difference in those without viability (7.7 vs. 6.2%, p-NS).[10] A Cleveland Clinic study suggested an equipoise for outcomes at 10% of hibernating myocardium, but beyond this there was incremental benefit from revascularization.[11] In the PET and Recovery Following Revascularization-2 (PARR-2) Randomized Controlled Trial (RCT), this figure stood at 7%.[12] Though this study found no benefit of FDG-PET imaging with primary composite end-point of cardiac mortality/MI/recurrent hospitalization at 1 year with FDG-PET Arm of 30% as against 36% with the control group [RR 0.82, 95% confidence interval (CI)—0.59-1.14, *p*—0.16];[13] at 5-years follow-up, there was a significant reduction in the primary end-point in the PET guided group [Hazard Ratio (HR)—0.73, 95% CI—0.54-0.99, *p*—0.042].[14] Even in the PARR-2 Ottawa 5 substudy, the outcomes were better in centers with ready access to 18F-FDG imaging and where advanced HF teams were in-charge of management of the cases.[15] Another RCT, the Heart Failure Revascularization Trial (HEART), was expected to provide the casting vote, but it was prematurely terminated because of recruitment issues and therefore analysis of just 180 patients out of the 800 intended led to a hugely underpowered conclusion of no benefit of revascularization.[16] In the viability substudy of the Surgical Treatment for Ischemic Heart Failure (STICH) trial, consisting of 601 patients, though the univariate analysis found SPECT or DSE based viability to the associated with a reduced mortality (HR 0.64, *p*—0.003), the same could not be confirmed on multivariate analysis [55.2% CABG vs. 72.1% optimum medical therapy (OMT), *p*—0.3903].[17] Even the AIMI-HF trial, presented at the American College of Cardiology 2023 meet, failed to show any advantage of advanced imaging modalities of PET or CMR compared with SPECT on cardiovascular composite end-points in patients with HF due to CAD. Both, the American[18] and the European guidelines[19] give a low class IIa (LOE "B") and IIb (LOE "B") recommendation respectively to viability-based decisions for myocardial revascularization. Notwithstanding the supra, viability testing is being utilized clinically by most physicians to predict outcomes and for decision making when faced with the dilemma of choosing conservative versus interventional management of CAD. Moreover, presence of viability is an important prognostic marker. In cases of ambiguity and equivocal results, decision favoring CABG should always factor in other astute observations of wisdom such as size and quality of the target coronary arteries, thickness of the ventricular myocardium of the subtended territory, pulmonary hypertension, and right heart function, regional wall motion abnormalities, intraventricular dys-synchrony, pulmonary venous hypertension, LV dilatation, and the risk assessment of the procedure itself, besides the quality of life and biological age of the individual.

In presence of angina, or angina equivalent, myocardial revascularization is clearly indicated. Only if the patient is having symptoms suggestive of predominant HF, viability studies assume special relevance. A classical phenotype is dyspnea, especially in diabetics with autonomic denervation, or those with atypical symptoms with clinical equipoise. In these situations, if there is critical coronary anatomy, good distal target vessels and sufficient thickness of myocardium, revascularization should always be offered, irrespective of the viability results. However, in generic terms, patients without demonstrable viability are likely to have inferior outcomes compared to those with viable myocardium. Cahill and Kharbanda suggest a simple algorithm for viability testing in ischemic cardiomyopathy **(Flowchart 1)**.[9] According to this algorithm, suitability for revascularization is judged essentially by coronary anatomy and amount of myocardium in jeopardy.

Flowchart 1: Decision making in ischemic cardiomyopathy.[9]

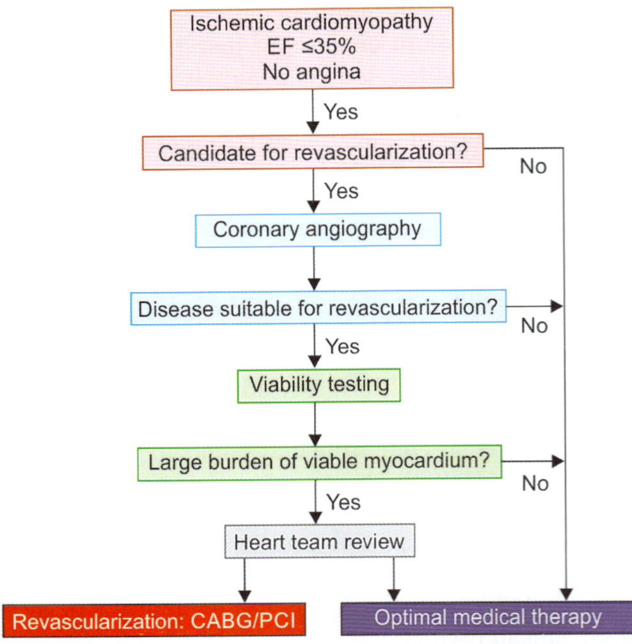

Flowchart 2: Benefits of revascularization.[21]

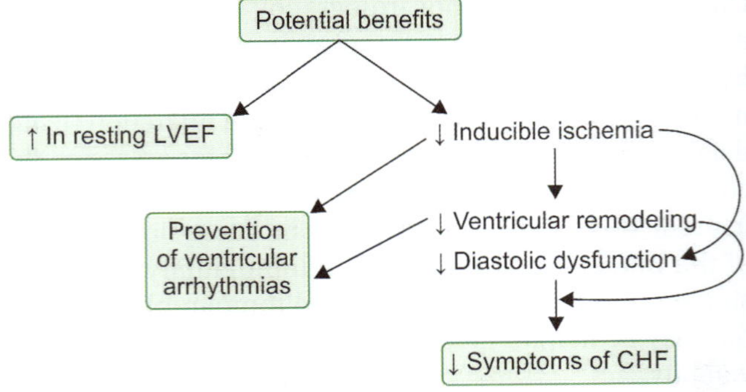

(CHF: congestive heart failure; LVEF: left ventricular ejection fraction)

CORONARY ARTERY BYPASS GRAFTING IN LEFT VENTRICULAR DYSFUNCTION–IS IT EFFECTIVE?

There is a great paucity of data of myocardial revascularization in HF. Majority of studies, including the well-planned RCTs like MASS-II (medicine, angioplasty, or surgery study), COURAGE (Clinical Outcomes Utilizing Revascularization and Aggressive Drug Evaluation), SYNTAX (Synergy Between Percutaneous Coronary Intervention With Taxus and Cardiac Surgery), FREEDOM (Future Revascularization Evaluation in Patients With Diabetes Mellitus: Optimal Management of Multivessel Disease) and ISCHEMIA, either excluded patients with LVEF <35%, or had <5% enrolment.

The most important goal of CABG in patients of HF is to improve survival, besides improving symptomatic state and quality of life. Even though patients with LV dysfunction and HF are a high-risk surgical group, with an in-hospital mortality of 4.6–11%,[20] the mid and long-term benefits of CABG over medical therapy alone are overwhelmingly superior **(Flowchart 2)**.[21] Therefore, patients with anatomy amenable to revascularization, and no other life-limiting comorbidity, irrespective of whether viability of myocardium can be demonstrated or not, should be offered CABG.[22]

The 10 year extended STICH trial (STICHES) demonstrated mortality benefits of CABG over OMT arm (58.9 vs. 66.1%, HR 0.84; *p*—0.02) with a number needed to treat (NNT) to prevent one death of 14 **(Figs. 1A to C)**.[23] Even at 5 years, though the STICH trial is traditionally presented as negative for revascularization, as the primary end-point of all-cause mortality was no different (CABG 36 vs. 41%; HR 0.86; *p*—0.12); secondary end-points of repeat revascularization plus mortality (CABG 39%, versus OMT 55%, $p < 0.001$) and cardiovascular hospitalization plus mortality, (CABG 58% vs. OMT 68%; $p < 0.001$) were in favor of CABG **(Figs. 2A to C)**.[24] Even PARR II Ottawa-Five Substudy support the role of CABG in patients with severe LV dysfunction.[15] These findings have been validated in a meta-analysis, where revascularization was associated with a significant reduction in mortality compared to OMT ($p < 0.001$) and there was a survival benefit (HR 0.82, $p < 0.001$).[25] Compared to either OMT or PCI, surgery always loses out early. For CABG to demonstrate its maximum potential of improving the most pithy of all end-points, viz. "survival," the follow-up has to be adequate, and probably >10 years.

TECHNIQUES IN CORONARY ARTERY BYPASS GRAFT

Off-pump versus On-pump Bypass Surgery

Off-pump coronary artery bypass (OPCAB) has been validated for high-risk cases as it reduces the operative mortality.[26] There is however, an equipoise between the "West" and the "East" on the use of off-pump strategy, with the Asian countries, especially India, China and Japan favoring it.

In a propensity score matched analysis of the patients with severe LV dysfunction in the Japanese National Database, Ueki et al. found lower 30-day mortality of 1.7% with off-pump CABG versus 3.7% with pump-CABG (*p*—0.01).[27] Even technically, the proponents of off-pump technique maintain that the reduced motion of the heart,

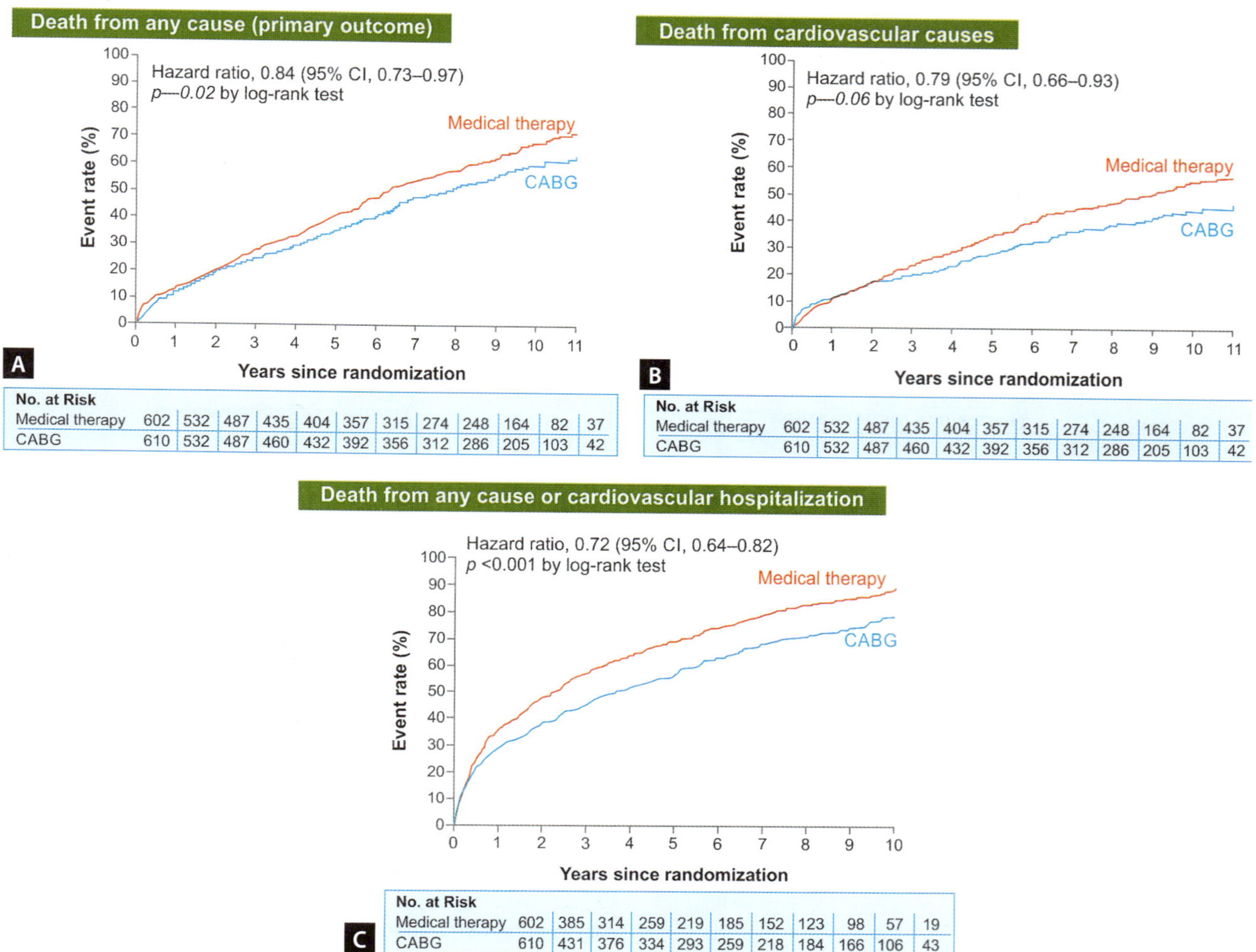

A — No. at Risk

Medical therapy	602	532	487	435	404	357	315	274	248	164	82	37
CABG	610	532	487	460	432	392	356	312	286	205	103	42

B — No. at Risk

Medical therapy	602	532	487	435	404	357	315	274	248	164	82	37
CABG	610	532	487	460	432	392	356	312	286	205	103	42

C — No. at Risk

Medical therapy	602	385	314	259	219	185	152	123	98	57	19
CABG	610	431	376	334	293	259	218	184	166	106	43

Figs. 1A to C: Kaplan–Meier estimates—STICHES trial.[23] (CABG: coronary artery bypass grafting)

and thus the reduced dp/dt, lead to better stabilization of the target coronary arteries, thereby making the surgery less demanding.

Having said that, there are contrarian view points with data supporting the contention that the quality of anastomosis is compromised and the patency rates of grafts in OPCAB is less. A meta-analysis comparing off-pump versus pump CABG found no significant mortality benefit of OPCAB (in-hospital mortality 4.4 vs. 5.4%, respectively).[28] The debate of off-pump versus pump CABG thus continues and even hybrid models like on-pump beating heart bypass have been suggested.[29]

All techniques are probably valid and it is the surgeon and ideology that he/she believe in, the experience, comfort, and the familiarity with the nuances of the techniques involved and decision making which are more important than the use or non-use of CPB support to carry out the procedure.

Use of Arterial Conduits

The moot primary question here is whether the natural history of reduced overall survival of patients with LV dysfunction, compared to those with preserved LV function, would allow sufficient time, long enough to be able to exhibit the benefits of multi- or total-arterial grafting strategies.

In a late breaking trial presentation at the recent Society of Thoracic Surgeons (STS) meeting, Sabik et al. looked at the STS Adult Cardiac Surgery Database of over 1 million patients undergoing CABG at 1,108 centers from 2008 to 2019 and found unequivocal benefit of multiarterial grafting irrespective of LV function.[30] However, Galbut et al. demonstrated survival advantage for bilateral IMAs over single IMA only for those with EF ≥ 30%,[31] while Mohammadi et al. failed to demonstrate any long-term survival advantage of bilateral IMAs.[32] Even the intention-to-treat analysis of arterial revascularization therapy (ART)

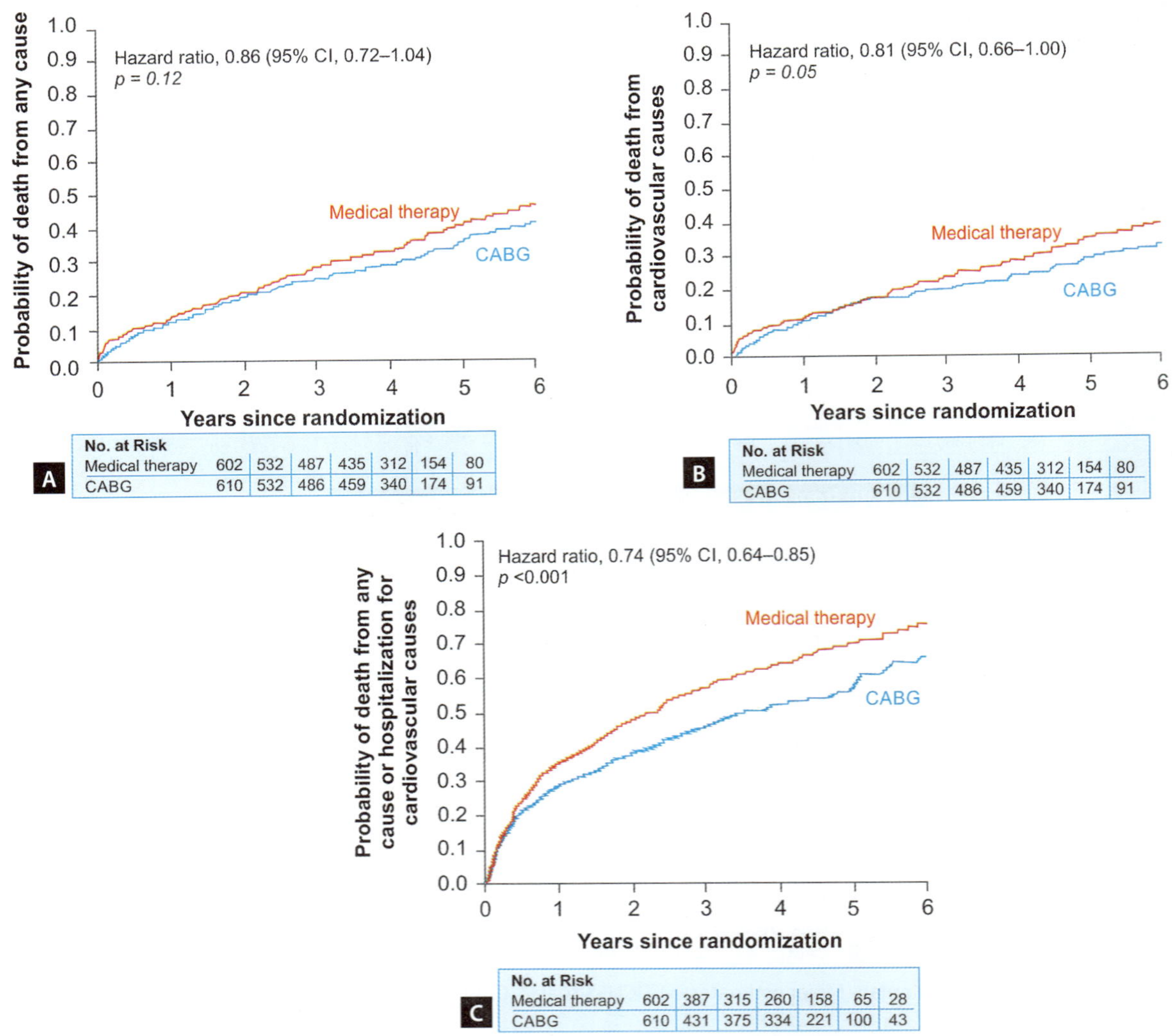

Figs. 2A to C: Intention to treat survival analysis—STICH trial.[24]

trial has failed to demonstrate any benefit of bilateral IMAs.[33] However, longer term (>10 years) follow-up and "as-treated" analysis has thrown early shoots of benefits for multi- and total arterial grafting.[34] Whether this holds true for patients with LV dysfunction is sub judice. Wisdom dictates, "what is good for the goose is good for the gander," or at the very least, cannot be bad. However, "Medicine" in contemporary era demands evidence base, which today stands at "LOE-C" for multiarterial strategy. Notwithstanding the supra, this author makes an impassioned plea that till more light is thrown on matters at hand, at the very minimum, an arterial graft to LAD should always be the default strategy. Additional arterial grafts should be prioritized after factoring in issues such as expected longevity of the patient, presence of comorbidities—specially obesity and DM, amount of myocardium in jeopardy, operative risk stratification, besides surgeon's comfort and experience with bilateral IMAs, keeping the age old adage—"primum non nocere," always the guiding principle.

Elective Use of Mechanical Support

Even though use of preoperative intraaortic balloon pump (IABP) has been shown to reduce in-hospital mortality and morbidity in high-risk patients undergoing cardiac surgery in multiple meta-analyses,[35,36] IABP SHOCK II trial was negative with no difference in either short-[37] or long-term[38] outcomes, especially mortality, with elective preoperative use of IABP in patients with acute coronary syndromes in cardiogenic shock undergoing myocardial revascularization. In such situations, the microaxial pump may provide better mechanical circulatory support (MCS) necessary to allow native heart recovery. "Recent evidence has demonstrated that preoperative optimization with MCS devices, especially in the setting of hemodynamic instability, can reduce perioperative morbidity and mortality."[39] However, most often the determining factor for choosing between IABP and temporary MCS is their availability, thus making this decision a no-choice in the developing world.

All patients with preoperative on-going ischemia should not be rushed to the operating theater. A brief period of stabilization and optimization of therapies, both pharmaceutical (intravenous nitrates, heparin, afterload reduction, diuretics for HF, etc.), and mechanical (IABP, MCS, extracorporeal membrane oxygenation, etc.) should be tried with a view to improving outcomes. In such a scenario, patient should be closely monitored while undergoing "goal-directed" therapy, with a surgical team and operation suite ready to offer myocardial revascularization at the first inkling of worsening, or realization of futility of conservative therapy. Even marginal improvement in ischemic LV dysfunction or reduction of LV end-diastolic pressure (LVEDP) and relief of ischemia can make the surgery more uneventful, more so when OPCAB is planned. However, in a stable patient undergoing CABG, use of IABP is not justified sheerly by the presence of LV dysfunction, as here the debatable "utilitarian" principle kicks in, especially in resource deficient countries. In such stable patients, IABP use should be dictated by patient's hemodynamic profile while manipulating the heart during off-pump surgery, and for those patients undergoing on-pump surgery, the call should be taken at the first failed attempt to come off CPB. There seems no debate, if indicated, it should be used earlier than later, and multiple attempts to come off CPB and delaying institution of counter-pulsation could actually be harmful.

ROLE OF SURGICAL VENTRICULAR RECONSTRUCTION/LEFT VENTRICULAR ANEURYSM SURGERY

Role of LV aneurysm surgery and surgical ventricular reconstruction (SVR) in LV dysfunction remains debatable. The STICH trial was neutral for benefits of SVR with concomitant CABG, compared with CABG alone.[40] National database of STS too did not find any benefit of SVR, with a 30-day mortality of 9.3%. Despite the controversies, SVR is an effective technique in patients with discrete scars and where postoperative LV end-systolic volume index (LVESVI) of <70 mL/m^2, along with maintenance of the elliptical shape of the LV, can be achieved.[22] The basic principles of LV aneurysm surgery, as enunciated by Chen et al.,[41] should always be guiding:

- Relief of ischemia by concomitant CABG.
- Reduction of LV volume (preferably <60 mL/m^2).
- Restoration of ventricular geometry to an ellipse.
- Mitral valve (MV) intervention to reduce LV volume overload, if there is associated mitral regurgitation (MR).

TACKLING CONCOMITANT MITRAL REGURGITATION

There is a widespread consensus to tackle severe concomitant MR during CABG. However, the issue of moderate MR (less than grade II), while undergoing CABG, is contentious. Currently, there is no conclusive evidence supporting surgical intervention for moderate MR in these patients, more so if the patient is undergoing off-pump surgery. Chan et al. conducted an RCT of adding mitral valve repair (MVr) to CABG in patients of moderate ischemic MR and concluded, "Adding mitral annuloplasty to CABG in patients with moderate ischemic MR may improve functional capacity, LV reverse remodeling, MR severity, and B-type natriuretic peptide levels, compared with CABG alone. The impact of these benefits on longer term clinical outcomes remains to be defined."[42] The trial was limited by its exclusion of severe LV dysfunction (<30%), structural abnormalities of the MV, advanced NYHA class IV symptoms, etc. Even in the Cardiothoracic Surgery Network (CTSN) randomized trial, in patients with moderate ischemic MR with multivessel CAD, though there was higher improvement in wall motion scores, there was no survival advantage.[43] However, in this trial too, the mean LVEF was >40% and therefore its validity and application for patients with severe LV dysfunction in HF is sub judice. A meta-analysis of observational trials too showed no survival advantage of adding a MV procedure to CABG (risk ratio—1.02; *p*—0.73).[44]

Probably a more nuanced and balanced outlook is required in the matter, and besides the degree of MR, one must also delineate the mechanism of MR. If papillary muscle ischemia with a tight lesion in the subtending coronary artery is noticed, and if the posterior wall thickness of the myocardium is satisfactory (>7–8 mm, preferably >10 mm) with no evidence of dyskinesia or akinesia, then myocardial revascularization itself may relieve ischemia and restore the tensing function of the papillary muscles and MR will reduce. However, if there is a structural defect in terms of ruptured chordae or even tethered posterior leaflets with grossly displaced papillary muscles, with thinning or aneurysmal posterobasal segment of LV, then MV intervention, should be considered. A prudent protocol is to do CABG first and then evaluate MR on transesophageal echocardiography, and take decision accordingly, guided by above basic principles.

Once the decision to intervene is made, the mode of intervention, viz., repair or replacement of the valve is the second bugbear a surgeon has to face. Durability of surgical MVr in patients with ischemic MR could not be demonstrated by the CTSN trial. It is suggested that MV replacement (MVR) with greater durability should be considered in these patients.[45] Robinson et al. opine, "in the absence of definitive data, concomitant mitral valve repair can be considered in the patients with reduced EF undergoing CABG in the presence of atrial arrhythmias, left atrial dilation or in setting of severe LV dilation. Replacement rather than repair should be considered in patients with limited viability in the posterolateral wall of the LV and the absence of adequate grafting targets in the posterolateral coronary territory."[39] When opting for MVR, every effort should be made to preserve the mitral subvalvular apparatus.

With the recent introduction of percutaneous techniques (Mitra Clip), probably they are the future and once transcatheter MV repair/replacement techniques evolve further, they may completely dispense with the need of surgical intervention in these patients.[45] Percutaneous therapies are being investigated in the ongoing Reshape-HF trial in Europe and COAPT trial in USA.

PERCUTANEOUS CORONARY INTERVENTION VERSUS CORONARY ARTERY BYPASS GRAFT

This polarized debate runs more on lines of turf protection, rather than on hard core science, as there is no compelling and conclusive data, one way or the other. Actually, the issue has not even been adequately examined, as most RCTs comparing PCI with CABG like the Bypass Angioplasty Revascularization Investigation (BARI), ARTS, FREEDOM, SYNTAX, etc., have excluded patients with LV dysfunction and HF, and therefore there is precious little data, other than observational and registry data, on the optimum revascularization strategy for these patients. However, there is consensus that completeness of myocardial revascularization should be a class I deciding factor for choosing any form of myocardial revascularization therapies.[19]

In a recent analysis of New York State Registry, PCI was validated in patients with LVEF ≤35% to be associated with a similar mortality as CABG (p—0.91), a lower risk of stroke, but an increased risk of MI and repeat revascularization.[46] To the contrary, in an analysis of British Cardiovascular Intervention Society data from 2006–2011, Mamas et al. found LV function an independent predictor of 30-day mortality after PCI in patients with LVEF <30% (HR—7.25; $p < 0.0001$).[47] Even in a meta-analysis of three real world registries by Kang et al., CABG reduced mid-term all-cause mortality (HR 0.43); cardiac mortality (HR 0.49) and need for repeat revascularization (HR 0.08; $p < 0.001$), compared to PCI.[48] Same findings were echoed in an independent meta-analysis by Cui et al.[49] Ngu et al. showed that there is greater improvement in EF with CABG.[50] These benefits get exaggerated in diabetics, with >60% relative risk reduction and 16% absolute risk reduction in 5-year mortality rate with CABG as against PCI.[51] This may even have a substantial public health impact. Survival benefit of CABG over PCI was also demonstrated by Wolff et al. in a meta-analysis of 21 studies (HR 0.82; 95% CI 0.75–0.90; $p < 0.001$).[25] Therefore CABG has been advocated to be a better method of revascularization in these patients (Class I recommendation) than PCI (Class IIa), albeit with "LOE-C" for both in the 2018 ESC/EACTS guidelines.[19] Surprisingly, the ACC/AHA/SCAI 2021 guidelines give CABG a Class IIb recommendation, and no recommendation at all for PCI,[52] thereby providing no guidance and in fact adding to the confusion. Till such time we have more definitive indicators, "The decision between percutaneous coronary intervention (PCI) and CABG should be based on the following: (1) Comorbidities, (2) coronary anatomy, (3) expected completeness of revascularization, and (4) patient's clinical status."[1] Though in a recent review and meta-analysis, Liga et al. found, "...surgical revascularization improves patients" prognosis at long-term follow-up, whereas evidence supports no benefit of percutaneous coronary intervention," they aver, "In patients deemed at higher risk for CABG, the SYNTAX score/SYNTAX score II may be also useful to tilt the balance toward PCI, which may remain an option, although not supported by clinical evidence, in patients at low anatomical complexity and low PCI procedural risk after multidisciplinary team discussion."[53] Their conclusion is supported by the REVIVED (Revascularization for Ischemic Ventricular Dysfunction)—BCIS II Study, which showed no difference in the primary outcomes between PCI and OMT.[54]

PHARMACOTHERAPY AND FOLLOW-UP

Recent advances in pharmaceuticals, especially the four foundational therapies for HF, have changed the natural history of LV dysfunction with HF and have contributed immensely to the improved outcomes of CABG in these patients **(Fig. 3)**.[1] The importance of rigorous prescription of OMT (lacking in almost one-thirds of patients post CABG), and diligent life-long compliance by the patients, can therefore not be overexaggerated. All patients, even after CABG, must be under regular follow-up of a HF

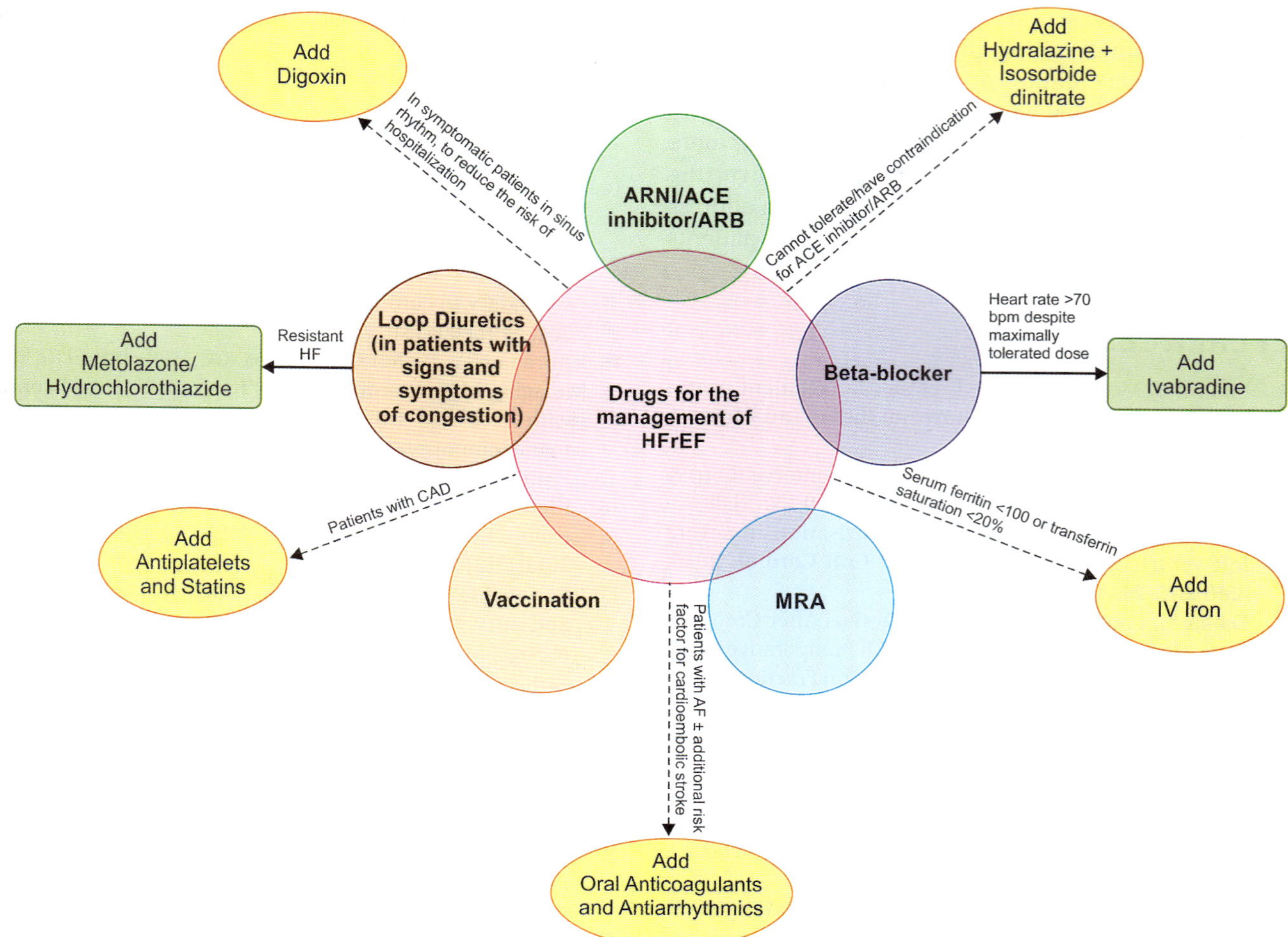

Fig. 3: Pharmaceutical armamentarium for heart failure with reserved ejection fraction (HFrEF).[1] (ACE: angiotensin converting enzyme; ARB: angiotensin receptor blockers; ARNI: angiotensin receptor neprilysin inhibitor; IV: intravenous; MRA: mineralocorticoid receptor antagonist)

specialist cardiologist, besides following a supervised and protocolized rehabilitation program, both of which elements are sadly missing in developing world.

Lately, use of angiotensin receptor neprilysin inhibitor (ARNI) has been found to be useful when used peri- and postoperatively. However, there are challenges associated with use of ARNI in the postoperative setting in form of hyperkalemia, hypotension, and potential for renal dysfunction, especially in patients with preexisting nephropathy. However, to the current date, though ARNI has been approved for regular management of patients with HFrEF (HF with reduced EF), they have not been validated for perioperative use. Moreover, a caveat is in order here—all renin angiotensin aldosterone system (RAAS) inhibitors, including angiotensin converting enzyme (ACE) inhibitors, angiotensin receptor blockers (ARBs), and ARNI have a tendency to produce intra-and postoperative vasoplegia with consequent need for higher inotropic support and therefore should be stopped 5 days prior to surgery.[55]

CONCLUSION

With improved techniques and technologies, operative morbidity and mortality of CABG in patients with LV dysfunction and HF have come down significantly. Even efficacy and survival benefits, compared to medical treatment, become discernible on longer term follow-ups. Viability testing, though not validated unequivocally, helps in prognostication, and must always be interpreted in light of clinical picture and coronary anatomy. Use of off-pump techniques and arterial conduits, in experienced hands, may contribute to improved short- and long-term outcomes. Both CABG and PCI have improved outcomes, but because of CABGs survival advantage and less MACCE, essentially driven by less follow-up spontaneous

MI and repeat revascularization, it may be preferred over PCI if countervailing increased cerebrovascular accidents are acceptable. Advances in contemporary pharmacotherapeutics have contributed immensely to the improved outcomes of these patients. However, more objective and evidence-based data is needed to firm up the recommendations, and RCTs should be set up to address the conundrum of the most optimum strategy for patients with LV dysfunction and HF.

REFERENCES

1. Mishra S, Mohan JC, Nair T, et al. Management protocols for chronic heart failure in India. Ind Heart J. 2018;70(1):105-27.
2. Kaul U, Bhatia V. Perspective on coronary interventions & cardiac surgeries in India. Ind J Med Res. 2010;132(5):88-93.
3. Velazquez EJ, Bonow RO. Revascularisation in severe left ventricular dysfunction, J Am Coll Cardiol. 2015; 65(6):615-24.
4. Dalén M, Lund LH, Ivert T, et al. Survival After Coronary Artery Bypass Grafting in Patients With Preoperative Heart Failure and Preserved vs Reduced Ejection Fraction. JAMA Cardiol. 2016;1(5):530-8.
5. Reynolds HR, Shaw LJ, Min JK, et al. Outcomes in the ISCHEMIA Trial Based on Coronary Artery Disease and Ischemia Severity. Circulation. 2022;146(1):e3.
6. Guha S, Harikrishnan S, Ray S, et al. CSI position statement on management of heart failure in India. Indian Heart J. 2018;70S:S1-S72.
7. Cheong BYC, Muthupillai R, Wilson JM, et al. Prognostic significance of delayed-enhancement magnetic resonance imaging: survival of 857 patients with and without left ventricular dysfunction. Circulation. 2009;120(21):2069-76.
8. Kwon DH, Halley CM, Carrigan TP, et al. Extent of left ventricular scar predicts outcomes in ischemic cardiomyopathy patients with significantly reduced systolic function: a delayed hyperenhancement cardiac magnetic resonance study. JACC Cardiovasc Imaging. 2009;2(1):34-44.
9. Cahill TJ, Kharbanda RK. Viability testing to guide myocardial revascularisation in patients with Heart Failure. Ind J Thorac Cardiovasc Surg. 2018;34(Suppl 3):S206-212.
10. Allman KC, Shaw LJ, Hachamovitch R, et al. Myocardial viability testing and impact of revascularization on prognosis in patients with coronary artery disease and left ventricular dysfunction: A meta-analysis. J Am Coll Cardiol. 2002;39(7):1151-58.
11. Ling LF, Marwick TH, Flores DR, et al. Identification of therapeutic benefit from revascularization in patients with left ventricular systolic dysfunction: Inducible ischemia versus hibernating myocardium. Circ Cardiovasc Imaging. 2013;6(3):363-72.
12. D'Egidio G, Nichol G, Williams KA, et al. Increasing benefit from revascularization is associated with increasing amounts of myocardial hibernation: a sub-study of the PARR-2 trial. J Am Coll Cardiol Img. 2009;2(9):1060-8.
13. Beanlands RS, Nichol G, Huszti E, et al. F-18-fluorodeoxyglucose positron emission tomography imaging-assisted management of patients with severe left ventricular dysfunction and suspected coronary disease. A randomized, controlled trial (PARR-2). J Am Coll Cardiol. 2007;50(20):2002-12.
14. Mc Ardle B, Shukla T, Nichol G, et al. Long-term follow-up of outcomes with f-18-fluorodeoxyglucose positron emission tomography imaging-assisted management of patients with severe left ventricular dysfunction secondary to coronary disease. Circ Cardiovasc Imaging. 2016;9(9):e004331.
15. Abraham A, Nichol G, Williams KA, et al. 18F-FDG PET imaging of myocardial viability in an experienced center with access to 18F-FDG and integration with clinical management teams: the Ottawa- FIVE substudy of the PARR 2 trial. J Nuclear Med. 2010;51(4):567-74.
16. Cleland JGF, Calvert M, Freemantle N, et al. The Heart Failure Revascularisation Trial (HEART). Eur J Heart Fail. 2011;13(2):227-33.
17. Bonow RO, Maurer G, Lee KL, et al. Myocardial viability and survival in ischemic left ventricular dysfunction. N Engl J Med. 2011;364(17):1617-25.
18. Yancy CW, Jessup M, Bozkurt B, et al. 2013 ACCF/AHA guideline for the management of heart failure. Circulation. 2013;128(16):e240-327.
19. Neumann FJ, Uva MS, Ahlsson A, et al. 2018 ESC/EACTS Guidelines on myocardial revascularisation. Eur Heart J. 2019;40(2):87-165.
20. Nagendran J, Norris CM, Graham MM, et al. Coronary revascularization for patients with severe left ventricular dysfunction. Ann Thorac Surg. 2013;96(6):2038-44.
21. Anavekar NS, Chareonthaitawee P, Narula J, et al. Revascularisation in patients with severe left ventricular dysfunction. Is the assessment of viability still viable. J Am Coll Cardiol. 2016;67(4):2874-87.
22. Garatti A, Castelvecchio S, Canziani A, et al. CABG in patients with left ventricular dysfunction: indications, techniques and outcomes. Ind J Thorac Cardiovasc Surg. 2018;34(Suppl 3):S279-286.
23. Velazquez EJ, Lee KL, Jones RH, et al. Coronary-artery bypass surgery in patients with ischemic cardiomyopathy. N Engl J Med. 2016;374:1511-20.
24. Velazquez EJ, Lee KL, Deja MA, et al. Coronary-artery bypass surgery in patients with left ventricular dysfunction. N Engl J Med. 2011;364:1607-16.
25. Wolff G, Dimitroulis D, Andreotti F, et al. Survival benefits of invasive versus conservative strategies in heart failure in patients with reduced ejection fraction and coronary artery disease: a meta-analysis. Circ Heart Fail. 2017;10(1):e003255.
26. Lemma MG, Coscioni E, Tritto FP, et al. On-pump versus off-pump coronary artery bypass surgery in high-risk patients: operative results of a prospective randomized trial (on-off study). J Thorac Cardiovasc Surg. 2012;143(3):625-31.
27. Ueki C, Miyata H, Motomura N, et al. off-pump versus on-pump coronary artery bypass grafting in patients with

left ventricular dysfunction. J Thorac Cardiovasc Surg. 2016;151(4):1092-98.
28. Kunadian V, Zaman A, Qiu W. Revascularization among patients with severe left ventricular dysfunction: a meta-analysis of observational studies. Eur J Heart Fail. 2011;13(7):773-84.
29. Al Jaaly E, Chaudhry UAR, Harling L, et al. Should we consider beating-heart on-pump coronary artery bypass grafting over conventional cardioplegic arrest to improve postoperative outcomes in selected patients?: Interact CardioVasc Thorac Surg. 2015;20(4):538-45.
30. Sabik JF, Mehaffey JH, Badhwar V, et al. Multi-arterial versus single-arterial coronary surgery: ten years follow-up of one million patients. Ann Thoracic Surg. 2024;117(4):780-8.
31. Galbut DL, Kurlansky PA, Traad EA, et al. Bilateral internal thoracic artery grafting improves long-term survival in patients with reduced ejection fraction: a propensity-matched study with 30-year follow-up. J Thorac Cardiovasc Surg. 2012;143(4):844-53.
32. Mohammadi S, Kalavrouziotis D, Cresce G, et al. Bilateral internal thoracic artery use in patients with low ejection fraction: is there any additional long-term benefit? Eur J Cardiothorac Surg. 2014;46(3):425-31.
33. Taggart DP, Benedetto U, Gerry S, et al. Bilateral versus Single Internal Thoracic Artery grafts at 10 years. N Engl J Med. 2019;380(5):437-46.
34. Taggart DP, Gaudino MF, Gerry S, et al. ART investigators. Effect of total arterial grafting in the Arterial Revascularization Trial. J Thorac Cardiovasc Surg. 2022;163(3):1002-9.e6.
35. Pilarczyk K, Boening A, Jakob H, et al. Preoperative intra-aortic counterpulsation in high-risk patients undergoing cardiac surgery: a meta-analysis of randomized controlled trials. Eur J Cardio-Thorac Surg. 2016;49(1):5-17.
36. Zangrillo A, Pappalardo F, Dossi R, et al. Preoperative intra-aortic balloon pump to reduce mortality in coronary artery bypass graft: a meta-analysis of randomized controlled trials. Crit Care. 2015;19(1):10.
37. Thiele H, Zeymer U, Neumann FJ, et al. Intra-aortic balloon counterpulsation in acute myocardial infarction complicated by cardiogenic shock (IABP-SHOCK II): final 12 month results of a randomised, open-label trial. Lancet. 2013;382(9905):1638-45.
38. Thiele H, Zeymer U, Thelemann N, et al. Intra aortic balloon pump in cardiogenic shock complicating acute myocardial infarction: long term 6 years outcome of the randomized IABP Shock II Trial. Circulation. 2018;139(3):395-403.
39. Robinson NB, Audisio K, Bakaeen FG, et al. Coronary artery bypass grafting in low ejection fraction: state of the art. Curr Opin Cardiol. 2021;36(6):740-7.
40. Jones RH, Velazquez EJ, Michler RE, et al. Coronary bypass surgery with or without surgical ventricular reconstruction. N Engl J Med. 2009;360(17):1705-17.
41. Chen WY, Wu FY, Shih CC, et al. Left ventricular aneurysm repair: a comparison of linear versus patch remodeling. J Chin Med Assoc JCMA. 2009;72(8):414-21.
42. Chan KM, Punjabi PP, Flather M, et al. on behalf of the RIME Investigators. Coronary Artery Bypass Surgery With or Without Mitral Valve Annuloplasty in Moderate Functional Ischemic Mitral Regurgitation: Final Results of the Randomized Ischemic Mitral Evaluation (RIME) Trial. Circulation. 2012;126(21):2502-10.
43. Michler RE, Smith PK, Parides MK, et al. Two-year outcomes of surgical treatment of moderate ischemic mitral regurgitation. N Engl J Med. 2016;374(20):1932-41.
44. Benedetto U, Melina G, Roscitano A, et al. Does combined mitral valve surgery improve survival when compared to revascularization alone in patients with ischemic mitral regurgitation? A meta-analysis on 2479 patients. J Cardiovasc Med (Hagerstown). 2009;10(2):109-14.
45. Acker MA, Parides MK, Perrault LP, et al. Mitral-valve repair versus replacement for severe ischemic mitral regurgitation. N Engl J Med. 2014;370:23-32.
46. Bangalore S, Guo Y, Samadashvili Z, et al. Revascularisation in patients with multivessel coronary artery disease and severe left ventricular systolic dysfunction: Everolimus eluting stents vs Coronary Artery bypass graft surgery. Circulation. 2016;133(22):2132-40.
47. Mamas MA, Anderson SG, O'Kane PD, et al. Impact of left ventricular function in relation to procedural outcomes following percutaneous coronary intervention: insights from the British Cardiovascular Intervention Society. Eur Heart J. 2014;35(43):3004-12.
48. Kang SH, Lee CW, Baek S, et al. Comparison of outcomes of coronary artery bypass grafting versus drug eluting stent implantation in patients with severe left ventricular dysfunction. Am J Cardiol. 2017;120(1):69-74.
49. Cui K, Zhang D, Lyu S, et al. Meta-analysis comparing percutaneous coronary revascularisation using drug eluting stents versus coronary artery bypass grafting in patients with left ventricular Systolic dysfunction. Am J Cardiol. 2018;122(10):1670-76.
50. Ngu JMC, Ruel M, Sun LY. Left ventricular function recovery after revascularization: comparative effects of percutaneous coronary intervention and coronary artery bypass grafting. Curr Opin Cardiol. 2018;33(6):633-37.
51. Nagendran J, Bozso SJ, Noris CM, et al. Coronary artery bypass surgery improves outcomes in patients with diabetes and left ventricular dysfunction. J Am Coll Cardiol. 2018;71(8):819-27.
52. Lawton JS, Tamis-Holland JE, Bangalore S, et al. 2021 ACC/AHA/SCAI Guideline for Coronary Artery Revascularization: A Report of the American College of Cardiology/American Heart Association Joint Committee on Clinical Practice Guidelines. JACC. 2022;79(2):e21-e129.
53. Liga R, Colli A, Taggart DP, et al. Myocardial Revascularization in patients with ischemic cardiomyopathy: for whom and how. J Am Heart Assoc. 2023;12:e026943: 1-13.
54. Perera D, Clayton T, O'Kane PD, et al. Percutaneous revascularization for ischemic left ventricular dysfunction. N Engl J Med. 2022;387:1351-60.
55. Sousa-Uva M, Head SJ, Milojevic M, et al. 2017 EACTS Guidelines on perioperative medication in adult cardiac surgery. Eur J Cardiothorac Surg. 2018;53(1):5-33.

SECTION 5

HFpEF and Arrhythmia

77. HFpEF and Atrial Fibrillation: A Dual Challenge
78. SGLT2i in HFpEF with AF with Stroke, Peripheral Vascular Disease
79. Lower Heart Rate Associated with Lower All-cause Mortality in HFpEF

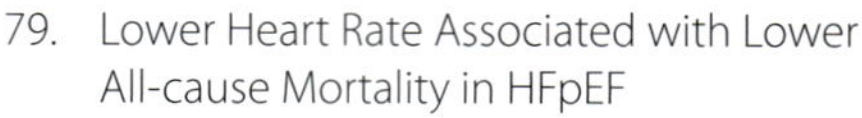

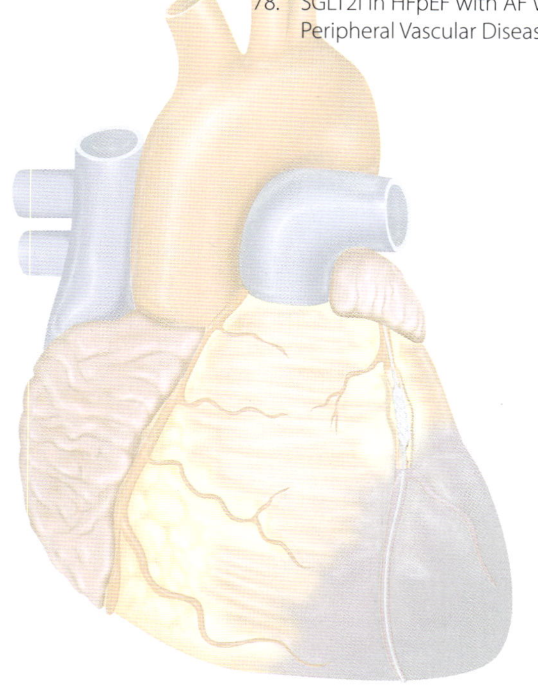

HFpEF and Atrial Fibrillation: A Dual Challenge

Arshad Nazir, Aditya Kapoor

INTRODUCTION

Atrial fibrillation (AF) is common in patients with heart failure with preserved ejection fraction (HFpEF) defined as left ventricular ejection fraction (LVEF) ≥50%, with a prevalence ranging around 40–60%. Patients with HFpEF and AF often have multiple comorbidities, such as advanced age, diabetes, ischemic heart disease, and other noncardiovascular conditions. HFpEF and AF predispose to each other and frequently coexist. In patients with dyspnea and no features of obvious volume overload, traditional echocardiographic indices may be difficult to interpret if there is associated AF, and a diagnosis of HFpEF may often be missed. Since AF and HFpEF may manifest with similar symptoms, diagnostic dilemmas can exist due to their interrelations that can affect the results of echocardiography and natriuretic peptides. The presence of AF in HFpEF is associated with poor atrial compliance and increased pulmonary vascular load that leads to pulmonary congestion, which further impairs cardiac output and exercise capacity.[1] Understanding and managing this complex relationship between HFpEF and AF is crucial for improving patient outcomes and ensuring better quality of life (QoL).

Clinical events are common despite anticoagulation and other medical therapies needed for heart failure (HF). This chapter enumerates salient management points for AF and HFpEF.

MANAGEMENT

Since many noncardiac conditions are common causes of morbidity and mortality in patients having HFpEF-AF, focusing on the management of these important noncardiovascular comorbidities can often help alter disease progression in HFpEF-AF patients.

Lifestyle and General Management for Atrial Fibrillation in Heart Failure with Preserved Ejection Fraction

Lifestyle changes are recommended for HFpEF-AF patients for optimal treatment. It was shown in a randomized control *RACE 3 trial* that targeted therapy of underlying comorbid conditions such as hypertension, hyperlipidemia, obesity, and HF leads to improvement in sinus rhythm maintenance in persistent AF patients.[2] The trial randomized 245 patients with early persistent AF and mild-to-moderate HF to conventional therapy (n = 126) versus targeted therapy (n = 119) of underlying conditions, with the primary endpoint being sinus rhythm at 1 year (with 7 days of Holter monitoring). Cardiac rehabilitative therapy included physical activity, dietary restrictions, and counseling. At 1 year, sinus rhythm was present in 75% versus 63% of patients in the intervention versus conventional group (odds ratio 1.765; lower limit of 95% confidence interval 1.021; $p = 0.042$). The trial concluded that targeted therapy of underlying conditions improves sinus rhythm maintenance in patients with persistent AF and associated HF.

Weight Loss

Weight loss is an important factor in obese HFpEF-AF patients. Obesity and diabetes are both risk factors for AF as well as HFpEF. The *LEGACY trial* explored the relationship between metabolic surgery and incident major adverse cardiovascular events in patients with type 2 diabetes and obesity. Metabolic surgery is usually defined as procedures that induce weight loss and alter gastrointestinal physiology. It was shown in the *LEGACY trial* that a 10% reduction in weight leads to a sixfold reduction in the probability of AF recurrence. Favorable effects were seen on resting and exercise hemodynamics, epicardial fat, and risk of incident HFpEF and AF due to substantial weight loss.[3]

Physical Activity

It was shown in a meta-analysis of six randomized controlled trials (RCTs) that exercise training in HFpEF patients leads to improved cardiorespiratory fitness and QoL.[4] The *TOPCAT trial* showed that every 10-fold increase in physical activity was associated with a 42.8% risk reduction of AF occurrence, concluding that a higher physical activity level is associated with a lower risk of AF in HFpEF patients.[5]

Sleep Apnea

A high incidence of sleep apnea is associated with AF-HFpEF patients. But the role of continuous positive airway pressure therapy in AF-HFpEF patients is of unproven value, and neither decrement in AF occurrence nor improvement in HFpEF was seen.[6]

Iron Deficiency Anemia Correction

A prospective cohort study, *DAMOCLES trial*, found that iron deficiency anemia was associated with decreased QoL and worse exercise capacity in HFpEF patients.[7]

Medical Therapy for Heart Failure with Preserved Ejection Fraction with Atrial Fibrillation

SGLT2 Inhibitors

As shown in the *PRESERVED-HF* and *EMPEROR Preserved trials*, SGLT2 inhibitors were efficacious in HFpEF in terms of decrease in HF hospitalization, improvement in QoL, and increase in 6-minute walk distance with no interaction by AF status,[8] and the AF events were reduced in the *DECLARE-TIMI 58 trial*. The mechanisms behind it are not clear, but SGLT2 inhibitors lead to weight loss, epicardial fat reduction, and natriuresis that may reduce AF events. Based on the EMPEROR Preserved trial, the 2022 ACC/AHA/HFSA guidelines gave SGLT2i a *class IIa* recommendation for the management of HF.

Treatment with SGLT2 inhibitors resulted in a lower risk of worsening HF (defined as hospitalization or unexpected visit for HF) or cardiovascular death than placebo in the two trials of SGLT2 inhibitors in HFpEF.[8,9] It is relevant to note that SGLT2 inhibitors similarly improved prognosis whether patients had AF or not at enrolment.[8-10] For the composite endpoint of cardiovascular death or first hospitalization for HF, the effect was consistent for those with AF [hazard ratio (HR) 0.77; 95% CI 0.69–0.87] and those without (HR 0.83; 95% CI 0.72–0.95).

ARBs, ACE Inhibitors, or BBs

In general, most HFrEF drugs are not efficacious in the management of HFpEF, including ARNIs, ARBs, ACE inhibitors, or beta-blockers (BBs). In patients with HFpEF and AF, excessive rate control may lead to blunting of chronotropic reserve.[11]

Direct Oral Anticoagulants

There is always a high risk of embolic events in HFpEF-AF patients due to LA myopathy and rhythm disturbance. Even sinus rhythm, HFpEF patients have a high risk of silent cardioembolic events.[11,12] Therefore, HFpEF-AF patients should be given direct oral anticoagulants to reduce the risk of cardioembolic events.

LAAO Devices

As we all know the fact that the left atrial appendage is the most common site of thrombus formation in AF patients; therefore, left atrial appendage occlusion (LAAO) devices may be an alternate method for stroke prevention in HFpEF-AF. LAAO devices were noninferior in the efficacy of stroke prevention but did show increased implantation failure for patients with HF.[13]

Rhythm versus Rate Control Strategies in Heart Failure with Preserved Ejection Fraction

Due to lack of RCT, there is no guideline-directed specific therapy for HFpEF-AF patients. The *AFFIRM trial* showed better results in HFpEF-AF patients who were able to maintain sinus rhythm.[14] BBs and nondihydropyridine calcium channel blockers are recommended as first-line agents for adequate rate control in HFpEF-AF patients. The *RATE-AF*, an open-label trial, compared the use of bisoprolol to digoxin in elderly HFpEF-AF patients and showed a comparable primary outcome of QoL between the two groups at 6 months, but the secondary outcome parameters such as functional ability and decrease in NT-proBNP were better in digoxin arm at 12 months, with comparable decrease in heart rate in both groups. Adverse events such as dizziness, drowsiness, and hypotension were seen more with BBs than digoxin.[15]

Antiarrhythmic Medications versus AF Ablation

Randomized controlled trials did not demonstrate an advantage of rhythm control over rate control with antiarrhythmic medications. Recent RCTs showed rhythm control strategy with ablation may be a better alternative to antiarrhythmic medicines. AF ablation incorporating pulmonary vein isolation is now a *class I* indication for treatment of individuals with symptomatic paroxysmal AF that is refractory to at least one antiarrhythmic medication, and a *class IIa* recommendation for individuals with recurrent paroxysmal AF even prior to initiation of therapeutic trials of antiarrhythmic drug therapies.[16]

In the *EAST-AFNET4 trial*, it was reported that early rhythm-control therapy was associated with a lower risk of adverse cardiovascular outcomes than usual care among patients with recent AF (diagnosed within 1 year) and underlying cardiovascular conditions (HF $n = 798$, most of whom had HFpEF).[17] The primary outcome (composite endpoint of death from cardiovascular causes, stroke, hospitalization with worsening of HF, or acute coronary syndrome) occurred less frequently in HF patients randomly assigned to early rhythm control versus those assigned to usual care (HR 0.74; 95% CI 0.56–0.97; $p = 0.03$).[18] Patients with HFpEF had a lower risk for the first primary outcome compared with those with HFrEF. However, the highest improvement in NYHA class occurred in patients with HFpEF. The majority of patients in this trial were on antiarrhythmic drugs as the first-line early rhythm control option and only a few of them underwent AF ablation. The exploratory analyses of AF patients in the EAST-AFNET 4 study suggested that amiodarone, but not treatment with flecainide, propafenone, or dronedarone, was potentially associated with early HF hospitalizations in patients with HFpEF, suggesting that further clinical research is needed to define the optimal antiarrhythmic drug therapy in patients with HFpEF.

A post hoc analysis of the *CABANA clinical trial* comparing catheter ablation and antiarrhythmic drug therapy in HFpEF-AF patients (79% of patients in the trial had HFpEF) showed that catheter ablation was associated with a striking 36% relative reduction in the primary composite endpoint of death, disabling stroke, serious bleeding, or cardiac arrest and a 43% relative reduction in all-cause mortality compared to antiarrhythmic drug therapy.[19] However, the effects on HF hospitalizations were not significant and the authors concluded that the results should be reproduced in a confirmatory trial.

AV Node Ablation and Permanent Pacemaker Implantation

Atrioventricular node ablation and placement of a permanent pacemaker may be beneficial in patients of HFpEF with failed rate and rhythm control. The *APAF-CRT trial* showed reduction in all-cause mortality, irrespective of ejection fraction in hospitalized patients with permanent AF and HF with narrow QRS hospitalized for HF, irrespective of their baseline EF.[20]

The ABC (Atrial Fibrillation Better Care) Pathway

A. Avoidance of stroke with the use of anticoagulation
B. Better management of symptoms with symptom-directed patient-centric decisions on rate or rhythm control
C. Cardiovascular and coexisting-condition risk management, including attention to psychological factors and lifestyle

Adherence to the ABC pathway can be associated with better outcomes in patients with AF and HFpEF.

CONCLUSION

Patients with HFpEF-AF are increasing in number as the population ages with increased longevity and more comorbidities. Many patients with AF and a normal LVEF have underlying HFpEF that is frequently unrecognized and underdiagnosed.

Heart failure with preserved ejection fraction and AF often coexist and can severely impact QoL, leading to frequent hospitalizations and increased mortality. Patients with both HFpEF and AF are difficult to manage due to limited evidence-based clinical management.

An established fact is that careful management of *heart rate and rhythm* in AF, along with aggressive treatment of comorbidities such as CAD, diabetes, and obesity, is necessary to improve outcomes in patients with both conditions.

The role of catheter ablation in HFpEF with AF requires more dedicated randomized trials. While it has also been found that SGLT2 inhibitors are associated with the reduction of AF, possibly due to protective effects against the development of AF, more data is required in this context. Further research is needed to understand the complex interplay between AF and HFpEF to help determine the best management strategy.

Heart failure with preserved ejection fraction with AF represents a clinical situation where a holistic and multidisciplinary approach to target comorbidities and appropriate lifestyle modifications is recommended to address both the HF and arrhythmia aspects in managing this challenging combination.

REFERENCES

1. Reddy YN, Obokata M, Verbrugge FH, et al. Atrial dysfunction in patients with heart failure with preserved ejection fraction and atrial fibrillation. J Am Coll Cardiol. 2020;76(9):1051-64.
2. Rienstra M, Hobbelt AH, Alings M, et al. Targeted therapy of underlying conditions improves sinus rhythm maintenance in patients with persistent atrial fibrillation: results of the RACE 3 trial. Eur Heart J. 2018;39(32): 2987-96.
3. Aminian A, Zajichek A, Arterburn DE, et al. Association of metabolic surgery with major adverse cardiovascular outcomes in patients with type 2 diabetes and obesity. JAMA. 2019;322(13):1271-82.
4. Pandey A, Parashar A, Kumbhani DJ, et al. Exercise training in patients with heart failure and preserved ejection fraction: meta-analysis of randomized control trials. Circ Heart Fail. 2015;8(1):33-40.
5. Zhu W, Liang W, Ye Z, et al. Association of physical activity and risk of atrial fibrillation in heart failure with preserved ejection fraction. Nutr Metab Cardiovasc Dis. 2021;31(1):247-53.
6. McEvoy RD, Antic NA, Heeley E, et al. CPAP for prevention of cardiovascular events in obstructive sleep apnea. N Engl J Med. 2016;375(10):919-31.
7. Alcaide-Aldeano A, Garay A, Alcoberro L, et al. Iron deficiency: impact on functional capacity and quality of life in heart failure with preserved ejection fraction. J Clin Med. 2020;9(4):1199.
8. Anker SD, Butler J, Filippatos G, et al. Empagliflozin in heart failure with a preserved ejection fraction. N Engl J Med. 2021;385(16):1451-61.
9. Solomon SD, McMurray JJV, Claggett B, et al. Dapagliflozin in heart failure with mildly reduced or preserved ejection fraction. N Engl J Med. 2022;387:1089-98.
10. Vaduganathan M, Docherty KF, Claggett BL, et al. SGLT-2 inhibitors in patients with heart failure: a comprehensive meta-analysis of five randomised controlled trials. Lancet Lond Engl. 2022;400(10354):757-67.
11. Mulder BA, Van Veldhuisen DJ, Crijns HJ, et al. Lenient vs. strict rate control in patients with atrial fibrillation and heart failure: a post-hoc analysis of the RACE II study. Eur J Heart Fail. 2013;15(11):1311-8.
12. Cogswell RJ, Norby FL, Gottesman RF, et al. High prevalence of subclinical cerebral infarction in patients with heart failure with preserved ejection fraction. Eur J Heart Fail. 2017;19(10):1303-9.
13. Munir MB, Hsu JC. Left atrial appendage occlusion should be offered only to select atrial fibrillation patients. Heart Rhythm O2. 2022;3(4):448-54.
14. Wyse DG, Waldo AL, DiMarco JP, et al. A comparison of rate control and rhythm control in patients with atrial fibrillation. N Engl J Med. 2002;347(23):1825-33.
15. Kotecha D, Bunting KV, Gill SK, et al. Effect of digoxin vs bisoprolol for heart rate control in atrial fibrillation on patient-reported quality of life: the RATE-AF randomized clinical trial. JAMA. 2020;324(24):2497-508.
16. January CT, Wann LS, Alpert JS, et al. 2014 AHA/ACC/HRS guideline for the management of patients with atrial fibrillation: a report of the American College of Cardiology/American Heart Association Task Force on Practice Guidelines and the Heart Rhythm Society. J Am Coll Cardiol. 2014;64(21):e1-76.
17. Kirchhof P, Camm AJ, Goette A, et al. Early rhythm-control therapy in patients with atrial fibrillation. N Engl J Med. 2020;383(14):1305-16.
18. Rillig A, Magnussen C, Ozga AK, et al. Early rhythm control therapy in patients with atrial fibrillation and heart failure. Circulation. 2021;144(11):845-58.
19. Packer DL, Piccini JP, Monahan KH, et al. Ablation versus drug therapy for atrial fibrillation in heart failure: results from the CABANA trial. Circulation. 2021;143(14):1377-90.
20. Brignole M, Pentimalli F, Palmisano P, et al. AV junction ablation and cardiac resynchronization for patients with permanent atrial fibrillation and narrow QRS: the APAF-CRT mortality trial. Eur Heart J. 2021;42(46):4731-9.

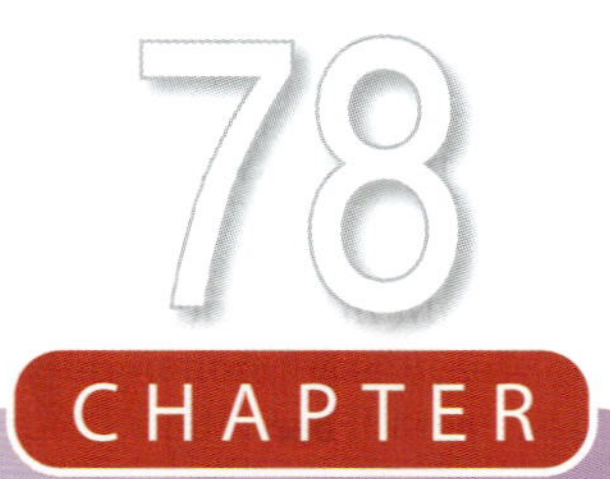

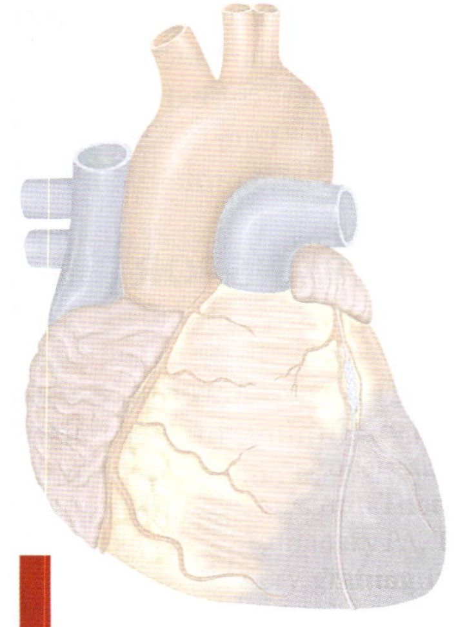

SGLT2i in HFpEF with AF with Stroke, Peripheral Vascular Disease

NN Khanna, Saurabh Bhardwaj

INTRODUCTION

Heart failure (HF) is a complex clinical syndrome resulting from structural and functional impairment of ventricular filling or ejection of blood.

While the clinical syndrome of HF may arise due to abnormalities or disorders involving all aspects of cardiac structure and function, most patients have impairment of myocardial function, ranging from normal ventricular size and function to marked dilation and reduced function.[1]

At the time of presentation, patients are clinically assessed and the objective of the assessment is to determine the clinical severity, find the underlying cause along with comorbidities, classify the type of HF, and form a plan of management.

After initial assessment, HF is classified as HF with preserved EF (HFpEF) with LVEF ≥50%, reduced EF (HFrEF) with LVEF ≤40%, mildly-reduced EF (HFmrEF) with LVEF 41–49%.

The HFpEF is a distinct entity with mechanisms of pathophysiology different from HFrEF. Hemodynamically, there is elevation of LV end-diastolic pressure (with resultant LA pressure elevation) at rest or with exertion and also have marked elevation in PCWP with minimal exertion.

The prevalence of HFpEF is increasing and is expected to exceed that of heart failure with reduced ejection fraction (HFrEF) in the near future. Using pooled data from the Cardiovascular Health Study (CHS) and multi-ethnic study of atherosclerosis (MESA), the estimated lifetime risk of HFpEF at age 45 years is >10% in both men and women. These data suggest that the total burden of HFpEF is projected to increase. Therefore, clinicians should have a low threshold for considering HFpEF as a potential (and increasingly common) diagnosis in patients with dyspnea or exercise intolerance.[2]

Epidemiological data also suggest important sex differences in HF subtypes. Although the incidence of HFpEF is similar among men and women, the prevalence of HFpEF is higher in women compared with men.[3]

Most traditional HF risk factors are shared and increase susceptibility for both HFpEF and HFrEF, including older age, hypertension, and ischemic heart disease. However, it is important to note that obesity, metabolic dysfunction, and physical inactivity appear to specifically predispose to HFpEF more so than HFrEF.[4]

It is also emphasized that HFpEF remains the most underdiagnosed entity in the heart failure spectrum, hence screening tools such as H2FPEF score and HFA-PEFF score have been formulated.[5]

Over the past decade, sodium-glucose cotransporter 2 (SGLT2) inhibitors have shown clinical benefit in patients with heart failure across the entire spectrum of ejection fraction, and among patients with worsening heart failure and acute heart failure. Several landmark trials, DELIVER, EMPEROR-Preserved, and SOLOIST-WHF, showed significant reductions in the composite of heart failure hospitalization/cardiovascular death with these agents in patients with HFpEF.

In the recently concluded ESC 2023 conference, updated ESC HF guidelines were published, which recommend Class 1A for the use of SGLT2i in treatment of HFpEF.[6]

We discuss here, the role of SGLT2i in HFPEF, with respect to the etiopathogenesis of the disease, pharmacodynamics of these agents and the clinical evidence available to date.

HEART FAILURE WITH PRESERVED EJECTION FRACTION

Zile et al.,[7] in their landmark study showed that diastolic dysfunction is the hallmark of HFpEF. There is impaired active relaxation and increased stiffness of the left ventricle. This is accompanied by neurohormonal activation, chronotropic incompetence, atrial arrhythmias, and renal dysfunction. The adverse remodeling is not just restricted to the LV but also involves atria and vasculature **(Table 1 and Fig. 1)**.

TABLE 1: Risk factors and mechanisms of heart failure with preserved ejection fraction (HFpEF).

Risk factors	*Mechanisms of HFpEF*
• Aging • Obesity • Metabolic syndrome • Diabetes • Hypertension • Renal disease • Smoking • Obstructed sleep apnea (OSA) • Myocardial infarction (MI)	• Cardiac remodeling and hypertrophy • Myofilament stiffness • Oxidative stress, inflammation, and fibrosis • Impaired energetics • Ionic imbalance

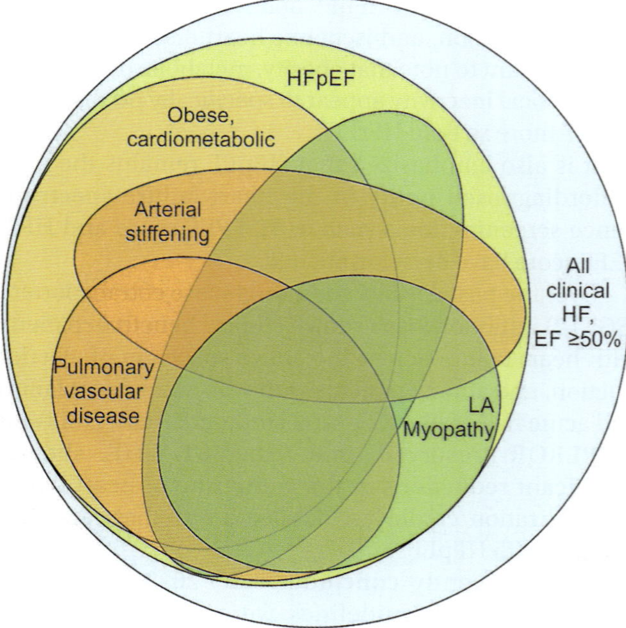

Fig. 1: Phenotypic spectrum of HF with normal EF. (EF: ejection fraction; HF: heart failure; HFpEF: heart failure with preserved ejection fraction; LA: left atrial)

Other important factors which contribute to the pathophysiology are cellular and molecular mechanisms;[8] changes to the cardiomyocyte structure, extracellular matrix, and cardiomyocyte energetics.[9] One key mediator of stiffness is dysregulation of cytoskeletal protein titin.[10]

SODIUM-GLUCOSE COTRANSPORTER 2 INHIBITORS

The SGLT2i, are a new class of glucose-lowering drugs. They work by blocking the low-affinity, high-capacity SGLT2 protein located in the proximal convoluted tubule of the nephron. The SGLT2 protein is responsible for the resorption of approximately 90% of filtered glucose while the remainder is reabsorbed by SGLT1 proteins found on the distal part of the proximal convoluted tubule. SGLT2 inhibition results in glycosuria (and natriuresis as the protein is a cotransporter), thereby lowering plasma glucose concentrations.[11]

The agents, though originally investigated for type 2 diabetes mellitus patients, were found to improve key outcomes including cardiovascular deaths and unexpectedly reduced heart failure hospitalizations in heart failure as well.[12-15]

Clinical evaluation of these agents proceeded to patients with HFrEF as well as those with chronic kidney disease (CKD). The SGLT2 inhibitors proved beneficial in HFrEF, reducing the composite of heart failure hospitalization/cardiovascular death in the EMPEROR-Reduced and DAPA-HF trials.[16,17] There was also scientific evidence which proved that these agents also slowed the rate of kidney function deterioration as well as improved heart failure outcomes in patients with CKD.[18-20]

The scientific data evolved over the time to study outcomes of these agents in patients with worsening/acute heart failure[21,22] and HFPEF. Land mark trials EMPEROR-Preserved and DELIVER trials both demonstrated significant reductions in their primary outcomes (cardiovascular death or hospitalization for heart failure) with SGLT2 inhibitors in HFpEF in addition to modest improvements in symptom burden measured by the Kansas City Cardiomyopathy Questionnaire score.[23,24]

SODIUM-GLUCOSE COTRANSPORTER 2 INHIBITORS AND HEART FAILURE WITH PRESERVED EJECTION FRACTION

As per the scientific data available over the past decade, SGLT2i, have remarkable impact on the management of heart failure across the spectrum from reduced LVEF to preserved LVEF. The likely mechanisms are multifactorial

BOX 1: Clinical effects of sodium-glucose cotransporter 2 inhibitors on heart.

- Diuresis and natriuresis
- Improved myocardial energetics
- Improved myocardial ionic homeostasis
- Autophagy
- Altered adipokine regulation
- Improved glycemic control and weight loss
- Increased red blood cell mass and hematocrit

which mau have direct and indirect myocardial effects related to metabolism, energetics, autophagic flux, ionic homeostasis, inflammation, oxidative stress, and cardiac remodeling **(Box 1)**.

The SGLT2i, have favorable effects on blood pressure and blood sugar level reductions.[25] The SGLT2 inhibitors have been shown to reduce systolic blood pressure by an average 4 mmHg as assessed using 24-hours ambulatory monitoring.[26]

Natriuresis/diuresis may be an important contributor to the clinical improvement observed with SGLT2i in patients with acute heart failure. Significant improvements compared with placebo in both clinical scores and markers (hematocrit and N-terminal pro-B-type natriuretic peptide) of congestion were also observed with empagliflozin by day 15.[27]

Sustained weight reduction with SGLT2i may instead be related to loss of calories through glycosuria and reduction in visceral fat.[28,29]

Studies have shown that epicardial fat has adverse effects on heart.[30,31] Adiponectin and leptin are cytokines that are released from adipocytes and their dysregulation has been implicated in the pathophysiology of heart failure.[32] SGLT2i increase the levels of adiponectin, an insulin sensitizing and anti-inflammatory hormone, and reducing levels of leptin, a hormone released by adipose tissue in states of nutritional excess.[33]

The cardio renal effects of these drugs are an important consideration given the strong association between CKD and HFpEF. SGLT2i have been shown to reduce the rate of decline in kidney function as well as to reduce kidney failure/death in patients with CKD with or without diabetes; the underlying mechanisms are believed to be a reduction in transglomerular pressure and regulation of tubule-glomerular feedback to protect kidney function. Cardio renal effects play a major role in heart failure: kidney dysfunction, perfusion and function.[18,34,35] DELIVER and EMPEROR-Preserved, trials have shown to improve cardiovascular outcomes throughout the spectrum of kidney function.[23,24]

Autophagy is the process by which cellular physiological equilibrium is maintained by removal of potentially dangerous constituents and recycling of cellular components as an adaptive response to metabolic stress including hypoxia and starvation.[36]

The pathways of autophagy induction involve activation of adenosine monophosphate-activated protein kinase (AMPK), sirtuin-1 (SIRT1), and hypoxia-inducible factors (HIF-1α and HIF-2α).[37] Induction of autophagy can also contribute to degradation of dysfunctional mitochondria and subsequent reduction in oxidative stress.[38] This cellular process is impaired in the failing myocardium, and induction of autophagy by SGLT2i may contribute to the improvements in cardiac function observed with these drugs.[39]

The SGLT2 inhibition enhances autophagic flux and induces a fasting/hypoxic mimicry state resulting in activation of mediators including AMPK, sirtuins, and HIF, which promote ketosis and erythropoiesis that lead to reductions in oxidative stress and inflammation as well as improved cellular function. This emerging mechanism may explain the beneficial effects of SGLT2 inhibitors on metabolism and cellular function in tissues/organs (such as the heart) that do not express the SGLT2 protein and could be a contributing factor to the reduction in oxidative stress and inflammation observed with these agents.[40]

A common comorbidity seen along with heart failure patients is iron deficiency anemia, which contributes to reduced functional outcomes.[41] SGLT2i have been shown to have favorable effects on iron homeostasis and erythrocytosis.[42] In the analysis of DAPA-HF and EMPEROR trial, SGLT2i were found to have reduced the circulating levels of both hepcidin and ferritin, while increasing levels of transferrin receptor protein 1.[43,44] These findings suggest that SGLT2i may reduce iron deficiency, and allowing iron mobilization and augmenting bioreactive cytosolic iron levels in erythroid precursors and cardiomyocytes.[42]

Another aspect that was highlighted in certain trials of SGLT2i, was the increase in levels of erythropoietin (EPO).[45,46] The DAPA-HF trial, treatment with dapagliflozin led to rises in hematocrit.[43]

Ionic homeostasis, especially calcium balance, is another important feature of SGLT2i.[47] These agents also reduce cardiac cytosolic sodium content by inhibiting sodium-hydrogen exchanger 1.[48,49]

The SGLT2i reduce levels of circulating proinflammatory factors such as C-reactive protein, tumor necrosis factor-α, and interleukin-6 along with markers of oxidative stress and reactive oxygen species including hydrogen peroxide in the myocardium.[50]

As discussed earlier, diastolic dysfunction in HFpEF has several components including intrinsic myofilament stiffness (related to titin regulation) as well as extracellular matrix related stiffness/myocardial fibrosis.[8-10] The IDDIA trial of patients with type 2 diabetes mellitus and at least grade 1 left ventricular diastolic dysfunction showed improvements in left ventricular diastolic function, including diastolic reserve, assessed by diastolic stress echocardiography after 24 weeks of treatment with dapagliflozin compared with placebo.[51] Beyond direct cardiomyocyte effects, SGLT2 inhibitors have been shown to reduce macrophage infiltration, regulate macrophage polarization, inhibit cardiac fibroblast differentiation, and suppress fibrotic markers such as type 1 collagen, resulting in attenuated fibrosis and adverse extracellular remodeling in the heart.[40,41]

HEART FAILURE WITH PRESERVED EJECTION FRACTION WITH ATRIAL FIBRILLATION AND SODIUM-GLUCOSE COTRANSPORTER 2 INHIBITORS

As mentioned previously, AF is the most common arrhythmia in patients with HFPEF and is an independent prognostic factor for morbidity.

A meta-analysis by Pandey et al.,[52] revealed that these agents reduced the rate of AF events in analyses of adverse event reporting from randomized controlled trials. DAPA-AF and EMPA-AF are two ongoing randomized trials, which will quantify the effects of SGLT2i on atrial fibrillation burden.[53,54]

SODIUM-GLUCOSE COTRANSPORTER 2 INHIBITORS AND PERIPHERAL VASCULAR DISEASE

As per observational studies, and meta-analyses; the safety and effectiveness of SGLT2i on PVD is still inconclusive. AS per the findings of CANVAS program[55] use of canagliflozin resulted in excess amputation rates. Preliminary evidence from observational research suggested that patients with PAD may even benefit from SGLT2 inhibitor treatment due to lower observed heart failure hospitalization rates.[56] A sub-analysis of EMPA-REG OUTCOME trial showed beneficial effects of empagliflozin in patients with type 2 diabetes mellitus (T2DM) and peripheral artery disease (PAD). There was reduction in mortality, and HF hospitalization, and progression of renal disease.[57] SGLT2i were associated with lower risks of CHF and adverse lower limb events compared with DPP4i among patients with T2DM and PAD.[58]

CONCLUSION

The SGLT2i have already been proven treatment for HF with reduced EF, but after the results of EMPEROR-Preserved and DELIVER trials their use has been consolidated for management of patients with HFpEF. With their pleiotropic effects they have benefits in patients with comorbidities of AF and PAD with reduction of mortality and HF hospitalizations.

REFERENCES

1. Januzzi JR JL, Mann Douglas L. Heart Failure. Braunwald's, 12th edition. Philadelphia: Elsevier; 2022.
2. Pandey A, Omar W, Ayers C, et al. Sex and race differences in lifetime risk of heart failure with preserved ejection fraction and heart failure with reduced ejection fraction. Circulation. 2018;137:1814-23.
3. Dunlay SM, Roger VL, Redfield MM. Epidemiology of heart failure with preserved ejection fraction. Nat Rev Cardiol. 2017;14(10):591-602.
4. Ho JE, Enserro D, Brouwers FP, et al. Predicting heart failure with preserved and reduced ejection fraction: the international collaboration on heart failure subtypes. Circ Heart Fail. 2016;9:e003116.
5. Selvaraj S, Myhre PL, Vaduganathan M, et al. Application of diagnostic algorithms for heart failure with preserved ejection fraction to the community. JACC Heart Fail. 2020;8(8):640-53.
6. McDonagh TA, Metra M, Adamo M, et al. ESC Scientific Document Group, 2023 Focused Update of the 2021 ESC Guidelines for the diagnosis and treatment of acute and chronic heart failure: Developed by the task force for the diagnosis and treatment of acute and chronic heart failure of the European Society of Cardiology (ESC) With the special contribution of the Heart Failure Association (HFA) of the ESC. Eur Heart J. 2023;44(37): 3627-39.
7. Zile MR, Baicu CF, Gaasch WH. Diastolic heart failure—abnormalities in active relaxation and passive stiffness of the left ventricle. N Engl J Med. 2004;350: 1953-9.
8. F Simmonds SJ, Cuijpers I, Heymans S, et al. Cellular and Molecular Differences between HFpEF and HFrEF: A Step Ahead in an Improved Pathological Understanding. Cells. 2020;9(1):242.
9. Henry JA, Couch LS, Rider OJ. Myocardial Metabolism in Heart Failure with Preserved Ejection Fraction. J Clin Med. 2024;13(5):1195.
10. Zile MR, Baicu CF, Ikonomidis JS, et al. Myocardial stiffness in patients with heart failure and a preserved ejection fraction: contributions of collagen and titin. Circulation. 2015;131:1247-59.
11. Joshi SS, Singh T, Newby DE, et al. Sodium- glucose cotransporter 2 inhibitor therapy: mechanisms of action in heart failure. Heart. 2021;107:1032-8.

12. Zinman B, Wanner C, Lachin JM, et al. Empagliflozin, cardiovascular outcomes, and mortality in type 2 diabetes. N Engl J Med. 2015;373(22):2117-28.
13. Neal B, Perkovic V, Mahaffey KW. Canagliflozin and cardiovascular and renal events in type 2 diabetes. N Engl J Med. 2017;377(7):644-57.
14. Wiviott SD, Raz I, Bonaca MP. Dapagliflozin and cardiovascular outcomes in type 2 diabetes. N Engl J Med. 2019; 380:347-57.
15. Cannon CP, Pratley R, Dagogo-Jack S. Cardiovascular outcomes with ertugliflozin in type 2 diabetes. N Engl J Med. 2020;383(15):1425-35.
16. McMurray JJV, Solomon SD, Inzucchi SE, et al. Dapagliflozin in patients with heart failure and reduced ejection fraction. N Engl J Med. 2019;381(21):1995-2008.
17. Packer M, Anker SD, Butler J, et al. Cardiovascular and renal outcomes with empagliflozin in heart failure. N Engl J Med. 2020;383(15):1413-24.
18. Heerspink HJL, Stefánsson BV, Correa-Rotter R, et al. Dapagliflozin in patients with chronic kidney disease. N Engl J Med. 2020;383(15):1436-46.
19. Mahaffey KW, Jardine MJ, Bompoint S, et al. Canagliflozin and cardiovascular and renal outcomes in type 2 diabetes mellitus and chronic kidney disease in primary and secondary cardiovascular prevention groups. Circulation. 2019;140(9):739-50.
20. Bhatt DL, Szarek M, Pitt B, et al. Sotagliflozin in patients with diabetes and chronic kidney disease. N Engl J Med. 2021;384(2):129-39.
21. Bhatt DL, Szarek M, Steg PG, et al. Sotagliflozin in patients with diabetes and recent worsening heart failure. N Engl J Med. 2021;384(2):117-28.
22. Voors AA, Angermann CE, Teerlink JR, et al. The SGLT2 inhibitor empagliflozin in patients hospitalized for acute heart failure: a multinational randomized trial. Nat Med. 2022;28(3):568-74.
23. Solomon SD, McMurray JJV, Claggett B, et al. Dapagliflozin in Heart Failure with Mildly Reduced or Preserved Ejection Fraction. N Engl J Med. 2022;387:1089-98.
24. Anker SD, Butler J, Filippatos G, et al. Empagliflozin in heart failure with a preserved ejection fraction. N Engl J Med. 2021;385(16):1451-61.
25. Bonora BM, Avogaro A, Fadini GP. Extraglycemic effects of SGLT2 inhibitors: a review of the evidence. Diabetes Metab Syndr Obes. 2020;13:161-74.
26. Baker WL, Buckley LF, Kelly MS, et al. Effects of sodium-glucose cotransporter 2 inhibitors on 24-hours ambulatory blood pressure: a systematic review and meta-analysis. J Am Heart Assoc. 2017;6:e005686.
27. Griffin M, Rao VS, Ivey-Miranda J, et al. Empagliflozin in heart failure. Circulation. 2020;142:1028-39.
28. Masson W, Lavalle-Cobo A, Nogueira JP. Effect of SGLT2-inhibitors on epicardial adipose tissue: a meta-analysis. Cells. 2021;10(8):2150.
29. Tosaki T, Kamiya H, et al. Sodium-glucose cotransporter 2 inhibitors reduce the abdominal visceral fat area and may influence the renal function in patients with type 2 diabetes. Intern Med. 2017;56(6):597-604.
30. Iacobellis G, Ribaudo MC, Zappaterreno A, et al. Relation between epicardial adipose tissue and left ventricular mass. Am J Cardiol. 2004;94(8):1084-7.
31. Iacobellis G, Bianco AC. Epicardial adipose tissue: emerging physiological, pathophysiological and clinical features. Trends Endocrinol Metab. 2011;22:450-7.
32. Ghantous CM, Azrak Z, Hanache S, et al. Differential role of leptin and adiponectin in cardiovascular system. Int J Endocrinol. 2015;2015:1-13.
33. Wu P, Wen W, Li J, et al. Systematic review and meta-analysis of randomized controlled trials on the effect of SGLT2 inhibitor on blood leptin and adiponectin level in patients with type 2 diabetes. Horm Metab Res. 2019;51:487-94.
34. Cherney DZ, Odutayo A, Aronson R, et al. Sodium glucose cotransporter-2 inhibition and cardiorenal protection: JACC review topic of the week. J Am Coll Cardiol. 2019; 74(20):2511-24.
35. Zelniker TA, Braunwald E. Mechanisms of cardiorenal effects of sodium-glucose cotransporter 2 inhibitors: JACC state-of-the-art review. J Am Coll Cardiol. 2020;75(4): 422-34.
36. Maiuri MC, Zalckvar E, Kimchi A, et al. Self-eating and self-killing: crosstalk between autophagy and apoptosis. Nat Rev Mol Cell Biol. 2007;8(9):741-52.
37. Luo G, Jian Z, Zhu Y, et al. Sirt1 promotes autophagy and inhibits apoptosis to protect cardiomyocytes from hypoxic stress. Int J Mol Med. 2019;43(5):2033-43.
38. Packer M. Autophagy stimulation and intracellular sodium reduction as mediators of the cardioprotective effect of sodium–glucose cotransporter 2 inhibitors. Eur J Heart Fail. 2020;22:618-28.
39. Lopaschuk GD, Verma S. Mechanisms of cardiovascular benefits of sodium glucose cotransporter 2 (SGLT2) inhibitors. JACC Basic Transl Sci. 2020;5(6):632-44.
40. Pandey AK, Bhatt DL, Lyon AR, et al. Mechanisms of benefits of sodium-glucose cotransporter 2 inhibitors in heart failure with preserved ejection fraction. Eur Heart J. 2023;44(37):3640-51.
41. Alnuwaysir RIS, Hoes MF, van Veldhuisen DJ, et al. Iron deficiency in heart failure: mechanisms and pathophysiology. J Clin Med. 2021;11(1):125.
42. Packer M. How can sodium–glucose cotransporter 2 inhibitors stimulate erythrocytosis in patients who are iron-deficient? Implications for understanding iron homeostasis in heart failure. Eur J Heart Fail. 2022;24(12): 2287-96.
43. Docherty KF, Welsh P, Verma S, et al. Iron deficiency in heart failure and effect of dapagliflozin: findings from DAPA-HF. Circulation. 2022;146:980-94.
44. Zannad F, Ferreira JP, Butler J, et al. Effect of empagliflozin on circulating proteomics in heart failure: mechanistic insights from the EMPEROR program. Eur Heart J. 2022;43(48):4991-5002.

45. Fuchs Andersen C, Omar M, Glenthøj A, et al. Effects of empagliflozin on erythropoiesis in heart failure: data from the Empire HF trial. Eur J Heart Fail. 2023;25(2):226-34.
46. Mazer CD, Hare GMT, Connelly PW, et al. Effect of empagliflozin on erythropoietin levels, iron stores, and red blood cell morphology in patients with type 2 diabetes mellitus and coronary artery disease. Circulation. 2020; 141:704-7.
47. Luo M, Anderson ME. Mechanisms of altered Ca^{2+} handling in heart failure. Circ Res. 2013;113(6):690-708.
48. Nakamura TY, Iwata Y, Arai Y, et al. Activation of Na^+/H^+ exchanger 1 is sufficient to generate Ca^{2+} signals that induce cardiac hypertrophy and heart failure. Circ Res. 2008;103:891-9.
49. Chung YJ, Park KC, Tokar S, et al. SGLT2 inhibitors and the cardiac Na^+/H^+ exchanger-1: the plot thickens. Cardiovasc Res. 2021;117: 2702-4.
50. Theofilis P, Sagris M, Oikonomou E, et al. Anti-inflammatory potential of SGLT2 inhibitors: a systematic review and meta-analysis of preclinical studies in rodents. Eur Heart J. 2022;43:2683.
51. Shim CY, Seo J, Cho I, et al. Randomized, controlled trial to evaluate the effect of dapagliflozin on left ventricular diastolic function in patients with type 2 diabetes mellitus. Circulation. 2021;143:510-2.
52. Pandey AK, Okaj I, Kaur H, et al. Sodium-glucose cotransporter inhibitors and atrial fibrillation: a systematic review and meta-analysis of randomized controlled trials. J Am Heart Assoc. 2021;10:e022222.
53. ClinicalTrials.gov. Use of Dapagliflozin to Reduce Burden of Atrial Fibrillation in Patients Undergoing Catheter Ablation of Symptomatic Atrial Fibrillation (DAPA-AF). NCT04792190. [online] Available from https://ctv.veeva.com/study/use-of-dapagliflozin-to-reduce-burden-of-atrial-fibrillation-in-patients-undergoing-catheter-ablatio [Last accessed January, 2025].
54. ClinicalTrials.gov. Empagliflozin and Atrial Fibrillation Treatment (EMPA-AF). NCT04583813. [online] Available from https://clinicaltrials.gov/ct2/show/NCT04583813 [Last accessed January, 2025].
55. Figtree GA, Rådholm K, et al. Effects of canagliflozin on heart failure outcomes associated with preserved and reduced ejection fraction in type 2 diabetes mellitus. Circulation. 2019;139(22):2591-3.
56. Marchiori E, Rodionov RN, Peters F, et al. SGLT2 Inhibitors and Peripheral Vascular Events: A Review of the Literature. Heart Fail Clin. 2022;18(4):609-23.
57. Verma S, Mazer CD, Al-Omran M, et al. Cardiovascular outcomes and safety of empagliflozin in patients with type 2 diabetes mellitus and peripheral artery disease: a subanalysis of EMPA-REG outcome. Circulation. 2018;137(4):405-7.
58. Lee HF, Chen SW, Liu JR, et al. Major adverse cardiovascular and limb events in patients with diabetes and concomitant peripheral artery disease treated with sodium glucose cotransporter 2 inhibitor versus dipeptidyl peptidase-4 inhibitor. Cardiovasc Diabetol. 2020;19(1): 160.

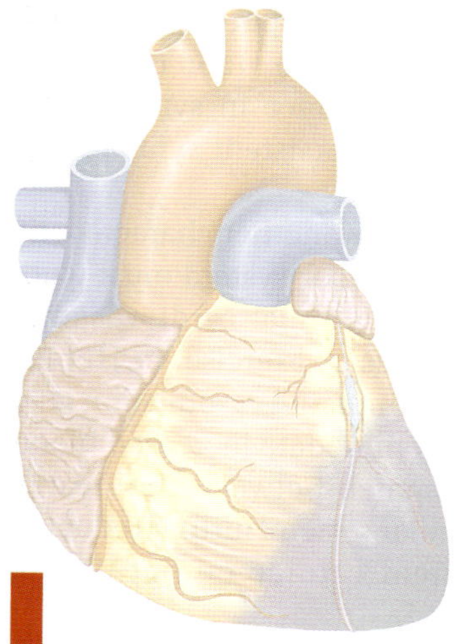

Lower Heart Rate Associated with Lower All-cause Mortality in HFpEF

Shraddha Ranjan, Kartikeya Bhargava

INTRODUCTION

The global prevalence of HF is projected to be 1–3% of the total population, amounting to an estimated 56.2 million people in 2019. In India, the incidence of HF is estimated to be between 0.5 and 1.7 cases per 1,000 persons, with 492,000 to 1.8 million new cases reported annually.[1-3] Patients with HFrEF respond well to typical pharmacological therapy regimens and have a better prognosis now. Patients with HFpEF have a reported 5-year survival rate of as low as 65%, and they have not been shown to respond well to typical pharmacological therapies.[4-6] This chapter aims to discuss HEpEF and its correlation with HR control.

PATHOPHYSIOLOGY

HFpEF refers to a group of disorders that can cause elevated left atrial pressures and clinical symptoms of HF when LVEF is ≥50%. Formerly known as "diastolic HF", this term is now acknowledged to be inaccurate because abnormalities in HFpEF also encompass structural and functional changes in the right side of the heart, lungs, blood vessels, metabolic processes, skeletal muscle, kidney, and liver in addition to diastolic function. HFpEF was initially thought to be a phenotype caused by increasing pressure load and subsequent eccentric ventricular hypertrophy, which resulted in diastolic abnormalities and myocardial restructuring.[7] Nevertheless, many normotensive patients can present with HFpEF, thus questioning this hypothesis. Therefore, a new theory has emerged suggesting that various pathophysiological mechanisms, such as microvascular inflammation, interstitial fibrosis, modified cardiomyocyte intracellular calcium cycling, and modified myofilament biochemical properties leading to increased myocardial stiffness.[8] These are usually influenced by frequent HFpEF comorbidities such hypertension, obesity, and diabetes. HFpEF is probably caused by many biochemical pathways, each with its own set of symptoms that require different treatments.[9-11] Identifying HFpEF phenotypes with distinct and therapeutically relevant pathophysiology is a significant focus of ongoing research in HFpEF.

INFLUENCE OF HEART RATE IN HEMODYNAMICS OF HFpEF

The hallmark of HFpEF is diastolic dysfunction, characterized by stiffening of the left ventricle and impaired filling during diastole. When the HR increases, diastolic filling time shortens, which worsens the problem in HFpEF. Normally, the heart compensates for shorter filling time during tachycardia by enhancing diastolic suction to draw more blood into the ventricles. However, this mechanism is impaired in HFpEF, where LV relaxation is delayed and ventricular stiffness is increased. As a result, higher HRs further reduce diastolic filling, contributing to elevated left atrial pressure and pulmonary congestion, worsening symptoms like dyspnea.

The effects of stimulation frequency on myocardial contraction and relaxation have been well characterized in isolated human myocardium. Isometrically contracting normal myocardium displays an increase in systolic force up to 130–150/min, above which the force declines.

As frequency increases, the relaxation rate also increases. When the diastolic interval becomes so short, the relaxation cannot be completed, which becomes more of a problem in already existing diastolic failure.[12] There is limited in vivo information about how isolated increases in HR, usually produced by atrial pacing, affect contraction–relaxation dynamics in normal hearts. Findings from animal studies are that higher HRs reduce left ventricular (LV) end-diastolic pressure and accelerate contraction and relaxation, reflected in a higher dP/dt and a shortened τ (time constant of isovolumic pressure decline).[13] Less well recognized is the fact that LV diastolic and systolic dimensions progressively decrease at higher HRs. At extremely high HRs, this leads to stroke volumes that approach zero, a physiological response commonly used during transcatheter aortic valve replacement procedures.

The hemodynamic effects of increasing HR to 120/min by atrial pacing in patients with HFpEF have been reported.[14] Compared with resting HR, LV end-diastolic pressure strikingly decreased (from 17 to 8 mm Hg) at 120/min while end-diastolic, end-systolic, and stroke volumes all declined. Compared with control subjects, as HR increased the rise in dP/dt was blunted, but shortening of τ was preserved. Given the critical contribution of diastole to ventricular filling and coronary perfusion, reduction of HR, with a view to prolonging diastole, especially in atrial fibrillation (AF), has been advocated as a therapeutic strategy to mitigate symptoms in HFpEF and has been endorsed by guideline. However, increased HR is the major physiological contributor that raises the cardiac output necessary to meet the metabolic demands of exercise, the capacity for which is reduced in both HFpEF and HFrEF. Because of these conflicting mechanisms, it is crucial to optimize and individualize the HR in these patients.

Chronotropic incompetence (the inability of the heart to adequately increase its rate during physical activity) is a common feature in these patients. There is inability to increase HR during exercise limiting the cardiac output. This, coupled with impaired stroke volume reserve because of HFpEF, further exacerbates the symptoms of fatigue and dyspnea during physical activity.[15,16] Chronotropic incompetence in HFpEF is mostly because of autonomic dysfunction. There is sympathetic dysfunction causing reduced responsiveness to β-adrenergic stimulation (which normally increases HR). This limits the heart's ability to increase its rate during exertion. Adjunctively, there is parasympathetic dysfunction also which causes impaired parasympathetic withdrawal during exercise. The withdrawal of parasympathetic activity normally helps to accelerate the HR. As a result, the HR increases slowly and inadequately during activity, causing reduced cardiac output and contributing to dyspnea and fatigue. Slow HR recovery is associated with poor outcomes in HFpEF and indicates an imbalance in sympathetic and parasympathetic tone, with persistent sympathetic overactivity.

Ventricular–arterial stiffening is another characteristic of HFpEF. The heart and the vascular system must work together efficiently to maintain normal cardiovascular function, especially during stress or exercise. In HFpEF, increased arterial stiffness and impaired vasodilation lead to an inability to properly accommodate increased blood flow. This worsens the mismatch between the heart's pumping ability and the vascular system, further reducing the heart's ability to augment cardiac output during exercise.[17,18]

PHARMACOLOGICAL THERAPY AND EVIDENCE

Since pathophysiology of HFpEF is still being understood, the management principles are also in a process of development. Guidelines now recommend that ARNI and SGLT2 inhibitors should be initiated in all HFpEF patients without contraindications. MRA may be beneficial in some HFpEF subsets with close monitoring of potassium and renal function. However, the role of rate-limiting drugs such as beta-blockers, calcium channel blockers (CCBs), or ivabradine is still not clear in HFpEF.[19]

Beta-blockers in HFpEF

In the E:LANDD study (Effects of Long-term Administration of Nebivolol on the Clinical Symptoms, Exercise Capacity, and Left Ventricular Function of Patients With Diastolic Dysfunction) which assessed the effect of nebivolol on clinical symptoms and exercise capacity in patients with diastolic dysfunction, β-blocker use was associated with a trend toward higher levels of natriuretic peptides.[20] Prolonged diastolic filling increases ventricular volumes and pressures, thus raising the ventricular load that in turn increases myocardial wall stress and provides an explanation for the elevated natriuretic peptide levels in patients receiving β-blockers in population studies.[21] Higher N-terminal-prohormone brain natriuretic peptide (NT-proBNP) levels were also reported in the CIBIS-ELD study (Cardiac Insufficiency Bisoprolol Study in Elderly) which evaluated the tolerability of β-blocker uptitration in HFpEF.[22] In addition to higher natriuretic peptide levels, neither study demonstrated any benefits of β-blockers. Finally, in the SWEDIC (Swedish Doppler-echocardiographic Study) echocardiographic study of patients with diastolic dysfunction randomized

TABLE 1: Legend to be provided.[29-35]

Trial/Study	*Drug used*	*Conclusion*
SENIORS Trial (2005)	Nebivolol	No definite benefit in composite outcome of all-cause mortality and cardiovascular hospitalizations in elderly patients
J-DHF Trial (2013)	Carvedilol	No significant reduction in the primary endpoint of all-cause mortality and hospitalization for cardiovascular causes
TOPCAT Trial (subanalysis, 2014)	β-blockers	β-blocker use was associated with no benefit and showed worse outcomes in terms of exercise capacity and overall quality of life
Hong Kong Heart Failure Registry (2017)	β-blockers	No significant reduction in mortality or HF hospitalizations in HFpEF patients and use was also associated with worsened exercise capacity
Swedish Heart Failure Registry (2011–2018)	β-blockers	No reduction in all-cause mortality or hospitalizations
PEP-CHF Trial (2006)	Primarily designed to test perindopril but many patients were on CCBs	No clear evidence that CCBs significantly reduced mortality or HF hospitalizations in HFpEF patients
REAL-WORLD STUDY (2017)	Calcium channel blockers	CCB therapy did not significantly alter CV outcomes, but it helped control hypertension and HR in patients with atrial fibrillation
EDIFY	Ivabradine	Did not prove to be improving E/e′ ratio, walk distance, or NT-proBNP levels

to carvedilol or placebo, BNP levels were higher with carvedilol, and the authors reported an unexpected worsening in HF symptoms.[23] Taken together, these studies raise the possibility that β-blockers exacerbate HFpEF. However, worse outcomes were not seen in the only two randomized, controlled, long-term trials of β-blockers in HFpEF (SENIORS and J-DHF). Recent trial REDUCE-AMI has shown that among patients with acute myocardial infarction who had a preserved LV ejection fraction (≥50%), long-term beta-blocker treatment did not lead to a lower risk of the composite primary end point of death from any cause than no beta-blocker use. The trials on beta blockers in HFpEF are summarized in **Table 1**.

Calcium Channel Blockers in HFpEF

These drugs are primarily used to manage hypertension and HR control, especially in patients with AF. Unlike in HFrEF, their use is not restricted due to negative inotropic effects and CCBs can be useful in specific situations in HFpEF. However, there is limited direct evidence that CCBs improve mortality or reduce HF hospitalizations in HFpEF, but they are beneficial in managing high blood pressure, which is a key risk factor **(Table 1)**.

Nondihydropyridine CCBs like diltiazem and verapamil are often used to control HR in HFpEF patients with AF. They slow down the HR by blocking calcium channels in the AV node, reducing the rapid ventricular response often seen in AF. These CCBs can be beneficial in managing symptoms of AF in HFpEF, especially when β-blockers are not well tolerated.

Ivabradine in HFpEF

Ivabradine has little in the way of cardiovascular effects other than HR lowering. The functional effects of selective HR lowering with ivabradine in patients with HFpEF were evaluated in two studies that showed contradictory results. The first found an improvement in functional capacity while the second demonstrated a reduction in exercise capacity.[24,25] The only randomized, placebo-controlled, long-term outcome trial of ivabradine in HFpEF, the EDIFY (Preserved Left Ventricular Ejection Fraction Chronic HF with Ivabradine Study), enrolled 179 patients with resting HRs above 70 bpm. An HR reduction of 8 per minutes failed to improve E/e′ ratio, walk distance, or NT-proBNP levels in patients with HFpEF.[26] The SHIFT trial primarily focused on HFrEF, but subgroup analyses have explored whether ivabradine's benefits might extend to patients with preserved ejection fraction, but with negative results.

CONCLUSION

The complex pathophysiology of HFpEF involves multiple factors beyond HR and that conundrum may not be addressed by HR reduction alone. Even in patients of post MI, one of the compelling indications of beta blockers, a recent trial (REDUCE-AMI) has shown no benefit if ejection fraction is preserved.[27] Nonetheless, there are selected indications for which pharmacological HR lowering is likely beneficial, including protection from excessive ventricular rates in AF, prophylaxis of tachyarrhythmias and symptomatic treatment of effort angina, albeit with uncertain effects on long-term outcomes. There also have been concerns about β-blocker safety in patients of HFpEF. However, a recent DELIVER trial subanalysis confirmed that its use was not associated with a higher risk of worsening HF or cardiovascular death.[28] The role of β-blockers in CV disease with normal or near-normal ejection fraction is getting limited and utmost care should be taken to avoid oversuppressing HR which may worsen exercise intolerance and quality of life in HFpEF patients. A recent quote in an article rightly states "β-blockers in HFpEF: Finding a role is easy... finding the evidence, Not So Much"

REFERENCES

1. Dassanayaka S, Jones SP. Recent Developments in Heart Failure. Circ Res. 2015;117(7):e58-63.
2. Khan MS, Shahid I, Bennis A, et al. Global epidemiology of heart failure. Nat Rev Cardiol. 2024;21(10):717-34.
3. Martinez-Amezcua P, Haque W, Khera R, et al. The Upcoming Epidemic of Heart Failure in South Asia. Circ Heart Fail. 2020;13(10):e007218.
4. Inamdar AA, Inamdar AC. Heart Failure: Diagnosis, Management and Utilization. J Clin Med. 2016;5(7):62.
5. Harper AR, Patel HC, Lyon AR. Heart failure with preserved ejection fraction. Clin Med (Lond). 2018;18(Suppl 2): s24-s9.
6. Omote K, Verbrugge FH, Sorimachi H, et al. Central haemodynamic abnormalities and outcome in patients with unexplained dyspnoea. Eur J Heart Fail. 2023;25(2): 185-96.
7. Borlaug BA. The pathophysiology of heart failure with preserved ejection fraction. Nat Rev Cardiol. 2014;11(9): 507-15.
8. Gevaert AB, Boen JRA, Segers VF, et al. Heart Failure With Preserved Ejection Fraction: A Review of Cardiac and Noncardiac Pathophysiology. Front Physiol 2019;10:638.
9. Shah SJ, Borlaug BA, Kitzman DW, et al. Research Priorities for Heart Failure With Preserved Ejection Fraction: National Heart, Lung, and Blood Institute Working Group Summary. Circulation. 2020;141(12):1001-26.
10. Paulus WJ, Zile MR. From Systemic Inflammation to Myocardial Fibrosis: The Heart Failure With Preserved Ejection Fraction Paradigm Revisited. Circulation Research. 2021;128(10):1451-67.
11. Shah SJ, Butler J, Shah SH, et al. Accelerating therapeutic discoveries for heart failure: a new public-private partnership. Nat Rev Drug Discov. 2022;21(11):781-2.
12. Runte KE, Bell SP, Selby DE, et al. Relaxation and the Role of Calcium in Isolated Contracting Myocardium From Patients With Hypertensive Heart Disease and Heart Failure With Preserved Ejection Fraction. Circ Heart Fail. 2017;10(8):e004311.
13. Karliner JS, Lewinter MM, Mahler F, et al. Pharmacologic and Hemodynamic Influences on the Rate of Isovolumic Left Ventricular Relaxation in the Normal Conscious Dog. J Clin Invest. 19771;60(3):511-21.
14. Wachter R, Schmidt-Schweda S, Westermann D, et al. Blunted frequency-dependent upregulation of cardiac output is related to impaired relaxation in diastolic heart failure. Eur Heart J. 2009;30(24):3027-36.
15. Duncker DJ, Bache RJ. Regulation of Coronary Blood Flow During Exercise. Physiol Rev. 2008;88(3):1009-86.
16. Borlaug BA, Melenovsky V, Russell SD, et al. Impaired Chronotropic and Vasodilator Reserves Limit Exercise Capacity in Patients With Heart Failure and a Preserved Ejection Fraction. Circulation. 2006;114(20):2138-47.
17. Pfeffer MA, Shah AM, Borlaug BA. Heart Failure With Preserved Ejection Fraction In Perspective. Circulation Research. 2019;124(11):1598-617.
18. Lam CSP, Roger VL, Rodeheffer RJ, et al. Cardiac Structure and Ventricular–Vascular Function in Persons With Heart Failure and Preserved Ejection Fraction From Olmsted County, Minnesota. Circulation. 2007;115(15):1982-90.
19. 2023 ACC Expert Consensus Decision Pathway on Management of Heart Failure With Preserved Ejection Fraction: A Report of the American College of Cardiology Solution Set Oversight Committee. J Am Coll Cardiol. 2023;81(18):1835-78.
20. Conraads VM, Metra M, Kamp O, et al. Effects of the long-term administration of nebivolol on the clinical symptoms, exercise capacity, and left ventricular function of patients with diastolic dysfunction: results of the ELANDD study. Eur J Heart Fail. 2012;14(2):219-25.
21. Meyer M, LeWinter MM. Heart Rate and Heart Failure With Preserved Ejection Fraction: Time to Slow β-Blocker Use? Circ Heart Fail. 2019;12(8):e006213.
22. Luchner A, Burnett JC, Jougasaki M, et al. Augmentation of the cardiac natriuretic peptides by beta-receptor antagonism: evidence from a population-based study. J Am Coll Cardiol. 1998;32(7):1839-44.
23. Edelmann F, Musial-Bright L, Gelbrich G, et al. Tolerability and Feasibility of Beta-Blocker Titration in HFpEF Versus HFrEF. JACC Heart Fail. 2016;4(2):140-9.
24. Kosmala W, Holland DJ, Rojek A, et al. Effect of If-Channel Inhibition on Hemodynamic Status and Exercise Tolerance in Heart Failure With Preserved Ejection Fraction. J Am Coll Cardiol. 2013;62(15):1330-8.
25. Pal N, Sivaswamy N, Mahmod M, et al. Effect of Selective Heart Rate Slowing in Heart Failure With Preserved Ejection Fraction. Circulation. 2015;132(18):1719-25.
26. Komajda M, Isnard R, Cohen-Solal A, et al. Effect of ivabradine in patients with heart failure with preserved ejection fraction: the EDIFY randomized placebo-controlled trial. Eur J Heart Fail. 2017;19(11):1495-503.
27. Troels Y, Bertil L, Katarina M, et al. Beta-Blockers after Myocardial Infarction and Preserved Ejection Fraction for

the REDUCE-AMI Investigators. N Engl J Med. 2024;390: 1372-81.
28. Peikert A, Bart B, B, Vaduganathan M, et al. Contemporary Use and Implications of Beta-Blockers in Patients With HFmrEF or HFpEF: The DELIVER Trial. JACC Heart Fail. 2024;12(4):631-44.
29. Flather MD, Shibata MC, Coats AJS, et al. Randomized trial to determine the effect of nebivolol on mortality and cardiovascular hospital admission in elderly patients with heart failure (SENIORS). Eur Heart J. 2005;26(3):215-25.
30. Yamamoto K, Origasa H, Hori M, on behalf of the J-DHF Investigators. Effects of carvedilol on heart failure with preserved ejection fraction: the Japanese Diastolic Heart Failure Study (J-DHF). Eur J Heart Fail. 2013;15(1):110-8.
31. Silverman DN, Plante TB, Infeld M, et al. Association of β-Blocker Use With Heart Failure Hospitalizations and Cardiovascular Disease Mortality Among Patients With Heart Failure With a Preserved Ejection Fraction: A Secondary Analysis of the TOPCAT Trial. JAMA Netw Open. 2019;2(12):e1916598.
32. Hai JJ, Chan PH, Huang D, et al. Clinical Characteristics, Management, and Outcomes of Hospitalized Heart Failure in a Chinese Population-The Hong Kong Heart Failure Registry. J Card Fail. 2016;22(8):600-8.
33. Meyer M, Du Fay Lavallaz J, Benson L, et al. Association Between β-Blockers and Outcomes in Heart Failure With Preserved Ejection Fraction: Current Insights From the SwedeHF Registry. J Card Fail. 2021;27(11):1165-74.
34. Cleland JG, Tendera M, Adamus J, et al. Perindopril for elderly people with chronic heart failure: the PEP-CHF study. The PEP investigators. Eur J Heart Fail. 1999;1:211-7.
35. Dalal J, Sawhney JP, Jayagopal PB, et al. A Retrospective, Observational, EMR-Based Real-World Evidence Study to Assess the Incidence of Pedal Edema in Essential Hypertensive Patients on Amlodipine or Cilnidipine. Int J Hypertens. 2022;2022:6868143.

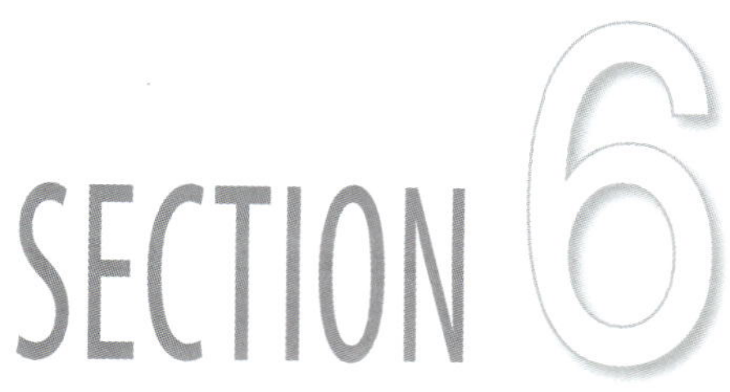

HFpEF and Hypertension

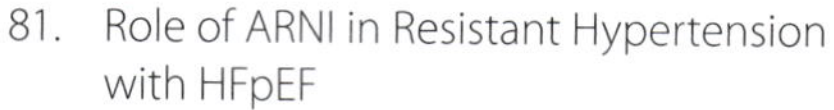

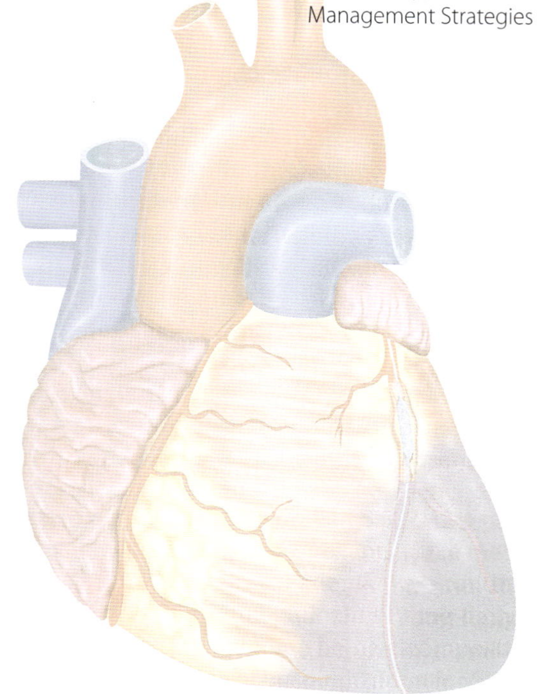

80. Resistant Hypertension and HFpEF: Management Strategies

81. Role of ARNI in Resistant Hypertension with HFpEF

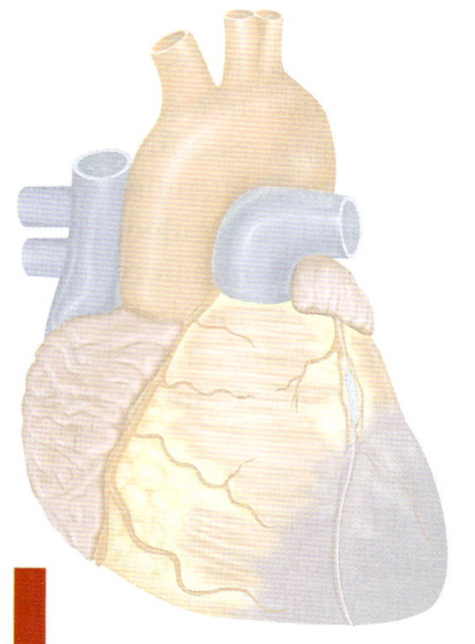

Resistant Hypertension and HFpEF: Management Strategies

Jostol Pinto, A George Koshy

INTRODUCTION

Resistant hypertension (RH) is defined as elevated systemic blood pressure (BP) despite appropriate lifestyle measures and the concurrent use of three classes of antihypertensives at maximally tolerated doses [often including a calcium channel blocker, an angiotensin-converting enzyme inhibitor or angiotensin receptor blocker (ACEi/ARB) and a diuretic] or controlled systemic BP requiring four or more classes of antihypertensives.[1,2] The latter condition was called "controlled RH" in the past. The term "refractory hypertension" (referring to uncontrolled BP despite five or more classes of anti-hypertensive medications) has not been included in current guidelines.[2] The diagnosis of true RH necessitates the exclusion of white-coat hypertension, nonadherence to prescribed medications, and erroneous BP measurement. Sometimes, RH remains undiagnosed as patients are continued on <3 classes of antihypertensives or under-dosed ≥3 classes despite uncontrolled hypertension (suboptimal therapy).

Resistant Hypertension and HFpEF

Heart failure with preserved ejection fraction (HFpEF) is a complex clinical syndrome with impaired ventricular structure or function causing impaired ventricular filling or ejection of blood with a left ventricular ejection fraction of ≥50% with spontaneous or provokable elevated left ventricular filling pressures characterized biochemically by raised natriuretic peptides. Hypertension is the most common phenotype in HFpEF. RH was noted in 15% of patients with HFpEF in the PARAGON-HF trial[3] and 17% of HFpEF patients in the Swedish registry.[4]

RELATED GUIDELINES

The first scientific statement on RH was issued by the American Heart Association (AHA) in 2008 and updated in 2018.[1,5] In 2017, the American College of Cardiology (ACC)/AHA released a guideline for the management of hypertension.[6] More pertinent to our discussion in this chapter, a position paper by the European Society of Hypertension was published in 2021 specifically on hypertension and HFpEF.[7] The latest guidelines on heart failure were published by the European Society of Cardiology (ESC) in 2021 and by the ACC/AHA in 2022. Finally, 2024 witnessed the ESC Guidelines published for the management of "elevated BP" and "hypertension."[2]

RATIONALE OF MANAGING RESISTANT HYPERTENSION WITH/WITHOUT HFpEF

The pathophysiological changes observed in RH include endothelial dysfunction, elevated systemic vascular resistance, and vascular disease (both peripheral and carotid).[8] Patients with RH also have attenuation of the normal nocturnal decline in BP which is called "nondipping"; in fact, some patients may have a paradoxical rise in nocturnal BP, which is then called "reverse dipping." RH is often associated with hyperuricemia, hyper-aldosteronism, and reduced renin levels.[1]

Managing RH is important per se and not only when associated with HFpEF. This is because RH entails increased risks of target organ damage, morbidity, and mortality despite ongoing therapy.[1] In a study involving over 4 lakh, patients, those with RH had a 46%, 32%, 24%, 14%, and 6% increased risk of developing heart failure, end-stage renal disease, a coronary event, a stroke, and death, respectively.[9] Furthermore, patients with RH are more likely to have adverse drug effects due to at least three medications they are taking (by definition) and also secondary causes of hypertension (diagnosed/undiagnosed). Managing RH need not necessarily resolve heart failure. In a study of over 1.18 lakh hypertensive patients, which included over 40,000 patients with RH, control of BP reduced the incidence of stroke and coronary events but not that of heart failure.[10]

MANAGEMENT OF RESISTANT HYPERTENSION AND HFpEF

Management of RH includes maximization of lifestyle interventions, use/modification of long-acting thiazide-like diuretics (chlorthalidone or indapamide), the addition of a mineralocorticoid receptor antagonist (spironolactone or eplerenone), and if BP remains elevated, stepwise addition of antihypertensive drugs with complementary mechanisms of action to lower BP **(Flowchart 1)**.[1] The first step in managing RH, however, is to exclude medication nonadherence as over 50% of patients on antihypertensives show suboptimal compliance.[11,12] Optimization of ongoing medications to maximally tolerated doses is often avoided for fear of drug-induced hypotension or drug-induced renal dysfunction. Furthermore, episodic hypotension due to dehydration or accidental overdosing (e.g., self-dosing of two tablets after missing one dose) often makes the patient and/or physician to limit to lower doses of antihypertensives in the future. Although the defined classes of drugs to treat RH include a CCB, a renin-angiotensin system (RAS) blocker and a diuretic, fine-tuning of each class is essential in this niche group of patients as opposed to the usual treatment of systemic hypertension as discussed below.

Control of RH begins with lifestyle modification which includes adequate sleep, control of obesity, reduction of alcohol intake, limitation of dietary sodium intake, and practice of regular aerobic exercise. Increasing the dose of medications without adhering to positive and sustained lifestyle changes often results in only ill-sustained results. Exercise capacity may be limited in patients with symptomatic HFpEF. Improving the quality of sleep has an important role in controlling RH. Quality of sleep has a greater correlation with RH than does obstructive sleep apnea (OSA). RH associated with OSA is only slightly reduced by continuous positive airway pressure (CPAP) therapy.[13] Before considering modification of antihypertensives, a review of potentially offending drugs must be done and such drugs should be avoided. These include steroids, nonsteroidal anti-inflammatory drugs (NSAIDs), oral contraceptive pills (OCPs), amphetamines, antidepressants, cocaine, cyclosporine, tacrolimus, erythropoietin, and vascular endothelial growth factor (VEGF) inhibitors.[1]

Sometimes diagnosis and management of an overlooked secondary cause of (resistant) hypertension is necessary. Thus, preexisting pheochromocytoma or paraganglioma, coarctation of the aorta, primary aldosteronism, Cushing syndrome, renal artery stenosis, renal parenchymal disease, thyroid disease, primary hyperparathyroidism, acromegaly, and other endocrine abnormalities should be looked for and treated. The management of RH also includes assessment of target organ damage by way of fundoscopy (for hypertensive retinopathy), echocardiography (for hypertensive heart disease and HFpEF), assessing proteinuria (for hypertensive nephropathy), and ankle-brachial index (for peripheral vascular disease). A significant challenge in managing RH is the presence of comorbidities that may include one or more of left ventricular hypertrophy, albuminuria, chronic kidney disease, obesity, and OSA.

Pharmacological therapy forms the mainstay in the management of RH as listed in **Flowchart 1**. As defined, the patient would already have been on a maximally tolerated dosage of a CCB, an ACEI/ARB, and a diuretic. Thus, the crux of further pharmacological treatment includes choosing the right diuretic, modifying the CCB/RAS blocking agent, and/or adding a further class of antihypertensive medication.

- When choosing or replacing the diuretic, it is worth noting that while hydrochlorothiazide does not offer predictable natriuresis below an estimated glomerular filtration rate (eGFR) of <45 mL/min/1.72 m^2, chlorthalidone does induce natriuresis even at an eGFR of 30 mL/min/1.72 m^2, and thiazide-like diuretics do so until 25 mL/min/1.72 m^2. At lower eGFRs, torsemide is recommended over shorter-acting agents such as furosemide or bumetanide.[14] Notably, chlorthalidone and indapamide have the greatest evidence for reducing cardiovascular outcomes.[15,16]
- Before choosing the fourth agent, optimizing the existing CCB and RAS blocker should also be done. For example, azilsartan medoxomil (the eighth ARB that is USFDA approved to treat hypertension) reduces systolic BP by an additional 4–8 mm Hg compared to

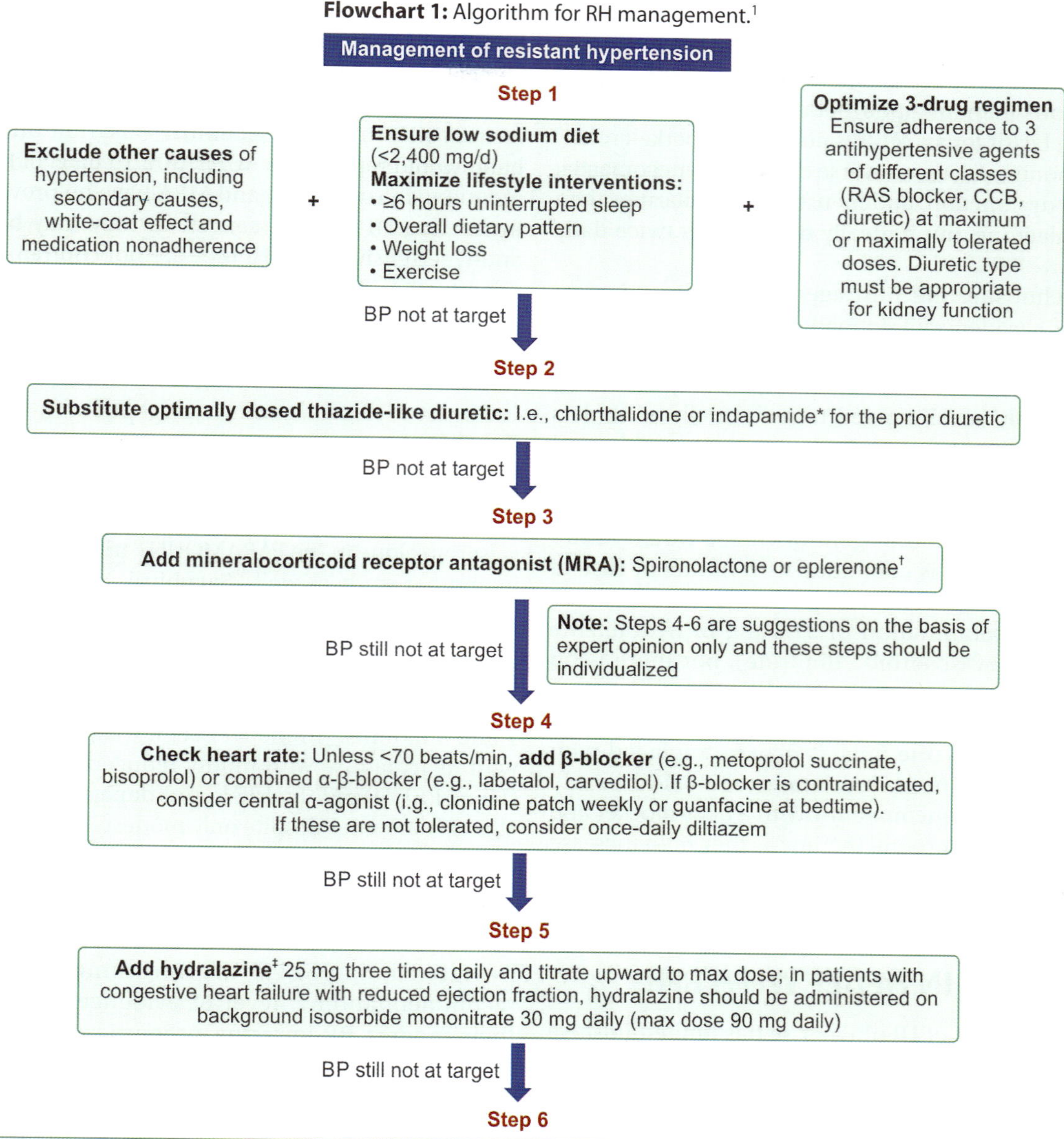

Flowchart 1: Algorithm for RH management.[1]

*Efficacious at an estimated glomerular filtration rate (eGFR) of 30 mL/min/1.72 m^2.
†Cautious if eGFR <30 mL/min/1.72 m^2.
‡Requires use of a beta-blocker and diuretic.
§Requires use of a beta-blocker and loop diuretic.
(RAS: renin–angiotensin system)

valsartan, olmesartan, and ramipril.[17] Among CCBs, long-acting dihydropyridines such as amlodipine and nifedipine are preferred. Furthermore, divided dosing to include a nocturnal dose may also be suggested despite the theoretical 24-hour pharmacodynamic effect with once-daily dosing in this niche group of patients.[18] For example, extended-release nifedipine may be administered as 30 mg twice a day instead of 60 mg in the morning, especially in a patient with "nondipping" or "reverse-dipping" RH.

- When choosing the fourth agent, it is prudent to consider the following: In the absence of volume overload, but presence of low-renin status or salt sensitivity, a mineralocorticoid receptor antagonist (MRA) such as spironolactone or eplerenone is more efficacious than an alpha/beta-blocker. However, the limiting factor for an MRA is potential hyperkalemia.[19] Eplerenone has lesser adverse effects of gynecomastia, erectile dysfunction, and menstrual irregularities than spironolactone, but it ideally necessitates twice daily dosing.

- While choosing the fifth agent ("refractory hypertension"), evidence of sympathetic drive (tachycardia) would suggest adding a beta-blocker or a centrally acting alpha-2 agonist. Clonidine, when prescribed, is preferably administered transdermally as tablets require frequent dosing and entail risk of rebound hypertension if a dose is missed. If BP remains uncontrolled and/or if there is no evidence of sympathetic drive, the agent of choice would rather be hydralazine. It is combined with nitrate in case of heart failure with reduced ejection fraction (HFrEF; fixed-dose combination of 37.5 mg of hydralazine with 20 mg of isosorbide dinitrate), but there is no such recommendation in HFpEF. A dose of over 150 mg/day of hydralazine risks development of lupus. If hydralazine fails, it may be replaced with minoxidil. Of note, hydralazine or minoxidil should always be used concomitantly with a beta-blocker and a diuretic as background therapy as they both increase sympathetic tone and sodium retention.

ROLE OF DRUGS FOR HFrEF (ARNI/MRA/SGLT2I) IN HFpEF WITH RH?

Although treatment of HFpEF per se has limited positive outcome data for guideline-directed medical therapy, controlling BP is often regarded as a central approach to its treatment.[7] With this rationale, the initial approach to treating HFpEF should be the treatment of hypertension, when present, and more importantly so when the hypertension is resistant. This approach could be modified in the future if/when HFpEF-directed specific therapies get established. In line with the hypertension management guidelines mentioned above, the first drug advised to treat hypertension, and by extrapolation to treat HFpEF, would then be an ACEi/ARB (RAS blocker). The modification advised in the 2021 position paper on hypertension and HFpEF quoted earlier[7] would be to incorporate an MRA like spironolactone, a sodium-glucose transport protein 2 inhibitor (SGLT2i) like dapagliflozin or empagliflozin and an angiotensin receptor neprilysin inhibitor (ARNI), which is sacubitril-valsartan; finerenone awaits outcome data. In this modification, MRA would be an add-on medication to the ongoing diuretic (loop/thiazide/thiazide-like) or a stand-alone diuretic depending on the clinical and biochemical circumstance; the SGLT2i would be an add-on medication to the ongoing three drugs to treat RH; the ARNI sacubitril-valsartan on the other hand would replace the ACEi/ARB. To date, of the above-mentioned drugs, ARNI and MRA have no proven benefit in treating HFpEF per se; but as they may be used as antihypertensives for RH, they are not contraindicated in this situation. To summarize, although these three classes of drugs are primarily indicated for the treatment of HFrEF based on trial evidence, their utility in HFpEF does exist when RH coexists considering the rationale above.

Trial Data

Sacubitril-valsartan reduces arterial stiffness more than that by ARBs[20] and also showed to control BP better than valsartan alone in the PARAMOUNT trial at 12 weeks[21] and in another study as well.[3] Sacubitril-valsartan also was a better antihypertensive than olmesartan within 8 weeks of therapy in a Japanese study.[22] Among patients of the PARAGON-HF trial having HFpEF, sacubitril-valsartan was more useful than valsartan alone in treating RH after 1 and 4 months.[3] In the DELIVER trial, 11.5% of patients with heart failure with mildly reduced ejection fraction (HFmrEF)/HFpEF had RH, and dapagliflozin improved clinical outcomes despite only modest reduction in BP.[23]

Guideline Recommendations

In the presence of HFpEF with concomitant systemic hypertension, SGLT2i are recommended (class of recommendation I, level of evidence A) considering their modest BP-lowering properties; however, ARBs and/or MRAs only have a lesser recommendation for reducing heart failure hospitalizations (class of recommendation IIb, level of evidence B).[2] In patients with HFmrEF, hypertension should be treated with heart failure medications also having antihypertensive actions, namely, ACEi/ARB or sacubitril-valsartan (ARNI), beta-blockers (metoprolol succinate/bisoprolol fumarate/carvedilol), MRA, and SGLT2i (class of recommendation I, level of evidence A).[2] Addition of an MRA as the fourth agent to treat RH receives a class of recommendation IIa, level of evidence B. One review article has recommended treating every HFpEF patient with a combination of MRA + sacubitril valsartan/ACEi/ARB.[24]

BEYOND PHARMACOTHERAPY

Device-based therapy tried for persistent RH includes renal nerve ablation/denervation and carotid baroreceptor activation therapy. The latter is also used to treat heart failure and arrhythmias. The failure of renal denervation to control RH in the first ever single-blinded, sham-controlled trial SYMPLICITY HTN-3 has prompted the design of newer catheters and trials and more extensive denervation.[25] However, to date, catheter-based renal denervation still only receives class of recommendation IIb, level of evidence B for treating RH.[2] Some newer therapies awaiting validation include central arteriovenous anastomosis ROX coupler device, ReCor Paradise endovascular ultrasonic renal denervation (USFDA approved on November 7, 2023) and median nerve stimulation that reduces sympathetic outflow by electroacupuncture.[26-28]

Alternative approaches needing further validation studies include yoga, acupuncture, transcendental meditation, device-guided slow-breathing, and isometric handgrip exercise.[1] In fact, a recent meta-analysis showed that isometric handgrip performed three to five times a week for 12 minutes each day lowered BP by 5.2/3.9 mm Hg.[29]

CONCLUSION

Resistant hypertension is a pretreated state by definition; thus, its treatment includes revising therapy, modifying ongoing medications, and adding on newer appropriate classes of medication. Treatment of HFpEF has limited options as of writing this chapter, with the only medication indicated being SGLT2i with a possible recommendation of ARNI in the future; however, any of ARNI, SGLT2i, and/or MRA may be advised if RH coexists as these medications may provide antihypertensive effect at least and treat HFpEF indirectly or directly at best. Nevertheless, CCB + ACEi/ARB + diuretic remains the cornerstone of therapy (as defined); MRA, ARNI, and SGLT2i are treatment options (as discussed).

REFERENCES

1. Carey RM, Calhoun AD, Bakris GL, et al. Resistant hypertension: detection, evaluation, and management: a scientific statement from the American Heart Association. Hypertension. 2018;72:e53-90.
2. McEvoy JW, McCarthy CP, Bruno RM, et al. 2024 ESC guidelines for the management of elevated blood pressure and hypertension: developed by the task force on the management of elevated blood pressure and hypertension of the European Society of Cardiology (ESC) and endorsed by the European Society of Endocrinology (ESE) and the European Stroke Organisation (ESO). Eur Heart J. 2024;45(38):3912-4018.
3. Jackson AM, Jhund PS, Anand IS, et al. Sacubitril-valsartan for resistant hypertension in HFpEF patients. Eur Heart J. 2021;42:3741-52.
4. Jackson AM, Benson L, Savarese G, et al. Apparent treatment-resistant hypertension across the spectrum of heart failure phenotypes in the Swedish HF registry. JACC Heart Fail. 2022;10:380-92.
5. Calhoun DA, Jones D, Textor S, et al. Resistant hypertension: diagnosis, evaluation, and treatment. A scientific statement from the American Heart Association Professional Education Committee of the Council for High Blood Pressure Research. Hypertension. 2008;51:1403-19.
6. Whelton PK, Carey RM, Aronow WS, et al. 2017 ACC/AHA/AAPA/ABC/ACPM/AGS/APhA/ASH/ASPC/NMA/PCNA guideline for the prevention, detection, evaluation, and management of high blood pressure in adults: a report of the American College of Cardiology/American Heart Association Task Force on clinical practice guidelines hypertension. 2018;71:e13-115.
7. Kasiakogias A, Rosei EA, Camafort M, et al. Hypertension and heart failure with preserved ejection fraction: position paper by the European Society of Hypertension. J Hypertens. 2021;39:1522-45.
8. Quinaglia T, Martins LC, Figueiredo VN, et al. Nondipping pattern relates to endothelial dysfunction in patients with uncontrolled resistant hypertension. J Hum Hypertens. 2011;25:656-64.
9. Sim JJ, Bhandari SK, Shi J, et al. Comparative risk of renal, cardiovascular, and mortality outcomes in controlled, uncontrolled resistant, and nonresistant hypertension. Kidney Int. 2015;88:622-32.
10. Egan BM, Kai B, Wagner CS, et al. Blood pressure control provides less cardiovascular protection in adults with than without apparent treatment-resistant hypertension. J Clin Hypertens (Greenwich). 2016;18:817-24.
11. Elliott WJ. What factors contribute to the inadequate control of elevated blood pressure? J Clin Hypertens (Greenwich). 2008;10:20-6.
12. Jung O, Gechter JL, Wunder C, et al. Resistant hypertension? Assessment of adherence by toxicological urine analysis. J Hypertens. 2013;31:766-74.
13. Gottlieb DJ, Punjabi NM, Mehra R, et al. CPAP versus oxygen in obstructive sleep apnea. N Engl J Med. 2014; 370:2276-85.
14. Goodfriend TL, Ball DL, Oelkers W, et al. Torsemide inhibits aldosterone secretion in vitro. Life Sci. 1998;63: PL45-50.
15. Roush GC, Sica DA. Diuretics for hypertension: a review and update. Am J Hypertens. 2016;29:1130-7.
16. DiNicolantonio JJ, Bhutani J, Lavie CJ, et al. Evidence-based diuretics: focus on chlorthalidone and indapamide. Future Cardiol. 2015;11:203-17.
17. Bakris GL, Sica D, Weber M, et al. The comparative effects of azilsartan medoxomil and olmesartan on ambulatory and clinic blood pressure. J Clin Hypertens (Greenwich). 2011; 13:81-8.

18. Sun Y, Yu X, Liu J, et al. Effect of bedtime administration of blood-pressure lowering agents on ambulatory blood pressure monitoring results: a meta-analysis. Cardiol J. 2016;23:473-81.
19. Williams B, MacDonald TM, Morant S, et al. Spironolactone versus placebo, bisoprolol, and doxazosin to determine the optimal treatment for drug-resistant hypertension (PATHWAY-2): a randomised, double-blind, crossover trial. Lancet. 2015;386:2059-68.
20. Schmieder RE, Wagner F, Mayr M, et al. The effect of sacubitril/valsartan compared to olmesartan on cardiovascular remodeling in subjects with essential hypertension: the results of a randomized, double-blind, active-controlled study. Eur Heart J. 2017;38:3308-17.
21. Solomon SD, Zile M, Pieske B, et al. The angiotensin receptor neprilysin inhibitor LCZ696 in heart failure with preserved ejection fraction: a phase 2 double-blind randomised controlled trial. Lancet. 2012;380:1387-95.
22. Rakugi H, Kario K, Yamaguchi M, et al. Efficacy of sacubitril/valsartan versus olmesartan in Japanese patients with essential hypertension: a randomized, double-blind, multicenter study. Hypertens Res. 2022;45:824-33.
23. Ostrominski JW, Vaduganathan M, Selvaraj S, et al. Dapagliflozin and apparent treatment-resistant hypertension in heart failure with mildly reduced or preserved ejection fraction: the DELIVER trial. Circulation. 2023; 148(24):1945-57.
24. Kjeldsen SE, von Lueder TG, Smiseth OA, et al. Medical therapies for heart failure with preserved ejection fraction. Hypertension. 2020;75:23-32.
25. Bhatt DL, Kandzari DE, O'Neill WW, et al. A controlled trial of renal denervation for resistant hypertension. N Engl J Med. 2014;370:1393-401.
26. Lobo MD, Sobotka PA, Stanton A, et al. Central arteriovenous anastomosis for the treatment of patients with uncontrolled hypertension (the ROX CONTROL HTN study): a randomised controlled trial. Lancet. 2015; 385:1634-41.
27. Mabin T, Sapoval M, Cabane V, et al. First experience with endovascular ultrasound renal denervation for the treatment of resistant hypertension. EuroIntervention. 2012;8:57-61.
28. Li P, Tjen-A-Looi SC, Guo ZL, et al. An arcuate-ventrolateral periaqueductal gray reciprocal circuit participates in electroacupuncture cardiovascular inhibition. Auton Neurosci. 2010;158:13-23.
29. Inder JD, Carlson DJ, Dieberg G, et al. Isometric exercise training for blood pressure management: a systematic review and meta-analysis to optimize benefit. Hypertens Res. 2016;39:88-94.

CHAPTER

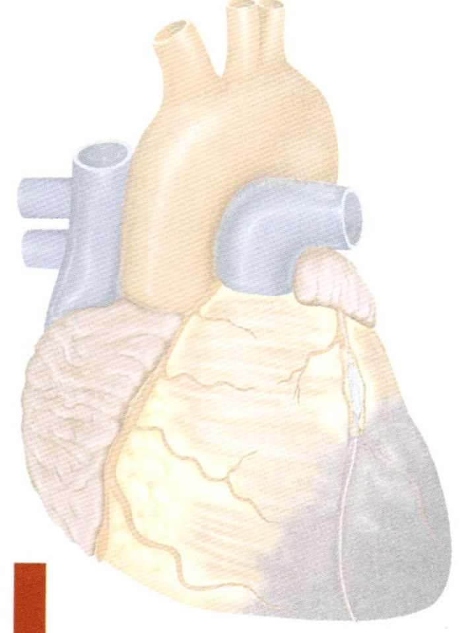

Role of ARNI in Resistant Hypertension with HFpEF

Rohan Patel, Rajiv Passey, Siddhant Passey

INTRODUCTION

Resistant hypertension is defined as failure to achieve target blood pressure (BP) goals despite treatment with optimal or maximal tolerated doses of at least three different classes of antihypertensive drugs (which should include a diuretic).[1] The prevalence of resistant hypertension has increased over the last decade. It is pathophysiologically closely related to heart failure with preserved ejection fraction (HFpEF), i.e., LVEF 50% or more. Resistant hypertension leads to development of left ventricular hypertrophy, impaired ventricular and active atrial relaxation and filling capacities, increased cardiomyocyte passive stiffness, reduced arterial compliance, and abnormal ventricular–arterial coupling, which finally lead to LV diastolic dysfunction and eventually to HFpEF.[2] The large proportion of patients with HFpEF have coexisting resistant hypertension.[3] The management of resistant hypertension and HFpEF represents "unmet need" in the cardiovascular disease.[4]

EFFECT OF ARNI ON RESISTANT HYPERTENSION WITH HFpEF

Sacubitril/valsartan (sac/val) is a combination of neprilysin inhibitor with angiotensin receptor blocker. It is recommended for the treatment of HFrEF to decrease cardiovascular mortality and heart failure hospitalization. Role of ARNI in HFpEF is not well established.[5] RCTs of angiotensin receptor–neprilysin inhibitor (ARNI) have been shown to significantly reduce both systolic and diastolic blood pressure as compared to comparator ACE inhibitors or ARB drugs.[6,7] A reasonable mechanism through which neprilysin inhibition produces a more marked BP reduction is the increased availability of natriuretic peptides (NP) and their binding with guanylate cyclase/cGMP-coupled receptors, which mediate vasodilation and natriuresis and contribute to the inhibition and counterbalance of the renin–angiotensin–aldosterone system (RAAS), the sympathetic nervous system (SNS), endothelin, and vasopressin.[8,9] The BP-lowering effect of ARNI in HFpEF patients was evaluated in the phase II PARAMOUNT (Prospective comparison of ARNI with ARB on Management Of heart failUre with preserved ejection fracTion) trial that randomized 301 participants to receive ARNI titrated to 200 mg twice daily or valsartan titrated to 160 mg twice daily. After 12 weeks of treatment, SBP reduction was significantly greater in the ARNI compared with the valsartan group (29.3 vs. 22.9 mm Hg, respectively), these results persisted at 36 weeks.[10]

A post-hoc analysis of data from the PARAGON-HF (Prospective Comparison of ARNI With ARB Global Outcomes in Heart Failure with Preserved Ejection Fraction) trial examined the effect of ARNI on BP control in HFpEF patients with apparent resistant hypertension [specifically defined as systolic BP (SBP) ≥140 mm Hg or ≥135 mm Hg if diabetic despite treatment with valsartan, a CCB, and a diuretic]. The summary of this analysis is as follows:

- There was a high prevalence of resistant hypertension in HFpEF patients, accounting for 15.2% of the overall population (731 patients). Moreover, 2.8% (135 patients) failed to achieve BP control despite treatment with a mineralocorticoid receptor antagonist (MRA), suggesting "apparent MRA-resistant" hypertension. These proportions might have been even underestimated since patients with SBP >180 mm Hg were excluded from the trial.

- The resistant hypertension had a negative prognostic effect on HFpEF. In fact, the rate of the primary composite outcome (total hospitalizations for HF and death from CV causes) was higher in patients with apparent resistant hypertension [17.3; 95% confidence interval (CI) 15.6–19.1 per 100 person-years], compared with those with controlled SBP (13.4; 95% CI 12.7–14.3 per 100 person-years), with an adjusted rate ratio (RR) of 1.29, 95% CI 1.05–1.58. Patients with apparent resistant hypertension also had a higher risk of the prespecified exploratory composite of CV death, HF hospitalization, myocardial infarction, and stroke. Patients with apparent resistant hypertension had an increased risk of cardiovascular mortality and HF rehospitalization despite lower median N-terminal pro-brain natriuretic peptide (NTproBNP) levels compared with those with controlled BP (744 vs. 962 pg/mL, respectively).
- ARNI appeared to be more effective than valsartan alone in treating resistant hypertension in HFpEF patients. Patients who were treated with ARNI had a mean of 4.8 mm Hg SBP reduction (–7.0 to –2.5 mm Hg) compared with 3.9 mm Hg (–6.6 to –1.3 mm Hg) in the valsartan group. Consistent results were obtained in individuals with apparent MRA-resistant hypertension [–8.8 mm Hg (–14.0 to –3.5 mm Hg) vs. –6.3 (–12.5 to –0.1 mm Hg) in the ARNI and valsartan groups, respectively]. ARNI improved the achievement of SBP control at 16 weeks by 22% compared with valsartan alone [47.9 vs. 34.3%; adjusted odds ratio (OR) 1.78; 95% CI 1.30–2.43]. In patients with apparent MRA resistant hypertension, the proportions were 43.6 vs. 28.4%, respectively, with an adjusted OR of 2.63 (95% CI 1.18–5.89). Although ARNI did not reduce the risk of the primary endpoint in the overall population of the PARAGON trial (RR 0.87; 95% CI 0.75–1.01; $p = 0.06$), its effects on clinical outcomes were not analyzed in the hypertensive subgroups.[11]

In this view, ARNI may represent a rational and viable therapeutic strategy in the management of resistant hypertension in HFpEF patients. The coexistence of resistant hypertension may play an independent role in influencing clinical outcomes in HFpEF, irrespective of pharmacological treatment, comorbidities, and biomarker levels. In this view, a more intensive BP-lowering strategy may effectively contribute to reduce outcomes in patients with HFpEF. However, specifically designed randomized clinical trials are required to support this indication. This relevant proportion of HFpEF patients with hypertension may benefit from ARNI treatment, though this hypothesis needs to be proven. On the other hand, the action of ARNI may be less relevant in patients with different prevalent etiologies of HFpEF, such as diabetes, obesity, renal dysfunction, or amyloidosis.[12]

In patients with resistant hypertension and HFpEF, there is a wide phenotypic heterogeneity that limits the use of a single therapeutic strategy for all patients. The analysis by Jackson et al. highlights favorable effects of ARNI on resistant hypertension in patients with HFpEF. ARNI may have a role in significant reduction of BP in patients with resistant hypertension and HFpEF, which may lead to favorable clinical outcomes.[13]

CONCLUSION

Although ARNI has not been approved for the treatment of resistant hypertension yet, existing post hoc analysis and data are encouraging, which show better BP control with ARNI in patients with resistant hypertension and HFpEF.

REFERENCES

1. Jin CN, Liu M, Sun JP, et al. The prevalence and prognosis of resistant hypertension in patients with heart failure. PLoS One. 2014;9(12):e114958.
2. Tadic M, Cuspidi C, Frydas A, et al. The role of arterial hypertension in development heart failure with preserved ejection fraction: just a risk factor or something more? Heart Fail Rev. 2018;23(5):631-9.
3. Zanchetti A, Cuspidi C, Comarella L, et al. Left ventricular diastolic dysfunction in elderly hypertensives: Results of the APROS-diadys study. J Hypertens. 2007;25(10): 2158-67.
4. Romano S, Idolazzi C, Fava C, et al. Prevalence and comorbidities of resistant hypertension: a collaborative population-based observational study. High Blood Press Cardiovasc Prev. 2018;25(3):295-301.
5. McDonagh TA, Metra M, Adamo M, et al. 2023 Focused Update of the 2021 ESC Guidelines for the diagnosis and treatment of acute and chronic heart failure: Developed by the task force for the diagnosis and treatment of acute and chronic heart failure of the European Society of Cardiology (ESC) With the special contribution of the Heart Failure Association (HFA) of the ESC. Eur Heart J. 2023;44(37):3627-39.
6. McMurray JJ, Packer M, Desai AS, et al. Angiotensin-neprilysin inhibition versus enalapril in heart failure. N Eng J Med. 2014;371(11):993-1004.
7. Solomon SD, McMurray JJ, Anand IS, et al.; PARAGON-HF Investigators and Committees. Angiotensin–neprilysin inhibition in heart failure with preserved ejection fraction. N Eng J Med. 2019;381(17):1609-20.

8. Volpe M, Carnovali M, Mastromarino V. The natriuretic peptides system in the pathophysiology of heart failure: from molecular basis to treatment. Clin Sci. 2016;130(2): 57-77.
9. Bavishi C, Messerli FH, Kadosh B, et al. Role of neprilysin inhibitor combinations in hypertension: insights from hypertension and heart failure trials. Eur Heart J. 2015; 36(30):1967-73.
10. Solomon SD, Zile M, Pieske B, et al.; Prospective comparison of ARNI with ARB on Management Of heart failUre with preserved ejectioN fracTion (PARAMOUNT) Investigators. The angiotensin receptor neprilysin inhibitor LCZ696 in heart failure with preserved ejection fraction: a phase 2 double-blind randomised controlled trial. Lancet. 2012;380(9851): 1387-95.
11. Jackson AM, Jhund PS, Anand IS, et al. Sacubitril-valsartan as a treatment for apparent resistant hypertension in patients with heart failure and preserved ejection fraction. Eur Heart J. 2021;42(36):3741-52.
12. Russo D, Musumeci MB, Volpe M. The neglected issue of cardiac amyloidosis in trials on heart failure with preserved ejection fraction in the elderly. Eur J Heart Fail. 2020;22:1740-1.
13. Volpe M, Gallo G. Sacubitril/valsartan for heart failure with preserved ejection fraction and resistant hypertension: One shot for a double strike? Eur Heart J. 2021; 42(36):3753-5.

SECTION 7

HFpEF and Pediatrics

82. HFpEF in Congenital Cyanotic Heart Diseases
83. Pediatric HFpEF
84. Prevention of HFpEF in Children
85. HFpEF Management in Children

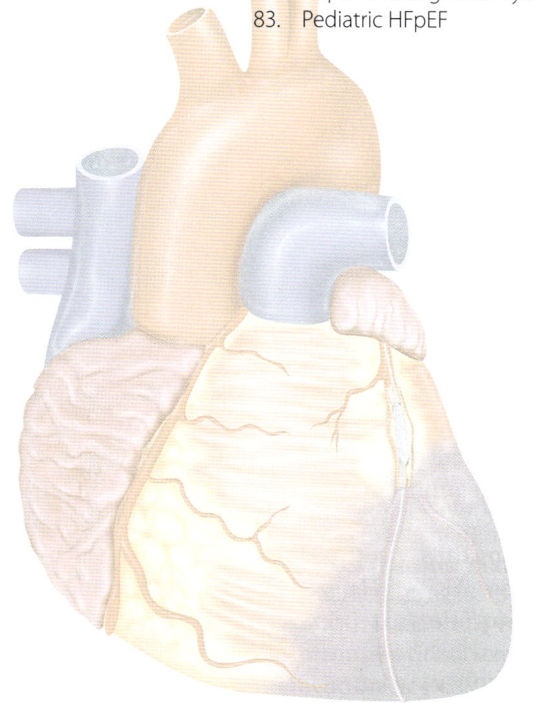

CHAPTER 82

HFpEF in Congenital Cyanotic Heart Diseases

Yasser Sedky, Sonia El-Saiedi

INTRODUCTION

Heart failure (HF) is usually due to impairment of ventricular contraction associated with reduced ejection fraction (EF). However, recently, HF with preserved EF (HFpEF) has become progressively reported in adults, with an incidence of 40–70% of total cases.[1] To date, HFpEF in pediatric patients is not well reported, and most cases of pediatric HFpEF were associated with congenital heart disease (CHD) and postcardiac surgery.[2] HFpEF defined as a left ventricular ejection fraction (LVEF) 50% associated with either elevated natriuretic peptide (NP) levels or other evidence of congestion.[3] The incidence rate of HFpEF is around 27 cases per 10,000 person-years.[4] Diastolic dysfunction (DD) points to functional or structural abnormality of the left ventricle, resulting in impaired filling of the heart. Severe DD can cause congestive HF even with normal systolic function. HFpEF accounts for almost half of the hospitalizations for acute HF in the adult population but the clinical recognition and understanding of HFpEF in children is poor.

DESCRIPTION

The HF is a common cause of morbidity and mortality in CHD, with rising prevalence due to advances in diagnosis and management options. The interplay between genetic factors and acquired postnatal factors in CHD might play a major role in progression to HF. Plasma N-terminal prohormone B-type natriuretic peptide (NT-proBNP) concentration is an HF biomarker in adults and children. Its prognostic value for HF associated cases has been established only in adults. HFpEF has been also reported in pediatric groups, including those with congenital aortic stenosis, hypertrophic cardiomyopathy, and restrictive cardiomyopathy.[5] DD has been reported in children suffering from restrictive cardiomyopathy, representing 5% of pediatric cardiomyopathy cases.[6] Restrictive cardiomyopathies may also be secondary to systemic diseases including infiltrative disease, collagen-vascular diseases. The common mechanism is the increasing myocardial stiffness, which decreases compliance.[6] The natural history of HFpEF differ depending upon the patient's age, sex, race, geographic location, nutritional status, biochemical risk factors, underlying heart disease, and genetic-environmental interaction. Pediatric HFpEF is different than that in adults. Advances in the noninvasive evaluation of the LV diastolic function by strain, and strain rate analysis with speckle-tracking echocardiography, tissue Doppler imaging, and cardiac magnetic resonance imaging have increased awarness of the HFpEF in children. There is limited available data on the epidemiology of HFpEF in pediatrics due to heterogeneous etiologies, and different genetic and biomarker profiles. A study of acute decompensated heart failure (ADHF) in pediatrics across 23 centers in the US showed 6% of 26,294 consecutive ICU admissions had either HFrEF or HFpEF requiring continuous vasoactive or diuretic infusion, respiratory support.[7]

ETIOLOGY

In general, HFpEF in children is a unique phenotype caused by heterogeneous etiologies such as HCM or

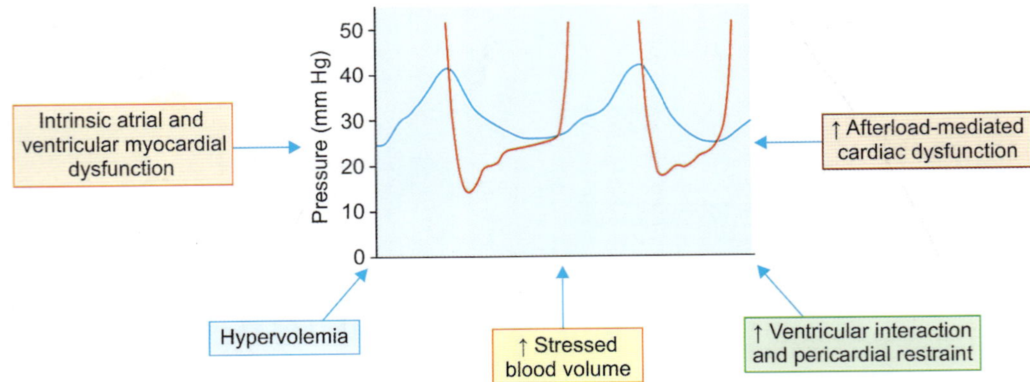

Fig. 1: Mechanisms of hemodynamic congestion in HFpEF increase in pulmonary capillary wedge pressure (blue) and left ventricular end diastolic pressure (red) develop through a variety of pathophysiological perturbations in HFpEF.[30]

RCM, CHD, cancer therapy including radiotherapy and chemotherapy, HIV infection, renal failure, and obesity. The major etiologies of HFpEF in children are complex CHD (53.4%), simple CHD (15.7%), and cardiomyopathies (7.4%).[8] The pathophysiological factors of HFpEF in CHD are multifactorial. They include ventricular fibrosis, pulmonary hypertension, valvular disease, scarring, arrhythmias, and cyanosis. There are five main types of CHD, which leads to DD:

1. Pressure-overload such as aortic stenosis.
2. Volume overload such as mitral regurgitation.
3. Mixed pressure and volume overloads, such as aortic stenosis and regurgitation.
4. Transposition of the great arteries (TGA)
5. Single ventricle CHD, especially after Fontan operation.

The TGA is one of the most common cyanotic CHD in neonates.The pulmonary artery (PA) is connected to the LV, and the aorta is connected to the RV. An arterial switch operation (ASO) is performed in TGA to convert the LV into the systemic ventricle, replacing the RV which was the systemic ventricle initially. The atrial switch[9,10] and later operation (ASO)[11] have had an impact on both survival and quality of life. Impairment of the DD of both LV and RV by TDI and conventional Doppler parameters of DD during the short- to mid-term follow-up of pediatric patients who underwent surgical correction for TGA has been reported.[12-14] In single ventricle, myocardial hypertrophy, fibrosis, and DD often result from multiple, cumulative insults, which include volume loading, pressure loading, chronic hypoxemia, coronary ischemia, chronic upregulation of the renin angiotensin aldosterone system, and chronic under-filling.[15] The Fontan patients with DD and normal EF had clinical evidence of decreased exercise tolerance suggestive of early HFpEF.[16] DD is a progressive phenomenon in patients with single ventricles. Several factors may contribute to this impairment, including chronic deprivation of preload with insufficient ventricular filling and resultant progressive myocardial stiffness **(Fig. 1)**. Alternatively, myocardial fibrosis may be a progressive phenomenon contributing to DD. Amino-terminal procollagen type III, a surrogate marker of fibrosis, is more prevalent with DD in patients with dilated cardiomyopathy.[17] Hypoxemia and volume overload before the Fontan procedure are associated with elevated amino-terminal procollagen type III levels, and preFontan amino-terminal procollagen type III levels correlate significantly with postFontan end-diastolic pressures.[17]

PATHOPHYSIOLOGY AND SYMPTOMS

The HFpEF is characterized by symptoms of HF due to increase in myocardial stiffness. The physiology and cellular mechanism of HFpEF depends on the cause and involves hypertrophy, fibrosis, and myocardial fibrosis also plays a role in DD as it increases ventricular rigidity and compromise the stretching capability of the myofibrils.[18] DD may be symptomless and may only be suspected during a routine imaging. Sometimes, it can cause dyspnea, atypical asthma, and syncope. The clinical signs that may suggest the presence of DD include increased jugular venous pressure, hepatomegaly, edema, and ascites.[6] Poor appetite, fatigue, and infection susceptibility are markers of HF exacerbation.

DIAGNOSIS

The gold standard to detect LV relaxation is cardiac catheterization. A catheter placed into the LV measure simultaneously LV volumes and pressure, pressure-volume loops reflect the filling and contractile properties.[19] Echocardiography is the primary testing modality for diagnosing LVDD in children. Doppler study of the

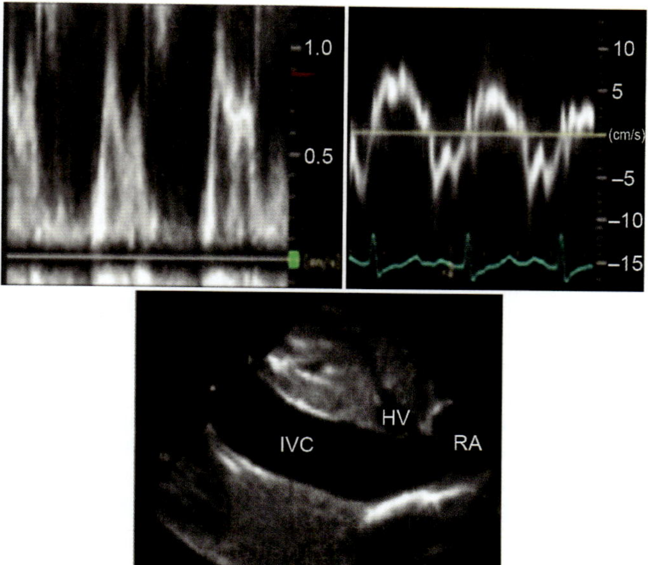

Fig. 2: Elevation in the E/e′ ratio and dilation/loss of collapsibility of the inferior cava.[30]

mitral inflow, there are four phases of diastole: Phase 1—isovolumic relaxation, Phase 2—rapid passive filling (E wave), Phase 3—slow filling and mild stasis, and Phase 4—active filling (A wave) due to atrial contraction. The LV diastolic function is better determined by TDI evaluating the longitudinal movement at the mitral, tricuspid, and septal annulus levels, calculating early (E′) and late diastolic (A′) velocities, respectively **(Fig. 2)**. TDI-based myocardial deformation imaging evaluate LV stiffness and LVDD in children with CHD. Lateral E:E′/end-diastolic volume (EDV) appeared to correlate well with LVEDP obtained by simultaneous cardiac catheterization in pediatric patients after Fontan surgery **(Table 1)**.[20] Strain imaging aims to provide a high-resolution, real-time measure of LV contractility, and relaxation in children with normal loading conditions.[21] Strain imaging can be used to distinguish between different diastolic dysfunctions. LA strain (LAS) has recently been proposed as a novel technique to be used in clinical practice. CMR provides important information to assess the etiology of HFpEF. Chronic hypoxemia, altered loading conditions, and genetic predisposition have been linked to diffuse myocardial fibrosis in CHD.[22] The application of CMR is crucial in evaluating DD in children with CHD, such as TGA and single ventricle.

TREATMENT

The treatment for HFpEF in children is extrapolated from adult clinical trials and is predominantly used for symptomatic relief. Diuretics are commonly used to relieve congestion in HFpEF. B-blockers are helpful by decreasing heart rate and increasing diastolic duration, and reducing myocardial oxygen consumption.[23] However, spironolactone may be effective in HFpEF treatment.[24] Effect of spironolactone may be due to the afterload reducing impact, changes in serum electrolytes (potassium-sparing effect), reduction in LV mass, and the antifibrotic action on the myocardium.[24] Milrinone is a phosphodiesterase-3 inhibitor, that increases cAMP, enhances myocardial contractility, promotes myocardial relaxation, and increases cardiac output. Angiotensin-converting enzyme inhibitors, angiotensin receptor blockers, and calcium channel blockers are only of limited use for symptomatic relief in pediatric HFpEF.[25] New therapies have been developed to interfere with the mediator pathways of HFpEF at the cellular and molecular level, including soluble guanyl atecyclase modulators and angiotensin receptor-neprilysin inhibitors (ARNI). ARNI is highly beneficial in treating adult HFrEF patients, but the PARAGON-HF trial revealed that it does not significantly lower the rate of total hospitalizations for HF and death from cardiovascular diseases in HFpEF patients.[26] A new class of sodium glucose transporter protein 2 (SGLT2) inhibitor drugs is beneficial in various trials in adults **(Table 2)**.[27] The role of left ventricular assist devices (LVAD) is limited in pediatric patients with HFpEF,[28] the therapeutic approach. For those with valvular

TABLE 1: Diagnostic approach for heart failure with preserved ejection fraction (HFpEF) in children.

Signs and symptoms of heart failure	*Dyspnea, fatigue, low exercise tolerance, lack of appetite, and infection susceptibility*
Suggestive TTE parameters	• LVEF >50% • No other cause of heart failure (absence of shunt or valvular disease) • DT <11 cm/s • LE enlargement >15 cm^2 • Low GLS
Elevated NT-proBNP levels29	• 0–2 days >12,000 pg/mL • 3–11 days >6,000 pg/mL • 1 month–1 year >650 pg/mL • 1–2 years >400 pg/mL 2–6 years >300 pg/mL • 6–18 years >160 pg/mL
Therapeutic testing	Symptoms improved by diuretics
Right heart catheterization	• LVEDP >15 mmHg • If doubtful, a rapid saline loading test may sensitive

(DT: mitral E wave deceleration time; GLS: global longitudinal strain; LVEF: left ventricular ejection fraction; LVEDP: left ventricular end diastolic pressure; NT-proBNP: N-terminal prohormone B-type natriuretic peptide; TTE: transthoracic echocardiographic)

TABLE 2: Different therapeutic options in Heart failure with preserved ejection fraction (HFpEF).

Drug	Effect
Diuretics	Relieve congestion
B-blockers	Decreasing heart rate and increasing diastolic duration, and reducing myocardial oxygen consumption
Spironolactone	Afterload reducing impact, changes in serum electrolytes
Milrinone	Phosphodiesterase-3 inhibitor, that increases cAMP, enhances myocardial contractility, promotes myocardial relaxation, and increases cardiac output
Angiotensin-converting enzyme inhibitors, angiotensin receptor blockers, and calcium channel blockers	Limited use for symptomatic relief
Angiotensin receptor-neprilysin inhibitors (ARNI)	Beneficial in treating adult HFrEF patients
Sodium glucose transporter protein 2 (SGLT2) inhibitor	Under trial in adult studies

diseases causing volume overload, such as in TOF, early intervention, including pulmonary valve replacement, may be beneficial.

CONCLUSION

The HFpEF is a rare and probably underdiagnosed condition in children. It can be caused by a variety of underlying conditions. Clinical presentation is not specific, and the diagnosis may be difficult. In pediatric CHD with HFpEF still the way to go.

REFERENCES

1. Lam CS, Donal E, Kraigher-Krainer E, et al. Epidemiology and clinical course of heart failure with preserved ejection fraction. Eur J Heart Fail. 2011;13(1):18-28.
2. Masutani S, Saiki H, Kurishima C, et al. Heart failure with preserved ejection fraction in children: hormonal imbalance between aldosterone and brain natriuretic peptide. Circ J. 2013;77(9):2375-82.
3. Bozkurt B, Coats AJS, Tsutsui H, et al. Universal definition and classification of heart failure: a report of the Heart Failure Society of America, Heart Failure Association of the European Society of Cardiology, Japanese Heart Failure Society and Writing Committee of the Universal Definition of Heart Failure: endorsed by Canadian Heart Failure Society, Heart Failure Association of India, the Cardiac Society of Australia and New Zealand, and the Chinese Heart Failure Association. Eur J Heart Fail. 2021;23:352-80.
4. Bhambhani V, Kizer JR, Lima JAC, et al. Predictors and outcomes of heart failure with midrange ejection fraction. Eur J Heart Fail. 2018;20(4):651-65.
5. Friedman KG, McElhinney DB, Rhodes J, et al. Left ventricular diastolic function in children and young adults with congenital aortic valve disease. Am J Cardiol. 2013;111(2):243-9.
6. Gewillig M, Mertens L, Moerman P, et al. Idiopathic restrictive cardiomyopathy in childhood: a diastolic disorder characterized by delayed relaxation. Eur Heart J. 1996;17(9):1413-20.
7. Lasa JJ, Gaies M, Bush L, et al. Epidemiology and outcomes of acute decompensated heart failure in children. Circ Heart Fail. 2020;13(4):e006101.
8. Pan B, Hu D, Sun H, et al. Pediatric diastolic heart failure: clinical features description of 421 cases. Front Pediatr. 2022;10:846408.
9. Senning A. Surgical correction of transposition of the great vessels. Surgery. 1959;45(6):966-80.
10. Mustard WT. Successful two-stage correction of transposition of the great vessels. Surgery. 1964;55:469-72.
11. Jatene AD, Fontes VF, Paulista PP, et al. Anatomic correction of transposition of the great vessels. J Thorac Cardiovasc Surg. 1976;72(3):364-70.
12. Öner T, Özdemir R, Guven B, et al. Evaluation of myocardial function in pediatric patients with transposition of great arteries after arterial switch operation. Anatol J Cardiol. 2016;16(1):55-61.
13. Wang C, Li VW-Y, So EK-F, et al. Left ventricular stiffness in adolescents and young adults after arterial switch operation for complete transposition of the great arteries. Pediatr Cardiol. 2020;41:747-54.
14. Hosny H, Sedky Y, Romeih S, et al. Revival and modification of the Mustard operation. J Thorac Cardiovasc Surg. 2020;159(1):241-9.
15. Hinton RB, Ware SM. Heart failure in pediatric patients with congenital heart disease. Circ Res. 2017;120(6):978-94.
16. Chowdhury SM, Graham EM, Taylor CL, et al. Diastolic dysfunction with preserved ejection fraction after the Fontan procedure. JAHA. 2022;10:e024095.
17. Sugimoto M, Masutani S, Seki M, et al. High serum levels of procollagen type III N-terminal amino-peptide in patients with congenital heart disease. Heart. 2009;95(24):2023-8.
18. Florianczyk T, Werner B. Assessment of left ventricular diastolic function in children after successful repair of aortic coarctation. Clin Res Cardiol. 2011;100(6):493-9.
19. Nagueh SF. Heart failure with preserved ejection fraction: insights into diagnosis and pathophysiology. Cardiovasc Res. 2021;117(4):999-1014.
20. Menon SC, Gray R, Tani LY. Evaluation of ventricular filling pressures and ventricular function by Doppler echocardiography in patients with functional single ventricle:

correlation with simultaneous cardiac catheterization. J Am Soc Echocardi ogr. 2011;24:1220-5.
21. Yuda S. Current clinical applications of speckle track ing echocardiography for assessment of left atrial function. J Echocardiogr. 2021;19(3):129-40.
22. Riesenkampff E, Messroghli DR, Redington AN, et al. Myocardial T1 mapping in pediatric and congeni tal heart disease. Circ Cardiovasc Imaging. 2015;8(2):e002504.
23. Cho MJ, Lim RK, Kwak MJ, et al. Effects of beta-block ers for congestive heart failure in pediatric and congenital heart disease patients-a meta-analysis of published studies. Minerva Cardioangio. 2015;63(6):495-505.
24. Edelmann F, Wachter R, Schmidt AG, et al. Effects of spironolactone on diastolic function and exercise capacity in patients with heart failure with preserved ejection function: the Aldo-DHF randomized controlled trial. JAMA. 2013;309(8):781-91.
25. liceto S. Left ventricular dysfunction: which role for calcium antagonists? Eur Heart J. Suppl A. 1997;18 Suppl A: A87-91.
26. Solomon SD, McMurray JJV, Anand IS, et al. Angiotensin Neprilysin inhibition in heart failure with preserved ejection fraction. N Engl J Med. 2019;381(17):1609-20.
27. Das SR, Everett BM, Birtcher KK, et al. 2020 expert con sensus decision pathway on novel therapies for cardiovascular risk reduction in patients with type 2 diabetes: a report of the American College of Cardiology Solution Set Oversight Com mittee. J Am Coll Cardiol. 2020;76(9):1117-45.
28. Grupper A, Park S, Pereira NL, et al. Role of ventricular assist therapy for patients with heart failure and restrictive physi ology: Improving outcomes for a lethal disease. J Heart Lung Transplant. 2015;34(8):1042-9.
29. Nir A, Lindinger A, Rauh M, et al. NT-Pro-B type natriuretic peptide in infants and children: reference values based on combined data from four studies. Pediatr Cardiol. 2009;30(1):3-8.
30. Borlaug BA, Sharma K, Shah SJ, et al. Heart Failure with Preserved Ejection Fraction: JACC Scientific Statement. J Am Coll Cardiol. 2023;81(18):1810-34.

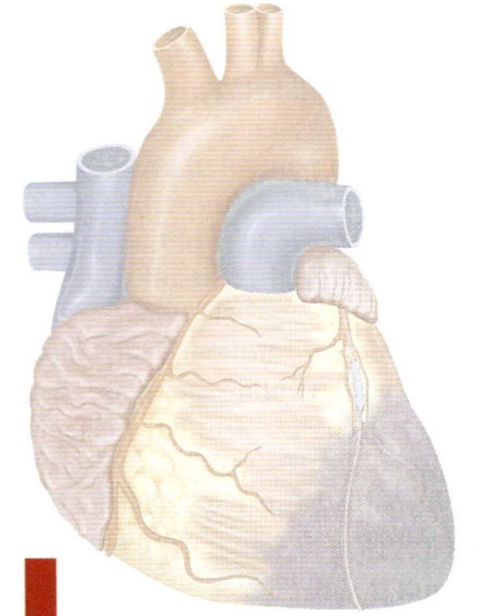

Pediatric HFpEF

Hala Elmarsafawy, Shaima Khaled Zakaria

INTRODUCTION

Left ventricular diastolic function plays an important role in determining the kinetics and quality of ventricular filling and thus stroke volume. *It can be defined as the ability of the heart to relax and expand during diastole*, resulting in filling of the left ventricular chamber to an adequate diastolic volume. Diastolic dysfunction is defined as the inability of the ventricle to fill even if the atrial pressure is normal. Diastolic dysfunction may result from *prolonged relaxation* and/or *increased ventricular stiffness*.[1]

Normal left ventricular function during diastole involves relaxation of its walls, allowing the ventricle to expand and accommodate incoming blood. This is facilitated by the normal functioning of the muscle cells within the ventricle, which contract during systole and then relax during diastole. However, in diastolic dysfunction, ventricular wall relaxation is impaired or slowed, resulting in decreased left ventricular filling.

At the cellular level, left ventricular relaxation during diastole is enabled by the dissociation of actin-myosin cross-bridges, which occurs after calcium uptake by the sarcoplasm. The ventricular network results in decreased cell tension. It is the main protein that regulates muscle cell stiffness. In addition, increased stiffness of the ventricular walls, due to conditions such as fibrosis or muscle hypertrophy, can also contribute to diastolic dysfunction by limiting the ventricle's ability to expand and accommodate blood.

Chamber stiffness is primarily determined by the stiffening properties of the sarcomeres, the interstitial space, the geometry of the left ventricular chamber, and wall thickness.[1] Another component that influences left ventricular filling and diastolic pressures is elastic recoil.

Early diastolic recoil, the ability of the left ventricle to "return" to its relaxed state, contributes to the rapid fall in left ventricular pressure during isovolumetric relaxation time (IVRT). In diastolic dysfunction, this recoil may be delayed or reduced, impeding the ventricle's ability to fill with blood during diastole.

Titin plays an important role in left ventricular dilatation. It is an elastic protein that holds the sarcomere unit together and acts as an elastic spring that is compressed during systole and rebounds during diastole.[2]

Left atrial pressure is closely related to left ventricular pressure and is used as a surrogate marker for left ventricular filling pressures. During diastole, as the left ventricle fills with blood, the pressure within the left ventricle increases. This increased pressure then travels backward into the left atrium, resulting in increased left atrial pressure. Therefore, in conditions where left ventricular diastolic function is impaired, there is an associated increase in left atrial pressure, reflecting elevated filling pressures within the left ventricle.

Today, the most commonly used definition is heart failure with a left ventricular ejection fraction (LVEF) >50% associated with evidence of spontaneous or provocatively increased left ventricular (LV) filling pressures.[2]

There is a fine line between heart failure with preserved ejection and diastolic dysfunction as patients with LV diastolic dysfunction are often asymptomatic at rest but have limitations during exercise.

CLINICAL MANIFESTATIONS

The clinical manifestations of heart failure with preserved ejection range from severe heart failure to *dyspnea on exertion*. While adults are able to describe the onset or worsening of dyspnea after a well-tolerated effort in the past, it may be difficult to identify poor exercise tolerance in children.

EPIDEMIOLOGY

Left ventricular diastolic dysfunction has been well studied and described in adults, with heart failure with preserved ejection fraction accounting for at least half of patients diagnosed with heart failure.[3] Risk factors in adults include age, obesity, hypertension, coronary artery disease, and diabetes.[4,5]

However, comprehensive studies have been conducted in elderly hypertensive and diabetic patients[6-8] and do not reflect the epidemiology and physiology of diastolic dysfunction in the pediatric population.

In fact, insights into the epidemiology and etiology of heart failure with preserved ejection fraction in children are scarce. Few studies have evaluated left ventricular diastolic function in children,[9-11] and examination of diastolic function is a challenge in the routine assessment of pediatric cardiologists.[12]

As a result, *the prevalence of HFpEF in children is unknown and may be underestimated.* Pan et al.[10] reported on 421 children with diastolic heart failure. This large cohort was collected between 2004 and 2014 at the Children's Hospital of Chongqing Medical University. Among a series of 3,907 pediatric hospital admissions to the Department of Cardiology that were retrospectively reviewed, only 18 patients were considered to have *HFpEF (0.5%).*[11]

PATHOPHYSIOLOGY

Heart failure with reduced ejection fraction is a heterogeneous group of diseases characterized by symptoms of heart failure due to increased myocardial stiffness.

The pathophysiology and cellular mechanism of heart failure with reduced ejection fraction depend on the cause and include, among others, cardiac hypertrophy and fibrosis,[13] intrinsic myocardial dysfunction,[14] impaired calcium handling,[15] titin sclerosis,[16] inflammatory state,[17] and large and small vessel diseases.[18]

In restrictive cardiomyopathy (RCM), the left ventricular wall thickness is mostly within normal limits, the pathophysiology of restrictive heart failure is associated with myocyte dysfunction such as myocyte hypertrophy, myocyte nuclei enlargement, irregularity, and hyperpigmentation.[19] *Genetic disorders leading to intracellular accumulation of material* such as Anderson-Fabry disease,[20] Danon disease,[21] and iron overload cardiomyopathy[22] are examples of restrictive physiology caused by myocytes.

In the study by Lombardi et al.,[23] a linear correlation was observed between aortic elasticity and left ventricular diastolic function.

Raising the hypothesis that just as in the elderly, aortic vascular stiffness leads to impaired left ventricular diastolic function. Indeed, with increasing vascular stiffness, the systolic pulse wave velocity increases and, consequently, the reflected wave returns to the heart earlier, during late systole, *increasing late systolic load, affecting the interactions of thin and thick myofilaments and the separation of the cross-bridge, leading to impaired relaxation.*

Interstitial myocardial fibrosis also plays a role in the pathogenesis of left ventricular diastolic dysfunction because it increases ventricular stiffness and impairs the extensibility of myofibers.[24] Collagen is a major component of the extracellular environment of the myocardium, and increased collagen deposition alters the viscoelasticity of the myocardium, impairing relaxation, diastolic rebound, and passive stiffness.[25] Fibrosis is a common endpoint of myocardial pathologic processes such as chronic ischemic heart disease or myocarditis.

ETIOLOGY

The causes of left ventricular diastolic dysfunction in children *differ significantly* from classical risk factors identified in adults.

Intrinsic abnormalities in the myocytes appear to be the main cause of diastolic dysfunction in children. Primary cardiomyopathies are diseases of the heart muscle in which myocardial dysfunction occurs in the absence of systemic, valvular, or congenital heart disease.[26] *Hypertrophic, dilated, and restrictive cardiomyopathies* are primary cardiomyopathies that can lead to diastolic dysfunction. There are two main clinical categories of left ventricular diastolic dysfunction in children: congenital, related to a genetic or metabolic disorder and acquired, i.e., secondary to another cause.[27] In this review, we chose not to describe transient diastolic dysfunction associated with a congenital heart defect because it almost always disappears after cardiac surgery.

Congenital: Hereditary hypertrophic cardiomyopathies, restrictive cardiomyopathies, and inherited infiltrative cardiomyopathies

Dilated cardiomyopathy (DCM) is defined by the presence of a dilated ventricular heart with systolic dysfunction without any hemodynamic, physiological, ischemic, or anatomical cause.[28] DCM accounts for approximately 50% of pediatric cardiomyopathies.[26]

Patients with dilated cardiomyopathy initially present with heart failure with reduced ejection fraction, but progression of cell death and extension of left ventricular fibrosis often leads to diastolic dysfunction.

The occurrence of diastolic dysfunction with high filling pressures is associated with a poor prognosis in these cases.[29]

Hypertrophic cardiomyopathy (HCM) is defined as ventricular hypertrophy and non-dilatation in the absence of a hemodynamic cause of wall thickening, excluding physiological hypertrophy (secondary to physical activity) and pathological hypertrophy (secondary to aortic stenosis, aortic valve stenosis, and hypertension).[28] HCM is the second most common cardiomyopathy in children (*40%* of patients).[26] Diastolic dysfunction is common and varies in severity. Impaired calcium handling, myocyte hypertrophy, and disorder, ischemia, and fibrosis are the causes of diastolic dysfunction.[30]

Diastolic dysfunction has been described mainly in children with restrictive cardiomyopathy, which accounts for <5% of pediatric cardiomyopathies.[19,26] Leading mutations associated with restrictive cardiomyopathy are *MYH7, TNNI3, TNNT2, MYL2,* and *DES.*[31] Restrictive cardiomyopathies may also be secondary to systemic diseases including infiltrative disorder, collagen vascular disease,[9] neoplastic process,[32] thoracic radiation, chemotherapy, bone marrow transplantation,[26,32,33] and endocardial disease with or without eosinophilia leading to endocardial fibrosis. Left heart obstruction such as aortic stenosis and aortic valve stenosis can lead to a restrictive left ventricular physiology that persists after repair.[18,34,35] *A common mechanism in these cardiomyopathies is increased myocardial stiffness, which reduces compliance.*

Acquired: Relaxation disorders secondary to cardiac remodeling and fibrosis reducing relaxation capacity, left ventricular diastolic dysfunction has been described in patients with aortic stenosis or aortic coarctation[18,23,24,35] even after successful repair. In the study of Moskowitz et al.,[35] variable slow relaxation was found in children who underwent successful repair of aortic coarctation and late diastolic filling pressures were affected by left ventricular mass suggesting that cardiac hypertrophy rather than increased afterload is the primary determinant of left ventricular diastolic dysfunction.

Some exogenous factors have also been described in children such as inflammatory diseases: Acute myocarditis,[36] Kawasaki shock syndrome,[37] and more recently multisystem inflammatory syndrome in children (MISC) due to severe acute respiratory syndrome coronavirus 2 (SARS-CoV-2).[38] Graft rejection is also a cause of left ventricular diastolic dysfunction in pediatric heart recipients.[39-44] Myocardial edema secondary to inflammation causes impaired ventricular compliance.

Temporary left ventricular diastolic dysfunction can be observed in acute settings, such as tachycardia, during the early postoperative period or during sepsis. It is important to note that at birth (within the first 7 days/2 months in premature infants), the diastolic properties of the left ventricle are severely impaired without pathological significance.

Pulmonary hypertension includes pulmonary hypertension associated with left heart disease including heart failure with reduced ejection fraction, heart failure with reduced ejection fraction, valvular heart disease, and congenital heart disease. Despite similar hemodynamic profiles, there are significant variations between these patient groups in terms of comorbidities and clinical phenotypes.[45-50] The hemodynamic definition of group 2 pulmonary hypertension was proposed at the 6th World Symposium on Pulmonary Hypertension as *a mean pulmonary artery pressure >20 mm Hg* and a pulmonary artery wedge pressure >15 mm Hg.[51] HFpEF associated with pulmonary hypertension can be divided into isolated post-capillary pulmonary hypertension (IPH) and combined pre-capillary pulmonary hypertension (CPH).

Diagnosis is based on measurement of pulmonary vascular resistance (PVR) during RHC: <3 Wood units (WU) for IPH or ≥3 WU for CPH. This distinction is important because it affects therapeutic strategies.[52]

Abnormal relaxation and increased left ventricular stiffness lead to increased left ventricular and left atrial pressures.[53] Elevated left atrial pressures expose the pulmonary veins to increased pressure[54] and cause stress failure of the alveolar-capillary junction leading to pulmonary edema and inflammation. Inflammatory mediators increase endothelin-1 depression and decrease nitric oxide and natriuretic peptide activity. Fibroblast proliferation is activated, leading to lumen obstruction and thickening of alveolar septa.[55] This structural change associated with pulmonary edema compresses small pulmonary arteries and induces precapillary pulmonary hypertension.

Thus, as diastolic disease progresses, pulmonary hypertension can progress from precapillary pulmonary hypertension to combined (pre- and postcapillary) pulmonary hypertension. *The pulmonary hemodynamic profiles in heart failure with preserved ejection have received little attention*, but the development of pulmonary hypertension with increased pulmonary vascular resistance in heart failure with preserved ejection is recognized as an important contributor to morbidity and mortality.

Pulmonary hemodynamic *profiles have not yet been studied in children with heart failure with preserved ejection fraction*, but pulmonary hypertension has been well described in children with RCM as a relevant proportion of them develops pulmonary heart failure without response to vasodilators and are contraindicated for orthotopic heart transplantation.[56] Up to half of children with RCM have pulmonary hypertension at diagnosis[57] and this is a factor in poor prognosis and therapeutic solutions are concerns.[58]

DIAGNOSIS

Clinical recognition and understanding of heart failure with preserved ejection fraction in children are poor. This may be due to the rarity of the condition but also because the diagnosis of diastolic dysfunction in children is difficult in clinical practice. Symptoms may be subtle and can vary depending on the severity of the condition.

The agreed definition of HFpEF is presence of signs and symptoms of heart failure, and left ventricular ejection fraction > 50% associated with evidence of spontaneous or provocative increased left ventricular filling pressure.[3]

The gold standard for characterizing left ventricular relaxation is cardiac catheterization. A high-resolution catheter is placed in the left ventricle measures left ventricular volumes and pressures simultaneously. Left ventricular pressure loops reflect the filling and contraction characteristics of the left ventricle.[5] Commonly measured parameters are: (1) The relaxation time constant (tau or τ) which reflects the rate of decline of left ventricular pressure during the isovolumetric relaxation period (IVRT). The normal duration of tau is 30–40 ms;[1] (2) The pulmonary capillary wedge pressure (PCWP) is the pressure measured in the pulmonary artery during diastole, which reflects the pressure in the left atrium and left ventricle; (3) Left ventricular end-diastolic pressure (LVEDP) is the pressure measured directly within the left ventricle at the end of diastole.

Rapid saline loading during RHC can also be used to assess the left ventricular response and elucidate the pathophysiology of heart failure.[59] Indeed, an increase in PCWP in response to increased afterload may indicate that diastolic dysfunction is associated with increased ventricular stiffness.

Due to its invasive nature, technical complexity, and cost, cardiac catheterization is impractical for the routine assessment of left ventricular filling pressures, which are almost *always estimated by transthoracic echocardiography (TTE)*. H2FpEF[60] and the HFA-PEFF diagnostic algorithm[61] have been proposed to assess left ventricular filling pressure in adults but precise thresholds are missing in the pediatric population.[12] Indeed, in children, cardiac arrhythmias and pediatric characteristics make Doppler measurements difficult and adult cut-off values for these various parameters are inappropriate.[62]

Previous studies have attempted to identify specific TTE parameters to facilitate estimation of ventricular end-diastolic pressure (LVEDP).[63,64] Dragulescu et al. found that *mitral E-wave deceleration time (DT)* (153 ± 23 ms in control patients versus 97 ± 27 ms in RCM patients) and *early diastolic tissue velocity of the mitral lateral peak (normal if >11 cm/s)* were the most discriminating parameters.[12]

Late diastolic peak mitral filling velocities (A) vary significantly throughout childhood, and this influences the ratio of early to late mitral filling velocity (E/A) and this parameter should not be considered without taking into account the patient's age.[65]

In contrast, isovolumetric relaxation time appeared to be stable with age, making it an excellent parameter in children. Sasaki et al. compared echocardiographic findings of 9 RCM patients with 27 controls and concluded that left atrial size differentiated patients with and without diastolic dysfunction with minimal interference as the *indexed left atrial area was significantly larger* in the RCM group: mean 22.8 cm^2/m^2 (range 16.9–28.6) versus 10.3 cm^2/m^2 (range 8.3–12.3) in the control group.[66]

By providing a quantitative analysis of longitudinal left ventricular function, speckle tracking derived from global longitudinal stress (GLS) is accurate in early detection of subclinical changes in longitudinal left ventricular function.[63]

There is no clear threshold for normal global longitudinal stress in children.[64] In the study by McAree et al.,[67] patients with MISC appeared to have a lower mean GLS than controls [*−20.4 (±2.8) vs. −22.0 (±1.9)*].

B-type natriuretic peptide (BNP) and its precursor hormone NT-proBNP (amino-terminal B-type natriuretic peptide) are produced by the ventricles in response to increased pressure or volume loads. It is normally released when muscle cells are stretched or under stress.[68]

NT-proBNP levels can be elevated in children with left ventricular diastolic dysfunction because increased pressure or volume in the heart leads to the release of NT-proBNP. Higher levels of NT-proBNP can therefore, be a marker of diastolic dysfunction and can be used to help diagnose this condition.

However, NT-proBNP levels are *age-dependent*, and to a *lesser* extent sex-dependent in the pediatric population.

In the review by Nir et al.,[69] data from four studies involving patients taking NT-proBNP for reasons other than heart failure, considering the 95th percentile as the upper limit of normal. They proposed a normal NT-proBNP threshold for age. Inspired by the H2FpEF[60] and the HFA-PEFF diagnostic algorithm[61] used in adults, we propose a stepwise diagnostic approach that is a compilation of published criteria **(Table 1)**.

Another relevant biomarker is aldosterone, in fact, in the study of Masutani et al.[11] The aldosterone/BNP ratio was significantly higher in patients with preserved ejection compared with patients with preserved ejection (38 ± 63 vs. 1.7 ± 1.9, $p < 0.05$) and "ROC curve analysis showed that an aldosterone/BNP ratio of 10.3 or higher better predicted heart failure with preserved ejection [area under the curve (AUC) = 0.89], with a sensitivity of 0.67 and a specificity of 1.0."

Cardiac magnetic resonance imaging (CMRI) is a noninvasive imaging modality that can provide valuable information about the structure and function of the heart. By providing details about the myocardial phenotype such as the location of myocardial hypertrophy (septal or apical) in HCM or specific myocardial structures such as the presence of fibrosis, edema, fat and iron overload (by T2* imaging) in patients with hemochromatosis.[70]

Cardiac magnetic resonance imaging is useful for accessing the etiology of HFpEF. *CMRI* allows characterization of myocardial tissue and the extent of fibrosis making it the preferred method in the diagnosis and follow-up of cardiomyopathies. In fact, intravenous gadolinium-based contrast administration is the gold standard for identifying and quantifying the extent of myocardial fibrosis.[71]

In the absence of focal LGE, T1 relaxation times and extracellular volume assessment confirm the diagnosis of diffuse fibrosis.[72] The extent of myocardial fibrosis assessed by late gadolinium enhancement (LGE) correlates significantly with the degree of diastolic dysfunction.[25]

The amount of fibrosis, maximum wall thickness, and left ventricular mass are markers of sudden cardiac death risk that can be obtained with ventricular MRI. Another important feature of ventricular MRI is its ability to provide information about blood flow patterns in the heart. Analysis of left ventricular filling velocity and volume flow, and volumetric assessment of the left ventricle and left atrium make ventricular MRI a highly accurate and reproducible noninvasive technique for assessing diastolic function.[73]

Wave intensity represents the energy flux per unit area carried by waves traveling in the cardiovascular network and is derived from ventricular MRI flow data.[74] There are two main wave patterns during systole: the front pressure wave at systolic ejection (FCW) and the front expansion wave (FEW) at end-systole. The *FCW/FEW* ratio was significantly lower in patients with preserved ejection heart failure, while the peak FCW was lower in patients with left ventricular diastolic dysfunction.

Cardiac MRI is useful in assessing graft function in pediatric heart transplant recipients.[75]

Clinical course and outcomes: The clinical course of children with diastolic dysfunction varies depending on the underlying cardiac condition. The overall prognosis of HFpEF in children is uncertain, especially since this term refers to a heterogeneous group of patients.

PROGNOSIS

There is limited literature on the prognosis of HFpEF in children beyond the HCM and RCM phenotypes. There are no well-defined predictors of survival after diagnosis, but the prognosis for RCM appears to be grim, with the risk of sudden death and development of pulmonary hypertension leading to early transplantation,[76] and younger age at diagnosis, recurrent admissions for heart failure, use of diuretics, and isolated RCM are risk factors for mortality.[76,77]

In the National Heart, Lung, and Blood Institute (NHLBI) Pediatric Cardiomyopathy Registry, children with congestive cardiomyopathy who had congestive heart failure and a low fractional shortening Z score at diagnosis had the worst prognosis. The occurrence of left ventricular diastolic dysfunction in patients with dilated cardiomyopathy is an indicator of poor prognosis[29,78] but there are no specific studies in children. Masutani et al.[11] compared the clinical course of 18 children with heart failure with reduced ejection fraction with 22 children with heart failure with reduced ejection fraction and observed that mortality from heart failure was significantly lower in patients with heart failure with reduced ejection fraction than in patients with heart failure with reduced ejection fraction (22% vs. 41%). Future work should focus on patients with isolated left ventricular diastolic dysfunction (and preserved ejection fraction) to identify appropriate predictors of outcome.

TREATMENT

It is important for children with left ventricular diastolic dysfunction to receive appropriate treatment in a timely manner to help prevent any long-term complications. To date, there is no pharmacological agent that facilitates myocardial relaxation or improves ventricular compliance. Pharmacological treatment of heart failure with preserved myocardial contractility in children is also being extrapolated from adult clinical trials.

Lifestyle management in children includes control of obesity and poor diet, control of blood pressure, and physical activity.

Medical management strategies include diuretics to relieve symptoms of congestive heart failure. In adult patients, careful monitoring of lung pressures with a device, the CardioMEMS sensor, allows for efficient titration of diuretics. It has been shown to reduce hospitalizations for heart failure in patients with heart failure with preserved ejection.[79,80] *Beta-blockers* may be useful because they increase diastolic duration by slowing the heart rate.[81] *Spironolactone* appears to improve prognosis in obese and diabetic adult patients with heart failure with preserved ejection.[15,82] However, these results are not transferable to pediatric patients. Angiotensin-converting enzyme inhibitors and sartans are prescribed to treat and prevent both systolic and diastolic dysfunction in cardiomyopathy and after repair of aortic stenosis, but there is *no evidence* of their effectiveness on diastolic function. Empagliflozin and sacubitril/valsartan[83] have shown promising results in adults, but data *in children are not yet available*. To date, no clinical trial has shown any benefit in treating patients with heart failure with preserved ejection associated with pulmonary hypertension using approved therapies for pulmonary hypertension.[84] In patients with postcapillary pulmonary hypertension and symptoms of heart failure, *the atrial inflow pacemaker*, a recently available interatrial shunt device, ***has been shown to be effective in treating symptoms and safe, including in the pediatric population.***[85-87]

CONCLUSION

Heart failure with preserved ejection is a rare condition and is probably underdiagnosed in children. It can be caused by a variety of underlying conditions. The clinical presentation is not specific, and diagnosis can be difficult. We have proposed a diagnostic algorithm that is easy to use in clinical practice. Prognosis is based on the cause, but the onset of associated hypertension represents a turning point in disease progression. Specific therapies are limited.

REFERENCES

1. Nagueh SF. Left ventricular diastolic function. JACC Cardiovasc Imaging. 2020;13(1):228-44. doi: 10.1016/j.jcmg.2018.10.038
2. Fukuda N, Terui T, Ishiwata S, et al. Titin-based regulations of diastolic and systolic functions of mammalian cardiac muscle. J Mol Cell Cardiol. 2010;48(576):876
3. Heidenreich PA, Bozkurt B, Aguilar D, et al. 2022 AHA/ACC/HFSA Guideline for the Management of Heart Failure: a report of the American College of Cardiology/American Heart Association Joint Committee on Clinical Practice Guidelines. Circulation. 2022;145(18):e895-1032.
4. Dunlay SM, Roger VL, Redfield MM. Epidemiology of heart failure with preserved ejection fraction. Nat Rev Cardiol. 2017;14(10):591-602.
5. Nagueh SF. Heart failure with preserved ejection fraction: insights into diagnosis and pathophysiology. Cardiovasc Res. 2021;117(4):999-1014.
6. Mishra S, Kass DA. Cellular and molecular pathobiology of heart failure with preserved ejection fraction. Nat Rev Cardiol. 2021;18(6):400-23.
7. Gevaert AB, Boen JRA, Segers VF, et al. Heart failure with preserved ejection fraction: a review of cardiac and noncardiac pathophysiology. Front Physiol. 2019;10:638.
8. Arques S, Quennelle F, Roux E. Accuracy of peak mitral e-wave velocity in the diagnosis of heart failure with preserved ejection fraction in older patients with acute dyspnea. Ann Cardiol Angeiol. 2021;70(5):281-5.
9. Das BB, Taylor AL, Yetman AT. Left ventricular diastolic dysfunction in children and young adults with Marfan syndrome. Pediatr Cardiol. 206; 27(2):256-8.
10. Pan B, Hu D, Sun H, et al. Pediatric diastolic heart failure: clinical features description of 421 cases. Front Pediatr. 2022;10:846408.
11. Masutani S, Saiki H, Kurishima C, et al. Heart failure with preserved ejection fraction in children: hormonal imbalance between aldosterone and brain natriuretic peptide. Circ J. 2013; 77(9):2375-82.
12. Dragulescu A, Mertens L, Friedberg MK. Interpretation of left ventricular diastolic dysfunction in children with cardiomyopathy by echocardiography: problems and limitations. Circ Cardiovasc Imaging. 2013;6(2):254-61.
13. Nakamura M, Sadoshima J. Mechanisms of physiological and pathological cardiac hypertrophy. Nat Rev Cardiol. 2018;15(7):387-407.
14. Rapezzi C, Aimo A, Barison A, et al. Restrictive cardiomyopathy: Definition and diagnosis. Eur Heart J. 2022; 43(45):4679-93.
15. Cohen JB, Schrauben SJ, Zhao L, et al. Clinical phenogroups in heart failure with preserved ejection fraction. JACC Heart Failure. 2020;8(3):172-84.
16. Zile MR, Baicu CF, Ikonomidis J, et al. Myocardial stiffness in patients with heart failure and a preserved ejection fraction: contributions of collagen and titin. Circulation. 2015;131(14):1247-59.
17. Murdoch CE. Endothelial NADPH oxidase-2 promotes interstitial cardiac fibrosis and diastolic dysfunction through proinflammatory effects and endothelialmesenchymal transition. J Am Coll Cardiol. 2014;63(24):8.
18. Dusenbery SM, Jerosch-Herold M, Rickers C, et al. Myocardial extracellular remodeling is associated with ventricular diastolic dysfunction in children and young adults with congenital aortic stenosis. J Am Coll Cardiol. 2014;63(17):1778-85.
19. Gewillig M, Mertens L, Moerman P, et al. Idiopathic restrictive cardiomyopathy in childhood: a diastolic

disorder characterized by delayed relaxation. Eur Heart J. 1996;17(9):1413-20.

20. Zarate YA, Hopkin RJ. Lysosomal storage disease 3 Fabry's disease. Lancet. 2008;372(9647):1427-35.
21. Yang Z, McMahon CJ, Smith LR, et al. Danon disease as an underrecognized cause of hypertrophic cardiomyopathy in children. Circulation. 2005;112(11):1612-7.
22. Murphy CJ, Oudit GY. Iron-overload cardiomyopathy: pathophysiology, diagnosis, and treatment. J Card Fail. 2010;16(11):888-900.
23. Lombardi KC, Northrup V, McNamara RL, et al. Aortic stiffness and left ventricular diastolic function in children following early repair of aortic coarctation. Am J Cardiol. 2013;112(11):1828-33.
24. Florianczyk T, Werner B. Assessment of left ventricular diastolic function in children after successful repair of aortic coarctation. Clin Res Cardiol. 2011;100(6):493-9.
25. Moreo A, Ambrosio G, De Chiara B, et al. Influence of myocardial fibrosis on left ventricular diastolic function: non-invasive assessment by CMR and ECHO. Circ Cardiovasc Imaging. 2009;2(6):437-43.
26. Choudhry S, Puri K, Denfield SW. An update on pediatric cardiomyopathy. Curr Treat Options Cardio Med. 2019;21(8):36.
27. Knudson JD, Cabrera AG. The pathophysiology of heart failure in children: the basics. CCR. 2016;12(2):99-103.
28. Lipshultz SE, Law YM, Asante-Korang A, et al. Cardiomyopathy in children: classification and diagnosis: A Scientific Statement from the American Heart Association. Circulation. 2019;140(1):e9-68.
29. Reichart D, Magnussen C, Zeller T, et al. Dilated cardiomyopathy: from epidemiologic to genetic phenotypes: a translational review of current literature. J Intern Med. 2019;286(4):362-72.
30. Menon SC, Eidem BW, Dearani JA, et al. Diastolic dysfunction and its histopathological correlation in obstructive hypertrophic cardiomyopathy in children and adolescents. J Am Soc Echocardiogr. 2009;22(12):1327-34.
31. Hershberger RE. Genetic evaluation of cardiomyopathy: a clinical practice resource of the American College of Medical Genetics and Genomics (ACMG). Genet Med. 2018; 20(9):11.
32. Minotti G, Reggiardo G, Camilli M, et al. From cardiac anthracycline accumulation to real-life risk for early diastolic dysfunction. JACC CardioOncology. 2022;4(1):139-40.
33. Dorup I, Levitt G, Sullivan I, et al. Prospective longitudinal assessment of late anthracycline cardiotoxicity after childhood cancer: the role of diastolic function. Heart. 2004;90(10):1214-6.
34. Tede NH, Child JS. Diastolic dysfunction in patients with congenital heart disease. Cardiol Clin. 2000;18(3):491-9.
35. Moskowitz WB, Schieken RM, Mosteller M, et al. Altered systolic anddiastolic function in children after "successful" repair of coarctation of the aorta. Am Heart J. 1990;120(1):103-9.
36. Shin JH, Choi HJ. Heart failure with preserved ejection fraction in children without congenital heart disease. J Cardiovasc Dis Diagn. 2018;S2:004.
37. Selamet Tierney ES, Newburger JW, Graham D, et al. Diastolic function in children with kawasaki disease. Int J Cardiol. 2011;148(3):309-12.
38. Matsubara D, Kauffman HL, Wang Y, et al. Echocardiographic findings in pediatric multisystem inflammatory syndrome associated with COVID-19 in the United States. J Am Coll Cardiol. 2020;76 (17):1947-61.
39. Putzer GJB, Cooper D, Keehn C, et al. An improved echocardiographic rejection-surveillance strategy following pediatric heart transplantation. J Heart Lung Transplant. 2000;19(12):1166-74.
40. Asante-Korang A, Fickey M, Boucek MM, et al. Diastolic performance assessed by tissue Doppler after pediatric heart transplantation. J Heart Lung Transplant. 2004;23(7): 865-72.
41. Ten Harkel ADJ, Cransberg K, Van Osch-Gevers M, et al. Diastolic dysfunction in paediatric patients on peritoneal dialysis and after renal transplantation. Nephrol Dial Transplant. 2009;24(6):1987-91.
42. Schoenmaker NJ, Kuipers IM, van der Lee JH, et al. Diastolic dysfunction measured by tissue Doppler imaging in children with end-stage renal disease: a report of the RICH-Q study. Cardiol Young. 2014;24 (2):236-44.
43. Mitsnefes MM. Cardiovascular disease in children with chronic kidney disease. J Am Soc Nephrol. 2012;23(4): 578-85.
44. Mitsnefes MM, Kimball TR, Border WL, et al. Impaired left ventricular diastolic function in children with chronic renal failure. Kidney Int. 2004 65(4):1461-6.
45. Bartkowiak J, Spitzer E, Kurmann R, et al. The impact of obesity on left ventricular hypertrophy and diastolic dysfunction in children and adolescents. Sci Rep. 2012; 11(1):13022.
46. Saiedi SAE, Mira MF, Sharaf SA, et al. Left ventricular diastolic dysfunction without left ventricular hypertrophy in obese children and adolescents: A tissue Doppler imaging and cardiac troponin I study. Cardiol Young. 2018;28(1):76-84.
47. Kozák-Bárány A, Jokinen E, Kero P, et al. Impaired left ventricular diastolic function in newborn infants of mothers with pregestational or gestational diabetes with good glycemic control. Early Hum Dev. 2004;77(1): 13-22.
48. Mehta S, Nuamah I, Kalhan S. Altered diastolic function in asymptomatic infants of mothers with gestational diabetes. Diabetes. 1991;40(Supplement_2):56-60.
49. Zablah JE, Gruber D, Stoffels G, et al. Subclinical decrease in myocardial function in asymptomatic infants of diabetic mothers: a tissue Doppler study. Pediatr Cardiol. 2017;38(4):801-6.
50. Guazzi M, Ghio S, Adir Y. Pulmonary hypertension in HFpEF and HFrEF: jACC review topic of the week. J Am Coll Cardiol. 2020;76(9):1102-11.

51. Galiè N, McLaughlin VV, Rubin LJ, et al. An overview of the 6th world symposium on pulmonary hypertension. Eur Respir J. 2019;53(1):1802148.
52. Inampudi C, Silverman D, Simon MA, et al. Pulmonary hypertension in the context of heart failure with preserved ejection fraction. Chest. 2021;160(6):2232-46.
53. Røe ÅT, Aronsen JM, Skårdal K, et al. Increased passive stiffness promotes diastolic dysfunction despite improved Ca_{2+} handling during left ventricular concentric hypertrophy. Cardiovasc Res. 2017;113(10):1161-72.
54. Inciardi RM, Rossi A, Bergamini C, et al. Mitral regurgitation, left atrial structural and functional remodelling and the effect on pulmonary haemodynamics. Eur J Heart Fail. 2020;22(3):499-506.
55. Obokata M, Kane GC, Reddy YNV, et al. The neurohormonal basis of pulmonary hypertension in heart failure with preserved ejection fraction. Eur Heart J. 2019;40(45):3707-17.
56. Ditaranto R, Caponetti AG, Ferrara V, et al. Pediatric restrictive cardiomyopathies. Front Pediatr. 2022;9:745365.
57. Weller RJ, Weintraub R, Addonizio LJ, et al. Outcome of idiopathic restrictive cardiomyopathy in children. Am J Cardiol. 2002;90 (5):501-6.
58. Schlein J, Riebandt J, Laufer G, et al. Reversal of pulmonary hypertension in paediatric patients with restrictive cardiomyopathy. Interact Cardiovasc Thorac Surg. 2021;33(5):834-6.
59. Fujimoto N, Borlaug BA, Lewis GD, et al. Hemodynamic responses to rapid saline loading: the impact of age, sex, and heart failure. Circulation. 2013;127(1):55–62.
60. Reddy YNV, Carter RE, Obokata M, et al. A simple, evidence-based approach to help guide diagnosis of heart failure with preserved ejection fraction. Circulation. 2018;138(9):861-70.
61. Pieske B, Tschöpe C, de Boer RA, et al. How to diagnose heart failure with preserved ejection fraction: the HFA-PEFF diagnostic algorithm: A consensus recommendation from the Heart Failure Association (HFA) of the European-society of cardiology (ESC). Eur Heart J. 2019;40(40):3297-317.
62. Recher M, Botte A, Baudelet JB, et al. Évaluation de la function diastolique du ventricule gauche en réanimation pédiatrique: Quelles indications, quells paramètres mesurer? Méd Intensive Réa. 2019;28(2):144-56.
63. Mor-Avi V, Lang RM, Badano LP, et al. Current and evolving echocardiographic techniques for the quantitative evaluation of cardiac mechanics: ASE/EAE Consensus Statement on Methodology and Indications Endorsed by the Japanese Society of Echocardiography. J Am Soc Echocardiogr. 2011;24(3):277-313.
64. Galderisi M, Cosyns B, Edvardsen T, Cardim N, Delgado V, Di Salvo G, et al. Standardization of adult transthoracic echocardiography reporting in agreement with recent chamber quantification, diastolic function, and heart valve disease recommendations: an expert consensus document of the European association of cardiovascular imaging. Eur Heart J Cardiovasc Imaging. (2017) 18(12):1301–10. doi: 10.1093/ehjci/jex244
65. Eidem BW, McMahon CJ, Cohen RR, et al. Impact of cardiac growth on Doppler tissue imaging velocities: a study in healthy children. J Am Soc Echocardiogr. 2004;17(3):212-21.
66. Sasaki N, Garcia M, Ko HH, et al. Applicability of published guidelines for assessment of left ventricular diastolic function in adults to children with restrictive cardiomyopathy: an observational study. Pediatr Cardiol. 2015;36(2):386-92.
67. McAree D, Hauck A, Arzu J, et al. Clinical predictors of subacute myocardial dysfunction in multisystem inflammatory syndrome in children (MIS-C) associated with COVID-19. Pediatr Cardiol. 2022;1-12.
68. Cowie MR, Mendez GF. BNP and congestive heart failure. Prog Cardiovasc Dis. 2022;44(4):293-321.
69. Nir A, Lindinger A, Rauh M, et al. NT-Pro-Btype natriuretic peptide in infants and children: reference values based on combined data from four studies. Pediatr Cardiol. 2009;30(1):3-8.
70. Treibel TA, White SK, Moon JC. Myocardial tissue characterization: histological and pathophysiological correlation. Curr Cardiovasc Imaging Rep. 2014;7(3): 9254
71. Messroghli DR, Moon JC, Ferreira VM, et al. Clinical recommendations for cardiovascular magnetic resonance mapping ofmT1, T2, T2* and extracellular volume: a consensus statement by the society for cardiovascular magnetic resonance (SCMR) endorsed by the European association for cardiovascular imaging (EACVI). J Cardiovasc Magn Reson. 2017;19(1):75.
72. Rao S, Tseng SY, Pednekar A, et al. Myocardial parametric mapping by cardiac magnetic resonance imaging in pediatric cardiology and congenital heart disease. Circ Cardiovasc Imaging. 2022;15(1):e012242.
73. Paelinck BP, Lamb HJ, Bax JJ, et al. Assessment of diastolic function by cardiovascular magnetic resonance. Am Heart J. 2002;144(2):198-205.
74. Ntsinjana HN, Chung R, Ciliberti P, et al. Utility of cardiovascular magnetic resonance-derived wave intensity analysis as a marker of ventricular function in children with heart failure and normal ejection fraction. Front Pediatr. 2017;5:65.
75. Belay W, Godown J, Chan KC, et al. Cardiac magnetic resonance diastolic indices correlate with ventricular filling pressures in pediatric heart transplant recipients. Pediatr Transplant. 2022:e14332.
76. Webber SA, Lipshultz SE, Sleeper LA, et al. Outcomes of restrictive cardiomyopathy in childhood and the influence of phenotype: Na report from the Pediatric Cardiomyopathy Registry. Circulation. 2012;126 (10):1237-44.
77. Wittekind SG, Ryan TD, Gao Z, et al. Contemporary outcomes of pediatric restrictive cardiomyopathy: a single-center experience. Pediatr Cardiol. 2019;40(4):694-704.
78. Dujardin KS, Tei C, Yeo TC, et al. Prognostic value of a Doppler index combining systolic and diastolic performance in idiopathic-dilated cardiomyopathy. Am J Cardiol. 1998;82(9):1071-6.

79. Adamson PB, Abraham WT, Bourge RC, et al. Wireless pulmonary artery pressure monitoring guides management to reduce decompensation in heart failure with preserved ejection fraction. Circ Heart Fail.2014;7(6):935-44.
80. Heywood JT, Jermyn R, Shavelle D, et al. Impact of practice-based management of pulmonary artery pressures in 2000 patients implanted with the CardioMEMS sensor. Circulation. 2017;135(16):1509-17.
81. Rai P, Okhomina VI, Kang G, et al. The effects of cardio-selective beta blockade on diastolic dysfunction in children with sickle cell disease. Haematol. 2022;108(2):594-8.
82. Pitt B, Pfeffer MA, Assmann SF, et al. Spironolactone for heart failure with preserved ejection fraction. N Engl J Med. 2014;370(15):1383-92.
83. Packer M, Butler J, Zannad F, et al. Effect of empagliflozin on worsening heart failure events in patients with heart failure and preserved ejection fraction: EMPEROR-Preserved Trial. Circulation. 2021;144(16):1284-94.
84. Vachiéry JL, Tedford RJ, Rosenkranz S, et al. Pulmonary hypertension due to left heart disease. Eur Respir J. 2019;53(1):1801897.
85. Paitazoglou C, Bergmann MW, Özdemir R, et al. One-year results of the first-in-man study investigating the atrial flow regulator for left atrial shunting in symptomatic heart failure patients: the PRELIEVE study. Eur J Heart Fail. 2021;23(5):800-10.
86. Paitazoglou C, Bergmann MW. The atrial flow regulator: current overview on technique and first experience. Ther Adv Cardiovasc Dis. 2022;14:1753944720919577.
87. Hansmann G, Sabiniewicz A, Sabiniewicz R. Atrial flow regulator for postcapillary pulmonary hypertension. JACC Case Rep. 2022;4(14):878-84.

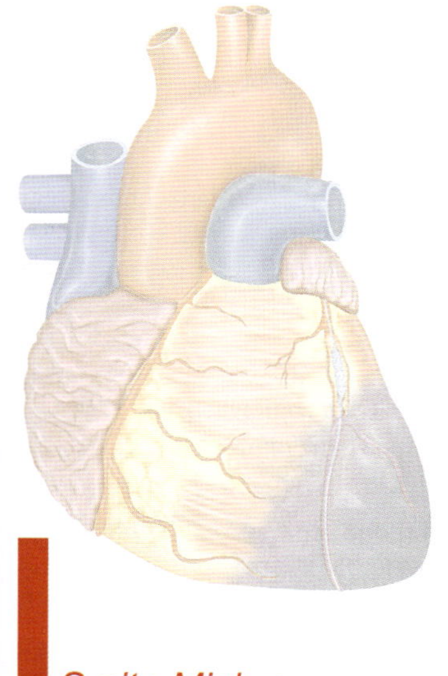

Prevention of HFpEF in Children

Smita Mishra

INTRODUCTION

Heart failure is a clinical syndrome consisting of diverse etiology due to abnormal cardiac structure or function leading to failure to meet tissue metabolic demand with existing cardiac output and normal filling pressures. HFpEF is a subset of HF, which presents with a constellation of HF-related symptoms, and neurohormonal changes with abnormal filling pressure, despite the preserved systolic function ejection fraction (LVEF >50%); it is ascribed to reduced compliance of left or right or both ventricles.[1]

The clinical course of children with HFpEF depends on the underlying cardiac condition, which usually, is a heterogeneous group of disorders. Therefore, the natural history and global prognosis of HFpEF in children are undefined. As in the adult population, pediatric HFpEF in association with restrictive cardiomyopathies, seems to have a grim prognosis due to the risk of sudden death, the progressive nature of pulmonary hypertension, and the subsequent need for a heart-lung transplant.

This article will discuss the spectrum of HFpEF and how we can prevent, revert, or delay the eventual adverse outcome.

CARDIAC CYCLE AND HEART FAILURE WITH PRESERVED EJECTION FRACTION (FIG. 1)

The cardiac cycle has two stages **(Fig. 1)**:

1. The diastolic phase consists of isovolumic relaxation (due to elastic recoil), ventricular rapid filling, a plateau, and late filling assisted by atrial contraction;
2. The systolic phase consists of isovolumic contraction and rapid ventricular ejection; stroke volume and cardiac output depend on preload (capacity of ventricles to relax during diastole and receive the desired volume of blood), afterload (pressure against which ventricle contracts). HFpEF is due to loss of the innate ability of the ventricular myocardium to relax (lusitropy) and distend, secondary to hypertrophy and fibrotic changes.[2]

Definition of HFpEF: So far, no separate definition for the pediatric age group has been suggested. ESC guidelines 2016 defines HFpEF based on the following criteria[3]: (1) Features suggestive of HF in the presence of LEF >50%; (2) Presence of high natriuretic hormones (BNP >35 pg/mL or NT-proBNP >125 pg/mL); (3) Relevant structural heart disease: (i) LV hypertrophy and/or LA enlargement-LAE; (ii) Abnormal left ventricular diastolic dimension; (iii) LA volume index >34 mL/m^2; (iv) Left ventricular mass index (LVMI) ≥115/95 g/m^2 (Men or Women); (v) Abnormal inflow indices (E/e′ ≥13, mean e′<9 cm/sec).

EPIDEMIOLOGY

Due to the lack of well-designed registries and less standardized diagnostic procedures in children, pediatric HFpEF remains underestimated and least studied.[4] Obesity, hypertension, coronary artery disease, and diabetes mellitus, usual risk factors in adults, have little contribution in the pediatric age group. In a series of 421 children with HFpEF, the top three cardiovascular causes were complex congenital heart disease (53.4%), and simple congenital heart defect (15.7%), while cardiomyopathy (7.4%)

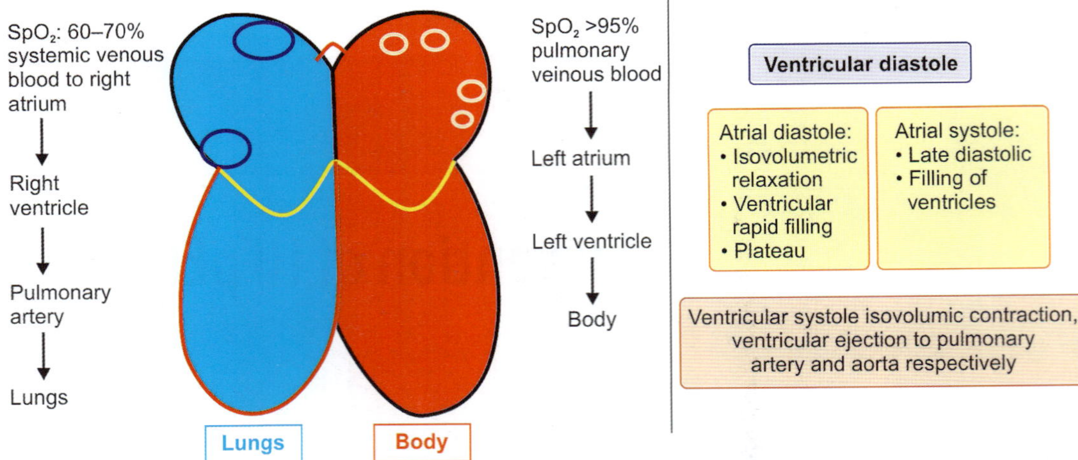

Fig. 1: Stages of cardiac cycle.

was 3rd common cause in the series.[5] With the present lifestyle of adolescents and young adults clinical obesity or metabolic syndrome may present with an underlying syndrome of HFpEF.

PATHOPHYSIOLOGY (FIG. 2)

It is well known that a mathematical relationship exists between myocardial force-velocity and instantaneous ventricular pressure-volume curve.[6] At the cellular level, both the contraction and relaxation phases are active, energy-dependent processes. During contraction, calcium influx, an ATP-requiring process, leads to calcium binding to troponin C altering the troponin–tropomyosin complex; interaction of myosin cross bridges with actin, initiates contraction. The diastole of the ventricle is marked by the detachment of actin-myosin cross bridges, which is preceded by calcium uptake by the sarcoplasmic reticulum (SR). These diastolic events also depend upon factors such as the viscoelastic myocardial forces, myocardial stress-strain relationship, ventricular interdependence, pericardial restraint, and atrial contraction.

Is HFpEF a coronary microvascular disease?: Recently, the pathophysiology of HFpEF has been explained based on maladaptive ventricular-vascular remodeling in response to multiple comorbidities.[7] In these patients, coronary microvascular dysfunction has been seen, even in the absence of coronary artery blockage.[8] It is speculated that the comorbidities induce low-grade subclinical systemic inflammation, provoking endothelial dysfunction and leading to suboptimal production and bioavailability of nitric oxide, for the microvasculature of both, systemic and coronary circulations. The triad of myocardial hypertrophy, stiffness, and interstitial fibrosis results from abnormal

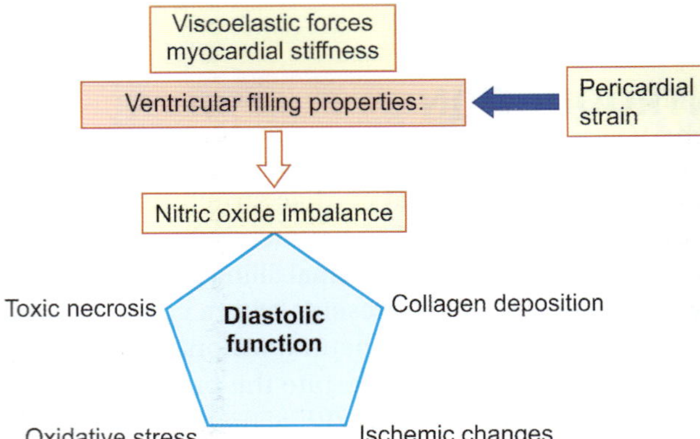

Fig. 2: Controlling factors of diastolic function.

actions of NO-cyclic guanosine monophosphate (cGMP) signaling pathway, and reduced protein kinase G (PKG) within the myocytes. These changes increase ventricular and arterial stiffness.[4,7]

CARDIAC FIBROSIS AS A PRECURSOR OF HEART FAILURE WITH PRESERVED EJECTION FRACTION (FLOWCHART 1)

Persistent myocardial damage provokes fibrosis once the limited regenerative mechanism of the myocardium is exhausted. Adaptive fibrotic process in these situations manifests with excess deposits of extracellular matrix, hampering normal myocytic function, and predisposing myocardium for intractable arrhythmias. It is a matter for future research if contextual factors activating excessive fibrotic response and initiating maladaptive processes can be targeted therapeutically.[9]

Flowchart 1: Etiology of heart failure wth preserved ejection fraction (HFpEF) in children.

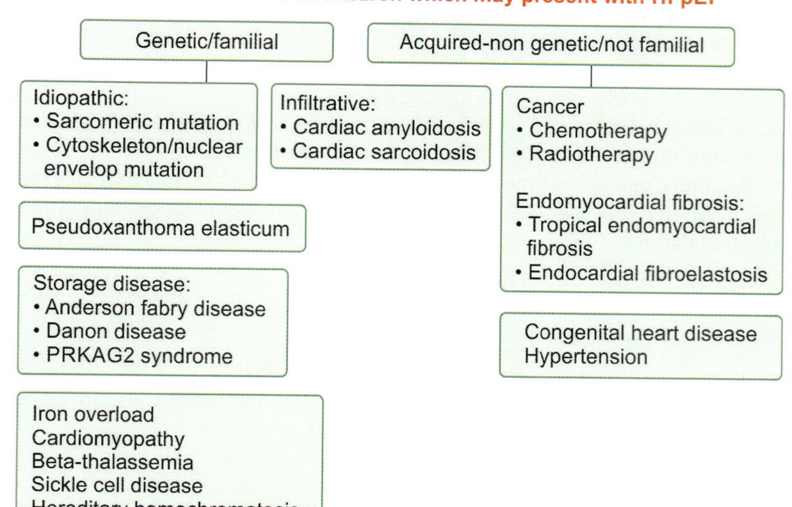

Moskowitz et al., reported HFpEF in children having high LV mass postrepair of coarctation of the aorta and poor relaxation capacity of ventricles.[10] Ventricular compliance may also be reduced in inflammatory diseases such as Kawasaki Disease, myocarditis, and severe acute respiratory syndrome coronavirus 2 (SARS-CoV-2). HFpEF is also seen in postradiation cancer, posttransplant cases, and in patients having renal insufficiency.[2,10-13]

CARDIOMYOPATHIES

Hypertrophic cardiomyopathy (HCM) is the second most common pediatric CMP, that presents with varying degrees of HFpEF;[1,2,4] it is attributed to impaired calcium handling, hypertrophy, disarray of myocytes, ischemia, and fibrosis. HCM-related mutations have been identified, in cardiac isoforms of myosin (MYH6/7/8), MyBP-C (MYBPC3), TnI (TNNI3), TnT (TNNT2), TnC (TNNC1), actin (ACTC1), Tm (TPM1), and MLC (MYL2).[10,11]

Dilated cardiomyopathy also tends to develop myocardial fibrosis in late phases.

Heart Failure with Preserved Ejection Fraction—Restrictive Cardiomyopathy in Pediatrics

Primary RCM is often due to the involvement of multiple mutations such as MYH7, MYL2, TNNI3, TNNT2, and DES. It contributes 5% of cases to the total CMP burden. Secondary RCM may be seen in children with CHDs, infiltrative and systemic diseases, and endomyocardial fibrosis associated with eosinophilia.[12] Transient restrictive patterns may be found in neonates born to diabetic mothers due to RV hypertrophy. Transient LV restrictive patterns may be seen in the postoperative period, and during tachyarrhythmias and sepsis.

DIAGNOSIS OF HEART FAILURE WITH PRESERVED EJECTION FRACTION

Diagnostic evaluation of HFpEF is given in **Table 1**. Echocardiographic criteria for pediatric diastolic dysfunction are not well established.[1,2,11-17] Therefore, it is an area open to further investigation.

MANAGEMENT PLAN (TABLES 2 AND 3)

Suboptimal myocardial lusitropy secondary to myocardial fibrosis is the cause of altered myocyte deformation and ventricular reserve category. Myocardial recovery is possible when the source of insult is removed, as in the case of aortic stenosis, aortic valvuloplasty takes away pressure overload, and myocardial recovery ensues. However, researchers are trying to correct the molecular pathobiology by pharmacotherapy or genomic modulation to attain "reverse remodeling", i.e., a sustained alteration in the size of myofibrils by targeting the fibrotic process and achieving normal ventricular geometry.

The understanding of the pathophysiology of HFpEF has changed and it is now described as a multi-organ involvement systemic syndrome, likely triggered by inflammation initiated due to lifestyle factors, genetic predisposition, and multiple comorbidities. So far, there

TABLE 1: Diagnosis of heart failure with preserved ejection fraction (HFpEF)—relevant investigations.[2,4,14-16]

Clinical features	Easy fatigability, lack of exercise intolerance, and other constitutional symptoms like lack of appetite
Echocardiography	Echo-Doppler criteria (ESC 2016): • *Grade I:* Mitral E/A ratio ≤0.8, E ≤50 cm/s, + Only one of the following three criteria is positive (E/e′ mean >14, LAVI >34 mL/m^2, TR_{max} > 2.8 m/s) • *Grade II:* Mitral E/A ratio ≥0.8 – <2 and E >50 cm/s, and two or three of the three criteria (E/e′ mean >14, LAVI >34 mL/m^2, TR_{max} >2.8 m/s) were positive • The isovolumic relaxation time appeared stable with age which makes it an excellent parameter in children • *Grade III:* When mitral E/A ratio ≥2, diastolic dysfunction global longitudinal strain (GLS): Low; Difficult to apply in pediatrics
Elevated NT pro-BNP levels (age appropriate)	• 0–2 days >12,000 pg/mL; 3–11 days >6,000 pg/mL • 1 month–1 year > 650 pg/mL; 1–2 years >400 pg/mL • 2–6 years >300 pg/mL; 6–18 years >160 pg/mL
Other biomarkers	Increased levels of soluble suppression of tumorigenesis 2 (sST2), hs-CRP, cystatin-C, TIMPs, N-terminal propeptide of type III procollagen (PIIINP), homocysteine, and resistin, alectin-3 (Gal-3), and growth differentiation factor 15 (GDF-15)
Therapeutic test	Diuretics causing improvement in symptoms
Cardiac magnetic resonance imaging	*Done for:* Accurate assessment of atrial and ventricular volumes, ejection fraction, and diastolic function; provides insights into myocardial stiffness evidenced by changes in blood flow patterns and myocardial strain; 4D-flow", (+AI assistance) is used for quantification of three-dimensional blood flow velocities throughout the cardiac cycle
Right heart catheterization (RHC)	(1) Simultaneously, left ventricle (LV) volumes and pressure (pressure-volume loops) measurement. Rate of decline of ventricular pressure (time constant of relaxation-tau or τ) during the IVRT. (Normal tau(τ) is 30–40 ms); (2) Pulmonary capillary wedge pressure (PCWP) akin to LA mean/LVEDP; (3) LVEDP (normal <15 mm H g) rapid saline loading during RHC can unmask restrictive pattern

TABLE 2: Etiology and possible management.[2,24-29]

Etiology		*Reason*	*Possible intervention*	*Comments*
Idiopathic—Sarcomere mutation (Cardiomyopathies RCM, HCM, DCM)		Possible role in abnormalities of relaxation and hypertrophy in HCM	Mavacamten (originally MYK-461) Aficamten; improved relaxation in HCM+ Supportive/ICD	Omecamtiv mercarbil and danicamtiv are other experimental drugs
Pseudoxanthoma elasticum		Autosomal recessive disorder caused by mutations in the ABCC6 gene	BP/Diabetes mellitus control/BMI and other lifestyle management	
Glycogen storage disorders	Anderson Fabry disease	Mutations in the GLA gene, deficiency of the enzymatic activity of α-galactosidase A	Drugs under evaluation: ERT with recombinant α-galactosidase A/Agalsidase alpha, beta, Migalastat	Only therapy available: lifestyle management/ICD/ supportive
	Danon disease	X-linked dominant/LAMP2 gene codes for 3 major LAMP2 protein isoforms	Lifestyle management/ICD/ supportive	
	PRKG2 syndrome	Early-onset autosomal dominant inherited disease	Lifestyle management	Implantable cardioverter-defibrillator (ICD) in selected cases
Endomyocardial fibrosis (EMF)		May present with tropical eosinophilia	In the early stage—treatment with steroids may help	
Iron overload due to hemolytic anemia		Thalassemia alfa, beta, traits; Sickle cell disease; Hemochromatosis	*Desferrioxamine:* Slow s.c. infusion over 8–12 hours of a 10% solution (Average dose 40 mg/kg), 5/7 days. Using an infusion pump	If started early, it can prevent the toxic effect of iron deposition + Lifestyle management/Supportive
Amyloidosis		Usually seen in the adult population	*Possible treatment:* Tafamidis	

Contd...

Contd...

Etiology	*Reason*	*Possible intervention*	*Comments*
Sarcoidosis	Etiology not known attributed to genetics, autoimmunity, etc.	*Early treatment:* Prednisone and repository corticotropin	Early diagnosis: HRCT, FDG-PET scanning, TBNA, and EBUS technologies
Radiation-induced heart disease (RIHD)	?Cardiac/coronary fibrosis secondary to endothelial injury, inflammation, and endoplasmic reticulum and mitochondrial dysfunction	*In (RCI) injection Primary preventive method:* To optimize radiation dose (dose reduction may not be possible) early diagnosis and use of drugs that may have	Possibly preventive role of drugs, including statins, ACE inhibitors, and antioxidants (secondary prophylaxis)
Chemotherapy	Oxidative injuries from oxygen radicals generated by chemotherapy	Cumulative anthracycline dose to be limited, the use of anthracycline structural analogs, and especially cardioprotective agents	Use of cardioprotection agent dexrazoxane Immune checkpoint inhibitors: Early detection and use of glucocorticoids
Congenital heart disease	*Substrate:* Common with CHD with pressure overload; complex CHD	Early valvuloplasty (PS, AS, Coarctation of aorta); Age-appropriate intervention of complex CHD	

TABLE 3: Probable pharmacotherapy of heart failure with preserved ejection fraction (HFpEF).[24-29]

Sodium-glucose cotransporter-2 inhibitors[23]	• Sodium-glucose cotransporter-2 inhibitors have shown protective effects in HFpEF • They are beneficial for adults with CHD even if the systemic ventricle is RV • In children efficacy and safety needs to be established.[23] They are beneficial for reverse remodeling	*Sirt1, Sirt1-mediated deacetylation of SMAD3 in HFpEF:* Downregulation of transforming growth factor-beta (TGF-β)-mediated fibrosis through inhibition of fibrotic transcriptional activity, and also by inhibiting myofibroblasts
Ivabradine[24]	Controls heart rate but *decreases* peak oxygen intake during exercise. Trials for the evaluation of benefits in the HFpEF group have shown contradictory results	Selectively inhibiting the sinoatrial node's funny current channels
β-blockers/Ca channel blockers/Digoxin[25]	"β-blockers" Conflicting data about the benefits	These drugs may be needed in the presence of arrhythmia-atrial fibrillation
Angiotensin-converting enzyme inhibitors (ACEi) and angiotensin II receptor blockers (ARB) ARNI, angiotensin receptor nepri-lysin inhibitor (ARNi) sacubitril-valsartan[26]	Conflicting data	However, ACEi, and ARBi may be helpful if HFpEF is associated with comorbidities diabetic nephropathy and when LVEF <60%
Mineralocorticoid receptor antagonist[25]	No benefits have been reported in HFpEF	
Lipid-lowering agents[27]	Lipid dysregulation may be a promoter of HFpEF in young adults. Early screening in susceptible populations—life style management statins and other drugs may be useful	

are no universally accepted pharmacotherapies, that can alter the clinical course of HFpEF.

Exercise limitations associated with HFpEF affect the quality of life (QOL) and are the hallmark of HFpEF which has been attributed to skeletal muscle changes (e.g., fat deposits) leading to a rapid depletion of high-energy phosphates early in exercise.[18] The progression of HFpEF may be arrested in children with timely intervention. Therefore, early diagnosis, and applying the best possible treatment plan (medical, surgical, or cath) are the only way forward. **Tables 2 and 3** provide brief information on the subject.

A group of instructions have been published to improve QOL of adult patients with HFpEF, few of them can be applicable to pediatric population also.

- Diuretics, sodium-restricted diet, weight management, BP monitoring, blood sugar, lipid profile for older age group, and nutritional support for adequate growth;
- Avoid juices, sugar-containing drinks, etc.
- Rhythm maintenance, physical activity chart;
- Psychological support to parents and family.

Maintaining life's simple 7 launched by American Heart Association in 2016 which includes: (1) Smoking, (2) Obesity, (3) Exercise, (4) Diet, (5) Blood pressure, (6) Cholesterol, and (7) Glucose.[19]

1. *Smoking:* Smoking may increase inflammation chronically and can result in significant acute diastolic dysfunction of the left ventricle, particularly in vulnerable populations. Alshehri et al., have established a relationship between cigarette smoking and diastolic heart failure has been established. Smoking is a common habit adopted in schools and colleges.[20]
2. *Obesity management:* Obesity is known to be associated with comorbidities such as hypertension, LV hypertrophy, diastolic dysfunction, renal impairment, and atrial fibrillation. Obesity often presents with fatigue, dyspnea, and ankle swelling, a clinical syndrome also associated with HFpEF. Obesity management has been associated with overall improvement.[21]
3. *Exercise training:* Four randomized controlled exercise intervention trials were designed to evaluate the role of physical training in the adult population with HFpEF; results were favorable as the distance walked in the 6-minute walk test improved and overall quality of life was impacted positively. Epigenetic modulation has been proved in animal experimental models. Differentially methylated genes were linked with myocardial fibrosis, myocyte hypertrophy, myocardial apoptosis, and myocardial energy metabolism.[22]
4. *Management of hypertension:* Systemic hypertension with metabolic syndrome, or in isolation, has shown a rising trend among adolescents and young adults. It leads to ventricular hypertrophy and myocardial stiffening. Thus, early detection and management of hypertension is important.[23] The recent guidelines recommended 6 monthly blood pressure monitoring after 5 years of age or earlier in vulnerable groups of children. Lifestyle management, meditation, diet regulation, salt restriction, and drugs must be appropriately used. The preferred drugs angiotensin-converting enzyme (ACE) inhibitors and calcium channel blockers are preferred over diuretics and β-blockers.
5. *Control of diabetes mellitus:* As advised by the ACC panel on HFpEF, the target for glycosylated hemoglobin HbA1c is <7–7.5% for individuals with lower comorbidity burden or less severe HF SGLT2 inhibitors should be first line for diabetic HFpEF.[27-29] Metformin may be considered if the estimated glomerular filtration rate (eGFR) is >30. Glucagon-like peptide-1 (GLP-1) agonists or GIP antagonists may be considered for obese individuals with diabetes mellitus and HFpEF. Dipeptidyl peptidase-4 (DPP4) inhibitors saxagliptin, alogliptin, and thiazolidinediones are contraindicated in HF. Agents slowing the progression for diabetic nephropathy include ACE inhibitors, ARBs, sodium-glucose cotransporter-2 (SGLT2) inhibitors, MRA (finerenone), ARNIs, and SGLT2 inhibitors.
6. *Arrhythmias and atrial fibrillation:* The supraventricular and ventricular tachycardias must be treated according to existing guidelines. Atrial fibrillation may have early onset in pediatric patients with HFpEF depending on underlying etiology. Though not beneficial in HFpEF, β-blockers, and nondihydropyridine calcium channel blockers, (with the addition of digoxin) have been recommended as the first-line drugs for rate control for AF-HFpEF. Anticoagulation should be considered based on CHA2DS2-VASc score.[29]
7. *Lipid profile:* As we discussed before, coronary microvasculature disease is now attributed to impaired lusitropy. In the presence of comorbidities, inducing systemic proinflammatory response, complex molecular pathways get activated to promote cardiac fibrosis and myocardium stiffening. The defective mitophagy in these situations aggravates undesired nonresolving inflammation. The overall effect of these activities leads to lipid dysregulation and atherosclerotic patches in the coronary and systemic arteries.[28-29]

The nonhigh-density lipoprotein (non-HDL-C) and low-density lipoprotein cholesterol (LDL-C) levels in childhood were associated with increased incidences of cardiovascular events in mid-life. Lifestyle changes and diet management are the first step but pharmacotherapy (statins and other drugs) may be indicated for more severe elevations.

CONCLUSION

Heart failure with preserved ejection fraction is less common in the pediatric age group and has heterogeneous etiologies; overall outcome in the pediatric age group may have multiple variables such as age of detection, availability of an appropriate method of management, e.g., enzyme replacement therapy or cardiac interventions for structural heart diseases, application of the timely treatment, superimposition of metabolic syndrome, obesity, or hypertension. Accordingly, an endpoint may be delayed or a status quo may be achieved. Like in HFrEF, a heart-lung transplant may be required particularly in genetically predisposed populations. Lifestyle management, prevention of subclinical inflammatory response, and prioritizing the advanced research on new candidates like bio-pathological factors responsible for exaggerated fibrotic signaling, are the recent recommendations on secondary prevention of HFpEF.

REFERENCES

1. Bozkurt B, Coats AJS, Tsutsui H, et al. Universal definition and classification of heart failure: a report of the Heart Failure Society of America, Heart Failure Association of the European Society of Cardiology, Japanese Heart Failure Society and Writing Committee of the Universal Definition of Heart Failure: Endorsed by the Canadian Heart Failure Society, Heart Failure Association of India, Cardiac Society of Australia and New Zealand, and Chinese Heart Failure Association. Eur J Heart Fail. 2021;23(3):352-80.
2. Fukuda N, Terui T, Ishiwata S, et al. Titin-based regulations of diastolic and systolic functions of mammalian cardiac muscle. J Mol Cell Cardiol. 2010;48(5):876-81.
3. Kim MN, Park SM. Heart failure with preserved ejection fraction: insights from recent clinical researches. Korean J Intern Med. 2020;35(3):514-34.
4. Quennelle S, Bonnet D. Pediatric heart failure with preserved ejection fraction, a review. Front Pediatr. 2023; 11:1137853.
5. Pan B, Hu D, Sun H, et al. Pediatric Diastolic Heart Failure: Clinical Features Description of 421 Cases. Front Pediatr. 2022;10:846408.
6. Suga H, Sagawa K. Mathematical interrelationship between instantaneous ventricular pressure-volume ratio and myocardial force-velocity relation. Ann Biomed Eng. 1972;1(2):160-81.
7. Tah S, Valderrama M, Afzal M, et al. Heart Failure With Preserved Ejection Fraction: An Evolving Understanding. Cureus. 2023;15(9):e46152.
8. Sweeney M, Corden B, Cook SA. Targeting cardiac fibrosis in heart failure with preserved ejection fraction: mirage or miracle? EMBO Mol Med. 2020;12(10):e10865.
9. Paulus WJ, Tschöpe C. A novel paradigm for heart failure with preserved ejection fraction: comorbidities drive myocardial dysfunction and remodeling through coronary microvascular endothelial inflammation. J Am Coll Cardiol. 2013;62(4):263-71.
10. Moskowitz WB, Schieken RM, Mosteller M, et al. Altered systolic and diastolic function in children after "successful" repair of coarctation of the aorta. Am Heart J. 1990;120(1):103-9.
11. Martin AA, Thompson BR, Hahn D, et al. Cardiac Sarcomere Signaling in Health and Disease. Int J Mol Sci. 2022;23(24):16223.
12. Zampieri M, Di Filippo C, Zocchi C, et al. Focus on Paediatric Restrictive Cardiomyopathy: Frequently Asked Questions. Diagnostics (Basel). 2023;13(24):3666.
13. Mitsnefes MM, Kimball TR, Border WL, et al. Impaired left ventricular diastolic function in children with chronic renal failure. Kidney Int. 2004;65(4):1461-6.
14. Dragulescu A, Mertens L, Friedberg MK. Misinterpretation of Left Ventricular Diastolic Dysfunction in Children With Cardiomyopathy by Echocardiography: Problems and Limitations. Circ Cardiovasc Imaging. 2013;6(2): 254-61.
15. Zhou Y, Zhao CM, Shen ZY, et al. Mitral early-diastolic inflow peak velocity (E)-to-left atrial strain ratio as a novel index for predicting elevated left ventricular filling pressures in patients with preserved left ventricular ejection fraction. Cardiovasc Ultrasound. 2021; 19(1):17.
16. Nir A, Lindinger A, Rauh M, et al. NT-pro-B-type natriuretic peptide in infants and children: reference values based on combined data from four studies. Pediatr Cardiol. 2009;30(1):3-8.
17. Huis In't Veld AE, de Man FS, van Rossum AC, et al. How to diagnose heart failure with preserved ejection fraction: the value of invasive stress testing. Neth Heart J. 2016;24(4):244-51.
18. Adam V. Linke A, Winzer E. Skeletal muscle alterations in HFrEF vs. HFpEF. Curr Heart Fail Rep. 2017;14:489-97.
19. Cilia L, Saeed A, Ganga HV, et al. Heart Failure With Preserved Ejection Fraction: Prevention and Management. Am J Lifestyle Med. 2017;13(2):182-9.
20. Alshehri AM, Azoz AM, Shaheen HA, et al. Acute effects of cigarette smoking on the cardiac diastolic functions. J Saudi Heart Assoc. 2013;25:173-9.
21. Bahrami H, Bluemke DA, Kronmal R, et al. Novel metabolic risk factors for incident heart failure and their relationship with obesity: the MESA (Multi-Ethnic Study of Atherosclerosis) study. J Am Coll Cardiol. 2008;51: 1775-83.
22. Liu K, Ju W, Ouyang S, et al. Exercise training ameliorates myocardial phenotypes in heart failure with preserved ejection fraction by changing N6-methyladenosine modification in mice model. Front Cell Dev Biol. 2022; 10:954769.

23. Kasiakogias A, Rosei EA, Camafort M, et al. Hypertension and heart failure with preserved ejection fraction: position paper by the European Society of Hypertension. J Hypertens. 2021;39(8):1522-45.
24. Wei W, Rao F, Liu F, et al. Involvement of Smad3 pathway in atrial fibrosis induced by elevated hydrostatic pressure. J Cell Physiol. 2018;233:4981-9.
25. Nadeem M, Hassib M, Aslam HM, et al. Role of Ivabradine in Patients with Heart Failure with Preserved Ejection Fraction. Cureus. 2020;12(2):e7123.
26. Palau P, Seller J, Domínguez E, et al. Effect of beta-blocker withdrawal on functional capacity in heart failure and preserved ejection fraction. J Am Coll Cardiol. 2021;78:2042-56.
27. Kataria R, G. Van Spall H. (2022). Pharmacologic Treatment For HFpEF: Role of Drug Therapies at the Higher End of LVEF Spectrum. [online] Available from https://www.acc.org/latest-in-cardiology/articles/2022/03/08/18/51/pharmacologic-treatment-for-hfpef [Last accessed January, 2025].
28. Leggat J, Bidault G, Vidal-Puig A. Lipotoxicity: a driver of heart failure with preserved ejection fraction? Clin Sci (Lond). 2021;135(19):2265-83.
29. Shore S. (2023). ACC Expert Consensus on Management of HFpEF: Key Points. [online] Available from https://www.acc.org/latest-in-cardiology/ten-points-to-remember/2023/04/17/16/40/2023-acc-expert-consensus-on-hfpef [Last accessed January, 2025].

CHAPTER 85

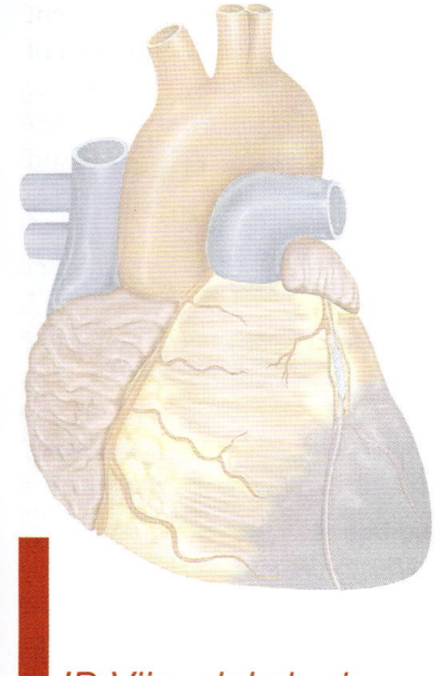

HFpEF Management in Children

IB Vijayalakshmi

INTRODUCTION

The heart failure (HF) is a complex clinical syndrome, caused by functional or structural heart disease hampering ventricular filling or ejection of blood into the pulmonary and/or systemic circulation. In HF with preserved ejection fraction (HFpEF), patients have signs and symptoms of HF due to high left ventricular (LV) filling pressure despite normal or near normal LV ejection fraction (LVEF).[1] HFpEF or diastolic dysfunction (DD) consists of elevated LV stiffness, prolonged isovolumetric LV relaxation, slow LV filling, and elevated LV end-diastolic pressure (LVEDP). Arterial hypertension (HT) occurs in majority of cases with HFpEF worldwide.[2] That means HFpEF is a type of HF where the LVEF is 50% or higher, but the LV filling pressure is high as LVEDP is high. The HFpEF is also known as diastolic heart failure (DHF). William Gaasch first described the pathophysiology of DHF in the early 1990s. Since then, DHF now known as HFpEF has emerged over the last two decades as a separate clinical entity and its diagnosis and treatment are more challenging than HF with reduced EF (HFrEF).

WHAT IS HEART FAILURE WITH PRESERVED EJECTION FRACTION?

Heart failure with preserved ejection fraction is abnormal cardiac relaxation, stiffness, or filling. Nearly half of the patients presenting with symptoms of congestive HF have near-normal LV systolic function at rest. This predominantly is due to HFpEF, which is generally considered to have a better prognosis than HFrEF. But frequency of hospitalizations is similar in both systolic and diastolic HF.[2] HFpEF is a clinical syndrome characterized by increased tissue fluid and decreased tissue and organ perfusion. It is often the cause of HF in obese, elderly, and women. It is estimated that 40–50% of patients with HF have HFpEF. These patients have high mortality rates and get hospitalized frequently. The HFpEF cases are associated with obesity, hypertension, aortic stenosis with cardiac hypertrophy, hypertrophic cardiomyopathy (HCM), restrictive cardiomyopathy, atrial fibrillation, diabetes, smoking or use of tobacco products, intake of alcohol, caffeine, aging, coronary artery disease (CAD) with history of heart attacks, sleep apnea, kidney dysfunction, some genetic disorders, physical inactivity, and some cancers. It is known that people with only DD with no CAD have near-normal lifespan like age-matched general population. Hence, DHF was neglected or ignored as insignificant in the past. Now, it is evident that there is no cure for HFpEF, but only symptoms can be managed. Therefore, equal importance is being given to HFpEF also.

American College of Cardiology (ACC) and American Heart Association (AHA) have described and defined the following stages of HF:[3]

- *Stage A:* It consists of patients at risk for HF without symptoms or structural heart disease or cardiac biomarkers of stretch or injury. Treatment at this stage is to modify underlying risk factors for the development of HF.
- *Stage B:* This stage of pre-HF consists of patients ith evidence of increased filling pressures by invasive or noninvasive methods or patients with risk factors and increased biomarkers of stretch or cardiac injury that are not explained by other diseases. Treatment at this stage is to treat risk factors and structural heart disease to prevent HF in future **(Figs. 1A to D)**.

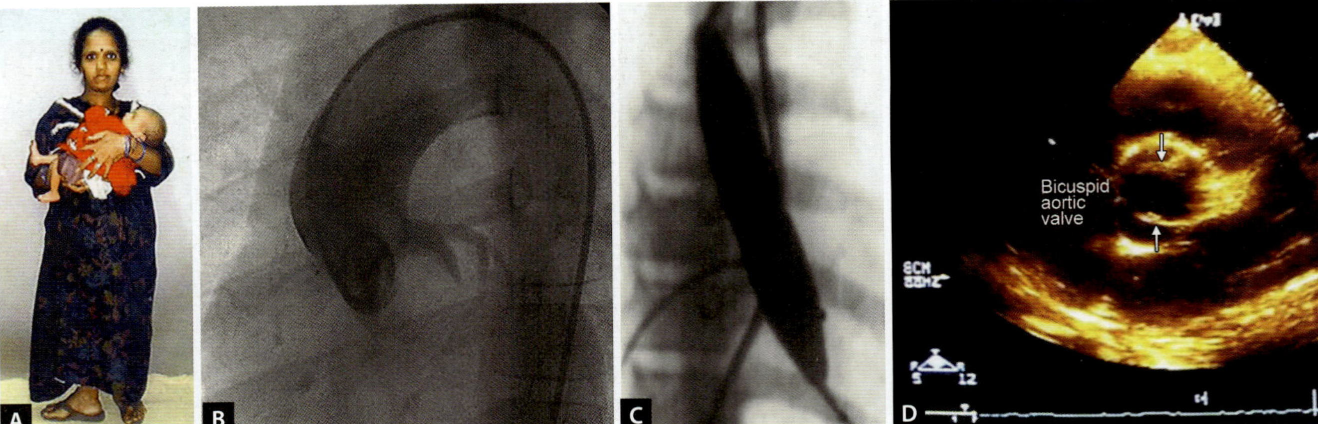

Figs. 1A to D: (A) Full-term pregnant achondroplasia patient with severe aortic stenosis after balloon dilatation of aortic valve and baby delivered by lower cesarian section; (B) Aortic root angiogram shows "Prussian helmet appearance" due to doming bicuspid aortic valve and negative shadow caused by blood entering aorta through the stenotic aortic valve; (C) Successful balloon dilatation with no waist; (D) Transthoracic echocardiogram in short axis shows well opened bicuspid aortic valve with good result of balloon dilatation.

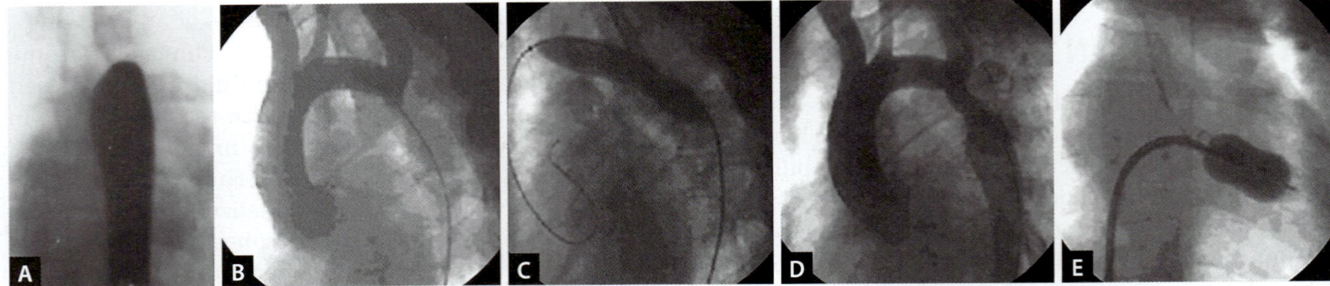

Figs. 2A to E: (A) Aortogram in AP view shows coarctation of aorta (COA); (B) Angiogram of ascending aorta shows tight COA; (C) Inflated balloon across COA with waist; (D) Check angiogram shows opened up COA; (E) Inoue balloon across stenosed mitral valve. Successful aortoplasty and balloon mitral valvotomy were both done in the same sitting in 16 years old boy of COA and RHD with MS with atrial fibrillation and pulmonary edema but normal LVEF.

- *Stage C:* It consists of patients with structural heart disease with current or previous symptoms of HF. Management at this stage aims to reduce symptoms, morbidity, and mortality **(Figs. 2A to E)**.
- *Stage D:* It consists of patients with marked symptoms of advanced HF that interfere with daily life and are accompanied by recurrent hospitalizations despite attempts to optimize guideline-directed medical therapy **(Figs. 3A and B)**. The intervention at this stage is to reduce symptoms, morbidity, and mortality.[3]

PATHOPHYSIOLOGY OF HEART FAILURE WITH PRESERVED EJECTION FRACTION IS BEYOND DIASTOLIC DYSFUNCTION

The clinical manifestations of HFpEF are due to complex pathophysiological processes in hemodynamic derangements due to changes in cardiomyocyte structure and function.[4] But the pathophysiology of HFpEF is not limited to only the cardiomyocyte. Many mechanisms have been proposed for DHF. Recently, cardiac oxidative stress has been associated with DD. Increased levels of cardiac reactive oxygen species (ROS) are used to explain changes in Ca^{2+} handling proteins and the increased Ca^{2+} sensitivity of myofilaments in DHF.

The phenotypes of HFpEF are shown in **Figure 4**.

GRADING OF HEART FAILURE WITH PRESERVED EJECTION FRACTION

Grading of HFpEF is as follows:

- *Grade I:* Impaired relaxation and decreased suction of the LV
- *Grade II:* Pseudonormalization, increased stiffness of the LV, and elevated filling pressure

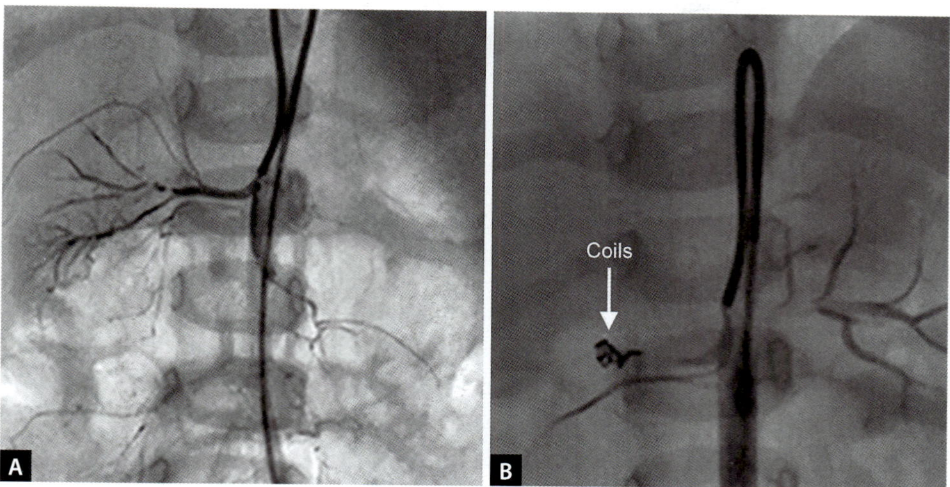

Figs. 3A and B: (A): Selective right renal angiogram; (B) Nonsurgical nephrectomy done with 5 × 3 and 3 × 4 embolization coils with complete closure of right renal artery in a 4-year-old boy with hypertensive crisis despite treatment with 3 drugs to control hypertension with nonfunctioning right kidney. Post coil closure blood pressure dropped from 240/120 to 140/90 mm Hg.

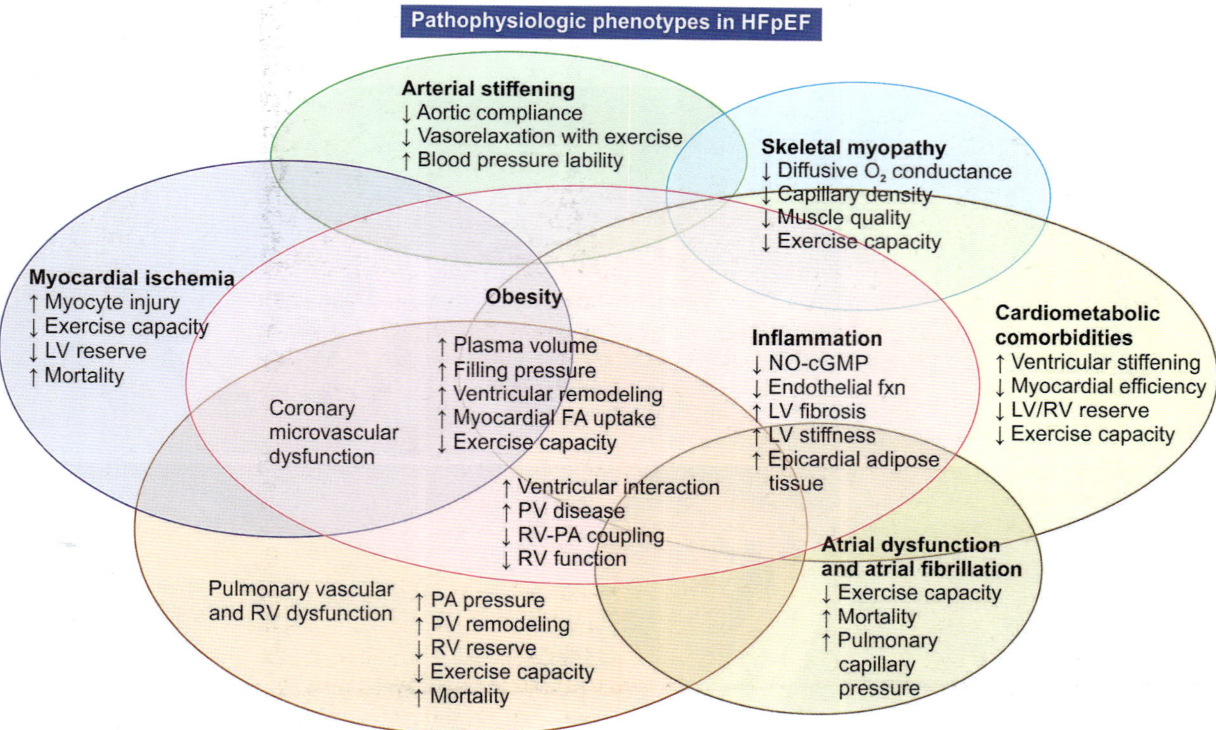

Fig. 4: Phenotypes of HFpEF.
Source: Obakata et al. (2020).

- *Grade III:* Restrictive filling with elevated filling pressure and noncompliant LV

The HFpEF may be reversible with reduction of preload or irreversible with no benefit from reduction of preload.[5] Elevated filling pressures are the main pathophysiological consequences of advanced DD.[6] Filling pressures represent the left atrial pressure (LAP) and the LVEDP, which are considered elevated when the mean pulmonary capillary wedge pressure is >12 mm Hg or when the LV end-diastolic pressure (left ventricular filling pressure [LVFP]) is >16 mm Hg (hemodynamic method).[7]

DIAGNOSTIC PARAMETERS

The diagnosis of HFpEF can be challenging, particularly in patients with overt signs and symptoms of HF.

Laboratory Testing

Initial basic evaluation includes:

- Complete blood count
- Serum electrolytes, including sodium, potassium, calcium, and magnesium
- Serum creatinine and blood urea nitrogen
- Serum glucose
- Lipid profile
- Liver function tests
- Iron studies, including serum iron, ferritin, and transferrin saturation,
- Thyroid-stimulating hormone
- *New biomarkers:* cMyBP-C is peptide (BNP) or N-terminal prohormone of B-type natriuretic peptide (NT-proBNP). Many of both cardiac and noncardiac conditions can cause increase in BNP levels, including advancing age, atrial fibrillation, and chronic kidney disease (CKD) which are actually responsible for HFpEF. The NT-proBNP and BNP appear to be the most reliable biomarkers in chronic HFpEF. The NT-proBNP shows higher specificity but BNP shows higher sensitivity. Although Gal-3 appears more reliable than ST2 in HFpEF diagnosis, the conclusions have limitations as only three studies were included in meta-analysis.[8]

1. 12-lead electrocardiogram (ECG)
2. Chest X-ray
3. Transthoracic echocardiography (TTE):

TTE is perhaps the most useful and essential tool in diagnosis of HFpEF.[3] To categorize HF, the TTE is indicated **(Figs. 5A to F)**.[9] The assessment of LVEF is the critical step for classifying HF in order to give appropriate evidence-based therapy.[3] The normal diastolic function is characterized by predominantly early diastolic mitral inflow when velocities E wave exceeds A-wave velocity.

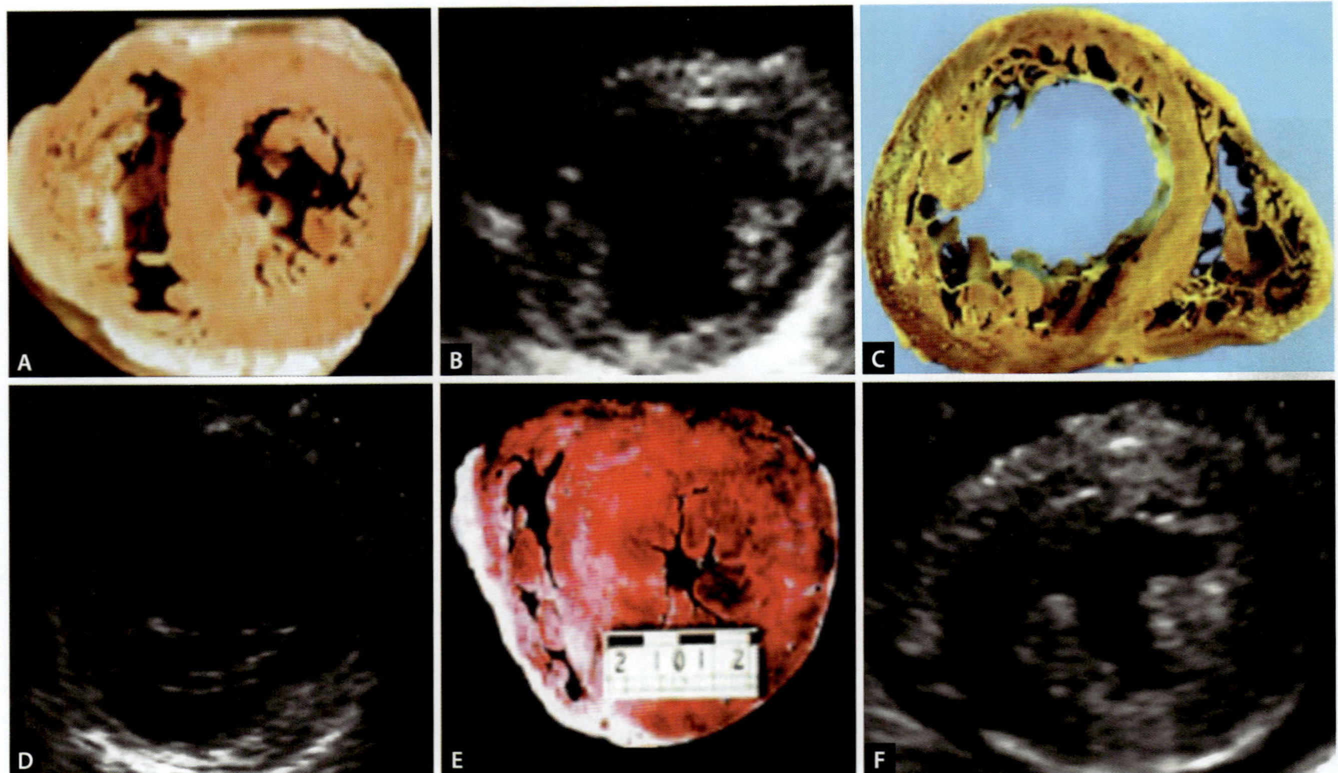

Figs. 5A to F: (A) Cut section of normal heart in short axis in autopsy, with normal ventricles and normal cavity; (B) TTE in short axis at papillary muscle level showing normal cavity and walls; (C) Cut section of heart in the short axis showing dilated ventricles with thin walls in autopsy of the patient with dilated left ventricle comparing with (D) TTE in short axis at mitral valve level that shows dilated LV with reduced EF in a case of dilated cardiomyopathy; (E) Cut section of hypertrophied heart in short axis in autopsy with thickened walls of ventricles and small cavity in a hypertensive patient with LF hypertrophy; and (F) TTE in short axis at papillary muscle shows hypertrophy of LV muscle with normal EF in a hypertensive patient with preserved EF.

When ventricular relaxation is impaired, atrial kick or boost contributes to ventricular filling that corresponds to early flow during LV relaxation and the subsequent contribution from atrial contraction (A wave > E wave velocity, with prolonged deceleration of the E wave, usually >240 milliseconds). This usually occurs with increasing age; hence, identifying patients at risk of HFpEF in elderly population is important. The mitral E and A waves that flow in pulmonary vein are also measured in 2 phases—systolic and diastolic. Newer modalities that are not as well validated include color M-mode of the mitral flow propagation wave and Doppler tissue imaging (diastolic velocities of the myocardial tissue itself). When ventricular diastolic pressure increases so much that atrial boost contributes little to filling, then "E" wave again becomes prominent but with rapid deceleration **(Figs. 6A and B)**, first in a pseudonormal pattern and ultimately, in a restrictive pattern (high "E" wave velocity is usually more than twice the velocity of "A" wave). Both E and A filling patterns are associated with diastolic-dominant pulmonary vein flow in aged patients. The two waves of pulmonary venous flow are during systole and diastole, similar to the "x" and "y" descents in jugular veins. Elevated left atrial pressure impairs atrial filling during descent of the base in ventricular systole, and pulmonary vein flow occurs mostly during diastole when the mitral valve is open. This pattern can be seen with both systolic heart failure (SHF) and HFpEF.

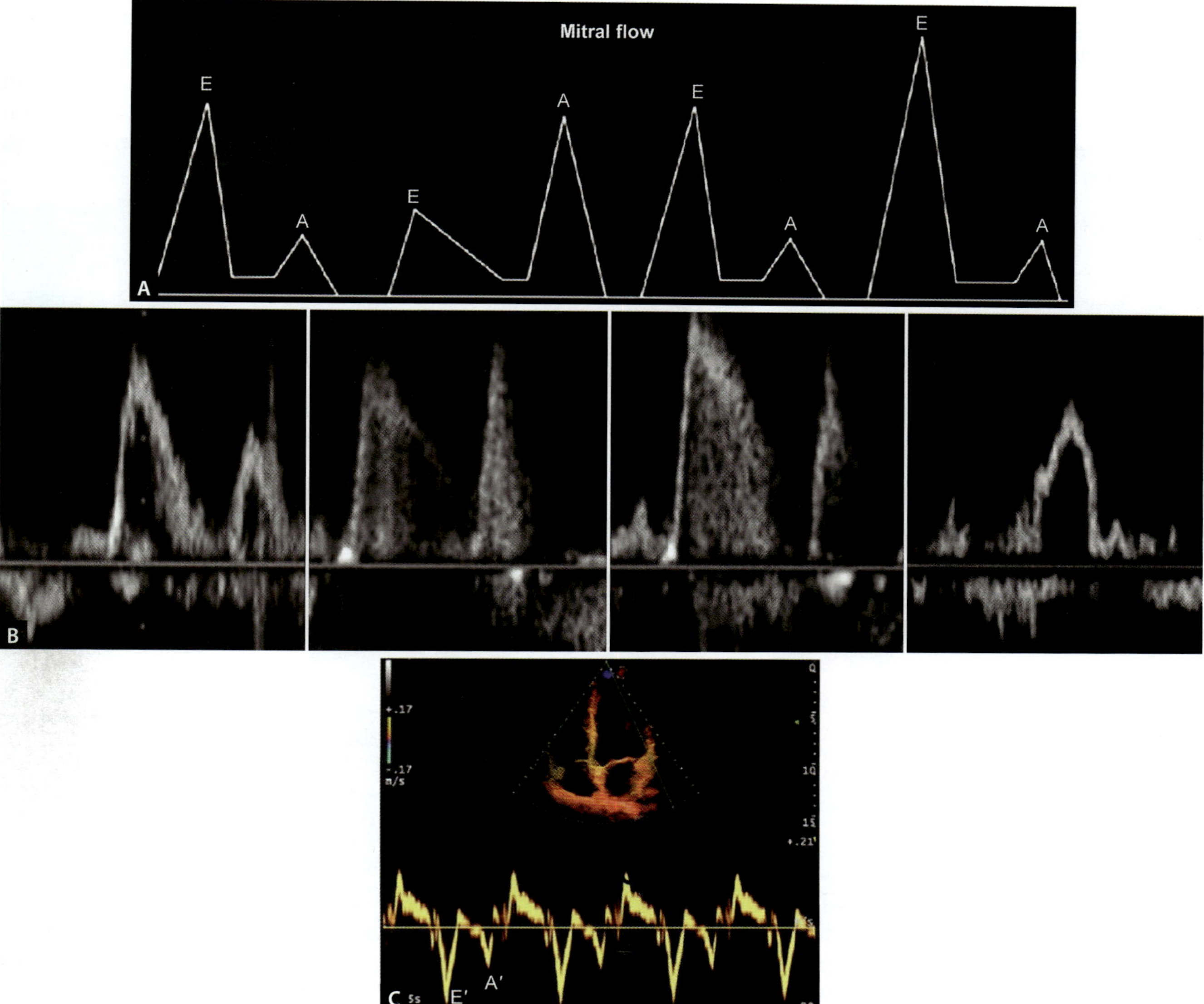

Figs. 6A to C: (A) Diagram of E and A waves in normal and three grades of diastolic dysfunction; (B) Real Doppler images of E and A in normal and three grades of HFpEF; (C) Tissue Doppler in early diastole (E') and late diastole (A').

Mitral annular plane systolic excursion (MAPSE) is a cardiac measurement that can be used to assess left ventricular diastolic dysfunction (LVDD) **(Fig. 6C)**. The MAPSE is measured using echocardiography by placing the cursor on the mitral valve annulus and pressing the M-mode button. The excursion is the distance from the lowest point to the highest point. A normal MAPSE is 12–15 mm. But a decreased MAPSE indicates longitudinal systolic dysfunction. A MAPSE of ≤10 mm is a cutoff value that can detect systolic dysfunction and/or DD. A MAPSE of ≤1.45 cm is an optimal threshold point for diagnosing LVDD in obese adults. Grading of DD can be done by tissue Doppler and MAPSE indicating reduced LV Global longitudinal strain (GLS) **(Figs. 7A to C)**. GLS measurement of how much the heart muscle lengthens and shortens during a cardiac cycle provides insight into the overall function of the left ventricle. GLS is considered a more sensitive indicator of early heart muscle dysfunction when compared to just looking at EF.

Pulmonary Venous Systolic/Diastolic (S/D) Ratio

The normal pulmonary venous flow usually shows a tri- or quadriphasic pattern, consisting of a pulmonary venous first systolic wave (S1), second systolic wave (S2) (S wave velocity is made by adding S1 and S2), pulmonary venous early diastolic wave (D), and pulmonary venous atrial reversed flow wave.

For example, in a 58-year-old patient with HFpEF due to diabetic nephropathy, CKD and systemic hypertension, TTE showed the fulfillment of HFA PEFF score with following major criteria of >5 points (each of the following has 2 points).

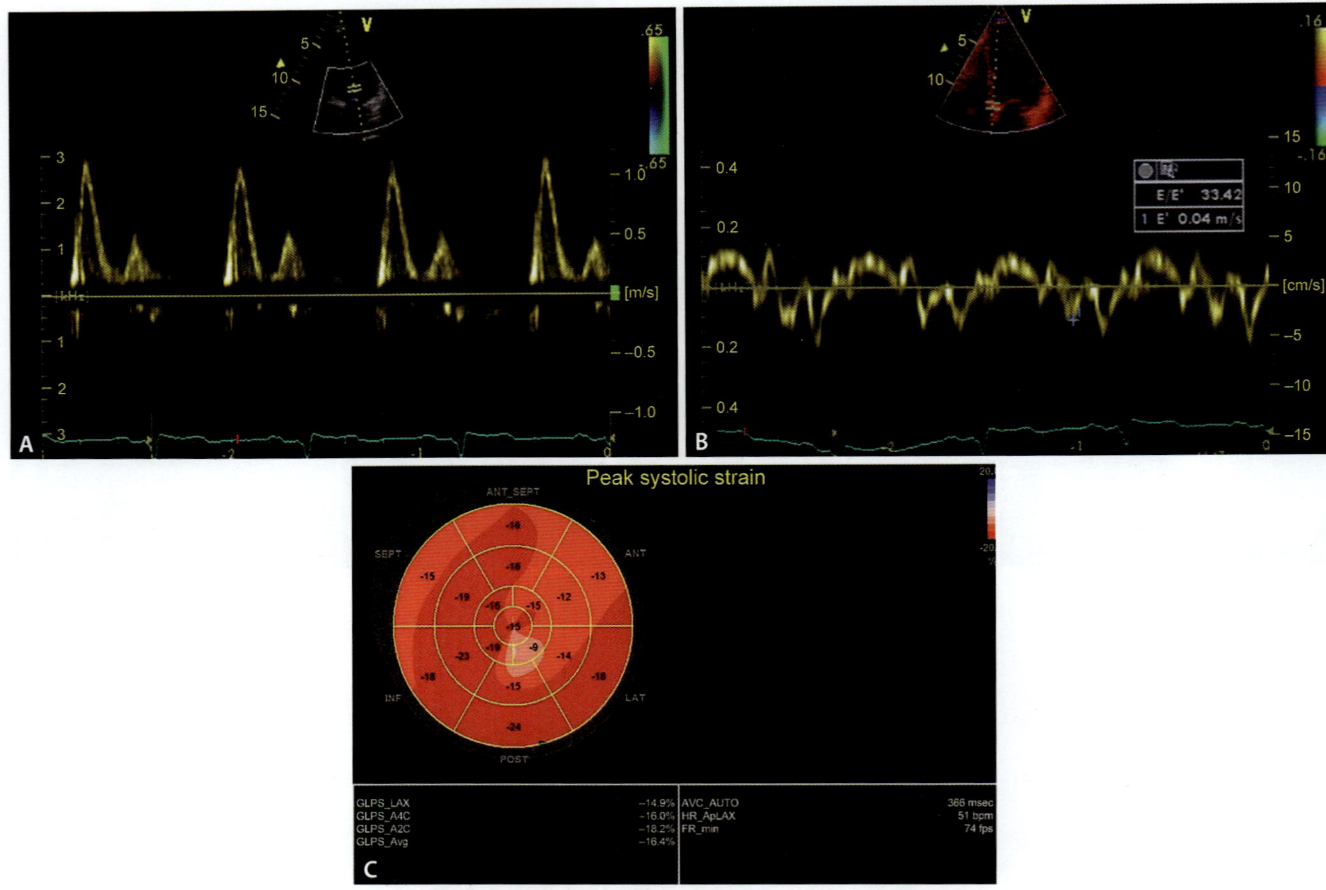

Figs. 7A to C: (A) M-mode Doppler of the mitral flow shows prominent "E" more than twice the velocity of "A" wave but with rapid deceleration; (B) Tissue Doppler shows mitral annular plane systolic excursion indicating grade 2 diastolic dysfunction; and (C) Reduced LV GLS.
Courtesy: Dr Satish Govind, Bengaluru.

- *Functional score* **(Fig. 8A):**
  - Septal e' <7 cm/sec and lateral e' <10 cm/sec
  - Average E/e' >15
  - TR velocity >2.8 m/sec (PASP > 35 mm Hg)
- *Morphological score* **(Figs. 8B and C)**
  - LAVI > 34 mL/m^2
  - LVMI > 149 g/m^2 (M) >122 g/m^2 (F)
  - Relative wall thickness (RWT) >0.42 (RWT = 2 × LVPW thickness/LVIDd)
- *Biomarker score*
  - NT Pro BNP >220 pg/mL (SR) > 660 pg/mL (AF)
  - BNP >80 pg/mL (SR) >240 pg/mL (AF)

If TTE is not adequate then other cardiac imaging studies such as cardiac magnetic resonance (CMR), cardiac computed tomography (CT), or radionuclide imaging can be considered.[3] However, TTE provides abundant information, including the size, shape, function, motion, and geometry of all cardiac chambers and valves. It estimates atrial LV function, pulmonary artery pressure (PAP), and central venous pressure (CVP).

Assessing Left Ventricular Relaxation Directly

Speckle-tracking echocardiography is a new method that evaluates myocardial deformation. In this technique, distinct echocardiography patterns and speckles are followed to assess wall motion.

Cardiac Computed Tomography

Cardiac computed tomography (CT) can be used to assess HFpEF. Cardiac CT imaging shows good correlations for mitral septal tissue velocity and transmitral velocity estimation of LV filling pressures in DD when compared with 2D echocardiography.[9] Late gadolinium

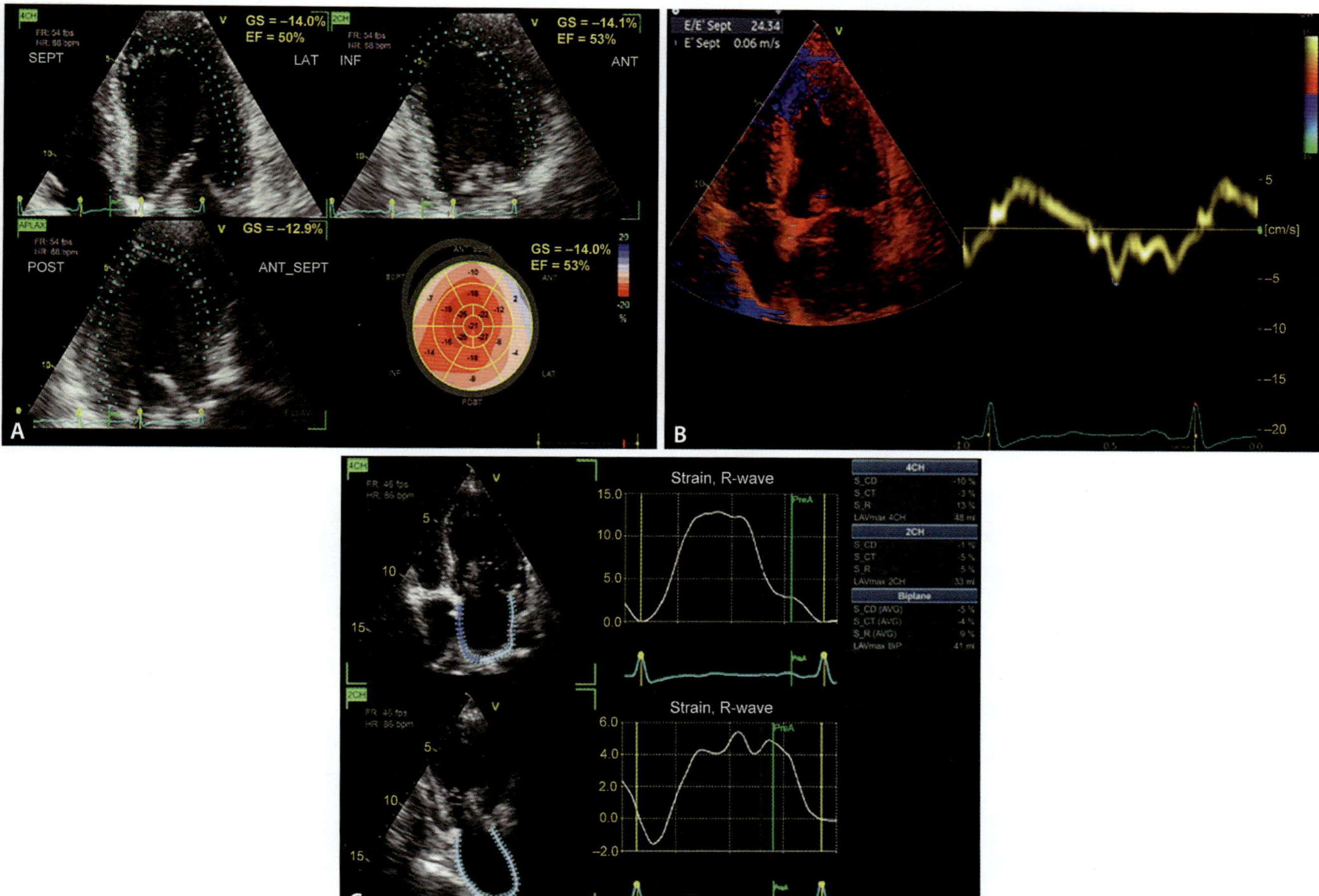

Figs. 8A to C: (A) LV strain imaging in HFpEF as GLS is < –15%; (B) E/e' 24; and (C) LA strain and volume in a 58-year-old patient with HFpEF due to diabetic nephropathy, CKD and systemic hypertension showing the fulfillment of HFA PEFF Score.
Courtesy: Dr Amuthan, Madurai.

enhancement (LGE) indicating fibrosis causing DD and gadolinium paramagnetic contrast can be used **(Figs. 9 and 10)**.

DEVICE-BASED THERAPIES

The device-based therapies can improve symptoms and quality of life (QoL) for patients with HFpEF. Examples include interatrial shunt, left atrial pacing, and implantable HF monitor. New diagnostic parameters like diastolic strain, strain rate, untwisting rate, and atrial strain are used for grading DD. CMR-T1-mapping imaging technique can help delineate the symptomatic phase in patients with HFpEF. CMR imaging can measure DF by labeling specific myocardial regions and analyzing them during diastole. LGE on a CMRI scan can be used to diagnose HFpEF by identifying areas of myocardial fibrosis (scarring) within the heart, which provides valuable information about the underlying pathology and potential prognosis of the patient with HFpEF **(Figs. 11 A to C)**.

Recent advances in diagnosis of DD include:

- Revised diagnostic criteria divide HFpEF into (a) definite, (b) probable, and (c) possible.
- Recognition of cytoskeletal proteins that can alter diastolic function
- ATP hydrolysis acts as energetic factor to alter diastolic function.
- DD can worsen leading to HF if not detected in time and treatment. Timely lifestyle modification and medications can prevent progression.

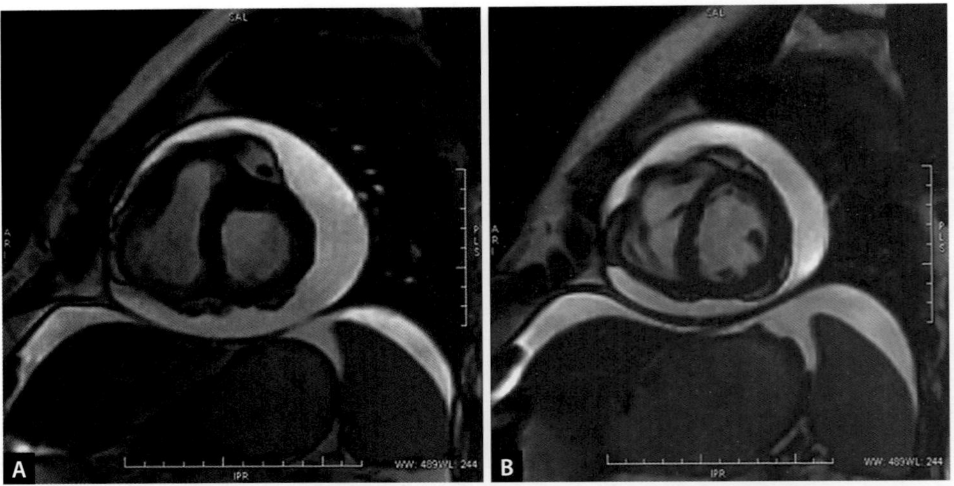

Figs. 9A and B: MRI in short-axis view shows mildly thickened LV wall of all segments with pericardial effusion.

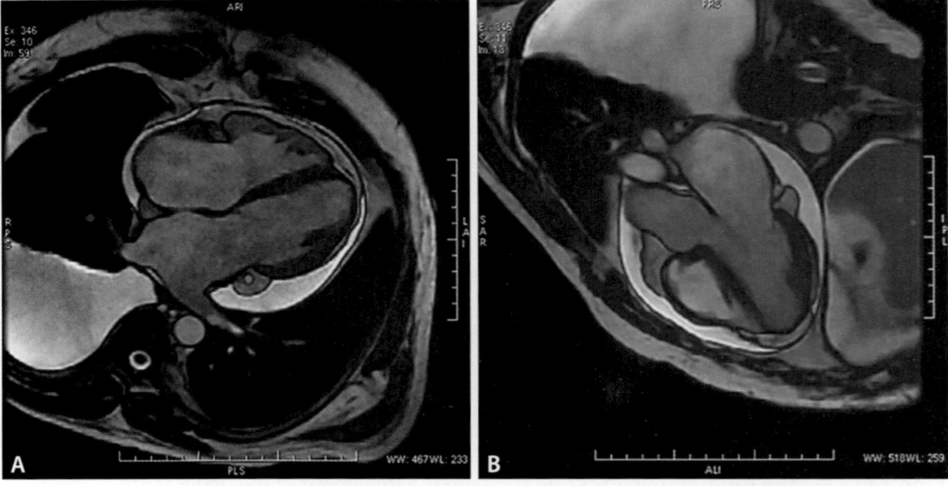

Figs. 10A and B: CMRI in horizontal long-axis view showing dilated RA and LA with small RV and LV cavities with mild pericardial effusion.

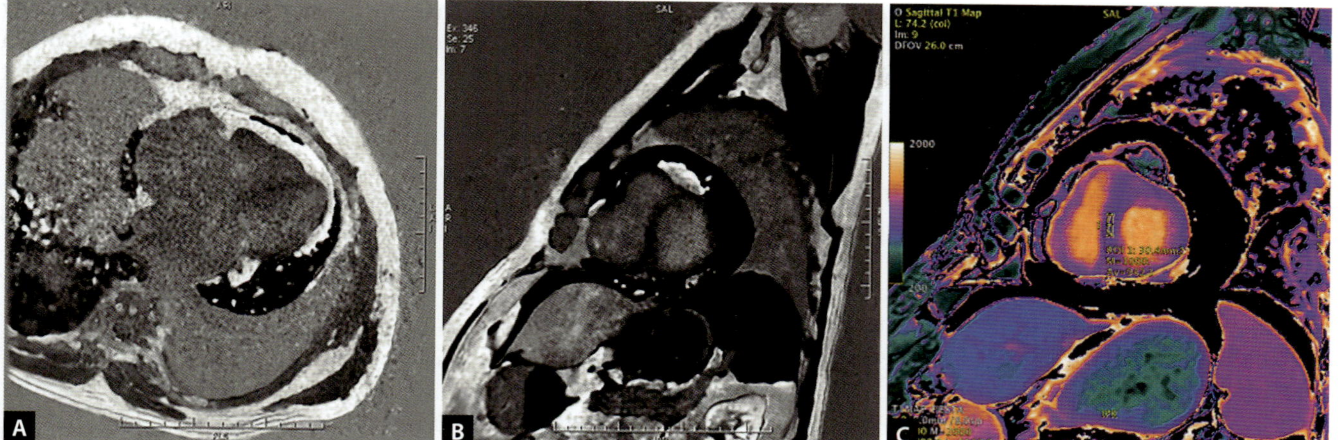

Figs. 11 A to C: CMRI in late gadolinium enhancement at LV apical and inferobasal region; RV anteroapical region. T1 map measures the rate of T1 relaxation time indicating fibrotic areas. RA free wall in LGE in a 45-year-old male with restrictive CMY with HFpEF. *Courtesy:* Dr Krishnam Raju.

- *Increased passive stiffness:* Apart from the active relaxation process, the ventricles also have passive compliance. As age advances, ventricles lose this compliance and become stiff. This appears to be due to diffuse fibrosis, as demonstrated by pathological studies, CT, CMR, and also by serum markers of collagen turnover. Passive stiffness is increased in patients with focal scar or aneurysm following myocardial infarction.
- Procollagen type-I C-terminal propeptide is released during the synthesis of collagen type I, and serum concentrations seem to increase in cardiac fibrosis.[10]
- Myocyte hypertrophy as in HCM and HT can increase both passive as well as active stiffness. Infiltrative cardiomyopathies such as amyloidosis increase passive myocardial stiffness and impair diastolic function in a similar fashion.
- Endocardial fibroelastosis and pericardial disorders like pericardial effusion with tamponade, constrictive pericarditis, and mitral stenosis cause increased resistance to diastolic filling.
- Microvascular flow and myocardial turgor both are responsible for DHF.

MECHANISMS OF HEART FAILURE WITH PRESERVED EJECTION FRACTION

Once LVH has occurred and LV diastolic pressure begins to rise, myocardial ischemia may play a role in worsening HFpEF, even without significant CAD. Extravascular compression caused by high LV diastolic pressure acts mainly on intramural coronary vessels and capillaries. Due to this, autoregulation gets disrupted and the vessels lose the ability to dilate.[11] Indeed, the LVH in HT patients is associated with decreased coronary flow reserve as compared to normal persons. It is a well-established fact that after balloon valvuloplasty or valve replacement of aortic stenosis, the LVH regresses with improvement of coronary flow reserve. HFpEF worsens due to LVH and high LVEDP that impair microvascular function that cause silent ischemia.[12] The myocardial turgor, due to engorgement of the microvasculature with blood, can lead to increase in diastolic stiffness. Clinically, this most likely occurs in association with right HF, as increased right atrial pressure leads to coronary venous engorgement.[13]

Neurohormonal Regulation

The higher renin–angiotensin system contributes to HFpEF due to development of hypertension and impaired myocardial relaxation.[14-16] Both endothelin and angiotensin II contribute to LVH. The DD correlates with reduced heart rate variability, suggesting autonomic imbalance.[17]

DIAGNOSIS

The HFpEF is suspected clinically by the presence of signs and symptoms of HF in the setting of increased ventricular filling pressure, with normal systolic function and normal EF. Ideally, there should also be objective evidence of DD by echocardiography or cardiac catheterization.[18,19] The specific lower limit of EF criteria is arbitrary; hence, distinction between HFpEF and SHF is often obscure. It is even more difficult in patients with both diastolic and systolic dysfunction. The HFpEF is even more difficult to identify in the compensated heart. Unlike SHF, in which a persistently decreased EF is evident, with control of blood pressure, there is relief of ischemia in patients with DHF.

Final Diagnostic Testing

The standard diagnostic test for HFpEF is cardiac catheterization, which illustrates increased ventricular EDP with normal ventricular volumes and preserved systolic function. The pressures in atria proximal to the affected ventricles are also elevated; for example, in patients with LVDD, there is increase in left atrial and pulmonary capillary wedge pressures.

TREATMENT

The morbidity and mortality can be reduced by pharmacological and nonpharmacological management. According to established clinical guidelines, the QoL can be improved, but there is no cure for DD, though symptoms can be reduced with lifestyle changes, medications, LV assist devices, or a heart transplant. The present recommendations for HFpEF treatment include control of blood pressure, control of heart rate in patients with atrial fibrillation, an attempt to establish sinus rhythm, and coronary revascularization procedures. It was considered that no medication or a group of medications can improve the survival of HFpEF patients in the past.[20] But today, studies have shown that the "fantastic four drugs" used in HFrEF are useful in HFpEF too.

1. Sodium–glucose transporter 2 inhibitors (SGLT2i) incorporated in treatment of HFpEF patients are well tolerated and have minimal side effects. SGLT2i provides a better therapy option for HF even in children that previously had few pharmacologic options. The EMPEROR-Preserved trial showed that empagliflozin is superior to placebo in improving HF outcomes among patients with symptomatic stable HFpEF on excellent baseline GDMT, irrespective of diabetes status.[21,22] Scientists have discovered potential new treatments for HFpEF. Studies have shown strong evidence that a glucagon-receptor blocker could work well to treat HFpEF. Repurposing this drug, which is already being tested in clinical trials for diabetes, could bypass the lengthy drug development process and provide quicker and more effective relief to millions of heart patients.[23] All SGLT2i are contraindicated in patients with end-stage renal disease who are on dialysis and in patients with history of type-1 diabetes or history of diabetic ketoacidosis.
2. *Beta-blockers:* The beta-blockers can be useful in treating HFpEF, especially when associated with HT. The long-term beta-blocker therapy can improve diastolic function by reducing blood pressure, which reduces myocardial hypertrophy and improves diastolic filling by increasing the duration of diastole.
3. *Angiotensin receptor–neprilysin inhibitors (ARNIs):* These are useful in treating HFpEF. ARNIs can improve QoL, reduce natriuretic peptide levels, and help the left ventricle work better, which pumps oxygen-rich blood to the body. ARNIs are generally safe and effective across all doses. The ACC guidelines recommend using ARNIs in HFpEF with a Class IIb recommendation. ARNIs reduce risk of ventricular arrhythmias. ARNIs basically function by getting rid of sodium from the body, leading to vasodilatation and diuresis.
4. *Mineralocorticoid receptor antagonists (MRAs):* It is a unique class of drugs that blocks the action of aldosterone and its harmful effects on the renal and extra renal system. They are usually used in the management of HF in hypertensive patients. Among patients with HF and diabetes mellitus or CKD, use of MRA lowers the incidence of repeated admissions to hospital despite greater risk of hyperkalemia and acute renal failure.[17] MRAs may help in HFpEF, but their efficacy is controversial. As MRAs may improve cardiac structure and function, decrease left ventricular filling pressure, reverse cardiac remodeling, and may also reduce the risk of hospitalization, they may also increase the risk of hyperkalemia and gynecomastia. They may also slightly decrease 6-minute-walk distance.
   - *Recommendations:* The 2017 ACC/AHA/HFSA guidelines recommend MRAs for appropriately selected HFpEF patients to decrease hospitalization. However, MRAs remain underutilized compared with other evidence-based therapies.
   - *Ongoing trials:* The SPIRRIT-HFpEF (Spironolactone Initiation Registry Randomized Interventional Trial in Heart Failure With Preserved Ejection Fraction) is an ongoing clinical trial of MRAs in HFpEF.

Heart failure with preserved ejection fraction is a diagnosis of exclusion, which is applied when a patient has symptoms of HF, but no evidence of reduced ejection fraction. In adults, it has been a subject of extensive research and generation of evidence-based guidelines, but there is a scarcity of evidence base in pediatric HF.[23]

HEART FAILURE WITH PRESERVED EJECTION FRACTION: KEY POINTS

- Approximately half of the patients presenting with symptoms of HF exhibit a near-normal LV systolic function at rest, which is thought to be caused by a predominant abnormality in diastolic function.

- Prevalence of DHF increases with age and is higher in women. It is associated with hypertension, hypertrophy, diabetes, aging, and ischemia.
- Mortality is somewhat lower but morbidity is similar in DHF versus SHF.
- Determinants of diastolic function include myocardial relaxation and passive properties of the ventricular wall.
- Myocardial relaxation is modulated by load, inactivation, and nonuniformity.
- Passive properties of the ventricular wall are influenced by myocardial stiffness (cytoskeleton and extracellular matrix), wall thickness, and chamber geometry.
- There is now evidence that diastolic stiffness is actively modulated by load and neurohumoral agents.
- The time constant of isovolumic relaxation, tau (τ), is the most widely used index to evaluate the rate of LV pressure fall, which is the hemodynamic manifestation of myocardial relaxation.
- Chamber stiffness can be quantified by examination of the end-diastolic pressure–volume relationship.
- Echocardiographic indices derived from Doppler mitral inflow velocities are load-dependent, but this limitation might be compensated by new indices derived from pulmonary venous flow, transmitral flow propagation, and tissue Doppler velocity.
- Virtually all patients with congestive heart failure and a normal ejection fraction exhibit evidence of DD.
- Until data from randomized clinical trials provide new evidence, treatment of DHF must be directed toward symptoms, etiology, and in the future, underlying mechanisms.
- Statin treatment may be associated with lower mortality in patients with DHF.
- In summary, DHF occurs in approximately half of all HF cases. This type of HF is caused by a failure of the myocardium to relax properly. Cardiac DD and subsequent HF appear to be distinct pathological entities from SHF. DD is accompanied by cardiac oxidation and oxidative modification of a cardiac contractile protein, MyBP-C. Oxidation of this protein appears to result in increased sensitivity to calcium and delayed and incomplete relaxation. Treatments that inhibit oxidation such as BH4 and mitochondria-target antioxidants can treat DD caused by hypertension or diabetes mellitus. Levels of modified MyBP-C may represent a new blood test for the presence of DD and a marker of therapy. These observations suggest that physicians may be able to diagnose DHF more accurately and dispense specific therapies in the future.

CONCLUSION

The clinical and echocardiographic criteria for the diagnosis of HFpEF are not perfect. But high index of suspicion is a must in a clinical presentation of HF in a patient with preserved systolic function. The echocardiography, CT angiography, and CMRI are handy in early diagnosis. The incorporation of serum BNP measurement in investigation increases the accuracy of the diagnosis. Until further evidence is available from randomized therapeutic trials, clinicians should focus on a few general principles in the treatment of HFpEF to reduce volume overload, slow the heart rate, control hypertension, and relieve myocardial ischemia. Agents that block the renin-angiotensin system and aldosterone are particularly attractive, on the basis of pathophysiological studies.

REFERENCES

1. Tah S, Valderrama M, Afzal M, et al. Heart failure with preserved ejection fraction: an evolving understanding. 2023;15(9):e46152.
2. Angeja BG, Grossman W. Evaluation and management of diastolic heart failure. Circulation. 2003;107:659-63.
3. Heidenreich PA, Bozkurt B, Aguilar D, et al.; ACC/AHA Joint Committee Members. 2022 AHA/ACC/HFSA guideline for the management of heart failure: A report of the American College of Cardiology/American Heart Association Joint Committee on Clinical Practice Guidelines. JACC. 2022;79(17):e263-421.
4. Obakata M, Reddy YNV, Borlaug BA, et al. Diastolic dysfunction and heart failure with preserved ejection fraction: Understanding mechanisms by using noninvasive methods. JACC Cardiovasc Imaging. 2020;13(1 Pt 2): 245-57.
5. Nagueh SF, Appleton CP, Gillebert TC, et al. Recommendations for the evaluation of left ventricular diastolic function by echocardiography: An Update from the American Society of Echocardiography and the European Association of Cardiovascular Imaging. J Am Soc Echocardiogr. 2009;29(4):277-314.
6. Reddy YNV, Kaye DM, Handoko ML, et al. Diagnosis of heart failure with preserved ejection fraction among patients with unexplained dyspnea. JAMA Cardiol. 2022;7(9):891-9.
7. Boogers MJ, van Werkhoven JM, Schuijf JD, et al. Feasibility of diastolic function assessment with cardiac CT: Feasibility study in comparison with tissue Doppler imaging. JACC Cardiovasc Imaging. 2011;4(3): 246-56.
8. Chen H, Chhor M, Rayner BS. Evaluation of the diagnostic accuracy of current biomarkers in heart failure with preserved ejection fraction: A systematic review and meta-analysis. Arch Cardiovasc Dis. 2021;114(12): 793-804.

9. Ovchinnikov AG, Ageev FT, Alekhin MN, et al. The role of diastolic transthoracic stress echocardiography with incremental workload in the evaluation of heart failure with preserved ejection fraction: Indications, methodology, interpretation. Expert consensus developed under the auspices of the National Medical Research Center of Cardiology, Society of Experts in Heart Failure (SEHF), and Russian Association of Experts in Ultrasound Diagnosis in Medicine (REUDM)]. Kardiologiya. 2021;60(12):48-63.
10. Kittleson MM, Panjrath GS, Amancherla K, et al. 2023 ACC expert consensus decision pathway on management of heart failure with preserved ejection fraction: A report of the American College of Cardiology Solution Set Oversight Committee. JACC. 2023;81(18):1835-78.
11. He J, Ogden LG, Bazzano LA, et al. Risk factors for congestive heart failure in US men and women: NHANES I epidemiologic follow-up study. Arch Intern Med. 2001; 161(7):996-1002.
12. Narita K, Amiya E. Social and environmental risks as contributors to the clinical course of heart failure. Heart Fail Rev. 2022;27(4):1001-16.
13. White-Williams C, Rossi LP, Bittner VA; American Heart Association Council on Cardiovascular and Stroke Nursing; Council on Clinical Cardiology; and Council on Epidemiology and Prevention. Addressing social determinants of health in the care of patients with heart failure: A scientific statement from the American Heart Association. Circulation. 2020;141(22):e841-63.
14. Anker SD, Usman MS, Anker MS, et al. Patient phenotype profiling in heart failure with preserved ejection fraction to guide therapeutic decision making. A scientific statement of the Heart Failure Association, the European Heart Rhythm Association of the European Society of Cardiology, and the European Society of Hypertension. Eur J Heart Fail. 2023;25(7):936-55.
15. Savarese G, Becher PM, Lund LH, et al. Global burden of heart failure: A comprehensive and updated review of epidemiology. Cardiovasc Res. 2023;118(17):3272-87.
16. Lee MP, Glynn RJ, Schneeweiss S, et al. Risk factors for heart failure with preserved or reduced ejection fraction among medicare beneficiaries: Application of competing risks analysis and gradient boosted model. Clin Epidemiol. 2020;12:607-16.
17. Eaton CB, Pettinger M, Rossouw J, et al. Risk factors for incident hospitalized heart failure with preserved versus reduced ejection fraction in a multiracial cohort of postmenopausal women. Circ Heart Fail. 2016;9(10).
18. Chin CWL, Ding ZP, Lam CSP, et al. Paradoxical low-gradient aortic stenosis: The HFpEF of aortic stenosis. J Am Coll Cardiol. 2016;67(20):2447-8.
19. Bozkurt B, Ahmad T, Alexander KM, et al.; Writing Committee Members. Heart failure epidemiology and outcomes statistics: A report of the Heart Failure Society of America. J Card Fail. 2023;29(10):1412-51.
20. Miljkovik LV, Spiroska V. Heart failure with preserved ejection fraction: Concept, pathophysiology, diagnosis and challenges for treatment. Open Access Maced J Med Sci. 2015;3(3):521-7.
21. Doehner W, Anker SD, Butler J, et al. Uric Acid and SGLT2 inhibition with empagliflozin in heart failure with preserved ejection fraction: The EMPEROR-Preserved Trial. JACC Heart Fail. 2024; 2024;12(12):2057-70.
22. Gao C, Xiong Z, Liu Y, et al. Glucagon receptor antagonist for heart failure with preserved ejection fraction. Circ Res. 2024;135(5):614:28.
23. Golla MSG, Shams P. Heart failure with preserved ejection fraction (HFpEF). In: StatPearls [Internet]. Treasure Island (FL): StatPearls Publishing; 2025. [online] Available from https://www.ncbi.nlm.nih.gov/books/NBK599960/ [Last accessed January, 2025].

SECTION 8

HFpEF and Renal Disease

86. Sodium-glucose Cotransporter 2 Inhibitors in Chronic Kidney Disease and HFpEF
87. Cardiovascular–Kidney–Metabolic Syndrome: Management Strategies
88. Efficacy and Safety of Spironolactone in Patients with HFpEF and CKD
89. Current Management of HFpEF in Chronic Kidney Disease: An Overview
90. Renal Safety and Efficacy of ARNI in HFpEF
91. Cardiorenal Syndrome in HFpEF
92. SGLT2i in HFpEF in Patient with Diabetes and Chronic Kidney Disease
93. Heart Failure in Chronic Kidney Disease: Conclusions from a KDIGO Controversies Conference
94. Role of New Antihyperkalemic Agents in the Treatment of Patients with HFpEF and Chronic Kidney Disease
95. Efficacy and Safety of Steroidal MRAs in Patients with HFpEF and Chronic Kidney Disease
96. Efficacy and Safety of Novel Nonsteroidal MRAs in Patients with HFpEF and Chronic Kidney Disease
97. Role of IV Iron in Management of Patients with HFpEF and Chronic Kidney Disease
98. Emerging Strategies in the Management of HFpEF in CKD: What does the Future Hold?

CHAPTER

Sodium-glucose Cotransporter 2 Inhibitors in Chronic Kidney Disease and HFpEF

Vishwas Gulati, Sunil Prakash

INTRODUCTION

Sodium-glucose cotransporter 2 (SGLT2) inhibitors, originally developed as antidiabetic agents, have rapidly gained recognition for their broad therapeutic benefits beyond glycemic control. These medications have revolutionized the management of chronic kidney disease (CKD) and heart failure with preserved ejection fraction (HFpEF), offering novel treatment avenues for conditions previously considered challenging to manage. This chapter will delve into the pharmacological action of SGLT2 inhibitors, their clinical efficacy in CKD and HFpEF, and their impact on current treatment paradigms.

CHRONIC KIDNEY DISEASE AND HEART FAILURE: A CLINICAL CHALLENGE

Chronic Kidney Disease: Epidemiology and Pathophysiology (Table 1)

Chronic kidney disease is a global health burden, affecting an estimated 10–15% of the population worldwide.[1] CKD is characterized by a progressive loss of kidney function, defined by a persistent reduction in glomerular filtration rate (GFR) below 60 mL/min/1.73 m^2, or the presence of kidney damage, usually identified by albuminuria, over 3 months or more.[2]

TABLE 1: Shared pathophysiology between heart failure with preserved ejection fraction (HFpEF) AND chronic kidney disease (CKD).[9]

Patho-physiological process	*Mechanism*	*Impact on HFpEF*	*Impact on CKD*
Systemic inflammation	Chronic low-grade inflammation due to obesity, diabetes mellitus (DM), and other factors	Endothelial dysfunction, myocardial fibrosis, and left ventricle (LV) stiffness	Glomerular and interstitial fibrosis, impaired kidney function
Oxidative stress	Over activation of mineralocorticoid receptors (MR) leading to increased reactive oxygen species (ROS) production	Increased LV diastolic dysfunction, myocardial stiffness	Glomerular damage, worsening CKD
Neurohormonal activation	Activation of RAAS and sympathetic nervous system	Contributes to cardiac remodeling, fluid retention	Sodium retention, fluid overload, hypertension
Venous congestion	Impaired natriuresis and extracellular fluid expansion due to reduced glomerular filtration rate (GFR)	LV hypertrophy, fixed stroke volume, worsening heart failure symptoms	Further reduced kidney perfusion, worsening of CKD
Iron deficiency	Poor nutritional intake, malabsorption, inflammation, leading to iron deficiency	Decreased exercise capacity, quality of life	Anemia, impaired mitochondrial function, contributing to CKD progression

The pathophysiology of CKD is multifactorial, involving a complex interplay between systemic hypertension, diabetes mellitus, and other metabolic disorders. In diabetic nephropathy, hyperglycemia triggers glomerular hyperfiltration and increased production of advanced glycation end products (AGEs), leading to glomerular damage and fibrosis.[3] Hypertension further exacerbates kidney injury by increasing intraglomerular pressure, leading to nephron loss over time.[4]

The CKD is also closely linked with cardiovascular disease (CVD), creating a vicious cycle where each condition accelerates the progression of the other. Risk of developing CVD in CKD patients is more than that of developing ESRD.[5] This cardiorenal syndrome underscores the need for treatments that can concurrently address both renal and cardiovascular outcomes.

HEART FAILURE WITH PRESERVED EJECTION FRACTION: AN ELUSIVE SYNDROME

Heart failure with preserved ejection fraction constitutes approximately half of all heart failure cases.[6] HFpEF is a syndrome characterized by symptoms and signs of heart failure, despite a normal or near-normal left ventricular ejection fraction (LVEF). The pathophysiology of HFpEF is distinct from heart failure with reduced ejection fraction (HFrEF), with the primary defect being diastolic dysfunction rather than systolic dysfunction.

In HFpEF, the left ventricle becomes stiff and noncompliant, leading to elevated filling pressures during diastole. This impaired filling results in pulmonary congestion and systemic venous hypertension, contributing to the clinical manifestations of HFpEF, such as dyspnea and fatigue. The etiology of HFpEF is often multifactorial, involving comorbid conditions such as hypertension, diabetes, obesity, and CKD.

The management of HFpEF has historically been challenging due to the lack of therapies that effectively target the underlying pathophysiology. Until recently, treatment options were limited to symptom management, with no therapies proven to reduce morbidity and mortality in HFpEF patients **(Figs. 1 and 2)**.

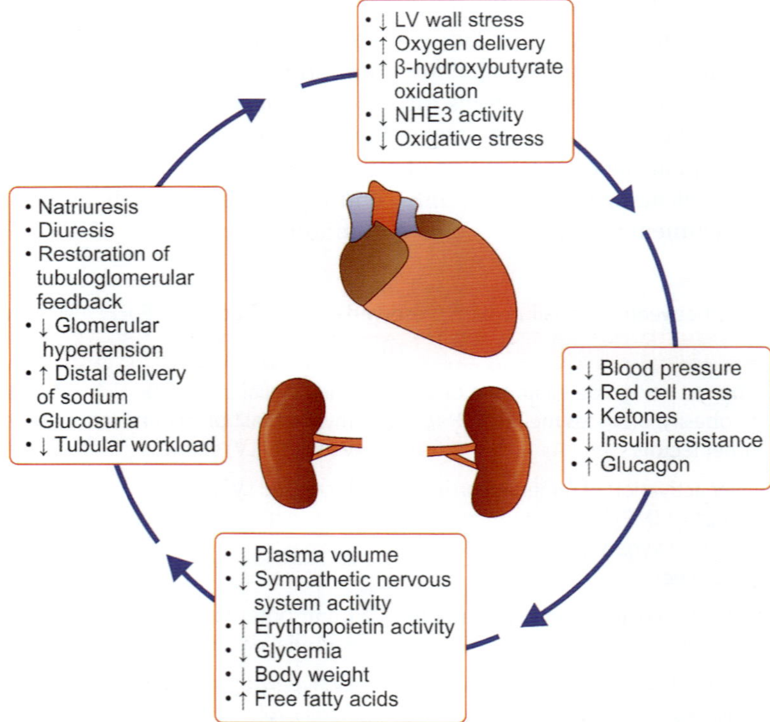

Fig. 1: The kidney-heart connection for organ protection. (LV: left ventricular; NHE3: sodium–hydrogen exchanger 3)
Courtesy: Reproduced courtesy of Emily J. Cox, PhD; original graphic © 2020 E.J. Cox.[7]

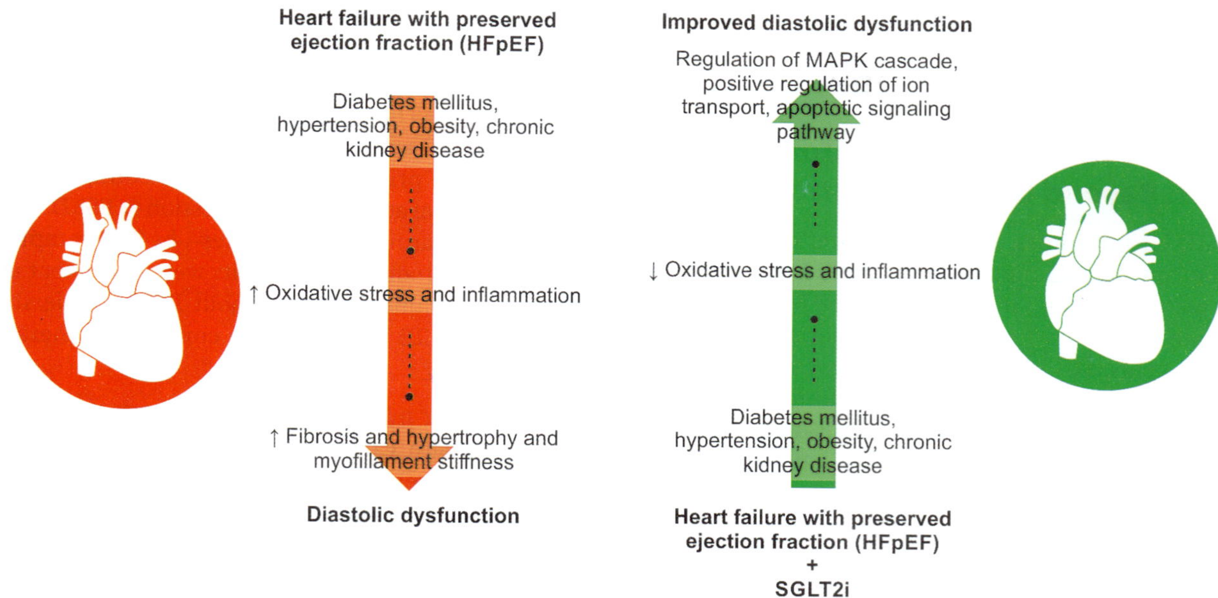

Fig. 2: Effect of sodium-glucose cotransporter 2 inhibitors (SGLT2i) for the treatment of type 2 diabetes (T2D) in patients with heart failure with preserved ejection fraction (HFpEF): The use of SGLT2i has shown improvement in diastolic dysfunction in patients with HFpEF or HF and reduced oxidative stress, inflammation, fibrosis, and myofilament stiffness when compared with patients not using SGLT2i.[8]

ROLE OF SODIUM-GLUCOSE COTRANSPORTER 2 INHIBITORS IN CHRONIC KIDNEY DISEASE AND HEART FAILURE WITH PRESERVED EJECTION FRACTION: MECHANISTIC INSIGHTS

Sodium-glucose Cotransporter 2 Inhibitors: A Paradigm Shift in Chronic Kidney Disease and Heart Failure with Preserved Ejection Fraction Management

The SGLT2 inhibitors, including empagliflozin, dapagliflozin, and canagliflozin, inhibit the SGLT2 in the proximal convoluted tubule of the kidney. By blocking this transporter, SGLT2 inhibitors prevent the reabsorption of glucose and sodium, leading to glycosuria and natriuresis. While initially developed to lower blood glucose levels in type 2 diabetes mellitus (T2DM), these drugs have demonstrated significant benefits in reducing the progression of CKD and the incidence of heart failure, including HFpEF.

The mechanisms by which SGLT2 inhibitors confer renoprotection and cardioprotection are complex and multifactorial. These include hemodynamic effects, such as reductions in blood pressure and intraglomerular pressure, as well as metabolic and anti-inflammatory effects. Additionally, SGLT2 inhibitors have been shown to modulate neurohormonal pathways, including the renin-angiotensin-aldosterone system (RAAS) and sympathetic nervous system, both of which play critical roles in the progression of CKD and HFpEF.

Hemodynamic Effects: Reducing Pressure and Volume Overload

One of the primary mechanisms by which SGLT2 inhibitors benefit patients with CKD and HFpEF is through their hemodynamic effects. By promoting the excretion of glucose and sodium, these drugs induce osmotic diuresis and natriuresis, leading to a reduction in plasma volume. This volume reduction translates into lower blood pressure and reduced cardiac preload and afterload, which are beneficial in both CKD and HFpEF.

In CKD, the reduction in intraglomerular pressure is particularly important, as hyperfiltration is a key driver of kidney damage. By decreasing sodium reabsorption in the proximal tubule, SGLT2 inhibitors increase sodium delivery to the macula densa, triggering tubuloglomerular feedback that results in afferent arteriolar constriction and reduced glomerular hyperfiltration. This mechanism helps to preserve kidney function and slow the progression of CKD.[10]

In HFpEF, where fluid overload and increased filling pressures are common, the diuretic effect of SGLT2 inhibitors helps alleviate symptoms of congestion without the risk of electrolyte imbalance often associated with traditional diuretics.[11] This property makes SGLT2 inhibitors particularly valuable in managing HFpEF, where maintaining hemodynamic stability is crucial.

Metabolic and Anti-inflammatory Effects: Beyond Glycemic Control

The SGLT2 inhibitors also exert beneficial effects on metabolism and inflammation, which are key contributors to the pathophysiology of both CKD and HFpEF. By shifting substrate utilization from glucose to ketone bodies and free fatty acids, SGLT2 inhibitors improve cellular energy efficiency, particularly in the myocardium and kidneys. This metabolic shift may reduce oxidative stress and improve organ function, offering protection against the progression of CKD and HFpEF.[12]

Moreover, SGLT2 inhibitors have been shown to reduce systemic inflammation, which is increasingly recognized as a driving factor in the development and progression of both CKD and HFpEF. Chronic low-grade inflammation contributes to endothelial dysfunction, fibrosis, and organ damage in these conditions. By attenuating inflammatory pathways, SGLT2 inhibitors may help to mitigate these deleterious effects and improve clinical outcomes.

CLINICAL EVIDENCE SUPPORTING SODIUM-GLUCOSE COTRANSPORTER 2 INHIBITORS IN CHRONIC KIDNEY DISEASE

Key Clinical Trials in Chronic Kidney Disease

The efficacy of SGLT2 inhibitors in CKD has been demonstrated in several landmark clinical trials, which have collectively transformed the treatment landscape for this condition.

CREDENCE trial: The CREDENCE (Canagliflozin and Renal Events in Diabetes with Established Nephropathy Clinical Evaluation) trial was a pivotal study that evaluated the renoprotective effects of canagliflozin in patients with T2DM and CKD. The trial enrolled over 4,400 participants with an estimated GFR between 30 and 90 mL/min/1.73 m^2 and albuminuria. Canagliflozin significantly reduced the risk of the composite primary endpoint, which included end-stage kidney disease (ESKD), doubling of serum creatinine, and renal or cardiovascular death, by 30% compared to placebo. The trial was terminated early due to the overwhelming efficacy of canagliflozin, marking a significant advance in the treatment of diabetic kidney disease.[13]

DAPA-CKD trial: The DAPA-CKD (Dapagliflozin and Prevention of Adverse Outcomes in Chronic Kidney Disease) trial extended the benefits of SGLT2 inhibition to a broader CKD population, including patients without diabetes. In this study, dapagliflozin significantly reduced the risk of the primary composite outcome—sustained decline in GFR of at least 50%, progression to ESKD, or death from renal or cardiovascular causes—by 39% compared to placebo. Importantly, the benefits were consistent across subgroups, including those without T2DM, underscoring the role of SGLT2 inhibitors as a cornerstone therapy for CKD.[14]

EMPA-KIDNEY trial: The EMPA-KIDNEY (Empagliflozin in Patients with Chronic Kidney Disease) trial further confirmed the renoprotective effects of SGLT2 inhibitors. Empagliflozin reduced the risk of the primary composite outcome, which included a decline in GFR, ESKD, or death from renal or cardiovascular causes, by 28% compared to placebo. This trial provided additional evidence supporting the use of SGLT2 inhibitors in CKD patients, regardless of their diabetic status.[15]

CLINICAL IMPLICATIONS IN CHRONIC KIDNEY DISEASE MANAGEMENT

The findings from these trials have had profound implications for the management of CKD. SGLT2 inhibitors are now recommended as a first-line therapy for patients with CKD, particularly those with T2DM, to slow disease progression and reduce the risk of ESKD and cardiovascular events. The extension of their benefits to nondiabetic CKD patients further highlights their potential as a universal therapy for CKD.

CLINICAL EVIDENCE SUPPORTING SODIUM-GLUCOSE COTRANSPORTER 2 INHIBITORS IN HEART FAILURE WITH PRESERVED EJECTION FRACTION

Key Clinical Trials in Heart Failure with Preserved Ejection Fraction

The role of SGLT2 inhibitors in heart failure, particularly HFpEF, has been evaluated in several major clinical trials, which have provided compelling evidence for their use in this challenging condition.

EMPEROR-Preserved trial: The EMPEROR-Preserved (Empagliflozin Outcome Trial in Patients with Chronic Heart Failure with Preserved Ejection Fraction) trial was the first large-scale study to demonstrate the efficacy of SGLT2 inhibitors in HFpEF. Empagliflozin significantly reduced the risk of the primary composite outcome—time to first hospitalization for heart failure or cardiovascular death—by 21% compared to placebo. The benefits were consistent across key subgroups, including those with and without diabetes, indicating that empagliflozin's effects extend beyond glucose control.[16]

DELIVER trial: The DELIVER (Dapagliflozin Evaluation to Improve the Lives of Patients with Preserved Ejection Fraction Heart Failure) trial evaluated dapagliflozin in patients with HFpEF. Similar to EMPEROR-Preserved, the DELIVER trial found that dapagliflozin reduced the risk of the composite primary endpoint of worsening heart failure or cardiovascular death by 18% compared to placebo. These results provided further support for the use of SGLT2 inhibitors in HFpEF, reinforcing their role as a novel therapeutic option for this condition.[17]

CLINICAL IMPLICATIONS IN HEART FAILURE WITH PRESERVED EJECTION FRACTION MANAGEMENT

The results of these trials represent a significant breakthrough in the management of HFpEF, a condition that has historically been difficult to treat. Until the advent of SGLT2 inhibitors, there were no therapies proven to improve outcomes in HFpEF patients. The findings from the EMPEROR-Preserved and DELIVER trials have established SGLT2 inhibitors as a new standard of care for HFpEF, offering hope to patients with this debilitating condition.

The mechanisms underlying the benefits of SGLT2 inhibitors in HFpEF are thought to include their hemodynamic effects, such as reducing plasma volume and lowering blood pressure, as well as their ability to improve myocardial energetics and reduce inflammation. By addressing multiple pathophysiological pathways in HFpEF, SGLT2 inhibitors offer a comprehensive approach to managing this complex syndrome.

SGLT2 INHIBITORS: SAFETY PROFILE AND CONSIDERATIONS

Safety and Tolerability

The SGLT2 inhibitors are generally well-tolerated, including those with CKD and HFpEF. The most common side effects include genital mycotic infections, urinary tract infections, and volume depletion, which are typically mild and manageable.[18] However, clinicians should be aware of the potential for more serious adverse events, such as diabetic ketoacidosis (DKA), particularly in patients with type 1 diabetes or those with low insulin reserves.[19]

In patients with CKD, the risk of acute kidney injury (AKI) with SGLT2 inhibitors is low, and these drugs have been shown to reduce the long-term risk of renal events.[20] Nevertheless, caution is advised in patients with advanced CKD (eGFR <30 mL/min/1.73 m^2), where the use of SGLT2 inhibitors may be less effective and requires careful monitoring.

In HFpEF, the safety profile of SGLT2 inhibitors is similar to that observed in other populations, with no significant increase in adverse events related to heart failure. The diuretic effect of SGLT2 inhibitors may be particularly beneficial in HFpEF, where fluid overload is common, but clinicians should monitor for signs of dehydration and hypotension, especially in elderly patients or those with baseline hypotension.

CONCLUSION

Sodium-glucose cotransporter 2 inhibitors have emerged as a cornerstone in the management of CKD and HFpEF. Their unique mechanisms of action provide benefits that extend beyond glycemic control, offering protection against the progression of kidney disease and heart failure. The clinical evidence supporting their use in these conditions is robust, with several landmark trials demonstrating significant reductions in renal and cardiovascular events.

The renoprotective and cardioprotective effects of SGLT2 inhibitors are mediated through multiple pathways, including hemodynamic, metabolic, and anti-inflammatory mechanisms. These drugs have transformed the treatment landscape for CKD and HFpEF, offering new hope to patients who previously had limited therapeutic options.

As the understanding of SGLT2 inhibitors continues to evolve, their role in the management of CKD and HFpEF is likely to expand, potentially benefiting an even broader range of patients. The integration of SGLT2 inhibitors into clinical practice represents a major advance in the care of patients with these challenging conditions, underscoring the importance of continued research and innovation in this field.

REFERENCES

1. Lv JC, Zhang LX. Prevalence and disease burden of chronic kidney disease. Adv Exp Med Biol. 2019;1165: 3-15.
2. Pub Med Central. Chapter 1: Definition and classification of CKD. Kidney Int Suppl (2011). 2013; 3(1):19-62.

3. Agarwal R. Pathogenesis of Diabetic Nephropathy. In: Chronic Kidney Disease and Type 2 Diabetes. Arlington (VA): American Diabetes Association; 2021.
4. Metcalfe W. How does early chronic kidney disease progress? A Background Paper prepared for the UK Consensus Conference on Early Chronic Kidney Disease. Nephrol Dial Transplant. 2007;22(suppl_9):ix26-ix30.
5. Tonelli M, Wiebe N, Culleton B, et al. Chronic kidney disease and mortality risk: a systematic review. J Am Soc Nephrol. 2006;17(7):2034-47.
6. Dunlay SM, Roger VL, Redfeld MM. Epidemiology of heart failure with preserved ejection fraction. Nat Rev Cardiol. 2017;14(10):591-602.
7. Tuttle KR, Brosius FC, Cavender MA, et al. SGLT2 Inhibition for CKD and Cardiovascular Disease in Type 2 Diabetes: Report of a Scientific Workshop Sponsored by the National Kidney Foundation. Am J Kidney Diseases. 2020;77(1):94-109.
8. Muscoli S, Barillà F, Tajmir R, et al. The new role of SGLT2 inhibitors in the management of heart failure: current evidence and future perspective. Pharmaceutics. 2022;14(8):1730.
9. Patel RN, Sharma A, Prasad A, et al. Heart failure with preserved ejection fraction with CKD: a narrative review of a multispecialty disorder. Kidney Med. 2023;5(12): 100705.
10. Koh ES, Kim GH, Chung S. Intrarenal mechanisms of sodium-glucose cotransporter-2 inhibitors on tubulo-glomerular feedback and natriuresis. Endocrinol Metab (Seoul). 2023;38(4):359-72.
11. Aguilar-Gallardo JS, Correa A, Contreras JP. Cardio-renal benefits of sodium-glucose co-transporter 2 inhibitors in heart failure with reduced ejection fraction: mechanisms and clinical evidence. Eur Heart J-Cardiovasc Pharmacother. 2021;8:311-21.
12. Gao YM, Feng ST, Wen Y, et al. Cardiorenal protection of SGLT2 inhibitors-perspectives from metabolic reprogramming. E BioMedicine. 2022;83:104215.
13. Perkovic V, Jardine MJ, Neal B, et al. Canagliflozin and renal outcomes in type 2 diabetes and nephropathy. N Engl J Med. 2019;380(24):2295-306.
14. Heerspink HJL, Stefánsson BV, Correa-Rotter R, et al. Dapagliflozin in patients with chronic kidney disease. N Engl J Med. 2020;383(15):1436-46.
15. The EMPA-KIDNEY Collaborative Group, Herrington WG, Staplin N, Wanner C, et al. Empagliflozin in patients with chronic kidney disease. N Engl J Med. 2023;388(2): 117-27.
16. Anker SD, Butler J, Filippatos G, et al. Empagliflozin in heart failure with a preserved ejection fraction. N Engl J Med 2021; 385(16):1451-61.
17. Solomon SD, McMurray JJV, Claggett B, et al. Dapagliflozin in heart failure with mildly reduced or preserved ejection fraction. N Engl J Med. 2022;387(12):1089-98.
18. Lega IC, Bronskill SE, Campitelli MA, et al. Sodium glucose cotransporter 2 inhibitors and risk of genital mycotic and urinary tract infection: a population-based study of older women and men with diabetes. Diabetes Obes Metab. 2019;21:2394-404.
19. Wiviott SD, Raz I, Bonaca MP, et al. Dapagliflozin and cardiovascular outcomes in type 2 diabetes. N Engl J Med. 2018;380:347-57.
20. Iskander C, Cherney DZ, Clemens KK, et al. Use of sodium-glucose cotransporter-2 inhibitors and risk of acute kidney injury in older adults with diabetes: a population-based cohort study. CMAJ. 2020;192:E351-E360.

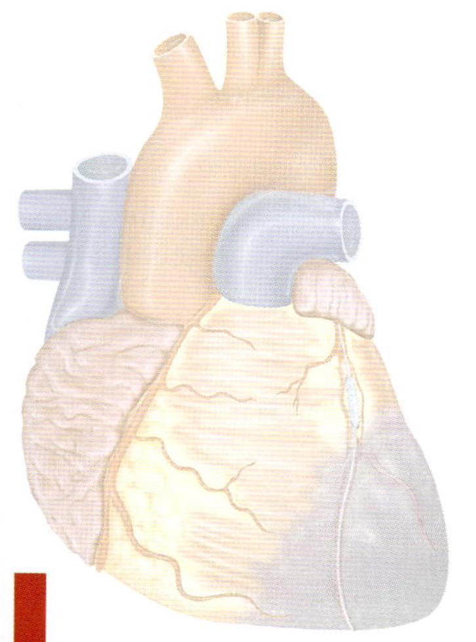

Cardiovascular–Kidney–Metabolic Syndrome: Management Strategies

Deodatta Chafekar, Neelima Chafekar

INTRODUCTION

"Cardiovascular-kidney-metabolic (CKM) syndrome" includes patients having metabolic dysfunction, such as obesity and type-2 diabetes mellitus (T2DM), chronic kidney disease (CKD), and cardiovascular disease (CVD) or ischemic heart disease since some pathophysiological factors are common to them.[1] The American Heart Association (AHA) in 2023 defined CKM as "a systemic disorder characterized by interactions in-between multiple metabolic risk factors including cardiovascular risk factors such as hypertension, hyperlipidemia and hyperglycemia, and chronic kidney disease that has the potential to lead into high rates of major adverse cardiovascular events".[2] Furthermore, the development of metabolic dysfunction-associated fatty liver disease (MAFLD) intensifies systemic inflammation and insulin resistance and is associated with CKM syndrome. Given the strong association between metabolic risk factors and this condition, the American Association for the Study of Liver Diseases recommends screening in individuals with established metabolic risk factors.[3]

The CKM syndrome is strongly associated with multiple comorbidities including atherosclerotic vascular diseases, ischemic cardiovascular diseases, congestive heart failure (HF), nonhemorrhagic cerebrovascular diseases, T2DM, CKD, end-stage kidney disease (ESKD), dyslipidemia, nonalcoholic fatty liver disease, and polycystic ovary disease with a considerable increase in the associated disability-adjusted life-years lost over the decades.[2] CKM health refers to the clinical manifestation of pathophysiological interactions between metabolic risk factors, including obesity and diabetes, CKD, and CVD.[3]

The CKM disease is categorized into four distinct stages, from stage 0 to stage 4 **(Fig. 1)**.[4] It is a progressive condition driven by hereditary, social, and environmental risk factors. It leads to excess, dysfunctional fatty tissue and elevated blood glucose levels, resulting in inflammation, insulin resistance, and oxidative stress. Furthermore, CKM syndrome can cause kidney failure, stroke, and CVD.[3,5]

IDENTIFICATION AND SCREENING

Detecting conditions with serious negative clinical impacts at an early stage is a critical preventive public health priority, mainly, when multiple effective treatments exist. The staging helps in identifying CKM patients at varying levels of severity, giving an opportunity for preventive intervention to slow or even reverse its course.

The AHA has launched a new risk calculator designed to estimate the likelihood of developing CVD over 10 years and 30 years, beginning at age of 30 years.[6] The CKM-staging framework identifies key risk factors, such as hypertension, diabetes, and dyslipidemia, and emphasizes early intervention to improve clinical outcomes.[3]

The core screening elements for metabolic risk factors involve measuring blood pressure, lipids, blood glucose, BMI, and waist circumference as anthropometric indicators **(Box 1)**. Healthy young adults are advised to undergo screening for traditional risk factors every 4–6 years. Since obesity is central to CKM syndrome, annual BMI assessments are commonly recommended.[7]

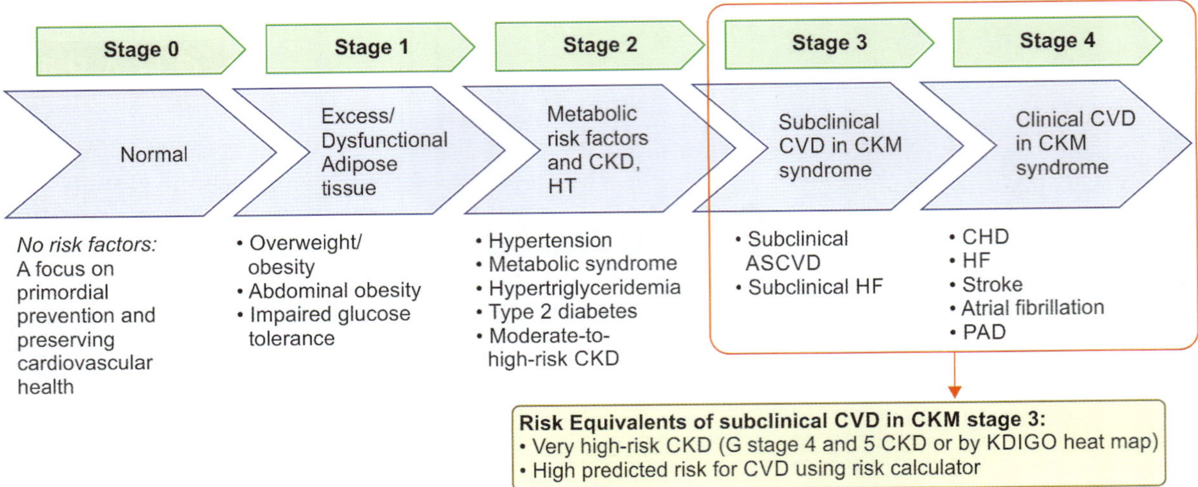

Fig. 1: Five stages of CKM syndrome.[4] (ASCVD: atherosclerotic cardiovascular disease; CHD: coronary heart disease; CKD: chronic kidney disease; CKM: cardiovascular–kidney–metabolic; CVD: cardiovascular disease; HF: heart failure; HT: hypertriglyceridemia; KDIGO: Kidney Disease Improving Global Outcomes; PAD: peripheral artery disease)

BOX 1: Cardiovascular–kidney–metabolic (CKM) identification and its screening.

CKM Identification

- *Risk-enhancing factors for CKM syndrome:*
  - High-risk demographic groups (e.g., South Asian ancestry and lower socioeconomic status)
  - Chronic inflammatory conditions (e.g., psoriasis, RA, lupus, and HIV/AIDS)
  - High burden of adverse
  - Social determinants of health (SDOH) mental health disorders (e.g., depression and anxiety)
  - Sleep disorders (e.g., obstructive sleep apnea)
  - Sex-specific risk enhancers (beyond gestational diabetes consideration in stage 1)
  - History of premature menopause (age <40 years)
  - History of adverse pregnancy outcomes (e.g., hypertensive disorders of pregnancy, preterm birth, and small for gestational age)
  - Polycystic ovarian syndrome erectile dysfunction
  - Elevated high-sensitivity C-reactive protein (>2.0 mg/L if measured)
  - Family history of kidney failure
  - Family history of diabetes

CKM Screening

- *Stage 1:*
  - BMI/waist circumference
  - *Screening for DM-FBS/PPBS/HbAIC*
- *Stage 2:*
  - Lipid profile
  - Blood pressure measurements
  - Liver function tests including screening for liver fibrosis
  - Renal function eGFR/S creatinine/Cystatin C and UACR
  - Screening for DM—FBS/PPBS/HbAIC
- *Stage 3:*
  - Coronary artery calcium screening
  - Subclinical HF screening with echo/ECG
  - Elevated cardiac biomarkers (NT-proBNP and high sensitivity troponin)
  - Renal function eGFR/S creatinine/Cystatin C, and UACR
- *Stage 4:*
  - Stage 3 parameters
  - SDOH screening can be done by various toolkits

Newer risk calculator which takes consideration of all the above together.

(BMI: body mass index; DM: diabetes mellitus; ECG: electrocardiogram; FBS: fasting blood sugar; FPG: fasting plasma glucose; GFR: glomerular filtration rate; HF: heart failure; HbA1c: hemoglobin A1c; HIV: human immunodeficiency virus; PPBS: postprandial blood sugar; RA: rheumatoid arthritis; UACR: urine albumin-creatinine ratio)

Evaluating kidney function adds valuable prognostic insight and helps inform treatment strategies.

The PREVENT (AHA Predicting Risk of CVD Events) equations provide accurate and precise estimates of both short-term and long-term CVD risk for adults aged 30–79 years. These equations were developed and validated using data from 46 observational cohort studies and electronic medical records (EMR) involving 6,612,004 US adults in this age group. They predict the risk of total CVD, including a composite of atherosclerotic cardiovascular disease (ASCVD) and HF, in the general primary prevention population.[8]

MANAGEMENT OF CARDIOVASCULAR–KIDNEY–METABOLIC SYNDROME

The core principles of management emphasize interdisciplinary care and the consideration of social determinants of health (SDOH). *Stagewise management for CKM syndrome:* For individuals at stage 0, the Life's Essential 8 framework offers a comprehensive approach to achieving and maintaining cardiovascular health. This framework emphasizes key factors such as managing body weight and BMI, controlling blood pressure and blood glucose levels, adhering to a balanced diet, engaging in regular physical activity, optimizing lipid levels, avoiding tobacco use, and ensuring sufficient, high-quality sleep. Stage 1, characterized by dysfunctional adiposity, is managed through lifestyle modifications, pharmacotherapy for obesity, bariatric surgery, and the use of metformin for impaired glucose tolerance (IGT).[6]

The management of stage-2 CKM is given in **Figure 2**.

For considering metformin coutilization in diabetes: If HbA1c >7.5% or consider insulin coutilization of metformin and cardioprotective antihyperglycemics and if HbA1c <7.5%, consider cardioprotective antihyperglycemics without metformin initiation (continue metformin if already using).[6]

The management of stage-3 CKM is given in **Figure 3**.

In stage 4 of CKM syndrome with established CVD, specific management strategies are applied based on the presence of HF or ASCVD. For HF, guideline-directed medical therapy (GDMT) includes aspirin, PCSK9 inhibitors, ezetimibe, and sodium–glucose transport protein 2 inhibitors (SGLT2i), with GLP1RA recommended for those with a BMI over 35 kg/m^2. Additional treatments include finerenone, while thiazolidinediones and DPP-4 inhibitors should be avoided. For ASCVD, SGLT2i and GLP1RA (for those with elevated BMI) are advised. In cases of diabetes with CVD, a combination of SGLT2i and GLP1RA may be utilized for optimal management.[6] Combination therapy with SGLT2i, RAAS blockers, statins, aspirin, finerenone, and other MRAs offers comprehensive protection in both diabetic and nondiabetic CKM patients. This approach reduces HF hospitalizations, slows CKD progression, lowers cardiovascular risk, and minimizes thrombotic events.[3]

It is advised that a CKM coordinator assumes primary responsibility for overseeing interdisciplinary care, coordinating across primary care, nephrology, cardiology, and endocrinology. The interdisciplinary team meets regularly to create tailored clinical protocols for patient management, with support from community health workers, nurse coordinators, and pharmacy services.

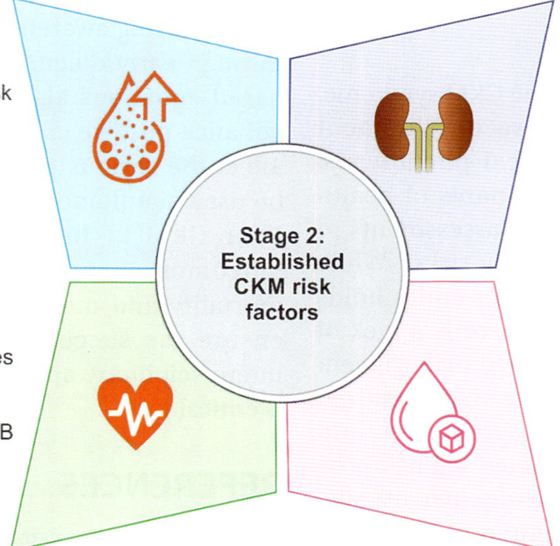

Fig. 2: Management of stage-2 CKM. (ACEi: angiotensin-converting enzyme inhibitor; ARB: angiotensin II receptor blocker; ASCVD: atherosclerotic cardiovascular disease; BMI: body mass index; BP: blood pressure; CKD: chronic kidney disease; CKM: cardiovascular–kidney–metabolic; DKD: diabetic kidney disease; GLP-1RA: glucagon-like peptide-1 receptor agonist; HbA1c: hemoglobin A1c; HTN: hypertension; MetS: metabolic syndrome; SGLT2i: sodium–glucose transport protein 2 inhibitors; TG, triglycerides; UACR: urine albumin–creatinine ratio)

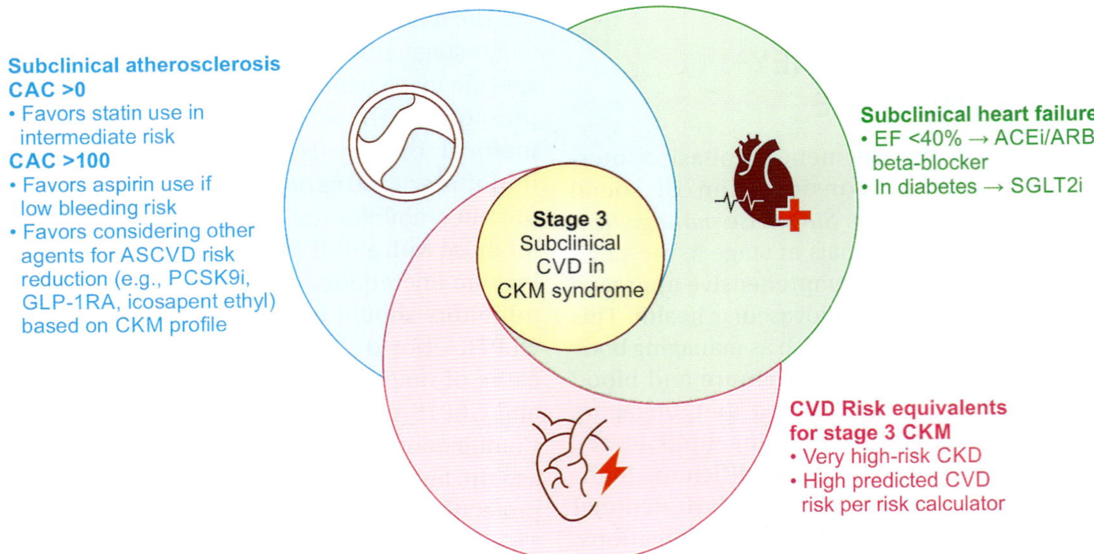

Fig. 3: Management of stage-3 CKM. (ACEi: angiotensin-converting enzyme inhibitor; ARB: angiotensin II receptor blocker; ASCVD: atherosclerotic cardiovascular disease; CAC: coronary artery calcium; CKM: cardiovascular–kidney–metabolic; CVD: cardiovascular disease; EF: ejection fraction; GLP-1RA: glucagon-like peptide-1 receptor agonist; PCSK9i: proprotein convertase subtilisin/kexin type 9 inhibitor; SGLT2i: sodium–glucose transport protein 2 inhibitors)

Regular reassessment by the team is also recommended to monitor and review treatment progress. CKM education plays a crucial role in raising awareness and improving risk prediction for early diagnosis. Implementing public policy measures that promote healthy lifestyles within communities, along with addressing social factors, will significantly help reduce the risk of CKM syndrome.

LIMITATIONS

Significant knowledge gaps exist regarding CKM syndrome, particularly in understanding disease development mechanisms, variability among clinical phenotypes, the interaction between social determinants of health and biological risk factors, and precise assessments of disease incidence considering competing risks.[3] While recognizing CKM syndrome as a distinct entity holds promise, several challenges remain. There is a lack of large-scale, long-term studies on integrated management approaches, which limits the development of standardized care protocols. Disparities in healthcare access and infrastructure, especially in resource-limited settings, pose additional barriers to implementing interdisciplinary care. Furthermore, uncertainties regarding the mechanisms and progression of CKM syndrome, along with inconsistent attention to SDOH, complicate management. Early diagnosis also relies on comprehensive screening, which may not be accessible or uniformly applied across healthcare systems.

CONCLUSION

Establishing a well-defined CKM syndrome with appropriate staging is essential for developing effective strategies to prevent and manage the risk of progressive organ failure. However, aspect of MAFLD also should be included, calling it "CKM(L)" syndrome. A key aspect of management is CKM(L) education, which will play a vital role in raising awareness and enhancing risk prediction through early diagnosis. Staging and using PREVENT-based equations also help for proper management to enhance positive clinical outcomes. Multiple drugs that affect the various pathophysiological mechanisms can be used simultaneously for treating CKM(L) syndrome. Poor CKM(L) health is linked to adverse clinical outcomes, including increased rates of premature mortality and morbidity due to CVD progression. To ensure the success of this initiative, a coordinated interdisciplinary approach, led by a CKM (L) specialist, is critical.

REFERENCES

1. Georgopoulou T, Petrakis I, Dermitzaki K, et al. Cardiorenal syndrome: challenges in everyday clinical practice and key points towards a better management. J Clin Med. 2023;12(12):4121.
2. Kanbay M, Guldan M, Ozbek L, et al. Exploring the nexus: The place of kidney diseases within the cardiovascular-

kidney-metabolic syndrome spectrum. Eur J Intern Med. 2024;127:1-14.

3. Ndumele CE, Neeland IJ, Tuttle KR, et al. A synopsis of the evidence for the science and clinical management of cardiovascular-kidney-metabolic (CKM) syndrome: A scientific statement from the American Heart Association. Circulation. 2023;148(20):1636-64.
4. Aggarwal R, Ostrominski JW, Vaduganathan M, et al. Prevalence of cardiovascular-kidney-metabolic syndrome stages in US Adults, 2011-2020. JAMA. 2024;331(21):1858-60.
5. Jaradat JH, Nashwan AJ. Cardiovascular-kidney-metabolic syndrome: Understanding the interconnections and the need for holistic intervention. J Med Surg Public Health. 2023;1:100028.
6. Ndumele CE, Rangaswami J, Chow SL, et al. Cardiovascular-kidney-metabolic health: A presidential advisory from the American Heart Association. Circulation. 2023;148(20):1606-35.
7. Visseren FLJ, Mach F, Smulders YM, et al.; ESC Scientific Document Group. 2021 ESC Guidelines on cardiovascular disease prevention in clinical practice. Eur Heart J. 2021;42(34):3227-37.
8. Khan SS, Matsushita K, Sang Y, et al. Development and validation of the American Heart Association's PREVENT Equations. Circulation. 2024;149(6):430-49.

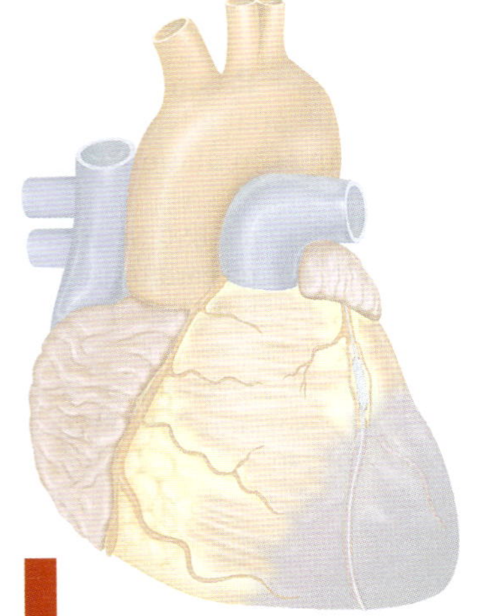

Efficacy and Safety of Spironolactone in Patients with HFpEF and CKD

Muthu Jayaraman, Rajeevalochana Parthasarathy

INTRODUCTION

Heart failure with preserved ejection fraction (HFpEF) is a syndrome with multiple phenotypic variants. The phenotype of HFpEF associated with chronic kidney disease (CKD) is common, complicated, and is being recognized as an important entity in the management of both.[1] Both CKD and HFpEF share risk factors such as obesity, hypertension, diabetes mellitus, and metabolic syndrome. This eventually leads to increased systemic inflammation and oxidative stress, elevated neurohormones and mineralocorticoid receptor (MR) activation and increased venous congestion. The diagnosis and management of patients when both these entities coexist can be challenging, needing a multidisciplinary approach. There is recent evidence on the beneficial effects of sodium-glucose cotransporter 2 inhibitors (SGLT2i), glucagon-like peptide-1 (GLP-1) agonists, and mineralocorticoid receptor antagonists (MRAs) in HFpEF, CKD, and metabolic syndrome. This chapter delves into the efficacy and safety of spironolactone in patients with both HFpEF and CKD, analyzing clinical evidence, potential benefits, and safety concerns.[2]

PATHOPHYSIOLOGY OF HEART FAILURE WITH PRESERVED EJECTION FRACTION AND CHRONIC KIDNEY DISEASE

The central issue in HFpEF is diastolic dysfunction due to impaired left ventricular dysfunction caused by fibrosis and pathological cardiac remodeling. Any stress such as tachycardia or hypertension will worsen the end-diastolic filling pressures, resulting in an inappropriate response.[3,4]

The heart and kidneys work in bidirectional harmony to maintain fluid homeostasis and blood pressure. In normal physiology, autoregulation prevents renal and cardiac injury. Acute or chronic deterioration of any of the organs or both impairs this homeostasis. In CKD, impaired natriuresis, abnormal renin secretion, and left ventricular hypertrophy lead to fluid overload. This can cause heart failure (HF) or worsen preexisting diastolic dysfunction, leading to fluid overload. The shared risk factors such as diabetes mellitus and metabolic syndrome stimulate sympathetic nervous system (SNS) and renin-angiotensin-aldosterone system (RAAS) pathway, leading to further stress on the ventricles and nephrons.[5] **Figure 1** shows the common risk factors and pathophysiological mechanisms of HFpEF and CKD.

Mineralocorticoid receptor/ligand activation in both these entities further leads to a cascade of proinflammatory, profibrotic pathways leading to negative ventricular remodeling and fluid overload[6-8] **(Flowchart 1)**. Spironolactone functions primarily as a steroidal MRA. Aldosterone, a hormone secreted by the adrenal cortex, promotes sodium and water retention while facilitating potassium excretion. Spironolactone counteracts these effects by blocking aldosterone receptors, reducing sodium and water retention, and is a potassium-sparing diuretic.[9]

Heart failure with preserved ejection fraction is now considered a systemic disorder because of the multiple physiological perturbations, and when it manifests in CKD, it shares many common diagnostic and management issues.[2]

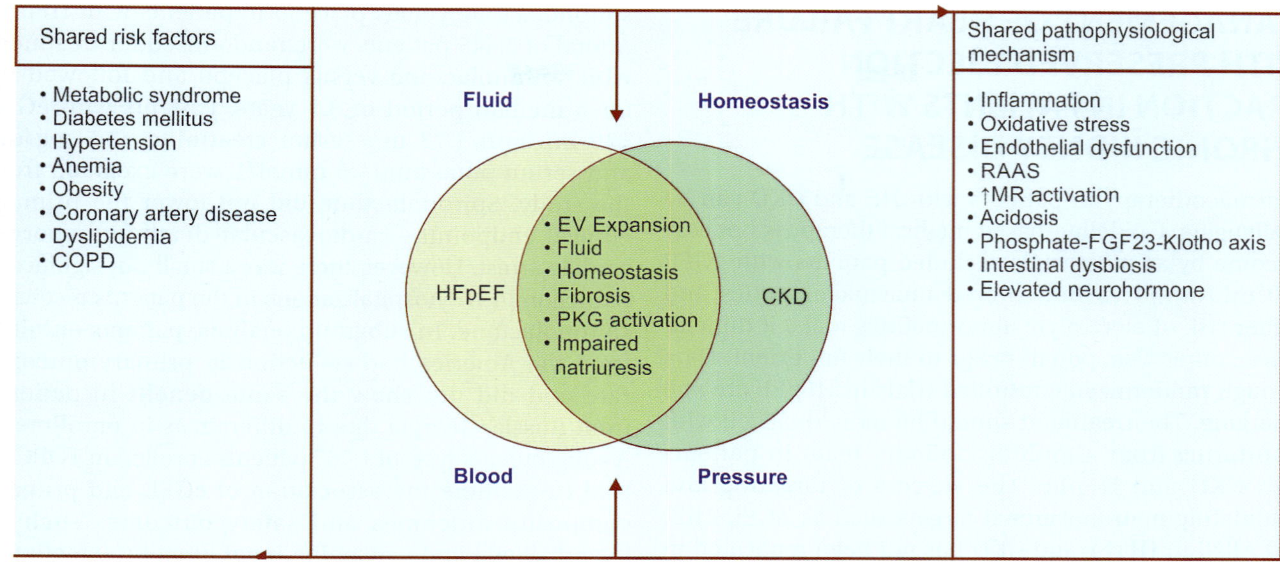

Fig. 1: Risk factors and pathophysiology of CKD and HFpEF. (CKD: chronic kidney disease; COPD: chronic obstructive pulmonary disease; EV: extracellular volume; FGF23: fibroblast growth factor 23; HFpEF: heart failure with preserved ejection fraction; MRA: mineralocorticoid receptor; PKG: protein kinase G; RAAS: renin–angiotensin–aldosterone system)

Flowchart 1: Mineralocorticoid receptor activation in CKD and HFpEF.

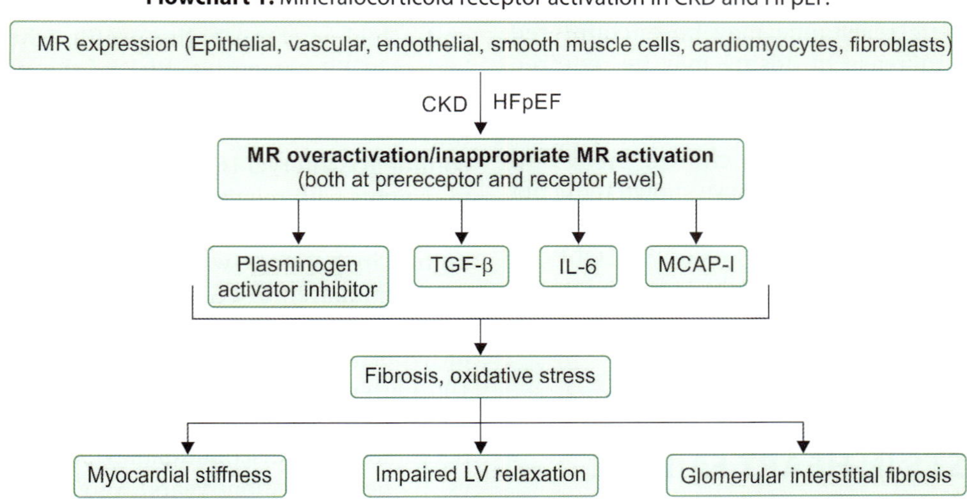

EPIDEMIOLOGY AND PROGNOSIS OF PATIENTS WITH CHRONIC KIDNEY DISEASE AND HEART FAILURE WITH PRESERVED EJECTION FRACTION

In large cohort studies, CKD [defined as estimated glomerular filtration rate (eGFR) <60 mL/min/1.73 m^2 and albuminuria] was present in up to 26–49% of patients with HFpEF.[10,11] CKD was more common in patients with HFpEF compared to heart failure with reduced ejection fraction (HFrEF).[12] Diuretic resistance is present in >20% of patients in this subgroup.[13] These patients have a poorer quality of life, and there is progressive decline in both kidney and cardiac functions.

Patients with HFpEF and CKD have a poor quality of life with worsening of renal and cardiac functions. Physiological decline of eGFR over time is 0.6–1 mL/min/1.73 m^2 per year and is worsened in patients with HFpEF, where the decline can be >5 mL/min/1.73 m^2 per year.[14] Decreased kidney function is associated with higher all-cause and cardiovascular mortality in all types of HF.[15]

MANAGEMENT OF HEART FAILURE WITH PRESERVED EJECTION FRACTION IN PATIENTS WITH CHRONIC KIDNEY DISEASE

Pharmacotherapy in patients with HF and CKD can be challenging. Guideline-based medical therapy is not easy to come by as most trials excluded patients with eGFR <30 mL/min/1.73 m^2. Altered pharmacokinetics and higher risk of electrolyte abnormalities make it difficult to use, otherwise, potent drugs to their full extent. Data through randomized controlled trials in HFpEF are still emerging. The treatment should be individualized with monitoring from a multidisciplinary team in patients with CKD and HFpEF. The success of targeting and modulating neurohormonal targets such as ACEi, ARB, and ARNI in HFrEF and CKD has not been replicated in patients with HFpEF. The goals of treatment in HFpEF include reduction of HF symptoms, improve functional status, and reduce hospitalization. Emphasis should be placed on lifestyle modifications and weight loss. Management of fluid overload with appropriate dose of loop diuretic therapy is indicated with salt and fluid restriction. Diuretic resistance may be encountered, and appropriate increase in dosing may be required. SGLT2i, which address metabolic syndrome, altered natriuresis, hypertension, and other pathophysiological pathways, have shown benefits in clinical trials. Both empagliflozin[16] and dapagliflozin[17] have shown reduction of cardiovascular death and HF hospitalizations in HFpEF. Glucagon-like peptide-1 receptor (GLP-1R) agonists with their effects on weight loss, pleiotropic effects, and improvement in insulin resistance are showing promise in patients with HFpEF and CKD.[18]

MINERALOCORTICOID RECEPTOR ANTAGONISTS IN HEART FAILURE WITH PRESERVED EJECTION FRACTION AND CHRONIC KIDNEY DISEASE

Targeting MR overactivation in patients with HFpEF and CKD is showing promise. In ALDO-DHF study, 25 mg of spironolactone a day led to improvement of diastolic dysfunction and ventricular remodeling. However, there was no improvement in quality of life parameters or exercise capacity.[19] The TOPCAT (Treatment of Preserved Cardiac Function Heart Failure With an Aldosterone Antagonist) study[20] was an international double-blind, placebo-controlled, parallel group study of the use of spironolactone versus placebo in patients with HFpEF. A total of 3,445 patients were randomized for treatment with spironolactone versus placebo and followed up for a median period of 3.3 years. Patients with eGFR <30 mL/min/1.73 m^2, serum creatinine >2.5 mg/dL, and serum potassium <5 mmol/L were excluded from the study. Spironolactone did not lower the primary clinical endpoints—cardiovascular death and aborted cardiac arrest. However, there was a small but significant reduction in HF hospitalizations in the patients receiving spironolactone. In subgroup analysis, patients enrolled from the America had reduction in primary outcome rate and did not show the same benefit in patients from Russia/Georgia due to differences in enrollment. A subgroup analysis of 1,767 patients enrolled in TOPCAT trial to examine the association of eGFR and primary composite outcomes and safety outcomes such as hyperkalemia and worsening renal function (creatinine >3 mg/dL) drug discontinuation due to adverse events was done.[21] The median eGFR at baseline was 57.9 mL/min/1.73 m^2, and 46.6% of the patients had eGFR >60 mL/min/1.73 m^2 and 23.3% of the patients had an eGFR between 30 and 45 mL/min/1.73 m^2. The patients in the lower eGFR category were commonly older women and a higher comorbidity profile when compared to higher eGFR categories. Risk of the primary outcome was higher for patients with severe renal dysfunction [eGFR <45 mL/min/1.73 m^2: hazard ratio (HR): 1.99; 95% confidence interval (CI): 1.62–2.45; p <0.001] compared to patients with relatively preserved eGFR (>60 mL/min/1.73 m^2). The rates of hyperkalemia were threefold higher in patients with eGFR <45 mL/min/1.73 m^2 when compared to eGFR >60 mL/min/1.73 m^2 (5.3 per 100 patient-years vs. 1.4 per 100 patient-years). Rates of hypokalemia (11.4 per 100 patient-years vs. 9.8 per 100 patient-years), worsening renal function (6.1 per 100 patient-years vs. 3.6 per 100 patient-years), and permanent drug discontinuation (9.4 per 100 patient-years vs. 1.7 per 100 patient-years) were also increased. There was a nominal statistical interaction between treatment and eGFR with regard to the composite endpoint of aborted cardiac arrest and sudden death, with lower risk noted among those assigned to spironolactone in higher, but not lower, eGFR categories (p for interaction = 0.03). Absolute risk differences between spironolactone and placebo over 4-year follow-up were examined, and the efficacy of spironolactone remained consistent across the full range of eGFR (absolute risk difference for total population: –6%; 95% CI: –11 to –0.2%; p for interaction = 0.23).[21] The subgroup analysis of the TOPCAT trial[21] showed that the adverse events and drug discontinuation were more pronounced in lower eGFR categories.

Based on these results, clinical guidelines have been updated to provide a IIB recommendation for the use of MRAs in HFpEF, indicating that it "may be considered" to reduce HF hospitalizations among patients with symptomatic HFpEF, elevated natriuretic peptides, eGFR >30 mL/min/1.73 m^2, creatinine <2.5 mg/dL, and potassium <5.0 mEq/L.[22-24]

DOSING OF SPIRONOLACTONE OUTCOMES IN HEART FAILURE WITH PRESERVED EJECTION FRACTION WITH CHRONIC KIDNEY DISEASE

Few studies have examined the relationship between spironolactone dosing and outcomes in patients with lower eGFR and HFpEF. Li et al.[25] studied the effect of low dose versus high dose (>40 mg/day) in 4,321 symptomatic patients with HFpEF and eGFR <60 mL/min/1.73 m^2. Primary outcome was a composite of all-cause death, HF hospitalization, and nonfatal stroke. The key safety outcome was hyperkalemia rates during the follow-up period. The primary outcome event rates in patients with or without spironolactone were 12.74 and 21.45 per 100 person-years, respectively. Compared with patients not taking spironolactone, the adjusted HR (95% CI) was 0.55 (0.38–0.79) with spironolactone group for primary outcomes. After grouped by the daily dose of spironolactone, low-dose group (≤40 mg) was associated with lower relative risk for the primary efficacy outcome [adjusted HR (95% CI) was 0.43 (0.23–0.81), 0.50 (0.33–0.76), and 0.74 (0.36–2.79) with <40, 40, and >40 mg, respectively]. During 3-year follow-up, the risk for hyperkalemia was amplified in the higher dose group (>40 mg) while showed no significant difference compared with low-dose group ($p = 0.425$). This suggested the use of low-dose (<40 mg/day) spironolactone as initial optimal therapy for patients with reduced GFR.[25]

SPIRONOLACTONE IN CHRONIC KIDNEY DISEASE STAGE 5 (END-STAGE RENAL DISEASE HEMODIALYSIS PATIENTS)

A 2-year multicentric, randomized, placebo-controlled study by Liu et al.[26] was to evaluate the long-term effects and adverse effects of spironolactone on hemodialysis patients without HF. In total, 253 non-HF dialysis patients with ESRD were randomly assigned to the spironolactone group (25 mg/day, $n = 125$) or the placebo group ($n = 128$). During the 2-year follow-up, in the spironolactone group, LVMI decreased by 8.7 g/m^2, LVEF increased by 5.1%, and the incidence of death due to cardiovascular, cerebrovascular events, or any cause in dialysis patients with ESRD was significantly reduced. Drug reaction, intolerance, gynecomastia, and hypotension were the adverse events seen in this subgroup.

More evidence is required to demonstrate the benefit of spironolactone on exercise tolerance and quality of life in patients with HFpEF and CKD. The ASIAN-HF registry[27] is relatively small ($n = 5,239$, 1,332 HFpEF), and the association of CKD and mortality was stronger in the HFrEF group than in the HFpEF group. eGFR <30 mL/min/1.73 m^2 worsened outcomes in patients with HFpEF. The HF registry of India[28] has done a multicentric study between 2019 and 2020 and collected data of 108,514 HF patients that were classified as HFrEF (65.2%), HFmrEF (22%), and HFpEF (12.7%). The main etiology of HF was ischemic heart disease. CKD was not highlighted in the analysis. In this complex kind of HF, further work to define the phenotypes of the population and then selection of appropriate therapy, perhaps by phenogroup, are directions that may help to improve clinical outcomes. Will these turned out to be different in Asia? We do not know currently, but databases such as ASIAN-HF may be valuable steps in finding that answer.

APPROACH FOR SPIRONOLACTONE DOSING IN CHRONIC KIDNEY DISEASE

Based on the current evidence, we propose the following protocols for spironolactone monitoring and dosing in CKD:

- *Renal function assessment:* Before starting spironolactone, assess kidney function, typically via serum creatinine and potassium levels.
- *Starting dose:* For patients with CKD, it is often recommended to start with a lower dose. A typical starting dose might be 25 mg daily.
- *Dose adjustment:* Depending on the patient's response and tolerability, the dose may be adjusted. In CKD, doses are often adjusted based on the eGFR) and serum potassium levels.
- *Mild CKD (eGFR ≥60 mL/min/1.73 m^2):* Doses can range from 25 to 50 mg daily.
- *Moderate CKD (eGFR 30–59 mL/min/1.73 m^2):* Lower doses, generally 25 mg every other day to 25 mg daily, are recommended.
- *Severe CKD (eGFR <30 mL/min/1.73 m^2):* Use with caution, often avoiding spironolactone or using it at very low doses. Regular monitoring of potassium and renal function is essential.

- *Monitoring:* Regular monitoring of serum potassium levels and kidney function is crucial to avoid hyperkalemia and worsening renal function. Typically, you should check these levels 1–2 weeks after in
- *Combination therapy:* If spironolactone is used in combination with other medications (such as ACE inhibitors or ARBs), the risk of hyperkalemia increases. Regular monitoring is even more critical in such cases of titrating or adjusting the dose and then periodically thereafter.[29]

CONCLUSION

Heart failure with preserved ejection fraction should be considered a systemic rather than a purely cardiovascular disorder. Association of kidney disease leads to greatest morbidity and mortality and sets up a vicious cardiorenal interactions. An integrated multidisciplinary approach is required to promote risk factor reduction and increase the adoption of newer therapeutics. In conclusion, while MRA remains an important pillar of HFrEF treatment, caution should be exercised in the complex patient group with both CKD and HF, and close biochemical monitoring is important during treatment.

REFERENCES

1. Lazzeri C, Valente S, Tarquini R, et al. Cardiorenal syndrome caused by heart failure with preserved ejection fraction. Int J Nephrol. 2011;2011:634903.
2. Patel RN, Sharma A, Prasad A, et al. Heart failure with preserved ejection fraction with CKD: a narrative review of a multispecialty disorder. Kidney Med. 2023;5(12):100705.
3. Kawaguchi M, Hay I, Fetics B, et al. Combined ventricular systolic and arterial stiffening in patients with heart failure and preserved ejection fraction: implications for systolic and diastolic reserve limitations. Circulation. 2003;107:714-20.
4. Abudiab MM, Redfield MM, Melenovsky V, et al. Cardiac output response to exercise in relation to metabolic demand in heart failure with preserved ejection fraction. Eur J Heart Fail. 2013;15(6):776-85.
5. Ter Maaten JM, Damman K, Verhaar MC, et al. Connecting heart failure with preserved ejection fraction and renal dysfunction: the role of endothelial dysfunction and inflammation. Eur J Heart Fail. 2016;18(6):588-98.
6. Buonafine M, Bonnard B, Jaisser F. Mineralocorticoid receptor and cardiovascular disease. Am J Hypertens. 2018;31(11):1165-74.
7. Jia G, Jia Y, Sowers JR. Role of mineralocorticoid receptor activation in cardiac diastolic dysfunction. Biochim Biophys Acta Mol Basis Dis. 2017;1863(8):2012-18.
8. Luther JM, Fogo AB. The role of mineralocorticoid receptor activation in kidney inflammation and fibrosis. Kidney Int Suppl (2011). 2022;12(1):63-8.
9. Cosimato C, Agoritsas T, Mavrakanas TA. Mineralocorticoid receptor antagonists in patients with chronic kidney disease. Pharmacol Ther. 2021;219:107701.
10. Unger ED, Dubin RF, Deo R, et al. Association of chronic kidney disease with abnormal cardiac mechanics and adverse outcomes in patients with heart failure and preserved ejection fraction. Eur J Heart Fail. 2016;18(1):103-12.
11. Gori M, Senni M, Gupta DK, et al. Association between renal function and cardiovascular structure and function in heart failure with preserved ejection fraction. Eur Heart J. 2014;35(48):3442-51.
12. Lofman I, Szummer K, Dahlstrom U, et al. Associations with and prognostic impact of chronic kidney disease in heart failure with preserved, mid-range, and reduced ejection fraction. Eur J Heart Fail. 2017;19(12):1606-14.
13. Sharma A, Patel R, Prasad A, et al. Diuretic resistance in acute decompensated HFpEF vs. HFrEF. Clin Nephrol. 2023;100:47-50.
14. Bonacchi G, Rossi VA, Garofalo M, et al. Pathophysiological link and treatment implication of heart failure and preserved ejection fraction in patients with chronic kidney disease. Biomedicines. 2024;12(5):981.
15. Hillege HL, Nitsch D, Pfeffer MA, et al. Renal function as a predictor of outcome in a broad spectrum of patients with heart failure. Circulation. 2006;113(5):671-8.
16. Anker SD, Butler J, Filippatos G, et al. Empagliflozin in heart failure with a preserved ejection fraction. N Engl J Med. 2021;385(16):1451-61.
17. Solomon SD, McMurray JJV, Claggett B, et al. Dapagliflozin in heart failure with mildly reduced or preserved ejection fraction. N Engl J Med. 2022;387(12):1089-98.
18. Kosiborod MN, Abildstrøm SZ, Borlaug BA, et al. Semaglutide in patients with heart failure with preserved ejection fraction and obesity. N Engl J Med. 2023;389:1069-84.
19. Edelmann F, Wachter R, Schmidt AG, et al. Effect of spironolactone on diastolic function and exercise capacity in patients with heart failure with preserved ejection fraction: the Aldo-DHF randomized controlled trial. JAMA. 2013;309(8):781-91.
20. Pitt B, Pfeffer MA, Assmann SF, et al. Spironolactone for heart failure with preserved ejection fraction. N Engl J Med. 2014;370(15):1383-92.
21. Beldhuis IE, Myhre PL, Claggett B, et al. Efficacy and safety of spironolactone in patients with HFpEF and chronic kidney disease. JACC Heart Fail. 2019;7(1):25-32.
22. Ezekowitz JA, O'Meara E, McDonald MA, et al. 2017 comprehensive update of the Canadian Cardiovascular Society guidelines for the management of heart failure. Can J Cardiol. 2017;33:1342-433.
23. Yancy CW, Jessup M, Bozkurt B, et al. 2017 ACC/AHA/HFSA focused update of the 2013 ACCF/AHA guideline for the management of heart failure. J Am Coll Cardiol. 2017;70:776-803.

24. Ponikowski P, Voors AA, Anker SD, et al. 2016 ESC guidelines for the diagnosis and treatment of acute and chronic heart failure. Eur J Heart Fail. 2016;18: 891-975.
25. Li JF, Qu X, Gao Z, et al. Association between dosing of spironolactone and outcomes in heart failure with preserved ejection fraction patients combined with chronic kidney disease------Balance of efficacy and risk. Front Pharmacol. 2023;14:1084442.
26. Liu J, Jia W, Yu C. Safety and efficacy of spironolactone in dialysis-dependent patients: meta-analysis of randomized controlled trials. Front Med. 2022;9.
27. MacDonald MR, Tay WT, et al. Regional variation of mortality in heart failure with reduced and preserved ejection fraction across Asia: outcomes in the ASIAN-HF registry. J Am Heart Assoc. 2020;9(1).
28. Harikrishnan S, Bahl A, Roy A, et al. Clinical profile and 90 day outcomes of 10 851 heart failure patients across India: National Heart Failure Registry. ESC Heart Fail. 2022;9(6):3898-908.
29. Pérez-Gordillo FL, Serrano-Morillas N, Acosta-García LM, et al. Novel 1,4-dihydropyridine derivatives as mineralocorticoid receptor antagonists. Int J Mol Sci. 2023; 24(3):2439.

CHAPTER

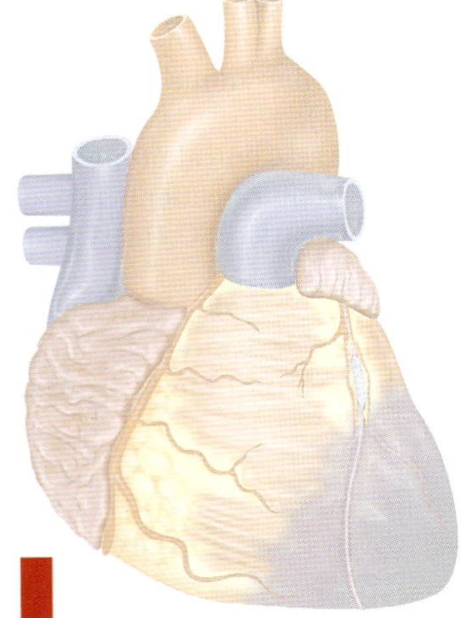

Current Management of HFpEF in Chronic Kidney Disease: An Overview

Dinesh Khullar, Narinder Pal Singh, Kulwant Singh, Simran Kaur, Anish Kumar Gupta

INTRODUCTION

Heart failure (HF) is a syndrome characterized by symptoms arising from a structural or functional heart abnormality, along with either elevated natriuretic peptide levels or evidence of cardiogenic pulmonary or systemic congestion. It is classified into three types: HF with reduced ejection fraction (HFrEF, ≤40%), mildly reduced ejection fraction (HFmrEF, 41–49%), and preserved ejection fraction (HFpEF ≥50%). HFpEF is frequently underdiagnosed and underreported, making it difficult to accurately estimate its prevalence globally. Over recent decades, the prevalence of HFpEF has risen in comparison to HFrEF, particularly in older adults, where myocardial stiffness increases. Inflammation, driven by metabolic risk factors such as hypertension, diabetes, atrial fibrillation, and renal insufficiency, tends to occur with age, leading to left ventricular wall thickening without dilation (cardiomyocyte hypertrophy). Women are twice as likely as men to develop HFpEF. Furthermore, about 20–30% of heart failure treatments result in acute kidney injury (AKI), and 50–66% of heart failure patients have reduced kidney function with an estimated glomerular filtration rate (eGFR) below 60 mL/min/1.73 m^2. Approximately 26–49% of the HFpEF patients have chronic kidney disease (CKD). In patients with CKD, 17–21% develop new-onset heart failure, and 44% of those with end-stage renal disease (ESRD) also have heart failure, highlighting the strong interconnection between heart and kidney health, where each condition profoundly influences the other.[1] Despite the high prevalence of HF in CKD, majority of HF clinical trials have informed current pharmacological treatment strategies excluded individuals with severe renal impairment, defined as an eGFR of ≤30 mL/min/1.73 m^2. In this review, we explore the current management of HF patients with preserved ejection fraction and/or CKD.

CHRONIC KIDNEY DISEASE AND HEART FAILURE WITH PRESERVED EJECTION FRACTION

The HFpEF has been classified into three biological phenogroups—the natriuretic peptide deficiency group (young individuals), cardiometabolic group (old individuals), and cardio abdominal-renal syndrome group (CKD patients). HF disrupts normal kidney function and leads to cardio renal syndrome that further promotes HF progression. HFpEF and CKD share common risk factors, including diabetes, hypertension, and obesity, but a number of pathophysiological processes contribute to the interplay between cardiac and renal dysfunction involve inflammation, oxidative stress, and neurohormonal activation, such as activation of the sympathetic nervous system (SNS), the renin-angiotensin-aldosterone system (RAAS), and natriuretic peptide system (NPS). Additionally, CKD can contribute to the development of HF by causing venous congestion due to salt and water retention as well as changes in hemodynamics. As a result, CKD and HF frequently coexist, with each condition acting as a risk factor for the other.

As per American College of Cardiology/American Heart Association (ACC/AHA) and European Society of

Cardiology (ESC) guidelines, diagnosis of HFpEF includes preserved ejection fraction, elevated left ventricular (LV) filling pressures, and elevated natriuretic peptides.[2] The recommended levels to qualify for diagnosing HFpEF is NT-proBNP >125 pg/mL or BNP >35 pg/mL in sinus rhythm. In patients of CKD, these levels may be spuriously elevated and hence makes the diagnosis challenging. To overcome this, H2FPEF score (parameters involved obesity, hypertension, atrial fibrillation, pulmonary hypertension (PASP >35 mmHg), age (>60 years), and diastolic function (E/e >9) and HFA-PEFF [parameters involved functional aspects—Diastolic function (E/e ≥15, GLS (<16%), and morphological aspects and natriuretic peptides] algorithm have been developed as per American and European guidelines. Additionally, there is a clear need for treatment that addresses both renal and cardiac pathophysiology, while also effectively managing the frequently coexisting comorbidities.

MANAGEMENT OF AND HEART FAILURE WITH PRESERVED EJECTION FRACTION PATIENTS WITH CHRONIC KIDNEY DISEASE

The ACC consensus document and the accompanying JACC scientific statement on HFpEF recommend several key treatment strategies, including managing comorbidities such as hypertension, diabetes mellitus, obesity, atrial fibrillation, CKD, and obstructive sleep apnea. Additionally, lifestyle modifications such as dietary modifications, regular physical exercise, and weight loss are emphasized. The approach also involves both symptomatic management and the use of disease-modifying therapies to improve patient outcomes.[3,4]

Multitargeted Therapy

Research indicates that angiotensin receptor neprilysin inhibitors (ARNI), sodium-glucose cotransporter 2 inhibitors (SGLT2i), nonsteroidal mineralocorticoid receptor antagonist (MRA, finerenone), and selective β1-blockers (bisoprolol), are beneficial in treating HF in patients with CKD stages 1–3. However, caution is advised when using these treatments in CKD stages 4 and 5, and consultation with a nephrologist is recommended. Studies have shown that combining ARNi with SGLT-2i or β-blockers is safe for renal function in patients with HF and/or CKD. These therapies are believed to offer both complementary and independent benefits to the heart and kidneys, enhancing renal blood flow, eGFR, cardiac output (CO), and mean arterial pressure (MAP), while preserving the filtration fraction.

Sodium-glucose Cotransporter 2 Inhibitors

The SGLT2 inhibitors are now considered the first line drug for treating HFpEF. These drugs have demonstrated efficacy and safety in treating HFpEF in patients with comorbid CKD, with and without diabetes. The extraglycemic pleiotropic effects of SGLT2 inhibitors play an important role in managing comorbidities associated with HFpEF. These drugs promote glomerular longevity by reducing the intraglomerular pressure through tubuloglomerular feedback.

Conclusive results in favor of SGLT2 inhibitors was provided by trials—EMPEROR PRESERVED,[5] and DELIVER trials.[6] Both these trials included patients with LVEF >40% and showed that empagliflozin and dapagliflozin significantly reduced CV death and hospitalizations due to heart failure when compared with placebo. DELIVER trial included both diabetic and nondiabetic patients.

As per 2023 focused update of the 2021 ESC guidelines, SGLT2i are recommended in HFpEF patients to reduce the risk of hospitalizations due to HF or CV death (Class IA recommendation). In patients of CKD and T2D, SGLT2i are recommended to reduce the risk of HFH or CV deaths (Class IA). According to the 2022 AHA/ACC guideline for the management of HF, SGLT2i are recommended for patients with HFpEF with a class 2A recommendation. Indian guidelines by the HF association of India have recommended the use of SGLT2i in both diabetic and nondiabetic patients of HFpEF. The Kidney Disease Improving Global Outcomes (KDIGO) guideline (2022) and the American Diabetes Association (ADA) guidelines (2023) recommended SGLT2i for patients with T2D and CKD with an eGFR of at least 20 mL/min/1.73 m^2 (class 1A).[7,8]

Diuretics

The use of loop diuretics such as furosemide and torsemide has been recommended in all patients with symptomatic HFpEF based in consensus among experts as Class I indication.[9]

Angiotensin Receptor Neprilysin Inhibitor

The ARNI play an important role in managing patients of heart failure **(Flowchart 1)**. Apart from this, these drugs have a beneficial impact on renal function in patients of HFpEF. Sacubitril stimulates the synthesis of c GMP, which increases the GFR and renal blood flow by promoting vasodilatation of afferent arterioles and myocardial relaxation.

Flowchart 1: Managing patients of heart failure.

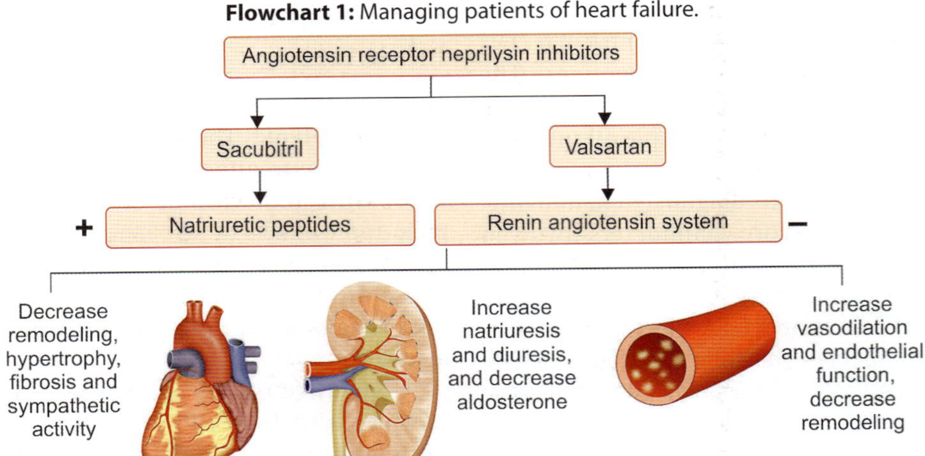

Landmark trials such as PARAMOUNT (2012),[10] PARAGON-HF (2019)[11] and PARALLAX (2021)[12] trial have provided valuable insights into use of ARNI in HFpEF patients. PARAMOUNT trial included patients with LVEF >45% and showed that significant decrease in NT-proBNP levels was achieved by sacubitril/valsartan as compared to valsartan by week 12, however, this difference became insignificant by 36 weeks. PARAGON HF trial was able to demonstrate decreased CV mortality and hospitalizations due to heart failure in sacubitril/valsartan group as compared to valsartan alone, however, this difference was not statistically significant. As per the 2024 ACC/AHA guidelines for management of HFpEF, ARNI have class IIb recommendation. The Chinese expert consensus on the use of ARNi in CKD patients also recommends the use of ARNi in nondialysis CKD patients with HF (grade IA) or hypertension (grade IB) or in hemodialysis patients with HF (grade IB) or hypertension (grade 2D).

No dose adjustment for sacubitril/valsartan is needed when eGFR ≥30 mL/min/1.73 m^2. In patients with moderate to severe renal impairment (eGFR <30 mL/min/1.73 m^2), 20–50 mg twice daily is recommended based on the patient's blood pressure. Thereafter, the dose is doubled every 2–4 weeks until a target maintenance dose of 200 mg twice daily is reached. The use of RAASi/ARNI in CKD should not be determined by a specific serum creatinine level, but rather by monitoring trends in serum creatinine and potassium levels. Unlike ACE inhibitors, ARNI carries a lower risk of causing hyperkalemia. The decision to use RAASi/ARNI in preserving GFR should be individualized for each case. It is advisable to initiate treatment with a low dose and not be overly concerned about an initial decline in eGFR. However, continuous monitoring is essential, and caution is warranted if there is a persistent decline in GFR. Frequent monitoring of serum potassium levels is also crucial throughout the treatment.

β-blockers

Bisoprolol, being a cardio-selective β-1 blocker, offers a range of benefits in patients of CKD and HF by reducing the cardiac workload, improving the cardiac performance, and by reducing the myocardial oxygen demand. Inspite of this, bisoprolol has some limitations and considerations, especially in CKD patients. It has been associated with decline in renal function, and hence is not suitable for all CKD patients. As per ESC 2023 update and ACC/AHA heart failure guidelines, β blockers have been recommended in the management of HFmrEF (Class IIb). The dose of BBs such as acebutolol, atenolol, bisoprolol, and nadolol should be reduced by 50% when GFR is <30 mL/min/1.73m^2.

Mineralocorticoid Receptor Antagonist

The MRAs offer substantial clinical benefit in patients with HFrEF, more than in patients with HFpEF. Aldosterone plays an important role in the pathogenesis of HFpEF, and hence MRA are useful in preventing the pathological alterations in HFpEF. Spironolactone, nonselective steroidal MRA, is recommended in patients of HFrEF. Trials conducted in HFpEF patients have not yet proven definite role of spironolactone in HFpEF. The Aldo-DHF trial included patients with LVEF >50% and showed that long-term aldosterone receptor blockade improved left ventricular diastolic function but did not affect maximal exercise capacity, patient symptoms, or quality of life in patients with HFpEF. TOPCAT (Treatment of Preserved

Cardiac Function Heart Failure with an Aldosterone Antagonist) trial[13] included patients with LVEF >45%, and showed that in HFpEF, treatment with spironolactone did not significantly reduce the incidence of the primary composite outcome of death from cardiovascular causes, aborted cardiac arrest, or hospitalization for the management of heart failure. In the 2022 ACC/AHA guidelines, MRAs hold class IIB recommendations and may be considered to decrease hospitalizations in patients of HFpEF.

Finerenone is a highly selective MRA and is more potent than steroidal MRA. It has lower risk of hyperkalemia when compared to spironolactone. FIDELITY pooled analysis of trials FIDELIO-DKD and FIGARO-DKD trials (excluded patients of HFrEF) concluded that finerenone reduced the risk of clinically important cardiovascular and kidney outcomes versus placebo across the spectrum of CKD in patients with type 2 diabetes. KDIGO 2024 guidelines suggest a nonsteroidal MRA with proven kidney or cardiovascular benefit for adults with T2D, an eGFR >25 mL/min per 1.73 m^2, normal serum potassium concentration, and albuminuria [>30 mg/g (>3 mg/mmol)] despite maximum tolerated dose of RAS inhibitor (RASi) (class IIA recommendation). Recently published landmark trails—FINEARTS-HF (2024)[14] included patients with LVEF >40%, with a mean LVEF of 53%. This study showed that finerenone resulted in significantly lower rate of worsening heart failure events and death from cardiovascular causes.

MANAGEMENT OF SPECIFIC CONDITIONS (FLOWCHART 2)

Hyperkalemia

Patients taking RAASi/ARNI face an increased risk of hyperkalemia, especially as their renal function declines. However, a recent meta-analysis by Feng et al. found no significant difference in hyperkalemia rates between ARNi and ACEI/ARB groups, suggesting that ARNi may have a favorable impact on potassium levels and a comparable hyperkalemia risk to ACEI/ARB use. Additionally, the safety analysis from the FIDELITY study indicates that finerenone has a low rate of discontinuation due to hyperkalemia, comparable to that of the placebo group. The FINEARTS-HF trial also showed a higher incidence of hyperkalemia with finerenone (9.7 vs. 4.2% in the placebo group), though this did not result in significant hospitalizations or deaths. Additionally, finerenone was associated with a lower risk of hypokalemia.

Recent advancements in hyperkalemia management with medications such as patiromer and sodium zirconium cyclosilicate allow for the safe continuation of RAASi, enabling dose optimization without hyperkalemia concerns, although cost considerations may be relevant when these drugs become available. In cases of severe hyperkalemia, characterized by ECG changes or potassium levels exceeding 6.5 mEq/L (even without ECG changes), immediate action is crucial. Treatment typically

Flowchart 2: Heart failure with preserved ejection fraction treatment.

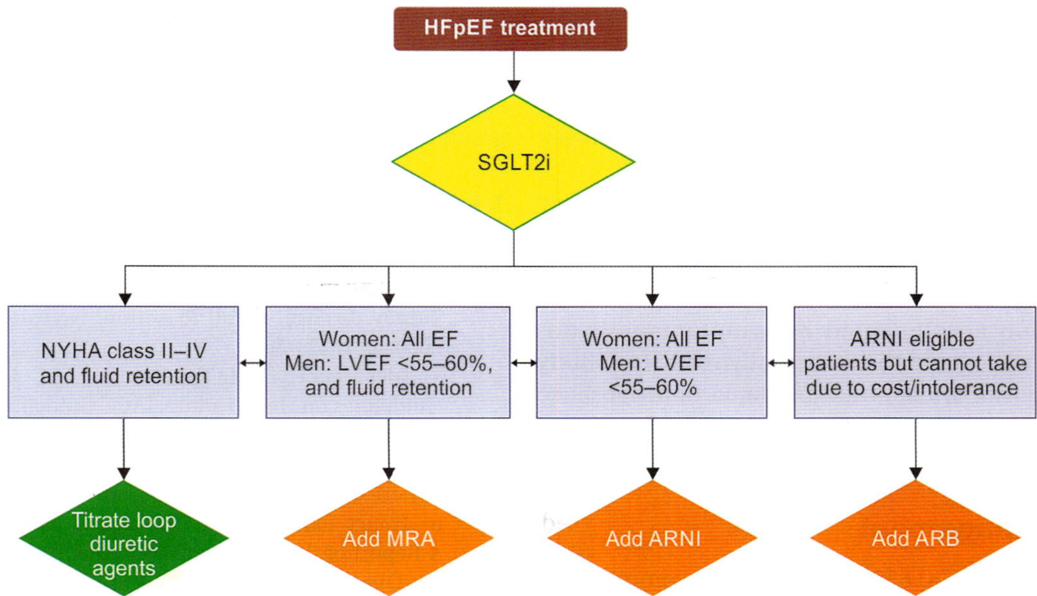

starts with administering calcium gluconate to stabilize cardiomyocyte membranes. Subsequently, insulin and β-agonist injections are recommended. High doses of diuretics may be necessary in cases of fluid retention. The initiation, titration, and maintenance of RAASi/ARNI treatment should remain a priority, even during concurrent illnesses or worsening heart failure.

Worsening Renal Function

Worsening renal function (WRF) is typically characterized by a 20–30% decline in eGFR or an increase in serum creatinine of 0.3 mg/dL or more within 15–30 days after a medical intervention. WRF following the initiation or dose adjustment of β-blockers may signify reduced cardiac output and is linked to a poorer prognosis. In contrast, medications such as RAASi, ARNI, and SGLT-2i cause acute eGFR reduction due to changes in renal hemodynamics. Typically, the eGFR stabilizes after the acute phase, indicating a slower progression of CKD. Renal function should be closely monitored during the initiation and titration of RAASi. According to the "Heart Failure Working Group of the French Society of Cardiology"[15] following should be considered:

- After starting RAASi, an increase in creatinine up to 50% and a rise in potassium to 5.5 mmol/L or lower are permissible.
- An increase in creatinine of 50–100% warrants a systematic evaluation of the clinical context, including factors such as congestion, dehydration, blood pressure, and medication interactions. Adjustments to medication doses, potentially halving the usual dose, may be necessary. Close patient monitoring is crucial.
- If potassium levels exceed 5.5 mmol/L, creatinine rises by >100%, or creatinine levels exceed 3.5 mg/dL, or eGFR drops below 20 mL/min, discontinue current MRA/ARNI/ACEI/ARBs, and consult a nephrologist for further guidance.
- A rise in creatinine exceeding 100%, the presence of underlying CKD with an abrupt eGFR reduction to below 20 mL/min, acutely decompensated heart failure, significant electrolyte imbalances, severe dehydration accompanied by symptomatic hypotension, cardiogenic shock, hemodynamic instability associated with urinary tract problems, or the absence of improvement after 48 hours of outpatient treatment requires an urgent hospital referral.

Anemia Management

The combination of CKD, HF, and anemia is common and linked to high morbidity and mortality. While anemia raises risks, intensive treatment with EPO or ESAs offers limited benefit due to potential confounding factors or adverse side effects. Iron-replacement therapy is now prioritized, as many CKD and HF patients are iron-deficient, and high-dose IV iron has shown improved outcomes, as seen in the PIVOTAL trial.[16] Additionally, SGLT-2 inhibitors, which improve CKD and HF prognosis, have been found to raise hemoglobin levels by increasing EPO and red blood cell mass, offering a potential anemia treatment that may also enhance renal and cardiac protection.[17]

CONCLUSION

Heart failure and CKD form a dangerous duo, each worsening the other's prognosis and creating a serious health burden, particularly in India. As these two conditions often go hand in hand, the need for effective treatment strategies is more urgent than ever. The use of drugs like ARNI, SGLT2 inhibitors, and bisoprolol has emerged as a game changer, as they target shared pathways and significantly reduce the neurohormonal activity that drives both heart and kidney dysfunction. Beyond their traditional role, these medications offer remarkable cardio renal and metabolic benefits for CKD patients, even those without HF, diabetes, or hypertension.

Imagine a carefully designed, protocol-driven approach where treatment is fine-tuned based on clinical assessments, echocardiograms, NT-proBNP levels, and eGFR to guide care. This precision could dramatically reduce morbidity and mortality, offering a beacon of hope for CKD patients living with HF. On the horizon, promising trials such as FINEOAVTE and THUNDERBALL CKD are set to further revolutionize care, potentially positioning finerenone as a cornerstone therapy in the battle against heart failure in CKD patients. The future of heart and kidney care is evolving, with new pathways unlocking greater potential for survival and quality of life.

REFERENCES

1. Romero-González G, Ravassa S, González O, et al. Burden and challenges of heart failure in patients with chronic kidney disease. A call to action. Nefrologia (Engl Ed). 2020;40(3):223-36.
2. Van der Meer P, Gaggin HK, Dec GW. ACC/AHA Versus ESC Guidelines on Heart Failure: JACC Guideline Comparison. J Am Coll Cardiol. 2019;73(21):2756-68.
3. Kittleson MM, Panjrath GS, Amancherla K, et al. 2023 ACC Expert Consensus Decision Pathway on Management of Heart Failure With Preserved Ejection Fraction: A Report of the American College of Cardiology Solution Set Oversight Committee. J Am Coll Cardiol. 2023 May 9;81(18):1835-1878.

4. Borlaug B, Sharma K, Shah S. Heart failure with preserved ejection fraction: JACC Scientific Statement. JACC. 2023;81(18):1810-34.
5. Packer M, Anker SD, Butler J, et al. Cardiovascular and renal outcomes with empagliflozin in heart failure. N Engl J Med. 2020;383(15):1413-24.
6. Solomon SD, Vaduganathan M, Claggett BL, et al. Baseline Characteristics of Patients With HF With Mildly Reduced and Preserved Ejection Fraction: DELIVER Trial. JACC Heart Fail. 2022;10(3):184-97.
7. Kidney Disease: Improving Global Outcomes (KDIGO) Diabetes Work Group. KDIGO 2022 Clinical Practice Guideline for Diabetes Management in Chronic Kidney Disease. Kidney Int. 2022;102(5S):S1-S127.
8. American Diabetes Association. Standards of Care in Diabetes-2023. Abridged for Primary Care Providers. Clin Diabetes. 2023;41(2):328.
9. Desai AS, Lam CSP, McMurray JJV. How to Manage Heart Failure With Preserved Ejection Fraction: Practical Guidance for Clinicians. JACC Heart Fail. 2023; 11(6):619-36.
10. Solomon SD, Zile M, Pieske B, et al. The angiotensin receptor neprilysin inhibitor LCZ696 in heart failure with preserved ejection fraction: a phase 2 double-blind randomised controlled trial. Lancet. 2012;380(9851): 1387-95.
11. Vaduganathan M, Mentz RJ, Claggett BL, et al. Sacubitril/valsartan in heart failure with mildly reduced or preserved ejection fraction: a pre-specified participant-level pooled analysis of PARAGLIDE-HF and PARAGON-HF. Eur Heart J. 2023;44(31):2982-93.
12. Pieske B, Wachter R, Shah SJ, et al. Effect of Sacubitril/Valsartan vs Standard Medical Therapies on Plasma NT-proBNP Concentration and Submaximal Exercise Capacity in Patients With Heart Failure and Preserved Ejection Fraction: The PARALLAX Randomized Clinical Trial. JAMA. 2021;326(19):1919-29.
13. Pfeffer MA, Claggett B, Assmann SF, et al. Regional variation in patients and outcomes in the Treatment of Preserved Cardiac Function Heart Failure With an Aldosterone Antagonist (TOPCAT) trial. Circulation. 2015;131(1):34-42.
14. Solomon SD, McMurray JJV, Vaduganathan M, et al. Finerenone in Heart Failure with Mildly Reduced or Preserved Ejection Fraction. N Engl J Med. 2024 Sep 1. doi: 10.1056/NEJMoa2407107.
15. Mewton N, Girerd N, Boffa JJ, et al. Practical management of worsening renal function in outpatients with heart failure and reduced ejection fraction: Statement from a panel of multidisciplinary experts and the Heart Failure Working Group of the French Society of Cardiology. Arch Cardiovasc Dis. 2020;113(10):660-70.
16. Macdougall IC, White C, Anker SD, et al. Intravenous Iron in Patients Undergoing Maintenance Hemodialysis. N Engl J Med. 2019;380(5):447-58.
17. Packer M. Mechanistic and clinical comparison of the erythropoietic effects of SGLT2 inhibitors and prolyl hydroxylase inhibitors in patients with chronic kidney disease and renal anemia. Am J Nephrol. 2024;55(2):255-9.

CHAPTER

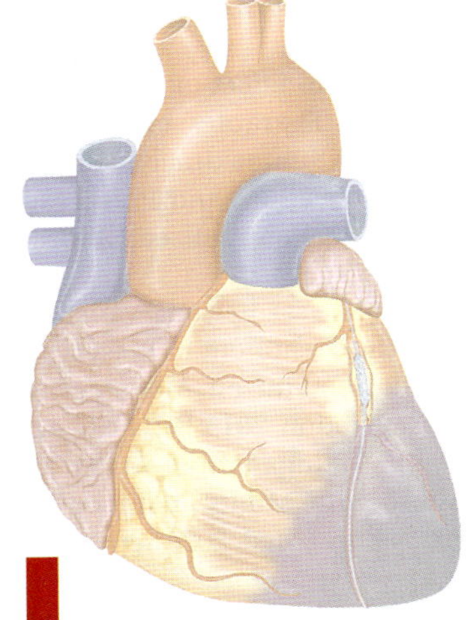

Renal Safety and Efficacy of ARNI in HFpEF

M Edwin Fernando, M Karthikeyan

INTRODUCTION

Chronic kidney disease (CKD) is characterized by progressive decline in glomerular filtration rate (GFR) and there is always tight link between CKD and cardiovascular disease (CVD). Hypertension, diabetes, obesity, and dyslipidemia are major risk factors for both CKD and CVD.[1] Baseline renal dysfunction and worsening of renal function over time are observed frequently in patients with heart failure (HF). Prevalence of CKD and worsening renal function was present in 32% and 23% of HF patients, respectively and both were associated with poor survival and outcomes.[2] Angiotensin receptor-neprilysin inhibitor (ARNi) which has the dual action of angiotensin receptor II type I blockade and neprilysin inhibition. Sacubitril/valsartan, a combined ARNI is one of the cornerstone therapies for HF. ARNI prevent worsening of renal function and progression of CKD when compared with renin-angiotensin system (RAS) inhibitors alone in HF patients. They improve ventricular function by preventing the degradation of endogenous natriuretic peptides (NPs) due to neprilysin inhibition and counteracting the detrimental effects of RAS activation.[3] CKD and CVD are a vicious cycle where CKD is a risk factor for CVD and CVD causes renal dysfunction and progression to CKD.[4] Based on this, sacubitril/valsartan will be able to protect kidney function by ameliorating heart failure.[5]

RENAL SAFETY AND EFFICACY OF ANGIOTENSIN RECEPTOR-NEPRILYSIN INHIBITOR IN HEART FAILURE WITH PRESERVED EJECTION FRACTION

Natriuretic peptides (NPs) are produced by the atria and left ventricle in response to excess preload and afterload. They are atrial, brain, and c-type NPs that help patients with heart failure to maintain fluid and sodium balance by natriuresis and diuresis in the kidney.[6] They reduce renal and systemic vascular resistance in heart failure despite excess RAS activation. NPs are degraded by neprilysin present in brush borders of proximal tubules, intestines, adipose tissues, adrenal gland, brain, and endothelial cells. Neprilysin inhibitors prevent this breakdown of NPs by inhibiting neprilysin and increases its bioavailability.[7] ARNi have the combined benefits of RAS and neprilysin inhibition without excess risk of angioedema.

To understand the renal effects of ARNi in heart failure, we look back to a study by Merril AJ in 1946. He measured renal plasma flow (RPF) and GFR in 37 patients with heart failure using inulin clearance and para-aminohippurate, and found that RPF was reduced from one-third to one-fifth compared to normal when cardiac output was reduced below one-half of the resting value. In heart failure, there is diversion of blood from the kidneys which receive 20% of cardiac output.[8] Despite a decrease in RPF, GFR is maintained by increasing intraglomerular pressure mediated by efferent arteriole vasoconstrictive action of RAS. This adaptive mechanism is compromised when using RAS inhibitors which prevent the angiotensin II mediated vasoconstriction which leads to fall in glomerular pressure and rise in serum creatinine.

Neprilysin inhibitors combined with RAS inhibition in ARNi, have increased the NPs bioavailability, which further reduces systemic BP and renal perfusion pressure. However, it causes vasodilation of the afferent arteriole and relative vasoconstriction of efferent arteriole, leading to increase in filtration fraction and GFR. This hypothesis has to be confirmed by direct measure of kidney perfusion and filtration, as alteration of renal hemodynamics has long-term kidney outcomes independent of HF.[9,10]

Recent trials have revealed the beneficial effect of ARNi on heart failure with preserved ejection fraction. The renal outcomes of ARNi in patients with HFpEF were reported in four randomized clinical trials which had a total of 8,005 participants.

PARAMOUNT-HF TRIAL (2012)[11]

149 patients randomly assigned to sacubitril/valsartan and 152 to the valsartan group and followed up for 8 months. Renal outcomes are defined as a rise in serum creatinine ≥0.3 mg/dL from baseline and or >25% between 2 time points. The baseline estimated glomerular filtration rate (eGFR) was 66.5 ± 19.4 in the sacubitril/valsartan group and 64.3 ± 21.3 in the valsartan group. The primary outcome was impact on NT-proBNP levels and there was greater impact found in sacubitril/valsartan on NT-proBNP levels.

Secondary analysis was done by Voor et al., to study the effect of ARNI on eGFR fall and urine albumin-creatinine ratio (UACR) in HFpEF patients. There was a greater decrease of eGFR in the valsartan group when compared to the sacubitril/valsartan group at 36 weeks (–15.2 mL/min/1.73 m^2 vs. –1.6 mL/min/1.73 m^2, respectively, p-value = 0.007). But there was a greater increase in UACR from baseline in the sacubitril/valsartan group at 36 weeks (1.9 mg/mmol at baseline and 2.9 mg/mmol at week 36) compared to valsartan (2.0 mg/mmol at baseline and 36 weeks).

The PARAMOUNT trial concluded that sacubitril/valsartan has a role in eGFR preservation compared to valsartan therapy in patients with HFpEF over 36 weeks but associated with increased UACR.[10]

PARAGON-HF TRIAL (2019)[12]

4,822 patients with New York Heart Association (NYHA) Class III–V heart failure, EF of 45% or higher with elevated levels of NPs randomized to receive sacubitril/valsartan (target dose of 97 mg of sacubitril and 103 mg of valsartan twice daily) or valsartan (target dose of 160 mg twice daily) followed up for 35 months. The primary outcome was CV death or heart failure hospitalization.

Renal outcome studied in secondary analysis defined as death from end stage renal failure or a 50% fall in eGFR.

The composite renal outcome occurred in 1.4% of patients on sacubitril/valsartan (n = 33) and 2.7% on valsartan (n = 64) [hazard ratio, 0.50 (95% CI, 0.33–0.77)]; p-value = 0.001). As like the PARAMOUNT study, less decline in eGFR in the intervention group than control group. It concluded that patients with HFpEF, sacubitril/valsartan reduced the risk of renal events and slowed the decline in eGFR in comparison with the valsartan group.[13]

PARALLAX-HF (2020)[14]

This RCT included 2,572 patients with heart failure and left ventricular ejection fraction higher than 40% and treated with sacubitril/valsartan or standard treatment with enalapril, valsartan, or placebo. The primary outcome was change in NT-proBNP levels at week 12 from baseline and 6 minute walk test distance at week 24.

In the secondary analysis, the annual decline in eGFR and the monthly change in eGFR slope were analyzed. There was a significantly lower monthly change in eGFR from baseline in sacubitril/valsartan group at week 24 from baseline compared to individualized medical therapy (–0.25 vs. –0.43 mL/min/1.73 m^2 respectively; p-value = 0.02). Slow decline in annual eGFR in sacubitril/valsartan group compared to other arm (–2.95 mL/min/1.73 m^2 vs. –5.14 mL/min/1.73 m^2; p-value = 0.01).

PARAGLID-HF TRIAL (2023)

This recent trial included 466 patients, were randomized to receive sacubitril/valsartan or valsartan and followed up for 20 months to assess change in NT-proBNP levels in primary outcome. It showed that sacubitril/valsartan had lower incidence of renal function worsening despite a higher incidence of symptomatic hypertension in this group compared to valsartan.[15]

Overall, sacubitril/valsartan have good renal outcomes in patients with HFpEF in terms of slower decline in GFR as compared with RAS inhibitors alone. Increase in albuminuria in ARNi group in HF patients are not due to glomerular hyperfiltration and podocyte injury. Studies showed that there is relaxation of contractile mesangial cells in the space between capillary endothelium and podocytes. This leads to expansion of capillary surface area available for filtration and there is attenuation of proximal tubular protein reabsorption.[16,17] This could be possible reason that albuminuria worsening is not associated with eGFR decline instead slower decline of eGFR in sacubitril/valsartan group.

LIMITATIONS

These trials have studied the effects of ARNi on cardiovascular events as primary outcomes in HFpEF and renal efficacy found in secondary analysis only. It is also difficult to determine the long term renal outcomes of sacubitril/valsartan in HFpEF as the longest follow up among these trials was 35 months. The adverse events of ARNI could not be evaluated in these trials apart from symptomatic hypotension.

CONCLUSION

The effectiveness of ARNI and its renal outcomes in individuals with HFpEF reviewed based upon randomized trials showed that sacubitril/valsartan delayed decline in eGFR and delayed the progression of renal disease when compared to RAS inhibitors alone. We need to have larger clinical trials which study the impact of ARNI on both cardiovascular and renal outcomes with longer duration of follow-up.

REFERENCES

1. Parikh NI, Hwang SJ, Larson MG, et al. Cardiovascular disease risk factors in chronic kidney disease: overall burden and rates of treatment and control. Arch Intern Med. 2006;166(17):1884-91.
2. Damman K, Valente MA, Voors AA, et al. Renal impairment, worsening renal function, and outcome in patients with heart failure: an updated meta-analysis. Eur Heart J. 2014; 35(7):455-69.
3. Mangiafico S, Costello-Boerrigter LC, Andersen IA, et al. Neutral endopeptidase inhibition and the natriuretic peptide system: an evolving strategy in cardiovascular therapeutics. Eur Heart J. 2013;34(12):886-93.
4. Go AS, Chertow GM, Fan D, et al. Chronic kidney disease and the risks of death, cardiovascular events, and hospitalization. New Engl J Med. 2004;351(13):1296-305.
5. Spannella F, Marini M, Giulietti F, et al. Renal effects of Sacubitril/Valsartan in heart failure with reduced ejection fraction: a real life 1-year follow-up study. Intern Emerg Med. 2019;14(8):1287-97.
6. Wilkins MR, Redondo J, Brown LA. The natriuretic-peptide family. Lancet. 1997;349(9061):1307-10.
7. Daniels LB, Maisel AS. Natriuretic peptides. J Am Coll Cardiol. 2007;50(25):2357-68.
8. Merrill AJ. Edema and decreased renal blood flow in patients with chronic congestive heart failure: evidence of "forward failure" as the primary cause of edema. J Clin Invest. 1946;25(3):389-400.
9. Ruggenenti P, Porrini EL, Gaspari F, et al. Glomerular hyperfiltration and renal disease progression in type 2 diabetes. Diabetes Care. 2012;35(10):2061-8.
10. Voors AA, Gori M, Liu LC, et al. Renal effects of the angiotensin receptor neprilysin inhibitor LCZ696 in patients with heart failure and preserved ejection fraction. Eur J Heart Fail. 2015;17(5):510-7.
11. Solomon SD, Zile M, Pieske B, et al. The angiotensin receptor neprilysin inhibitor LCZ696 in heart failure with preserved ejection fraction: a phase 2 double-blind randomised controlled trial. Lancet. 2012;380(9851):1387-95.
12. Solomon SD, McMurray JJ, Anand IS, et al. Angiotensin-neprilysin inhibition in heart failure with preserved ejection fraction. New Engl J Med. 2019;381(17):1609-20.
13. Mc Causland FR, Lefkowitz MP, Claggett B, et al. Angiotensin-neprilysin inhibition and renal outcomes in heart failure with preserved ejection fraction. Circulation. 2020;142(13):1236-45.
14. Pieske B, Wachter R, Shah SJ, et al. Effect of sacubitril/valsartan vs standard medical therapies on plasma NT-proBNP concentration and submaximal exercise capacity in patients with heart failure and preserved ejection fraction: the PARALLAX randomized clinical trial. JAMA. 2021;326(19):1919-29.
15. Mentz RJ, Ward JH, Hernandez AF, et al. Angiotensin-neprilysin inhibition in patients with mildly reduced or preserved ejection fraction and worsening heart failure. J Am Coll Cardiol. 2023;82(1):1-2.
16. Mullens W, Martens P. Exploiting the natriuretic peptide pathway to preserve glomerular filtration in heart failure. JACC: Heart Failure. 2018;6(6):499-502.
17. Jacobs EM, Vervoort G, Branten Aj, et al. Atrial natriuretic peptide increases albuminuria in type 1 diabetic patients: evidence for blockade of tubular protein reabsorption. Eur J Clin Invest. 1999;29(2):109-15.

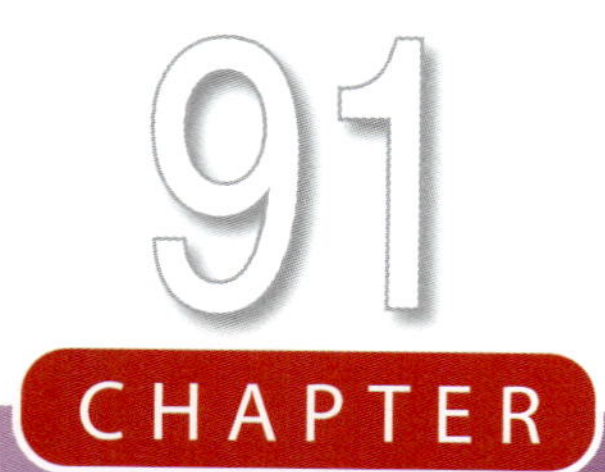

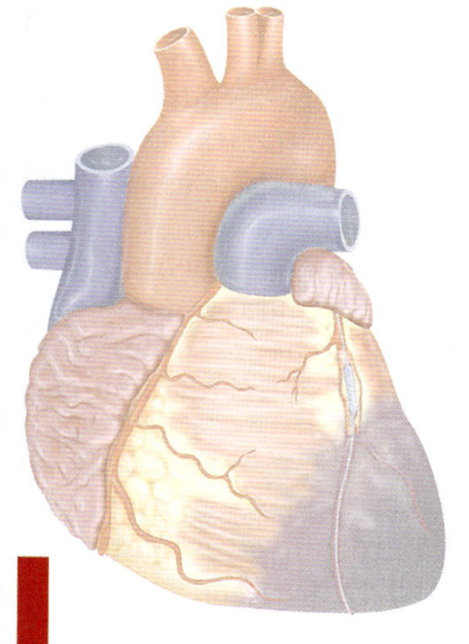

Cardiorenal Syndrome in HFpEF

Vineet Behera, Madhuri Matta

INTRODUCTION

Heart failure with preserved ejection fraction (HFpEF) is a subtype of heart failure characterized by preserved left ventricular systolic function but impaired diastolic function. Cardiorenal syndrome (CRS) with preserved ejection fraction (PEF) is a complex condition characterized by the coexistence of HFpEF and kidney dysfunction. The interplay between the heart and kidneys in HFpEF involves multiple factors, including hemodynamic abnormalities, neurohormonal activation, inflammation, and endothelial dysfunction.

PATHOPHYSIOLOGY

- *Elevation of intra-abdominal and central venous pressure:* HFpEF is predominantly a diastolic disorder, wherein the heart's ability to relax and fill is impaired, leading to increased left ventricular end-diastolic pressure. Elevated filling pressures result in increased venous congestion, which affects renal perfusion. Increased renal venous pressure decreases the filtration gradient in the glomerulus, leading to reduced glomerular filtration rate (GFR) and contributing to renal dysfunction.
- *Vascular stiffness:* Increased arterial stiffness reduces the ability of the arteries to buffer pressure fluctuations, leading to increased afterload on the heart and decreased renal blood flow. The stiff left ventricle in HFpEF results in inefficient ventricular–arterial coupling, leading to systemic hypertension, which can further exacerbate renal injury. This hemodynamic interplay is a key contributor to the development of CRS in HFpEF patients.
- *Neurohormonal activation:* The renin–angiotensin–aldosterone system (RAAS), sympathetic nervous system (SNS), and arginine vasopressin pathways are activated in both heart failure and renal dysfunction. In HFpEF, these systems are chronically upregulated due to the pressure overload, reduced cardiac output, and decreased effective arterial blood volume. The persistent activation of these pathways leads to sodium and water retention, worsening both heart failure and renal function. RAAS activation increases angiotensin II levels, promoting vasoconstriction and inflammation, which exacerbate both cardiac and renal dysfunction. Additionally, elevated aldosterone levels contribute to fibrosis in the heart and kidneys, further impairing their function **(Fig. 1)**.
- *Endothelial dysfunction and oxidative injury:* Endothelial dysfunction plays a significant role in HFpEF and contributes to CRS by impairing vasodilation and promoting inflammation. HFpEF patients exhibit increased oxidative stress, which reduces the bioavailability of nitric oxide, a key vasodilator. The resultant endothelial dysfunction worsens systemic and renal microvascular blood flow, leading to further organ damage. Increased oxidative stress damages cellular components, including proteins, lipids, and DNA, in both cardiac and renal tissues.
- *Inflammation:* Inflammatory markers, such as C-reactive protein (CRP), interleukins (IL-6, IL-1β), and tumor necrosis factor-α (TNF-α), are elevated in both HFpEF and CRS. Inflammation is linked to worsening

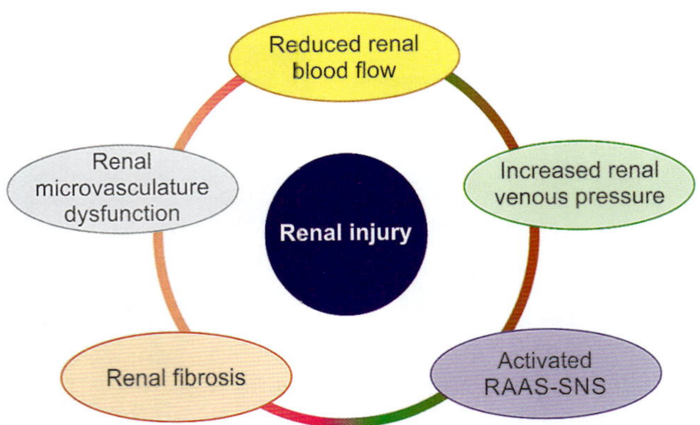

Fig. 1: Modes of renal injury in cardiorenal syndrome in HFpEF. (RAAS-SNS: renin–angiotensin–aldosterone system-sympathetic nervous system)

renal function, and chronic low-grade inflammation in HFpEF exacerbates kidney injury.

- *Renal microvascular dysfunction:* Reduced renal blood flow and increased renal vascular resistance contribute to kidney damage and fibrosis.

CLINICAL PRESENTATION

Patients with HFpEF and CRS often present with overlapping symptoms of both heart failure and renal dysfunction. Symptoms include:

- *Volume overload:* Peripheral edema, ascites, and pulmonary congestion
- *Renal impairment:* Elevated serum creatinine, urea, cystatin C levels, and albuminuria
- *Hypertension:* Systemic and renal hypertension
- *Electrolyte disturbances:* Hyponatremia, hyperkalemia, or metabolic acidosis

DIAGNOSIS

- *Echocardiography:* This is critical in diagnosing HFpEF and assessing left ventricular diastolic dysfunction. Key findings include PEF (≥50%) and evidence of abnormal relaxation, elevated filling pressures, or left atrial enlargement.
- *Cardiac biomarkers:* Natriuretic peptides (BNP and NT-proBNP) are elevated in HFpEF and provide useful prognostic information. However, their levels may be confounded by renal dysfunction, as they are partially cleared by the kidneys.
- *Biochemical markers kidney injury:* Serum creatinine and cystatin C are commonly used to assess renal function. Albuminuria and urinary sodium excretion can indicate early renal injury.
- *Renal imaging:* Renal ultrasonography can be helpful in identifying structural abnormalities in the kidneys, while Doppler imaging may assess renal blood flow. Advanced imaging techniques, such as magnetic resonance imaging (MRI), may be used to assess renal perfusion and fibrosis in research settings.
- *Additional tests:* These include assessment of fluid status using IVC collapsibility on ultrasound, VExUS; cardiac catheterization to measure pulmonary capillary wedge pressure (PCWP) and cardiac output.

MANAGEMENT

The management of CRS in HFpEF involves addressing the underlying mechanisms of both heart and kidney dysfunction while preventing further deterioration **(Fig. 2)**. Treatment must be individualized, often requiring a multidisciplinary approach between cardiologists and nephrologists. Treatment strategies for HFpEF-induced CRS focus on:

- *Volume management:* Diuretics, fluid restriction, and ultrafiltration
- *Blood pressure control:* RAAS blockers, beta-blockers, and calcium channel blockers
- *Neurohormonal modulation:* Aldosterone antagonists and ivabradine
- *Inotrope therapy:* Phosphodiesterase inhibitors (e.g., milrinone)
- *Renal replacement therapy:* Hemodialysis or peritoneal dialysis in advanced cases
- *Lifestyle modifications:* Salt restriction, exercise, and weight management

Diuretic Therapy

Diuretics are the cornerstone of managing volume overload in CRS, particularly loop diuretics such as furosemide, torsemide, or bumetanide. However, excessive diuretic use can precipitate intravascular volume depletion and worsen renal function, creating a delicate balance in managing fluid status. Monitoring weight, urine output, and renal function is essential in titrating diuretics.

RAAS Inhibition

RAAS blockers, such as angiotensin-converting enzyme (ACE) inhibitors, angiotensin receptor blockers (ARBs), and mineralocorticoid receptor antagonists (MRAs), are commonly used in HF. However, their use in HFpEF is controversial, as large clinical trials have shown limited benefit in this population. Additionally, these agents may

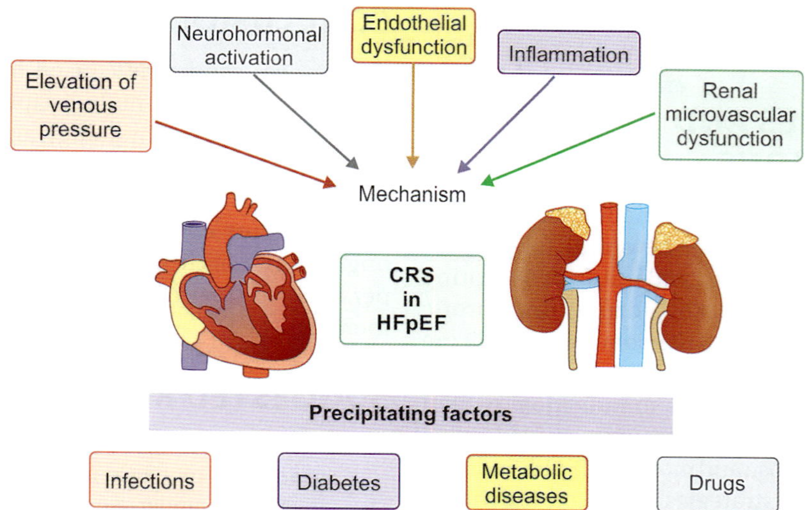

Fig. 2: Mechanisms and precipitating factors of cardiorenal syndrome in HFpEF. (CRS: cardiorenal syndrome; HFpEF: heart failure with preserved ejection fraction)

worsen renal function or cause hyperkalemia in patients with CRS.

Neprilysin Inhibitors

Sacubitril/valsartan, a neprilysin inhibitor combined with an ARB, has shown benefits in heart failure with reduced ejection fraction (HFrEF). Although its role in HFpEF remains under investigation, sacubitril/valsartan may help modulate the neurohormonal axis and reduce volume overload, with potential renal benefits.

Sodium–Glucose Cotransporter-2 Inhibitors

Sodium-glucose cotransporter-2 (SGLT2) inhibitors, originally developed for diabetes, have emerged as promising agents in the management of HF and CRS. These agents, such as empagliflozin and dapagliflozin, improve both cardiovascular and renal outcomes by promoting osmotic diuresis, reducing sodium reabsorption, and modulating RAAS activation. Recent studies have demonstrated that SGLT2 inhibitors reduce hospitalization for heart failure and slow the progression of kidney disease in HFpEF.

Vasodilators

Vasodilators, such as nitrates or hydralazine, may be used to reduce afterload and improve renal perfusion in select patients. However, their benefit in HFpEF is limited due to the already stiff left ventricle, and careful monitoring for hypotension is necessary.

Ultrafiltration

In cases of severe fluid overload that are refractory to diuretic therapy, ultrafiltration may be considered. This extracorporeal therapy mechanically removes excess fluid, offering a more controlled approach to fluid management.

Management of Comorbidities

- *Hypertension:* Optimal control of blood pressure is crucial in managing CRS in HFpEF. Target BP levels are often individualized based on patient comorbidities and tolerance.
- *Diabetes:* Tight glycemic control is essential in slowing the progression of both HFpEF and renal dysfunction.
- *Atrial fibrillation (AF):* It is common in HFpEF and is associated with worse outcomes. Management includes rate or rhythm control and anticoagulation for stroke prevention.

Strategies to Improve Cardiac Output

Efforts must be made to correct the primary cardiac conditions such as coronary revascularization in coronary artery disease, pacemaker implantation for chronotropic incompetence, valve repair, or replacement for valvular heart disease.

Acute versus Chronic Cardiorenal Syndrome

The cornerstone of acute management of CRS in HFpEF includes ultrafiltration and diuretics whereas chronic management includes pharmacological agents like

ACE inhibitors/ARBs, mineralocorticoid antagonists, sacubitril–valsartan, or SGLT2 inhibitors.

NOVEL THERAPIES AND FUTURE DIRECTIONS

Emerging therapies targeting inflammation, fibrosis, and endothelial dysfunction may offer new hope for patients with CRS in HFpEF. Ongoing trials are investigating agents such as anti-inflammatory drugs, antifibrotic agents, and nitric oxide donors. Personalized medicine approaches, including the use of biomarkers and genomic profiling, may help tailor therapies to individual patient characteristics. Ongoing research focuses on identifying novel biomarkers to diagnose and monitor HFpEF-induced CRS, tailoring treatment strategies based on individual patient characteristics, and exploring device therapy like implantable devices, such as cardiac resynchronization therapy (CRT).

PROGNOSIS

Cardiorenal syndrome in HFpEF is associated with poor outcomes, including increased mortality and frequent hospitalizations. The combination of heart and renal dysfunction creates a vicious cycle that accelerates the progression of both conditions. Patients with CRS tend to have a higher burden of comorbidities, such as hypertension, diabetes, and AF, which further complicates their management. Despite advances in the understanding of HFpEF and CRS, effective treatments remain limited, and the prognosis for these patients is often grim. Early identification and a multidisciplinary approach are critical in improving outcomes.

CONCLUSION

Cardiorenal syndrome caused by HFpEF is a complex condition requiring a multidisciplinary approach. Understanding the pathophysiology and clinical presentation is crucial for diagnosis and management. While current treatment strategies focus on volume management, blood pressure control, and neurohormonal modulation, ongoing research aims to identify novel biomarkers, personalize treatment, and develop innovative device therapies.

SUGGESTED READING

1. Agrawal A, Naranjo M, Kanjanahattakij N, et al. Cardiorenal syndrome in heart failure with preserved ejection fraction-an under-recognized clinical entity. Heart Fail Rev. 2019;24(4):421-37.
2. Mitsas AC, Elzawawi M, Mavrogeni S, et al. Heart Failure and Cardiorenal Syndrome: A Narrative Review on Pathophysiology, Diagnostic and Therapeutic Regimens-From a Cardiologist's View. J Clin Med. 2022;11(23):7041.
3. Méndez AB, Azancot MA, Olivella A, et al. New aspects in cardiorenal syndrome and HFpEF. Clin Kidney J. 2022;15(10):1807-15.
4. Patel RN, Sharma A, Prasad A, et al. Heart Failure With Preserved Ejection Fraction With CKD: A Narrative Review of a Multispecialty Disorder. Kidney Med. 2023;5(12):100705.
5. Rangaswami J, Bhalla V, Blair JEA, et al; American Heart Association Council on the Kidney in Cardiovascular Disease and Council on Clinical Cardiology. Cardiorenal Syndrome: Classification, Pathophysiology, Diagnosis, and Treatment Strategies: A Scientific Statement From the American Heart Association. Circulation. 2019;139(16):e840-78.

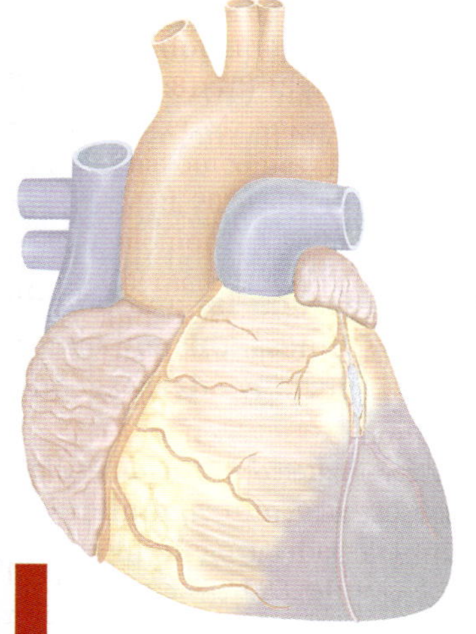

SGLT2i in HFpEF in Patient with Diabetes and Chronic Kidney Disease

Garima Aggarwal, Amit Malik

INTRODUCTION

There is a substantial health cost associated with the combination of diabetes mellitus (DM), chronic kidney disease (CKD), and heart failure with preserved ejection fraction (HFpEF). The risk of death or hospitalization for heart failure (HF) is more than doubled for patients with both DM and CKD compared to those without both disorders. Patients with diabetes often have undiagnosed HF and develop chronic HF at earlier ages. Up to one-third of diabetics were found to have previously undiagnosed HF. Because CKD restricts therapy options and deteriorates outcomes, the interaction of HF, diabetes, and CKD makes care more difficult. This emphasizes the need for focused therapeutic approaches in this population.

Sodium-glucose cotransporter-2 (SGLT2) inhibitors were first created to treat type 2 diabetes, but they also demonstrated an unexpected and noteworthy decrease in cardiovascular outcomes, particularly a decrease in the number of patients admitted to hospitals for HF.[1] Furthermore, independent of DM, studies such as DAPA-HF and EMPEROR-Reduced showed that these medications significantly reduce the risk of cardiovascular death and hospitalization in patients with HFpEF and heart failure with reduced ejection fraction (HFrEF). Because of these complex consequences, SGLT2 inhibitors are now a must in all current HF therapy guidelines.

PATHOPHYSIOLOGY OF HFpEF IN PATIENTS WITH DIABETES AND CHRONIC KIDNEY DISEASE

The complicated disorder known as HFpEF is typified by increased left ventricular (LV) stiffness and poor ventricular filling.

Myocardial stiffness, endothelial dysfunction, diastolic impairment, volume overload, insulin resistance, inflammation, oxidative stress, and renal dysfunction all interact in a complex way to cause HFpEF in patients with diabetes and CKD.[2]

HFpEF in Diabetic Patients

Heart failure with preserved ejection fraction develops and progresses in patients with diabetes due to a number of factors given as follows:

- Insulin resistance is a metabolic disorder that can affect heart function by increasing fatty acid oxidation and decreasing glucose utilization in the myocardium.
- *Inflammation:* Diabetes is linked to a persistent inflammatory condition that can encourage fibrosis and remodeling of the heart, which makes it even more rigid.
- *Oxidative stress:* High reactive oxygen species levels can harm heart cells and worsen endothelial dysfunction, which can lead to microvascular and macrovascular problems.
- *Microvascular dysfunction:* Coronary microvascular dysfunction (CMD), which is frequently brought on

by diabetes, affects how blood flow is regulated in response to myocardial oxygen needs. Even in the absence of coronary artery disease, this may cause symptoms of angina or HF.

HFpEF in Chronic Kidney Disease Patients

The pathogenesis of HFpEF is greatly impacted by CKD as follows:

- *Volume status:* Fluid retention due to kidney dysfunction might make volume overload symptoms worse. This leads to pulmonary congestion and raises LV filling pressures.
- *Electrolyte imbalance:* CKD can lead to electrolyte abnormalities that impact myocardial rhythm and contractility, such as calcium and potassium imbalances.
- *Cardiorenal syndrome:* Renal function can be further compromised by developing HF, and the reduction in renal function might hasten the progression of HF.

Relationship Between Vascular, Heart, and Kidney Health

Both diabetes and CKD cause neurohumoral activation, such as the renin–angiotensin–aldosterone system, which makes fluid retention worse and raises vascular resistance, putting additional pressure on the heart.

Systemic Inflammation

Systemic inflammation exacerbates the effects on heart function in both situations by contributing to endothelial dysfunction in several organ systems.

SODIUM–GLUCOSE COTRANSPORTER-2 INHIBITORS MECHANISM OF ACTION IN RELATION TO HFpEF, DIABETES, AND CHRONIC KIDNEY DISEASE

Sodium–glucose cotransporter-2 inhibitors (SGLT2is) work through a variety of intricate and interconnected routes given as follows:[3]

- *Natriuresis and diuresis:* SGLT2 inhibitors enhance urine glucose, sodium excretion, and diuresis by blocking glucose and sodium reabsorption in the proximal renal tubules.
- *Decreased afterload and preload:* The resulting drop in blood volume reduces afterload and preload, which eases the heart's effort without leading to serious electrolyte imbalances.
- *Utilization of ketones and metabolic effectiveness enhanced myocardial energetics:* SGLT2 inhibitors cause the metabolism of the heart to change in favor of ketone usage, which is a more effective energy source than glucose. By boosting cardiac energetics and myocardial function, this metabolic flip helps patients with HF.
- *Antifibrotic and anti-inflammatory properties:* SGLT2 inhibitors have anti-inflammatory qualities that reduce cardiac fibrosis and vascular inflammation. By reducing cardiac muscle stiffness, this enhances diastolic function, which is especially advantageous for individuals with HFpEF.
- *Mechanisms of renal protection reduced intraglomerular pressure:* SGLT2 inhibitors reduce intraglomerular pressure and albuminuria by lessening hyperfiltration in the kidneys. For individuals with CKD, this nephroprotective effect is essential in maintaining renal function over time. By addressing the cardiorenal syndrome frequently observed in patients with diabetes and HFpEF, these advantages also include improved interactions between kidney function and heart health.

IMPORTANT CLINICAL TRIALS ENDORSING THE USE OF SODIUM–GLUCOSE COTRANSPORTER-2 INHIBITORS IN HFpEF WITH DIABETES AND CKD

The effectiveness of SGLT2 inhibitors in patients with HFpEF, especially those with diabetes and CKD, has been shown in a number of significant clinical trials. Notable trials that offer strong evidence in favor of the usage of these medicines in this patient population include the EMPEROR-Preserved and DELIVER trials **(Figs. 1 and 2)**.[4,5]

Other Important Trials

The PRESERVED-HF trial demonstrated that 12 weeks of dapagliflozin treatment significantly improved symptoms, physical limitations, and exercise function in patients with HFpEF.[6] These advantages held true for both individuals with and without diabetes, and they were clinically significant.

In the SOLOIST-WHF (Effect of Sotagliflozin on Cardiovascular Events in Participants With Type 2 Diabetes Post Worsening Heart Failure) trial, recently hospitalized individuals with T2DM, regardless of LVEF, were enrolled before or shortly after discharge. The results showed that sotagliflozin, an inhibitor of both SGLT1 and SGLT2 and not yet approved by the Food and Drug Administration (FDA), significantly reduced the overall

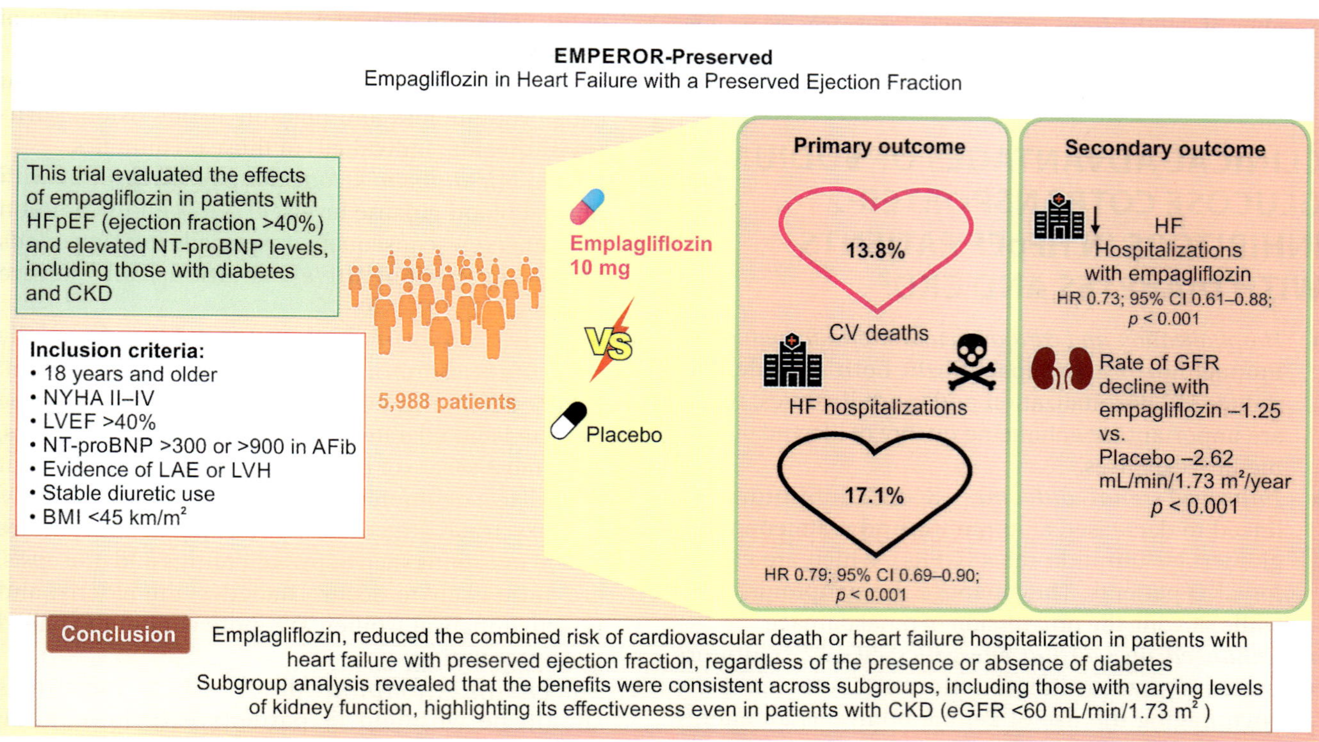

Fig. 1: EMPEROR-Preserved trial visual abstract.
Source: Anker et al.[4]

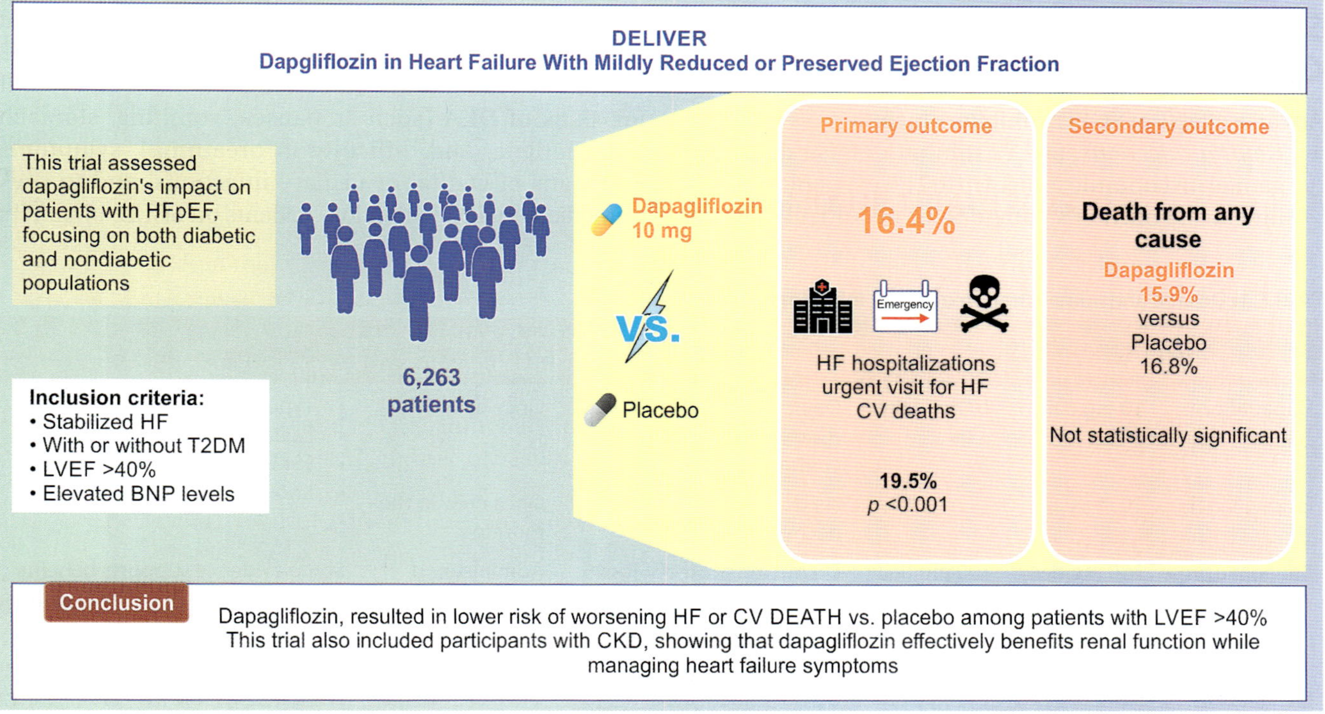

Fig. 2: DELIVER trial visual abstract.
Source: Solomon et al.[6]

number of deaths from cardiovascular causes as well as hospitalizations and urgent visits for HF compared to placebo.[7]

CLINICAL ADVANTAGES OF SODIUM–GLUCOSE COTRANSPORTER-2 INHIBITORS IN HFpEF PATIENTS WITH DIABETES AND CKD[2]

- *Hospitalization and cardiovascular mortality reduction:* Empagliflozin and dapagliflozin both considerably reduce HF hospitalization and mortality rates, which are important for enhancing quality of life and cutting medical expenses.
- *Improved renal outcomes:* SGLT2 inhibitors are linked to decreased albuminuria and maintenance of glomerular filtration rates (GFRs), which are crucial for CKD patients. They manage the symptoms of HF while slowing the progression of renal damage.
- *Enhanced myocardial energetics:* SGLT2 inhibitors increase myocardial function and efficiency by encouraging the use of ketone bodies as an energy source. This enhances exercise tolerance and quality of life.
- *Glycemic and metabolic effects:* SGLT2 inhibitors lower weight and HbA1c while improving insulin sensitivity.

SAFETY PROFILE AND PRACTICAL CONSIDERATIONS

Adverse effects of SGLT2 inhibitors include:

- *Genital infections:* SGLT2 inhibitors raise the risk of genital mycotic infections. Up to 11% of people get these illnesses. Fournier's gangrene or necrotizing fasciitis of the perineum is an uncommon but potentially fatal consequence.
- *Dehydration:* SGLT2 inhibitors' diuretic action might cause volume loss and possibly hypotension, particularly in older individuals or those on diuretics.
- *Euglycemic diabetic ketoacidosis (eDKA):* Even with normal blood glucose levels, eDKA is an uncommon but dangerous consequence especially during periods of fasting, perioperative conditions, and severe illnesses.
- *Acute reductions in eGFR:* SGLT2 inhibitors usually result in a brief drop in eGFR, which is usually transient. A 20% decline in eGFR in the first month may be expected and tolerated after starting SGLT2 inhibitors, but a more severe or prolonged decline should prompt referral to a nephrologist.
- Urinary tract infections (UTIs), particularly more severe infections such as pyelonephritis and urosepsis, are more likely to occur. Diabetics, the elderly, and postmenopausal women are more at risk, thus need close monitoring.
- *Lower limb amputations:* SGLT2 inhibitors should be withheld in patients with lower limb infections or ulcers. Peripheral vascular disease, neuropathy, diabetic foot ulcer history, and prior amputation history are factors that raise the risk of amputation.

Patients who are severely ill, have decreased oral intake, are fasting, or are undergoing surgery should be advised beforehand to temporarily stop using SGLT2 inhibitors. Patients should be taught to keep an eye out for signs of DKA (such as nausea, vomiting, stomach pain, fatigue, and difficulty in breathing), symptoms and signs of genital or urinary infections, and to seek immediate medical attention. Patients on SGLT2 inhibitors

TABLE 1: Dosage and administration of SGLT2 inhibitors.

SGLT2 inhibitor	*Starting dose*	*Target dose*	*Dose modification with eGFR (in mL/min/1.73 m²)*	*Administration*	*Contraindication*
Dapagliflozin	10 mg daily	10 mg daily	Do not initiate if eGFR <25 If already taking may continue until dialysis	Once daily	• Type 1 DM • Lactating mothers • ESKD on dialysis • Known hypersensitivity
Empagliflozin	10 mg daily	10 mg daily	No dosage adjustment necessary for eGFR >20	Once daily in the morning	
Canagliflozin	100 mg daily	100 mg daily	Do not initiate if eGFR <45 Discontinue if eGFR <30	Administered before first meal of the day	Some evidence supports benefits of canagliflozin for patients with *HFrEF*, though it is used less frequently for this indication
Ertugliflozin	5 mg daily	15 mg daily	Do not initiate if eGFR <45	Once daily in the morning	Ertugliflozin's role in *heart failure* is not as well established as dapagliflozin or empagliflozin

TABLE 2: Guideline recommendations on SGLT2 inhibitor use in the management of HFpEF.

Guideline	*Recommendation*	*Strength/class of recommendation*
2023 ACC Expert Consensus Decision Pathway on management of heart failure with preserved ejection fraction[8]	SGLT2 inhibitors should be initiated in all individuals with HFpEF lacking contraindications	2A
2023 focused update of the 2021 ESC guidelines for the diagnosis and treatment of acute and chronic heart failure[9]	An SGLT2 inhibitor (dapagliflozin or empagliflozin) is recommended in patients with HFpEF to reduce risk of HF hospitalization or CV death	1A
2022 AHA/ACC/HFSA guideline for management of heart failure[10]	In patients with HFpEF, SGLT2 inhibitors can be beneficial in decreasing HF hospitalizations and CV mortality	2A
2021 ESC guidelines for the diagnosis and treatment of acute and chronic heart failure[11]	SGLT2 inhibitors (canagliflozin, dapagliflozin, empagliflozin, ertugliflozin, sotagliflozin) are recommended in patients with diabetes at high risk of CV disease or with CV disease in order to prevent HF hospitalizations	1A

need to be closely monitored during clinic visits for the following:

- Volume status
- Renal functions at baseline and monitor regularly
- Signs and symptoms of genital infections and UTIs
- Consider ketone testing for patients who are at high risk of developing DKA
- Monitor for hypoglycemia in patients also taking insulin or insulin secretagogues

GUIDELINES AND RECOMMENDATIONS FOR SGLT2 INHIBITOR USE

The guidelines and recommendations for SGLT2 inhibitor use are given in **Tables 1 and 2**.

CONCLUSION

Through their diuretic effects, augmentation of myocardial energetics via ketone consumption, anti-inflammatory properties, and renal protective mechanisms, SGLT2 inhibitors offer a variety of benefits pertinent to HFpEF, diabetes, and CKD. Patients with these interrelated illnesses benefit from better clinical outcomes as a result of these multifactorial interventions.

REFERENCES

1. Nassif ME, Windsor SL, Borlaug BA, et al. The SGLT2 inhibitor dapagliflozin in heart failure with preserved ejection fraction: a multicenter randomized trial. Nat Med. 2021;27(11):1954-60.
2. Singh P, Goyal L, Mallick DC, et al. Role of sodium-glucose co-transporter 2 inhibitors in chronic kidney disease, congestive heart failure and stroke—a review and clinical guide for healthcare professionals. J Clin Med. 2023;12(19):6202.
3. Padda IS, Mahtani AU, Parmar M. Sodium-glucose transport protein 2 (SGLT2) inhibitors. In: StatPearls [Internet]. Treasure Island (FL): StatPearls Publishing; 2024.
4. Anker SD, Butler J, Filippatos G, et al. Empagliflozin in heart failure with a preserved ejection fraction. N Engl J Med. 2021;385(16):1451-61.
5. Anker SD, Butler J, Usman MS, et al. Efficacy of empagliflozin in heart failure with preserved versus mid-range ejection fraction: a pre-specified analysis of EMPEROR-Preserved. Nat Med. 2022;28(12):2512-20.
6. Solomon SD, McMurray JJ, Claggett B, et al. Dapagliflozin in heart failure with mildly reduced or preserved ejection fraction. N Engl J Med. 2022;387:1089-98.
7. Bhatt DL, Szarek M, Steg PG, et al. Sotagliflozin in patients with diabetes and recent worsening heart failure. N Engl J Med. 2021;384(2):117-28.
8. Kittleson MM, Panjrath GS, Amancherla K, et al. 2023 ACC Expert Consensus Decision Pathway on management of heart failure with preserved ejection fraction: a report of the American College of Cardiology Solution Set Oversight Committee. J Am Coll Cardiol. 2023;81(18):1835-78.
9. McDonagh TA, Metra M, Adamo M, et al. 2023 focused update of the 2021 ESC guidelines for the diagnosis and treatment of acute and chronic heart failure. Eur Heart J. 2023;44(37):3627-39.
10. Heidenreich PA, Bozkurt B, Aguilar D, et al. 2022 AHA/ACC/HFSA guideline for the management of heart failure: A report of the American College of Cardiology/American Heart Association joint committee on clinical practice guidelines. Circulation. 2022;145(18):e895-1032.
11. McDonagh TA, Metra M, Adamo M, et al. 2021 ESC guidelines for the diagnosis and treatment of acute and chronic heart failure. Eur Heart J. 2021;42(36):3599-726.

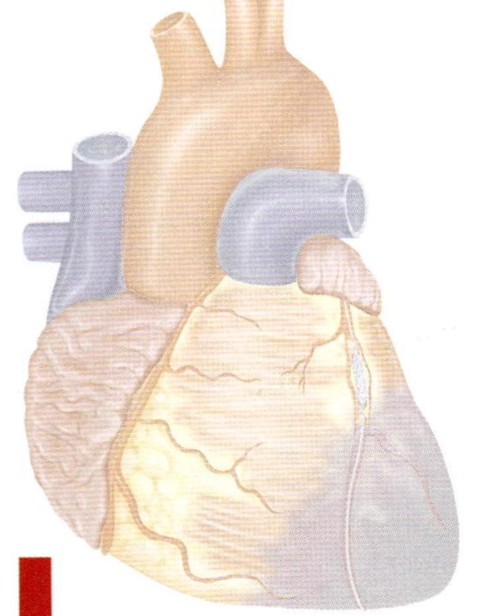

Heart Failure in Chronic Kidney Disease: Conclusions from a KDIGO Controversies Conference

Arunkumar S, Sandeep Mahajan

INTRODUCTION

Chronic kidney disease (CKD) and heart failure (HF) frequently coexist, creating a complex interplay that significantly impacts patient outcomes. Approximately, 40–70% of patients with CKD also suffer from cardiovascular disease (CVD), with HF being a significant component of this burden. CKD patients are predisposed to HF due to factors like volume overload, hypertension, and uremic toxicity, while HF patients face an elevated risk of renal dysfunction. HF manifests commonly with symptoms such as shortness of breath and fatigue, alongside physical signs like edema and lung crepitations. While these symptoms and signs can indicate HF, they are also common among individuals with kidney disease, even when HF is absent. Moreover, an improved understanding of kidney function over both short and long terms is essential to comment on the prognosis in HF patients, especially in relation to guideline-recommended medical treatments.

The Kidney Disease: Improving Global Outcomes (KDIGO) Controversies Conference brought together leading experts to examine recent advancements and persistent challenges in the understanding and treatment of HF in patients with CKD. Since the initial conference on this topic in 2017, substantial progress has been made in comprehending HF's pathophysiology, diagnostic methods, and treatment strategies.[1] The most recent conference, held in March 2024 in Vancouver, Canada, sought to explore these advancements and challenges in understanding the interplay between CKD disease and HF. This chapter summarizes the conference's key findings, highlighting pathophysiological links between CKD and HF, diagnostic complexities, therapeutic approaches, and directions for future research.

HEART FAILURE IN CHRONIC KIDNEY DISEASE: DEFINITIONS AND EPIDEMIOLOGY

The relationship between CKD and HF is characterized by a bidirectional influence where each condition exacerbates the other. There is a stepwise increase in the incidence of HF and consequent mortality risk with the stage of CKD. CKD significantly heightens cardiovascular risk. Key indicators of CKD, such as albuminuria, reduced glomerular filtration rate (GFR), or a combination of both, are linked to a progressively higher risk of major atherosclerotic events, HF, and cardiovascular mortality. As a result, HF and atherosclerotic cardiovascular disease (ASCVD) are the leading causes of death among individuals with both diabetes and CKD. Patients with CKD stage 3 or higher (eGFR <60 mL/min/1.73 m^2) have a threefold higher risk of HF. This risk escalates as kidney function worsens, with over 50% of individuals in CKD stages 4–5 experiencing both HF and CVD. Conversely, HF patients often develop renal dysfunction. In the Acute Decompensated Heart Failure National Registry (ADHERE), 30% of patients hospitalized for HF showed varying levels of renal impairment.[2]

Heart failure is traditionally classified based on ejection fraction (EF):

- *Heart failure with reduced ejection fraction (HFrEF):* EF <40%

- *Heart failure with preserved ejection fraction (HFpEF):* EF ≥50%
- *Heart failure with mildly reduced ejection fraction (HFmrEF):* EF 41–49%

While these classifications are useful, they may not fully capture the complexity of HF in patients with CKD. The KDIGO conference highlighted the need for more inclusive classification systems that consider the following:

- *Kidney function:* Incorporating measures like estimated glomerular filtration rate (eGFR) and urine albumin-creatinine ratio (UACR) could provide a more comprehensive view of patient status. This is important as albuminuria and eGFR are independent predictors of HF outcome.
- *Symptomatology:* Classifying patients based on symptom burden rather than solely on EF may better reflect their clinical condition.

Suggested updates to the classification systems include the following parameters to enhance their comprehensiveness:

- Staging based on both cardiac function and kidney status
- Differentiation between acute versus chronic kidney impairment
- Consideration of comorbidities that influence prognosis

CARDIOVASCULAR–KIDNEY–METABOLIC SYNDROME

The cardiovascular-kidney-metabolic (CKM) syndrome is defined as a systemic disorder characterized by pathophysiological interactions among metabolic risk factors, CKD, and the cardiovascular system, leading to multiorgan dysfunction and a high rate of adverse cardiovascular outcomes.[3] CKM syndrome includes both individuals at risk for CVD due to the presence of metabolic risk factors, CKD, or both and individuals with existing CVD that is potentially related to or complicates metabolic risk factors or CKD. CKM staging helps in categorizing patients based on CVD risk and need for optimized individual care **(Fig. 1)**.

Evaluating CKM risk factors such as diet, physical activity, sleep duration, body mass index (BMI), blood pressure, lipid levels, and nicotine exposure helps categorize patients within these parameters. Currently, the Predicting Risk of Cardiovascular Disease EVENTS (PREVENT) equation is the most comprehensive tool for cardiovascular risk assessment that integrates kidney health into CVD risk calculations.[4] Key CKM risk factors, like BMI and eGFR, are part of this equation. Additionally, social determinants of health are included, with albuminuria as an optional component, highlighting the role of kidney function metrics in predicting future CVD risk.[5]

DECISION-MAKING AND CO-MANAGEMENT OF HEART FAILURE AND CHRONIC KIDNEY DISEASE

Chronic kidney disease is characterized by a persistent eGFR <60 mL/min/1.73 m^2 or by the presence of at least one marker of kidney damage lasting more than 3 months. HF can lead to secondary CKD and both conditions may also coexist due to common risk factors or underlying

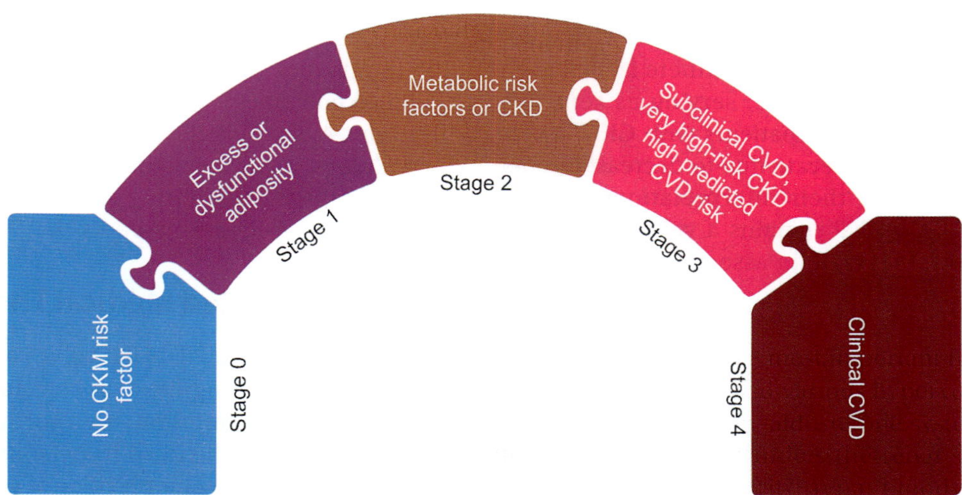

Fig. 1: Staging of CKM syndrome. (CKD: chronic kidney disease; CKM: cardiovascular–kidney–metabolic syndrome; CVD: cardiovascular disease)

systemic diseases. Determining which condition is primary and which is secondary can often be complex.

Diagnosis of Heart Failure in Chronic Kidney Disease

Diagnosing HF in patients with CKD presents unique challenges due to overlapping symptoms such as dyspnea, fatigue, and edema. There are currently no established definitions or criteria for diagnosing HF in patients with CKD. Additionally, both intravascular and extravascular volume overload may occur even when structural heart disease is not present. A thorough symptom assessment is critical for differentiating between fluid overload due to HF versus kidney disease. Echocardiographic assessments are valuable for evaluating cardiac structure and function but may be limited by fluid overload or other confounding factors in CKD patients. In dialysis patients, echocardiography should be done on a nondialysis day, especially when the patient is close to the dry weight.[6]

Biomarkers

Biomarkers are essential for the identification, evaluation, and management of HF, especially in patients with CKD. In the context of HF, these biomarkers can provide insights into cardiac stress, myocardial damage, and fluid overload. Incorporating these biomarkers into clinical practice has the potential to enhance risk stratification and inform treatment decisions. Key biomarkers that have been extensively studied include N-terminal pro-B-type natriuretic peptide (NT-proBNP), B-type natriuretic peptide (BNP), cardiac troponins, and various inflammatory markers.[7]

Among these, NT-proBNP and BNP are the most established biomarkers for diagnosing and managing HF. These peptides are released when there is increased ventricular volume and pressure, serving as sensitive indicators of HF. However, in patients with CKD, levels of these biomarkers may elevate due to decreased renal clearance, complicating their interpretation. Despite this challenge, NT-proBNP remains a valuable tool for assessing risk; higher levels are associated with poorer clinical outcomes in CKD patients.

Cardiac troponins—specifically troponin I and troponin T—are indicators of myocardial injury. In CKD patients, troponin levels can be elevated even without acute coronary syndrome due to underlying cardiac conditions such as left ventricular hypertrophy and diastolic dysfunction. Monitoring troponin levels can help identify patients at greater risk for HF exacerbations and assist in guiding treatment strategies.

Inflammation is a significant factor in both HF and CKD. Biomarkers like high-sensitivity C-reactive protein (hs-CRP) and interleukins have been investigated for their prognostic significance in these populations. Ongoing research aims to discover novel biomarkers that could provide further insights into HF within the context of CKD. Potential candidates include markers related to fibrosis, myocardial strain, and neurohormonal activation, such as galectin-3 and soluble ST2. These emerging biomarkers may enhance our understanding of different HF phenotypes and aid in developing targeted therapies.

MANAGEMENT STRATEGIES

The management of HF in CKD requires a comprehensive and nuanced approach. Guideline-directed medical therapy, including the strategic use of mineralocorticoid receptor antagonists (MRAs), angiotensin receptor-neprilysin inhibitors (ARNIs), and glucagon-like peptide-1 (GLP-1) receptor agonists, offers promise for improving outcomes in this complex patient population. KDIGO Controversies Conference has shed light on current strategies for managing HF in CKD, highlighting the importance of guideline-directed medical therapy (GDMT) and the potential roles of emerging pharmacological agents, including MRAs, ARNIs, and GLP-1 receptor agonists. The various components of management strategy are:

- *Risk assessment and stratification:* Identifying patients at high risk for adverse outcomes is crucial. Risk factors such as diabetes, hypertension, obesity, and previous cardiovascular events should be assessed. Tools like the PREVENT equations can aid in stratifying risk and guiding management decisions.[5]
- *Multidisciplinary care:* A collaborative approach involving nephrologists, cardiologists, dietitians, and primary-care providers is essential for optimizing patient outcomes.
- *Patient education:* Educating patients about their conditions, medication adherence, dietary restrictions, and symptom monitoring empowers them to participate actively in their care.

Guideline-directed Medical Therapy

Managing HF through GDMT involves a comprehensive strategy, encompassing lifestyle changes, medications, and vigilant renal function monitoring. The KDIGO guidelines highlight the need to personalize treatments to address the unique complexities of CKD, where core GDMT components play essential roles across both HF and CKD management **(Fig. 2)**.[8]

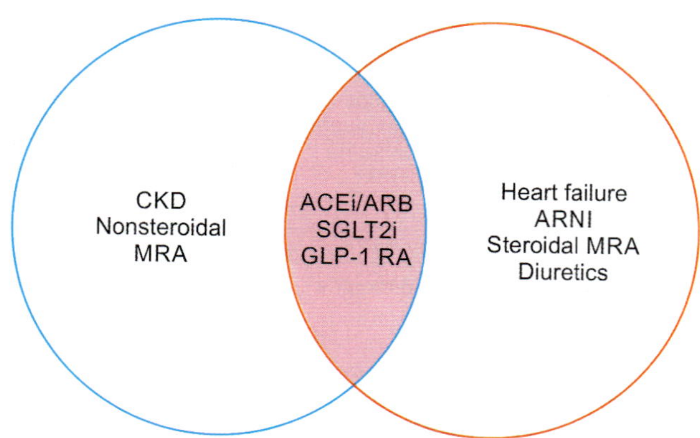

Fig. 2: Components of GDMT in kidney disease and heart failure. (ACEi: angiotensin-converting enzyme inhibitor; ARB: angiotensin receptor blocker; ARNI: angiotensin receptor–neprilysin inhibitors; CKD: chronic kidney disease; GDMT: guideline-directed medical therapy; GLP-1RA: glucagon-like peptide-1 receptor agonists; MRA: mineralocorticoid receptor antagonists; SGLT2i, sodium–glucose cotransporter 2 inhibitor)

- *Loop diuretics:* Loop diuretics are often the first line of treatment for managing volume overload in HF. They promote diuresis and help alleviate symptoms related to fluid retention. However, the dose may need adjustment based on renal function and response, with the goal of achieving euvolemia without causing electrolyte imbalances.
- *Angiotensin-converting enzyme (ACE) inhibitors and angiotensin II receptor blockers (ARBs):* These are foundational therapies for HFrEF. These agents are renoprotective and are associated with improved cardiovascular outcomes. Their use in advanced CKD is limited due to risks of worsening renal function and hyperkalemia, requiring close and careful monitoring.
- *Sodium-glucose cotransporter-2 inhibitors (SGLT2i):* Emerging evidence supports the use of SGLT2i for improving HF outcomes in patients with CKD. These agents have shown benefits in reducing hospitalization rates for HF and slowing kidney disease progression. SGLT2i help enhance the tolerability of RAS blockade and MRAs in CKD patients by reducing the risk of hyperkalemia.
- *MRAs*, such as spironolactone and eplerenone, have been shown to provide significant benefits for patients with HFrEF. They work by antagonizing aldosterone, leading to reduced cardiac fibrosis and improved ventricular remodeling. The KDIGO Controversies Conference highlighted the need for cautious use of MRAs in CKD patients due to the risk of hyperkalemia and worsening renal function.
- *ARNIs*, such as sacubitril/valsartan, represent a breakthrough in HF management. By simultaneously blocking the angiotensin II receptor and inhibiting neprilysin, ARNIs improve outcomes in HFrEF patients by reducing hospitalizations and mortality. The evidence presented suggests that ARNIs may be safe and beneficial in patients with CKD, particularly when initiated at low doses and titrated gradually.
- *GLP-1 receptor agonists*, such as liraglutide and semaglutide, have garnered attention for their potential cardiovascular benefits, particularly in diabetic patients with HF. These agents not only assist in glycemic control but also contribute to weight loss and improved cardiovascular outcomes. The KDIGO conference addressed the role of these agents in CKD, highlighting their nephroprotective effects and favorable safety profile in patients with moderate-to-advanced renal impairment.

Traditionally, the stepwise addition of these drugs results in a delay of 9–12 months before a patient receives the full set of GDMT components. An accelerated approach could reduce this to around 6 months. For patients at highest risk, a rapid sequence method—adding all medications within 2–4 months—might offer the greatest benefits in a shorter timeframe **(Fig. 3)**.[9]

CONCLUSION AND FUTURE DIRECTIONS

Clinical evidence of HF in CKD necessitates a multidisciplinary approach with repeated assessments to deliver personalized care. The management plan involves carefully evaluating the potential reversibility of both heart and kidney disease through guideline-recommended medical treatments, weighing the risks and benefits of each therapy, and incorporating patient-centered choices. Conference discussions revealed significant knowledge gaps, particularly in HFpEF and CKD. KDIGO called for research focused on personalized therapy trials that can account for diverse patient needs. Additional research is needed to address the existing knowledge gaps and formulate a standardized protocol for diagnosing and managing HF in CKD.

Heart failure in CKD presents a considerable clinical challenge, defined by the intricate interplay between these two common conditions. Insights from the KDIGO Controversies Conference highlight the critical need to address this dual burden in patients and to apply evidence-based therapies that meet their specific requirements. Emphasizing a multidisciplinary approach and advancing research into effective treatments can greatly enhance outcomes for this vulnerable group.

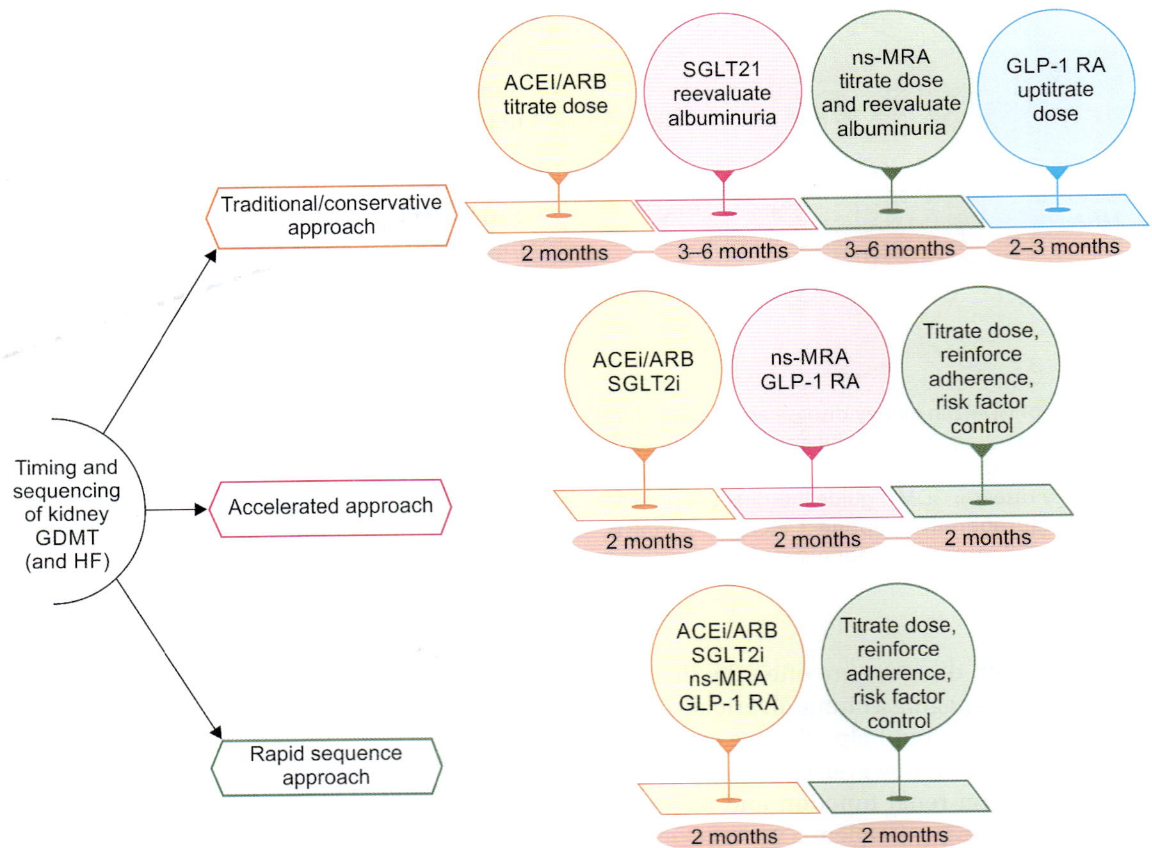

Fig. 3: Approaches to implementing GDMT in CKD and heart failure. (ACEi: angiotensin-converting enzyme inhibitor; ARB: angiotensin receptor blocker; CKD: chronic kidney disease; GDMT: guideline-directed medical therapy; GLP-1RA: glucagon-like peptide-1 receptor agonists; HF: heart failure; ns-MRA: nonsteroidal mineralocorticoid receptor antagonists; SGLT2i: sodium–glucose cotransporter 2 inhibitor)

REFERENCES

1. House AA, Wanner C, Sarnak MJ, et al; Conference Participants. Heart failure in chronic kidney disease: Conclusions from a Kidney Disease: Improving Global Outcomes (KDIGO) Controversies Conference. Kidney Int. 2019;95(6):1304-17.
2. Schefold JC, Filippatos G, Hasenfuss G. et al. Heart failure and kidney dysfunction: Epidemiology, mechanisms, and management. Nat Rev Nephrol. 2016;12(10):610-23.
3. Ndumele CE, Neeland IJ, Tuttle KR, et al; American Heart Association. A Synopsis of the Evidence for the Science and Clinical Management of Cardiovascular-Kidney-Metabolic (CKM) Syndrome: A scientific statement from the American Heart Association. Circulation. 2023;148(20):1636-64.
4. Khan SS, Matsushita K, Sang Y, et al; Chronic Kidney Disease Prognosis Consortium and the American Heart Association Cardiovascular-Kidney-Metabolic Science Advisory Group. Development and Validation of the American Heart Association's PREVENT Equations. Circulation. 2024;149(6):430-49.
5. Garba DL, Razavi AC, Blumenthal RS, et al. Advances in predicting cardiovascular risk: Applying the PREVENT equations. Am J Prev Cardiol. 2024;19:100705.
6. Ponikowski P, Voors AA, Anker SD, et al; ESC Scientific Document Group. 2016 ESC Guidelines for the diagnosis and treatment of acute and chronic heart failure: The Task Force for the diagnosis and treatment of acute and chronic heart failure of the European Society of Cardiology (ESC) Developed with the special contribution of the Heart Failure Association (HFA) of the ESC. Eur Heart J. 2016;37(27):2129-200.
7. Colbert G, Jain N, de Lemos JA, et al. Utility of traditional circulating and imaging-based cardiac biomarkers in patients with predialysis CKD. Clin J Am Soc Nephrol. 2015;10(3):515-29.
8. Guaricci AI, Sturdà F, Russo R, et al. Assessment and management of heart failure in patients with chronic kidney disease. Heart Fail Rev. 2024;29(2):379-94.
9. Neuen BL, Tuttle KR, Vaduganathan M. Accelerated Risk-Based Implementation of Guideline-Directed Medical Therapy for Type 2 Diabetes and Chronic Kidney Disease. Circulation. 2024;149(16):1238-40.

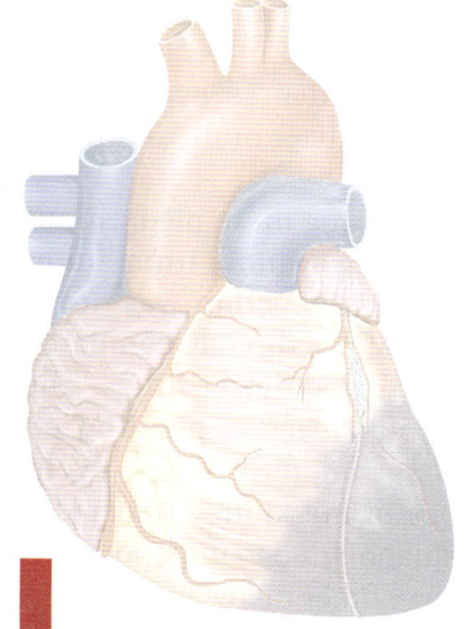

Role of New Antihyperkalemic Agents in the Treatment of Patients with HFpEF and Chronic Kidney Disease

N Ramachandran, Sreejith Parameswaran

INTRODUCTION

Up to 45–70% of heart failure (HF) patients have CKD with GFR <60 mL/min/1.73 m^2.[1,2] The frequency of HF rises in tandem with the severity of CKD. The presence of either CKD or HF increases the risk of development and worsening of the other condition. Patients with both HF and CKD have a higher chance of hospitalization, intensive care admission, undergoing renal replacement therapy, and death than patients with HF without CKD with a progressive rise in death due to HF with advancing stages of CKD.[3]

HYPERKALEMIA IN HEART FAILURE AND CHRONIC KIDNEY DISEASE

Patients with HF and CKD who develop hyperkalemia have higher mortality compared to patients with HF and CKD without hyperkalemia.[4] In patients with HFrEF, therapy with angiotensin-converting enzyme inhibitors (ACEI), β-blockers, mineralocorticoid receptor antagonists (MRAs), and angiotensin receptor neprilysin inhibitors (ARNI) improve patient outcomes.[5] However, there is no medication that can effectively lower the morbidity and mortality in CKD with HFpEF (left ventricular EF ≥50%).

Although the treatment of HF is similar in patients with CKD, or without the presence of CKD presents unique challenges. As the GFR decreases, there is a progressively higher risk of hyperkalemia, especially if it is <30 mL/min per 1.73 m^2. ACEIs, ARBs, and ARNI can decrease GFR in patients with HFpEF. However, worsening azotemia alone should not lead to withdrawal of these drugs, as stopping these drugs may lead to worse patient outcomes. MRAs are typically just as effective in patients with HF and CKD G3a-G3b, as they are in those without CKD.[6] Due to the risk of hyperkalemia, there is a notable reduction in utilization of renin-angiotensin-aldosterone system inhibitors and a high discontinuation rate of these drugs in patients with HF and CKD.[7] In some patients with a kidney transplant, management of HF is complicated by persistent, severe hyperkalemia mainly due to calcineurin inhibitors that may hinder the utilization of ACEIs, ARBs, and MRAs.

RISK FACTORS FOR HYPERKALEMIA

Risk of worsening hyperkalemia in HF patients is inversely related to GFR, with significant risk in patients with GFR <30 mL/min/1.73 m^2, patients with diabetes, decompensated HF, AKI, and use medications such as ACE/ARBs/MRAs/ARNI/use of potassium-sparing diuretics, NSAIDs, digoxin, and calcineurin inhibitors in postrenal transplant patients.

MANAGEMENT OF HYPERKALEMIA

Management of hyperkalemia includes dietary management, antihyperkalemic drugs, intensified use of diuretics (especially loop diuretics), and renal replacement therapy. Food with high potassium content such as seaweed, molasses, dried figs, wheat germ, bran cereals, nuts, dried fruits, avocados, carrots, beets, tomatoes, spinach, potatoes, cauliflower, bananas, mangoes, oranges, kiwis, and meat should be avoided. Pharmacological management depends on the extent of the rise in potassium levels, particularly when accompanied by significant changes in ECG and severe weakness of muscles.

PROBLEMS WITH CURRENTLY USED ANTIHYPERKALEMIC DRUGS

Calcium polystyrene sulfonate (30–60 g) and sodium polystyrene sulfonate (SPS) are commonly used as non-specific potassium binding resins. Their onset of action varies from 1 to 2 hours and action last up to 4–6 hours. Due to the nonspecific nature of cation binding, SPS can produce significant dyselectrolytemia, including hypomagnesemia, hypokalemia, hypocalcemia, and metabolic alkalosis. Besides GI side effects including bitter taste, SPS can produce fatal GI injuries. Newer drugs (patiromer and sodium zirconium cyclosilicate) have lower incidences of these adverse events. The summary of these newer drugs is given in the following **Table 1**.

Incidentally, all the trials involving these medications were conducted without any separation from other drugs, and no evidence of drug interaction was noted in these trials. As of now, no trial has directly compared the efficacy and tolerability of these newer drugs. The frequency of monitoring should vary depending on patient comorbidities and serum potassium levels. The use of these newer drugs in the kidney transplant population needs further evaluation due to their potential for interfering with absorption of other medications.

TABLE 1: Antihyperkalemic drugs.

	Patiromer (Veltassa)	*Sodium zirconium cyclosilicate—(SZC) (Lokelma)*
Contents of drugs with quantity	• Sodium—Nil • Calcium—1.6 g per 8.4 g • Sorbitol—4,000 mg per 8.4 g	• Sodium—400 mg per 5 g dose • Calcium—Nil • Sorbitol—Nil
Compound	• Nonabsorbed • Organic polymer and sorbitol complex	• Nonabsorbed • Inorganic crystal
FDA approval	2015	2018
Formulation	Oral suspension	Oral suspension
Route	Oral	Oral
Selectivity for potassium	Nonselective cation binding	Highly selective for potassium
Site of action	Predominantly distal colon	Small and large bowel
Mechanism of action	Increases excretion of fecal potassium by binding potassium in the bowel in exchange for calcium	Increases excretion of fecal potassium by binding potassium in the bowel in exchange for H^+ and Na^+
Onset of action	7 hours	1 hour
Initial starting dose	8.4 g oral	10 g oral
Maximum dose for maintenance	25.2 g (based on serum potassium levels dose can be increased further)	15 g
Dosing	Once or twice a day	Once a day
Timing of medication	separated from other medications for 3 hours	separated from other medications for 2 hours
Adverse effects:	• Abdominal discomfort • Constipation • Diarrhea • Nausea • Flatulence • *Dyselectrolytemia:* Hypomagnesemia	• Abdominal discomfort • Constipation • Diarrhea • Nausea • Sodium retention leading to pedal edema
Storage	2–8°C (To be used within 3 months if stored at room temperature)	15–30°C
Use in emergency	Not suitable as a treatment in emergency due to delayed onset of action	Not suitable as a treatment in emergency due to delayed onset of action
Contraindications	Bowel obstruction, severe constipation	None

ADVANTAGES OF NEWER AGENTS

Newer antihyperkalemic drugs are safe, effective, and well-tolerated. They may facilitate more opportunities to optimize ACEI/ARB/MRA/ARNI. In terms of safety, using a potassium binder is better option instead of increasing the dosage of loop diuretics to manage hyperkalemia. Moreover, in a trial where there was a placebo-controlled withdrawal of Patiromer, no rapid increase in serum potassium was noted after stopping Patiromer.[8]

STUDIES ON THE NEWER ANTIHYPERKALEMIC DRUGS

In PEARL-HF (phase 2 trial), in patients with chronic HF and GFR <60 mL/min/1.73 m^2 and receiving ACEI or ARB with serum K$^+$ between 4.3 and 5.2 mEq/L and indication to initiate spironolactone, it was found that at 28 days, Patiromer significantly reduced the hyperkalemia.[9] In AMBER trial (phase 2 trial), when spironolactone and Patiromer was added for patients with resistant hypertension, CKD, and serum K$^+$ between 4.3 and 5.1 mEq/L, significant number (86%) of patients remained on spironolactone in Patiromer group compared to placebo group (66%).[10]

HARMONIZE-OLE and HARMONIZE-Global studies showed benefit of long-term (11 months) SZC and hyperkalemia correction in outpatients with serum K$^+$ >5.1 mEq/L.[11,12] Summary of the important phase 3 studies on these newer antihyperkalemic drugs are given in **Table 2**.

TABLE 2: Phase 3 studies on newer antihyperkalemic drugs.

S. No.	*Study design/ setting*	*Study population*	*LVEF in study population*	*Intervention*	*Primary outcome*
1.	*Patiromer:* OPAL-HK[8]	*4-week treatment phase:* CKD patients on RAAS inhibitors with mild (*Serum potassium:* 5.1–5.5 mEq/L) or moderate to severe (serum potassium 5.5–6.5 mEq/L) hyperkalemia (*n* = 237)	85% of the patients had an eGFR of 15–60 mL per min per 1.73 m^2; All the patients were on RAAS inhibitors and 9% were on aldosterone antagonist 42% had heart failure. Mean eGFR–35.4 mL/ min/1.73 m^2+16	Patiromer 4.2 g BID and 8.4 g BID for mild and moderate to severe hyperkalemia, respectively	*Mean change in serum potassium at week 4:* *−0.65 mEq/L in mild hyperkalemia:* −1.23 mEq/L in moderate-to-severe hyperkalemia *−1.01 mEq/L:* Overall (*p* <.001 vs. baseline)
		8-week randomized withdrawal phase: Serum potassium of 5.5 mmol/L or higher at baseline of the initial phase		Patiromer at same dose or placebo (Serum potassium: 3.8–5.1 mEq/L)	*Median change in serum potassium to week 4:* 0 mEq/L with patiromer and + 0.72 mEq/L with placebo (*p* <.001 vs. placebo)
2.	*SZC:* Randomized, placebo-controlled, double-blind study in two stages (14 days)[13]	*Correction phase:* Patients with serum potassium of 5.0–6.5 mEq/L (*n* = 754)	Approximately 40% of patients in SZC had heart failure and up to 70% patients were on RAAS inhibitors	*Correction phase:* SZC 1.25, 2.5, 5, or 10 g TID or placebo for 48 hours	*Exponential rate of change in mean serum potassium at 48 hours:* −0.30%,−0.21%, and −0.16% with SZC 10 g, 5g, and 2.5 g. −0.09% with placebo (*p* <.001 vs. placebo for three highest doses)
		Maintenance phase: Patients with serum K$^+$ of 3.5–4.9 mmol/L at 48 hours in SZC group were randomized to receive either their original dose of SZC or placebo once a day on days 3–14		*Maintenance phase:* Same dose of SZC or placebo QD (*Serum potassium:* 3.5–4.9 mEq/L for 14 days)	*Exponential rate of change in mean serum potassium:* +0.14% vs. +1.04% per hour with SZC 10 g and placebo (*p* <.001) + 0.09% vs. + 0.47% per hour with SZC 5 g and placebo (*p* = 0.008)

Contd...

Contd...

S. No.	Study design/ setting	Study population	LVEF in study population	Intervention	Primary outcome
3.	HARMONIZE[14] Randomized, placebo-controlled, double-blind study in two stages (28 days)	Outpatients with hyperkalemia (Two consecutive serum potassium values, 60 minutes apart ≥5.1 mEq/L) ($n = 258$)	Up to 44% of patients in SZC had heart failure and up to 75% of the patients had eGFR <60 mL/min/1.73 m^2	*Open-label initial phase:* SZC10 g TID for 48 hours	*Mean change in serum potassium over 48 hours:* −1.1 mEq/L (p <.001 vs. baseline)
				Double-blind maintenance phase: SZC 5, 10, or 15 g or placebo QD for 28 d (K^+ 3.5–5 mEq/L)	*Mean serum potassium during days 8–29:* 4.8, 4.5, and 4.4 mEq/L with SZC 5 g QD, 10 g QD, and 15 g QD, respectively 5.1 mEq/L with placebo (p <.001 vs. placebo for each dose)

CONCLUSION

Hyperkalemia due to the use of ACEI/ARB/MRA/ARNI in HFrEF and CKD can be reduced with newer antihyperkalemic drugs. The usefulness of these drugs with or without the antihyperkalemic agents in patients with CKD and HFpEF is yet to be proven. Further evidence is needed to assess the efficacy as well as safety of the newer antihyperkalemic drugs in patients with HFpEF and advanced CKD and recipients of kidney transplant.

REFERENCES

1. Ahmed A, Rich MW, Sanders PW, et al. Chronic kidney disease associated mortality in diastolic versus systolic heart failure: a propensity matched study. Am J Cardiol. 2007;99(3):393-8.
2. Cobo Marcos M, de la Espriella R, Gayán Ordás J, et al. Prevalence and clinical profile of kidney disease in patients with chronic heart failure. Insights from the Spanish cardiorenal registry. Rev Esp Cardiol (Engl Ed). 2024;77(1):50-9.
3. McAlister FA, Ezekowitz J, Tarantini L, et al. Renal dysfunction in patients with heart failure with preserved versus reduced ejection fraction: impact of the new Chronic Kidney Disease-Epidemiology Collaboration Group formula. Circ Heart Fail. 2012;5:309-14.
4. Collins AJ, Pitt B, Reaven N, et al. Association of serum potassium with all-cause mortality in patients with and without heart failure, chronic kidney disease, and/or diabetes. Am J Nephrol. 2017;46(3):213-21.
5. House AA, Wanner C, Sarnak MJ, et al. Heart failure in chronic kidney disease: conclusions from a Kidney Disease: Improving Global Outcomes (KDIGO) controversies conference. Kidney Int. 2019;95:1304-17.
6. Eschalier R, McMurray JJ, Swedberg K, et al. Safety and efficacy of eplerenone in patients at high risk for hyperkalemia and/or worsening renal function: analyses of the EMPHASIS-HF study subgroups (Eplerenone in Mild Patients Hospitalization And Survival Study in Heart Failure). J Am Coll Cardiol. 2013;62:1585-93.
7. Epstein M, Reaven NL, Funk SE, et al. Evaluation of the treatment gap between clinical guidelines and the utilization of renin-angiotensin aldosterone system inhibitors. Am J Manag Care. 2015;21(11 suppl):S212-20.
8. Weir MR, Bakris GL, Bushinsky DA, et al.; OPAL-HK Investigators. Patiromer in patients with kidney disease and hyperkalemia receiving RAAS inhibitors. N Engl J Med. 2015;372(3):211-21.
9. Pitt B, Anker SD, Bushinsky DA, et al. Evaluation of the efficacy and safety of RLY5016, a polymeric potassium binder, in a double-blind, placebo-controlled study in patients with chronic heart failure (the PEARL-HF) trial. Eur Heart J. 2011;32(7):820-8.
10. Agarwal R, Rossignol P, Romero A, et al. Patiromer versus placebo to enable spironolactone use in patients with resistant hypertension and chronic kidney disease (AMBER): a phase 2, randomised, double-blind, placebo-controlled trial. Lancet. 2019;394(10208):1540-50.
11. Roger SD, Spinowitz BS, Lerma EV, et al. Efficacy and Safety of Sodium Zirconium Cyclosilicate for Treatment of Hyperkalemia: An 11-Month Open-Label Extension of HARMONIZE. Am J Nephrol. 2019;50(6):473-80.
12. Zannad F, Hsu BG, Maeda Y, et al. Efficacy and safety of sodium zirconium cyclosilicate for hyperkalaemia: the randomized, placebo-controlled HARMONIZE-Global study. ESC Heart Fail. 2020;7(1):54-64.
13. Packham DK, Rasmussen HS, Lavin PT, et al. Sodium zirconium cyclosilicate in hyperkalemia. N Engl J Med. 2015;372(3):222-31.
14. Kosiborod M, Rasmussen HS, Lavin P, et al. Effect of Sodium Zirconium Cyclosilicate on Potassium Lowering for 28 Days Among Outpatients With Hyperkalemia: The HARMONIZE Randomized Clinical Trial. *JAMA.* 2014;312(21):2223-33.

CHAPTER

Efficacy and Safety of Steroidal MRAs in Patients with HFpEF and Chronic Kidney Disease

Vaishnavi Venkatasubramanian, Sahil Garg, Jasmine Sethi

INTRODUCTION

Heart failure (HF) is characterized by the hyperactivation of the mineralocorticoid receptor, resulting in sodium and water retention with the resultant adverse cardiac remodeling. Mineralocorticoid receptor antagonists (MRAs) are recommended for the treatment of heart failure with reduced ejection fraction (HFrEF), still these drugs are underutilized due to the concerns regarding hyperkalemia and their use in impaired renal function. Also, there is some uncertainty regarding their efficacy in heart failure with preserved ejection fraction (HFpEF). The recent American College of Cardiology (ACC) guidelines recommend the following agents for patients with heart failure with preserved ejection fraction (HFpEF): (1) Angiotensin receptor blocker (ARB), (2) mineralocorticoid receptor antagonist (MRA), (3) angiotensin receptor-neprilysin inhibitor (ARNI), and (4) sodium-glucose cotransporter 2 inhibitor (SGLT2i).[1] There is ample evidence to suggest that MRA use in HFpEF can lead to reduced frequency of HF-related hospitalizations, improve patient symptoms, and in addition, slow the disease progression.[2] While MRAs have demonstrated potential benefits in HFpEF, the efficacy of these agents in patients with reduced glomerular filtration rate (GFR) still remains doubtful.[3] Considering the increased risk of further worsening of renal function and hyperkalemia, it is advised to avoid using MRAs in patients with a GFR below 30 mL/min/1.73 m^2 or those with hyperkalemia (serum potassium ≥5.0 mmol/L).

The coexistence of chronic kidney disease (CKD) and HFpEF is a common clinical scenario, with CKD serving as a risk factor for the development of HFpEF. Individuals with both conditions are typically older, exhibit elevated natriuretic peptide levels, are more likely to have comorbidities like diabetes mellitus (DM) and hypertension and demonstrate a lower New York Heart Association (NYHA) functional class.[4] These patients are particularly at increased risk of fluid overload, resistance to diuretic agents, and a decline in renal function indices following diuresis. Also, CKD in the presence of HFpEF is associated with an increased risk of hospitalization and up to a threefold increased risk of mortality. This risk of increased mortality directly correlates with the severity of kidney disease.[5,6] The potential for improved cardiac function and reduced morbidity associated with MRAs may outweigh the transient GFR decline, particularly in patients exhibiting permissive hypercreatinemia. Vigilant monitoring of renal function and serum potassium is of paramount importance to ensure the safe and effective use of MRAs in this patient population.

MINERALOCORTICOID RECEPTOR ANTAGONISTS: STEROIDAL AND NONSTEROIDAL

Diuretics are one of the most important treatments for HF, hypertension, CKD, and various hypervolemic disorders. The renin-angiotensin-aldosterone system (RAAS) is the main pathway that handles the renal sodium balance, fluid balance, osmolarity, renal blood flow, and blood pressure. Many antihypertensive and diuretic medications primarily target RAAS.[7] The main hormone of this RAAS pathway is aldosterone. The mineralocorticoid hormone is produced by the adrenal cortex. The principal cells of the kidney in the collecting ducts are the main target of aldosterone, which increases the number of epithelial sodium channels (ENaC) and activates the basolateral Na^+/K^+ ATPase pump. This pump activation increases potassium secretion, sodium reabsorption, and effective circulating volume.[8] Along with regulatory action on the kidney, this mineralocorticoid also stimulates similar types of receptors present in the myocardium. It is presumed that aldosterone directly promotes the proliferation of cardiomyocytes and fibroblasts in response to damage or inflammation.[9] The level of aldosterone increases by up to 20% in patients having HF. This increased level of aldosterone provides an opportunity for RAAS inhibitors to decrease the deleterious effects of aldosterone. One of the main diuretics that inhibits the action of aldosterone is the MRA. This class of drugs is categorized into two types: Steroidal (nonspecific) and nonsteroidal (specific); based on their chemical class nonspecific MRAs were initially used due to their metabolic regulatory effects as moderate antiandrogens, strong antimineralocorticoids, and weak antisteroidogenesis agents. The main drawback of these agents was the blocking of androgen receptors stimulated by testosterone and dihydrotestosterone, which led to breast tenderness, gynecomastia, and feminization.[7] Various studies have shown the beneficial effects of spironolactone in hyperaldosteronism, HFrEF, and refractory hypertension. Although the data on the use of spironolactone in HFpEF is limited, studies suggest a possible benefit. Another use of MRA is in CKD where it has shown antiproteinuric effects. Along with antiandrogenic side effects, steroidal MRAs also cause hyperkalemia. To improve the side effect profile of nonspecific MRAs, specific or nonsteroidal MRAs were designed to ideally provide the same antimineralocorticoid effects while minimizing the side effects. To tackle the side effects of nonspecific MRAs, a novel agent called finerenone, originally named BAY 94-8862, was designed, which showed selective and stronger antimineralocorticoid activity compared with eplerenone and spironolactone. Because finerenone has a high affinity for protein binding, its effectiveness can be influenced by serum albumin levels, making conditions like nephrotic syndrome and malnutrition important considerations for dosing. Overall, finerenone has a more favorable side effect profile than earlier MRAs.[10]

ROLE OF MRA IN HFpEF

Heart failure with preserved ejection fraction is characterized by symptoms of HF resulting from elevated left ventricular (LV) filling pressures, despite a normal or near-normal LV ejection fraction (LVEF ≥50%). The primary goals in treating HFpEF patients are to enhance their functional capacity and alleviate the severity of symptoms. The management of chronic therapy includes loop diuretics and SGLT2 inhibitors as the initial therapy **(Fig. 1)**. GLP1 analogs and MRAs should be used as additional therapy after SGLT2 inhibitors or diuretics. In patients receiving optimal treatment with a diuretic and an SGTL2 inhibitor with or without semaglutide and who have persistent NYHA class II–III HF symptoms, MRAs are usually added.[11] The potassium level and estimated glomerular filtration rate (eGFR) play an important role in deciding the addition of MRAs like spironolactone or eplerenone. The starting dose of spironolactone is 12.5 mg once daily and it is titrated as tolerated every 2 weeks to the maximum tolerated dose that is either 25 mg or 50 mg. Key factors that limit dosage include hyperkalemia, declining kidney function, or hypotension. Similarly, eplerenone begins at 25 mg daily and is titrated to 50 mg over a 4-week period as tolerated.

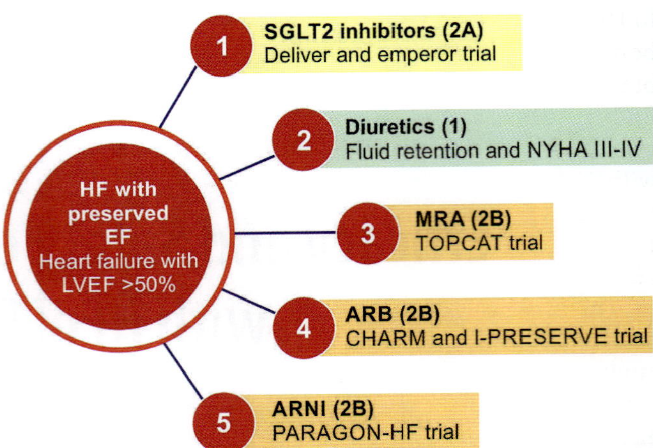

Fig. 1: Medical management of Heart failure with preserved Ejection fraction (HFpEF) as per recent American College of Cardiology Guidelines (ACC). (ARB: angiotensin receptor blocker; ARNI: angiotensin receptor–neprilysin inhibitor; LVEF: left ventricular ejection fraction; MRA: mineralocorticoid receptor antagonist; NYHA: New York heart association; SGLT2i: Sodium–glucose cotransporter inhibitor)
Note: Yellow denotes Class 2A evidence, orange denotes Class 2B, and green denotes class 1 evidence.

Two trials showed the efficacy of MRAs in HFpEF, out of which one trial, the TOPCAT trial, used spironolactone, and the other, the FINEART trial, used finerenone. The TOPCAT trial, which included patients with HFpEF, found that spironolactone led to a nonsignificant reduction in the composite outcome of aborted cardiac arrest, death, and HF hospitalizations [hazard ratio (HR): 0.89]. However, it did show a significant reduction in hospitalizations due to HF (HR: 0.83). A post hoc analysis indicated potential benefits for patients in the American cohort (HR: 0.83) but not in the Russian–Georgian cohort (HR: 1.10). These findings suggest a possible advantage of spironolactone in carefully selected HFpEF patients, particularly those with LVEF ≥45%, elevated BNP levels, a history of HF hospitalization within the past 1 year, eGFR >30 mL/min/1.73 m^2, creatinine <2.5 mg/dL, and serum potassium <5.0 mEq/L).[2]

The American College of Cardiology guidelines give a class 2b recommendation for MRAs in HFpEF treatment, advising close monitoring of potassium levels, kidney function, and diuretic dosages at the start of treatment and during follow-up. While research has not conclusively shown that MRAs improve exercise tolerance or quality of life in HFpEF patients, many will still benefit from their use to achieve balanced diuresis, implement sequential nephron blockade, control blood pressure, and reduce hospitalizations related to HF.

The approach to medical management of HFpEF as per recent ACC guidelines is given in **Figure 1**.

CURRENT EVIDENCE OF USE OF STEROIDAL MRA IN CKD

All the pivotal trials that evaluated the use of steroidal MRAs in HFpEF—namely, Randomized Aldactone Evaluation Study (RALES), Eplerenone Post-Acute Myocardial Infarction Heart Failure Efficacy and Survival Study (EPHESUS), and Eplerenone in Mild Patients Hospitalization and Survival Study in Heart Failure (EMPHASIS-HF) included patients with a serum creatinine level of <2.5 mg/dL or an eGFR of at least 30 mL/min/1.73 m^2. In a combined analysis by Ferreira et al., which included 12,700 participants, only 331 (2.6%) had an eGFR of ≤30 mL/min/1.73 m^2. The study found that MRAs, compared to placebo reduced the composite outcome of cardiovascular (CV) death or HF hospitalization, but the advantage diminished as eGFR decreased. For those with an eGFR of ≤30 mL/min/1.73 m^2, the hazard ratio was 0.96 (95% confidence interval (CI): 0.70–1.32). Additionally, they reported hyperkalemia and worsening renal function was observed to be 2- to 3 times more frequent among patients using MRAs, with risk of hyperkalemia worsening as eGFR declined (p = 0.002). They concluded that the diminishing benefits and increased safety concerns may restrict the use of MRAs in patients with lower eGFR, especially those with values ≤30 mL/min/1.73 m^2.[12]

Several smaller randomized studies, employing either crossover or parallel group designs, have been conducted involving patients with diabetic nephropathy (characterized by UACR ≥30 mg/g) who were already receiving angiotensin-converting enzyme inhibitors (ACEIs) or angiotensin receptor blockers (ARBs). These studies were analyzed collectively in a meta-analysis comprising 16 trials that assessed the effects of adding spironolactone to standard antidiabetic, renoprotective, or antihypertensive therapies, with durations ranging from 2 to 18 months. The analysis revealed a statistically significant decrease in 24-hour urinary albumin/protein excretion at the end of treatment, with a mean difference of –61.48 (95% CI: –96.74 to –26.23; p = 0.0006). However, a significant concern arose from a more than fivefold increase in the risk of hyperkalemia, particularly among patients with existing renal impairment.[13] Another meta-analysis, which included both diabetic and nondiabetic patients with CKD stages 1–4 and assessed both selective and nonselective steroidal MRAs, found a 38.7% reduction in weighted mean protein/albumin excretion. Nonetheless, this was accompanied by a threefold higher relative risk of trial withdrawal due to hyperkalemia.[14]

The MRAs are generally not recommended for use in late-stage CKD. A 2016 meta-analysis, which focused on patients undergoing dialysis, included nine trials with a total of 829 participants. The analysis found that MRAs reduced CV mortality in dialysis patients by 66%, but also led to a threefold increase in the risk of hyperkalemia compared to control groups. However, the overall quality of evidence was deemed low due to methodological issues present in many of the studies included.[15] Following this meta-analysis, the multicenter feasibility study known as SPin-D, which investigated the safety and CV efficacy of spironolactone in patients with end-stage renal disease (ESRD) requiring dialysis, did not find any CV benefit associated with spironolactone. The incidence of hyperkalemia (potassium levels exceeding 6.5 mmol/L) was comparable between the placebo and the 25 mg dose of spironolactone, while the 50 mg dose resulted in a higher rate of hyperkalemia.[16]

The significant adverse effect of hyperkalemia limits the use of MRAs in patients with advanced CKD. However, the introduction of new potassium binders may help manage potassium levels effectively, potentially allowing for the safe use of MRAs. The AMBER randomized trial enrolled patients with resistant hypertension, eGFR between 25 and 45 mL/min/1.73 m^2, and serum potassium levels ranging from 4.3 to 5.1 mmol/L. Participants were randomly assigned to receive either patiromer (8.4 g daily) or a placebo, in addition to open-label spironolactone (up to 50 mg daily) and their usual antihypertensive medications. The results indicated that patiromer allowed a greater proportion of patients to continue taking spironolactone compared to the placebo group: 86% versus 66%, with a between-group difference of 19.5% (95% CI 10.0–29.0%, $p < 0.001$).[17]

With the advent of nonsteroidal MRAs and their benefits in reducing CV death and CKD progression, the role of steroidal MRAs is restricted to CKD patients with refractory hypertension, hyperaldosteronism, and HF. The risk of hyperkalemia and reversible decline in glomerular filtration among patients with lower eGFR should be considered as suggested by the KDIGO 2024 CKD guidelines.[18]

CONCLUSION

Mineralocorticoid receptor antagonists offer significant potential benefits for patients with HFpEF and CKD. Although their use may be associated with a temporary and transient decline in GFR, the overall balance of benefits and risks should be carefully considered. Hyperkalemia is one of the main reasons for MRA withdrawal. One strategy to reduce the risk of hyperkalemia is to use a lower the dose of MRA and in CKD, submaximal doses of MRA are suggested, i.e., <25 mg daily for spironolactone and <50 mg daily for eplerenone. Additionally, patients at high risk of hyperkalemia are advised for a reduced potassium intake of ≤2–3 g per day. Recently, newer potassium binders like patiromer and sodium zirconium cyclosilicate have come up and can mitigate the risks of hyperkalemia associated with the use of drugs in the presence of CKD. To conclude, key considerations for the use of MRA in the presence of CKD include the concept of permissive hypercreatinemia, close monitoring of serum potassium and renal function, and lastly individual variability in the responses to MRAs.

REFERENCES

1. Kittleson MM, Panjrath GS, Amancherla K, et al. 2023 ACC Expert Consensus Decision Pathway on Management of Heart Failure With Preserved Ejection Fraction: A Report of the American College of Cardiology Solution Set Oversight Committee. J Am Coll Cardiol. 2023;81(18):1835-78.
2. Pitt B, Pfeffer MA, Assmann SF, et al.; TOPCAT Investigators. Spironolactone for heart failure with preserved ejection fraction. N Engl J Med. 2014;370(15):1383-92.
3. Edelmann F, Wachter R, Schmidt AG, et al. Effect of spironolactone on diastolic function and exercise capacity in patients with heart failure with preserved ejection fraction: The Aldo-DHF randomized controlled trial. JAMA. 2013;309(8):781-91.
4. Vijay K, Neuen BL, Lerma EV. Heart Failure in Patients with Diabetes and Chronic Kidney Disease: Challenges and Opportunities. Cardiorenal Med. 2022;12(1):1-10.
5. Khan YH, Sarriff A, Adnan AS, et al. Chronic kidney disease, fluid overload and diuretics: A complicated triangle. PLoS One. 2016;11(7):e0159335.
6. Damman K, Valente MA, Voors AA, et al. Renal impairment, worsening renal function, and outcome in patients with heart failure: an updated meta-analysis. Eur Heart J. 2014;35(7):455-69.
7. Rico-Mesa JS, White A, Ahmadian-Tehrani A, et al. Mineralocorticoid receptor antagonists: a comprehensive review of finerenone. Curr Cardiol Rep. 2020;22(11):140.
8. Butterworth MB. Regulation of the epithelial sodium channel (ENaC) by membrane trafficking. Biochim Biophys Acta. 2010;1802(12):1166-77.
9. Delcayre C, Swynghedauw B. Molecular mechanisms of myocardial remodeling. The role of aldosterone. J Mol Cell Cardiol. 2002;34(12):1577-84.
10. Solomon SD, McMurray JJV, Vaduganathan M, et al. Finerenone in heart failure with mildly reduced or preserved ejection fraction. N Engl J Med. 2024;391(16):1475-85.
11. Heidenreich PA, Bozkurt B, Aguilar D, et al. 2022 AHA/ACC/HFSA Guideline for the Management of Heart Failure: A Report of the American College of Cardiology/American Heart Association Joint Committee on Clinical Practice Guidelines. Circulation. 2022;145(18):e895-e1032.
12. Ferreira JP, Pitt B, McMurray JJV, et al. Steroidal MRA across the spectrum of renal function: a pooled analysis of RCTs. JACC Heart Fail. 2022;10(11):842-50.
13. Hou J, Xiong W, Cao L, et al. Spironolactone add-on for preventing or slowing the progression of diabetic nephropathy: A meta-analysis. Clin Ther. 2015;37(9):2086-103.e10.
14. Currie G, Taylor AH, Fujita T, et al. Effect of mineralocorticoid receptor antagonists on proteinuria and progression of chronic kidney disease: A systematic review and meta-analysis. BMC Nephrol. 2016;17(1):127.
15. Quach K, Lvtvyn L, Baigent C, et al. The Safety and Efficacy of Mineralocorticoid Receptor Antagonists in Patients Who Require Dialysis: A Systematic Review and Meta-analysis. Am J Kidney Dis. 2016;68(4):591-8.
16. Charytan DM, Himmelfarb J, Ikizler TA, et al. Safety and cardiovascular efficacy of spironolactone in dialysis-dependent ESRD (SPin-D): a randomized, placebo-controlled, multiple dosage trial. Kidney Int. 2019;95(4):973-82.
17. Agarwal R, Rossignol P, Romero A, et al. Patiromer versus placebo to enable spironolactone use in patients with resistant hypertension and chronic kidney disease (AMBER): a phase 2, randomised, double-blind, placebo-controlled trial. Lancet. 2019;394(10208):1540-50.
18. Kidney Disease: Improving Global Outcomes (KDIGO) CKD Work Group. KDIGO 2024 Clinical Practice Guideline for the Evaluation and Management of Chronic Kidney Disease. Kidney Int. 2024;105(4S):S117-314.

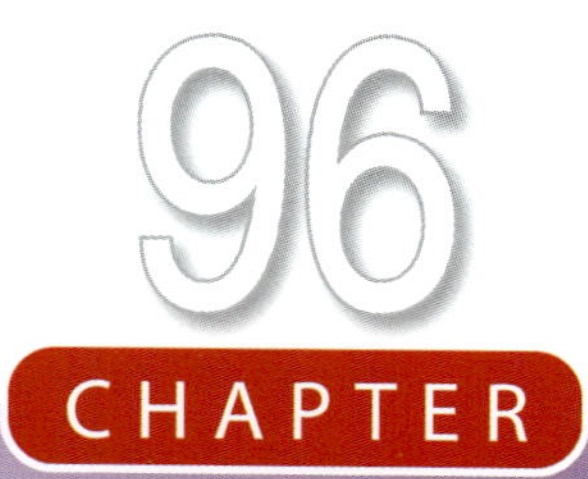

Efficacy and Safety of Novel Nonsteroidal MRAs in Patients with HFpEF and Chronic Kidney Disease

Dinesh Khullar, Rahul Grover, Abhishek, Deepak Panigrahi, Anish Kumar Gupta

INTRODUCTION

Current global guidelines recommend the use of steroidal mineralocorticoid receptor antagonists (MRAs) for patients with HFrEF.[1,2] However, the broader use of steroidal MRA in HF has been limited and there is mixed data on the efficacy and safety of steroidal MRA in patients with HFpEF.[3,4] However, their use has been linked to increased risks of hyperkalemia, acute kidney injury (AKI), and gynecomastia.[5] The lack of long-term follow-up and insufficient power to detect benefits on critical clinical outcomes, such as kidney failure and major adverse CV events (MACE), leave the risk-benefit ratio of steroidal MRAs uncertain.

Finerenone, a selective nonsteroidal MRA was approved in 2021 to reduce the risk of kidney disease progression and cardiovascular events in patients with chronic kidney disease (CKD) and T2D. The approval was based on the results of two major trials: FIDELIO-DKD[6] (Finerenone in Reducing Kidney Failure and Disease Progression in Diabetic Kidney Disease), which showed an 18% reduction in CKD progression and a 14% reduction in cardiovascular events, and FIGARO-DKD[7] (Finerenone in Reducing Cardiovascular Mortality and Morbidity in Diabetic Kidney Disease), which demonstrated a 13% reduction in cardiovascular risks and a notable 29% decrease in heart failure hospitalizations.

A pooled analysis of these trials, known as FIDELITY,[8] confirmed that finerenone offers benefits across different stages of CKD severity, improving both kidney and cardiovascular outcomes. Finerenone provides a new treatment option, particularly for patients with cardio-kidney-metabolic comorbidities, and offers potential advantages over traditional therapies like spironolactone.

With ongoing uncertainties about the role of MRAs in heart failure with HFmrEF or HFpEF, the FINEARTS-HF trial[9] was conducted to test finerenone's ability to reduce heart failure events and cardiovascular deaths in this population. The results suggest finerenone could play a significant role in addressing unmet needs in heart failure management, especially in patients with CKD. In this review, we explore the efficacy and safety of finerenone demonstrated by current clinical landmark trials in a cohort of HF patients with preserved or mild reduced ejection fraction and/or CKD with T2D.

METHODS

Data sources: We searched major electronic databases, including PubMed, Embase, Scopus, and the Cochrane Library, from their inception until September, 2024.

Search strategy: Keywords and MeSH terms used in various combinations were: "finerenone," "heart failure with preserved ejection fraction," "chronic kidney disease," "heart failure with chronic kidney disease," "mineralocorticoids receptor antagonists," "nonsteriodial MRAs," and "landmark clinical trials."

FINERENONE: HOW IS IT A DISTINCT ENTITY?

Finerenone, the first nonsteroidal MRA, blocks the binding of aldosterone and cortisol to the mineralocorticoid

Flowchart 1: Mineralocorticoid (MR) over activation on kidney, blood vessels, and heart.

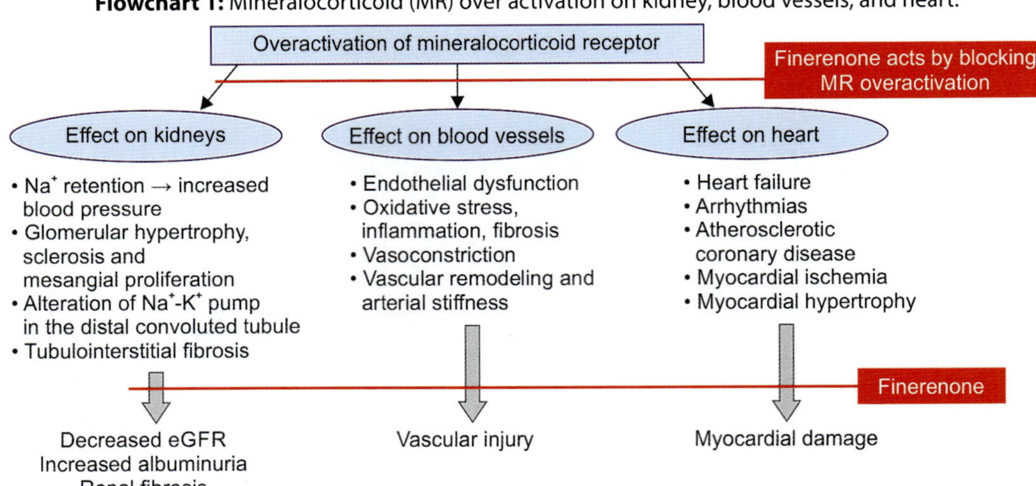

receptor, preventing the activation of genes involved in hypertrophy, inflammation, and fibrosis **(Flowchart 1)**. Unlike traditional steroidal MRAs such as spironolactone and eplerenone, finerenone offers superior MR selectivity, ensuring more targeted action and reducing off-target effects. It is characterized by balanced distribution across both cardiac and renal tissues, a shorter half-life, no active metabolites, and stronger receptor-binding affinity, making it more effective and better tolerated in managing conditions such as heart failure and chronic kidney disease.

EFFICACY AND SAFETY OF FINERENONE IN PATIENTS WITH HEART FAILURE AND CHRONIC KIDNEY DISEASE

Numerous preclinical and clinical studies have suggested that finerenone provides significant benefits for cardiovascular and renal health, underscoring its potential as an effective treatment option in a broad spectrum of HF populations, including those with HFmrEF and HFpEF. Ongoing research endeavors, such as the FINEOVATE program are investigating the definitive role of finerenone in patients across the spectrum of HF, T2D, and kidney disease, respectively. FINEARTS-HF (patients with symptomatic HF, LVEF ≥40%, NCT04435626), REDEFINE-HF (patients hospitalized for HF, LVEF ≥40%, NCT06008197), CONFIRMATION-HF (patients hospitalized for HF independent of LVEF in combination with SGLT2i, NCT06024746), and FINALITY-HF (Patients with HFrEF not on steroidal MRAs, NCT06033950) trials involving over 15,000 patients with HF across clinical settings. FIDELITY-CKD (pooled analysis of FIDELIO-DKD and FIGARO-DKD), ReFineDR (nonproliferative diabetic retinopathy, NCT04477707), CONFIDENCE (combination therapy of finerenone and SGLT2i in patients with CKD and T2D, NCT05254002), FINE-ONE (In CKD patients with T1D, NCT05901831), and FIND-CKD (albuminuric CKD in patients without diabetes, NCT05047263) trials aim to examine cardio-renal outcomes in cohort of CKD and/or T2D/T1D.

Finerenone has undergone testing in various rodent models relevant to HF. Finerenone has shown significant anti-inflammatory and antifibrotic effects in preclinical studies.[10,11] It reduces cardiac macrophage accumulation and exhibits potent antifibrotic actions in various rodent models. Additionally, it diminishes cardiac hypertrophy, reduces plasma prohormone of brain natriuretic peptide, and improves parameters related to diastolic dysfunction and early signs of systolic dysfunction. The risk of electrolyte disturbances was low.[11] Although its antihypertensive effects in clinical studies are modest compared to placebo and spironolactone, preclinical findings suggest promising potential for finerenone as a therapeutic option in HF, awaiting confirmation in future clinical trials.

FIDELIO-DKD ("Finerenone in Reducing Kidney Failure and Disease Progression in Diabetic Kidney Disease")[6] and FIGARO-DKD ("Finerenone in Reducing Cardiovascular Mortality and Morbidity in Diabetic Kidney Disease")[7] trials demonstrated that finerenone, compared to placebo, improved composite CV outcomes, including time to CV death, nonfatal myocardial infarction, stroke, or HHF, and was well tolerated in patients with albuminuric CKD and T2D. The FIDELITY analysis, a pooled data review from both trials involving 13,026 patients,[8] showed that finerenone reduced the composite CV outcome by 14% and the composite kidney outcome by 23%.

Both the FIDELIO-DKD and FIGARO-DKD trials assessed finerenone's efficacy in DKD patients, with or without HF. Notably, these studies excluded patients with symptomatic HFrEF (NYHA class II–IV), so the HF patients included had either asymptomatic HFrEF, HFrEF (NYHA class I), HFmrEF, or HFpEF at baseline. In the FIDELIO-DKD trial, 7.7% of the participants had a history of HF, and over a median follow-up of 2.6 years, finerenone significantly reduced the composite CV outcomes regardless of HF history. Similar results were observed in the FIGARO-DKD trial, where 7.8% of the patients had a history of HF, and finerenone significantly reduced the risk of developing new-onset HF. The FIDELITY analysis further confirmed finerenone's role in preventing HHF in patients with DKD, demonstrating a reduced risk of the first hospitalization for HF, cardiovascular death or initial hospitalization, recurrent HF hospitalizations, as well as cardiovascular death or recurrent HF. These benefits were observed consistently across different eGFR levels and UACR values **(Table 1)**. Both preclinical and clinical data emphasize finerenone's therapeutic potential in HFpEF, which remains an area for further exploration.

TABLE 1: Landmark trials on finerenone.

Parameter	*FIDELIO-DKD; 2020*[6]	*FIGARO-DKD; 2021*[7]	*FIDELITY; 2022 (Pooled analysis)*[8]	*FINEARTS-HF 2024*[9]
Phase	III	III	Pooled analysis of FIGARO-DKD and FIDELIO-DKD	III
Study population	T2D, advanced CKD treated with ACEi/ARBs, and severely increased albuminuria	Patients with T2D and CKD (stage 2–4, moderately elevated albuminuria) and/or CKD (stage 1–2) with significantly increased albuminuria	T2D with a wide spectrum of CKD	Aged ≥40 years, NYHA Class II–IV, LVEF ≥40%, Structural heart abnormalities, diuretics within 30 days
Sample size (n)	5,674	7,352	13,026	6,001
Male gender n (%)	3,983 (70.2%)	5,105 (69.4%)	9,088 (69.8%)	3,269 (54.5%)
Mean age (years)	65.6	64.1	64.8	72
Mean BMI (kg/m²)	31.1 ± 6.0	31.4 ± 6.0	31.3 ± 6.0	30.0 ± 6.1
Intervention arm	Finerenone 10–20 mg/day vs. placebo	Finerenone 10–20 mg/day vs. placebo	Finerenone 10–20 mg/day vs. placebo	Finerenone 10, 20, 40 mg based on eGFR
Control arm	Placebo	Placebo	Placebo	Placebo
Mean serum potassium (mEq/L)	4.4 ± 0.5	4.3 ± 0.4	4.35 ± 0.4	4.4 ± 0.5
Mean glycated Hemoglobin (%)	7.7 ± 1.3	7.7 ± 1.4	7.7 ± 1.4	7.2
Mean eGFR	44.3 ± 12.6	67.8 ± 21.7	57.6 ± 21.7	62.0 ± 20.0
UACR (Median IQR)	852 (446–1,634)	308 (108–740)	515 (198–1,147)	18 (7–67)
Composite endpoints	Kidney failure, eGFR reduction (≥40%) for ≥4 weeks, or death due to kidney disease	Death from CV causes, nonfatal MI, stroke, or HHF	CV death, nonfatal MI, stroke, HHF, kidney failure, eGFR reduction (≥57%), or death due to kidney disease	CV deaths, total HF events, KCCQ-TSS, improvement in NYHA class, composite kidney outcome
Composite CV event	0.86 (0.75–0.99)	0.87 (0.76–0.98)	0.86 (0.78–0.95)	0.84 (0.74–0.95)
Death due to CV event	0.86 (0.68–1.08)	0.90 (0.74–1.09)	0.88 (0.76–1.02)	0.93 (0.78–1.11)
MI (nonfatal)	0.80 (0.58–1.09)	0.99 (0.76–1.31)	0.91 (0.74–1.12)	-
Stroke (nonfatal)	1.03 (0.76–1.38)	0.97 (0.74–1.26)	0.99 (0.82–1.21)	-
HHF	0.86 (0.68–1.08)	0.71 (0.56–0.90)	0.78 (0.66–0.92)	-
Total HF events	-	-	-	0.82 (0.71–0.94)
Composite kidney outcome	-	-	-	1.33 (0.94–1.89)

The FINEARTS-HF (NCT04435626) trial,[9] a double-blind, randomized, event-driven study, enrolled 6,001 high-risk HF patients to assess the efficacy and safety of finerenone (at a maximum dose of 20–40 mg daily alongside standard care) compared to a placebo. The trial included individuals with HFmrEF or HFpEF, structural heart disease, and elevated natriuretic peptide levels (mean age 72 years, with 36% having an ejection fraction below 50%). The primary endpoint was a composite measure of "worsening heart failure," which encompassed CV death and total HF events. Secondary endpoints evaluated improvements in NYHA functional class, a kidney composite outcome, and all-cause mortality.

After a median follow-up of 32 months, results from FINEARTS-HF showed that finerenone significantly lowered the risk of the primary composite endpoint, which included worsening HF events (unplanned hospitalizations or urgent visits for HF) or CV death (rate ratio 0.84, $p = 0.007$). The reduction was mainly attributed to fewer worsening HF events (rate ratio 0.82, $p = 0.006$), although the difference in CV death rates between the finerenone and placebo groups was not statistically significant (8.1% vs. 8.7%; hazard ratio 0.93). When evaluating the composite of the first worsening HF event or CV death, the finerenone group showed a reduced risk compared to the placebo group (RR 0.84). However, finerenone did not significantly reduce the risk of the kidney composite outcome (2.5% in finerenone vs. 1.8% in placebo; hazard ratio 1.33) in this population, which had a low risk of kidney disease progression, minimal albuminuria, and a small number of kidney events.

Several larger, ongoing landmark trials have been initiated to further assess the efficacy and safety of finerenone across various HF populations. REDEFINE-HF (NCT06008197), is a phase III, randomized, double-blind, placebo-controlled, multicenter, event-driven trial designed to evaluate the efficacy and safety of finerenone, in addition to standard of care (SoC), compared to placebo. This trial will involve over 5,200 patients and aims to assess the reduction in total HF events (first and subsequent) and CV death in individuals hospitalized with acute decompensated HF, and mildly reduced or preserved left ventricular ejection fraction (LVEF).

FINALITY-HF (NCT06033950) is another phase III, randomized, double-blind, placebo-controlled, multicenter, event-driven trial that will examine the efficacy and safety of finerenone, in addition to SoC, compared to placebo. This study will enroll over 2,600 patients with symptomatic HFrEF who are intolerant of, contraindicated for, or ineligible for treatment with steroidal MRAs, such as spironolactone or eplerenone. As in the REDEFINE-HF trial, patients with eGFR below 25 mL/min/1.73 m^2 or serum/plasma potassium levels above 5.0 mmol/L will not be eligible for participation.

The ongoing phase III, CONFIRMATION-HF study (NCT06024746) is a randomized, controlled, open-label trial that aims to assess finerenone combined with an SGLT2 inhibitor in approximately 1,500 patients who have been recently hospitalized for HF, irrespective of their left ventricular ejection fraction (LVEF). The primary outcomes, evaluated over a six-month period, include a hierarchical composite of clinical benefits measured using the win-ratio, which considers time to death from any cause, the number of HF events, and the time to the first HF event.

SAFETY PROFILE OF FINERENONE

The safety analysis from the FIDELITY study indicates that finerenone has a low rate of discontinuation due to hyperkalemia, comparable to that of the placebo group. The occurrence of treatment-emergent adverse events (TEAEs) was similar between patients receiving finerenone and those on placebo, with no increase in sex hormone-related side effects or any significant impact on HbA1c levels. Additionally, the safety profile of finerenone in patients with stage 4 CKD was consistent with its profile in earlier CKD stages.[8] In the FIDELIO-DKD study, adverse events such as diarrhea, nausea, vomiting, and hypovolemia occurred at comparable rates in both the finerenone and placebo groups.

While traditional steroidal MRAs are often limited by their potential to cause hyperkalemia, finerenone offers a promising alternative for managing patients with T2D and CKD or CVD. However, hyperkalemia remains a key concern with finerenone. Although hyperkalemia-related events were more frequent in the finerenone group compared to placebo, these events were generally mild, with few cases leading to treatment discontinuation or hospitalization.[8] The FINEARTS-HF trial also showed a higher incidence of hyperkalemia with finerenone (9.7% vs. 4.2% in the placebo group), though this did not result in significant hospitalizations or deaths. Additionally, finerenone was associated with a lower risk of hypokalemia.[9]

CONCLUSION

Finerenone, a novel nonsteroidal mineralocorticoid receptor antagonist, has shown significant promise in improving cardiovascular and renal outcomes in patients with CKD and type 2 diabetes, as demonstrated in the FIDELIO-DKD and FIGARO-DKD trials. These studies also suggest potential benefits for HFpEF. Finerenone's selective action on the heart and kidneys offers advantages over traditional steroidal MRAs, with a lower risk of hyperkalemia and kidney dysfunction. The FINEARTS-HF trial showed that finerenone reduces the risk of worsening heart failure events or cardiovascular death in patients with HFmrEF or HFpEF. Ongoing trials such as REDEFINE-HF, FINALITY-HF, and CONFIRMATION-HF are further investigating its efficacy and potential in combination with other therapies for a broad range of heart failure conditions.

REFERENCES

1. McDonagh TA, Metra M, Adamo M, et al.; ESC Scientific Document Group. 2021 ESC Guidelines for the diagnosis and treatment of acute and chronic heart failure. Eur Heart J. 2021;42:3599-726.
2. Writing Committee Members, Yancy CW, Jessup M, Bozkurt B, Butler J, et al. 2013 ACCF/AHA guideline for the management of heart failure: a report of the American College of Cardiology Foundation/American Heart Association Task Force on practice guidelines. Circulation. 2013;128:e240-327.
3. Pfeffer MA, Claggett B, Assmann SF, et al. Regional variation in patients and outcomes in the Treatment of Preserved Cardiac Function Heart Failure With an Aldosterone Antagonist (TOPCAT) trial. Circulation. 2015;131:34-42.
4. Xiang Y, Shi W, Li Z, et al. Efficacy and safety of spironolactone in the heart failure with mid-range ejection fraction and heart failure with preserved ejection fraction: a meta-analysis of randomized clinical trials. Medicine (Baltimore). 2019;98:e14967.
5. Ferreira JP, Pitt B, McMurray JJV, et al. Steroidal MRA across the spectrum of renal function: A pooled analysis of RCTs. JACC Heart Fail. 2022;10:842-50.
6. Bakris GL, Agarwal R, Anker SD, et al. FIDELIO-DKD Investigators. Effect of finerenone on chronic kidney disease outcomes in type 2 diabetes. N Engl J Med 2020;383:2219-29.
7. Pitt B, Filippatos G, Agarwal R, et al.; FIGARO-DKD Investigators. Cardiovascular events with finerenone in kidney disease and type 2 diabetes. N Engl J Med. 2021;385:2252-63.
8. Agarwal R, Filippatos G, Pitt B, et al.; FIDELIO-DKD and FIGARO-DKD Investigators. Cardiovascular and kidney outcomes with finerenone in patients with type 2 diabetes and chronic kidney disease: The FIDELITY pooled analysis. Eur Heart J. 2022;43:474-84.
9. Solomon SD, McMurray JJV, Vaduganathan M, et al. Finerenone in Heart Failure with Mildly Reduced or Preserved Ejection Fraction. N Engl J Med. 2024.
10. Grune J, Beyhoff N, Smeir E, et al. Selective mineralocorticoid receptor cofactor modulation as molecular basis for Finerenone's antifibrotic activity. Hypertension. 2018;71(4):599-608.
11. Kolkhof P, Delbeck M, Kretschmer A, et al. Finerenone, a novel selective nonsteroidal mineralocorticoid receptor antagonist protects from rat cardiorenal injury. J Cardiovasc Pharmacol. 2014;64(1):69-78.

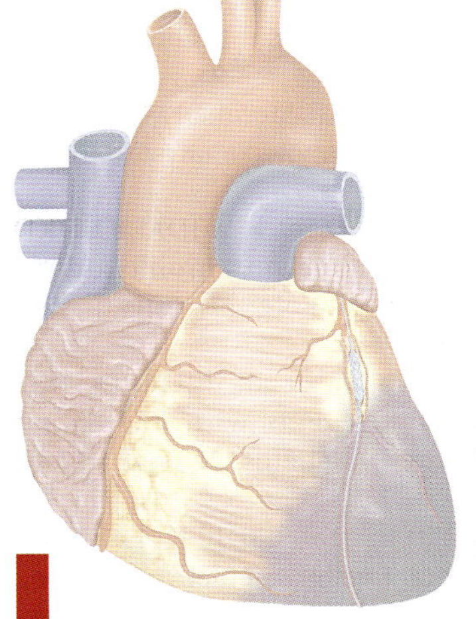

Role of IV Iron in Management of Patients with HFpEF and Chronic Kidney Disease

Megha Saigal, Priti Meena

INTRODUCTION

Anemia is frequently observed in both heart failure (HF) and chronic kidney disease (CKD) and is associated with a diminished quality of life (QoL) and poorer clinical outcomes **(Fig. 1)**. Compared to nonanemic individuals with HF, those with anemia tend to be older, more often female, and more likely to have diabetes, CKD, more severe HF with reduced functional capacity, lower exercise tolerance, worse health-related QoL, lower blood pressure, a higher reliance on diuretics, and heightened activation of neurohormonal and proinflammatory pathways.[1]

Iron deficiency stands out as the primary factor contributing to anemia in these patients. Iron is crucial for mitochondrial function, especially in the final step of adenosine triphosphate (ATP) synthesis from glucose, fatty acids, or ketones. Organs such as the heart and kidneys, which have high energy demands, rely heavily

Iron therapy in Heart failure and chronic kidney disease

- Oxidative stress, fibrosis, mineralocorticoid excess,
- SNS overactivity, RAAS activation, inflammation, endothelial dysfunction, volume expansion

Kidneys

Heart

Fibrosis, ischemia, adverse cardiovascular remodeling leading to impaired left ventricular relaxation and reduced ventricular compliance

- Diabetes
- Obesity
- Vascular calcification
- Hypertension
- Metabolic syndrome

IV iron

Decrease all-cause mortality, CV deaths, and hospitalizations due to HF, along with improvements in functional capacity, symptoms, and quality of life

Anemia

Poor quality of life, hypoxia, higher mortality, increased hospitalization, decreased exercise capacity, more edema, hypotension and heart failure exacerbations

Fig. 1: Complex relationship between heart failure, chronic kidney disease, and anemia.

on mitochondria. Consequently, iron deficiency leads to structural and functional mitochondrial impairments in these organs. Iron deficiency can also be observed in patients who do not have anemia.[2] Cardiorenal iron deficiency syndrome is a complex interplay of iron deficiency, HF, anemia, and CKD.[3] Overlapping biomarker profiles suggest shared pathophysiological pathways in these conditions. Several mechanisms contribute to iron deficiency in these patients, including poor dietary intake, gastrointestinal malabsorption, and inflammation driven by mediators like hepcidin and IL-6, which inhibit iron absorption and the release of iron from its stores. Additionally, blood loss in hemodialysis patients also leads to iron deficiency. These mechanisms lead to iron-restricted erythropoiesis and impair hemoglobin synthesis. Anemia in the cardiorenal syndrome worsens both CKD and CVD by reducing erythropoietin (EPO) production, impairing oxygen delivery, and promoting tissue hypoxia, which triggers peripheral vasodilation and enhances neurohormonal activation, perpetuating the cardiorenal cycle. The inflammatory cytokines released in CKD and cardiovascular conditions increase hepcidin-25 levels, further limiting iron absorption and mobilization from stores. Studies have shown that iron supplementation in patients with HF and advanced CKD can improve outcomes, including reducing mortality and major cardiovascular events.[4]

TREATMENT OF IRON DEFICIENCY ANEMIA IN HFpEF AND CHRONIC KIDNEY DISEASE

Intravenous iron therapy has emerged as an important treatment option for patients with HF and CKD [who suffer from iron deficiency anemia (IDA)]. While erythropoiesis-stimulating agents (ESAs) have traditionally been used to manage anemia in these patients, studies have shown that ESAs alone do not significantly improve outcomes in HF and are instead associated with worsened outcomes, including an increased risk of stroke.[5] Iron deficiency has been shown to be associated with increased mortality, independent of anemia. Poor absorption of oral iron, especially in CKD patients with elevated hepcidin levels, makes IV iron the preferred treatment option.

Absolute iron deficiency is defined by serum ferritin levels below 100 ng/mL and transferrin saturation (TSAT) <20%, while functional iron deficiency, commonly observed in HF due to chronic inflammation and elevated hepcidin levels, is characterized by ferritin levels between 100 and 299 ng/mL and TSAT <20%.[6]

The KDIGO guidelines recommend iron supplementation for treating anemia in CKD patients when TSAT is <30% and ferritin is below 500 ng/mL.[7] In patients with iron deficiency, IV iron is often preferred over oral iron to reduce pill burden, enhance absorption, and bypass functional iron deficiency.

Two randomized controlled trials (RCTs), FAIR-HF and CONFIRM-HF, highlighted the positive effects of IV ferric carboxymaltose (FCM) in HF patients with iron deficiency.[8,9] In the FAIR-HF trial, 6 months of FCM treatment resulted in improvements in QoL, NYHA functional class, and exercise capacity in both anemic and nonanemic individuals. Similarly, the CONFIRM-HF trial demonstrated better exercise capacity, symptom relief, and QOL, while also reducing hospitalizations related to HF exacerbations. A sub-analysis of FAIR-HF further suggested that IV iron therapy may improve kidney function.[10] A meta-analysis confirmed these benefits, showing a decrease in all-cause mortality, cardiovascular deaths, and hospitalizations due to HF, along with improvements in functional capacity, symptoms, and QOL.[4] The FERRIC-HF trial also found that IV iron sucrose significantly enhanced exercise tolerance and symptom relief, particularly in HF patients.[11]

The IV formulations of iron that have been used across various trials are FCM, iron–sucrose, ferumoxytol, low-molecular-weight iron dextran, iron isomaltoside, and ferric gluconate. Out of these, the first two are most commonly available and used; however, no difference has been seen across trials between different preparations.[4] IV iron formulations such as FCM and iron sucrose are widely used in clinical practice, with no significant differences in efficacy across different preparations. While iron therapy is generally well tolerated, mild-to-moderate side effects such as gastrointestinal disturbances and injection-site reactions can occur.

Many trials for the use of IV iron in patients with CKD and HFrEF have been done, which have shown positive results. However, only two RCTs have been conducted for the use of IV iron therapy in patients with HFpEF and CKD—FAIR-HFpEF published in 2024.

The FAIR-HFpEF trial was a multicenter RCT investigating the effects of IV FCM versus placebo in patients with symptomatic HFpEF and iron deficiency. Participants received 1000–2000 mg of FCM or saline at the start of the trial, with additional doses of 500–1000 mg administered at weeks 16 and 32.[12] Treatment continued at these intervals unless ferritin levels exceeded 800 ng/mL, ferritin was greater than 500 ng/mL with TSAT above 50% or hemoglobin levels surpassed 16.0 g/dL during follow-up. The trial found that patients receiving IV iron showed improvements in the 6-minute-walk test at both 24 and 32 weeks, although these benefits diminished by 52 weeks. Additionally, the treatment was associated with fewer serious adverse events.

The use of IV iron in patients with HF and iron deficiency is supported by strong evidence, particularly in those with HFrEF. The potential benefits of IV iron therapy in HFpEF are being explored in ongoing trials such as the Iron-MET-HFpEF study (NCT04945707). While early results are promising, further research is needed to confirm these findings in larger cohorts and RCTs.

CHALLENGES IN MANAGING IRON DEFICIENCY IN HEART FAILURE AND CHRONIC KIDNEY DISEASE

Managing IDA in patients with CKD and HF presents a unique challenge due to ferritin's dual role as an indicator of iron stores and a marker of inflammation. Elevated ferritin levels are strongly linked to higher mortality rates, but this association is significantly reduced when accounting for malnutrition–inflammation complex syndrome, a common issue in these populations. Studies suggest that while IV iron doses above 400 mg per month are associated with increased mortality, moderate doses of IV iron have been linked to improved survival rates. The common markers used to assess iron status, ferritin, and TSAT, lack the accuracy to reliably guide treatment decisions.[13] The European Society of Cardiology (ESC) recently updated its clinical guidelines to recommend IV FCM for symptomatic patients with HFrEF and iron deficiency.[14] This treatment aims to enhance symptoms, improve exercise capacity, and elevate overall QoL, underscoring the importance of iron supplementation in HF management while highlighting the need to carefully balance iron dosing for optimal outcomes.

CONCLUSION

An integrated multidisciplinary approach is required to promote risk factor reduction and increase the adoption of newer therapeutics. Though we have achieved many important milestones in understanding the benefits of IV iron therapy in HFrEF, the journey to uncover its potential in HFpEF is just beginning and the results still leave a lot to be desired; however, future RCTs should not only confirm this positive signal of IV iron therapy on exercise capacity but also reassess its benefits on health-related QoL, morbidity, and mortality. ESC has added many new therapies in their armamentarium in treatment of HFpEF, such as SGLT2 inhibitors and GLP1-receptor agonists. We are hopeful that this favorable journey will continue and that IV iron therapy will eventually be added to the list of successes in HFpEF therapy.

REFERENCES

1. Anand IS, Gupta P. Anemia and iron deficiency in heart failure: Current concepts and emerging therapies. Circulation. 2018;138(1):80-98.
2. Fischer C, Valente de Souza L, Komlódi T, et al. Mitochondrial respiration in response to iron deficiency anemia: Comparison of peripheral blood mononuclear cells and liver. Metabolites. 2022;12(3):270.
3. Alnuwaysir RIS, Grote Beverborg N, Hoes MF, et al. Additional burden of iron deficiency in heart failure patients beyond the cardio-renal anaemia syndrome: Findings from the BIOSTAT-CHF study. Eur J Heart Fail. 2022;24(1):192-204.
4. Yamani N, Ahmed A, Gosain P, et al. Effect of iron supplementation in patients with heart failure and iron deficiency: A systematic review and meta-analysis. Int J Cardiol Heart Vasc. 2021;36:100871.
5. Koulouridis I, Alfayez M, Trikalinos TA, et al. Dose of erythropoiesis-stimulating agents and adverse outcomes in CKD: A metaregression analysis. Am J Kidney Dis. 2013; 61(1):44-56.
6. Rohr M, Brandenburg V, Brunner-La Rocca HP. How to diagnose iron deficiency in chronic disease: A review of current methods and potential marker for the outcome. Eur J Med Res. 2023;28(1):15.
7. Drüeke TB, Parfrey PS. Summary of the KDIGO guideline on anemia and comment: Reading between the (guide) line(s). Kidney Int. 2012;82(9):952-60.
8. Anker SD, Comin Colet J, Filippatos G, et al. Ferric carboxymaltose in patients with heart failure and iron deficiency. N Engl J Med. 2009;361(25):2436-48.
9. Ponikowski P, van Veldhuisen DJ, Comin-Colet J, et al. Beneficial effects of long-term intravenous iron therapy with ferric carboxymaltose in patients with symptomatic heart failure and iron deficiency†. Eur Heart J. 2015;36(11): 657-68.
10. Ponikowski P, Filippatos G, Colet JC, et al. The impact of intravenous ferric carboxymaltose on renal function: An analysis of the FAIR-HF study. Eur J Heart Fail. 2015; 17(3):329-39.
11. Okonko DO, Grzeslo A, Witkowski T, et al. Effect of intravenous iron sucrose on exercise tolerance in anemic and nonanemic patients with symptomatic chronic heart failure and iron deficiency FERRIC-HF: A randomized, controlled, observer-blinded trial. J Am Coll Cardiol. 2008;51(2):103-12.
12. Von Haehling S, Doehner W, Evertz R, et al. Ferric carboxymaltose and exercise capacity in heart failure with preserved ejection fraction and iron deficiency: The FAIR-HFpEF trial. Eur Heart J. 2024;45(37):3789-800.
13. Packer M, Anker SD, Butler J, et al. Redefining iron deficiency in patients with chronic heart failure. Circulation. 2024;150(2):151-61.
14. McDonagh T, Damy T, Doehner W, et al. Screening, diagnosis and treatment of iron deficiency in chronic heart failure: Putting the 2016 European Society of Cardiology heart failure guidelines into clinical practice. Eur J Heart Fail. 2018;20(12):1664-72.

CHAPTER

Emerging Strategies in the Management of HFpEF in CKD: What does the Future Hold?

Manisha Sahay

INTRODUCTION

The prevalence of heart failure with preserved ejection fraction (HFpEF) in chronic kidney disease (CKD) is increasing due to increasing age and comorbidities such as diabetes, hypertension, dyslipidemia, metabolic syndrome, and obesity.[1] The American College of Cardiology (ACC), American Heart Association (AHA),[2] and European Society of Cardiology[3] have provided recommendations for the diagnosis and management of HFpEF.

Lifestyle modifications, including physical activity, achievement of ideal body weight, and salt restriction, are cornerstones of treatment. As per the ACC/AHA guidelines, RAAS blockers (level 2a), sodium-glucose cotransporter-2 inhibitors (SGLT2i) (level 1 recommendation), MRAs and sacubitril/valsartan (2a recommendation) in HFpEF, and GLP1Ra have become standard therapies for the management of HFpEF and have been discussed in previous chapters. This chapter focuses on the probable role of newer drugs, stem cell therapy, and device therapy in HFpEF.

NOVEL THERAPIES

Several novel therapies are being tried for HFpEF **(Table 1)**. These include drugs, cell therapies, and devices.

Drug Therapy

Recent advances in the understanding of pathophysiology of HFpEF have demonstrated the role of inflammation,[4,5] fibrosis, mitochondrial dysfunction, and reduction in NO levels in the pathogenesis **(Fig. 1)**. This has opened new vistas for the treatment targeting these pathways.

TABLE 1: Novel drug therapies and ongoing trials.

Novel drug therapies	*Trials*
Anti-inflammatory	
IL-1	DHART2
IL-18	ColpEFF
TNF-α	RENEWAL ATTACH
Antifibrotic	
Pirfenidone	PIROUETTE
ARNI	ARNI-CHF
Spironolactone	SPIRIT-HF
Finerenone	FINEARTS-HF
Mitochondrial therapies	
AMPK	GRAPEVINE-HF
ETC	RESTORE-HF
Adenosine-receptor agonist	PANACHE HF
Calcium dynamics	
Calcium channel nifedipine	DEMAND-HF (Nifedipine)
Sodium channel	RALI-HF, RAZE (Ranolazine)
Sodium pump, IC calcium	DIG PEF (Digoxin)
PDE-5 inhibitors	
Sildenafil	SOCRATES PRESERVED
Udenafil	ULTIMATE HEF
	PASSION

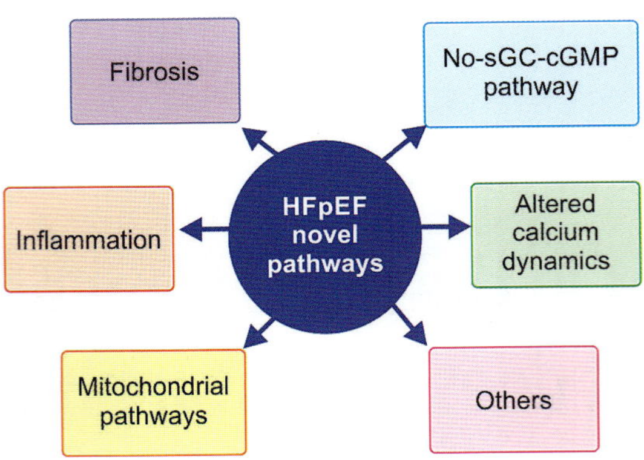

Fig. 1: Pathophysiology of HFpEF.

Anti-inflammatory Agents

In HFpEF, the exposure of cardiac proteins by damaged or dead cardiomyocytes may break immune tolerance and result in the activation of autoreactive T and B cells and inflammatory cascade. Many therapies are directed to reduce inflammation and improve the cardiac function given as follows:

- *Anti-TNF-alpha therapy:* It was evaluated in the RENEWAL (Randomized Etanercept Worldwide Evaluation) trial,[6,7] which studied the effects of etanercept, a decoy TNF-alpha receptor. Another trial, the ATTACH (Anti-TNF Therapy Against Congestive Heart Failure) trial analyzed the effects of infliximab, a neutralizing antibody, in patients with HFpEF.[8] However, there was no benefit, and on the contrary, there was an increase in mortality. Hence, no further studies were carried out.
- *Anti-IL-1 and IL-6:* The effect of IL-1 blocker anakinra was tested in the DHART2 study, but there was no improvement in peak VO_2 and VE/VCO_2 slope in obese HFpEF patients in this trial.[9] Anti-IL-6 therapy is currently used in autoimmune disease, but there are very few studies on this drug in heart failure (HF).
- *Rituximab:* It is anti-CD20 antibody targeting the B cells and has been tried for HFpEF.
- *Colchicine:* It has anti-inflammatory actions. It suppresses tubulin polymerization and inhibits the inflammasome. The production of IL-1β and IL-18 is reduced. Colchicine improves diastolic dysfunction in animal models of heart failure rats with preserved ejection fraction (EF) induced by a high-salt diet.[10] The COLpEF trial is evaluating the effect on NT-proBNP and troponin in patients with HFpEF.
- *Sodium-glucose cotransporter-2 inhibitors (SGLT2i):* Dapagliflozin and empagliflozin have been studied in the large randomized controlled trials (RCTs) and are strongly recommended for the treatment of HF.[2,3] The reduction in cardiovascular (CV) mortality and hospitalizations with SGLT2i is also seen in HFpEF.[11] A recent study on HFpEF patients with empagliflozin demonstrated a reduction in ICAM and VCAM, decrease in TNF-alpha and IL-6, which are proinflammatory cytokines, and also reduction in oxidative stress in myocardial fibers.[12] Thus, SGLT2i is useful in HFpEF by its potent anti-inflammatory action.
- *Intravenous immunoglobulin (IVIg):* It is hypothesized that the binding of autoantibodies to cardiac-specific antigens on cardiomyocytes may induce cardiac dysfunction. IVIg may prevent binding of the antibodies and may improve cardiac function.
- *Sitagliptin:* In a study in animal models, sitagliptin was found to reduce TNF-alpha and IL-6 and reduced fibrosis.[13]
- *Metformin:* It is known to be anti-inflammatory. The effect of metformin on peak oxygen capacity during exercise and the inflammatory biomarkers in HFpEF patients aged older than 60 years is being tested in a clinical trial.[8-10, 14-17, 19]

Novel Trials Related to the NO-sGC-cGMP Pathway

- *Soluble guanylate cyclase stimulators:* Vericiguat and riociguat stimulate the sGC enzyme and also sensitize sGC to low levels of NO. These improve biventricular and left atrial filling pressures; however, benefits on hard outcomes have not been reported. These trials included approximately 50% subjects with CKD. The SOCRATES-PRESERVED was a phase 2b trial, which showed no reduction of NT-proBNP or left atrial dimensions with vericiguat.[18] Vericiguat was well tolerated, and there was an improvement in the quality of life. Another trial, VITALITY-HFpEF, did not demonstrate any improvement in the physical limitation score.[19]
  The CAPACITY HFpEF trial[20] with praliciguat tested its effects on functional capacity. However, there was no significant differences in VO_2 peak compared to placebo. Riociguat in the haemoDYNAMIC trial improved exercise capacity in pulmonary hypertension and improved cardiac output.[21] However, there were many dropouts, and patients with HFpEF did not show any symptomatic improvement.
- *Phosphodiesterase inhibitors:* Reduced level of cGMP is an important factor in the pathophysiology of HFpEF. Phosphodiesterase type 5 (PDE5) inhibitors such as sildenafil reduce cGMP degradation. The SIDAMI trial with sildenafil showed improvement in hemodynamics.[22] However, there was no benefit

seen in other trials. The ACC/AHA 2022 recommends avoidance of routine use of PDE5 inhibitors (class of recommendation 3: no benefit). Ongoing trials using PDE5 inhibitors are the ULTIMATE-HFpEF trial with udenafil, another trial with sildenafil, and the PASSION trial.

- *Nitric oxide donors:* Many benefits have been attributed to nitrates in previous CV trials. However, the NEAT-HFpEF trial[23] showed that isosorbide mononitrate, a long working organic nitrate, did not improve quality of life and exercise capacity. Similarly, in the INDIE-HFpEF trial, inhaled nebulized inorganic nitrate did not improve exercise capacity. The ACC/AHA 2022 recommends avoidance of routine use of nitrates in HFpEF (class of recommendation 3: no benefit). However, other trials are in progress to analyze the effect of nitrates in HFpEF.

Calcium Dynamics Approach Therapies

- *Calcium channel blockers:* Nifedipine inhibits calcium entry and reduces calcium overload. The DEMAND study with nifedipine 10–60 mg once a day showed that there was an improvement in LV filling pressures. However, the complete results are not yet available.
- *Ranolazine:* This drug inhibits the late sodium current and prevents NCX calcium entry. In the RALI-DHF study, ranolazine was shown to improve diastolic relaxation parameters. The RAZE study showed some improvement in exercise capacity, but the results were inconclusive.
- *Istaroxime:* It is a Na/K ATPase inhibitor. It is a steroidal agent, which stimulates the sarcoplasmic reticulum calcium ATPase isoform 2a (SERCA2a). SERCA2a pumps calcium into the sarcoplasmic reticulum, which improves cardiac relaxation and contraction. It is being tested in HFpEF.[24]
- *Digoxin:* It did not show any reduction in mortality or CV hospitalizations in patients with EF >45%, sinus rhythm, and on angiotensin-converting enzyme inhibitors and diuretics in the DIG-PEF study.

Antifibrotic Molecules

- *Pirfenidone:* The PIROUETTE (Pirfenidone in Patients with Heart Failure and Preserved Left Ventricular Ejection Fraction) was a phase 2 trial with pirfenidone, an antifibrotic agent which is approved for idiopathic pulmonary fibrosis.[25] This randomized, placebo-controlled trial included symptomatic patients with HFpEF within 12 months of diagnosis, with LVEF >45%. The myocardial fibrosis was assessed by cardiac magnetic resonance (CMR). There was a reduction in cardiac fibrosis in 1 year. Phase III trial is required for confirmation.
- *Spironolactone:* It is useful in HFrEF due to its hormonal effects and antifibrotic properties. The TOPCAT study initially revealed no significant benefit in HFpEF patients treated with spironolactone;[26] however, later analysis revealed a difference in results when considering the geographical region from where patients were recruited.[27] The clinical impact on outcomes requires further study. The SPIRIT-HF trial is ongoing in which spironolactone is compared with placebo in patients with HFpEF and HFmrEF in reducing the composite endpoint of recurrent HF hospitalizations and CV mortality. Two phase III clinical trials (SPIRRIT-HFpEF[28] comparing spironolactone or eplerenone and FINEARTS-HF) are ongoing to test the efficacy of MRAs. The FIDELITY trial with finerenone showed CV benefits in patients with diabetic kidney disease.[29]
- *Sacubitril/valsartan:* Several trials have demonstrated the benefits of this drug in HFrEF as mentioned in other chapters. Currently, the ARNI-CHF trial is underway to assess the efficacy of this combination in reducing fibrosis by CRM in HFpEF.
- *Drugs (such as nintedanib and pamrevlumab):* These are antifibrotic drugs used for other diseases, but these need to be studied in HFpEF.
- *Salinomycin:* It is an anticoccidial drug but is also shown to prevent fibroblast activation and promote survival of cardiomyocyte in mice.[30]
- *Galectin-3 inhibitors:* These are antifibrotic drugs and may be useful in HFpEF, but presently no compound of this class is available.[31]

Mitochondrial Therapies

- *Perhexiline:* This drug is a carnitine palmitoyltransferase-1 inhibitor. It shifts the metabolism of the heart toward the use of carbohydrates. This results in enhancement of mechanical efficiency of the heart and hence may be useful in HFpEF.[32]
- *Resveratrol:* It exerts a protective action against HFpEF-induced adverse cardiac remodeling by decreasing Smad3 acetylation and transcriptional activity via activating Sirt1. Resveratrol, which is a polyphenol found in red wine, is also found to stimulate mitochondrial biogenesis through AMPK and NO-dependent mechanisms. Due to these positive effects on heart function, it is currently being tested for HFpEF in the GRAPEVINE-HF trial.[33]

- *Elamipretide:* Mitochondrial abnormalities contribute to impaired oxygen utilization and exercise intolerance in HFpEF. Cardiolipin is a lipid component of inner membrane of the mitochondria. It anchors to cytochrome c and helps in electron transport between complex III and IV in the electron transport chain (ETC). Cardiolipin is reduced in HF. This increases ROS by decoupling ETC. Elamipretide acts on the inner mitochondrial membrane and increases cardiolipin and restores mitochondrial bioenergetics. It is currently being tested in the RESTORE-HF trial.
- *Neladenoson:* It is a partial adenosine A1 receptor agonist. Some preclinical studies showed that it has beneficial effects on mitochondrial function and energy utilization. However, the PANACHE trial with this drug in HFpEF failed to show any benefit.[34]

Other Miscellaneous Therapies

- *Iron supplementation:* The PIVOTAL (Proactive IV IrOn Therapy in HaemodiaLysis Patients) trial demonstrated the efficacy of high-dose intravenous iron,[35] with reduction in HF events [hazard ratio (HR) 0.66; 95% CI 0.46–0.94].
  Intravenous ferric carboxymaltose was found to be useful in patients with HFrEF. The FAIR-HFpEF and PREFER-HF are two currently ongoing RCTs that are evaluating the efficacy and safety of intravenous ferric carboxymaltose in HFpEF.
- *Paricalcitol and cinacalcet:* The PRIMO (Paricalcitol in Renal Failure-Induced Cardiac Morbidity) study was an RCT that studied the effect of paricalcitol on cardiac function in CKD. However, it showed no effect on LVMI or other echocardiographic measures of diastolic function.[36] In the post hoc analysis of the EVOLVE (Evaluation of Cinacalcet Hydrochloride Therapy to Lower Cardiovascular Events) trial, the use of the calcimimetic, cinacalcet, was shown to significantly decrease the risk of HF.[37]
- *Semaglutide:* The STEP-HFpEF trial in patients with DM is underway for determining the efficacy of semaglutide in HFpEF.
- *Tirzepatide:* Trials with this drug in Heart Failure with Preserved Ejection Fraction and Obesity (SUMMIT) are currently ongoing.
- *Inhibitors of advanced glycation end products (AGEPs):* AGEPs are associated with HFpEF. Aminoguanidine, benfotiamine, and alagebrium, which inhibit the AGEPs, have been tried in HFpEF.
- *Recombinant HDL:* Increased apoA-I/HDL levels show a protective effect on vascular function by down-regulation of the angiotensin-1 receptor, and infusion of recombinant HDL is being tried in HFpEF in animal models.

CELL THERAPY

Cell therapy is a novel therapy where stem cells, progenitor cells, primary cells, or genetically modified cells are used to repair a damaged tissue or organ. These cells can be given intravenously or transplanted into the affected region. The cells can be derived from embryonic or adult stem cell lines.[38] Adult stem cells include those from bone marrow, fibroblasts, skeletal muscle, adipose tissue, and umbilical cord. The REGRESS-HFpEF phase 2 trial is currently testing the role of intracoronary treatment with allogeneic cardiosphere-derived cells in HFpEF. HFpEF patients have a lower level of circulating $CD34^+$ cells, which are inversely correlated with diastolic dysfunction, and these can be repleted using cell therapy. Regulatory T cells may also provide a new vista of treatment in HFpEF.

DEVICE-BASED THERAPIES

In HFpEF, the size of LV may be small, and there is poor filling of LV. The high LV end-diastolic pressure is transmitted to the left atrium (LA) in a retrograde fashion, which is then transmitted to the pulmonary circulation. This leads to pulmonary congestion and remodeling. Device therapies have been designed, which can normalize hemodynamics by reducing LA pressure **(Fig. 2)**.

The devices used are as follows:

- *Interatrial shunt devices (IASDs):*
  - *Transcatheter atrial shunt:* They are installed percutaneously. These form a shunt pathway between the LA and another cavity and hence reduce LA pressure. A left–right interatrial shunt is created, which decreases LA pressure, but increases the pressures in the right side of the heart. Newer devices to circumvent this problem are being developed, which connect LA to the coronary sinus. This will prevent the atrial arrhythmias and thromboembolism.[39]
  - *V-wave shunts:* These are percutaneously placed devices, which allow flow from the LA to RA when the pressure gradient is >5 mm Hg.
  - *Atrial flow regulator (AFR):* The AFR is self-expanding device that provides an opening diameter of 6–10 mm, which allows a bidirectional interatrial flow. They are also installed percutaneously.
- *Left ventricular expander (LVE) devices*: These devices assist in early ventricular filling.[40]
  - LVEs are spring-like devices. During systole, elastic energy is stored by these devices and transferred

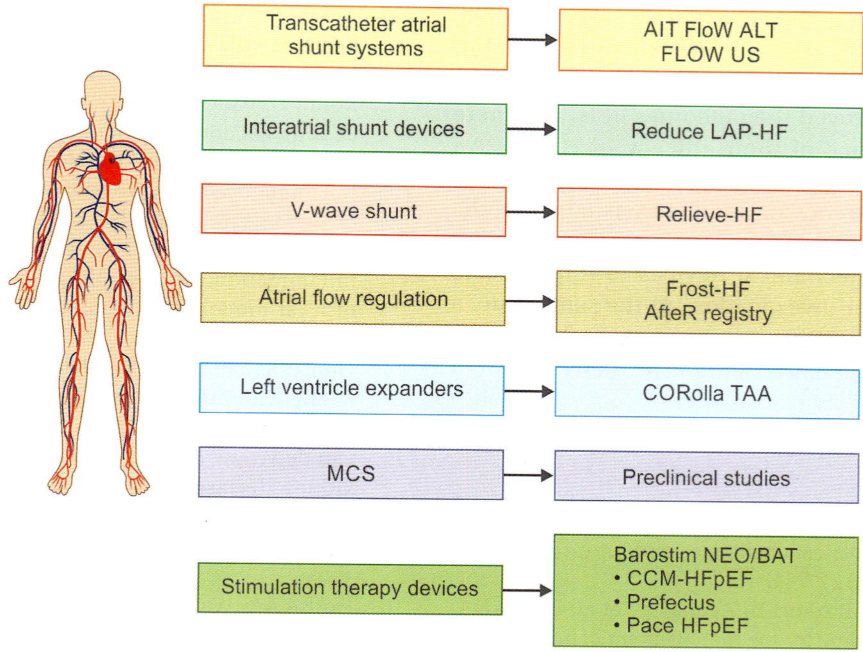

Fig. 2: Device therapies and trials.

to the LV during diastole, thus improving the filling in the early phase of the cardiac cycle. ImCardia and the CORolla transapical approach (CORolla TAA) devices are currently available. These can be implanted at the level of the pericardium and endocardium, respectively.[41] The CORolla TAA is superior to ImCardia as it can be installed by a minimally invasive technique through an intercostal incision.

- *Mechanical circulatory support devices:* These devices are the continuous flow rotodynamic blood pumps (RBPs), which act by decompressing the LA. This restores the cardiac output.
  - *Left atrial decompression pumps (synergy pump):* In this device, the blood flow from the LA or left ventricle is ejected directly into the aorta.
  - The CoPulse is valveless pulsatile pump device, which is implanted in the apex of the heart. It has an air chamber and a blood chamber separated by a flexible polyurethane membrane. During the diastole, the blood flow enters the chamber and is expelled during systole.
  - *Left atrial assist device (LAAD):* The LAAD is a continuous pump device, which is implanted in the mitral valve. It transfers the blood flow from the LA to left ventricle.[42]
- *Neurohumoral devices:* These devices act by modifying the autonomic nervous system response in patients with HFpEF. These include:
  - *Barostim Neo system:* This system works by activating the baroreceptors in the carotid artery wall. This increases parasympathetic tone and decreases sympathetic stimuli. This subcutaneous device is installed next to the carotid artery under ultrasound guidance.
  - *Cardiac contractility modulation (CCM):* By using this device, high-voltage nonexcitatory biphasic electrical signals are delivered during the absolute refractory period of the action potential in the right ventricular septum. There is a consequent increase in the calcium influx into the cardiomyocytes, which increases contractility. There is, however, no increase in the myocardial oxygen consumption. Prolonged use of this device may cause changes in gene expression with improved myocardial contractility.
  - *Cardiac resynchronization therapy (CRT):* The PROSPECT (Predictors of Response to CRT) trial of CRT was performed in patients with HFrEF. A subgroup analysis of the same trial showed a similar improvement in patients with LVEF >35%.
  - *Left bundle branch pacing (LBBP):* This therapy can be done in emergency setting and improves heart function. It is an effective alternative to CRT.

CONCLUSION

Heart failure with preserved ejection fraction is thought to be a systemic disease and is associated with multiple comorbidities such as diabetes, hypertension, metabolic syndrome, and CKD. HFpEF with CKD has a high morbidity and mortality. Though SGLT2i, MRA, ARNI, and RAASi have improved the outcomes in HFrEF, there is less robust evidence of their efficacy in HFpEF. An increased understanding of the pathophysiology of HFpEF in CKD has paved the way for interventions targeting the inflammatory, fibrotic, and other pathways. In addition, cell therapies and mechanical devices to improve the LV function are under investigation. At the same time, a multidisciplinary approach to management and strategies for risk reduction are essential for holistic management of HFpEF.

REFERENCES

1. Zakeri R, Cowie MR. Heart failure with preserved ejection fraction: controversies, challenges and future directions. Heart. 2018;104(5):377-84.
2. Heidenreich PA, Bozkurt B, Aguilar D, et al. 2022 AHA/ACC/HFSA guideline for the management of heart failure: a report of the American College of Cardiology/American Heart Association Joint Committee on Clinical Practice Guidelines. Circulation. 2022;145(18):e895-1032.
3. McDonagh TA, Metra M, Adamo M, et al. 2021 ESC guidelines for the diagnosis and treatment of acute and chronic heart failure. Eur Heart J. 2021;42(36):3599-726.
4. Youn JC, Ahn Y, Jung HO. Pathophysiology of heart failure with preserved ejection fraction. Heart Fail Clin. 2021;17(3):327-35.
5. Pfeffer MA, Shah AM, Borlaug B. Heart failure with preserved ejection fraction in perspective. Circ Res. 2019;124(11):1598-617.
6. Parra-Lucares A, Romero-Hernández E, Villa E, et al. New opportunities in heart failure with preserved ejection fraction: from bench to bedside... and back. Biomedicines. 2022;11(1):70.
7. Mann DL, McMurray JJV, Packer M, et al. Targeted anticytokine therapy in patients with chronic heart failure: results of the Randomized Etanercept Worldwide Evaluation (RENEWAL). Circulation. 2004;109(13):1594-602.
8. Chung ES, Packer M, Lo KH, et al. Randomized, double-blind, placebo-controlled, pilot trial of infliximab, a chimeric monoclonal antibody to tumor necrosis factor-alpha, in patients with moderate-to-severe heart failure: results of the anti-TNF Therapy Against Congestive Heart Failure (ATTACH) trial. Circulation. 2003;107(25):3133-40.
9. Murphy SP, Kakkar R, McCarthy CP, et al. Inflammation in heart failure: JACC state-of-the-art review. J Am Coll Cardiol. 2020;75(11):1324-40.
10. Shen S, Duan J, Hu J, et al. Colchicine alleviates inflammation and improves diastolic dysfunction in heart failure rats with preserved ejection fraction. Eur J Pharmacol. 2022;929:175126.
11. Anker SD, Butler J, Filippatos G, et al. Empagliflozin in heart failure with a preserved ejection fraction. N Engl J Med. 2021;385(16):1451-61.
12. Kolijn D, Pabel S, Tian Y, et al. Empagliflozin improves endothelial and cardiomyocyte function in human heart failure with preserved ejection fraction via reduced pro-inflammatory-oxidative pathways and protein kinase Gα oxidation. Cardiovasc Res. 2020;117(2):495-507.
13. Esposito G, Cappetta D, Russo R, et al. Sitagliptin reduces inflammation, fibrosis and preserves diastolic function in a rat model of heart failure with preserved ejection fraction. Br J Pharmacol. 2017;174(22):4070-86.
14. Dunlay SM, Roger VL, Redfield MM. Epidemiology of heart failure with preserved ejection fraction. Nat Rev Cardiol. 2017;14(10):591-602.
15. van de Wouw J, Broekhuizen M, Sorop O, et al. Chronic kidney disease as a risk factor for heart failure with preserved ejection fraction: a focus on microcirculatory factors and therapeutic targets. Front Physiol. 2019;10:1108.
16. House AA, Wanner C, Sarnak MJ, et al. Heart failure in chronic kidney disease: conclusions from a Kidney Disease: Improving Global Outcomes (KDIGO) Controversies Conference. Kidney Int. 2019;95(6):1304-17.
17. Cameron AR, Morrison VL, Levin D, et al. Anti-inflammatory effects of metformin irrespective of diabetes status. Circ Res. 2016;119(5):652-65.
18. Cleland JGF, Mueller C. What can we learn from SOCRATES: more questions than answers? Eur Heart J. 2017;38(15):1128-31.
19. Armstrong PW, Lam CSP, Anstrom KJ, et al. Effect of vericiguat vs placebo on quality of life in patients with heart failure and preserved ejection fraction: the VITALITY-HFpEF Randomized Clinical Trial. JAMA. 2020;324(15):1512-21.
20. Udelson JE, Lewis GD, Shah SJ, et al. Effect of praliciguat on peak rate of oxygen consumption in patients with heart failure with preserved ejection fraction: the CAPACITY HFpEF randomized clinical trial. JAMA. 2020;324(15):1522-31.
21. Dachs TM, Duca F, Rettl R, et al. Riociguat in pulmonary hypertension and heart failure with preserved ejection fraction: the haemoDYNAMIC trial. Eur Heart J. 2022;43(36):3402-13.
22. Andersen MJ, Ersbøll M, Axelsson A, et al. Sildenafil and diastolic dysfunction after acute myocardial infarction in patients with preserved ejection fraction: the Sildenafil and Diastolic Dysfunction After Acute Myocardial Infarction (SIDAMI) trial. Circulation. 2013;127(11):1200-8.
23. Redfield MM, Anstrom KJ, Levine JA, et al. Isosorbide mononitrate in heart failure with preserved ejection fraction. N Engl J Med. 2015;373(24):2314-24.
24. Torre E, Arici M, Lodrini AM, et al. SERCA2a stimulation by istaroxime improves intracellular Ca2+ handling and diastolic dysfunction in a model of diabetic cardiomyopathy. Cardiovasc Res. 2021;118(4):1020-32.

25. Lewis GA, Dodd S, Clayton D, et al. Pirfenidone in heart failure with preserved ejection fraction: a randomized phase 2 trial. Nat Med. 2021;27(8):1477-82.
26. Savill P. Spironolactone in heart failure with preserved ejection fraction. Practitioner. 2014;258:10.
27. de Denus S, O'Meara E, Desai AS, et al. Spironolactone metabolites in TOPCAT—new insights into regional variation. N Engl J Med. 2017;376(17):1690-2.
28. Cortes LT, Hong L. Heart failure with preserved ejection fraction—out with the old and out with the new? Front Cardiovasc Med. 2022;9:943572.
29. Patel RN, Sharma A, Prasad A, et al. Heart failure with preserved ejection fraction with CKD: a narrative review of a multispecialty disorder. Kidney Med. 2023;5(12):100705.
30. Burke RM, Dirkx RA, Quijada P, et al. Prevention of fibrosis and pathological cardiac remodeling by salinomycin. Circ Res. 2021;128(11):1663-78.
31. Yu L, Ruifrok WPT, Meissner M, et al. Genetic and pharmacological inhibition of galectin-3 prevents cardiac remodeling by interfering with myocardial fibrogenesis. Circ Heart Fail. 2013;6(1):107-17.
32. Singh S, Beadle R, Cameron D, et al. Randomized double-blind placebo-controlled trial of perhexiline in heart failure with preserved ejection fraction syndrome. Future Cardiol. 2014;10(6):693-8.
33. Kumar AA, Kelly DP, Chirinos JA. Mitochondrial dysfunction in heart failure with preserved ejection fraction. Circulation. 2019;139(11):1435-50.
34. Shah SJ, Voors AA, McMurray JJV, et al. Effect of neladenoson bialanate on exercise capacity among patients with heart failure with preserved ejection fraction: a randomized clinical trial. JAMA. 2019;321(21):2101-12.
35. Macdougall IC, White C, Anker SD, et al. Intravenous iron in patients undergoing maintenance hemodialysis. N Engl J Med. 2019;380(5):447-58.
36. Thadhani R, Appelbaum E, Pritchett Y, et al. Vitamin D therapy and cardiac structure and function in patients with chronic kidney disease: the PRIMO randomized controlled trial. JAMA. 2012;307(7):674-84.
37. EVOLVE trial investigators, Chertow GM, Block GA, et al. Effect of cinacalcet on cardiovascular disease in patients undergoing dialysis. N Engl J Med. 2012;367(26): 2482-94.
38. Buzhor E, Leshansky L, Blumenthal J, et al. Cell-based therapy approaches: the hope for incurable diseases. Regen Med. 2014;9(5):649-72.
39. Hasenfuß G, Hayward C, Burkhoff D, et al. A transcatheter intracardiac shunt device for heart failure with preserved ejection fraction (REDUCE LAP-HF): a multicentre, open-label, single-arm, phase 1 trial. Lancet. 2016;387(10025): 1298-304.
40. Feld Y, Reisner Y, Meyer-Brodnitz G, et al. The CORolla device for energy transfer from systole to diastole: a novel treatment for heart failure with preserved ejection fraction. Heart Fail Rev. 2023;28(2):307-14.
41. Burkhoff D, Maurer MS, Joseph SM, et al. Left atrial decompression pump for severe heart failure with preserved ejection fraction: theoretical and clinical considerations. JACC Heart Fail. 2015;3(4):275-82.
42. Moscato F, Wirrmann C, Granegger M, et al. Use of continuous flow ventricular assist devices in patients with heart failure and a normal ejection fraction: a computer-simulation study. J Thorac Cardiovasc Surg. 2013;145(5): 1352-8.

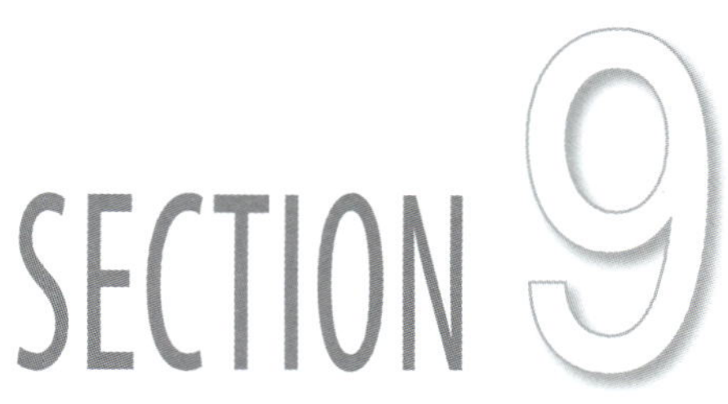

SECTION 9

HFpEF, Critical and Emergency Care

99. Role of ARNI in Critical Care Patients with HFpEF

100. HFpEF Care in an Intensive Care Unit

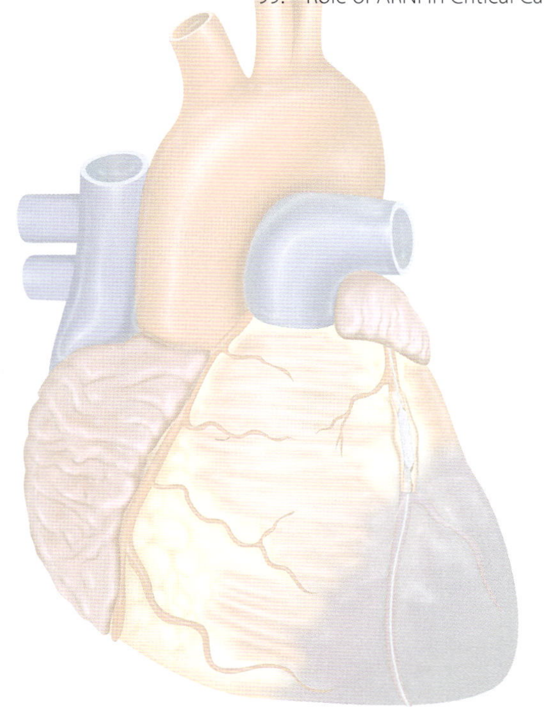

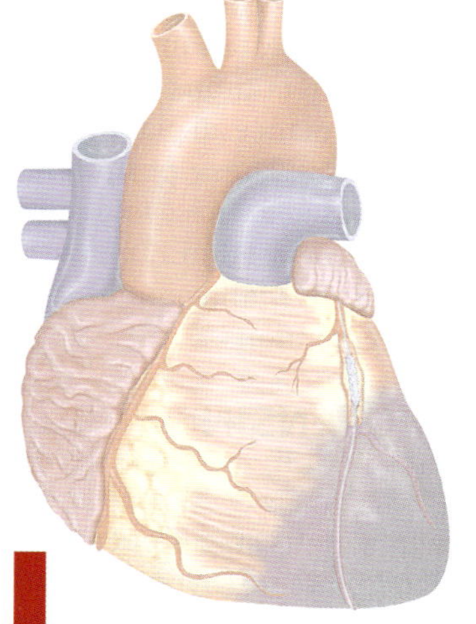

Role of ARNI in Critical Care Patients with HFpEF

Aashish Jain, Yatin Mehta

INTRODUCTION

Heart failure with preserved ejection fraction (HFpEF) is increasingly recognized as a significant public health challenge, particularly among the aging population.[1] HFpEF is mainly characterized by diastolic relaxation abnormality and inefficient stroke volume generation. In HFpEF, the overactivity of renin-angiotensin-aldosterone system (RAAS) leads to several problems: It causes the heart muscle to become stiff and fibrous, disrupts normal heart function, raises blood pressure, and contributes to issues with blood vessel elasticity.[2]

The HFpEF manifests through symptoms such as dyspnea, fatigue, and congestion. The complexity of this condition poses considerable challenges in critical care settings, where timely and effective management strategies heavily influence patient outcomes.[3]

The risk of heart failure (HF) increases with increasing age. HF is frequently a progressive disease process and is associated with decreased survival, irrespective of the underlying etiology.

The recent introduction of angiotensin receptor-neprilysin inhibitors (ARNI), particularly sacubitril/valsartan, has transformed the therapeutic landscape for HF, primarily focusing on patients with HF with reduced ejection fraction (HFrEF).[4] However, emerging evidence suggests that ARNI may also offer benefits for patients with HFpEF, a subgroup that has historically been difficult to treat effectively.[5]

The mechanisms underlying HFpEF involve a multifactorial interplay of comorbidities, including hypertension, obesity, and diabetes, which contribute to increased left ventricular filling pressures and subsequent HF symptoms. ARNI works by enhancing the natriuretic peptide system while inhibiting the RAAS, leading to vasodilation, reduced blood pressure, and improved renal function.[6] These pharmacological effects can potentially alleviate the congestion and fluid overload commonly seen in HFpEF patients, thereby improving their functional capacity and quality of life.

Recent clinical trials, such as the PARAGON-HF study, have provided compelling evidence that ARNI can reduce the risk of cardiovascular death and hospitalizations due to HF in patients with HfpEF.[7] The study demonstrated that sacubitril/valsartan significantly improved outcomes compared to traditional therapies, which often provide limited relief for this patient population. The favorable safety profile and tolerability of ARNI further underscore its potential role in managing HFpEF in critical care settings.

CLASSIFICATION

The American College of Cardiology and the American Heart Association (ACC/AHA) have established a comprehensive framework for understanding HF, categorizing it into four distinct stages: A, B, C, and D.[8] Each stage reflects the progression of HF and informs therapeutic interventions to mitigate risks and improve patient outcomes.

Stage A identifies individuals at risk for HF but without any symptoms or structural heart disease. Here, the focus is on modifying underlying risk factors. *Stage B* encompasses patients with evidence of structural heart disease or increased filling pressures, albeit without overt symptoms. Therapeutic efforts at this stage aim to manage risk factors and treat existing structural abnormalities. *Stage C* marks the onset of symptomatic HF, where patients exhibit structural heart disease along with current or previous symptoms. At this juncture, therapeutic interventions aim to alleviate symptoms, reduce morbidity, and lower mortality rates. *Stage D* represents advanced HF, characterized by severe symptoms that significantly impair daily activities and frequent hospitalizations despite optimal medical therapy. Therapeutic strategies here are focused on symptom relief and improving quality of life.

The ACC, AHA, and Heart Failure Society of America (HFSA) guidelines categorize HF into four types:[9] HF with reduced ejection fraction (HFrEF), HF with improved ejection fraction (HFimpEF), HF with mildly reduced ejection fraction (HFmrEF), and HFpEF. Notably, HFpEF constitutes approximately 50% of HF cases and presents unique challenges in diagnosis and management. While all HF patients exhibit some degree of diastolic dysfunction, not all with diastolic dysfunction meet the criteria for HFpEF.

The diagnosis of HFpEF can be challenging, particularly in patients with overt signs or symptoms of congestion. However, approximately 50% of patients with HF are classified as HFpEF; not all patients with HFpEF will progress to HFrEF. HFpEF is a heterogeneous clinical syndrome with many phenotypes, and the underlying pathophysiological processes of HFpEF differ from those of HFrEF.

While there are clear treatment guidelines for HFrEF, specific recommendations for treating HFpEF are limited, largely due to insufficient scientific evidence. However, there is general agreement that managing symptoms and risk factors, like controlling blood pressure, is important for HFpEF patients. The lack of effective treatments that can improve outcomes for those with HFpEF represents a significant public health challenge.

PATHOPHYSIOLOGY OF HEART FAILURE

The pathophysiology of HFpEF is multifaceted, involving a constellation of factors that contribute to both diastolic and systolic dysfunction. Central to this process are abnormalities such as chronotropic incompetence, left atrial dysfunction, and atrial fibrillation, alongside arterial stiffening, autonomic imbalance, and endothelial dysfunction. These interrelated factors collectively impair cardiac output reserve, thereby exacerbating LV filling pressures and culminating in symptomatic HF.[10]

Moreover, peripheral impairments cannot be overlooked in the context of HFpEF. Deterioration in endothelial function, alterations in body composition, and compromised skeletal muscle performance all play pivotal roles in the disease's manifestation. These peripheral abnormalities contribute to a decreased exercise tolerance and exacerbate the challenges posed by HFpEF, necessitating a comprehensive approach to management that transcends traditional cardiac interventions.[11]

ROLE OF RENIN ANGIOTENSIN SYSTEM (FLOWCHART 1)

The RAAS is often overactive in various stages of cardiovascular disease, from high blood pressure (hypertension) to HF. This makes RAAS a key focus for treatment in cardiovascular medicine, especially for HF patients.[12]

In patients experiencing HFpEF, the activation of the RAAS contributes to cardiac fibrosis and rigidity, impaired diastolic function, and corresponding alterations in myocardial function. It also leads to elevated systolic and diastolic blood pressures, unfavorable interaction between arterial and ventricular pulsatile load, and arterial stiffening accompanied by decreased arterial compliance, as evidenced by increased pulse wave velocity.

ROLE OF ANGIOTENSIN RECEPTOR NEPRILYSIN INHIBITORS THERAPY IN HEART FAILURE WITH PRESERVED EJECTION FRACTION

The ARNI is a revolutionary treatment that combines the benefits of angiotensin receptor blockade with neprilysin inhibition **(Flowchart 2)**.

Mechanism of Action

- *ARNI combines two drugs:* Sacubitril and valsartan.
- Sacubitril inhibits neprilysin, an enzyme that breaks down natriuretic peptides, leading to vasodilation and sodium excretion.

Flowchart 1: Renin-angiotensin-aldosterone system.

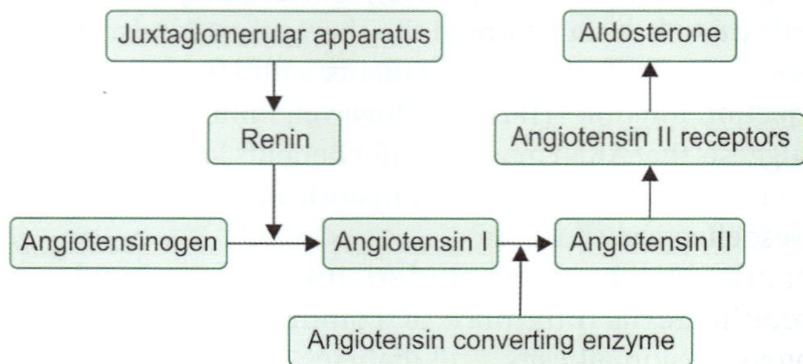

Flowchart 2: Angiotensin receptor neprilysin inhibitors therapy.

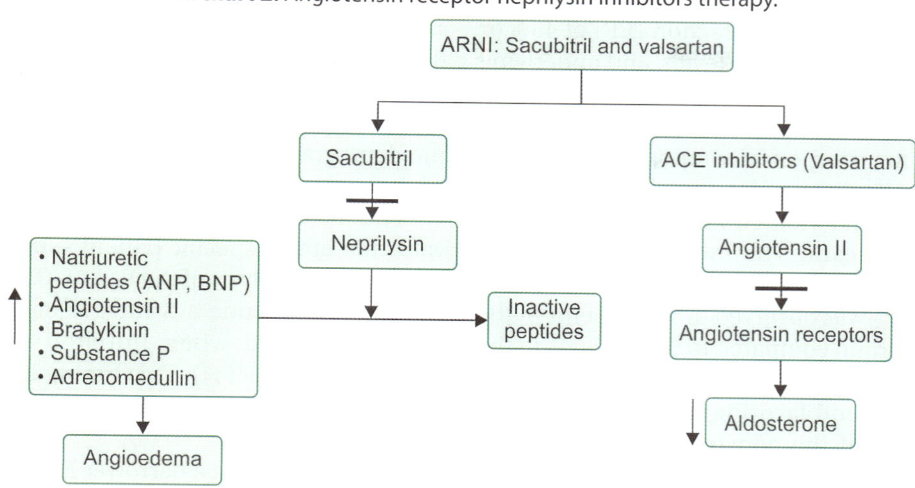

(ACE: angiotensin-converting enzyme; ANP: atrial natriuretic peptide; BNP: B-type natriuretic peptide)

- Valsartan is an angiotensin II receptor blocker (ARB) that prevents blood vessel constriction, reducing blood pressure.

At present, the sacubitril and valsartan combination is the only available ARNI. The medication is approved by the Food and Drug Administration (FDA) to treat patients with HFrEF with NYHA class II, III, or IV symptoms.

Sacubitril cannot be used alone. Sacubitril mediates inhibition of neprilysin which leads to the accumulation of angiotensin II and bradykinin. Sacubitril cannot be used with an angiotensin-converting enzyme inhibitors (ACEI). Both of these mechanisms build up bradykinin and therefore lead to an increased risk of angioedema. Also, a washout period of 36 hours is a must while switching between ACEI and ARNI, to decrease the risk of angioedema. ARNi is contraindicated in case of a known hypersensitivity, history of angioedema, confirmed pregnancy, and in patients on aliskiren; a renin inhibitor.

Sacubitril/valsartan is taken orally and converted into LBQ657. The oral bioavailability of sacubitril is at least 60%. About 52–68% of sacubitril (as LBQ657) and 13% of valsartan are excreted in the urine, while 37–48% of sacubitril and 86% of valsartan are eliminated through feces.

GUIDELINE-DIRECTED MEDICAL THERAPY FOR HEART FAILURE WITH PRESERVED EJECTION FRACTION

Guideline-directed medical therapy (GDMT) for HFpEF primarily focuses on managing symptoms and underlying conditions, as there are currently no specific therapies proven to improve outcomes specifically for HFpEF patients. However, some key components of GDMT include controlling hypertension, managing heart rate, optimizing volume status, and treating comorbidities such as diabetes, anemia, and obesity. Sodium-glucose cotransporter-2 (SGLT2) inhibitors and ARNIs have shown some benefit in certain cases, but the overall management still requires a comprehensive approach tailored to each patient.[13]

Angiotensin Receptor Neprilysin Inhibitors in Heart Failure-trials and Outcomes

The HF in critical care can lead to congestion, low cardiac output, and hemodynamic instability. Diagnostic tests include ECG, chest X-ray, biomarkers, and echocardiogram. Treatment involves prioritizing life-threatening concerns, with medication prescribed according to the standard guidelines, including ACC and AHA. Over 50% of cases are HFpEF. Once acute decompensated heart failure (ADHF) patients are stabilized in critical care units, it is crucial to prioritize minimizing the risk of morbidity, mortality, and hospital readmissions.[14]

PARAGON-HF Trial: Evaluating Angiotensin Receptor Neprilysin Inhibitors versus Angiotensin-receptor Blockers in Heart Failure with Preserved Ejection Fraction[15]

The prospective comparison of ARNI with angiotensin-receptor blockers (ARB) global outcomes in HF with preserved ejection fraction (PARAGON-HF) trial represents a significant investigation into therapeutic options for patients with HFpEF. This randomized, double-blind, active-comparator trial enrolled 4,822 patients exhibiting NYHA class II–IV HF, an ejection fraction (EF) of 45% or greater, elevated natriuretic peptide levels, and underlying structural heart disease. Participants were assigned to receive either sacubitril-valsartan or valsartan, with the primary outcome focusing on a composite of total HF hospitalizations and cardiovascular mortality.

Results from the trial yielded insightful data albeit not statistically significant. The incidence of primary events—a composite of HF hospitalization and cardiovascular death—was observed in 526 patients in the sacubitril-valsartan group compared to 557 patients in the valsartan group. The rate ratio of 0.87 (95% CI, 0.75–1.01; $p = 0.06$) indicated a trend favoring sacubitril-valsartan, although it fell short of the conventional significance threshold. Notably, cardiovascular mortality rates were 8.5% for the sacubitril-valsartan cohort versus 8.9% in the valsartan group (hazard ratio, 0.95; 95% CI, 0.79–1.16). Furthermore, significant differences emerged concerning hospitalizations for HF, showcasing 690 events in the sacubitril-valsartan group against 797 in the valsartan group (rate ratio, 0.85; 95% CI, 0.72–1.00).

The secondary outcomes highlighted improvements in functional status, with 15.0% of the sacubitril-valsartan group experiencing NYHA class improvement, compared to 12.6% in the valsartan group (odds ratio, 1.45; 95% CI, 1.13–1.86). Additionally, renal function was more stable in the sacubitril-valsartan cohort, exhibiting a lower rate of worsening renal function (1.4% vs. 2.7%; hazard ratio, 0.50; 95% CI, 0.33–0.77). The Kansas City Cardiomyopathy Questionnaire (KCCQ) clinical summary score revealed a modest mean increase of 1.0 point (95% CI, 0.0–2.1) for those receiving sacubitril-valsartan.

Regarding safety, an increased incidence of hypotension and angioedema was noted in the sacubitril-valsartan group, while hyperkalemia rates decreased. Reassuringly, potential benefits were suggested across specific subgroups, including those with lower ejection fractions and female patients. In patients with HFpEF, sacubitril-valsartan resulted in a lower level of N-terminal pro-B-type natriuretic peptide (NT-proBNP), a larger reduction in left atrial size, and greater improvement in the NYHA functional class than valsartan.

In conclusion, while sacubitril-valsartan demonstrated favorable trends and safety profiles relative to valsartan in patients with HFpEF, it did not significantly reduce total hospitalizations or cardiovascular mortality. These results warrant further investigation into the nuanced effects of ARNI in various patient demographics and highlight the complexity of managing HHpEF. The PARAGON-HF trial, has undoubtedly added valuable data to the ongoing discourse on HF management in clinical practice.

The recent expansion of the US FDA approval of sacubitril/valsartan marks a significant development in the management of HF with preserved ejection fraction (HFpEF), particularly for patients with an EF in the range of 0.45–0.57. This designation is especially pertinent given the demographic composition of HFpEF patients, where women represent a substantial proportion.

The evidence suggesting benefits of sacubitril/valsartan in this specific patient subgroup is compelling. The posthoc analysis of the PARAGON-HF study indicates that the therapeutic advantages of sacubitril/valsartan are accentuated when initiated shortly after a HF hospitalization (HFH). This timing is crucial; it targets a vulnerable cohort that experiences a higher risk of short-term morbidity.

The emphasis on a narrower EF threshold, specifically below 0.60, highlights a focused approach to treatment that may improve clinical outcomes for a traditionally challenging patient population.

PARAGLIDE-HF Trial: Implications of Sacubitril/Valsartan in Heart Failure with Preserved Ejection Fraction Management[16]

The PARAGLIDE-HF clinical trial, spearheaded by Mentz et al. investigated the efficacy of sacubitril/valsartan compared to valsartan alone in patients with HFpEF who experienced a recent worsening HF event. This double-blind, multicenter study enrolled 466 patients who were stabilized postdecompensation. The primary objective was to ascertain the impact of sacubitril/valsartan on the reduction of NT-proBNP levels, a key biomarker in HF management.

The study was meticulously designed to detect a statistically significant relative reduction of 23% in NT-proBNP levels in the sacubitril/valsartan group compared to the valsartan monotherapy group. Ultimately, the findings revealed a nominally significant 15% greater reduction in NT-proBNP levels for patients receiving sacubitril/valsartan, with a 95% confidence interval of 0–27% and a p-value of 0.049. This outcome demonstrates the potential of sacubitril/valsartan not only to improve clinical markers of HF but also to offer a therapeutic advancement in the management of HFpEF.

In conclusion, the PARAGLIDE-HF trial results contribute valuable insights into the treatment of HFpEF, evidencing that sacubitril/valsartan can significantly reduce NT-proBNP levels following a worsening HF event. This finding holds implications for clinical practice, suggesting that incorporating sacubitril/valsartan in the therapeutic arsenal for HFpEF may enhance patient outcomes and warrant further investigation into its broader applications in HF management.

Prospective Comparison of Angiotensin Receptor—Neprilysin Inhibitors with Angiotensin-receptor Blockers on Management of HFpEF (PARAMOUNT) Trial[17]

The HFpEF represents a significant clinical challenge, characterized by a complex interplay of hemodynamic and neurohormonal alterations. The PARAMOUNT study, a phase 2 trial, investigated the efficacy of sacubitril-valsartan, an ARNI, in comparison to valsartan, in patients diagnosed with HFpEF. The findings of this study have provided a critical foundation for further exploration of ARNI therapy within this patient population.

In the PARAMOUNT study, sacubitril-valsartan demonstrated superior efficacy over valsartan in achieving significant reductions in levels of NT-proBNP. Over a 12-week period, patients receiving sacubitril-valsartan exhibited pronounced improvements, suggesting a more effective modulation of the neurohormonal pathways involved in HFpEF. This outcome is pivotal, given that elevated NT-proBNP levels correlate with disease severity and prognosis.

The rationale for pursuing ARNI therapy in HFpEF is rooted in the multifaceted pathophysiology of the condition, which involves not only fluid overload but also inflammation, fibrosis, and altered neurohormonal regulation. By simultaneously inhibiting neprilysin and blocking angiotensin II receptor activity, sacubitril-valsartan addresses these divergent mechanisms more comprehensively than ARBs alone.

Furthermore, the results of PARAMOUNT strengthen the argument for moving towards larger-scale trials to assess the long-term implications of ARNI use in HFpEF management. Such studies could potentially elucidate the role of ARNI in improving clinical outcomes, functional capacity, and overall quality of life in this often under-treated population.

New research has found that ARNi medications sacubitril and valsartan can improve quality of life and renal function in patients with ADHF and HFpEF. Results from a study of over 4800 patients showed that these medications were safe and well-tolerated, with positive outcomes in reducing NT-proBNP levels. The PIONEER-HF trial found that sacubitril/valsartan was superior to enalapril in reducing NT-proBNP levels and the risk of serious clinical events by 46%, with no significant difference in adverse events or laboratory abnormalities.

A publication from India provides practical recommendations for the use of ARNi in HF. ARNi medications like sacubitril and valsartan can be crucial in treating HF patients with reduced, preserved, or improved EF. Transthoracic echocardiography (TTE) and biomarkers can be used to diagnose HF. GDMT should be more widely utilized by following these recommendations. Sacubitril/valsartan has been recommended as a replacement for an ACE inhibitor.

Hot trials 2023 is a great resource for staying up-to-date on ongoing critical care trials, including ARNI. Featured trials include PILOT NITRIC, FIRST-ABC, and PLUS. These trials assess the safety and effectiveness of sacubitril/valsartan in treating HF patients.

Expanded Approval of ENTRESTO®: A Milestone in Heart Failure Management[18]

The approval of ENTRESTO® (sacubitril/valsartan) by the FDA in February 2021 represents a pivotal advancement in the treatment landscape for HF. This expansion of the medication's indications to include all patients with chronic HF, regardless of their left ventricular ejection fraction (LVEF), addresses a longstanding deficiency in therapeutic options, particularly for individuals diagnosed with HFpEF.

Traditionally, treatment strategies for HF have predominantly focused on patients with reduced ejection fraction (HFrEF), often neglecting the significant clinical needs of those suffering from HFpEF. These patients, despite their substantial prevalence, have been largely underrepresented in treatment protocols, thereby highlighting the urgent requirement for more inclusive medical approaches. The FDA's decision to include HFpEF patients in the ENTRESTO® eligible population marks a momentous shift in this paradigm, recognizing the multifaceted nature of HF as a syndrome that transcends LVEF metrics. This recommendation should be considered carefully because it is based on a subgroup analysis that involves a trial that did not reach its primary endpoint.

This regulatory change is anticipated to improve clinical outcomes and enhance the quality of life for millions of patients who previously lacked access to effective treatment options. Moreover, it has the potential to alleviate the broader healthcare burden associated with managing HF, thus benefiting both patients and healthcare systems alike.

CONCLUSION

The ACC/AHA staging system, combined with the NYHA classification and LVEF stratification, provides a robust framework for understanding HF. This multifaceted approach allows for tailored therapeutic interventions that address the specific needs of patients at various stages of HF, ultimately aiming to enhance their quality of life and reduce the burden of this prevalent condition.[19]

While HFpEF remains a complex and challenging condition, the advent of ARNI offers a promising avenue for improving patient outcomes. By addressing the underlying pathophysiology of HFpEF and providing symptomatic relief, ARNI can enhance the quality of care for critical care patients suffering from this debilitating condition. Continued research and clinical application of ARNI in HFpEF will be crucial in refining treatment protocols and improving the prognosis for these patients.[20]

REFERENCES

1. Campbell P, Rutten FH, Lee MM, et al. Heart failure with preserved ejection fraction: everything the clinician needs to know. Lancet. 2024;403(10431):1083-92.
2. LeWinter MM, Meyer M. Mechanisms of diastolic dysfunction in heart failure with a preserved ejection fraction: If it's not one thing it's another. Circ Heart Fail. 2013;6(6):1112-5.
3. Bozkurt B, Coats AJS, Tsutsui H, et al. Universal Definition and Classification of Heart Failure. J Cardiac Failure. 2021;27(4):387-413.
4. Greenberg B. Angiotensin Receptor-Neprilysin Inhibition (ARNI) in Heart Failure. Int J Heart Fail. 2020;2(2):73-90.
5. Morin-Grandmont A, Walsh-Wilkinson E, Thibodeau SÈ, et al. A murine model of hypertensive heart disease in older women. PeerJ. 2024;12:(e17434).
6. Lin Y, Fu S, Yao Y, et al. Heart failure with preserved ejection fraction based on aging and comorbidities. J Transl Med. 2021;19(1):291.
7. Gronda E, Vanoli E, Iacoviello M. The PARAGON-HF trial: the sacubitril/valsartan in heart failure with preserved ejection fraction. Eur Heart J Suppl. 2020;22(Suppl L): L77-L81.
8. Bozkurt B, Hershberger RE, Butler J, et al. 2021 ACC/AHA Key Data Elements and Definitions for Heart Failure: A Report of the American College of Cardiology/American Heart Association Task Force on Clinical Data Standards (Writing Committee to Develop Clinical Data Standards for Heart Failure. Circulation: Cardiovascular Quality and Outcomes. J Am Coll Cardiol. 2021;77(16): 2053-150.
9. Behnoush AH, Khalaji A, Naderi N, et al. ACC/AHA/HFSA 2022 and ESC 2021 guidelines on heart failure comparison. ESC Heart Fail. 2023;10(3):1531-44.
10. Golla MSG, Shams P. Heart Failure With Preserved Ejection Fraction (HFpEF). In: StatPearls. Treasure Island (FL): StatPearls Publishing; 2024.
11. Saw EL, Ramachandran S, Valero-Muñoz M, et al. Skeletal muscle (dys) function in heart failure with preserved ejection fraction. Curr Opin Cardiol. 2021;36(2):219-26.
12. Ames MK, Atkins CE, Pitt B. The renin-angiotensin-aldosterone system and its suppression. J Vet Intern Med. 2019;33(5):2551.
13. Zhang Z, Wang C, Tu T, et al. Advancing Guideline-Directed Medical Therapy in Heart Failure: Overcoming Challenges and Maximizing Benefits. Am J Cardiovasc Drugs. 2024;24(3):329-42.
14. Malik A, Brito D, Vaqar S, et al. Congestive Heart Failure. In: StatPearls. Treasure Island (FL): StatPearls Publishing; 2024.
15. Solomon SD, McMurray JJV, Anand IS. Angiotensin–Neprilysin Inhibition in Heart Failure with Preserved Ejection Fraction. New Engl J Med. 2019;381(17):1609-20.
16. Vaduganathan M, Mentz RJ, Claggett BL, et al. Sacubitril/valsartan in heart failure with mildly reduced or preserved ejection fraction: a pre-specified participant-level pooled analysis of PARAGLIDE-HF and PARAGON-HF. Eur Heart J. 2023;44(31):2982-93.
17. Biering-Sørensen T, Lassen MCH, Shah A, et al.; PARAMOUNT Investigators. The Effect of Sacubitril/Valsartan on Left Ventricular Myocardial Deformation in Heart Failure with Preserved Ejection Fraction (PARAMOUNT trial). J Card Fail. 2023;29(6):968-73.
18. Khalil P, Kabbach G, Said S, et al. Entresto, a New Panacea for Heart Failure? Cardiovasc Hematol Agents Med Chem. 2018;16(1):5-11.
19. Joglar JA, Chung MK, Armbruster AL, et al. 2023 ACC/AHA/ACCP/HRS Guideline for the Diagnosis and Management of Atrial Fibrillation: A Report of the American College of Cardiology/American Heart Association Joint Committee on Clinical Practice Guidelines. Circulation. 2024;149(24):e1413.
20. Sapna F, Raveena F, Chandio M, et al. Advancements in Heart Failure Management: A Comprehensive Narrative Review of Emerging Therapies. Cureus. 2023;15(10): e46486.

CHAPTER

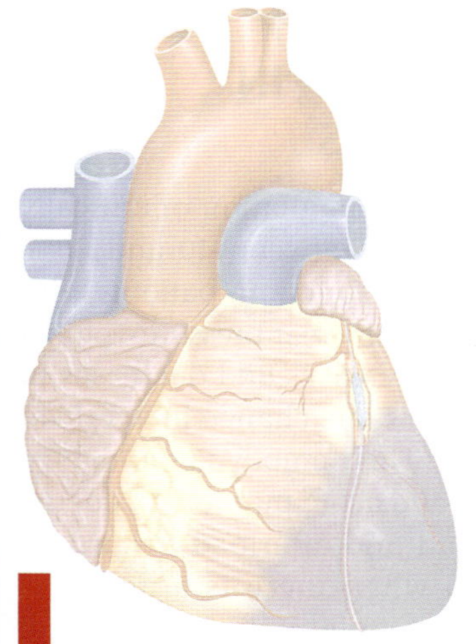

HFpEF Care in an Intensive Care Unit

Bhavik Shah, Girish Sabnis, Sadanand Shetty

INTRODUCTION

Since its first description in 1998, the grave impact of left ventricular diastolic dysfunction (DD) on the outcome of patients with heart failure has been well established. However, the relevance of DD for critically ill patients admitted to the intensive care unit (ICU) has seen growing interest in the recent years.[1] Acute deterioration in myocardial function is a common finding in critically ill patients. Cardiac dysfunction in such patients may contribute to multiorgan failure leading to increased mortality. Heart failure with preserved ejection fraction (HFpEF) can be the reason for ICU admission itself or can result from another critical illness.[2] In this chapter, the authors illustrate a holistic approach toward understanding the complexities of HFpEF in ICU with the current guidelines and their intrinsic limitations.

DIAGNOSTIC DILEMMA OF HFpEF IN ICU

Echocardiography is essential for the noninvasive evaluation of left ventricular diastolic function in an ICU. It comprehends a number of mechanisms and measurements including active myocardial relaxation, left ventricular compliance, and estimation of left atrial pressure as pathophysiological consequences of worsening left ventricular DD. Besides, these variables do not show a linear trajectory with worsening of dysfunction as it happens for changes in left ventricular ejection fraction to describe the systolic function. Such a nonlinear change in the variables is due to activation of compensatory mechanisms.[1]

In the context of ICU patients, it is worth noting that a crucial aspect of HFpEF is the question of whether the left ventricular filling pressure is increased or not, with an understanding of the repercussions on pulmonary circulation and respiratory function. Over the years, we have seen evolution in the diagnosis and grading of DD. The 2016 American Society of Echocardiography (ASE) guidelines have proposed an algorithmic approach that includes mainly four parameters for the assessment of DD on echocardiography. This algorithm relies on the e' values, mitral E/e' ratio, left atrial volume, and tricuspid regurgitation jet velocity.[3] ICU clinicians understanding the relevance of DD for the outcome of their critically ill patients are often left puzzled questioning the use of these parameters and their cutoffs suggested by the current guidelines in the ICU setting.

It should be considered that parameters used for the assessment of HFpEF become more challenging when applied to critically ill patients due to fluid shifts with variation in preload, changes in afterload, and use of vasoactive drugs, just to name a few. Thus, a fair number of patients may remain in a gray zone between normal and abnormal DD. Besides, knowing whether an increase in left atrial pressure or the left ventricular filling pressure has led to DD in critically ill patients would be helpful to the clinician for devising a further plan of action in the ICU. Addressing such questions is far more complex with echocardiography, yet the answer has significant clinical implications, with consequences on the interpretation of hemodynamic and respiratory parameters, on the appropriateness of performing fluid challenges, or to apply a rather restrictive approach.

The cutoffs validated for self-breathing patients cannot be easily translated into the typical ICU patients supported with inotropes or vasopressors, sedated and ventilated, and exposed to large fluid shifts. In critically ill and mechanically ventilated patients, the cutoff values of the *E/e′* ratio to predict an increase in left atrial pressure have consistently differed from those suggested in outpatients, and a ratio of 8 seems the most likely appropriate threshold in predicting an increase in left atrial pressure rather than the current cutoff ranging between 13 and 15 used for the outpatient population.[4] The guidelines are based on a cross-sectional approach of assessing the DD rather than identifying acute deterioration of it, and ICU patients suffering from acute conditions may experience rapid clinical evolutions that cannot be detected by the conventional ranges of these parameters.

It needs to be reminded that even though left ventricular filling pressure and left atrial pressure are frequently used interchangeably, they do not, from a physiological standpoint, convey the same information. The closest estimate of left ventricular preload serving as a proxy for left ventricular end-diastolic volume is provided by the end-diastolic pressure, which also gives information regarding left ventricular compliance. Patients with similar end-diastolic pressure can experience significantly varying left atrial pressure. This idea is extremely important in the ICU, because fluid challenges and modifications to mechanical ventilator settings can result in changes to left atrial compliance. Hence, a more detailed study of the left atrium may be desirable to manage critically ill patients.

CLINICAL IMPLICATIONS OF DIASTOLIC DYSFUNCTION IN CRITICALLY ILL PATIENTS

The incidence of DD in selected population of critically ill patients is estimated to vary between 40 and 80%. Compared with normal diastolic function, patients with DD have a deviation in the left ventricular pressure–volume curve leading to exaggerated increases and decreases in left ventricular pressure for the same change in afterload and preload **(Figs. 1A and B)**.[5] This hemodynamic change results in hypertensive crisis and acute pulmonary edema when an increase in preload and afterload occurs, or hypotension and azotemia when there is a decrease in preload or afterload. There are a number of clinical situations where DD could play a key role in critically ill patients, worsening the evolution and prognosis. Some of these conditions have been addressed in detail in the following text.

Acute Pulmonary Edema

The apparent diagnosis of acute pulmonary edema due to HFpEF requires the presence of signs and symptoms of heart failure, normal systolic function including left ventricular end-diastolic volume index <97 mL/m^2, and evidence of DD. The deviation in left ventricular pressure–volume curve in DD may lead to abrupt pulmonary edema secondary to various precipitating factors such as volume overload, tachycardia, rhythm disturbances, or hypertensive crisis. Hypertensive acute pulmonary edema is the usual presentation in ICU patients. Gandhi et al. demonstrated isolated variations in diastolic function with

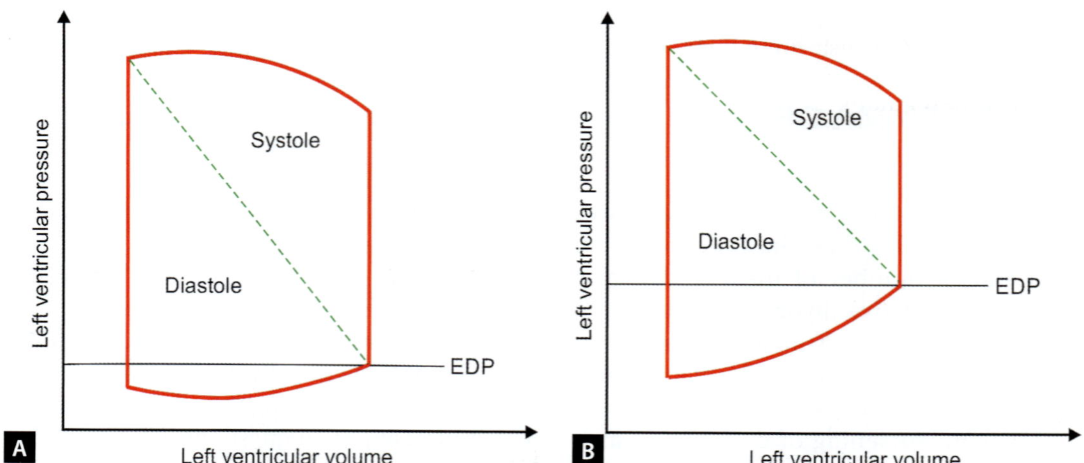

Figs. 1A and B: Pressure–volume curve of (A) a healthy subject compared to (B) a critically ill patient with HFpEF. Note the increase of end-diastolic pressure (EDP) for the same end-diastolic volume in case of diastolic dysfunction.

no variation in parameters of systolic function in patients presenting with acute pulmonary edema as a consequence of severe arterial hypertension.[6] These findings suggest that DD was the sole mechanism of decompensation. Apparently, 50% of patients presenting with acute pulmonary edema had a preserved ejection fraction.[5]

Myocardial Ischemia

Myocardial ischemia, along with hypertensive crisis, is one of the main precipitating mechanisms of DD. Myocardial ischemia and derived arrythmias may lead to a significant decrease in myocardial relaxation and aggravate the degree of DD. Physiological studies in animal models undergoing induced ischemia have evidenced that DD was present even before systolic dysfunction. If no severe myocardial injury has been established, the DD normalized after reperfusion. On the other hand, patients with myocardial infarction and preserved ejection fraction remained in impaired relaxation pattern and those with myocardial infarction and depressed ejection fraction showed a pseudonormal pattern secondary to reduced compliance and increased end-diastolic pressures.

Sepsis

Myocardial dysfunction is a common phenomenon in patients with sepsis or septic shock, characterized by deterioration of biventricular contractility and relaxation, thus altering systolic and diastolic function. This is the most complex sepsis-induced organ failure to characterize because of the dynamic evolution due to the adaptation of the cardiovascular system to the disease process and resuscitation treatment. The pathophysiology is rather complex and multifactorial including systemic, intra- and extracellular mechanisms like abnormal distribution of coronary blood flow due to nitric oxide metabolism deregulation, excess of proinflammatory cytokines, calcium metabolism deregulation, and hypoxia. These changes finally lead to an impairment in the contractility and relaxation of both ventricles.

The incidence of DD related to septic shock is around 20–56% and is considered an independent predictor of early mortality.[7,8] Left ventricular DD can complicate hemodynamic management of patients with severe sepsis or septic shock due to a poor clinical response to fluid challenges. While fluids are one of the most important therapies to improve hemodynamic in sepsis, the positive fluid balance in patients with DD may aggravate lung congestion and noncardiogenic pulmonary edema leading to pulmonary hypertension and hypoxemia. According to Mahjoub et al., a significant increase in *E/e'* after volume expansion in patients with sepsis-induced DD and nonresponders to fluid challenges points toward an increase in left ventricular filling pressures, whereas patients with DD and responders to fluid challenge showed an increase in *e'* but not in *E/e'*, suggesting that left ventricular relaxation can be improved in preload-dependent patients.[9]

Weaning from Mechanical Ventilation

Many asymptomatic patients attending outpatient clinics with early stages of DD develop symptoms due to a deterioration of diastolic function during exercise. Similarly, spontaneous breathing trial (SBT) with low levels of pressure support may cause symptoms of heart failure even in patients with early stages of DD. Pulmonary artery catheterization remains the gold standard to clearly identify such a scenario of heart failure during SBT. However, advances in echocardiography in critically ill during the past decade have replaced the pulmonary artery catheterization in this setting.[10] Classically, weaning-induced pulmonary edema has been related to systolic dysfunction. However, a few studies have concluded that the presence of DD before SBT can predict weaning failure where $E/e' > 7.8$.[5] According to Moschietto et al., patients who failed the weaning process had a lower *e'* and slightly higher *E/e'* before SBT than patients who successfully passed the SBT.[11] Ten minutes after starting the SBT, weaning was successful when the patients were capable to maintain the *E/e'* ratio, thanks to a proportional increase in both *E* and *e'*. On the contrary, patients who failed weaning could not face the increase in *E* (due to an increased venous return) with a potential increase in *e'* (due to a DD) resulting in an elevated *E/e'* suggestive of an increase in left ventricular filling pressures.[5]

"CHEOPS" BUNDLE

The Doppler echocardiography has been considered the "Rosetta Stone" for studying DD. Apart from the left atrial volume, all currently used variables for the assessment of left ventricular DD are based on Doppler echocardiography. Hence, Sanfilippo et al. proposed a bundle based on Doppler echocardiography that could be useful for managing DD in critically ill patients.[1] The bundle with its aspects is summarized under the acronym of CHEOPS, the famous ancient Egyptian Pharaoh (also known as Khufu) of the Fourth Dynasty living in the first half of the 26th century before Christ. The CHEOPS bundle has been summarized in short in **Table 1**.

Due to its complex nature, left ventricular DD in critically ill patients should be managed by a multifaceted

TABLE 1: CHEOPS bundle for managing DD in critically ill patients.

Items of CHEOPS bundle	*Clinical Implications*
Chest ultrasound	The use of echocardiography is mandatory for evaluation of DD and for the non-invasive evaluation of LV filling pressure
HEmodynamics	Assessment of hemodynamics to achieve: • Heart rate as low as reasonable • Prevent atrial fibrillation • Maintain adequate afterload
OPtimize PEEP	Ensure positive effects of mechanical ventilation and PEEP on biventricular function: • To set PEEP in order to facilitate left ventricular ejection and decrease preload • To favor alveolar recruitment with beneficial effects on pulmonary vascular resistance • Avoid right ventricular dilatation
Stabilization and fluid removal	For the clinical stabilization, consider fluid administration cautiously due to a high risk of congestion. Once stabilized, start personalized fluid removal to reduce ventricular filling pressures.

(DD: diastolic dysfunction; LV: left ventricular; PEEP: positive end-expiratory pressure)

proactive approach. This CHEOPS bundle includes the use of *C*hest ultrasound; *HE*modynamics considerations on heart rate and rhythm, as well as on afterload; *OP*timization of mechanical ventilation and pulmonary circulation; and *S*tabilization and fluid removal with a personalized approach targeting negative fluid balance. However, whether any dedicated management of patients with left ventricular DD improves outcomes remains an area that deserves further research.

MANAGEMENT OF HFpEF IN ICU

No treatment has yet been shown to reduce morbidity and mortality in patients with HFpEF. Treatment should rather be targeted toward reducing symptoms by decreasing cardiac preload. This target can be achieved by lowering left ventricular volume, blunting neurohormonal activation, maintaining atrial contraction, and preventing tachycardia. Besides, management of concomitant cardiovascular as well as noncardiovascular diseases and their precipitating causes is of utmost importance. In the acute setting of critically ill patients, no specific studies focused on the treatment of HFpEF. Its treatment is still based on a reduction in pulmonary congestion and correction of precipitating factors.

CONCLUSION

- HFpEF is a common feature in ICU patients. Echocardiography plays a key role in the diagnosis of DD in critically ill patients.
- Use of routine echocardiography can help to identify early stages of DD and repeated echocardiography throughout the ICU stay could help to adjust the therapy and improve the prognosis of critically ill patients.
- Epidemiological studies regarding DD are needed in ICU patients in order to know the magnitude of the problem and to better understand those scenarios where DD could worsen the patients' outcome.

REFERENCES

1. Sanfilippo F, Messina A, Scolletta S, et al. The "CHEOPS" bundle for the management of Left Ventricular Diastolic Dysfunction in critically ill patients: an experts' opinion. Anaesth Crit Care Pain Med. 2023;42(6):101283.
2. Cavefors O, Ljung Faxén U, Bech-Hanssen O, et al. Isolated diastolic dysfunction is associated with increased mortality in critically ill patients. J Crit Care. 2023;76:154290.
3. Gonzalez FA, Santonocito C, Maybauer MO, et al. Diastology in the intensive care unit: Challenges for the assessment and future directions. Echocardiography. 2024;41(2):e15773.
4. La Via L, Merola F, Schembari G, et al. The interplay between left ventricular diastolic and right ventricular dysfunction: challenges in the interpretation of critical care echocardiography studies. Egypt Heart J. 2023;75(1):7.
5. Suárez JC, López P, Mancebo J, et al. Diastolic dysfunction in the critically ill patient. Med Intensiva. 2016;40(8):499-510.
6. Gandhi SK, Powers JC, Nomeir AM, et al. The Pathogenesis of Acute Pulmonary Edema Associated with Hypertension. N Engl J Med. 2001;344(1):17-22.
7. Bouhemad B, Nicolas-Robin A, Arbelot C, et al. Isolated and reversible impairment of ventricular relaxation in patients with septic shock. Crit Care Med. 2008;36(3):766-74.
8. Landesberg G, Gilon D, Meroz Y, et al. Diastolic dysfunction and mortality in severe sepsis and septic shock. Eur Heart J. 2012;33(7):895-903.
9. Mahjoub Y, Benoit-Fallet H, Airapetian N, et al. Improvement of left ventricular relaxation as assessed by tissue Doppler imaging in fluid-responsive critically ill septic patients. Intensive Care Med. 2012;38(9):1461-70.
10. Lamia B, Maizel J, Ochagavia A, et al. Echocardiographic diagnosis of pulmonary artery occlusion pressure elevation during weaning from mechanical ventilation. Crit Care Med. 2009;37(5):1696-701.
11. Moschietto S, Doyen D, Grech L, et al. Transthoracic Echocardiography with Doppler Tissue Imaging predicts weaning failure from mechanical ventilation: evolution of the left ventricle relaxation rate during a spontaneous breathing trial is the key factor in weaning outcome. Crit Care. 2012;16(3): R81.

SECTION 10

HFpEF: Cardio-obstetrician and Gynecology

101. Role of the ARNI and SGL2i in Women with HFpEF
102. Estrogen Deficiency in Postmenopausal Women: Harbinger to HFpEF
103. Gender Differences in HFpEF Pathophysiology
104. Obesity is Culprit in Heart Failure: Do not Miss HFpEF especially in Obese Women
105. HFpEF Risk Decreased with More Physical Activity Among Older Women
106. Heart Failure in Women

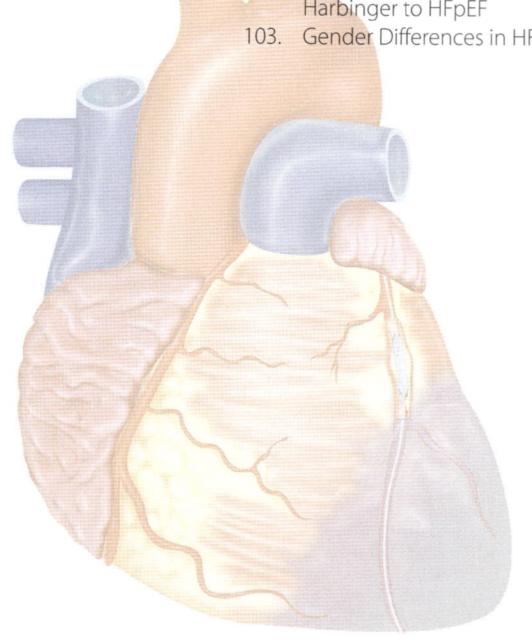

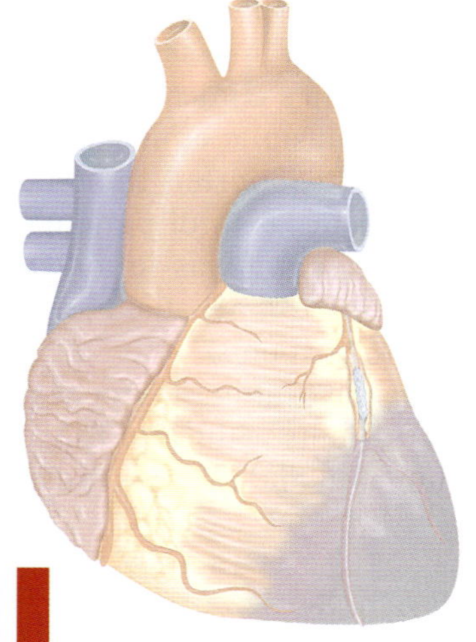

Role of the ARNI and SGL2i in Women with HFpEF

Mohan Bhargava, Sneha Garg

INTRODUCTION

According to the ACC/AHA 2022 guidelines, heart failure (HF) is defined as "a complex clinical syndrome with symptoms and signs that result from any structural or functional impairment of ventricular filling or ejection of blood."[1] Left ventricular ejection fraction (LVEF) is important in HF patients because of prognosis and response to treatments. Diastolic HF defined by the ACC/AHA as heart failure with preserved ejection fraction (HFpEF) has LVEF >50% with evidence of spontaneous/provokable increased LV filling pressures. Diastolic HF accounts for 50% of cases of HF. Women are at increased risk of HFpEF.

The score proposed to diagnose diastolic HF is given in **Table 1**.

A score, including six variables, was used to create the weighted amalgamated score. It ranged from 0 to 9.

TABLE 1: H_2FPEF score: Diagnosis of diastolic heart failure.[2]

	Clinical variable	*Values*	*Points*
H_2	Heavy	Body mass index >30 kg/m^2	2
	Hypertensive	Two or more antihypertensive	1
F	Atrial fibrillation	Paroxysmal or persistent	3
P	Pulmonary hypertension	Pulmonary artery systolic pressure >35 mm Hg (echocardiographic)	1
E	Elder	Age >60 years	1
F	Filling pressure	E/é >9 (echocardiographic)	1

The odds of HFpEF doubled for every 1-unit score increase. The scores <2 and >6 showed low and high likelihood for HFpEF, respectively. Scores between 2 and 5 required further evaluation. Most commonly HFpEF is found in elderly women with comorbid conditions, such as ischemic heart disease (35–70%) that may be occult, hypertension with LV hypertrophy (60–80%), atrial fibrillation (AF) (15–65%), diabetes mellitus (20–45%), obesity (32–46%), renal disease (51–58%), and obstructive lung disease (24–30%) **(Box 1)**.

PATHOPHYSIOLOGICAL MECHANISMS OF DIASTOLIC HEART FAILURE

Diastolic dysfunction of LV in patients with HFpEF results from increased diastolic ventricular stiffness slowing LV relaxation, increasing LV diastolic filling pressures, and limiting cardiac output (CO). **Box 2** shows different pathophysiologic mechanisms that are hypothesized as mechanisms of HFpEF.[3]

BOX 1: Etiology of diastolic heart failure.

Conditions that contribute to heart failure with preserved ejection fraction:

- Obesity
- Hypertension
- Coronary artery disease
- Atrial fibrillation
- Diabetes mellitus
- Chronic obstructive pulmonary disease
- Obstructive sleep apnea

BOX 2: Hypothesis of mechanisms of diastolic heart failure.

- Cardiomyocyte titin hypophosphorylation
- Vascular endothelial cell inflammation and dysfunction
- Abnormal calcium homeostasis
- Increased ventricular matrix formation
- Obesity

BOX 3: Echocardiographic indices of diastolic dysfunction.

- E/A ratio ≥2
- An E/e′ ratio 10 = mild and E/e′ ratio >14 = significant LV dysfunction. If the lateral mitral annulus e′ velocity is not quantifiable, the septal mitral annular e′ velocity can be used. In this case, the E/e′ is increased if the ratio is >15
- Lateral mitral annular e′ velocity <10 cm/s or septal e′ mitral annular velocity <7 cm/s
- PASP >35 mm Hg indicative of PAH. PASP = 4 × (peak tricuspid regurgitation velocity) 2 + estimated RA pressure. Should not be used in patients with significant pulmonary disease
- An echocardiographic determination of global longitudinal strain of −16.05 ± 2.16. This measurement can separate patients with HFpEF from patients with hypertension and normal controls in whom the global longitudinal strain measurements are −18.58 ± 2.84 and −19.59 ± 1.49, respectively

DIAGNOSIS

The HFpEF diagnosis is based on clinical history, laboratory data, examination, echocardiogram, and cardiac catheterization when needed.

In patients with HFpEF, chest radiographs show cardiomegaly and evidence of pulmonary congestion. ECG is suggestive of nonspecific ST-T wave changes or old ischemic changes. AF is present frequently. Markers such as N-terminal pro-BNP (NT-proBNP) or brain natriuretic peptide (BNP) are increased mildly. Usual values are NT-proBNP >300 pg/mL or BNP >100 pg/mL. In HFrEF, higher values are found. But, these values are predictors of MACE in patients with HFpEF independently. In the present scenario, natriuretic peptides and troponins measurements have recommendations for the diagnosis as well as prognosis of patients with HF. For additional risk stratification and prognosis suppression of tumorgenicity 2 (systemic inflammation marker) and galectin-3 (cardiac fibrosis marker), measurements are advised.

A very useful tool is echocardiography for the diagnosis of HFpEF. It is suggestive of LV hypertrophy/concentric LV remodeling with an EF ≥50% and an LV volume index of <97 mL/m^2. LA enlargement with an LA volume index of >34 mL/m^2 is present in patients without AF. Common echocardiographic parameters of significant LVDD are given in **Box 3**.

However, in isolation, echocardiographically measured E/A and E/e′ ratios must not be used in assessing but rather must be used with the patient's clinical features and laboratory data to diagnose diastolic abnormality accurately. The I-PRESERVE study reported that the LVEDV was in the normal range in >95% of patients, LV hypertrophy/concentric remodeling was found in 50–60%, diastolic dysfunction was in >70% of patients, and LA area enlargement was in >65% of patients.

The extracellular matrix of the myocardium is measured with CMR T1 mapping. In patients with HFpEF, it is used to predict diastolic dysfunction and LV myocardial stiffness.

TREATMENT

Role of Sodium–Glucose Cotransporter 2 Inhibitors

EMPEROR-Preserved (Empagliflozin Outcome Trial in Patients with Chronic HFpEF) demonstrated a significant benefit of empagliflozin, an SGLT2i, in symptomatic HF patients with ejection fraction (EF) >40% and elevated natriuretic peptides. It also led to a significant decrease in HF hospitalizations, modest quality of life (QoL) improvement, and decreased eGFR decline slope at 52 weeks. It is important to note that the benefit was similar regardless of the presence/absence of diabetes at diagnosis.[4]

Role of Angiotensin Receptor-neprilysin Inhibitors

Trials with RAAS inhibition did not show much benefit in HFpEF patients. In CHARM-Preserved (Candesartan in Patients with Chronic HF and Preserved LVEF) trial, patients with EF of >40% were randomized into candesartan or the placebo group. The primary endpoint (CV death or HF hospitalization) was not significantly different between the two.[5] An analysis post hoc of CHARM trials showed that the improvement in results with candesartan was more at the lower end of the ejection fraction spectrum.

In the phase II RCT in patients with HFpEF (LVEF ≥45%), i.e., PARAMOUNT-HF (Prospective Comparison of ARNi with ARB on Management of HFpEF) trial, sacubitril–valsartan resulted in a lower value of NT-proBNP after 12 weeks of treatment in comparison with valsartan. In 4,822 patients of HFpEF (LVEF ≥45%, raised natriuretic peptide levels or HF admission within 9 months, and eGFR ≥30 mL/min/1.73 m^2) that is the PARAGON-HF (Prospective Comparison of Angiotensin Receptor-Neprilysin Inhibitor with Angiotensin Receptor Blocker

Global Outcomes in HFpEF) trial, sacubitril–valsartan was compared with valsartan; however, it did not result in a significant reduction in the primary composite. Thus, there was no mortality benefit but showed benefit for the ARNI for HF hospitalizations.[6]

Others

In patients with HFpEF, the treatment with nonsignificant coronary artery disease (CAD) includes weight management and blood pressure control.

The prevalence of obesity in HFpEF is >80%. A diet with caloric restriction is safe and feasible in HFpEF in older and obese patients. This improves the patient's difficulty in breathing, oxygen consumption (peak), and QoL significantly. Along with endurance exercise, the outcomes are additive, such as walking exercise for 1 hour ≥3 times/week. With the cardiac rehabilitation program, the exercise training improves the maximum HR and LV diastolic function (as measured by E/A ratio and the E/e′ ratio).

Systemic inflammatory biomarker concentration in the body attributes to increased skeletal muscle and increased peripheral microvascular function. Weight management and peak O_2 consumption increase result in decreased systemic inflammatory biomarkers.

The importance of BP control is well known for the prevention of HF as well as for decreasing other MACE and HF mortality. More aggressive BP control in patients with high CV risk significantly decreases HF, and other MACE was established by the SPRINT (Systolic Blood Pressure Intervention) trial and meta-analyses. BP targets for HFpEF, according to ACC/AHA 2022 guidelines, are extrapolated from those for the management of hypertension patients in general.[7]

In present times, AF comprehensive care is being extrapolated from the routine clinical guidelines, with strategy individualization for rate/rhythm control in patients with diastolic HF. The RATE-AF trial compared the use of bisoprolol to digoxin in elderly patients with HF symptoms and AF (most with preserved LVEF). The primary endpoint QoL was comparable between the two groups at 6 months. However, many secondary QoL endpoints, reduction in NT-proBNP, and functional capacity favored digoxin at the end of 12 months. Heart rate reduction was comparable in both groups.

Mineralocorticoid receptor antagonists improve diastolic function in patients with diastolic HF. The TOPCAT trial studied the effects of spironolactone in patients with HFpEF. There was a small reduction (HR, 0.89) in the composite of death, averted cardiac death, and HF hospitalization that were not significant statistically.

Flowchart 1: ACC/AHA 2022 recommendations for the treatment of HFpEF.[1]

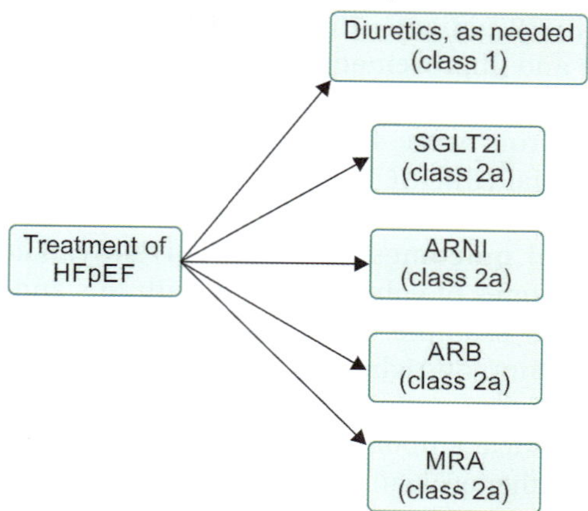

There was a decrease in the number of HF hospitalizations. Adverse effects of hyperkalemia and rising creatinine levels were more common in the treatment group. A benefit possibility in selected patients appropriately with symptomatic HFpEF (LVEF ≥45%, HF admission within 1 year, elevated BNP level, eGFR >30 mL/min/1.73 m^2, Cr <2.5 mg/dL, and K^+ <5.0 mEq/L).[8]

The NEAT-HFpEF (Nitrate's Effect on Activity Tolerance in HFpEF) trial randomized 110 patients with EF of ≥50% on stable HF GDMT, not including nitrates, and with activity limited by fatigue, dyspnea, or chest pain, to either isosorbide mononitrate or placebo. It found no significant beneficial effects on QoL, activity levels, exercise tolerance, and NT-proBNP levels. The RELAX (Phosphodiesterase-5 Inhibition to Improve Clinical Status and Exercise Capacity in HFpEF) trial randomized patients (n = 216) with EF of ≥50% on stable HF GDMT and with decreased exercise tolerance (peak VO_2 <60% of predicted) to PDE-5 inhibition with sildenafil versus placebo. This study did not show improvement in O_2 consumption or exercise tolerance **(Flowchart 1)**.

Medical Devices

Rate-adaptive atrial pacing is being tested in patients with HFpEF and chronotropic incompetence. Patients with HFpEF can develop a marked increase in LA pressures and PAH with exercise because of a reduction in LV diastolic compliance. This is usually presented as exertional dyspnea. New medical devices placed into patients with HFpEF in trials have shown some promise in improving patient symptoms.

Interatrial Septostomy

A unidirectional interatrial left-to-right shunt device of 8 mm in HFpEF patients has shown to reduce LA pressure by 3–11 mm Hg and provide symptomatic relief from dyspnea. In a REDUCE-LA Pressure in HF Randomized Trial I in 39 patients, the reduction in PCWP during exercise and improvement in workload-corrected PCWP, exercise duration, and peak exercise workload compared with controls were better in the treatment group. A larger trial (REDUCE LAP-HF II; Governmental Trial NCT03088033) is studying the effects of an IAS device on clinical outcomes and QoL currently. The long-term outcomes of volume loading with this and similar devices, for example, the V-Wave device and the atrial flow regulator, on right heart dimensions and function, cardiac rhythm, pulmonary circulation, and potential for paradoxical embolism in older patients with HFpEF, require further evaluation.

CONCLUSION

The ACC, AHA, and Heart Failure Society recommended the following treatments for women with diastolic HF (HFpEF) and its symptoms and signs:

- Hypertension treatment in all HFpEF patients with angiotensin-converting enzyme inhibitors, angiotensin receptor blockers, beta-adrenergic receptor blocking drugs, or calcium channel blockers
- Treatment with diuretics in HFpEF with volume overload
- In HFpEF patients with raised BNP, Cr <2.5 mg/dL, eGFR >30 mL/min/1.73 m^2, and potassium <5 mEq/L, treatment with a MRA
- Heart rate control with medications in AF patients
- In patients with HFpEF and type 2 diabetes mellitus, an SGLT-2 inhibitor such as empagliflozin must be considered
- Treatment of patients with obstructive CAD with symptoms and myocardial ischemia that contribute to HF with coronary revascularization.

REFERENCES

1. Heidenreich PA, Bozkurt B, Aguilar D, et al. 2022 AHA/ACC/HFSA guideline for the management of heart failure: a report of the American College of Cardiology/American Heart Association Joint Committee on clinical practice guidelines. J Am Coll Cardiol. 2022;79(17):e263-421.
2. Reddy YNV, Carter RE, Obokata M, et al. A simple, evidence-based approach to help guide diagnosis of heart failure with preserved ejection fraction. Circulation. 2018;138(9):861-70.
3. Westermann D, Kasner M, Steendijk P, et al. Role of left ventricular stiffness in heart failure with normal ejection fraction. Circulation. 2008;117(16):2051-60.
4. Anker SD, Butler J, Filippatos G, et al. Empagliflozin in heart failure with a preserved ejection fraction. N Engl J Med. 2021;385(16):1451-61.
5. Yusuf S, Pfeffer MA, Swedberg K, et al. Effects of candesartan in patients with chronic heart failure and preserved left-ventricular ejection fraction: the CHARM-Preserved trial. Lancet. 2003;362(9386):777-81.
6. Solomon SD, Zile M, Pieske B, et al. The angiotensin receptor neprilysin inhibitor LCZ696 in heart failure with preserved ejection fraction: a phase 2 double-blind randomised controlled trial. Lancet. 2012;380(9851):1387-95.
7. Whelton PK, Carey RM, Aronow WS, et al. 2017 ACC/AHA/AAPA/ABC/ACPM/AGS/APhA/ASH/ASPC/NMA/PCNA guideline for the prevention, detection, evaluation, and management of high blood pressure in adults: a report of the American College of Cardiology/American Heart Association Task Force on clinical practice guidelines. J Am Coll Cardiol. 2018;71(19):e127-248.
8. Edelmann F, Wachter R, Schmidt AG, et al. Effect of spironolactone on diastolic function and exercise capacity in patients with heart failure with preserved ejection fraction: the Aldo-DHF randomized controlled trial. JAMA. 2013;309(8):781-91.

CHAPTER

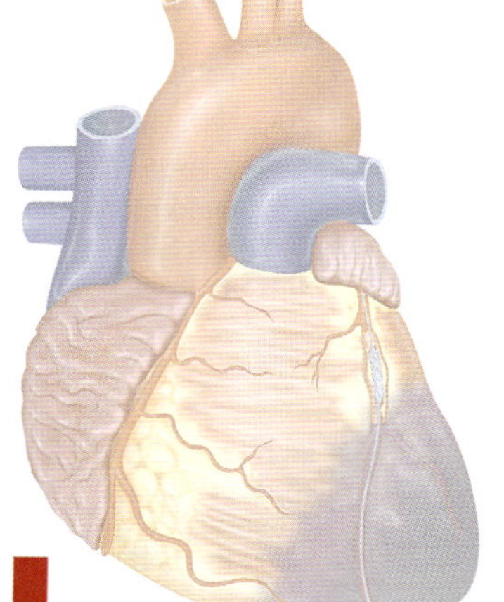

Estrogen Deficiency in Postmenopausal Women: Harbinger to HFpEF

Shibba Takkar Chhabra, Prerna Goyal

INTRODUCTION

Heart failure (HF) remains a major global concern owing to its high mortality and morbidity and encompasses three distinct phenotypes based on left ventricular functionality/ ejection fraction (EF). Out of this, heart failure with preserved ejection fraction (HFpEF) (EF ≥50%) accounts for nearly 50% of HF patients and presents primarily with diastolic dysfunction and impaired ventricular filling. Overall, females, especially postmenopausal females, are predominantly affected by HFpEF in unison with age-related surge in diabetes, hypertension, obesity, and dyslipidemia.[1] Current precision-based medicine underscores the role of pathophysiological-based phenotyping of HFpEF which can expand the horizon of therapeutic considerations, unlike other phenotypes. For this purpose, one such pathophysiological type of HFpEF seen in postmenopausal women has been explored vastly, and this chapter is an attempt to elucidate the mechanistic insights of menopausal-related HFpEF secondary to estrogen (E2) depletion along with current and futuristic therapeutic options.

PATHOPHYSIOLOGY OF MENOPAUSE-RELATED HFpEF

As age advances, the gap between gender-associated trajectories of cardiovascular diseases (CVDs) starts narrowing down; elderly females almost match or even surpass the age-matched males in the prevalence and morality rates of CVDs. This has been attributed to loss of cardioprotective effects of E2 in the elderly females. E2 in interaction with estrogen receptors (ERs), namely ERα, Erβ, and G protein-coupled ER (GPER) present in cardiomyocytes, fibroblasts, and vasculature, plays a crucial role in modulating fibrotic, inflammatory, apoptotic, oxidative, and calcium hemostasis via a variety of distinct signaling pathways **(Flowchart 1)**. ERα and ERβ mediate several biological functions directly or indirectly by affecting a variety of gene transcription and expression. ERα in health is responsible for preventing cardiac apoptosis and hypertrophy and promotes vasodilatation by its action on Akt, nitric oxide synthetase (NOS), and superoxide mutase. ERβ and GPER function to prevent fibrosis and inflammation in fibroblasts and vascular smooth muscle cells. Besides this, there is an extensive interplay between E2/ER axis and β adrenergic

Flowchart 1: Estrogen-mediated actions on the cardiovascular system via different subtypes of estrogen receptors.

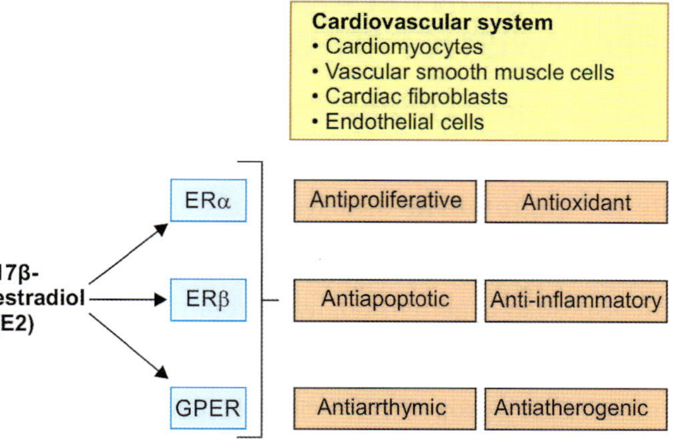

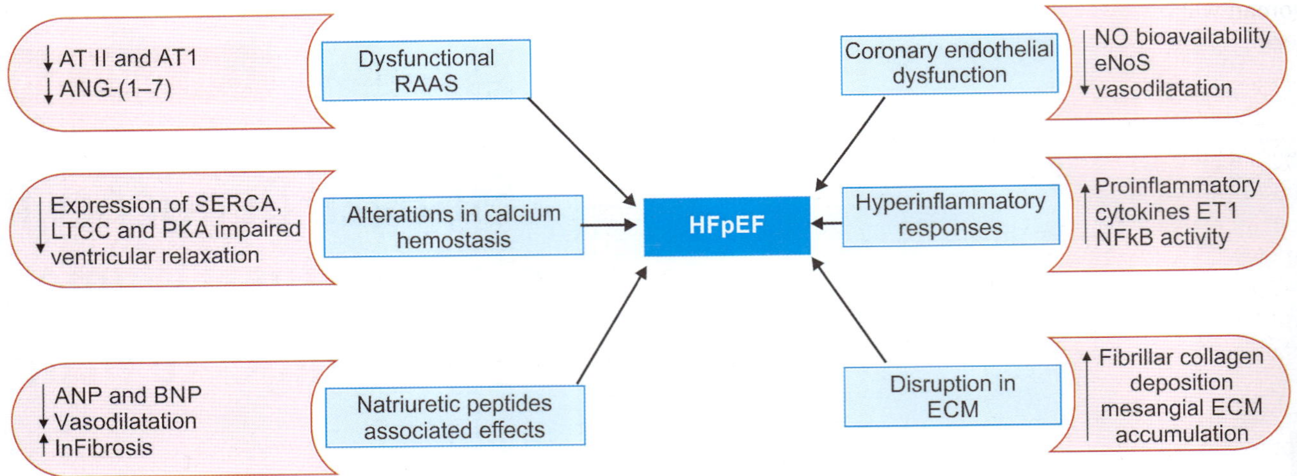

Fig. 1: Estrogen-mediated mechanistic pathways to HFpEF.

receptors (βARs), namely β_1AR and β_2AR also present in cardiac fibroblasts, cardiomyocytes, and vasculature. Under physiological conditions, E2 actively modulates the expression of pleotropic responses of catecholamines mediated by βARs. The characteristic diastolic incompliance seen in HFpEF occurs on the scaffolding of distorted myocardial architecture due to inflammation and fibrosis-associated alterations in extracellular matrix (ECM), cytoskeleton proteins, endothelium, and vasculature leading to poor ventricular relaxation. This whole phenomenon gets primed up by estrogenic deficiency in menopause along with unprotected βARs' hyperstimulation which cascades the sequence of cardiac structural and functional maladaptive pathways and hence expedites the onset and progression of HFpEF in postmenopausal females. A detailed discussion of various mechanistic pathways involved in the pathogenesis of HFpEF secondary to deficiency of E2 is given below and shown in **Figure 1**.

ESTROGEN IN RELATION TO MECHANISTIC PATHWAYS TO HFpEF

Dysfunctional Renin–Angiotensin–Aldosterone Axis

Renin-angiotensin-aldosterone-derived potent vasoconstrictors, namely angiotensin (ANG) II and aldosterone, have been implicated in HFpEF as they predispose to hypertension, hypertrophy, inflammation, oxidative radical formation, and vascular proliferation. On the other hand, ANG(1-7) display antioxidant and anti-inflammatory properties. Various epidemiological and clinical trials have confirmed the effect of E2 in attenuating the effects of proinflammatory angiotensin-converting enzyme, ANG II, and angiotensin type II receptor type 1 (AT1) and augmenting the anti-inflammatory ANG(1-7) production, thereby modulating the pathogenetic pathways to HFpEF.

Alterations in Calcium Hemostasis

E2/ER can influence cardiac contractility and relaxation coupling by its effects on calcium receptors and various downstream proteins, namely L-type calcium channel (LTCC), protein kinase A (PKA), sarcoplasmic reticulum Ca^{2+} ATPase (SERCA), ryanodine receptor (RyR), etc.[2] E2 conduces regulated gated movement of calcium in cardiomyocytes by enhancing expression of SERCA, phosphorylation of cardiac troponin I and myosin binding protein-C by PKA and reduces the sensitivity of myofilaments to calcium, all of which fortify the premenopausal females with appropriate diastolic relaxation.

Natriuretic Peptide-associated Effects

There are gender differences in atrial natriuretic peptide (ANP) and B-type natriuretic peptide (BNP). Younger females and females of all ages have higher levels of ANP and BNP levels, respectively, as compared to men. Nevertheless, E2 has been positively correlated with the natriuretic system in various clinical models, where E2 supplementation upregulated natriuretic peptides and conferred natriuretic, diuretic, vasodilatory, antifibrotic, antiproliferative, and antihypertrophic benefits.[3] Therefore, it can be considered that a postmenopausal woman will be devoid of such E2-associated benefits and hence might be at an increased risk of HFpEF.

Disruption in Extracellular Matrix

Extracellular matrix in healthy heart is made up of different kinds of proteins which are primarily regulated by balanced activity of TIMPs (tissue inhibitor of metalloproteinases) and MMPs (matrix metalloproteinases). ERs and βARs are well expressed on fibroblasts and control their proliferation and hence preserve ECM composition. In menopausal-related HFpEF, E2 deficiency results in ECM remodeling via upregulation of genes expressing collagens I and III, increased deposition, and cross-linkage of fibrillar collagen along with downregulation of MMPs, ultimately leading to ventricular stiffness and diastolic incompliance.[4]

Coronary Microvascular Endothelial Dysfunction

Endothelial dysfunction (ED) in HFpEF is the outcome of microvascular inflammation and oxidative stress. In premenopausal women, E2 plays a crucial role as free radicals scavenger by reducing the formation of reactive oxygen species (ROS) through action on mitochondrial proteins.[5] This is critical to suppress trafficking of leukocytes to subendothelial cells and to increase nitric oxide (NO) bioavailability. Additionally, ERs present in coronary endothelium promote the production of NO by modulating tetrahydrobiopterin, an important cofactor of enzyme endothelial NOS,[6] and thus indirectly facilitates the coronary circulation. NO plays a vital role in maintaining coronary vascular tone, angiogenesis, endothelial cell proliferation, and platelet functioning. Furthermore, E2-mediated downregulation of AT1 coupled with decreased production of tumor necrosis factor alpha (TNF-α) controls the oxidative and inflammatory forces in premenopausal women, but this is negated in postmenopausal group due to E2 deficiency and hence predispose to cardiac remodeling and HFpEF.

Hyperinflammatory Responses

Besides aforementioned effects on eNOS and ROS, numerous other physiological anti-inflammatory effects of E2 are mediated via a myriad of protective channels; important ones are reduction of endothelin, interleukin-6, intercellular adhesion molecule-1, vascular cell adhesion molecule-1, and E-selectin.[7] Above all, E2 has been found to repress the expression of the central regulatory gene, named nuclear factor kappa-light-chain-enhancer of activated B cells (NFκB), which controls all the inflammatory responses in health. Not just that, in adipose tissue, E2 enhances the effect of anti-inflammatory leptins, mitigates proinflammatory adipokines, regulates fat distribution, and prevents abdominal obesity. Substantial weight gain seen in postmenopausal females in synergy with E2 decline may exaggerate the cytokine production via activation of various transcription factors and expedite the onset of HFpEF in postmenopausal females.

THERAPEUTICS OPTIONS OF MENOPAUSE-RELATED HFpEF: CURRENT AND FUTURE

Decades of research into putative mechanisms for HFpEF have paved interest into diverse classes of therapeutic agents with different modes of action. Similarly, E2 deficiency in menopause-associated HFpEF has sparked interest in the potential role of E2 and hormone replacement therapy (HRT) in the treatment paradigm besides traditional four pillars and lifestyle modification.

Four Pillars in Menopause-associated HFpEF: Gender-specific Outcomes

The current evidence of pharmacological therapy in HFpEF, whether it aligns with similar effects in menopausal-induced HFpEF, is immature and has been interpreted from few available trials incorporating a considerable strength of women population with HFpEF. There have been neutral results with RAS modulators—candesartan, perindopril, and irbesartan—in HFpEF. Sacubitril/valsartan has shown some hope in HFpEF as it led to reduction in BNP levels[8] and blood pressure, which can translate into a lesser hospitalization rate. For aldosterone antagonists, a gender analysis of spironolactone in the TOPACT trial failed to show significant reduction in the composite of CV deaths, HF hospitalization, and cardiac arrest except a significant decline in all-cause mortality in women population.[9] On the contrary, finerenone has been recently found to improve diastolic functions in obese female mice with metabolic syndrome and HFpEF and also prevented the progression of diastolic incompliance after ovariectomy when used on a long-term basis in female mice.[10] Similar findings have been reported in another paper where finerenone improved CV dysfunction and exercise capacity in ovariectomy-induced HFpEF mice.[11] More concrete evidence in future can provide us more insights about this class of drugs in HFpEF. SGLT2 inhibitors have been given class 2a recommendation for HFpEF by the American Heart Association with proven benefits in a population cohort including 24% women.[12] Ironically though sympathetic activation has been implicated in the pathogenesis of menopausal-related HFpEF, limited data available on beta blockers (BB) failed to show any significant improvement in exercise capacity, NYHA class, and BNP levels.[13] The potential role of BB specifically in a female cohort of HFpEF needs further exploration.

Estrogen and Hormone Replacement Therapy

Aforementioned elaboration on menopausal -linked HFpEF based on maladaptive cardiac structural and functional changes induced by E2 deficiency has stimulated researchers to explore E2/ER axis for the prevention and management of CVDs. Overall, the beneficial effects of HRT for CVD have remained incongruous and indecisive in various randomized controlled trials,[14] largely explained by the timings of initiation, pharmacological preparation used (conjugated equine E2 in combination with medroxyprogesterone acetate), and failure to mimic the endogenous hormonal milieu of a postmenopausal woman as well as superseding the risk of increased clotting and inflammation.[15] A recent systemic pooled analysis of five RCTs did not find any beneficial effect of E2 therapy in preventing first hospitalization due to HF and hospital admissions in postmenopausal women.[16]

Phytoestrogens (PhE), plant-derived estrogens, have recently gained momentum to circumvent the harmful effects of pharmacological estrogenic preparations. PhE, namely glycitein and genistein, have been implicated in CVD risk. A meta-analysis on PhE supplementation showed modest CV benefits with some favorable alterations in lipids, obesity, and blood pressure.[17] However, controversy regarding the durability and adverse effects remains unaddressed. Isoflavones and lignans are a specific group of plants which contain a maximum amount of PhE and are present in three commercially available food grains, namely flaxseed (*Linum usitatissimum* L.), soybean (*Glycine max* L.), and red clover (*Trifoliump ratense* L.) All have shown positive effects on lipids and markers of inflammation through modulation of various enzymatic pathways involved in cholesterol biosynthesis.[18] Therefore, these phytochemicals can be investigated further to prevent CVD and HFpEF in postmenopausal females.

CONCLUSION

Estrogen confers various CV benefits beyond endocrine functions. Menopausal transition in a woman's lifespan can cast deleterious transformation in cardiac health subsequent to drop in E2 levels. Experimental models have confirmed the critical role of E2/ER in the pathogenesis and rising incidence of HFpEF in postmenopausal females to the extent that HFpEF in them can be considered as one of the elements of postmenopausal syndrome. Despite this, the beneficial effects on E2 replacement/HRT in preventing and treating the postmenopausal HFpEF remains elusive. Future research can focus on developing newer formulations of estrogen preparations or advanced molecules that can target ERs and help in maintaining the cardiac integral hemostatic and structural domains. Also, we need more well-designed trials in future to see the outcomes of already available pharmacotherapies, particularly in this specific postmenopausal group of HFpEF population, so that management guidelines of menopausal-related HFpEF can be made more distinctive in the coming years.

REFERENCES

1. Özlek B, Özlek E, Kahraman S, et al. Gender disparities in heart failure with mid-range and preserved ejection fraction: results from APOLLON study. Anatol J Cardiol. 2019;21:242-52.
2. Machuki JO, Zhang HY, Zhang HY, et al. Estrogen regulation of cardiac cAMP-L-type Ca(2+) channel pathway modulates sex differences in basal contraction and responses to β(2)AR-mediated stress in left ventricular apical myocytes. Cell Commun Signal. 2019;17:34.
3. Lam CSP, Cheng S, Choong K, *et al.* Influence of sex and hormone status on circulating natriuretic peptides J Am Coll Cardiol. 2011;58:618-26.
4. Petrov G, Regitz-Zagrosek V, Lehmkuhl E, et al. Regression of myocardial hypertrophy after aortic valve replacement: faster in women? Circulation. 2010;122:S23-8
5. Lancaster TS, Jefferson SJ, Craig Hunter J, et al. Quantitative proteomic analysis reveals novel mitochondrial targets of estrogen deficiency in the aged female rat heart. Physiol Genomics. 2012;44:957-69.
6. Silberman GA, Fan THM, Liu H, et al. Uncoupled cardiac nitric oxide synthase mediates diastolic dysfunction Circulation. 2010;121:519-28.
7. Silvestri A, Gebara O, Vitale C, et al. Increased levels of C-reactive protein after oral hormone replacement therapy may not be related to an increased inflammatory response. Circulation. 2003;107: 3165-9.
8. Pieske B, Wachter R, Shah SJ, et al. Effect of Sacubitril/Valsartan vs. Standard Medical Therapies on Plasma NT-proBNP Concentration and Submaximal Exercise Capacity in Patients With Heart Failure and Preserved Ejection Fraction: The PARALLAX Randomized Clinical Trial. JAMA. 2021;*326*:1919-29.
9. Merrill M, Sweitzer NK, Lindenfeld JA, et al. Sex Differences in Outcomes and Responses to Spironolactone in Heart Failure With Preserved Ejection Fraction: A Secondary Analysis of TOPCAT Trial. JACC Heart Fail. 2019;7: 228-38.

10. Monmirel M, Frimat C, Charrabi A, et al. Finerenone improves HFpEF in obese female mice and slows down its acceleration after a postmenopausal transition. Arch Cardiovasc Dis. 2024;117:S192.
11. Pieronne-Deperrois M, Guéret A, Djerada Z, et al. Mineralocorticoid receptor blockade with finerenone improves heart function and exercise capacity in ovariectomized mice. ESC Heart Fail. 2021;8(3):1933-43.
12. Packer M, Anker SD, Butler J, et al. Cardiovascular and Renal Outcomes with Empagliflozin in Heart Failure. N Engl J Med. 2020;383:1413-24.
13. Fukuta H, Goto T, Wakami K, et al. Effect of beta-blockers on heart failure severity in patients with heart failure with preserved ejection fraction: A meta-analysis of randomized controlled trials. Heart Fail Rev. 2021;26:165-71.
14. Iorga A, Cunningham C, Moazeni S, et al. The protective role of estrogen and estrogen receptors in cardiovascular disease and the controversial use of estrogen therapy. Biol Sex Differ. 2017;8:33.
15. Gersh FL, Lavie CJ. Menopause and hormone replacement therapy in the 21st century. Heart. 2020;106:479-81.
16. Chen Z, Wu C, Huang Z, et al. Association between estrogen replacement therapy and heart failure in postmenopausal women: A systematic review and meta-analysis. Prev Med. 2024;181:107909.
17. Wolters M, Dejanovic GM, Asllanaj E, et al. Effects of phytoestrogen supplementation on intermediate cardiovascular disease risk factors among postmenopausal women: A meta-analysis of randomized controlled trials. Menopause. 2020;27:1081-92.
18. Campos JR, Severino P, Ferreira CS, et al. Linseed Essential Oil—Source of Lipids as Active Ingredients for Pharmaceuticals and Nutraceuticals. Curr Med Chem. 2019;26:4537-58.

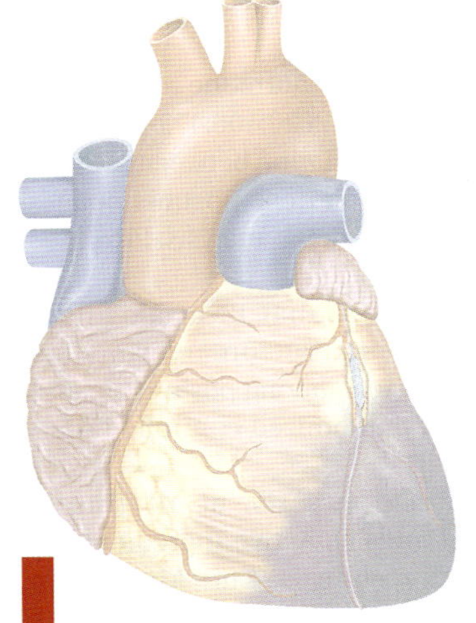

Gender Differences in HFpEF Pathophysiology

Rupender Saha, Vijay Kumar, Bhanu Duggal

INTRODUCTION

Heart failure is broadly classified into two categories: (1) Heart failure with reduced ejection fraction (HFrEF) and (2) heart failure with preserved ejection fraction (HFpEF). Each category has different epidemiology, risk factors, and management. The "Framingham Heart Study" shows a decline in the incidence of HFrEF but an increase in HFpEF over the last twenty years. There are significant sex differences in incidence, pathophysiology, and management between these two types of heart failure. For example, the "Framingham Heart Study" found that females had more than two times higher risk of HFpEF than males. Women have a higher frequency of HFpEF, which becomes more prevalent with age, 10% in females and 6% in males for individuals over 80 years old.[1] Heart failure is supposed to affect >64 million people worldwide.[2] Meanwhile, it affects 1% of the population in India; however, the prevalence of heart failure increases with age.[3] The lifetime risk of getting heart failure is believed to be roughly 20% for both men and women. In a few South Asian countries, including India, findings from the International REPORT-HF revealed that the proportions of Heart failure with reduced ejection fraction, moderately reduced ejection fraction, and preserved ejection fraction were 59, 18, and 23%, respectively. Among the heart failure registries, women constitute a stark difference of 55% of patients with HFpEF; on the other hand, only 29% of patients with HFrEF.[4]

Various characteristics found in the leading trials for HFpEF throughout recent years are discussed in **Table 1**.

PATHOPHYSIOLOGY AND RISK FACTORS

Immune System and Inflammation

It is hypothesized that chronic inflammation is considered one of the causes of the development of HFpEF. In human and animal models numerous studies have demonstrated myocardial inflammation and raised inflammatory markers in HFpEF with diastolic dysfunction. Women generally suffer more frequently from rheumatological diseases such as rheumatoid arthritis, which are associated with chronic inflammatory state and diastolic dysfunction. This suggests a connection between HFpEF and elevated immune responses. Systemic inflammation is more significant in females due to higher amounts of proinflammatory genes, inflammatory cytokines, and activated CD4 and CD8 T-cells. C-reactive protein levels are more substantial in women than in males. Gene expression in human hearts is sexually dimorphic, particularly for nuclear factor κB and Kruppel-like factor 4. These genes impact proinflammatory signaling, myocardial hypertrophy, cell survival and proliferation, stress response, and cardiac mitochondrial function. Other comorbidities that can damage the myocardium and induce inflammation that are more frequent in women are preeclampsia, diabetes, obesity, iron deficiency, hypertension, and chronic renal disease.[5]

Mitochondrial Genetics

A genomic investigation was done on mice after inducing heart failure by isoproterenol. It showed that many genes

TABLE 1: Sex differences in recent HFpEF treatment trials.

Trial Name	*Population*	*% of female*	*Drug*	*Ejection fraction Cut-off*	*Baseline characteristics differences (women versus men)*	*Gender difference*
"TOPCAT" (2019)	1767	50	Spironolactone	45%	• Older age, fewer comorbidities higher LV contractility, blood pressure, greater NYHA class • BMI, Less GFR, hemoglobin • Lower KCCQ score	Spironolactone lowers mortality in females but not in males
"PARAGON-HF" (2020)	4796	52	Sacubitril-Valsartan	45%	• Higher BMI, fewer comorbidities, more aged, reduced KCCQ score, reduced median NT-proBNP, higher LVEF, higher NYHA class, less likely on MRA • Lower GFR	Women were more likely to be hospitalized in the control group and had lower rates of cardiovascular mortality, which was primarily associated with heart failure
"EMPEROR PRESERVED" (2021)	5988	45%	Empagliflozin	40%	-	There is no distinction between males and women
"DELIVER" (2022)	6,263	44%	Dapagliflozin	40%	-	There is no distinction between males and women
"STEP-HFpEF STEP-HFpEF DM," (2023)	1,145	50%	Semaglutide	45%	• More obese • Higher LVEF • Higher NYHA class • Lower KCCQ score • Lower 6MWD • Higher baseline CRP • Less incidence of concomitant atrial fibrillation and CAD	Men and women had equal effects on HF effects, despite women losing more weight than men
"FINEARTS-HF" (2024)	6001	45%	Finerenone	40%	-	Females had a lower rate of adverse effects on finerenone than males

(CAD: coronary artery disease; CRP: C-reactive protein; GFR: glomerular filtration rate; HFpEF: heart failure with preserved ejection fraction; LVEF: left ventricular ejection fraction; KCCQ: Kansas City Cardiomyopathy Questionnaire; MRA: mineralocorticoid receptor antagonists)

responsible for diastolic function are present within the mitochondrial genome. A link between many diastolic dysfunction parameters and mitochondrial copy number was also discovered. To study whether the diastolic function differences in the two genders are due to hormonal misbalance or differences in mitochondrial properties, gonadectomy was done in a set of mice. Gonadectomies were associated with reduced mitochondrial functionality and diastolic dysfunction in males while enhanced mitochondrial replication, protein synthesis, and better diastolic function in females. However, the same female mice who had ovariectomy in the long term will develop diastolic dysfunction due to overstimulation of the renin-angiotensin-aldosterone system (RAAS) and reduced Nitric oxide signaling. It has also been shown that overexpression of the *Acsl6 gene* encoding a mitochondrial protein improves the diastolic function in males much more compared to female mice. Thus, though human studies are lacking, the relation between mitochondrial protein synthesis and plasma levels of sex hormones can be utilized clinically to assess diastolic dysfunction.[6]

Structural Differences

Even after considering body size, the general population has varying left ventricular measurements, capacities, and volumes corresponding to gender. Despite females having smaller left ventricle (LV) chambers than males, women have faster resting heart rates, maintaining a comparable cardiac output. Women exhibit greater diastolic and systolic LV compliance (stiffness) than men at any age. In aged people, these differences become more noticeable, with women seeing quicker increases in LV elastance than males. Both sexes have an increase in LV ejection fraction (EF) with age, with women experiencing a more significant rise.

Women age with slower systolic long-axis contraction velocity but with improved contractility due to an increased apical rotation. At birth, both genders have an equal number of cardiomyocytes. Women progressively experience a reduction in the total number of cardiomyocytes and their mass as they age, but the reduction is less than in males. Women also have a reduced propensity for eccentric left ventricular hypertrophy compared to men, but concentric hypertrophy with diastolic dysfunction is more abundant in females with HFpEF than males; thus, cardiac aging increases the likelihood of HFpEF in older females.

Exercise intolerance is a result of reduced chronotropic and myocardial reserve, as well as more significant LV diastolic elastance in women than in men with HFpEF. Because of their smaller LV chamber diameters, women with HFpEF needed to exercise at a higher heart rate to meet the demands of their cardiac output. This implies that women's reduced peak oxygen consumption may be more significantly caused by chronotropic incompetence than by males. When examining gender variations in peak oxygen demand, other parameters, such as peripheral oxygen handling and elevated pulmonary capillary wedge pressure (PCWP) should be considered. It is established that LA pathology plays a significant part in HFpEF pathophysiology. However, there is no proof of substantial gender variations in the anatomy or function of the left atrium (LA).[7]

Structural differences between male and a female heart responsible for diastolic dysfunction are discussed in **Table 2**.

Women are predisposed to LV diastolic failure with aging, but the cellular or molecular processes are unknown. Menopause stimulates the renin-angiotensin-aldosterone system, collagen formation, increasing reactive oxygen species causing diastolic failure. Rat models with ovariectomy cause cardiac myocyte enlargement with profuse myocardial fibrosis, which contributes to diastolic dysfunction. Estradiol decreases myocardial collagen synthesis by the angiotensin-II pathway. Cardiomyocyte stiffness affects diastolic function and is influenced by structural proteins like titin. Titin's mechanical characteristics are affected by whether it is phosphorylated or not and can be positively modified with the help of protein kinases A and G. Estrogen has been shown to decrease the activity of protein kinase A. Progesterone activates Kinase 2 regulated by extracellular signals, leading to cardiac remodeling in pregnancy and potentially influencing titin phosphorylation. Females have reduced calcium currents and decreased gain from excitation-contraction coupling compared to males, which may alter the calcium handling properties. Differential metabolism of various myocardial substrates according to gender differences may also contribute. Females have reduced glucose absorption with decreased utilization, thus resulting in metabolic inefficiency and greater lipid intake.[8]

TABLE 2: Structural differences between male and a female heart responsible for diastolic dysfunction.

Structural difference in women	*Structural difference in men*
Smaller Left ventricular cavity, and mass	Has a relatively large left ventricular cavity and LV mass
Cardiac output is maintained by a faster resting heart rate, so it is more symptomatic in chronotropic incompetence	Cardiac output is maintained till the very last due to larger cavity size and lesser dependence on heart rate
Slower systolic long-axis contraction velocity and an increased apical rotation with increased EF	More significant systolic long-axis contraction but reduced apical rotation
More prone to concentric left ventricular remodeling	More prone to eccentric left ventricular remodeling
Since EF is already increased in baseline, during exercise, peak oxygen consumption is more dependent on heart rate	Peak oxygen consumption is less dependent on heart rate and more on increasing contractility

Peripheral Circulation

The pathophysiology of HFpEF includes modifications of vascular and cardiac function, comprising diminished endothelial function and heightened arterial stiffness. Increased afterload, hypertension, reduced coronary blood flow, blood pressure instability, and earlier, greater arterial wave reflection all predisposes to HFpEF. Early arterial wave reflection in a smaller arterial system leads to systolic wave reflection than in diastole and as a result, myocardial relaxation is affected. Thus, afterload-induced diastolic dysfunction happens. Regardless of body size and heart rate, women have more significant pulse pressure, stiffer aortic arch, quicker wave reflection, and stronger arterial elastance than males. Regardless of age, female's aortic root diameters are smaller than their counterparts and the aortic arch has undergone less outward remodeling in response to hemodynamic demand so that pulse pressure may rise. Small vessel arteriolar function is affected in females due to inadequate dilation of the brachial arteries, reduced flow velocity, and diminished amplitude of the peripheral pulses. Due to worse LV relaxation brought on by higher load, women are more susceptible than males to the detrimental effects of arterial stiffness and early wave reflection on LV diastolic performance. Enhanced stiffness of arteries requires a compensatory rise in elastance of left ventricular systole to maintain stable cardiac output and coupling between arteries and ventricles. In men, arterial-ventricular coupling remains stable as they age, while it decreases in women. Older women may be more prone to HFpEF, characterized by a lack of arterial-ventricular coupling reserve during exercise.

Pulmonary arterial hypertension is essential in the constellation of symptoms of HFpEF. Pulmonary hypertension in HFpEF is primarily caused by higher LV filling and LA pressure, although other variables affecting pulmonary circulation, especially in women, may also play a role. A fraction of HFpEF patients develop combined pre- and postcapillary PH, which is linked to old age and valvular lesions, especially mitral regurgitation, predominant in females. Women have a four times higher incidence of pulmonary hypertension than males, which is characterized by pulmonary vasoconstriction and intrinsic pulmonary artery remodeling. This may indicate sex variations in pulmonary vascular remodeling and responsiveness.

A study found that >80% of patients having concomitantly significant pulmonary hypertension and heart failure with preserved ejection fraction belong to the female gender, highlighting the link between pulmonary vascular function and gender. Older women are likely to have higher left and right atrial pressure when loaded rapidly with saline. If plotted in a graph, the mean pressure of the pulmonary artery curve compared with the volume of normal saline loaded was sharper in women across all ages, indicating a lesser capacity for adjustment of pulmonary artery than in males.[9]

Pregnancy and Reproductive Health

Pregnancy hypertensive disorders, such as preeclampsia increase the risk of developing cardiovascular disease, particularly HFpEF. Preeclampsia was linked to a fourfold increase in future incidence of heart failure. A study showed that women suffering from preeclampsia are twice as likely to suffer from HFpEF.[10] Both traditional and gender-specific cardiovascular risk factors may interact reciprocally. Hypertensive and diabetic females have a higher chance of manifesting preeclampsia and individuals with preeclampsia have a greater chance of acquiring diabetes and hypertension later on. This highlights the need to detect and monitor high-risk women for future cardiovascular complications. Preeclampsia and microvascular dysfunction can cause diastolic failure, which can persist till one year after birth for almost half of the pregnant mothers.

The main hypotheses explaining these correlations are endothelial dysfunction, poor nitric oxide bioavailability, and LV remodeling. It was found that women who had preeclampsia had reduced endothelium-dependent flow-mediated dilation, indicated endothelial dysfunction, and had a threefold greater prevalence of HF. Adverse events of pregnancy, including preterm delivery, intrauterine growth restriction, and preeclampsia, can raise the risk of future hypertension, concentric LV remodeling, and endothelial dysfunction.

Proteomic analysis reveals elevated inflammatory markers and procoagulation state in women with HFpEF. In addition, normotensive pregnancies with fetal growth restriction can lead to decreased myocardial relaxation. It was seen that one-third of women with a history of intrauterine growth restriction of the fetus experience diastolic dysfunction, while hypertensive disorders in pregnancy are found to be most strongly associated with HFpEF. Other pregnancy-related factors, such as parity, are linked to diastolic function. Grand parity (defined as more than four pregnancies) is also connected to an increased risk of diastolic failure. The reason for such an increased risk is still not well understood. On the other hand, nulliparity is also associated with an increased risk of HFpEF. The reason for such occurrence is attributed to reduced exposure to pregnancy-specific hormones. Infertility also, on the other hand, is another risk factor for dysfunction. The Women's Health Initiative found a strong link between infertility and incident HFpEF (20% increased risk) **(Fig. 1)**.[11]

TRADITIONAL RISK FACTORS

Hypertension

Hypertensive females are thrice more likely to suffer from heart failure, hypertensive males are only twice more likely to suffer from heart failure. Women may have a more extensive augmentation index between central and peripheral blood pressure, leading to extensive end-organ damage and concentric remodeling. Females also show a link between carotid augmentation index and diastolic dysfunction. Compared to males, women react to pressure stress differently, undergoing greater concentric remodeling and having a stronger reaction to obesity and hypertension.[12]

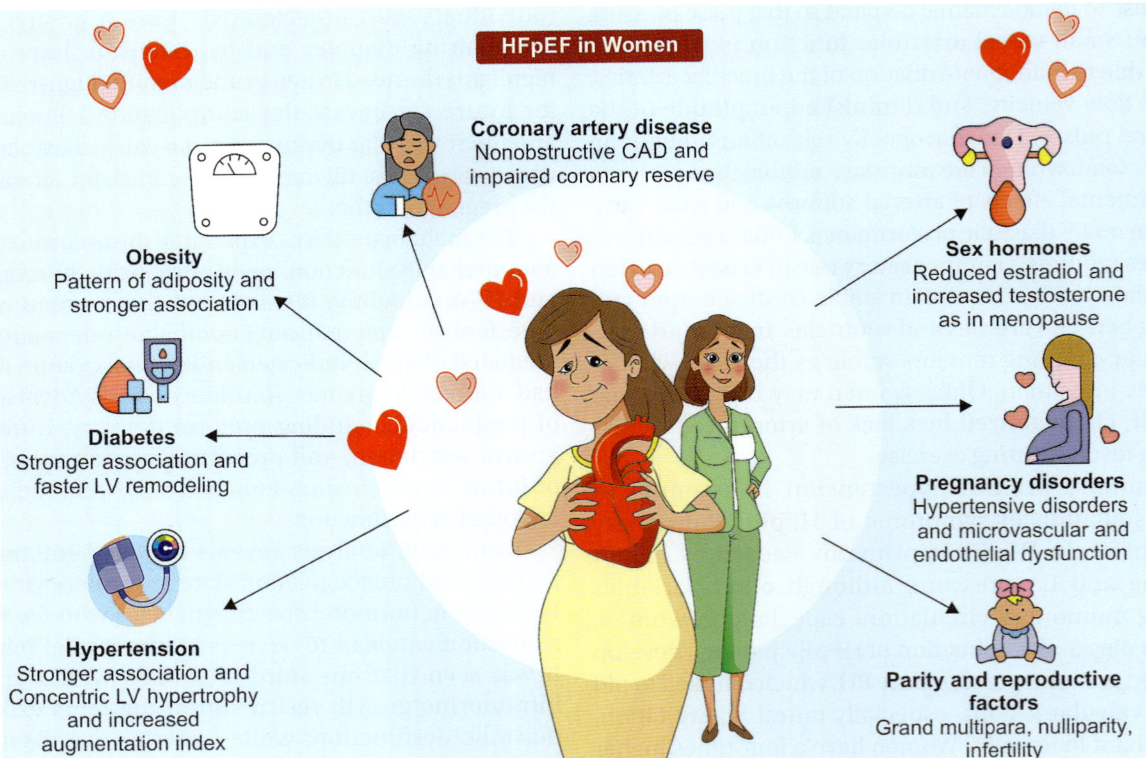

Fig. 1: Diagram summarizing main risk pathophysiology of gender difference in heart failure with preserved ejection fraction (HFpEF).

Diabetes Mellitus

Women who have diabetes mellitus have a five-fold increased risk of heart failure compared to twice the increased risk in males. According to the HFpEF hypothesis, endothelial dysfunction and vascular inflammation are the essential reasons for HFpEF in people with diabetes and other cardiometabolic risk factors. In cardiomyocytes, soluble guanylate cyclase and protein kinase G (PKG) action are reduced producing reactive oxygen metabolites and decreasing nitric oxide bioavailability. Reduced cardiac relaxation and increased cardiomyocyte hypertrophy result from inadequate PKG activation. Compared to males, women go through this phase earlier during their illness.[13]

Obesity

Obesity increases the risk of heart failure and has lately been linked to HFpEF. Obesity is more prevalent in females with HFpEF than males respectively (46 vs. 35%), according to the "Irbesartan in Heart Failure with Preserved Ejection Fraction (I-PRESERVE) trial."[14] In a study of twenty-two thousand patients, obesity was more commonly associated with HFpEF than HFrEF.[15]

Obesity is linked to HFpEF through cardiometabolic variables such as insulin resistance, which causes inflammation, endothelial dysfunction, and myocyte remodeling. Additionally, males and women have different fat distribution patterns. Women before attaining menopause exhibit higher subdermal and lower central obesity than males. Decreased estrogen levels in the perimenopausal period led to increased visceral adiposity. Estrogen may regulate gene expression in adipocytes and cardiomyocytes via promoting noncoding ribonucleic acid (RNA) expression, including microRNAs and long noncoding RNAs.

Abdominal fat tissue is linked to concentrated LV hypertrophy and exercise intolerance, which are symptoms of individuals with HFpEF having significantly more intra-abdominal fat than healthy controls. Fat is also an accurate marker of maximum oxygen consumption, which measures exercise efficiency. Physical function tests, such as peak oxygen consumption and 6-minute walk distance, showed inverse relationships with intra-abdominal fat levels.[16]

Atrial Fibrillation

Atrial fibrillation affects 25–39% of all patients having HFpEF and has common risk factors of age and hypertension. Research indicates that AF is linked to HF hospitalization and death in HFpEF patients. Although men develop AF more commonly than women with HFpEF, women with both conditions have worse outcomes. In the TOPCAT (Treatment of Preserved Cardiac Function Heart Failure with an Aldosterone Antagonist) trial, women with HFpEF had a stronger association with AF and hospitalization compared to men.[17]

Coronary Artery Disease

Ischemic heart disease was more prevalent in males with HFpEF than in women (30.6 vs 17.5%). Research has shown that men with HFpEF symptoms are hospitalized for CAD, coronary angioplasty, or coronary artery bypass grafting more likely than women. On the other hand, nonobstructive CAD and microvascular syndrome are more prevalent in women. Generalized microvascular dysfunction, as determined by peripheral arterial tonometry testing, was linked to 75% of coronary microvascular dysfunction in HFpEF patients. In a study including people with noncritical coronary artery diseases, coronary microvascular dysfunction checked by a raised coronary flow reserve was found to be associated with diastolic failure and peripheral artery disease. Lastly, a review of 6,809 healthy adults in the Multiethnic Study of Atherosclerosis (MESA) revealed that CT coronary artery calcium score levels greater than three hundred have a greater chance of causing HFpEF in females.[18]

Iron Deficiency Anemia

Across a range of ejection fractions, anemia has been independently linked to an increased risk of mortality and HF hospitalization, making it a prevalent comorbidity in HF. Higher levels of systemic inflammation and unfavorable LV remodeling neurohormonal activation are potential explanations. In the HFrEF and HFpEF subgroups of the "Get With the Guidelines-Heart Failure registry," females had more anemia than males.[19] Regarding the adverse effects on oxidation mechanisms and immunological responses, it has been hypothesized that a higher frequency of iron deficiency in women exposes them to a greater chance of HFpEF. Furthermore, the relationship between anemia and outcomes varied according to sex in the "Japanese Acute Decompensated Heart Failure Syndromes registry." Anemia causes significant all-cause mortality in HFpEF in females and HfrEF in males.[20]

Management Differences

As evident from the previously summarized table on trials on HfpEF, various treatment modalities have contrasting effects on gender differences in HfpEF. Mineralocorticoid receptor antagonists of both steroidal spironolactone type and nonsteroidal type finerenone had a more beneficial effect on the female gender. Sacubitril-valsartan also had a better impact on women suffering from HFpEF. It was proposed that females had higher left ventricular diastolic pressures, which have fewer cyclic guanosine monophosphate (cGMP) signaling, and lower BNP levels relative to the intensity of symptoms. BNP levels are lowered by overall adiposity, which is more common in women. Therefore, all of the processes that raise BNP are more beneficial to women, which brings us to the gender-specific contribution of antagonists of the mineralocorticoid receptor and ARNI. To prove this hypothesis indirectly, sodium-glucose cotransporter-2 (SGLT2) inhibitors do not have a gender-specific effect on HFpEF patients.[21]

CONCLUSION

A multitude of variables contribute to the disproportionate frequency of HFpEF in women, including risk factors, different sex-specific effects, and distinct pathophysiological effects that increase the risk of these conventional risk factors for women. Even though women make up the bulk of HFpEF patients, their presence in clinical studies is still insufficient. More research is required to develop more precise risk classification algorithms that consider both conventional and gender-specific risk markers, given the variability of HFpEF. Furthermore, how men and women respond differently to comorbidities and pathophysiological pathways is poorly understood.

REFERENCES

1. Ho JE, Gona P, Pencina MJ, et al. Discriminating clinical features of heart failure with preserved vs. reduced ejection fraction in the community. Eur Heart J. 2012; 33(14):1734-41.
2. GBD 2017 Disease and Injury Incidence and Prevalence Collaborators. Global, regional, and national incidence, prevalence, and years lived with disability for 354 diseases and injuries for 195 countries and territories, 1990-2017: a systematic analysis for the Global Burden of Disease Study 2017. Lancet. 2018;392(10159):1789-858.
3. Huffman MD, Prabhakaran D. Heart failure: epidemiology and prevention in India. Natl Med J India. 2010;23(5): 283-8.
4. Stolfo D, Uijl A, Vedin O, et al. Sex-based differences in heart failure across the ejection fraction spectrum: phenotyping, and prognostic and therapeutic implications. JACC Heart Fail. 2019;7(6):505-15.
5. InanlooRahatloo K, Liang G, Vo D, et al. Sex-based differences in myocardial gene expression in recently

deceased organ donors with no prior cardiovascular disease. PLoS One. 2017;12(8):e0183874.

6. Cao Y, Vergnes L, Wang YC, et al. Sex differences in heart mitochondria regulate diastolic dysfunction. Nat Commun. 2022;13(1):3850.
7. Zhao Z, Wang H, Jessup JA, et al. Role of estrogen in diastolic dysfunction. Am J Physiol Heart Circ Physiol. 2014;306(5):H628-40.
8. Beale AL, Meyer P, Marwick TH, et al. Sex Differences in Cardiovascular Pathophysiology: Why Women Are Overrepresented in Heart Failure With Preserved Ejection Fraction. Circulation. 2018;138(2):198-205.
9. Thenappan T, Shah SJ, Gomberg-Maitland M, et al. Clinical characteristics of pulmonary hypertension in patients with heart failure and preserved ejection fraction. Circ Heart Fail. 2011;4(3):257-65.
10. Williams D, Stout MJ, Rosenbloom JI, et al. Preeclampsia predicts risk of hospitalization for heart failure with preserved ejection fraction. J Am Coll Cardiol. 2021;78(23): 2281-90.
11. Lau ES, Wang D, Roberts M, et al. Infertility and risk of heart failure in the women's health initiative. J Am Coll Cardiol. 2022;79(16):1594-603.
12. Kuch B, Muscholl M, Luchner A, et al. Gender specific differences in left ventricular adaptation to obesity and hypertension. J Hum Hypertens. 1998;12(10):685-91.
13. Paulus WJ, Tschöpe C. A novel paradigm for heart failure with preserved ejection fraction: comorbidities drive myocardial dysfunction and remodeling through coronary microvascular endothelial inflammation. J Am Coll Cardiol. 2013;62(4):263-71.
14. Carson PE, Anand IS, Win S, et al. The Hospitalization Burden and Post-Hospitalization Mortality Risk in Heart Failure With Preserved Ejection Fraction: Results From the I-PRESERVE Trial (Irbesartan in Heart Failure and Preserved Ejection Fraction). JACC Heart Fail. 2015;3(6):429-41.
15. Savji N, Meijers WC, Bartz TM, et al. The association of obesity and cardiometabolic traits with incident HFpEF and HFrEF. JACC Heart Fail. 2018;6(8):701-9.
16. Haykowsky MJ, Nicklas BJ, Brubaker PH, et al. Regional adipose distribution and its relationship to exercise intolerance in older obese patients who have heart failure with preserved ejection fraction. JACC Heart Fail. 2018;6(8):640-9.
17. Pitt B, Pfeffer MA, Assmann SF, et al. Spironolactone for heart failure with preserved ejection fraction. N Engl J Med. 2014;370(15):1383-92.
18. Sharma K, Al Rifai M, Ahmed HM, et al. The usefulness of coronary artery calcium to predict heart failure with preserved ejection fraction in men versus women (from the multi-ethnic study of atherosclerosis). Am J Cardiol. 2017;120(10):1847-53.
19. Vaduganathan M, Greene SJ, Zhang S, et al. Applicability of US Food and Drug Administration Labeling for Dapagliflozin to Patients With Heart Failure With Reduced Ejection Fraction in US Clinical Practice: The Get With the Guidelines-Heart Failure (GWTG-HF) Registry. JAMA Cardiol. 2021;6(3):267-75.
20. Kajimoto K, Minami Y, Sato N, et al. Gender Differences in Anemia and Survival in Patients Hospitalized for Acute Decompensated Heart Failure With Preserved or Reduced Ejection Fraction. Am J Cardiol. 2017;120(3):435-42.
21. McMurray JJV, Jackson AM, Lam CSP, et al. Effects of Sacubitril-Valsartan Versus Valsartan in Women Compared With Men With Heart Failure and Preserved Ejection Fraction: Insights From PARAGON-HF. Circulation. 2020; 141(5):338-51.

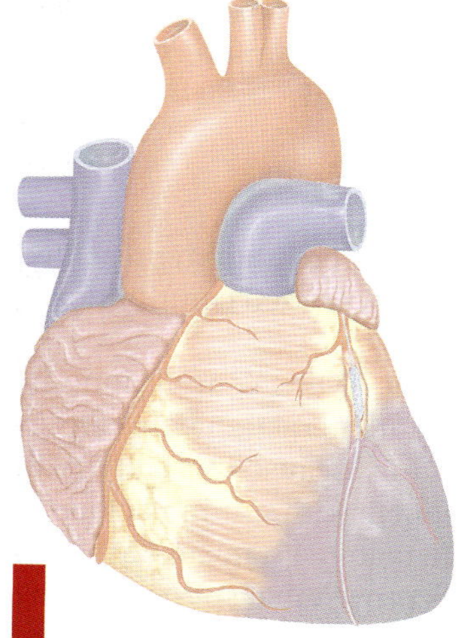

Obesity is Culprit in Heart Failure: Do not Miss HFpEF especially in Obese Women

RJ Cecily Mary Majella, Suriyakanth, Geetha Subramanian

INTRODUCTION

Obesity was once considered a disease in high-income countries but as of now, the prevalence of obesity is increasing rapidly in middle-income countries. Globally, the obesity pandemic is increasing over the last two decades. The percentage of adults >18 years and older living with obesity doubled from 7 to 16%. By 2025, the prevalence of obesity will reach 18% in men and 21% in women.[1]

According to ICMR-INDIAB study 2015, prevalence rate of obesity and central obesity varies from 11.8–31.3% and 16.9–36.3% respectively.[2] According to National Family Health Survey 5 (NFHS-5), one in every four Indian is now obese.

In this chapter, we are going to emphasize the impact of obesity in cardiovascular health, in particular about heart failure with preserved ejection fraction (HFpEF) in women.

OBESITY IN WOMEN

Apart from the traditional risk factors like type-2 diabetes, systemic hypertension, dyslipidemia, and obstructive sleep apnea, there are certain changes that are unique to women contributing to obesity.

- *Pregnancy:* Obesity during pregnancy causes endothelial dysfunction, insulin resistance, and a low-grade inflammatory state, which predisposes to vascular disease.[3]
    - A small group study demonstrated adverse cardiometabolic profile (increased DBP and LDL) among postpartum women who have not achieved adequate weight loss following pregnancy.
- *Preeclampsia:* Various postulates and links are described in literature regarding preeclampsia, which exaggerates the "physiological" manifestations of pregnancy like insulin resistance, hyperlipidemia, and hypercoagulability, which in turn can lead to "metabolic syndrome" in pregnancy.[4]
- *Postmenopausal and HRT:* Even in patients with normal BMI, CVD risk increases during menopause, and risk will be higher in women with truncal obesity. Beneficial role of HRT and its timeline is a long-term debate.

PATHOGENESIS OF OBESITY AND HEART FAILURE

World Health Organization describes overweight and obesity as "abnormal or excessive fat accumulation that presents a risk to health". The excess adiposity poses effects on the structure of cardiac myocytes and vasculature **(Table 1)**.

Mechanisms of heart failure in obesity are given in **Flowchart 1**.

CLINICAL FEATURES

The HFpEF has a little varied presentation in women compared to men. Women generally exhibit worsened quality of life (QoL) due to greater fatigue, dyspnea, and decreased exercise capacity compared with their male counterparts.

TABLE 1: Hemodynamic, structural, and autonomic changes.

Hemodynamic changes	*Structural alteration*	*Autonomic changes*
• Increased blood volume • Increased CO	Increased LA volume	Sympathovagal imbalance
• Increased O_2 consumption • AV O_2 difference increases • Leftward shift of Frank–Starling curve	• LV hypertrophy (both eccentric and concentric patterns) • RV dilatation and hypertrophy	Decreased NO availability
• Increased peripheral vascular resistance • Increased aortic stiffness • Hypoxia-induced pulmonary vasoconstriction • Pulmonary hypertension	• Increased epicardial fat (fatty infiltration in atrial and ventricular myocardium especially in RV/cardiac skeleton)	• Increased catecholamines • Increased FFA (myocardial irritability)
	• Myocardial fibrosis • Medial hypertrophy of intramyocardial coronary arteries	• Infiltration into conduction system • Increased incidence of AF

Flowchart 1: Mechanisms of heart failure in obesity.[2]

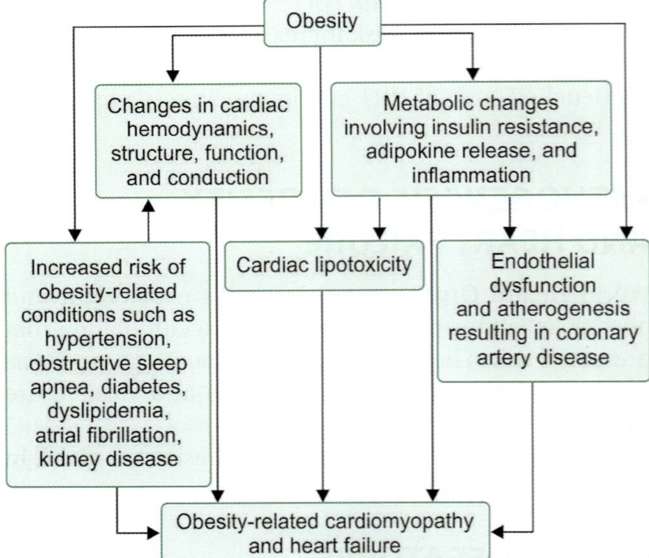

Source: Ebong IA, et al. Mechanisms of heart failure in obesity. Obes Res Clin Pract. 2014;8(6):e540-8.

Study done by Kim et al. showed that the prevalence of diastolic dysfunction was greater in women than in men with metabolic syndrome.[5]

According to Savji et al., women demonstrated a strong correlation between obesity and parameters such as insulin resistance, with incident HFpEF.

DATA FROM MAJOR TRIALS

In previous age-old trials, women were underrepresented but in newer trials, around 40–50% women contribution is present.

The post hoc analysis of the TOPCAT trial done by Merril et al. reported a significant interaction between sex and treatment arm in regards to all-cause mortality, with women exhibiting a greater benefit with spironolactone.[6]

In ALDO DHF trial, 50% females with mean BMI of 28 were part of the study. Results proved that spironolactone has significant improvement in LV diastolic function but not in QoL.

Obokata et al.[7] supported obese HFpEF as a valid HFpEF phenotype and effectively ushered obese HFpEF from pariah to its rightful place as a central player in the HFpEF syndrome. They provided insights into the pathophysiology of obese HFpEF and also the unique mechanisms of the symptomatology of obese HFpEF patients. Compared with both nonobese patients with HFpEF and controls, obese patients with HFpEF had increased plasma volume and more concentric left ventricular remodeling, RV dilatation, and RV dysfunction. Obese individuals have increased epicardial fat thickness and total epicardial heart volume, which cause pericardial restraint and increased ventricular interdependence. During exercise, obese-HFpEF individuals have much lower exercise capacity, higher LV and RV filling pressures, and lower pulmonary artery vasodilator reserve. In obese-HFpEF subjects, increased filling pressures correlated with increased BMI and plasma volume. Obese-HFpEF individuals have worse derangements despite lower NT-proBNP levels.

Excess adipose tissue can produce impairments relevant to HFpEF by two general categories of mechanisms—local/mechanical and systemic/metabolic. Examples of local/mechanical mechanisms include enhanced pericardial restraint suggested by Obokata, decreased oxygen diffusion from capillaries to working skeletal muscle cells suggested by Haykowsky, accelerated coronary atherosclerosis linked to epicardial adipose, and accelerated renal dysfunction linked to perirenal fat. Excess adipose tissue can also produce a plethora of adverse systemic/metabolic effects. Adipose tissue is metabolically active and produces an array of powerful vasoconstrictors, including angiotensin-II and inflammatory cytokines. Excess adipose tissue has been linked with capillary rarefaction, which can impair critical tissue perfusion.

Capillary rarefaction has been demonstrated in both the myocardium and skeletal muscle in HFpEF and is associated with worse clinical outcomes and worse objectively measured exercise capacity. Excess adipose tissue is also associated with impaired mitochondrial function, which is present in patients with HFpEF and contributes to their severe exercise intolerance. Excess adiposity could exacerbate capillary rarefaction and mitochondrial dysfunction, and thereby contribute to the more severe exercise intolerance and hemodynamic derangements in obese-HFpEF individuals.

It should now be apparent that obese patients with HFpEF do not get dyspneic merely because they are carrying excess weight (a common misconception), but because of their excess adipose tissue, which results in a plethora of adverse consequences that produce genuine HF. This theory is further supported by the fact that with caloric restriction in HFpEF, the improvements in symptoms, QoL, and exercise capacity do not result merely from removing mechanical weight and that bariatric surgery reduces clinical HF events in both reduced EF and HFpEF.

HFpEF IN ASIANS: DIFFERENCES

Further support for important adverse consequences of relative excess adipose tissue for HFpEF derives from observations in Asian populations. In contrast to Western populations, most Asian patients with HFpEF are normal weight or even underweight. However, for any given BMI, Asian populations have a significantly higher percentage of body fat (particularly intra-abdominal fat) compared with white populations, supporting the concept that the relative amount of excess adipose (body composition) tissue is the critical factor and highlighting the limitations of BMI as a surrogate for body composition. In asymptomatic Asians with normal left ventricular EF and relatively low BMI, larger waist circumference was associated with unfavorable left ventricular remodeling, impaired diastolic function, and worse global myocardial deformation. In a large population-based cohort of Asian patients with HF (22% HFpEF), only 19% were obese by BMI criteria; however, 57% had diabetes mellitus. Furthermore, the rate of diabetes mellitus in these Asian patients with HF was strikingly high for any given BMI: 40% for BMI $\leq$20 kg/m^2 and >60% for BMI >30 kg/m^2. Diabetes mellitus rates were three-fold higher than in white patients, and diabetes mellitus in Asians was more strongly associated with poor outcomes. These cross-ethnic data support the concept that the relative amount of excess adipose tissue (i.e., body composition) and its numerous adverse metabolic consequences (including diabetes mellitus), rather than merely weight (mechanical load), are the key contributors to the metabolic/obese HFpEF phenotype.

But what about reports, including our own, suggesting that obesity paradoxically confers a survival advantage in HFpEF?

All such studies to date have key limitations, including not accounting for unintentional weight loss such as that due to occult malignancy. An obesity-related survival advantage had previously been strongly suggested in the literature for obese older people in general until recently reported randomized trials showed that intentional weight loss in overweight/obese older persons improves long-term survival. Similar results would seem likely for obese older patients with HFpEF, particularly given observed significant improvements in clinical cardiovascular outcomes from bariatric surgery.

CONCLUSION

Despite the relatively specific findings in obese HFpEF demonstrated by Obokata, obese and nonobese HFpEF should still be viewed as phenotypes of the same disorder (HFpEF) and not as separate or distinct diseases. Reconciling these two common phenotypes into a single disorder is facilitated by our evolving understanding of HFpEF as a systemic disorder, likely triggered by circulating systemic factors, such as inflammatory cytokines and other as-yet-unidentified factors, and resulting in capillary rarefaction, arterial dysfunction, fibrosis, mitochondrial dysfunction, and other widespread abnormalities. Identifying the fundamental trigger(s) for HFpEF could dramatically advance our understanding by linking together the seemingly disparate major HFpEF phenotypes and lead to interventions that improve all HFpEF. Indeed, the only intervention definitively proven in multiple randomized trials to improve HFpEF (exercise training) is effective for both nonobese and obese HFpEF. Likewise, reducing adipose tissue by caloric restriction appears effective even in modestly obese patients.

As we work to differentiate and better understand specific mechanisms of the various HFpEF phenotypes, including obese HFpEF, even greater rewards may result from efforts to identify the fundamental factors that underlie the HFpEF syndrome and unite its phenotypes.

REFERENCES

1. NCD Risk Factor Collaboration (NCD-RisC). Trends in adult body-mass index in 200 countries from 1975 to 2014: a pooled analysis of 1698 population-based measurement studies with 19·2 million participants. Lancet. 2016;387:1377-96.

2. Ahirwar R, Mondal PR. Prevalence of obesity in India: A systematic review. Diabetes Metab Syndr. 2019;13(1): 318-21.
3. Ramsay JE, Ferrell WR, Crawford L, et al. Maternal obesity is associated with dysregulation of metabolic, vascular, and inflammatory pathways. J Clin Endocrinol Metab. 2002; 87(9):4231-7.
4. Rodie VA, Freeman DJ, Sattar N, et al. Pre-eclampsia and cardiovascular disease: Metabolic syndrome of pregnancy? Atherosclerosis. 2004;175(2):189-202.
5. Kim HL, Kim MA, Oh S, et al. Sex difference in the association between metabolic syndrome and left ventricular diastolic dysfunction. Metab Syndr Relat Disord. 2016; 14:507-12.
6. Merrill M, Sweitzer NK, Lindenfeld J, et al. Sex differences in outcomes and responses to spironolactone in heart failure with preserved ejection fraction: a secondary analysis of TOPCAT trial. JACC Heart Fail. 2019;7(3): 228-38.
7. Obokata M, Reddy YN, Pislaru SV, et al. Evidence supporting the existence of a distinct obese phenotype of heart failure with preserved ejection fraction. Circulation. 2017;136(1):6-19.

CHAPTER

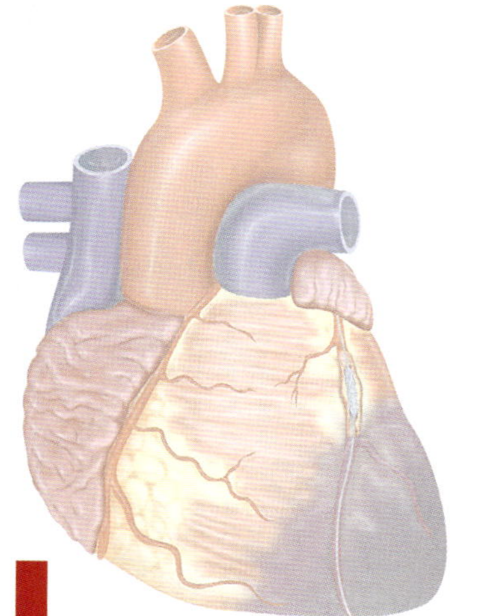

HFpEF Risk Decreased with More Physical Activity Among Older Women

Geetha Subramanian, J Cecily Mary Majella, Karthikaa Saminathan, Pavithra Arumugam, Ganesan Manohar

INTRODUCTION

Heart failure with preserved ejection fraction (HFpEF) is a common type of heart failure (HF) in older people, accounting for almost 90% of new cases in elderly women. The prevalence of HFpEF increases with age, from <0.5% in individuals aged 20–39 years to >10% in individuals aged >80 years. There is an increased risk of HFpEF in elderly women with a more sedentary lifestyle. The Physical Activity Guidelines evidence report from the United States in 2018 reported that 150 minutes of moderate to vigorous physical activity in a week is linked to a 10% lower risk of incident HF as compared to no physical activity. HFpEF is a common problem in the elderly due to cellular aging, stiffness of the myocardium, and comorbidities. Older women are under-represented in trials. Screening and management of hypertension (HTN), coronary artery disease (CAD), valvular heart disease (VHD), amyloidosis, and comorbidities such as diabetes mellitus, iron deficiency, obesity, and thyroid dysfunction are the main lines of management of HFpEF. Even in the elderly, exercise enhances 6-minute walking distance, peak and submaximal exercise capacity, and quality of life compared to other nonpharmacological measures. Exercise training under supervision (either resistance or endurance) has clearly been shown to improve exercise capacity [peak oxygen uptake (VO_2)] and reverse remodeling of the atrium and left ventricular diastolic dysfunction.

PATHOPHYSIOLOGY (FIG. 1)

Ventricular stiffness and a rise in diastolic pressures are common in elderly patients. Pulmonary edema can occur when physiological stressors, such as hypertensive crisis, exceed compensatory mechanisms. The risk factors involve the presence of obesity, diabetes, atrial fibrillation (AF), and dyslipidemia which are proved by larger trials. HTN remains the far most important cause. In aged patients, there are notable age-related elevations that specifically occur in sympathetic nerve activity, left ventricular wall thickness, myocardial fibrosis, and apoptosis, as well as micro- and macrovascular coronary disease and aortic stiffness. These patients experience both systolic heart failure (SHF) as well as diastolic heart failure (DHF). In older patients, especially in women, there is a distinct shift in the relationship between systolic and DHF and is in favor of DHF. Both systolic and diastolic dysfunction are related to increased rates of mortality and morbidity, particularly in the elderly.[1]

Figure 2 depicts aging and HFpEF.

DIAGNOSIS OF HEART FAILURE WITH PRESERVED EJECTION FRACTION IN THE ELDERLY (FIG. 3)

In a patient with suspected HF, the systematic use of clinical scoring is helpful. In a patient with dyspnea, H2FPEF,[2] and HFA-PEFF[3] algorithms evaluate the likelihood of HFpEF in a dyspneic person. H2FPEF is far more useful and comes from the gold-standard reference of invasive exercise hemodynamic measures. It is composed of the following six elements: (1) A body mass index (BMI) >30 kg/m^2, (2) elderly people (over 60 years old), (3) pulmonary HTN (anticipated pulmonary artery systolic

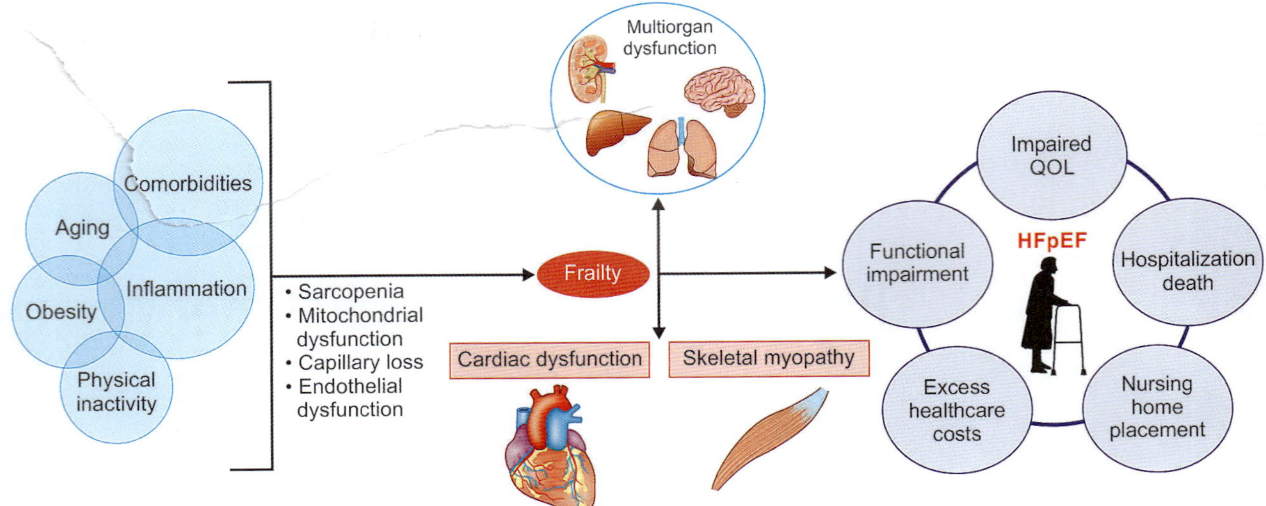

Fig. 1: Pathophysiology and outcomes in heart failure with preserved ejection fraction.
Source: Pandey A, Shah SJ, Kellogg D, et al. Exercise Intolerance in Older Adults With Heart Failure With Preserved Ejection Fraction: JACC State-of-the-Art Review. J Am Coll Cardiol. 2022;78(11):1166-87.

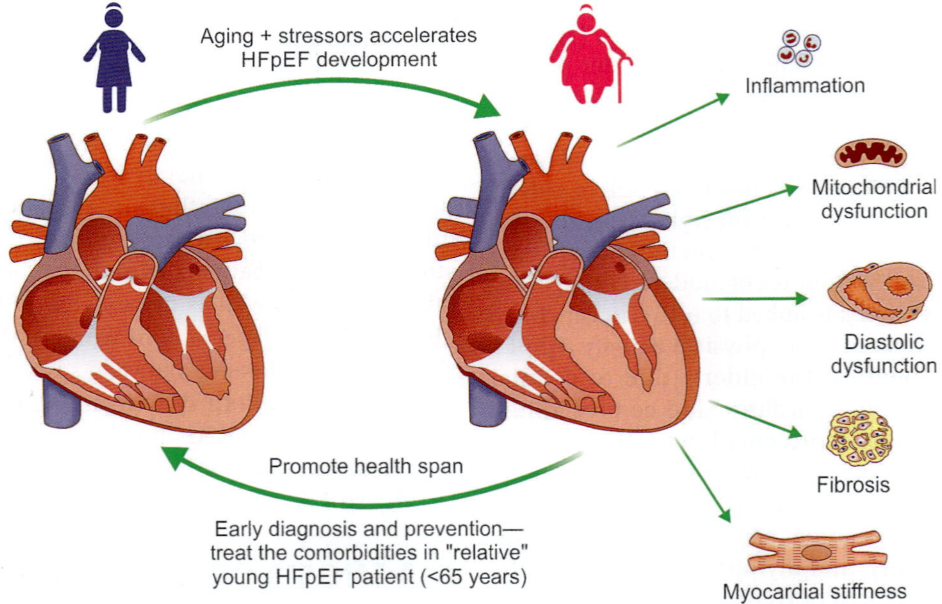

Fig. 2: Aging and heart failure with preserved ejection fraction (HFpEF).

pressure >35 mm Hg on Doppler echocardiography), (4) AF, (5) HTN (on two or more antihypertensive drugs), and (6) filling pressures (E/e' > 9 on Doppler echocardiogram). A score of six or higher strongly suggests HFpEF.

The HFA-PEFF algorithm is based on expert consensus including potential hemodynamic assessment. There are four steps:

1. The first step is the pretest examination, employing clinical assessment as well as standard diagnostic methods such as natriuretic peptides, electrocardiograms, and echocardiograms to identify persons potentially suffering from HF.
2. The second step is the echocardiographic and natriuretic peptide scoring system, which allocates points according to the concentrations of natriuretic peptide and echocardiographic parameters.
3. The third step includes performing functional testing in instances of ambiguity. This stage may involve invasive

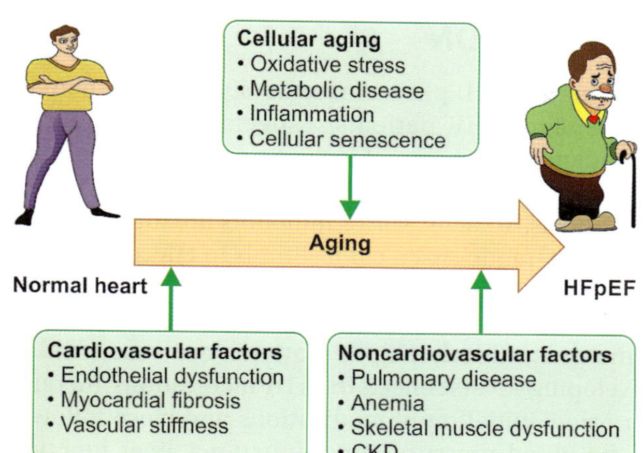

Fig. 3: Interaction and triggers between age and heart failure with preserved ejection fraction (HFpEF).[4]
Source: Adapted from Sauer AJ. Empagliflozin and Elderly Patients With Preserved Ejection Fraction Heart Failure: Is Age Just a Number? J Am Coll Cardiol. 2022;80(1):19-21.

hemodynamic assessments following a diastolic stress test using exercise stress echocardiography.

4. The fourth step is final etiology, which involves testing of exclusion of other cardiac disorders such as pericardial disease, valvular disease, and infiltrative/restrictive cardiomyopathy that may be the cause of dyspnea and/or edema.

PHYSICAL ACTIVITY AND HEART FAILURE WITH PRESERVED EJECTION FRACTION IN ELDERLY

To evaluate if increased levels of physical activity are linked with reduced HF risk, data from the Objective Physical Activity and Cardiovascular Health (OPACH)[5] study ancillary to the Women's Health Initiative (WHI) Long-Life Study was done from 2012 to 2014. Women (n = 5,951) aged between 63 to 99 years without known HF wore a triaxial accelerometry device on their hip for 7 consecutive days. Risk for incident HF through 2022 was evaluated based on their physical activity.

The women had a mean age of 78.6 years, they had a BMI of 28.1, 49.2% were white, 70.2% did not use an assistive walking device, 17.8% had no comorbidities, 51.3% had self-rated good health, and they engaged in a median of 3,133 (IQR: 2,303–4,547) steps per day. Higher usual levels of light physical activity (PA), moderate-to-vigorous physical activity (MVPA), and steps per day measured by accelerometry were associated with lower risks of incident overall HF and HFpEF in women aged 63–99 years. Physical activity was positively related to physical function and high-density lipoprotein cholesterol levels and negatively related with BMI, blood pressure, glucose, total cholesterol, triglycerides, and C-reactive protein levels (all $p < 0.001$).

With every 90-minute increase in physical activity daily, the risk for incident HF [adjusted hazard ratio (aHR): 0.85; 95% confidence interval (CI): 0.75–0.95] and HFpEF (aHR: 0.78; 95% CI: 0.67–0.91) was decreased. No effects on HFrEF were observed. Similarly, with every 3,600 steps per day increase, the risk for incident HF (aHR: 0.74; 95% CI: 0.63–0.88) and HFpEF (aHR: 0.71; 95% CI: 0.57–0.88) was significantly lower. With an additional 102 minutes spent sedentary per day, the risk for incident HF (aHR: 1.17; 95% CI: 1.04–1.33) and HFpEF (aHR: 1.29; 95% CI: 1.10–1.51) was significantly greater.

Stratified by physical activity groups, compared with the most sedentary group, a dose-dependent relationship was observed between greater physical activity and lower HF and HFpEF risk. The major limitation of this study was that physical activity data was only collected in a single week.

Exercise training can improve exercise capacity and quality of life for people with HFpEF, especially in the elderly.

- *Aerobic exercise:* At least 20–30 minutes, 3 days a week, at 50–80% of VO_2 max, such as walking, swimming, stationary cycling, rowing, and water aerobics.
- *Resistance exercise:* Two to three times a week, with 8–10 exercises. For upper body exercises, use an intensity of 30–70% of one repetition maximum (1RM). For lower body exercises, use an intensity of 40–80% of 1RM.
- *Exercise intensity and duration:* Start at 40–50% of your heart rate reserve for the first 2 weeks and gradually increase the duration and intensity.

Exercise training can improve exercise capacity without significantly changing the structure or function of the left ventricle. It can also reverse remodeling of the atrium and left ventricular diastolic dysfunction.

MANAGEMENT

The three main areas of management for HFpEF are (1) risk assessment and management of cooccurring conditions, such as diabetes, obesity, obstructive sleep apnea, CAD, chronic kidney disease (CKD), and AF; (2) nonpharmacological management, such as the application of wireless, implantable pulmonary artery monitors, and the role of exercise and weight loss; and (3) symptom management as well as disease-modifying therapy with loop diuretic agents, sodium-glucose cotransporter-2 inhibitors (SGLT2is), angiotensin receptor blockers (ARBs), mineralocorticoid antagonists (MRAs), and angiotensin receptor–neprilysin inhibitors (ARNIs).[6]

NONPHARMACOLOGICAL APPROACHES (PHYSICAL ACTIVITY)

Even among the elderly, exercise training has been shown to enhance peak and submaximal exercise capacity, 6-minute walking distance, and overall quality of life compared to nonpharmacological treatments. Supervised exercise training (either resistance or endurance) was shown to improve exercise capacity (peak VO_2) and reverse remodeling of the atrium and left ventricular diastolic dysfunction in all patients above and above the benefits gained from standard medical therapy. In the REHAB-HF (Rehabilitation Therapy in Older Acute Heart Failure Patients) trial, Kitzman et al. demonstrated the benefit of a supervised exercise program in improving the functional capacity of elderly patients after admission for acute HF, including HFpEF patients.

Device Therapy

Hospitalizations for HF (including HFpEF) were significantly reduced using the wireless implantable hemodynamic monitoring system (CardioMEMS) of the pulmonary artery pressure. The benefit extended over a mean follow-up period of 13 months. Another emerging device is the interatrial shunt device. It is a percutaneously inserted interatrial conduit that aims to decompress the left side of the heart, reducing the left atrial pressure and the pulmonary capillary wedge pressure whenever they are high. The evidence on this device is still controversial without a significant improvement in cardiovascular (CV) morbidity and mortality.

Guideline-directed Medical Therapy for Heart Failure with Preserved Ejection Fraction

Guideline-directed medical therapy (GDMT) can be started safely and effectively in acute and long-term care settings. Apart from judicious utilization of diuretics, beta blockers are to be used with caution even in patients with myocardial infarction (MI), and AF with monitoring of exercise tolerance, and chronotropic competence. Elderly patients are generally at higher risk of side effects from HF medications due to a higher prevalence of polypharmacy, cognitive impairment, and reduced liver and kidney functions.

CONCLUSION

Treatment of HFpEF remains a significant challenge in managing HF patients, especially in the elderly. The management should focus on addressing the causes of HFpEF and the associated comorbidities in the affected individuals. To date, SGLT2 inhibitors are the only agents proven by randomized clinical trials to effectively reduce the hard endpoints of CV mortality and HF hospitalizations. Exercise training and loop diuretics can improve HF symptoms. Elderly HFpEF patients are susceptible to developing adverse effects from HF medications; therefore, very slow initiation of medications and close follow-up of the blood pressure, renal functions, liver functions, and electrolytes are mandatory. Adjustments in the prescriptions should be considered on a case-to-case basis. Higher usual levels of light physical activity, moderate-to-vigorous physical activity, and steps per day measured by accelerometry are associated with lower risks of incident overall HF and HFpEF in women aged 63–99 years in the community setting. A sedentary lifestyle is associated with higher risks. Physical activity, weight reduction, volume restriction, and comorbidities management are essential. Exercise training under supervision (either resistance or endurance) has been shown to improve exercise capacity (peak VO_2) and reverse remodeling of the atrium and left ventricular diastolic dysfunction.

REFERENCES

1. Pandey A, Shah SJ, Kellogg D, et al. Exercise Intolerance in Older Adults With Heart Failure With Preserved Ejection Fraction: JACC State-of-the-Art Review. J Am Coll Cardiol. 2022;78(11):1166-87.
2. Ariyaratnam JP, Mishima RS, Kadhim K, et al. Utility and Validity of the HFA-PEFF and H2FPEF Scores in Patients With Symptomatic Atrial Fibrillation. JACC Heart Fail. 2024;12(6):1015-25.
3. Mert GO, Özlek B, Özlek E, et al. Comparing the Diagnostic Performance of HFA-PEFF and H2FPEF Scoring Systems in Heart Failure with Preserved Ejection Fraction Patients: Insights from the APOLLON Registry. Anatol J Cardiol. 2023;27(9):539-48.
4. Sauer AJ. Empagliflozin and Elderly Patients With Preserved Ejection Fraction Heart Failure: Is Age Just a Number? J Am Coll Cardiol. 2022;80(1):19-21.
5. LaMonte MJ, LaCroix AZ, Nguyen S, et al. Accelerometer-measured physical activity, sedentary time, and heart failure risk in women aged 63 to 99 years. JAMA Cardiol. 2024;9(4):336-45.
6. Gharagozloo K, Mehdizadeh M, Heckman G, et al. Heart Failure With Preserved Ejection Fraction in the Elderly Population: Basic Mechanisms and Clinical Considerations. Can J Cardiol. 2024;40(8):1424-1444.

Heart Failure in Women

Harshit Khare, Roopali Khanna

INTRODUCTION

The risk of developing heart failure (HF) is similar between men and women, but there are marked sex differences in the etiology, presentation, and pathophysiology of developing HF. The existence of gender differences across various aspects of HF as a disease, per se, has always intrigued the medical community. It becomes even more relevant if we consider the low percentage of women population enrolment in most of the HF trials. At the same time, all evidence for guidelines and recommendations from them extended their results to the underrepresented women population. There is a paucity of data regarding the sex-specific mechanisms of HF, optimal dosing of drugs, and the role of device therapy in women.

In this article, we explore the gender differences in risk factors, diagnosis, clinical manifestation, and heart failure outcomes while trying to understand the pathophysiology behind these differences.

EPIDEMIOLOGY AND PRESENTATION

The fact that the incidence of HF is higher in men misleadingly paints an unfair picture of the distribution of HF burden. Women form almost 50% of the population with HF symptoms, making the prevalence of HF equal in men and women.[1] This means that HF is equally prevalent in women despite being more incident in men after age adjustment. This is explained by the fact that the overall survival of women is better than men.

The gender differences prevail even in HF presentations, with women presenting more with preserved left ventricular ejection fraction (LVEF) phenotype, and even when having HF with reduced ejection fraction (HFrEF), women tend to have higher LVEF as supported by the HF study cohort from Framingham Heart Study, later in Candesartan in Heart failure Assessment of Reduction in Mortality and morbidity study (CHARM study), further in Irbesartan in heart failure with Preserved ejection fraction study (I-Preserve), and then in Treatment of Preserved Cardiac Function Heart Failure with an Aldosterone Antagonist study (TOPCAT study) .[2-6]

The comorbidities such as hypertension and hypothyroidism are more prevalent in women with HF. Women with HF are older and have higher body mass index (BMI) and higher ejection fraction (EF) when compared to men with HF. Diabetes, hypertension, and renal dysfunction are more prevalent in women. The most common risk factor for developing HF in women is hypertension, whereas it is coronary artery disease in women. The other nontraditional cardiovascular risk factors such as anxiety, depression, caregiver stress, and low household income also contribute more in women **(Table 1)**.[3]

As far as epidemiological data from the Indian perspective is concerned, the INDUS study from Northern India, the first of its kind, comprising both rural community and tertiary care-level community population, determined the HF prevalence in rural communities to be 1.2/1,000 was relatively low compared to western data. The sex ratio of women to men was 1.9:1 in this study, with rheumatic heart disease as the most common etiology.[7]

TABLE 1: Differences in epidemiology and clinical presentation among men and women.

	Women compared to men
Age of presentation	*Older*
Risk factors: • BMI • Hypertension • CAD • Atrial fibrillation	 • Higher • Major risk factor • Less common • Higher predictive in developing HFpEF
HF phenotype: • HFpEF • PPCM • Stress cardiomyopathy	 • HFpEF more common • Specific to women • More
Symptoms: Dyspnea, edema	More symptomatic
Pathological changes: • Macrovascular CAD • Microvascular endothelial dysfunction	 • Less common • More common
Anatomical changes: • Left ventricular mass • Contractility • Cell turnover/apoptosis • Coronary vessel caliber • Blood pressure • Resting heart rate • Catecholamine-mediated vasoconstriction	 • Lower • Greater • Lower • Smaller • Lower • Higher • Less
Survival: HF hospitalisation and life expectancy	Better
Treatment: • Drug therapy • Device therapy • ICD • CRT	 • Summarized in **Table 2** • Underrepresentation of women in trials • Significant benefit in men but trends toward benefit in women

DIAGNOSIS, ETIOLOGY, AND SURVIVAL DIFFERENCES

The echocardiographic confirmation of heart failure with decreased left ventricular systolic function occurs in only around 17–25%, and in the majority of women, LVEF is largely preserved, and even in those with HFrEF, women have higher LVEF (Framingham heart study and Olmsted County data[8]). This forms the basis of the hypothesis that better LVEF in women with HF probably results in higher survival for women than men. The data from the real-world comes from the OPTIMIZE-HF registry, where acute HF in women resulted in lower 1-year mortality even when they were less likely to receive GDMT.[9]

The diagnosis of HF has been a clinical diagnosis from the beginning, based on the presence of symptoms and signs of congestion or impaired ventricular compliance. Women with HF may have more congestive symptoms when the presentation is chronic.

The reasons for these sex differences have been variously speculated, and studies have come up with two main hypotheses: the difference in their systolic function and their etiology for HF. Since women with HF have better LVEF, whether in HFrEF or HFpEF phenotype, they have better survival. Secondly, due to the lesser incidence of ischemic cardiomyopathy in women, they may have better survival. Both above-mentioned hypotheses have been questioned in different studies, and the survival differences are often also dependent on parameters being studied for correlation with survival. For example, while both brain natriuretic peptide and cardiopulmonary exercise have performed better as predictors of mortality in women with HF in most of the recent studies, LV systolic function has not always been consistent as a marker of survival, questioning our first hypothesis of gender differences in HF.[10]

Elaborating on the etiology of HF across both genders, women have a higher likelihood of having hypertension and valvular disease and a lesser likelihood of having coronary artery disease (CAD).[3,11] Complications during pregnancy such as gestational diabetes, preeclampsia, and premature birth are emerging as important risk factors for developing cardiovascular disease. Preeclampsia increases the incidence of essential hypertension by four times and the risk of CAD and stroke by two times, which increases the likelihood of developing HF by 80%. Other significant causes of HF in women include chemotherapy-related cardiac toxicity and peripartum cardiomyopathy (PPCM).

Sex-specific Etiologies of Heart Failure

Peripartum Cardiomyopathy

Peripartum cardiomyopathy is defined as ventricular systolic dysfunction, occurring either in the last month of pregnancy or 5 months within the postpartum period, not attributable to known existing cardiac diseases. The causes for PPCM have been variously speculated as myocarditis, abnormal immunologic response, myocytic apoptosis, genetic cause, and oxidative cleavage of prolactin. The different risk factors include advanced age, higher parity, multiple or twin pregnancy, use of tocolytics, and poor socioeconomic status. The diagnosis is often difficult because the hemodynamics of pregnancy masks congestive signs and symptoms of HF. More than half the patients recover their LV systolic function postpartum over 3–6 months, while one-fifth continue to have poor LV systolic function. Studies suggest LVEF in following pregnancies is determined by residual LVEF following episodes of PPCM. The goals of therapy include symptomatic treatment, recovery of LV function, and prevention of thromboembolic episodes and other complications. Treatment modalities include early initiation of GDMT HF therapy, with caution to fetal safety and lactation. Another therapeutic option is bromocriptine; however, the lack of supporting evidence for bromocriptine limits its use in clinical practice.[12]

Chemotherapy-induced Cardiomyopathy

Chemotherapy-induced HF needs special mention in the women subgroup due to the higher incidence of breast cancer. Patients with early breast cancer (EBC) develop HF mainly after anthracycline and trastuzumab treatment and have fewer comorbidities than those who develop HF from other etiologies. When comparing HF related to trastuzumab therapy with anthracyclines, trastuzumab-related HF, had a lesser risk of future HF hospitalization. The morality and clinical outcome associated with EBC chemotherapy-induced HF are lesser when compared with those in HF from other etiologies, likely due to the reversible nature of the former with GDMT.

Most of the data on chemotherapy-induced HF is from anthracycline-associated HF, reporting mortality as high as 3.5-fold compared to outcomes with idiopathic cardiomyopathy. The best clinical practice includes close follow-up with these cardiotoxic chemotherapies and early detection with early institution of GDMT.[13]

THERAPY

Primary Prevention of Heart Failure

Due to differences in predisposing risk factors and etiologies for developing HF in women, targeted and sex-specific strategies are needed to increase awareness and optimal control of risk factors for HFrEF and HFpEF. Screening of risk factors during pregnancy and the need for close surveillance of women with predisposing risk factors will help in reducing the burden of HF.

The current guideline recommendations for HF therapy derive evidence from clinical trials where women were hugely underrepresented **(Table 2)**. Therefore, we must use caution in exercising these recommendations freely in the female population.

Angiotensin-converting Enzyme Inhibitors

Although there was an under-representation of women in most trials of angiotensin-converting enzyme (ACE) inhibitors, the benefit of mortality reduction in HFrEF can be extrapolated to women by data from various meta-analyses. In their landmark meta-analysis, Garg and Yusuf showed lower mortality with ACEIs in HF across both gender[14,] and the study of Shekelle et al. further supported this.[15] They obtained gender-stratified results from seven studies on ACE inhibitors [Survival And Ventricular Enlargement (SAVE), Studies Of Left Ventricular Dysfunction (SOLVD) Prevention, SOLVD Treatment, Cooperative North Scandinavian Enalapril Survival Study (CONSENSUS), Survival of Myocardial Infarction Long-term Evaluation (SMILE), Acute Infarction Ramipril Efficacy (AIRE) and Trandolapril Cardiac Evaluation (TRACE)]. The difference in effect between men and women approached statistical significance for the relative risk reduction ($p = 0.07$).

TABLE 2: Female representation in major heart failure trials and gender-based mortality or HF hospitalization benefit in major HF therapy trials.

Study	*% women represented*	*Endpoint*	*HR/OR/RH with confidence interval (CI) women*	*HR/OR/RH with confidence interval (CI) men*
ACEI meta-analysis[14]	20–24	Mortality	OR 0.79 (0.59–1.06)	OR 0.76 (0.65–0.88]
Val-HeFT[16]	20	Mortality	HR 0.93 (0.68–1.27)	HR 1.04 (0.90–1.19)
Val-HeFT[16]	20	HF hospital stays	HR 0.74 (0.55–0.98)	HR 0.73 (0.62–0.86)
CIBIS-II[18]	19	Mortality	RH 0.53 (0.42–0.67)	RH 0.37 (0.19–0.69)
SCD-HeFT[26]	24	Mortality	HR 0.96 (0.58–1.61)	HR 0.73 (0.57–0.93)
CARE-HF[24]	27	Mortality + hospital stay	HR 0.64 (0.42–0.97)	HR 0.62 (0.49–0.79)

(OR: odds ratio; HR: hazard ratio; RH: relative hazards)

They further showed that while the male population benefited from ACE inhibitor, whether symptomatic or asymptomatic, the female population benefitted most when symptomatic or having LV dysfunction, and the benefit, however, was less compared to the male population.

Angiotensin Receptor Blocker

Angiotensin receptor blockers (ARBs) are a good choice for ACE inhibitor-intolerant patients, but gender-based differences for ARBs have not been largely explored. Much of the data for benefit in women with HF is with candesartan and valsartan. Data from CHARM trials show benefit in the combined endpoint of hospitalization and mortality with candesartan, while data from Val-HeFT (Valsartan Heart failure trial) showed benefit only in HF hospitalization and the secondary endpoint of cardiac events including cardiac arrest, stay of HF hospital, or use of intravenous inotropes.[16]

Beta-blockers

Post hoc analysis from landmark randomized control trials of all 3 β-blockers studied, namely, carvedilol, bisoprolol, and metoprolol succinate, suggested that adding β-blockers to the regimen of ACE inhibitor in women patients of HF, had added beneficial effect, despite their low representation in these studies.

Carvedilol studied in the COPERNICUS trial, showed improved survival in women population as well, and the benefit was more in those with more severe LV dysfunction.[17]

Similarly, Bisoprolol in the CIBIS II trial improved survival in women with HF.[18] This metoprolol studied in the MERIT-HF trial reduced HF hospital stays significantly in the women subgroup. Therefore, the benefit of β-blockers in women with HF is quite substantial and irrefutable.[19]

Aldosterone Antagonists

The mortality benefits of mineralocorticoid receptor antagonists for the women subgroup with HF are well supported by post-hoc analyses from both RALES and EPHESUS trials. The RALES trial enrolled a substantial subgroup of women with HF. It showed significant mortality reduction with spironolactone in both ischemic and nonischemic cardiomyopathies with NYHA class III to IV with LVEF <35%.[20] The EPHESUS trial showed similar mortality benefit post-MI patients with LVEF <40%.[21]

Digoxin

Digoxin, in general, is a class-IIb recommendation for patients with HFrEF, as digoxin reduces HF hospital stay but has no beneficial effect on survival. Higher levels of digoxin in women HFrEF were linked to increased rates of mortality, but at lower therapeutic levels, digoxin was shown to be safe and tolerable in women (DIG trial).[22]

Cardiac Resynchronization Therapy

Cardiac resynchronization therapy (CRT) is recommended in patients of HF in NYHA class-III–IV with LVEF <35%, despite GDMT and a wide QRS, to improve functional capacity and reduce mortality, based on various trial data. In the COMPANION study, CRT lowered the combined endpoint of mortality or hospital stay, and the result was also consistent in the women subgroup. Similarly, CARE-HF, which enrolled around 200 women with HF, again showed reduced mortality and hospital stay combined.[23,24]

Implantable Cardioverter-defibrillator

The women population in Implantable cardioverter-defibrillator ICD trials was remarkably low. The landmark MADIT-II trial had only 119 women of ICMP with LVEF <30%, and it showed a trend toward lowering mortality in the women subgroup.[25] Similarly SCDHeFT trial, which enrolled around 588 women with LVEF <35%, was not powered enough to detect gender differences.[26]

Ventricular Assist Device

Ventricular assist device (VAD) data for outcomes in women with HF are limited. Firstly, we have limited representation of women in studies using VADs. Secondly, women with smaller builds may have further limited options, as LVADs need a minimum body surface to be placed properly. Studies show women have a worse prognosis compared with men with LVADs.[27]

Heart Transplantation

Heart transplantation data from the US population show women comprised one-fourth population of donors, and nearly one-fourth of the transplant population were women. The outcomes, i.e., survival rates, were lower for the women subgroup than men. However, long-term survival data for 10 and 15 years was similar, and coronary allograft vasculopathy was lower for the women subgroup.[28]

CONCLUSION

Women comprise the majority of the HF population, with a higher incidence at an older age. The HFpEF phenotype is more prevalent in women, and HF in women is more likely to be associated with co-morbidities such as hypertension and hypothyroidism and less likely associated with CAD. The clinical outcomes are better in women with HF compared to men, and likely reasons include differences in etiology and survival data for women.

Despite robust data for various therapies from different landmark trials in HF, the data analysis for the women subgroup remains scarce, and there is limited exploration of these gender differences in basic sciences. We need to elaborate more on these differences and investigate into pathophysiology behind these differences besides recruiting more women with HF in trials. In the past, female representation in HF trials was a meager 19%, which has marginally increased to 28% in recent trials such as CHARM and COMPANION, and this explains the work that's still needed in this area. This is why present data results for therapeutic recommendations had to be extrapolated from post-hoc analysis and various meta-analyses. The need indicates that investigators in upcoming HF trials may try to elaborate more on these gender-based differences. We may have better-designed trials enrolling at least 40% women sub-group. The change is almost imminent.

REFERENCES

1. Lindenfeld J, O'Connor CM. Heart failure in women. JACC Heart Fail. 2019;7(3):274-75.
2. Mahmood SS, Levy D, Vasan RS, et al. The Framingham Heart Study and the epidemiology of cardiovascular disease: A historical perspective. Lancet. 2014;383(9921): 999-1008.
3. Ho KK, Pinsky JL, Kannel WB, et al. The epidemiology of heart failure: the Framingham Study. J Am Coll Cardiol. 1993;22(4 Suppl A):6A-13.
4. Ostergren JB. Angiotensin receptor blockade with candesartan in heart failure: findings from the Candesartan in Heart failure—assessment of reduction in mortality and morbidity (CHARM) programme. J Hypertens Suppl. 2006;24(1):S3-7.
5. Carson P, Massie BM, McKelvie R, et al; I-PRESERVE Investigators. The irbesartan in heart failure with preserved systolic function (I-PRESERVE) trial: rationale and design. J Card Fail. 2005;11(8):576-85.
6. Pitt B, Pfeffer MA, Assmann SF, et al; TOPCAT Investigators. Spironolactone for heart failure with preserved ejection fraction. N Engl J Med. 2014;370(15):1383-92.
7. Chaturvedi V, Parakh N, Seth S, et al. Heart failure in India: The INDUS (INDia Ukieri Study) study. J Pract Cardiovasc Sci 2016;2:28-35.
8. Roger VL, Weston SA, Redfield MM, Hellermann-Homan JP, Killian J, Yawn BP, Jacobsen SJ. Trends in heart failure incidence and survival in a community-based population. JAMA. 2004 Jul 21;292(3):344-50.
9. Fonarow GC, Stough WG, Abraham WT, et al; OPTIMIZE-HF Investigators and Hospitals. Characteristics, treatments, and outcomes of patients with preserved systolic function hospitalized for heart failure: a report from the OPTIMIZE-HF Registry. J Am Coll Cardiol. 2007; 50(8):768-77.
10. Johnstone D, Limacher M, Rousseau M, et al. Clinical characteristics of patients in studies of left ventricular dysfunction (SOLVD). Am J Cardiol. 1992;70(9): 894-900.
11. He J, Ogden LG, Bazzano LA, et al. Risk factors for congestive heart failure in US men and women: NHANES I epidemiologic follow-up study. Arch Intern Med. 2001; 161(7):996-1002.
12. Abboud J, Murad Y, Chen-Scarabelli C, et al. Peripartum cardiomyopathy: a comprehensive review. Int J Cardiol. 2007;118(3):295-303.
13. Abdel-Qadir H, Tai F, Croxford R, et al. Characteristics and Outcomes of Women Developing Heart Failure After Early Stage Breast Cancer Chemotherapy: A Population-based Matched Cohort Study. Circ Heart Fail. 2021;14(7): e008110.
14. Garg R, Yusuf S. Overview of randomized trials of angiotensin-converting enzyme inhibitors on mortality and morbidity in patients with heart failure. Collaborative Group on ACE Inhibitor Trials. JAMA. 1995;273(18): 1450-6. Erratum in: JAMA 1995;274(6):462.
15. Shekelle PG, Rich MW, Morton SC, et al. Efficacy of angiotensin-converting enzyme inhibitors and beta-blockers in the management of left ventricular systolic dysfunction according to race, gender, and diabetic status: A meta-analysis of major clinical trials. J Am Coll Cardiol. 2003;41(9):1529-38.
16. Latini R, Masson S, Anand I, et al; Valsartan Heart Failure Trial Investigators. Effects of valsartan on circulating brain natriuretic peptide and norepinephrine in symptomatic chronic heart failure: the Valsartan Heart Failure Trial (Val-HeFT). Circulation. 2002 ;106(19):2454-8.
17. Eichhorn EJ, Bristow MR. The Carvedilol Prospective Randomized Cumulative Survival (COPERNICUS) trial. Curr Control Trials Cardiovasc Med. 2001;2(1):20-23.
18. The Cardiac Insufficiency Bisoprolol Study II (CIBIS-II): A randomised trial. Lancet. 1999 Jan 2;353(9146):9-13. PMID: 10023943.
19. Wikstrand J. MERIT-HF--description of the trial. Basic Res Cardiol. 2000;95 Suppl 1:I90-7.
20. Kulbertus H. L'étude clinique du mois. L'étude RALES (randomized aldactone evaluation study) [Study of the month. The RALES study (randomized aldactone evaluation study]. Rev Med Liege. 1999;54(9):770-2.
21. Pitt B, Williams G, Remme W, et al. The EPHESUS trial: eplerenone in patients with heart failure due to systolic

dysfunction complicating acute myocardial infarction. Eplerenone Post-AMI Heart Failure Efficacy and Survival Study. Cardiovasc Drugs Ther. 2001;15(1):79-87
22. Collins JF, Egan D, Yusuf S, Garg R, Williford WO, Geller N; DIG Investigators. Overview of the DIG trial. Control Clin Trials. 2003 Dec;24(6 Suppl):269S-276S. doi: 10.1016/s0197-2456(03)00104-1. PMID: 14643073.
23. Anand IS, Carson P, Galle E, et al. Cardiac resynchronization therapy reduces the risk of hospitalizations in patients with advanced heart failure: Results from the Comparison of Medical Therapy, Pacing and Defibrillation in Heart Failure (COMPANION) trial. Circulation. 2009;119(7):969-77.
24. Cleland JG, Daubert JC, Erdmann E, et al. Cardiac Resynchronization-Heart Failure (CARE-HF) Study Investigators. The effect of cardiac resynchronization on morbidity and mortality in heart failure. N Engl J Med. 2005;352: 1539-1549.
25. Coats AJ. MADIT II, the Multi-center Autonomic Defibrillator Implantation Trial II stopped early for mortality reduction, has ICD therapy earned its evidence-based credentials? Int J Cardiol. 2002;82(1):1-5.
26. Bardy GH, Lee KL, Mark DB, et al. Sudden Cardiac Death in Heart Failure Trial (SCD-HeFT) Investigators. Amiodarone or an implantable cardioverter-defibrillator for congestive heart failure. N Engl J Med. 2005;352(3):225-37. Erratum in: N Engl J Med. 200519;352(20):2146.
27. Morgan JA, Weinberg AD, Hollingsworth KW, et al. Effect of gender on bridging to transplantation and posttransplantation survival in patients with left ventricular assist devices. J Thorac Cardiovasc Surg. 2004; 127(4):1193-5.
28. Chambers DC, Cherikh WS, Harhay MO, et al; International Society for Heart and Lung Transplantation. The International Thoracic Organ Transplant Registry of the International Society for Heart and Lung Transplantation: Thirty-sixth adult lung and heart-lung transplantation Report-2019; Focus theme: Donor and recipient size match. J Heart Lung Transplant. 2019;38(10):1042-55.

SECTION 11

HFpEF: Cardio-ophthalmology

107. Retinal Microvascular Impairment in HFpEF

108. Impact of Diabetic Retinopathy on Prognosis of Patients with HFpEF

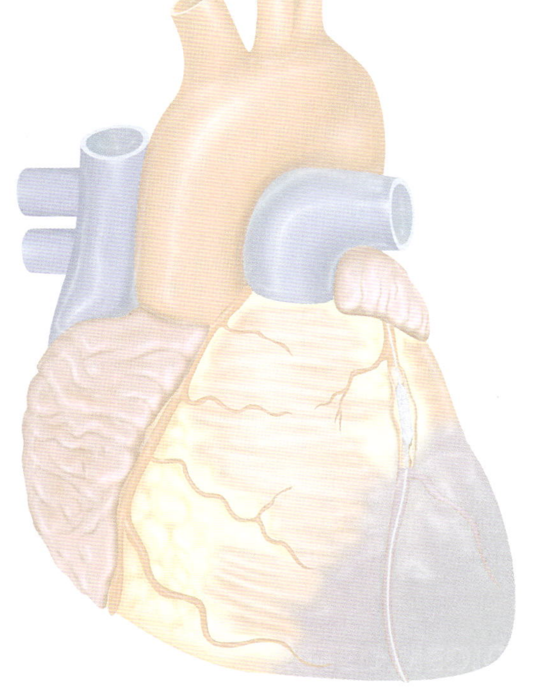

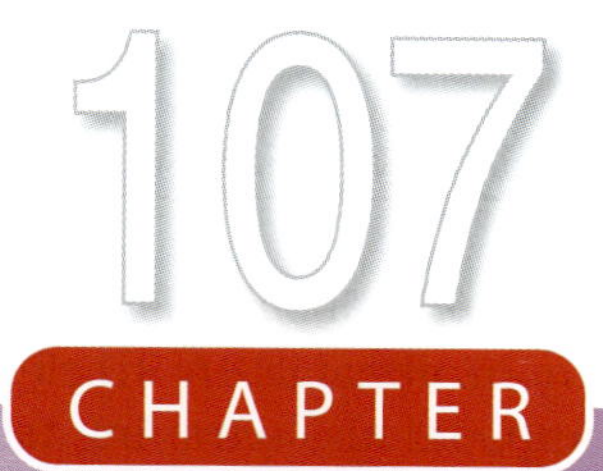

Retinal Microvascular Impairment in HFpEF

Krishna Vaitheeswaran, Preetinder Kaur, Monika Nadar

INTRODUCTION

Endothelial cells play a central role in blood vessel physiology by regulating vessel wall integrity, vasodilatation, and blood coagulation. Impairment of endothelial function (endothelial dysfunction) plays an important role in the development and progression of heart failure (HF) and is considered an important marker of elevated cardiovascular risk.[1] Microvascular alteration in the body results from endothelial dysfunction due to systemic disease and precedes the development of more well-known macrovascular changes that are therapeutic targets used conventionally in the management of vascular disorders, including those associated with HF.

Retinal microcirculation may be rapidly assessed and imaged with current imaging modalities, which are readily available such as the wide-field imaging systems, nonmydriatic systems, and ubiquitous smartphone fundus evaluation and provide a window of opportunity to evaluate the risk of HF as well as stratify risk and prognosis of patients with HF.

The microvascular complications that are revealed by retinal imaging are better correlated in patients with heart failure with preserved ejection fraction (HFpEF) rather than heart failure with reduced ejection fraction (HFrEF).[2]

Retinal diseases have been long associated with hypertension, and retinal imaging has been used to assess and monitor retinal microcirculation. This allows an easy and noninvasive modality to assess systemic microcirculation, which would reflect and indicate severity of diseases in many organs, including the heart.

Advances in retinal imaging and easy availability of the acquisition devices have allowed the integration of the techniques with other cardiac evaluation techniques such as cardiac imaging, electrophysiology, and biomarkers to stratify persons at high risk of developing HF as well as prognosticate those with HF, particularly those with HFpEF where the retinal alterations may be more marked.

ASSESSMENT OF RETINAL MICROVASCULAR STRUCTURE AND FUNCTION

Retinal structural evaluation in patients with left ventricular remodeling and HF involves the following:

- Static assessment, including measurements of retinal vascular caliber
    - Central retinal arterial equivalent (CRAE)
    - Central retinal venular equivalent (CRVE)
    - Arteriolar to venular ratio (AVratio)
- Focal arteriolar narrowing
- Generalized arteriolar narrowing
- Retinal vascular geometry
- Specific background signs:
    - Retinal microaneurysms
    - Hemorrhages
    - Cotton-wool spots (soft exudates)
    - Hard exudates
    - Venous beading
    - Neovascularization
    - AV shunts
    - Microaneurysms

- *Optical coherence tomography:* Cross-sectional image of retinal layers in selected location
- Confocal scanning laser ophthalmoscopy to obtain images for retinal vascular caliber measurements
- *OCT angiography:* This provides a 3D depth-encoded retinal blood flow image with a view of the retinal capillary flow. This may allow the assessment of microvascular function, including a differential flow rate in the superficial and deep capillary plexus as well as characterization of vascular structures and exploration of anomalous capillary and microvascular circulation. Retinal perfusion maps allow the demonstration of areas of retinal vascular perfusion and its alterations such as vascular remodeling, areas of generalized or focal nonperfusion as well as development of microaneurysms.
- *Ultra-wide-field imaging:* This provides a panretinal view of the retinal vasculature. While conventional imaging evaluates mainly the macular area, the retinal periphery can be visualized with ultra-wide-field technology. Wide-field angiography may allow detailed evaluation of the peripheral blood supply and microcirculation. While the retinal angiography is performed using intravenous injection of dyes, oral fluorescein angiography to assess the circulation is also possible with current day high-resolution machines.

RETINAL MICROVASCULAR FUNCTION

Retinal dynamic vessel analysis (RVA) is another method of detecting endothelial dysfunction using a combination of retinal vessel analyzer and a fundus camera.

After dilatation, retinal arteriolar and venular caliber are assessed after provocation by optoelectronic flicker light. This causes vessel dilatation through nitric oxide release in retinal vascular smooth vessels.

Videos of selected segments are compared with the baseline, and the percentage of flicker-induced dilatation (FID) of retinal arterioles and retinal venules (FID_{art} and FID_{ven}, respectively) is calculated.

Reduced FID values in arterioles and venules suggest impaired retinal microcirculation and endothelial dysfunction.

The effect of mydriatic drugs may affect the retinal vessel caliber and is a confounding factor for which the examination is done at a fixed time after dilatation (20 minutes).

In addition, poor fixation may enhance variability and give inaccurate results.

The normal and cutoff values for the abnormal in different conditions are not yet determined for all systemic and ocular conditions, limiting its use clinically.

However, it has been shown that abnormal FID_{art} and FID_{ven} were significantly higher in HF patients than patients with other cardiovascular morbidities.[3] Furthermore, FID_{art} was found to be more impaired in ischemic than in nonischemic cardiomyopathy, suggesting that FID_{art} may be a marker of atherosclerotic burden.[3]

OCULAR ELECTROPHYSIOLOGY IN HEART FAILURE WITH PRESERVED EJECTION FRACTION

Electrophysiology may be used in the diagnosis of HFpEF to detect microvascular alterations.

The main tests are electroretinogram (ERG), electro-oculogram (EOG), and visual evoked potential (VEP).

While ERG assesses the retinal function, EOG is used for retinal pigment epithelial function as well as photoreceptor interaction. VEP evaluates the visual pathways up to the visual cortex.

Together, these may be used to evaluate the existing microvascular changes induced by the systemic condition.

The changes in ERG, more evident in flicker ERG and the oscillatory potentials, often predate the structural changes and actual development of clinical retinopathy. In addition, these may reverse or stabilize with appropriate treatment even though the retinopathy may continue to be visualized.

Of late, mfERG has been used to detect maculopathy much earlier than the observation of macular edema in vascular conditions involving the posterior pole. In addition, localized areas of neuroretinal dysfunction were demonstrable even with just systemic deviations of blood biochemistry such as poor glycemic control.

The various ERG techniques that may be used are:
- Standard full-field ERG
- Flicker ERG
- mfERG
- Pattern ERG (PERG)
- Focal ERG

Visual evoked potential has also been demonstrated to have changes in patients with DM and HF. These are detected before anatomical abnormalities can be seen. These may be due to a reversible or an irreversible change in ganglion cells due to the vascular alterations.

Damage to central neurons is very early compared to retinal ones, and VEP may be able to pick this up earlier than structural or functional assessment of the retina.

Recently, the use of multifocal VEP (mfVEP) has been shown to have differences between normal and patients with diabetes and diabetic retinopathy. The areas with diabetic retinopathy had significant differences compared to areas without retinopathy.

The use of visual electrophysiology techniques may support diagnosis of microvascular and vascular events associated with systemic disease such as HF even before the occurrence of demonstrable structural changes. The use of flash/flicker ERG with PERG along with VEP will allow localization of the alterations that may be coincident with the systemic disease.

CURRENT EVIDENCE LINKING RETINOPATHIES AND HEART FAILURE

Retinal Artery Narrowing

Asymptomatic left ventricular hypertrophy was independently associated with narrowing of retinal arterioles and presence of retinopathy. This was found in patients who did not have hypertension, diabetes, or coronary calcification, suggesting that retinal microcirculatory damage may reflect subclinical dysfunction of systemic and cardiac circulation.[4]

A subsequent study also demonstrated that CRAE narrowing and dilatation of CRVE could predict an increase in left ventricular size and mass.[5]

Retinal microvascular changes have been shown to be associated with subclinical systolic and diastolic dysfunction. A decreased CRAE and increased CRVE were associated with both left ventricular systolic and diastolic dysfunction.[5]

Decreased retinal venular branching and fractal dimension were also observed with left ventricular and left atrial dysfunction.[6]

Diabetic retinopathy has been shown to have echocardiographic parameters of left ventricular diastolic dysfunction.[7]

Therefore, retinal photography may serve as a useful biomarker of left ventricular diastolic function, wall stress, inflammation, and metabolic insult to the cardiac muscles leading to maladaptive left ventricular modeling.

SYMPTOMATIC HEART FAILURE

Retinal microvascular lesions have been demonstrated in patients with incident HF in population-based studies.[8]

Wong et al. suggested that the presence of retinopathy is a predictor of developing HF within 7 years, independent of demographics or cardiovascular risk factors. This was also significant in patients who did not have hypertension, DM, or coronary artery disease, suggesting retinal microvascular anomalies pose an increased risk of HF even in healthy individuals.

Chandra et al.[5] demonstrated that after adjusting for demographics and CVD risks, CRVE remained significant in predicting incident HF. Venular dilatation could represent asymptomatic elevated systemic venous pressure.

Diabetic retinopathy has been shown to be an independent predictor of HF[9] with moderate-to-severe diabetic retinopathy associated with a twofold increase of HF independent of cardiovascular risks, atherosclerotic burden, and glycemic control.[2]

Retinopathy and retinal microvascular complications in patients with diabetes may play a greater role in HFpEF rather than HFrEF.[2]

CURRENT STATUS AND FUTURE DIRECTIONS

The current evidence points to the role of retinal microcirculation in assessing HF. However, applications are limited primarily to research initiatives due to heterogeneity of patient characteristics, retinal imaging techniques as well as definition of outcome assessments and parameters of interest.

Again, the equipment used in research articles such as dynamic vessel assessments is not readily available clinically, and optical coherence tomograms and widefield imaging systems that are routinely used clinically have not been studied extensively with a lack of robust data for algorithm development and classification.

Though diagnostic data exist, comparison of retinal imaging for prognostication for HF is insufficient, which limits wide clinical application in the presence of more classical biomarkers such as echocardiography and natriuretic peptide.

The acquisition and assessment of retinal images by trained staff are also a challenge currently, which are offset by smartphone-based fundus cameras and deep learning-based image analysis, which address most concerns of widespread application and universal clinical application for patients with HF.

Deep learning retinal image analysis integrated into fundus imaging devices has the capability to perform automated image analysis using recurrent convolutional or deep convolutional networks with multiple levels of abstraction using supervised, unsupervised, or reinforcement algorithms.

CONCLUSION

Future applications of retinal imaging and analysis could be given as follows:

- Predicting the risk of developing HF
- Identifying patients with stage B HF
- Stratifying prognosis in patients with stage C HF
- Defining HF phenotypes
- Monitoring HF treatment response

- Identifying genetic determinants of cardiovascular and cerebrovascular abnormalities using microvascular changes identified by retinal imaging.[10]
- Telemedicine applications and community screening of population by a simple optometric evaluation are the major applications, which may enhance early detection for intervention in population at risk for cardiovascular disorders, including HF. This may be included in routine cardiovascular epidemiological screening protocols, which require further research and data input.

REFERENCES

1. Deanfield JE, Halcox JP, Rabenik TJ. Endothelial function and dysfunction: testing and clinical relevance. Circulation. 2007;115:1285-95.
2. Tromp J, Lim SL, Tay WT, et al. Microvascular disease in patients with reduced ejection fraction versus preserved ejection fraction. Diabetes Care. 2019;42:1792-9.
3. Nagele MP, Barthelmes J, Ludovici V, et al. Retinal microvascular dysfunction in heart failure. Eur Heart J. 2017;39:47-56.
4. Cheung N, Bluemke DA, Klein R, et al. Retinal arteriolar narrowing and left ventricular remodeling: the multi-ethnic study of atherosclerosis. J Am Coll Cardiol. 2007; 50:48-55.
5. Chandra A, Seidelmann SB, Claggett BL, et al. The association of retinal vessel calibres with heart failure and long-term alterations in cardiac structure and function: the Atherosclerosis Risk in Communities (ARIC) study. Eur J Heart Fail. 2019;21:1207-15.
6. Huang L, Chen WQ, Aris IM, et al. Associations between cardiac function and retinal microvascular geometry among Chinese adults. Sci Rep. 2020;10:14797.
7. Takeda Y, Sakata Y, Mano T, et al. Diabetic retinopathy is associated with impaired left ventricular relaxation. J Card Fail. 2011;17:556-60.
8. Wong TY, Rosamond W, Chang PP, et al. Retinopathy and risk of congestive heart failure. JAMA. 2005;293: 63-9.
9. Cheung N, Wang JJ, Rogers SL, et al. Diabetic retinopathy and risk of heart failure. J Am Coll Cardiol. 2008;51: 1573-8.
10. Zekavat SM, Raghu VK, Trinder M, et al. Deep learning of the retina enables phenome- and genome-wide analysis of the microvasculature. Circulation. 2022;145:134-50.

CHAPTER

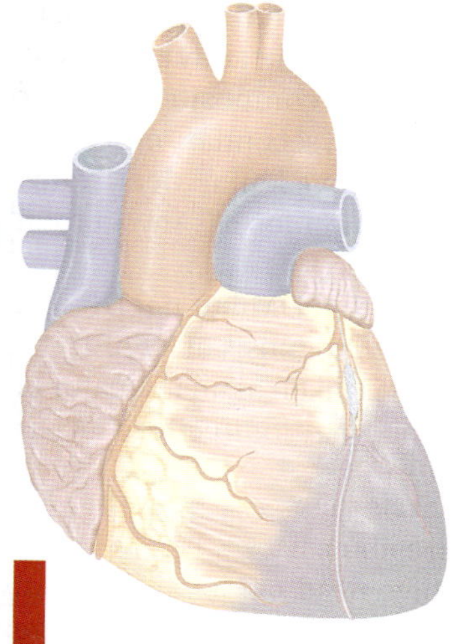

Impact of Diabetic Retinopathy on Prognosis of Patients with HFpEF

Monika Nadar, Krishna Vaitheeswaran, Preetinder Kaur

INTRODUCTION

Heart failure is a chronic phase of cardiac functional impairment and may be associated with the metabolic derangement in diabetes. HF is associated with a higher prevalence of DM as compared to those without HF.[1] A higher risk of HF was also observed in patients with DM ranging from 10 to 30%.[2]

Heart failure with preserved ejection fraction (HFpEF) accounts for nearly 50% of all cases of heart failure and this proportion is increasing. The disorder is a heterogeneous syndrome of multiple discrete phenotypes mediated by different comorbid conditions[3] which provide predictive values for the prognosis of heart failure. Diabetes is a common concomitant disease and is reported to increase the HF related hospitalization and death.[4]

Diabetic retinopathy (DR) is the most common microvascular complication of diabetes characterized by increased vascular permeability and retinal ischemia potentially causing and leading to blindness.

Estimated 40% of DM2 patients and 86% of DM1 patents would have some form of DR,[5] with the presence of DR indicating a more severe stage of DM. The presence of DR increases the risk of HF irrespective of other known risk factors such as age, sex, BMI, duration of DM, smoking, and medications for DM.[1]

STAGES OF DIABETIC RETINOPATHY

Broadly, there are following stages of DR:

- *Nonproliferative retinopathy:* This is a mild form of retinopathy where the blood vessels swell and leak. This causes retinal edema particularly in the region of the macular giving rise to diabetic macular edema and decreased vision.
  - *Mild NPDR:* These are characterized by micro aneurysms and macula edema without any major symptoms.
  - *Moderate NPDR:* Presence of retinal hemorrhages, micro aneurysms, hard exudates, and macular edema with symptoms of decreased vision, micropsia, macropsia, and metamorphopsia.
  - *Severe NPDR:* The presence of four quadrant hemorrhages and microaneurysms, venous beading in at least two quadrants and the presence of intraretinal microvascular anomalies (IRMAs) in one quadrant indicates severe form of NPDR and the danger of development of blinding PDR if prompt intervention is not made available.
- *Proliferative diabetic retinopathy:* The presence of new blood vessels on the disc or elsewhere, retinal and vitreous hemorrhages leading to the development of retinal traction by fibrous bands progressing to tractional retinal detachment and blindness.

DIABETIC RETINOPATHY AND CARDIAC STRUCTURE AND FUNCTION

- Left ventricular diastolic function:
  - Studies have shown an association between diastolic function of the left ventricle and the severity of DR. Assessment using pulsed wave Doppler evaluation of the mitral valve E/A ratio[6]

have shown an increased late diastolic peak transmitral A wave velocity reflecting a greater contribution of atrial systole to LV diastolic filling.

- Left atrial diameter is larger with worsening retinopathy. Left atrial enlargement, as a consequence of elevated LV diastolic pressure due to abnormalities of diastole and LV compliance, has been shown to be a marker of diastolic dysfunction severity.[7] The association of a larger atrial diameter and the severity of retinopathy indicates a microvascular process in the development of diastolic dysfunction.

- *Left ventricular mass:* The left ventricular mass increased as a function of increasing severity of retinopathy and independent of hypertension or any other cardiovascular disorders. It was shown that there was a concentric cardiac remodeling as assessed by magnetic resonance imaging. The cause of the left ventricular mass increase could be due to obesity and associated hypertension but the changes were seen even after accounting for the confounding variables. The reason could be due to increased arterial stiffness which has been demonstrated in increasing amount with increasing retinopathy.

The presence of DR is associated with an enhanced risk heart failure particularly HFpEF which suggests a strong contribution of microvascular disease to the development of HFpEF.

Retinopathy and retinal microvascular complications in patients with diabetes may play a greater role in HFpEF rather than heart failure with reduced ejection fraction (HFrEF).[8]

PROGNOSIS OF PATIENTS WITH RETINOPATHY AND HEART FAILURE WITH PRESERVED EJECTION FRACTION

The prognosis of HFpEF in patients with diabetes and DR was assessed in a large, international population suffering from HFpEF ($n = 3{,}442$) based on the Treatment of Preserved Cardiac Function Heart Failure with an Aldosterone Antagonist (TOPCAT) trial.[9] The associations of baseline DR with clinical outcomes were expressed as adjusted hazard ratios (HRs) and 95% confidence intervals (CIs) using the Cox proportional hazard regression models. The crude incidence rates of all the outcomes studied were significantly increased when DM patients with or without DR compared to those without DM (all $p < 0.05$), whereas there were no differences between DM patients without DR versus those with DR (all $p > 0.05$). In the multivariate cox regression analysis, DR was not significantly associated with increased risks of the primary composite outcome [HR, 1.178 (95% CI, 0.870–1.596)] and secondary outcomes including all-cause death, cardiovascular death, all-cause hospitalization, hospitalization for HF, myocardial infarction, and stroke (all $p > 0.05$).

The inference of this trial was that DM but not DR was an independent risk factor for the prognosis of HFpEF.

However, the presence of DR is taken as an indicator of the severity of diabetes and hence may indirectly reflect as a risk factor in clinical trials.

REFERENCES

1. Echouffo-Tcheugui JB, Xu H, DeVore AD, et al. Temporal trends and factors associated with diabetes mellitus among patients hospitalized with heart failure: Findings from Get With The Guidelines-Heart Failure registry. Am Heart J. 2016;182:9-20.
2. Kelly McHugh, Adam D. DeVore, Jingjing Wu, et al. Hernandez. Heart Failure With Preserved Ejection Fraction and Diabetes: JACC State-of-the-Art Review. J Am Coll Cardiol. 2019;73:602-11.
3. Jose M Mostaza, Carmen Suarez, Luis Manzano, et al.; on behalf of the MERITO study group. Sub-clinical vascular disease in type 2 diabetic subjects: relationship with chronic complications of diabetes and the presence of cardiovascular disease risk factors. Eur J Intern Med. 2008; 19:255-60.
4. Boonman-de Winter LJ, Rutten FH, Cramer MJ, et al. High prevalence of previously unknown heart failure and left ventricular dysfunction in patients with type 2 diabetes. Diabetologia. 2012;55(8):2154-62.
5. Ogurtsova K, da Rocha Fernandes JD, Huang Y, et al. IDF Diabetes Atlas: Global estimates for the prevalence of diabetes for 2015 and 2040. Diabetes Res Clin Pract. 2017;128:40-50.
6. Annonu AK, Fattah AA, Mokhtar MS, et al. Left ventricular systolic and diastolic functional abnormalities in asymptomatic patients with non-insulin-dependent diabetes mellitus. J Am Soc Echocardiogr. 2001;14(9): 885-91.
7. Pritchett AM, Mahoney DW, Jacobsen SJ, et al. Diastolic dysfunction and left atrial volume: a population-based study. J Am Coll Cardiol. 2005;45:87-92.
8. Tromp J, Lim SL, Tay WT, et al. Microvascular disease in patients with reduced ejection fraction versus preserved ejection fraction. Diabetes Care. 2019;42:1792-9.
9. Yang Y, Zhou Y, Cao Y, et al. Impact of diabetic retinopathy on prognosis of patients with heart failure with preserved ejection fraction. Nutr Metab Cardiovasc Dis. 2022;32(7): 1711-8.

SECTION 12

HFpEF and Cardiodermatology

109. Skin Autofluorescence as a Predictor of First Heart Failure Hospitalization in Patients with HFpEF

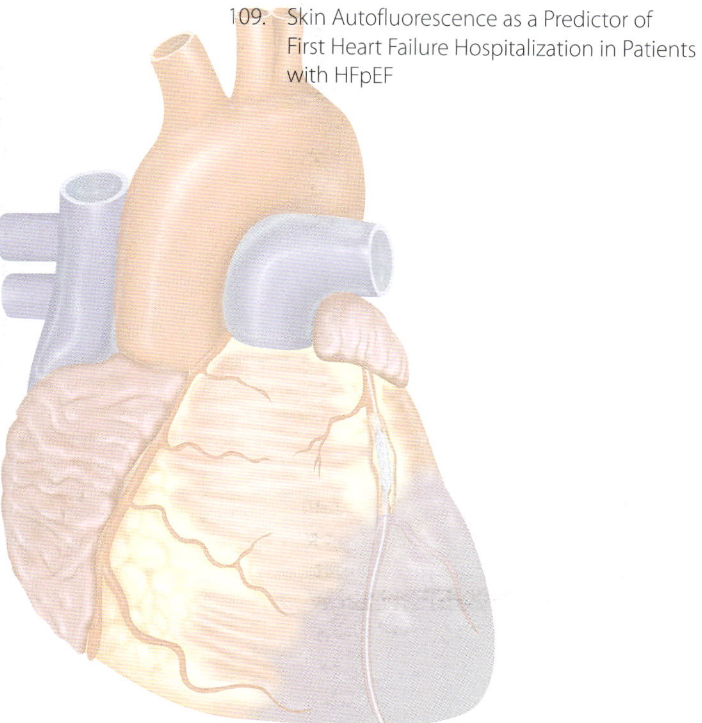

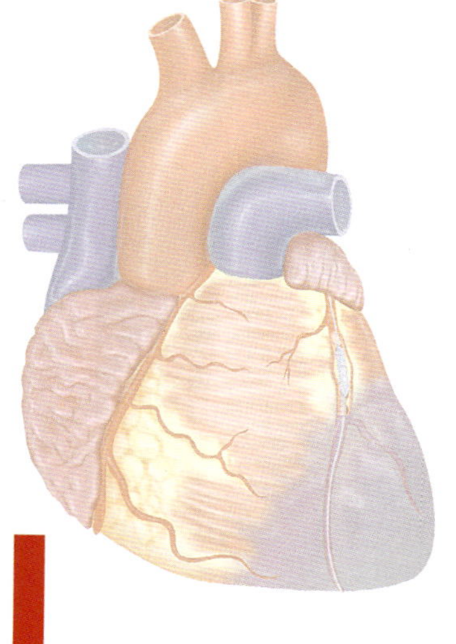

Skin Autofluorescence as a Predictor of First Heart Failure Hospitalization in Patients with HFpEF

Payal Gupta

INTRODUCTION

Skin autofluorescence (SAF) is a noninvasive way to measure the amount of advanced glycation end products (AGEs) in the skin, indicating high oxidative stress and inflammation, a key process in heart failure. Heart failure with preserved ejection fraction (HFpEF) is increasingly recognized as a significant public health concern, characterized by a complex interplay of comorbidities and pathophysiological mechanisms. Early identification of patients at risk for heart failure hospitalization is crucial for optimizing management and improving outcomes. Recent research has highlighted SAF as a potential noninvasive biomarker for assessing underlying metabolic and cardiovascular risks.

Early identification of patients at high risk for heart failure hospitalization is crucial for effective management and intervention. Traditional risk stratification approaches often rely on clinical parameters and biomarker assessments that may not adequately capture the intricate interplay of metabolic and cardiovascular factors. In this context, SAF has emerged as a promising noninvasive biomarker that could help predict hospitalizations due to heart failure in patients with HFpEF.[1]

SKIN AUTOFLUORESCENCE: AN OVERVIEW

Skin autofluorescence is a measurement technique that quantifies the natural fluorescence emitted by skin tissues when exposed to specific wavelengths of light, typically ultraviolet (UV) light. The primary contributors to this autofluorescence are AGEs, which are formed through nonenzymatic glycation of proteins and lipids in the presence of elevated blood glucose levels and oxidative stress **(Figs. 1 and 2)**.

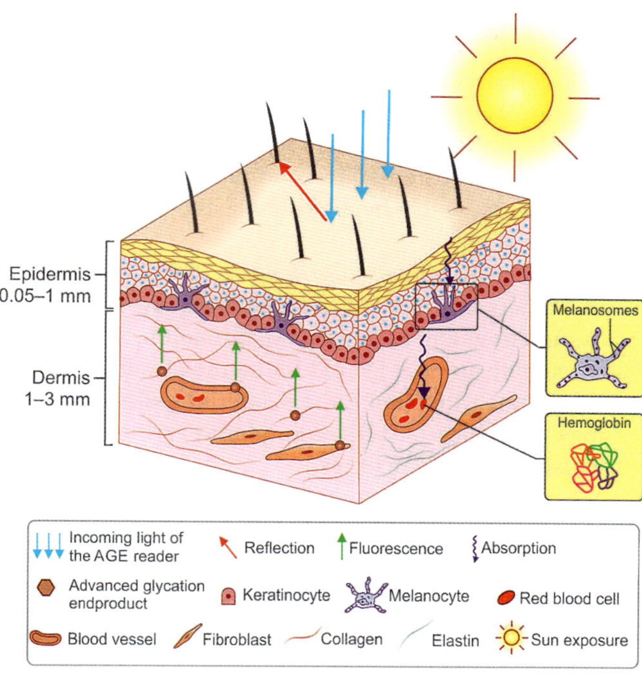

Fig. 1: This figure shows light of the advanced glycation end products (AGE) reader illuminating the skin. Skin autofluorescence (SAF) is subsequently calculated by the ratio of skin fluorescence and reflectance. Absorption of light is mainly due to the main absorbers melanin and hemoglobin. Also, the localization of AGEs is shown.

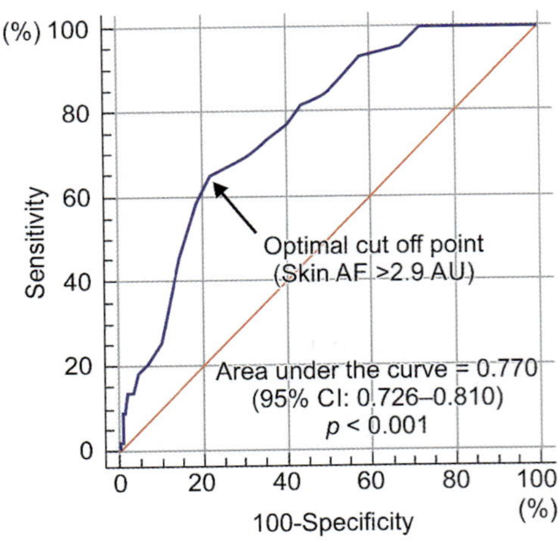

Fig. 2: Prediction of first heart failure hospitalization at follow-up period using skin autofluorescence. Receiver operating characteristics to determine the optimal cutoff point of skin AF for the first heart failure hospitalization. The area under curve was 0.770 ($p < 0.001$). Maximum Youden index indicated that a skin AF > 2.9 arbitrary units was optimal cutoff point to predict the first heart failure hospitalization, indicating a sensitivity of 65.1% and a specificity of 78.1%. Arrow indicates the optimal cutoff point. (AF: autofluorescence; AU: arbitrary units; CI: confidence interval)

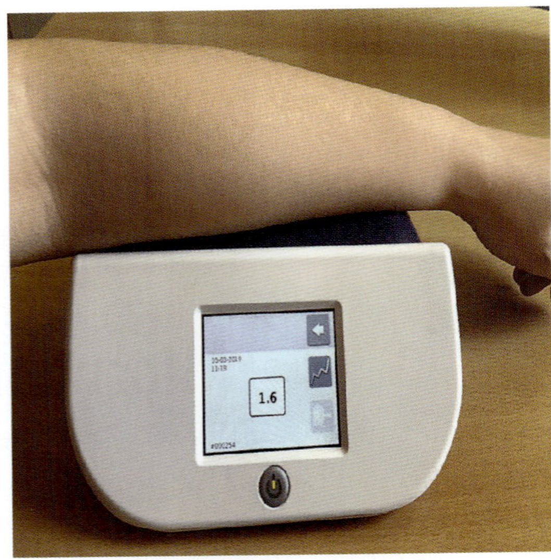

Fig. 3: Skin autofluorescence, as measured by the autofluorescence reader AGE reader mu connect (Diagnoptics, NL). Local creams should not have been applied for 12 hours. The examinee places the forearm of his/her dominant upper limb on the silicone armrest of the device. In this armrest, there is a small examination window for selection of a skin area. The elbow should be aligned with the edge of the armrest and no movements should be made during measurement. The examiner switches on the device using the power button. Activation is performed through the menu on the touch screen. AGEs result is shown on the screen. Approximate measurement duration is 30 seconds. Interpretation of results may be facilitated by available age- and sex-adjusted normative data.

MECHANISM OF ACTION

- *AGE formation:* AGEs are generated when reducing sugars react with amino groups in proteins, leading to structural alterations and functional impairments. This process is exacerbated in conditions such as diabetes and obesity, where hyperglycemia and oxidative stress are prevalent.
- *Impact on cardiovascular health:* The accumulation of AGEs contributes to vascular stiffness, endothelial dysfunction, and increased inflammation, all of which are significant risk factors for cardiovascular disease. In patients with HFpEF, the deleterious effects of AGEs may precipitate adverse remodeling of the heart and worsen clinical outcomes.
- *Measurement technique:* The measurement of SAF involves a specialized device that emits UV light onto the skin and captures the resultant fluorescence. SAF was defined as the average light intensity per nanometer in the spectrum 300–420 nm. The emitted light is analyzed to quantify the levels of AGEs, providing an indirect assessment of oxidative stress and metabolic dysfunction.

Skin autofluorescence is measured using an autofluorescence reader (e.g., AGE reader mu connect; Diagnoptics, NL) **(Fig. 3)**, which illuminates a small portion of the skin (approximately 4 cm^2) on the volar side of the patients forearm.[2] The device produces light on the selected area with an excitation light source of ~370 nm. The emission light and reflected excitation light emanating from the skin is then measured. Then with the help of a computer and different calculations values in arbitrary units (AU) are given. Williams et al.[3] have shown that measurements by the AGE reader exhibited adequate correlations with readings from skin biopsies for specific AGEs, such as pentosidine, CML and carboxyethyl lysine (CEL). The AGE levels in skin biopsy are taken as gold standard.

The AGEs assessment with the newer, fast, and simple method of SAF has recently gained special interest because of its noninvasive, highly reproducible nature, and its acceptable correlation with the reference method of skin biopsy.[4]

CLINICAL RELEVANCE OF SKIN AUTOFLUORESCENCE IN HEART FAILURE WITH PRESERVED EJECTION FRACTION

Unlike heart failure with reduced ejection fraction (HFrEF), HFpEF is characterized by the inability of the heart to properly fill with blood, despite normal contractile function. Patients with HFpEF often present with a complex constellation of symptoms, including shortness of breath, fatigue, and fluid retention, which can significantly impair quality of life.[5] HFrEF is often preceded by the acute or chronic loss of cardiomyocytes whereas the clinical course of HFpEF is frequently complicated by the presence of comorbidities such as obesity, hypertension, diabetes, and chronic kidney disease.

Recent studies have suggested that SAF may serve as an important predictor of cardiovascular outcomes, including hospitalization for heart failure.[6] A recent study found that an SAF level greater than 2.9 arbitrary units was the optimal cutoff point to predict first heart failure hospitalization. The predictive value of SAF arises from its association with systemic inflammation, oxidative stress, and the burden of cardiovascular comorbidities. High SAF values reflect left ventricular diastolic dysfunction which is an important factors of prognosis in HFpEF patients. Also some studies indicate significant association in inflammatory markers like hs-CRP levels.

KEY FINDINGS FROM CLINICAL STUDIES

- *Cohort studies:* Several cohort studies have investigated the relationship between SAF and hospitalization in patients with HFpEF. One study found that patients with elevated SAF levels (>2.5 μg/mL) had a significantly higher risk of hospitalization for heart failure compared to those with lower SAF levels. This association persisted even after adjusting for traditional risk factors such as age, gender, diabetes, hypertension, and renal function.
- *Longitudinal observations:* In a longitudinal analysis of patients with HFpEF, elevated SAF levels were linked to an increased rate of adverse cardiovascular events over a follow-up period of 2 years. The study emphasized that SAF could serve as an early warning signal for clinicians to initiate more aggressive monitoring and management strategies in at-risk populations.

LIMITATIONS

Despite the promise of SAF as a predictive tool for heart failure hospitalization, several limitations must be considered:

- *Variability in measurement:* The accuracy and reproducibility of SAF measurements can be influenced by various factors, including skin type, hydration status, and environmental conditions during testing. This variability may lead to inconsistent results across different populations and settings. For example in dark skin the SAF was lower compared to lighter skin due to melanin which also absorbs light emission.[7]
- *Lack of standardization:* Currently, there is no universally accepted protocol for SAF measurement, resulting in significant variability in methodologies used across studies. Standardizing measurement techniques would enhance the reliability and comparability of findings.
- *Confounding factors:* While SAF is a valuable marker, it does not account for acute changes in clinical status, such as recent infections or changes in medication that may impact heart failure risk. Additional research is needed to disentangle the effects of SAF from other clinical variables.
- *Generalizability:* Most studies examining SAF in relation to heart failure hospitalization have focused on specific cohorts, often with homogeneous characteristics. The findings may not be generalizable to diverse populations, particularly those with varying ethnic backgrounds or unique comorbidity profiles.
- *Need for longitudinal studies:* While cross-sectional studies have established a relationship between SAF and heart failure hospitalization, longitudinal studies are necessary to better understand the temporal dynamics and causative pathways involved.

CONCLUSION

Skin autofluorescence represents a novel and noninvasive biomarker with significant potential for predicting first heart failure hospitalization in patients with HFpEF. The correlation between elevated SAF levels and increased hospitalization risk highlights its potential role in risk stratification and early intervention. As healthcare moves toward a more personalized approach, incorporating SAF into routine clinical assessments could enhance the ability to identify at-risk patients, leading to timely and effective management strategies.

However, further research is warranted to validate the findings across diverse populations, standardize measurement techniques, and explore the underlying mechanisms linking SAF to heart failure outcomes. As our understanding of the pathophysiology of HFpEF evolves, SAF may play an integral role in shaping future clinical practices and improving patient outcomes.

REFERENCES

1. Kunimoto M, Yokoyama M, Shimada K, et al. Relationship between skin autofluorescence levels and clinical events in patients with heart failure undergoing cardiac rehabilitation. Cardiovasc Diabetol. 2021;20:208.
2. Papachristou S, Pafili K, Panas N, et al. Skin AGEs and diabetic neuropathy. BMC Endocrine Disorders. 2021;21:28.
3. Williams LM, Green JR, Salah HM, et al. Non-invasive Biomarkers in Heart Failure: A Focus on Skin Autofluorescence. Eur J Heart Fail. 2023;25(1):56-67.
4. Zhang Y, Lee S. Predictive Models for Hospitalization in Heart Failure Patients. Am Heart J. 2020;220:1-10.
5. Lee JH, Kim SW. Advanced Glycation End Products and Heart Failure: Implications for Clinical Practice. Cardiovasc Res. 2023;119(4):870-82.
6. Hitsumoto T. Skin Autofluorescence as a Predictor of First Heart Failure Hospitalization in Patients With Heart Failure With Preserved Ejection Fraction. Cardiol Res. 2020;11(4):247-55.
7. IM Atzeni, SC van de Zande, J Westra, et al. The AGE Reader: A non-invasive method to assess long-term tissue damage. Methods. 2022;203:533-41.

SECTION 13

HFpEF, Cardio-ENT and Cardiopulmonary Disease

110. Pulmonary Hypertension in HFpEF: Management Strategies
111. Pulmonary Hypertension in HFpEF: Current Challenges and Promising New Therapies
112. Obstructive Sleep Apnea and Hypertension to HFpEF: Management Strategies
113. Noise Pollution, Hypertension, and HFpEF

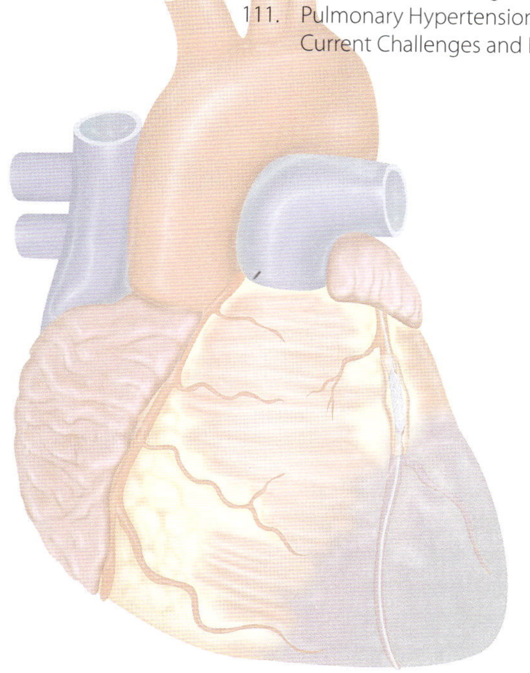

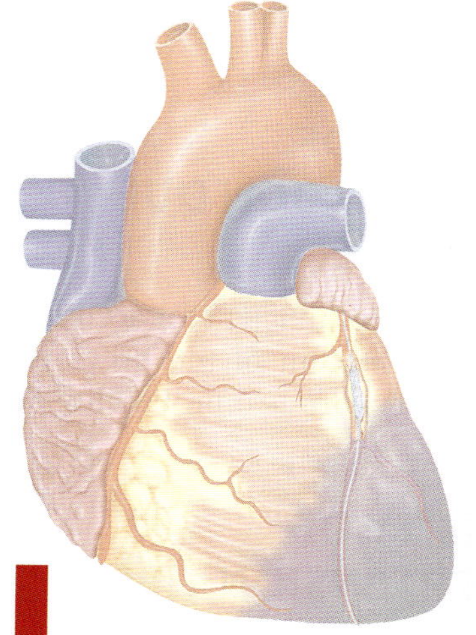

Pulmonary Hypertension in HFpEF: Management Strategies

Bhagwan Mantri, Tanymol Saju, Leyla Kedir Bereka

INTRODUCTION

Pulmonary hypertension due to left-sided heart disease (PH-LHD), classified by the World Health Organization (WHO) as postcapillary or group 2 pulmonary hypertension, is the most common cause of pulmonary hypertension. It is defined by a mean pulmonary arterial pressure (mPAP) >20 mm Hg and pulmonary capillary wedge pressure (PCWP) >15 mm Hg.[1]

It is subclassified as isolated postcapillary (IPC-PH) when pulmonary vascular resistance (PVR) <2 wood units (WU) or combined pre- and postcapillary (CPC-PH) when PVR ≥2 WU.

Pulmonary hypertension-LHD is categorized by the underlying etiology as follows:

- Left ventricular systolic dysfunction
  - With a preserved ejection fraction
  - With reduced or mildly reduced ejection fraction
- Left ventricular diastolic dysfunction
- Valvular Heart disease (VHD)
- Congenital/acquired left heart inflow/outflow tract obstruction and congenital cardiomyopathies[2]

Table 1 discusses about PH-LHD hemodynamic phenotypes.

EPIDEMIOLOGY

Heart failure with preserved ejection fraction (HFpEF) is a common form of disease occurring in about one-half of patients with Heart Failure globally. Recent reports have highlighted that the prevalence of PH in HFpEF is as high as 50%, occurring mostly among elderly obese females. Risk factor for PH-HFpEF includes Obesity, female gender, microvascular coronary disease, atrial fibrillation (AF), chronic kidney disease, and chronic obstructive pulmonary disease.[3]

PATHOPHYSIOLOGY

The pathophysiology of PH-LHD is complex and features both a passive and an active mechanism of changes to the pulmonary vasculature. There is increasing focus on the pathophysiology of PH in HfpEF, aiming for the development of preventive and therapeutic strategies.

In HFpEF, PH initially occurs only during exercise as a result of a steep increase in left atrial pressure (LAP) with increasing cardiac output. Consequently, right ventricle (RV) afterload increases at low workload and an apparently normal RV at echocardiography at rest

TABLE 1: PH-LHD hemodynamic phenotypes.

Phenotype	*mPAP (mm Hg)*	*PAWP (mm Hg)*	*PVR (WU)*
Non-PH-LHD phenotype:			
• PAH	>20	<15	>2
PH-LHD phenotypes:			
• Ipc-PH	>20	>15	<2
• Cpc-PH	>20	>15	>2
• PH-LHD associated with VHD	>20	>15	>or <2

(Cpc-PH: combined pre- and postcapillary pulmonary hypertension; Ipc: isolated postcapillary; PAH: pulmonary arterial hypertension; PAWP: pulmonary arterial wedge pressure; PH: pulmonary hypertension; LHD: left heart disease)

becomes insufficiently coupled to its hydraulic load during exercise, which contributes to low cardiac output and limited exercise capacity. When present at rest, PH associated with HFpEF mainly reflects evolutive disease with chronically elevated LAP and Ipc-PH. RV systolic dysfunction may already be present, reducing survival probability. With time, Cpc-PH may also emerge in HFpEF with a particularly detrimental impact on the RV. Indeed, RV stroke volume reserve becomes very limited with Cpc-PH, and a prominent increase in right atrial pressure can be seen first during exercise and then at rest. Already-enlarged right-sided chambers then further dilate within a restricted pericardial space, resulting in increasing encroachment of the left ventricle (LV), blunted cardiac output, and further increase in LV filling pressures. As a consequence of hemodynamic and functional perturbations, PH-HFpEF develops as a more advanced corollary of diastolic HF, leading to abnormal phenotypes of the lung microcirculation, the arterial system, and right heart function **(Fig. 1)**.[4,5]

DIAGNOSTIC APPROACH

Pulmonary hypertension in HFpEF represents the most complex situation, as it may be misdiagnosed with group 1 PH. Although, right heart catheterization (RHC) is the gold standard for the diagnosis of PH, it is not sufficient to make a clear distinction between idiopathic PAH (IPAH) and PH-LHD, especially when risk factors or documented history of cardiovascular disease (CVD) coexist.[6]

A pretest probability assessment of LHD should be part of the diagnostic approach of PH.

PRETEST PROBABILITY OF PULMONARY HYPERTENSION DUE TO LEFT HEART DISEASE

As a single variable will unlikely be sufficient for accurate differential diagnosis, a combination of the previous features may help to determine a pre-test probability of group 2 PH.

PRETEST PROBABILITY OF PULMONARY HYPERTENSION-HEART FAILURE WITH PRESERVED EJECTION FRACTION

See **Flowcharts 1A and B**.

THERAPEUTIC PERSPECTIVES

The obvious first step in treating PH-LHD is to optimize the management of the underlying cardiac disease. This must include the appropriate use of guideline-directed medical therapies (GDMT) together with the treatment of comorbidities notably associated with HFpEF, primarily, diabetes, obesity, and hypertension.

As discussed in the previous sections, the primary driver of PH-LHD is the upstream transmission of the

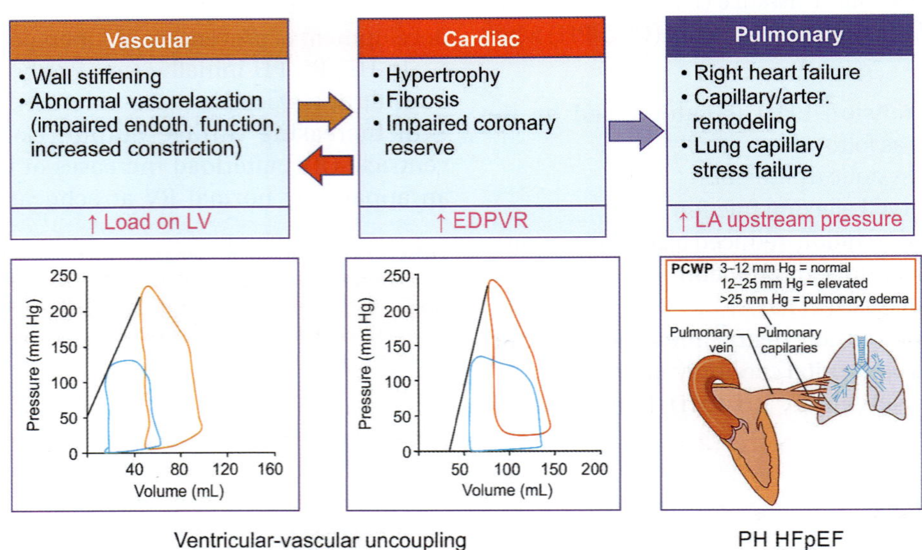

Fig. 1: From HFpEF to PH HFpEF: Hemodynamic components and pathophysiological correlates. In HFpEF, the central pathophysiological role is played by the impaired LV filling mechanics that can arise both from intrinsic structural and molecular alterations in the LV (stiff heart).[4] (EDPVR: end-diastolic pressure–volume relationship; HFpEF: heart failure with preserved ejection fraction; LA: left atrium; LV: left ventricle; PH: pulmonary hypertension)

Flowcharts 1A and B: Hemodynamic assessment of PH due to HFpEF. (A) Pretest probability of PH-LHD is based on the features presented in **Table 2**. RHC is recommended in intermediate probability when risk factors of pulmonary arterial hypertension/CTEPH are present and/or if there is evidence of right ventricle abnormality. If the probability is high, patients should be managed according to recommendations for LHD. (B) For the assessment of PH, RHC should be performed at expert centers. In patients with intermediate/ high probability **(Table 2)** and PAWP between 13- and 15-mm Hg, PH-HFpEF is not excluded; provocative testing be considered. For patients with systemic sclerosis, risk factors for CTEPH and/or unexplained dyspnea and if PAWP >15 mm Hg, LVEDP validation should be considered.

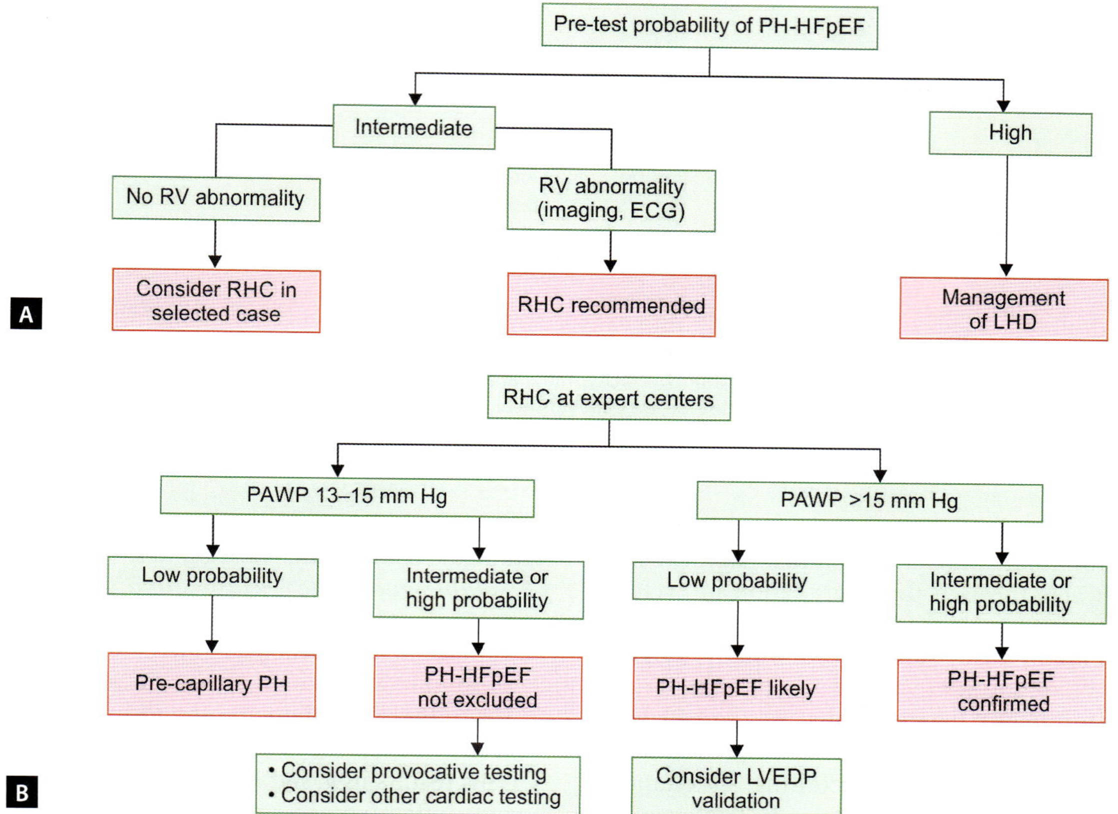

(CTEPH: chronic thromboembolic pulmonary hypertension; HFpEF: heart failure with preserved ejection fraction; LHD: left heart disease; LVEDP: left ventricular end-diastolic pressure; PAWP: pulmonary arterial wedge pressure; PH: pulmonary hypertension; RV: right ventricular; RHC: right heart catheterization)[6]

elevated LA pressure to the pulmonary circulation, promoting an increase in the pulsatile afterload of the RV by reducing PA compliance (Ipc-PH). In a subset of patients, chronic pulmonary arterial wedge pressure (PAWP) elevation results in progressive PVD, with the subsequent elevation in PVR leading to a further rise in RV afterload (Cpc-PH). Therefore, therapy for PH-LHD should, first, aim to decrease PAWP to improve PA compliance and prevent PVD and, second, to reduce PVR in the case of established PVD, with the final goal to prevent or treat RV-PA uncoupling.[5]

The following are the pharmacological therapy according to the current evidence-based practice.

- *Endothelin receptor antagonists (ERAs):* PH is associated with an increased expression of endothelin-1 in endothelial cells. This high expression is associated with increased PVR, specifically in PAH. ERAs act by blocking endothelin-1 receptors on endothelial vascular smooth muscle, leading to vasodilation, and their use is recommended for the management of PAH. Recent studies show that elevated plasma endothelin-1 correlates with the severity of PH and is associated with poor prognosis in heart failure patients.[7,8]

  Endothelin receptor antagonists in patients with HFpEF-related PH have been evaluated in many studies and has been found that endothelin receptor blockade in patients with PH-HFpEF has no beneficial effects and could even be detrimental and may be associated with significant side effects, primarily increased congestion and liver toxicity in comparison to a placebo.[9,10]

TABLE 2: Pretest probability of LHD phenotype.

Feature	*High probability*	*Intermediate probability*	*Low probability*
Age	>70 years	60–70 years	<60 years
Obesity, systemic hypertension, dyslipidemia, glucose intolerance/ diabetes	More than two factors	One to two factors	None
Previous cardiac intervention*	Yes	No	No
Atrial fibrillation	Current	Paroxysmal	No
Structural LHD	Present	No	No
ECG	LBBB or LVH	Mild LVH	Normal or signs of RV strain
Echocardiography	LA dilation; grade >2 mitral flow	No LA dilation; grade <2 mitral flow	No LA dilation; E/e' <13
CPET	Mildly elevated V'E/V'CO_2 slope; EOV	Elevated V'E/V'CO_2 slope or EOV	High V'E/V'CO_2 slope; no EOV
Cardiac MRI	LA strain or LA/RA >1		No left heart abnormalities

*Coronary artery and/or valvular surgical and/or non-surgical procedures, including percutaneous interventions

(CPET: cardiopulmonary exercise testing; E/e': early mitral inflow velocity/mitral annular early diastolic velocity ratio; EOV: exercise oscillatory ventilation; LBBB: left bundle branch block; LHD: left heart disease; LVH: left ventricular hypertrophy; MRI: magnetic resonance imaging; RA: right atrial; RV: right ventricular; LA: left atrial; V'E: minute ventilation; V'CO_2: carbon dioxide production)

- *Phosphodiesterase-5 inhibitors (PDE5i):* PDE5 is the most abundant phosphodiesterase isoform in the lung. It acts through the degradation of cyclic guanosine monophosphate (cGMP), thereby reducing cGMP-dependent vasodilation. Additionally, PDE5 may promote pulmonary vascular remodeling and is unregulated in the hypertrophied RV, and PDE5 inhibition has been associated with improved RV inotropism PDE5 inhibitors, including sildenafil, tadalafil, and vardenafil, are effective in decreasing PAP and pulmonary vascular remodeling, specifically in group 1 PAH.[11,12]

Studies evaluating PDE5i in patients with HFpEF-related PH yielded conflicting results. In three randomized controlled trials of RCTs with sildenafil, no significant improvement in hemodynamic variables (PCWP and PAP) or exercise capacity [6-minute walking distance (6MWD), peak oxygen consumption]. In marked contrast, another study assessed sildenafil therapy in two RCTs, including only HFpEF patients with Cpc-PH and RV failure reported significant reductions in PAP and improved RV function and exercise capacity, as well as clinical amelioration [New York Heart Association (NYHA) class].[13,14]

Overall, current evidence does not support the general use of PDE5i for PH-LHD, related to HFpEF, especially for patients with Ipc-PH, no RV dysfunction, and chronic AF. It remains possible that PDE5i may exert some positive effects in patients with Cpc-PH and RV, and in patients with persisting high PVR undergoing LVAD therapy, but additional studies are required to confirm such possibilities.[5]

- *Soluble guanylate cyclase stimulators (SGCSs):* SGC stimulators, including the drugs riociguat, vericiguat, and praliciguat, increase the sensitivity of soluble guanylate cyclase (sGC) to nitric oxide (NO), thereby enhancing the formation of cyclic GMP, the major second messenger of NO signaling. This results in vasodilation and antiproliferative, anti-inflammatory, and antifibrotic effects. This is of particular interest when the availability of NO is reduced as a consequence of endothelial dysfunction (reduced NO biosynthesis) or oxidative stress (direct NO inactivation), which prevails in the context of heart failure. The SGC riociguat is approved for the therapy of PAH and chronic thromboembolic PH (CTPEH).[15]

A multicentric RCT with riociguat showed significant improvement in resting cardiac output (primary outcome), and it significantly decreased PVR while not changing PAWP, as assessed by right heart catheterization, especially in the Cpc-PH phenotype. However, due to significant adverse events, there were more dropouts from the study.[16,17]

To sum up current knowledge, it appears that SGCSs are generally well tolerated and provide favorable hemodynamic effects in HFpEF patients, with a significant increase in cardiac output and reduction in PVR. Additional studies specifically

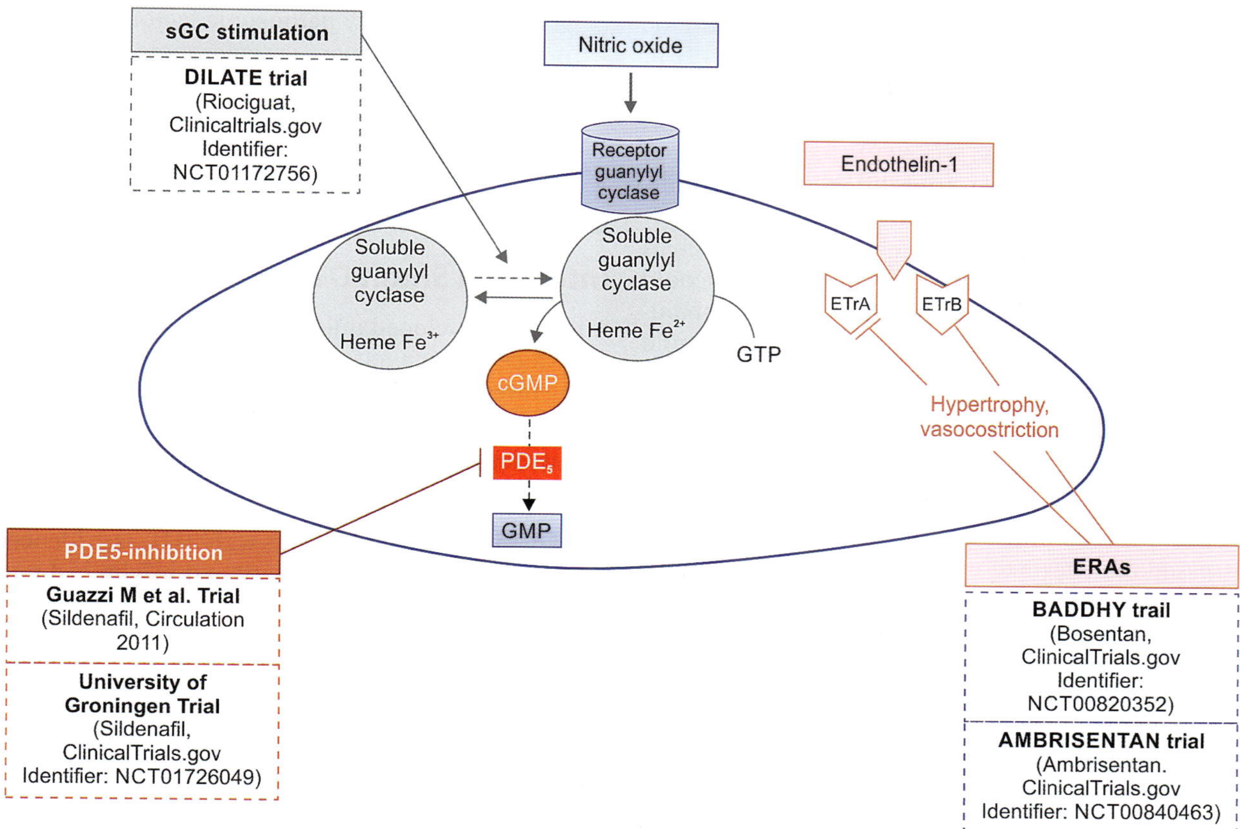

Fig. 2: Summarizes pathways, pharmacological agents, and relative ongoing and published trials relative to PH-HfpEF. (cGMP: cyclic guanosin-monofosphate; ERAs: endothelin receptor antagonists; ETrA: endothelin receptor A; ETrB: endothelin receptor B; GTP: guanosintrifosphate; PDE5: phosphodiesterase-5; sGC: soluble guanilate cyclase)

exploring these effects in patients with a Cpc-PH profile should be conducted.[5]

Prostacyclin analogs: Prostacyclin [prostaglandin I2 (PGI2)] is a prostanoid produced via PGI2 synthase in vascular endothelial cells which acts on specific receptors in platelet and endothelial cells. It promotes potent vasodilator effects decreasing both pulmonary and systemic vascular resistance, reduces platelet aggregation, and displays antiproliferative actions.

Various prostacyclin analogs, including beraprost, treprostinil, iloprost, and epoprostenol, are recommended in patients with PAH. A few studies have evaluated the role of these therapeutic approaches in patients with PH-LHD.[18]

In summary, only limited information currently exists regarding prostacyclin analogs for the treatment of PH-LHD. In HFpEF, some encouraging experimental data have been produced using treprostinil, but no clinical data have so far confirmed these promising effects **(Fig. 2)**.[5]

- *Sodium-glucose cotransporter 2 inhibitors (SGLT-2i):* SGLT-2 inhibitors (gliflozins), a novel hypoglycemic agent, which are effective in the treatment of type 2 diabetes, have recently been associated with clinical benefits in patients with heart failure and have been incorporated in the GDMTs. This hypothesis was recently addressed in the EMBRACE-HF trial, which randomized HF patients to receive either empagliflozin or a placebo. Results indicated that empagliflozin significantly reduced PAP, which appeared independent of diuretic management. These promising findings suggest that SGLT-2 inhibitors could offer novel opportunities to control PA pressure in heart failure patients.[5,12]
- *Angiotensin receptor–neprilysin inhibitor (ARNI):* The paradigm- HF trial showed that a combination of valsartan with sacubitril, an inhibitor of neprilysin, improved outcomes in patients with HFrEF. Since neprilysin degrades natriuretic peptides (NP), which possess inherent pulmonary vasodilating properties, treatment with sacubitril could theoretically enhance such vasodilation. A retrospective study on HFrEF patients reported that the transition from an angiotensin-converting enzyme (ACE) inhibitor or an angiotensin receptor blocker (ARB) to sacubitril/

valsartan resulted in a significant reduction in PAP. However, there is limited data on its role in PH in HFpEF.[5]

- *Levosimendan:* Levosimendan (Levo) is a calcium sensitizer, potassium ATP (KATP) channel activator, and phosphodiesterase-3 inhibitor with inotropic, vasodilatory, and cardioprotective activity. It is widely used in the treatment of acute and advanced heart failure. Experimental data showed that Levo could attenuate pulmonary vascular remodeling in an animal model of PH, attributed to antiproliferative and anti-inflammatory effects mediated by KATP channel activation.[19] In humans, some limited evidence suggests that Levo may reduce PAP and PVR and improve RV function in patients with PAH.[20,21]

  The effects of Levo have also been evaluated in HFpEF patients in the phase II HELP Study, which assessed the effects of intravenous infusions of Levo and showed improvement in 6MWD. Although Levo was associated with a reduction in resting PAWP, there was no significant difference in the primary outcome which was a reduction in the increase in PAWP upon a 25-week exercise challenge. In contrast, patients receiving Levo displayed a significant improvement in the secondary outcome which is 6MWD, which is comparable to that reported for approved pulmonary vasodilators for PH. Interestingly, there were no effects of Levo on PAP, PVR, and systemic vascular resistance, but there was a decrease in resting central venous pressure and PAWP, suggestive of a reduction in venous return related to venodilation.[22,23] Although preliminary, these data are important given the lack of available effective therapy for patients with HFpEF-related PH-LHD. Further studies are now required to confirm these promising effects of Levo.
- *β3-adrenoreceptor agonists:* Beta-3 adrenergic receptor (β3AR) agonists represent a new class of drugs approved for the clinical treatment of overactive bladder. In the cardiovascular system, β3AR stimulation promotes NO-dependent signaling and indirectly activates cardiac myocyte Na^+/K^+-ATPase. An RCT (SPHERE-HF) was conducted with Cpc-PH, mostly in HFpEF, comparing the effect of oral mirabegron with a placebo. The trial was negative for its primary outcome (no reduction in PVR), but it reported a significant improvement in RV function (secondary outcome).[24]

  It has been speculated that β3AR agonists could exert some benefits in PH-LDH. Additional studies are required to confirm this hypothesis.
- *Activin receptor type IIA-Fc fusion protein (ACTRIIA-Fc):* Activin receptor type IIA-Fc fusion protein (ActRIIA-Fc) including Sotatercept has proven to be efficacious in group 1 PAH. A key pathogenic factor in PH-LHD is progressive pulmonary vascular remodeling. Studies are ongoing to address the role of ActRIIA-Fc in pulmonary vascular remodeling, thereby alleviating PH in PH-LHD.

OTHER THERAPEUTIC OPTIONS

Interatrial Shunt Devices

A recently developed interatrial shunt device (IASD) able to reduce LAP via left atrial decompression is currently being investigated in the treatment of heart failure.

Pulmonary Artery Denervation

Increased activity of the sympathetic nervous system has been demonstrated in patients with PAH, as evidenced by elevated plasma catecholamines and heightened muscle sympathetic nerve activity.

Although more studies on this issue are needed, these promising results suggest that percutaneous pulmonary artery denervation (PADN) might soon find a place in the management of PAH in general, and in PH-LHD in particular.[5]

LIMITATIONS

We have highlighted the available pharmacologic strategies for the treatment of PH in patients with HFpEF; however, more studies need to be done and guidelines need to be established so that these drugs can be used in routine clinical practice.

CONCLUSION

Pulmonary hypertension related to left heart disease[25] represents the most frequent form of PH, which will continue to pose significant challenges in terms of public health and economic burden in years to come. Key issues in future trials will be the proper selection of patients, according to the nature of heart failure (preserved or reduced ejection fraction), the phenotype of PH (Ipc-PH vs. Cpc-PH), and the degree of RV dysfunction, as well as the clear definition of outcome variables (hemodynamic and clinical). Multiple trials of therapies specifically targeting the pulmonary vasculature, such as phosphodiesterase (PDE) inhibitors, prostacyclin analogs, endothelin receptor antagonists (ERA), and soluble guanylate cyclase stimulators have also been conducted. However, these therapies demonstrated a lack of consistency in improving hemodynamics or functional outcomes in PH-HFpEF. The mainstay of therapy remains the treatment of the underlying HFpEF condition. Additionally, studies will need to address the role of pulmonary vasodilators in the context of new heart failure therapies, including angiotensin receptor–neprilysin inhibitors and SGLT2 inhibitors.

Some novel strategies may prove beneficial to patients with PH-LHD. As an example, the recent observation of clinical improvement in patients treated with oral levosimendan is an encouraging development. Positive results obtained with pulmonary artery denervation are also of considerable interest, and this approach could represent a breakthrough in years to come. Finally, the improved understanding of the molecular mechanisms of pulmonary vascular remodeling may permit us to envision novel specific targeted therapies for the future.

REFERENCES

1. Simonneau G, Robbins IM, Beghetti M, et al. Updated clinical classification of pulmonary hypertension. J Am Coll Cardiol. 2009;54(1 Suppl):S43-54.
2. Barot N, Nguyen P, Kamangar N. (2024). Group 2 Pulmonary Hypertension. [Online] Available from https://emedicine.medscape.com/article/2500055-overview?form=fpf [Last accessed January, 2025].
3. Guazzi M, Ghio S, Adir Y. Pulmonary Hypertension in HFpEF and HFrEF: JACC Review Topic of the Week. J Am Coll Cardiol. 2020;76(9):1102-11.
4. Guazzi M. Pulmonary hypertension in heart failure preserved ejection fraction: prevalence, pathophysiology, and clinical perspectives. Circ Heart Fail. 2014;7(2):367-77.
5. Guazzi M, Dixon D, Labate V, et al. RV Contractile Function and its Coupling to Pulmonary Circulation in Heart Failure With Preserved Ejection Fraction: Stratification of Clinical Phenotypes and Outcomes. JACC Cardiovasc Imaging 2017;10(10 Pt B):1211-21.
6. Vachiéry J-L, Tedford RJ, Rosenkranz S, et al. Pulmonary hypertension due to left heart disease. Eur Respir J. 2019;53(1):1801897.
7. Cody RJ, Haas GJ, Binkley PF, et al. Plasma endothelin correlates with the extent of pulmonary hypertension in patients with chronic congestive heart failure. Circulation. 1992;85(2):504-9.
8. Pousset F, Isnard R, Lechat P, et al. Prognostic value of plasma endothelin-1 in patients with chronic heart failure. Eur Heart J. 1997;18(2):254-8.
9. Koller B, Steringer-Mascherbauer R, Ebner CH, et al. Pilot Study of Endothelin Receptor Blockade in Heart Failure with Diastolic Dysfunction and Pulmonary Hypertension (BADDHY-Trial). Heart Lung Circ. 2017;26(5):433-41.
10. Vachiéry JL, Delcroix M, Al-Hiti H, et al. Macitentan in pulmonary hypertension due to left ventricular dysfunction. Eur Respir J. 2018;51(2):1701886.
11. Barnes H, Brown Z, Burns A. Phosphodiesterase 5 inhibitors for pulmonary hypertension. Cochrane Database Syst Rev. 2019;1:CD012621.
12. Sebkhi A, Strange JW, Phillips SC, et al. Phosphodiesterase type 5 as a target for the treatment of hypoxia-induced pulmonary hypertension. Circulation. 2003;107(25):3230-35.
13. Guazzi M, Vicenzi M, Arena R, Guazzi MD. Pulmonary hypertension in heart failure with preserved ejection fraction: a target of phosphodiesterase-5 inhibition in a 1-year study. Circulation. 2011;124(2):164-74.
14. Redfield MM, Chen HH, Borlaug BA, et al. Effect of phosphodiesterase-5 inhibition on exercise capacity and clinical status in heart failure with preserved ejection fraction: a randomized clinical trial. JAMA. 2013;309(12):1268-77.
15. Emdin M, Aimo A, Castiglione V, et al. Targeting Cyclic Guanosine Monophosphate to Treat Heart Failure: JACC Review Topic of the Week. J Am Coll Cardiol. 2020;76(15):1795-807.
16. Pieske B, Maggioni AP, Lam CSP, et al. Vericiguat in patients with worsening chronic heart failure and preserved ejection fraction: results of the SOluble guanylate Cyclase stimulatoR in heArT failurE patientS with PRESERVED EF (SOCRATES-PRESERVED) study. Eur Heart J. 2017;38(15):1119-27.
17. Dachs TM, Duca F, Rettl R, et al. Riociguat in pulmonary hypertension and heart failure with preserved ejection fraction: The haemoDYNAMIC trial. Eur Heart J. 2022;43(36):3402-13.
18. Humbert M, Kovacs G, Hoeper MM, et al. 2022 ESC/ERS Guidelines for the diagnosis and treatment of pulmonary hypertension. Eur Heart J. 2022;43(38):3618-731.
19. Revermann M, Schloss M, Mieth A, et al. Levosimendan attenuates pulmonary vascular remodeling. Intensive Care Med. 2011;37(8):1368-77.
20. Jiang R, Zhao QH, Wu WH, et al. Efficacy and safety of a calcium sensitizer, levosimendan, in patients with right heart failure due to pulmonary hypertension. Clin Respir J. 2018;12(4):1518-25.
21. Kleber FX, Bollmann T, Borst MM, et al. Repetitive dosing of intravenous levosimendan improves pulmonary hemodynamics in patients with pulmonary hypertension: Results of a pilot study. J Clin Pharmacol. 2009;49(1):109-115.
22. Burkhoff D, Borlaug BA, Shah SJ, et al. Levosimendan improves hemodynamics and exercise tolerance in PH-HFpEF: Results of the randomized placebo-controlled HELP trial. JACC Heart Fail. 2021;9(5):360-70.
23. McMurray JJ, Packer M, Desai AS, et al. Angiotensin-neprilysin inhibition versus enalapril in heart failure. N Engl J Med. 2014;371(11):993-1004.
24. García-Álvarez A, Blanco I, García-Lunar I, et al. β3 adrenergic agonist treatment in chronic pulmonary hypertension associated with heart failure (SPHERE-HF): A double blind, placebo-controlled, randomized clinical trial. Eur J Heart Fail. 2023;25(3):373-85.
25. Ltaief Z, Yerly P, Liaudet L. Pulmonary hypertension in left heart diseases: pathophysiology, hemodynamic assessment and therapeutic management. Int J Mol Sci. 2023;24(12):9971.

Pulmonary Hypertension in HFpEF: Current Challenges and Promising New Therapies

Agam Vora, Mangesh Tiwaskar

INTRODUCTION

According to the European Society of Cardiology (ESC) and European Respiratory Society (ERS) guidelines, pulmonary hypertension (PH) is defined as a mean pulmonary artery pressure (PAPm) ≥25 mm Hg at rest, measured by right heart catheterization (RHC). This includes pulmonary arterial hypertension [PAH, World Health Organization (WHO) Group 1] and PH due to left heart disease (LHD, WHO Group 2); both conditions elevate pulmonary artery pressure (PAP), affecting the right ventricle (RV) and potentially leading to right heart failure (HF). RHC is currently the only method to differentiate between PH subgroups through direct hemodynamic measurements. In PAH, a diagnosis requires PAPm ≥25 mm Hg at rest, pulmonary arterial wedge pressure (PAWP) ≤15 mm Hg, and pulmonary vascular resistance (PVR) >3 Wood units (WU), with the absence of chronic lung diseases, chronic thromboembolic PH, or other rare conditions. PAH involves elevated pressures in the pulmonary arteries, while left atrial pressures (LAPs) remain normal.[1]

Heart failure with preserved ejection fraction (HFpEF) is characterized by impaired myocardial relaxation and stiffness, partly due to increased left ventricular load from arterial stiffness, leading to ventricular–vascular uncoupling.[2] Hemodynamic and structural abnormalities in HFpEF contribute to the development of PH. HFpEF-related PH is associated with symptoms such as dyspnea, reduced aerobic capacity, ventilatory impairments, high-symptom burden, increased hospitalizations, and higher mortality.[3] HFpEF is a leading cause of PH. As summarized in **Table 1**, PH-HFpEF is classified as WHO Group II PH due to left heart disease (PH-LHD) and carries a high healthcare burden with significant morbidity and mortality.[4] PH due to HFpEF typically presents as isolated postcapillary PH (IpcPH), though it can also manifest as combined pre- and postcapillary PH (CpcPH).[1] Current guidelines distinguish IpcPH by a diastolic pressure gradient (DPG, the gradient between diastolic PAP and PAWP) <7 mm Hg and/or PVR ≤3 WU, while CpcPH is defined by a DPG ≥7 mm Hg and/or PVR >3 WU.[5] CpcPH is linked to reduced RV function and increased morbidity and mortality compared to IpcPH.[3] The 6th World Symposium on Pulmonary Hypertension recently recommended lowering the mPAP threshold from 25 to 20 mm Hg and incorporating PVR into the PH definition, though these changes have not yet been adopted in international guidelines.[6] The American Heart Association (AHA) has called for further research due to the lack of evidence-based treatments for PH-HFpEF, largely stemming from limited understanding of its pathophysiology.[4]

PREVALENCE AND CLINICAL CHARACTERISTICS OF PULMONARY HYPERTENSION IN HEART FAILURE WITH PRESERVED EJECTION FRACTION

Pulmonary hypertension is common in patients with HFpEF and is linked to worsened symptoms and increased mortality.[7] Approximately 50% of HFpEF patients develop PH, often in conjunction with various clinical

TABLE 1: Definitions of pulmonary hypertension by the World Health Organization.

Group				
PAH; WHO Group 1	*PH-LHD; WHO Group II*	*PH due to chronic lung disease and/or hypoxia; WHO Group III*	*CTEPH; WHO Group IV*	*PH secondary to other diseases; WHO Group V*
Examples Idiopathic PAH, heritable PAH, drug and toxin-induced veno-occlusive disease, secondary to portal hypertension, congenital heart diseases, human immunodeficiency virus infection, connective tissue disease subtypes	Left ventricular systolic dysfunction, left ventricular diastolic dysfunction, valvular disease, congenital cardiac anomalies/outflow tract obstruction	Chronic obstructive pulmonary disease, interstitial lung disease, obstructive sleep apnea, alveolar hypoventilation disorders	CTEPH	Chronic hemolytic anemia, splenectomy, sarcoidosis, metabolic disorders
Idiopathic/heritable pathophysiology	Isolated postcapillary PH/ combined pre- and postcapillary PH	Nonsevere PH/severe PH	NA	Hematologic/systemic disorders
• Increased vasoconstrictors, decreased vasodilators • Extracellular matrix remodeling, vascular proliferation, and inflammatory cell infiltration • Right ventricular dysfunction	• Elevated left heart pressure transmitted to pulmonary vasculature leading to pulmonary–vascular remodeling • Molecular mechanisms behind pulmonary–vascular remodeling largely unknown • Right ventricular dysfunction	• Chronic hypoxia leading to pulmonary vasoconstriction, which leads to increased pulmonary vascular resistance and PH • Inflammation and fibrosis contribute to remodeling • Right ventricular dysfunction	• Persistent clotting • Pulmonary vascular remodeling • Right ventricular dysfunction	Variable pathophysiology

Note: Pulmonary hypertension (PH) refers to any cause of high blood pressure in the lungs. The WHO defines five major groups of PH based on different etiologies.

(CTEPH: chronic thromboembolic pulmonary hypertension; NA: not applicable; PAH: pulmonary arterial hypertension; PH-LHD: PH due to left heart disease)

Source: Adapted from Aradhyula et al.[4]

conditions.[2] PH-HFpEF is the most prevalent among elderly women with metabolic syndrome, and its severity worsens with coexisting obesity. Additional risk factors include microvascular coronary disease, atrial fibrillation (AF), chronic kidney disease, and chronic obstructive pulmonary disease.[8]

The prevalence of PH in HFpEF ranges widely, from 30 to 80%, depending on the population, study design, PH definition, and diagnostic methods, with the most data derived from echocardiographic measurements, particularly elevated PAP values.[3] A population-based study of 244 HFpEF patients reported echocardiographic signs of PH in 83%, with systolic PAP identified as a mortality predictor (hazard ratio 1.3 per 10 mm Hg increase; $p < 0.001$).[1,5] Moreover, randomized clinical trials highlighted by the American College of Cardiology (ACC)/AHA hypertension treatment guidelines indicate that treating hypertension can reduce HFpEF incidence by up to 40% over 2–8 years.[4]

PATHOBIOLOGY OF PULMONARY HYPERTENSION RELATED TO LEFT HEART DISEASE

The pathobiology of PH related to left HF is complex and not fully understood. PH mainly arises from the passive backward transmission of elevated left-sided filling pressures due to systolic or diastolic LV dysfunction **(Fig. 1)**. Furthermore, functional mitral regurgitation (MR) can also elevate LAP and PAP, particularly worsening during exercise. In addition to LV remodeling and dysfunction, increased left atrial (LA) size (an indicator of morbidity and mortality in HF), interstitial fibrosis leading

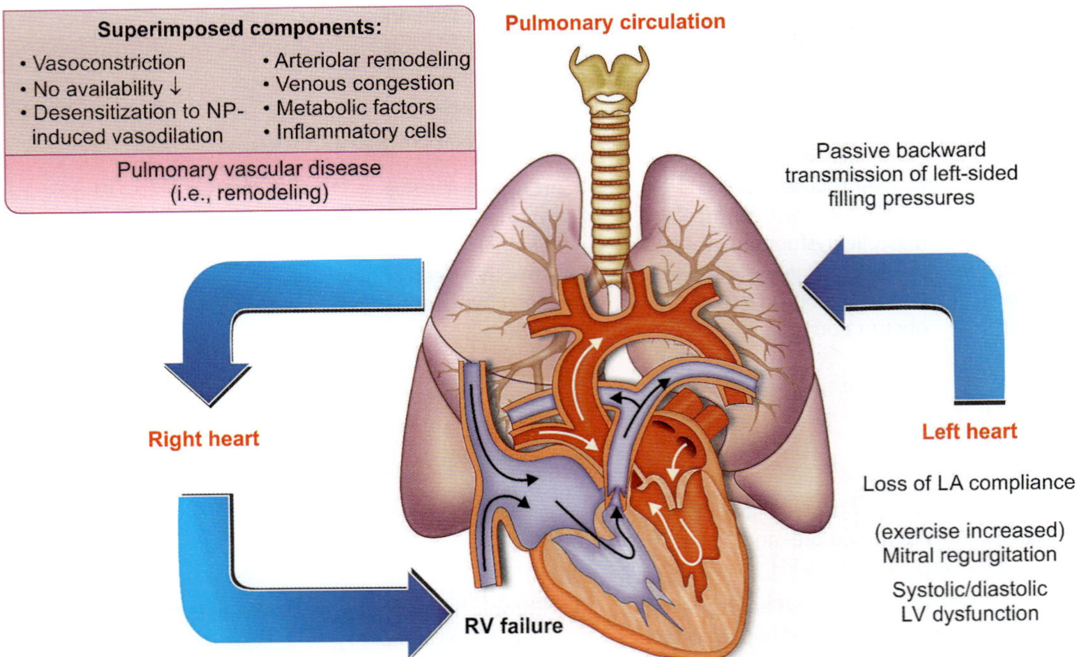

Fig. 1: Cardiopulmonary interaction and pathobiology of pulmonary hypertension (PH) in left ventricular heart failure. Shown are (1) the backward transmission of elevated left ventricular filling pressures into the pulmonary circulation (postcapillary hemodynamic profile), (2) potential superimposed components contributing to the extent of PH (leading to a precapillary component) which may be associated with (3) pulmonary vascular remodeling in some patients, thus leading to (4) right ventricular (RV) strain and dysfunction over time. RV dilation and increase in wall stress/tension (internal RV afterload) result in elevated myocardial oxygen consumption, which, along with concomitant reduction in coronary perfusion gradient, leads to RV ischemia and progressive RV failure.
Source: Adapted from Rosenkranz et al.[9]

to LA stiffness, reduced LA compliance, and impaired LA contractility contribute to pathogenic changes that further disrupt the pulmonary circuit and impact right heart function.[9]

DIAGNOSIS OF HEART FAILURE WITH PRESERVED EJECTION FRACTION ASSOCIATED WITH PULMONARY HYPERTENSION

Diagnosing HFpEF associated with PH requires a thorough clinical, echocardiographic, and hemodynamic evaluation, as it can easily be misdiagnosed as PAH. Key factors suggesting PH due to LHD include AF, LA enlargement, age over 60 years, coronary artery disease, and a BMI over 30 kg/m^2, which help in assessing the pretest probability of LHD-related PH **(Table 2)**. Physical examination and chest X-rays can reveal fluid retention or signs of RV failure. Transthoracic echocardiography is an effective screening tool and is the first step in the evaluation of patients suspected of PH. Although elevated PA systolic pressures

TABLE 2: Examples of key factors suggestive of group 2 pulmonary hypertension.

Clinical presentation	*Echocardiography*	*Other features*
Age >65 years	Structural left heart abnormality • Disease of left heart valves • LA enlargement (>4.2 cm) • Bowing of the IAS to the right • LV dysfunction • Concentric LV hypertrophy and/or increased LV mass	ECG • LVH and/or LAH • AF/Afib • LBBB • Presence of Q waves
Symptoms of left heart failure	Doppler indices of increased filling pressures • Increased E/e' • >Type 2–3 mitral flow abnormality	Other imaging • Kerley B lines • Pleural effusion • Pulmonary edema • LA enlargement

Contd...

Contd…

Clinical presentation	*Echocardiography*	*Other features*
Features of metabolic syndrome	Absence of • RV dysfunction • Mid-systolic notching of the PA flow • Pericardial effusion	
History of heart disease (past or current)		
Persistent atrial fibrillation		

(AF: atrial flutter; Afib: atrial fibrillation; ECG: electrocardiogram; IAS: interatrial septum; LA: left atrium; LAH: left atrial hypertrophy/dilation; LBBB: left bundle branch block; LV: left ventricle; LVH: left ventricular hypertrophy; PA: pulmonary artery; RV: right ventricle)
Source: Adapted from Galiè et al.[10]

measured by Doppler echocardiography correlate with high pulmonary pressures, the accuracy of these estimates varies across studies. Transthoracic echocardiography is the recommended screening tool; however, RHC remains the gold standard for diagnosis and accurate phenotyping. The role of fluid loading and exercise testing in identifying PH-LHD in patients with HFpEF is not yet standardized, and established normal values are needed to guide clinical recommendations. Additionally, some evidence suggests that patients diagnosed with PAH may exhibit an abnormal increase in PAWP in response to fluid loading.[3,4,10]

CURRENT CHALLENGES IN TREATING PULMONARY HYPERTENSION-HEART FAILURE WITH PRESERVED EJECTION FRACTION

Currently, no approved pharmacologic agents specifically target PH in the context of HFpEF, largely due to disappointing results from multiple studies. Loop diuretics remain the mainstay of therapy in HFpEF for managing volume overload, alongside treatment for comorbidities and HFpEF associated with PH. Diuresis helps normalize intracardiac and pulmonary pressures, relieving symptoms, and improving pulmonary arterial compliance (PAC), which in turn reduces the pulsatile load on the RV. Pulmonary artery monitoring devices may also aid in achieving and maintaining euvolemia.[3]

While pulmonary vasodilators are essential in the treatment of PAH, their efficacy has not been consistently demonstrated in patients with PH-LHD. Despite this, some patients with PH-HFpEF receive these therapies due to severe symptoms and poor prognosis. Trials of phosphodiesterase-5 inhibitors (PDE5i), soluble guanylate cyclase (sGC) stimulators, endothelin receptor antagonists (ERAs), and prostacyclin have shown mixed outcomes.[7] Studies have shown that nitric oxide-mediated pulmonary vasodilation is impaired in HF and contributes to endothelial dysfunction, which has further led to the investigation of PDE5i and sGC stimulators as potential treatment options for PH-LHD, but results remain inconsistent.[7]

Guazzi et al. studied sildenafil (50 mg, three times daily) in a 12-month randomized trial involving 44 HFpEF patients with PH and showed improvements in PA pressures, PVR, and RV function.[7,11] However, the RELAX study, which used sildenafil (60 mg, three times daily) in HFpEF patients with EF >50%, failed to show significant effect in the primary endpoint of change in peak oxygen consumption after 24 weeks of therapy.[7,12] Other studies also reported limited effects: A 12-week sildenafil study, phosphodiesterase-5 (PDE5) inhibitor, in 52 patients showed no improvement in hemodynamics or exercise capacity,[5,13] and the DILATE-1 trial found no significant hemodynamic changes after 6-hour treatment with riociguat (sGC stimulator) in stable patients.[5,14] Similarly, in the SOCRATES PRESERVED trial, vericiguat did not improve NT-proBNP and LA volume in patients with EF ≥45%.[7,15] The MELODY-1 trial observed no improvement in PVR or mean right atrial pressure with macitentan (endothelin receptor antagonist) in patients with CpcPH at 12 weeks, and adverse events were more frequent compared to placebo.[3,7,16]

Thus, current evidence discourages using targeted PAH therapies in PH related to left HF. Selected patients with Cpc-PH and/or RV phenotypes should be referred to specialized centers with expertise in both HF and PH, and considered for clinical trials whenever possible.[9]

FUTURE THERAPIES BEYOND TRADITIONAL PULMONARY VASODILATORS

There is growing interest in understanding the cardiac and vascular changes in PH-HFpEF to guide potential therapies beyond traditional pulmonary vasodilators.[7,17] Future treatment targets include vascular remodeling, oxidative stress from metabolic syndrome, and fibrosis. The vascular changes in PH-HFpEF differ from those in idiopathic PAH and PH-HFrEF, leading to varied responses to existing treatments.[7,18] With the rise in obesity and metabolic-related HFpEF, weight loss and aerobic exercise have become essential interventions, both shown to improve exercise tolerance and reduce body weight in HFpEF.[3,19]

Levosimendan, an intravenous calcium sensitizer and inodilator, was studied in PH-HFpEF patients (mean PA ≥35 mm Hg, PCWP ≥20 mm Hg, EF ≥40%). While 6 weeks of weekly infusions did not reduce peak exercise PCWP, it did decrease resting PCWP and improved 6-minute walk distance compared to placebo.[7,20] Metformin is currently in a phase 2 trial for PH-HFpEF (NCT03629340), supported by data suggesting benefits in HF outcomes among type 2 diabetes patients, reductions in cardiac workload, and improved metabolism in skeletal and pulmonary vascular muscle through the SIRT3-AMPK-Glut4 pathway.[3,21]

Sodium-glucose cotransporter-2 (SGLT2) inhibitors, such as empagliflozin and dapagliflozin, have shown benefits in HF outcomes for patients with type 2 diabetes, regardless of LV ejection fraction or prior HF history. The EMPEROR and DELIVER trials highlight their potential as a treatment option for HFpEF, where other therapies have had limited success. Although promising, further research is needed to optimize their use specifically for PH-HFpEF patients.[3,6,22,23] Nitrite, reduced to nitric oxide by hemoglobin, is under investigation in an oral formulation for PH-HFpEF (NCT03015402) after showing promise in an inhaled form by improving PAC. However, a broader HFpEF study (not limited to PH patients) found no improvement in exercise capacity as measured by cardiopulmonary exercise testing and 6-minute walk distance.[3,24]

CONCLUSION

Pulmonary hypertension-HFpEF presents significant diagnostic and therapeutic challenges due to its complex pathophysiology and limited treatment options. Current therapies primarily focus on symptom management rather than addressing the underlying mechanisms. While traditional pulmonary vasodilators have shown inconsistent results, emerging agents such as SGLT2 inhibitors, levosimendan, and metformin present new opportunities for improving patient outcomes. Ongoing research is crucial to better understand PH-HFpEF and develop targeted, evidence-based interventions that can effectively mitigate its high morbidity and mortality.

REFERENCES

1. Ruocco G, Gavazzi A, Gonnelli S, et al. Pulmonary arterial hypertension and heart failure with preserved ejection fraction: are they so discordant? Cardiovasc Diagn Ther. 2020;10(3):534-45.
2. Guazzi M. Pulmonary hypertension in heart failure preserved ejection fraction: prevalence, pathophysiology, and clinical perspectives. Circ Heart Fail. 2014;7(2):367-77.
3. Inampudi C, Silverman D, Simon MA, et al. Pulmonary hypertension in the context of heart failure with preserved ejection fraction. Chest. 2021;160(6):2232-46.
4. Aradhyula V, Vyas R, Dube P, et al. Novel insights into the pathobiology of pulmonary hypertension in heart failure with preserved ejection fraction. Am J Physiol Heart Circ Physiol. 2024;326(6):H1498-514.
5. Hoeper MM, Lam CSP, Vachiery JL, et al. Pulmonary hypertension in heart failure with preserved ejection fraction: a plea for proper phenotyping and further research. Eur Heart J. 2017;38(38):2869-73.
6. Macera F, Vachiéry JL. Management of pulmonary hypertension in left heart disease. Methodist Debakey Cardiovasc J. 2021;17(2):115-23.
7. Moles VM, Grafton G. Pulmonary hypertension in heart failure with preserved ejection fraction. Cardiol Clin. 2022;40(4):533-40.
8. Guazzi M, Ghio S, Adir Y. Pulmonary hypertension in HFpEF and HFrEF: JACC review topic of the week. J Am Coll Cardiol. 2020;76(9):1102-11.
9. Rosenkranz S, Gibbs JSR, Wachter R, et al. Left ventricular heart failure and pulmonary hypertension. Eur Heart J. 2016;37(12):942-54.
10. Galiè N, Humbert M, Vachiéry JL, et al. 2015 ESC/ERS guidelines for the diagnosis and treatment of pulmonary hypertension: the joint task force for the diagnosis and treatment of pulmonary hypertension of the European Society Of Cardiology (ESC) and the European Respiratory Society (ERS): endorsed by: Association for European Paediatric and Congenital Cardiology (AEPC), International Society for Heart and Lung Transplantation (ISHLT). Eur Respir J. 2015;46(4):903-75.
11. Guazzi M, Vicenzi M, Arena R, et al. Pulmonary hypertension in heart failure with preserved ejection fraction: a target of phosphodiesterase-5 inhibition in a 1-year study. Circulation. 2011;124(2):164-74.
12. Redfield MM, Chen HH, Borlaug BA, et al. Effect of phosphodiesterase-5 inhibition on exercise capacity and clinical status in heart failure with preserved ejection fraction: a randomized clinical trial. JAMA. 2013;309(12):1268-77.
13. Hoendermis ES, Liu LCY, Hummel YM, et al. Effects of sildenafil on invasive haemodynamics and exercise capacity in heart failure patients with preserved ejection fraction and pulmonary hypertension: a randomized controlled trial. Eur Heart J. 2015;36(38):2565-73.
14. Bonderman D, Pretsch I, Steringer-Mascherbauer R, et al. Acute hemodynamic effects of riociguat in patients with pulmonary hypertension associated with diastolic heart failure (DILATE-1): a randomized, double-blind placebo-controlled, single-dose study. Chest. 2014;146(5):1274-85.
15. Pieske B, Maggioni AP, Lam CSP, et al. Vericiguat in patients with worsening chronic heart failure and preserved

ejection fraction: results of the soluble guanylate cyclase stimulator in heart failure patients with PRESERVED EF (SOCRATES-PRESERVED) study. Eur Heart J. 2017;38(15):1119-27.

16. Vachiéry JL, Delcroix M, Al-Hiti H, et al. Macitentan in pulmonary hypertension due to left ventricular dysfunction. Eur Respir J. 2018;51(2):1701886.
17. Vachiéry JL, Tedford RJ, Rosenkranz S, et al. Pulmonary hypertension due to left heart disease. Eur Respir J. 2019;53(1):1801897.
18. Fayyaz AU, Edwards WD, Maleszewski JJ, et al. Global pulmonary vascular remodeling in pulmonary hypertension associated with heart failure and preserved or reduced ejection fraction. Circulation. 2018;137(17):1796-810.
19. Kitzman DW, Brubaker P, Morgan T, et al. Effect of caloric restriction or aerobic exercise training on peak oxygen consumption and quality of life in obese older patients with heart failure with preserved ejection fraction: a randomized clinical trial. JAMA. 2016;315(1):36-46.
20. Burkhoff D, Borlaug BA, Shah SJ, et al. Levosimendan improves hemodynamics and exercise tolerance in PH-HFpEF: results of the randomized placebo-controlled HELP trial. JACC Heart Fail. 2021;9(5):360-70.
21. Sanders-van Wijk S, Tromp J, Beussink-Nelson L, et al. Proteomic evaluation of the comorbidity-inflammation paradigm in heart failure with preserved ejection fraction: results from the PROMIS-HFpEF study. Circulation. 2020;142(21):2029-44.
22. Anker SD, Butler J, Filippatos G, et al. Empagliflozin in heart failure with a preserved ejection fraction. N Engl J Med. 2021;385(16):1451-61.
23. Solomon SD, McMurray JJV, Claggett B, et al. Dapagliflozin in heart failure with mildly reduced or preserved ejection fraction. N Engl J Med. 2022;387(12):1089-98.
24. Borlaug BA, Anstrom KJ, Lewis GD, et al. Effect of inorganic nitrite vs placebo on exercise capacity among patients with heart failure with preserved ejection fraction: the INDIE-HFpEF randomized clinical trial. JAMA. 2018;320(17):1764-73.

112

CHAPTER

Obstructive Sleep Apnea and Hypertension to HFpEF: Management Strategies

Chanchal Pal

INTRODUCTION

Snoring and obstructive sleep apnea (OSA) have become quite prevalent in the last few decades. OSA and heart failure commonly overlap and have been studied vastly in the past three decades.[1] Heart failure with preserved ejection fraction (HFpEF), is also not uncommon but less understood,[2] and studies on effects of OSA on it were done only recently,[3] OSA also has been detected in 50% of heart failure with preserved ejection fraction (HFpEF).[4]

PATHOPHYSIOLOGY

Pathophysiology of HFpEF is heterogeneous in nature with traditional models focused on increased left ventricular overload resulting in left ventricular hypertrophy (LVH) and diastolic dysfunction. However, emerging studies attribute HFpEF development to proinflammatory changes secondary to comorbidities like hypertension and OSA and resultant changes in passive ventricular stiffness, ventricular-arterial coupling, peripheral microvascular function, and systolic reserve.[2] There are many similarities between the pathological effects of OSA and other known etiologies of HFpEF.[5]

Several mechanisms have been suggested to explain the relationship between OSA and HFpEF.

Studies have shown that OSA is associated with a higher degree of diastolic dysfunction,[6] reduced left ventricular diastolic function due to arterial stiffness, increased sympathetic nerve activity, and raised blood pressure, all leading to HFpEF,[7-9] OSA due to intermittent hypoxia also stimulates the sympathetic nervous system and induces oxidative stress and renin–angiotensin–aldosterone system. This results in systemic inflammatory state as happens in cases of other risk factors of HFpEF. The final pathway is the development of structural changes in collagen and myocardial fibrosis resulting in myocardial stiffening.[5] Additionally, oxidative stress and increased inflammatory factors are caused by worsening cardiovascular function and risk of arrhythmias.[10,11] OSA resulting in myocardial damage due to intermittent hypoxia-led sympathetic activity and transmural pressures, low-grade vascular inflammation, and oxidative stress was also documented in another study.[1] OSA affects hemodynamics with its effect on intrathoracic pressures.[4] On the other hand, in case of heart failure, pharyngeal collapse worsens from the fluid accumulation in the neck as a result of daytime fluid retention and night fluid shift from the leg,[1] thus worsening the OSA.

Fluid retention in heart failure can cause airway obstruction. Nocturnal oxygen desaturation affects ventricular relaxation during diastole, and therefore predisposes to HFpEF. In patients with heart failure, the coexistence of OSA may be associated with higher sympathetic nerve activity; consequently, the nocturnal and daytime BP may be higher in these patients. OSA could lead to the progression of heart failure through various pathophysiological mechanisms:[1] (1) By increasing sympathetic activity to the heart, kidney, and resistance vessels during wakefulness and sleep; (2) by increasing left ventricular afterload both acutely/intermittently and chronically; (3) by inducing hypoxia, increasing pulmonary artery pressure, and secondary increases in right ventricular afterload; and (4) by increasing the risk of myocardial ischemia and infarction.[8] Treatment with continuous positive airway pressure (CPAP) may benefit patients with OSA and all phenotypes of heart failure, namely, HfrEF/HfmrEF/HfpEF.[4]

MANAGEMENT

Management strategies for HFpEF are decided by its heterogeneous nature. There is no uniform therapy for all, it has to be tailor-made for each patient depending on comorbidities like OS and hypertension. Controlling OSA and hypertension remains a cornerstone of HFpEF management. Tailoring antihypertensive therapy to specific phenotypes of HFpEF is an important strategy. Antihypertensive therapies lead to LVH regression and improvement in diastolic dysfunction. However, no therapy has definite mortality benefit. Nonpharmacologic management for hypertension like dietary modification, exercise, and treating OSA may provide morbidity benefits. Further research may identify effective and more specific treatments.[2] A review of a diverse range of studies by Polecka et al. found the effect of positive airway pressure (PAP), sodium-glucose cotransporter-2 inhibitors (SGLT2i), and sacubitril/valsartan on OSA. PAP improved apnea-hypopnea index, left ventricular ejection fraction, and oxygen saturation, thus overall quality of life. SGLT2i and sacubitril/valsartan influenced OSA outcomes through weight loss, improved metabolism, and direct effect on upper airway muscles.[12] The largest analysis exploring the association between OSA therapy and patients with HFpEF observed that adherence to PAP therapy is associated with improvements in healthcare resource use, including reductions in hospitalization rate, ER visits, and cardiovascular hospitalizations, thus demonstrating both clinical and economic benefits associated with treating OSA in HFpEF, particularly among patients adherent to therapy.[13] Similar benefits of PAP for OSA were seen in patients with HFrEF in a separate study;[14] benefit of adherence to PAP therapy for OSA in HFpEF is independent of other comorbidities[13] and similar results are expected from OSA control by surgical correction of upper airway obstruction like LASER palatopharyngoplasty, and Transoral robotic surgery (TORS).

The PAP therapy prevents upper airway collapse, reducing ill effects of OSA,[15-17] by controlling blood pressure, better sleep efficiency, and reversing diastolic abnormalities.[18-20] One of the largest analyses on OSA therapy for patients with HFpEF observed that adherence to PAP therapy also helped in optimizing use of healthcare resources.[13]

Recent studies also showed that OSA control by PAP adherence reduces the risk of cardiovascular events. In a cohort of older patients with cardiovascular disease and comorbid OSA, PAP adherence helped low readmission rates and a 40% reduction in healthcare costs.[21,22] LASER sleep surgeries for OSA also give good results in reversing the ill effects of OSA on HFpEF.

Recent literature highlights new therapeutic options for HFpEF particularly, SGLT2 inhibitors, which when given in combination with mineralocorticoid receptor antagonists such as spironolactone, improve underlying OSA in patients with resistant hypertension[23] and help in controlling HFpEF.

Addition of loop diuretic can improve upper airway edema, reducing upper airway obstruction in OSA.[24,25]

LIMITATIONS

There is limited data on the effects of existing HFpEF therapies on sleep-disordered breathing.

More studies are needed to establish the relation.

As OSA also causes hypertension by same pathophysiological pathways, its role as independent player for HFpEF can not be established.

There are limited data on effect of LASER sleep surgeries for OSA, which at times give very good results to reverse the ill effects of OSA on HFpEF.

CONCLUSION

Considering the pathophysiology of OSA and HFpEF, OSA is very much likely to be a significant risk factor for HFpEF. In patients referred for sleep study and echocardiogram, markers of diastolic dysfunction are associated with OSA severity.

The OSA prevalence and severity are associated with increased H_2FPEF scores. Clinicians should have low thresholds for referring patients with HFpEF for sleep study and with OSA for cardiac workup.[3] Review studies suggest heart failure management strategies should include control of OSA. A multifaceted approach is the need of the day, seeing the complex interplay between the two.[12]

The PAP treatment has shown good results as adjuvant to heart failure pharmacotherapy.[12] These findings encourage further study of OSA in HFpEF.[13]

REFERENCES

1. Lévy P, Naughton MT, Tamisier R, et al. Sleep apnoea and heart failure. Eur Respir J. 2022;59(5):2101640.
2. Tam MC, Lee R, Cascino TM, et al. Current perspectives on systemic hypertension in heart failure with preserved ejection fraction. Curr Hypertens Rep. 2017;19(2):12.
3. Connolly JE, Genuardi MV, Mora JI, et al. Heart failure with preserved ejection fraction risk is associated with

prevalence and severity of obstructive sleep apnea. J Clin Sleep Med. 2024;20(3):381-7.
4. Sanzgiri P, Shingare V, Thanki F, et al. Sleep-disordered breathing and cardiac disorders. Int J Head Neck Surg. 2019;10(3):51-4.
5. Sanderson JE, Fang F, Lu M, et al. Obstructive sleep apnoea, intermittent hypoxia and heart failure with a preserved ejection fraction. Heart. 2021;107:190-4.
6. Sidana J, Aronow WS, Ravipati G, et al. Prevalence of moderate or severe left ventricular diastolic dysfunction in obese persons with obstructive sleep apnea. Cardiology. 2005;104(2):107-9.
7. Caples SM, Gami AS, Somers VK. Obstructive sleep apnea. Ann Intern Med. 2005;142(3):187-97.
8. Drager LF, Diegues-Silva L, Diniz PM, et al. Obstructive sleep apnea, masked hypertension, and arterial stiffness in men. Am J Hypertens. 2010;23(3):249-54.
9. Leung RS, Bradley TD. Sleep apnea and cardiovascular disease. Am J Respir Crit Care Med. 2001;164(12):2147-65.
10. Jelic S, Le Jemtel TH. Sleep-disordered breathing in acute decompensated heart failure. Curr Heart Fail Rep. 2009;6:169-75.
11. May AM, Van Wagoner DR, Mehra R. OSA and cardiac arrhythmogenesis: mechanistic insights. Chest. 2017;151:225-41.
12. Polecka A, Olszewska N, Danielski Ł, et al. Association between obstructive sleep apnea and heart failure in adults—a systematic review. J Clin Med. 2023;12(19):6139.
13. Cistulli PA, Malhotra A, Cole KV, et al. Positive airway pressure therapy adherence and health care resource use in patients with obstructive sleep apnea and heart failure with preserved ejection fraction. J Am Heart Assoc. 2023;12(14):e028733.
14. Malhotra A, Cole KV, Malik A, et al. Abstract 13554: Effect of positive airway pressure therapy for obstructive sleep apnea in heart failure patients with reduced ejection fraction—implications for healthcare resource utilization. Circulation. 2022;146:A13554.
15. Javaheri S, Barbe F, Campos-Rodriguez F, et al. Sleep apnea: Types, mechanisms, and clinical cardiovascular consequences. J Am Coll Cardiol. 2017;69:841-58.
16. Pépin JL, Bailly S, Rinder P, et al. Relationship between CPAP termination and all-cause mortality: A French nationwide database analysis. Chest. 2022;161:1657-65.
17. Yeghiazarians Y, Jneid H, Tietjens JR, et al. Obstructive sleep apnea and cardiovascular disease: A scientific statement from the American Heart Association. Circulation. 2021;144:e56-67.
18. Montesi SB, Edwards BA, Malhotra A, et al. The effect of continuous positive airway pressure treatment on blood pressure: a systematic review and meta-analysis of randomized controlled trials. J Clin Sleep Med. 2012;8:587-96.
19. Pengo MF, Soranna D, Giontella A, et al. Obstructive sleep apnoea treatment and blood pressure: which phenotypes predict a response? A systematic review and meta-analysis. Eur Respir J. 2020;55(5):1901945.
20. Colish J, Walker JR, Elmayergi N, et al. Obstructive sleep apnea: Effects of continuous positive airway pressure on cardiac remodeling as assessed by cardiac biomarkers, echocardiography, and cardiac MRI. Chest. 2012;141(3):674-81.
21. Bailey MD, Wickwire EM, Somers VK, et al. Adherence to continuous positive airway pressure reduces the risk of 30-day hospital readmission among older adults with comorbid obstructive sleep apnea and cardiovascular disease. J Clin Sleep Med. 2022;18:2739-44.
22. Bock JM, Needham KA, Gregory DA, et al. Continuous positive airway pressure adherence and treatment cost in patients with obstructive sleep apnea and cardiovascular disease. Mayo Clin Proc Innov Qual Outcomes. 2022;6:166-75.
23. Gaddam K, Pimenta E, Thomas SJ, et al. Spironolactone reduces severity of obstructive sleep apnoea in patients with resistant hypertension: a preliminary report. J Hum Hypertens. 2010;24:532-7.
24. White LH, Bradley TD. Role of nocturnal rostral fluid shift in the pathogenesis of obstructive and central sleep apnoea. J Physiol. 2013;591:1179-93.
25. Kasai T, Bradley TD, Friedman O, et al. Effect of intensified diuretic therapy on overnight rostral fluid shift and obstructive sleep apnoea in patients with uncontrolled hypertension. J Hypertens. 2014;32:673-80.

113

CHAPTER

Noise Pollution, Hypertension, and HFpEF

Nidhi Dhawan, HK Chopra

INTRODUCTION

Hitherto, it has been assumed that noise is simply sound that is annoying.[1] In 2023 June, however, the International Congress on Biological Effects of Noise (ICBEN), in its 14th iteration, adopted a new and more nuanced definition of noise. The word harmful was added to the previous definition that stated simply "unwanted".[2] Daniel Fink categorically states that the addition of the words "and/or harmful" is significant, important, and needed. While the phrase "sitting is the new smoking" may have gained momentum and popularity in the past few years, it is important to consider that noise may really be the more important equivalent to smoking in its impact on heart health and hypertension. In fact, Dr William Stewart, the former Surgeon General, US, remarked that considering noise a nuisance alone is akin to considering smog simply an inconvenience.[3] He goes on to emphasize that noise must be considered a public health hazard and be treated like one in policy and legal frameworks.

WHAT IS SOUND AND WHAT IS NOISE?

Sound has been traditionally defined as a signal that makes sense, as vibration that travels through a medium and results in auditory perception as it enters the ear of a biological entity as a mechanical energy that needs a medium to travel and produces an acoustic result in the ear.[2,4,5]

Noise, then, is defined as unwanted sound. Additionally, in terms of physics or engineering, noise implies a signal varying over time, without meaning. This assumption presupposes that noise is a mere nuisance and not a really harmful phenomenon.[1] It is important to note that desired, nonannoying sound can have its biological effects and that the harm is dose-dependent and preventable.

Certain sounds and noises in nature—the sound/noise of a stream in the mountains, of rain falling, or the ocean waves can be deeply calming and anti-inflammatory. While many man-made sounds or noises, such as traffic, aircraft, and machines, can have significant biological effects even when we "psychologically" do not get actively annoyed by them.

Ingoon Song et al., in a study of 26 university students published in August 2023, found that nature sounds like water, birds, and forest and environmental sounds of insects and crickets not only promote the parasympathetic response but also promote recovery from stress states induced by urban noises like traffic, aircraft, and machines.[6,7] Contrarily, as per World Health Organization (WHO) and European Environmental Agency estimates, EU initiative [Environmental Noise Directive (END)] of measuring noise and its impact in Europe has revealed shockingly alarming figures—over a hundred million people are exposed to harmful levels of noise. It is estimated that nearly 48,000 new cases of heart disease and 12,000 premature deaths are attributable, at least in part, to noise.

EFFECTS OF NOISE

Noise and Inflammation

Li Yang et al., in a systematic review of 811 potentially relevant studies came to the conclusion that noise affects the function of the immune system and its components through its effect on central nervous system (CNS), circulatory system, and the heart, auditory system, gut as well as the auditory system. The central common pathway appears to be the oxidative injury involving the NADPH oxidase and the ROS.[8] They report that noise impacts all critical organs and organ systems, including the liver, kidneys, pancreas, lungs, and GI tract.

Lee et al., found that stress hormone levels were significantly increased in saliva and serum as result of exposure to sounds at 75 dB and that this was dose-dependent.

Babisch proposed a Noise-Stress Model in 2002 to explain the systemic effects of noise, especially on the cardiovascular system.[9,10] Changes in salivary and serum stress hormone levels have been well documented in subjects exposed to acute and chronic noise environments. It is proposed that this may be mediated via the pituitary-adrenal-medullary axis.

Noise and Hypertension

Li Yang et al.[11] also established a strong association between noise exposure and hypertension with as little, as an increment of 5 dB, increase in noise levels with an odds ratio of 1.034, rising to a relative risk of 1.36 with a 10 dB rise in traffic or occupational noise levels. According to WHO and European Environmental Agency, there is an 8% increase in risk of CHD with every 10 dB rise in environmental noise.

Several large prospective studies have demonstrated that traffic, aircraft, and rail noise exposure is associated with significantly increased risk of hypertension.[12-14]

EPIDEMIOLOGY

Of the estimated 220 million Indians with diagnosed hypertension, an abysmal 12% have satisfactory control of their blood pressure. This means one in four adults in India have hypertension and only about one in ten of those have satisfactory BP control.[15] Hypertension is a major contributor to the patient pool with heart failure. The natural history of heart failure is one of transition from longstanding hypertension to heart failure.[16] In the Framingham Heart Study Cohort, 91% of patients with heart failure had previous history of hypertension, a twofold increase in risk in males, and a threefold increase in risk in females of developing heart failure compared to normotensive individuals.

World Health Organization estimates for Europe:[17] Even very conservative assumptions are shocking in terms of disease burden—estimated DALYs lost due to environmental noise exceed a million healthy life years, 6,100 from ischemic heart disease, 45,000 from childhood cognitive impairment, 903,000 lost to sleep disturbances, and >587,000 due to annoyance. Nearly 22,000 years lost to tinnitus make it a significant pathology to tackle in public health and policy initiatives.

Further, European studies emphasize the seriousness of noise as a public health problem stating that noise is responsible annually for nearly 1.7 million cases of hypertension, 18,000 cases of premature deaths, and 80,000 hospitalizations.

PATHOPHYSIOLOGY

Munzel et al., have emphasized that >75% of all non-communicable disease burden and disability is associated with ambient noise and air pollution, making them number one cause of this critical mass.[18-20] 17 out of the top 30 cities for premature cardiovascular mortality are in Asia and account for nearly 7% of global burden of disease attributable to outdoor air pollution and noise. Environmental factors greatly modify the levels of noise and include noise barriers such as vegetation and trees, road conditions as well as surrounding buildings. Eriksson et al. investigated the effect of noise exposure on body mass index, waist circumference, and type 2 diabetes. They found an increase of 1.5 cm waist circumference with 5 dB increase in noise levels. This is consistent with the hypothesis that (aircraft) noise stimulates the release of cortisol, contributing to central obesity and metabolic syndrome.[21,22]

Current research unequivocally suggests that air and noise pollution induce low-grade inflammation, oxidative stress, and vascular dysfunction. The impact of dysautonomia is a further factor to consider toward disease burden. The impact of these environmental factors may be much larger than anticipated as they may act independently as well as through the traditional risk factors.

Munzel et al., also found that long-term exposure to noise greater than 55 dB has strong correlation with cardiovascular disease (CVD). They found this effect kicks in with as little as 5 dB increments in evening noise levels.[18] They propose four pathways, possibly not mutually exclusive, that could explain causal cascade between air pollution, noise exposure, and CVD.

These are as follows:

1. Activation of the sympathoadrenal axis with an autonomic dysfunction
2. Inflammation via inflammatory mediators, modified lipids/phospholipids, and activated leukocytes
3. Oxidative stress-induced endothelial dysfunction
4. Activation of prothrombotic pathways

Babisch et al.,[9,18,20] theorized two principal pathways to explain adverse health effects of noise: Direct and Indirect. The direct pathway is activated by the immediate effect of interaction between auditory nerve and its CNS connections. The indirect pathway addresses the cognitive perception of sound and its cortical ramifications. It is important to note that adverse effects of noise are completely independent of quality of sleep or perceived annoyance. The immune system and the body keep the score.

Both, the direct and the indirect pathways work through the hypothalamus–pituitary–adrenal axis and the sympathetic–adrenal–medulla axis with activation of the hypothalamus, limbic system, and the autonomic nervous system. The resultant rise in the level of stress hormones (cortisol, noradrenalin, and adrenalin) mediates not just the inflammation but also the rise in the heart rate and the spiral toward heart failure.

Furthermore, the disturbed sleep–wake cycle, circadian rhythm disturbances, and disturbed or interrupted recovery phases escalate the inflammatory response.

Hypertension and environmental noise near airports (HYENA) study done across six European countries explored whether the noise and its associated annoyance together can predict arterial hypertension as an outcome. The more annoyed a subject, the more likely the arterial hypertension. However, road traffic noise does not show this correlation to be valid.[23,24]

However, several epidemiological studies have shown beyond doubt that exposure to environmental noise is associated with arterial hypertension, myocardial infarction, and even stroke. This effect is particularly significant for nighttime noise exposures.[25] Not only are single events of noise exposure significant in their effect on cardiovascular health, but also, the authors note a priming effect, i.e., the subjects who have been previously exposed to noise show greater effect.[24] These effects are also stronger in middle-aged subjects and in males.

Noise by itself, due to the CNS connections of auditory pathways that span the limbic system and serve the areas of cognition, language, and memory, can have deep-seated effects on these functions.

Several possible mechanisms can explain the effect of noise on the development of hypertension and subsequent transition into heart failure, with or without preserved ejection fraction.

- *Stress-hormone-mediated metabolic syndrome* with central obesity, disturbed lipid and glucose metabolism, and manifold increased risk of CVD[14,18,20]
- *Oxidative endothelial damage and dysfunction* are mediated through ROS and NADPH pathways.[20,26] In the Swiss Cohort Study on Air pollution and Lung and Heart diseases, adults clearly demonstrated that nighttime noise exposure is associated with increased arterial stiffness in a dose-dependent manner.[27] Munzel et al., found demonstrable disturbance of vascular function within 4 days of exposure with elevated blood pressure and even alteration in gene expression in the vascular wall.
- *CNS inflammation and centrally driven dysregulation:* As aforementioned, the areas of the brain serving reception and processing of sound are the ones also serving emotions, memory, and language. Direct stimulation of the limbic system, amygdala, and higher cortical areas of auditory cortex by noise, especially in sleep and recovery time of the body leads to increased activity in the said areas. These are evolutionarily areas to process threats and seek safety. Thus, excessive noise exposure causes stress, anxiety, and fear with its attendent hormonal and chemical changes.
- Prothrombotic pathway activation further increases the stasis and the stress on the heart leading to heart failure.

MITIGATION OF RISK AND PREVENTION STRATEGIES

Efforts to mitigate the risk of noise and air pollution are complex problems. They require far-reaching and interconnected sources and effects to be identified and disconnected from the chain of events. Most efforts need to start with individual efforts, and that requires advocacy and awareness campaigns.

Prevention of noise pollution is a major public health problem. Industrialization, heavy reliance on transportation, and the constant sources of noise even in our domestic environments have made need for global initiatives and policy decisions a necessity.

World Health Organization has acknowledged the need to lay standards of noise to prevent coronary heart disease. These standards vary for the day and the night—nighttime exposures being more critical to prevent.[28]

- *Aircraft noise:* Daytime 45 dB and nighttime 40 dB
- *Road traffic:* Daytime 53 dB and nighttime 45 dB
- *Rail traffic:* Daytime 54 dB and nighttime 44 dB

Introduction of efficient and convenient public transport, reducing need for individual transportation, and shifting to electric vehicles with more stringent noise and emission standards will help reduce both noise and air pollution. India is moving in this direction quite rapidly.

Creating green belts and noise barriers between roads and residential areas can also help reduce noise exposure.

Urban planning and zoning and separation of commercial, roads, and residential areas need to be a government and planning initiative. One often ignored source of noise in our surroundings is from poor quality roads—development of better quality road surfaces and quieter tire technology is no longer science fiction.

Personal commitment to preventing exposure can include responsible usage of transportation, refraining from usage of horns unnecessarily, and personal noise protection.

Advocacy to make the public aware of ill-effects of noise exposure and creating campaigns for quiet public spaces would improve our environment and our quality of life immensely.

It is important to emphasize that several studies have demonstrated clearly an independent improvement in quality of life and life expectancy upon reducing exposure to noise.

CONCLUSION

Noise has become a grave and great public health problem and is all around us. WHO has included a new category of intervention and diagnosis—recreational noise exposure. Hearing loss, hypertension, mental health issues, and CVD are occurring sooner, in younger populations and are more severe than ever before.

This chapter has sought to bring a surface awareness of the studies that have begun to uncover the hitherto ignored source of aging and ill-health.

We need a paradigm shift in human activity and concerted action on both individual and collective fronts. Given that there is now a large body of evidence to prove that noise and air pollutions are significant modifiable factors for prevention of CVD and hypertension, it would bode us well to create, publicize, and implement standards and guidelines to tackle this problem.

REFERENCES

1. Basner M, Babisch W, Davis A, et al. Auditory and non-auditory effects of noise on health. Lancet. 2014;383(9925):1325-32.
2. Fink D. (2019). A new definition of noise: Noise is unwanted and/or harmful sound. Noise is the new 'secondhand smoke'. [online] Available from https://pubs.aip.org/asa/poma/article/39/1/050002/838992/A-new-definition-of-noise-noise-is-unwanted-and-or [Last accessed January, 2025].
3. United States Environmental Protection Agency. (1978). Noise: A health problem. [online] Available from https://www.nonoise.org/library/epahlth/epahlth.htm [Last accessed January, 2025].
4. Dictionary.com. (2025). Definition of sound. [online] Available from https://www.dictionary.com/browse/sound [Last accessed January, 2025].
5. Kryter KD. Handbook of Hearing and Effects of Noise: Physiology, Psychology, and Public Health. Leiden, Netherlands: Brill Publishers; 1994.
6. Song I, Baek K, Kim C, et al. Effects of nature sounds on the attention and physiological and psychological relaxation. Urban Forestry & Urban Greening. 2023:86.
7. European Environment Agency. (2020). Health risks caused by environmental noise in Europe. [online] Available from https://www.eea.europa.eu/publications/health-risks-caused-by-environmental- [Last accessed January, 2024].
8. Abouee-Mehrizi A, Rasoulzadeh Y, Kazemi T, et al. Inflammatory and immunological changes caused by noise exposure: A systematic review. J Environ Sci Health C Toxicol Carcinog. 2020;38(1):61-90.
9. Babisch W. The noise/stress concept, risk assessment and research needs. Noise Health. 2002;4(16):1-11.
10. Lee SH, Kim AR, Lee J. Effects of noise exposure on stress hormone changes during task performance in young Korean men: quasi-experimental study. J Toxicol Environ Health A. 2024;87(15):605-15.
11. Yang L, Gutierrez DE, Guthrie OW. Systemic health effects of noise exposure. J Toxicol Environ Health B Crit Rev. 2024;27(1):21-54.
12. Thacher JD, Poulsen AH, Raaschou-Nielsen O, et al. Exposure to transportation noise and risk for cardiovascular disease in a nationwide cohort study from Denmark. Environ Res. 2022;211:113106.
13. Seidler A, Wagner M, Schubert M, et al. Myocardial infarction risk due to aircraft, road, and rail traffic noise. Dtsch Arztebl Int. 2016;113(24):407-14.
14. Eriksson C, Rosenlund M, Pershagen G, et al. Aircraft noise and incidence of hypertension. Epidemiology. 2007;18(6):716-21.
15. Geldsetzer P, Manne-Goehler J, Theilmann M, et al. Diabetes and hypertension in India: A nationally representative study of 1.3 million adults. JAMA Intern Med. 2018;178(3):363-72.
16. Messerli FH, Rimoldi SF, Bangalore S. The transition from hypertension to heart failure: Contemporary Update. JACC Heart Fail. 2017;5(8):543-1.
17. World Health Organization. (2011). Burden of disease from environmental noise-quantification of healthy life years lost in Europe. [online] Available from https://www.who.int/publications/i/item/burden-of-disease-from-environmental-noise-quantification-of-healthy-life-years-lost-in-europe [Last accessed January, 2025].
18. Münzel T, Sørensen M, Gori T, et al. Environmental stressors and cardio-metabolic disease: Part I–epidemiologic evidence supporting a role for noise and air pollution and effects of mitigation strategies. Eur Heart J. 2017;38(8):550-6.
19. European Environmental Agency. (2018). European Topic Centre on Air Pollution and Climate Change Mitigation (ETC/ACM 2014-2018). [online] Available from http://geografia.uab.cat. [Last accessed January, 2025].

20. Münzel T, Sørensen M, Gori T, et al. Environmental stressors and cardio-metabolic disease: Part II-mechanistic insights. Eur Heart J. 2017;38(8):557-64.
21. Lelieveld J, Evans JS, Fnais M, et al. The contribution of outdoor air pollution sources to premature mortality on a global scale. Nature. 2015;525:367-71.
22. Eriksson C, Hilding A, Pyko A, et al. Long-term aircraft noise exposure and body mass index, waist circumference, and type 2 diabetes: A prospective study. Environ Health Perspect. 2014;122(7):687-94. Erratum in: Environ Health Perspect. 2014;122(7):693.
23. Tetreault LF, Perron S, Smargiassi A. Cardiovascular health, traffic-related air pollution and noise: Are associations mutually confounded? A systematic review. Int J Public Health. 2013;58(5):649-66.
24. Floud S, Blangiardo M, Clark C, et al. Exposure to aircraft and road traffic noise and associations with heart disease and stroke in six European countries: A cross-sectional study. Environ Health. 2013;12:89.
25. Münzel T, Gori T, Babisch W, et al. Cardiovascular effects of environmental noise exposure. Eur Heart J. 2014;35(13): 829-36.
26. Schmidt F, Kolle K, Kreuder K, et al. Nighttime aircraft noise impairs endothelial function and increases blood pressure in patients with or at high risk for coronary artery disease. Coin Res Cardiol. 2015;104(1):23-30.
27. Foraster M, Eze IC, Schaffner E, et al. Exposure to road, railway, and aircraft noise and arterial stiffness in SAPALDIA Study: Annual Average noise levels and temporal noise characteristics. Environ Health Perspect. 2017;125(9):097004.
28. World Health Organization. (2018). Environmental noise guidelines for the European region. [online] Available from https://www.who.int/europe/publications/i/item/9789289053563 [Last accessed January, 2025].

SECTION 14

HFpEF, Cardiodiabetes and Metabolic Disease

114. Metabolic Syndrome and HFpEF: Management Strategies
115. Diabetes and HFpEF: New Insights
116. SGLT2i and Semaglutide in Cardiometabolic Syndrome with HFpEF
117. Obesity and HFpEF
118. Management of HFpEF: A Recent Approach
119. Interplay Between HFpEF and Hypothyroidism
120. Role of Sodium–Glucose Cotransporter-2 Inhibitors in Patients with HFpEF
121. Effect of SGLT2i on Cardiovascular Outcomes and Mortality in Type 2 DM with HFpEF
122. Cardiovascular Outcome Studies with SGLT2 Inhibitors on HFpEF

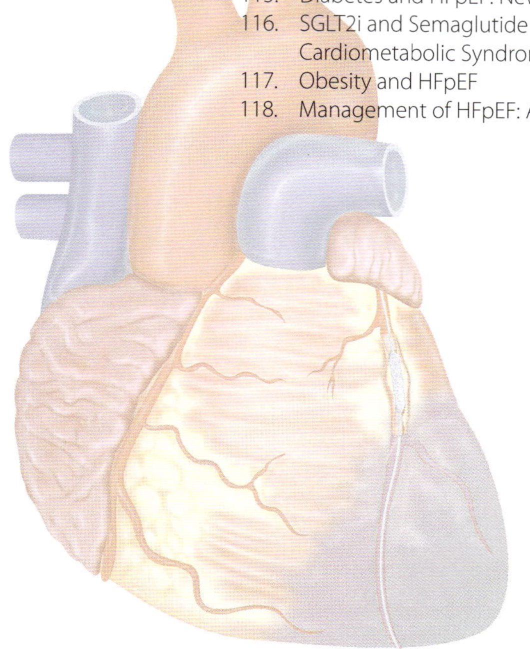

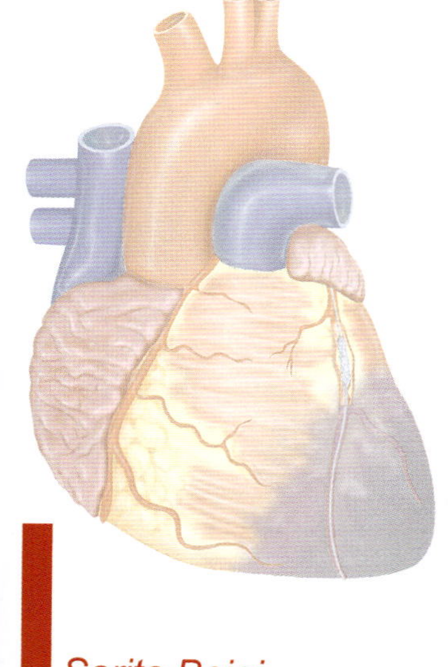

Metabolic Syndrome and HFpEF: Management Strategies

Sarita Bajaj

INTRODUCTION

Heart failure is a growing health problem affecting over 30 million people worldwide. There are two major phenotypes of heart failure—heart failure with reduced ejection fraction (HFrEF) and heart failure with preserved ejection fraction (HFpEF). HFpEF accounts for 50% of all heart failure cases and its prevalence is increasing at a rate 10% higher than that of HFrEF.[1] This is due to the aging population and the increase in the incidence of the predisposing conditions leading to the development of HFpEF, especially obesity and metabolic syndrome. HFpEF is a heterogeneous disorder in which multiple comorbidities differentially contribute to the overall clinical presentation resulting in various phenotypes of HFpEF. The four commonly discussed phenotypes of HFpEF are—the aging phenotype, the coronary artery disease (CAD) phenotype, the pulmonary hypertension (PH) phenotype, and the obesity phenotype, also known as the cardiometabolic HFpEF.[2] Though there is overlap in the presentation and pathogenesis of all these different phenotypes, cardiometabolic HFpEF is the most common. Presently, the average body mass index (BMI) of HFpEF patients in the US is >35 kg/m.

OBESITY PARADOX IN HEART FAILURE WITH PRESERVED EJECTION FRACTION

It was earlier thought that obesity protects against adverse outcomes in HFpEF even though it is a well-known predisposing factor for HPpEF. However, the basis for this paradox is mostly observational studies. A study using Mendelian randomization of >100,000 individuals found that obesity not only increases the incidence of HFpEF but also increases heart failure mortality (HR = 1.18) and all-cause mortality (HR = 1.02) causation.[3] The effect of obesity on HFpEF outcomes in various studies depends also on the parameter used. While higher BMI was associated with better outcomes, larger waist circumference is associated with worse outcomes.[4]

Obese HFpEF patients present with worse functional parameters as well as increased risk of poor outcomes compared to their lean HFpEF counterparts. Cardio-metabolic stress due to obesity, metabolic syndrome, and in most cases, type 2 diabetes, leads to increased proinflammatory state and microvascular endothelial dysfunction. This contributes to impaired myocardial relaxation and compliance which are the major drivers of pathophysiology of HFpEF. This is further evidenced by the fact that improvement in metabolic parameters through lifestyle changes (such as diet, exercise, etc.) or therapeutic options (SGLT2 inhibitors, GLP-1 agonists, and bariatric surgery) lead to improvement in HFpEF clinical outcomes.

Even though HFpEF is increasing in incidence and is associated with high symptom- and mortality burden, it has been historically been difficult to treat due to its complexity and lack of effective options. However, recent clinical trials have introduced new pharmacological treatments which show promise in reducing hospitalizations and improving quality of life. **Flowchart 1** shows the pathophysiology and the treatment options for cardiometabolic HFpEF.

Flowchart 1: Pathophysiology and available treatment options for cardiometabolic heart failure with preserved ejection fraction (HFpEF).

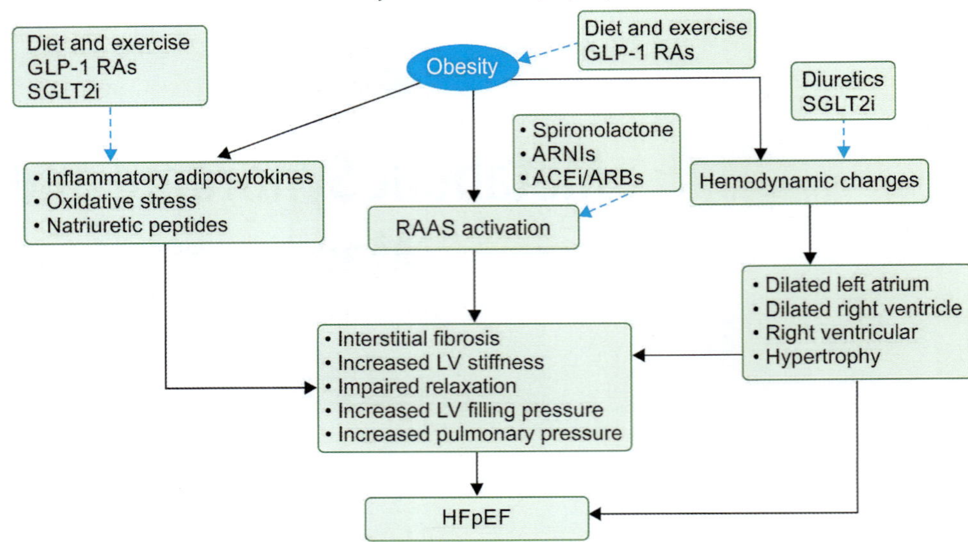

(ACEi: angiotensin-converting enzyme inhibitor; ARB: angiotensin receptor blocker; ARNI: angiotensin receptor–neprilysin inhibitor; LV: left ventricular: GLP-1 RAs: glucagon-like peptide-1 receptor agonists; RAAS: renin-angiotensin-aldosterone system; SGLT2i: sodium-glucose cotransporter-2 inhibitor)

TREATMENT

Diet and lifestyle changes play a pivotal role in the prevention and treatment of cardiovascular diseases associated with metabolic syndrome. Moderate weight loss of 5–10 kg through dietary and exercise interventions results in a clinically meaningful reduction of cardiometabolic risk.

DIETARY STRATEGIES

Calorie restriction (CR) by 30–40% results in weight loss thereby leading to decreased oxidative stress and systemic inflammation and improved insulin sensitivity. Improvement in VO_2 was seen in a study done on 100 obese patients with HFpEF treated with CR and aerobic exercise training for 20 weeks.[5] Another study in which 38 obese and hypertensive HFpEF patients underwent a 6-month CR diet program leading to a >5 kg weight loss, resulted in decrease in NT-proBNP circulating levels and improvement in diastolic function and 6 minute walk distance (6MWD).[6] Furthermore, calorie restriction shows significant cardiometabolic benefits such as improving cardiorespiratory fitness, reducing body weight, ameliorating insulin sensitivity and glucose metabolism, improving lipid profile, and reducing systemic inflammation. Low carbohydrate diet of <130 g of carbohydrates per day has also been shown to improve insulin sensitivity and oxygen saturation in HF patients.[7]

The GOURMET-HF trial showed that the Dietary Approach to Stop Hypertension (DASH) diet reduced rehospitalization at 30 days in both HFrEF and HFpEF patients.[8]

Mediterranean diet was associated with a significant reduction in HF hospitalizations but not with reduced long-term mortality in MEDIT-AHF trial.[9] The Hellenic Heart Failure Study, in which 38% of patients had HFpEF, showed improved long-term outcomes with better long-term results in patients with HFpEF compared to HFrEF.[10]

PHYSICAL ACTIVITY

The American College of Cardiology (ACC)/American Heart Association (AHA) guidelines recommend exercise training in patients with HF as a class 1 recommendation, without a distinction between HFpEF and HFrEF, although the association between physical activity and HFpEF is stronger than with other forms of HF.[11] Exercise training in HFpEF improves diastolic function, cardiorespiratory fitness, and exercise capacity as evidenced by improved VO_2 peak and 6MWD, and quality of life. While all forms of exercise modalities have some benefit, high intensity interval training (HIIT) has shown better results compared to moderate intensity continuous training (MICT) and low intensity training in some studies.[7]

PHARMACOLOGICAL TREATMENT

Diuretics

While diuretics reduce filling pressure and congestion, and hence, symptoms in patients with HFpEF, they are more poorly tolerated in obese HFpEF patients as compared to nonobese patients. Obese HFpEF patients have increased risk of renal dysfunction with diuretics compared to nonobese HFpEF despite having more marked volume expansion.[4] Hence, diuretics are used with caution in cardiometabolic HFpEF patients with volume overload.

Angiotensin-converting Enzyme Inhibitors and Angiotensin Receptor Blockers

Angiotensin-converting enzyme inhibitors (ACEis) and angiotensin receptor blockers (ARBs) have not shown reduction in all-cause or CV mortality in HFpEF. The CHARM-Preserved trial showed that while candesartan did decrease HF hospitalizations, there was no decrease in CV mortality. Moreover, the decreased HF hospitalizations were seen in patients at the lower end of the ejection fraction spectrum. These agents are recommended mainly as first-line agents for blood pressure control in HFpEF patients with hypertension.[11]

Mineralocorticoid Receptor Antagonists

MRAs, like spironolactone, may have greater benefit in cardiometabolic HFpEF patients as compared to nonobese patients as evidenced in the posthoc analysis of TOPCAT trial which showed that patients with lower NT-proBNP levels, a marker of central adiposity in HFpEF, had a better response to spironolactone.[12] The results of the recently published FINEARTS-HF trial conducted on over 6,000 HF patients with LVEF >40% show that finerenone use in such patients was associated with reduced CV mortality and reduced worsening of heart failure (WHF), especially in patients with recent WHF.[13]

Neprilysin Inhibitors

Sacubitril-valsartan use was associated with decreased HF hospitalizations and CV death in PARAGON-HF trial though it fell slightly short of the significant level of difference.[14] There have been no subgroup analyses of the trial on the basis on BMI. However, ARNis are approved for use in HFpEF patients, especially those with LVEF on the lower end of the spectrum.

Sodium-glucose Cotransporter-2 Inhibitors

Epicardial fat deposition leading to inflammation and oxidative stress is one of the proposed pathogeneses of cardiometabolic HFpEF. SGLT2 inhibitors cause increased glucose uptake by adipocytes, decrease in epicardial fat deposition, and decrease in inflammatory markers, and oxidative stress. Hence, SGLT2 inhibitors are now considered the cornerstone of treatment in patients with HFpEF.

The landmark trials examining the use of SGLT2 inhibitors in patients with HFpEF are EMPEROR-Preserved, which evaluated empagliflozin, and DELIVER, which assessed dapagliflozin. The EMPEROR-Preserved trial showed that empagliflozin significantly decreased the combined risk of CV death or hospitalizations due to HF in patients with HFpEF, irrespective of the presence of type 2 diabetes mellitus (T2DM) but the trial excluded patients with BMI >30 kg/m.[15] The results of the DELIVER trial showed that dapagliflozin reduced the combined risk of worsening heart failure or cardiovascular death among patients with HFpEF.[16] The BMI cutoff for inclusion in the DELIVER trial was <50 kg/m^2. However, because of high NT-proBNP cutoffs for inclusion into the study, several obese patients were excluded from the study because, as already mentioned, obese patients tend to have lower NT-proBNP levels. Hence, there is a need to study the effect of SGLT2 inhibitors specifically on cardiometabolic HFpEF.

Glucagon-like Peptide-1 Receptor Agonists

Over the past decade, GLP-1 RAs have emerged as highly effective treatment for individuals with T2DM, obesity, or both. T2DM as an associated comorbidity in patients with HFpEF, especially cardiometabolic HFpEF, is associated with worse hemodynamic and clinical features, including increased symptom burden, and reduced functional capacity compared to patients without T2DM. Both obesity and diabetes induce a proinflammatory state that can contribute to endothelial dysfunction and coronary microvascular impairment, finally resulting in HFpEF. Since GLP-1 RAs directly targets obesity and has shown benefit in many associated comorbidities such as T2DM and metabolic dysfunction associated fatty liver disease (MAFLD), it is now being studied as a potential treatment option for HFpEF in obese patients and the results of these trials have been promising.

The SELECT trial (Semaglutide Effects on Cardiovascular Outcomes in People with Overweight or Obesity) assessed 17,604 overweight or obese patients with preexisting cardiovascular disease over a 5-year period. It was found that weekly subcutaneous administration of semaglutide reduced the risk of cardiovascular death, nonfatal myocardial infarction, or nonfatal stroke by 20%. Additionally, the trial also showed an 18% reduction in composite HF outcomes which was a secondary endpoint for the trial. However, only 24% of the patients in this trial had heart failure at baseline.[17] STEP-HFpEF trial conducted on 529 obese patients with BMI >30 kg/m^2 and HFpEF, showed that once weekly 2.4 mg semaglutide injection for 52 weeks improved quality of life and functional capacity as evidenced by Kansas City Cardiomyopathy Questionnaire clinical summary score (p <0.001) and improvement in 6MWD (p <0.001).[18] A prespecified analysis of the STEP-HFpEF trial based on obesity class found semaglutide improved physical limitations and quality of life and reduced body weight across the spectrum of obesity categories. Furthermore, in patients treated with semaglutide, greater degree of weight loss was associated with more improvement in symptoms, physical limitations and inflammation, even after adjusting for relevant baseline characteristics such as age, sex, and baseline body weight.[19]

This recently published evidence has given promising results in terms of efficacy and safety of GLP-1RAs in obese HFpEF patients. This can be further extended to other GLP-1 based agents and trials are underway with other drugs in this category. The phase 3 results of SUMMIT trial, assessing the use of tirzepatide, a dual GLP-1 and GIP agonist, in HFpEF have also been very promising showing a significant 38% reduction in the risk of a composite HF endpoint.[20]

CONCLUSION

Traditionally, HFpEF has been challenging to treat due to the lack of effective therapies, particularly for patients with obesity and T2DM. SGLT2 inhibitors have shown efficacy in reducing heart failure hospitalization and improving clinical outcomes in various heart failure populations, including those with HFpEF. This class of medications has become the mainstay of treatment in patients with HFpEF. Moreover, recent research has highlighted the potential of GLP-1-based agents, such as semaglutide and tirzepatide, as valuable additions to the treatment arsenal. These agents not only support weight loss but also demonstrate cardioprotective effects. Their dual action could lead to improved outcomes in both heart failure symptoms and metabolic control. The move toward personalized medicine is critical, given the heterogeneous nature of cardiometabolic HFpEF. Tailoring treatment plans based on individual patient profiles, including their metabolic status, comorbidities, and specific heart failure characteristics, can significantly enhance patient outcomes.

REFERENCES

1. Dunlay SM, Roger VL, Redfield MM. Epidemiology of heart failure with preserved ejection fraction. Nat Rev Cardiol. 2017;14(10):591-602.
2. Samson R, Jaiswal A, Ennezat PV, et al. Clinical phenotypes in heart failure with preserved ejection fraction. J Am Heart Assoc. 2016;5(1):1-15.
3. Benn M, Marott SCW, Tybjærg-Hansen A, et al. Obesity increases heart failure incidence and mortality: observational and Mendelian randomization studies totalling over 1 million individuals. Cardiovasc Res. 2023;118(18):3576-85.
4. Borlaug BA, Jensen MD, Kitzman DW, et al. Obesity and heart failure with preserved ejection fraction: new insights and pathophysiological targets. Cardiovasc Res. 2022;118(18):3434-50.
5. Kitzman DW, Brubaker P, Morgan T, et al. Effect of Caloric Restriction or Aerobic Exercise Training on Peak Oxygen Consumption and Quality of Life in Obese Older Patients With Heart Failure With Preserved Ejection Fraction. JAMA. 2016;315(1):36.
6. Cocco G, Chu D. Weight reduction decreases NT-proBNP levels in obese coronary patients with chronic diastolic heart failure. Arch Med Sci. 2007;3(2):112-6.
7. Vacca A, Wang R, Nambiar N, et al. Lifestyle interventions in cardiometabolic HFpEF: dietary and exercise modalities. Heart Fail Rev; 2024.
8. Hummel SL, Karmally W, Gillespie BW, et al. Home-Delivered Meals Postdischarge From Heart Failure Hospitalization. Circ Heart Fail. 2018;11(8).
9. Miró Ò, Estruch R, Martín-Sánchez FJ, et al. Adherence to Mediterranean Diet and All-Cause Mortality After an Episode of Acute Heart Failure. JACC Heart Fail. 2018;6(1):52-62.
10. Kouvari M, Chrysohoou C, Aggelopoulos P, et al. Mediterranean diet and prognosis of first-diagnosed Acute Coronary Syndrome patients according to heart failure phenotype: Hellenic Heart Failure Study. Eur J Clin Nutr. 2017;71(11):1321-8.
11. Heidenreich PA, Bozkurt B, Aguilar D, et al. 2022 AHA/ACC/HFSA Guideline for the Management of Heart Failure: A Report of the American College of Cardiology/American Heart Association Joint Committee on Clinical Practice Guidelines. Circulation. 2022;145(18).
12. Anand IS, Claggett B, Liu J, et al. Interaction Between Spironolactone and Natriuretic Peptides in Patients With Heart Failure and Preserved Ejection Fraction. JACC Heart Fail. 2017;5(4):241-52.

13. Desai AS, Vaduganathan M, Claggett BL, et al. Finerenone in Patients With a Recent Worsening Heart Failure Event. J Am Coll Cardiol; 2024.
14. Solomon SD, Rizkala AR, Gong J, et al. Angiotensin Receptor Neprilysin Inhibition in Heart Failure With Preserved Ejection Fraction. JACC Heart Fail. 2017;5(7):471-82.
15. Anker SD, Butler J, Filippatos G, et al. Empagliflozin in Heart Failure with a Preserved Ejection Fraction. New Engl J Med. 2021;385(16):1451-61.
16. Solomon SD, McMurray JJV, Claggett B, et al. Dapagliflozin in Heart Failure with Mildly Reduced or Preserved Ejection Fraction. New Engl J Med. 2022;387(12):1089-98.
17. Lincoff AM, Brown-Frandsen K, Colhoun HM, et al. Semaglutide and Cardiovascular Outcomes in Obesity without Diabetes. New Engl J Med. 2023;389(24):2221-32.
18. Kosiborod MN, Abildstrøm SZ, Borlaug BA, et al. Semaglutide in Patients with Heart Failure with Preserved Ejection Fraction and Obesity. New Engl J Med. 2023;389(12):1069-84.
19. Borlaug BA, Kitzman DW, Davies MJ, et al. Semaglutide in HFpEF across obesity class and by body weight reduction: a prespecified analysis of the STEP-HFpEF trial. Nat Med. 2023;29(9):2358-65.
20. Lilly. Lilly's tirzepatide successful in phase 3 study showing benefit in adults with heart failure with preserved ejection fraction and obesity. [online] Available from https://investor.lilly.com/news-releases/news-release-details/lillys-tirzepatide-successful-phase-3-study-showing-benefit [Last accessed January, 2025].

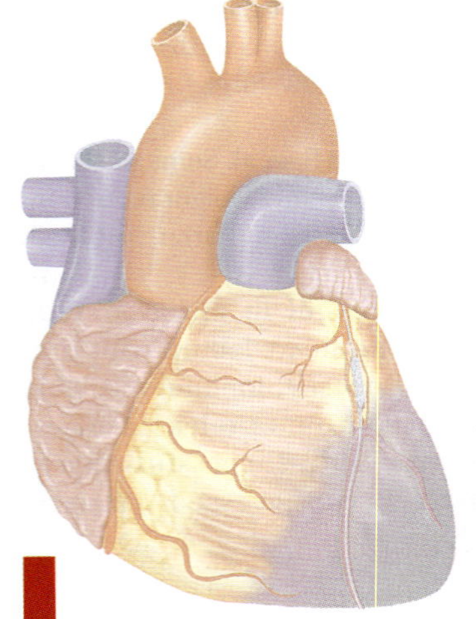

Diabetes and HFpEF: New Insights

Varun Anil Damle, Viswanathan Mohan

INTRODUCTION

Diabetes mellitus is known to affect 537 million people worldwide.[1] In India alone, there are 101 million people with diabetes and 136 million people with prediabetes.[2] Diabetes can affect the cardiovascular system in many ways, and heart failure is one of them. In the earlier days, heart failure was defined as "the inability of the heart to pump blood to the body at a rate commensurate to its needs or to do so only at the cost of high filling pressures." This definition only focuses on the pumping ability and ejection fraction of the heart.[3] In the 1980s, case reports emerged that heart failure could occur in the absence of overt reduction in left ventricular ejection fraction (LVEF). Hence, the term "heart failure with preserved ejection fraction" was (HFpEF) coined.

According to 2016 guidelines of the European Society of Cardiology (ESC), HFpEF is defined as heart failure in which LVEF is >50%. When the LVEF is between 40 and 50%, it is termed HF with mid-range EF.[4] The most common comorbidity in HF is diabetes mellitus, and conversely one of the common cardiovascular complications of diabetes mellitus is heart failure. Hence, it is clear that these two conditions often coexist.

Diabetes and HFpEF are common conditions which have significant overlap in pathophysiology and clinical outcomes. This chapter deals with the connection between diabetes and HFpEF. The focus is on epidemiology, pathophysiology, clinical features, and management strategies including the use of newer antidiabetic agents such as sodium-glucose co-transporter 2 (SGLT2) inhibitors and GLP1 receptor agonists (RAs).

EPIDEMIOLOGY

The prevalence of diabetes in those with HFpEF is high, ranging from 30 to 50%, which is far higher than that in the general population.[5] Conversely, patients with diabetes have an increased risk of developing HFpEF, especially in the presence of obesity.[6,7] Both conditions share common risk factors such as obesity, hypertension, and dyslipidemia.

PATHOPHYSIOLOGY OF DIABETES AND HEART FAILURE WITH PRESERVED EJECTION FRACTION

The pathophysiology linking diabetes and HFpEF involves multiple mechanisms including chronic inflammation, oxidative stress, endothelial dysfunction, myocardial fibrosis, and impaired myocardial energetics.[8] Additionally, insulin resistance and hyperglycemia contribute to myocardial stiffness, impaired relaxation, and diastolic dysfunction, all of which are characteristic features of HFpEF.[8] Additionally, neurohormonal activation adipokine dysregulation and altered cardiac metabolism combine to produce a vicious cycle of cardiovascular dysfunction leading to HFpEF.

Diabetes is also associated with increased concentration of serum inflammatory markers such as C-reactive protein, soluble suppression of tumorgenesis and 2, and galectin 3, among others. These inflammatory markers are postulated to lead to myocardial fibrosis and thus to worse outcomes in individuals with diabetes and HFpEF.

The lifetime risk for HFpEF is higher in white than in black individuals, but black individuals have worse heart failure readmissions as compared to white individuals. The lifetime risk of HFpEF is similar in both men and women, but female sex is associated with worse outcomes, probably due to hormonal factors.[9]

DIAGNOSIS OF HEART FAILURE WITH PRESERVED EJECTION FRACTION

Diagnosing HFpEF is often a clinical challenge, and this is especially true at an early stage of the disease when there are no overt signs of heart failure.[10,11] At that point, the diagnosis can be easily missed, as a normal ejection fraction and no evidence of signs of fluid retention may shift attention toward other causes of dyspnea, such as pulmonary disease, obesity, or even poor physical fitness.

For diagnosing HFpEF, three criteria have to be fulfilled:[12] (1) Signs and/or symptoms of heart failure, (2) no impaired systolic LV function (LV ejection fraction > 50 % and indexed LV end-diastolic volume < 97 mL/m^2), and (3) evidence of LV diastolic dysfunction. Regarding evidence of diastolic dysfunction, the guideline by Paulus et al.[12] states that either invasive hemodynamic measurements [pulmonary capillary wedge pressure (PCWP) >15 mm Hg or LV end-diastolic pressure >12 mm Hg at rest] or tissue Doppler measurements (E/e′ >15) provide sufficient evidence of diastolic dysfunction. E/e′ in the range of 8–15 or high NT-pro B-type natriuretic peptide (NT-proBNP) levels (>220 pg/mL or BNP >200 pg/mL) need to be accompanied by at least one additional sign of diastolic dysfunction, including a low E/A ratio combined with a high deceleration time, pulmonary venous flow patterns suggestive of diastolic dysfunction, high indexed left atrial volume, presence of atrial fibrillation, and/or LV hypertrophy

IMPACT OF DIABETES ON SERUM BIOMARKERS IN HEART FAILURE WITH PRESERVED EJECTION FRACTION

The presence of diabetes is associated with higher levels of cardiac, profibrotic, and proinflammatory biomarkers in HFpEF such as high-sensitivity C-reactive protein (hs-CRP), high-sensitivity troponin T (hs-TnT), matrix metalloproteinase 2 (MMP2), matrix metalloproteinase 9 (MMP-9), N-terminal pro-B-type natriuretic peptide (NT-proBNP), pro-collagen type I carboxy-terminal peptide (PICP), pro-collagen type III terminal peptide (PIIINP), and soluble ST2 (sST2) or tissue inhibitor of metalloproteinase (TIMP1).[13]

CURRENT MANAGEMENT OF DIABETES WITH HEART FAILURE WITH PRESERVED EJECTION FRACTION

Current management of heart failure with preserved ejection fraction deals with controlling hypertension mainly by the use of ACE/ARBs and mineralocorticoid receptor antagonists, relieving lung tachycardia by the use of beta blockers and congestion by diuresis. Hypertension is a major risk factor for HFpEF.[14] Blood pressure management is paramount, and an ACE inhibitor or ARB is appropriate. Diuresis helps lower left ventricular pressures, reducing pulmonary congestion and improving symptoms.[15] Furosemide (frusemide), a loop diuretic, is most commonly used.

Aside from their cholesterol-lowering benefits, statins also target systemic inflammation.[16] This is an important contributor to the pathogenesis of HFpEF. Their use has been associated with lower mortality in these patients, even in those without coronary artery disease.[17] Sacubitril with valsartan inhibits both neprilysin and angiotensin AT1 receptor. In addition, neprilysin inhibition increases natriuretic and vasoactive peptides, leading to natriuresis, diuresis, and vasodilation.[18]

When HFpEF is associated with type 2 diabetes, good glycemic control is important. Metformin is the most commonly used first-line oral hypoglycemic drug in treating type 2 diabetes.[19] SGLT2 inhibitors have shown significant benefits in HFrEF as well as HFpEF by reducing mortality in patients with and without diabetes.[20]

There is evidence of cardioprotective effect of SGLT2 inhibitors in patients of diabetes with HFpEF as shown by several randomized controlled trials.[21] These are summarized in **Table 1**.

It can be seen that most of the SGLT2 inhibitors, namely empagliflozin, dapagliflozin, and canagliflozin, have been shown to have beneficial effects in treating heart failure.

HOW DO SGLT2 INHIBITORS WORK?

These agents work through multiple mechanisms and are illustrated in **Figure 1**.

CURRENT GUIDELINES FOR USING SGLT2 INHIBITORS IN HEART FAILURE

The American Diabetes Association (ADA) recommends the addition of SGLT2 inhibitors in the management of T2DM with HF or patients at high risk of HF.[23] The most recent ESC 2021[24] and the American Heart Association/ American College of Cardiology/Heart Failure Society

TABLE 1: Summary of trials on SGLT2 inhibitors in HFpEF.[21]

Trial	*Trial population*	*Primary findings*	*Adverse events*
EMPEROR-Preserved (*n* = 5,988)	• All patients LVEF >40% • 66% with LVEF >50% • 49% with diabetes • Mean age 71 years • Mean eGFR 60 mL/min/1.73 m^2	Empagliflozin 10 mg reduced the risk of cardiovascular death or HF hospitalization, mainly driven by a 29% reduction in hospitalizations	*Most common ADEs:* • Hypotension • Acute kidney injury • Uncomplicated genital and urinary tract infections
PRESERVED-HF (*n* = 324)	• HFpEF, LVEF >45% (mean EF = 60%), elevated natriuretic peptides (NT-proBNP or BNP) • 55% with diabetes • Median age 70 years • Baseline eGFR = 55 mL/min/ 1.73 m^2	Dapagliflozin 10 mg improved symptoms and physical limitations in HF in 12 weeks. as measured by KCCQ-CS	*Most common ADEs:* • Volume depletion • Acute kidney injury • No DKA, severe hypoglycemia, or amputations
CHIEF-HF (*n* = 448)	• 59.6% with HFpEF (EF >50%) • 27.9% with diabetes • >50% of patients aged >65 years	Canagliflozin 100 mg resulted in rapid improvement of HF symptoms as evaluated using the KCCQ	9.9% of all participants had serious ADEs (hospitalization or ED visit)
DELIVER (*n* = 6,263)	• LVEF >40% • Patients aged >40 years • NYHA class 2 to 5 symptoms • 45% had diabetes	Dapagliflozin 10 mg reduced composite endpoint of HF hospitalizations and cardiovascular death by 18%	• *Serious ADEs (including death)* • 43.5% of dapagliflozin patients and 45.5% of placebo patients

(ADEs: adverse events; BNP: brain natriuretic peptide; ED: emergency department; EF: ejection fraction; eGFR: estimated glomerular filtration rate; HF: heart failure; HFpEF: heart failure with preserved ejection fraction; KCCQ-CS: Kansas City Cardiomyopathy Questionnaire-clinical summary; LVEF: left ventricular ejection fraction; NYHA: New York Heart Association; NT-proBNP: N-terminal prohormone BNP)

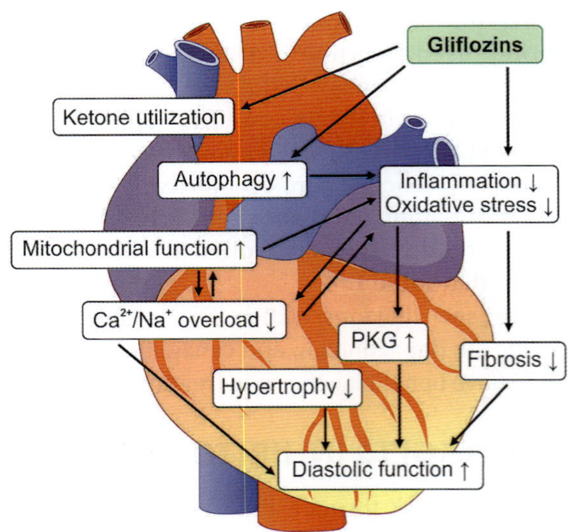

Fig. 1: Mechanisms by which SGLT2 inhibitors (gliflozins) work in heart failure.[22]

of America (AHA/ACC/HFSA) 2022[25] HF guidelines recommend the use of SGLT2 inhibitors (currently only dapagliflozin and empagliflozin) in the management of chronic, stable HFrEF (class 1 recommendation for a reduction in cardiovascular death and HF hospitalizations) irrespective of baseline diabetes status.

The drug is prescribed as part of a single-dose daily regimen (10 mg for both dapagliflozin and empagliflozin) with no need for dose titration and no routine laboratory monitoring required. Experts advocate for the initiation of SGLT2 inhibitors in those hospitalized for HF as part of an aggressive approach of rapid, simultaneous optimization of medical therapies.[26,27]

EMERGING ROLE OF GLP1 RECEPTOR AGONISTS IN HEART FAILURE

Recently, a lot of trials are focusing on the effect of GLP1 RAs on cardiovascular outcomes. GLP1 RAs are incretin hormones which help in achieving glycemic control by increasing insulin secretion after meals and slowing gastric emptying, thereby increasing satiety.

Mechanism of Action of GLP1 Receptor Agonists on Cardiovascular System

GLP1 analogs mainly exert cardioprotective effects by inhibiting RAAS pathway and stimulating AMPK/mTOR pathway. Due to this, there is reduction in angiotensin 2 and AT1R levels and increase in AMPK phosphorylation leading to a decrease in cardiac hypertrophic markers, further resulting in a decrease in cardiomyocyte hypertrophy and myocardial fibrosis.[28] GLP1 analog exenatide was shown to slow gastric emptying and increase satiety and thereby help in reducing obesity which prevented accumulation of adipose tissue in the epicardium, left atrium, and ventricular remodeling, thereby preventing heart failure.[29]

TRIALS ON CARDIOPROTECTIVE EFFECTS OF GLP1 AGONISTS

The recent STEP HF trial was done in nondiabetic individuals. Injectable Semaglutide 2.4 mg once weekly demonstrated a change in the Kansas City Cardiomyopathy Questionnaire score by 16.6 as compared with placebo which showed a change of 8.7 at the end of 52 weeks.[30] The mean change in 6-minute walk distance was 21.5 meters with semaglutide and 1.2 meters with placebo. Hence, in patients with heart failure with preserved ejection fraction and obesity, treatment with semaglutide led to larger reductions in symptoms, physical limitations, and greater improvement in exercise function.

In the Step-HF DM trial, a total of 616 participants underwent randomization. The mean change in the KCCQ-CSS was 13.7 points with semaglutide and 6.4 points with placebo ($p < 0.001$) and the mean percentage change in body weight was –9.8% with semaglutide and –3.4% with placebo ($p < 0.001$). The results for the confirmatory secondary end points also favored semaglutide over placebo. Serious adverse events were reported in 55 participants (17.7%) in the semaglutide group and 88 (28.8%) in the placebo group.

Among patients with obesity-related HFpEF and type 2 diabetes, semaglutide led to larger reductions in heart failure–related symptoms and physical limitations and greater weight loss than placebo at 1 year.[31] Earlier trials using lixisenatide (ELIXA trial), liraglutide (LEADER trial), semaglutide (SUSTAIN-6 trial), exenatide (EXSCEL trial), albiglutide (HARMONY trial), oral semaglutide (PIONEER trial), and dulaglutide (REWIND trial) also showed beneficial results, but these are not discussed in detail here.

CONCLUSION

None of the GLP1 agonists has demonstrated either a decreased or an increased risk of heart failure in patients with type 2 diabetes. Certain GLP1 agonists have shown benefit when compared with placebo in decreasing the risk of composite cardiovascular outcomes in those with type 2 diabetes. Current guidelines have changed to recommend GLP1 agonist as the preferred therapy after metformin in type 2 diabetes individuals with established cardiovascular diseases. There are ongoing trials of GLP1 agonists to further understand the cardiovascular benefits in diabetics with acute or chronic heart failure.

Currently, the guidelines suggest the use of SGLT2 inhibitors in diabetic individuals with HFpEF due to their proven cardioprotective effect. However, newer trials of GLPI analogs have certainly shown cardioprotective benefit and in the future they may also become the cornerstone of treatment in treating obese type 2 diabetes individuals with HFpEF, due to their effects on achieving glycemic control and reducing weight and cardioprotective effects.

In conclusion, diabetes and HFpEF are interrelated conditions. Presence of either condition should prompt us to look for the other. With the newer antidiabetic agents such as SGLT2 inhibitors and GLP1 RAs showing cardioprotection, the field of cardiodiabetology is rapidly evolving with more collaboration between cardiologists and diabetologists.

REFERENCES

1. International Diabetes Federation. (2021). IDF Diabetes Atlas, 10th edn. International Diabetes Federation, Brussels. [online] Available from https://diabetesatlas.org/atlas/tenth-edition/ [Last accessed January, 2025].
2. Anjana RM, Unnikrishnan R, Deepa M, et al.; ICMR-INDIAB Collaborative Study Group. Metabolic non-communicable disease health report of India: the ICMR-INDIAB national cross-sectional study (ICMR-INDIAB-17). Lancet Diabetes Endocrinol. 2023;11:474-89.
3. Libby P, Mann DL, Tomaselli GF, et al. Braunwald's Heart Disease: A Textbook of Cardiovascular Medicine, 12th edition. Philadelphia: Elsevier; 2021.
4. Harper AR, Patel HC, Lyon AR. Heart failure with preserved ejection fraction. Clin Med (Lond). 2018;18(Suppl 2): s24-s29.
5. Boonman-de Winter LJ, Rutten FH, Cramer MJ, et al. High prevalence of previously unknown heart failure and left ventricular dysfunction in patients with type 2 diabetes. Diabetologia. 2012;55:2154-62.
6. Dei Cas A, Fonarow GC, Gheorghiade M, et al. Concomitant diabetes mellitus and heart failure. Curr Probl Cardiol. 2015;40:7-43.
7. Nichols GA, Gullion CM, Koro CE, et al. The incidence of congestive heart failure in type 2 diabetes: an update. Diabetes Care. 2004;27:1879-84.
8. Mishra S, Kass DA. Cellular and molecular pathobiology of heart failure with preserved ejection fraction. Nat Rev Cardiol. 2021;18:400-23.
9. Tadic M, Cuspidi C, Plein S, et al. Sex and heart failure with preserved ejection fraction: from pathophysiology to clinical studies. J Clin Med. 2019;8:792.
10. Hancock HC, Close H, Mason JM, et al. High prevalence of undetected heart failure in long-term care residents: findings from the Heart Failure in Care Homes (HFinCH) study. Eur J Heart Fail. 2013;15:158-65.

11. Penicka M, Bartunek J, Trakalova H, et al. Heart failure with preserved ejection fraction in outpatients with unexplained dyspnea: a pressure-volume loop analysis. J Am Coll Cardiol. 2010;55:1701-10.
12. Paulus WJ, Tschöpe C, Sanderson JE, et al. How to diagnose diastolic heart failure: a consensus statement on the diagnosis of heart failure with normal left ventricular ejection fraction by the Heart Failure and Echocardiography Associations of the European Society of Cardiology. Eur Heart J. 2007;28:2539-50.
13. Biasucci LM, Maino A, Grimaldi MC, et al. Novel biomarkers in heart failure: new insight in pathophysiology and clinical perspective. J Clin Med. 2021;10:2771.
14. Dunlay SM, Roger VL, Redfield MM. Epidemiology of heart failure with preserved ejection fraction. Nat Rev Cardiol. 2017;14:591-602.
15. Borlaug BA. The pathophysiology of heart failure with preserved ejection fraction. Nat Rev Cardiol. 2014;11: 507-15.
16. Quist-Paulsen P. Statins and inflammation: an update. Curr Opin Cardiol. 2010;25:399-405.
17. Marume K, Takashio S, Nagai T, et al. Effect of statins on mortality in heart failure with preserved ejection fraction without coronary artery disease-report from the JASPER study. Circ J. 2019;83:357-67.
18. Gori M, D'Elia E, Senni M. Sacubitril/valsartan therapeutic strategy in HFpEF: Clinical insights and perspectives. Int J Cardiol. 2019;281:158-65.
19. Atherton JJ, Sindone A, De Pasquale CG, et al. NHFA CSANZ Heart Failure Guidelines Working Group. National Heart Foundation of Australia and Cardiac Society of Australia and New Zealand: Guidelines for the prevention, detection, and management of heart failure in Australia 2018. Heart Lung Circ. 2018;27:1123-208.
20. Lytvyn Y, Bjornstad P, Udell JA, et al. Sodium glucose cotransporter-2 inhibition in heart failure: potential mechanisms, clinical applications, and summary of clinical trials. Circulation. 2017;136:1643-58.
21. Mann L, Smith A. Investigating SGLT2 Inhibitors in Heart Failure. US Pharm. 2023;48:45-8.
22. Pabel S, Hamdani N, Luedde M, et al. SGLT2 inhibitors and their mode of action in heart failure-has the mystery been unravelled? Curr Heart Fail Rep. 2021;18:315-28.
23. American Diabetes Association. 9. Pharmacologic approaches to glycemic treatment: Standards of Medical Care in Diabetes-2020. Diabetes Care. 2020;43:S98-110.
24. McDonagh TA, Metra M, Adamo M, et al. 2021 ESC guidelines for the diagnosis and treatment of acute and chronic heart failure. Eur Heart J. 2021;42:3599-726.
25. Heidenreich PA, Bozkurt B, Aguilar D, et al. 2022 AHA/ ACC/HFSA guideline for the management of heart failure: a report of the American College of Cardiology/American Heart Association Joint Committee on Clinical Practice Guidelines. Circulation. 2022;145:e895-1032.
26. Packer M, McMurray JJ. Rapid evidence-based sequencing of foundational drugs for heart failure and a reduced ejection fraction. Eur J Heart Fail. 2021;23:882-94.
27. Greene SJ, Butler J, Fonarow GC. Simultaneous or rapid sequence initiation of quadruple medical therapy for heart failure-optimizing therapy with the need for speed. JAMA Cardiol. 2021;6:743-4.
28. Skov J, Dejgaard A, Frøkiær J, et al. Glucagon-like peptide-1 (GLP-1): effect on kidney hemodynamics and renin-angiotensin-aldosterone system in healthy men. J Clin Endocrinol Metab. 2013;98:E664-71.
29. Dutour A, Abdesselam I, Ancel P, et al. Exenatide decreases liver fat content and epicardial adipose tissue in patients with obesity and type 2 diabetes: a prospective randomized clinical trial using magnetic resonance imaging and spectroscopy. Diabetes Obes Metab. 2016;18: 882-91.
30. Kosiborod MN, Abildstrøm SZ, Borlaug BA, et al. STEP-HFpEF Trial Committees and Investigators. Semaglutide in patients with heart failure with preserved ejection fraction and obesity. N Engl J Med. 2023;389: 1069-84.
31. Kosiborod MN, Petrie MC, Borlaug BA, et al.; STEP-HFpEF DM Trial Committees and Investigators. Semaglutide in patients with obesity-related heart failure and type 2 diabetes. N Engl J Med. 2024;390:1394-407.

CHAPTER

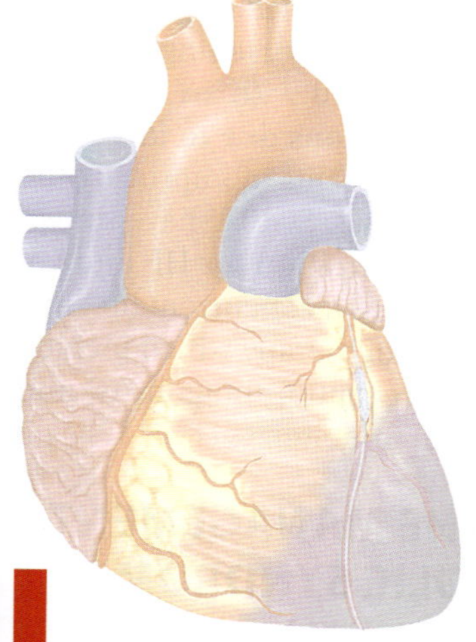

SGLT2i and Semaglutide in Cardiometabolic Syndrome with HFpEF

Simran Thakkar, SK Wangnoo

INTRODUCTION

Cardiometabolic syndrome (CMS) is a multifaceted disorder that represents a cluster of metabolic abnormalities associated with an increased risk for cardiovascular disease and type 2 diabetes mellitus. Heart failure with preserved ejection fraction (HFpEF) is often concurrent with CMS and poses significant management challenge due to its multifactorial nature. This chapter explores the role of sodium glucose cotransporter-2 inhibitor (SGLT2i) and semaglutide, a glucagon-like peptide-1 (GLP-1) analogue in the management of CMS and HFpEF.

DEFINING CARDIOMETABOLIC SYNDROME AND HEART FAILURE WITH PRESERVED EJECTION FRACTION

Metabolic syndrome is defined as clustering of varying clinical abnormalities that often develop diabetes mellitus, cardiovascular disease, and chronic renal failure. Central adiposity, elevated triglycerides level, reduced high-density lipoprotein cholesterol levels, elevated blood pressure, and raised plasma glucose form the core elements in defining CMS.[1] Other components that often coexist include endothelial dysfunction, oxidative stress, increased inflammation, microalbuminuria, coagulation abnormalities, dysfunction of the renin-angiotensin-aldosterone system, and metabolic dysfunction associated steatotic liver disease.[2]

The HFpEF, characterized by signs and symptoms of heart failure (HF), with normal or mildly abnormal systolic function (left ventricular ejection fraction >50%), with evidence of left ventricular diastolic dysfunction.[3,4]

ROLE OF SODIUM GLUCOSE COTRANSPORTER-2 INHIBITOR IN HEART FAILURE WITH PRESERVED EJECTION FRACTION

The SGLT2i, primarily approved as antidiabetic drugs, have gained significant attention for their cardiovascular (CV) and renoprotective benefits. They have recently been included in the treatment guidelines owing to reduced hospitalization for HF and reduced CV mortality in patients with HFpEF.[5] These agents work by inhibiting the reabsorption of glucose in the proximal renal tubules, increased urinary glucose excretion, natriuresis, and thereby improving glycemic control and promoting weight loss.

Potential mechanisms proposed by which SGLT2i confer cardiovascular benefits have been summarized in **Box 1**.

Various clinical trials have investigated the impact of SGLT2i on patients with HFpEF. EMPEROR-Preserved trial was the first landmark trial demonstrating 29% lower risk of hospitalization for HFpEF (LVEF >40%) as well as 21% lower relative risk of composite primary outcome, irrespective of the presence or absence of diabetes.[6] Patients with HFpEF have a poor quality of life owning to the high symptom burden and functional limitations. Kansas City Cardiomyopathy Questionnaire Clinical Summary Score (KCCQ-CS) has been used to study the benefit of dapagliflozin and canagliflozin on patient lifestyle outcomes.[7,8] Both drugs showed an improvement in KCCQ-total symptom score (KCCQ-TSS), KCCQ-physical limitation (KCCQ-PL) score, quality of life as well as total daily step score.[7,8] Another recent trial, dapagliflozin in heart failure with mildly reduced or preserved ejection fraction (DELIVER), supported the use of SGLT2i in the patients with HFpEF.[9] Dapagliflozin 10 mg was compared against placebo and a significant reduction of 18% in HF hospitalizations was noted in the dapagliflozin group. Key trials demonstrating the role of SGLT2i in HFpEF have been summarized in **Table 1**. A dual SGLT1/SGLT2i, sotagliflozin, has been approved by the FDA across all spectrums of HF based on its phase 3 clinical trial in patients with T2D with worsening HF.[10]

The SGLT2i have been associated with an increased incidence of genital mycotic infections due to increased glucosuria, however, the overall benefits in improving the survival appear to outweigh the risks. SGLT2i have shown a significant reduction in hospitalization for HF and CV deaths and should be considered as a concurrent first line therapy with other major pillars of therapy which include β-blockers, mineralocorticoid receptor antagonists, and angiotensin receptor-neprilysin inhibitor.

BOX 1: Potential mechanism of action of sodium glucose cotransporter-2 inhibitor (SGLTi2) which confer cardiovascular benefit.

- *Natriuresis and diuresis:* Reduction of extracellular fluid volume, systolic blood pressure reduction.[17,18]
- Enhancement of myocardial energy metabolism by promoting ketogenesis and induction of autophagy.[19-21]
- Reduction of myocardial oxygen demand and ventricular hypertrophy/left ventricle (LV) mass.[22]
- Reduction in markers of systemic inflammation and oxidative stress.[23,24]

SEMAGLUTIDE IN THE MANAGEMENT OF CARDIOMETABOLIC SYNDROME AND HEART FAILURE WITH PRESERVED EJECTION FRACTION

Majority of patients with HFpEF have obesity and this visceral adiposity may play a pivotal role in progression and adverse outcomes of HFpEF as adiposity has been associated with increased inflammation, insulin resistance, and systolic as well as diastolic left ventricular dysfunction.[11] Hence, pharmacotherapy for obesity could potentially improve the cardiovascular outcomes in a patient with HF. Semaglutide is a glucagon-like peptide-1 (GLP) analogue which shares 94% structural homology with the human GLP. It leads to increased glucose-dependent insulin secretion, suppresses glucagon release,

TABLE 1: Role of sodium glucose cotransporter-2 inhibitor (SGLT2i) in heart failure with preserved ejection fraction (HFpEF).

Trial (year)	*Drug studied*	*Population characteristics*	*Primary outcomes*
Emperor-Preserved (2021)[6]	Empagliflozin 10 mg versus placebo	• All patients had LVEF >40% • Nearly 66% had LVEF >50% • Nearly 50% T2D • 50% eGFR<60 mL/min/1.73 m^2	21% lower relative risk in the composite of cardiovascular death or hospitalization for heart failure, 29% lower risk of hospitalization for heart failure with empagliflozin
Preserved-HF (2021)[7]	Dapagliflozin 10 mg versus placebo	• Median age—70 years • 56%—T2D; 53%—AF • Median LVEF—60% • Elevated NT-proBNP • Baseline median eGFR 56 mL/min/ 1.73 m^3	Dapagliflozin improved KCCQ-CS at 12 weeks (KCCQ-TSS as well as KCCQ-PL)
CHIEF-HF (2022)[8]	Canagliflozin 100 mg versus placebo	• Mean age—63.4 years • T2D—27.9% • HFpEF—59.7%	12-week change in KCCQ TSS was 4.3 points (95% confidence interval, 0.8–7.8; $p=0.016$) higher with canagliflozin than with placebo
DELIVER (2022)[9]	Dapagliflozin 10 mg versus placebo	• Age >40 years • NYHA class II–IV • LVEF >40% • T2D—45%	Dapagliflozin reduced composite endpoint of HF hospitalization and CV death by 18%

(CV: cardiovascular; eGFR: estimated glomerular filtration rate; HF: heart failure; HFpEF: heart failure with preserved ejection fraction; KCCQ-TSS: Kansas City Cardiomyopathy Questionnaire-total symptom score; LVEF: left ventricular ejection fraction; NT-proBNP: N-terminal pro b-type natriuretic peptide; T2D: type 2 diabetes)

TABLE 2: Role of semaglutide for patients with obesity related heart failure.

Trial (year)	*Drug studied*	*Population characteristics*	*Outcomes*
STEP-HFpEF (2023)[13]	Semaglutide 2.4 mg subcutaneously once a week versus placebo	• Median age 69 years • Median BMI 37 kg/m^2 • Median LVEF 57% • NYHA II 66%; NYHA III–IV—33%	Mean change in KCCQ-TSS at 52 weeks was 16.2 points versus 8.7 points in placebo % change in body weight—13.2 % in semaglutide versus—2.6% in placebo (estimated difference, −10.7 percentage points; 95% CI, −11.9 to −9.4; $p < 0.001$)
STEP-HFpEF DM (2024)[14]	Semaglutide 2.4 mg subcutaneously once a week versus placebo	• Median age 69 years • Median BMI 36.9 kg/m^2 • Median duration of diabetes 8 years • Median HbA1c 6.8%	• Mean change in the KCCQ-CSS at week 52 was 13.7 points in the semaglutide group and 6.4 points in the placebo group. • Mean percentage change in body weight at week 52 was −9.8% in the semaglutide group and −3.4% in the placebo group (estimated difference, −6.4 percentage points; 95% CI, −7.6 to −5.2; $p < 0.001$)
SELECT trial (2024)[15]	Semaglutide 2.4 mg s/c versus placebo	• Mean age 61.6 years • Mean BMI 33.4 kg/m^2 53% had HFpEF	Improvement of MACE and all-cause mortality (HR 0.69, CI 0.51–0.91 for MACE; HR 0.75, CI 0.52–1.07 for the composite heart failure endpoint)

(BMI: body mass index; CI: confidence interval; HFpEF: heart failure with preserved ejection fraction; LVEF: left ventricular ejection fraction; KCCQ-TSS: Kansas City Cardiomyopathy Questionnaire-total symptom score)

slows gastric emptying, and mitigates the hunger sense. The role of semaglutide for patients with obesity related HF has been studied and these findings are summarized in **Table 2**. In the STEP-HFpEF and STEP-HFpEF DM trials, the GLP-1 receptor agonist semaglutide improved symptoms, physical limitations, bodyweight, and exercise function in people with obesity-related HFpEF.[12-14] Moreover, in SELECT, the benefits of semaglutide on MACE, HF composite, and cardiovascular death in patients with HFpEF were demonstrated.[15]

FUTURE DIRECTIONS

Tirzepatide, a dual agonist for GLP-1 and glucose-dependent insulinotropic polypeptide (GIP) receptors, is a novel agent approved by FDA for T2DM and obesity. It is currently being studied for patients with HFpEF and obesity.[16] Tirzepatide represents a promising therapeutic option in addressing the metabolic dysfunctions associated with HFpEF. While clinical evidence specifically linking tirzepatide to improved outcomes in HFpEF is still emerging, its established benefits in managing obesity and diabetes make it a compelling candidate for further investigation.

CONCLUSION

The SGLT2i have become one of the most important pillars in the management of CMS and HFpEF and is currently recommended as a first line agent for the management of HFpEF. With ongoing large-scale investigations into the pathobiology of HFpEF, a variety of clinical trials assessing new therapeutic approaches, there is emerging optimism for a future characterized by lower prevalence, reduced morbidity, and decreased mortality related to HFpEF.

REFERENCES

1. Grundy SM, Brewer HB, Cleeman JI, et al. Definition of Metabolic Syndrome: Report of the National Heart, Lung, and Blood Institute/American Heart Association Conference on Scientific Issues Related to Definition. Circulation. 2009;109(3):433-8.
2. Castro JP, El-Atat FA, McFarlane SI, et al. Cardiometabolic syndrome: Pathophysiology and treatment. Curr Hypertens Rep. 2003;5(5):393-401.
3. Paulus WJ, Tschöpe C, Sanderson JE, et al. How to diagnose diastolic heart failure: a consensus statement on the diagnosis of heart failure with normal left ventricular ejection fraction by the Heart Failure and Echocardiography Associations of the European Society of Cardiology. Eur Heart J. 2007;28(20):2539-50.
4. Shah SJ, Borlaug BA, Kitzman WE, et al. Research Priorities for Heart Failure With Preserved Ejection Fraction: National Heart, Lung, and Blood Institute Working Group Summary. Circulation. 2020;141(12):1001-1026.
5. Heidenreich PA, Bozkurt B, Aguilar D, et al. 2022 AHA/ACC/HFSA Guideline for the Management of Heart Failure: A Report of the American College of Cardiology/

American Heart Association Joint Committee on Clinical Practice Guidelines. Circulation. 2022;145(18): e876-94.

6. Anker SD, Butler J, Filippatos G, et al. Empagliflozin in Heart Failure with a Preserved Ejection Fraction. N Engl J Med. 2021;385(16):1451-61.
7. Nassif ME, Windsor SL, Borlaug BA, et al. The SGLT2 inhibitor dapagliflozin in heart failure with preserved ejection fraction: a multicenter randomized trial. Nat Med. 2021;27(11):1954-60.
8. Spertus JA, Birmingham MC, Nassif M, et al. The SGLT2 inhibitor canagliflozin in heart failure: the CHIEF-HF remote, patient-centered randomized trial. Nat Med. 2022; 28(4):809-13.
9. Solomon SD, McMurray JJV, Claggett B, et al. Dapagliflozin in Heart Failure with Mildly Reduced or Preserved Ejection Fraction. N Engl J Med. 2022;387(12):1089-98.
10. Bhatt DL, Szarek M, Steg PG, et al. Sotagliflozin in Patients with Diabetes and Recent Worsening Heart Failure. N Engl J Med. 2021;384(2):117-28.
11. Kitzman DW, Nicklas BJ. Pivotal Role of Excess Intra-Abdominal Adipose in the Pathogenesis of Metabolic/Obese HFpEF. JACC Heart Fail. 2018;6(12):1008-10.
12. Butler J, Shah SJ, Petrie MC, et al. Semaglutide versus placebo in people with obesity-related heart failure with preserved ejection fraction: a pooled analysis of the STEP-HFpEF and STEP-HFpEF DM randomised trials. The Lancet. 2024;403(10437):1635-48.
13. Kosiborod MN, Abildstrøm SZ, Borlaug BA, et al. Semaglutide in Patients with Heart Failure with Preserved Ejection Fraction and Obesity. N Engl J Med. 2023; 389(12):1069-84.
14. Kosiborod MN, Petrie MC, Borlaug BA, et al. Semaglutide in Patients with Obesity-Related Heart Failure and Type 2 Diabetes. N Engl J Med. 2024;390(15):1394-407.
15. Deanfield J, Verma S, Scirica BM, et al. Semaglutide and cardiovascular outcomes in patients with obesity and prevalent heart failure: a prespecified analysis of the SELECT trial. The Lancet. 2024;404(10454):773-86.
16. NCT04847557. A Study of Tirzepatide (LY3298176) in Participants With Heart Failure With Preserved Ejection Fraction and Obesity (SUMMIT). [online] Available from https://clinicaltrials.gov/show/NCT04847557 [Last accessed January, 2025].
17. Damman K, Beusekamp JC, Boorsma EM, et al. Randomized, double-blind, placebo-controlled, multi-centre pilot study on the effects of empagliflozin on clinical outcomes in patients with acute decompensated heart failure (EMPA-RESPONSE-AHF). Eur J Heart Fail. 2020;22(4):713-22.
18. Iqbal F, Shuja MH, Azam L, et al. Effect of Sodium-Glucose Cotransporter 2 Inhibitors on the 24-Hour Ambulatory Blood Pressure in Patients With Type 2 Diabetes Mellitus and Hypertension: An Updated Meta-Analysis. Endocr Pract Off J Am Coll Endocrinol Am Assoc Clin Endocrinol. 2024;30(5):481-9.
19. Gao YM, Feng ST, Wen Y, et al. Cardiorenal protection of SGLT2 inhibitors-Perspectives from metabolic reprogramming. EBioMedicine. 2022;83:104215.
20. Hoong CWS, Chua MWJ. SGLT2 Inhibitors as Calorie Restriction Mimetics: Insights on Longevity Pathways and Age-Related Diseases. Endocrinology. 2021;162(8): bqab079.
21. Packer M. Autophagy stimulation and intracellular sodium reduction as mediators of the cardioprotective effect of sodium–glucose cotransporter 2 inhibitors. Eur J Heart Fail. 2020;22(4):618-28.
22. Verma S, Mazer CD, Tan AT, et al. Effect of Empagliflozin on Left Ventricular Mass in Patients With Type 2 Diabetes Mellitus and Coronary Artery Disease. Circulation. 2019;140(21):1693-702.
23. Elrakaybi A, Laubner K, Zhou Q, et al. Cardiovascular protection by SGLT2 inhibitors – Do anti-inflammatory mechanisms play a role? Mol Metab. 2022;64:101549.
24. Xing Y jie, Liu B hu, Wan SJ, et al. A SGLT2 Inhibitor Dapagliflozin Alleviates Diabetic Cardiomyopathy by Suppressing High Glucose-Induced Oxidative Stress in vivo and in vitro. Front Pharmacol. 2021;12:708177.

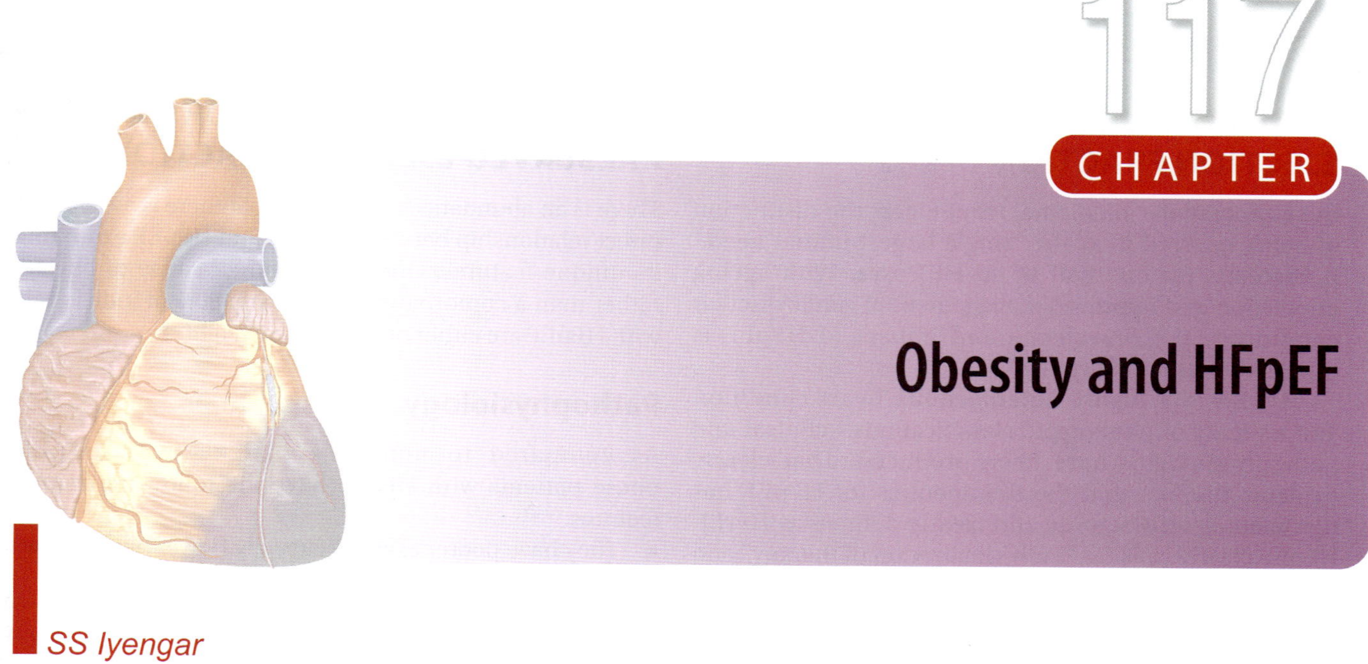

117

CHAPTER

Obesity and HFpEF

SS Iyengar

"Obesity and heart failure with preserved ejection fraction (HFpEF) represent two intermingling epidemics driving perhaps the greatest unmet health problem in cardiovascular medicine in the 21st century."[1]

INTRODUCTION

Both "obesity"—a heavy problem—and "heart failure" (HF)—where we have faced some failures—are posing a threat to global health. Both are essentially preventable diseases. The WHO estimates that there are about 2 billion adults who are overweight, and 650 million of them meet criteria for obesity. If preventive measures are not implemented now, 2.7 billion adults are likely to be overweight and over 1 billion, obese by 2025. Prevalence of HF is increasing, and heart failure with preserved ejection fraction (HFpEF) accounts for 50% of HF cases and is associated with significant mortality and morbidity.

Obesity increases the risk of HF and it has a specific and independent association with HFpEF with unique clinical and hemodynamic features, prompting many to suggest that it is a direct cause of HFpEF. Nonpharmacologic, pharmacologic, and interventional modalities of treatment are finding their ways into the therapeutics of "Obesity with HFpEF."

OBESITY

Obesity is defined as a chronic, complex, and metabolic disease, characterized by excessive fat accumulation, adipose tissue dysfunction, and abnormal fat mass, resulting in adverse metabolic, biomechanical, and psychosocial health consequences.[2]

In clinical practice, BMI is used to diagnose obesity, though this metric has certain flaws.

BMI is calculated by dividing body weight (kg) by height squared (m^2). A BMI >30 kg/m^2 indicates obesity and a BMI between 25 and 29.9 kg/m^2 overweight. An Indian Consensus Group classified a BMI of ≥23 kg/m^2 and ≥25 kg/m^2 as overweight and obese, respectively, for Asian Indians residing in India.[3] However, several patients can have excess adipose tissue causing a deterioration in health with BMIs below these cut-points, while others may have BMIs above the cut-points without excess adipose tissue causing a worsening of health. Hence, there is a need to embrace other metrics such as waist measurement, waist-to-hip ratio or body roundness index, which better reflects visceral adiposity.[4]

Obesity is associated with insulin resistance, hypertension, dyslipidemia, sleep disorders, depression, and musculoskeletal problems. Obesity during adolescence has also been associated with an increased risk of mortality from cardiovascular disease and type 2 diabetes in adulthood. Obesity reduces life expectancy because of its association with diabetes and cardiovascular disease. Excess of visceral fat indicates likelihood of accumulation of fat in heart, kidneys, liver, pancreas and skeletal muscle.[5] The adipose tissue (AT) is not merely an energy storage organ but is an active endocrine organ that secretes numerous bioactive molecules.[6]

Obesity is associated with a number of risk factors for HF. But it is independently associated with HF, with a relative risk of 1.41 per 5-U increment in BMI.[7] More than 80% of patients with HFpEF are overweight or obese.[8]

HEART FAILURE WITH PRESERVED EJECTION FRACTION

In cardiovascular medicine, HFpEF gets the distinction of being referred to as the "single largest unmet need." It accounts for one-half of all HF cases. With ageing population and improved management of cardiovascular conditions, the prevalence and impact of HFpEF is expected to rise significantly.[9]

HFpEF is a highly heterogenous heart condition and a plenty of phenotypic classifications—clinical and pathophysiologic—have been produced. That clearly explains the fact that the therapeutics for HFpEF has not been as satisfactorily and clearly defined as HFrEF. HFpEF clearly calls for "individualization of therapy" and not "one size fits all" approach.

One has to follow the universal definition of HF,[10] and refine it further with clinical scoring systems to diagnose HFpEF.[11,12]

As shown in **Flowchart 1,** there are multiple pathophysiologically distinct phenogroups of HFpEF with considerable overlap.[13]

Rohan Samson et al.[14] describe basically four phenotypes—aging phenotype, obesity phenotype, pulmonary hypertension (PH) phenotype and coronary artery disease (CAD) phenotype. They consider hypertension as the underpinning, and atrial fibrillation, anemia, chronic obstructive pulmonary disease (COPD), frailty, diabetes, obstructive sleep apnea, and chronic kidney disease (CKD) as comorbidities. There are many phenotypic classifications with large overlaps. However, in all the phenotypic classifications of HfpEF, obesity finds a prominent place. From initial focus on hypertension and LVH, there is a shift toward multiple morbidities as the mechanism for HFpEF, notably obesity, diabetes and metabolic syndrome with elements of inflammation, endothelial dysfunction, myocardial energetics, and skeletal muscle abnormalities.[15,16] The prevalence of HFpEF is higher in women than men.[17]

OBESITY AND HEART FAILURE WITH PRESERVED EJECTION FRACTION

There is an abundance of evidence that there is a clear and direct relationship between obesity and HFpEF exhibiting its unique features. Obesity is a direct cause of obesity rather than a comorbidity.[1,18-20] Nearly 80% of individuals with HFpEF are either obese or overweight.[20]

Pathophysiology

As compared to nonobese patients with HFpEF, obese patients with HFpEF have the following unique features:[20-22]

- They have poorer exercise capacity (lower peak oxygen consumption) and worse 6-minute walk test
- The biventricular filling pressures are higher.
- Pulmonary artery vasodilatory reserve is diminished.
- They are more likely to have RV dysfunction.
- There is cardiomegaly due to increased epicardial fat, leading to enhanced pericardial restraint. That contributes to myocardial stiffness.
- Systemic inflammation is much higher.

Obesity through enhanced systemic inflammation and neurohormonal activation and the restraint imposed by the epicardial fat lead to myocardial stiffness. Obesity also leads to increase in blood and plasma volume, and this relationship is greater in women than men.

Management (Flowchart 2)

Management of "obesity with HFpEF" has to focus on the following:

- Lifestyle intervention paying attention to weight loss (with diet and exercise)
- Guideline-directed medical therapy including loop diuretics and disease-modifying drugs like GLP1receptor analogs, SGLT2 inhibitors, MRAs, and ARNI/ARBs.

Flowchart 1: Phenotypes of HFpEF.[13]

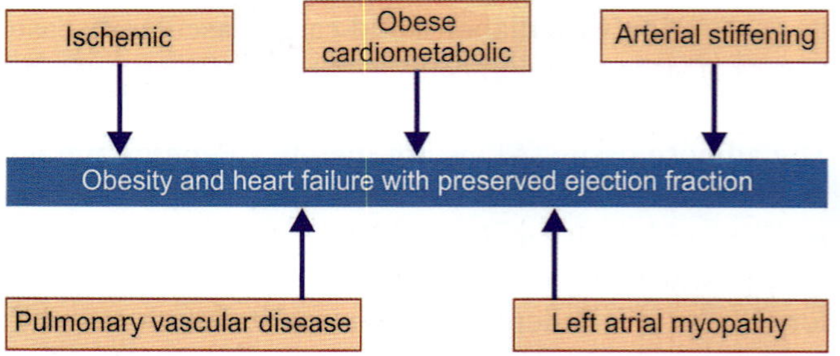

Flowchart 2: Obesity with HFpEF treatment.[30]

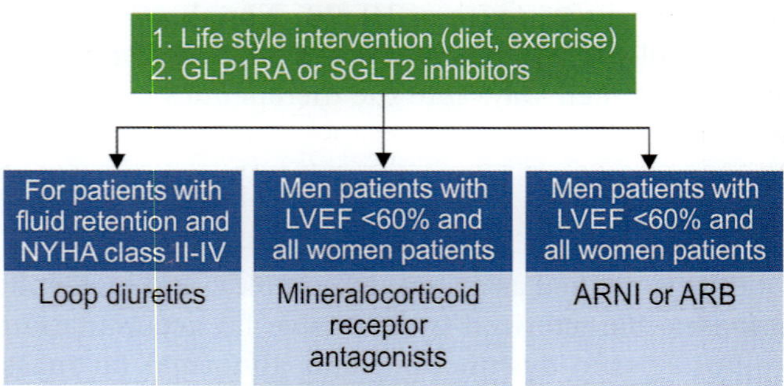

- Management of comorbidities, including hypertension, DM, AF, CAD, CKD, arrhythmias, iron deficiency, and obstructive sleep apnea

It is important to institute specific treatment of obesity-related HFpEF, as these patients have unique features such as increased epicardial fat, limited cardiac reserve, greater biventricular remodeling, and worse pulmonary vascular disease as compared to those without concomitant obesity.[20]

Weight Loss Measures

The options available for treating obesity are lifestyle modifications (dietary changes, increased physical activity, and cognitive behavioral therapy), pharmacotherapy, and bariatric surgery. Double-digit weight loss has been shown to result in significant improvement. This can be achieved by lifestyle modification (improved nutritional content of the diet and modest increases in physical activity and fitness).

Studies have shown that weight loss programs lead to significant improvements in quality of life and exercise capacity. It has also shown improvement in parameters such as left ventricular or right ventricular hypertrophy, diastolic parameters, and aortic stiffness. Bariatric surgery has shown similar benefits.[23-25]

In a systematic review and meta-analysis of 375 participants of 3–6-month duration, patients with HFpEF showed significant weight loss with, lifestyle intervention significant favorable effects on blood pressure, aerobic capacity, the NYHA class, and quality of life.

The authors concluded that weight loss in isolation, using nonpharmacological methods, improves intermediate markers of cardiovascular risk, functional status, and health-related quality of life in HFpEF population.[26]

Antiobesity medications such as orlistat, phentermine/topiramate extended release (ER), lorcaserin, naltrexone sustained-release (SR)/bupropion SR, setmelanotide, and liraglutide have been approved for use. The FDA is currently considering semaglutide 2.4 mg once weekly for approval.

Bariatric surgery is the most effective treatment for obesity in reducing symptoms, long-term weight loss, attenuation of complications, improvement of quality of life improvement, and overall mortality reduction. The current indications for bariatric surgery are patients with a BMI ≥40.0 kg/m^2 or with BMI between 35.0 and 39.9 kg/m^2 and obesity complications.[27]

Guideline-directed Medical Therapy for HFpEF[28]

Initial trials were negative and discouraging to be replaced recently by some positive trials.

- Loop diuretics are used to reduce congestion and improve symptoms.
- *SGLT2 inhibitors:* Both DELIVER (Dapagliflozin Evaluation to Improve the LIVEs of Patients With PReserved Ejection Fraction Heart Failure) and EMPEROR-Preserved (Empagliflozin Outcome Trial in Patients with Chronic Heart Failure with Preserved Ejection Fraction) trials have clearly shown to reduce the risk of hospitalization for HF and cardiovascular death across all EF subgroups in diabetics and nondiabetics.[29,30]
- *MRAs:* MRAs have been shown to control hypertension and reduce HF hospitalizations, though they may not improve quality of life or exercise tolerance.[29]
- *Angiotensin receptor–neprilysin inhibitors (ARNI):* There was a benefit in those patients with LVEF between 45 and 57% and women showed a greater benefit compared with men.[31]
- *ARBs:* ARBs may be used as an alternative to ARNI.[32]
- *Comorbidities:* Hypertension, coronary artery disease, atrial fibrillation, sleep apnea, and chronic kidney disease should be appropriately managed.

SEMAGLUTIDE STUDIES

The following two studies showed beneficial effects of semaglutide in obese patients with HFpEF:[33,34]

1. 529 patients who had HFpEF and a BMI of 30 kg/m^2 or more to received once-weekly semaglutide (2.4 mg) or placebo for 52 weeks. In patients with HFpEF and obesity, treatment with semaglutide (2.4 mg) led to larger reductions in symptoms and physical limitations, greater improvements in exercise function, and 11% greater weight loss than placebo.
2. 616 diabetics with a median BMI of 36.9 (64.3% of them having a BMI of 35 or more) participated in the study. The weight loss was 4.7 percentage points among participants who received SGLT2 inhibitor therapy at baseline and 7.2 percentage points among those who did not receive SGLT2 inhibitor therapy at baseline. The authors concluded that among patients with obesity-related HFpEF and type 2 diabetes, semaglutide reduced HF-related symptoms and physical limitations and resulted in greater weight loss than placebo at 1 year.

Does "obesity paradox" exist?

A post-hoc analysis of the Treatment of Preserved Cardiac Function Heart Failure with an Aldosterone Antagonist (TOPCAT) study showed an association between weight loss and an increased risk of subsequent mortality.[35]

This paradox is usually observed in situations where there is unintentional weight loss because of advanced HF or cancer. There are two important biases which may also contribute to this paradox—collider bias and lead time bias. The survival benefit claimed by obesity is not seen in individuals with a better physical fitness status and when waist circumference is used instead of BMI for assessing obesity. Hence, it is important to impress on the fact that weight loss is beneficial in individuals with obesity.[1,36-38]

CONCLUSION

Obesity with HFpEF is a distinct phenotype. With recent clinical trials, newer pharmacotherapies are available. The scenario also emphasizes the importance of prevention, early detection, and treatment of obesity.

"The HFpEF obesity phenotype: the elephant in the room."[22]

REFERENCES

1. Borlaug BA, Jensen MD, Kitzman DW, et al. Obesity and heart failure with preserved ejection fraction: new insights and pathophysiological targets. Cardiovascular Research 2022;118:3434-50.
2. Pilitsi E, Farr OM, Polyzos SA, et al. Pharmacotherapy of obesity: available medications and drugs under investigation. Metabolism. 2019;92:170-92.
3. Misra A, Chowbey P, Makkar BM, et al. Consensus statement for diagnosis of obesity, abdominal obesity and the metabolic syndrome for Asian Indians. J Assoc Physicians India. 2009;57:163-70.
4. Zhang X, Ma N, Lin Q, et al. Body roundness index and all-cause mortality among US adults. JAMA Network Open. 2024;7(6):e2415051.
5. Després JP, Carpentier AC, Tchernof A, et al. Management of obesity in cardiovascular practice. J Am Coll Cardiol. 2021;78:513-31.
6. Kershaw EE, Flier JS. Adipose tissue as an endocrine organ. J Clin Endocrinol Metab. 2004;89:2548-56.
7. Aune D, Sen A, Norat T, et al. Body mass index, abdominal fatness, and heart failure incidence and mortality: a systematic review and dose-response meta-analysis of prospective studies. Circulation. 2016;133:639-49.
8. Owan TE, Hodge DO, Herges RM, et al. Trends in prevalence and outcome of heart failure with preserved ejection fraction. N Engl J Med. 2006;355:251-9.
9. Lewis GA Schelbert, EB, Williams SG, et al. Biological phenotypes of heart failure with preserved ejection fraction. J Am Coll Cardiol. 2017;70:2186-200.
10. Bozkurt B, Coats AJ, Tsutsui H, et al. Universal definition and classification of heart failure. J Card Fail. 2021:S1071-9164(21)00050-6.
11. Reddy YNV, Carter RE, Obokata M, et al. A simple, evidence-based approach to help guide diagnosis of heart failure with preserved ejection fraction. Circulation. 2018;138:861-70.
12. Pieske B, Tschope C, de Boer RA, et al. How to diagnose heart failure with preserved ejection fraction: the HFA-PEFF diagnostic algorithm: a consensus recommendation from the Heart Failure Association (HFA) of the European Society of Cardiology (ESC). Eur J Heart Fail. 2020;22: 391-412.
13. Borlaug BA, Sharma K, Shah SJ, et al. Heart failure with preserved ejection fraction: JACC Scientific Statement. J Am Coll Cardiol. 2023;81:1810-34.
14. Samson R, Jaiswal A, Ennezat PV, et al. Clinical phenotypes in heart failure with preserved ejection fraction. J Am Heart Assoc. 2016;5:e002477.
15. Paulus WJ, Tschope C. A novel paradigm for heart failure with preserved ejection fraction: comorbidities drive myocardial dysfunction and remodeling through coronary microvascular endothelial inflammation. J Am Coll Cardiol. 2013;62:263-71.
16. Schiattarella GG, Rodolico D, Hill JA. Metabolic inflammation in heart failure with preserved ejection fraction. Cardiovasc Res. 2021;117:423-34.
17. Ho JE, Enserro D, Brouwers FP, et al. Predicting heart failure with preserved and reduced ejection fraction: The International Collaboration on Heart Failure Subtypes. Circ Heart Fail. 2016;9(6):e003116.
18. Pandey A, Parashar A, Kumbhani DJ, et al. Exercise training in patients with heart failure and preserved ejection fraction: meta-analysis of randomized control trials. Circ Heart Fail. 2015;8:33-40.
19. Anker SD, Usman MS, Anker MS, et al. Patient phenotype profiling in heart failure with preserved ejection fraction to guide therapeutic decision making. A scientific statement of the Heart Failure Association, the European Heart Rhythm Association of the European Society of Cardiology, and the European Society of Hypertension. Eur J Heart Fail. 2023;25:936-55.
20. Obokata M, Reddy YN, Pislaru SV, et al. Evidence supporting the existence of a distinct obese phenotype of heart failure with preserved ejection fraction. Circulation. 2017;136:6-19.
21. Kitzman DW, Shah SJ. The HFpEF obesity phenotype: The elephant in the room. J Am Coll Cardiol. 2016;68:200-3.
22. Koepp KE, Obokata M, Reddy YNV, et al. Hemodynamic and functional impact of epicardial adipose tissue in heart failure with preserved ejection fraction. J Am Coll Cardiol HF. 2020;8:657-666.
23. Rider OJ, Francis JM, Ali MK, et al. Beneficial cardiovascular effects of bariatric surgical and dietary weight loss in obesity. J Am Coll Cardiol. 2009;54:718-26.
24. Hajj EC, Hajj MC, Sykes B et al. Pragmatic weight management program for patients with obesity and heart failure with preserved ejection fraction. J Am Heart Assoc. 2021; 10:e022930.
25. Mikhalkova D, Holman SR, Jiang H, et al. Bariatric surgery-induced cardiac and lipidomic changes in obesity related heart failure with preserved ejection fraction. Obesity (SilverSpring). 2018;26:284-90.

26. Lee VYJ, Lauren Houston L, Adam Perkovic A, et al. The effect of weight loss through lifestyle interventions in patients with heart failure with preserved ejection fraction: a systematic review and meta-analysis of randomised controlled trials. Heart Lung Circ. 2024;33:197-208.
27. Busetto L, Dicker D, Azran C, et al. Practical recommendations of the obesity management task force of the European Association for the Study of obesity for the post-bariatric surgery medical management. Obesity Facts. 2017;10: 597-632.
28. Kittleson MM, Panjrath GS, Amancherla K, et al. ACC Expert Consensus Decision Pathway on Management of HFpEF. J Am Coll Cardiol. 2023; 81:1835-78.
29. Solomon SD, McMurray JJV, Claggett B, et al. Dapagliflozin in heart failure with mildly reduced or preserved ejection fraction. N Engl J Med. 2022;387: 1089-98.
30. Anker SD, Butler J, Filippatos G, et al. Empagliflozin in heart failure with a preserved ejection fraction. N Engl J Med. 2021;385:1451-61.
31. McMurray JJV, Jackson AM, Lam CSP, et al. Effects of sacubitril-valsartan versus valsartan in women compared with men with heart failure and preserved ejection fraction: insights from PARAGON-HF. Circulation. 2020; 141:338-51.
32. Yusuf S, Pfeffer MA, Swedberg K, et al. Effects of candesartan in patients with chronic heart failure and preserved left-ventricular ejection fraction: the CHARM-Preserved trial. Lancet. 2003;362:777-81.
33. Kosiborod MN, Abildstrøm SZ, Borlaug BA, et al. Semaglutide in patients with heart failure with preserved ejection fraction and obesity. N Engl J Med. 2023;389: 1069-84.
34. Kosiborod MN, Petrie MC, Borlaug BA, et al. Semaglutide in patients with obesity-related heart failure and type 2 diabetes. N Engl J Med. 2024;390:1394-407.
35. Ferreira JP, Rossignol P, Claggett BL, et al. Weight changes in heart failure with preserved ejection fraction: findings from TOPCAT. Clin Res Cardiol. 2022;111:451-9.
36. Khalid U, Ather S, Bavishi C, et al. Pre-morbid body mass index and mortality after incident heart failure: the ARIC study. J Am Coll Cardiol. 2014;64: 2743-49.
37. Lavie CJ, McAuley PA, Church TS, et al. Obesity and cardiovascular diseases: implications regarding fitness, fatness, and severity in the obesity paradox. J Am Coll Cardiol. 2014;63:1345-54.
38. Tsujimoto T, Kajio H. Abdominal obesity is associated with an increased risk of all-cause mortality in patients with HFpEF. J Am Coll Cardiol. 2017;70:2739-49.

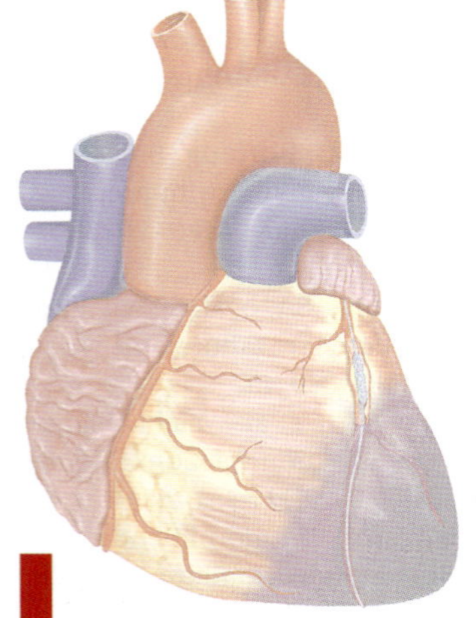

Management of HFpEF: A Recent Approach

Siddant Trehan, Rajeev Chawla

INTRODUCTION

Heart failure (HF) is a global epidemic affecting millions of individuals, with a prevalence that continues to rise due to aging populations and improvements in survival rates from other cardiovascular conditions. Historically, HF was categorized based on ejection fraction (EF) into reduced (HFrEF) and preserved ejection fraction (HFpEF). HFpEF, which comprises approximately 50% of HF cases, has emerged as a major public health problem. Unlike HFrEF, where evidence-based therapies have significantly improved patient outcomes, HFpEF remains a challenging condition with limited treatment options. Recent advances in understanding the pathophysiology of HFpEF and the development of novel therapeutic strategies have provided some hope for managing this complex syndrome. This chapter of ours reviews the recent approach to the management of HFpEF, emphasizing key clinical trials, emerging therapies, and evidence-based strategies.

PATHOPHYSIOLOGY OF HEART FAILURE WITH PRESERVED EJECTION FRACTION

The pathophysiology of HFpEF is complex and multifactorial, involving several cardiac and extracardiac mechanisms. At its core, HFpEF is characterized by the presence of symptoms and signs of HF despite normal or near-normal left ventricular ejection fraction (LVEF), typically defined as EF ≥50%. The main contributing factors include:

- *Left ventricular diastolic dysfunction:* HFpEF is primarily driven by impaired relaxation and increased stiffness of the left ventricle, leading to elevated filling pressures and pulmonary congestion during diastole.
- *Ventricular-arterial coupling:* Altered interactions between the left ventricle and the arterial system contribute to increased afterload and worsened systolic and diastolic function.
- *Endothelial dysfunction and systemic inflammation:* Comorbidities such as hypertension, obesity, diabetes, and chronic kidney disease promote a systemic inflammatory state, which contribute to endothelial dysfunction and increased myocardial stiffness.
- *Atrial and ventricular remodeling:* Structural changes, including atrial enlargement and ventricular hypertrophy, are common in HFpEF and contribute to the syndrome's progression.
- *Extracardiac factors:* HFpEF is associated with noncardiac comorbidities, including renal dysfunction, pulmonary hypertension (PH), and obesity, which complicate management.

CLINICAL PRESENTATION AND DIAGNOSIS

The HFpEF presents with typical symptoms of HF, including dyspnea, fatigue, and exercise intolerance, often in older adults with multiple comorbidities. Diagnosis is challenging and requires careful evaluation of clinical features, echocardiographic evidence of diastolic dysfunction, and exclusion of other causes of HF. Key diagnostic tools include:

- *Echocardiography:* It plays a pivotal role in assessing left ventricular filling pressures, atrial size, and diastolic function. The E/A ratio, tissue Doppler imaging, and left atrial volume index are useful markers.
- *Invasive hemodynamic monitoring:* In complex cases, right heart catheterization may be required to measure pulmonary capillary wedge pressure (PCWP) and confirm elevated left ventricular filling pressures.
- *Biomarkers:* B-type natriuretic peptide (BNP) and N-terminal proBNP (NT-proBNP) levels are often elevated in HFpEF, although typically lower than in HFrEF.

MANAGEMENT OF HEART FAILURE WITH PRESERVED EJECTION FRACTION: RECENT APPROACHES

Unlike HFrEF, where therapies targeting neurohormonal pathways have been highly successful, treatment options for HFpEF are limited, and no single drug has proven to significantly reduce mortality in this population. The management of HFpEF focuses on symptomatic relief, comorbidity management, and lifestyle interventions. Recent advances in clinical trials and emerging therapies have provided some promising avenues for managing HFpEF.

Pharmacologic Therapies

Diuretics

Diuretics remain the cornerstone of symptomatic management in HFpEF, particularly for managing volume overload. Loop diuretics (e.g., furosemide) are commonly used to reduce pulmonary and systemic congestion. Thiazide diuretics or mineralocorticoid receptor antagonists (MRAs) may be added for patients with resistant hypertension or persistent symptoms. Although diuretics improve symptoms, they do not modify the disease's progression or mortality.

Mineralocorticoid Receptor Antagonists

The MRAs, such as spironolactone and eplerenone, have been evaluated in HFpEF due to their ability to reduce fibrosis and improve diastolic function. The *TOPCAT trial* (Treatment of Preserved Cardiac Function Heart Failure with an Aldosterone Antagonist) assessed spironolactone in HFpEF patients. While the trial did not demonstrate a significant reduction in the primary composite outcome of cardiovascular death, hospitalization for HF, or aborted cardiac arrest, a subgroup analysis suggested potential benefit in certain populations, particularly those from the Americas.

Sodium-Glucose Cotransporter-2 Inhibitors

The SGLT2 inhibitors, initially developed for the treatment of type 2 diabetes, have recently emerged as promising agents in the management of HF. The *EMPEROR-preserved trial* evaluated empagliflozin in patients with HFpEF and demonstrated a significant reduction in the combined endpoint of cardiovascular death or hospitalization for HF, particularly through a reduction in HF hospitalizations. This marked the first major breakthrough in HFpEF management, leading to the approval of SGLT2 inhibitors for HFpEF treatment.

Angiotensin Receptor-Neprilysin Inhibitors

The ARNIs, which combine an angiotensin receptor blocker (ARB) with a neprilysin inhibitor, have shown substantial benefits in HFrEF. The *PARAGON-HF trial* tested sacubitril/valsartan in HFpEF patients but did not meet its primary endpoint of reducing cardiovascular death or HF hospitalization. However, a trend toward benefit was observed in certain subgroups, such as women and those with LVEF in the lower range of normal.

β-blockers and Calcium Channel Blockers

β-blockers and calcium channel blockers are commonly used to manage comorbidities such as hypertension and atrial fibrillation (AF) in HFpEF. However, their role in improving outcomes specifically related to HFpEF remains unclear. These agents can reduce heart rate and improve diastolic filling, but they have not been shown to reduce mortality or hospitalizations in HFpEF patients.

Nitric Oxide Pathway Modulation

The HFpEF is associated with endothelial dysfunction and impaired nitric oxide (NO) bioavailability, contributing to increased vascular stiffness and impaired exercise tolerance. Phosphodiesterase-5 (PDE5) inhibitors, such as sildenafil, have been evaluated in HFpEF to enhance NO signaling and improve hemodynamics. However, clinical trials, including the *RELAX trial*, have not demonstrated significant benefits in improving exercise capacity or quality of life in HFpEF patients.

Nonpharmacologic Therapies

Lifestyle Modifications

Lifestyle interventions, including weight loss, dietary modifications (e.g., low sodium intake), and regular physical activity, are crucial components of HFpEF management. Exercise training has been shown to improve exercise capacity, quality of life, and diastolic function in

HFpEF patients. Cardiac rehabilitation programs tailored to HFpEF may provide additional benefits, particularly in frail and elderly patients.

Management of Comorbidities

The HFpEF is often accompanied by multiple comorbidities, including hypertension, diabetes, AF, obesity, and chronic kidney disease. Aggressive management of these conditions is essential to improving outcomes in HFpEF. Antihypertensive therapy, including RAAS inhibitors and ARBs, can help reduce afterload and improve diastolic function. Blood pressure control is particularly important in HFpEF, as elevated systolic blood pressure is a key driver of left ventricular stiffness.

Atrial Fibrillation Management

Atrial fibrillation is common in HFpEF and is associated with worse outcomes, including increased risk of HF hospitalizations and mortality. Rate control, rhythm control, and anticoagulation therapy are critical components of AF management in HFpEF. Catheter ablation may be considered in select patients with symptomatic AF and preserved ventricular function.

Pulmonary Hypertension Management

Pulmonary hypertension is frequently observed in HFpEF and is associated with poor prognosis. PH-targeted therapies, such as pulmonary vasodilators, have been evaluated in HFpEF with mixed results. Inhaled nitric oxide and sildenafil have shown limited success in improving pulmonary pressures and right ventricular function in this population. However, ongoing studies are investigating novel therapies for PH in HFpEF.

Device Therapy

Cardiac devices, such as pacemakers or cardiac resynchronization therapy (CRT), are generally not indicated for HFpEF patients unless there are specific indications, such as advanced atrioventricular block or ventricular dyssynchrony. Left atrial pressure monitoring devices, such as the *CardioMEMS*™ system, have shown promise in reducing HF hospitalizations by enabling remote monitoring and early intervention for rising filling pressures.

Emerging Therapies and Future Directions

The treatment landscape for HFpEF is rapidly evolving, with several novel therapeutic strategies under investigation. Key areas of focus include:

Anti-inflammatory Therapies

Given the role of systemic inflammation in the pathogenesis of HFpEF, targeting inflammatory pathways is a promising therapeutic approach. Novel agents, such as interleukin-1 (IL-1) inhibitors and colchicine, are being investigated for their potential to reduce inflammation and improve outcomes in HFpEF.

Myocardial Metabolic Modulation

Modulating myocardial energetics and metabolism is another area of active research. Trimetazidine and ranolazine, which improve myocardial energy efficiency, are being evaluated for their potential to improve diastolic function and reduce symptoms in HFpEF.

Gene Therapy and Precision Medicine

Advances in genomics and molecular biology have opened the door to precision medicine approaches in HFpEF. Identifying specific molecular subtypes of HFpEF based on genetic, proteomic, and metabolomic profiles may enable the development of personalized therapies targeting underlying disease mechanisms.

CONCLUSION

The HFpEF remains a challenging syndrome with limited therapeutic options compared to HFrEF. However, recent advances in our understanding of its pathophysiology and the development of novel therapies have provided some hope for improved management. Diuretics continue to play a key role in symptomatic relief, while emerging therapies, such as SGLT2 inhibitors, have shown promise in reducing HF hospitalizations. Lifestyle modifications, comorbidity management, and nonpharmacologic interventions are essential components of HFpEF care. Ongoing research into novel therapeutic targets, including anti-inflammatory agents, metabolic modulators, and precision medicine approaches, may provide further advancements in the management of this complex condition. Future studies will continue to refine the optimal approach to treating HFpEF and improving patient outcomes.

SUGGESTED READING

1. Ahmed A, Rich MW, Zile MR, et al. Renin-Angiotensin inhibition in diastolic heart failure and chronic kidney disease. Am J Med. 2013;126(2):150-61.
2. Anker SD, Butler J, Filippatos G, et al. Empagliflozin in Heart Failure with a Preserved Ejection Fraction. N Engl J Med. 2021;385(16):1451-61.

3. Borlaug BA. The pathophysiology of heart failure with preserved ejection fraction. Nat Rev Cardiol. 2014;11(9): 507-15.
4. Guazzi M, Vicenzi M, Arena R, et al. Pulmonary hypertension in heart failure with preserved ejection fraction: A target of phosphodiesterase-5 inhibition in a 1-year study. Circulation. 2011;124(2):164-74.
5. Komajda M, Lam CSP. Heart failure with preserved ejection fraction: a clinical dilemma. Eur Heart J. 2014; 35(16):1022-32.
6. Lam CSP, Donal E, Kraigher-Krainer E, et al. Epidemiology and Clinical Course of Heart Failure with Preserved Ejection Fraction. Eur J Heart Fail. 2011;13(1):18-28.
7. Maeder MT, Kaye DM. Heart failure with normal left ventricular ejection fraction. J Am Coll Cardiol. 2009;53(11):905-18.
8. Massie BM, Carson PE, McMurray JJ, et al. Irbesartan in patients with heart failure and preserved ejection fraction. N Engl J Med. 2008;359:2456-67.
9. Packer M, Anker SD, Butler J, et al. Empagliflozin in Patients with Heart Failure and Preserved Ejection Fraction. N Engl J Med. 2022;43(5):416-26.
10. Paulus WJ, Tschöpe C. A novel paradigm for heart failure with preserved ejection fraction: Comorbidities drive myocardial dysfunction and remodeling through coronary microvascular endothelial inflammation. J Am Coll Cardiol. 2013;62(4):263-71.
11. Pfeffer MA, Shah AM, Borlaug BA. Heart Failure With Preserved Ejection Fraction In Perspective. Circ Res. 2019;124(11):1598-617.
12. Redfield MM, Anstrom KJ, Levine JA, et al. Effect of Phosphodiesterase-5 inhibition on exercise capacity and clinical status in heart failure with preserved ejection fraction. JAMA. 2013;309(12):1268-77.
13. Shah AM, Claggett B, Kitzman D, et al. Contemporary assessment of diastolic dysfunction in heart failure with preserved ejection fraction: Role of echocardiography and invasive hemodynamics. J Am Coll Cardiol. 2018.
14. Shah SJ, Kitzman DW, Borlaug BA, et al. Phenotype-Specific Treatment of Heart Failure With Preserved Ejection Fraction. Circulation. 2016;134(1):73-90.
15. Shah SJ. Precision Medicine for Heart Failure With Preserved Ejection Fraction. Circulation. 2016;10(3): 233-44.
16. Solomon SD, Claggett B, Lewis EF, et al. Influence of Ejection Fraction on Outcomes in Patients with Heart Failure Treated with Sacubitril/Valsartan. Eur J Heart Fail. 2016;37(5):455-62.
17. Solomon SD, McMurray JJV, Anand IS, et al. Angiotensin–neprilysin inhibition in heart failure with preserved ejection fraction. N Engl J Med. 2019;381(17):1609-20.
18. Verma S, McMurray JJV. The Serendipitous Story of SGLT2 Inhibitors in Heart Failure. Circulation. 2019;139(22):2537-41.
19. Yancy CW, Jessup M, Bozkurt B, et al. 2017 ACC/AHA/HFSA Focused Update of the 2013 ACCF/AHA Guideline for the Management of Heart Failure. J Am Coll Cardiol. 2017;70(6):776-803.
20. Zile MR, Baicu CF, Gaasch WH. Diastolic heart failure - abnormalities in active relaxation and passive stiffness of the left ventricle. N Engl J Med. 2004;350(19):1953-9.

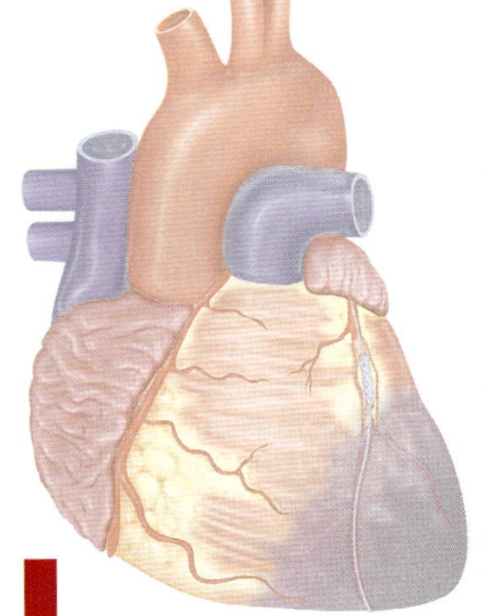

Interplay Between HFpEF and Hypothyroidism

Vinod M Vijan, Vikrant V Vijan, Gulshan B Tolani

INTRODUCTION

Every cell and organ's growth, development, and metabolism are significantly impacted by thyroid hormones (THs). Moreover, they are essential for cardiovascular (CV) homeostasis and regulation of vital pathways that preserve ventricular contractility, electrophysiological activities, and cardiac structure. Any disruption in the TH levels is known to have a profound impact on cardiac function.[1]

Thyroid hormones exert their effects by binding to nuclear receptors in cardiomyocytes, leading to the transcription of genes that modulate calcium handling, adrenergic receptor expression, and energy metabolism. Insufficient TH is known to lead to hyperlipidemia and ventricular arrhythmias, whereas excess may lead to atrial arrhythmias, and both are known to cause hypertension and heart failure (HF).[2]

Hypothyroidism, i.e., low levels of thyroid hormones, significantly alters the cardiac function, including bradycardia, decreased contractility, and increased systemic vascular resistance. Subclinical hypothyroidism with thyroid stimulating hormone (TSH) levels >10 mIU/L has been associated with increased risk of ischemic heart disease, and subclinical hypothyroidism with TSH levels >7 mIU/L has been associated with increased CV mortality. Subclinical thyroid dysfunction with TSH values >10 mIU/L or below 0.1 mIU/L has also been associated with a higher risk of incident HF.[3]

Hypothyroidism is known to increase the stiffness of arterial walls, increasing vascular resistance and afterload. These changes may exacerbate the symptoms of HF, particularly in patients with HF with preserved ejection fraction (HFpEF) with a higher mortality **(Fig. 1)**.[4]

UNDERSTANDING HEART FAILURE WITH PRESERVED EJECTION FRACTION

Heart failure with preserved ejection fraction is characterized by the presence of HF symptoms despite a normal or near-normal left ventricular ejection fraction (LVEF) of ≥50%. HFpEF is predominantly a disease of diastolic dysfunction. The heart's ability to relax and fill during diastole is impaired, leading to elevated filling pressures, congestion, and the classic symptoms of HF, such as dyspnea, fatigue, and edema despite a normal morphology. The pathophysiology of HFpEF is complex and involves multiple interrelated processes:

- *Left ventricular hypertrophy (LVH):* Chronic pressure overload, often due to hypertension, leads to LVH, which increases myocardial stiffness and contributes to diastolic dysfunction.
- *Endothelial dysfunction:* Impaired nitric oxide (NO) signaling and increased oxidative stress contribute to the increased vascular stiffness and impaired coronary microcirculation.
- *Fibrosis:* Myocardial fibrosis, driven by chronic inflammation and neurohormonal activation, further stiffens the myocardium, exacerbating diastolic dysfunction.
- *Comorbidities:* HFpEF is associated with comorbidities such as obesity, diabetes, and chronic kidney disease, which may additionally contribute to the systemic inflammation and neurohormonal dysregulation.

The presence of multiple comorbidities in HFpEF patients further complicates management and contributes to the overall burden of the disease.[6]

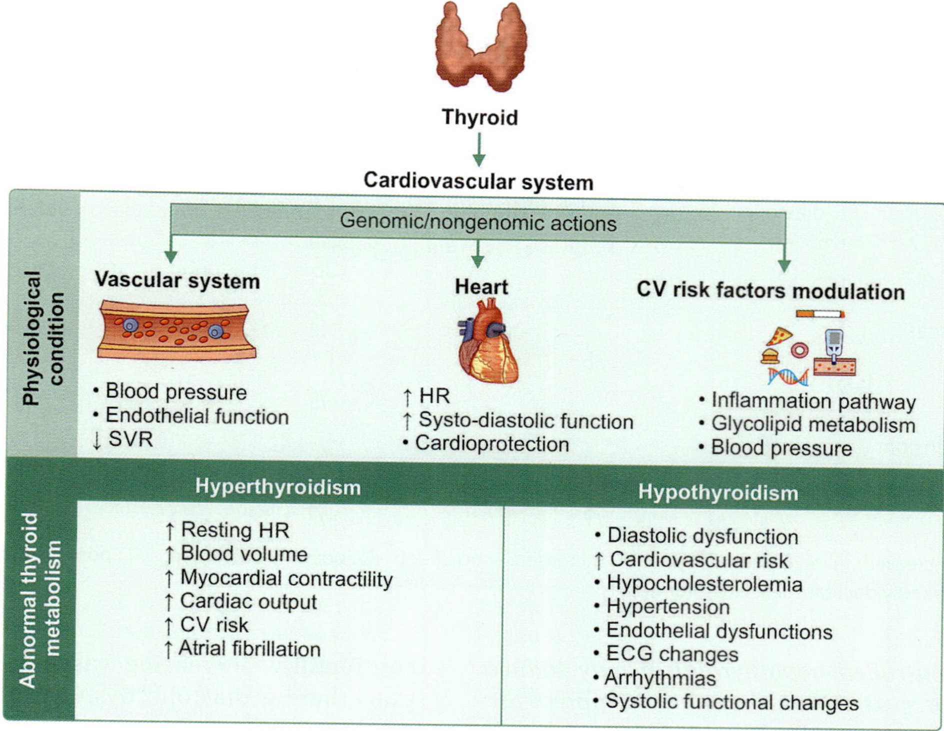

Fig. 1: Thyroid and impact on heart.[5]

ASSOCIATION OF HEART FAILURE WITH PRESERVED EJECTION FRACTION AND HYPOTHYROIDISM

The coexistence of hypothyroidism and HFpEF is not uncommon, and the two conditions share several pathophysiological mechanisms. Hypothyroidism may exacerbate the symptoms of HFpEF and contribute to its progression through several mechanisms **(Table 1)**:

- *Diastolic dysfunction:* It impairs myocardial relaxation and increases myocardial stiffness (central features of HFpEF). The reduced expression of calcium-handling proteins in hypothyroidism leads to prolonged relaxation time and decreased compliance of the left ventricle.
- *Increased vascular resistance:* It promotes vasoconstriction and increases arterial stiffness. This adds to the hemodynamic burden in HFpEF patients, leading to elevated left ventricular filling pressures and worsening symptoms.
- *Hypercholesterolemia:* It is associated with lipid abnormalities, including elevated levels of low-density lipoprotein (LDL) cholesterol and triglycerides. Lipid abnormalities accelerate the development of atherosclerosis, increasing the risk of coronary artery disease (CAD) and further compromising myocardial perfusion and function in HFpEF.[7]

MECHANISMS LINKING HYPOTHYROIDISM AND HEART FAILURE WITH PRESERVED EJECTION FRACTION

Several mechanisms have been proposed to explain the link between hypothyroidism and HFpEF, which are as follows:[9,10]

- *Altered gene expression:* Hypothyroidism leads to altered gene expression, resulting in impaired myocardial relaxation, increased stiffness, and reduced contractility.
- *Increased myocardial fibrosis* is associated with increased myocardial fibrosis, driven by chronic inflammation and neurohormonal activation. Fibrosis increases myocardial stiffness, contributing to diastolic dysfunction and elevated filling pressures in HFpEF.
- *Impaired calcium handling:* Thyroid hormones modulate the expression of calcium-handling proteins such as SERCA2a and phospholamban. In hypothyroidism, the reduced expression of these proteins impairs calcium reuptake into the sarcoplasmic reticulum, leading to prolonged relaxation time and impaired diastolic function.
- *Increased oxidative stress:* It contributes to endothelial dysfunction, vascular stiffness, and impaired coronary microcirculation which may exacerbate the diastolic dysfunction.

TABLE 1: Cardiovascular changes and thyroid abnormalities.[8]

	Overt hypothyroidism	*Subclinical hypothyroidism*	*Subclinical hyperthyroidism*	*Overt hyperthyroidism*
Systolic dysfunction	↑↑	↑	↓/↑	↓/↑
Diastolic dysfunction	↑↑	↑↑	↓/↑	↓/↑
Heart rate	↓↓	↓	↓	↑↑
Hypertension	↑ (diastolic)	↑ (diastolic)	↑ (systolic)	↑ (systolic)
Dyslipidemia	↑↑	↑	↓	↓
Heart failure	↑↑	↑	–/↑	↑↑
Coronary artery disease	↑↑	↑	–/↑	–/↑
Atrial fibrillation	–/↓	–/↓	↑	↑↑
Atherosclerosis	↑↑	↑	–/↑	–/↑
Pulmonary hypertension	–	–	–	↑
Cardiovascular mortality	↑	–/↑	–/↑	↑
All-cause mortality	↑	–/↑	–/↑	↑

Note: ↑↑: markedly increased; ↑: increased; –/↑: possibly increased; –: no effect; –/↓: possibly decreased; ↓/↑: possibly decreased or increased; ↓: decreased; ↓↓: markedly decreased. See text for details.

Chronic uncontrolled hypothyroidism may induce myocardial fibrosis, as thyroid hormones suppress the pro-α1 collagen gene expression. It is associated with loss in small coronary arteries, thus reducing coronary blood flow. Levels of TSH in patients with metabolic syndrome were related directly with circulating endothelin-1s and inversely with nitroxide serum concentration.[11,12]

HYPOTHYROIDISM AND HEART FAILURE WITH PRESERVED EJECTION FRACTION EXACERBATION

Hypothyroidism may exacerbate the symptoms and progression of HFpEF through several pathways:

- *Worsening diastolic dysfunction:* The impaired myocardial relaxation and increased stiffness associated with hypothyroidism exacerbate the diastolic dysfunction seen in HFpEF, leading to increased filling pressures and worsening symptoms.
- *Increased vascular resistance:* The increased systemic vascular resistance associated with hypothyroidism adds to the hemodynamic burden in HFpEF patients, leading to elevated left ventricular filling pressures and worsening symptoms.
- *Exacerbation of comorbidities:* Hypothyroidism can worsen the comorbidities associated with HFpEF, such as hypertension, diabetes, and hyperlipidemia. These comorbidities contribute to the overall burden of disease and complicate management.
- *Reduced exercise tolerance:* Hypothyroidism reduces exercise tolerance by impairing myocardial contractility, increasing vascular resistance, and exacerbating diastolic dysfunction. This leads to increased symptoms and reduced quality of life in HFpEF patients.

CHALLENGES

Though low thyroid hormone levels are known to lead to both systolic and diastolic dysfunction, clinical studies have highlighted predominance of diastolic abnormalities, thus the coexistence of hypothyroidism and HFpEF presents several challenges in clinical practice:

- *Diagnostic challenges:*
  - *Overlapping symptoms:* The symptoms of hypothyroidism and HFpEF can overlap, making it difficult to distinguish between the two conditions. Routine screening for thyroid function in patients with HFpEF is essential to identify hypothyroidism and initiate appropriate treatment.[13]
- *Management challenges:* Hypothyroidism in HFpEF requires careful titration of thyroid hormone replacement therapy. Over-replacement may lead to hyperthyroidism, which may further exacerbate HF symptoms and increase the risk of arrhythmias.[14]
- *Prognostic challenges:* The coexistence of hypothyroidism and HFpEF may worsen the prognosis, leading to increased morbidity and mortality. A TSH ≥7 mIU/L was linked to a higher risk of a composite end outcome in patients with HFrEF and HFpEF, including the insertion of ventricular assist devices, heart transplantation, or death in the Penn Heart Failure Study.[15]

BLOOD TESTS FOR DIAGNOSIS AND MONITORING[15,16]

Blood tests for diagnosis and monitoring are as follows:

- *Thyroid-stimulating hormone (TSH):* It is the most sensitive marker for diagnosing hypothyroidism. Elevated TSH levels indicate primary hypothyroidism, while low or normal TSH levels may indicate secondary or central hypothyroidism.
- *Free thyroxine (free T4):* It helps to confirm the diagnosis of hypothyroidism and assess the severity of the condition. Low free T4 levels indicate hypothyroidism.
- *Free triiodothyronine (Free T3):* Often measured in cases of suspected central hypothyroidism or to assess the adequacy of thyroid hormone replacement therapy.
- *Lipid profile:* Hypothyroidism is associated with lipid abnormalities, including elevated LDL cholesterol and triglycerides. A lipid profile can help assess the cardiovascular risk and guide management in HFpEF patients with hypothyroidism. We recommend a nonfasting full lipid profile (which includes an extended lipid profile that incorporates Apo(B), LP(a), and even hs-CRP).

Thyroid disorders and diagnostic levels are given in **Table 2**.

TABLE 2: Thyroid disorders and diagnostic levels.

Clinical condition	*TSH*	*Free T4*	*Associated abnormality*
Subclinical hypothyroidism	↑	Normal	Impaired systolic and diastolic cardiac function, increased carotid artery intima–media thickness, vascular dysfunction, and higher blood pressure[17]
Overt hypothyroidism	↑↑	↓	Increased risk of HF, coronary artery disease, and all-cause and cardiovascular mortality[18]
Subclinical hyperthyroidism	↓↓	Normal	Higher risk of cardiovascular disease, including coronary events, HF, and atrial fibrillation[19]
Overt hyperthyroidism	↓↓	↑↑	Hyperdynamic state, characterized by tachycardia, increased cardiac preload and contractility, and diminished systemic vascular resistance[18,20]

Source: Neves et al. (2020).

MANAGING HEART FAILURE WITH PRESERVED EJECTION FRACTION WITH HYPOTHYROIDISM

Diastolic dysfunction in hypothyroidism or subclinical hypothyroidism is reversible with thyroid hormone supplementation and usually, the management of HFpEF in patients with hypothyroidism requires a comprehensive and individualized approach.[18]

- *Thyroid hormone replacement therapy:* The cornerstone of treatment for hypothyroidism is thyroid hormone replacement therapy. Levothyroxine (T4) forms the standard of care.[21] The goal is to achieve and maintain euthyroidism and benefits are not restricted to only cardiac but include decreased adiposity, decreased epicardial adiposity, improved endothelial function, arterial compliance, lipid profiles, and skeletal muscle function.[22,23]
- *Management of comorbidities:* Optimal management of comorbid conditions such as hypertension, diabetes, and hyperlipidemia is essential in HFpEF patients. For dyslipidemia in Indian patients, it is highly recommended to follow LAI recommendations.[24,25] An interesting approach to alleviate the hypersympathetic response is the administration of β- blockers.[26]
- *Lifestyle modifications:* Lifestyle interventions, including dietary changes, weight management, and regular physical activity, are important components of managing HFpEF and hypothyroidism. These interventions can help reduce the overall burden of disease and improve quality of life.
- *Pharmacological management:* In addition to thyroid hormone replacement therapy, pharmacological management of HFpEF may include the use of diuretics, ACE inhibitors, angiotensin II receptor blockers (ARBs), beta-blockers, and mineralocorticoid receptor antagonists. The choice of therapy should be individualized based on the patient's clinical profile and comorbidities.[27]

  The impact of correction of hypothyroidism is given in **Figure 2**.

PROGNOSIS

The prognosis of HFpEF in patients with hypothyroidism depends on several factors, including the severity of diastolic dysfunction, the presence of comorbidities, and the adequacy of thyroid hormone replacement therapy. Evidence from trials in HFrEF, and trials in patients without HF, suggest a positive impact of thyroid hormone supplementation in diastolic function.[28] *Risk of cardiovascular events:*

- Higher TSH, higher FT4, and lower TT3 were each associated with more severe symptoms of HF at

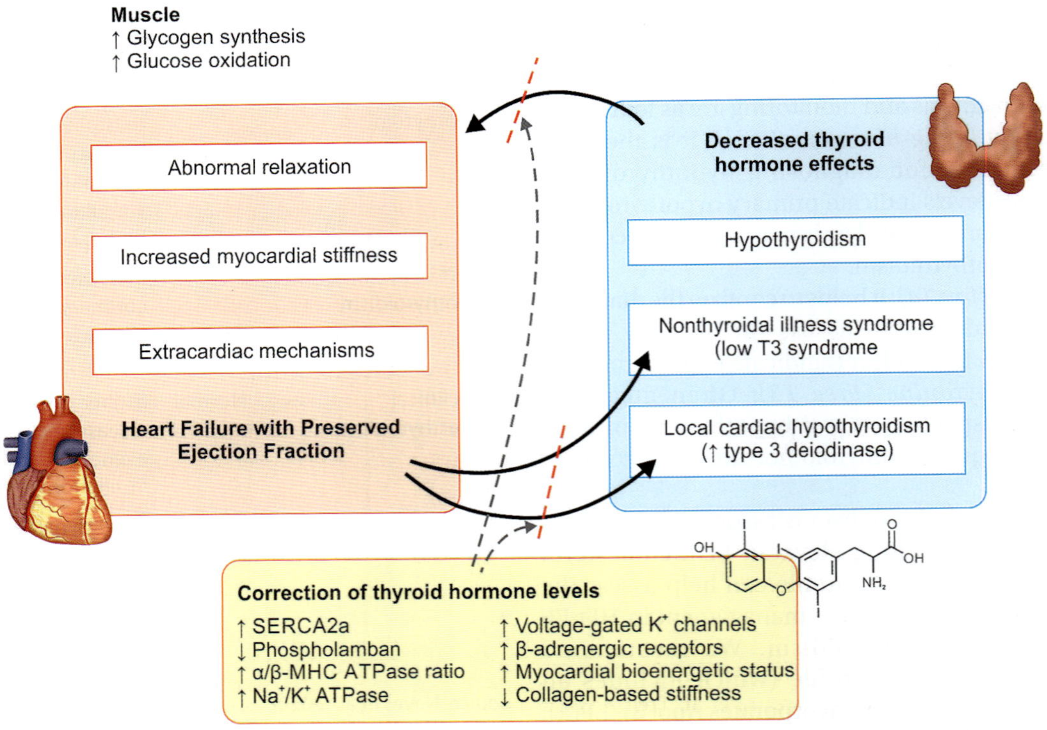

Fig. 2: Impact of correction of hypothyroidism. (MHC: myosin heavy chain; SERCA2a: sarco/endoplasmic reticulum calcium-ATPase; T3: triiodothyronine)
Source: Neves et al. (2020).

baseline and also with an increased risk of a composite outcome of VAD placement, cardiac transplant, or all-cause mortality.

- Severe subclinical hypothyroidism was associated with a >threefold risk and low T3 syndrome with a >twofold risk of incident VAD placement, cardiac transplantation, or all-cause mortality. TSH values >10.0 mIU/L or <0.1 mIU/L are associated with an increased risk of incident HF.[3]
- In patients with HF, low T3 levels has been associated with myocardial fibrosis and abnormalities in myocardial perfusion and metabolism.[29]

The coexistence of HFpEF and hypothyroidism significantly impacts the quality of life. Addressing both conditions through appropriate treatment and lifestyle modifications improves functional status and overall well-being.

FUTURE DIRECTIONS AND RESEARCH

Several areas of future research are needed to better understand the relationship between HFpEF and hypothyroidism and to improve the management of these conditions:

- *Long-term outcomes:* Long-term studies are needed to evaluate the impact of thyroid hormone replacement therapy on the prognosis of HFpEF patients with hypothyroidism. These studies should assess the effects on mortality, hospitalization rates, and quality of life. A lot of our understanding is currently based on animal models.
- *Biomarkers:* Identifying biomarkers that predict the development of HFpEF in patients with hypothyroidism could help in early diagnosis and intervention. Additionally, biomarkers that track the response to thyroid hormone replacement therapy may guide treatment decisions and improve patient outcomes.
- *Novel therapies:* The development of novel therapies targeting the specific pathophysiological mechanisms linking hypothyroidism and HFpEF is a promising area of research. These may include drugs that modulate thyroid hormone signaling, reduce myocardial fibrosis, or improve endothelial function.

CONCLUSION

- HFpEF is a complex syndrome characterized by diastolic dysfunction, and hypothyroidism can exacerbate the symptoms and progression of the condition.
- Routine screening for thyroid function in patients with HFpEF is essential for identifying hypothyroidism and initiating appropriate treatment.

- Subclinical hypothyroidism with TSH ≥7 mIU/L and low T3 syndrome are poor prognostic indicators in ambulatory patients with HF.
- Future research should focus on understanding the molecular mechanisms linking hypothyroidism and HFpEF, identifying biomarkers for early diagnosis, and developing novel therapies to improve patient outcomes.

REFERENCES

1. Jabbar A, Pingitore A, Pearce SH, et al. Thyroid hormones and cardiovascular disease. Nat Rev Cardiol. 2017;14(1): 39-55.
2. Klein I, Danzi S. Thyroid disease and the heart. Circulation. 2007;116(15):1725-35.
3. Gencer B, Collet TH, Virgini V, et al; Thyroid Studies Collaboration. Subclinical thyroid dysfunction and the risk of heart failure events: an individual participant data analysis from 6 prospective cohorts. Circulation. 2012; 126(9):1040-9.
4. Gerdes AM, Lervasi G. Thyroid replacement therapy and heart failure. Circulation. 2010;122(4):385-93.
5. Pingitore A, Mastorci F, Lazzeri MFL, et al. Thyroid and heart: a fatal pathophysiological attraction in a controversial clinical liaison. Endocrines. 2023;4(4):722-74.
6. Paulus WJ, Tschöpe C. A novel paradigm for heart failure with preserved ejection fraction: Comorbidities drive myocardial dysfunction and remodeling through coronary microvascular endothelial inflammation. J Am Coll Cardiol. 2013;62(4):263-71.
7. Saravanan P, Chau WF. The impact of hypothyroidism on the cardiovascular system. Clinical Endocrinology. 2020;93(3):297-308.
8. JS Neves, C Vale, von Hafe M, et al. Thyroid hormones and modulation of diastolic function: a promising target for heart failure with preserved ejection fraction. Ther Adv Endocrinol Metab. 2020;11:1-12
9. Zúñiga D, Balasubramanian S, Mehmood KT, et al. Hypothyroidism and Cardiovascular Disease: A Review. Cureus. 2024;16(1):e52512.
10. Patrizio A, Ferrari SM, Elia G, et al. Hypothyroidism and metabolic cardiovascular disease. Front Endocrinol. 2024;15:1408684.
11. Ahirwar AK, Singh A, Jain A, et al. Raised TSH is associated with endothelial dysfunction in metabolic syndrome: A case control study. Rom J Intern Med. 2017;55(4):212–21.
12. Biondi B, Galderisi M, Pagano L et al. Endothelial-mediated coronary flow reserve in patients with mild thyroid hormone deficiency. Eur J Endocrinol. 2009;161:323-9.
13. Gazewood JD, Turner PL. Heart Failure with Preserved Ejection Fraction: Diagnosis and Management. Am Fam Physician. 2017;96(9):582-8.
14. Okosieme OE. Thyroid hormone replacement: current status and challenges. Expert Opin Pharmacother. 2011; 12(15):2315-28.
15. Kannan L, Shaw PA, Morley MP, et al. Thyroid dysfunction in heart failure and cardiovascular outcomes. Circ Heart Fail. 2018;11(12):e005266.
16. Rodondi N, den Elzen WP, Bauer DC, et al; Thyroid Studies Collaboration. Subclinical hypothyroidism and the risk of coronary heart disease and mortality. JAMA. 2010;304(12):1365-74.
17. Biondi B, Fazio S, Palmieri EA, et al. Left ventricular diastolic dysfunction in patients with subclinical hypothyroidism. J Clin Endocrinol Metab. 1999;84(6):2064-7.
18. Cappola AR, Ladenson PW. Hypothyroidism and atherosclerosis. J Clin Endocrinol Metab. 2003;88:2438-44.
19. Walsh JP, Bremner AP, Bulsara MK, et al. Subclinical thyroid dysfunction as a risk factor for cardiovascular disease. Arch Intern Med. 2005;165(21):2467–72.
20. Siu CW, Yeung CY, Lau CP, et al. Incidence, clinical characteristics and outcome of congestive heart failure as the initial presentation in patients with primary hyperthyroidism. Heart. 2007;93(4):483-7
21. Jonklaas J, Bianco AC, Bauer AJ, et al. Guidelines for the treatment of hypothyroidism: Prepared by the American thyroid association task force on thyroid hormone replacement. Thyroid. 2014;24(12): 1670-751.
22. Caraccio N, Ferrannini E, Monzani F. Lipoprotein profile in subclinical hypothyroidism: response to levothyroxine replacement, a randomized placebo-controlled study. J Clin Endocrinol Metab. 2002;87(4):1533-8.
23. Razvi S, Ingoe L, Keeka G, et al. The beneficial effect of L-thyroxine on cardiovascular risk factors, endothelial function, and quality of life in subclinical hypothyroidism: randomized, crossover trial. J Clin Endocrinol Metab. 2007;92(5):1715-23.
24. Puri R, Bansal M, Mehta V, et al. Lipid Association of India 2023 update on cardiovascular risk assessment in Indian patients. Consensus statement IV. J Clin Lipidol. 2014;18(3):e351-e373.
25. Puri R, Mehta V, Bansal M, et al. Does adopting Western low-density lipoprotein cholesterol targets expose Indians to a higher risk of cardiovascular events? Expert opinion from the lipid association of India. J Assoc Physicians India. 2024;72(10):71-76.
26. Ortiz VD, Turck P, Teixeira R, et al. Carvedilol and thyroid hormones co-administration mitigates oxidative stress and improves cardiac function after acute myocardial infarction. Eur J Pharmacol. 2019;854:159-66.
27. Stoicescu L, Crişan D, Morgovan C, et al. Heart Failure with Preserved Ejection Fraction: The Pathophysiological Mechanisms behind the Clinical Phenotypes and the Therapeutic Approach. Int J Mol Sci. 2024;25(2):794
28. Virtanen VK, Saha HH, Groundstroem KW, et al. Thyroid hormone substitution therapy rapidly enhances left-ventricular diastolic function in hypothyroid patients. Cardiology. 2001;96(2):59-64.
29. Wang W, Guan H, Fang W, et al. Free Triiodothyronine Level Correlates With Myocardial Injury And Prognosis In Idiopathic Dilated Cardiomyopathy: Evidence from Cardiac MRI and SPECT/PET Imaging. Sci Rep. 2016;6:39811.

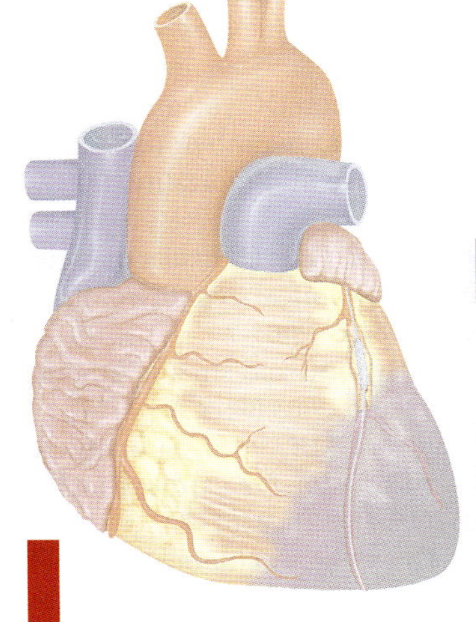

Role of Sodium–Glucose Cotransporter-2 Inhibitors in Patients with HFpEF

Vinod Mittal

INTRODUCTION

Heart failure with preserved ejection fraction (HFpEF) is a clinical syndrome characterized by signs and symptoms of heart failure (HF) due to elevated left ventricular (LV) filling pressure, despite a normal or near-normal LV ejection fraction (LVEF; ≥50%).[1-5] Most patients with HFpEF exhibit normal LV volumes and an abnormal diastolic filling pattern, indicative of diastolic dysfunction.[1-5]

The global prevalence and clinical significance of HFpEF highlight the public health challenge posed by HF. In 2019, there were 56.19 million HF cases worldwide, with an increasing trend, especially in low-income countries, since 1990.[6] The age-standardized prevalence of HF varies widely across regions. According to the 2019 Global Burden of Disease study, Asia reported 31.89 million HF cases with an age-standardized rate of 722.45 per 100,000 population.[7]

Current HFpEF management focuses on risk stratification and comorbidity control, nonpharmacological approaches, and symptom management, with disease-modifying treatments. Guideline-directed medical therapy (GDMT) includes loop diuretics, SGLT2 inhibitors (SGLT2i), mineralocorticoid receptor antagonists (MRAs), angiotensin receptor-neprilysin inhibitors (ARNIs), and angiotensin receptor blockers (ARBs). The GDMT is essential for reducing morbidity and mortality, improving symptoms, and enhancing functional ability in HFpEF patients. The SGLT2i should be initiated in all individuals with HFpEF without contraindications, as they reduce hospitalization and cardiovascular (CV) death risk across all EF subgroups. Recent trials have shown benefits from SGLT2i, leading to a class 2a recommendation in 2022 guidelines and suggesting their potential for stronger future endorsements.[8,9] Therefore, this chapter focuses on the mechanism, pathophysiology, and effect of SGLT2i in HFpEF management.

PATHOPHYSIOLOGY OF HEART FAILURE WITH PRESERVED EJECTION FRACTION

The HFpEF involves various structural and functional cardiac changes. Typically, patients exhibit concentric LV hypertrophy, but some may have normal geometry or eccentric hypertrophy. These variations arise from microscopic differences in cardiomyocytes and age-related ventricular wall thickening.[10] A hallmark of HFpEF is diastolic dysfunction, where the heart has trouble filling properly and experiences elevated filling pressures.[11] Despite having normal QRS complexes on an electrocardiogram, patients often suffer from ventricular dyssynchrony, leading to mechanical inefficiency in heart function.[12] Atrial dysfunction and atrial fibrillation (AF) frequently occur in HFpEF,[13] increasing pulmonary pressures and causing right ventricular dysfunction.[14] Pulmonary hypertension and RV disease often co-occur, raising mortality risks.[15] High filling pressures are worsened by pericardial restraint, especially in obese patients or in those with pulmonary hypertension.[16] Vascular stiffness and endothelial dysfunction, often due to reduced nitric oxide bioavailability, exacerbate diastolic dysfunction and predict poor outcomes.[17] Chronotropic incompetence, where the heart cannot adequately increase its rate during exercise, reduces exercise capacity.[18] Aging accelerates these heart dysfunctions, particularly in women and obese individuals. In HFpEF, hypervolemia or excess fluid tends to accumulate in the tissues rather than the blood vessels.[19] This complicates treatment with diuretics but responds well to SGLT2i. The pathophysiology of HFpEF is depicted in **Figure 1**.

Associated Comorbidities

The 2021 European Society of Cardiology guidelines emphasize the importance of screening and treating both CV and non-CV comorbidities in HFpEF patients.[20] Major CV factors include hypertension, AF, diabetes, and obesity. Hypertension is prevalent in 55–90% of HFpEF patients, leading to LV dysfunction and systemic inflammation.[21-23] The AF, present in 15–40%, complicates HFpEF diagnosis and worsens prognosis.[24] Diabetes, affecting about one-third of HFpEF patients, contributes to oxidative stress and endothelial dysfunction.[25] Obesity, present in nearly 80% of HFpEF patients, is linked to increased HFpEF risk and complex pathophysiology, including inflammation and altered fat distribution.[26] Chronic kidney disease (CKD) affects 26–49% of HFpEF patients and is associated with poor prognosis and cardiorenal syndrome.[22] Other notable comorbidities include chronic obstructive pulmonary disease (COPD), iron deficiency, and anemia, all impacting HFpEF progression. Specific secondary causes of HFpEF, such as amyloidosis and restrictive cardiomyopathies, require targeted treatments.[27] Comorbidities associated with the HFpEF are depicted in **Figure 2**.

MULTIFACETED MECHANISMS UNDERLYING HFpEF BENEFITS OF SGLT2i

The overall mechanism of action of SGLT2i is depicted in **Figure 3**. For HFpEF, inhibiting SGLT2 and Na^+/H exchanger 3 (NHE3) in the proximal tubule improves hemodynamic outcomes by causing glycosuria, natriuresis, and osmotic diuresis.[28,29] The process of natriuresis lowers filling pressures and plasma volume, which may assist in preventing diuretic resistance. By reducing glomerular hyperfiltration and delaying the development of CKD, blocking NHE3 in the proximal tubule improves sodium supply to the macula densa.[30] Furthermore, a persistently negative sodium balance can lessen aortic stiffness, which will reduce symptoms and delay the advancement of HFpEF.[29,31] In order to relieve cardiac congestion and move the end-diastolic pressure–volume relationship to the right, glycosuria and the osmotic diuresis it is linked with increase plasma oncotic pressure.[32]

Moreover, glucosuria induces a glucose-deficient state that raises glucagon levels and causes the breakdown of adipose tissue in the epicardial cavity. It is possible to improve the end-diastolic pressure–volume relationship and minimize pericardial restriction by reducing epicardial adipose tissue.[29] Moreover, adipokines released by epicardial adipose tissue are inhibited and counteracted by SGLT2i. The inhibition of glucose causes the sirtuins (Sirt1, Sirt3, Sirt6) to become active.[28,33] When Sirt1 is activated, the heart experiences less oxidative stress, more ketone synthesis occurs, and these actions may have anti-inflammatory and energy-efficient benefits.[34] Furthermore, by blocking xanthine oxidase, Sirt1 lowers

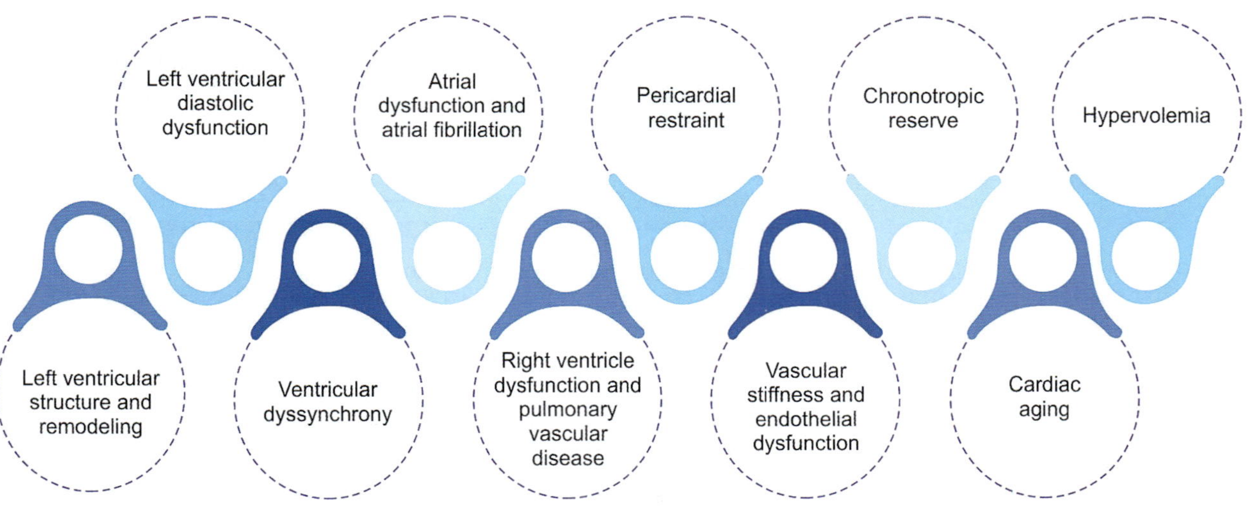

Fig. 1: Pathophysiology of HFpEF. (HFpEF: heart failure with preserved ejection fraction)

the formation of reactive oxygen species and uric acid while also raising hemoglobin levels through increased erythropoietin synthesis. Moreover, Sirt1 inhibits fibrosis mediated by tumor necrosis factor-B, which may inhibit AF and cardiac remodeling.[35,36] Elevated levels of Sirt3 have a positive effect on the metabolic pathways in the heart and skeletal muscle, which helps to prevent hypertrophy, fibrosis, and coronary microvascular rarefaction as well as relieve symptoms of HFpEF.[37,38] Moreover, sirtuins prevent hypertrophy by inhibiting the insulin-like growth factor/protein kinase B signaling pathway. For many years, HFpEF has been difficult to treat.[39]

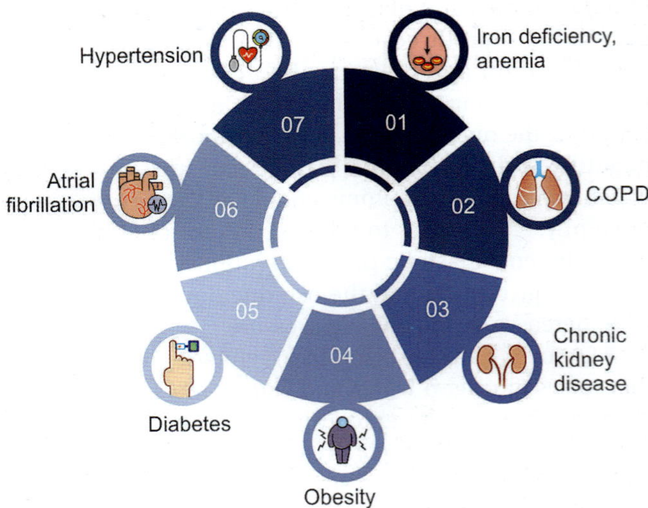

Fig. 2: Comorbidities associated with HFpEF. (COPD: chronic obstructive pulmonary disorder; HFpEF: heart failure with preserved ejection fraction)

MANAGEMENT OF HEART FAILURE WITH PRESERVED EJECTION FRACTION

Current treatment strategies for HFpEF focus on three main areas: Risk stratification and management of comorbidities (e.g., hypertension, diabetes, obesity, AF, coronary artery disease, CKD, obstructive sleep apnea); nonpharmacological management (e.g., exercise, weight loss, and use of wireless, implantable pulmonary artery monitors); and symptom management and disease-modifying therapy. Medications used include loop diuretics, SGLT2i, MRAs, ARNIs, and ARBs.[8]

Management of HFpEF using GDMT

Patients with HF benefit from SGLT2i, which reduces hospitalization and CV death risk across all EF subgroups. Therefore, SGLT2i should be initiated in all individuals with HFpEF who lack contraindications. Treating HFpEF has been historically challenging, but recent trials show that GDMT is beneficial for these patients. The use of GDMT drugs is essential for reducing HF-related morbidity and mortality, improving symptoms, and

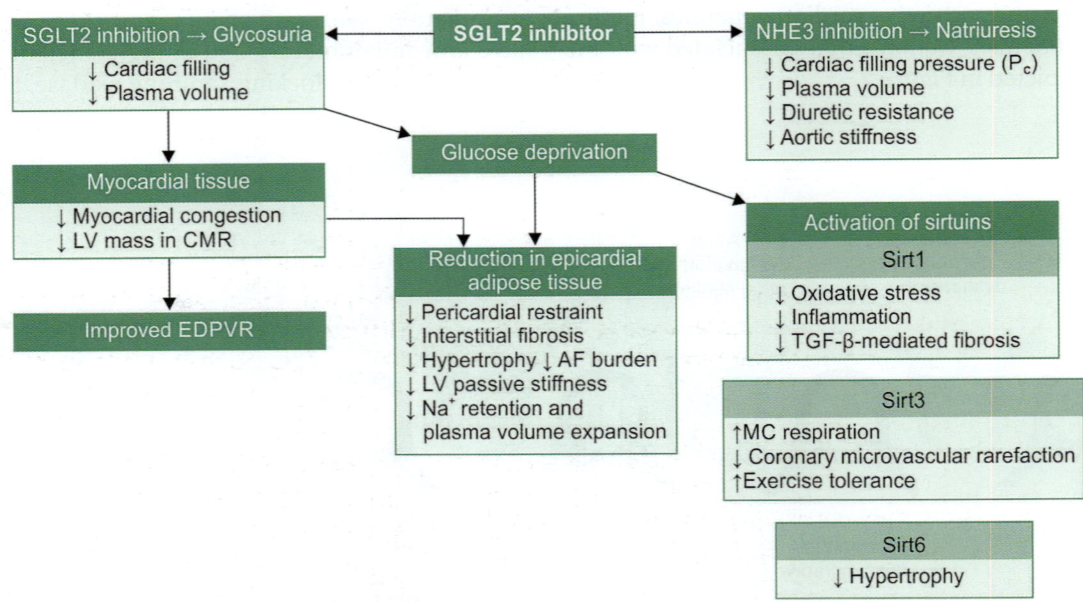

Fig. 3: Mechanism of action in SGLT2i. (AF: atrial fibrillation; CKD: chronic kidney disease; CMR: cardiac magnetic resonance; EDPVR: end-diastolic pressure–volume relationship; LV: left ventricular; MC: mitochondrial; NHE3: Na^+/H exchanger 3; SGLT2: sodium–glucose cotransporter 2; TGF-β: transforming growth factor-β)

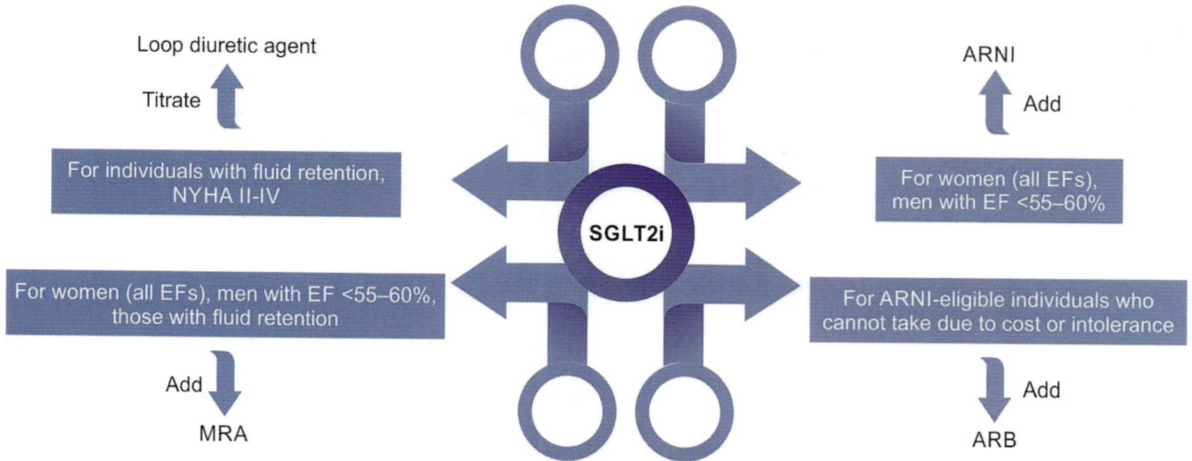

Fig. 4: Guideline-directed medical therapy for HFpEF. (ARNI: angiotensin receptor/neprilysin inhibitor; EF: ejection fraction; HF: heart failure; HFrEF: heart failure with reduced ejection fraction; MRA: mineralocorticoid receptor antagonists; NYHA: New York Heart Association; SGLT: sodium–glucose cotransporter)

enhancing functional ability. GDMT can be started in acute and chronic care settings, and it is both safe and effective. When administering GDMT in HFpEF, clinicians should also consider cautions and contraindications and follow suggested starting and target doses. According to GDMT, starting treatment with an SGLT2i in HFpEF patients is classified as Class 2a therapy. For NYHA class II–IV patients with fluid retention, titrating SGLT2i with a loop diuretic is considered class 1 therapy. Adding an MRA is class 2b therapy for women (all EF) and men with EF <55–60% who have fluid retention. Adding an ARNI is class 2b therapy for women (all EF) and men with EF <55–60%. If ARNI is not an option due to cost or intolerance, adding an ARB is class 2b therapy.[8] **Figure 4** outlines the approach to GDMT initiation and titration.

CLINICAL EFFICACY OF SGLT2 INHIBITORS IN HFpEF MANAGEMENT

Several clinical trials showed the effectiveness of SGLT2i in HFpEF patients which is depicted in **Table 1**. The EMPEROR-Preserved trial showed that empagliflozin, starting as early as 18 days into the trial and continuing throughout the follow-up period, significantly decreased the incidence of outpatient visits for worsening HF, including urgent care visits. Furthermore, empagliflozin was linked to a lower chance of hospitalization for HF needing intensive care, vasopressor or inotropic medication, and a reduced need for higher diuretic therapy in the outpatient context.[40] Empagliflozin became the first SGLT2i to be designated as a breakthrough therapy by the FDA, for the treatment of HFpEF.[41] The FDA then authorized the extension of the HF indication for empagliflozin to cover both HF with reduced ejection fraction and HFpEF.

The SGLT2i dapagliflozin improved symptoms, physical limits, and 6-minute walking distance in patients with HFpEF in the PRESERVED-HF trial. Regardless of diabetes, improvements were seen in just 12 weeks among 324 individuals in the experiment who had a median EF of 60%. The Kansas City Cardiomyopathy Questionnaire (KCCQ)-Total Symptom Score increased by 5.8 points [95% CI (2.0–9.6); $p = 0.003$) and the physical limitations score increased by 5.3 points [95% CI (0.7–10.0); $p = 0.026$] for the treatment group, resulting in a 5.8-point increase in the clinical summary score [95% CI (2.3–9.2); $p = 0.001$]. Furthermore, there was an improvement of 20.1 meters [95% CI (5.6–34.7); $p = 0.007$] in the 6-minute walk test and a 4.5-point [95% CI (1.1–7.8); $p = 0.009$] rise in the KCCQ-Overall Summary Score.[6]

Empagliflozin was found to have a nonsignificant 2.0-point increase in the KCCQ-Total Symptom Score in the EMPERIAL-Preserved trial, although there was no significant difference in the 6-minute walk test.[6,42] On the other hand, the PRESERVED-HF trial showed significant improvements, perhaps as a result of enrolling patients who had higher levels of functional impairment and severe symptoms at baseline, as well as higher rates of AF and loop diuretic use. More women, African-Americans, and patients with higher BMI were included in PRESERVED-HF, which more accurately reflected the demographics of the United States.[43,44] Canagliflozin, independent of diabetes status, was found to enhance symptoms and quality of life in HFpEF patients, according to the CHIEF-HF trial. Within 2 weeks, there was a 4.5-point increase in the KCCQ-Total Symptom Score, and this improvement

TABLE 1: Summary of clinical trial of SGLT2 inhibitors in HFpEF.

Trial name	*Study intervention*	*Study endpoints*	*Study outcome*
Soloist-WHF[54]	In a study involving 256 participants with an EF of 50% or higher and diabetes, sotagliflozin was compared to a placebo.	Composite of CV death, HHF and urgent HF visits	*HR 0.48; 95%CI [0.27-0.86]
Preserved-HF[6]	In a study involving 315 participants with a median EF of 60%, including 267 participants with and without diabetes, dapagliflozin was compared to a placebo.	Change from baseline in KCCQ-CS	*5.8 points; 95%CI [2.3-9.2]
EMPERIAL-Preserved[42]	In a study involving 315 participants with an EF of 40% or higher, both with and without diabetes, empagliflozin was compared to a placebo.	Change from baseline in 6 MWT	4.0 m; 95%CI [-5.0,13.0]
EMPEROR-Preserved[48]	In a study involving 5,988 participants with an EF of 40% or higher, both with and without diabetes, empagliflozin was compared to a placebo.	Composite of CV death or HHF	*HR 0.79; 95%CI [0.69-0.90]
CHIEF-HF[38]	In a study involving 267 participants with an EF of 40% or higher, both with and without diabetes, canagliflozin was compared to a placebo.	Change from baseline in KCCQ-CS	*4.5 points; 95%CI [0.3-9.4]
DELIVER[55]	In a study involving 6,263 participants with an EF of 40% or higher, both with and without diabetes, dapagliflozin was compared to a placebo.	Composite of CV death, HHF and urgent HF visits	mean LVEF: 54.2 (8.8)%

*Significant.

(6MWT: 6-minute walk test; CV: cardiovascular; EF: ejection fraction; HF: heart failure; HHF: hospitalization for heart failure; KCCQ-CS: Kanas City Cardiomyopathy Questionnaire-clinical summary score; KCCQ-TSS: Kanas City Cardiomyopathy Questionnaire-total symptom score; RCTs: randomized controlled trials)

persisted for 3 months.[38] However, the statistics are less persuasive because CHIEF-HF included individuals who had HFmrEF, which is a clinically more similar condition to HFrEF; therefore, data are less convincing for those with EF ≥50.[45]

The DELIVER trial, involving 6,263 HFpEF patients (EF >40%), aimed to assess the impact of dapagliflozin on reducing CV death, hospitalization for HF, and urgent HF visits.[46] This trial evaluates the effect of SGLT2i on mortality in HFpEF, addressing uncertainties from previous studies like SOLOIST-WHF and EMPEROR-Preserved, which showed benefits primarily in reducing hospitalizations.[47,48] DELIVER is notable for its large sample size and inclusion of diverse EF ranges (41–49%, 50–59%, ≥60%), particularly focusing on patients at the higher end of the EF spectrum. Dapagliflozin was associated with a reduced risk of worsening HF or CV death, fewer incidents of worsening HF and CV deaths, and a lower symptom burden, all without an increase in adverse events. These findings were consistent across all prespecified subgroups, including those categorized by LVEF.[49] The EMPULSE trial's analysis has already suggested the benefits of empagliflozin in acute HF regardless of EF.[37]

The CAMEO-DAPA trial (NCT04730947) was a double-blind study with 46 participants, evaluating the change in pulmonary capillary wedge pressure in patients with EF ≥50, BMI ≥30 kg/m^2, and elevated wedge pressure (≥25 mm Hg) during exercise at baseline. In patients with HFpEF, dapagliflozin treatment lowers resting and exercise pulmonary capillary wedge pressure and has beneficial effects on plasma volume and body weight. These results offer new insights into the hemodynamic benefits of SGLT2i in managing HFpEF.[50]

The SAK HFpEF trial (NCT05138575) is a randomized crossover study with 53 participants, testing whether empagliflozin, alone or with potassium nitrate, improves exercise endurance, muscle oxidative capacity, and perfusion in HFpEF patients. It aims to uncover SGLT2 inhibitors' metabolic impacts on skeletal muscle.[51]

The STADIA-HFpEF trial (NCT04475042) is a quadruple-masked crossover study with 26 participants aimed at exploring the effects of dapagliflozin on LV stiffness in early HFpEF. It will be the first study to assess the direct impact of dapagliflozin on reducing LV stiffness using histological phenotyping to gain a deeper understanding of early HFpEF.[52]

GUIDELINES AND RECOMMENDATION FOR HFpEF

According to the updated 2021 ESC guidelines for HFpEF and the 2022 AHA/ACC/HFSA guidelines, SGLT2i, specifically dapagliflozin or empagliflozin, are recommended to reduce the risk of hospitalizations for heart failure (HHF) or CV death, with a class IA recommendation.[52] The 2023 ACC Expert Consensus also supports the use of SGLT2i for all HFpEF patients, advising that these medications, administered at 10 mg once daily, should be initiated in patients without contraindications, ideally once they are stable during hospitalization for the index event.[53]

CONTRAINDICATIONS

Sodium–glucose cotransporter 2 inhibitors are contraindicated in patients with type 1 diabetes mellitus, lactation, dialysis, and known hypersensitivity. Precautions are necessary for patients with kidney impairment (eGFR <25 mL/min/1.73 m^2 for dapagliflozin, eGFR <20 mL/min/1.73 m^2 for empagliflozin) and during pregnancy. Additional caution is advised for those at an increased risk of mycotic genital infections, volume depletion, hypotension, ketoacidosis (including euglycemic), acute kidney injury, and necrotizing fasciitis of the perineum (Fournier's gangrene), a rare but serious condition.[8]

FUTURE PERSPECTIVES AND CHALLENGES

Treatment challenges persist even when HFpEF is diagnosed, as clinicians must consider comorbidities that impact symptoms and prognosis, utilize nonpharmacological approaches for symptom relief, and implement GDMT to enhance quality of life, reduce hospitalizations for both HF and non-HF conditions, and improve survival rates. Effective management requires multidisciplinary cooperation to deliver high-quality care, and there is a crucial opportunity to re-evaluate the care strategies for individuals with HFpEF given the diagnostic complexities and advancements in treatment.

CONCLUSION

Heart failure with preserved ejection fraction is a growing public health concern marked by elevated LV filling pressures and diastolic dysfunction, despite normal ejection fraction. Its prevalence is rising globally, especially in low-income countries, due to aging populations, comorbidities, and improved diagnostics. Management focuses on comorbidities, nonpharmacological interventions, and symptom relief. SGLT2i like empagliflozin and dapagliflozin have shown promise in reducing hospitalizations and improving symptoms. Empagliflozin's success in the EMPEROR-Preserved trial has led to FDA approval for HFpEF, while dapagliflozin has shown similar benefits. Updated guidelines from the ESC and AHA/ACC/HFSA recommend SGLT2i for reducing hospitalization and CV death in HFpEF patients. Despite this progress, optimizing HFpEF management remains challenging, requiring attention to comorbidities, diagnostics, and multidisciplinary care.

REFERENCES

1. Paulus WJ, Tschöpe C, Sanderson JE, et al. How to diagnose diastolic heart failure: a consensus statement on the diagnosis of heart failure with normal left ventricular ejection fraction by the Heart Failure and Echocardiography Associations of the European Society of Cardiology. Eur Heart J. 2007;28(20):2539-50.
2. Sharma K, Kass DA. Heart failure with preserved ejection fraction: mechanisms, clinical features, and therapies. Circ Res. 2014;115(1):79-96.
3. Borlaug BA, Paulus WJ. Heart failure with preserved ejection fraction: pathophysiology, diagnosis, and treatment. Eur Heart J. 2011;32(6):670-9.
4. Andersen MJ, Borlaug BA. Heart failure with preserved ejection fraction: current understandings and challenges. Curr Cardiol Rep. 2014;16(7):501.
5. Reddy YN, Borlaug BA. Heart failure with preserved ejection fraction. Curr Probl Cardiol. 2016;41(4):145-88.
6. Nassif ME, Windsor SL, Borlaug BA, et al. The SGLT2 inhibitor dapagliflozin in heart failure with preserved ejection fraction: a multicenter randomized trial. Nat Med. 2021;27(11):1954-60.
7. Feng J, Zhang Y, Zhang J. Epidemiology and burden of heart failure in Asia. JACC: Asia. 2024;4(4):249-64.
8. Kittleson MM, Panjrath GS, Amancherla K, et al. 2023 ACC Expert Consensus Decision Pathway on Management of Heart Failure With Preserved Ejection Fraction: A Report of the American College of Cardiology Solution Set Oversight Committee. J Am Coll Cardiol. 2023;81(18):1835-78.
9. Heidenreich PA, Bozkurt B, Aguilar D, et al. 2022 AHA/ACC/HFSA Guideline for the Management of Heart Failure: A Report of the American College of Cardiology/American Heart Association Joint Committee on Clinical Practice Guidelines. Circulation. 2022;145(18):e895-e1032.
10. Borlaug BA. The pathophysiology of heart failure with preserved ejection fraction. Nat Rev Cardiol. 2014;11(9):507-15.
11. Borlaug BA, Redfield MM, Melenovsky V, et al. Longitudinal changes in left ventricular stiffness: a community-based study. Circ Heart Fail. 2013;6(5):944-52.
12. Santos AB, Kraigher-Krainer E, Bello N, et al. Left ventricular dyssynchrony in patients with heart failure and preserved ejection fraction. Eur Heart J. 2014;35(1):42-7.
13. Chen X, Savarese G, Dahlström U, et al. Age-dependent differences in clinical phenotype and prognosis in heart failure with mid-range ejection compared with heart failure with reduced or preserved ejection fraction. Clin Res Cardiol. 2019;108(12):1394-405.
14. Vanderpool RR, Saul M, Nouraie M, et al. Association Between Hemodynamic Markers of Pulmonary

Hypertension and Outcomes in Heart Failure With Preserved Ejection Fraction. JAMA Cardiol. 2018;3(4): 298-306.
15. Gorter TM, Hoendermis ES, van Veldhuisen DJ, et al., Right ventricular dysfunction in heart failure with preserved ejection fraction: a systematic review and meta-analysis. Eur J Heart Fail. 2016;18(12):1472-87.
16. Borlaug BA, Jaber WA, Ommen SR, et al. Diastolic relaxation and compliance reserve during dynamic exercise in heart failure with preserved ejection fraction. Heart. 2011;97(12):964-9.
17. Borlaug BA, Olson TP, Lam CSP, et al. Global cardiovascular reserve dysfunction in heart failure with preserved ejection fraction. J Am Coll Cardiol. 2010;56(11):845-54.
18. Abudiab MM, Redfield MM, Melenovsky V, et al. Cardiac output response to exercise in relation to metabolic demand in heart failure with preserved ejection fraction. Eur J Heart Fail. 2013;15(7):776-85.
19. Stoicescu L, Crişan D, Morgovan C, et al. Heart failure with preserved ejection fraction: the pathophysiological mechanisms behind the clinical phenotypes and the therapeutic approach. Int J Mol Sci. 2024;25(2):794.
20. McDonagh TA, Metra M, Adamo M, et al. 2021 ESC Guidelines for the diagnosis and treatment of acute and chronic heart failure. Eur Heart J. 2021;42(36):3599-726.
21. Bhatia RS, Tu JV, Lee DS, et al. Outcome of heart failure with preserved ejection fraction in a population-based study. N Engl J Med. 2006;355(3):260-9.
22. Yancy CW, Lopatin M, Stevenson LW, et al. Clinical presentation, management, and in-hospital outcomes of patients admitted with acute decompensated heart failure with preserved systolic function: a report from the Acute Decompensated Heart Failure National Registry (ADHERE) Database. J Am Coll Cardiol. 2006;47(1):76-84.
23. Lee DS, Gona P, Vasan RS, et al. Relation of disease pathogenesis and risk factors to heart failure with preserved or reduced ejection fraction: insights from the framingham heart study of the national heart, lung, and blood institute. Circulation. 2009;119(24):3070-7.
24. Lam CSP, Donal E, Kraigher-Krainer E, et al. Epidemiology and clinical course of heart failure with preserved ejection fraction. Eur J Heart Fail. 2011;13(1):18-28.
25. Lam CS. Diabetic cardiomyopathy: an expression of stage B heart failure with preserved ejection fraction. Diab Vasc Dis Res. 2015;12(4):234-8.
26. Kitzman DW, Brubaker P, Morgan T, et al. Effect of Caloric Restriction or Aerobic Exercise Training on Peak Oxygen Consumption and Quality of Life in Obese Older Patients With Heart Failure With Preserved Ejection Fraction: A Randomized Clinical Trial. JAMA. 2016;315(1):36-46.
27. Yeo TJ, Yeo PSD, Wong RCC, et al. Iron deficiency in a multi-ethnic Asian population with and without heart failure: prevalence, clinical correlates, functional significance and prognosis. Eur J Heart Fail. 2014;16(10):1125-32.
28. Packer M. Differential pathophysiological mechanisms in heart failure with a reduced or preserved ejection fraction in diabetes. JACC Heart Fail. 2021;9(8):535-49.
29. Mullens W, Martens P. Empagliflozin-induced changes in epicardial fat: the centerpiece for myocardial protection? JACC Heart Fail. 2021;9(8):590-3.
30. Hallow KM, Gebremichael Y, Helmlinger G, et al., Primary proximal tubule hyperreabsorption and impaired tubular transport counterregulation determine glomerular hyperfiltration in diabetes: a modeling analysis. Am J Physiol Renal Physiol. 2017;312(5):F819-35.
31. Karagodin I, Aba-Omer O, Sparapani R, et al. Aortic stiffening precedes onset of heart failure with preserved ejection fraction in patients with asymptomatic diastolic dysfunction. BMC Cardiovasc Disord. 2017.17(1):62.
32. Mullens W, Martens P. Empagliflozin and renal sodium handling: an intriguing smart osmotic diuretic. Eur J Heart Fail. 2021;23(1):79-82.
33. Lee IH. Mechanisms and disease implications of sirtuin-mediated autophagic regulation. Exp Mol Med. 2019;51(9):1-11.
34. Lopaschuk GD, Karwi QG, Tian R, et al. Cardiac energy metabolism in heart failure. Circ Res. 2021;128(10): 1487-513.
35. Hajjar RJ, Leopold JA. Xanthine oxidase inhibition and heart failure: novel therapeutic strategy for ventricular dysfunction? Circ Res. 2006;98(2):169-71.
36. McNally JS, Saxena A, Cai H, et al. Regulation of xanthine oxidoreductase protein expression by hydrogen peroxide and calcium. Arterioscler Thromb Vasc Biol. 2005;25(8): 1623-8.
37. Kosiborod MN, Angermann CE, Collins SP, et al. Effects of Empagliflozin on Symptoms, Physical Limitations, and Quality of Life in Patients Hospitalized for Acute Heart Failure: Results From the EMPULSE Trial. Circulation. 2022;146(4):279-88.
38. Nassif M, Birmingham MC, Lanfear DE, et al. Recruitment Strategies of a Decentralized Randomized Placebo Controlled Clinical Trial: The Canagliflozin Impact on Health Status, Quality of Life and Functional Status in Heart Failure (CHIEF-HF) Trial. J Card Fail. 2023;29(6):863-9.
39. Sundaresan NR, Vasudevan V, Zhong L, et al. The sirtuin SIRT6 blocks IGF-Akt signaling and development of cardiac hypertrophy by targeting c-Jun. Nat Med. 2012; 18(11): 1643-50.
40. Packer M, Butler J, Zannad F, et al. Effect of Empagliflozin on Worsening Heart Failure Events in Patients With Heart Failure and Preserved Ejection Fraction: EMPEROR-Preserved Trial. Circulation. 2021;144(16):1284-94.
41. FDA grants Jardiance® Breakthrough Therapy designation for heart failure with preserved ejection fraction September 9, 2021. [online] Available from https://investor.lilly.com/news-releases/news-release-details/fda-grants-jardiancer-breakthrough-therapy-designation-heart [Last accessed January, 2025].
42. Abraham WT, Lindenfeld J, Ponikowski P, et al. Effect of empagliflozin on exercise ability and symptoms in heart failure patients with reduced and preserved ejection fraction, with and without type 2 diabetes. Eur Heart J. 2021;42(6):700-10.

43. Reddy YNV, Obokata M, Verbrugge FH, et al. Atrial dysfunction in patients with heart failure with preserved ejection fraction and atrial fibrillation. J Am Coll Cardiol. 2020;76(9):1051-64.
44. Dunlay SM, Roger VL, Redfield MM. Epidemiology of heart failure with preserved ejection fraction. Nat Rev Cardiol. 2017;14(10):591-602.
45. Li P, Zhao H, Zhang J, et al., Similarities and differences between HFmrEF and HFpEF. Front Cardiovasc Med. 2021;8:678614.
46. Solomon SD, McMurray JJV, Claggett B, et al. Dapagliflozin in heart failure with mildly reduced or preserved ejection fraction. N Engl J Med. 2022;387(12):1089-98.
47. Bhatt DL, Szarek M, Steg G, et al. Sotagliflozin in patients with diabetes and recent worsening heart failure. N Engl J Med. 2021;384(2):117-28.
48. Anker SD, Butler J, Filippatos G, et al. Empagliflozin in heart failure with a preserved ejection fraction. N Engl J Med. 2021;385(16):1451-61.
49. Solomon SD, Vaduganathan M, Claggett BL, et al., Baseline Characteristics of Patients With HF With Mildly Reduced and Preserved Ejection Fraction: DELIVER Trial. JACC Heart Fail. 2022;10(3):184-97.
50. Borlaug BA, Reddy YNV, Braun A, et al. Cardiac and Metabolic Effects of Dapagliflozin in Heart Failure With Preserved Ejection Fraction: The CAMEO-DAPA Trial. Circulation. 2023;148(10):834-44.
51. ClinicalTrials.gov. Dapagliflozin Evaluation to Improve the LIVEs of Patients With PReserved Ejection Fraction Heart Failure. (DELIVER). [online] Available from https://clinicaltrials.gov/study/NCT03619213 [Last accessed January, 2025].
52. McDonagh TA, Metra M, Adamo M, et al. 2023 Focused update of the 2021 esc guidelines for the diagnosis and treatment of acute and chronic heart failure. Eur Heart J. 2023;44(37):3627-39.
53. American College of Cardiology. 2023 ACC Expert Consensus on Management of HFpEF: Key Points. [online] Available from https://www.acc.org/Latest-in-Cardiology/ten-points-to-remember/2023/04/17/16/40/2023-acc-expert-consensus-on-hfpef [Last accessed January, 2025].
54. Deschaine B, Verma S, Rayatzadeh H. Clinical evidence and proposed mechanisms of sodium-glucose cotransporter 2 inhibitors in heart failure with preserved ejection fraction: a class effect? Card Fail Rev. 2022;8:e23.
55. Solomon SD, de Boer RA, DeMets D, et al. Dapagliflozin in heart failure with preserved and mildly reduced ejection fraction: rationale and design of the DELIVER trial. Eur J Heart Fail. 2021;23(7):1217-25.

CHAPTER

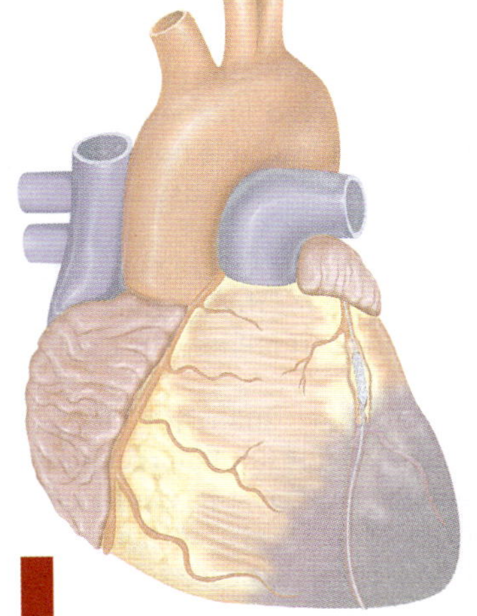

Effect of SGLT2i on Cardiovascular Outcomes and Mortality in Type 2 DM with HFpEF

Namrata Gaur, Dushyant Singh Gaur, Anu Gaur

INTRODUCTION

The sodium-glucose cotransporter-2 (SGLT2) inhibitors are a boon, and a new ray of hope for the treatment of metabolic disease spectrum with the potential to impact maximum lives.

The SGLT2 inhibitors resemble two wonder drugs in medicine which have a universal appeal and have been on top of game.

Metformin has no clear mechanism of action but is beyond question in its efficacy and safety in diabetes.

β-blockers evolved as antihypertensives contra-indicated in setting of heart failure. Later they became a benchmark of care in heart failure.

The SGLT2 as antidiabetic drugs enhance renal glycosuria and reduce glucose levels. FDA mandates all antidiabetic drugs to produce cardiovascular safety evidence before getting approval for clinical use. Surprisingly, SGLT2 inhibitors surpassed all expectations especially in heart failure and chronic kidney disease subsets. It even surpassed status of GLP agonists in atherosclerotic cardiovascular disease population.[1]

Role of SGLT2 inhibitors in heart failure and CKD is beyond expectations in terms of benefits. And benefits occur without much reduction in myocardial infarction and stroke events.

Another striking observation about SGLT2 inhibitors is the equivalence of degree of benefit in all stages of CKD which means that if GFR drops below 30, the glycemic benefits disappear but the cardiovascular benefit is retained indicating a different dose response curve to it.

Effect of SGLT2 inhibitors in suppression of insulin secretion and the increased ketogenesis can cause diabetic ketoacidosis. However, the baseline risk of diabetic ketoacidosis was low across all trails (0.2 per 1,000 patient years in the combined placebo group) and simple measures to stop SGLT2 inhibitors use in patients on insulin or secretagogues if their food intake or medications are altered (e.g., surgery or diarrheal issues) can further mitigate the risk.

The SGLT2 inhibitors can cause dehydration due to natriuretic and diuretic effect and gastrointestinal effects in case of nonselective SGLT2 inhibitors and may require dose adjustments of other diuretic medications.

They have emerged as novel therapy for management of patients with CKD. The efficiency was initially observed in CREDENCE trials which primarily evaluated Reno protective effects of SGLT2 inhibitors. Canaglifozin was found significantly reduce major cardiovascular events in pts with type 2 DM.[1] DAPA CKD in study of heart and kidney patients[2] and EMPA kidney trails demonstrated similar benefits irrespective of DM.[3]

The SGLT2 inhibitors are pioneer metabolic drugs. They may cause a modest decrease in HBA1c, but their cardio protective effects irrespective of DM are very encouraging.

There are many ongoing trials that have demonstrated their cardio protective role but recently their role in heart failure has gained a lot of significance **(Table 1)**.

TABLE 1: Phase III randomized controlled trials with SGLT2 inhibitors.

Study	*Details*	*Primary endpoint*	*Results*
Soloist-WHF	Sotagliflozin versus placebo, $n = 256$, EF ≥50%, with diabetes	Composite of CV death, HHF and urgent HF visits	*HR 0.48; 95% CI (0.27–0.86)
EMPERIAL-Preserved	Empagliflozin versus placebo, $n = 315$, EF >40%, with and without diabetes	Change from baseline in 6MWT	4.0 m; 95% CI (−5.0, 13.0)
EMPEROR-Preserved	Empagliflozin versus placebo, $n = 5,988$, EF >40%, with and without diabetes	Composite of CV death or HHF	*HR 0.79; 95% CI (0.69–0.90)
Preserved-HF	Dapagliflozin versus placebo, $n = 267$, median EF 60%, with and without diabetes	Change from baseline in KCCQ-CS	*5.8 points; 95% CI (2.3–9.2)
CHIEF-HF	Canagliflozin versus placebo, $n = 267$, EF >40%, with and without diabetes	Change from baseline in KCCQ-TSS	*4.5 points; 95% CI (−0.3, 9.4)
ELIVER	Dapagliflozin versus placebo, 6,263 enrolled, EF >40%, with and without diabetes	Composite of CV death, HHF and urgent HF visits	Results pending; estimated completion March 2022

*Significant.

(6MWT: 6-minute walk test; CV: cardiovascular; EF: ejection fraction; HF: heart failure; HHF: hospitalization for heart failure; KCCO-CS: Kansas City Cardiomyopathy Questionnaire-Clinical Summary Score; KCCO-TSS: Kansas City Cardiomyopathy Questionnaire - Total Symptom Score; RCTs: randomized controlled trials)

MECHANISM OF ACTION OF SODIUM-GLUCOSE COTRANSPORTER-2 IN HEART FAILURE WITH PRESERVED EJECTION FRACTION

In the healthy kidney, most filtered glucose is reabsorbed in the proximal tubule by SGLT2 and most filtered sodium is reabsorbed by Na^+/H^+ exchanger 3 (NHE3). SGLT2 colocalizes with NHE3 thereby SGLT2 inhibitor also interferes with the function of NHE3. SGLT2 direct inhibition of SGLT2 and indirect inhibition of NHE3 induces glycosuria, osmotic diuresis, and natriuretic—mechanisms commonly proposed as providing potential benefit in HFpEF.

The glucose lowering and weight loss properties of SGLT2i alone cannot explain the CV benefits seen in HFpEF since glycemic control and other antihyperglycemics that promote weight loss do not appear to decrease CV death or HF hospitalizations in HFpEF.[4]

The osmotic diuresis with resultant free water loss has been projected to explain the beneficial relatively higher interstitial versus intravascular fluid losses with a reduced reflexive neurohormonal activation thought to make SGLT2i unique when compared to conventional diuretic.

The SGLT2i induced osmotic diuresis may improve myocardial edema by increasing plasma oncotic pressure and stimulating plasma refill, thereby pulling fluid from the cardiac interstitium through Starling's forces. A reduction in myocardial edema is associated with rightward shift in end diastolic pressure volume relationship with decrease left ventricular mass on cardiac magnetic resonance and may be contributing in the early improvement of functional status demonstrated by PRESERVED and CHIEF-HF trails, and may also partly explain EMPEROR-preserved reaching significance in just 18 days with a reduction in worsening HF events. SGLT2i are novel because the fluid response can vary depending on the baseline volume status of the patient with less extracellular fluid loss in patients without fluid retention, potentially helping maintain a suitable body fluid status with lower risk of volume depletion.

The SGLT2i induced natriuresis via inhibition of NHE3 which is up regulated in HF and implicated in diuretic resistance may explain the reduced need for increasing outpatient diuretic therapy demonstrated in EMPEROR preserved trail. Natriuresis may also be partly responsible for the reduced progression of kidney disease seen in people with diabetes, by increasing the sodium load to the macula densa with a resultant afferent arteriolar constriction and reduced glomerular hyperfiltration via tubule-glomerular feedback.

SGLT2i (dapaglifozin) are also displaying prevention against the progression of chronic kidney disease in people without diabetes.[5] Thus by kidney protection, cardiac benefit is conferred indirectly but this is speculative. Progression and symptoms of HFpEF may also reduce due to long-term negative sodium balance associated with natriuresis, which reduces aortic stiffness.

The SGLT2i induced natriuresis and diuresis may partly explain the reduced hospitalization and the easing of symptoms and physical limitations seen in HFpEF patients. But evidence suggests that SGLT2i mechanisms acting more directly on the heart may also play a significant role in their CV protection.

The SGLT2i activate sirtuins, reduce epicardial adipose tissue and its associated pro inflammatory adipokines, promote cardio myocyte sodium and calcium homeostasis and relieve the right ventricle of pulmonary hypertension.

The SGLT2i create a "starvation" kind of state through glycosuria and calorie loss. Nutrient deprivation activates proteins called sirtuins (SIRT1, SIRT3, and SIRT6).[6] Sirtuins are NAD dependent deacetylases involved in regulating autophagy. Metabolism and mitochondrial function thereby helping to alleviate cellular stress and inflammation. Autophagy protects the cells from oxidative stress which is dysfunctional in the hearts of patients with HFpEF.[7]

Increase in sirtuin activity are complex but there may be relationship between nutrient deprivation and a rise in NAD levels that activate sirtuins. Patients with HFpEF have reduced availability of NAD and impaired actions of SIRT1, SIRT3, and SIRT6. SGLT2i induce abundance and activity of SIRT1, SIRT3, and SIRT6 in numerous tissues and this may be the reason behind their clinical benefits in HFpEF.

The SGLT2i inhibition of NHE1 in the heart either directly or indirectly produces cardio protective effect. Enhanced activity of NHE1 has been noticed in patients with HFpEF such as pressure overload and hypertensive hypertrophy. Studies show that dapaglifozin corrects diastolic dysfunction possibly by its effect on coronary endothelium. Empaglifozin has also shown to modulate cardio myocyte stiffness.[8]

Similarly, pulmonary artery vasculature may be affected thus reducing pulmonary hypertension SGLT2i act just such as sodium nitroprusside and relax pulmonary vasculature in a dose dependent manner.

Thus SGLT2i mechanism of action has multiple pathways and benefits. It is a complex mechanism and needs further evaluation through long-term follow-up although presently the reports are very encouraging.[9]

SODIUM-GLUCOSE COTRANSPORTER-2 IN HEART FAILURE

Heart failure is a significant health issue affecting millions of people worldwide. Current HF prevention guidelines recommend aggressive management of risk factors including treatment of asymptomatic left ventricular dysfunction (with angiotensin converting enzyme inhibitors (ACEis) hypocholesterolemia (with statins) and hypertension [with diuretics, ACEis, and angiotensin receptor blockers (ARBs)], smoking cessation, and reduction of alcohol intake. Effective treatment options are limited for HFpEF.

Several CV outcome trials have focused on glucose lowering therapies and their impact on CV outcomes.[10] SGLT2i have demonstrated beneficial effects on CV outcomes in long-term studies of patients with type-2 DM with established CV disease and/or a broad range of CV risk factors.

Recent studies have extended these findings to patients with HF, with and without type-2 DM and found SGLT2i are effective therapeutic interventions for the treatment and prevention of HF.[11]

Dapaglifozin was the first to receive US FDA approval for treatment of HF, to reduce the risk of CV deaths and hospitalization.[12] Recently, FDA has also approved empaglifozin for this indication. EMPEROR-PRESERVED study of empaglifozin in patients with HFpEF has shown promise on the utility of SGLT2i.[13]

As with general CV and renal effects, the beneficial effects of SGLT2i on HF outcomes specifically are thought to be due to nonglycemic mechanisms. The cardio protective effects of SGLT2i have been in part attributed to SGLT2i associated reductions in proximal renal tubule burden and central sympathetic over activity. A mild ketosis also contributes to a reduction in sympathetic tone; decreased sympathetic outflow from the brain to kidney alters the pressure natriuresis relationship with more renal excretion of sodium and water at a given pressure, thereby improving fluid retention SGLT2i may also modulate the renal renin angiotensin system and attenuate renal neprilysin activity. There is growing evidence that SGLT2i can be used safely as a complementary therapy to existing guidelines.

EMPEROR-PRESERVED study has shown that role of empaglifozin in HFpEF is encouraging with or without DM.

A therapeutic framework considering DM and CV risk factors would be an effective tool to guide therapy. A disease management approach has been proposed as a framework for guiding cardiologists through patient selection, initiation of SGLT2i therapy, and long-term

TABLE 2: Completed and ongoing studies involving sodium-glucose cotransporter-2 (SGLT2) inhibitors on heart failure.

	Trial Name (Date published)							
	EMPA-REG OUTCOME (2015)	*Canvas (2017)*	*DECLARE-TIMI 58 (2019)*	*VERTIS CV (2020)*	*DAPA-HF (2019)*	*EMPEROR-Reduced (2020)*	*SOLOIST-WHF (2021)*	*EMPEROR-Preserved (2021)*
Focus of trial	CV outcomes	CV outcomes	CV outcomes	CV outcomes	HF outcomes	HF outcomes	HF outcomes	HF outcomes
Interventions	Empagliflozin Placebo	Canagliflozin Placebo	Dapagliflozin Placebo	Ertugliflozin Placebo	Dapagliflozin Placebo	Empagliflozin Placebo	• Sotagliflozin • Placebo	• Empagliflozin • Placebo
Population	Patients with T2D and CVD (n = 7,020)	Patients with T2D and with or at risk of CVD (n= 10,142)	Patients with T2D and with or at risk of CVD (n = 17,160)	Patients with T2D and CVD (n = 8,246)	Patients with NYHA class II–IV HFrEF (n = 4,744)	Patients with NYHA class II–IV HFrEF (n = 3,730)	Patients with T2D, hospitalized forsigns/symptoms of HF and treated with IV diuretic (n = 1,222)	Patients with NYHA class II–IV HFpEF (n = 5,988)
Median follow-up	3.1 years	126.1 weeks	4.2 years	3.0 years	18.2 months	16 months	9 months	26.2 months
History of CVD, n (%)	6,964 (99.2)	6,656 (65.6)	6,974 (40.6)	8,246 (100)	2,674 (56.3)	1,929 (51.2)	NR	2,117 (35.4)
History of HF, n (%)	706 (10.1)	1,461 (10.4)	1,742 (10)	1,958 (23.7)	4,744 (100)	3,730 (100)	1,222 (100)	5,987 (100
Outcomes (HR, 95% CI)								
MACE	0.86 (0.74–0.99)	0.86 (0.75–0.97)	0.93 (0.84–1.03)	0.97 (0.85–1.11)	NR	NR	NR	NR
CV death/HHF	0.65 (0.50–0.85)	0.78 (0.67–0.91)	0.83 (0.73–0.95)	0.88 (0.75–1.03)	0.75 (0.65–0.85)	0.75 (0.65–0.86)	NR	0.79 (0.69–0.90)
HHF	0.65 (0.50–0.85)	0.67 (0.52–0.87)	0.73 (0.61–0.88)	0.70 (0.54–0.90)	0.70 (0.59–0.83)	0.69 (0.59–0.81)	NR	0.71 (0.60–0.83)
CV death	0.62 (0.49–0.77)	0.87 (0.72–1.06)	0.98 (0.82–1.17)	0.92 (0.77–1.11)	0.82 (0.69–0.98)	0.92 (0.75–1.12)	0.84 (0.58–1.22)	0.91 (0.76–1.09)
Worsening HF/CV death	NR	NR	NR	NR	0.74 (0.65–0.85)	NR	NR	NR
Deaths from CV causes, HHF, and urgent visits for HF	NR	NR	NR	NR	NR	NR	0.67 (0.52–0.85)	NR
Deaths from CV causes, HHF, and urgent visits for HF/HF events during hospitalization	NR	NR	NR	NR	NR	NR	0.68 (0.54–0.86)	NR
Death from CV causes/HHF/ nonfatal MI/nonfatal strokes	NR	NR	NR	NR	NR	NR	0.72 (0.56–0.92)	NR
HHF and urgent visits for HF	NR	NR	NR	NR	NR	NR	0.64 (0.49–0.83)	NR

(CV: cardiovascular; CVD: Cardiovascular disease; HFrEF: Heart failure with reserved ejection fraction; HF: heart failure; T2D: Type-2 diabetes) monitoring of patients. Another practical consideration for introducing SGLT2i therapy in HF patients is the potential for SGLT2i related adverse events.

Genitourinary infections are mild and treatable, but there are rare yet serious adverse events that should be kept in mind while initiating therapy in patients with comorbidities and concomitant medications. These are diabetic ketoacidosis, renal injury, volume depletion, and lower limb amputation.

SCORED trail of sotaglifozin has shown some significant adverse events like diarrhea, genital mycotic infections, volume depletion, and DKA.

The use of SGLT2i as sole therapy has not been associated with hypoglycemia but its combination with insulin and insulin secretagogues (e.g., sulfonylurea has the risk). There was a concern about SGLT2i causing hypoglycemia in nondiabetic patients but so far evidence suggests no major hypoglycemia risk. Also DKA is not seen in patients without DM and in diabetic patients too it is a rare event.[14]

Insulin/pancreatic deficiency, low carbohydrate intake, postoperative stress, and excessive alcohol intake can cause DKA in DM patients on SGLT2i. Additionally, possibility of euglycemic DKA should also be kept in mind where sugar is normal but urine and serum has ketones.

Thus, treating physicians must do a risk assessment and identification of patients at low risk before initiating SGLT2i therapy. Regular follow-ups and careful monitoring is required to avoid any adverse event. Patients with multiple comorbidities will need SGLT2i with other CV therapy. There are very few reported drug interactions with SGLT2i.

Patients may require dose adjustment while they are on combination therapy of SGLT2i and diuretics and ARNI.[15]

In spite of encouraging results and growing evidence, there are still knowledge gaps in assessment of SGLT2i for HF therapy. The effect of SGLT2i in HFrEF and HFpEF need further clarification.

Historically treatments that have shown efficacy in HFrEF have not been effective in HFpEF. There are multiple pathways involved in mechanism of disease in HFrEF and HFpEF and they need to be studied to be clarified to develop a treatment and dosage strategy.

HFpEF is a distinct entity, where LV wall thickness increases, with increased LA size as a sign of increased filling pressures as well as diastolic dysfunction.

Diabetic patients with HFpEF have a higher risk of mortality, hospitalization, and CV events compared to nondiabetic patients. SGLT2i reduced overall risk of mortality but with no significant difference between HFrEf and HFpEF.

However, a meta-analysis of eight studies concluded that SGLT2i have an affinity for lowering risk of CV events in patients with HFpEF.

There are ongoing randomized trials that aim to further clarify these unsolved queries. Clinicians need evidence based options when considering use of SGLt2i for patients with HF. There is a need of long-term study as evidence for their safety in patients with HF but all trials have been short term (medium follow-up of 26 months) compared to trails on SGLT2i and DM patients (median follow-up of 4.2 years).

Additional evidence through ongoing trails is needed to consolidate the beneficial effects of SGLT2i in patients with HF irrespective of DM as well as demonstrating that SGLT2i are effective in both HFpEF and HFrEF **(Table 2)**.

CONCLUSION

The SGLT2i are hailed as blockbusters in the management of patients with DM and their role in management of heart failure has been very encouraging as per recent data.

The limitation is that most of studies need a follow-up on human beings and the cost of medication may compel the patient to drop out of study or not take the medication regularly due to finance constraints.

The treating physician needs to make customized plan for patients and switch over to newer regime should be monitored closely and counseling the patient about possible dehydration, volume depletion, genital and urinary infections is important.

A multidisciplinary approach with cardiologists, nephrologists, diabetologist, nutritionists, physician, matters. The patient needs to understand the treatment benefits and side effects to help them continue the regime.

Heart failure with preserved ejection fraction is a complex condition and needs attention especially in diabetic patients.

The SGLT2i show a lot of promise and hopefully will bring in the much needed change in cardiovascular disease management in patients with DM.

REFERENCES

1. Arnott C, Li Q, Kang A, et al. Sodium-glucose cotransporter 2 inhibitor for the prevention of cardiovascular events in patients with type 2 diabetic mellitus: a systematic review and Meta-Analysis. J Am Heart Assoc. 2020;9:e014908.
2. Petrie MC, Verma S, Docherty KF, et al. Effect of Dapagliflozin in worsening heart failure and cardiovascular death in patients with heart failure with or without diabetes. JAMA. 2020;323(14):1353-68.
3. Verma S, Mazer CD, Yan AT, et al. Effect of Empagliflozin on Left Ventricular Mass in Patients With Type 2 Diabetes

Mellitus and Coronary Artery Disease: The EMPA HEART CardioLink-6 Randomised Clinical Trial. Circulation. 2019;140(21):1693-702.

4. Lu Y, Li F, Fan Y, et al. Effect of SGLT2i on cardiovascular outcomes in heart failure patients: a meta-analysis of randomized controlled trails. Euro J Intern Med. 2021; 87:20-8.
5. Solini A, Giannini L, Seghieri M, et al. Dapaglifozin acutely improves endothelial dysfunction reduces aortic stiffness and renal resistive index in type 2 diabetic patients: a pilot study. Cardiovasc Diabetol. 2017:16(1):138.
6. Packer M. Do sodium-glucose-transporter-2 inhibitors prevent heart failure with a preserved ejection fraction by counterbalancing the effects of leptin? A novel hypothesis. Diabetes Obes Metab. 2018;20(6):1361-6.
7. Yaribeygi H, Atkin SL, Butler AE, et al. Sodium–glucose cotransporter inhibitors and oxidative stress: an update. J Cell Physiol. 2019;234(4):3231-7.
8. Sattar N, McLaren J, Kristensen S, et al. SGLT2i and cardiovascular events: why did EMPA REG outcomes surprise and what were the likely mechanisms? Diabetologia. 2016;59(7):1333-9.
9. Inzucchi SE, Zinman B, Fitcett D, et al. How Does Empaglifozin Reduce Cardiovascular Mortality, Insights from a Mediation Analysis of the EMPA-REG OUTCOME Trial. Diabetes Care. 2018;41(2):356-63.
10. Wanner C, Lachin JM, Inzucchi SE, et al. Empaglifozin and Clinical Outcomes in Patients With Type 2 Diabetes Mellitus, Established Cardiovascular Disease and Chronic Kidney Disease. Circulation. 2018;137(2):119-29.
11. Rau M, Thiele K, Hartmann NUK, et al. Empaglifozin does not change cardiac index nor systemic vascular resistance but rapidly improves left ventricular filling pressure in patients with type 2 diabetes: a randomized controlled study. Cardiovasc Diabetol. 2021;20(1):6.
12. Kolijin D, Pabel S, Tian Y, et al. Empaglifozin improves endothelial and cardio myocyte function in human heart failure with preserved ejection fraction via reduced pro-inflammatory–oxidative pathways and protein kinase Gα oxidation. Cradiovasc Res. 2021;117(2):495-507.
13. Sato T, Aizawa Y, Yuasa S, et al. Effect of dapaglifozin treatment on epicardial adipose tissue volume. Cardiovasc Diabetol. 2018;17(1):6.
14. Kappel BA, Lehrke M, Schutt K, et al. Effect of Empaglifozin on the Metabolic Signature of Patients With Type 2 Diabetes Mellitus and Cardiovascular disease. Circulation. 2017;136(10):969-72.
15. Anker SD, Butler J, Filippatos G, et al. Effect of Empaglifozin on Cardiovascular and Renal Outcomes In Patients With Heart Failure by Baseline Diabetes Status: Results From the EMPEROR–Reduced Trail. Circulation. 2021;143(4):337-49.

122

CHAPTER

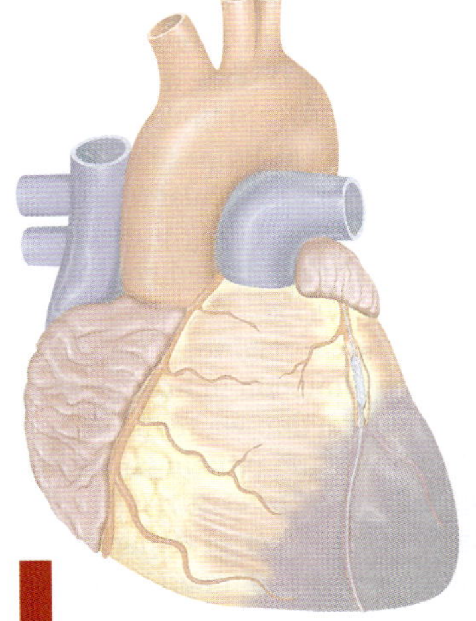

Cardiovascular Outcome Studies with SGLT2 Inhibitors on HFpEF

Neeru Gera, Monashis Sahu

INTRODUCTION

Heart failure (HF) societies have classified HF with respect to ejection fraction (EF) criteria as HF with reduced EF—HFrEF (LVEF <40%), HF with mildly reduced EF—HFmrEF (LVEF = 41–49%), and HF with preserved EF—HFpEF (LVEF >50%). Patients presenting with clinical features of HF and echocardiographic evidence of structural heart disease, especially left atrial enlargement and LVEF >50% are considered to have true HFpEF. Overall prevalence of HF is rising among people with type-2 diabetes and is thought to be primarily driven by HFpEF.

Therapeutically, patients with HFmrEF respond to the four foundational treatments of HF similar to HFrEF. Treatment of HFpEF is an unmet need in cardiovascular (CV) medicine. Recent large randomized controlled trials (RCTs) on SGLT2 inhibitors (SGLT2i), i.e., EMPEROR-Preserved (empagliflozin outcome trial in patients with chronic heart failure with preserved ejection fraction) and DELIVER (Dapagliflozin Evaluation to improve the LIVEs of patients with preserved ejection fraction heart failure) have demonstrated benefits of SGLT2i in the management of HFpEF among people with diabetes as well as nondiabetics.

STUDIES WITH SGLT2 INHIBITORS

Empagliflozin

EMPEROR-Preserved, a large double-blind, parallel-group, placebo-controlled, event-driven study with empagliflozin 10 mg, enrolled 4,005 (67% of total) patients with baseline EF of >50% (n = 2,502 in empagliflozin arm and n = 2,003 in placebo arm) and 1,983 (33% of total) with LVEF of 41–49%. Baseline characteristics of HFpEF patients were mean age of 73 years (range 63.6–82 years), 50% women, mean BMI = 30, history of smoking in 45%, and hypertension in 91% which was also the major (42%) cause for HF. Other comorbidities were diabetes (48%), CKD (55%), anemia (52%), and AF (55%). Patients were predominantly (81%) in NYHA class II with median NT-pro BNP of 946 pg/mL. Majority (81%) of patients were on diuretics (apart from MRA), RAAS blockers (77%), beta blockers (84%), and MRA (33 %). These characteristics were well balanced between empagliflozin and placebo arms and significantly different from HFmrEF patients.[1,2]

Primary composite outcome of cardiovascular death or hospitalization for heart failure (HHF) occurred in lesser number of patients in empagliflozin group as compared to placebo resulting in 17% relative risk reduction (HR 0.83, CI 0.71–0.98, p = 0.024). This outcome was mainly driven by reduction in first HHF (RRR 22%; HR 0.78, CI 0.64–0.95, p = 0.013). Neither cardiovascular death (HR 0.89, CI 0.7–1.13, p = 0.34) nor total mortality (HR 1.02, CI 1.02–1.21, p = 0.84) were affected by empagliflozin. Number needed to treat first HHF over 2.15 years was 44 (CI 24–248) and for total (first and recurrent) HHF was 38 (CI 15–68) with empagliflozin compared to placebo. Empagliflozin cohort had 32% higher chances of improving NYHA class at year 1 (OR 1.32, CI 1.1–1.56, p = 0.0033) and 26% lesser chances of worsening NYHA class at year 1 (OR 0.74, CI 0.54–1.01, p = 0.0606) compared to placebo cohort. However, subgroup with higher LVEF >65–<70% had an attenuated cardiovascular response for primary composite outcome (HR 1.34, CI 0.84–2.12, p = 0.91), first HHF (HR 1.55, CI 1.02–3.2, p = 0.29), and total HHF (HR 1.81, CI 1.02–3.2, p = 0.29).[1-3]

Above were the results in chronic ambulatory HF patients. Combined analysis of HF with EF >40% was also done for hospital care settings. Empagliflozin group was associated with lower risk of any cause of death or HHF (15%, HR 0.85, CI 0.76–0.95, p = 0.005), cardiovascular hospitalization (11%; HR 0.89, CI 0.81–0.98, p = 0.014), any cause hospitalization (8%; HR 0.92, CI 0.85–0.99, p = 0.025), time to first cardiovascular hospitalization (15%, HR 0.85, CI 0.77–0.94, p = 0.002), time to first any cause hospitalization (8%, HR 0.92, CI 0.85–0.99, p = 0.032), total cardiovascular hospitalization (16%, HR 0.84, CI 0.74–0.95, p = 0.005), and total any cause hospitalization (7%, HR 0.93, CI 0.85–1.01, p = 0.1). This lower risk was not associated with longer hospital stays. Time to first statistical significance for the primary endpoint was observed by day 18 with empagliflozin compared to placebo (HR at 18 days: 0.41, 95% CI 0.17–0.99; p=.0476).[4]

Dapagliflozin

DELIVER, a phase 3 multicenter event-driven trial enrolled 6,263 patients randomized to 10 mg dapagliflozin (n = 3,131) and placebo (n = 3,132). Out of total population, 65.9% (n = 2,064) in dapagliflozin arm and 66.6% (n = 2,083) in placebo arm had HFpEF (LVEF >50 %). Proportion of patients having type-2 diabetes was similar in both trial arms (44.7% in dapagliflozin and 44.9% in placebo group). Patients with HFpEF had mean age of ~73 years, 90% had history of hypertension, and 60% had history of AF. Among HFpEF group, 54.4% of patients had LVEF 50–59% and 45.6% had LVEF >60%, with median NT-pro BNP of 1,024 pg/mL and 912 pg/mL, respectively. More than 70% of HFpEF patients were on loop diuretics and beta blockers.[5,6]

The primary composite endpoint, defined as time to first event of worsening HF or CV death occurred significantly lesser in dapagliflozin group with 18% relative risk reduction (HR 0.82, 95% CI 0.73–0.92, p < 0.001), primarily driven due to reduction in worsening of HF, i.e., RRR of 21% in worsening of HF (HR 0.79, 95% CI 0.69–0.91) and 12% RRR in CV death (HR 0.88, 95% CI 0.74–1.05). Presence or absence of diabetes did not impact primary outcome, i.e., 17% RRR among diabetics (HR 0.83, CI 0.70–0.97), and 19% RRR among nondiabetics (HR 0.81, CI 0.68–0.96). There was also no heterogeneity in primary outcome based on baseline LVEF, i.e., 21% RRR among LVEF 50–59% (HR 0.79, CI 0.65–0.97), 22 % RRR among LVEF >60% (HR 0.78, CI 0.62–0.98). There was no observation on any attenuation of benefit with increasing EF in DELIVER, a finding that stands inexplicably in contrast to EMPEROR-Preserved. Time to first nominal statistical significance for the primary endpoint was observed to be as early as 13 days with dapagliflozin treatment (HR 0.45, 95% CI 0.20–0.99, p = .046).[5,7]

A subgroup analysis of DELIVER trial by baseline glycemic status provided further clinical relevance for use of SGLT2i in type-2 diabetes with HFpEF. The reported mean age among diabetes subgroup was 71 years and had median diabetes duration of 9.2 (3.8–17) years. The subgroup analysis reported a higher incidence rate of primary composite outcome among type-2 diabetics versus normoglycemics (10.1 per 100 patient-years in type-2 diabetes subgroup vs. 6.9 per 100 patient-years in normoglycemic subgroup, p < 0.0001 for trend). This translated into higher absolute risk reduction (ARR) of primary outcomes among diabetics subgroup (2·2 per 100 patient-years; numbers needed to treat = 46; HR 0·81, 95% CI 0·69–0·95, log-rank p = 0·0077) compared to normoglycemics (ARR of 1·8 per 100 patient-years; numbers needed to treat = 56; HR 0·77, 95% CI 0·57–1·04, log-rank p = 0·088). Post hoc analysis revealed no heterogeneity in primary outcomes irrespective of duration of diabetes (less than or more than 10 years) or severity of diabetes (HbA1c less or higher than 7.1%).[8]

Sotagliflozin

SOLOIST WHF (Sotagliflozin on Cardiovascular Events in Patients with Type-2 Diabetes Post Worsening Heart Failure Trial), unlike DELIVER and EMPEROR-Preserved enrolled patients only with type-2 diabetes with recent hospitalization for acute decompensated HF. Out of 1,222 patients enrolled, approximately 21% had LVEF >50%. The primary endpoint of total number of CV deaths and hospitalizations and urgent visits of HF was significantly lower with sotagliflozin compared to placebo over a median 9 months follow-up (HR 0.67, 95% CI 0.52–0.85, p < 0.001), without any heterogeneity across prespecified subgroups of baseline LVEF [HR 0.48 (0.27–0.86), for LVEF >50%; HR 0.72 (0.56–0.94), for LVEF <50%).[9]

Pooled data from SCORED (Sotagliflozin on Cardiovascular and Renal Events in Patients with Type 2 Diabetes and Moderate Renal Impairment who are at Cardiovascular Risk) and SOLOIST WHF trial for HFpEF patients (n = 739, median follow up 9 months, all enrolled patients had type-2 diabetes) demonstrated significant reduction of 37% (HR 0.63, CI 0.45–0.89, p = 0.009) in composite end point of cardiovascular mortality, total HHF, or urgent visits for HF.[10]

Pooled Analysis of SGLT2 Inhibitors in HFpEF

A meta-analysis based on HFpEF RCTs (where HF was diagnosed based on clinical examination, biochemistry, and echocardiography) and CVOTs (where HF diagnosis was based on medical history only) was performed.

This included 14,034 patients from three HF-RCTs (EMPEROR Preserved, DELIVER, SOLOIST-WHF) and four CVOTs (EMPA-REG, DECLARE TIMI 58, VERTIS-CV, SCORED). SGLT2i reduced the risk of cardiovascular death or HHF in all RCTs pooled together (HR 0.75, 95% CI 0.63–0.89, NNT 19), in HF-RCTs (HR 0.71, 95% CI 0.52–0.97, NNT 13), and CVOTs (HR 0.78, 95% CI 0.60–0.99, NNT 26). SGLT2i also decreased the risk of HHF in all RCTs (risk ratio 0.81, 95% CI 0.73–0.90, NNT 45), in HF-RCTs (risk ratio 0.81, 95% CI 0.72–0.93, NNT 37), and in CVOTs (risk ratio 0.78, 95% CI 0.61–0.99, NNT 46). There was no benefit of SGLT2i compared to placebo for cardiovascular death or all-cause death in all RCTs, HF-RCTs, or CVOTs. Further the type of RCT (HF-RCT vs. CVOT) did not influence the SGLT2i effect.[11]

Although there was an attenuation of observed benefit in EF >65% at EMPEROR-Preserved; however, in a pooled analysis of EMPEROR-Preserved and DELIVER comprising 12,251 participants wherein approximately half of trial patients had type-2 diabetes, there was no change in HR for primary outcome as per EF status (HR 0·78, 95% CI 0·67–0·90 for LVEF <50%; HR 0·79, 95% CI 0·68–0·93 for LVEF 50–59%, and HR 0·81, 95% CI 0·69–0·96 for LVEF >60%).[12]

CONCLUSION

Prevalence of HFpEF is increasingly becoming more prevalent than other forms of HF in type-2 diabetes mellitus. The serendipitous observation of benefit with SGLT2i in reducing HHF from initial CVOT, and further, in trials of HFrEF, led to the design of well powered CV outcome studies in HFpEF. Till date, only two CV outcome studies with SGLT2i in the setting of HFpEF have been carried out, namely, EMPEROR-Preserved with empagliflozin and DELIVER with dapagliflozin. Both trials had comparable trial population, with similar proportion having type-2 diabetes (approximately 45% in DELIVER and 49% in EMPEROR-Preserved) and approximately two-thirds having EF >50%. Both trials demonstrated clear benefits on the reduction of primary composite endpoint (21% RRR in EMPEROR-Preserved and 18% RRR in DELIVER), driven primarily due to reduced HF events. Prespecified analysis in both trials demonstrated significant reduction of primary outcome in HF patients with LVEF >50%. Taking both the trial results into consideration, ESC guidelines updated itself to incorporate the use of SGLT2i (dapagliflozin or empagliflozin) as Class I recommendation in patients with symptomatic chronic HFpEF to reduce the risk of HHF or CV death.[13]

All CV outcome studies in HFpEF conducted till date had also people with HFmrEF, and analysis in diabetes with HFpEF remains a subgroup analysis, thus marking a need for future CV outcome studies for assessment of outcomes in exclusive population of type-2 diabetes with symptomatic HF and preserved ejection fraction.

REFERENCES

1. Anker SD, Butler J, Filippatos G, et al. Empagliflozin in heart failure with a preserved ejection fraction. New Eng J Med. 2021;385:1451-61.
2. Anker SD, Butler J, Usman MS, et al. Efficacy of empagliflozin in heart failure with preserved versus mid-range ejection fraction: a pre-specified analysis of EMPEROR-Preserved. Nat Med. 2022;28(12):2512-20.
3. Butler J, Packer M, Filippatos G, et al. Effect of empagliflozin in patients with heart failure across the spectrum of left ventricular ejection fraction. Eur Heart J. 2022;43(5):416-26.
4. Packer M, Butler J, Zannad F, et al. Effect of Empagliflozin on Worsening Heart Failure Events in Patients With Heart Failure and Preserved Ejection Fraction: EMPEROR-Preserved Trial. Circulation. 2021;144(16):1284-94.
5. Solomon SD, McMurray JJV, Claggett BL, et al. Dapagliflozin in Heart Failure with Mildly Reduced or Preserved Ejection Fraction. N Eng J Med. 2022;387:1089-98.
6. Solomon SD, Vaduganathan M, Claggett BL, et al. Baseline Characteristics of Patients with HF With Mildly Reduced and Preserved Ejection Fraction: DELIVER Trial. JACC Heart Fail. 2022;10(3):184-97.
7. Vaduganathan M, Claggett BL, Jhund P, et al. Time to Clinical Benefit of Dapagliflozin in Patients With Heart Failure With Mildly Reduced or Preserved Ejection Fraction: A Prespecified Secondary Analysis of the DELIVER Randomized Clinical Trial. JAMA Cardiol. 2022; 7(12):1259-63.
8. Kato ET, Silverman MG, Mosenzon O, et al. Effect of dapagliflozin on heart failure and mortality in type 2 diabetes mellitus. Circulation. 2019;139(22):2528-36.
9. Bhatt DL, Szarek M, Steg PG, et al. Sotagliflozin in patients with diabetes and recent worsening heart failure. New Engl J Med. 2021;384:117-28.
10. Bhatt, D. Szarek M, Steg G, et al. Benefits of SGLT1/2 inhibition with sotagliflozin in heart failure with preserved ejection fraction. In: The American College of Cardiology (ACC) 70th Annual Scientific Session and Expo Virtual Experience; 2021. [online] Available from https://www.acc.org/~/media/35FE8CDA17FF4648995E0E17021FDB79.pdf [last accessed January, 2025].
11. De Marzo V, Savarese G, Porto I, et al. Efficacy of SGLT2-inhibitors across different definitions of heart failure with preserved ejection fraction. J Cardiovasc Med (Hagerstown). 2023;24(8):537-43.
12. Vaduganathan M, Docherty KF, Claggett BL, et al. SGLT-2 inhibitors in patients with heart failure: A comprehensive meta-analysis of five randomised controlled trials. Lancet. 2022;400:757-67.
13. McDonagh TA, Metra M, Adamo M, et al; ESC Scientific Document Group. 2023 Focused Update of the 2021 ESC Guidelines for the diagnosis and treatment of acute and chronic heart failure. Eur Heart J. 2023;44(37):3627-39.

SECTION 15

HFpEF and Cardiolipidology

123. HFpEF and Cardiolipidology

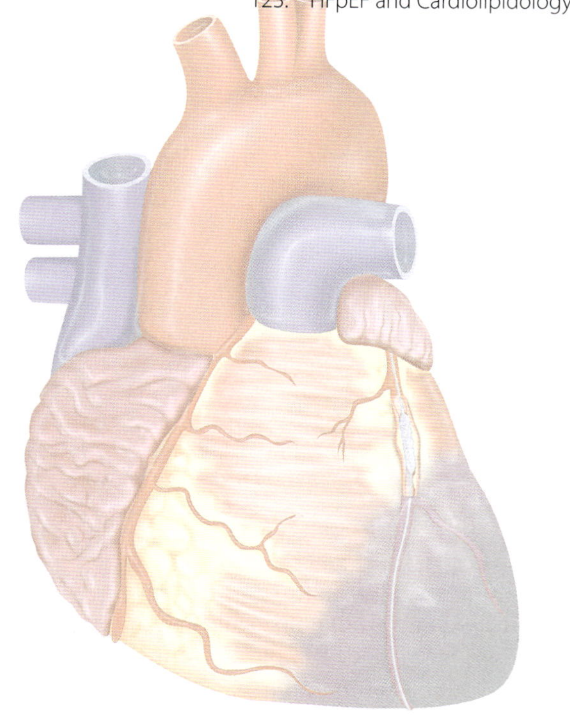

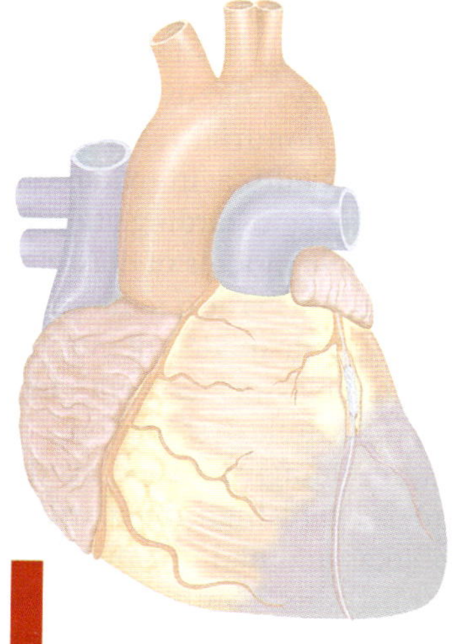

HFpEF and Cardiolipidology

Juhi Singh, Rohan Patel, JPS Sawhney

INTRODUCTION AND PREVALENCE

Heart failure (HF) is defined as a clinical syndrome with symptoms and/or signs (e.g., elevated jugular venous pressure, pulmonary congestion, and peripheral edema) due to structural and/or functional cardiac abnormality resulting in elevated intracardiac pressures and/or inadequate cardiac output at rest and/or during exercise. Based on left ventricular ejection fraction (EF) measurement, HF has been classified into as HF with reduced EF (HFrEF), mildly reduced EF (HFmrEF), and preserved EF (HFpEF) with EF ranges ≤40%, 41–49%, and ≥50%, respectively.[1]

Globally, HF affects >64 million people, thus, a major concern for public health worldwide.[2] With increase in the aging of the population, improved survival following myocardial infarction (MI) and better treatment modalities, there is increase in the prevalence of HF. Due to mortality and morbidity, poor quality-of-life and functional capacity, HF poses a burden on healthcare system.

According to Trivandrum HF registry (THFR) for HF (834 men, 69%) with mean age of 61.2 years, ischemic heart disease (IHD) was the most common etiology of HF in 72% study population.[3] Approximately 26% of the study population was found to have HFpEF, although this figure may be underestimated. Many patients continue to seek care from nephrologists or pulmonologists for their symptoms, as the clinical manifestations of HFpEF, such as dyspnea and fluid retention, are often mistaken for kidney or pulmonary conditions. The registry also noted that HF patients were younger and had a higher prevalence of coronary artery disease (CAD) compared to other populations.

The Asian Sudden Cardiac Death in Heart Failure (ASIAN-HF) registry, comprising 5,000 patients with symptomatic HF (stage C) and left ventricular systolic dysfunction (EF ≤40%), was conducted across 44 centers in 11 Asian regions, including India. The study aimed to assess the mortality and morbidity burden of HF in Asian patients, patients from Southeast Asia (particularly low-income countries with the youngest patients) had the poorest outcomes regardless of LVEF. Ethnic differences revealed a poorer prognosis in Indians, primarily due to a higher burden of diabetes and atherosclerotic vascular disease.[4]

RISK FACTORS ASSOCIATED WITH HEART FAILURE

- *Ischemic heart disease:* The IHD is one of the major risk factors for HF with population-attributable risk around 65% for men and 48% for women.[5] OPTIMIZE-HF registry showed hospitalization in 15% of HF patients was due to IHD and was associated increased risk of mortality following discharge.[6] In another registry, IHD was the primary HF etiology in 49% of patients with HFrEF, 42% in HFmrEF, and 24% in HFrEF.[7] In the ASIAN-HF registry showed that ischemic etiology was more common in Southeast Asia (62%) as compared to South Asia (35%) and Northeast Asia (30%) and in HFrEF than HFpEF.[8]

  Risk factors for IHD such as obesity and dyslipidemia (81.2%) is on rise in India as per the recent Indian Council of Medical Research–India Diabetes (ICMR-INDIAB) study.[9]

High prevalence rates of both generalized (28.6%) and abdominal obesity (39.5%) were observed in urban areas compared with rural areas. The prevalence of hypertriglyceridemia and low HDL cholesterol was high in all the regions of India.

- *Age:* Age is another most important risk factor for development of HF of any type. In a UK based study, 20% of the community surveyed were above 65 years of age had 80% of incident HF.[10] In India, the prevalence of old age >65 years is about 5.5% or about 70 million individuals.[11]
- *Hypertension:* Overall, hypertensive heart disease is the HF etiology in 15% of the population.[12] In hypertension was a leading cause for HF in 17%, 22%, and 31% of patients with HFrEF, HFmrEF, and HFrEF, respectively in OPTIMIZE-HF registry.[6] The prevalence of hypertension was 35·5% which was higher in urban areas and among males as per ICMR-INDIAB study.[9]
- *Diabetes mellitus:* Diabetes is another important risk factor for HF with an estimated prevalence of 30% in patients with HFrEF and HFpEF.[13] In India overall weighted prevalence of diabetes was 11.4% as per ICMR-INDIAB study, with significantly higher prevalence in urban compared with rural areas.[9]
- *Chemotherapy and radiotherapy induced cardiomyopathy:* Radiotherapy and chemotherapy, particularly with anthracyclines, can lead to long-term cardiovascular (CV) complications, including HF with acute toxicity occurring in about 1% of cases (usually reversible) while chronic toxicity can affect up to 7.1% of patients and is often irreversible.[14,15] Additionally, up to 10% of patients receiving radiotherapy may develop HF, and 64% of women who undergo thoracic radiation for breast cancer are at risk of developing HFpEF.[16]

LIPID AND HEART FAILURE

As per the recent Indian Council of Medical Research–India Diabetes (ICMR-INDIAB) study of 113,043 individuals (79,506 from rural areas and 33,537 from urban areas), an estimated prevalence dyslipidemia is on the rise (81.2%) as evident from the ICMR-INDIAB study.[9] The prevalence of total cholesterol ≥200 mg/dL ranges from 4.6–7.9% to 45.6–50.3%; LDL cholesterol ≥130 mg/dL from 4.6–6.2% to 46.8–52.1%; triglycerides (TGs) ≥150 mg/dL from 21.2–22.7% to 43.4–47.9%; and low HDL cholesterol ranges from 51.8 to 83.1%.

LIPOTOXICITY AND HEART FAILURE

Heart is a metabolically demanding organ, derives energy (0.5 μmol/g/s of ATP) from oxidative phosphorylation for continuous cardiac contraction. About 70–90% ATP is derived from the oxidation of energy-dense fatty acids (FAs) in the fasted state.[17] In systolic dysfunction and HFrEF, there is reduced mitochondrial respiration along with deceased in myocardial fatty acid oxidation (FAO). However, there is little evidence regarding HFpEF. Studies based on surgical and genetic models of diastolic dysfunction suggest that myocardial FAO is also reduced in HFpEF.[18] Observation study from genetic models of murine obesity and diabetes have shown the association with left ventricle hypertrophy (LVH) and diastolic dysfunction.[19]

Cardiac magnetic resonance imaging based study showed HFpEF patients had 2.3-fold high myocardial lipid content than control subjects and had independent association with diastolic strain rate.[20] Similar studies have shown HFpEF patients have significantly greater intramyocardial fat relative to both non-HF and HFrEF patients that independently correlates with both E:e′ ratio and left atrial volume index, and that women with subclinical HFpEF have greater intramyocardial fat than reference controls.[21] Hence, HFpEF is associated with myocardial lipid accumulation, but could these lipids have a causative role in the pathogenesis of the condition. Thus, myocardial lipid burden is associated with diastolic dysfunction suggesting that myocardial lipotoxicity may be pivotal in the pathogenesis of HFpEF. TGs are relatively inert, thus do not mediate lipotoxicity themselves, but rather it is the accumulation of reactive lipid intermediates such as diacylglycerols (DAG), ceramides, and acylcarnitines that is responsible.

Mechanism underlying the pathogenesis of HFpEF remain contentious, impaired lipid handling, and subsequent lipotoxicity in both cardiomyocytes and coronary ECs play a key role in mediating diastolic dysfunction. Whether lipids drive this phenotype independently of, or synergistically with systemic inflammation is still unknown in the pathogenesis of HFpEF **(Flowchart 1)**.

HEART FAILURE MANAGEMENT

Management of HFpEF includes screening for, and treatment of, etiologies, and CV and non-CV comorbidities is recommended in patients with HFpEF.

As per European Society of Cardiology (ESC) for HF 2023:[22]

- Diuretics are recommended in congested patients with HFpEF.
- Management of hypertension to prevent or delay the onset of HF, and to prevent HF hospitalizations.
- Statins in patients at high risk or with CVD.
- SGLT2 inhibitors (canagliflozin, dapagliflozin, empagliflozin, ertugliflozin, and sotagliflozin) in diabetes at high risk or with CVD.

- Counseling against sedentary habit, obesity, cigarette smoking, and alcohol abuse is recommended to prevent or delay the onset of HF.
- In patients with T2DM and CKD, finerenone is recommended to reduce the risk of HF hospitalization.

MANAGEMENT OF DYSLIPIDEMIA IN HEART FAILURE WITH PRESERVED EJECTION FRACTION

There are no separate guidelines for management of dyslipidemia in HF. Recently, Cardiological Society of India (CSI) has published guidelines for management of dyslipidemia.[23] Risk stratification is important to guide lipid lowering therapy and to identify goals for which five categories has been identified as shown in **Flowchart 2**.

These are:

1. *Low-risk group*—General population without any risk factor.
2. *Moderate-risk group*—Presence of at least one of the standard risk factors such as smoking/tobacco use, hypertension, diabetes, or family history of premature CAD (men <55 and women <60 years).
3. *High-risk group*—Presence of ≥2 risk factors in absence of atherosclerotic cardiovascular disease (ASCVD), chronic kidney disease, long-standing diabetes >10 years, or heterozygous familial hypercholesterolemia (HeFH).
4. *Very high-risk group*—Clinical evidence of ASCVD, atherosclerotic disease in other vascular beds, diabetes >20 years, HeFH with ASCVD, or coronary imaging showing >50% lesion in 2 coronary vessels. ASCVD includes coronary artery, cerebrovascular, and peripheral vascular disease.
5. *Extremely high-risk group*—Individuals with recurrent vascular events and ASCVD with genetic dyslipidemias [FH and High Lp(a)].

- In acute coronary syndrome (ACS) patients, a nonfasting lipid profile is acceptable as the goal is to achieve LDL cholesterol below 55 mg/dL as early as possible **(Flowchart 3)**. High dose of statins with ezetimibe at initiation of treatment is recommended.
- Addition of another non-statin drug if LDL cholesterol target of <55 mg/dL is not achieved at 4 weeks (bempedoic acid, PCSK9 inhibitors, or inclisiran) is recommended.

Flowchart 1: Role of cardiac lipid accumulation in the pathophysiology of heart failure.

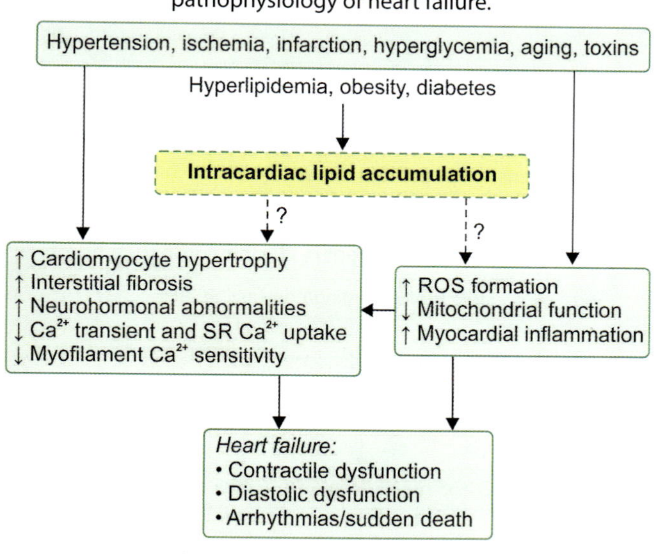

(ROS: reactive oxygen species)

Flowchart 2: Cardiovascular risk estimation and lipid management goals.

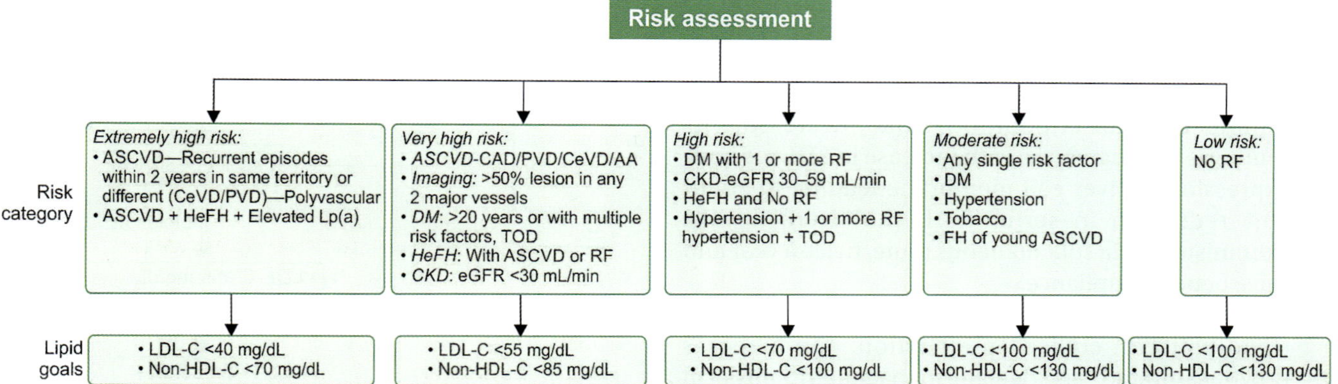

(ASCVD: atherosclerotic cardiovascular disease; CKD: chronic kidney disease; CVD: cardiovascular disease; DM: diabetes mellitus; HeFH: Heterozygous familial hypercholesterolemia; HDL-C: high-density lipoprotein cholesterol; LDL-C: low-density lipoprotein cholesterol; Lp(a): lipoprotein)

Flowchart 3: Lipid management in the setting of acute coronary syndromes (ACS).

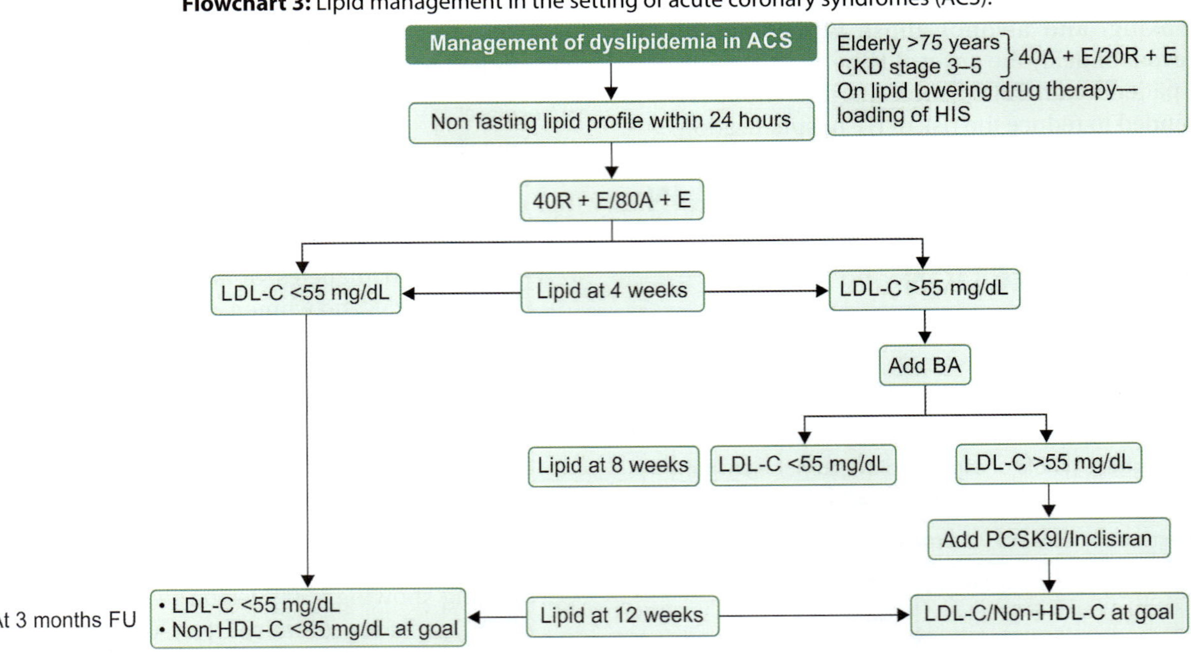

(HDL-C: high-density lipoprotein cholesterol; LDL-C: low-density lipoprotein cholesterol)

- In chronic coronary syndrome (CCS), goal is to achieve LDL cholesterol <55 mg/dL and non-HDL cholesterol <85 mg/dL **(Flowchart 4)**.
- Statins are the drugs of choice for management if dyslipidemias, particularly useful in lowering total and LDL cholesterol and TGs in high dose.
- Newer lipid lowering agents such as ezetimibe, bempedoic acid, PCSK9 (proprotein convertase subtilisin/kexin type 9) inhibitors, and inclisiran can be combined with statins.
- Although, statins are safe and well tolerated, but are associated with (usually reversible) muscle and liver toxicity. Thus, should be promptly detected and treated.
- The statin-ezetimibe combination is recommended to achieve LDL cholesterol target early after acute coronary events and in HeFH as an initial therapy.
- Inclisiran long-acting small interfering RNA (siRNA), inhibits the transcription of PCSK9, decreasing its synthesis in hepatocytes with increase in LDL receptor expression in liver cell membrane leading to about 50% reduction in serum LDL cholesterol levels. Administered via subcutaneous route, twice a year and thus, better compliance.
- Lifestyle management includes dietary habits (food patterns, choices, preparation, and omega-3 polyunsaturated fats), weight management, physical activity (moderate-to-vigorous intensity physical activity for at least 5 days/week to achieve the target of 150 min/week), and yoga practice **(Flowchart 5)**.

Flowchart 4: Lipid management in chronic coronary syndromes.

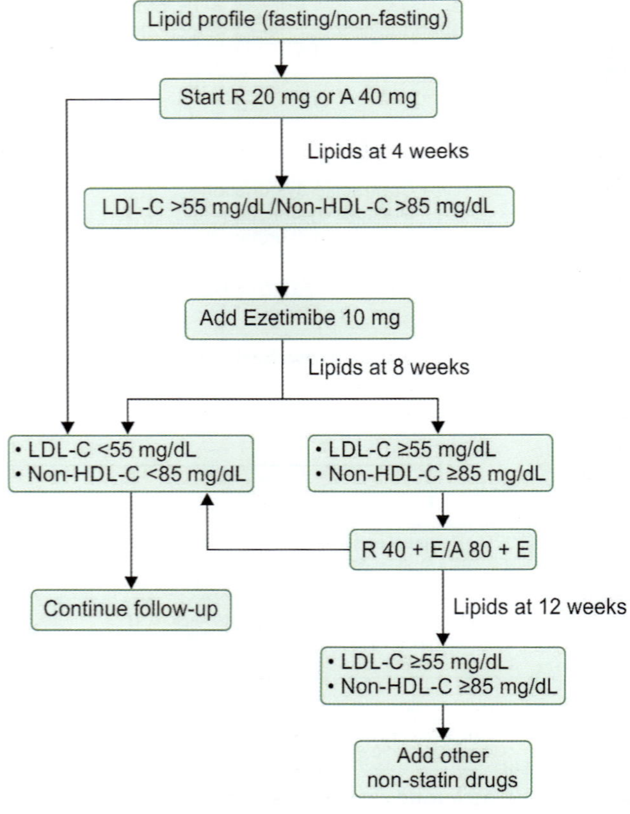

(HDL-C: high-density lipoprotein cholesterol; LDL-C: low-density lipoprotein cholesterol)

Flowchart 5: Management of hypertriglyceridemia.

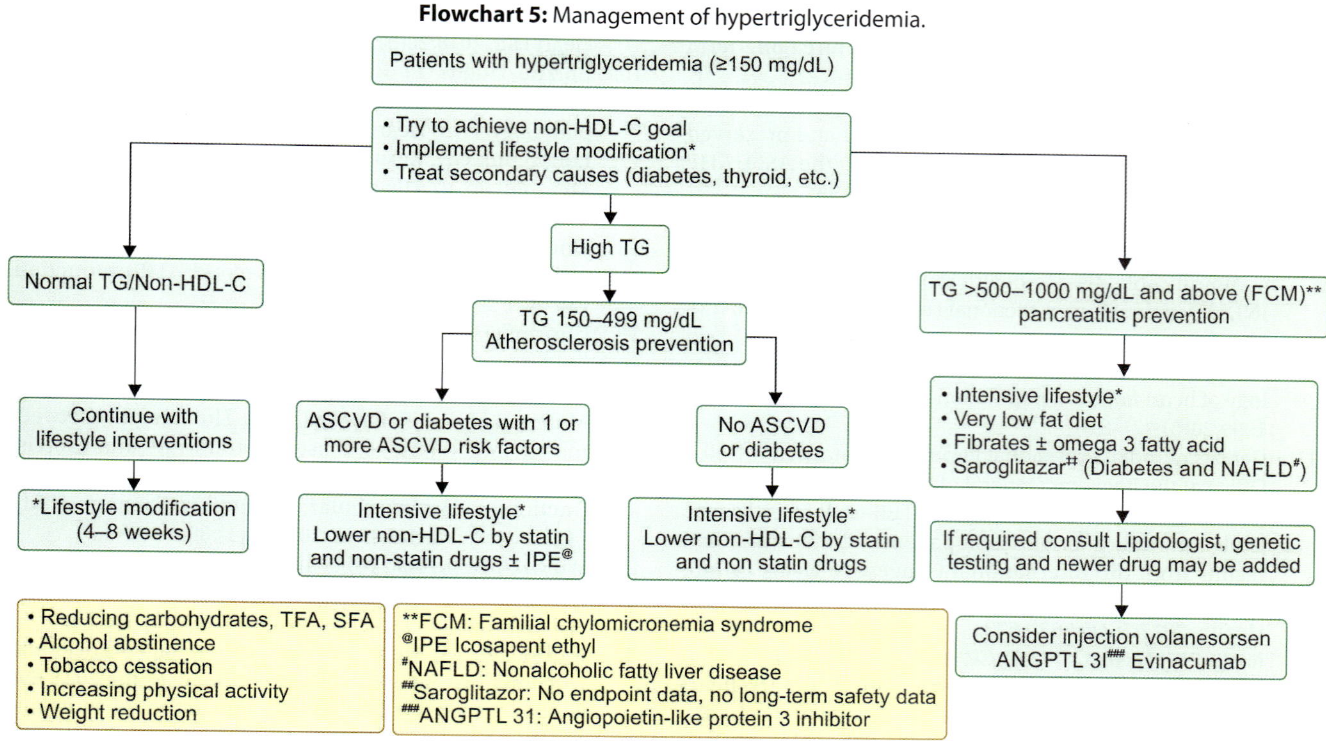

(HDL-C: high-density lipoprotein cholesterol; LDL-C: low-density lipoprotein cholesterol; TFA: transfatty acid; SFA: saturated fatty acid)

CONCLUSION

Heart failure particularly, HFpEF is an emerging public health concern with increasing prevalence due to aging population and CV risk factors. Dyslipidemia contributes to the pathogenesis of HFpEF through myocardial lipotoxicity and diastolic dysfunction, though the precise underlying mechanisms remains unclear. A comprehensive approach targeting risk factors including lifestyle changes, lipid-lowering therapies, and risk stratification, is essential. Further research is needed to understand the role of lipid metabolism and inflammation in HFpEF and develop targeted therapies.

REFERENCES

1. Bozkurt B, Coats AJS, Tsutsui H, et al. Universal definition and classification of heart failure: a report of the Heart Failure Society of America, Heart Failure Association of the European Society of Cardiology, Japanese Heart Failure Society and Writing Committee of the Universal Definition of Heart Failure: endorsed by the Canadian Heart Failure Society, Heart Failure Association of India, Cardiac Society of Australia and New Zealand, and Chinese Heart Failure Association. Eur J Heart Fail. 2021;23(3):352-80.
2. GBD 2017 Disease and Injury Incidence and Prevalence Collaborators. Global, regional, and national incidence, prevalence, and years lived with disability for 354 diseases and injuries for 195 countries and territories, 1990–2017: a systematic analysis for the Global Burden of Disease Study 2017. Lancet. 2018;392(10159):1789-858.
3. Harikrishnan S, Sanjay G, Anees T, et al.; Trivandrum Heart Failure Registry. Clinical presentation, management, in-hospital and 90-day outcomes of heart failure patients in Trivandrum, Kerala, India: the Trivandrum Heart Failure Registry. Eur J Heart Fail. 2015;17(8):794-800.
4. Lam CS, Anand I, Zhang S, et al. Asian Sudden Cardiac Death in Heart Failure (ASIAN-HF) registry. Eur J Heart Fail. 2013;15(8):928-36.
5. Vedin O, Lam CSP, Koh AS, et al. Significance of ischemic heart disease in patients with heart failure and preserved, midrange, and reduced ejection fraction: a nationwide cohort study. Circ Heart Fail. 2017;10(6):e003875.
6. Fonarow GC, Stough WG, Abraham WT, et al; OPTIMIZE-HF Investigators and Hospitals. Characteristics, treatments, and outcomes of patients with preserved systolic function hospitalized for heart failure: a report from the OPTIMIZE-HF Registry. J Am Coll Cardiol. 2007;50(8):768-77.
7. Chioncel O, Lainscak M, Seferovic PM, et al. Epidemiology and one-year outcomes in patients with chronic heart

failure and preserved, mid-range and reduced ejection fraction: an analysis of the ESC Heart Failure Long-term Registry. Eur J Heart Fail. 2017;19(12):1574-85.

8. MacDonald MR, Tay WT, Teng TK, et al. Regional variation of mortality in heart failure with reduced and preserved ejection fraction across Asia: outcomes in the ASIAN-HF registry. J Am Heart Assoc. 2020;9(1):e012199.
9. Anjana RM, Unnikrishnan R, Deepa M, et al.; ICMR-INDIAB Collaborative Study Group. Metabolic non-communicable disease health report of India: the ICMR-INDIAB national cross-sectional study (ICMR-INDIAB-17). Lancet Diabetes Endocrinol. 2023;11(7):474-89.
10. Cowie MR, Wood DA, Coats AJ, et al. Incidence and aetiology of heart failure: a population-based study. Eur Heart J. 1999;20(6):421-8.
11. Census of India. Provisional Population Totals. New Delhi: Office of the Registrar General of India; 2011.
12. Dokainish H, Teo K, Zhu J, et al; INTER-CHF Investigators. Global mortality variations in patients with heart failure: results from the International Congestive Heart Failure (INTER-CHF) prospective cohort study. Lancet Glob Health. 2017;5(7):e665-e672.
13. Rashid M, Kwok CS, Gale CP, et al. Impact of co-morbid burden on mortality in patients with coronary heart disease, heart failure, and cerebrovascular accident: a systematic review and meta-analysis. Eur Heart J Qual Care Clin Outcomes. 2017;3(1):20-36.
14. Bloom MW, Hamo CE, Cardinale D, et al. Cancer therapy-related cardiac dysfunction and heart failure: part 1: definitions, pathophysiology, risk factors, and imaging. Circ Heart Fail. 2016;9(1):e002661.
15. Fornaro A, Olivotto I, Rigacci L, et al. Comparison of long-term outcome in anthracycline-related versus idiopathic dilated cardiomyopathy: a single centre experience. Eur J Heart Fail. 2018;20(5):898-906.
16. Belzile-Dugas E, Eisenberg MJ. Radiation-induced cardiovascular disease: review of an underrecognized pathology. J Am Heart Assoc. 2021;10(18):e021686.
17. Lopaschuk GD, Karwi QG, Tian R, et al. Cardiac Energy Metabolism in Heart Failure. Circ Res. 2021;128(10):1487-513.
18. Doenst T, Nguyen TD, Abel ED. Cardiac metabolism in heart failure: implications beyond ATP production. Circ Res. 2013;113(6):709-24.
19. Christoffersen C, Bollano E, Lindegaard ML, et al. Cardiac lipid accumulation associated with diastolic dysfunction in obese mice. Endocrinology. 2003;144(8):3483-90.
20. Mahmod M, Pal N, Rayner J, et al. The interplay between metabolic alterations, diastolic strain rate and exercise capacity in mild heart failure with preserved ejection fraction: a cardiovascular magnetic resonance study. J Cardiovasc Magn Reson. 2018;20(1):88.
21. Wu CK, Lee JK, Hsu JC, et al. Myocardial adipose deposition and the development of heart failure with preserved ejection fraction. Eur J Heart Fail. 2020;22(3):445-54.
22. McDonagh TA, Metra M, Adamo M, et al.; ESC Scientific Document Group. 2023 Focused Update of the 2021 ESC Guidelines for the diagnosis and treatment of acute and chronic heart failure: Developed by the task force for the diagnosis and treatment of acute and chronic heart failure of the European Society of Cardiology (ESC) With the special contribution of the Heart Failure Association (HFA) of the ESC. Eur J Heart. 2023;44(37):3627-39.
23. Sawhney JP, Ramakrishnan S, Madan K, et al. CSI clinical practice guidelines for dyslipidemia management: executive summary. Indian Heart J. 2024;76(Suppl 1):S6-S19.

SECTION 16

HFpEF and Cardionutrition

124. Iron Deficiency and HFpEF with Atrial Fibrillation
125. Malnutrition and HFpEF
126. Ideal Edible Oil for Heart Health Among Indians

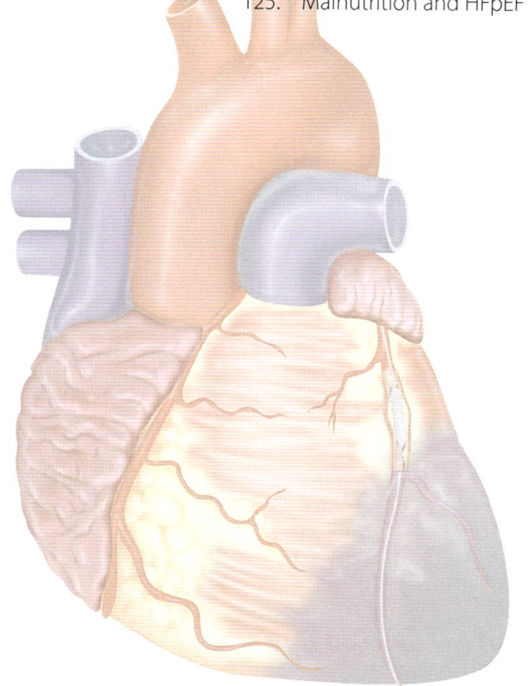

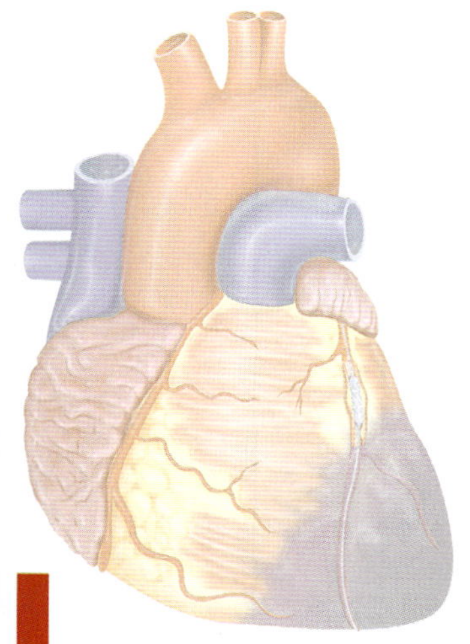

CHAPTER

Iron Deficiency and HFpEF with Atrial Fibrillation

Rabindra Nath Chakraborty, Debopriyo Mondal

INTRODUCTION

Heart failure with preserved ejection fraction (HFpEF) is a complex clinical syndrome characterized by the presence of heart failure (HF) symptoms despite a normal or near-normal left ventricular ejection fraction. HFpEF is increasingly recognized as a major public health issue due to its high prevalence and significant morbidity and mortality rates. The pathophysiology of HFpEF is multifactorial, involving diastolic dysfunction, systemic and pulmonary hypertension, vascular stiffening, and comorbid conditions such as obesity and diabetes.

Atrial fibrillation (AF) frequently coexists with HFpEF, further complicating its management and prognosis. AF is a common arrhythmia that is associated with increased risks of stroke, HF, and mortality. The coexistence of AF and HFpEF presents a therapeutic challenge, as the presence of AF can exacerbate HF symptoms and vice versa.

Iron deficiency (ID) is another prevalent comorbidity in HFpEF that can exacerbate symptoms and outcomes. ID is a common nutritional deficiency that can lead to anemia, but even in the absence of anemia, ID can impair physical performance and quality of life. This manuscript explores the relationship between ID and HFpEF with AF, focusing on the pathophysiological mechanisms, clinical implications, and potential therapeutic strategies.

PATHOPHYSIOLOGY OF IRON DEFICIENCY IN HFpEF WITH ATRIAL FIBRILLATION

Iron plays a crucial role in oxygen transport and energy metabolism.[1] In HFpEF, ID is prevalent due to factors such as inadequate dietary intake, malabsorption, chronic inflammation, and increased hepcidin levels. Hepcidin, a liver-produced hormone, regulates iron homeostasis. Inflammatory conditions, common in HFpEF, can increase hepcidin levels, reducing iron absorption and mobilization.

The AF further complicates iron metabolism by causing rapid atrial rates, which increase metabolic demand and contribute to iron depletion. The increased heart rate in AF leads to higher myocardial oxygen consumption, which can exacerbate the effects of ID. In HFpEF, ID impairs myocardial oxygen delivery, leading to reduced exercise capacity and increased fatigue. Additionally, ID affects skeletal muscle function, contributing to the exercise intolerance often seen in HFpEF patients.

In AF, ID may contribute to arrhythmogenesis through systemic inflammation and altered cardiac electrophysiology. Iron is essential for maintaining the function of iron-containing enzymes involved in cellular respiration and energy production. An ID can lead to oxidative stress and mitochondrial dysfunction, promoting arrhythmias (**Fig. 1**).

CLINICAL IMPLICATIONS

Iron deficiency in HFpEF patients with AF can lead to worsening HF symptoms, reduced exercise capacity, and poor quality of life. It is associated with increased hospitalization rates and mortality. Recognizing and treating ID is vital for improving patient outcomes. Iron supplementation has emerged as a validated therapeutic approach for HF patients with concurrent ID. Up to 50%

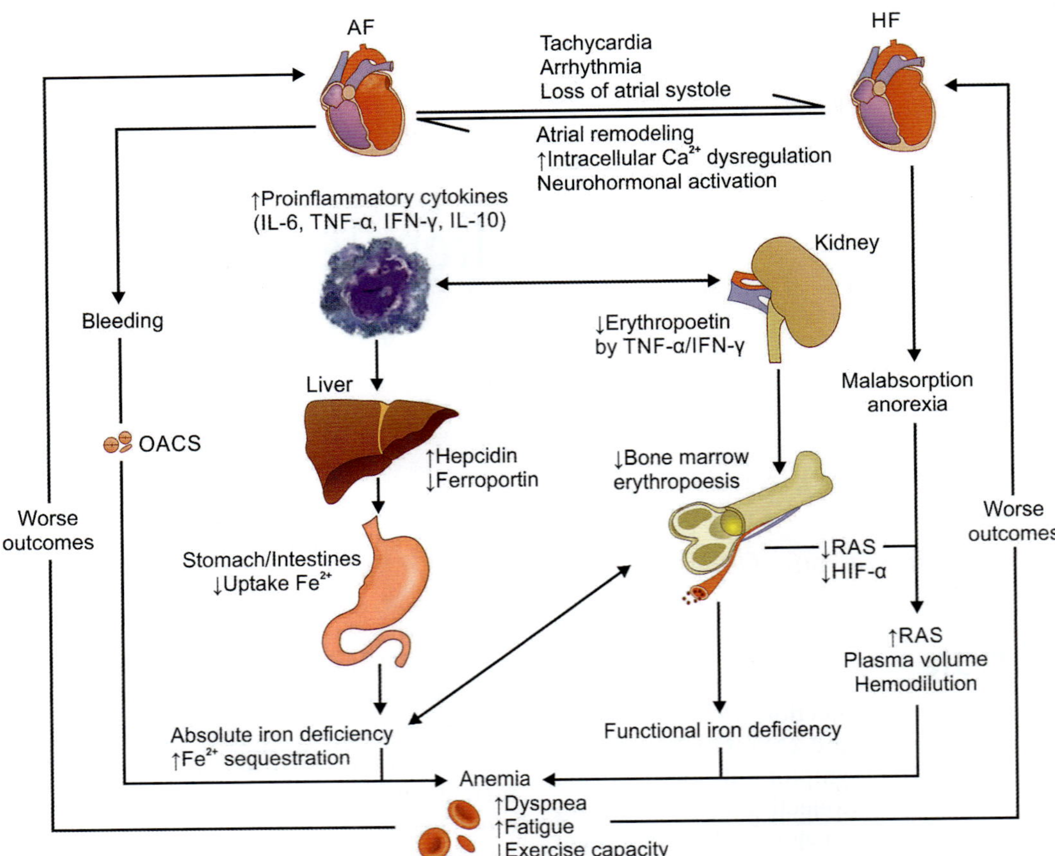

Fig. 1: Potential mechanisms linking atrial fibrillation, heart failure, iron deficiency, and anemia. (AF: atrial fibrillation; HF: heart failure; TNF-α: tumor necrosis factor α; RBC: red blood cell; IFN-γ: interferon γ; DMT-1: divalent metal transporter 1; IL-6/10 interleukin-6/10; RAS: renin angiotensin system; HIF-α: hypoxia-inducible factor α; GI: gastrointestinal; OACS: oral anticoagulants)

of HF patients with reduced ejection fraction (HFrEF) exhibit ID, with even higher prevalence in HFpEF patients, approaching 60%. Notably, this high prevalence persists even without anemia.

While erythropoietin and oral iron have not shown benefit, intravenous iron therapy has consistently yielded positive outcomes. Intravenous iron bypasses the gastrointestinal tract, ensuring better absorption and faster replenishment of iron stores. Clinical trials have demonstrated the efficacy of intravenous iron in improving symptoms and functional capacity in HF patients.

The FAIR-HF trial demonstrated significant improvements in patient global assessment, 6-minute walk test, and quality of life with intravenous ferric carboxymaltose, regardless of anemia status. Similarly, the CONFIRM-HF trial reported enhancements in the 6-minute walk test, NYHA class, patient global assessment, and health-related quality of life with ferric carboxymaltose. The EFFECT-HF trial highlighted the maintenance of peak oxygen consumption in the treatment group versus a decline in controls over 24 weeks. A meta-analysis confirmed that intravenous iron reduces cardiac-related hospitalizations, mortality, and all-cause mortality. The AFFIRM-AHF trial further supported these findings by showing reduced recurrent hospitalizations postdischarge after acute HF with intravenous iron therapy.

DIAGNOSTIC APPROACHES

Diagnosis of ID involves evaluating serum ferritin and transferrin saturation (TSAT) levels. A ferritin level <100 ng/mL or 100–299 ng/mL with TSAT <20% indicates ID. Ferritin is an acute-phase reactant and can be elevated in the presence of inflammation, which is common in HFpEF. Therefore, it is crucial to interpret ferritin levels in conjunction with other markers of iron status.

Additional tests, such as soluble transferrin receptor and hepcidin levels, can provide further insights. Soluble transferrin receptor levels increase in ID and are not affected by inflammation, making them a useful marker

TABLE 1: Diagnostic criteria for iron deficiency in HFpEF with AF.

Parameter	Criteria
Serum ferritin	<100 ng/mL or 100–299 ng/mL with TSAT <20%
Transferrin saturation	<20%
Soluble transferrin	Elevated
Hepcidin	Variable

(AF: atrial fibrillation; HFpEF: heart failure with preserved ejection fraction; TSAT: transferrin saturation)

in this context. Hepcidin levels, although not routinely measured in clinical practice, can help elucidate the underlying cause of ID, particularly in cases of inflammation-induced iron sequestration **(Table 1)**.

THERAPEUTIC STRATEGIES

Iron supplementation, particularly intravenous iron, has shown benefits in HFpEF patients with ID.[2] Studies demonstrate improvements in exercise capacity, quality of life, and reduced hospitalizations. The role of oral iron remains less clear due to variable absorption and gastrointestinal side effects. Oral iron supplementation is often poorly tolerated due to gastrointestinal side effects, such as constipation, nausea, and abdominal pain, which can limit adherence to therapy.

Intravenous iron formulations, such as ferric carboxymaltose and iron sucrose, have been shown to effectively replenish iron stores and improve clinical outcomes in HF patients.[3] The choice of formulation and dosing regimen should be tailored to the individual patient's needs and tolerance.

In clinical practice, it is essential to monitor iron status regularly and adjust therapy accordingly. Follow-up assessments of serum ferritin and TSAT can help guide the duration and intensity of iron supplementation. It is also important to address potential underlying causes of ID, such as gastrointestinal bleeding or malabsorption, to ensure sustained improvement in iron status.

LIMITATION

There is a lack of extensive data on ID in patients with AF. A retrospective study in Turkey analyzed ID in 101 AF patients, finding a 47.6% prevalence using ferritin levels below 100 μg/L or 100–299 μg/L with transferrin saturation below 20%. The prevalence was higher in permanent AF compared to paroxysmal or persistent AF. The study's limitations included small sample size and lack of medication data.

A larger National Inpatient Sample analysis found that 2.5% of hospitalized AF patients had ID anemia, associated with longer hospital stays and worse outcomes, though likely underestimated due to reliance on hospital coding data. These findings highlight the need for more comprehensive studies to better characterize the prevalence and impact of ID in AF and HFpEF patients.

Further studies are needed to evaluate the combined effects and establish optimal treatment protocols. Additionally, long-term safety and efficacy data for intravenous iron therapy are lacking. The potential for iron overload and adverse effects with long-term intravenous iron therapy necessitates careful monitoring and judicious use of this treatment modality.

TABLE 2: Future research directions.

Area	Goals
Incidence and prevalence	Additional studies on the incidence and prevalence of anemia and iron deficiency in different atrial fibrillation (AF) subpopulations, including by age, gender, AF type, anticoagulation use, ethnicity, and setting (outpatient, inpatient)
Symptoms	• Impact of anemia and iron deficiency on AF symptoms • Impact of anemia and iron deficiency on exercise/functional capacity and peak oxygen consumption in patients with AF
Complications	• Confirmation of reported associations of anemia, stroke, and bleeding in patients with AF • Impact of iron deficiency on future complications such as stroke, bleeding, heart failure, and mortality
Pathophysiology	Assessment of iron deficiency and other causes as contributors to anemia in patients with AF
Therapy	Evaluation of investigation and treatment of anemia and iron deficiency in patients with AF

FUTURE RESEARCH DIRECTIONS

- Large-scale epidemiological studies to determine the prevalence of ID in AF and HFpEF patients.
- Randomized controlled trials to evaluate the efficacy and safety of different iron supplementation strategies.
- Long-term follow-up studies to assess the durability of benefits and potential risks associated with intravenous iron therapy.
- Investigations into the underlying mechanisms linking ID, inflammation, and arrhythmogenesis in AF **(Table 2)**.

CONCLUSION

Iron deficiency is a significant comorbidity in HFpEF patients with AF, adversely affecting clinical outcomes. Early diagnosis and appropriate treatment of ID can improve symptoms, exercise capacity, and reduce hospitalizations. Optimizing iron status in these patients represents a valuable therapeutic target that can enhance their quality of life and overall prognosis. Further research is needed to establish comprehensive management guidelines, evaluate long-term outcomes, and identify the most effective and safe iron supplementation strategies for this patient population.

REFERENCES

1. Anker SD, Comin Colet J, Filippatos G, et al. Iron deficiency in heart failure. Lancet. 2009;373(9673):1254-60.
2. Ponikowski P, Mentz RJ, Hernandez AF, et al. Beneficial effects of long-term intravenous iron therapy with ferric carboxymaltose in patients with symptomatic heart failure and iron deficiency. Eur Heart J. 2015;36(11):657-68.
3. van Veldhuisen DJ, Pellicori P, Kalra PR, et al. Intravenous iron in patients with heart failure: an updated review. J Am Coll Cardiol. 2016;68(5):544-55.

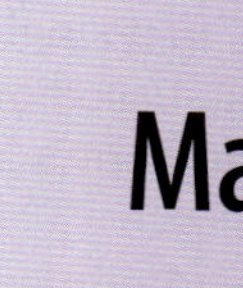

125
CHAPTER

Malnutrition and HFpEF

Preetinder Kaur, Krishna Vaitheeswaran, Monika Nadar

INTRODUCTION

Heart failure with preserved ejection fraction (HFpEF) accounts for over 50% of all heart failure subtypes in the world with over 3 million people being affected in the United States.[1] Today, HFpEF has been accepted as a geriatric syndrome,[2] with mean age of incidence being 76 years[3] and prevalence increasing exponentially with advancing age.[4]

Advancing age also is associated with many comorbid conditions with deficits ranging from cognitive impairment, physical and mobility limitation, and socio-economic isolation.[4] These comorbid conditions may be associated with prognostic associations.[5] In addition, malnutrition has also been shown to be an important detrimental prognostic factor in geriatric patients with HFpEF.[6]

Malnutrition arises from an imbalance of anabolic and catabolic states of metabolism, typically with a protein-calorie deficit.[7] In addition, deficiency of other micro and macro nutrients may also exist, compounding the malinfluence on bodily structure and function.

The etiology of malnutrition may be multifactorial and may not be just a reduced intake. The proposed mechanisms include:

- *Reduced intake:* Socio-economic isolation and hampered self-care due to physical and mobility limitations may reduce the intake in the geriatric population.
- *Decreased absorption:* This may be an age associated reduced function of the GI tract. In addition, in the setting of an HFpEF, there may be intestinal edema which may further impair absorption at multiple levels including active transport of nutrients. The malnutrition itself would further lead to further reduction in the processes of active and passive intestinal transport.
- Cytokine dysregulation
- Abnormal internal milieu resulting from alterations in the regulatory loops involving cortisol, renin, angiotensin, aldosterone, epinephrine, and tumor necrosis factor alpha.[8]

The effects of malnutrition are well known in the general geriatric population and may involve loss of muscle mass, adipose tissue, and bone mass affecting adversely in turn metabolic processes as well as predisposing to adverse events with clinical outcomes involving increased mortality and morbidity.[9]

In patients with heart failure and reduced ejection fraction (HFrEF), epidemiological data has revealed that malnutrition may onset simultaneously with heart failure. The blood stasis in congestive heart failure (CHF) in the systemic and pulmonary circulation, slows gastrointestinal peristalsis, reduces digestive enzymes, and enhances the metabolism due to cytokine release further giving rise to dystrophic absorption. Despite being in state of high catabolism due to the underlying heart failure, the intake is reduced giving rise to a worsening clinical prognosis. According to reports, the all-cause mortality rate of malnutrition within 12 months is 5.0–30.0%, and the 1-year hospitalization rate is 18.9–65.0%.[10]

In patients with HFpEF, the data was less clear due to divergent results reported by various authors. In a subgroup analysis of the Aldosterone Antagonist Therapy for Adults with Heart Failure and Preserved Systolic Function (TOPCAT) trial, malnutrition, based on the Geriatric Nutritional Risk Index (GNRI) criteria, was found to be associated with a myriad of adverse outcomes including cardiovascular death, all-cause death, hospitalization for any reason, and hospitalization for noncardiovascular reasons over a 3-year follow-up.[11] Meanwhile, in a single center study from Spain (n = 555), malnutrition, based on the MNA-SF, was not associated with adverse outcomes at 2 years.[12]

The data examined by Zainul et al. showed clinical outcomes similar to that seen in HFrEF.[13] The differences reported in previous studies were probably due to the different scoring systems used by different authors as well as interventional confounding effects due to nutritional counselling and support seen in various countries and regions for the geriatric population. They reported a prevalence of malnutrition of 42% (n = 97). The MNA-SF scores did not significantly correlate with body mass index (R = –0.02, p = 0.71).

At the 6-month follow-up in this study, 62 patients (26.8%) were hospitalized and 4 patients died (1.7%). In a fully-adjusted analysis, malnutrition was independently associated with the composite outcome of all-cause mortality and all-cause hospitalization [HR 1.94 (95% CI: 1.17–3.20), p = 0.01]. They concluded that despite a high prevalence of obesity, 2 out of 5 ambulatory adults with HFpEF are malnourished. Malnutrition was independently associated with adverse outcomes at 6 months.

The various tools used to assess the extent of malnutrition in studies include the following:

- Nutritional risk screening (NRS2000)
- Nutritional status control (CONUT)
- Mini nutritional assessment (MNA)
- Mini-nutritional assessment short form (MNA-SF)
- Geriatric nutritional risk index (GNRI)
- Nutritional risk index (NRI)
- Prognostic nutritional index (PNI)
- Anthropometry:
    - Body mass index (BMI)
    - Upper arm circumference
    - Skinfold thickness
- Biomarkers (albumin, lymphocyte count)

CONCLUSION

The prevalence of malnutrition and its association with adverse outcomes underscore the importance of considering malnutrition when evaluating adults with HFpEF. While previously nutritional status was assessed using anthropometric data such as BMI, frailty, and sarcopenia, it is required to assess the malnutrition using specialized tools such as MNF, MNF-SF, or any of the others to determine a prognostic value imparted by the nutritional status. Despite having obesity as a factor in the premorbid condition of a patient with HFpEF, the presence of malnutrition needs to be evaluated using scores and correction instituted early in the course of the disease to modify the prognosis and improve clinical outcomes.

REFERENCES

1. Tsao CW, Aday AW, Almarzooq ZI, et al. Heart Disease and Stroke Statistics-2022 Update: A Report From the American Heart Association. Circulation. 2022;145(8):e153-e639.
2. Goyal P, Zainul O BS, MD, et al. Geriatric Domains in Patients with Heart Failure with Preserved Ejection Fraction. Cardiol Clin. 2022;40(4):517-32.
3. Goyal P, Almarzooq ZI, Horn EM, et al. Characteristics of Hospitalizations for Heart Failure with Preserved Ejection Fraction. Am J Med 2016;129(6):635. e15-26.
4. Kitzman DW, Gardin JM, Gottdiener JS, et al. Importance of heart failure with preserved systolic function in patients > or = 65 years of age. CHS Research Group. Cardiovascular Health Study. Am J Cardiol. 2001;87(4):413-9.
5. Gulea C, Zakeri R, Quint JK. Differences in Outcomes between Heart Failure Phenotypes in Patients with Coexistent Chronic Obstructive Pulmonary Disease: A Cohort Study. Ann Am Thorac Soc. 2022;19(6):971-80.
6. Evans C. Malnutrition in the elderly: a multifactorial failure to thrive. Perm J. 2005;9(3):38-41.
7. Norman K, Haβ U, Pirlich M. Malnutrition in Older Adults-Recent Advances and Remaining Challenges. Nutrients. 2021;13(8).
8. Rahman A, Jafry S, Jeejeebhoy K, et al. Malnutrition and Cachexia in Heart Failure. J Parenter Enteral Nutr. 2016;40(4):475-86.
9. Lane JS, Magno CP, Lane KT, et al. Nutrition impacts the prevalence of peripheral arterial disease in the United States. J Vasc Surg. 2008;48(4):897-904.
10. Kelly JP, Hammill BG, Doll JA, et al. The potential impact of expanding cardiac rehabilitation in heart failure. J Am Coll Cardiol. 2016;68(9):977-8.
11. Minamisawa M, Seidelmann SB, Claggett B, et al. Impact of Malnutrition Using Geriatric Nutritional Risk Index in Heart Failure With Preserved Ejection Fraction. JACC Heart Fail. 2019;7(8):664-75.
12. Joaquín C, Alonso N, Lupón J, et al. Mini Nutritional Assessment Short Form is a morbi-mortality predictor in outpatients with heart failure and mid-range left ventricular ejection fraction. Clin Nutr. 2020;39(11):3395-401.
13. Zainul O, Perry D, Pan M, et al. Malnutrition in heart failure with preserved ejection fraction. J Am Geriatr Soc. 2023;71(11):3367-75.

Ideal Edible Oil for Heart Health Among Indians

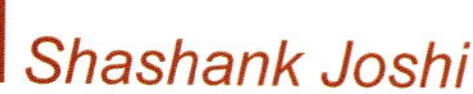
Shashank Joshi

INTRODUCTION

Burden of Noncommunicable Diseases: Global and India

Centre for Disease Control and Prevention (CDC) characterizes noncommunicable diseases (NCDs) as chronic conditions that do not result from an (acute) infectious process, and hence are "not communicable". NCDs have a prolonged course, not resolving spontaneously with rare cures.[1]

The burden of NCDs has increased even in the developing countries now, which earlier were linked with economic growth and were called "diseases of the rich".[2] More than 74% of total deaths are due to NCDs yearly and cardiovascular diseases (CVDs) account for over 31% of total deaths by NCDs, followed by cancer, chronic respiratory diseases (chronic obstructive pulmonary diseases and asthma), and diabetes.[3] The proportional causal factors for deaths due to NCDs (in millions) are depicted in **Figure 1**. Heart attack and stroke caused 85% of deaths due to CVDs.[4]

RISK FACTORS OF NONCOMMUNICABLE DISEASES

Risk factor is an aspect of personal behavior or lifestyle, an environmental exposure, or a hereditary characteristic that is associated with an increase in the occurrence of a particular disease, injury, or other health condition.[1] There are several *modifiable* and *nonmodifiable* risk factors that can attribute to developing NCDs **(Box 1)**. While the *non-modifiable factors* such as the genetic makeup of an individual, race, ethnicity, and age are uncontrollable, there are several *modifiable* lifestyle habits like diet, physical activity, and stress that can be addressed to avert the risk of NCDs.[2]

Modifiable risk factors include behaviors that can be controlled by intervention, thereby reducing the probability of disease. WHO has prioritized physical inactivity, tobacco use, alcohol use, and unhealthy diets as the primary modifiable factors, which if controlled can help manage NCDs.[1,5] The American Heart Association (AHA) has devised *Life's Essential* eight key measures as *health behaviors* and *health factors* to improve and maintain cardiovascular health (CVH) and overall NCDs.

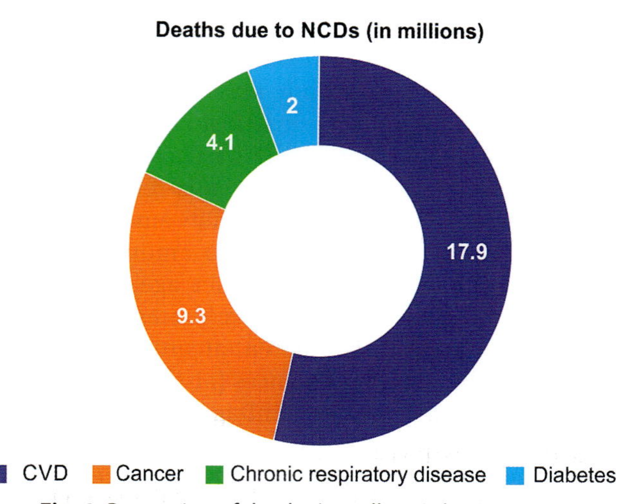

Fig. 1: Proportion of deaths (in millions) due to NCDs.
Source: World Health Organization (WHO). (2023).

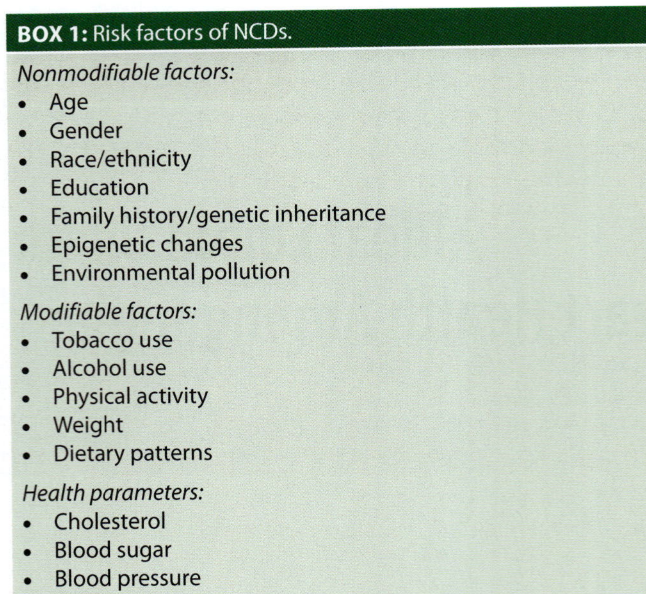

BOX 1: Risk factors of NCDs.

Nonmodifiable factors:
- Age
- Gender
- Race/ethnicity
- Education
- Family history/genetic inheritance
- Epigenetic changes
- Environmental pollution

Modifiable factors:
- Tobacco use
- Alcohol use
- Physical activity
- Weight
- Dietary patterns

Health parameters:
- Cholesterol
- Blood sugar
- Blood pressure
- Stress

Source: Budreviciute et al. (2020).

A better CVH helps reduce the risk of CVDs. The *health behaviors* include being more active, quitting tobacco, getting healthy sleep, and the *health factors* are managing weight, cholesterol, blood sugar, and blood pressure.[6]

INDIANS AND CARDIOVASCULAR DISEASE

Nearly a quarter of the world's population reside in South Asia.[7] India, due to its high population density, shows a large prevalence of NCDs. The overall prevalence of diabetes was 11.4%, prediabetes 15.3%, hypertension 35.5%, generalized obesity 28.6%, abdominal obesity 39.5%, and dyslipidemia 81.2% **(Fig. 2)**. Further analysis of the target population revealed that urban Indians are younger with higher body mass index (BMI), waist circumference, blood pressure, fasting blood glucose, and lipid parameters (total and LDL cholesterol) despite higher educational status.[7] Dyslipidemia-related CVDs are the leading cause of death and disability among Indians.[8]

The peculiarity of the scenario among Indians is relatively higher risk, earlier onset age, higher case fatality, and higher premature death rates as compared to other countries. This differential situation is due to the inherent biological differences (also called *biological risk*) in lipid, glucose, and inflammatory states and the early life influences during prenatal and neonatal stages, coupled with the *population levels changes* including epidemiological, demographic, nutritional, environmental, social-cultural, and economic influences.

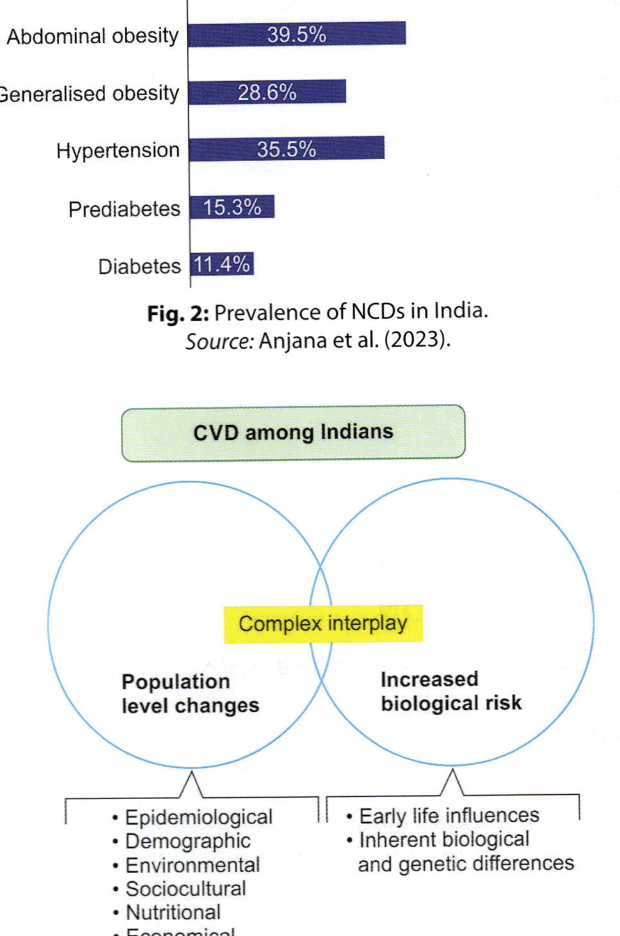

Fig. 2: Prevalence of NCDs in India. *Source:* Anjana et al. (2023).

Fig. 3: Risk factors of CVD in India. *Source:* Kalra et al. (2023).

The complex interplay of these factors decides the course of CVDs in India **(Fig. 3)**.[8]

DIET AND DISEASE

Imbalanced diets lead to 50% of the NCD deaths.[8] A long-term analysis (1990–2016) showed that heart diseases cause the most deaths while dietary iron deficiency is the biggest contributor to disability. High prevalence of both anemia and heart diseases shows the rising problem of the *double burden of undernutrition and overnutrition in India*. Unhealthy diets including insufficient intakes of fruits, whole grains, vegetables, legumes, fish, nuts, seeds and phytonutrients, intake of trans fat and sugar-sweetened drinks, and excess consumption of foods high in saturated fat, added sugar, and sodium are a major contributor to this syndemic.[2,9-11]

Whole grains are high in fiber and vitamins and are known to maintain cholesterol, blood sugar levels, and gut health. Good-quality proteins are essential for bone and muscle development and maintenance, and maintaining adequate weight in terms of lean muscle mass and further monitoring glucose metabolism are essential. Unsaturated fats are healthier and associated with lowering LDL cholesterol (LDL-c).[12]

Fat as Important Part of Diet

Fats are an important component of a balanced diet. They are a source of readily available and stored energy, a structural and functional component of cell membranes, cell signaling molecules, and are vital for the absorption of fat-soluble vitamins in the body.[2,13]

Dietary fats are categorized into: Saturated fatty acids (SFA), cisunsaturated fatty acids, and transunsaturated fatty acids (TFA). Cisunsaturated fatty acids can be further divided into monounsaturated fatty acids (MUFA) and polyunsaturated fatty acids (PUFA).[14]

Saturated fatty acids are found in dairy, meat, and tropical plant oils like palm and coconut oil. Sources of MUFA include oils of olive, canola, and peanuts; meat; and dairy. PUFA are classified as omega 6 (n-6) and omega 3 (n-3). They are essential fatty acids (EFA), which cannot be synthesized in the body and are obtained from the diet. Alpha-linolenic acid (ALA) is a n-3 PUFA, which is converted to long chain n-3 PUFAs (LCFAs) as eicosapentaenoic acid (EPA) and docosahexaenoic acid (DHA). Linoleic acid (LA) is a n-6 PUFA that is converted to long-chain n-6 PUFA and arachidonic acid (AA). LCFAs are needed to form membrane phospholipids for brain development during early life and heart health in later life stages. ALA is mainly obtained from nuts and seeds, deep-sea fatty fish like salmon, and some vegetable oils such as soybean and flaxseed. LA is mainly found in vegetable oils.[2] Indian diets are deficient in n-3 FA, which may be a major reason for higher rates of CVDs. Trans fatty acids (TFA) are found in highly processed foods, dairy, and meat. Repeated frying of oil also leads to generation of TFA.[15,16]

Linkage of dietary fats to incidence of CVDs since long has led to dietary guidance emphasizing limited intakes of SFA and cholesterol. It was hypothesized that a diet rich in fat increases serum cholesterol which in turn are associated with CVD.[17,18] Recent evidence indicates that increased consumption of MUFA and PUFA instead of low-fat diets can prevent and reduce the risk of CVDs.[11,19] Replacement of carbohydrates with SFA increases the cardiac parameters like total cholesterol, LDL-c, and triglycerides, and decreases HDL-c. While replacement with MUFA and PUFA showed marked improvement in these parameters,[20] a diet with low MUFA and high TFA is a reported as a leading modifiable risk factor for several NCDs.[21] Therefore, the guidance is shifting to emphasize increased consumption of MUFA and n-3 PUFAs, substitution of SFA with unsaturated fatty acids, and avoidance of TFA.[16,22,23]

RECOMMENDED FAT INTAKE VERSUS ACTUAL INTAKE IN INDIA

Indian Council of Medical Research, National Institute of Nutrition (ICMR-NIN) "My Plate" recommends a maximum of 30% of energy (30% E) from total fat in the diet (about 67 g/d), of which visible fat ranges from 25–30 g/d. SFA should be <10 g/d; n-6 PUFA, 6.6 g; n-3 PUFA, 2–4 g; and MUFA, 20–31 g/d. The average consumption of fats among rural and urban Indians is 36 g/d and 55 g/d, respectively.[12,22,24] Therefore, quality of fat in the diet is equally important as the quantity.

Edible oils are major sources of fats in diet followed by nuts and seeds, animal foods, and cereals. They also contain minor components such as tocopherols, tocotrienols, and sterols, which keep them shelf stable by preventing rancidity. These bioactives have also been proven to impart heart health benefits. Hence, a careful selection of edible oils is important. No single oil seed has all the fatty acids **(Fig. 4)** and bioactive compounds in recommended amounts.[12,22] The ICMR and AHA recommend consuming various oils either by rotating oils or blending to obtain the benefits of more than one with respect to a balanced fatty acid profile and bioactives in the diet.[22,25]

MULTISOURCED EDIBLE OILS AS POSSIBLE SOLUTION OF OIL PROBLEM FOR INDIANS

Multisourced edible oils (MSEOs) are the admixtures of 2 or 3 edible oils, scientifically formulated to have a better balance of fatty acids and bioactive compounds to confer shelf stability during tropical climates, reduce formation of harmful chemicals (e.g., acrylamide) during high-temperature treatments, and health benefits. MSEOs, like other similar stringent categories of baby foods and packaged water, are strictly governed by Food Safety and Standards Authority of India (FSSAI) and AGMARK for controlled quality and safety measures. Indian food standards by FSSAI (2011) allow minimum of 20% of each seed oil in double-blend MSEOs and minimum of 5% of chia or flax seeds in triple-blend MSEOs. The introduction of triple blend is to increase the intake of n-3 fatty acids as ALA.[26]

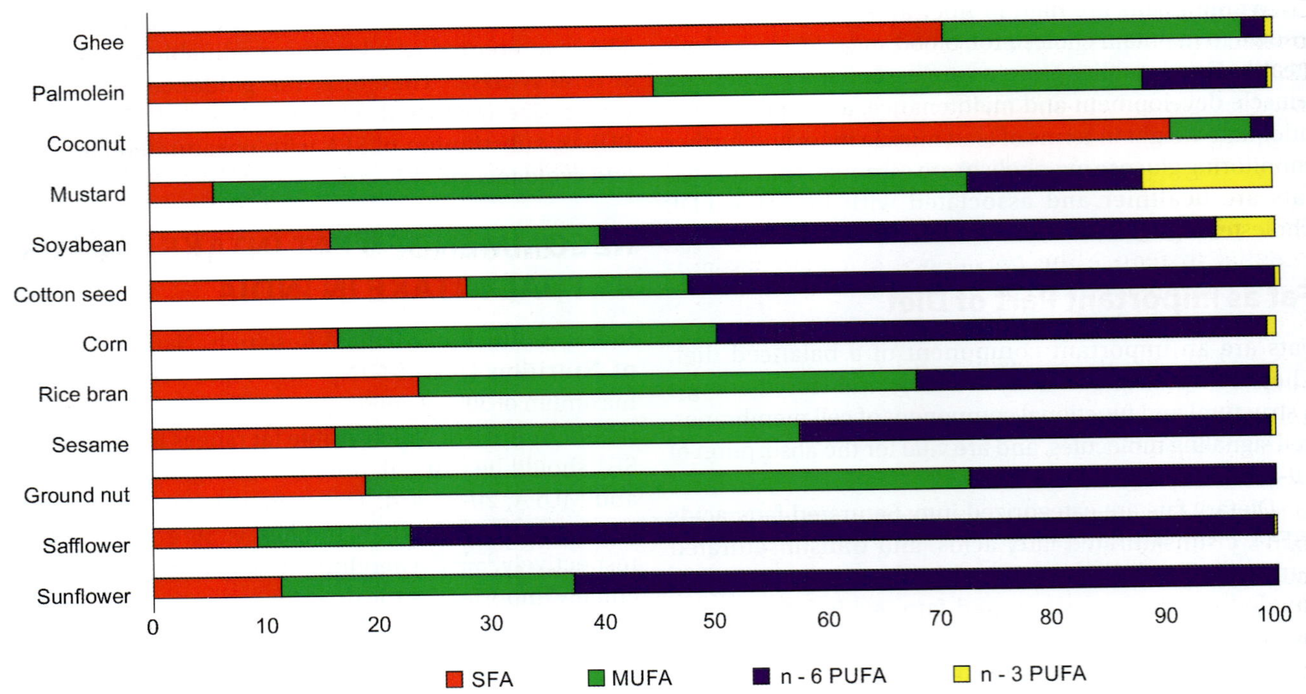

Fig. 4: Fatty acid composition of edible vegetable oils (g/100 g oils).
Source: ICMR-National Institute of Nutrition. (2024).

TABLE 1: Nonglyceride components of various oils.

Nonglyceride components	*Oil*	*Functional benefits*
Plant sterols	All oils	↓ LDL-c
Oryzanol	Rice bran	↓ LDL-c + Antioxidant
Sesamin, sesamol, and sesamolin	Sesame	↓ LDL-c + Antioxidant + Anti-inflammatory
Vitamin E	Rice bran, and sunflower	Antioxidant
Tocotrienols	Rice bran	Vitamin + Antioxidant
Carotenes	Red palm	Provitamin + Antioxidant
Hydroxytyrosol and phenolic acid	Olive	Antioxidant
Sitosterol	Safflower	↓ LDL-c

Source: Indian Council of Medical Research, National Institute of Nutrition. (2020).[22]

- *Fatty acid profile of MSEOs:* MSEOs are designed to have a better balance of fatty acids. Oils high in MUFA (e.g., rice bran or groundnut oil) are blended with those with high PUFA (e.g., safflower or sunflower oil) to obtain an adequate balance of the fatty acids. The recommended fatty acids consumption is 1:1.5:1 as SFA:MUFA:PUFA.[22] Regular consumption of MSEOs could help Indians get closer to this recommendation.
- *Non-glyceride/bioactive components and their nutritional and health-promoting effects:* Vegetable oils contain several nonglyceride components which have proven functional benefits **(Table 1)**.[22]
- *Proven health benefits of MSEOs:* MSEOs of several single oils like rice bran oils (RBO), sesame oil (SO), soyabean oil (SBO), sunflower oil (SNO), safflower oil (SFO), groundnut oil (GO), and canola oil (CO) have proven to be efficacious in managing lipid markers like reducing the LDL-c, triglycerides and total cholesterol (TC); increasing HDL-c; and reducing inflammatory markers like apolipoprotein b (apo-b), homocysteine, C reactive protein (CRP). They are also proven to manage blood sugar levels by reducing HbA1C.

A blend of 70:30 RBO and SFO was effective in improving the lipid markers and the inflammatory markers.[27,28]

Consumption of another blend of 80:20 RBO and SO lowered hyperglycemia and improved the lipid profile in T2DM patients.[29,30] CO and SO blend also has been shown to reduce hypertension in subjects over 9 weeks.[31]

CONCLUSION

Dietary management with appropriate fat quality is essential to reduce the prevalence of CVDs. Indians should consume fatty acids in a defined ratio of 1:1.5:1 (SFA: MUFA: PUFA). Since edible oils are the major source of fats in our diets, their quality in turn decides the fat quality in diet. MSEOs are scientifically formulated to complement the fatty acid ratios to help come close to the recommended fatty acid balance. MSEOs are also formulated with precision to include various bioactive components in appropriate amounts to improve their stability during shelf storage and high-temperature cooking apart from imparting health benefits in managing CVDs. Hence, MSEOs come as an overall convenient solution for Indian scenario in terms of maintaining shelf and cooking stability and managing CVDs.

REFERENCES

1. Overview of Noncommunicable Diseases and Related Risk Factors, Centers for Disease Control and Prevention. https://www.cdc.gov/globalhealth/healthprotection/fetp/training_modules/new-8/overview-of-ncds_ppt_qa-revcom_09112013.pdf
2. Budreviciute A, Damiati S, Sabir DK, et al. Management and prevention strategies for non-communicable diseases (NCDs) and their risk factors. Front Public Health. 2020;8:574111.
3. World Health Organization. (2024). Noncommunicable Diseases. [online] Available from https://www.who.int/news-room/fact-sheets/detail/noncommunicable-diseases [Last accessed January, 2025].
4. World Health Organization. (2021). Cardiovascular diseases (CVDs). [online] Available from https://www.who.int/news-room/fact-sheets/detail/cardiovascular-diseases-(cvds) [Last accessed January, 2025].
5. World Health Organization. (2024). Preventing non-communicable diseases. [online] Available from https://www.who.int/activities/preventing-noncommunicable-diseases#:~:text=Reducing%20the%20major%20risk%20factors,to%20prevent%20deaths%20from%20NCDs. [Last accessed January, 2025].
6. Lloyd-Jones DM, Allen NB, Anderson CAM, et al. Life's Essential 8: Updating and enhancing the American Heart Association's construct of cardiovascular health: A presidential advisory from the American Heart Association. Circulation. 2022;146(5):e18-e43.
7. Anjana RM, Unnikrishnan R, Deepa M, et al. Metabolic non-communicable disease health report of India: The ICMR-INDIAB national cross-sectional study (ICMR-INDIAB-17). Lancet Diabetes Endocrinol. 2023;11(7):474-89.
8. Kalra A, Jose AP, Prabhakaran P, et al. The burgeoning cardiovascular disease epidemic in Indians: Perspectives on contextual factors and potential solutions. Lancet Reg Health Southeast Asia. 2023;12:100156.
9. Sharma M, Kishore A, Roy D, et al. A comparison of the Indian diet with the EAT-Lancet reference diet. BMC Public Health. 2020;20(1):812.
10. Mozaffarian D. Identifying nutritional priorities for global health: Time for a more PURE focus on protective foods. Eur Heart J. 2023;44(28):2580-2.
11. Billingsley HE, Carbone S, Lavie CJ. Dietary fats and chronic noncommunicable diseases. Nutrients. 2018;10(10):1385.
12. ICMR-National Institute of Nutrition. (2024). Dietary guidelines for Indians. [online] Available from https://www.nin.res.in/dietaryguidelines/pdfjs/locale/DGI07052024P.pdf [Last accessed January, 2024].
13. Field CJ, Robinson L. Dietary Fats. Adv Nutr. 2019;10(4):722-4.
14. Lichtenstein AH, Jones PJH. Lipids: Absorption and transport. In: Present Knowledge in Nutrition. Washington DC, US: International Life Sciences Institute Press; 2022. pp. 118-31.
15. Mozaffarian D, Aro A, Willett WC. Health effects of trans-fatty acids: Experimental and observational evidence. Eur J Clin Nutr. 2009;63 Suppl 2:S5-21.
16. Schwingshack L, Heseker H, Kiesswetter E, et al. Reprint of: Dietary fat and fatty foods in the prevention of non-communicable diseases: A review of the evidence. Trends Food Sci Technol. 2022;130:20-31.
17. Forouhi NG, Krauss RM, Taubes G, et al. Dietary fat and cardiometabolic health: Evidence, controversies, and consensus for guidance. BMJ. 2018;361:k2139.
18. Kannel WB, Castelli WP, Gordon T, et al. Serum cholesterol, lipoproteins, and the risk of coronary heart disease. The Framingham study. Ann Internal Med. 1071;74(1):1-12.
19. Howard BV, Van Horn L, Hsia J, et al. Low-fat dietary pattern and risk of cardiovascular disease: The Women's Health Initiative Randomized Controlled Dietary Modification Trial. JAMA. 2006;295(6):655-66.
20. Mensink RP. Effects of saturated fatty acids on serum lipids and lipoproteins: A systematic review and regression analysis. Geneva: World Health Organization; 2016.
21. Afshin A, Sur PJ, Fay KA, et al. Health effects of dietary risks in 195 countries, 1990-2017: A systematic analysis for the global burden of disease study 2017. Lancet. 2019;393:1958-72.
22. Indian Council of Medical Research, National Institute of Nutrition (ICMR-NIN) (2020). Recommended Dietary Allowances and Estimated Average Requirements Nutrient Requirements for Indians-2020: A Report of the Expert Group Indian Council of Medical Research National Institute of Nutrition. [online] Available from https://www.ijfcm.org/html-article/18750 [Last accessed January, 2025].

23. Understanding the Scientific Process, Guidelines, and Key Recommendations. Snetselaar LG, de Jesus JM, DeSilva DM, et al. Dietary Guidelines for Americans, 2020-2025. Nutr Today. 2021;56(6):287-95.
24. Hemalatha A, Laxmaiah A, Sriswan MR, et al. (2020). What India Eats. [online] Available from https://www.nin.res.in/nutrition2020/what_india_eats.pdf [Last accessed January, 2025].
25. American Heart Association. (2025). Healthy Cooking Oils. [online] Available from https://www.heart.org/en/healthy-living/healthy-eating/eat-smart/fats/healthy-cooking-oils [Last accessed January, 2025].
26. Food Safety and Standards Authority of India (FSSAI). (2023) Chapter 2: Food Products Standard. [online] Available from https://www.fssai.gov.in/upload/uploadfiles/files/Chapter%202_2_Fats_oil_fat%20emulsions.pdf. Accessed on 13.08.2024 [Last accessed January, 2025].
27. Sugano M, Tsuji E. Rice bran oil and cholesterol metabolism. Journal Nutr. 1997;127(3):521S-4S.
28. Upadya H, Devaraju CJ, Joshi SR. Anti-inflammatory properties of blended edible oil with synergistic antioxidants. Indian J Endocrinol Metab. 2015;19(4):511-9.
29. Devarajan S, Chatterjee B, Urata H, et al. A blend of sesame and rice bran oils lowers hyperglycemia and improves the lipids. Am J Med. 2016;129(7):731-9.
30. Hota D, Srinivasan A, Sahoo JP, et al. Possible anti-diabetic and anti-hyperlipidemic efficacy of blended rice bran oil with sesame oil in comparison with soybean oil: A Clinical investigation in pre-diabetic and diabetic individuals. J Clin Trials. 2020;10:419.
31. Amiri M, Raeisi-Dehkordi H, Moghtaderi F, et al. The effects of sesame, canola, and sesame–canola oils on cardiometabolic markers in patients with type 2 diabetes: A triple-blind three-way randomized crossover clinical trial. Eur J Nutr. 2022;61(7):3499-516.

SECTION 17

HFpEF and Cardio-oncology

127. The Role of ARNI in Doxorubicin-induced Cardiotoxicity and HFpEF

128. HFpEF After Chemotherapy: Management Strategies

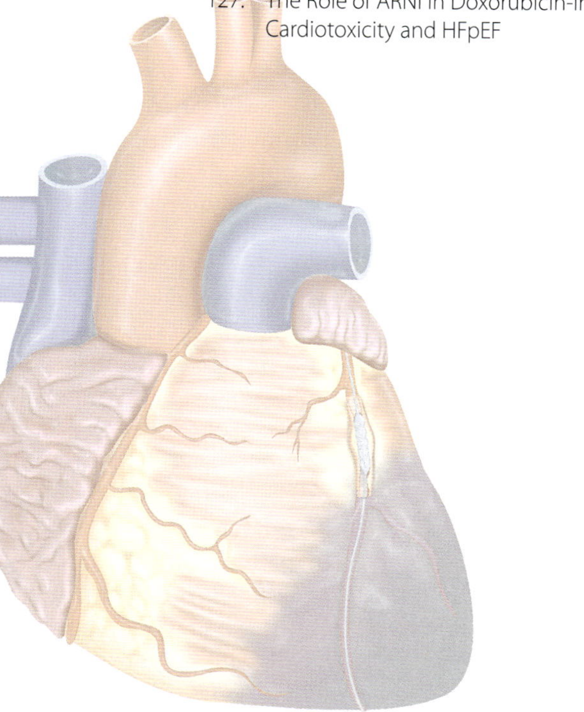

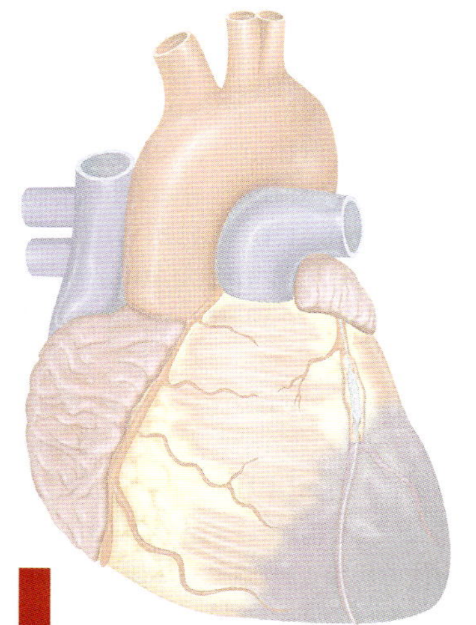

CHAPTER

The Role of ARNI in Doxorubicin-induced Cardiotoxicity and HFpEF

Indu Bansal, Vikas Goyal, Harmesh Aggarwal

INTRODUCTION

Cardiotoxicity is a serious side effect of anthracycline chemotherapy agents such as doxorubicin and poses significant risks to cancer patients. Heart failure with preserved ejection fraction (HFpEF) represents a complex clinical syndrome, characterized by the heart's inability to relax and fill properly, despite normal contraction. Sacubitril/valsartan [an angiotensin receptor-neprilysin inhibitor (ARNI)] has emerged as a promising therapeutic approach to mitigate cardiotoxicity and improve outcomes in HFpEF patients. This chapter explores the mechanisms, efficacy, and clinical guidelines associated with the use of ARNI in these contexts, drawing from recent studies and clinical trials.

Chemotherapy is a very integral part of cancer treatment, and many patients face cardiotoxicity as a consequence of cancer treatment. A number of drugs cause cardiotoxicity including anthracyclines and doxorubicin is one of them. In the year 2022, the International Cardio-oncology Society described "cancer therapy-related cardiac dysfunction" (CTRCD) as symptomatic heart failure (HF) and asymptomatic cardiac dysfunction related to chemotherapy.[1] Asymptomatic cardiac dysfunction is further defined as: Severe—a decrease in LVEF to <40%, moderate—40–49%, and mild as preserved left ventricular ejection fraction (LVEF) ≥50% with >15% reduction in global longitudinal strain (GLS) relative to baseline or a new rise in cardiac troponins and/or natriuretic peptides (NPs).[1]

The preferred imaging modality to diagnose and monitor CTRCD is 3-dimensional transthoracic echocardiography (TTE) or two-dimensional TTE or cardiac magnetic resonance (CMR).[2] These guidelines define anthracycline-induced cardiotoxicity (AIC) as CTRCD or other toxicities as myocarditis and cardiac arrhythmias, which can manifest clinically or get detected during surveillance imaging.[2,3]

Doxorubicin-induced cardiotoxicity can be detected early by a drop in LVEF from baseline.[4] As per European Society of Cardiology, a 10% point decline in LVEF from baseline to below 50% is an indicator of cardiotoxicity.[4,5] Similarly, the European Society of Cardiology and European Association of Cardiovascular Imaging describes a 10% point decline in LVEF from baseline to below 53% as clinical cardiotoxicity while subclinical cardiotoxicity is preserved LVEF with a 15 % reduction in GLS with or without an increase in cardiac serum biomarkers.[6]

Anthracycline-induced cardiotoxicity can be acute, occurring within days of anthracycline administration, and is usually reversible.[4] It may present as chest pain and palpitations and may lead to myopericarditis, involve cardiac conducting system, or lead to development of arrhythmias.[4] The chronic AIC may occur later after stoppage of treatment and present as CTRCD in form of HFrEF or may be asymptomatic, which is detected on cardiac imaging. It may be early-onset chronic cardiotoxicity (occurring within the 1st year of the treatment completion or late-onset (occurring many years after chemotherapy completion).[7] Hence, it is very important to serially monitor left ventricular systolic function before and after completion of doxorubicin-based chemotherapy with either cardiac biomarkers (troponin-I and NT-pro-BNP), 2D echocardiography, or 2-D speckle tracking echocardiography to measure GLS.[4]

The incidence of chronic AIC depends on the cumulative dose of anthracyclines received. As per the studies by Von Hoff et al. (1979) and Swain et al. (2003), the risk of developing congestive heart failure (CHF) was dependent on cumulative dose of doxorubicin received: 3–5% at a dose of 400 mg/m^2, 16% at 500 mg/m^2, 7–26% at 550 mg/m^2, and 18–48% at 700 mg/m^2.[8,9] The other risk factors for cardiotoxicity are enumerated in **Box 1**.

BOX 1: Risk factors for anthracycline cardiotoxicity.

Risk factors for anthracycline cardiotoxicity:
- Age >65 years or <18 years
- African–American descent
- Female sex
- Hypertension
- Coronary artery disease (CAD)
- Obesity
- Type-2 diabetes mellitus (T2DM)
- CHF
- Valve diseases
- Baseline LV function
- Renal failure
- Electrolyte imbalance (hypokalemia and hypomagnesemia)
- Type and cumulative dose of chemotherapy
- Regimen and route of administration
- Combination with other cardiotoxic drugs or with radiation therapy on the chest area
- Prior therapy with anthracyclines or radiation therapy
- Concomitant use of other anticancer drugs (cyclophosphamide, methotrexate, trastuzumab, and others)
- Genetic and environmental risk factors

Doxorubicin-induced cardiotoxicity is primarily mediated through oxidative stress, inflammation, and apoptosis. These processes lead to myocardial damage, manifesting as reduced cardiac function and progressive systolic dysfunction of the left ventricle (LV) leading to subsequent development of CHF with its life-long consequences.[3] The different mechanisms of doxorubicin-induced cardiotoxicity are well enumerated in **Flowchart 1**.

Heart failure is a clinical syndrome occurring because of structural and functional abnormalities in the myocardium, which leads to impaired filling or ejection of blood from the ventricles. Impaired relaxation or contractility of the heart leads to elevated cardiac filling pressure, elevated jugular venous pressure (JVP), physical symptoms, and lung crackles. Heart failure can be classified into different categories based on the LVEF. HFrEF is heart failure with reduced ejection fraction (LVEF ≤40%), HFpEF represents heart failure with preserved ejection fraction (LVEF ≥50% or higher) and HFmrEF is heart failure with mildly reduced ejection fraction (LVEF between 41% and 49%).[10] The mechanism of HFpEF is shown in **Table 1**.

ANGIOTENSIN RECEPTOR-NEPRILYSIN INHIBITOR AND CARDIOTOXICITY

A number of treatments available for HFrEF include ARNIs, SGLT2i, ACEIs, ARBs, beta-blockers, aldosterone antagonists, loop diuretics, hydralazine/isosorbide dinitrate, and ivabradine, except for loop diuretics, which have been proven to improve symptoms, reduce hospital stays, and increase survival rates in clinical trials.[10]

Flowchart 1: Mechanism of doxorubicin-induced cardiotoxicity.

Doxorubicin

One electron reduction ↓ Production of reactive oxygen species (ROS) Superoxide anion and hydrogen peroxide ↓ ROS react with iron (Fe^{2+} and Fe^{3+}) ↓ Production of highly toxic hydroxyl radical ↓ Toxic hydroxyl radical promotes oxidative stress ↓ Damage to DNA, proteins, and lipids ↓ Leading to cell death	Increases intracellular iron concentration ↓ Through inhibition of iron regulatory protein-1 (IRP-1) ↓ IRP-1 regulates the expression of genes involved in iron metabolism and homeostasis ↓ Increased intracellular iron levels ↓ Reduces the expression of antioxidative enzymes (glutathione and catalase) ↓ Leads to oxidative stress	Other mechanisms • Targeting signal molecules in apoptotic signaling as p53 • Promotes dysfunction of mitochondria • Causes DNA damage through topoisomerase II alpha *Cardioprotective strategies* • Less dose • Slow administration • Liposomal doxorubicin • Dexrazoxane • Angiotensin-converting enzyme (ACE) inhibitors

"ROS and iron" hypothesis

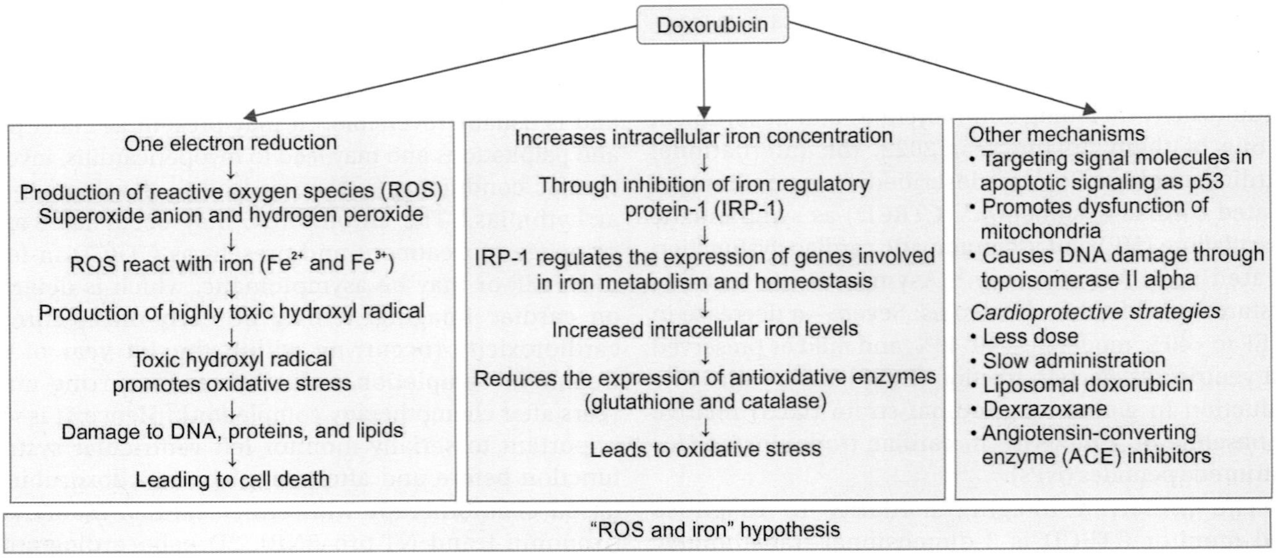

TABLE 1: The mechanism of HFpEF.

Parameter	*HFpEF*	*HFrEF*
Cardiac fibrosis and rigidity, impaired diastolic function	Activation of the RAAS	Alterations in myocardial systolic function
Arterial stiffening and decreased arterial compliance		↑ Systolic and diastolic blood pressures
	↑ Pulse wave velocity	

After the promising results of PARADIGM-HF trial, the ARNI has been incorporated into HF management and has shown its effectiveness in not just reducing cardiovascular death or heart failure hospitalization but also an improvement in quality of life and diminution of risk of ventricular arrhythmias. ARNIs are a very vital component of treatment for HFrEF, HFpEF, as well as for HFimpEF.[3]

Angiotensin receptor-neprilysin inhibitor administration leads to a number of cardioprotective effects such as amelioration of oxidative stress levels, the inhibition of myocardial inflammatory response, decreased mitochondrial damage and endothelial dysfunction, reduction of endoplasmic reticulum stress, and improvement in the RAAS imbalance. Several reports of ARNI administration in animal models of AIC have shown promising results; however, there is not enough data on ARNI's effectiveness in the prevention of AIC.[7]

Neprilysin [neutral endopeptidase (NEP), CD10] is a zinc-dependent metalloproteinase involved in the regulation of the activity of endocrine system and is expressed in a variety of organs/systems, such as kidneys, heart, brain, lungs, gastrointestinal system, adrenal glands, reproductive system, and placenta, etc.[11] The heart, especially LV in the setting of HF, is a major source of soluble circulating NEP. NEPs have twofold actions—degradation of cardioprotective agents such as natriuretic peptides (NPs) and also the modulation of RAAS activation. The administration of NEP inhibitors (NEPi) alone lead to unopposed Ang II/ATR1 signaling activation, which lead to failure of monotherapy with NEPi. The combination of NEPi with ACEi has been tried to counter the overactivation of the RAAS, which provides a survival benefit to HF patients, but also leads to an increased risk of angioedema. So, a combination drug of NEPi–sacubitril and ARB–valsartan was introduced [sacubitril/valsartan, (LCZ696)], offering the inhibition of both NEP and RAAS, without causing significant side effects.[7]

Sacubitril/valsartan has shown potential in attenuating doxorubicin-induced cardiotoxicity. The drug sacubitril/valsartan is a combination of two active drugs in equal amounts—valsartan and sacubitril. It is a unique crystalline salt combination having high stability and favorable physicochemical and pharmacokinetic properties. It targets two aspects of heart failure: The NPs system through sacubitril, and the RAAS through valsartan.[12] Studies indicate that this ARNI combination exerts protective effects through its anti-inflammatory, antioxidant, and antiapoptotic properties. It also interferes with oxidative stress pathways and reduces caspase-3-mediated apoptosis, thereby preserving myocardial integrity.[10]

CLINICAL EVIDENCE: PARAGLIDE-HF AND PARAGON-HF TRIALS

The ACC guidelines have given a Class IIb recommendation for using ARNI in HFpEF. PARAGLIDE-HF and PARAGON-HF trials investigated the efficacy of sacubitril/valsartan in patients with HFpEF. Both trials demonstrated significant reductions in NPs and favorable outcomes in reducing cardiovascular and renal events compared to valsartan alone. These trials also highlighted the ARNI's role in reducing total worsening HF events and cardiovascular deaths, particularly in patients with mildly reduced or preserved ejection fraction.[10,13,14]

In the PARAGON-HF trial, 4,822 patients with New York Heart Association (NYHA) class II–IV HF were taken with LVEF ≥45% or higher, increased levels of NP, and structural heart disease. The patients were treated with either sacubitril/valsartan (97 mg sacubitril with 103 mg valsartan twice daily) or with only valsartan (160 mg twice daily). There was no significant difference between the rate of cardiovascular deaths or hospitalizations due to HF in sacubitril/valsartan group (12.8 events per 100 patient-years) and the valsartan group (14.6 events per 100 patient-years), which was the primary outcome of the trial. Secondary outcomes confirmed a significant improvement in NYHA class (15.0% improvement in NYHA class in the sacubitril/valsartan group compared to 12.6% in the valsartan group) and renal function (1.4% in the sacubitril/valsartan group as against 2.7% in the valsartan group), with more benefits seen in female patients and patients with EF between 45% and 57%, highlighting need for personalized therapy with ARNI in HFpEF. The timing of initiating sacubitril/valsartan after a HF hospitalization was very important. Early initiation within 30 days led to an absolute 6.4% reduction in cardiovascular death or hospitalization while the reduction was 4.6% when initiated after 30–90 days and only 3.4% when initiated after 91–180 days, and no significant benefit if initiated >180 days after the index hospitalization.[15]

The PARADIGM-HF (Angiotensin–Neprilysin Inhibition versus Enalapril in Heart Failure) study demonstrated reduced mortality and HF hospitalization with sacubitril/valsartan over enalapril in 2014.[16] While the PARADIGM-HF trial showed potential benefits across various subgroups, the PARAGON-HF trial identified only two subgroups: (1) Patients with an ejection fraction between 45% and 57% and (2) women, that showed a possible treatment advantage.[16-18]

DOSE ADJUSTMENTS

As per Dalal et al., the suggested initial dose of sacubitril/valsartan is 50 mg, to be taken orally twice daily. After a period of 2–4 weeks, the dosage can be increased to 100 mg and further escalated to 200 mg if the individual tolerates the drug. The dose titration may be done over 3 weeks (for 100 mg BID starting dose) or at 6 weeks (for 50 mg BID starting dose). However, in a few patients not currently receiving an ACEI or ARB, patients with severe renal or moderate hepatic impairment, and if the blood pressure is below 90/60, the starting dose may be reduced.[19] If a patient has severe hepatic impairment, ARNI should not be prescribed. In a patient with moderate hepatic impairment (Child–Pugh B), the loading dose of ARNI should be halved and the subsequent doses should be gradually increased to reach the maximum tolerated dose, but no dose adjustment is required for mild hepatic impairment (Child–Pugh A). ARNI dose adjustment is not required in HF patients with mild-to-moderate renal impairment. In patients with CKD, ARNI can be prescribed to nondialysis patients as it leads to reduction of cardiovascular risk and improvement in eGFR compared to ACEI/ARBs. Depending on the patient's blood pressure, a loading dose of 25–50 mg BID is advised in severe renal impairment. The dose of ARNI should be gradually increased every 2–4 weeks to reach the maintenance dose of 200 mg BID (maximum tolerated dose).[10] The guidelines for use of ARNI in AIC are enumerated in **Table 2**.

TABLE 2: Guidelines for use of ARNI in anthracycline-induced cardiotoxicity.

Patient selection	• Consider ARNI for patients undergoing anthracycline chemotherapy with high risk for cardiotoxicity • Use in patients with HFpEF with recent hospitalization for worsening heart failure
Dosage and administration	Start with a low dose of sacubitril/valsartan and titrate based on tolerance and renal function
Monitoring and follow-up	• Regularly monitor renal function, electrolytes, and blood pressure • Use echocardiography to assess left ventricular function periodically
Management of side effects	• Address hypotension and hyperkalemia promptly • Adjust dosages or switch to alternative therapies if adverse effects are significant

PREVENTION OF ANTHRACYCLINE-INDUCED CARDIOTOXICITY

The European Society of Cardiology Guidelines on cardiovascular disease (CVD) suggest taking primary as well as secondary measures to prevent the development of AIC. The suggested preventive measures are to avoid risk factors such as obesity, cigarette smoking, and alcohol consumption, manage arterial hypertension, encourage physical activity, and, encourage use of the liposomal doxorubicin, dexrazoxane, ACEi, ARB, beta-adrenergic receptor antagonists, and statins in high-risk patients.[2] As a secondary preventive measure, LVEF assessment before and within 12 months after the administration of anthracyclines should be done with additional assessments throughout the treatment for high-risk patients.[2,7] Although there is not much human-derived data available on the use of ARNI in AIC primary prevention, currently, a multicenter, randomized, placebo-controlled, double-blind phase-2 clinical trial (Prevention of Cardiac Dysfunction During Breast Cancer Therapy (PRADA II)] aimed at assessing the efficacy of ANRI during anthracycline-containing chemotherapy for breast cancer is ongoing and the trial results are expected by late 2025.

LIMITATIONS

Despite the promising results, there are notable limitations. The methodology of some studies has been questioned, particularly the lack of quantitative histological data and imaging tools to assess left ventricular functions comprehensively. Additionally, the generalizability of trial results to broader populations and long-term safety data remains limited. Further research is needed to confirm these findings and establish robust clinical guidelines.

CONCLUSION

Sacubitril/valsartan represents a significant advancement in the management of doxorubicin-induced cardiotoxicity and HFpEF. Its multifaceted mechanisms, encompassing anti-inflammatory, antioxidant, and antiapoptotic effects, offer a protective shield against myocardial damage. Clinical trials such as PARAGLIDE-HF and PARAGON-HF provide compelling evidence supporting their efficacy in improving cardiovascular outcomes. However, further studies are essential to refine patient selection, optimize dosing strategies, and fully understand the long-term implications of ARNI therapy.

REFERENCES

1. Herrmann J, Lenihan D, Armenian S, et al. Defining cardiovascular toxicities of cancer therapies: an International Cardio-Oncology Society (IC-OS) consensus statement. Eur Heart J. 2021;43:280-99.
2. Lyon AR, López-Fernández T, Couch L, et al. 2022 ESC Guidelines on Cardio-Oncology Developed in Collaboration with the European Hematology Association (EHA), the European Society for Therapeutic Radiology and Oncology (ESTRO) and the International Cardio-Oncology Society (IC-OS). Developed by the Task Force on Cardio-Oncology of the European Society of Cardiology (ESC). Eur Heart J. 2022;43(41):4229-361.
3. Hahn VS, Sharma K. Angiotensin receptor-neprilysin inhibition for doxorubicin-mediated cardiotoxicity: time for a paradigm shift. JACC CardioOncol. 2020;2(5):788-90.
4. Belger C, Abrahams C, Imamdin A, et al. Doxorubicin-induced cardiotoxicity and risk factors. Int J Cardiol Heart Vasc. 2023;50:101332.
5. Zamorano JL, Lancellotti P, Rodriguez Muñoz D, et al. ESC Position Paper on cancer treatments and cardiovascular toxicity developed under the auspices of the ESC Committee for Practice Guidelines: The Task Force for cancer treatments and cardiovascular toxicity of the European Society of Cardiology (ESC). Eur Heart J. 2016;37(36):2768-801.
6. Plana JC, Galderisi M, Barac A, et al. Expert consensus for multimodality imaging evaluation of adult patients during and after cancer therapy: a report from the American Society of Echocardiography and the European Association of Cardiovascular Imaging. J Am Soc Echocardiogr. 2014;27(9):911-39.
7. Sobiborowicz-Sadow AM, Kamińska K, Cudnoch-Jędrzejewska A. Neprilysin inhibition in the prevention of anthracycline-induced cardiotoxicity. Cancers. 2023; 15(1):312.
8. Von Hoff DD, Layard MW, Basa P, et al. Risk factors for doxorubicin-induced congestive heart failure. Ann Intern Med. 1979;91:710-7.
9. Swain SM, Whaley FS, Ewer MS. Congestive heart failure in patients treated with doxorubicin: a retrospective analysis of three trials. Cancer. 2003;97:2869-79.
10. Dalal J, Chandra P, Ray SP, et al. Practical recommendations for the use of angiotensin receptor-neprilysin inhibitors (ARNI) in heart failure: Insights from Indian Cardiologists. Cardiol Ther. 2023;12(3):445-71.
11. Feygina EE, Katrukha AG, Semenov AG. Neutral endopeptidase (Neprilysin) in therapy and diagnostics: Yin and Yang. Biochemistry. 2019;84(11):1346-58.
12. Pascual-Figal D, Bayés-Genis A, Beltrán-Troncoso P, et al. Sacubitril-valsartan, clinical benefits and related mechanisms of action in heart failure with reduced ejection fraction. A review. Front Cardiovasc Med. 2021;8: 754499.
13. Visseren FLJ, Mach F, Smulders YM, et al.; ESC National Cardiac Societies; ESC Scientific Document Group. 2021 ESC guidelines on cardiovascular disease in prevention in clinical practice. Eur. Heart J. 2021;42:3227-337.
14. Massari F, Scicchitano P, Iacoviello M, et al. Multiparametric approach to congestion for predicting long-term survival in heart failure. J Cardiol. 2020;75(1):47-52.
15. Gronda E, Vanoli E, Iacoviello M. The PARAGON- HF trial: the sacubitril/valsartan in heart failure with preserved ejection fraction. Eur Heart J Suppl. 2020;22(Suppl L): L77-81.
16. Krum H. Prospective comparison of ARNi with ACEI to determine impact on global mortality and morbidity in heart failure (PARADIGM-HF): paragon of a study or further investigation paramount? Circulation. 2015;131(1): 11-2.
17. Gulati G, Heck LS, Ree AH, et al. Prevention of cardiac dysfunction during adjuvant breast cancer therapy (PRADA): a 2 × 2 factorial, randomized, placebo-controlled, double-blind clinical trial of candesartan and metoprolol. Eur Heart J. 2016;37(21):1671-80.
18. Vaduganathan M, Mentz RJ, Claggett BL, et al. Sacubitril/valsartan in heart failure with mildly reduced or preserved ejection fraction: a pre-specified participant-level pooled analysis of PARAGLIDE-HF and PARAGON-HF. Eur Heart J. 2023;44(31):2982-93.
19. Senni M, McMurray JJV, Wachter R, et al. Initiating sacubitril/valsartan (LCZ696) in heart failure: results of TITRATION, a double-blind, randomized comparison of two uptitration regimens. Eur J Heart Fail. 2016;18: 1193-202.

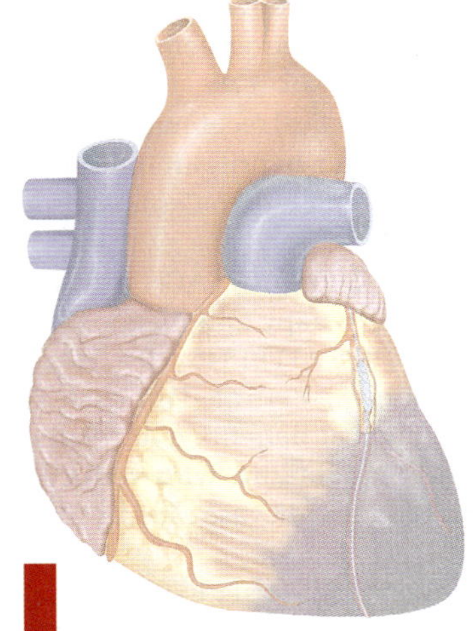

HFpEF After Chemotherapy: Management Strategies

Kanika Sood Sharma, Aditi Tanwar, Jishnu Prem

INTRODUCTION

Heart failure with preserved ejection fraction (HFpEF) poses a significant challenge in both cardiology and oncology, particularly among patients undergoing cancer treatment. Traditional management of cardiotoxicity in patients receiving chemotherapy and radiotherapy has primarily focused on heart failure with reduced ejection fraction (HFrEF), termed "cancer therapy-related cardiac dysfunction". Much of the research and clinical monitoring of cardiotoxicity associated with agents like anthracyclines and trastuzumab have concentrated on asymptomatic reductions in left ventricular ejection fraction (LVEF) and the development of HFrEF. However, emerging evidence suggests that many cancer therapies also induce cardiovascular effects—including myocardial, vascular, and metabolic changes—that may predispose patients to HFpEF. Cancer patients, particularly those with preexisting cardiovascular risk factors or cancer-related cardiometabolic alterations, are already at a heightened risk for HFpEF. Despite the limited focus on HFpEF outcomes in oncology trials, healthcare providers should recognize that cancer treatments can increase the risk for both HFrEF and HFpEF. This chapter aims to summarize the latest advances in HFpEF management, particularly in the context of cancer therapy and its cardiovascular implications.

DESCRIPTION

Anthracyclines are well documented for causing left ventricular systolic dysfunction and HFrEF. Additionally, anthracycline treatment has been linked to increased aortic stiffness and diastolic dysfunction, suggesting a possible risk for HFpEF. Several cohort studies highlight significant changes in echocardiographic measures of diastolic function in breast cancer patients treated with anthracyclines. In one study, diastolic dysfunction was found in over 50% of patients within the first year of treatment. SEER-Medicare data has shown an increased risk of heart failure in older breast cancer survivors, although it does not always distinguish between HFrEF and HFpEF. Further research is needed to clarify the long-term effects of anthracycline-induced diastolic and vascular dysfunction on clinical outcomes. A study conducted by Lagoeiro et al. showcased the interplay between cancer treatments and cardiovascular risks, particularly HFpEF. It emphasized the importance of oncologist–cardiologist collaboration for early detection and personalized management of cardiotoxicity.

Most breast cancer patients receiving chemotherapy also receive adjuvant radiation therapy. Radiation therapy also carries profound cardiovascular risks, leading to microvascular endothelial damage, inflammation, fibrosis, and capillary loss, affecting multiple cardiac structures. Long-term cardiovascular effects include coronary artery disease, valvular disorders, arrhythmias, and heart failure. One population-based study identified a higher mean radiation dose to the heart as significantly associated with an increased risk of HFpEF after breast cancer treatment. Therefore, the HFpEF or any cardiotoxicity will be higher in this subgroup of patients, particularly patients receiving radiation to the left side of chest. A similar situation may be encountered in patients receiving thoracic radiation, especially with concurrent taxane-based chemotherapy.

Hematopoietic cell transplantation (HCT) presents a considerable risk for heart failure and atherosclerotic events. Pre- and post-transplant cancer treatments, combined with pre-existing cardiac risk factors, compound the risk of heart failure. VEGF inhibitors, including monoclonal antibodies and tyrosine kinase inhibitors (TKIs), often cause hypertension, increasing the risk of cardiomyopathy and heart failure. Sunitinib, an anti-VEGF TKI, has been shown to increase vascular stiffness and disrupt diastolic function, suggesting a heightened risk of HFpEF.

Additionally, carfilzomib, a proteasome inhibitor used in multiple myeloma treatment, has been linked to elevated heart failure rates, particularly HFpEF. Multiple myeloma patients are already at an increased risk for heart failure due to cardiac amyloidosis, prevalent cardiac and renal diseases, and treatment-related factors.

Tyrosine kinase inhibitors used in chronic myeloid leukemia (CML), such as ponatinib, nilotinib, and dasatinib, are associated with increased risks of atherosclerosis and heart failure. Dasatinib, in particular, can induce pulmonary hypertension and pleural or pericardial effusions, which may clinically resemble HFpEF. Immune checkpoint inhibitors, used in many cancer therapies, have been associated with myocarditis, which can present with preserved LVEF despite changes in global longitudinal strain.

Advanced age, presence of cardiovascular disease risk factors, and previous anthracycline treatment predispose to trastuzumab-induced cardiotoxicity (TIC), with anthracycline exposure being the most significant contributary factor. Cardiac biomarkers such as troponins and pro-BNP and imaging assessments such as echocardiogram before and during trastuzumab therapy may help in early identification of TIC. Camilli et al. discussed early detection of anthracycline-induced cardiotoxicity through biomarkers like troponin and BNP, and the importance of multidisciplinary teams in implementing cardioprotective strategies, such as ACE inhibitors and β-blockers. Ky et al. have also emphasized the importance of biomarkers for early detection of cardiotoxicity than LVEF, in patients undergoing doxorubicin and trastuzumab-based treatment.

Cardiopulmonary exercise testing in newly diagnosed breast cancer patients shows significant reductions in exercise capacity even before cancer treatment starts. Similar findings have been noted across other cancers, highlighting the importance of structured exercise interventions in maintaining cardiopulmonary fitness during and after treatment. Nair et al. have highlighted the importance of aerobic exercise in reducing the risk of chemotherapy-induced cardiomyopathy, potentially delaying HFpEF progression. The study emphasized the role of exercise as a preventive strategy in anthracycline-treated patients.

HFpEF management in cancer patients often mirrors approaches used in noncancer populations, including diuretic therapy, risk factor management, and evaluating coronary artery disease and arrhythmias.

In patients undergoing chest radiation, conditions such as constrictive pericarditis, coronary artery disease, valvular disorders, and restrictive cardiomyopathy should be considered alongside HFpEF as potential cardiovascular outcomes. A study conducted by Saiki et al. addressed the gap in understanding HFpEF risk older women following radiation for breast cancer. They identified cardiovascular comorbidities like hypertension and diabetes, as well as the duration since radiotherapy, as the key factors contributing to HFpEF. Hence, an aggressive management of cardiovascular risk factors and routine cardiac function assessment are essential for mitigating these risks in cancer survivors **(Flowchart 1)**.

Flowchart 1: Risk factors for HFpEF after oncological treatment.

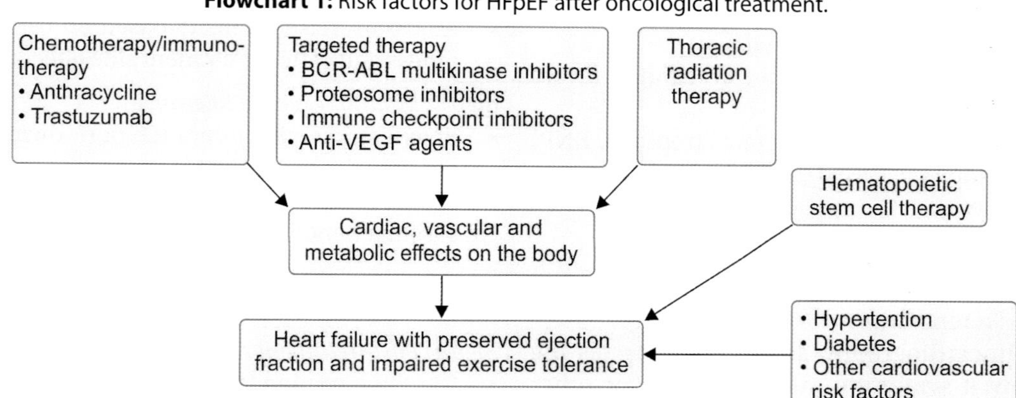

LIMITATIONS

Despite significant advancements, predicting and preventing HFpEF in cancer patients remain challenging. The heterogeneity of HFpEF and the diverse effects of different cancer therapies make it difficult to establish universal treatment guidelines. Many studies focus on small sample sizes, and larger randomized controlled trials are necessary to validate findings related to biomarkers and cardioprotective strategies.

ALGORITHM FOR MANAGING HFpEF IN CANCER PATIENTS

Pretreatment Risk Stratification

Step 1: Baseline cardiovascular assessment

- Conduct a thorough history and physical examination.
- Review any preexisting cardiovascular risk factors (e.g., hypertension, diabetes, obesity, coronary artery disease, atrial fibrillation).
- Assess prior cancer treatments (e.g., anthracyclines, radiation therapy, VEGF inhibitors).

Step 2: Diagnostic testing

- Perform baseline echocardiography to evaluate LVEF and diastolic function.
- Conduct baseline biomarker assessment [e.g., troponin I, BNP, myeloperoxidase (MPO)].

Step 3: Risk stratification

- Categorize patients into low, moderate, or high cardiovascular risk groups based on:
  - Cardiovascular comorbidities
  - Type and dosage of cancer therapy
  - Age and functional status
- Consider early cardiology consultation for moderate- to high-risk patients.

Cardiotoxicity Monitoring

Step 1: Routine monitoring during treatment

- Regularly monitor LVEF with echocardiography (every 3–6 months during treatment).
- Perform serial biomarker testing (e.g., troponin, BNP) at predefined intervals based on risk (every 1–3 months during treatment).

Step 2: Symptom-based monitoring

- Assess for symptoms of heart failure (e.g., dyspnea, fatigue, fluid retention).
- Repeat echocardiography and biomarker testing immediately if symptoms suggest HFpEF or other cardiac dysfunction.

Step 3: Monitoring for radiation effects

- Evaluate for late cardiac effects in patients receiving chest radiation, with echocardiography or CT/MRI at 6–12 months post treatment.

Intervention

Step 1: Early detection of cardiotoxicity

- If biomarkers (troponin, BNP) or LVEF changes occur, initiate early cardioprotective treatment.

Step 2: Cardioprotective strategies

- *For HFpEF prevention*:
  - Initiate ACE inhibitors, ARBs, or β-blockers in patients with rising biomarkers or declining LVEF.
- *For patients with diabetes or prediabetes*:
  - Consider SGLT2 inhibitors based on recent clinical trial data (e.g., EMPEROR-Preserved, DELIVER trials).
- *Other therapies*:
  - Use diuretics for symptomatic fluid overload.
  - Evaluate for coronary artery disease and treat with appropriate revascularization if needed.

Step 3: Managing advanced cardiotoxicity

- For persistent cardiac dysfunction, escalate therapy to include aldosterone antagonists and advanced HF management (e.g., CRT, ICDs).
- Multidisciplinary management between oncology and cardiology teams.

Exercise Prescription

Step 1: Pretreatment exercise evaluation

- Assess baseline cardiopulmonary fitness using cardiopulmonary exercise testing (CPET) or a 6-minute walk test.

Step 2: Tailored exercise intervention

- Prescribe individualized aerobic exercise programs for all patients (e.g., moderate-intensity aerobic activity, 150 min/wk).
- Adjust exercise intensity based on cardiopulmonary fitness and cancer treatment side effects.

Step 3: Monitor exercise tolerance

- Reassess exercise tolerance periodically and adjust the program accordingly.
- Include resistance training for additional cardiovascular benefits.

Long-term Follow-up

Step 1: Post-treatment surveillance

- Continue routine follow-up with cardiac imaging and biomarker monitoring at 6–12-month intervals.

Step 2: Preventive cardiovascular care

- Optimize management of hypertension, diabetes, and other cardiovascular risk factors.
- Encourage long-term adherence to exercise and healthy lifestyle modifications.

Step 3: Consideration of late cardiovascular effects

- Monitor for delayed onset of cardiotoxicity, especially in patients with a history of chest radiation or anthracycline therapy.

ALGORITHM SUMMARY

		Recommendations
1.	Pretreatment	• Baseline cardiovascular assessment (echocardiography, biomarkers) • Risk stratification (low/moderate/high)
2.	During treatment	• Routine echocardiography and biomarker monitoring • Cardiotoxicity management based on LVEF/biomarker changes
3.	Interventions	• Early initiation of cardioprotective medications • Adjust therapy for biomarkers or symptom changes
4.	Exercise program	• Cardiopulmonary fitness evaluation • Tailored aerobic exercise regimen
5.	Long-term follow-up	• Surveillance for delayed cardiovascular effects • Continued cardiovascular risk management

CONCLUSION

Managing heart failure with preserved ejection fraction (HFpEF) in cancer patients undergoing chemotherapy and radiotherapy is a complex challenge requiring a multidisciplinary approach. Traditionally, research and management of cancer-related cardiotoxicity have focused on heart failure with reduced ejection fraction (HFrEF). However, emerging evidence highlights that many cancer therapies, such as anthracyclines, radiation, VEGF inhibitors, and proteasome inhibitors, can contribute to HFpEF by inducing diastolic dysfunction and vascular changes. These effects are exacerbated by preexisting cardiovascular risk factors such as hypertension, diabetes, and obesity, commonly seen in cancer patients.

Early detection through biomarkers such as troponin, BNP, and MPO offers a promising method to identify subclinical myocardial injury before symptomatic heart failure develops. Combined with regular echocardiographic monitoring, these biomarkers enable earlier interventions and may help reduce HFpEF progression. Cardioprotective therapies like ACE inhibitors, β-blockers, and SGLT2 inhibitors are increasingly showing potential in managing HFpEF and improving patient outcomes. Structured aerobic exercise programs have also been shown to mitigate chemotherapy-induced cardiomyopathy, enhancing cardiopulmonary fitness.

Successful management of HFpEF in cancer patients requires close collaboration between oncologists and cardiologists to ensure comprehensive care that balances cancer treatment with cardiovascular protection. Despite advancements, ongoing challenges remain due to the heterogeneity of HFpEF and the long-term cardiovascular effects of newer therapies. Continued research, including larger trials, will be crucial in shaping future guidelines and optimizing outcomes for cancer survivors.

SUGGESTED READING

1. Camilli M, CM Cipolla, Dent S, et al. Anthracycline Cardiotoxicity in Adult Cancer Patients. JACC: CardioOncol. 2024. 6(5):655-77.
2. Dempsey N, Rosenthal A, Dabas N, et al. Trastuzumab-induced cardiotoxicity: a review of clinical risk factors, pharmacologic prevention, and cardiotoxicity of other HER2-directed therapies. Breast Cancer Res Treat. 2021; 188:21-36.
3. Jasinska-Piadlo A, Campbell P. Management of patients with heart failure and preserved ejection fraction. Heart. 2023;109(11):874-83.
4. Jorge AJL, Villacorta H, Danzmann LC, et al. Heart Failure with Preserved Ejection Fraction and Cancer. ABC Heart Fail Cardiomyop. 2022;2(4):343-53.
5. Ky B, Putt M, Sawaya H, et al. Early increases in multiple biomarkers predict subsequent cardiotoxicity in patients with breast cancer treated with doxorubicin, taxanes, and trastuzumab. J Am Coll Cardiol. 2014;63(8):809-16.
6. Nair N, Gongora E. Heart failure in chemotherapy-related cardiomyopathy: Can exercise make a difference? BBA Clin. 2016;6:69-75.
7. Qiu Y, Jiang P, Huang Y, et al. Anthracycline-induced cardiotoxicity: mechanisms, monitoring, and prevention. Front Cardiovasc Med. 2023;10:1242596.
8. Saiki H, Petersen IA, Scott CG, et al. Risk of Heart Failure With Preserved Ejection Fraction in Older Women After Contemporary Radiotherapy for Breast Cancer. Circulation. 2017;135(15):1388-96.
9. Zambelli A, Della Porta, Eleuteri E, et al. Predicting and preventing cardiotoxicity in the era of breast cancer targeted therapies. Novel molecular tools for clinical issues. Breast. 2011;20(2):176-83.

SECTION 18

HFpEF and ECMO

129. Extracorporeal Membrane Oxygenation and HFpEF

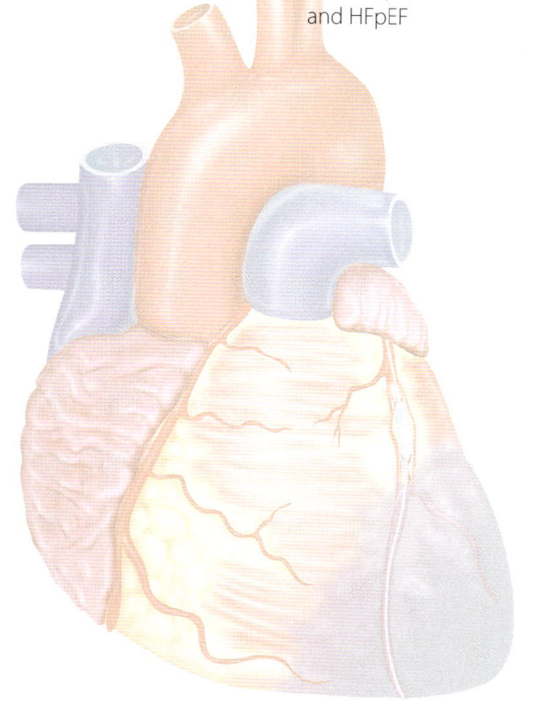

CHAPTER

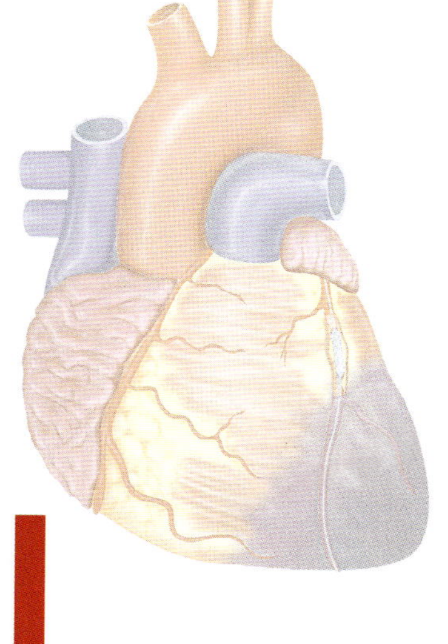

Extracorporeal Membrane Oxygenation and HFpEF

Poonam Malhotra Kapoor

INTRODUCTION

Heart failure with preserved ejection fraction (HFpEF) accounts for almost half of all heart failure cases, particularly affecting elderly patients and those with significant comorbidities such as hypertension, diabetes, and obesity. HFpEF is characterized by preserved left ventricular ejection fraction (LVEF ≥50%) with the presence of clinical symptoms of heart failure, including breathlessness, fatigue, and exercise intolerance. Unlike heart failure with reduced ejection fraction (HFrEF), where systolic dysfunction dominates, HFpEF involves primarily diastolic dysfunction, along with abnormalities in ventricular stiffness, microvascular dysfunction, and systemic inflammation.

Extracorporeal membrane oxygenation (ECMO) is an advanced life support modality that is used to manage patients with life-threatening cardiac or respiratory failure. While ECMO has been primarily employed for patients with severe systolic HF or cardiogenic shock, its use in HFpEF is emerging, albeit less commonly due to the complex pathophysiology of HFpEF. Whether to use peripheral versus central VA ECMO, is dependent on stage of diastolic shock. In the ICUs, it is recently been observed that mortality with central ECMO, remains higher than peripheral ECMO in cardiogenic shock **(Fig. 1)**.[1] This chapter explores the growing intersection between ECMO therapy and HFpEF, including patient selection, potential benefits, risks, and current evidence from the latest studies **(Fig. 2)**.

EXTRACORPOREAL MEMBRANE OXYGENATION IN PRESERVED HEART FAILURE

Extracorporeal membrane oxygenation is a form of mechanical circulatory and respiratory support that can

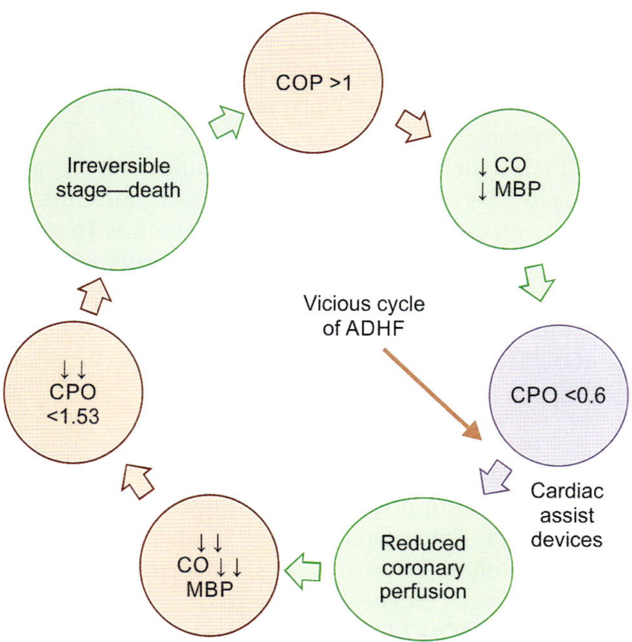

Fig. 1: Course of hemodynamic compromise in heart failure with preserved ejection fraction. (CO: cardiac output; MBP: mean blood pressure; CPO: cardiac power output infraction; PCI: percutaneous coronary intervention)

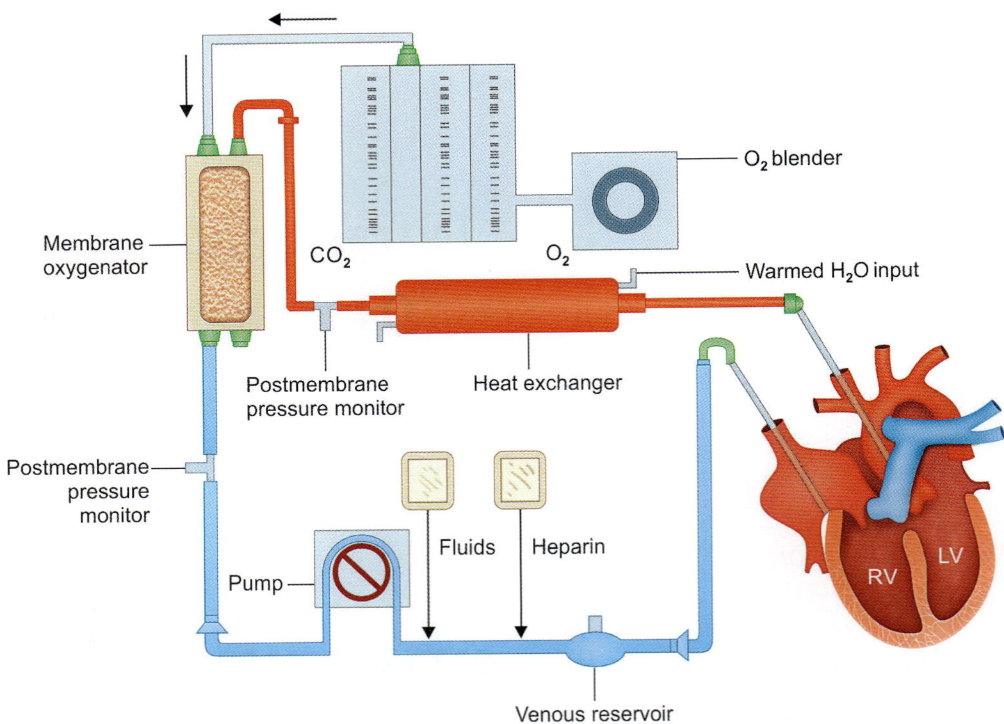

Fig. 2: Extracorporeal membrane oxygenation (ECMO) system.

temporarily stabilize patients with refractory cardiac or respiratory failure. ECMO provides oxygenation and/or hemodynamic support by removing blood from the venous system, oxygenating it through an external circuit, and reinfusing the blood back into either the venous or arterial system.[2]

ECMO, which is a partial cardiopulmonary bypass (CPB), provides good LV unloading and is a good choice in patients with low cardiac output in heart failure. There are two types of ECMO, venoarterial and venovenous ECMO. For HF patients, it is VA ECMO, which is used mainly and is the main temporary bypass employed in main ICUs. An ECMO CPR (E-CPR) used to resuscitate patients on ECMO is salvage in acute emergency situations.[3]

The two main types of ECMO are:

1. *Venoarterial (VA) ECMO:* Provides both cardiac and respiratory support by bypassing the failing heart and lungs. This is typically used in cardiogenic shock, where both the heart and lungs are unable to meet the body's oxygen and perfusion needs.
2. *Venovenous (VV) ECMO:* Provides respiratory support alone and is primarily used for severe respiratory failure without direct cardiac support. The major differences between the two types are enumerated in **Table 1 (Figs. 3A and 3B)**.

Given the preserved ejection fraction in HFpEF, VA-ECMO is the primary modality used in this population, particularly when patients experience acute decompensations that progress to cardiogenic shock or severe right HF. VA-ECMO can provide temporary hemodynamic

TABLE 1: Extracorporeal membrane oxygenation (ECMO) types and their differences.

Property	*Venoarterial (VA) ECMO*	*Venovenous (VV) ECMO*
Cannulation site	IJV/FV and RCC/Ax/FA/Ao	IJV alone/IJV-FV/FV-FV/Saph-saph/RA
PaO_2	60–150 mm Hg	45–80 mm Hg
Indicator of O_2 sufficiency	Mixed venous saturation or PaO_2	Combination of SaO_2, PaO_2, cerebral ven sat and pre membr sat trend
Cardiac effect	↓ preload; ↑afterload; pulse pr ↓; coronary oxygen by left ventricular (LV) blood; "Cardiac stun"	Negligible effects; may improve coronary oxygen; may reduce right ventricular (RV) afterload
O_2 delivery capacity	High	Moderate, ↑cephalad drain
Circulatory support	Partial to complete	*Indirect:* ↑ delivery of O_2 to coronary and pulmonary circulation

(FA: femoral artery; FV: femoral vein; IJV: internal jugular vein)

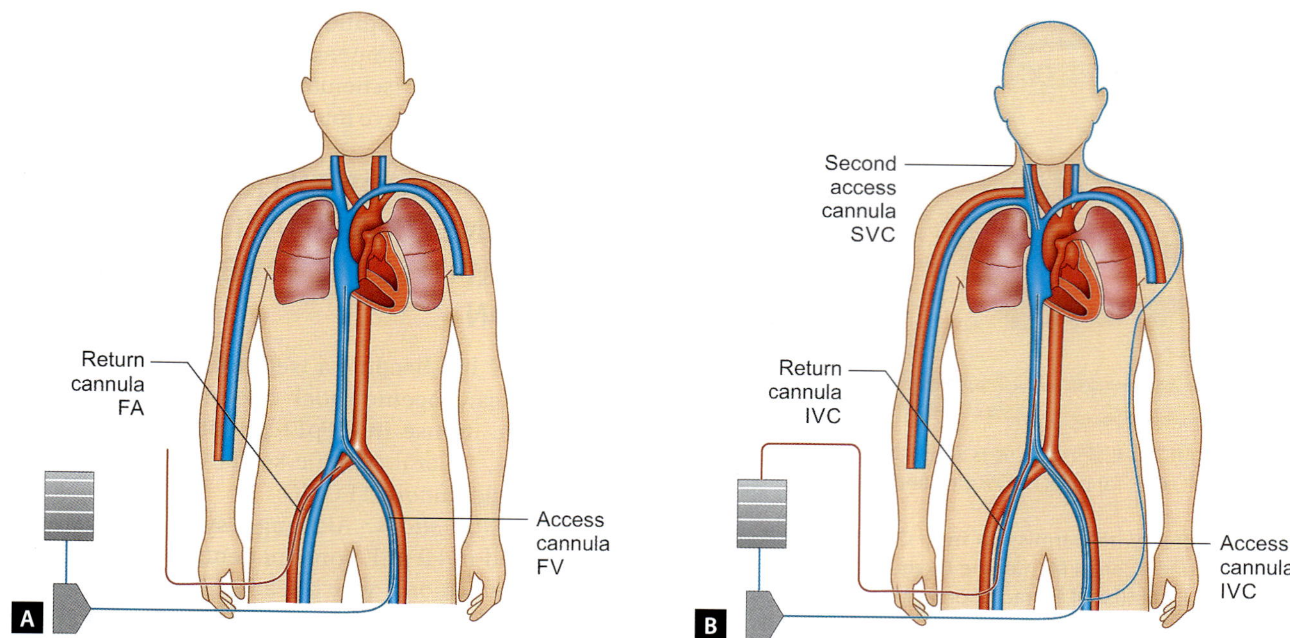

Figs. 3A and 3B: (A) A peripheral venoarterial ECMO with access cannula in femoral vein and return cannula in femoral artery; (B) Venovenous ECMO with access cannula in IVC and return cannula in IVC/SVC. (ECMO: extracorporeal membrane oxygenation; FA: femoral artery; IVC: inferior vena cava; SVC: superior vena cava)

support to stabilize the patient and bridge them to recovery or definitive therapy.

The debate over hemodynamic effects of VA-ECMO continuous. Recent literature has concluded that high-flow VA-ECMO support, significantly reduces LV end-diastolic pressure and volume, along with stroke work, with higher diastolic velocities and mean arterial pressure.[4]

CARDIOHELP EXTRACORPOREAL MEMBRANE OXYGENATION SYSTEM FOR VENOVENOUS AND VENOARTERIAL TYPES

The modern CARDIOHELP machine is an upgraded form of an ECMO. It is lightweight and sleek for easy portability and can be easily used in changing scenarios in a hospital set-up. This new machine is most suitable in providing all of patients' needs for ECMO and in one single platform; it carries all range of ECMO features for cardiac insufficiency as well as respiratory distress.

In both VV and VA types of ECMO and also in percutaneous as well as centrally cannulated patients of ECMO, the CARDIOHELP works well to remove carbon dioxide efficiently and provide ideal "Protective Ventilation Protocols" **(Box 1)**. Cost efficiency, improved mobility and portability, and improved clinical performance are the advantages of CARDIOHELP **(Fig. 4 and Box 2)**. The CARDIOHELP system delivers optimal care for the ECMO patients, with the improved features of protective ventilation and carbon dioxide removal.[2]

BOX 1: Pump-assisted protection.

- *Possible fields of application:* Respiratory failure, such as ARDS, ALI, VILI
- *Patient and user values:* Extracorporeal CO_2 removal enables protective ventilation
- *Special feature:* Support of gas exchange for up to 30 days without exchanging components with focus on low flow and CO_2 removal instead of oxygenation
- *Cannulation:* Percutaneous cannulation of either jugular, subclavian, or femoral vein

(ALI: acute lung injury; ARDS: acute respiratory distress syndrome; VILI: ventilator-induced lung injury)

PATHOPHYSIOLOGY OF HEART FAILURE WITH PRESERVED EJECTION FRACTION AND ITS CHALLENGES

Mechanisms of Heart Failure with Preserved Ejection Fraction

The HFpEF is fundamentally a disease of diastolic dysfunction, where the left ventricle (LV) fails to relax adequately during diastole, leading to increased filling pressures. This is often caused by structural changes in the myocardium, including hypertrophy, fibrosis, and

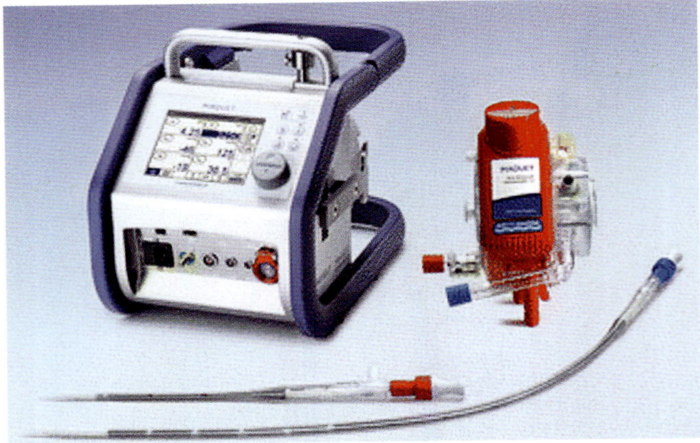

Fig. 4: The CARDIOHELP machine is lighter and easily portable and used for ECMO CPR for both in-hospital and out of hospital cardiac arrest.
Source: Adopted with permission from Ch 40. Cardio Help: The Future of Extracorporeal Membrane Oxygenation. In: Kapoor PM, Hasija S (Eds). Manual of Extracorporeal Membrane Oxygenation (ECMO) in the ICU. New Delhi: Jaypee Publishers; 2014. pp. 243-8.

BOX 2: CARDIOHELP bedside adaption and transportation.

- Different windows for optimized visualization enable the user to only see what he wants to see; separate lab value screen displaying hemoglobin, venous saturation, hematocrit, and temperature readings (venous and arterial)
- All alarms are indicated with colors and sound patterns, enabling the user to identify different alarm priorities
- The CARDIOHELP device alarm header will tell the user what the problem is, no hidden views, windows for fastest reaction time, and maximum patient safety. The ward call allows alarms to be indicated even in remote locations
- Continuous storage of data in 3 seconds–10 minutes steps
- Fast and simple start-up procedure with automated self-test and calibration
- User-defined start-up configuration

increased collagen deposition, which stiffen the ventricular walls. Additional factors contributing to HFpEF include:

- *Endothelial dysfunction:* Microvascular and endothelial dysfunction lead to impaired vasodilation, systemic inflammation, and increased ventricular afterload.
- *Pulmonary hypertension (PH):* Increased left-sided filling pressures in HFpEF can lead to secondary pulmonary hypertension and right ventricular dysfunction, complicating clinical management.
- *Comorbidities:* HFpEF is frequently associated with metabolic syndromes, such as obesity, diabetes mellitus, and hypertension, which contribute to systemic inflammation and vascular stiffness.

These complexities make managing HFpEF more challenging than HFrEF, as there are currently no therapies that have consistently demonstrated survival benefits in HFpEF patients. Additionally, HFpEF patients often experience acute decompensations triggered by stressors such as arrhythmias, ischemia, or infection, necessitating urgent and often invasive interventions.

INDICATIONS FOR EXTRACORPOREAL MEMBRANE OXYGENATION IN HEART FAILURE WITH PRESERVED EJECTION FRACTION

While ECMO has become a well-established therapy in HFrEF and cardiogenic shock due to profound systolic dysfunction, its use in HFpEF is still relatively novel. Nonetheless, several specific scenarios in HFpEF may warrant consideration of ECMO:

- *Cardiogenic shock:* Although systolic function is preserved in HFpEF, some patients experience acute decompensations, which lead to cardiogenic shock. This may occur due to acute ischemia, arrhythmias, or significant volume overload that overwhelms diastolic function. VA-ECMO can stabilize hemodynamics by decreasing the workload of the heart and ensuring end-organ perfusion during periods of shock.[5,6]
- *Right ventricular failure and pulmonary hypertension:* Many HFpEF patients develop secondary pulmonary hypertension, which can lead to right ventricular (RV) failure. In cases of acute RV failure and hemodynamic collapse, ECMO can offload the failing RV and maintain oxygenation.[7]
- *Severe decompensated HF with multiorgan failure:* When HFpEF leads to progressive HF and subsequent multiorgan dysfunction (renal, hepatic, or respiratory failure), ECMO may be used as a temporary support to allow time for recovery or assessment for more definitive therapies (e.g., heart transplant or durable ventricular assist devices).[8]
- *Bridge to transplant or bridge to decision:* For patients with advanced HFpEF awaiting heart transplantation, ECMO can serve as a bridge to transplant. Additionally, it may serve as a bridge to the decision in cases where clinicians need time to determine the viability of recovery or other long-term therapies.[9]

CLINICAL OUTCOMES OF EXTRACORPOREAL MEMBRANE OXYGENATION IN HEART FAILURE WITH PRESERVED EJECTION FRACTION

Despite its growing use, the outcomes of ECMO in patients with HFpEF remain underexplored, as most ECMO studies

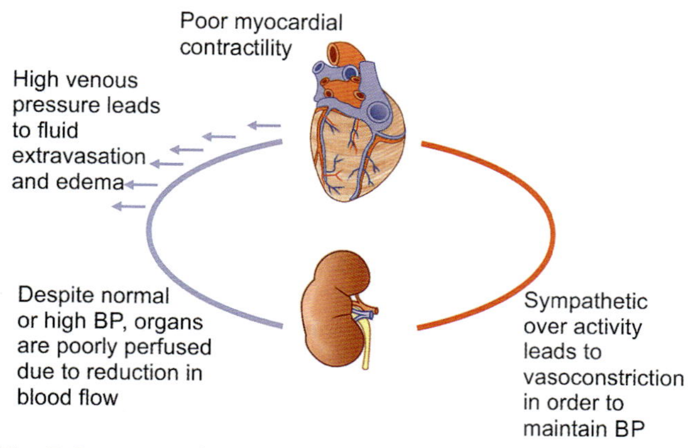

Fig. 5: Sequence of events leading to cardiogenic shock.
Source: Adopted with permission from Ch 32. Extracorporeal Membrane Oxygenation in Cardiogenic Shock. In: Sharma J, Mehta Y (Eds). Manual of Extracorporeal Membrane Oxygenation (ECMO) in the ICU. New Delhi: Jaypee Publishers; 2014. pp. 193-8.

focus on patients with HFrEF or cardiogenic shock due to acute myocardial infarction. However, a few recent studies have begun to shed light on the utility of ECMO in this patient population.

EXTRACORPOREAL MEMBRANE OXYGENATION FOR CARDIOGENIC SHOCK IN HEART FAILURE WITH PRESERVED EJECTION FRACTION (FIG. 5)

A retrospective study by Patel et al. (2023) examined outcomes in patients with HFpEF who underwent VA-ECMO for cardiogenic shock. The study found that while short-term survival rates were lower than those of patients with HFrEF, ECMO provided a critical bridge to recovery or decision in a subset of patients. Early initiation of ECMO in patients who had not yet progressed to irreversible organ failure was associated with better outcomes.[10,11]

EXTRACORPOREAL MEMBRANE OXYGENATION IN PULMONARY HYPERTENSION AND RIGHT HEART FAILURE

Given the association between HFpEF and pulmonary hypertension, ECMO has also been explored in HFpEF patients with right ventricular failure. In a study by Nakamura et al. (2022), patients with combined HFpEF and pulmonary hypertension who developed RV failure were supported with ECMO. The study showed that while ECMO successfully stabilized the patients, mortality remained high due to the advanced stage of right HF at the time of initiation. Early identification and intervention with ECMO were key factors in improving survival.[12]

PROGNOSIS AND LONG-TERM OUTCOMES

The long-term prognosis of HFpEF patients on ECMO is highly variable. While ECMO can provide life-saving support in the acute setting, patients with HFpEF often have multiple comorbidities, such as diabetes, obesity, and chronic kidney disease, which can complicate recovery. Additionally, the underlying diastolic dysfunction that characterizes HFpEF is not directly addressed by ECMO, meaning that patients may remain at high risk for recurrent HF hospitalizations after ECMO weaning.

A systematic review of ECMO in HFpEF by Ahmad et al. (2022) noted that while ECMO can stabilize hemodynamics in acute decompensations, the overall survival rate remains lower than in HFrEF patients. The review highlighted the need for careful patient selection and early initiation of ECMO before the onset of irreversible multiorgan dysfunction.[13]

DEVICE THERAPY FOR ACUTE DECOMPENSATED HEART FAILURE

Mechanical-assist device may be considered in those cases of acute decompensated heart failure (ADHF) which are not amenable to drugs alone. IABP assists in adequate unloading of the heart and so does ECMO and ventricular assist devices (VADs) such as the Tandem heart[14] **(Figs. 6 and 7) (Box 3)**.

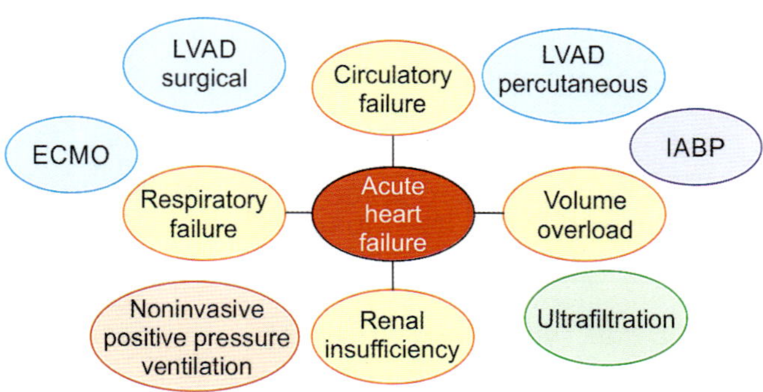

Fig. 6: Overview of the devices available for managing acute heart failure. (ECMO: extracorporeal membrane oxygenation; LVAD: left ventricular assist device; IABP: intra-aortic balloon pump)

WHEN BLEEDING ON EXTRACORPOREAL MEMBRANE OXYGENATION PERSISTS

Ultra-fractionated used on all types of ECMO. It is a prodrug which acts through antithrombin III. In an ECMO patient bleeding is common. If it continues, then heparin is the major anticoagulant. ATIII concentrate is given if the ATIII activity drops below 70%. It is advisable to perform beyond ACT and antithrombin III levels, a routine activated partial thromboplastin time with kaolin (aPTT) → (normal 50–80 seconds on ECMO) and serum fibrinogen levels as well (>1.5 g/L). Point-of-care viscoelastic tests such as ROTEM/TEG (rotational thromboelastometry/thromboelastography) or Sonoclot can be done if bleeding persists. These tests provide prompt action as they have shorter turnaround time and guides the intensivist, as to how to give the correct blood, component therapy.[15,16] Patients on arteriovenous ECMO are ventilated with conventional settings, with a FiO_2 to achieve an acceptable PaO_2 (at least 60 mm Hg). Inotropic support can be slowly weaned off but a more potent inodilator which has strong vasodilator effects at the tissue level like milrinone can be continued.[17] Fluid management is aimed at preserving renal function and ensuring a stable circulation. Comprehensive bleeding assessment during surgery is challenging due to the dynamic coagulation cascade. A multimodal approach, supported by institutional protocols and point-of-care testing, is vital, especially in India with limited resources[18-26] **(Flowchart 1 and Fig. 8)**.

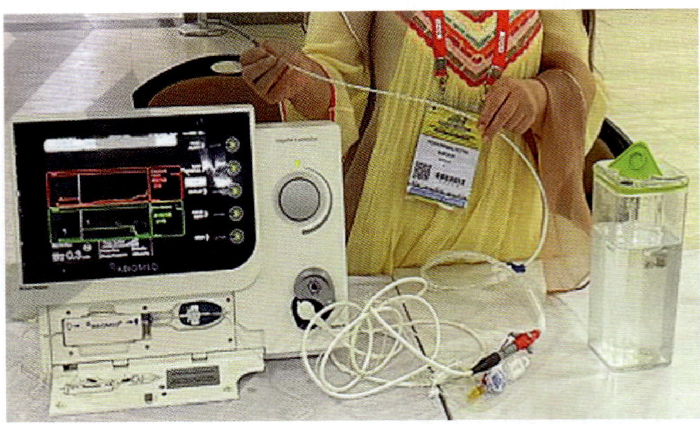

Fig. 7: Impella device placement with extracorporeal membrane oxygenation (ECMO) in a failing heart in cardiogenic shock.

BOX 3: Advantages of extracorporeal membrane oxygenation (ECMO) in acute decompensated heart failure (ADHF) patients.

- ECMO can be inserted at the bedside
- It is relatively cheap [as compared to the implantable left ventricular assist device (LVAD)]
- Gives the treating physicians some time to wait for recovery or a more stable condition
- Portable, can be inserted in Cath lab
- 17–21 Fr cannulas
- Intra-aortic balloon pump (IABP) to reduce afterload
- Centrifugal pump at 2–4 L/min
- Bridge to surgical ventricular assist device (VAD), transplant, or recovery

Flowchart 1: New cyanotic POC All India Institute of Medical Sciences algorithm to implement blood conservation strategy.[27]

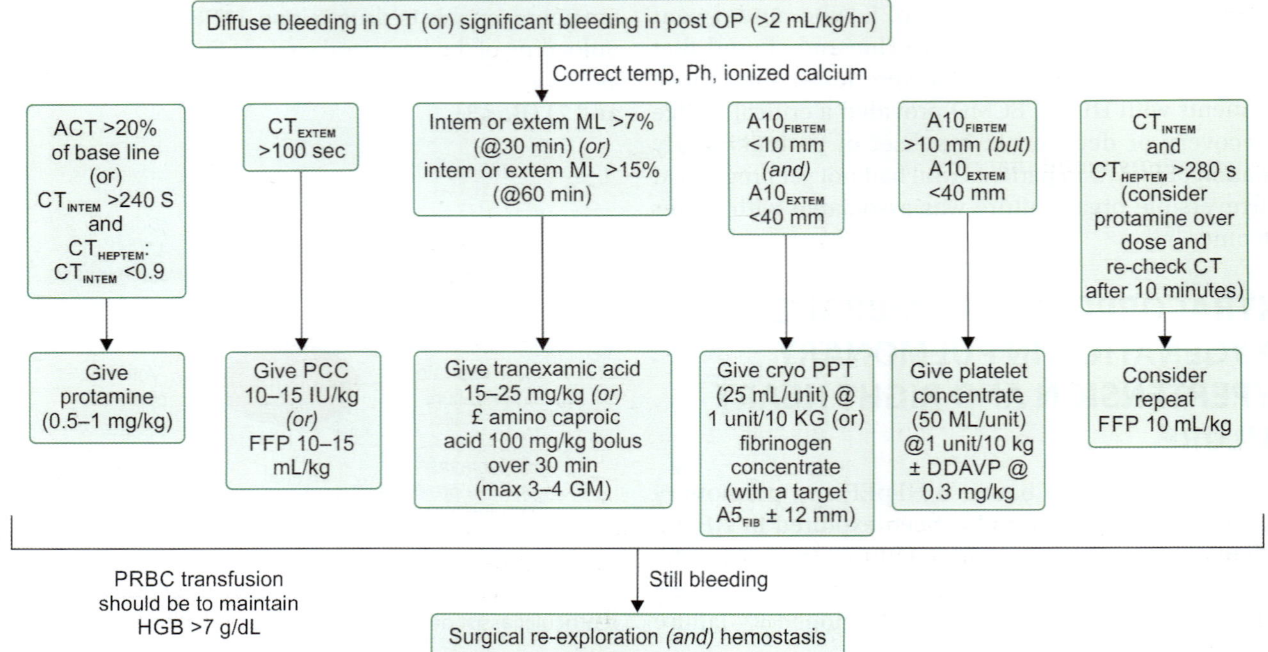

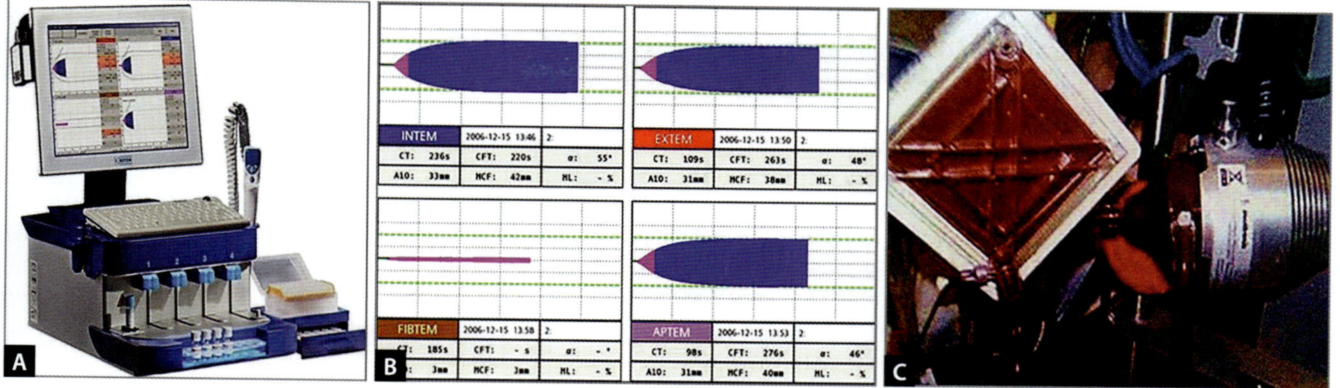

Figs. 8A to C: (A) The Rotem machine with four channels for anticoagulation in ECMO; (B) Point-of-care testing graphs of fibrinogen deficiency with ROTEM machine; (C) Hemolysis leading to thrombosis to the ECMO leads to ECMO failure and extensive bleeding.

USE OF ANGIOTENSIN RECEPTOR NEPRILYSIN INHIBITOR ON EXTRACORPOREAL MEMBRANE OXYGENATION

Angiotensin receptor neprilysin inhibitor (ARNI) reduces the need for device therapy. HK Chopra et al. have recommended that all the foundational pillars of HFrEF therapy, which include ARNI, β-blockers, SGLT2 inhibitors, and MRAs should be tried in maximally tolerated dosages for at least 3–6 months, and then the LVEF should be reassessed by three-dimensional echocardiography and/or cardiac magnetic resonance imaging before deciding for cardioverter defibrillator/cardiac resynchronization therapy implant.[28]

Treating Heart Failure in Postoperative Congenital Cardiac Repair in Children

Experience from AIIMS on an anomalous left coronary artery from the pulmonary artery (ALCAPA) patient with HF, the authors found that treating HF in postoperative congenital cardiac repair in children with an ALCAPA is a daunting task. Regular antifailure measures with angiotensin-converting enzyme (ACE) inhibitors may become inadequate or resistant in certain situations. ARNI in place of ACE inhibitors can be an alternative to help these postcardiac surgical children convalesce better. Sacubitril/valsartan is an ARNI-approved treatment for HF in adults, and in pediatric HF patients, it is showing promising benefits. However, in postcardiac surgical children with HF, its effects are not well known. Meera Rajeev et al. ARNI in postcardiac surgical infants with ALCAPA repair in HF patients, described. Overlapping dobutamine infusions with ARNI in place of ACE inhibitors helped in weaning the respiratory support and recovery of the child on VA-ECMO post-ALCAPA repair.[29]

RIGHT CHOICE OF MECHANICAL CIRCULATORY SUPPORT DEVICES IN HEART FAILURE AND CARDIOGENIC SHOCK IS VENOARTERIAL EXTRACORPOREAL MEMBRANE OXYGENATION

The VA-ECMO has slowly become the MCS device of choice for postcardiotomy cardiogenic shock (PCCS) in the contemporary era. This is attributed to the improvements Ho circuit technologies, ease of bedside cannulation, improvement in percutaneous access techniques, and the evolution of critical care cardiologists capable of managing these circuits.[30] VA-ECMO may be inserted either centrally (right atrium and aortic cannulation) or peripherally (via femoral artery and vein cannulation or axillary artery and femoral vein), with the femoral access being more common in the recent times. VA-ECMO typically comprises an arterial limb, a venous limb, a membrane oxygenator, and a centrifugal pump. It is capable of providing nearly 4–5 L of cardiac output support, biventricular support (indirect support), and respiratory support.[31]

Temporal for postcardiac cardiogenic shock (PCCS) VA-ECMO for PCCS have been studied from multiple registries and national databases. Typically the use of ECMO in PCCS has been reported between 0.4 and 3.7%.[32] In the Extracorporeal Life Support Organization (ELSO) registry, the use of VA-ECMO for PCCS has increased exponentially from 2 to 3% in 2000 to nearly 30% in 2015.[33] Similarly, using the National Inpatient Sample database, (Chung et al. noted about 40% of all postsurgical ECMO in the United States to be used in PCCS).[34]

Similarly, in all-comer cardiogenic shock being bridged to durable LVAD, VA-ECMO use being use increased from 4% to nearly 10% suggestive of the preference for the VA-ECMO as the device of choice for bridging.[35] In recent times, there is renewed enthusiasm for the use of the VA-ECMO in combination with either an IABP or Impella to assist with increasing circulatory support and providing reliable LV unloading.[36,37] Despite the significant improvement in VA-ECMO technology, it continues to be associated with important complications, such as intracranial hemorrhage, limb ischemia, and hematological issues.

The universal initial therapy for cardiogenic shock in stage D HF consists of inotropic therapy, often combined with vasodilators (to decrease afterload). However, these agents can be ineffective, increase myocardial oxygen consumption, impair tissue perfusion, and increase the risk of arrhythmias.[38] Accordingly, in many cases medical therapy alone is unlikely to suffice as a bridge to durable treatment for cardiogenic shock in advanced HF various temporary MCS options exist to support patients with cardiogenic shock and stage D HF. The goal of temporary MCS is to primarily serve as a bridge to advanced HF therapies (durable LVAD/transplant) and in a small percentage of patients serves as a bridge to recovery from cardiogenic shock. **Figure 9** shows the interplay between outpatient and inpatient evaluation for advanced HF therapies such as durable MCS/LVAD.

Wang et al. generated a predictive tool that incorporates a PC-ECMO score to stratify the risk of mortality after postcardiotomy VA-ECMO. In patients undergoing coronary artery bypass grafting, a scoring system has been devised to stratify the risk hospital mortality in patients undergoing VA-ECMO following surgery.[39] Age, left main disease, inotropic support, as creatinine kinase, serum creatinine, and thrombocytopenia were identified as independent predictors of hospital mortality (Wang et al. 2019). Using these variables, the authors devised the REMEMBER score for predicting mortality in patients with postcardiotomy cardiogenic shock requiring ECMO. The diverse nature of the patients and the rarity of needing postcardiotomy ECMO make these risk models difficult to apply broadly. Thus, the current risk models that predict which patients may benefit from postcardiotomy ECMO support need to be used with caution **(Table 2)**.[40,41]

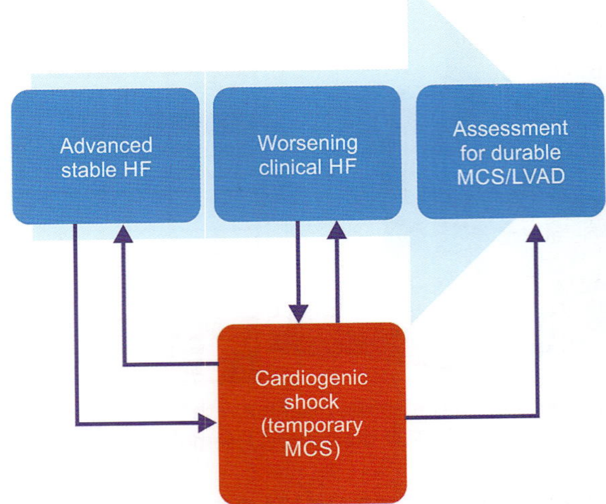

Fig. 9: Patients with progressive advanced HF, classified as ACC/AHA stage C and stage D HF may worsen clinically and need evaluation for durable mechanical circulatory support devices (MCS) in the outpatient setting. These patients may also deteriorate and require hospital admission for cardiogenic shock where temporary MCS may be required. The figure shows multiple possible outcomes where temporary MCS may serve as a bridge to durable MCS or allow for recovery and subsequent outpatient evaluation for durable MCS.

CHALLENGES AND LIMITATIONS OF EXTRACORPOREAL MEMBRANE OXYGENATION IN HEART FAILURE WITH PRESERVED EJECTION FRACTION

Left Ventricular Distension

One of the primary challenges in using ECMO for HFpEF patients is the risk of left ventricular distension. Since HFpEF patients retain normal or near-normal systolic function, VA-ECMO may increase afterload, causing the LV to become distended due to the high filling pressures. Left ventricular distension can worsen diastolic dysfunction and contribute to pulmonary congestion. This challenge often requires additional interventions, such as left ventricular venting or the use of devices like the Impella to decompress the LV. Echocardiography should be done twice a day, while on ECMO, to know the filling pressures, velocities, IVRT, deceleration time, and biventricular function. LV distension on ECMO is common and often seen. Echocardiography aids in deciphering thrombosis, ECMO flow obstruction and tamponade while on ECMO **(Figs. 10 to 16)**.

Echocardiography aids in deciphering thrombosis, ECMO flow obstruction and tamponade on ECMO.

COMPLICATIONS ASSOCIATED WITH EXTRACORPOREAL MEMBRANE OXYGENATION

Like all forms of mechanical support, ECMO carries a risk of complications, including bleeding, thrombosis, infection, and vascular injury. The need for systemic anticoagulation to prevent thrombotic events on ECMO increases the risk of bleeding, particularly in elderly HFpEF patients who may have underlying coagulopathies or be on anticoagulant

TABLE 2: Globally available percutaneous and surgically implanted temporary mechanical circulatory support devices.

	IABP	*Impella CP*	*Impella 5.0*	*VA-ECMO*	*CentrMag/RotaFlow*
Maximal flow (LPM)	0.5–1	4	5	4–6	10
Pump	Pneumatic pump	Axial flow	Axial flow	Centrifugal flow	Centrifugal flow
Bedside implantation	Yes	No	No	Yes	No
Circuit/location	Descending aorta	LV/LVOT	LV/LVOT	FV to FA	LA/LV to ascending aorta
Catheter size	8F	9F	9F	18–21 F inflow 15–22 F outflow	32–36 F inflow 22 F outflow
Pump size	25–50 cc balloon	14F	21F	EC	EC
Sheath size	8F	14F	22F	18–21 F (FV) 15–22F (FA)	N/A
Hemodynamic support	Low	Moderate-high	High	High	High
Implantation time	+	++	+++	+++	++++
Anticoagulation required	Very low	Low	Low	High	High
Hemolysis risk	Very low	Low	Low-moderate	Low	Low
Limb ischemia risk	Very low	Low	Moderate	High	N/A
Cost (approximate)	$1,000	$20,000–$25,000	$15,000	$5,000/$3000	Cost (approximate)

(CP: cardiac power; EC: extracorporeal; FA: femoral artery; FV: femoral vein; IABP: intra-aortic balloon pump; LA: left atrium; LPM: liters per minute; LV: left ventricle; LVOT: left ventricular outflow tract; VA-ECMO: venoarterial extracorporeal membrane oxygenation)

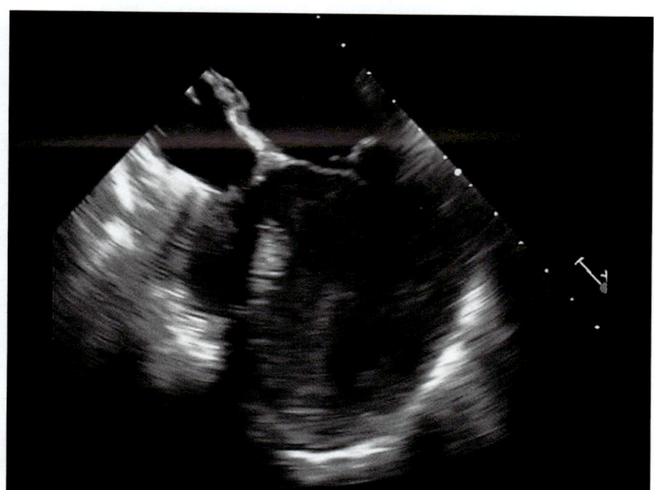

Fig. 10: Left ventricular (LV) distension as seen on transesophageal echocardiogram.

therapy for other conditions. Additionally, cannulation for ECMO can be technically challenging in HFpEF patients who often have vascular disease, further increasing the risk of access-site complications.

PROGNOSTIC FACTORS

Studies have shown that patient selection is critical for determining outcomes in ECMO-supported HFpEF patients. Those with fewer comorbidities, better baseline functional status, and earlier initiation of ECMO tend to have improved outcomes compared to patients with more advanced multiorgan failure or significant right ventricular dysfunction. Age and the presence of severe comorbidities such as diabetes or chronic kidney disease also play significant roles in determining ECMO success.

RECENT ADVANCES IN EXTRACORPOREAL MEMBRANE OXYGENATION (FIG. 17)

Dual-lumen cannula (V-V), single access site, less recirculation, ambulation/rehab potential, HFO oxygenator, can last for weeks, lower surface area and pressure, gradient, improved tubing, thicker PVC decreases rupture or, breach, heparin-bonding, centrifugal pumps, no more tube-crimping roller pumps, portability—<30 kg.

FUTURE DIRECTIONS

As the understanding of HFpEF continues to evolve, so too will the role of ECMO in its management. Future research is needed to better define the optimal timing and patient selection for ECMO in HFpEF. Additionally, advancements in ECMO technology, such as portable ECMO devices and improved biocompatible circuits, may make ECMO more accessible and safer for this patient population. Integrating ECMO with other advanced therapies, such as ventricular

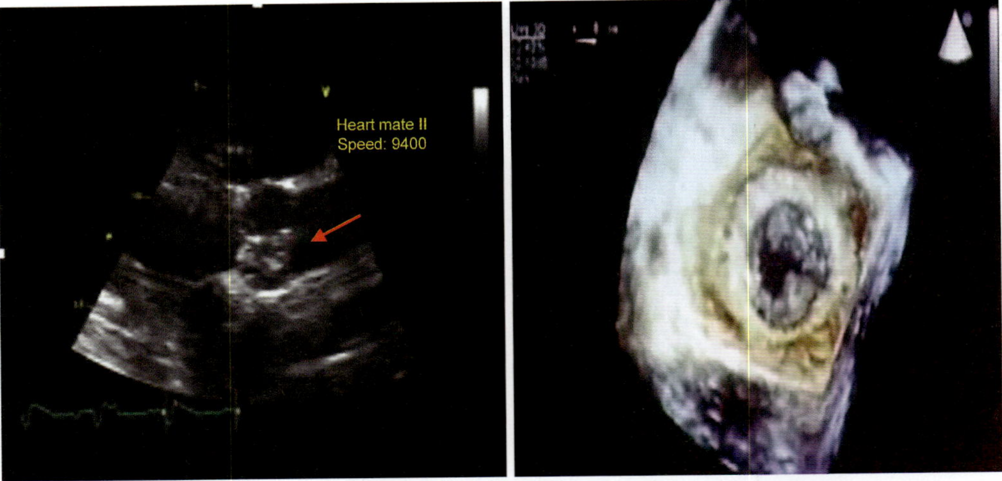

Fig. 11: Thrombosis on extracorporeal membrane oxygenation (ECMO).

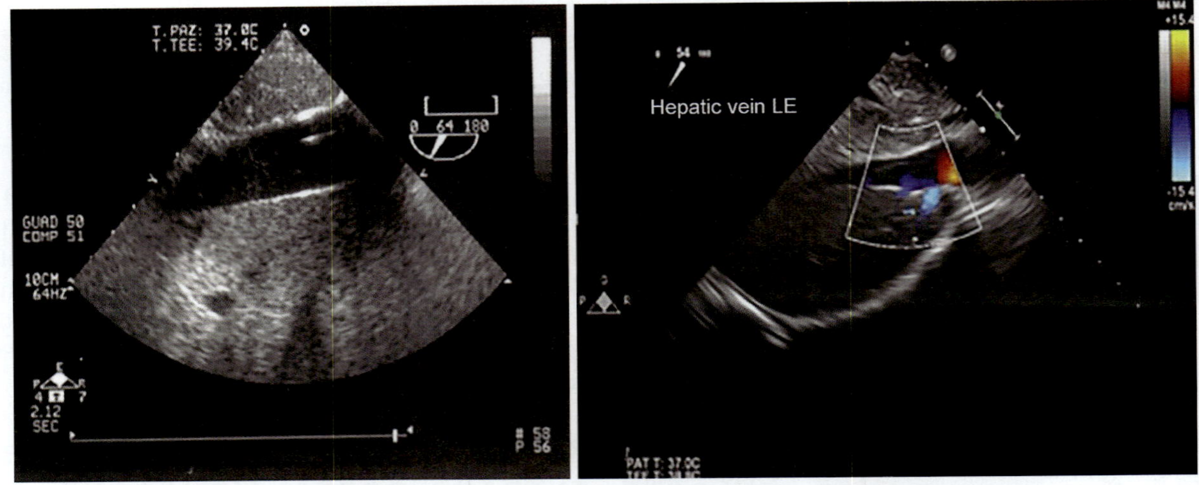

Fig. 12: Extracorporeal membrane oxygenation (ECMO) complications—flow obstruction.

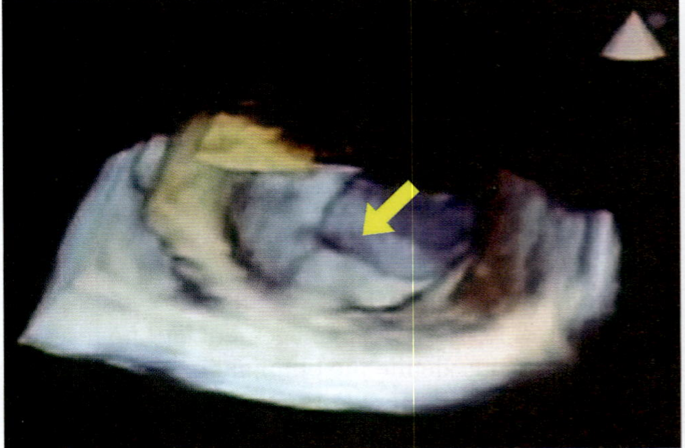

Fig. 13: Bleeding tamponade.

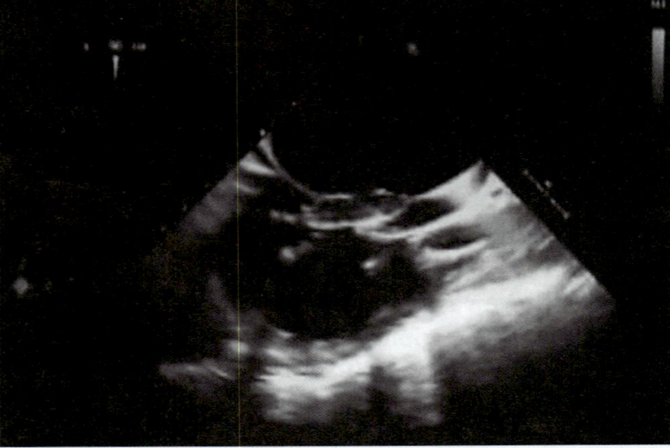

Fig. 14: Balloon atrial septostomy to decompress left atrium, left ventricle.

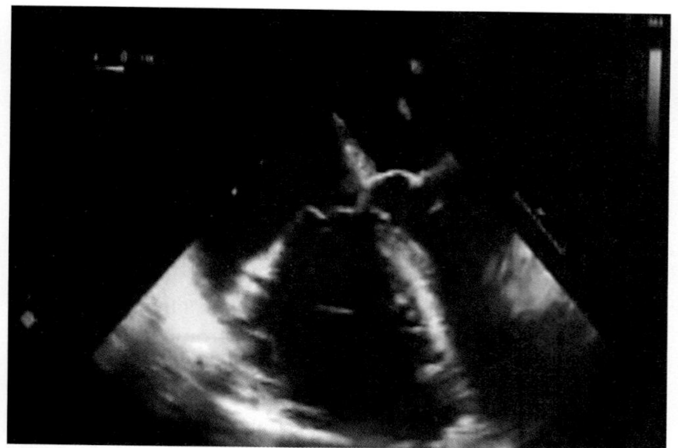

Fig. 15: Severe right ventricular (RV) dysfunction at time of initiation.

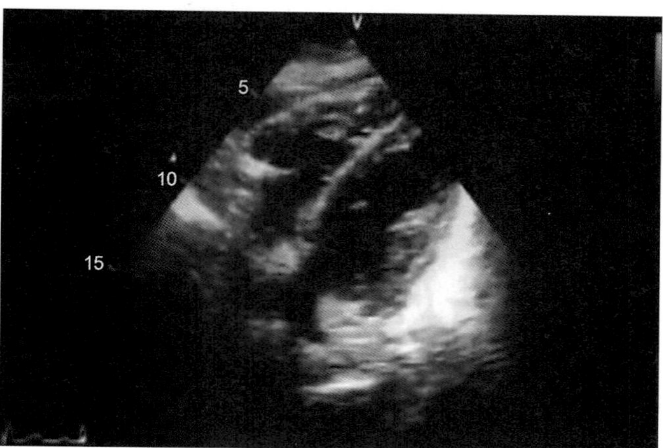

Fig. 16: Normalization of right ventricular (RV) function at time weaning.

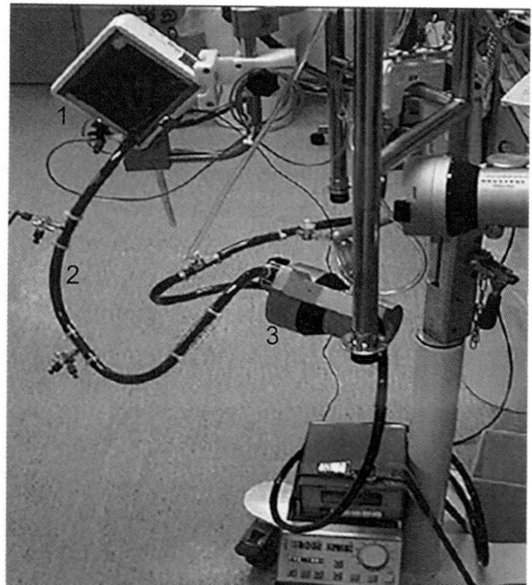

Fig. 17: Cannula used in extracorporeal membrane oxygenation.

assist devices and pharmacological treatments targeting diastolic dysfunction, will also be crucial.

Further studies are also warranted to evaluate long-term outcomes and quality of life in HFpEF patients after ECMO support, as well as the development of strategies to mitigate complications such as left ventricular distension and right ventricular failure.

CONCLUSION

The use of ECMO in patients with HFpEF is a developing area of research and clinical practice. While ECMO can provide life-saving hemodynamic support in acute decompensations of HFpEF, its use is associated with unique challenges, including left ventricular distension and high rates of comorbidities. Despite these challenges, ECMO offers a potential bridge to recovery, decision, or transplant for carefully selected HFpEF patients. Future research will be essential to refine patient selection criteria, improve outcomes, and integrate ECMO with other advanced HF therapies.

REFERENCES

1. Antonopoulos M, Koliopoulou A, Elaiopoulos D, et al. Central versus peripheral VA ECMO for cardiogenic shock: an 8-year experience of a tertiary cardiac surgery center in Greece. Hellenic J Cardiol. 2024:S1109-9666(24):00207-0.
2. Chopra HK, Kapoor PM. Chapter 45. Importance of mechanical-assist devices in acute decompensated heart failure. Textbook of cardiac critical care; 2023. pp. 453-61.
3. Kapoor PM. Angiotensin Receptor Neprilysin Inhibitor (ARNI) and Extracorporeal Membrane Oxygenation. In: HK Chopra (Ed). Advances and Revolutions in Heart Failure (ARHF): A textbook of cardiology. New Delhi: Jaypee Publishers Medical Publisher Pvt Ltd; 2024. pp. 763-9.
4. Kalra R, Alexy T, Bartos JA, et al. Left ventricular hemodynamics with veno-arterial extracorporeal membrane oxygenation. Catheter Cardiovasc Interv. 2024;103(3):472-81.
5. Beghini A, Sammartino AM, Papp Z, et al. 2024 update in heart failure, ESC Heart Failure. 2024.
6. De Backer D, Donker DW, Combes A, et al. Mechanical circulatory support in cardiogenic shock: microaxial flow pumps for all and VA-ECMO consigned to the museum? J Crit Care. 2024;28(203):1-4.
7. Chowdhury UK, George N, Sushamagayatri B, et al. Atrial correction (modified senning) of transposition of the great arteries and intact atrial septum with regressed left ventricle and pulmonary hypertension: a video presentation. J Card Crit Care TSS. 2023;7:59-64.
8. Truby LK, Rogers JG. Advanced heart failure: epidemiology, diagnosis, and therapeutic approaches. JACC Heart Fail. 2020;8(7):523-36.

9. Kapoor PM, Sharan S, Choudhury M. TIVA for ECMO and VAD. J Card Crit Care. 2021;5(1);60-9.
10. Ahmad T, Wang TS, Desai NR. Outcomes of extracorporeal membrane oxygenation in heart failure with preserved ejection fraction: a systematic review and meta-analysis. J Cardiac Fail. 2022;28(4):548-56.
11. Nakamura K, Tanaka Y, Inoue Y. ECMO in Patients with right ventricular failure and pulmonary hypertension: an emerging role in HFpEF. J Crit Care Med. 2022;45(6):220-8.
12. Patel N, Shaheen M, Hammond M. Cardiogenic shock in HFpEF: role of VA-ECMO in stabilizing hemodynamics. Circulation: Heart Failure. 2023;16(1):25-31.
13. Morrow DA, Braunwald E. Advances in the treatment of cardiogenic shock and acute heart failure: the role of ECMO. Circulation. 2023;147(2):123-31.
14. Chandra D, Kar B, Idelchik G, et al. The usefulness of percutaneous left ventricular assist device as a bridge to recovery from myocarditis. Am J Cardiol. 2007;99(12):1755-6.
15. Malhotra KP, Karanjkar A, Bhardwaj V. Evaluation of coagulopathy on veno-arterial ECMO (VA) extracorporeal membrane oxygenation using platelet aggregometry and standard tests: a narrative review. Egyptian J Crit Care Med. 2018;6(3):73-8.
16. Malhotra KP, Garg S, Prakash M, et al. Viscoelastic testing on venoarterial extracorporeal membrane oxygenation: need or greed? J Card Crit Care TSS. 2023;7:118-28.
17. Poonam MK. Patient Blood Management in Cardiac Surgery and ECMO: The Indian Scenario in 2021. 2021;5(3): 181-3.
18. Görlinger K, Kapoor P. Massive transfusion/hemorrhage protocols versus goal-directed bleeding management: science gone eerie? J Cardiac Crit Care TSS. 2024;8:16-27.
19. Gandhi A. Patient blood management: moving above and beyond the optimal use of blood! J Card Crit Care TSS. 2024;8:28-32.
20. Singh S, Solanki Y, Kapoor P. Thromboelastography in venovenous extracorporeal membrane oxygenation for acute respiratory distress syndrome. J Cardiac Crit Care TSS. 2017;01:101-4.
21. Karanjkar A, Bhardwaj V, Kapoor P. Is rotational thromboelastometry the answer for rapid prediction of coagulopathy on extracorporeal membrane oxygenation? J Cardiac Crit Care TSS. 2017;01:108-10.
22. Kapoor P. Anticoagulation during ECMO: will the tight rope be tighter in 2018? J Cardiac Crit Care TSS. 2017;01:55-6.
23. Bhardwaj V, Kapoor PM, Karanjkar A, et al. Congenital cyanotic cardiac surgery in children: is algorithm-based point-of-care testing essential to prevent bleeding? J Cardiac Crit Care TSS. 2019;03(01):1692118.
24. Sandeep S, Gandhi A, Kapoor PM. Utility of platelet function tests: a recent review round up. J Card Crit Care TSS. 2020;3:24-7.
25. Sharan S, Kapoor PM, Choudhury M, et al. Platelet function test in coronary artery bypass grafting: does it predict postoperative bleeding? J Cardiac Critical Care TSS. 2021;05:186-95.
26. Görlinger K. Implementation of patient blood management: a long and winding road but worth doing! J Card Crit Care TSS. 2024;8:1-4.
27. Chakraborty S, Malhotra Kapoor P, Rajashekar P, et al. Prospective Interventional Cohort Study using AIIMS Simplified POC Algorithm for Restricted Blood Transfusion in Cyanotic Children. J Card Crit Care TSS. 2024;8:195-204.
28. Chopra HK, Wander GS, Ponde CK, et al. The Power and Promise of Angiotensin Receptor Neprilysin Inhibitor (ARNI) in Heart Failure Management: National Consensus Statement. J Assoc Physicians India. 2023;71(2):11-2.
29. Rajeev M, Sahu MK; Singh U, et al. Successful use of angiotensin receptor–neprilysin inhibitor along with intravenous inotropes, in a postcardiac surgery child with an anomalous left coronary artery from the pulmonary artery repair. J Pract Cardiovasc Scien. 2023;9(3):206-9.
30. Lorusso R, Whitman G, Milojevic M, et al. 2020 EACTS/ELSO/STS/AATS expert consensus on post-cardiotomy extracorporeal life support in adult patients. J Thorac Cardiovasc Surg. 2021;161(4):1287-331.
31. Kapur NK, Esposito ML, Bader Y, et al. Mechanical circulatory support devices for acute right ventricular failure. Circulation. 2017;136(3):314-26.
32. Lorusso R, Raffa GM, Alenizy K, et al. Structured review of post-cardiotomy extracorporeal membrane oxygenation: part 1-Adult patients. J Heart Lung Transplant. 2019;38(11): 1125-43.
33. Whitman GJ. Extracorporeal membrane oxygenation for the treatment of postcardiotomy shock. J Thorac Cardiovasc Surg. 2017;153(1):95-101.
34. Chung M, Zhao Y, Strom JB, et al. Extracorporeal membrane oxygenation use in cardiogenic shock: impact of age on in-hospital mortality, length of stay, and costs. Crit Care Med. 2019;47(3):e214-e221.
35. Vallabhajosyula S, Arora S, Lahewala S, et al. Temporary mechanical circulatory support for refractory cardiogenic shock before left ventricular assist device surgery. J Am Heart Assoc. 2018;7(22):e010193.
36. Vallabhajosyula S, O'Horo JC, Antharam P, et al. Concomitant intra-aortic balloon pump use in cardiogenic shock requiring veno-arterial extracorporeal membrane oxygenation. Circ Cardiovasc Interv. 2018;11(9):e006930.
37. Vallabhajosyula S, O'Horo JC, Antharam P, et al. Venoarterial extracorporeal membrane oxygenation with concomitant impella versus venoarterial extracorporeal membrane oxygenation for cardiogenic shock. ASAIO J. 2020;66(5):497-503.
38. Schumann J, Henrich EC, Strobl H, et al. Inotropic agents and vasodilator strategies for the treatment of cardiogenic shock or low cardiac output syndrome. Cochrane Database Syst Rev. 2018;1:CD009669.
39. Wang L, Yang F, Wang X, et al. Predicting mortality in patients undergoing VA-ECMO after coronary artery bypass grafting: the REMEMBER score. Crit Care. 2019;23(1):11.
40. Granholm A, Perner A, Jensen AKG, et al. Important methodological flaws in the recently published clinical prediction model the REMEMBER score. Crit Care. 2019;23(1):71.
41. Chopra HK, Kapoor PM. Ch 31. Role of extracorporeal membrane oxygenation for acute decompensated heart failure. Manual of ECMO in the ICU. New Delhi: Jaypee Publishers; 2014; pp. 188-92.

SECTION 19

HFpEF and Therapeutics

HFpEF and ARNI

130. Angiotensin Receptor Blocker and Neprilysin Inhibitor in HFpEF
131. Top 10 Take-home Messages from the ACC/AHA and HFSA on SGLT2 Inhibitor/ARN Inhibitor in HFpEF
132. Angiotensin Receptor-Neprilysin Inhibitor in HFpEF: Outcome Data
133. Patiromer in Hyperkalemia in HF and CKD and ARNI Use in HFpEF
134. ARNI as In-hospital Therapy in HFpEF
135. ARNI and MRA Combination in PARAGON-HF: Odd Couple or Dynamic Duo in HFpEF

HFpEF and SGLT2i

136. Role of SGLT2 Inhibitors in HFpEF
137. SGLT2 Inhibitors in Acute HFpEF: Is It Time to Broaden the Horizon?
138. Role of SGLT2 Inhibitors in HFpEF with Diabetes Mellitus
139. Indication, Contraindication and Uniqueness of SGLT2i and ARNI in HFpEF
140. Role of SGLT2i in HFpEF with Takotsubo Syndrome
141. SGLT2i in HFpEF: Fighting the Enemy with a Newly Crafted Weapon
142. Dapagliflozin with Sitagliptin in HFpEF and Diabetes
143. SGLT2 Inhibitor and DPP-4 Inhibitor Combination in Diabetes Mellitus with HFpEF
144. Left Atrial Failure in HFpEF: The Role of SGLT2is, ARNI, Bisoprolol, and MRAs
145. Development of Treatment Selection Algorithm for SGLT2 Inhibitors in HFpEF
146. Role of SGLT2 Inhibitors in Cardiac Remodeling Reversal: Beyond Glycemic Control in HFpEF
147. Role of SGLT2i in all Spectrum of HFpEF Management

HFpEF and Beta-blockers

148. ACC/AHA Guidelines on Beta-blocker Use in HFpEF
149. Role of Bisoprolol in HFpEF with AF, Stroke, and Hypertension
150. Morbidity and Mortality Benefits of SGLT2i, ARNI, and Bisoprolol in HFpEF with Atrial Fibrillation
151. Promise of Bisoprolol in HFpEF: Present Status
152. Role of Bisoprolol in Patients with HFpEF
153. Beta-blockers in the Management of HFpEF: What is the Consensus?
154. Use of Beta-blockers in Patients with HFpEF and Comorbidities

HFpEF and MRA

155. Mineralocorticoid Receptor Antagonist in HFpEF and Atrial Fibrillation

HFpEF and FCM

156. Global Data on Ferric Carboxymaltose in HFpEF

HFpEF and Semaglutide

157. Semaglutide in Patients with Obesity and HFpEF with or without Diabetes and Prespecified Pooled Analysis of STEP-HFpEF and STEP-HFpEF-DM Trials
158. Semaglutide in Obesity, HFpEF, and Diabetes Mellitus: STEP-HFpEF Trial

HFpEF and Finerenone

159. Finerenone in HFpEF with Chronic Kidney Disease: Hope or Hype

HFpEF and Device Therapy

160. Heart Support Devices in HFpEF
161. MitraClip in Heart Failure in Patients on Angiotensin Receptor Neprilysin Inhibitors: When and How?
162. Stage D HFpEF, Heart Transplantation, and Mechanical Circulatory Support
163. Drug Switch or Device: How do I Decide in HFpEF?
164. Implant or No-implant, Interatrial Shunt for HFpEF Patients
165. Renal Denervation: A Novel Treatment for Hypertension

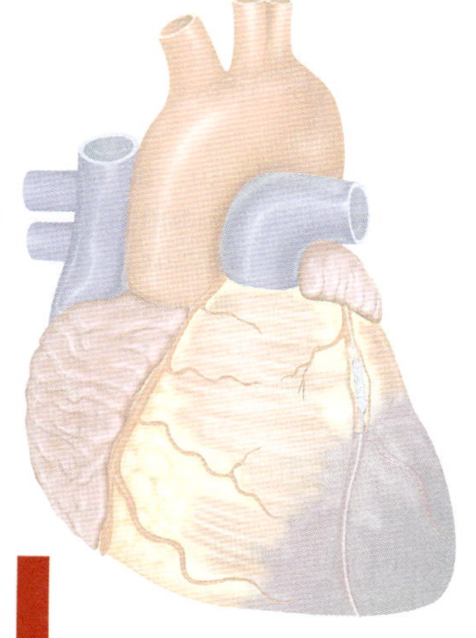

Angiotensin Receptor Blocker and Neprilysin Inhibitor in HFpEF

Bhavna Mastebhakti, Nilashish Dey, Peeyush Jain

INTRODUCTION

Heart failure with preserved ejection fraction (HFpEF) is a complex clinical syndrome characterized by the presence of diastolic dysfunction (DD) and elevated left ventricular (LV) filling pressure, in the setting of an LV ejection fraction (LVEF) ≥50%.[1] HFpEF is a prevalent condition, accounting for around 50% of all patients with heart failure (HF), and is associated with significant morbidity and mortality.[2] It is a heterogenous disorder, contributed to by comorbidities such as hypertension, diabetes, obesity, coronary artery disease (CAD), chronic kidney disease (CKD), and specific causes such as cardiac amyloidosis.[2] Despite its high epidemiological prevalence, a prompt diagnosis is often challenging, and many uncertainties exist as it is characterized by different phenotypes driven by various cardiac and noncardiac comorbidities. This is also the reason why several HFpEF clinical trials in the past did not reach strong outcomes to recommend therapies for this syndrome which show a mortality benefit.[3]

FOUNDATIONAL THERAPIES FOR HEART FAILURE

Foundational therapies are the key life-saving pharmacological treatments with mortality benefit which form the foundations of management of patients with HF and are strongly recommended in international guidelines for all patients who can tolerate it.[4] Currently, in patients with HF, especially "heart failure with reduced ejection fraction (HFrEF)", such a therapy consists of angiotensin receptor blocker and neprilysin inhibitor (ARNI), beta-blocker, mineralocorticoid receptor antagonist (MRA) and a sodium-glucose cotransporter 2 (SGLT2) inhibitor,[2] whereas in HFpEF patients, only SGLT2 inhibitors have recently shown to have a mortality benefit.[5] Our chapter focusses on the role of ARNI in the management of patients with HFpEF.

PATHOPHYSIOLOGICAL BASIS OF ANGIOTENSIN RECEPTOR BLOCKER AND NEPRILYSIN INHIBITOR IN HFrEF

In the early stages of HF, neurohormonal activation compensates to maintain the perfusion to vital organs whereas chronic activation of these compensatory mechanisms leads to vascular and cardiac remodeling, inappropriate increases in preload and afterload, cardiomyocyte apoptosis, and oxidative stress.[6] With time, persistent activation of the renin-angiotensin-aldosterone system (RAAS) contributes to the cardiotoxic effects through mechanisms involving the upregulation of mineralocorticoid receptors and elevation of aldosterone levels resulting in a subsequent increase in aldosterone signaling leading to myocardial inflammation, vascular remodeling, and interstitial fibrosis, thereby deteriorating the cardiac function.[6] Another mechanism implicated in the cardiotoxic effects is the upregulation of angiotensin-1 (AT_1) receptors which aggravates myocardial fibrosis by inducing fibroblast hypertrophy and collagen deposition.[6]

The renal and vascular effects of RAAS are opposed by natriuretic peptides which include atrial natriuretic peptide (ANP) and B-type natriuretic peptide (BNP).[7] ANP is a counterregulatory peptide released from the atria in response to atrial stretch due to elevated atrial intramural pressure or increased intravascular volume,[8] and it inhibits sodium reabsorption, thereby promoting natriuresis and diuresis in the renal medullary collecting tubules.[9] This effect works synergistically by ANP's ability to suppress renin release, thereby inhibiting RAAS-mediated sodium reabsorption.[9] ANP also exhibits systemic vasodilation and increases vascular permeability which aids in reducing blood pressure.[9] BNP is released in response to ventricular stretch and exhibits effects similar to those of ANP along with its cardioprotective effect to abrogate myocardial apoptosis and fibrosis.[10] Importantly, these cardiotoxic effects of RAAS predominate as the cardiac and renal protective effects of ANP gradually diminish.[6] Taken together, these events result in ventricular remodeling.

Natriuretic peptides function mainly through two different natriuretic peptide receptors, NPR-A and NPR-B. Natriuretic peptide is broken down by neprilysin, a zinc-dependent type II integral membrane metalloprotease, which also metabolizes other substances such as bradykinin, angiotensin II, and amyloid-β. Neprilysin is a highly abundant enzyme primarily expressed in the proximal renal tubules, as well as in other sites such as cardiomyocytes, fibroblasts, vascular smooth muscle cells, endothelial cells, and neuronal cells.[9] ARNIs' dual

Flowchart 1: Pathophysiology of HFrEF and pathophysiological basis of ARNI in HFrEF.

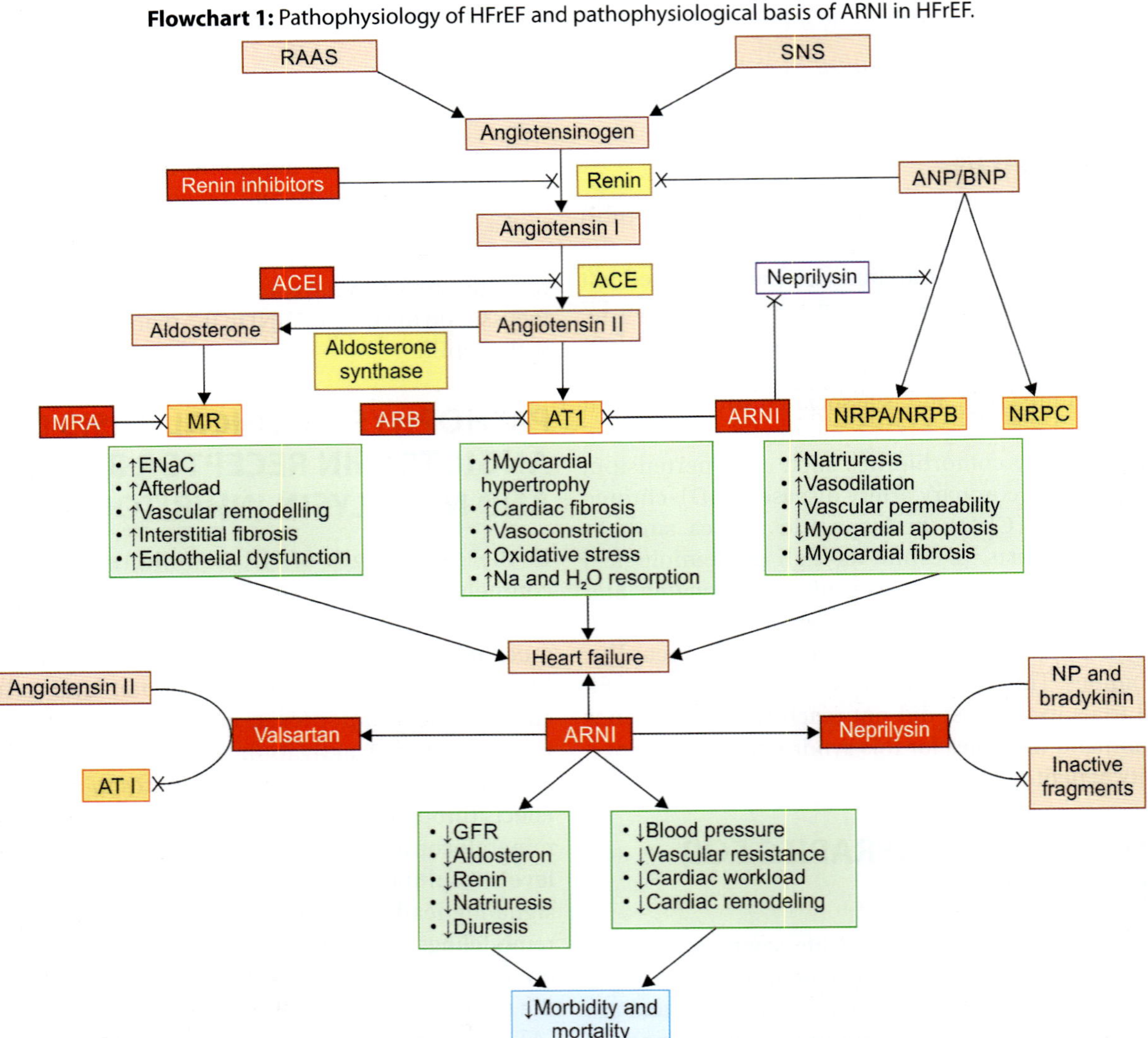

(ACE: angiotensin-converting enzyme; ACEI: angiotensin-converting enzyme inhibitors; ANP: atrial natriuretic peptide; ARNI: angiotensin receptor blocker neprilysin inhibitor; AT1: angiotensin 1 receptor; BNP: brain natriuretic peptide; NRPA/NRPB/NRPC: natriuretic peptide receptors A/B/C; eNaC: epithelial sodium channels; MR: mineralocorticoid; MRA: mineralocorticoid receptor antagonist; NP: natriuretic peptide; RAAS: renin–angiotensin–aldosterone system; SNS: sympathetic nervous system)

inhibition **(Flowchart 1)** of AT_1 and neprilysin exerts beneficial effects on both the heart and the kidneys, collectively reducing the rates of HF-related morbidity and mortality. Angioedema, resulting from bradykinin accumulation, and hypotension are potential side effects of ARNIs that might limit their use in high-risk populations.[6]

PATHOPHYSIOLOGICAL BASIS OF HFpEF

The myocardial remodeling and dysfunction in HFpEF result from a sequence of the following events[11] **(Flowchart 2)**:

- Comorbidities and especially obesity induce a systemic proinflammatory state.
- This proinflammatory state causes the coronary microvascular endothelial cells to produce reactive oxygen species (ROS), which limit nitric oxide (NO) bioavailability for adjacent cardiomyocytes.
- The resultant limited NO bioavailability decreases protein kinase G (PKG) activity in cardiomyocytes through a decrease in the cyclic guanosine monophosphate (cGMP).
- Low PKG activity removes the brake on cardiomyocyte hypertrophy, thereby inducing concentric LV remodeling, and stiffens the cardiomyocyte because of hypophosphorylation of the giant cytoskeletal protein titin.
- Both the stiff cardiomyocytes and increased collagen deposition by myofibroblasts cause diastolic LV dysfunction, the major cardiac functional deficit in HFpEF.
- In addition, decrease in cGMP leads to endothelial dysfunction, hypertrophy, and pathological signals of fibrosis through the calcineurin pathway, wherein dephosphorylation of nuclear factor of activated T cells (NFAT) allows its nuclear translocation and transcriptional activation of hypertrophic genes.

DIFFERENCE BETWEEN PATHOPHYSIOLOGY OF HFrEF AND HFpEF

In HFpEF, myocardial dysfunction and remodeling are driven by endothelial inflammation and oxidative stress. In HFrEF, oxidative stress originates in the cardiomyocytes because of ischemia, infection, or toxic agents. These ROS trigger cardiomyocyte autophagy, apoptosis, or necrosis. The latter attracts leukocytes. Dead cardiomyocytes are then replaced by fibrous tissue.[11]

PATHOPHYSIOLOGICAL BASIS OF ARNI IN HFpEF

Neprilysin is an enzyme that degrades NPs and vasoactive peptides. Sacubitril is further metabolized to sacubitrilat that inhibits neprilysin, which increases NPs. After combining with the NPR, a rise in the second messenger cGMP levels is caused by NPs signaling via membrane-bound particulate guanylate cyclase (pGC). cGMP heightens the activity of PKG enzymes, mediating phosphorylation of titin. Also, the calcineurin/NFAT pathway is directly inhibited by NPs, leading to a reduction in cardiac stiffness and hypertrophy[12] **(Flowchart 2)**. Valsartan exhibits its role by preventing the binding of angiotensin I to AT1 receptors, thereby resulting in a decreased sympathetic tone, decreased aldosterone secretion, decreased blood pressure, decreased myocardial fibrosis. and decreased ventricular hypertrophy.

STUDIES ON THE USE OF NEPRILYSIN INHIBITORS IN HFpEF

Table 1 summarizes the important clinical trials which studied ARNIs in patients with HFpEF.

PLEIOTROPIC EFFECTS OF ANGIOTENSIN RECEPTOR BLOCKER AND NEPRILYSIN INHIBITOR

- *Hypertension:* The PARAMETER study (Prospective Comparison of Angiotensin Receptor Neprilysin Inhibitor with Angiotensin Receptor Blocker Measuring Arterial Stiffness in the Elderly), for the first time, demonstrated superiority of sacubitril/valsartan versus olmesartan in reducing clinic and ambulatory central aortic and brachial pressures in elderly patients with systolic hypertension and stiff arteries.[13]
- *Post myocardial infarction:* The risk of fatal and nonfatal ischemic events continues to increase following MI. Sacubitril/valsartan group compared with a placebo demonstrated lower cardiac weight and reduced fibrosis in the peri-infarct and remote myocardium. The sacubitril/valsartan group also had a lower LV end-diastolic diameter, a higher LVEF, and higher circular and diastolic wall strain, confirming improved LV function 4 weeks after treatment.[14]
- *Renal impairment:* Studies have found no clinically significant changes in creatinine, potassium, blood urea nitrogen, and eGFR of patients with renal impairment treated with ARNIs. Besides, there was a

Flowchart 2: Pathophysiology of HFpEF and pathophysiological basis of ARNI in HFpEF.

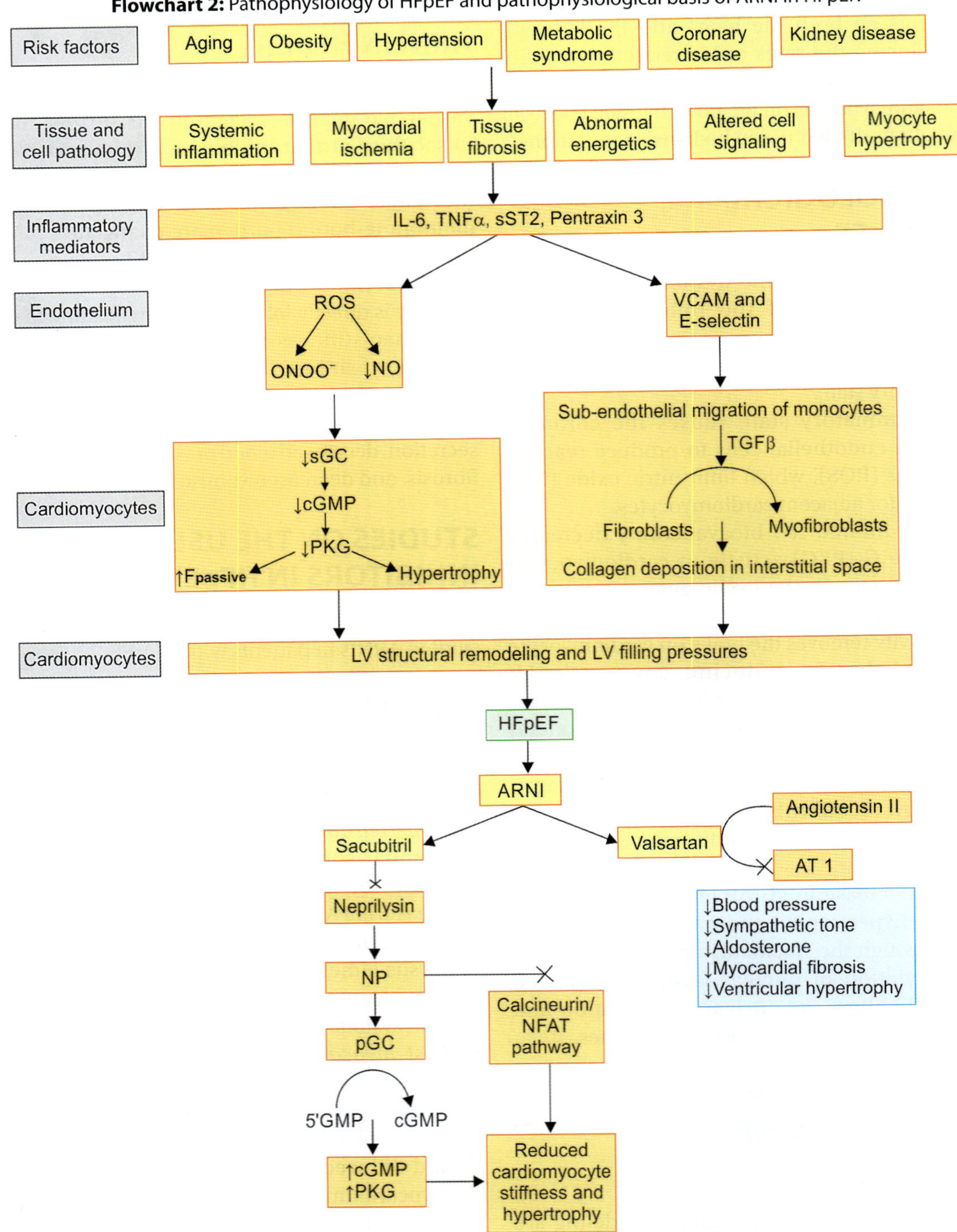

(ARNI: angiotensin receptor blocker neprilysin inhibitor; AT1: angiotensin 1 receptor; cGMP: cyclic guanosine monophosphate; IL-6: interleukin 6; LV: left ventricular; NFAT: nuclear factor of activated T cells; NP: natriuretic peptides; NPR: natriuretic peptide receptors; pGC: particulate guanylate cyclase; PKG: phosphokinase G; ROS: reactive oxygen species; sGC: soluble guanylate cyclase; TNFα: tumor necrosis factor α; VCAM: vascular cell adhesion molecule)

reduction in the urinary albumin-to-creatinine ratio (UACR). Moreover, re-analysis of the data from the PARAMOUNT study revealed better eGFR progression and a greater decrease in BP and serum creatinine levels in patients on sacubitril-valsartan when compared to valsartan.[14]

TABLE 1: Trials comparing ARNI in patients with HFpEF.

	Trial design	*Sample size*	*Inclusion criteria*	*Comparator arm*	*Outcome*
PARAMOUNT (2012)	Phase 2, randomized, parallel group, double-blind, multicenter trial	$n = 301$ (1:1 randomization)	NYHA classes II–III HF, LVEF ≥45%, and NT-proBNP ≥400 pg/mL	S/V titrated to 200 mg BD or valsartan titrated to 160 mg BD for 36 weeks	GCS significantly improved at 36 weeks in the ARNI group when compared with the valsartan group (4.42, 95% CI 0.67–8.17, $p = 0.021$), with no significant difference observed in GLS (0.25, 95% CI 1.19–1.70, $p = 0.73$)
PARALLAX (2020)	Randomized, parallel, double-blind, stratification	$n = 2,572$	≥45 years of age, LVEF >40%, NYHA classes II–IV, LAE/LVH, patients treated with ACE inhibitor or ARB for hypertension, KCCQ-CSS <75, NT-proBNP >220 pg/mL if not in atrial fibrillation or >600 pg/mL if atrial fibrillation	• S/V 93/103 mg BD versus enalapril 10 mg BD • S/V 93/103 mg BD versus valsartan 160 mg BD • S/V 93/103 mg twice daily versus placebo	The primary co-outcome, NT-proBNP change from baseline to week 12, favored sacubitril/valsartan versus individualized medical therapy ($p < 0.0001$). The primary co-outcome, 6-minute walk distance change from baseline to week 24, was similar between sacubitril/valsartan versus individualized medical therapy ($p = 0.24$)
PARAGON (2024)	Randomized, parallel, blinded	$n = 4,822$	≥50 years of age in NYHA classes II-IV, LVEF ≥45%, elevated level of natriuretic peptides, structural heart disease	S/V 97/103 mg twice daily ($n = 2,419$) versus valsartan 160 mg twice daily ($n = 2,403$)	The primary outcome, rate of cardiovascular deaths or hospitalizations for HF, was 12.8 events per 100 patient-years in the sacubitril/valsartan group versus 14.6 events per 100 patient-years in the valsartan group (p = not significant)

(GCS: global circumferential strain; GLS: global longitudinal strain; HF: heart failure; KCCQ-CSS: Kansas City Cardiomyopathy Questionnaire clinical summary score; LAE: left atrial enlargement; LVEF: left ventricular ejection fraction; LVH: left ventricular hypertrophy; NT-proBNP: N-terminal pro-brain natriuretic peptide; NYHA: New York Heart Association; S/V: sacubitril/valsartan)

- *Diabetes:* In a post hoc analysis of the PARADIGM-HF trial, 3778 patients with HFrEF and known diabetes or HbA_{1c} ≥6.5% at screening who were randomly assigned to treatment with sacubitril/valsartan or enalapril found that during the first year of follow-up, HbA_{1c} concentrations decreased by 0.16% in the enalapril group and 0.26% in the sacubitril/valsartan group. The HbA_{1c} concentrations were persistently lower in the sacubitril/valsartan group than in the enalapril group over the 3-year follow-up.[15] ARNIs through their action via sacubitril also increase secretion of insulin and increase insulin sensitivity.[6]
- *Dyslipidemia:* There are studies that show that the SNS, insulin regulation, and NP activity play crucial roles in lipid metabolism inhibiting neprilysin results in increased lipolysis, lipid oxidation, and brown adipose tissue.[12]
- *Arrhythmias:* ARNI reverses electrical and structural remodeling and the inflammatory responses caused by HF, which accounts for its role in suppression of ventricular arrhythmia.[16]

CURRENT RECOMMENDATIONS FOR ANGIOTENSIN RECEPTOR BLOCKER AND NEPRILYSIN INHIBITOR IN HFpEF

Although RAAS inhibition strategies have been successful in the treatment of HFrEF, and RAAS activation is suggested in HFpEF, clinical trials with RAAS inhibitors have not showed mortality benefit in patients HFpEF.[2] Currently, ARNIs are a Class 2b recommendation along with beta blockers and MRA, in patients with HFpEF, whereas, the SGLT2 inhibitors are the only drug group to have a class I recommendation in HFpEF patients.[5]

In patients with HFrEF and NYHA classes II–III, ARNIs along with beta blockers, MRA, and SGLT2 inhibitors, are class 1 recommendation and have shown to reduce morbidity and mortality.[2]

CONCLUSION

Heart failure is a disease encompassing multiple etiologies and comorbidities. The congestive pathophysiology and the inflammatory responses occur across the spectrum of LVEF. Regardless of LVEF, HF implies major adverse impacts on both the quality and the longevity of life. As more attention was paid to the HFrEF subset of patients in the trials from the past, the randomized trial evidence on which to base therapeutic decisions for those with preserved LVEF is much more limited and less definitive. This paradigm is now changing and patients with HFpEF are currently considered an unmet need in cardiology. Drugs like SGLT2 inhibitors and ARNIs have been studied in various HFpEF subsets. ARNI is a unique drug in simultaneously blocking the RAAS while augmenting the body's intrinsic NP system through neprilysin inhibition which presents a beneficial therapeutic approach for a range of cardiovascular diseases, including HF and hypertension in which vasoconstriction, volume overload, and neurohormonal activation play a part in pathophysiology. In addition, the appropriateness of testing new therapies against placebo in HFpEF population, rather than comparing against known multiple proven agents and devices, has enhanced the appeal to conduct major randomized clinical trials in these patients, and many are currently underway. More specific phenotyping and genotyping of subpopulations may lead to improvements in outcomes from future trials, further diminishing the burden of HFpEF.

REFERENCES

1. Gori M, D'Elia E, Zambelli G, Senni M. [Heart failure with preserved ejection fraction: an update on diagnosis and treatment]. G Ital Cardiol 2006. 2020;21(2):119-27.
2. Heidenreich PA, Bozkurt B, Aguilar D, et al. 2022 AHA/ACC/HFSA Guideline for the Management of Heart Failure: A Report of the American College of Cardiology/American Heart Association Joint Committee on Clinical Practice Guidelines. Circulation. 2022;145(18):e895-1032.
3. Balestrieri G, Limonta R, Ponti E, et al. The Therapy and Management of Heart Failure with Preserved Ejection Fraction: New Insights on Treatment. 2023. [online] Available from https://www.cfrjournal.com/articles/therapy-and-management-heart-failure-preserved-ejection-fraction-new-insights-treatment [Last accessed January, 2025].
4. McMurray JJV, Docherty KF. Insights into foundational therapies for heart failure with reduced ejection fraction. Clin Cardiol. 2022;45(Suppl 1):S26.
5. European Society of Cardiolo. 2023 Focused Update of the 2021 ESC Guidelines for the diagnosis and treatment of acute and chronic heart failure. [online] Available from https://www.escardio.org/Guidelines/Clinical-Practice-Guidelines/Focused-Update-on-Heart-Failure-Guidelines [Last accessed January, 2025].
6. Nasrallah D, Abdelhamid A, Tluli O, et al. Angiotensin receptor blocker-neprilysin inhibitor for heart failure with reduced ejection fraction. Pharmacol Res. 2024;204:107210.
7. Manolis AA, Manolis TA, Manolis AS. Neurohumoral Activation in Heart Failure. Int J Mol Sci. 2023;24(20):15472.
8. Richards AM. The renin-angiotensin-aldosterone system and the cardiac natriuretic peptides. Heart. 1996;76(3 Suppl 3):36.
9. Salazar J, Rojas-Quintero J, Cano C, et al. Neprilysin: A Potential Therapeutic Target of Arterial Hypertension? [online] Bentham Science Publishers; 2020. Available from https://www.ingentaconnect.com/content/ben/ccr/2020/00000016/00000001/art00006 [Last accessed January, 2025].
10. Fu S, Ping P, Wang F, et al. Synthesis, secretion, function, metabolism and application of natriuretic peptides in heart failure. J Biol Eng. 2018;12(1):2.
11. Paulus WJ, Tschöpe C. A Novel Paradigm for Heart Failure With Preserved Ejection Fraction: Comorbidities Drive Myocardial Dysfunction and Remodeling Through Coronary Microvascular Endothelial Inflammation. J Am Coll Cardiol. 2013;62(4):263-71.
12. Jia R, Ji Y, Sun D. Progress and prospects of Sacubitril/Valsartan: Based on heart failure with preserved ejection fraction. Biomed Pharmacother. 2022;155:113701.
13. Dargad RR, Prajapati MR, Dargad RR, et al. Sacubitril/valsartan: A novel angiotensin receptor-neprilysin inhibitor. Indian Heart J. 2018;70:S102-10.
14. von Lueder TG, Wang BH, Kompa AR, et al. Angiotensin Receptor Neprilysin Inhibitor LCZ696 Attenuates Cardiac Remodeling and Dysfunction After Myocardial Infarction by Reducing Cardiac Fibrosis and Hypertrophy. Circ Heart Fail. 2015;8(1):71-8.
15. Seferovic JP, Claggett B, Seidelmann SB, et al. Effect of sacubitril/valsartan versus enalapril on glycaemic control in patients with heart failure and diabetes: a post-hoc analysis from the PARADIGM-HF trial. Lancet Diabetes Endocrinol. 2017;5(5):333-40.
16. Tsai YN, Cheng WH, Chang YT, et al. Mechanism of angiotensin receptor-neprilysin inhibitor in suppression of ventricular arrhythmia. J Cardiol. 2021;78(4):275-84.

CHAPTER

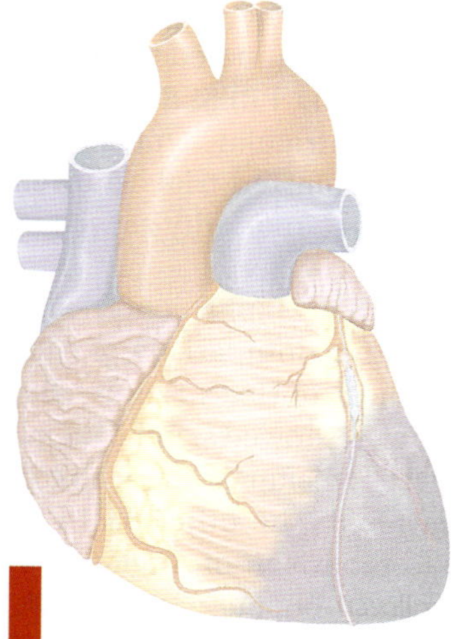

Top 10 Take-home Messages from the ACC/AHA and HFSA on SGLT2 Inhibitor/ARN Inhibitor in HFpEF

Satyendra Tewari, Harshit Khare

INTRODUCTION

The recently published 2022 ACC/AHA/HFSA guidelines for the management of heart failure (HF) present an update to the earlier HF guidelines of 2013 and 2017. Besides, management of atrial fibrillation (AF) and secondary mitral regurgitation (MR) in HF, they emphasize on prevention of HF, treatment strategies for symptomatic HF and newer treatment modalities such as sodium-glucose cotransport protein 2 (SGLT2) inhibitors and angiotensin receptor-neprilysin (ARN) inhibitors.[1]

DISCUSSION

Heart failure classification now includes[1]:

- Heart failure with reduced ejection fraction (HFrEF), with left ventricle ejection fraction (LVEF) ≤40%
- Heart failure with improved EF (HFimpEF), with previous LVEF ≤40% and on follow up, ≥40 %
- Heart failure with mildly reduced EF (HFmrEF), with LVEF 40–49%
- Heart failure with preserved EF (HFpEF), with LVEF ≥50%.
- While the SGLT2 inhibitor, ARN inhibitor, mineralocorticoid receptor antagonist (MRA) and beta-blocker (BB) therapies form the four pillars of HFrEF treatment, the therapeutic options in HFpEF are still in infancy.

Sodium–glucose Cotransporter-2 Inhibitor

The novel SGLT2 inhibitor therapy for HF has class I recommendations for treatment in symptomatic HFrEF patients to reduce hospitalization for HF (HHF) and cardiovascular (CV) mortality, irrespective of the presence of type 2 diabetes.[1] These recommendations for HFrEF, stem from the landmark trials - DAPA-HF and EMPEROR-REDUCED.[2,3] More specifically, both the DAPA-HF trial, enrolling HFrEF patients irrespective of diabetes status, and EMPEROR-REDUCED trial, found a relative risk reduction of around 25% in the primary endpoint of CV death or HHF with gliflozin molecules, when compared to standard care therapy.

However, there are fewer prospective trials exploring the clinical outcomes with SGLT2 inhibitor in HFpEF patients. Two such trials exploring efficacy of SGLT2 inhibitor in HFpEF are EMPEROR-PRESERVED and DELIVER.[4,5]

EMPEROR-PRESERVED enrolled around 5,988 patients with LVEF >40%, with majority in the New York Heart Association (NYHA) class II. They were randomly assigned in 1:1 manner to receive either 10 mg empagliflozin once a day or placebo and followed for a median of 26.2 months. The primary outcome comprised of composite of CV death or HHF. There was relative risk reduction of 21% for primary endpoint with empagliflozin group compared to placebo [hazard ratio 0.79; 95% confidence interval (CI), 0.69–0.90; $p < 0.001$]. This result, however, was mainly driven by 29% lower HHF in the empagliflozin group. Further this effect was independent of diabetes status. Although EMPEROR-PRESERVED trial failed to demonstrate mortality benefit with empagliflozin, it showed effectiveness of this group of molecules across different spectrums of LVEF, with a caveat that there was decrease in efficacy with higher LVEF.[4] The 2022 ACC/AHA/HFSA guidelines for HF were drafted before the results of DELIVER trial which evaluated Dapagliflozin in patients with HFpEF. In view of the EMPEROR-PRESERVED results, the guidelines gave a class 2a recommendation for use of SGLT2 inhibitor in HFpEF patients, with level of evidence (LOE) B-R.[1] DELIVER trial evaluated the efficacy of dapagliflozin in patients with HFpEF as well as HFmrEF, and HFimpEF. The results were similar to EMPEROR-PRESERVED, with significant reduction in composite primary endpoint of CV death or HHF. Further its prespecified subgroup analyses showed extension of these benefits to both LVEF ≥60% and HFimpEF groups. Moreover, unlike EMPEROR-PRESERVED, it showed that these benefits extended to even patients with a body mass index (BMI) ≥30 and NYHA class III or IV.[5]

Despite all the progress made with SGLT2 inhibitor in patients HFpEF, the trials are yet to show reduction in CV mortality. Can these results of SGLT2 inhibitor trials in HFpEF be replicated in trials enrolling patients with cardiomyopathies (like hypertrophic cardiomyopathy, viral myocarditis, amyloidosis, cardiac sarcoidosis, etc.), remains to be seen?

Renin–angiotensin–aldosterone System Inhibition

The renin–angiotensin–aldosterone system (RAAS) inhibition strategies have fared well in clinical trials of HFrEF patients. However, the trial results of RAAS inhibition in HFpEF have not been encouraging. Pooled analyses from earlier studies evaluating ACE inhibitors suggested that ACE inhibitor had no effect on CV mortality, all-cause mortality, and HHF.[6]

Early large trials evaluating the role of angiotensin receptor blockers (ARBs) in HFpEF include Digitalis Investigation Group in HFpEF (DIG-PEF), Candesartan in Heart Failure: Assessment of Reduction in Mortality and Morbidity in HFpEF (CHARM-PRESERVED), and Irbesartan in Heart Failure with Preserved Systolic Function trial (I-PRESERVE). The patient cohorts in these studies differed in terms of LVEF. While the DIG-PEF cohort had an LVEF >45% and CHARM-PRESERVED patients had an LVEF >40, the most strictly recruited cohort of HFpEF was in I-PRESERVE study with median LVEF of 59%.[7-9] Among these, the DIG-PEF trial failed to show any effect on natural history of HFpEF patients, with no effect on all-cause mortality or HHF.[7] The CHARM-PRESERVED, however, was first to show significant reduction in HHF with candesartan compared to placebo.[8] But in I-PRESERVE trial, again there was no difference in HHF or CV mortality with irbesartan compared to placebo.[9] In fact, these trials were criticized for selection bias with inclusion of relatively healthier HFpEF patients; clearly, the patients enrolled were having HF-PEF syndrome with diastolic dysfunction and had poor prognosis compared to general population. In fact, poor outcomes in I-PRESERVE cohort could not be attributed to left ventricular hypertrophy alone. Metaanalysis of these randomized trials showed that ARB did not affect CV, all-cause mortality as well as HHF.[6]

Two large trials evaluated ARNI in HFpEF cohort. First was PARAMOUNT-HF (Prospective Comparison of ARN inhibitor with ARB on Management of Heart Failure with Preserved Ejection Fraction) trial. It showed significant fall in NT-pro-BNP levels after 12 weeks therapy with sacubitril-valsartan compared to valsartan.[10] The other trial was PARAGON-HF (Prospective Comparison of Angiotensin Receptor Neprilysin Inhibitor with Angiotensin Receptor Blocker Global Outcomes in Heart Failure and Preserved Left Ventricular Ejection Fraction), which showed no benefit with sacubitril-valsartan compared to valsartan, in terms of composite of CV mortality or HHF. However, in secondary analyses, there were trends toward significance for reduced HHF.[11] The metaanalyses of these two trials suggest that although there is no mortality benefit with ARNI, it may result in reduction in HHF.

Overall, the RAAS inhibition has only been shown to reduce HHF in HFpEF cohort to some extent, with no added mortality benefit. This has resulted in class 2b recommendations for ACE inhibitor, ARB, and even ARNI in HFpEF management, with LOE B-R.[1]

GUIDELINES

From the above discussion, the following top-10 take-home messages can be derived **(Fig. 1)**:

1. Medication classes for HF now include SGLT2 inhibitor, ARN inhibitor (or ACEi or ARB), BB, and MRAs.
2. Newer classification for HF includes HFmrEF and HFimpEF.
3. When LVEF >40%, supporting evidence for increased LV filling pressures is required to make diagnosis of HF.
4. Recommendation for SGLT2 inhibitor in HFpEF is class 2a (LOE B-R).
5. Recommendation for ARN inhibitor in HFpEF is class 2b (LOE B-R).
6. New recommendations for HFmrEF include use of SGLT2 inhibitor (class 2a).
7. Diuretics are recommended in HFpEF to achieve state of decongestion, class of recommendation 1.
8. For most treatments, a value statement has been quoted. High-value treatment modalities include ARN inhibitor, ACE inhibitor, ARB, BB, MRA,

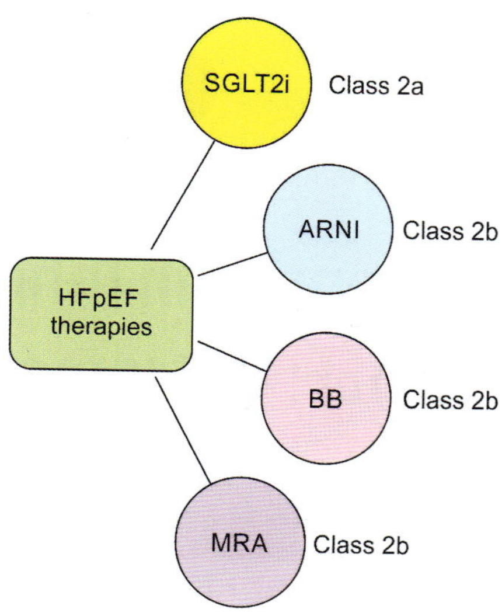

Fig. 1: Guideline recommendations in HFpEF.

implantable cardioverter-defibrillator, and cardiac resynchronization therapy. Intermediate-value therapies include SLGT2 inhibitor and cardiac transplantation.

9. Patients with HFimpEF need to continue their HFrEF treatment.
10. Patients with advanced HF need to be treated by HF specialty team.

LIMITATIONS

The recommendations in the 2022 ACC/AHA/HFSA guidelines for treatment in HFpEF are based on data from limited number of clinical trials on HFpEF and few systematic reviews. Moreover, these trial data suffer from selection bias and most of them had very few event rates over the duration of follow-up. Perhaps, more intuitively designed trials evaluating soft clinical end points such as quality of life, NYHA class and biomarker levels instead of hard endpoints of CV mortality will perform better and yield additional insights into the action of these medication classes.

CONCLUSION

There is paucity of treatment modalities available for HFpEF, which can alter the natural history of this entity. At present, the available medication recommendations are derived from limited trial data and extrapolated mainly from HFrEF and HFmrEF cohorts. Although, the addition of SGLT2 inhibitor to this group has revolutionized the management of HFpEF, other groups of medications have not been able to make a mark. Probably, larger and more stringent studies are warranted to observe the effect of other treatment modalities, before any newer recommendations come.

REFERENCES

1. Writing Committee Members; ACC/AHA Joint Committee Members. 2022 AHA/ACC/HFSA Guideline for the Management of Heart Failure. J Card Fail. 2022;28(5):e1-167.
2. McMurray JJV, Solomon SD, Inzucchi SE, et al. Dapagliflozin in patients with heart failure and reduced ejection fraction. N Engl J Med. 2019;381:1995-2008.
3. Packer M, Anker SD, Butler J, et al. Cardiovascular and renal outcomes with empagliflozin in heart failure. N Engl J Med. 2020;383:1413-24.
4. Anker SD, Butler J, Filippatos G, et al. Empagliflozin in heart failure with a preserved ejection fraction. N Engl J Med. 2021;385:1451-61.
5. Solomon SD, McMurray JJV, Claggett B, et al. Dapagliflozin in heart failure with mildly reduced or preserved ejection fraction. N Engl J Med. 2022;387:1089-98.
6. Martin N, Manoharan K, Davies C, et al. Beta-blockers, and inhibitors of the renin-angiotensin aldosterone system for chronic heart failure with preserved ejection fraction. Cochrane Database Syst Rev. 2021;5(5):CD012721.
7. Ahmed A, Rich MW, Fleg JL, et al. Effects of digoxin on morbidity and mortality in diastolic heart failure: The ancillary digitalis investigation group trial. Circulation. 2006;114:397.
8. Yusuf S, Pfeffer MA, Swedberg K, et al. Effects of candesartan in patients with chronic heart failure and preserved left-ventricular ejection fraction: the CHARM-Preserved Trial. Lancet. 2003;362(9386):777-81.
9. Massie BM, Carson PE, McMurray JJ, et al. Irbesartan in patients with heart failure and preserved ejection fraction. N Engl J Med. 2008;359(23):2456-67.
10. Solomon SD, McMurray JJV, Anand IS, et al. Angiotensin-neprilysin inhibition in heart failure with preserved ejection fraction. N Engl J Med. 2019;381:1609-20.
11. Solomon SD, Vaduganathan M, B LC, et al. Sacubitril/valsartan across the spectrum of ejection fraction in heart failure. Circulation. 2020;141:352-61.

132

CHAPTER

Angiotensin Receptor-Neprilysin Inhibitor in HFpEF: Outcome Data

Venugopal Krishnan Nair, Sunil Roy Thottuvelil

INTRODUCTION

Heart failure with preserved ejection fraction (HFpEF) is a significant public health concern, and considerable uncertainties persist regarding its pathophysiology and treatment.[1] HFpEF affects approximately 32 million individuals globally and exhibits a mortality rate of 15–19% per annum.[2] HFpEF is characterized by the presence of diastolic dysfunction (DD) and elevated left ventricular (LV) filling pressure in the context of an LV ejection fraction (LVEF) of ≥50%.[3] HFpEF demonstrates profound clinical and pathophysiological heterogeneity, which accounts for the challenge of identifying a singular pharmacological intervention.[4] HFpEF is present in nearly half of patients with heart failure (HF). The prevalence increases more rapidly than in patients with HFrEF. According to data from registries, such as the Trivandrum Heart Failure Registry[5] and ASIAN-HF,[6] the prevalence of HFpEF in India ranges from approximately 19% to 25%, substantially lower than that observed in Western populations.[7]

Significant uncertainties persist in the pathophysiology and treatment of HFpEF. The differential effectiveness of HFrEF therapies in HFpEF may be attributed to the heterogeneity among patients with HFpEF. RAAS upregulation has been identified as a crucial pathological process in fibrosis, cardiomyocyte abnormalities, inflammation, and endothelial dysfunction, all of which are associated with the progression of HFpEF.[8] Animal models and clinical trials have demonstrated that RAAS inhibition improves cardiac diastolic function and mitigates these deleterious effects.[9] However, in clinical trials, ACEI/ARBs have not been shown to confer mortality benefits in patients with HFpEF. Spironolactone, β-blockers, digoxin, ivabradine, and calcium channel blockers have also not demonstrated significant efficacy in clinical trials. The patterns of neurohormonal activation differ in HF cohorts according to LVEF. Sympathetic and RAAS activation, resulting in elevated levels of plasma renin activity, aldosterone, catecholamines, and N-terminal pro-B-type natriuretic peptide NT-proBNP, are key features of HFrEF; however, only a small proportion of patients with HFpEF exhibit the same activation cascade.[10]

The CHARM-Preserved Trial,[11] conducted in patients with an ejection fraction (EF) >40%, reported no significant difference between candesartan and placebo regarding cardiovascular mortality and the combined outcome of hospitalization due to HF (HHF). The I-PRESERVE trial[12] performed in patients with an EF ≥45% demonstrated no significant difference between irbesartan and placebo in terms of the primary outcome of death from any cause or hospitalization for cardiovascular causes. Similarly, the PEP-CHF trial[13] reported that perindopril could reduce HHF; however, it did not affect the primary outcomes of unplanned HHF and cardiovascular death. An international multicenter study of the clinical effects of spironolactone on HFpEF (TOPCAT)[14] enrolled 3,455 HF patients with EF ≥45%, demonstrating that spironolactone did not reduce the incidence of cardiac arrest, CV death, or hospital readmission due to worsening HF in patients with HFpEF. The J-DHF study enrolled a small sample of patients with HFpEF and found that carvedilol did not improve the incidence of CV death or HF readmission in this patient population.[15]

ROLE OF ANGIOTENSIN RECEPTOR-NEPRILYSIN INHIBITOR IN HEART FAILURE WITH PRESERVED EJECTION FRACTION

Sacubitril inhibits neprilysin, an enzyme that deactivates several critical vasoactive peptides that contribute to the pathogenesis and progression of HF, including natriuretic peptides, bradykinin, and substance P. Combination with valsartan is essential because neprilysin inhibition elevates angiotensin levels, which could potentially counteract the vasodilatory effect of sacubitril, unless simultaneously inhibited.[16] Sacubitril/valsartan (ARNI) provides a modest additional benefit compared to valsartan in individuals with HFpEF. The roles of ARNI in HFpEF and heart failure with mildly reduced ejection fraction (HFmrEF) remain under investigation. Given the complexities of HFpEF treatment, recent studies have focused on the role of ARNI as a promising therapeutic option.

The PARAGON-HF trial[17] compared ARNI with valsartan in 4,822 patients with HFpEF. The study involved 4,822 patients with New York Heart Association class II to IV HF, an EF of 45% or higher, elevated natriuretic peptide levels, and structural heart disease. The primary outcome was a composite of total hospitalizations for HF and deaths due to cardiovascular causes. ARNI did not result in a significantly lower rate of total hospitalizations for HF or death from cardiovascular causes among patients with HF and an EF ≥45%. The ARNI group had a higher incidence of hypotension and angioedema, whereas the valsartan group had a lower incidence of hyperkalemia. The mean change in the KCCQ clinical summary score at 8 months was higher in the ARNI group. The trial did not meet the primary endpoint of reducing cardiovascular death or hospitalization for HF. However, it showed a trend toward benefit with ARNI, especially in women and those with lower LVEF. It did suggest benefits in patients with an EF in the lower range and in women who represent a high proportion of patients with HFpEF. This suggests that ARNI may be more beneficial in these subgroups and warrants further investigation.

The PARAMOUNT-HF trial[18] was a phase II trial designed to assess the effects of ARNI against ARB in patients with HFpEF and 301 patients with HFpEF with NYHA II–IV patients. ARNI was superior to valsartan in reducing NT-proBNP levels at 12 weeks, lowering left atrial size, and improving NYHA class at 36 weeks of treatment. Moreover, BP reductions were also more significant at both 12 and 36 weeks of treatment in the group of patients receiving ARNI than in those assigned to valsartan. A further subanalysis of the trial demonstrated a decrease in high-sensitive troponin I (hsTnI) levels in HFpEF patients treated with ARNI with regard to ARB, suggesting that ARNI has the potential to ameliorate myocardial injury in HFpEF patients.[19] This finding opens a new perspective on the benefits of ARNI in HFpEF management and encourages further research in this area.

The PARAGLIDE-HF study[20] reported the primary findings of a randomized, double-blind, multicenter clinical trial comparing ARNI and valsartan alone in patients with HFpEF (>0.40) and a recent worsening HF event. The study enrolled 466 patients and found a 23% greater reduction in the primary endpoint of time-averaged reduction in NT-proBNP in the ARNI group than in the valsartan group. This study met its primary endpoint, demonstrating a nominally significant reduction of 15% in the ARNI arm. However, win ratio analysis did not suggest any benefits for these patients. Safety analyses also revealed a 50% higher rate of symptomatic hypotension in the ARNI group than in the valsartan group.

The PARALLAX trial[21] tested the effects of ARNI versus optimal individualized background therapy, which could be the ACE inhibitor enalapril, ARB valsartan, or placebo, an optimal individualized background therapy in patients with HF. The trial involved 2,572 patients, 51% of whom were women, with a mean age of 73 years. The trial met the first primary endpoint, showing a 16.4% greater reduction in NT-proBNP after 12 weeks compared to patients treated with optimal individualized medical therapy. However, the second primary endpoint, quality of life, and NYHA functional class showed no significant differences between the two groups. Overall, except for HF events, serious adverse events were reported in similar proportions in both the groups. The patients in the ARNI group also showed a significantly lower decline in renal function at 24 weeks.

The PARAGLIDE-HF trial demonstrated reductions in natriuretic peptides with ARNI compared with valsartan in patients with HF with mildly reduced or preserved EF who had experienced a recent worsening HF event. Although the study lacked sufficient power to examine clinical outcomes, a hierarchical secondary endpoint was prespecified for analysis using a win ratio, which encompassed cardiovascular death, number and timing of worsening HF events, and meaningful changes in time-averaged NT-proBNP. The win ratio analysis (1.19; 95% CI 0.93–1.52) did not indicate any benefits for these patients. However, combined analyses of PARAGLIDE-HF and PARAGON-HF studies demonstrated that ARNI decreased cardiovascular and renal incidents in patients with HF with slightly diminished or maintained EFs.[22] These findings support the use of ARNI in individuals experiencing HF with mildly reduced or preserved EF, particularly in those whose LVEF is below normal, irrespective of the treatment setting.

ARNICFH, a randomized, open-label trial that aimed to assess the effect of ARNI on cardiac fibrosis in patients with HFpEF, is currently in phase 2 with an estimated population of 60 participants.[23] The PARABLE trial[24] will examine the hypothesis that ARNI can improve left atrial structure and function and LV structure and function in asymptomatic patients with HFpEF (stage A/B). This interventional, randomized, double-blind, controlled trial recruited 250 participants.

The ARNI-PRESERVED study[25] was a retrospective single-center study that examined the efficacy and safety of ARNI in Indian patients with HFpEF. The study analyzed data from 154 patients aged 65.6 ± 18.4 years, with 56.5% of them being female. Significant symptomatic clinical improvement was demonstrated with a substantial decrease in NYHA class ($p = 0.018$). A reduction in NYHA class resulted in symptomatic clinical improvement, rales, and peripheral edema ($p < 0.001$). NT-proBNP levels were also significantly lower ($p < 0.001$). Echocardiographic parameters for diastolic function (E/A and E/E' ratios) improved. Consequently, in Indian patients with HFpEF, the ARNI demonstrated a significant decrease in NYHA class, as well as reduced fluid retention and peripheral edema. However, the small sample size and limited follow-up duration, biomarkers, and echocardiographic characteristics limited this retrospective observational study. Furthermore, the absence of a control group precluded determination of therapeutic benefits attributable to ARNI in the examined patients.

In summary, in patients with HFpEF, ARNI frequently demonstrates the benefit of reduced NT-proBNP levels; however, this effect attenuates over time. The cardiovascular benefits of ARNI on HFpEF may be more pronounced in female patients and in those with moderate EF decline. Additionally, ARNI exhibits a significant antihypertensive effect in patients with HFpEF; nevertheless, vigilance is required regarding the potential occurrence of hypotension. Furthermore, although NT-proBNP decreased significantly, indicators of clinical symptoms, such as NYHA, KCCQ, and 6-minute walking distance, and improvements in echocardiographic measures, may not be sufficiently sensitive to reflect the benefits in patients treated with ARNI.[26] Consequently, more extended observations are necessary to identify the potential benefits that may exist. This analysis was based on the notable consistency and complementarity of the results of the PARAMOUNT, PARAGON-HF, and PARALLAX trials.

ROLE OF ANGIOTENSIN RECEPTOR-NEPRILYSIN INHIBITOR IN HEART FAILURE WITH MILDLY REDUCED PRESERVED EJECTION FRACTION

The efficacy of ARNI was not evaluated in a dedicated HFmrEF trial. Nevertheless, some data were available from the PARADIGM-HF[27] and PARAGON-HF trials,[17] which included patients with LVEF between 40% and 49%. In the PARADIGM-HF trial, ARNI reduced the primary endpoint of cardiovascular death or HF hospitalization by 13% and all-cause mortality by 19% in the HFmrEF subgroup compared with ACEi. In the PARAGON-HF trial, ARNI reduced the primary endpoint of cardiovascular death or HF hospitalization by 28% in the HFmrEF subgroup compared with valsartan.[28] These findings suggest that ARNI may be efficacious in HFmrEF; however, additional evidence is required to support its use in this population. Another clinical trial, PARALLAX, examined the effects of ARNI in patients with HFmrEF or HFpEF. The study demonstrated that ARNI decreased NT-proBNP levels; however, there was no observed improvement in the 6-minute walk distance compared with individualized medical therapy. Finally, the PARAGLIDE-HF clinical trial investigated the effect of ARNI on changes in NT-proBNP outcomes and safety in patients with HFpEF.

A meta-analysis of studies evaluating the use of ARNI therapy for different types of HF provides valuable insights into its overall effectiveness.[29] The meta-analysis included studies on HF with reduced EF (HFrEF), preserved EF, and mildly reduced EF. The results of the meta-analysis indicated that ARNI therapy significantly reduced mortality and hospitalizations across all types of HF. Moreover, ARNI therapy was associated with improvements in symptoms, functional capacity, quality of life, physical examination findings, and cardiac parameters, such as NT-proBNP. Furthermore, ARNI therapy demonstrated positive effects on cardiac parameters, including NT-pro-BNP and troponin levels, as well as echocardiographic measures such as EF, ventricular volume, and global longitudinal strain.

Notably, the guidelines for the utilization of ARNI in HFpEF are different. In Europe, ARNI may be considered in HFmrEF with a class IIb recommendation but not in HFpEF,[30] whereas in US guidelines,[31] they are also considered in HFpEF, with a class IIb recommendation "particularly at the lower end of this spectrum". Lifestyle modifications and control of risk factors are deemed significant in managing HFpEF and are accorded class I recommendations in both guidelines including the Indian guideline.[7] SGLT2 inhibitors and diuretics are the only currently available pharmacological agents that have demonstrated benefits, primarily in reducing hospitalization in both diabetic and nondiabetic patients with HFpEF. Spironolactone and ARNI have shown efficacy in certain subsets of patients with HFpEF and a lower EF range.

CONCLUSION

In conclusion, the efficacy of ARNIs in HFpEF and heart failure with midrange ejection fraction (HFmrEF) remains a subject of ongoing scientific inquiry. While clinical trials have yielded heterogeneous results, evidence suggests potential therapeutic benefits, particularly in reducing NT-pro BNP levels and improving outcomes in specific patient subgroups, notably in women and individuals with lower EFs. The effectiveness of ARNIs appears to vary across the spectrum of HF, with more consistent benefits observed in HFrEF. Despite the challenges in treating HFpEF owing to its heterogeneous etiology, ARNIs have emerged as a promising therapeutic modality. As research progresses, healthcare professionals should consider the potential benefits of ARNIs in managing patients with HFpEF and HFmrEF while remaining cognizant of potential adverse effects such as hypotension.

REFERENCES

1. Lam CS, Donal E, Kraigher-Krainer E, et al. Epidemiology and clinical course of heart failure with preserved ejection fraction. Eur J Heart Fail. 2011;13(1):18-28.
2. Tsao CW, Lyass A, Enserro D, et al. Temporal trends in the incidence of and mortality associated with heart failure with preserved and reduced ejection fractions. JACC Heart Fail. 2018;6:678-85.
3. Dunlay SM, Roger VL. Redfield MM. Epidemiology of heart failure with preserved ejection fraction. Nat Rev Cardiol. 2017;14(10):591-602.
4. Xanthopoulos A, Triposkiadis F, Starling RC. Heart failure with preserved ejection fraction: Classification based upon phenotype is essential for diagnosis and treatment. Trends Cardiovasc Med. 2018;28(6):392-400.
5. Sanjay G, Jeemon P, Agarwal A, et al. In-Hospital and Three-Year Outcomes of Heart Failure Patients in South India: The Trivandrum Heart Failure Registry. J Card Fail. 2018;24(12):842-8.
6. Lam CS, Anand I, Zhang S et al. Asian Sudden Cardiac Death in the Heart Failure (ASIAN-HF) Registry. Eur J Heart Fail. 2013;15(8):928-36.
7. Harikrishnan S, Oomman A, Jadhav UM, et al. Heart Failure with Preserved Ejection Fraction: Management Guidelines (From Heart Failure Association of India, Endorsed by Association of Physicians of India). J Assoc Physicians India. 2022;70(8):11-2.
8. Sharma K, Kass DA. Heart failure with preserved ejection fraction: Mechanisms, clinical features, and therapies. Circ Res. 2014;20;115(1):79-96.
9. Sciarretta S, Paneni F, Palano F, et al. Role of the renin-angiotensin-aldosterone system and inflammatory processes in the development and progression of diastolic dysfunction. Clin Sci (Lond). 2009;116(6):467-77.
10. Fragasso G. The Concept of "Heart Failure with Preserved Ejection Fraction": Time for a Critical Reappraisal. Rev Cardiovasc Med. 2023;24(7):202.
11. Yusuf S, Pfeffer MA, Swedberg K, et al.; CHARM Investigators and Committees. Effects of candesartan in patients with chronic heart failure and preserved left ventricular ejection fraction: The CHARM-Preserved Trial. Lancet. 2003;362(9386):777-81.
12. McMurray JJ, Carson PE, Komajda M, et al. Heart failure with preserved ejection fraction: Clinical characteristics of 4133 patients enrolled in the I-PRESERVE trial. Eur J Heart Fail. 2008;10(2):149-56.
13. Cleland JG, Tendera M, Adamus J, et al. PEP-CHF Investigators. Perindopril in elderly people with chronic heart failure (PEP-CHF). Eur Heart J. 2006;27(19):2338-45.
14. Pitt B, Pfeffer MA, Assmann SF, et al.; TOPCAT Investigators. Spironolactone for heart failure with preserved ejection fraction. N Engl J Med. 2014;370(15):1383-92.
15. Yamamoto K, Origasa H, Suzuki Y, et al.; J-DHF Investigators. Relationship of risk factors with response to carvedilol in heart failure with preserved ejection fraction: a report from the Japanese Diastolic Heart Failure Study (J-DHF). J Cardiol. 2014;63(6):424-31.
16. Jia R, Ji Y, Sun D. Progress and prospects of Sacubitril/Valsartan: Based on heart failure with preserved ejection fraction. Biomed Pharmacother. 2022;155:113701.
17. Solomon SD, McMurray JJV, et al.; PARAGON-HF Investigators and Committees. Angiotensin-Neprilysin Inhibition in Heart Failure with Preserved Ejection Fraction. N Engl J Med. 2019;381(17):1609-20.
18. Solomon SD, Zile M, Pieske B, et al. Prospective comparison of ARNI with ARB on Management Of heart failure with preserved ejection fraction (PARAMOUNT). The angiotensin receptor neprilysin inhibitor LCZ696 in heart failure with preserved ejection fraction: a phase 2 double-blind, randomized controlled trial. Lancet. 2012;380(9851):1387-95.
19. Biering-Sørensen T, Lassen MCH, Solomon SD, et al.; PARAMOUNT Investigators. Effect of Sacubitril/Valsartan on Left Ventricular Myocardial Deformation in Heart Failure with Preserved Ejection Fraction (PARAMOUNT trial). J Card Fail. 2023;29(6):968-73.
20. Mentz RJ, Ward JH, Braunwald E; PARAGLIDE-HF Investigators. Angiotensin-Neprilysin Inhibition in Patients With Mildly Reduced or Preserved Ejection Fraction and Worsening Heart Failure. J Am Coll Cardiol. 2023;82(1):1-12.
21. Pieske B, Wachter R, Shah SJ, et al.; PARALLAX Investigators and Committee members. Effect of Sacubitril/Valsartan vs. Standard Medical Therapies on Plasma

NT-proBNP concentration and Submaximal Exercise Capacity in Patients With Heart Failure and Preserved Ejection Fraction: The PARALLAX Randomized Clinical Trial. JAMA. 2021;326(19):1919-29.
22. Vaduganathan M, Mentz RJ, Claggett BL, et al. Sacubitril/valsartan in heart failure with mildly reduced or preserved ejection fraction: a pre-specified participant-level pooled analysis of PARAGLIDE-HF and PARAGON-HF. Eur Heart J. 2023;44(31):2982-93.
23. Ventura HO, Lavie CJ, Mehra MR. Angiotensin-neprilysin inhibition in heart failure with preserved ejection fraction: You win some, you lose some. J Am Coll Cardiol. 2023;82(1):13-5.
24. Ledwidge M, Dodd JD, Ryan F, et al. Effect of Sacubitril/Valsartan vs Valsartan on Left Atrial Volume in Patients With Pre-Heart Failure With Preserved Ejection Fraction: The PARABLE Randomized Clinical Trial. JAMA Cardiol. 2023;8(4):366-75.
25. Jariwala P, Punjani A, Harikishan B, et al. Safety and Effectiveness of Angiotensin Receptor-Neprilysin Inhibitors (ARNI) in Indian Patients with Heart Failure with Preserved Ejection Fraction (HFpEF) – 'ARNI-PRESERVED' study. Heart India. 2021;9(3):179-83.
26. Balestrieri G, Limonta R, Ponti E, et al. The Therapy and Management of Heart Failure with Preserved Ejection Fraction: New Insights on Treatment. Card Fail Rev. 2024;10:e05.
27. McMurray JJ, Packer M, Desai AS, et al. Angiotensin-neprilysin inhibition versus enalapril in heart failure. N Engl J Med. 2014;371(11):993-1004.
28. Leite M, Sampaio F, Saraiva FA. The impact of heart failure therapy in patients with mildly reduced ejection fraction: a network meta-analysis. ESC Heart Fail. 2023;10(3):1822-34.
29. Lin Y, Cai Z, Yuan J, et al. Effect of pharmacological treatment on outcomes of heart failure with preserved ejection fraction: an updated systematic review and network meta-analysis of randomized controlled trials. Cardiovasc Diabetol. 2022;21(1):237.
30. McDonagh TA, Metra M, Adamo M, et al. ESC Scientific Document Group, 2023 Focused Update of the 2021 ESC Guidelines for the diagnosis and treatment of acute and chronic heart failure: Developed by the task force for the diagnosis and treatment of acute and chronic heart failure of the European Society of Cardiology (ESC) With the special contribution of the Heart Failure Association (HFA) of the ESC. Eur Heart J. 2023;44(37):3627-39.
31. Heidenreich PA, Bozkurt B, Aguilar D, et al. 2022 AHA/ACC/HFSA Guideline for the Management of Heart Failure: A Report of the American College of Cardiology/American Heart Association Joint Committee on Clinical Practice Guidelines. J Am Coll Cardiol. 2022;79(17):e263-e421.

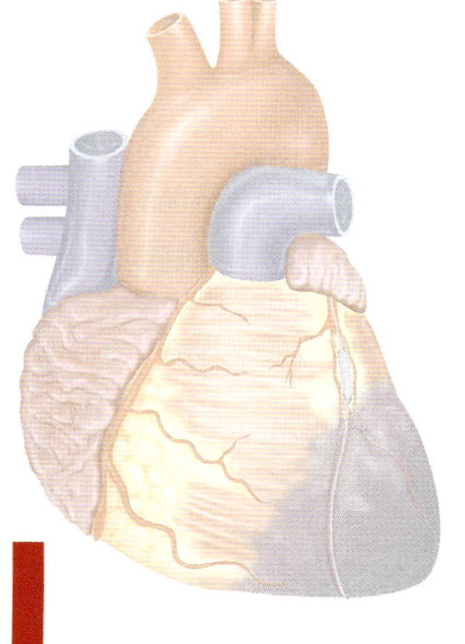

CHAPTER 133

Patiromer in Hyperkalemia in HF and CKD and ARNI Use in HFpEF

Asesh Haldar, DP Sinha

INTRODUCTION

Heart failure (HF) is a global pandemic affecting >64 million people all around the world.[1] It is not only associated with significantly increased mortality, morbidity, and impaired quality of life but also imparts a great economic burden. Though the prevalence is 1–3% in general adult population, it increases to >10% beyond the age of 70 years. The prevalence of different phenotypes also varies; in outpatient settings, 60% patients have HFrEF, 24% have HFmrEF, and 16% have HFpEF (ESC long-term registry). Studies done in in-hospital settings suggest a little different picture (50% patients have HFrEF and rest 50% have HFpEF and HFmrEF).[1,2]

Renin–angiotensin–aldosterone system (RAAS) plays a pivotal role in the pathophysiology of HF. RAAS inhibitors [angiotensin-converting enzyme inhibitors (ACEi), angiotensin II receptor blockers (ARB), mineralocorticoid receptor antagonists (MRA), and angiotensin receptor-neprilysin inhibitors (ARNI)] decrease mortality, reduce hospitalization, and improve quality of life of the patients with HF and are standard of guideline-directed medical therapy over the last few years. Dyskalemia is common in HF and it is certainly arduous for the physician to implement guideline-directed medical therapy, specifically RAAS inhibitor in the context of hyperkalemia. Potassium is found in the intracellular compartment almost exclusively (98%) and kidney has an integral role in maintaining potassium homeostasis. 30–40% patients of HF have concomitant chronic kidney disease (CKD). The reason for hyperkalemia is multifactorial—renal dysfunction, severity of HF, aging, diabetes mellitus, and use of RAAS inhibitor. Hyperkalemia is classified as mild [serum potassium (K^+) 5.1–5.5 mEq/L], moderate (serum K^+ 5.6–6.0 mEq/L), or severe (serum K^+ >6.0 mEq/L). Serum potassium has a very narrow margin of safety (3.5–5.5 mEq/L) and follows the "U" shaped relationship with mortality.[3,4]

Various studies comparing effect of different drugs and RAASi in hyperkalemia are given in **Table 1**.

DOES HYPERKALEMIA INCREASE MORTALITY?

Hyperkalemia enhances the risk of arrhythmia, hospitalization, and mortality.

In REVOLUTIONIZE III[14] study, recurrent hyperkalemia (serum K^+ ≥5.1 mEq/L, ≥2 events within 1 year) was associated with 30% higher risk of all-cause mortality ($p < 0.001$) and 45% higher risk ($p < 0.001$) of major adverse cardiovascular events (MACE) + (MACE+: All-cause mortality or inpatient admission with myocardial infarction, stroke, or HF) compared to normokalemia in patients with HF and stage 3–4 CKD.

Palaka et al.[15] in their review article showed that in patients with HF with serum K^+ >6 mmol/L, the hazard ratio (HR) for all-cause mortality and cardiovascular mortality was 4.89 and 3.33, respectively compared to normokalemic patients. In presence of serum K 5.5–6 mmol/L and HF, the HR for all-cause mortality and cardiovascular mortality was 2.94 and 1.88, respectively. Not only that, in HF patients with serum potassium of >6 mmol/L, the chance of hospitalization increases by 5 times.

TABLE 1: Various studies comparing effect of different drugs and RAASi in hyperkalemia.

Study		*RAASi*	*Hyperkalemia*	*p-value*
CONSENSUS[5]	Enalapril vs. placebo	*Spironolactone:* 50%	7.1 vs. 4%	
SOLVD[6]	Enalapril vs. placebo	*K-sparing diuretics:* 9.2%	*K >5.5:* 6.4 vs. 2.5%	<0.01
CHARM alternative[7]	Candesartan vs. placebo	*Spironolactone:* 23%	1.9 vs. 0.3%	0.0005
CHARM-added[8]	Candesartan vs. placebo	• *ACEi:* 100% • *Spironolactone:* 17%	3.4 vs. 0.7%	<0.0001
RALES[9]	Spironolactone vs. placebo	*ACEi:* 95%	*K >6:* 2 vs. 1%	0.42
EPHESUS[10]	Eplerenone vs. placebo	*ACE or ARB:* 86%	*K >6:* 5.5 vs. 3.9%	0.002
EMPHASIS-HF[11]	Eplerenone vs. placebo	*ACEi:* 78.3%, *ARB*: 19.1%	• *K >5.5:* 11.8 vs. 7.2% • *K >6:* 2.5 vs. 1.9%	• <0.001 • NS
TOPCAT[12]	Spironolactone. vs placebo	*ACEi/ARB:* 84%	18.7 vs. 9.1	
PARADIGM HF[13]	ARNI vs enalapril	*MRA:* 54%	• *K >5.5: 16.1 vs. 17.3%* • *K >6:* 4.3 vs. 5.6%	• 0.15 • 0.007

In-hospital mortality increases in patients admitted with acute HF with initial serum K^+ of >4.8 mEq/L.

CONTINUATION VERSUS DISCONTINUATION OF RAAS INHIBITORS IN PRESENCE OF HYPERKALEMIA

One recent systematic review and meta-analysis[16] has shown that MRA use in HF patients was associated with 74% increased risk of hyperkalemia. There was 31% increased risk of mortality in patients who discontinued MRA (30% HF patients discontinued MRA) compared to the patients who continued receiving MRA.

In another study,[17] hyperkalemia-related RAAS inhibitor discontinuation/downtitration was associated with significantly increased risk of cardiorenal events (HF emergency visit, HF hospitalization, or progression to end-stage kidney disease) compared to patients who were receiving similar or uptitrated RAASi. In another similar study, hyperkalemia-related discontinuation of RAAS inhibitor was associated with higher risk of all-cause mortality in CKD (eGFR <60 mL/min/1.73 m^2). Irrespective of etiology (hyperkalemia, hypotension, or AKI), RAASi discontinuation was seen to be associated with increased risk of all-cause mortality, all-cause hospitalization, cardiac arrhythmia, HF hospitalization, and cardiac arrest.[18-20]

In nutshell, in HF patients with or without CKD, we should use RAASi in a way where we will achieve the best possible benefit of RAASi without exposing the patients to the hyperkalemia-related harms. So, we were in search of a molecule (without much drug-related adverse events) that will serve the purpose of a chronic use to maintain normokalemia so that RAASi use can be maintained or even escalated. In this regard, the role of sodium polystyrene sulfonate is limited because of lack of any large-scale randomized trials and chronic use and its association with gastrointestinal (GI) complications. Patiromer and sodium zirconium cyclosilicate are new-generation potassium-lowering agents that can be used to fulfil the gaps.

Patiromer is a nonabsorbed cation exchange polymer, which exchanges potassium for calcium ions instead of sodium ions. Therefore, it might be safer in situations where any extra sodium load is unwanted such as in severe hypertension (HTN), HF, and CKD.[21]

EVIDENCE WITH PATIROMER

PEARL-HF Trial[22,23]

In this randomized, double-blind, placebo-controlled study, efficacy and safety of RLY5016 were evaluated in 105 patients of chronic HF with history of hyperkalemia-related discontinuation of RAASi and/or beta-blocker (BB) or CKD with eGFR <60 mL/min/1.73 m^2 and receiving HF therapies (ACE-I, ARB, and BB). Spironolactone was added at a dose of 25 mg/day and dose was escalated if serum K^+ >3.5–≤5.1 mEq/L after 2 weeks. After 4 weeks, use of 30 g/day RLY5016 was associated with significant reduction of serum potassium level compared to placebo (serum K^+ difference between groups was –45 mEq/L, $p < 0.001$). There was lower incidence of hyperkalemia and spironolactone dose was escalated in greater proportion to the study drug. GI side effects were seen more commonly with RLY5016 compared to placebo.

DIAMOND Trial[24]

This prospective phase 3, multicenter, double-blind, randomized, placebo-controlled study was done on patients with HFrEF (LVEF ≤40%) with current or a history of RAASi-related hyperkalemia (two serum K^+ values of >5 mmol/L). During the run-in phase up to 12 weeks with patiromer (up to 3 packs/day, 8.4 g/pack), RAASi dose was optimized [≥50% recommended dose of ACEI/ARB/ARNI, and 50 mg of spironolactone or eplerenone]. Patients with eGFR <30 mL/min/1.73 m^2 were excluded from the study. Prespecified target dose of RAASi was achieved in 84.6% patients. After this initial run-in phase, eligible patients were randomized into 1:1 ratio so that in one group, patiromer was continued and in another group study drug was switched to placebo. At the end of study (median 27 weeks), the primary endpoint of difference in the adjusted mean change in serum potassium between 2 groups was significantly different (adjusted mean change in potassium was +0.03 mmol/L and +0.13 mmol/L in the patiromer group and in the placebo group, respectively; difference in the adjusted mean change between two groups was −0.10 mmol/L, $p < 0.001$). 13.9% in the patiromer group and 19.4% in the placebo group had hyperkalemia events (serum K^+ of >5.5 mmol/L) [hazard ratio (HR) 0.63; 95% CI 0.45, 0.87; $p = 0.006$]. MRA dose reduction or discontinuation was seen in 13.9% in the patiromer and 18.9% in the placebo group (HR 0.62; 95% CI 0.45, 0.87; $p = 0.006$. Total adjusted hyperkalemia events per 100 person-years (77.7 vs. 118.2; HR 0.66; 95% CI 0.53, 0.81; $p < 0.001$) were significantly lower with patiromer. Both hyperkalemia-related morbidity-adjusted events (win ratio 1.53, $p < 0.001$) and total RAASi use score (win ratio 1.25, $p = 0.048$) were favorable in the patiromer arm. Cardiovascular death, all-cause death, HF hospitalization, and adverse events were not different between groups.

AMETHYST-DN Trial[25]

This was a phase-2 multicenter, open-label, randomized clinical trial that was done to assess the long-term safety and efficacy of patiromer in patients with diabetes and CKD (eGFR 15–59 cc/min/1.73 m^2) with mild-to-moderate hyperkalemia on RAASi. Patiromer was given at a dose of 4.2–12.6 mg twice daily to the patient having serum K^+ of 5.1–5.5 mEq/L (mild hyperkalemia) and the dose of patiromer was 8.4–16.8 mg twice daily if the serum K^+ was 5.6–5.9 mEq/L (moderate hyperkalemia). Throughout the maintenance phase, patients continued RAASi and patiromer dose was titrated to maintain serum K^+ ≤5 mEq/L. After 4 weeks of treatment, patiromer 4.2–16.8 g twice daily (8.4–33.6 g/d) resulted in statistically significant decreases in serum K+ which lasted 52 weeks. During the maintenance phase, 83.1–92.7% patients in the mild hyperkalemia group and 77.4–95.1% patients in the moderate hyperkalemia group maintained normokalemia (3.8–5 mEq/L).

OPAL HK Trial[26]

This study was conducted in two phases. In phase 1, patiromer was given to the patients of stage 3 or 4 CKD (eGFR15 to <60 mL/min/1.73 m^2 of body-surface area) with hyperkalemia (serum K^+ 5.1–6.5 mmol/L), all of them were receiving RAAS inhibitors. Potassium-related electrocardiographic changes, uncontrolled or unstable arrhythmias, or clinically significant ventricular arrhythmias were excluded concurrently. At the end of 4 weeks, target potassium level (3.8–<5.1 mmol/L) was reached in 74% patients with mild hyperkalemia (baseline K^+ 5.1–<5.5 mEq/L, treated with patiromer 4.2 g twice daily) and 77% patients with moderate-to-severe hyperkalemia (baseline K^+ 5.5–<6.5 mEq/L, treated with 8.4 gm patiromer twice daily). In the subsequent randomized withdrawal phase, patients who had a baseline K^+ of ≥5 mmol/L and achieved target K of 3.8–<5.1 mmol/L after 4 weeks of patiromer therapy were divided into 2 groups, one group continued patiromer but the other group was switched to placebo. After 4 weeks, the median increase in serum K^+ from the baseline of withdrawal phase was significantly lesser in the patiromer group compared to placebo. Recurrence of hyperkalemia was also found to be significantly lesser in the patiromer group.

AMBER Trial[27]

Spironolactone is used to treat resistant HTN which is quite common in presence of CKD. In this phase 2 multicenter, randomized, double-blind, placebo-controlled study, patiromer allowed more patients of CKD (eGFR 25–≤45 mL/min/1.73 m^2) and resistant HTN to remain on spironolactone. This trial demonstrated comparable safety and efficacy in different subgroups of CKD (eGFR 25–<30 and 30–≤45 mL/min/1.73 m^2).

In a recently published longitudinal observational study among US[28] veterans with CKD and hyperkalemia, all-cause mortality was reduced with long-term patiromer use.

The most frequent adverse event in relation to patiromer use is GI disorders namely constipation, diarrhea, and nausea. Hypokalemia and hypomagnesemia are among others.

TREATING HYPERKALEMIA WITH POTASSIUM BINDER IN PATIENTS RECEIVING RAAS INHIBITOR[29-31]

Firstly, exclude pseudo-hyperkalemia. Irrespective of etiology, it is extremely important to identify patients with hyperkalemic emergency [any one of these: (1) ECG changes or neuromuscular symptoms related to hyperkalemia; (2) K >6.5 mEq/L; (3) K >5.5 mEq/L with significant renal impairment and features of tissue breakdown like in rhabdomyolysis], so that rapidly-acting therapies (calcium gluconate and insulin + dextrose etc.) can be instituted without any delay and other medications enhancing excretion of potassium (diuretic, potassium binder, etc.) can be started subsequently. RAASi must be stopped in such scenario.

The following practical aspects should be followed while managing chronic hyperkalemia to ensure at least >50% RAASi dose continuation:

- *Serum K^+ 3.5–5 mEq/L:*
  - Initiate/uptitrate RAASi
  - Ensure following while treating/preventing hyperkalemia:
    - Exclude pseudo-hyperkalemia
    - Stop K supplementation, avoid taking potassium-rich food, NSAIDs
    - Oral sodium bicarbonate in case of metabolic acidosis
- *Serum K^+ 5.1–5.5 mEq/L:*
  - Initiate/uptitrate RAASi
  - *Consider K binder in specific situations:* In presence of history of RAASi-related hyperkalemia or in presence of HF ± CKD3b-4±DM or when regular monitoring is doubtful, patiromer 8.4 g once daily to maximum 25.2 g once daily targeting K^+ <5.1 mEq/L is required, titrate RAASi and reassess serum K^+ after 7 days.
- *Serum K+ 5.6–6 mEq/L:*
  - *Submaximal/<50% dose of RAASi:* Add K^+ binder/patiromer 8.4 g once daily to maximum 25.2 g once daily targeting K^+ <5.1 mEq/L; uptitrate RAASi to at least >50% of the recommended dose if serum K^+ <5.1 mEq/L.
  - *Maximally tolerated/guideline-recommended dose of RAASi:* Add K^+ binder/patiromer 8.4–25.2 g once daily and maintain RAASi dose; check serum K^+ after 7 days, if K^+ remains high, then downtitrate RAASi.
- *Serum K >6 mEq/L:* Add K binder/patiromer 8.4 g once daily to maximum dose of 25.2 g once daily and discontinue RAASi; check serum K after 7 days and restart RAASi preferably one at time if target K^+ is achieved.

How frequently do we monitor serum electrolytes?[29-31]

Serum K^+ and creatinine should be checked 3–7 days after starting or changing patiromer dose, repeat the tests after 1 week. Once the desired serum potassium level is achieved then measure serum K^+ at 1 month. Following this, 3 monthly monitoring is recommended.

Serum magnesium should also be measured for a month.

CONCLUSION

Hyperkalemia is a limiting factor of RAASi therapy, especially in patients with HF and CKD and discontinuation of RAASi certainly leads to adverse cardiovascular consequences. Use of patiromer facilitates the continuation of RAASi with a good safety profile.

REFERENCES

1. Savarese G, Becher PM, Lund LH, et al. Global burden of heart failure: a comprehensive and updated review of epidemiology. Cardiovasc Res. 2023;118(17):3272-87. Erratum in: Cardiovasc Res. 2023;119(6):1453.
2. McDonagh TA, Metra M, Adamo M, et al.; ESC Scientific Document Group. 2021 ESC Guidelines for the diagnosis and treatment of acute and chronic heart failure. Eur Heart J. 2021;42(36):3599-726.
3. ECC Committee, Subcommittees and Task Forces of the American Heart Association. 2005 American Heart Association Guidelines for cardiopulmonary resuscitation and emergency cardiovascular care. Part 10.1: Life-threatening electrolyte abnormalities. Circulation. 2005;112:IV121-5.
4. Silva-Cardoso J, Brito D, Frazão JM, et al. Management of RAASi-associated hyperkalemia in patients with cardiovascular disease. Heart Fail Rev. 2021;26(4):891-6.
5. CONSENSUS Trial Study Group. Effects of enalapril on mortality in severe congestive heart failure. Results of the Cooperative North Scandinavian Enalapril Survival Study (CONSENSUS). N Engl J Med. 1987;316(23):1429-35.
6. SOLVD Investigators; Yusuf S, Pitt B, Davis CE, et al. Effect of enalapril on survival in patients with reduced left ventricular ejection fractions and congestive heart failure. N Engl J Med. 1991;325(5):293-302.
7. Granger CB, McMurray JJ, Yusuf S, et al. Effects of candesartan in patients with chronic heart failure and reduced left-ventricular systolic function intolerant to angiotensin-converting-enzyme inhibitors: The CHARM-Alternative trial. Lancet. 2003;362:772-6.
8. McMurray JJ, Ostergren J, Swedberg K, et al; CHARM Investigators and Committees. Effects of candesartan in patients with chronic heart failure and reduced

left-ventricular systolic function taking angiotensin-converting-enzyme inhibitors: The CHARM-Added trial. Lancet. 2003;362(9386):767-71.

9. Vardeny O, Wu DH, Desai A, et al. Influence of baseline and worsening renal function on efficacy of spironolactone in patients with severe heart failure: Insights from RALES (Randomized Aldactone Evaluation Study). J Am Coll Cardiol. 2012;60:2082-9.
10. Pitt B, Williams G, Remme W, et al. The EPHESUS trial: Eplerenone in patients with heart failure due to systolic dysfunction complicating acute myocardial infarction. Eplerenone Post-AMI Heart Failure Efficacy and Survival Study. Cardiovasc Drugs Ther. 2001;15:79-87.
11. Eschalier R, McMurray JJ, Swedberg K, et al. Safety and efficacy of eplerenone in patients at high risk for hyperkalemia and/or worsening renal function: Analyses of the EMPHASIS-HF study subgroups (Eplerenone in Mild Patients Hospitalization and Survival Study in Heart Failure). J Am Coll Cardiol. 2013;62:1585-93.
12. Desai AS, Liu J, Pfeffer MA, et al. Incident hyperkalemia, hypokalemia, and clinical outcomes during spironolactone treatment of heart failure with preserved ejection fraction: Analysis of the TOPCAT trial. J Card Fail. 2018;24:313-20.
13. McMurray JJ, Packer M, Desai AS, et al.; PARADIGM-HF Investigators and Committees. Angiotensin-neprilysin inhibition versus enalapril in heart failure. N Engl J Med. 2014;371(11):993-1004.
14. Bakris G, Agiro A, Greatsinger A. et al. Mortality and cardiovascular outcomes in patients with heart failure and chronic kidney disease with recurrent hyperkalemia: Revolutionize III study. JACC. 2024;83(13_Suppl):331.
15. Palaka E, Grandy S, Darlington O, et al. Associations between serum potassium and adverse clinical outcomes: a systematic literature review. Int J Clin Pract. 2020; 74(1):e13421.
16. Siddiqi T, Usman M, Abid M, et al. Is stopping mineralo-corticoid receptor antagonists after hyperkalemia associated with increased mortality in heart failure? A systematic review and meta-analysis. JACC. 2022;79 (9_Suppl):406.
17. Kanda E, Rastogi A, Murohara T, et al. Clinical impact of suboptimal RAASi therapy following an episode of hyperkalemia. BMC Nephrol. 2023;24:18.
18. An J, Zhou H, Ni L, et al. Discontinuation of renin-angiotensin-aldosterone system inhibitors secondary to hyperkalemia translates into higher cardiorenal outcomes. Am J Nephrol. 2023;54(7-8):258-67.
19. Humphrey TJL, James G, Wittbrodt ET, et al. Adverse clinical outcomes associated with RAAS inhibitor discontinuation: Analysis of over 400,000 patients from the UK Clinical Practice Research Datalink (CPRD). Clin Kidney J. 2021;14 (10):2203-12.
20. Janse RJ, Fu EL, Clase CM, et al. Stopping versus continuing renin–angiotensin–system inhibitors after acute kidney injury and adverse clinical outcomes: an observational study from routine care data. Clin Kidney J. 2022;15(6):1109-19.
21. Li L, Harrison SD, Cope MJ, et al. Mechanism of action and pharmacology of patiromer, a nonabsorbed cross-linked polymer that lowers serum potassium concentration in patients with hyperkalemia. J Cardiovasc Pharmacol Ther. 2016;21(5):456-65.
22. Buysse JM, Huang IZ, Pitt B. PEARL-HF: Prevention of hyperkalemia in patients with heart failure using a novel polymeric potassium binder, RLY5016. Future Cardiol. 2012;8:17-28.
23. Pitt B, Anker SD, Bushinsky DA, et al.; PEARL-HF Investigators. Evaluation of the efficacy and safety of RLY5016, a polymeric potassium binder, in a double-blind, placebo-controlled study in patients with chronic heart failure (the PEARL-HF) trial. Eur Heart J. 2011;32: 820-8.
24. Butler J, Anker SD, Lund LH, et al. Patiromer for the management of hyperkalemia in heart failure with reduced ejection fraction: The DIAMOND trial. Eur Heart J. 2022;43:4362-73.
25. Bakris GL, Pitt B, Weir MR, et al. AMETHYST-DN Investigators. Effect of patiromer on serum potassium level in patients with hyperkalemia and diabetic kidney disease: The AMETHYST-DN randomized clinical trial. JAMA. 2015;314:151-61.
26. Weir MR, Bakris GL, Bushinsky DA, et al. OPAL-HK Investigators. Patiromer in patients with kidney disease and hyperkalemia receiving RAAS inhibitors. N Engl J Med. 2015;372:211-21.
27. Agarwal R, Rossignol P, Romero A, et al. Patiromer versus placebo to enable spironolactone use in patients with resistant hypertension and chronic kidney disease (AMBER): A phase 2, randomised, double-blind, placebo-controlled trial. Lancet. 2019;394:1540-50.
28. Obi Y, Thomas F, Dashputre AA, et al. Long-term patiromer use and outcomes among us veterans with hyperkalemia and CKD: A Propensity-Matched Cohort Study. Kidney Med. 2023;6(1):100757.
29. De Nicola L, Ferraro PM, Montagnani A, et al. Recommendations for the management of hyperkalemia in patients receiving renin-angiotensin-aldosterone system inhibitors. Intern Emerg Med. 2024;19(2): 295-306.
30. Almenar Bonet L, González-Franco Á; Working Group for the Study of Hyperkalemia. Consensus on the management of hyperkalemia in patients with heart failure: Recommendations from the SEC-SEMI. Rev Clin Esp (Barc). 2022;222(4):235-40.
31. Ferreira JP, Butler J, Rossignol P, et al. Abnormalities of potassium in heart failure: JACC State-of-the-Art Review. JACC. 2020;75(22):2836-2850. doi: 10.1016/j.jacc.2020.04.021. PMID: 32498812.

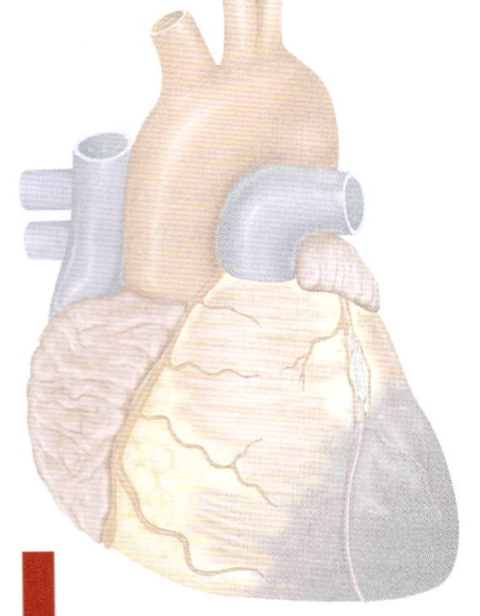

ARNI as In-hospital Therapy in HFpEF

Uday M Jadhav, Shilpa Deshmukh Kadam

INTRODUCTION

Heart failure (HF) is a clinical syndrome with symptoms and/or signs caused by a structural and/or functional cardiac abnormality and corroborated by elevated natriuretic peptide levels and/or objective evidence of pulmonary or systemic congestion.[1] Prevalence of HF is escalating rapidly, with a projected increase of 34% in upcoming decades.[2,3] HF is a syndrome that consumes substantial health care resources, inflicts considerable morbidity and mortality, and adversely affects quality of life.[4]

Sacubitril/valsartan is 1 of the "4 pillars" of medical care for HFrEF. The 2022 AHA/ACC/HFSA HF guideline recommends sacubitril/valsartan as a class I, level of evidence: A therapy to reduce the risk of HF hospitalization and CV mortality in patients with symptomatic chronic HFrEF.

Rapid optimization of quadruple foundational therapy for HF with reduced ejection fraction comprising β-blockers, angiotensin receptor neprilysin inhibitors, mineralocorticoid receptor antagonists (MRAs), and sodium-glucose cotransporter-2 inhibitors has been advocated recently. HF hospitalization has been identified as an optimal time for initiation and up titration of medications, not only because the patients are at a high risk but also because this encounter occurs in a setting of close surveillance under the care of a team of clinicians that lasts several days, all facilitating rapid initiation and titration of therapy.

The angiotensin receptor/neprilysin inhibitor (ARNi) is composed of angiotensin receptor blockers (ARB) and an inhibitor of neprilysin, an enzyme that degrades natriuretic peptides, bradykinin, adrenomedullin, and other vasoactive peptides. By inhibiting neprilysin, ARNI increases levels of beneficial peptides that promote vasodilation, natriuresis, and diuresis, while valsartan provides angiotensin II receptor blockade, mitigating its vasoconstrictive effects.

In PARADIGM-HF (Prospective Comparison of ARNi with ACEi to Determine Impact on Global Mortality and Morbidity in Heart Failure), an RCT that compared the first approved ARNi, sacubitril-valsartan, with enalapril in symptomatic patients with HFrEF tolerating an adequate dose of either ACEi or ARB, sacubitril-valsartan significantly reduced the composite endpoint of cardiovascular death or HF hospitalization by 20% relative to enalapril.[5]

The ARNIs have been associated with improvements in surrogates such as diastolic function, LV function, natriuretic peptide concentrations, burden of ventricular arrhythmias, and hard endpoints, including quality of life, costs, hospital days, and HF hospitalizations.

STRONG HF (Safety, Tolerability, and Efficacy of Rapid Optimization, Helped by N-terminal pro-b-type natriuretic peptide (NT-proBNP) Testing, of Heart Failure Therapies) trial demonstrated that for individuals hospitalized with acute HF, intensive and rapid initiation and titration of GDMT supported by in-person follow-up after hospitalization was safe, was tolerated, and resulted in a reduction in 180-day HF hospitalizations and/or CV deaths.[6,7]

When making the transition from an ACE inhibitor to an ARNI, a 36-hour washout period should be strictly observed (to avoid angioedema); this delay is not required when switching from an ARB to an ARNI.[8]

ANGIOTENSIN RECEPTOR NEPRILYSIN INHIBITOR IN HEART FAILURE WITH PRESERVED EJECTION FRACTION

PARAGON-HF trial failed to show that sacubitril/valsartan reduced adverse events among patients with Heart failure with preserved ejection fraction (HFpEF). Patients with HFpEF were randomized to sacubitril/valsartan 97/103 mg twice daily (n = 2,419) versus valsartan 160 mg twice daily (n = 2,403) in the PARAGON-HF trial.[9]

Primary outcome, rate of cardiovascular deaths or hospitalizations for HF, was 12.8 events per 100 patient-years in the sacubitril/valsartan group versus 14.6 events per 100 patient-years in the valsartan group (p = not significant). Secondary outcomes, New York Heart Association (NYHA) class improvement was noted 15.0% in the sacubitril/valsartan group versus 12.6% in the valsartan group (p <0.05). Renal composite outcome was 1.4% in the sacubitril/valsartan group versus 2.7% in the valsartan group (p <0.05). Sacubitril/valsartan was associated with a reduction of the primary outcome in women, but not in men.

Sacubitril/valsartan versus placebo was associated with an absolute 6.4% reduction in cardiovascular death or hospitalization for HF when initiated <30 days from index hospitalization, 4.6% when initiated 30–90 days after index hospitalization, 3.4% when initiated 91–180 days after index hospitalization, and no benefit when initiated >180 days after index hospitalization (p for interaction = 0.05).

On echocardiographic examination of patients with HFpEF, prevalence of LV hypertrophy was 21%, left atrial enlargement 83%, elevated E/e′ ratio 53%, and pulmonary hypertension 31% in the study.

NT-proBNP was associated with the primary endpoint, total HF hospitalizations and cardiovascular death [rate ratio (RR) 1.68 per log increase in NT-proBNP, p <0.001]. Relationship was stronger with atrial fibrillation (p for interaction <0.001) and weaker with obesity (p for interaction <0.001). Sacubitril/valsartan compared with valsartan reduced NT-proBNP by 19%. Patients with orthopnea appeared to derive greater benefit from sacubitril/valsartan (RR 0.67) compared with those without orthopnea (RR 0.97, p for interaction = 0.04).

Risk of cardiovascular death or first heart failure hospitalization among those with no deterioration in eGFR: 11.8 events per 100 person-years with sacubitril/valsartan versus 13.0 events per 100 person-years with enalapril (HR 0.89). Risk of cardiovascular death or first heart failure hospitalization among those with deterioration in eGFR <30 mL/min/1.73 m²: 28.1 events per 100 person-years with sacubitril/valsartan versus 33.9 events per 100 person-years with enalapril (HR 0.81, p for interaction = 0.64)

The mean change in mini-mental state examination (MMSE) from baseline to 96 weeks was –0.05 in the sacubitril/valsartan group versus –0.04 in the valsartan group.

POOLED ANALYSIS AND META-ANALYSIS OF ANGIOTENSIN RECEPTOR NEPRILYSIN INHIBITOR IN HEART FAILURE WITH PRESERVED EJECTION FRACTION

PARAGLIDE-HF trial demonstrated reductions in natriuretic peptides with sacubitril/valsartan compared with valsartan in patients with HF with mildly reduced or preserved ejection fraction who had a recent worsening HF event, but was not adequately powered to examine clinical outcomes. PARAGON-HF included a subset of PARAGLIDE-HF-like patients who were recently hospitalized for HF. Participant-level data from PARAGLIDE-HF and PARAGON-HF were pooled to better estimate the efficacy and safety of sacubitril/valsartan in reducing cardiovascular and renal events in HF with mildly reduced or preserved ejection fraction.[10]

PARAGLIDE-HF and PARAGON-HF were multicenter, double-blind, randomized, active-controlled trials of sacubitril/valsartan versus valsartan in patients with HF with mildly reduced or preserved left ventricular ejection fraction (LVEF >40% in PARAGLIDE-HF and ≥45% in PARAGON-HF). Prespecified primary analysis pooled participants in PARAGLIDE-HF (all of whom were enrolled during or within 30 days of a worsening HF event) with a "PARAGLIDE-like" subset of PARAGON-HF (those hospitalized for HF within 30 days) and also pooled the entire PARAGLIDE-HF and PARAGON-HF populations.

Primary endpoint for this analysis was the composite of total worsening HF events (including first and recurrent HF hospitalizations and urgent visits) and cardiovascular death. The secondary endpoint was the prespecified renal composite endpoint for both studies (≥50% decline in estimated glomerular filtration rate from baseline, end-stage renal disease, or renal death).

Compared with valsartan, sacubitril/valsartan significantly reduced total worsening HF events and cardiovascular death in both the primary pooled analysis of participants with recent worsening HF [n = 1,088; rate ratio (RR) 0.78; $p = 0.042$] and in the pooled analysis of all participants ($n = 5{,}262$; RR 0.86; $p = 0.027$). In the pooled analysis of all participants, first nominal statistical significance was reached by day 9 after randomization, and treatment benefits were larger in those with LVEF ≤60% (RR 0.78) compared with those with LVEF >60% (RR 1.09; $p = 0.021$). Sacubitril/valsartan was also associated with lower rates of the renal composite endpoint in the primary pooled analysis [hazard ratio (HR) 0.67; $p = 0.080$] and the pooled analysis of all participants (HR 0.60; $p = 0.002$).

Meta-analysis to comprehensively evaluate the efficacy and safety of sacubitril/valsartan compared to valsartan in HF with different LVEF categories was conducted.[11] Four RCTs were included in the analysis, with 3,375 patients in the sacubitril/valsartan group and 3,362 in the valsartan group.

Sacubitril/valsartan was associated with improvements in the HF outcomes of the Kansas City Cardiomyopathy Questionnaire Clinical Summary Score (KCCQ CSS), the NYHA class, and the composite outcome of hospitalization for HF and cardiovascular death when compared to valsartan. KCCQ CSS had significant but lesser mean difference of 1.13 ($p = 0.024$), improvement in the NYHA class (odds ratio or OR of 1.32, $p = 0.002$), and the composite outcome of hospitalizations for HF and cardiovascular death, with a relative risk (RR) of 0.86 ($p = 0.04$). Sacubitril/valsartan compared to valsartan did not demonstrate increase in the risk of hyperkalemia or worsening renal function.

ANGIOTENSIN RECEPTOR NEPRILYSIN INHIBITOR AND HYPOTENSION IN HEART FAILURE WITH PRESERVED EJECTION FRACTION

PARAGLIDE-HF participants experienced symptomatic hypotension at rates of 24% in the sacubitril/valsartan group versus 15% in the valsartan group.[12] When prescribing sacubitril/valsartan or valsartan for patients diagnosed with HFpEF or HFmrEF, consideration should be given to patients with higher LVEF (>60%) and lower baseline systolic BP (<120 mm Hg) at higher risk for symptomatic hypotension during treatment.

PARAGLIDE-HF study participants included 466 patients randomized to sacubitril/valsartan versus valsartan and this analysis found that 92 (19.7%) experienced symptomatic hypotension. This included 24% with sacubitril/valsartan and 15.5% with valsartan.

Factors that were associated with symptomatic hypotension included being White (odds ratio 1.87), having a lower baseline systolic BP (per 10 mm Hg increase: OR, 0.68), or having a left ventricular EF (LVEF) >60% (OR, 2.21). There were no differences in time-averaged changes in NT-proBNP with baseline systolic BP ≥128 mm Hg versus ≤128 mm Hg (interaction $p = 0.43$).

ANGIOTENSIN RECEPTOR NEPRILYSIN INHIBITOR EFFECT ON NATRIURETIC PEPTIDE AND LEFT ATRIAL FUNCTION

Randomized clinical trial of 250 asymptomatic patients, sacubitril/valsartan versus valsartan was associated with a reduction in blood pressure, pulse pressure, and N-terminal pro-b-type natriuretic peptide; an increase in maximal left atrial volume index measured by cardiac magnetic resonance imaging despite lower filling pressures; less decline in kidney function; and fewer serious adverse cardiovascular events.

Personalized prospective comparison of ARNI with ARB in Patients With Natriuretic Peptide Elevation (PARABLE) trial was a prospective, double-blind, double-dummy, randomized clinical trial.[13]

250 asymptomatic patients 40 years and older with hypertension or diabetes, elevated B-type natriuretic peptide (BNP) greater than 20 pg/mL or N-terminal pro-b-type natriuretic peptide greater than 100 pg/mL, left atrial volume index greater than 28 mL/m^2, and preserved ejection fraction greater than 50% were included.

Maximal left atrial volume index was increased in patients assigned to receive sacubitril/valsartan (6.9 mL/m^2) versus valsartan (0.7 mL/m^2, $p < .001$). Changes in pulse pressure and N-terminal pro-BNP were lower in the sacubitril/valsartan group (−4.2 mm Hg and −17.7%, respectively; $p < .001$) than the valsartan group (−1.2 mm Hg; and 9.4% respectively; $p < .001$). Major adverse cardiovascular events occurred in 6 patients (4.9%) assigned to sacubitril/valsartan and 17 (13.3%) assigned to receive valsartan (adjusted hazard ratio, 0.38; $p = .04$).

ANGIOTENSIN RECEPTOR NEPRILYSIN INHIBITOR IN HEART FAILURE WITH PRESERVED EJECTION FRACTION WITH CHRONIC KIDNEY DISEASE

Systematic review was conducted based on search in Embase, MEDLINE, and Cochrane databases to evaluate the efficacy and safety of sacubitril-valsartan versus standard care in patients with ESKD on dialysis.[14] No significant difference was noted in the change of LVEF between patients on PD and those on HD. PD subgroup mainly consisted of patients with HFpEF and the HD subgroup included both HFpEF and HFrEF patients.

Twelve studies involving 799 patients with ESKD demonstrated significant improvement in patients with LVEF <50% and heart failure with moderately reduced ejection fraction (HFmrEF) with sacubitril-valsartan compared to a control group. Patients with LVEF >50% (HFpEF) did not exhibit statistically significant effect (MD 2.6%). The complex pathophysiology of HFpEF may underline the lack of efficacy in these set of patients. No differences in incidence of hyperkalemia (OR 0.72) or hypotension (RR 1.03) was reported confirming the safety profile.

Effect of sacubitril-valsartan in patients with HFpEF and CKD on serum natriuretic peptides BNP or NT-proBNP is difficult to evaluate as renal failure can independently affect NT-proBNP concentrations.

ANGIOTENSIN RECEPTOR NEPRILYSIN INHIBITOR IN HEART FAILURE WITH PRESERVED EJECTION FRACTION: COST EFFECTIVENESS AND QUALITY OF LIFE

Economic evaluation using participant-level clinical trial data, sacubitril and valsartan increases quality-adjusted life-years (QALYs) at an incremental cost-effectiveness ratio consistent with high economic value for patients inclusive of reduced and mildly reduced ejection fractions (≤50%) and at least intermediate value at an ejection fraction of 60% or lower. Among 13,264 total patients whose data were analyzed, for those with EFs of 60% or less, sacubitril-valsartan was projected to add 0.53 QALYs at an incremental lifetime cost of $40 892 compared with RASi, yielding an ICER of $76 852 per QALY.[15]

Comparison of the annualized cost needed to treat (CNT) to prevent the composite outcome of total HF hospitalizations and CVD with dapagliflozin or sacubitril-valsartan based on data collected from the DELIVER trial for dapagliflozin and a pooled analysis of PARAGLIDE-HF and PARAGON-HF trials for sacubitril-valsartan was evaluated for real world evaluation. Dapagliflozin provided a better monetary value than sacubitril-valsartan in preventing the composite outcome of total HF hospitalizations and CVD among patients with HFmrEF or HFpEF.[16]

CONCLUSION

The ARNI is the mainstay of treatment in acute HFrEF and must be initiated in the hospital. Although PARAGON-HF trial failed to show that in sacubitril/valsartan reduced adverse events among patients with HFpEF, there was a reduction of the primary outcome in women. Sacubitril/valsartan versus placebo was associated with an absolute significant reduction in cardiovascular death or hospitalization for HF when initiated <30 days from index hospitalization. No deterioration in eGFR or hyperkalemia were noted with initiation of ARNI. Reduction of NT-proBNP and left atrial structure and function were noted with ARNI. ARNI reduced total worsening HF events and cardiovascular death in pooled analysis of participants with recent worsening HF. ARNI increases QALYs at an incremental cost-effectiveness ratio in heart failure.

REFERENCES

1. Bozkurt B, Andrew JS, Tsutsui H, et al. The Universal Definition of Heart Failure: Perspectives from Diverse Stakeholders. J Cardiac Failure. 2021;27(4):386-7.
2. Mohebi R, Chen C, Ibrahim NE, et al. "Cardiovascular disease projections in the United States based on the 2020 census estimates". J Am Coll Cardiol. 2022;80:565-78.
3. Bozkurt B, Ahmad T, Alexander KM, et al. Heart failure epidemiology and outcomes statistics: a report of the Heart Failure Society of America. J Card Fail. 2023;29:1412-51.
4. 2024 ACC Expert Consensus Decision Pathway for Treatment of Heart Failure With Reduced Ejection Fraction: A Report of the American College of Cardiology Solution Set Oversight Committee. JACC. 2024;83(15):1444-88.
5. McMurray JJ, Packer M, Desai AS, et al.; PARADIGM-HF Investigators and Committees. Angiotensin-neprilysin inhibition versus enalapril in heart failure. N Engl J Med. 2014;371:993-1004.
6. Mebazaa A, Davison B, Chioncel O, et al. Safety, tolerability, and efficacy of up-titration of guideline-directed medical therapies for acute heart failure (STRONG-HF): a multinational, open-label, randomised trial. Lancet. 2022;400(10367):1938-52.
7. Cotter G, Deniau B, Davison B, et al. Optimization of evidence-based heart failure medications after an acute heart failure admission: a secondary analysis of the STRONG-HF randomized clinical trial. JAMA Cardiol. 2024;9(2):114-24.
8. Dalal J, Chandra P, Ray S, et al. Practical Recommendations for the Use of Angiotensin Receptor-Neprilysin Inhibitors (ARNI) in Heart Failure: Insights from Indian Cardiologists. Cardiol Ther. 2023;12(3):445-71.
9. Solomon SD, McMurray JJV, Anand IS, et al., on behalf of the PARAGON-HF Investigators and Committees. Angiotensin–Neprilysin Inhibition in Heart Failure With Preserved Ejection Fraction. N Engl J Med. 2019; 381:1609-20.
10. Vaduganathan M, Mentz RJ, Claggett BL, et al. Sacubitril/valsartan in heart failure with mildly reduced or preserved ejection fraction: a pre-specified participant-level pooled

analysis of PARAGLIDE-HF and PARAGON-HF. Eur Heart J. 2023;44(31):2982-93.

11. Kommu S, Berg RL. The Efficacy and Safety of Sacubitril/Valsartan Compared to Valsartan in Patients with Heart Failure and Mildly Reduced and Preserved Ejection Fractions: A Systematic Review and Meta-Analysis of Randomized Controlled Trials. J Clin Med. 2024;13(6):1572.
12. Fudim M, Cyr DD, Ward JH, et al.; on behalf of the PARAGLIDE-HF Investigators. Association of Sacubitril/Valsartan versus Valsartan with Blood Pressure Changes, and Symptomatic Hypotension: The PARAGLIDE-HF Trial. J Card Fail. 2024;30(12):1568-77.
13. Ledwidge M, Dodd JD, Ryan F, et al. Effect of Sacubitril/Valsartan vs Valsartan on Left Atrial Volume in Patients With Pre–Heart Failure With Preserved Ejection Fraction: The PARABLE Randomized Clinical Trial. JAMA Cardiol. 2023;8(4):366-75.
14. Charkviani M, Krisanapan P, Thongprayoon C, et al. Systematic Review of Cardiovascular Benefits and Safety of Sacubitril-Valsartan in End-Stage Kidney Disease. Kidney Int Rep. 2023;9(1):39-51.
15. Bhatt AS, Vaduganathan M, Claggett BL, et al. Health and Economic Evaluation of Sacubitril-Valsartan for Heart Failure Management. JAMA Cardiol. 2023;8(11):1041-8.
16. Arbel R, Azab AN, Oberoi M, et al. Dapagliflozin versus sacubitril–valsartan for heart failure with mildly reduced or preserved ejection fraction. Front Pharmacol. 2024;15: 1357673.

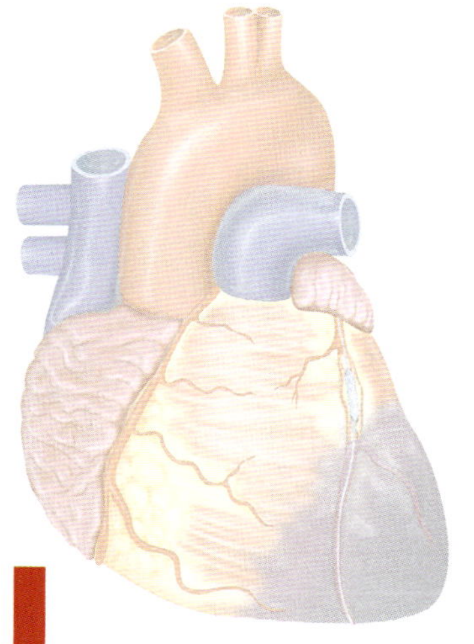

CHAPTER

ARNI and MRA Combination in PARAGON-HF: Odd Couple or Dynamic Duo in HFpEF

Suman Bhandari, Mohamad Akram

INTRODUCTION

Heart failure (HF) is a clinical syndrome that occurs due to structural and functional abnormalities in the myocardium, leading to the impaired filling or ejection of blood from the ventricles. Impaired relaxation or contractility of the heart leads to elevated cardiac filling pressure, elevated jugular venous pressure (JVP), physical symptoms, and lung crackles.[1]

Heart failure with preserved ejection fraction is defined as a left ventricular ejection fraction (LVEF) ≥50% further corroborated by either elevated natriuretic peptide (NP) levels or other evidence of congestion.[2]

ANGIOTENSIN RECEPTOR–NEPRILYSIN INHIBITORS IN HFpEF

The PARAGON-HF (Prospective Comparison of Angiotensin Receptor–Neprilysin Inhibitors (ARNI) with ARB Global Outcomes in HF with Preserved Ejection Fraction) study randomized 4,796 patients with an LVEF ≥45%, elevated N-terminal pro-B-type NP, and symptomatic HF to either sacubitril–valsartan 97/103 mg twice daily or valsartan 160 mg twice daily.[3]

Jering et al.[4] established that among prespecified cardiorenal composite endpoints, sacubitril–valsartan compared with valsartan was consistent in PARAGON-HF without regard to background mineralocorticoid receptor antagonists (MRA) use; however, the combination of sacubitril–valsartan with an MRA resulted in a potentially additive renoprotective benefit and appeared well-tolerated. Although renin–angiotensin-system blockers like angiotensin-converting enzyme inhibitors and angiotensin-receptor blockers have long been known to confer renal protection in patients with HF and or diabetes, the impact of MRA or angiotensin receptor-neprilysin inhibitors (ARNI), alone or in combination, on the progression of kidney disease is less certain. MRAs and ARNIs have renoprotective benefits as suggested by clinical and preclinical data.[5]

MINERALOCORTICOID RECEPTOR ANTAGONISTS IN HFpEF

The data from TOPCAT trial has led to incorporation of spironolactone into AHA/ACC/HFSA guidelines as a class IIb indication in HFpEF. Patients with evidence of chronic kidney disease demonstrated a reduced benefit–risk ratio compared with those with better renal function,[6] whereas patients with HF and LVEF 45–60% appeared to benefit the most from spironolactone in TOPCAT.[7] SPIRIT HF and SPIRRIT HFpEF are two recent ongoing trials that will give us a more clear picture about role of MRA in HFpEF **(Figs. 1 and 2)**.

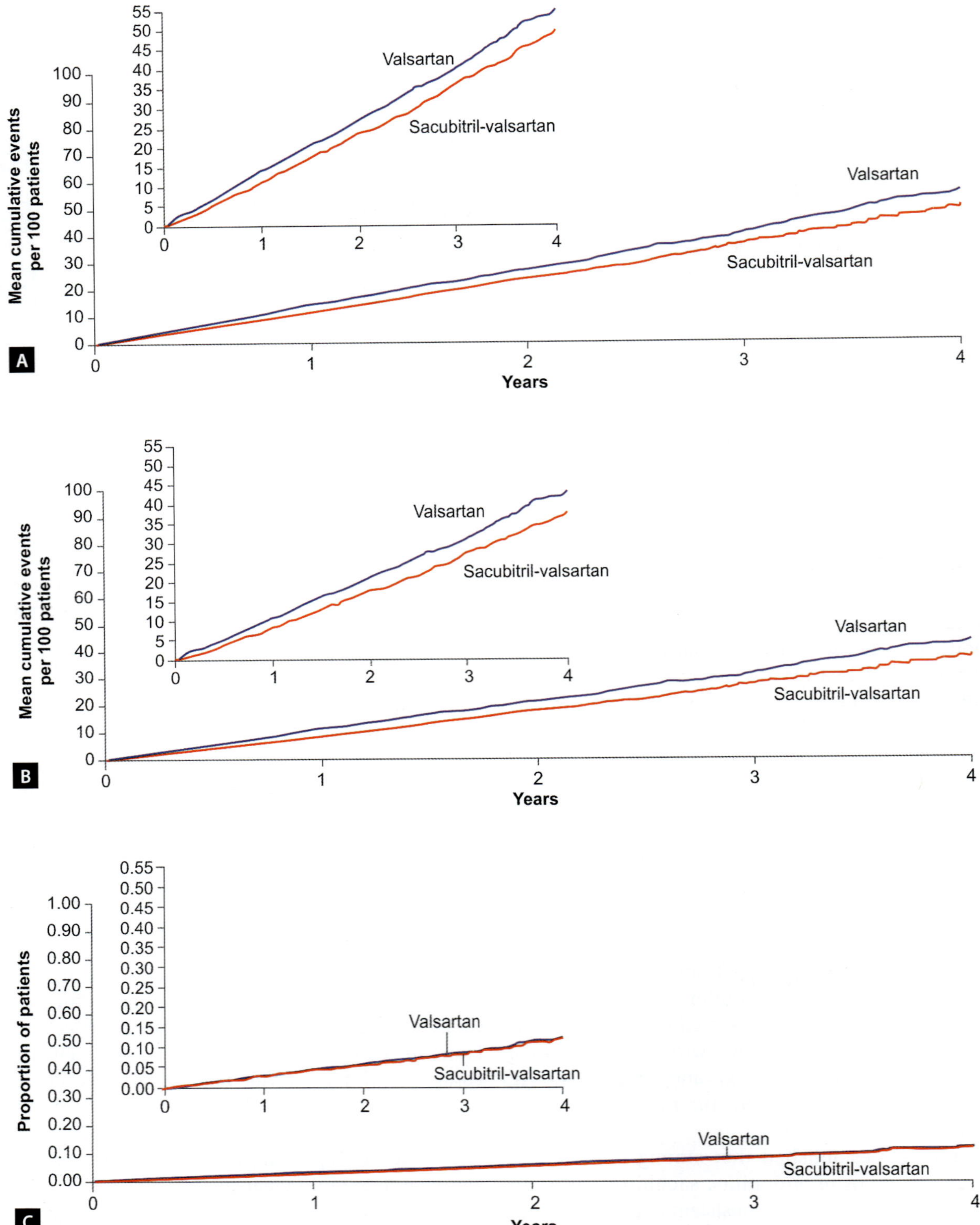

Figs. 1A to C: (A) Ghosh–Lin curves for the primary composite outcome of total hospitalizations for heart failure and death from cardiovascular causes; (B) Ghosh–Lin curves for total hospitalizations for heart failure; and (C) Kaplan–Meier curves for death from cardiovascular causes. Insets show the same data on an enlarged y-axis.
Source: PARAGON HF trial.

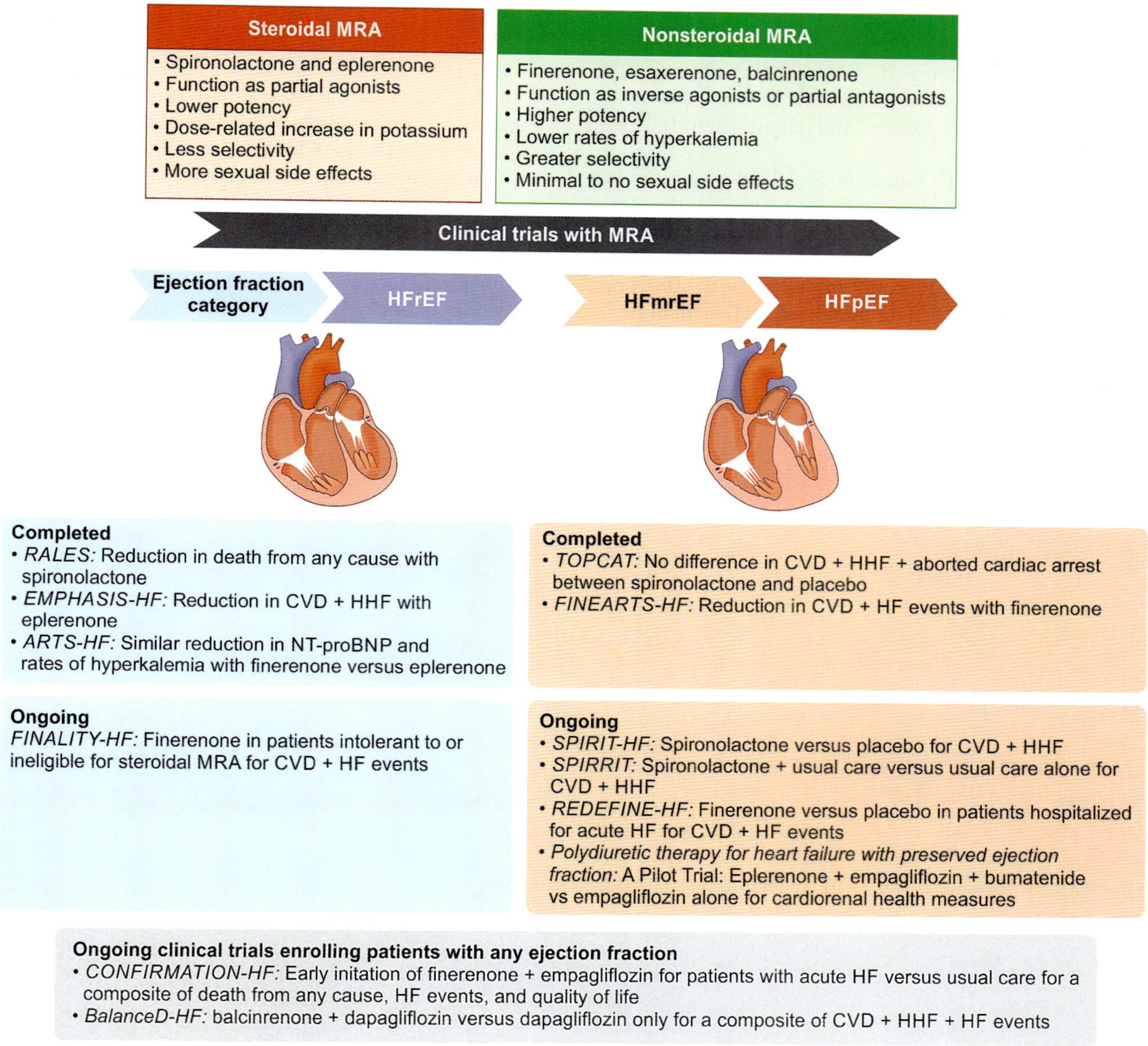

Steroidal MRA
- Spironolactone and eplerenone
- Function as partial agonists
- Lower potency
- Dose-related increase in potassium
- Less selectivity
- More sexual side effects

Nonsteroidal MRA
- Finerenone, esaxerenone, balcinrenone
- Function as inverse agonists or partial antagonists
- Higher potency
- Lower rates of hyperkalemia
- Greater selectivity
- Minimal to no sexual side effects

Clinical trials with MRA

Ejection fraction category — HFrEF | HFmrEF — HFpEF

HFrEF

Completed
- *RALES:* Reduction in death from any cause with spironolactone
- *EMPHASIS-HF:* Reduction in CVD + HHF with eplerenone
- *ARTS-HF:* Similar reduction in NT-proBNP and rates of hyperkalemia with finerenone versus eplerenone

Ongoing
FINALITY-HF: Finerenone in patients intolerant to or ineligible for steroidal MRA for CVD + HF events

HFmrEF / HFpEF

Completed
- *TOPCAT:* No difference in CVD + HHF + aborted cardiac arrest between spironolactone and placebo
- *FINEARTS-HF:* Reduction in CVD + HF events with finerenone

Ongoing
- *SPIRIT-HF:* Spironolactone versus placebo for CVD + HHF
- *SPIRRIT:* Spironolactone + usual care versus usual care alone for CVD + HHF
- *REDEFINE-HF:* Finerenone versus placebo in patients hospitalized for acute HF for CVD + HF events
- *Polydiuretic therapy for heart failure with preserved ejection fraction:* A Pilot Trial: Eplerenone + empagliflozin + bumatenide vs empagliflozin alone for cardiorenal health measures

Ongoing clinical trials enrolling patients with any ejection fraction
- *CONFIRMATION-HF:* Early initation of finerenone + empagliflozin for patients with acute HF versus usual care for a composite of death from any cause, HF events, and quality of life
- *BalanceD-HF:* balcinrenone + dapagliflozin versus dapagliflozin only for a composite of CVD + HHF + HF events

Fig. 2: Steroidal versus nonsteroidal MRA in clinical trials.
Source: Chang J, Ambrosy AP, Vardeny O, et al. Mineralocorticoid antagonism in heart failure: Established and emerging therapeutic role. JACC Heart Fail. 2024;12(12):1979-93.

CONCLUSION

The combination of ARNI and MRA may seem like an odd couple for broad management, but in selected patients, it may serve more like a dynamic duo considering the lack of proven HFpEF therapies including those known at a minimum to preserve kidney function. Should future clinical studies confirm that ARNI in combination with MRA has additive or synergistic effects on the progression of CKD, this would have important implications because the progression of CKD has long-term consequences for both cardiovascular and renal outcomes in patients with HFpEF. The failure of sacubitril–valsartan and MRA to alter cardiorenal outcomes in PARAGON-HF despite significantly attenuating a decline in renal function in comparison with sacubitril–valsartan without MRA and valsartan with or without MRA is possibly related to the duration of the trial. A beneficial effect on renal function, as evidenced by an attenuated eGFR decline, may require several years to impact cardiorenal endpoints. Thus, future studies attempting to evaluate the benefits of sacubitril–valsartan and MRA may require a far longer duration of follow-up than PARAGON-HF.[4]

REFERENCES

1. McDonagh TA, Metra M, Adamo M, et al. 2021 ESC Guidelines for the diagnosis and treatment of acute and chronic heart failure. Eur Heart J. 2021;42(36): 3599-726.
2. Bozkurt B, Coats AJS, Tsutsui H, et al. Universal definition and classification of heart failure: A report of the Heart Failure Society of America, Heart Failure Association of the European Society of Cardiology, Japanese Heart Failure Society and Writing Committee of the Universal Definition of Heart Failure: Endorsed by Canadian Heart Failure Society, Heart Failure Association of India, the Cardiac Society of Australia and New Zealand, and the Chinese Heart Failure Association. Eur J Heart Fail. 2021;23(3):352-80.
3. Solomon SD, McMurray JJV, Anand IS, et al. Angiotensin–neprilysin inhibition in heart failure with preserved ejection fraction. N Eng J Med. 2019;381(17):1609-20.
4. Jering KS, Zannad F, Claggett B, et al. Cardiovascular and renal outcomes of mineralocorticoid receptor antagonist use in PARAGON-HF. JACC Heart Fail. 2021;9(1):13-24.
5. Barrera-Chimal J, Girerd S, Jaisser F. Mineralocorticoid receptor antagonists and kidney diseases: Pathophysiological basis. Kidney Int. 2019;96(2):302-19.
6. Beldhuis IE, Myhre PL, Claggett B, et al. Efficacy and safety of spironolactone in patients with HFpEF and chronic kidney disease. JACC Heart Failure. 2019;7(1):25-32.
7. Solomon SD, Claggett B, Lewis EF, et al. Influence of ejection fraction on outcomes and efficacy of spironolactone in patients with heart failure with preserved ejection fraction. Eur Heart J. 2016;37(5):455-62.

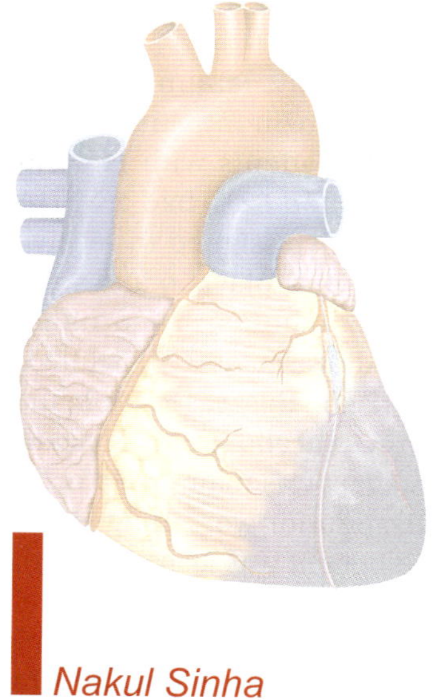

Role of SGLT2 Inhibitors in HFpEF

Nakul Sinha

INTRODUCTION

Heart failure (HF) is a common, progressive, and complex clinical syndrome characterized by the inability of the heart to pump sufficient blood to meet the body's needs. Heart failure with preserved ejection fraction (HFpEF) makes up around half of all HF cases. HF is classified according to the left ventricle's ejection fraction (EF). When a left ventricular ejection fraction (LVEF) is 50% or more and HF symptoms are present, this condition is known as HFpEF.[1] There are not many viable therapy choices for HFpEF, in contrast to heart failure with reduced ejection fraction (HFrEF), which has undergone substantial therapeutic advancements. The mechanics, clinical effectiveness, and growing role of sodium–glucose cotransporter-2 (SGLT2) inhibitors in the treatment of HFpEF are enumerated in this chapter.

The prevalence of patients with HFpEF increases as the population ages. Like HFrEF, HFpEF is also a progressive condition with an increase in mortality and a decrease in quality of life (QoL). Globally, HFpEF accounts for close to 50% of patients presenting with HF. Indian studies such as Trivandrum Heart registry[2] and ASIAN-HF[3] put the proportion of such patients at 19–25% approximately, which is much lower as compared to that of Western population. Moreover, the mean age of presentation of patients from India is around 58–68 years, which is about 10 years younger than the data reported from the West. According to the Trivandrum Heart Failure Registry,[2] among Indian patients, 33% of women had HFpEF, compared to 23% of men. The hospital readmission rates for HFrEF (30.1%) and HFpEF (31.6%) were similar, with no significant gender differences.

The SGLT2 inhibitors that were developed to lower blood glucose, hold great promise for the treatment of patients with HFpEF. Randomized trials have shown that in such patients they prevent hospitalization for HF and slow the progression of chronic kidney disease (CKD), especially in diabetics.

PATHOPHYSIOLOGY

Heart failure with preserved ejection is a multifaceted syndrome involving pathophysiological changes at both the cardiac and systemic levels, including diastolic dysfunction, comorbidities, endothelial dysfunction, and neurohormonal activation. Besides management of comorbid conditions like obesity, diabetes, hypertension, CKD, atrial fibrillation (AF), etc., pharmacological interventions targeting the abovementioned diverse mechanisms are needed to provide comprehensive management for HFpEF patients.

MECHANISMS OF ACTION OF SODIUM–GLUCOSE COTRANSPORTER-2 INHIBITORS

The SGLT2 inhibitors, which were first indicated for management of type 2 diabetes mellitus (T2DM), lower blood glucose levels by preventing the renal proximal tubules from reabsorbing glucose, which increases the excretion of glucose in the urine. However, SGLT2 inhibitors' pleiotropic effects go beyond glucose regulation, especially their possible advantages for the heart and kidneys. Patients with HFpEF may benefit from SGLT2 inhibitors through the following mechanisms:

- *Osmotic diuresis and natriuresis:* SGLT2 inhibitors cause osmotic diuresis by encouraging the excretion of sodium and glucose. Preload and afterload decrease as a result of the reduction in plasma volume and interstitial fluid overload. Lowering left ventricular filling pressures quickly can relieve symptoms and lessen the chance of HF hospitalization.
- *Blood pressure reduction:* Through vasodilation and volume reduction, SGLT2 inhibitors have modest antihypertensive effects that might lessen cardiac workload and improve outcomes in individuals with hypertension.
- *Metabolic shifts:* SGLT2 inhibitors promote a shift in myocardial energy substrate utilization from glucose to ketones and free fatty acids, which are more energy-efficient for the failing heart. The heart's energetics and function may be enhanced by this metabolic flexibility.
- *Anti-inflammatory effects:* By lowering biomarkers like interleukin-6 (IL-6) and tumor necrosis factor-alpha (TNF-α), which are linked to the pathophysiology of HFpEF, SGLT2 inhibitors reduce oxidative stress and proinflammatory pathways.
- *Decrease in myocardial fibrosis:* By blocking pathways linked to cardiac fibrosis, SGLT2 inhibitors may lessen myocardial stiffness and enhance diastolic performance.
- *Improvement in endothelial function:* By enhancing nitric oxide bioavailability and reducing endothelial dysfunction, SGLT2 inhibitors can improve vascular health by alleviating microvascular dysfunction.
- *Renal effects:* These include a decrease in albuminuria, intrarenal RAAS activation, glomerular pressure, and increase in tubuloglomerular feedback mechanism.
- SGLT2 inhibitors offer a little decrease in body weight, which is significant considering the high rate of obesity in HFpEF.
- Other mechanisms include an improved insulin sensitivity, activation of the fatty acid oxidation in the skeletal muscle, decrease in epicardial fat, enhanced erythropoietin levels, improved calcium hemostasis, and increased liver SIRT-1.

CLINICAL EVIDENCE FROM TRIALS

Robust clinical trials have begun to elucidate the benefits of SGLT2 inhibitors in patients with HFpEF, underscoring their potential to fill a significant therapeutic gap.

EMPEROR-Preserved Trial[4]

The EMPEROR-Preserved trial was a landmark study evaluating the efficacy of empagliflozin in patients with HFpEF. The trial enrolled 5,988 patients with HF and an EF of >40%. Most patients, around 82%, had a NYHA Class 2 HF. Patients were randomly assigned to receive either empagliflozin 10 mg daily or a placebo and were followed up for an average of 26 months. The primary outcome was a composite of cardiovascular (CV) death or hospitalization for worsening HF and this was lower in the empagliflozin group than in the placebo group—hazard ratio 0.79 (CI 0.69–0.90). This effect was mainly related to a 29% lower risk of hospitalization for worsening HF in the empagliflozin group.[1] The benefit was also seen with respect to the secondary outcome of the total number of hospitalizations for HF. There was a nonsignificant 9% lower risk of death from CV causes in the empagliflozin group compared to the placebo group—hazard ratio 0.91 (CI 0.76–1.09) while the effect on death from any cause was neutral—hazard ratio 1.00 (CI 0.87–1.15). These results were observed across various subgroups, irrespective of diabetes status, reinforcing the applicability of SGLT2 inhibitors in a broad HFpEF population.[1] In the EMPEROR-Preserved trial, empagliflozin generally appeared to be effective across the spectrum of EFs in subgroup analysis, but there may be a decrement of benefit in patients with the highest EFs. The observed number of adverse renal outcomes was relatively small in this trial. Nevertheless, these data suggest that empagliflozin has less kidney protective effect in patients with HFpEF compared to those with a HFrEF. It seems likely that renal protection is perhaps not the main mechanism by which empagliflozin prevents hospitalizations for HF.

DELIVER Trial[5]

In this randomized placebo-controlled trial involving more than 6,250 patients with HF and a mildly reduced or a preserved EF, dapagliflozin resulted in a lower risk of the primary composite outcome of worsening HF or CV death compared to placebo with no appreciable difference in benefit among patients with either a LVEF of 60% or more compared to those with the LVEF of <60%, or in other subgroups. The rationale for the dual primary analysis in this trial, i.e., evaluation of the primary outcome in patients with a LVEF <60%, in addition to the overall patient population, was based on concern about a potential declining benefit in patients with EF in the normal range that had been observed in previous EMPEROR-Preserved trial. The results showed no evidence of heterogeneity with respect to the LVEF with similar overall treatment effects among patients with EF of 60% or more compared with those with a 60% or less.[2] This finding suggests that the benefit of SGLT 2 inhibition is likely to extend throughout the full range of EF. Each of the three components of this composite outcome was less common in the dapagliflozin group than in the placebo group. In addition, dapagliflozin resulted in a fewer total HF events and CV deaths and a lower symptom burden than placebo. The incidence of adverse events was similar to that in the placebo group. The main features of the DELIVER trial that distinguish it from the EMPEROR-Preserved trial were the inclusion of patients who previously had an EF of 40% or less that had subsequently improved to more than 40%. (i.e., patients with HF and an improved LVEF). This group of patients also showed a similar benefit with the use of dapagliflozin additionally. There was also a clear benefit among patients with body mass index of 30 or higher and among those with more severe symptoms of NYHA class 3 or 4. The trialists agree that due to the use of very specific inclusion and exclusion criteria, the generalizability of the findings may be limited, especially since <5% of the patients enrolled were blacks. It is also unknown, whether similar benefits accrue or extend to patients with HFpEF because of certain cardiomyopathies like hypertrophic cardiomyopathy or restrictive cardiomyopathies caused due to amyloidosis or sarcoidosis.

SOLOIST-WHF Trial[6]

Although primarily targeting patients with worsening HF, the SOLOIST-WHF trial included subgroups with HFpEF and observed beneficial effects of sotagliflozin (a combined SGLT1 and SGLT2 inhibitor) in reducing the composite endpoint of CV death and hospitalization for HF. However, this trial was not designed to test sotagliflozin in patients with HFpEF. Moreover, the overall number of such patients enrolled was quite low.

PRESERVED-HF Trial[7]

This multicenter, double-blind, randomized, placebo-controlled trial explored the effects of dapagliflozin on HF biomarkers and health status and physical limitations as measured by KCCQ CS after 12 weeks of treatment in a population that was especially at a poor health status. Among patients with HFpEF, dapagliflozin was associated with reductions in N-terminal pro-B-type natriuretic peptide (NT-proBNP) levels and improvements in self-reported QoL, indicating a positive impact on both objective (6-minute-walk test) and subjective measures of HF status. Consistent with previous data from comparable trials, dapagliflozin treatment had no significant effect on natriuretic peptides. Although natriuretic peptide levels are predictive of prognosis in HFpEF, they are known to be considerably lower than in HFrEF, and previous studies have shown little or no relationship between natriuretic peptides and health status (DEFINE HF trial[8]).

POOLED ANALYSIS of DAPA HF and DELIVER (2022)[9]

In this pooled meta-analysis of >11,000 patients from the 2 trials, compared with placebo, Dapagliflozin 10 mg once a day reduced the risk of each of the prespecified endpoints, i.e., death from CV causes by 14% and death from any cause by 10%, total (i.e., first and repeat) hospital admissions for HF by 29%, and the composite of death from CV causes, MI, or stroke by 10% in patients with HF with no evidence of heterogeneity of the benefit across the range of EFs. The number of patients with HF who needed to be treated (NNT) for a median of 22 months to prevent one death from CV causes was 68 (95% CI. 39–281). The conclusion for death from any cause was similar, with a modest size benefit that was statistically significant. The reduction in MACE was of a borderline statistical significance. However, the beneficial effect on hospital admissions for HF was substantial as was observed in the individual trials also. The NYHA class and KCCQ-TSS score were dissociated across the spectrum of LVEF at baseline and the effect of dapagliflozin was consistent across the range of KCCQ-TSS scores included.

Meta-analysis by Vaduganathan et al.[10]

This included data from DELIVER as well as EMPEROR-Preserved study, which showed a robust reduction of composite CV death or first hospitalization for HF [hazard ratio (HR) 0.80], the benefits were consistent with reductions observed in both CV death (HR 0.88, 95% CI 0.77–1.00) and first hospitalization for HF (HR 0.74, 95% CI 0.67–0.83). The inclusion of data from additional trials such as DAPA-HF, EMPEROR-Reduced, and SOLOIST-WHF in this meta-analysis has provided the statistical power needed to confirm the efficacy of SGLT2 inhibitors. Extending to the broader context of five trials with 21,947 participants, SGLT2 inhibitors also reduced the risk of composite CV death or hospitalization for HF (HR 0.77, 95% CI 0.72–0.82), CV death (HR 0.87; 95% CI 0.79–0.95), first hospitalization for HF (HR 0.72, 95% CI 0.67–0.78), and all-cause mortality (HR 0.92, 95% CI 0.86–0.99). These beneficial treatment effects were consistently observed across the studied endpoints in both HFmrEF and HFpEF and all the five trials. The effects on the primary endpoint were generally consistent across the 14 subgroups examined, including age, sex, region, and those defined by EF.

DISCUSSION

The evolving landscape of HFpEF treatment is poised for a significant transformation with the introduction of SGLT2 inhibitors. The multidimensional mechanisms of these drugs address multiple pathophysiological aspects of HFpEF, providing a holistic approach to management. Key discussion points and possible limitations include:

- *Patient selection:* While the benefits of SGLT2 inhibitors are evident across various subgroups, optimal patient selection remains crucial. Factors such as comorbidities, baseline renal function, and concomitant therapies should also be considered to maximize therapeutic outcomes.
- *Measurement of LVEF* is highly dependent on the method used. Repeated measurements in the same patients with the use of the same methods routinely may vary by 7% or more. Moreover, differences between the values obtained by operators and those obtained by the core laboratory may vary by as much as 15%. Thus, the findings of the trial(s) should be interpreted with some caution because of the severe limitations encountered when LVEF cutoff levels are used to classify HF and guide treatment.
- *Patient subgroups:* At least in the DELIVER HF, the risk reduction was higher in patients with HF with an improved EF than in those without an improved EF. Moreover, before the recommendations are implemented and put into practice, the external validity of the trial results should be established across the heterogeneous real-world population of patients with HFpEF, including many patients who are older and have more coexisting conditions than those enrolled in these two large trials.
- *Combination therapy:* Currently, diuretic therapy is still considered to be the initial drug to be deployed to reduce symptoms of congestion in such patients with HF even before the EF has been measured. SGLT2 inhibitors may synergize with other HFpEF treatments, including mineralocorticoid receptor antagonists (MRAs), angiotensin-converting enzyme inhibitors (ACE inhibitors), and beta-blockers. Combination therapy could potentially enhance diuresis, reduce neurohormonal activation, and improve overall CV health.
- *Long-term outcomes:* The long-term impact of SGLT2 inhibitors on survival, QoL, and progression of HFpEF remains to be fully elucidated. Ongoing trials and extended follow-up periods will provide crucial data to inform clinical practice. We should advocate for thoughtful and systematic implementation of SGLT2 inhibitors with the use of cluster randomized strategies along with follow-up of patient outcomes through long-term healthcare registries.
- *Safety and adverse effects:* The safety profile of SGLT2 inhibitors is generally favorable; however, potential adverse effects, including genitourinary infections and euglycemic diabetic ketoacidosis, should be monitored. Educating patients on recognizing and managing these risks is essential.

CONCLUSION

Sodium-glucose cotransporter-2 inhibitors represent a significant advancement in the treatment of HFpEF. By engaging in various pathophysiological pathways, these drugs provide a comprehensive therapeutic approach that meets the complex requirements of HFpEF patients. Clinical trials like EMPEROR-Preserved and DELIVER have been crucial in demonstrating the efficacy and safety of SGLT2 inhibitors in this patient group. As our knowledge of HFpEF continues to expand, SGLT2 inhibitors are likely to become a cornerstone in improving outcomes and QoL for those suffering from this condition.

Given the paucity of therapeutic options that have proven themselves in the management of HFpEF and which are available at present, the use of SGLT2 inhibitors seems to be one of the initial and important treatment additions. Unlike other HF medications, SGLT2 inhibitors show a rapid onset of action in clinical endpoints. This rapid effect, combined with the findings from the STRONG-HF trial, suggests that SGLT2 inhibitors should be initiated as soon as the diagnosis of HF is made.

The unique CV benefits of SGLT2 inhibitors, which operate independently of their glucose-lowering properties, highlight their potential beyond managing diabetes. Their actions on cellular and molecular mechanisms at systemic, vascular, cardiac, and renal levels contribute to their wide-ranging benefits. Currently, over 50 Phase-3 randomized control trials are underway to explore these drugs' applications further. The SGLT2 inhibitors have been likened to the statins of the 21st century due to their anticipated widespread utility in various medical conditions. Ongoing research investigates their potential for treating acute HF, AF, valvular heart disease, cardiogenic shock, hypertrophic cardiomyopathy, and more. Additionally, their benefits in nephrology and hepatology, especially in CKD and nonalcoholic fatty liver disease, are promising. Future research should aim to refine patient selection criteria, enhance combination therapies, and explore the long-term benefits to fully integrate SGLT2 inhibitors into comprehensive HFpEF management strategies. The impact on weight reduction associated with SGLT2 inhibitors also warrants further detailed exploration in future studies.

In conclusion, SGLT2 inhibitors hold great promise for a wide array of CV and metabolic conditions, potentially transforming the landscape of treatment and improving patient outcomes across several fields of medicine.

REFERENCES

1. Das SR, Everett BM, Birtcher KK, et al. 2018 ACC Expert consensus decision pathway on novel therapies for cardiovascular risk reduction in patients with type 2 diabetes and atherosclerotic cardiovascular disease. J Am Coll Cardiol. 2018;72(24):3200-23.
2. Harikrishna S, Sanjay G. One-year mortality outcomes and hospital readmissions of patients admitted with acute heart failure: Data from the Trivandrum Heart Failure Registry in Kerala, India. Am Heart J. 2017;189: 193-9.
3. MacDonald MR, Tay WT, Teng TK, et al. Regional Variation of Mortality in Heart Failure with Reduced and Preserved Ejection Fraction Across Asia: Outcomes in the ASIAN-HF Registry. J Am Heart Assoc. 2020;9(1):e012199.
4. Anker SD, Butler J, Filippatos G, et al. Empagliflozin in heart failure with a preserved ejection fraction. N E J Med. 2021;385(16):1451-61.
5. McMurray JJV, Solomon SD, Inzucchi SE, et al. Dapagliflozin in patients with heart failure and reduced ejection fraction. N Eng J Med. 2019;381(21):1995-2008.
6. Bhatt DL, Szarek M, Steg PG, et al. Sotagliflozin in patients with diabetes and recent worsening heart failure. N Eng J Med. 2020;384(2):117-28.
7. Nassif ME, Windsor SL, Borlaug BA, et al. The SGLT2 inhibitor dapagliflozin in heart failure with preserved ejection fraction: a multicenter randomized trial. Nat Med. 2021;27(11):1954-60.
8. Nassif ME, Windsor SL, Tang F, et al. Dapagliflozin effects on Biomarkers, Symptoms, and Functional Status in Patients with Heart Failure with Reduced Ejection Fraction: The DEFINE-HF Trial. Circulation. 2019;140(18):1463-76.
9. Desai AS, Jhund PS, Claggett, et al. Effect of Dapagliflozin on Cause-Specific Mortality in Patients with Heart Failure Across the Spectrum of Ejection Fraction: A Participant-Level Pooled Analysis of DAPA-HF and DELIVER. JAMA Cardiol. 2022;7(12):1227-34.
10. Vaduganathan M, Docherty KF, Claggett BL, et al. SGLT-2 inhibitors in patients with heart failure: a comprehensive meta-analysis of five randomised controlled trials. Lancet. 2022;400(10354):757-67.

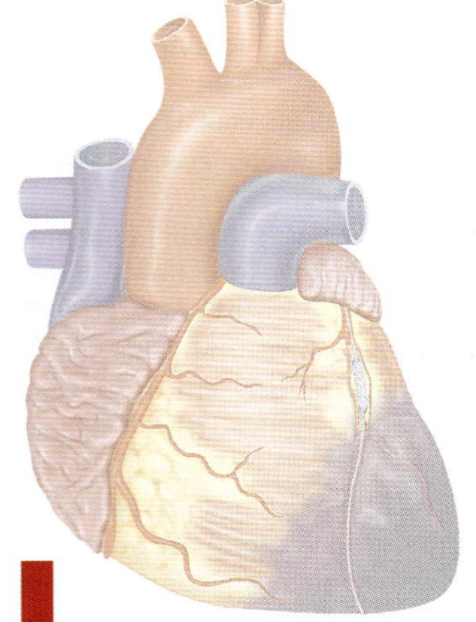

SGLT2 Inhibitors in Acute HFpEF: Is It Time to Broaden the Horizon?

Harshit Khare, Aditya Kapoor

INTRODUCTION

Acute heart failure (AHF) represents one end of the heart failure spectrum and is one of the leading causes of emergency admissions. At the other end of the spectrum lies the stable chronic heart failure (CHF). The two entities are quite different in terms of pathophysiology and management. Presently, there are four pillars of therapies recommended for CHF management. On the other hand, because of limited understanding, the therapy for AHF has not evolved over the past few decades.[1] The recent addition of sodium-dependent glucose-cotransport inhibitors (SGLT2i) to CHF therapy, irrespective of diabetes, renal function, and ejection fraction, has raised speculations about the effectiveness of this newer group of gliflozins in the management of AHF.[2] Recently, there have been studies in this regard that have closely examined and investigated this question.

MECHANISTIC EFFECTS OF SODIUM-DEPENDENT GLUCOSE-COTRANSPORT INHIBITORS IN HFpEF

Since their FDA approval, SGLT2i have continued to show their efficacy and safety in improving cardiovascular (CV) outcomes across most spectrums of HF, irrespective of the diabetes status and renal function.[2] The recent positive results of SGLT2i in HF with preserved ejection fraction (HFpEF) cohort have encouraged investigators to explore their effectiveness in the AHF subset of HFpEF patients, targeting different pathophysiologic mechanisms of AHF.[1] Various pathophysiological aspects of AHF that SGLT2i are expected to address include:

- Persistent intravascular congestion is seen in the postdischarge period of AHF patients. SGLT2i may increase the effectiveness of diuretic therapy.[1]
- Elevated ventricular filling pressures where SGLT2i can act to decrease intravascular volume by natriuresis, shifting the pressure-volume loop toward better hemodynamics.[1]
- Renal impairment resulting from central venous congestion due to altered neurohormonal axis. SGLT2i can improve renal function by decreasing the intraglomerular pressures by afferent arteriolar vasoconstriction, increasing the filtered sodium load at the proximal convoluted tubule. Moreover, they reduce renal inflammation and fibrosis.[3]
- Peripheral arterial stiffness leads to detrimental increased afterload in AHF. SGLT2i can decrease this by inhibiting sympathetic discharge mediated mainly through the crosstalk mechanism.[4]
- There is increased myocardial energetics in AHF either due to myocardial ischemia or elevated ventricular filling pressures, and SGLT2i can act as mitotropes, favoring better energetics via reduced afterload, lesser intravascular volume, lesser oxygen demand–supply mismatch, and lesser oxidative stress.[1]
- SGLT2i can also reduce endothelial dysfunction complicating the AHF by reducing both oxidative stress and inflammation.[1]

EVIDENCE FOR SODIUM-DEPENDENT GLUCOSE-COTRANSPORT INHIBITORS FROM TRIALS

EMPA-RESPONSE-AHF, a pilot study investigating empagliflozin in an AHF cohort, evaluated the change in visual analog scale (VAS) dyspnea score and diuretic response along with the changes in NT-proBNP levels and the length of hospital stay. The trial, however, failed to show any significant differences between the empagliflozin (EMPA) and placebo groups **(Table 1)**. Furthermore, there was significantly increased urinary output and more negative fluid balance with EMPA group, but without betterment in dyspnea score, NT-proBNP levels, and clinical outcomes at 30 days. This may be because of a lack of standardized protocol for diuretic therapy. Moreover, due to small study size, the number of clinical events was low, limiting its power to show clinical benefits. Even the reported result of significant reduction in combined clinical endpoint at 60 days is to be interpreted in view of the limited power of the study as discussed by the authors themselves.[5]

EMBRACE HF trial measured change in pulmonary artery pressures mainly diastolic pressure (PADP) in EMPA versus placebo group mainly in the CardioMEMS device cohort. Even though the trial results were reported positive at 12 weeks, the reduction in PADP started appearing only after the first week. The mechanism suggested included lowering of LV filling pressures and favorable modulation of endothelial function across pulmonary vasculature.[6]

The SOLOIST-WHF trial then followed, which was the largest trial studying sotagliflozin (a combined SGLT1 and 2 inhibitor) in the AHF cohort. Unfortunately, the trial had to be terminated prematurely due to loss of funding, limiting its power to differentiate the primary endpoint of the first occurrence of CV death or hospitalization for heart failure (HHF) between the study groups. So, the primary endpoint was changed to total number of CV deaths and hospitalizations and subsequent revisits. The trial showed significant reduction in the modified primary endpoint in the sotagliflozin group, and this was mainly driven by the number of total hospitalizations. The trial intended to study the response of combined SGLT1 and 2 inhibition in HFpEF subset also, but due to earlier termination, this could not be clearly opined. Furthermore, the primary events were not adjudicated and were investigator-defined events, raising questions about the generalizability of the reported results.[7]

While the aforementioned trials had suggested a role of SGLT2i in AHF, the benefit was clearly seen with higher doses (25 mg) of empagliflozin in EMPAG HF trial. The study showed a 25% increase in cumulative urine output of 5 days and further increased lowering of NT-proBNP levels in the EMPA group. This supported the earlier speculated mechanism and role of SGLT2i in the AHF cohort starting within 12 hours. The trial, however, did not study clinical endpoints.[8] The benefit in clinical endpoints was later suggested by EMPULSE trial, which showed a higher win ratio with the EMPA group, mainly driven by lower HHF rates. However, the trial was criticized for its randomization, which was initiated almost a day after hospital discharge.[9]

The most recently published DICTATE-AHF trial failed to meet its primary endpoint of diuretic response at 30 days with dapagliflozin compared to placebo, probably due to the utilization of lower doses of gliflozins and shorter follow-up period.[10]

INFERENCES

The above-mentioned trials **(Table 1)** when critically analyzed suggest a beneficial role of SGLT2i in AHF, especially in the HFpEF subset. These benefits were apparent as early as a few days after starting therapy. But there are some questions that need to be answered. Do these benefits, which are largely in terms of reduced HHF, appear as early as within 24–48 hours of gliflozin therapy? Perhaps, no. Does gliflozin therapy in acute settings produce an augmented diuretic response? Probably, yes. Does this augmented diuretic response culminate in better clinical outcomes? There is some suggestion that it does in some of the trials, namely, SOLOIST-WHF, EMPAG-HF, and EMPULSE trials, but the results are debatable. Then arises a key question: What about translation of this evidence into real-world scenario, where we have an all-comer cohort of AHF? The answer can be found in real-world registries. A large Japanese study, SAKURA-HF registry-2, presented this data.[11] They performed a post hoc analysis dividing a cohort of 118 AHF patients into the early dapagliflozin (DAPA) initiation group and late initiation group based on whether dapagliflozin was initiated within 6 days or not and compared them for HF characteristics and the length of the hospital stay. They observed that the early initiation group had a shorter length of hospital stay, despite the fact that NT-proBNP levels and NYHA class were similar in the two groups.[11]

FUTURE DIRECTIVES

The response with oral SGLT2i therapy in CHF is sufficiently supported by evidence; however, what is needed in the AHF setting is probably to develop intravenous gliflozins, which, when administered, will bring an early

TABLE 1: Trials of gliflozins in AHF.

Trial	*Study drug*	*Study period*	*Population size*	*Population characteristics*	*Study endpoints*	*Results*	*Remarks*
EMPA-RESPONSE-AHF[5]	Empagliflozin 10 mg daily dose versus placebo	December 2017–July 2019	Multicentric Netherlands-based, double-blind randomized trial enrolling 80 patients in 1:1 fashion with a follow-up of 60 days	• AHF patients with or without diabetes assessed for endpoints at 30 and 60 days • Mean age was 76 years, with predominant male population, with 47% having de novo HF and NT-proBNP (median) was 5,236 pg/mL	• Change in VAS dyspnea score, weight change with furosemide 40 mg (diuretic response), change in NT-proBNP, and length of stay • Secondary outcomes included worsening HF or rehospitalization or death and safety profile	• There was no difference between empagliflozin and placebo groups with respect to primary endpoints • Empagliflozin significantly reduced composite secondary endpoints at 60 days compared with placebo and had no adverse events related to hypotension or renal impairment	Increase in urinary output was significantly greater with empagliflozin after 4 days
EMBRACE HF[6]	Empagliflozin 10 mg daily dose versus placebo	July 2017–November 2019	Multicentric double-blind US-based study screening 93 patients of whom 65 were included for randomization in 1:1 with a follow-up of 12 weeks	• HF patients irrespective of their EF and diabetes status, who were previously implanted with CardioMEMS device • Mean age was 66 years with majority being males, with 52% having diabetes, with mean LVEF of 44%, with 54% in NYHA class III/IV, and median NT-proBNP levels of 637 pg/mL and mean PADP of 22 mm Hg • They were followed for 12 weeks	• Primary endpoint was changed in PADP • Secondary endpoint included KCCQ score, NT-Pro-BNP levels, and 6-MWD	Empagliflozin group had significantly lower PADP, as well as PA systolic and PA mean pressures beginning at 1 week and further declining with time	• PADP was lowered by 1.5 mm Hg between 8 and 12 weeks and by 1.7 mm Hg lower at 12 weeks • No difference was noted in mean loop diuretic doses • KCCQ score and 6MWD also did not differ

Contd...

Contd...

Trial	*Study drug*	*Study period*	*Population size*	*Population characteristics*	*Study endpoints*	*Results*	*Remarks*
SOLOIST-WHF[7]	Sotagliflozin 200–400 mg daily dose versus placebo	June 2018–March 2020	Multicentric double-blind trial screening 1,549 patients, enrolled 1,222 randomized in 1:1 fashion between the two groups with median follow-up of 9 months	Stabilized diabetic HF patients off oxygen and transitioned to oral diuretics with NT-proBNP >600 pg/mL	Primary outcome included the total number of CV deaths and hospitalizations and first and subsequent emergency visits for HF	• The number of primary events per 100 patient years was significantly lower in the sotagliflozin group compared with placebo group ($p < 0.001$) • The rate of CV death did not differ between the two groups • Diarrhea and severe hypoglycemia were more common with sotagliflozin while hypotension and AKI rates were also similar in the two groups	• The trial was initially designed to assess primary endpoint of the first occurrence of either CV death or HHF • But due to loss of funding enrolment ended in March 2020 • To increase study power executive committees and sponsors changed its primary endpoints
EMPAG-HF[8]	Empagliflozin 25 mg once daily dose versus placebo	September 2019–June 2021	Germany-based single-center, double-blind, randomized study, assigning 60 ADHF patients to either empagliflozin 25 mg daily or placebo in addition to decongestive measures including loop diuretics	60 patients with ADHF were randomized within 12 hours of admission	• The primary outcome was a cumulative urine output of 5 days • Secondary outcomes included diuretic efficiency, kidney function markers, and NT-proBNP	• There was a 25% increase in cumulative urine of 5 days ($p = 0.003$) in empagliflozin group, increasing the diuretic efficiency compared with placebo (14.1 mL increased urine for each milligram of furosemide ($p = 0.041$) without affecting renal function • Furthermore, there was greater decrease in NT-proBNP in the empagliflozin group compared with placebo ($p < 0.001$) • No difference in safety points was noted between two groups	

Contd...

Contd...

Trial	*Study drug*	*Study period*	*Population size*	*Population characteristics*	*Study endpoints*	*Results*	*Remarks*
EMPUSE[9]	Empagliflozin 10 mg once daily dosing versus placebo	May 2020–May 2021	530 patients with a primary diagnosis of acute de novo or decompensated CHF regardless of left ventricular ejection fraction were randomly assigned to receive empagliflozin 10 mg once daily or placebo and were treated and followed up to 90 days	Patients with AHF and ADHF after stabilization were randomized in-hospital (median time from admission to randomization, was of 3 days)	The primary outcome was assessed using win ratio and defined as hierarchical composite of all-cause death, number of HF events, and time to first HF event, or ≥5 points in the KCCQ score at 90 days	• Empagliflozin group showed greater clinical benefit compared with placebo (stratified win ratio, 1.36; $p = 0.0054$) • This was for both AHF and decompensated CHF and regardless of LVEF and diabetes status • Empagliflozin was well tolerated; serious adverse events were similar in both	
DICTATE-AHF[10]	Dapagliflozin 10 mg once daily versus placebo	April 2020–May 2023	• US-based multicentric open-label randomized trial enrolling around 240 ADHF patients in 1:1 fashion between the two groups • Majority were diabetics and 48% of patients had LVEF >40% with median follow-up of 30 days	ADHF patients diagnosed clinically or by measured PCWP >19 mm Hg plus one sign/symptom on/requiring IV loop diuretics with eGFR ≥25 mL/min/1.73 m^2	• Primary endpoint was diuretic response calculated by dividing cumulative weight change by cumulative dose of loop diuretic • Secondary and exploratory endpoints were worsening AHF, rehospitalization for AHF or diabetes at 30 day, change in NT-proBNP, and measures of natriuresis • Safety endpoints comprised hyper/hypoglycemia, ketoacidosis, renal impairment, hypovolemic hypotension, and mortality	• Diuretic response did not differ between the two groups at 30 days • Furthermore, the groups were similar in terms of glycemic, renal, and safety endpoints diabetic, renal, or cardiovascular safety events • However, among exploratory endpoints, dapagliflozin showed improved median 24-hour natriuresis ($p = 0.03$) as well as increased urine output ($p = 0.005$)	The protocol was amended in September 2021 to include patients without DM

(ADHF: acutely decompensated heart failure; AHF: acute heart failure: AKI: acute kidney injury; CHF: chronic heart failure; DM: diabetes mellitus; eGFR: estimated glomerular filtration rate; HF: heart failure; KCCQ: Kansas City Cardiomyopathy Questionnaire; LVEF: left ventricle ejection fraction; NT-proBNP: N-terminal pro-B type-natriuretic peptide; VAS: visual analog scale; 6MWD: 6-minute walk distance) and efficient response in such patients, targeting various pathophysiologic mechanisms. So, the answer to the aforementioned question "is it time to broaden our horizon" is perhaps affirmative and is to be directed at exploration and meticulously collecting more evidence for gliflozins in AHF rather than vaguely approving them for each and every HF subset.

CONCLUSION

There is enough evidence to suggest that oral SGLT2i therapy increases the natriuresis and diuretic response in AHF patients, often requiring only limited escalation in diuretic therapy during admission. This early initiation of gliflozins may help in a shorter length of hospital stay and later can reduce the recurrent HHF.

REFERENCES

1. Njoroge JN, Teerlink JR. Pathophysiology and therapeutic approaches to acute decompensated heart failure. Circ Res. 2021;128(10):1468-86.
2. Braunwald E. SGLT2 inhibitors: the statins of the 21st century. Eur Heart J. 2022;43(11):1029-30.
3. Bailey CJ, Day C, Bellary S. Renal protection with SGLT2 inhibitors: effects in acute and chronic kidney disease. Curr Diab Rep. 2022;22(1):39-52.
4. Herat LY, Magno AL, Rudnicka C, et al. SGLT2 inhibitor-induced sympathoinhibition: a novel mechanism for cardiorenal protection. JACC Basic Transl Sci. 2020;5(2): 169-79.
5. Damman K, Beusekamp JC, Boorsma EM, et al. Randomized, double-blind, placebo-controlled, multicentre pilot study on the effects of empagliflozin on clinical outcomes in patients with acute decompensated heart failure (EMPA-RESPONSE-AHF). Eur J Heart Fail. 2020; 22(4):713-22.
6. Nassif ME, Qintar M, Windsor SL, et al. Empagliflozin effects on pulmonary artery pressure in patients with heart failure: results from the EMBRACE-HF trial. Circulation. 2021;143(17):1673-86.
7. Bhatt DL, Szarek M, Steg PG, et al. Sotagliflozin in patients with diabetes and recent worsening heart failure. N Engl J Med. 2021;384(2):117-28.
8. Schulze PC, Bogoviku J, Westphal J, et al. Effects of early empagliflozin initiation on diuresis and kidney function in patients with acute decompensated heart failure (EMPAG-HF). Circulation. 2022;146(4):289-98.
9. Biegus J, Voors AA, Collins SP, et al. Impact of empagliflozin on decongestion in acute heart failure: the EMPULSE trial. Eur Heart J. 2023;44(1):41-50.
10. Cox ZL, Collins SP, Aaron M, et al. Efficacy and safety of dapagliflozin in acute heart failure: rationale and design of the DICTATE-AHF trial. Am Heart J. 2021;232: 116-24.
11. Mizobuchi S, Saito Y, Miyagawa M, et al. Early initiation of dapagliflozin during hospitalization for acute heart failure is associated with a shorter hospital stay. Intern Med. 2023;62(21):3107-17.

CHAPTER

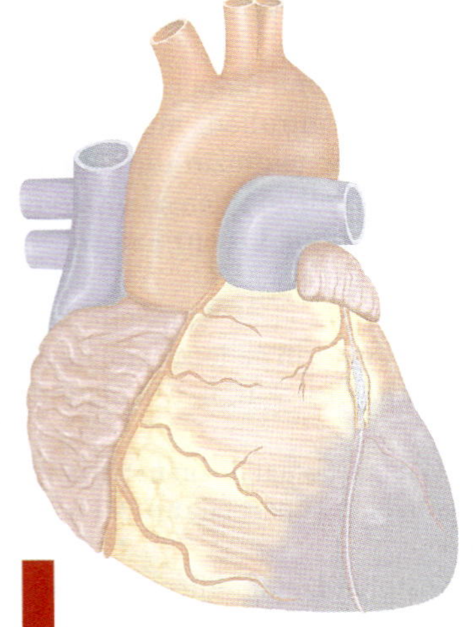

Role of SGLT2 Inhibitors in HFpEF with Diabetes Mellitus

Saumitra Ray, Mainak Mukhopadhyay

INTRODUCTION

Heart failure is a complex clinical syndrome that underlines the inability of the heart to perform its circulatory function with the desired efficiency due to structural and/or functional (systolic or diastolic) alterations. Based on left ventricular ejection fraction (LVEF), heart failure can be divided into 3 types: (1) Heart failure with reduced ejection fraction (HFrEF), which is characterized by LVEF below or equal to 40% and accounts for half of heart failure cases; (2) nearly one-tenth of heart failure cases are heart failure with mildly reduced ejection fraction (HFmrEF) in which the LVEF is 41–49%, whereas the remaining is (3) heart failure with preserved ejection fraction (HFpEF). The mortality and morbidity of HFpEF are like HFrEF. The estimated prevalence of heart failure in India is 1%.[1] In India, the prevalence of diabetes mellitus in the 20–70 years age group is around 8.8%.[2] Diabetes is the most commonly associated comorbidity in patients with heart failure. A double combination of diabetes and heart failure is prognostically worse. The risk of heart failure doubles in diabetics than in non-diabetics.[3] Heart failure in diabetics may present as a dilated phenotype (HFrEF) or restrictive phenotype (HFpEF).[4] Many of them are also having underlying epicardial or microvascular ischemic heart disease. Each 1% increase in HbA1c is associated with an 8% increase in risk of heart failure.[5] Response to protocol-based heart failure therapy is also worse in diabetic heart failure than nondiabetic heart failure.

HEART FAILURE WITH PRESERVED EJECTION FRACTION IN DIABETES: PATHOPHYSIOLOGY

Heart failure with preserved ejection fraction in diabetes mellitus is a complex condition with several interconnected pathophysiological mechanisms contributing to its development.[5,6] Here are some key aspects:

- *Diastolic dysfunction:* HFpEF is characterized by impaired relaxation and increased stiffness of the left ventricle during diastole. In diabetes, chronic hyperglycemia can lead to increased deposition of advanced glycation end-products (AGEs) in myocardial tissues. AGEs crosslink with collagen and other proteins, leading to myocardial fibrosis and increased stiffness of the myocardium, contributing to diastolic dysfunction.
- *Systemic inflammation and endothelial dysfunction:* Diabetes is associated with chronic low-grade inflammation and endothelial dysfunction, characterized by reduced nitric oxide bioavailability and increased oxidative stress. These factors contribute to impaired vasodilation and enhance vascular resistance, which can exacerbate diastolic dysfunction and contribute to the pathogenesis of HFpEF.
- *Insulin resistance:* Insulin resistance, a hallmark of type 2 diabetes, is associated with dysregulation of glucose and lipid metabolism. Insulin resistance can directly impact myocardial energetics and contractile function,

contributing to impaired relaxation and diastolic dysfunction seen in HFpEF.

- *Microvascular disease:* Diabetes is associated with microvascular disease, affecting small blood vessels throughout the body, including coronary microcirculation. Microvascular dysfunction can lead to impaired coronary flow reserve and subclinical myocardial ischemia, which contribute to myocardial fibrosis and impaired diastolic function in HFpEF.
- *Obesity and Adipokines:* Obesity, often associated with diabetes, is a risk factor for HFpEF. Adipose tissue secretes adipokines such as leptin, adiponectin, and resistin, which can have proinflammatory and profibrotic effects on the myocardium, contributing to myocardial stiffness and diastolic dysfunction.
- *Renin-angiotensin-aldosterone system (RAAS) activation:* Diabetes and HFpEF are associated with the activation of the RAAS. Increased aldosterone levels and aldosterone receptor activation can promote myocardial fibrosis, sodium retention, and increased vascular tone, all of which contribute to diastolic dysfunction and the pathophysiology of HFpEF.
- *Oxidative stress:* Diabetes is characterized by increased oxidative stress due to mitochondrial dysfunction and increased reactive oxygen species (ROS) production. Oxidative stress can promote inflammation, endothelial dysfunction, and fibrosis in the myocardium, exacerbating diastolic dysfunction in HFpEF.
- *Aging population:* Both diabetes and HFpEF are more prevalent in older adults, and the aging population is at increased risk for both conditions.
- *Hypertension:* Many individuals with diabetes also have hypertension (high blood pressure), which further stresses the heart and can contribute to the development of HFpEF.

Overall, the pathophysiology of HFpEF in diabetes involves a complex interplay of metabolic abnormalities, inflammation, endothelial dysfunction, myocardial fibrosis, and neurohormonal dysregulation. These mechanisms contribute to impaired diastolic function, leading to the clinical syndrome of HFpEF characterized by symptoms such as dyspnea on exertion, fatigue, and exercise intolerance.

HEART FAILURE WITH PRESERVED EJECTION FRACTION IN DIABETES: CLINICAL PRESENTATION

Clinical Assessment

Symptoms: Patients often present with symptoms such as exertional dyspnea, fatigue, and exercise intolerance. These symptoms may overlap with those of other cardiovascular or respiratory conditions.

Medical history: A detailed history is crucial, including any past cardiac conditions (like hypertension, atrial fibrillation, and ischemic heart disease), diabetes duration, obesity, or other relevant comorbidities, e.g., smoking.

Physical Examination

Signs such as elevated jugular venous pressure, pulmonary rales, or peripheral edema may be present. Precordial auscultation may reveal S3 or S4 and is important to rule out valvular heart disease as the cause of heart failure. However, it is important to note that signs may be subtle or absent in some patients, especially early in the disease process.

HEART FAILURE WITH PRESERVED EJECTION FRACTION IN DIABETES: DIAGNOSTIC WORKUP

Diagnosis of HFpEF can be challenging due to its diverse clinical presentations and overlapping symptoms with other conditions. Here are the key steps and considerations typically involved in making this diagnosis:

- *Laboratory tests:* Routine blood tests including complete blood count, electrolytes, renal function tests, glycemic control status, and thyroid function tests are important to assess for underlying conditions or contributing factors.
- *Imaging studies:*
    - *Echocardiography:* This is the primary imaging modality used to assess cardiac structure and function. Key findings suggestive of HFpEF include:
        - Left ventricular hypertrophy.
        - Normal or near-normal ejection fraction (usually ≥50%).
        - Evidence of diastolic dysfunction, such as abnormal relaxation patterns or elevated filling pressures.
        - Other imaging modalities such as cardiac MRI (CMRI) or CT scan may be used in specific cases to assess for myocardial fibrosis or other structural abnormalities. It is worth mentioning that few patients of diabetic HFpEF can have underlying cardiac amyloid, which can be picked up by echocardiographic strain imaging for its typical "Cherry-on-top" appearance or by CMRI by its diffuse subendocardial enhancement pattern along with T1 mapping.

- *Functional assessment:* Exercise testing (e.g., 6-minute-walk test and cardiopulmonary exercise testing) may help assess functional capacity and symptoms.
- *Additional testing:*
  - *Biomarkers:* Elevated levels of natriuretic peptides (BNP or NT-proBNP) may support the diagnosis, but levels can be influenced by other conditions as well.
  - *Invasive hemodynamic assessment:* In selected cases where the diagnosis remains uncertain, invasive hemodynamic assessment (right heart catheterization) can directly measure pressures. Also, coronary angiography is vital to rule out associated coronary artery disease.
- *Differential diagnosis consideration:* HFpEF shares symptoms with other conditions such as chronic lung disease, deconditioning, and other cardiac diseases (e.g., valvular heart disease), necessitating careful consideration and exclusion of these conditions.

Given the complexity and variability in presentation, the diagnosis of HFpEF often requires a comprehensive approach integrating clinical assessment, imaging, and functional testing. Collaboration between primary care physicians, cardiologists, and other specialists may be crucial in reaching an accurate diagnosis and developing an appropriate management plan.

ROLE OF SGLT2 INHIBITORS IN HFpEF WITH DIABETES

Diabetes mellitus, especially type 2 diabetes, is a major risk factor for developing HFpEF. Managing HFpEF in patients with diabetes involves controlling blood glucose levels, managing blood pressure, promoting weight loss if necessary, and addressing other risk factors such as smoking and cholesterol levels. Treatment strategies often include medications that can help manage symptoms and improve outcomes by targeting specific aspects of heart function and remodeling. Sodium-glucose cotransporter 2 inhibitors (SGLT2 inhibitors) are a relatively recent class of medications used primarily to treat type 2 diabetes mellitus. They have shown promising results in managing both HFpEF and HFrEF in diabetic patients. Studies like the DAPA-HF trial have demonstrated that dapagliflozin, an SGLT2 inhibitor, reduced the risk of worsening heart failure and cardiovascular death in patients with HFrEF regardless of diabetic status. Similar results were seen with dapagliflozin in HFpEF (DELIVER Trial) and with empagliflozin in HFrEF (EMPEROR Reduced) and HFpEF (EMPEROR Preserved) patients. This suggests that the benefits of SGLT2 inhibitors in heart failure are dependent neither on the diabetic status nor on the LVEF.

Discovery and Development

The SGLT2 transporter was discovered in the late 19th century, but its significance in glucose reabsorption in the kidneys was fully understood much later. The first SGLT2 inhibitor, phlorizin, was discovered in the 1930s. It inhibits both SGLT1 and SGLT2 transporters, leading to glucose excretion in urine. However, its clinical use was limited due to nonspecific effects and poor oral bioavailability. In the early 2000s, researchers began focusing on developing selective SGLT2 inhibitors that would specifically target the SGLT2 transporter in the kidneys. In 2008, the FDA approved the first SGLT2 inhibitor, dapagliflozin, developed by Bristol-Myers Squibb and AstraZeneca. This marked a significant advancement in diabetes treatment, as it provided a new mechanism of action to reduce blood glucose levels by increasing urinary glucose excretion. Following dapagliflozin, other SGLT2 inhibitors like canagliflozin and empagliflozin were subsequently developed and approved.

Mechanisms of Action

The SGLT2 inhibitors primarily work by inhibiting glucose reabsorption in the kidneys, leading to increased glucose excretion **(Fig. 1)**. This mechanism also results in natriuresis and osmotic diuresis, which can reduce plasma volume and cardiac preload. Additionally, SGLT2 inhibitors have been shown to benefit metabolic and inflammatory pathways relevant to heart failure.

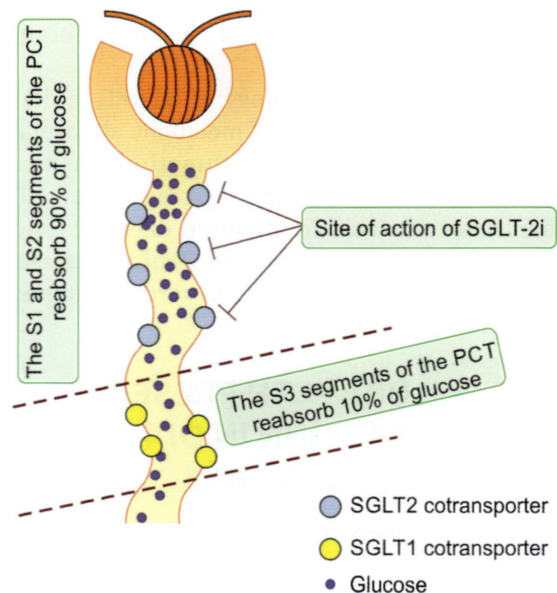

Fig. 1: SGLT2 inhibitor site of action.

Benefits Observed

- *Improved cardiovascular outcomes:* SGLT2 inhibitors have been shown to reduce the risk of hospitalization for heart failure and cardiovascular death in patients with type 2 diabetes, and these benefits extend to diabetic patients with HFpEF.
- *Reduced fluid retention:* These drugs promote diuresis (excretion of excess fluid through urine), which can help manage fluid overload, a common issue in HFpEF.
- *Renal protection:* SGLT2 inhibitors have nephroprotective effects, including reducing the risk of kidney disease progression, which is important since kidney dysfunction is often associated with heart failure.
- *Metabolic effects:* These drugs lower blood glucose levels and may have beneficial effects on other metabolic parameters, potentially impacting the underlying mechanisms of HFpEF.
- *Potential cardiac remodeling:* There is emerging evidence suggesting that SGLT2 inhibitors might directly benefit cardiac structure and function beyond their metabolic effects.

Evidence

The role of SGLT2 inhibitors in HFrEF was well established with DAPA HF and EMPEROR REDUCED trials.[7,8] A few small trials also addressed the role of these molecules in reverse remodeling; for example, EMPA TROPISM study showed the positive role of empagliflozin in reducing the LV volume and hypertrophy, whereas the EMPA HEART study showed the LV mass reduction in the diabetic population without heart failure.[9,10] The DAPA MODA study demonstrated the important beneficial effect of dapagliflozin on remodeling.[11] The landmark trials that established the importance of SGLT2 inhibitors in the therapy of HFpEF are EMPEROR PRESERVED and DELIVER trials.[12,13]

EMPEROR-Preserved Trial

The EMPEROR-Preserved trial was the first study that exclusively evaluated the efficacy of SGLT-2 inhibitors (empagliflozin) in patients with HFmrEF and HFpEF irrespective of the patient's diabetes status.

- *Design:*
  - *Type:* Phase 3, randomized, double-blind, placebo-controlled trial
  - *Participants:* Patients with LV ejection fraction >40%
  - *Intervention:* Patients were randomized to receive either empagliflozin or a placebo.
  - *Primary endpoint:* A composite of cardiovascular death or hospitalization for heart failure.
- *Results:*
  - *Efficacy:* Empagliflozin reduced the primary composite outcome of cardiovascular death and heart failure hospitalizations by 19%, driven by a significant 27% risk reduction in heart failure hospitalizations **(Fig. 2)**
  - *Safety:* Empagliflozin was well-tolerated, with a safety profile consistent with other SGLT2 inhibitors.
- *Conclusion:* The EMPEROR-Preserved trial confirmed that empagliflozin provides significant benefits for patients with HFpEF, making it a valuable treatment option for this condition. Primary endpoint reduction was seen 18 days post drug initiation. The treatment effect diminishes at LVEF >60%. The drug is possibly more effective at lower LVEF spectrum in HFpEF. Primary endpoint reduction is consistent regardless of baseline diabetes status **(Table 1)**.

DELIVER Trial

The DELIVER trial was a major clinical study evaluating the effectiveness of dapagliflozin, an SGLT2 inhibitor, in patients with heart failure. Here is a concise summary of the trial.

- *Objective:* To assess the efficacy and safety of dapagliflozin in patients with heart failure, with LVEF above 40%.
- *Design:*
  - *Type:* Phase 3, randomized, double-blind, placebo-controlled trial
  - *Participants:* Adult patients with heart failure and ejection fraction of >40%.
  - *Intervention:* Patients were randomized to receive either dapagliflozin or a placebo.
  - *Primary endpoint:* The primary outcome was a composite of cardiovascular death or worsening heart failure.

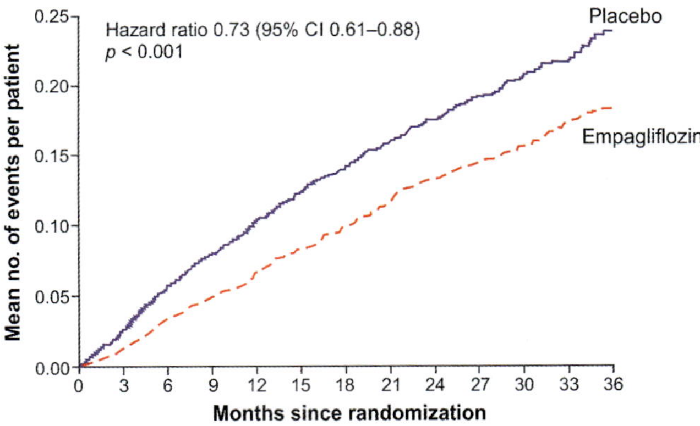

Fig. 2: Graph showing the event reduction of empagliflozin in EMPEROR-Preserved trial.

TABLE 1: Forest plot showing the primary composite outcomes in prespecified subgroups of EMPEROR-Preserved trial.

Subgroup	*Empagliflozin*	*Placebo*	*Hazard ratio (95% CI)*	
	Number of patients with events/total number			
Overall	415/2997	511/2991		0.79 (0.69–0.90)
Diabetes at baseline				
Yes	239/1466	291/1472		0.79 (0.67–0.94)
No	176/1531	220/1519		0.78 (0.64–0.95)
LVEF at baseline				
<50%	145/995	193/988		0.71 (0.57–0.88)
≥50% to <60%	138/1028	173/1030		0.80 (0.64–0.99)
≥60%	132/974	145/973		0.87 (0.69–1.10)
Age				
<70 years	134/1066	152/1084		0.88 (0.70–1.11)
≥70 years	281/1931	359/1907		0.75 (0.64–0.87)
Sex				
Male	253/1659	297/1653		0.81 (0.69–0.96)
Female	162/1338	214/1338		0.75 (0.61–0.92)
Race				
White	310/2286	370/2256		0.81 (0.69–0.94)
Black	24/133	28/125		0.73 (0.42–1.25)
Asian	54/413	77/411		0.65 (0.46–0.92)
Other	27/164	36/198		0.95 (0.58–1.57)
BMI at baseline				
<30	223/1654	292/1642		0.74 (0.62–0.88)
≥30	192/1343	219/1349		0.85 (0.70–1.03)

- *Results:*
  - *Efficacy:* Dapagliflozin significantly reduced the risk of the primary composite endpoint compared to placebo. It showed a beneficial effect on both cardiovascular death and heart failure hospitalization. Dapagliflozin was found to significantly reduce the primary composite endpoint by 18% compared to the placebo, driven largely by a significant 21% reduction in heart failure hospitalizations and urgent visits for heart failure **(Fig. 3)**. The reduction in the primary endpoint was consistent across patients with LVEF ≥60% (HR: 0.78), in contrast to what was observed in the EMPEROR-Preserved trial. But like EMPEROR-Preserved trial, diabetic status did not change the outcomes.
  - *Safety:* Dapagliflozin was well-tolerated, with a safety profile consistent with previous studies of SGLT2 inhibitors. The incidence of serious adverse events was low.
- *Conclusion:* The DELIVER trial demonstrated that dapagliflozin effectively improves outcomes in patients with heart failure across different ejection fraction categories irrespective of the diabetic status. It supports the use of dapagliflozin as a valuable treatment option in the management of heart failure. This trial contributes to the growing evidence supporting the role of SGLT2 inhibitors in heart failure management.

Safety and Tolerability

The SGLT2 inhibitors are generally well-tolerated with a safety profile that includes risks of volume depletion, urinary tract infections, and genital mycotic infections. The overall safety in patients with HFpEF appears to be consistent in the broader population of patients with type 2 diabetes or heart failure.

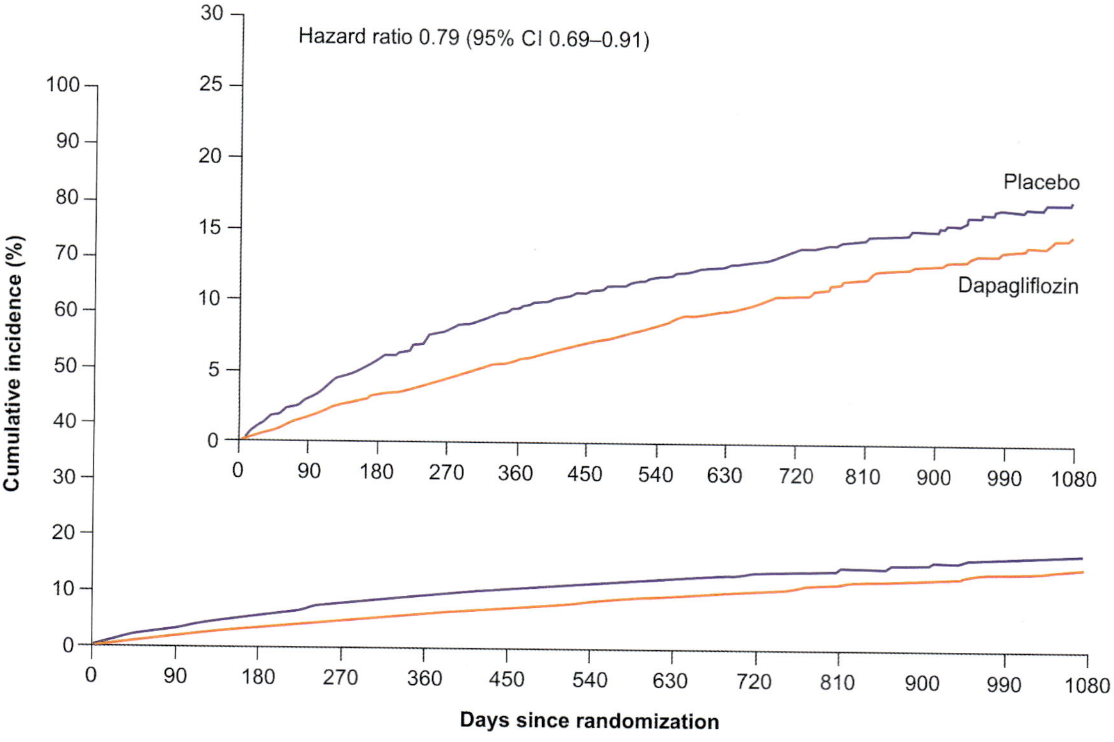

Fig. 3: Graph showing the event reduction with dapagliflozin in the DELIVER trial.

Guideline Recommendations

As of the latest ESC or ACC/AHA guidelines, SGLT2 inhibitors are recommended not only for patients of HFrEF but also their role in HFpEF has been established (Class I) irrespective of the diabetic status.[14-16]

CONCLUSION

Heart failure with preserved ejection fraction is an enigmatic disease due to the multifactorial pathophysiological process. It complicates the cardiovascular health of the diabetic population. Regular monitoring and early intervention are crucial in managing HFpEF in diabetic patients to improve quality of life and reduce the risk of complications. SGLT2 inhibitors represent a significant advancement in diabetes management, offering a novel approach to lowering blood glucose levels and potentially improving cardiovascular and renal outcomes in patients with type 2 diabetes mellitus. Their development and refinement continue to be an active area of pharmaceutical research and clinical investigation. SGLT2 inhibitors appear to be promising therapeutic options for diabetic patients with HFpEF due to their multifaceted benefits including improved cardiovascular outcomes, diuretic effects, renal protection, and potential cardiac remodeling effects.

REFERENCES

1. Chaturvedi V, Parakh N, Seth S, et al. Heart failure in India: The INDUS (INDia Ukieri Study) study. J Pract Cardiovasc Sci. 2016;2(1):28-35.
2. Kumar AS, Sinha N. Cardiovascular disease in India: a 360 degree overview. Med J Armed Forces India. 2020;76(1):1-3.
3. McAllister DA, Read SH, Kerssens J, et al. Incidence of hospitalization for heart failure and case-fatality among 3.25 million people with and without diabetes mellitus. Circulation. 2018;138:2774-86.
4. Seferović PM, Paulus WJ. Clinical diabetic cardiomyopathy: a two-faced disease with restrictive and dilated phenotypes. Eur Heart J. 2015;36(27):1718-27.
5. Iribarren C, Karter AJ, Go AS, et al. Glycemic control and heart failure among adult patients with diabetes. Circulation. 2001;103(22):2668-73.
6. Amato L, Paolisso G, Cacciatore F, et al. Congestive heart failure predicts the development of non-insulin-dependent diabetes mellitus in the elderly. The Osservatorio Geriatrico Regione Campania Group. Diabetes Metab. 1997;23:213-8.
7. McMurray JJV, Solomon SD, Inzucchi SE, et al. Dapagliflozin in patients with heart failure and reduced ejection fraction. N Engl J Med. 2019;381(21):1995-2008.
8. Packer M, Anker SD, Butler J, et al.; EMPEROR-Reduced Trial Investigators. Cardiovascular and renal outcomes with empagliflozin in heart failure. N Engl J Med. 2020; 383(15):1413-24.

9. Santos-Gallego CG, Vargas-Delgado AP, Requena-Ibanez JA, et al.; EMPA-TROPISM (ATRU-4) Investigators. Randomized trial of empagliflozin in nondiabetic patients with heart failure and reduced ejection fraction. J Am Coll Cardiol. 2021;77(3):243-55.
10. Verma S, Mazer CD, Yan AT, et al. Effect of empagliflozin on left ventricular mass in patients with type 2 diabetes mellitus and coronary artery disease: The EMPA-HEART CardioLink-6 Randomized Clinical Trial. Circulation. 2019;140(21):1693-702.
11. Pascual-Figal DA, Zamorano JL, Domingo M, et al.; DAPA-MODA Study Investigators. Impact of dapagliflozin on cardiac remodelling in patients with chronic heart failure: The DAPA-MODA study. Eur J Heart Fail. 2023;25(8):1352-60.
12. Anker SD, Butler J, Filippatos G, et al.; EMPEROR-Preserved Trial Investigators. Empagliflozin in heart failure with a preserved ejection fraction. N Engl J Med. 2021;385:1451-61.
13. Solomon SD, McMurray JJV, Claggett B, et al. Dapagliflozin in heart failure with mildly reduced or preserved ejection fraction. N Engl J Med. 2022;387(12):1089-98.
14. Heidenreich PA, Bozkurt B, Aguilar D, et al.; ACC/AHA Joint Committee Members. 2022 AHA/ACC/HFSA Guideline for the Management of Heart Failure: A Report of the American College of Cardiology/American Heart Association Joint Committee on Clinical Practice Guidelines. Circulation. 2022;145(18):e895-e1032.
15. Kittleson MM, Panjrath GS, Amancherla K, et al. 2023 ACC Expert Consensus Decision Pathway on Management of Heart Failure With Preserved Ejection Fraction: A Report of the American College of Cardiology Solution Set Oversight Committee. J Am Coll Cardiol. 2023;81(18):1835-78.
16. McDonagh TA, Metra M, Adamo M, et al.; ESC Scientific Document Group. 2023 Focused Update of the 2021 ESC Guidelines for the diagnosis and treatment of acute and chronic heart failure. Eur Heart J. 2023;44(37):3627-39.

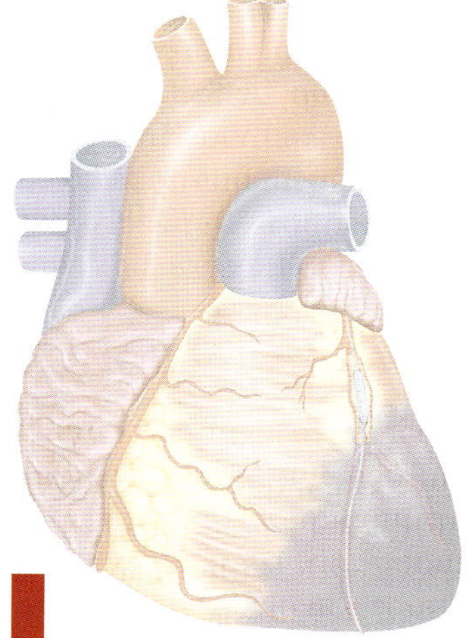

Indication, Contraindication and Uniqueness of SGLT2i and ARNI in HFpEF

HK Chopra, Md Inamul Haque, Sunil Raheja, Vidushi Bangia, NR Shastry

INTRODUCTION

Heart failure with preserved ejection fraction (HFpEF) is a prevalent and increasingly common condition characterized by the signs and symptoms of heart failure (HF), without reduction in left ventricular ejection fraction (LVEF). Sodium-glucose cotransporter-2 inhibitors (SGLT2is) and angiotensin receptor-neprilysin inhibitors (ARNIs) have both shown effectiveness in improving cardiovascular outcomes, such as reducing cardiovascular death (CVD) and heart failure hospitalization (HHF) in HFpEF patients.[1]

SODIUM–GLUCOSE COTRANSPORTER-2 INHIBITORS AND ANGIOTENSIN RECEPTOR-NEPRILYSIN INHIBITORS IN HEART FAILURE WITH PRESERVED EJECTION FRACTION

Sodium-glucose cotransporter-2 inhibitors and ARNIs have relatively well-understood mechanisms of action. SGLT2 inhibitors such as dapagliflozin and empagliflozin target myocardial cells; enhance cardiac function; and promote natriuresis, osmotic diuresis, and the excretion of glucose in the urine.[2]

Sacubitril/valsartan, a combination of the angiotensin receptor blocker (ARB) valsartan and the neprilysin inhibitor sacubitril, was the first ARNI to be developed.[3] It works by modulating the interaction between natriuretic peptides and the renin-angiotensin-aldosterone system (RAAS), which helps counteract the harmful effects of RAAS while enhancing the beneficial effects of the natriuretic peptide system. This interaction contributes to reversing cardiac remodeling and improving HF outcomes.

Since ARNI and SGLT2 inhibitors operate through distinct, nonoverlapping mechanisms, they can be used together. In the DAPA-HF study, a randomized controlled trial of dapagliflozin, 11% of participants were treated with a combination of ARNI and the SGLT2 inhibitor, demonstrating that this combination can be both safe and effective.[4]

SODIUM–GLUCOSE COTRANSPORTER-2 INHIBITORS

Sodium-glucose cotransporter-2 inhibitors were originally developed to control hyperglycemia in type 2 diabetes mellitus (T2DM) by inhibiting glucose reabsorption in the proximal tubule. In addition to their effects on glycemic control, SGLT2 inhibitors have also been shown to provide cardioprotective benefits through various mechanisms. Currently, there are four SGLT2 inhibitors approved by FDA for the use in the adults: (1) canagliflozin, (2) dapagliflozin, (3) empagliflozin, and (4) ertugliflozin **(Flowchart 1)**.[5]

The FDA-approved indications for SGLT2 inhibitors are given as follows:

- Improvement of glycemic control in T2DM (as an adjunct to diet and exercise)[6]
- Reduction in major adverse cardiovascular events (including nonfatal myocardial infarction, nonfatal

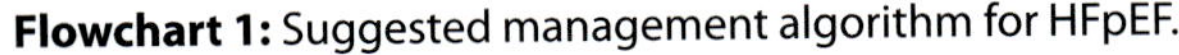

Flowchart 1: Suggested management algorithm for HFpEF.

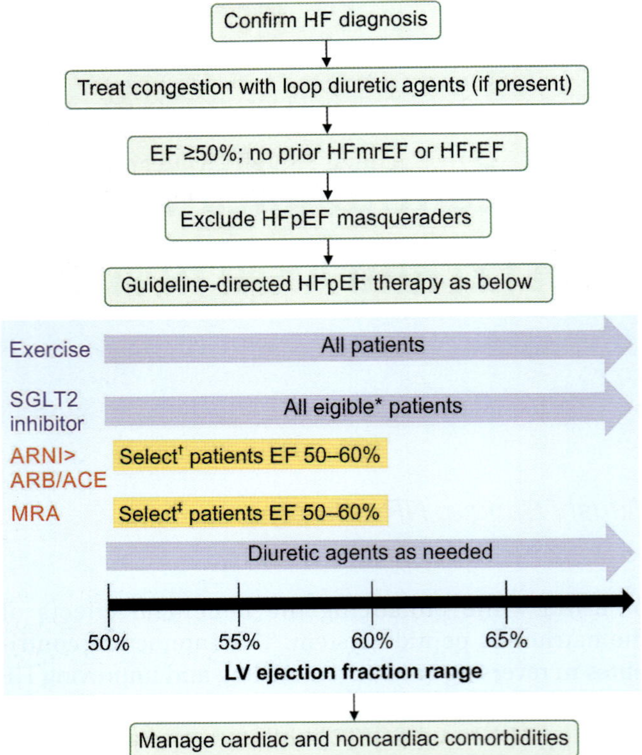

*No type 1 diabetes mellitus, estimated glomerular filtration rate (eGFR) >20 mL/min/1.73 m^2, no history of diabetic ketoacidosis (DKA).

†Elevated natriuretic peptides levels or at high risk of heart failure (HF) hospitalization or with need for additional blood pressure (BP) control.

‡Elevated natriuretic peptides levels or at high risk of HF hospitalization or with need for additional BP control with eGFR >30 mL/min/1.73 m^2 and K <5.0 and compliant with monitoring.

(ACE: angiotensin-converting enzyme; ARB: angiotensin receptor blocker; ARNI: angiotensin receptor neprilysin inhibitor; EF: ejection fraction; HFmrEF: heart failure with mildly reduced ejection fraction; HFpEF: heart failure with preserved ejection fraction; HFrEF: heart failure with reduced ejection fraction; LV: left ventricular; MRA: mineralocorticoid receptor antagonist; SGLT2: sodium-glucose cotransporter-2)

Source: Desai AS, Lam CSP, McMurray JJV, et al. How to manage heart failure with preserved ejection fraction: practical guidance for clinicians. JACC Heart Fail. 2023;11(6):619-36.

stroke, and CVD) in patients with T2DM and established cardiovascular disease[7]

- Reduction of the risk of cardiovascular hospitalization and death due to heart failure with reduced ejection fraction (HFrEF) [the New York Heart Association (NYHA) classes II–IV][8]
- Reduction of the risk of estimated glomerular filtration rate (eGFR) decline and hospitalization in patients with chronic kidney disease at risk of progression[9]
- Improvement of cardiovascular outcomes in patients with HFpEF[10]
- Dapagliflozin is now FDA approved for the treatment of HF across the full spectrum of LVEF, including HFrEF, HFpEF, and heart failure with mildly reduced ejection fraction (HFmrEF) (LVEF of 40–49%).[11]

Sodium–Glucose Cotransporter-2 Inhibitors in Heart Failure with Preserved Ejection Fraction

The common comorbidities associated with HFpEF include diabetes, hypertension, dyslipidemia, and obesity. Inhibition of SGLT2 transporters in the kidneys leads to glucosuria, natriuresis, and osmotic diuresis, resulting in lower blood glucose levels, reduced obesity, improved blood pressure (BP), and better lipid metabolism. Given these effects, it is reasonable to speculate that SGLT2 inhibitors could be beneficial for HFpEF patients, as their pleiotropic actions address the multifactorial pathophysiology of the disease.[12]

Heart failure with preserved ejection fraction has long been a challenging condition to treat. However, recent evidence from the landmark DELIVER and EMPEROR-Preserved trials has demonstrated that SGLT2 inhibitors can reduce the combined risk of HHF or CVD in patients with HFpEF.

Studies have shown that SGLT2 inhibitors can reduce inflammation and oxidative stress in HFpEF, leading to improvements in microcirculatory dysfunction, a reduction in vascular stiffness, and lower systemic BP. It has also been shown to reduce myofilament stiffness and prevent extracellular matrix remodeling and fibrosis in the heart, leading to improvements in diastolic function.

Overall, the 2022 guidelines from the American Heart Association, American College of Cardiology, and Heart Failure Society of America provide a class 2a recommendation for SGLT2 inhibitors in patients with HFpEF, suggesting that the potential benefits likely outweigh the risks provided there are no contraindications **(Flowcharts 2 and 3)**.[13]

UNIQUENESS OF SODIUM–GLUCOSE COTRANSPORTER-2 IN HEART FAILURE WITH PRESERVED EJECTION FRACTION

Effects of Sodium–Glucose Cotransporter-2 Inhibitors on Diastolic Function

At the myocardial level, HFpEF is characterized by diastolic dysfunction where impaired relaxation of the heart muscle leads to inadequate ventricular filling. In small, prospective clinical studies involving patients with T2DM and normal ejection fraction (EF), SGLT2 inhibitors were shown to improve diastolic function, as assessed by echocardiography, after 3[14] and 6 months[15] of treatment.

Flowchart 2: Summary of the pathophysiology of HFpEF and potential mechanisms by which SGLT2 inhibitors may improve outcomes. As comorbidities play a significant role in HFpEF, the positive effects of SGLT2 inhibitors on hypertension, diabetes, obesity, and dyslipidemia are particularly important. Additionally, SGLT2 inhibitors may directly impact the myocardial pathological processes underlying HFpEF.

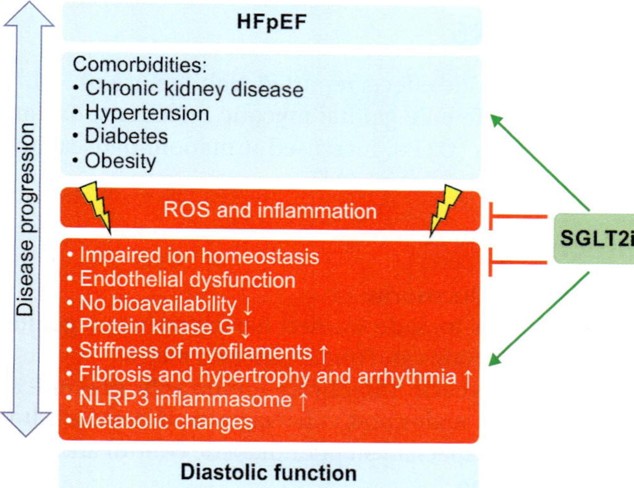

(HFpEF: heart failure with preserved ejection fraction; NO: nitric oxide; SGLT2i: sodium–glucose cotransporter-2 inhibitor)
Source: Adapted from JMCC.

Effects of Sodium–Glucose Cotransporter-2 Inhibitors on Myofilament Function

Myofilament function is critical in regulating diastolic cardiomyocyte stiffness, and in HFpEF patients, myofilament stiffness is often abnormally elevated.[16] Empagliflozin has been shown to reduce pathological cardiomyocyte stiffness in the myocardium of HFpEF patients.[17]

Effects of Sodium–Glucose Cotransporter-2 Inhibitors on Cardiac Hypertrophy

In patients with HFpEF, diastolic dysfunction and cardiac hypertrophy often occur together. The relationship between hypertrophy, diastolic function, and HFpEF is complex; increased left ventricular hypertrophy can impair chamber geometry, potentially leading to diastolic dysfunction.

A reduction in left ventricular mass following SGLT2 inhibitor therapy was also observed in echocardiographic measurements of patients with T2DM.[18] The mechanisms underlying the regression of hypertrophy still require further investigation, particularly in patients with HFpEF.

Renal Protective Effects of Sodium–Glucose Cotransporter-2 Inhibitors[19,20]

- Restore tubuloglomerular feedback, leading to afferent vasoconstriction
- Decrease intraglomerular pressure and hyperfiltration
- Slow the progression of renal disease
- Reduce renoglomerulosclerosis
- Reverse remodeling of afferent and efferent glomeruli
- Decrease proteinuria
- Improve the decline in eGFR

Flowchart 3: Algorithm for the initiation of SGLT2 inhibitor in HFpEF.

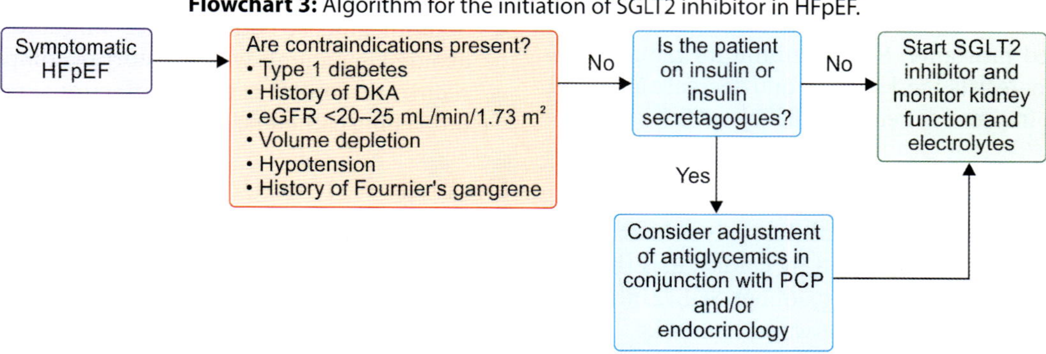

(DKA: diabetic ketoacidosis; eGFR: estimated glomerular filtration rate; HFpEF: heart failure with preserved ejection fraction; PCP: primary care physician)
Source: Adapted from AHA/ASA.

Metabolic Effects of Sodium–Glucose Cotransporter-2 Inhibitors[21,22]

Sodium-glucose cotransporter-2 inhibitors provide several metabolic benefits given as follows:

- Decrease excess glucose uptake by the heart
- Lower uric acid levels through uricosuric effects via the glucose transporter 9 (GLUT9)
- Increase glucagon release, promoting hepatic ketogenesis, which enhances cardiac inotropic and chronotropic effects
- Reduce plasma triglyceride levels
- Increase the ratio of low-density lipoprotein (LDL) to high-density lipoprotein (HDL) cholesterol

Glucosuric Effects of Sodium–Glucose Cotransporter-2 Inhibitors[23,24]

- Improvement in glycemic control, reflected by a reduction in glycated hemoglobin (HbA1c) by approximately 0.5–1%
- Promotes increased loss of calories, leading to a decrease in body weight
- Reduces the cardiac effects associated with glucose toxicity

Natriuresis and Blood Pressure Reduction[25]

- The osmotic diuretic effect of enhanced natriuresis leads to a negative salt and water balance, resulting in improved BP control and reversal of tubuloglomerular feedback stimulation.
- This reduction in plasma volume is associated with a decrease in BP, with a reduction of 3–6 mm Hg in systolic BP and 1–1.5 mm Hg in diastolic BP.

Decrease in Arterial Stiffness[26]

Arterial stiffness is a significant predictor of cardiovascular morbidity and mortality. SGLT2 inhibitors reduce peripheral vascular resistance, lower BP, and decrease afterload, which in turn improve subendocardial blood flow.

Weight Loss[27]

Initial weight loss with SGLT2 inhibitors is primarily due to volume contraction, followed by caloric loss through glucosuria. After 6–12 months of treatment, SGLT2 inhibitors typically induce weight loss of between 2 and 4 kg.

Antioxidant and Anti-inflammatory Effects

Sodium-glucose cotransporter-2 inhibitors reduce oxidative stress, proinflammatory and pro-oxidant factors. This helps decrease the formation of advanced glycation end products and improve endothelial function.

Shift in Fuel Energetics[28]

Glucosuria induces a state of relative glucose deprivation, prompting a shift toward using lipids as an energy substrate. This shift favors ketone production, which serves as a more efficient energy source for renal and myocardial cells. Additionally, it reduces cellular lipotoxicity and improves oxidative stress.

ADVERSE DRUG REACTIONS AND CONTRAINDICATIONS OF SODIUM–GLUCOSE COTRANSPORTER-2 INHIBITORS

The common side effects reported with the use of SGLT2 inhibitors are female genital mycotic infections, urinary tract infections (UTIs), increased urination, nausea, and constipation.[29]

Infection[23,30-32]

It is related to glucosuria.

- Risk factors include women having previous genital fungal infections and uncircumcised males.
- Genital mycotic infections commonly present as balanitis in males and vulvovaginitis in females. It is quite low, especially in poor diabetic control and poor local hygiene.
- Fournier's gangrene, a rare but severe complication, involves necrotizing fasciitis of the perineum. If this occurs, the SGLT2 inhibitor should be discontinued immediately, and treatment should begin with broad-spectrum antibiotics, along with surgical debridement if necessary.
- Sodium-glucose cotransporter-2 inhibitors should be avoided in patients with a history of complicated UTIs, recurrent genital mycotic infections, or those with indwelling catheters.

Diabetic Ketoacidosis[30,31,33,34]

Sodium-glucose cotransporter-2 inhibitors are contraindicated in patients with diabetic ketoacidosis (DKA).

Risk factors for DKA include:

- Hypovolemic states
- Acute illness or surgery
- Alcohol abuse
- Previous episodes of ketosis

Additionally, SGLT2 inhibitors are not approved for use in latent autoimmune diabetes in adults or type 1 diabetes.

It is also recommended that SGLT2 inhibitors should be stopped at least 48 hours before any surgical procedure to reduce the risk of complications.

Euglycemic Diabetic Ketoacidosis

Euglycemic DKA in the context of SGLT2 inhibitors is characterized by a triad of:

- Serum glucose <250 mg/dL
- Increased anion gap acidosis
- Presence of ketosis

This condition is thought to arise due to several factors, including:

- *Noninsulin-dependent glucose loss:* SGLT2 inhibitors promote urinary glucose excretion, leading to glucose loss via the kidneys.
- *Hyperglucagonemia:* Elevated glucagon levels increase hepatic glucose production, exacerbating hyperglycemia.
- *Volume depletion:* Osmotic diuresis resulting from increased urinary glucose excretion leads to dehydration and reduced intravascular volume.

Acute Kidney Injury[25,30]

Acute kidney injury (AKI) may occur with the initiation of SGLT2 therapy due to intravascular volume contraction. Risk factors include volume depletion, hypotension, diuretics, angiotensin-converting enzyme (ACE) inhibitors, ARBs, nonsteroidal anti-inflammatory drugs (NSAIDs), or nephrotoxic drugs. Close monitoring of kidney function is recommended, especially in patients with these risk factors, when starting or adjusting SGLT2 inhibitor therapy.

Hypoglycemia

The risk of hypoglycemia is increased with SGLT2 if combined with insulin secretagogues, such as sulfonylureas and insulin.

Lower Limb Amputation[35]

Sodium-glucose cotransporter-2 inhibitors cause volume depletion, hemoconcentration, and reduced BP, which may reduce lower limb perfusion and produce tissue ischemia.

Risk factors include peripheral vascular disease, neuropathy, history of diabetic foot ulcer, and previous history of amputations. It is, therefore, suggested to discontinue SGLT2 inhibitors in case of lower limb ulcers and infection.

Bone Fracture[36]

Sodium-glucose cotransporter-2 inhibitors are associated with an increased bone fracture, especially observed with canagliflozin.

Fracture is possibly related to the increased parathyroid hormone (PTH), fibroblast growth factor 23 (FGF23) excretion, orthostatic hypotension, and postural falls due to value depletion.

Bladder Cancer[37]

Dapagliflozin is associated with bladder cancer.

Sodium-glucose cotransporter-2 inhibitors, especially dapagliflozin, are not advised in patients with hematuria or a history of bladder cancer.

Sodium-glucose cotransporter-2 inhibitors are contraindicated in the following cases:

- History of type 1 diabetes mellitus
- History of DKA
- History of Fournier's gangrene
- Patient receiving dialysis eGFR <20 mL/min/1.73 m^2
- Hypersensitivity reactions such as anaphylaxis or angioedema to SGLT2 inhibitors
- Pregnancy (due to potential fetal risk during second and third trimesters)
- Breastfeeding
- Recurrent UTI is a relative contraindication
- Fungal infection in urine

INDICATION OF ANGIOTENSIN RECEPTOR-NEPRILYSIN INHIBITOR IN HEART FAILURE WITH PRESERVED EJECTION FRACTION

The incidence of HFpEF increases progressively with age, and the underlying mechanisms involve elevated left ventricular filling pressure, impaired left ventricular relaxation, reduced left atrial function, and increased vascular stiffness.[38]

Upregulation of the RAAS has been identified as a key pathological process in fibrosis, cardiomyocyte abnormalities, inflammation, and endothelial dysfunction, all of which contribute to the worsening of HFpEF.

In patients with HFpEF, sacubitril/valsartan resulted in a lower level of N-terminal pro-B-type natriuretic peptide (NT-proBNP), a larger reduction in left atrial size, and greater improvement in the NYHA functional class than valsartan.[39]

The ACC guidelines have issued a class 2b recommendation for the use of sacubitril/valsartan in HFpEF. Primary outcome of the PARADIGM-HF trial showed a nonsignificant reduction in CVDs or hospitalizations due to HF in the sacubitril/valsartan group. Secondary outcomes demonstrated a significant improvement in the NYHA class and renal function, with greater benefits observed in female patients. These findings emphasize the importance of personalized therapy with ARNI in HFpEF.[40,41]

The PARAGON-HF study demonstrated that sacubitril/valsartan was effective in reducing primary end point events and renal complications in patients with HFpEF. Following the outcomes of the PARAGON-HF trial, the FDA approved the use of sacubitril/valsartan for patients with HFpEF.[42]

UNIQUENESS OF ANGIOTENSIN RECEPTOR-NEPRILYSIN INHIBITOR

Cardiovascular Benefits of Sacubitril/Valsartan in Heart Failure with Preserved Ejection Fraction

Sacubitril/valsartan has consistently demonstrated efficacy in managing cardiovascular conditions in patients with HFpEF, as evidenced by several large clinical trials conducted over the years. These include the PARAMOUNT trial (2012), the PARAGON-HF trial (2019), and the PARALLAX trial (2021). All of these studies were double-blind, multicenter, randomized controlled trials.

The cardiovascular benefits of sacubitril/valsartan in HFpEF include:[43]

- Decrease left ventricular remodeling
- Reduce myocardial hypertrophy and fibrosis
- Reduce cardiomyocyte stiffness
- Reduce fibroblast proliferation
- Improvement of endothelial dysfunction
- Reduction in arterial stiffness

Renal Benefits of Angiotensin Receptor-Neprilysin Inhibitor in Heart Failure with Preserved Ejection Fraction

Heart failure and chronic kidney disease share several common risk factors, including traditional cardiovascular risks such as age, gender, hypertension, dyslipidemia, and diabetes. Beyond these shared etiological factors, there are also complex interactions between their underlying pathophysiology. In HF, when the cardiac cycle is impaired, the heart struggles to provide adequate tissue perfusion and effectively adapt to changes in venous return, leading to further complications.[44] Sacubitril/valsartan's benefit on renal function in HF populations may be partially attributed to improved cardiac function.[45]

The effects of ARNI on the kidneys include:

- Decreased renal sodium absorption
- Increased vasodilation of afferent arterioles
- Reduction in oxidative stress and inflammation

These actions contribute to improved renal hemodynamics and may help mitigate renal damage in patients with HF.

Metabolic Benefit of Angiotensin Receptor-Neprilysin Inhibitor in Heart Failure with Preserved Ejection Fraction

Diabetes and dyslipidemia are common in patients with HFpEF. Cardiac lipotoxicity and metabolic disturbances are associated with the development of HFpEF, contributing to its characteristic diastolic dysfunction.[46]

Effect on Lipid

In the PARAGON-HF study, sacubitril/valsartan reduces triglycerides, increases high-density lipoprotein cholesterol (HDL-C), and increases low-density lipoprotein cholesterol (LDL-C).[47]

Effect on Blood Glucose

Recent research indicated that sacubitril/valsartan may help improve blood glucose control in diabetes. This effect is thought to be partly due to an increase in glucagon-like peptide-1 (GLP-1), which in turn enhances insulin secretion.[48]

CONTRAINDICATIONS OF ANGIOTENSIN RECEPTOR-NEPRILYSIN INHIBITOR[49-51]

- History of angioedema related to previous treatment with an ACE inhibitor or another ARB
- Concomitant use with ACE inhibitors: A 36-hour washout period is required before switching from an ACE inhibitor to sacubitril/valsartan to avoid the risk of angioedema.
- Concomitant use of aliskiren in patients with diabetes due to an increased risk of hypotension, hyperkalemia, and renal impairment
- Pregnancy
- Breastfeeding

- Hypersensitivity reactions: Patients with known hypersensitivity (e.g., anaphylaxis or angioedema) to any component of sacubitril/valsartan
- Renal artery stenosis: Not recommended for use in patients with bilateral renal artery stenosis or renal artery stenosis in a solitary kidney due to the potential for renal impairment.
- Severe renal impairment (eGFR <30 mL/min/1.73 m^2)
- Hyperkalemia: Sacubitril/valsartan should be used with caution or avoided in patients with serum potassium levels >5.4 mEq/L.
- Severe (Child–Pugh C) hepatic impairment

CONCLUSION

Sodium–glucose cotransporter-2 inhibitors and ARNI (sacubitril/valsartan) offer significant benefits in treating HFpEF. SGLT2 inhibitors improve symptoms by targeting comorbidities such as hypertension, diabetes, and obesity while reducing HHFs. ARNI has shown effectiveness in reducing myocardial fibrosis and improving cardiac function. Both therapies address key pathophysiological mechanisms of HFpEF, offering a promising approach to improve patient outcomes. These treatments represent a valuable addition to the HFpEF therapeutic landscape. Both SGLT2 inhibitors and ARNI are iconic molecules of the century in the management of HFpEF with their uniqueness mentioned above.

REFERENCES

1. Ponikowski P, Voors AA, Anker SD, et al. 2016 ESC guidelines for the diagnosis and treatment of acute and chronic heart failure. Eur Heart J. 2016;37:2129-200.
2. Pradhan A, Vohra S, Vishwakarma P, et al. Review on sodium-glucose cotransporter 2 inhibitor (SGLT2i) in diabetes mellitus and heart failure. J Family Med Prim Care. 2019;8:1855-62.
3. Gu J, Noe A, Chandra P, et al. Pharmacokinetics and pharmacodynamics of LCZ696, a novel dual-acting angiotensin receptor-neprilysin inhibitor (ARNi). J Clin Pharmacol. 2010;50(4):401-14.
4. Docherty KF, Vaduganathan M, Solomon SD, et al. Sacubitril/valsartan: neprilysin inhibition 5 years after PARADIGM-HF. JACC Heart Fail. 2020;8:800-10.
5. Lopaschuk GD, Verma S. Mechanisms of cardiovascular benefits of sodium glucose cotransporter 2 (SGLT2) inhibitors. JACC Basic Transl Sci. 2020;5:632-44.
6. American Diabetes Association Professional Practice Committee. 9. Pharmacologic approaches to glycemic treatment: Standards of Medical Care in Diabetes-2022. Diabetes Care. 2022;45(Suppl 1):S125-43.
7. Zelniker TA, Wiviott SD, Raz I, et al. SGLT2 inhibitors for primary and secondary prevention of cardiovascular and renal outcomes in type 2 diabetes: a systematic review and meta-analysis of cardiovascular outcome trials. Lancet. 2019;393(10166):31-9.
8. Monzo L, Ferrari I, Cicogna F, et al. Sodium-glucose co-transporter-2 inhibitors eligibility in patients with heart failure with reduced ejection fraction. Int J Cardiol. 2021;341:56-9.
9. Kidney Disease: Improving Global Outcomes (KDIGO) Diabetes Work Group. KDIGO 2022 clinical practice guideline for diabetes management in chronic kidney disease. Kidney Int. 2022;102(5S):S1-127.
10. Pabel S, Hamdani N, Singh J, et al. Potential mechanisms of SGLT2 inhibitors for the treatment of heart failure with preserved ejection fraction. Front Physiol. 2021;12: 752370.
11. Solomon SD, McMurray JJV, Claggett B, et al. Dapagliflozin in heart failure with mildly reduced or preserved ejection fraction. N Engl J Med. 2022;387(12):1089-98.
12. Abdul-Ghani M, Del Prato S, Chilton R, et al. SGLT2 inhibitors and cardiovascular risk: lessons learned from the EMPA-REG OUTCOME study. Diabetes Care. 2016;39:717-25.
13. Heidenreich PA, Bozkurt B, Aguilar D, et al. 2022 AHA/ACC/HFSA guideline for the management of heart failure: A report of the American College of Cardiology/American Heart Association Joint Committee on clinical practice guidelines. Circulation. 2022;145(18):e895-1032.
14. Matsutani D, Sakamoto M, Kayama Y, et al. Effect of canagliflozin on left ventricular diastolic function in patients with type 2 diabetes. Cardiovasc Diabetol. 2018;17(1):73.
15. Shim CY, Seo J, Cho I, et al. Randomized, controlled trial to evaluate the effect of dapagliflozin on left ventricular diastolic function in patients with type 2 diabetes mellitus: the IDDIA trial. Circulation. 2021;143:510-2.
16. Pabel S, Wagner S, Bollenberg H, et al. Empagliflozin directly improves diastolic function in human heart failure. Eur J Heart Fail. 2018;20:1690-700.
17. Paulus WJ, Tschöpe C. A novel paradigm for heart failure with preserved ejection fraction: comorbidities drive myocardial dysfunction and remodeling through coronary microvascular endothelial inflammation. J Am Coll Cardiol. 2013;62 263-71.
18. Brown AJM, Gandy S, McCrimmon R, et al. A randomized controlled trial of dapagliflozin on left ventricular hypertrophy in people with type two diabetes: the DAPA-LVH trial. Eur Heart J. 2020;41:3421-32.
19. Layton AT, Vallon V, Edwards A. Modeling oxygen consumption in the proximal tubule: effects of NHE and SGLT2 inhibition. Am J Physiol Renal Physiol. 2015;308(12):F1343-57.
20. Staels B. Cardiovascular protection by sodium glucose cotransporter 2 inhibitors: potential mechanisms. Am J Cardiol. 2017;120(1S):S28-36.
21. Scheen AJ. Cardiovascular effects of new oral glucose-lowering agents: DPP-4 and SGLT-2 Inhibitors. Circ Res. 2018;122(10):1439-59.

22. Lytvyn Y, Bjornstad P, Udell JA, et al. Sodium glucose cotransporter-2 inhibition in heart failure: potential mechanisms, clinical applications, and summary of clinical trials. Circulation. 2017;136(17):1643-58.
23. Zinman B, Wanner C, Lachin JM, et al. Empagliflozin, cardiovascular outcomes, and mortality in type 2 diabetes. N Engl J Med. 2015;373(22):2117-28.
24. Abdul-Ghani MA, Norton L, DeFronzo RA. Role of sodium–glucose cotransporter 2 (SGLT2) inhibitors in the treatment of type 2 diabetes. Endocr Rev. 2011;32(4):515-31.
25. Neal B, Perkovic V, Mahaffey KW. Canagliflozin and cardiovascular and renal events in type 2 diabetes. N Engl J Med. 2017;377(21):644-57.
26. Baker WL, Smyth LR, Riche DM, et al. Effects of sodium-glucose co-transporter 2 inhibitors on blood pressure: a systematic review and meta-analysis. J Am Soc Hypertens. 2014;8(4):262-75.e9.
27. DeFronzo RA, Norton L, Abdul-Ghani M. Renal, metabolic and cardiovascular considerations of SGLT2 inhibition. Nat Rev Nephrol. 2017;13(1):11-26.
28. Flores E, Santos-Gallego CG, Diaz-Mejía N, et al. Do the SGLT-2 inhibitors offer more than hypoglycemic activity? Cardiovasc Drugs Ther. 2018;32(2):213-22.
29. Halimi S, Vergès B. Adverse effects and safety of SGLT-2 inhibitors. Diabetes Metab. 2014;40(6 Suppl 1):S28-34.
30. Scheen AJ. Pharmacodynamics, efficacy and safety of sodium-glucose co-transporter type 2 (SGLT2) inhibitors for the treatment of type 2 diabetes mellitus. Drugs. 2015;75(1):33-59.
31. Lupsa BC, Inzucchi SE. Use of SGLT2 inhibitors in type 2 diabetes: weighing the risks and benefits. Diabetologia. 2018;61(10):2118-25.
32. Thong KY, Yadagiri M, Barnes DJ, et al. Clinical risk factors predicting genital fungal infections with sodium-glucose cotransporter 2 inhibitor treatment: the ABCD nationwide dapagliflozin audit. Prim Care Diabetes. 2018;12(1): 45-50.
33. Rosenstock J, Ferrannini E. Euglycemic diabetic ketoacidosis: a predictable, detectable, and preventable safety concern with SGLT2 inhibitors. Diabetes Care. 2015;38(9):1638-42.
34. Heerspink HJ, Perkins BA, Fitchett DH, et al. Sodium glucose cotransporter 2 inhibitors in the treatment of diabetes mellitus: cardiovascular and kidney effects, potential mechanisms, and clinical applications. Circulation. 2016;134(10):752-72.
35. Mahaffey KW, Neal B, Perkovic V, et al. Canagliflozin for primary and secondary prevention of cardiovascular events: results from the CANVAS program (Canagliflozin Cardiovascular Assessment Study). Circulation. 2018; 137(4):323-34.
36. Watts NB, Bilezikian JP, Usiskin K, et al. Effects of canagliflozin on fracture risk in patients with type 2 diabetes mellitus. J Clin Endocrinol Metab. 2016;101(1):157-66.
37. García M, Arteche-Martinez U, Lertxundi U, et al. SGLT2 inhibitors and bladder cancer: analysis of cases reported in the European pharmacovigilance database. J Clin Pharmacol. 2021;61(2):187-92.
38. Tartière-Kesri L, Tartière JM, Logeart D, et al. Increased proximal arterial stiffness and cardiac response with moderate exercise in patients with heart failure and preserved ejection fraction. J Am Coll Cardiol, 2012;59(5):455-61.
39. Solomon SD, Zile M, Pieske B, et al. The angiotensin receptor neprilysin inhibitor LCZ696 in heart failure with preserved ejection fraction: a phase 2 double-blind randomised controlled trial. Lancet. 2012;380:1387-95.
40. Massari F, Scicchitano P, Iacoviello M, et al. Multiparametric approach to congestion for predicting long-term survival in heart failure. J Cardiol. 2020;75:47-52.
41. Krum H. Prospective comparison of ARNi with ACE-I to determine impact on global mortality and morbidity in heart failure (PARADIGM-HF): paragon of a study or further investigation paramount? Circulation. 2015;131: 11-12.
42. Solomon SD, McMurray JJV, Anand IS, et al. Angiotensin-neprilysin inhibition in heart failure with preserved ejection fraction. N Engl J Med. 2019;381(17):1609-20.
43. Gori M, D'Elia E, Senni M. Sacubitril/valsartan therapeutic strategy in HFpEF: clinical insights and perspectives. Int J Cardiol. 2019;281:158-65.
44. Hunt SA, Abraham WT, Chin MH, et al. 2009 focused update incorporated into the ACC/AHA 2005 guidelines for the diagnosis and management of heart failure in adults. Circulation. 2009;119(14):e391-479.
45. Pontremoli R, Borghi C, Filardi PP. Renal protection in chronic heart failure: focus on sacubitril/valsartan. Eur Heart J Cardiovasc Pharmacother. 2021;7(5):445-52.
46. Shah SJ, Kitzman DW, Borlaug BA, et al. Phenotype-specific treatment of heart failure with preserved ejection fraction: a multiorgan roadmap. Circulation. 2016;134(1): 73-90.
47. Selvaraj S, Claggett BL, Packer M, et al. Effects of sacubitril/valsartan on serum lipids in heart failure with preserved ejection fraction. J Am Heart Assoc. 2021;10(17): e022069.
48. Nougué H, Pezel T, Picard F, et al. Effects of sacubitril/valsartan on neprilysin targets and the metabolism of natriuretic peptides in chronic heart failure: a mechanistic clinical study. Eur J Heart Fail. 2019;21(5):598-605.
49. Kittleson MM, Panjrath GS, Amancherla K, et al. 2023 ACC Expert Consensus Decision Pathway on management of heart failure with preserved ejection fraction: a report of the American College of Cardiology Solution Set Oversight Committee. J Am Coll Cardiol. 2023;81(18):1835-78.
50. Fala L. Entresto (sacubitril/valsartan): first-in-class angiotensin receptor neprilysin inhibitor FDA approved for patients with heart failure. Am Health Drug Benefits. 2015;8(6):330-4.
51. Nicolas D, Kerndt CC, Patel P, et al. Sacubitril-Valsartan. In: StatPearls [Internet]. Treasure Island (FL): StatPearls Publishing; 2025.

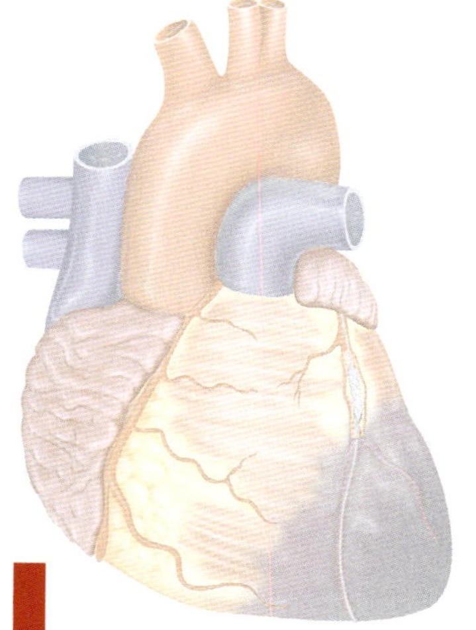

CHAPTER 140

Role of SGLT2i in HFpEF with Takotsubo Syndrome

Sandipta Ray, Mainak Mukhopadhyay, Kajal Ganguly

INTRODUCTION

Sodium-glucose cotransporter-2 inhibitor (SGLT2i) continues to be a promising treatment for heart failure (HF) irrespective of left ventricular ejection fraction (LVEF) and diabetic status. SGLTi is one of the foundational pharmacotherapies in patients with HF having LVEF of <40% along with renin-angiotensin-aldosterone (RAAS) blockade, mineralocorticoid receptor antagonist (MRA), and β-blockers (BB). In patients with heart failure and preserved ejection fraction (HFpEF), beneficial effects of SGLT2i are quite promising in recent randomized clinical trials (RCTs). Hence, this molecule has been placed as a class I recommendation in the medical management of HFpEF as per the European Society of Cardiology (ESC). This molecule has favorable effects on cardiac as well as vascular health. SGLT2i has a proinflammatory effect, reduces endothelial dysfunction, reduces cardiac stiffness, and prevents cardiac arrhythmia. Furthermore, it also reduces hospitalization due to heart failure (HFH), and cardiovascular as well as all-cause mortality.[1,2]

Takotsubo cardiomyopathy is stress-induced cardiomyopathy particularly common in postmenopausal women. It is a great mimicker of acute coronary syndrome (ACS) and myocarditis. Raised serum catecholamine level leads to apical hypokinesia or akinesia of the left ventricle (LV) with sparing of basal part. Cardiac biomarkers are often raised. A coronary angiogram may fail to demonstrate significant obstructive coronary artery disease (CAD). This is a form of reversible LV dysfunction, and most patients recover within 6–12 weeks.

There are case reports where the use of SGLT2i can lead to euglycemic diabetic ketoacidosis, increased catecholamine level, and the development of stress-induced cardiomyopathy (Takotsubo cardiomyopathy). Use of SGLT2i in patients with chronic thyroiditis can lead to the development of thyroid storm and catecholamine surge leading to stress-induced cardiomyopathy.

HFpEF AND SGLT2 INHIBITORS

Sodium-glucose cotransporter-2 inhibitors increase urine glucose excretion by inhibiting SGLT2 in the proximal tubule of the kidney, thereby lower blood glucose levels. Initially, SGLT2i was evaluated for its cardiovascular safety in type-2 diabetes mellitus (T2DM) patients with either established atherosclerotic cardiovascular disease or multiple cardiac risk factors. SGLT2i showed unexpected beneficial effects on the rate of major adverse cardiovascular events (MACE) consisting of cardiovascular events, cardiovascular death, and all-cause mortality, with benefits only seen in patients with atherosclerotic cardiovascular disease. The benefit of SGLT2i is predominantly a reduction in HFH. In HFpEF patients, SGLT2i decreases extracellular fluid (ECF) volume as can be measured by cardiac MRI. In addition to that, there is reduction in myocardial fibrosis, oxidative stress, and improvement in myocardial energetics.

The mechanism and rationale of SGLT2i in HF are given in **Flowchart 1**.

Flowchart 1: Mechanism and rationale of SGLT2i in heart failure.

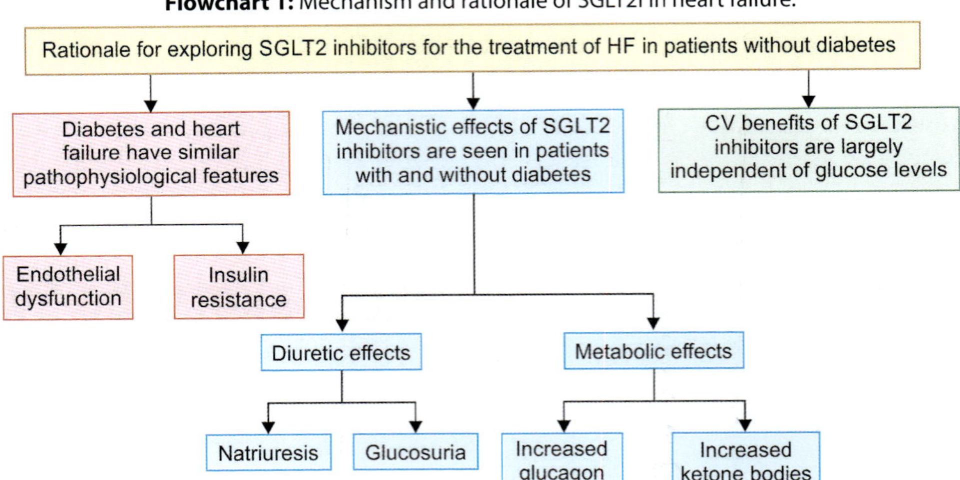

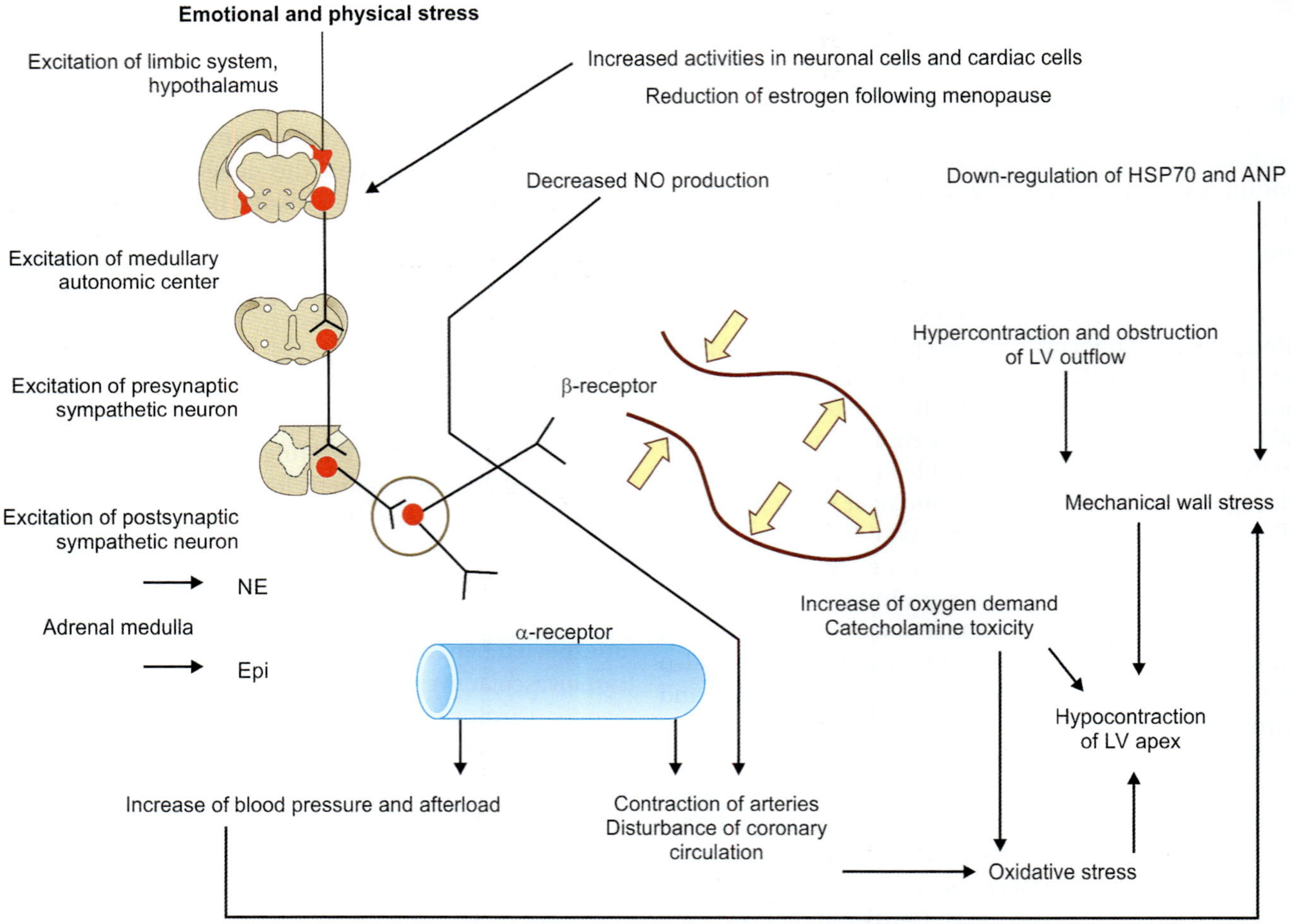

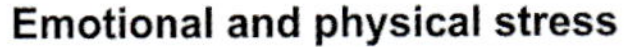

Fig. 1: Pathophysiology of takotsubo cardiomyopathy. (LV: left ventricular)

TAKOTSUBO CARDIOMYOPATHY

The pathophysiology of takotsubo cardiomyopathy is given in **Figure 1**.

It is one of the reversible cardiomyopathies of acute onset mostly secondary to emotional or physical trauma. Abnormal catecholamine dynamics play a pivotal role in pathogenesis. Symptoms may vary from HF to mechanical complications like free-wall rupture. HF is sometimes associated with fulminant pulmonary edema. These patients are prone to develop ventricular tachycardia secondary to QT prolongation. LV involvement in this type of cardiomyopathy is also variable. Commonly, LV apex is involved although mid-ventricular as well as basal involvement is also reported. Recurrent takotsubo does not involve the same segment of the myocardium by a unique mechanism like ischemic pre-conditioning.[3] Treatments are largely supportive. Guideline-directed medical therapy should be offered in the acute stage. Some patients may require a left ventricular assist device (LVAD). Although the disease is predominantly due to catecholamine surge, many patients do have normal plasma epinephrine and norepinephrine levels.

Combined β-blockers and α-blockers should be used in takotsubo cardiomyopathy particularly if it is secondary to pheochromocytoma of hyperthyroidism. Beta-blockers alone should be avoided as they may prolong the QT interval. Postmenopausal women may benefit from estrogen supplementation.

To understand the pathogenesis of stress-induced cardiomyopathy and to devise rational treatment and prevention strategies, more attention should be paid not only to the myocardium and coronary arteries but also to the integration of central neural, autonomic, endocrine, and circulatory systems in emotional distress.[4]

CONCLUSION

There are some case reports where the use of SGLT2i can lead to the development of stress-induced cardiomyopathy, particularly, in the elderly population along with underlying thyroid disorder or pheochromocytoma. Stress-induced cardiomyopathy, generally, has a favorable prognosis where LV function tends to normalize in around 6–10 weeks. SGLT2i can be used along with other guideline-directed therapy in patients with takotsubo cardiomyopathy presented with HFpEF. SGLT2i reduces oxidative stress, has got favorable effect on LV remodeling, and has antiarrhythmic properties, and hence can be considered in a stable phase of takotsubo cardiomyopathy. Some authorities have also proved that SGLT2i reduces central sympathetic overactivity, probably by suppressing renal afferent signaling to the brain.[5] This concept might usher a new horizon in its role in the management of takotsubo cardiomyopathy. A structured randomized trial is needed in the future for further evaluation of the role of SGLT2i in stress-induced cardiomyopathy.

REFERENCES

1. Bhatt DL, Szarek M, Steg PG, et al. Sotagliflozin in patients with diabetes and recent worsening heart failure. N Engl J Med. 2021;384:117-28.
2. Fitchett D, Zinman B, Wanner C, et al. Heart failure outcomes with empagliflozin in patients with type 2 diabetes at high cardiovascular risk: Results of the EMPA-REG OUTCOME trial. Eur Heart J. 2016;37(19):1526-34.
3. Kaushik M, Alla VM, Madan R, et al. Recurrent stress cardiomyopathy with variable regional involvement: insights into etiopathogenetic mechanisms. Circulation. 2011;124(22):e556-7.
4. Goldstein DS. Adrenaline and the Inner World: An Introduction to Scientific Integrative Medicine. Baltimore, Maryland: Johns Hopkins University Press; 2006.
5. Herat LY, Magno AL, Rudnicka C, et al. SGLT2 Inhibitor-Induced Sympathoinhibition: A Novel Mechanism for Cardiorenal Protection. JACC Basic Transl Sci. 2020; 5(2):169-79.

141

CHAPTER

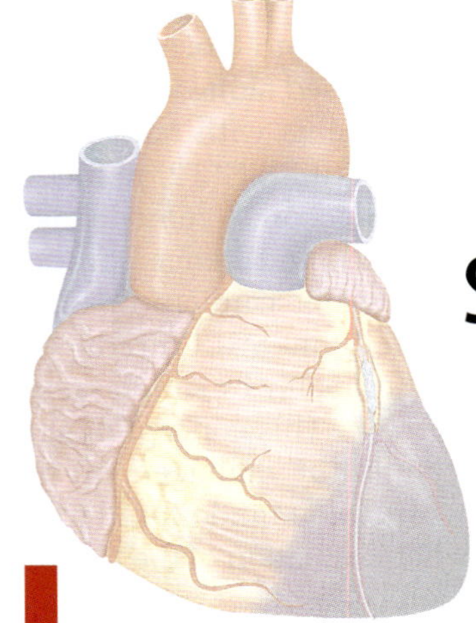

SGLT2i in HFpEF: Fighting the Enemy with a Newly Crafted Weapon

Ashokan Nambiar, Raghuram A Krishnan

INTRODUCTION

Heart failure with preserved ejection fraction (HFpEF) has become a growing focus in cardiovascular medicine, as it accounts for nearly half of all heart failure cases and presents unique therapeutic challenges. Unlike heart failure with reduced ejection fraction (HFrEF), where various pharmacological treatments have shown success, HFpEF has long been without effective, targeted therapies. Recently, sodium-glucose cotransporter-2 inhibitors (SGLT2i) have shown promise as a potential treatment for HFpEF, offering hope for improved outcomes. This chapter will explore the mechanism, clinical evidence, and guidelines of SGLT2i use in HFpEF, highlighting both the potential benefits and ongoing challenges.

UNDERSTANDING HEART FAILURE WITH PRESERVED EJECTION FRACTION

Heart failure with preserved ejection fraction is characterized by symptoms and signs of heart failure, a left ventricular ejection fraction (LVEF) of 50% or greater, and evidence of diastolic dysfunction. Unlike HFrEF, HFpEF patients exhibit normal or near-normal systolic function, but they suffer from increased ventricular stiffness, impaired relaxation, and increased left atrial pressure. These changes lead to pulmonary congestion and systemic symptoms. The pathophysiology of HFpEF is complex and involves multiple mechanisms including myocardial fibrosis, endothelial dysfunction, and systemic inflammation.

MECHANISM OF ACTION OF SODIUM–GLUCOSE COTRANSPORTER-2 INHIBITORS

The mechanism of action of SGLT2i in HFpEF[1] involves multiple pathways, primarily through their effects on the kidneys **(Flowchart 1)**:

- *SGLT2 inhibition in the kidneys:* SGLT2i block sodium and glucose reabsorption in the proximal tubule, promoting osmotic diuresis and natriuresis (sodium excretion), leading to a reduction in fluid retention.
- *Sodium-hydrogen exchanger 3 (NHE3) inhibition:* Indirectly, SGLT2 inhibition downregulates NHE3 activity, further enhancing sodium excretion.
- *Osmotic diuresis:* The reduction in glucose and sodium reabsorption causes increased water excretion, relieving congestion and reducing volume overload, improving symptoms in HFpEF.
- *Improved myocardial energy use:* By promoting the excretion of glucose, the heart shifts toward using free fatty acids and ketones as alternative energy sources, which are considered more efficient fuel sources for the failing heart.
- *Improved insulin sensitivity and reduced levels of hyperinsulinemia* can decrease the metabolic burden on the heart, potentially reducing inflammation and improving vascular health.
- *SGLT2i* have been shown to reduce inflammatory markers such as TNF-α and IL-6, which may help in reducing systemic inflammation that is often elevated in heart failure. This also reduces oxidative stress,

Flowchart 1: Mechanisms of SGLT2i in HFpEF and their effects on kidneys.

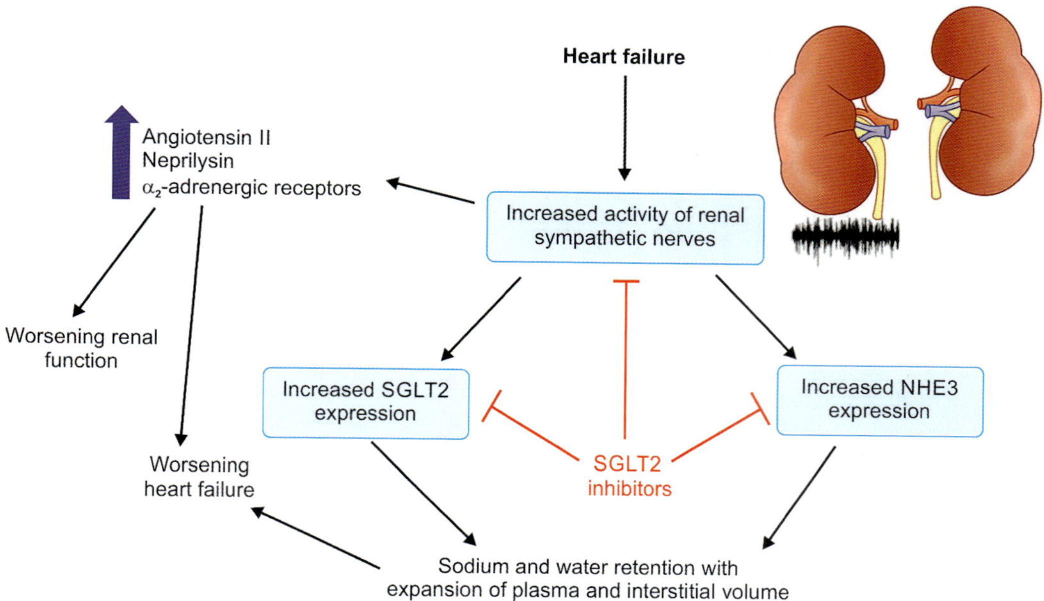

(HFpEF: heart failure with preserved ejection fraction; NHE3: sodium–hydrogen exchanger 3; SGLT2i: sodium–glucose cotransporter-2 inhibitors)

Source: Reproduced from Pandey et al.[2]

which helps in protecting the heart muscle and blood vessels from damage that exacerbates heart failure.

CLINICAL EVIDENCE SUPPORTING SODIUM–GLUCOSE COTRANSPORTER-2 INHIBITORS IN HEART FAILURE WITH PRESERVED EJECTION FRACTION

EMPEROR-Preserved Trial

The EMPEROR-Preserved trial[2] is one of the most pivotal studies investigating the efficacy of SGLT2i in HFpEF. This randomized, double-blind trial evaluated empagliflozin in patients with HFpEF (defined as an ejection fraction of 40% or higher). The primary endpoint was a composite of cardiovascular death or hospitalization for heart failure.

Results from the EMPEROR-Preserved trial demonstrated that empagliflozin significantly reduced the risk of the primary endpoint by 21% compared to placebo. This benefit was primarily driven by a reduction in heart failure hospitalizations, with a 29% relative risk reduction. These findings marked a major advancement, providing robust evidence for the use of SGLT2i in HFpEF.

DELIVER Trial

The DELIVER trial[3] assessed the effects of dapagliflozin in a broad spectrum of heart failure patients, including those with mildly reduced and preserved ejection fraction. Similar to EMPEROR-Preserved, this trial aimed to evaluate the impact on cardiovascular death and heart failure hospitalizations.

Dapagliflozin demonstrated a significant reduction in the combined risk of cardiovascular death or worsening heart failure events by 18% compared to placebo. This study reinforced the beneficial effects of SGLT2i across a wide range of heart failure phenotypes, including HFpEF.

The estimated cumulative incidence of the primary outcome in the two groups is shown in **Figure 1**.

GUIDELINES

The latest American College of Cardiology guidelines and expert consensus for the management of HFpEF assign specific recommendation classes to the use of SGLT2i as follows:

- *Class 1 recommendation (first-line treatment):* SGLT2i are strongly recommended as a first-line therapy for all patients with HFpEF who do not have contraindications.
- *Class 1 recommendation (management of comorbidities):* For patients with HFpEF and concurrent diabetes, SGLT2i are emphasized due to their dual benefits in managing both heart failure and diabetes.
- *Class 2a recommendation (symptom management and mortality reduction):* SGLT2i are suggested for reducing

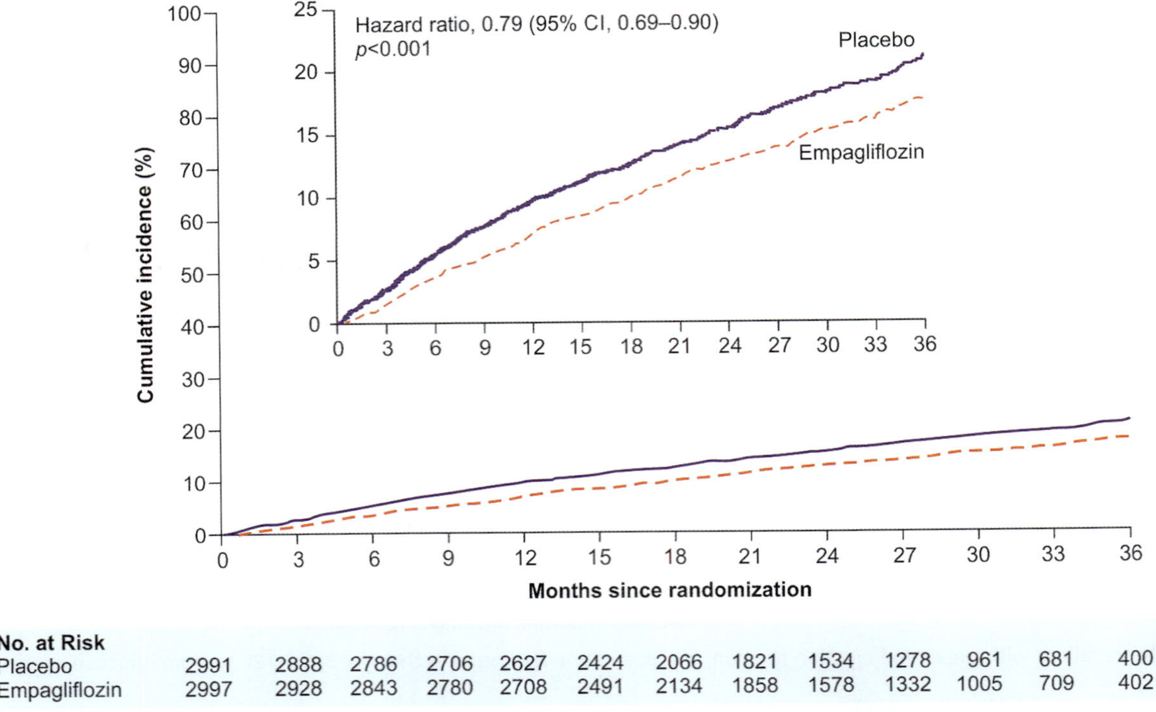

Fig. 1: Primary outcome, a composite of cardiovascular death or hospitalization for heart failure.
Source: Reproduced from Anker et al.[4]

symptoms and improving outcomes, particularly in reducing the risk of hospitalization due to heart failure. Although the evidence is strong, the class 2a designation reflects the need for further studies to confirm these benefits across all HFpEF subgroups.

LIMITATIONS

There are specific subgroups within the HFpEF population where the benefits of SGLT2i are less evident or the supporting evidence is less robust.[5]

- *Patients with very high ejection fraction (≥60%):* In patients with very high ejection fractions, the effectiveness of SGLT2i is often diminished. These individuals typically have different underlying pathophysiological mechanisms, such as increased left ventricular stiffness and diastolic dysfunction, which may not respond as well to SGLT2i.
- *Patients with significant right ventricular dysfunction:* For HFpEF patients with substantial right ventricular dysfunction or pulmonary hypertension, the benefits of SGLT2i may be reduced. This is because these drugs primarily target left ventricular function and fluid balance, rather than right ventricular issues.
- *Patients with severe kidney disease:* While SGLT2i are generally beneficial for patients with mild-to-moderate chronic kidney disease (CKD), their efficacy in HFpEF patients with advanced CKD (e.g., with an eGFR <30 mL/min/1.73 m^2) is less clear. These patients were often excluded from major clinical trials, leading to a gap in the available evidence.
- *Elderly patients with multiple comorbidities:* In elderly HFpEF patients who have multiple comorbid conditions, the benefits of SGLT2i may be less pronounced. The complex interplay of various health issues in these patients can dilute the effectiveness of SGLT2i on heart failure outcomes.

CONCLUSION

Sodium-glucose cotransporter-2 inhibitors represent a significant advancement in the treatment of HFpEF, a condition that has historically been difficult to manage effectively. The positive outcomes observed in recent clinical trials highlight their potential to fill a crucial therapeutic gap. As our understanding of their mechanisms and effects continues to evolve, SGLT2i may become a cornerstone in the management of HFpEF.[6] Future research should focus on elucidating the precise pathways through which these drugs exert their benefits, identifying patient subgroups that may derive the most benefit, and ensuring long-term safety and efficacy in diverse patient populations.

REFERENCES

1. Vaduganathan M, Januzzi JL, et al. Sodium-glucose cotransporter-2 inhibitors in heart failure: expanding indications and mechanisms. J Am Coll Cardiol. 2022; 79(22):2277-87.
2. Pandey AK, Bhatt DL, Pandey A, et al. Mechanisms of benefits of sodium-glucose cotransporter-2 inhibitors in heart failure with preserved ejection fraction. Eur Heart J. 2023;44(37):3640-51.
3. Solomon SD, McMurray JJV, Claggett B, et al. Dapagliflozin in heart failure with mildly reduced or preserved ejection fraction. N Engl J Med. 2022;387(12):1089-98.
4. Anker SD, Butler J, Filippatos G, et al. Empagliflozin in heart failure with a preserved ejection fraction. N Engl J Med. 2021;385(16):1451-61.
5. Packer M. Do sodium-glucose co-transporter-2 inhibitors prevent heart failure with a preserved ejection fraction by counterbalancing the effects of leptin? A novel hypothesis. Diabetes Obes Metab. 2018;20(6):1361-6.
6. Heidenreich PA, Bozkurt B, Aguilar D, et al. 2022 AHA/ACC/HFSA guideline for the management of heart failure: a report of the American College of Cardiology/American Heart Association Joint Committee on clinical practice guidelines. J Am Coll Cardiol. 2022;79(17):e263-421.

CHAPTER

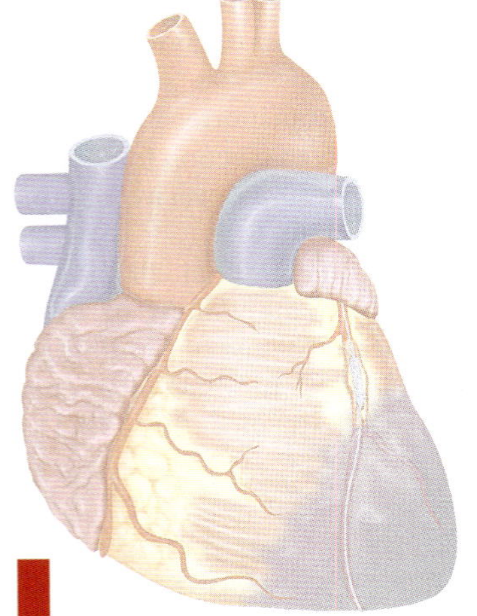

Dapagliflozin with Sitagliptin in HFpEF and Diabetes

Mohit Tayal, Ankit Tandon, Rohit Tandon

INTRODUCTION

Heart failure (HF) is broadly categorized into three subcategories:

1. Heart failure with reduced ejection fraction [HFrEF (EF <40%)],
2. Heart failure with mid-range ejection fraction [HFmrEF (EF = 40–50%)], and
3. Heart failure with preserved ejection fraction HFpEF (EF >50%).[1]

The HFpEF now accounts for >50% of cases of HF, with comparable outcomes.

Multiple registries report incidence of HFrEF, HFmrEF, and HFpEF to be approximate 54%, 21%, and 24%, respectively. Prevalence of HFpEF relative to HFrEF may continue to increase due to, increasing age, and increased prevalence of obesity and reduction in death from other comorbidities.[2]

Identifiable risk factors are old age, hypertension, obesity, diabetes, and coronary artery disease. Incidence of HFpEF is significantly higher in women than in men. Diabetes mellitus especially is also associated with increased left ventricular (LV) stiffness through cardiomyocyte hypertrophy and myocardial deposition of collagen and advanced glycation end products, leading to HF.[3]

INTRIGUING INSIGHTS IN PATHOPHYSIOLOGY OF HFpEF (FIG. 1)

Multiple mechanisms lead to HFpEF. These include dysfunctional atrial and ventricular active relaxation, increased passive stiffness of left ventricle, and reduction in arterial compliance, endothelial oxidative stress associated with a decreased nitric oxide bioavailability, causes vasoconstriction, and enhances a proinflammatory and prothrombotic state. Cardiac remodeling is affected by changes in the composition and structure of the extracellular matrix with fibrillar collagen deposition.[4]

The LV diastolic dysfunction is the final disease expression of heterogeneous phenotypes and clinical presentations.

Four clinically recognized phenotypes in HFpEF are:

1. Aging phenotype
2. Obesity phenotype
3. Ischemic heart disease phenotype
4. Pulmonary artery hypertension phenotype.[5]

EMERGING ROLE OF DAPAGLIFLOZIN IN HFpEF

Despite advances in management of HFrEF, there is no approved targeted therapy for treatment of HFpEF. Currently physician has to rely on management of comorbidities. However various drugs including ARNI, MRA, ARBs, sodium-glucose cotransporter 2 (SGLT2) inhibitors are being investigated, of which SGLT2 inhibitors have gained most significance.

The SGLT2 is responsible for reabsorption of 90% of the urinary glucose in the proximal tubule. Inhibition of SGLT2 induces glucosuria, which is more pronounced in hyperglycemic individuals owing to the higher amounts of filtered glucose. The effect of glucosuria diminishes with normalizing of blood glucose levels. In addition dapagliflozin also enhance natriuresis, it changes tissue sodium handling, lower systolic blood pressure, and reduce body mass **(Fig. 2)**.

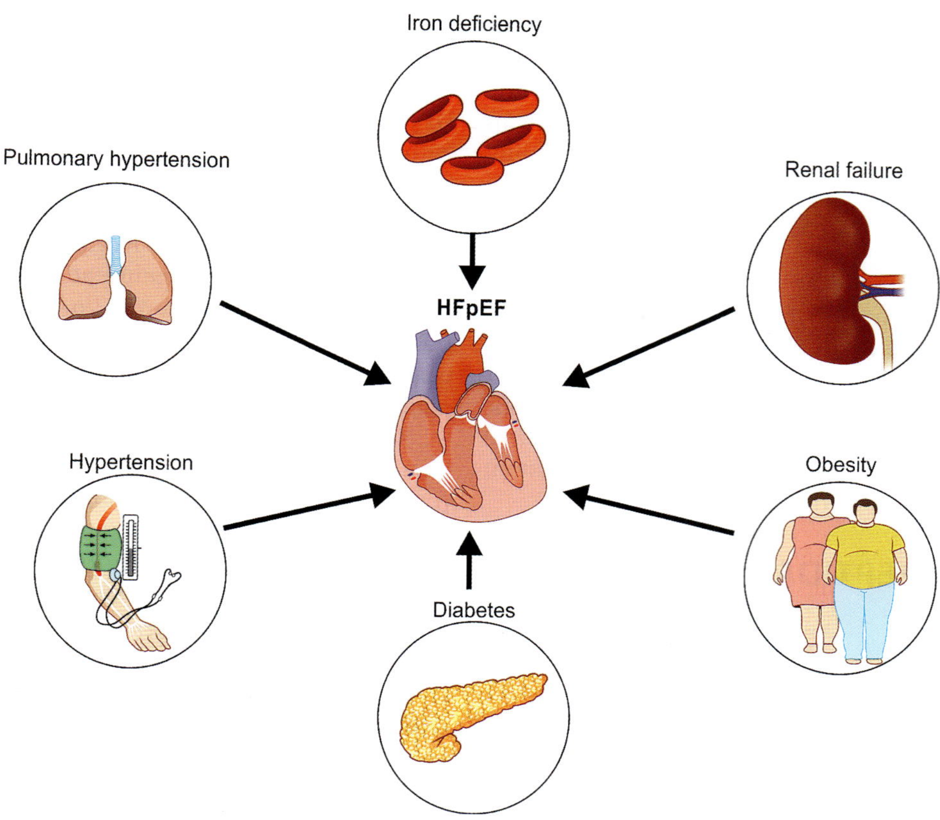

Fig. 1: Effects of comorbidities in heart failure with preserved ejection fraction.

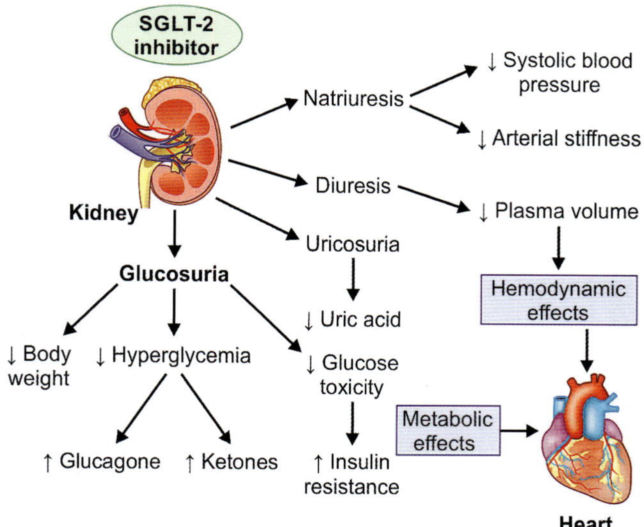

Fig. 2: Primary mechanisms of action of sodium-glucose cotransporter 2 (SGLT2) inhibitors and their hemodynamic and metabolic effects resulting in improved myocardial function and a reduced risk of heart failure.

Two randomized clinical trials of 5,988 (EMPEROR-preserved) and 6,263 (DELIVER trial) patients demonstrated benefit of SGLT2 inhibitors (empagliflozin or dapagliflozin 10 mg orally once daily) versus placebo in patients with HFpEF. Both studies demonstrated an 18–21% reduction in the rate of HF hospitalization or cardiovascular death and benefit was due to lower rates of HF hospitalizations, with no significant reduction in cardiovascular mortality.

The results of DELIVER trial indicate that dapagliflozin is superior to placebo in improving HF outcomes among patients with symptomatic stable mildly reduced or preserved LVEF (EF >40%), irrespective of diabetes status, duration of HF baseline diuretic use, and baseline NT-proBNP levels. Benefit is primarily driven by a reduction in HF hospitalizations, not mortality. The benefit of dapagliflozin was consistent across the range of frailty, baseline SBP, and BMI categories. Improvement in health-related quality of life with dapagliflozin occurred early and was greater among patients with greater frailty and higher BMI.

Recently DAPA-MODA trial results showed that initiation of dapagliflozin in patients with stable chronic HF is associated with a reduction of LAVI, LV mass, and natriuretic peptides after 6 months. These findings support the concept of left atrium as part of global adverse remodeling in HF, regardless of LVEF, and suggest that dapagliflozin may have the ability to reverse cardiac remodeling as part of its benefit in HF patients. This trial was specifically designed to assess effects of dapagliflozin on left atrial (LA) remodeling based on principle that left atrium plays a critical role in cardiac function, particularly in LV filling during diastole and atrial dysfunction can directly lead to pulmonary congestion. LA remodeling occurs in HF irrespective of the degree of LV systolic dysfunction, and can be observed in the presence of preserved or reduced LVEF.[4,5] The geometry of the left atrium is a predictor for the development of HF in high-risk patients, and has been consistently linked to higher rates of hospitalization and death in patients with HF. This trial supported the promising results of the randomized IDDIA (The Impact of Dapagliflozin on Left Ventricular Diastolic Dysfunction in Patients with Type 2 Diabetes Mellitus) trial done only on 60 patients, which showed that treatment with dapagliflozin improved LV diastolic dysfunction.

DIPEPTIDYL PEPTIDASE-4 IN HFpEF (FIG. 3)

Like SGLT2 inhibitors, dipeptidyl peptidase-4 (DPP-4) inhibitors are important drugs for DM control. DPP-4 inhibitors block proteolytic DPP-4 enzyme activity, which results in an increase in glucagon-like peptide 1 and thus lowers blood glucose levels. Initially, beneficial effects of DPP-4 inhibitors on CV diseases were not established in clinical trials (SAVOR-TIMI trial using saxagliptin). Recently, conclude TECOS trial using sitagliptin, EXAMINE trial using alogliptin, and CARMELINA trial using linagliptin, however did not report increase in heart failure hospitalizations.[6,7]

There are no trials to assess the relationship between DPP-4 inhibitors and long-term prognosis in patients with established HF except for small scale single-center observational study indicating beneficial effects of DPP-4 inhibitors in HF patients.

Recently data taken from JROADHF (Japanese Registry of Acute Decompensated Heart Failure) registry a retrospective, multicenter, nationwide registry of hospitalized patients with HF showed DPP-4 inhibitor use was associated with better long-term outcomes in HFpEF patients with DM.[8]

Subgroup analysis of the PROLOGUE trial that focused on the effect of sitagliptin on echocardiographic parameters of diastolic function. The key finding of the study was that addition of sitagliptin to conventional diabetic care significantly attenuated the increase in echocardiographic parameters of diastolic function (E/e), relative to conventional treatment alone. Use of DPP-4 inhibitors was significantly associated with reduced risk of cardiovascular events including mortality in patients with diabetes who underwent PCI in which insulin-like growth factor-1, one of the substrates of catalytic degradation of DPP-4, may play a part and also favorable prognostic impact of DPP-4 inhibitors was further enhanced in individuals who are not overweight [body mass index (BMI <25 kg/m^2)] compared with those who are overweight (BMI >25 kg/m^2).[9]

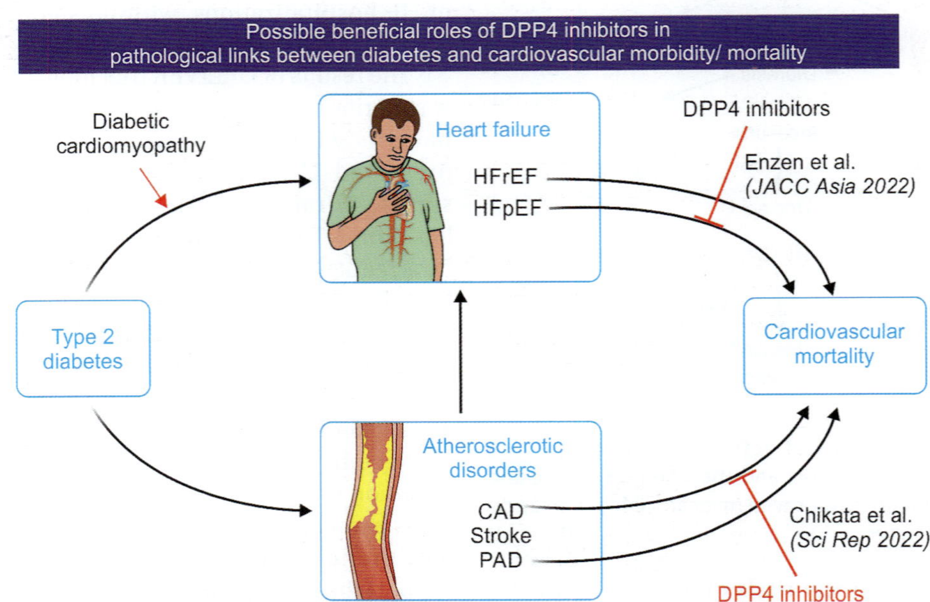

Fig. 3: Beneficial roles of dipeptidyl peptidase-4 (DPP-4) inhibitors in pathological link between diabetes mellitus (DM) and cardiovascular (CVS) morbidity/mortality. (DPP-4: dipeptidyl peptidase-4; HFrEF: heart failure with reduced ejection fraction; HFpEF: heart failure with preserved ejection fraction)

COMBINED USE OF SITAGLIPTIN AND DAPAGLIFLOZIN—A SHORT EXPERIENCE (FLOWCHART 1)

Reported clinical evidence suggest utility of fixed-dose combination of dapagliflozin and sitagliptin shown to be effective in uncontrolled T2DM or T2DM with multiple cardiovascular risk factors. Dapagliflozin reported to be effective as add-on therapy to sitagliptin with or without metformin in a 24-week, multicenter, randomized, double-blind, and placebo-controlled study. As reported, in patients with type 2 diabetes, inadequately controlled on sitagliptin with or without metformin, add-on treatment with dapagliflozin provides additional clinical benefit with well tolerability. Around 432 patients were randomized in the study to receive dapagliflozin 10 mg/day or placebo added to sitagliptin (100 mg/day) ± metformin (≥1,500 mg/day). In this trial, baseline HbA1c and FPG levels were 7.9% (63.0 mmol/mol) and 162.2 mg/dL (9.0 mmol/L) for the dapagliflozin group and 8.0% (64.0 mmol/mol) and 163 mg/dL (9.0 mmol/L) for placebo. At week 24, dapagliflozin significantly reduced mean HbA1c levels [-0.5% (-4.9 mmol/mol)] versus placebo [0.0% (+0.4 mmol/mol)]. Dapagliflozin reduced body weight versus placebo (-2.1 and -0.3 kg) and reduced HbA1c levels in patients with baseline values ≥8.0% [-0.8% (8.7 mmol/mol) and 0.0% (0.3 mmol/mol)] and fasting plasma glucose levels [-24.1 mg/dL (-1.3 mmol/L) and 3.8 mg/dL (0.2 mmol/L)]. Similar results were observed when data were stratified by background therapy. Glycemic and weight benefits observed at week 24 were maintained through week 48. Changes from baseline in systolic blood pressure at week 8 were not significantly different between treatment groups. Over 48 weeks, fewer patients receiving dapagliflozin were discontinued or rescued for failing to achieve glycemic targets compared with placebo. Adverse events were balanced between groups, and discontinuation rates were low. At week 48, signs and symptoms suggestive of genital infection were more frequent with dapagliflozin (9.8%) than with placebo (0.4%). Signs and symptoms suggestive of urinary tract infection were balanced between dapagliflozin (6.7%) and placebo (6.2%).[10]

Flowchart 1: Pharmacological benefits of dipeptidyl peptidase-4 (DPP-4) inhibitors and sodium-glucose cotransporter 2 (SGLT2) inhibitors on cardiovascular system (CVS).

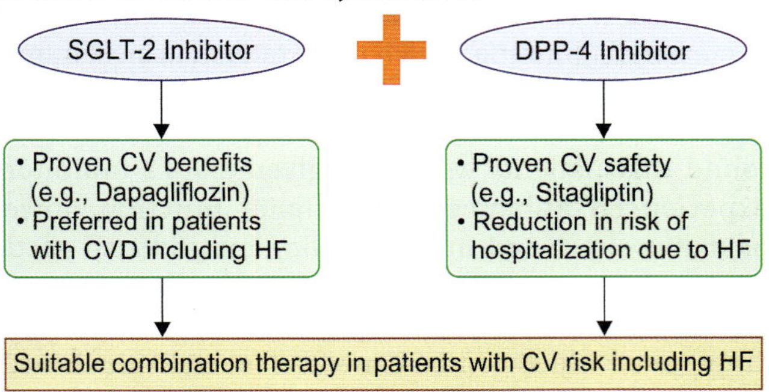

(CVD: cardiovascular disease; HF: heart failure)

CONCLUSION

Primary goal of treatment for a diabetic patient with or without HFpEF is adequate glucose control. Both dapagliflozin and sitagliptin have been tried individually and in combination in various trials with evident benefits regarding cardiovascular outcomes. Thus, so far it looks imperative that physicians should be encouraged to employ this combination in a typical patient of diabetic HFpEF.

REFERENCES

1. Escobar C, Palacios B, Varela L, et al. Prevalence, characteristics, management and outcomes of patients with heart failure with preserved, mildly reduced, and reduced ejection fraction in spain. J Clin Med. 2022; 11(17):5199.
2. Oktay AA, Rich JD, Shah SJ. The emerging epidemic of heart failure with preserved ejection fraction. Curr Heart Fail Rep. 2013;10(4):401-10.
3. Gupta M, Rao S, Manek G, et al. The role of dapagliflozin in the management of heart failure: an update on the emerging evidence. Ther Clin Risk Manag. 2021;17:823-30.
4. Strachinaru M, Roussoulières A, Manintveld OC, et al. Sodium-glucose cotransporter 2 inhibitors for chronic heart failure: The ultimate solution. Eur J Heart Fail. 2023; 25(8):1361-3.
5. Volpe M, Gallo G. Cardiometabolic phenotype of heart failure with preserved ejection fraction as a target of sodium-glucose co-transporter 2 inhibitors and glucagon-like peptide receptor agonists. Cardiovasc Res. 2021;117(9): 1992-4.
6. Scirica BM, Bhatt DL, Braunwald E, et al. Saxagliptin and cardiovascular outcomes in patients with type 2 diabetes mellitus. N Engl J Med. 2013;369(14):1317-26.
7. White WB, Cannon CP, Heller SR, et al. Alogliptin after acute coronary syndrome in patients with type 2 diabetes. N Engl J Med. 2013;369(14):1327-35.
8. Yamada H, Tanaka A, Kusunose K, et al. Effect of sitagliptin on the echocardiographic parameters of left ventricular diastolic function in patients with type 2 diabetes: a subgroup analysis of the PROLOGUE study. Cardiovasc Diabetol. 2017;16(1):63.
9. Chikata Y, Iwata H, Miyosawa K, et al. Dipeptidyl peptidase-4 inhibitors reduced long-term cardiovascular risk in diabetic patients after percutaneous coronary intervention via insulin-like growth factor-1 axis. Sci Rep. 2022;12(1):5129.
10. Jabbour SA, Hardy E, Sugg J, et al. Dapagliflozin is effective as add-on therapy to sitagliptin with or without metformin: a 24-week, multicenter, randomized, double-blind, placebo-controlled study. Diabetes Care. 2014;37(3):740-50.

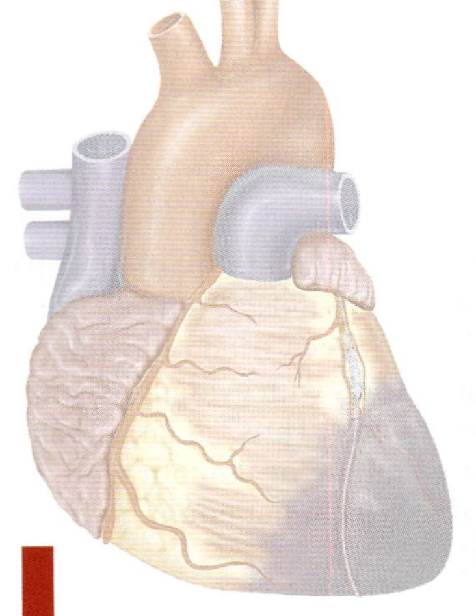

SGLT2 Inhibitor and DPP-4 Inhibitor Combination in Diabetes Mellitus with HFpEF

Sunil Modi, Ranjan Modi

INTRODUCTION

Both preclinical and clinical investigations have demonstrated substantial beneficial effects of sodium-glucose cotransporter 2 (SGLT2) inhibitors on several organs and tissues, including the kidney, liver, pancreas, blood plasma, blood vessels, and adipose tissue. These effects lead to a decrease in the workload of the heart, a reduction in tissue scarring, a decrease in oxygen demand, and a decrease in the enlargement of the left ventricle. SGLT2 inhibitors exert their impact by targeting SGLT2, a sodium-glucose cotransporter found on the apical membrane of the renal proximal convoluted tubules. The majority of glucose reabsorption in the kidney, over 90%, is carried out by this component, whereas the remaining portion is accomplished by SGLT1 in the descending section of the loop of Henle.[1] The disparity in glucose concentration between the cytoplasm and plasma facilitates the passive transport of glucose through the basolateral membrane. The occurrence of glucosuria as a result of SGLT2 inhibition is directly proportional to the concentration of glucose in the bloodstream. SGLT2 inhibitors demonstrate a moderate effectiveness in decreasing plasma glucose levels, resulting in a reduction in HbA1c by around 0.5–1%.

DISCUSSION

The SGLT2 inhibitors have a diuretic and natriuretic action, causing a reduction in plasma volume. This reduction is crucial in preventing fluid retention and worsening of heart failure. In contrast to conventional diuretics, these drugs have demonstrated the ability to decrease both intravascular volume and interstitial fluid. This method can have negative consequences on patients with heart failure who already have reduced intravascular volume, potentially leading to resistance to diuretic treatment.

The diuretic impact of SGLT2 inhibitors is linked to a decrease in preload and left ventricular filling pressure, as well as stretching of the heart muscle and the development of fibrous tissue in the heart's interstitial space. Moreover, the drop in extracellular fluid volume is linked to a decrease in blood pressure,[2,3] which is further intensified by the decrease in body mass caused by SGLT2 inhibitors.[3] This weight loss is associated with elevated glucose excretion in the urine and depletion of extracellular fluid. In their study, Böhm et al. found that the SGLT2 inhibitor empagliflozin decreased the likelihood of heart failure, as well as cardiovascular and renal complications, regardless of the average systolic blood pressure seen during the trial.[4] These findings indicate that empagliflozin has a cardiovascular and heart failure impact that is not dependent on blood pressure.

Research has demonstrated that SGLT2 inhibitors decrease albuminuria, which is the ratio of urine albumin to creatinine, and impede the advancement from microalbuminuria to macroalbuminuria.[5] Studies have found that patients who were given SGLT2 inhibitors experienced enhanced endothelial function, lower oxidative stress and inflammation, and reduced aortic stiffness.[6] These mechanisms are linked to a decrease in central blood pressure, pulse pressure, and forward wave amplitude,[7] which can be beneficial for individuals with heart failure. Recent investigations have uncovered a decrease in the sympathetic nervous system in individuals who have been treated with SGLT2 inhibitors.[8] This finding may partially account for the positive effects observed in patients with heart failure.

SODIUM-GLUCOSE COTRANSPORTER 2 INHIBITORS IN HEART FAILURE WITH PRESERVED EJECTION FRACTION

There is a lack of data on the use of SGLT2 inhibitors in heart failure with preserved ejection fraction (HFpEF), and the existing studies have a small sample size. From a pathophysiological standpoint, the prescription of these drugs can be justified due to their favorable impact on reducing left ventricular filling pressure and improving left ventricular diastolic function. These are crucial factors in the treatment of HFpEF. The network meta-analysis, which was recently published, demonstrated that SGLT2 inhibitors exhibited the most significant decrease in the probability of hospitalization for heart failure when compared to a placebo.[9] Furthermore, there was a notable decrease in risk when comparing SGLT2 inhibitors to both GLP-1R agonists and Dipeptidyl peptidase-4 (DPP-4) inhibitors. A study showed that SGLT2 inhibitors have a 99.6% likelihood of being the most effective medication for reducing the risk of heart failure, followed by GLP-1 agonists (0.27%) and DPP-4 inhibitors (0.1%).[9]

A recent study found that a 6-month treatment with dapagliflozin led to a significant improvement in left ventricular diastolic function (measured by E/e' and left atrial volume index) in patients with HFpEF and diabetes mellitus (DM), despite no significant change in B-type natriuretic peptide (BNP) levels.[10] Upon reevaluation of the data, it was shown that there was a significant improvement in both left ventricular diastolic function and left ventricular longitudinal strain. However, this improvement was observed only in patients with HFpEF, and not in subjects with HFrEF.[11] The enhancement in left ventricular longitudinal strain was not influenced by demographic, clinical, or echocardiographic factors related with E/e' following the injection of dapagliflozin.[11]

The EMPEROR-Preserved study, which is currently the largest trial on this subject, included 5,988 symptomatic HF patients with a left ventricular ejection fraction (LVEF) >40%, some of whom had type 2 DM. One-third of the patients had an LVEF between 40 and 50%, indicating heart failure with mid-range LVEF, while two-thirds had an LVEF greater than 50%, indicating HFpEF.[12] Comorbidities such as diabetes (49%) and chronic kidney disease (50%) were frequently observed among the patients. The majority of the patients were treated with angiotensin-converting enzyme inhibitors/angiotensin receptor blockers/ angiotensin receptor-neprilysin inhibitors (80%), and β-blockers (86%). Additionally, 37% of the patients were prescribed mineralocorticoid receptor antagonists.[12] This trial yielded significant insights into the efficacy of SGLT2 inhibitors, specifically dapagliflozin, in relation to outcomes and left ventricular remodeling in patients with HFpEF and heart failure with mid-range ejection fraction (HFmrEF).

ROLE OF DIPEPTIDYL PEPTIDASE-4 INHIBITORS IN CARDIOVASCULAR SYSTEM

The DPP-4 inhibitors are enzymes that break down two hormones, GLP-1 and GIP, which are produced in the gut and help regulate insulin release in response to glucose. DPP-4 inhibitors have gradually supplanted sulfonylureas as a treatment for type 2 DM in some countries. This is because DPP-4 inhibitors do not cause hypoglycemia or weight gain, and they have a favorable safety profile. Additionally, they can be used comfortably even in patients with chronic renal failure.[13] While DPP-4 inhibitors primarily utilize the GLP-1 route, they do not exhibit the same level of cardiovascular protection as GLP-1R antagonists.[13] The reasons likely stem from the fact that other substances regulated by DPP-4, such as stromal cell-derived factor-1 and brain natriuretic peptide, also have an effect on the heart. This is why there are disagreements about the role of DPP-4 inhibitors in worsening heart failure and increasing hospitalizations in these patients. The majority of studies demonstrated that DPP-4 inhibitors were only equivalent to other treatments in terms of significant adverse cardiovascular events, such as stroke, nonfatal myocardial infarction, and cardiovascular death.[14-16] The provided results are derived from significant trials that examined the impact of saxagliptin, alogliptin, sitagliptin, and linagliptin.[15-17] Nevertheless, there was some apprehension due to certain studies indicating a higher incidence of hospitalization caused by heart failure.[14] However, a research examining the impact of sitagliptin on individuals with DM did not discover any rise in hospitalizations caused by heart failure.[18] This also substantiates the continuing debates regarding the effectiveness of DPP-4 inhibitors in patients with DM who also have cardiovascular problems.

DIPEPTIDYL PEPTIDASE-4 INHIBITORS IN HEART FAILURE

A comprehensive assessment, involving over 500,000 individuals with DM, half of whom received treatment with DPP-4 inhibitors, compared the effects of DPP-4 inhibitors with sulfonylurea. The study found no discernible difference in the incidence of heart failure between these two groups.[19] The scientists conducted a comparison of various DPP-4 inhibitors and discovered that sitagliptin and linagliptin were linked to a reduced risk of hospitalization for heart failure compared to sulfonylurea. Vildagliptin and saxagliptin demonstrated a decreased incidence of heart failure when compared to sulfonylurea, however these changes did not reach statistical significance.[19]

A randomized placebo-controlled trial done in individuals with DM and HFrEF found that vildagliptin did not have any effect on LVEF after a 12-month period of treatment.[20] Nevertheless, patients who received vildagliptin experienced a notable increase in left ventricular volume during the end-diastolic phase. The CARMELINA trial demonstrated that linagliptin had no impact on the occurrence of hospitalization due to heart failure, the combined outcome of cardiovascular death and hospitalization due to heart failure, or the likelihood of recurring heart failure events when compared to a placebo.[21] The meta-analysis, which combined data from five studies, demonstrated a slightly elevated risk of hospital admission for heart failure in patients who were treated with DPP-4 inhibitors[22] compared to the control group. However, this finding was only marginally significant.[23] However, it is challenging to account for all potential confounding factors in a meta-analysis, which may lead to uncertainty regarding its ultimate findings.

Additional meta-analyses, which examined the impact of saxagliptin, alogliptin, sitagliptin, and linagliptin on hospitalization rates for heart failure (HF), separately analyzed patients with and without a history of HF. These analyses concluded that DPP-4 inhibitors did not increase the risk of hospitalization for HF in patients with prior HF. However, in diabetic patients without a history of HF, DPP-4 inhibitors were found to elevate the risk of hospitalization for HF.[23] The study found that GLP-1 receptor antagonists had a little helpful effect, but SGLT2 inhibitors had a considerable good effect, on reducing hospitalization in both groups, regardless of whether they had a history of heart failure or not. Authorities issued a caution about the careful prescribing of DPP-4 inhibitors in patients with type 2 DM and a history of heart failure or kidney impairment due to inconsistent findings. The warning specifically pertained to saxagliptin and alogliptin, excluding other DPP-4 inhibitors. However, it is important to note that this group of medications is quite diverse. The European Society for Heart Failure has highlighted a significant difference between saxagliptin, which may increase the risk of hospitalization for heart failure, and other DPP-4 inhibitors such as alogliptin, sitagliptin, vildagliptin, and linagliptin, which do not have a negative impact on hospitalization rate.

The TOPLEVEL trial of tenegliptin was done which targeted LV diastolic dysfunction in T2DM patients. This study demonstrated the effectiveness of DDP-4 inhibitors on LV diastolic dysfunction, an important surrogate end point to predict the CV outcomes of HFpEF.[24] A study conducted on animals found that inhibiting DPP-4 had no impact on LV hypertrophy, although it did enhance cardiac function and reduce myocardial and perivascular fibrosis.[25] The results suggest that inhibiting DPP-4 slows down the evolution of heart failure by altering the characteristics and amount of cardiac fibrosis. This could explain why these drugs are used in patients with HFpEF.

CONCLUSION

Novel antidiabetic medications are gradually improving the course of DM treatment; nevertheless, their impact on CV result, and especially on the effects in patients with HF, is still mainly unknown and may perhaps be overestimated. The information now available about the use of SGLT2 inhibitors in HFrEF patients is highly positive, but more research is needed to determine how they affect HFpEF patients. Particularly with regard to the latter class of drugs, the effects of GLP-1R agonists and DPP-4 inhibitors on patients with heart failure have been far less studied and the findings are debatable. Thus, further data regarding the effects of these drugs in patients with HF, and especially in those with HFpEF, should come from currently active trials. Preclinical research revealed beneficial effects of novel antidiabetic medications in HFpEF, which is extremely important from a clinical standpoint because there are currently few effective treatment options for this sizable population of HF patients. At present though individually both SGLT2i and DDP 4i have shown ground breaking advantages but we do not have enough data on FDC fixed dose combination of dapagliflozin and linagliptin in HFpEF in diabetic patients. We are awaiting the newer trials to answer the question soon.

REFERENCES

1. Wojcik C, Warden BA. Mechanisms and evidence for heart failure benefits from SGLT2 inhibitors. Curr Cardiol Rep. 2019;21(10):130.
2. Kario K, Okada K, Kato M, et al. 24-Hour blood pressure-lowering effect of an SGLT-2 Inhibitor in patients with diabetes and uncontrolled nocturnal hypertension: results from the randomized, placebo-controlled SACRA study. Circulation. 2018;139(18):2089-97.

3. Teo YH, Teo YN, Syn NL, et al. Effects of sodium/glucose cotransporter 2 (SGLT2) Inhibitors on cardiovascular and metabolic outcomes in patients without diabetes mellitus: a systematic review and meta-analysis of randomized-controlled trials. J Am Heart Assoc. 2021;10(5):e019463.
4. Böhm M, Fitchett D, Ofstad AP, et al. Heart failure and renal outcomes according to baseline and achieved blood pressure in patients with type 2 diabetes: results from EMPA-REG OUTCOME. J Hypertens. 2020;38(9): 1829-40.
5. Bae JH, Park EG, Kim S, et al. Effects of sodium-glucose cotransporter 2 inhibitors on renal outcomes in patients with type 2 diabetes: a systematic review and meta-analysis of randomized controlled trials. Sci Rep. 2019;9(1): 13009.
6. Ugusman A, Kumar J, Aminuddin A, et al. Endothelial function and dysfunction: Impact of sodium-glucose cotransporter 2 inhibitors. Pharmacol Ther Mar. 2021;1: 107832.
7. Papadopoulou E, Loutradis C, Tzatzagou G, et al. Dapaglifozin decreases ambulatory central blood pressure and pulse wave velocity in patients with type 2 diabetes: a randomized, double-blind, placebo-controlled clinical trial. J Hypertens. 2021;39(4):749-58.
8. Matthews VB, Elliot RH, Rudnicka C, et al. Role of the sympathetic nervous system in regulation of the sodium glucose cotransporter 2. J Hypertens. 2017;35(10):2059-68.
9. Kramer CK, Ye C, Campbell S, et al. Comparison of new glucose-lowering drugs on risk of heart failure in type 2 diabetes: a network meta-analysis. JACC Heart Fail. 2018;6(10):823-30.
10. Otagaki M, Matsumura K, Kin H, et al. Effect of tofoglifozin on systolic and diastolic cardiac function in type 2 diabetic patients. Cardiovasc Drugs Ther. 2019;33(4):435-42.
11. Tanaka H, Soga F, Tatsumi K, et al. Positive effect of dapaglifozin on left ventricular longitudinal function for type 2 diabetic mellitus patients with chronic heart failure. Cardiovasc Diabetol. 2020;19(1):6.
12. Anker SD, Butler J, Filippatos G, et al.; EMPEROR-Preserved Trial Committees and Investigators. Baseline characteristics of patients with heart failure with preserved ejection fraction in the EMPEROR-Preserved trial. Eur J Heart Fail. 2020;22(12):2383-92.
13. Scheen AJ. Cardiovascular efects of new oral glucose lowering agents: DPP-4 and SGLT-2 inhibitors. Circ Res. 2018;122(10):1439-59.
14. Scirica BM, Bhatt DL, Braunwald E, et al.; SAVOR-TIMI 53 Steering Committee and Investigators. Saxagliptin and cardiovascular outcomes in patients with type 2 diabetes mellitus. N Engl J Med. 2013;369(14):1317-26.
15. White WB, Cannon CP, Heller SR, et al.; EXAMINE Investigators. Alogliptin after acute coronary syndrome in patients with type 2 diabetes. N Engl J Med. 2013;369(14): 1327-35.
16. Green JB, Bethel MA, Armstrong PW, et al.; TECOS Study Group. Effect of sitagliptin on cardiovascular outcomes in type 2 diabetes. N Engl J Med. 2015;373(3):232-42.
17. Mulvihill EE, Drucker DJ. Pharmacology, physiology, and mechanisms of action of dipeptidyl peptidase-4 inhibitors. Endocr Rev. 2014;35(6):992-1019.
18. Rosenstock J, Kahn SE, Johansen OE, et al. CAROLINA Investigators. Effect of linagliptin vs glimepiride on major adverse cardiovascular outcomes in patients with type 2 diabetes: The CAROLINA Randomized Clinical Trial. JAMA. 2019;322(12):1155-66.
19. Kim YG, Yoon D, Park S, et al. Dipeptidyl peptidase-4 inhibitors and risk of heart failure in patients with type 2 diabetes mellitus: a population based cohort study. Circ Heart Fail. 2017;10(9):e003957.
20. McMurray JJV, Ponikowski P, Bolli GB, et al. VIVIDD Trial Committees and Investigators. Efects of vildagliptin on ventricular function in patients with type 2 diabetes mellitus and heart failure: a randomized placebo-controlled trial. JACC Heart Fail. 2018;6(1):8-17.
21. McGuire DK, Alexander JH, Johansen OE, et al. CARMELINA Investigators. Linagliptin effects on heart failure and related outcomes in individuals with type 2 diabetes mellitus at high cardiovascular and renal risk in CARMELINA. Circulation. 2019;139(3):351-61.
22. Li L, Li S, Deng K, et al. Dipeptidyl peptidase-4 inhibitors and risk of heart failure in type 2 diabetes: systematic review and meta-analysis of randomized and observational studies. BMJ. 2016;352:i610.
23. Pan X, Xu S, Li J, et al. The Effects of DPP-4 Inhibitors, GLP-1RAs, and SGLT-2/1 inhibitors on heart failure outcomes in diabetic patients with and without heart failure history: insights from CVOTs and drug mechanism. Front Endocrinol (Lausanne). 2020;11:599355.
24. Imazu M, Nakano A, Ito S, et al.; TOPLEVEL investigators and study coordinators. Effects of teneligliptin on the progressive left ventricular diastolic dysfunction in patients with type 2 diabetes mellitus in open-label, marker-stratified randomized, parallel-group comparison, standard treatment-controlled multicenter trial (TOPLEVEL Study): rationale and study design. Cardiovasc Drugs Ther. 2019;33(3):363-70.
25. Hirose M, Takano H, Hasegawa H, et al. The effects of dipeptidyl peptidase-4 on cardiac fibrosis in pressure overload-induced heart failure. J Pharmacol Sci. 2017; 135(4):164-73.

CHAPTER

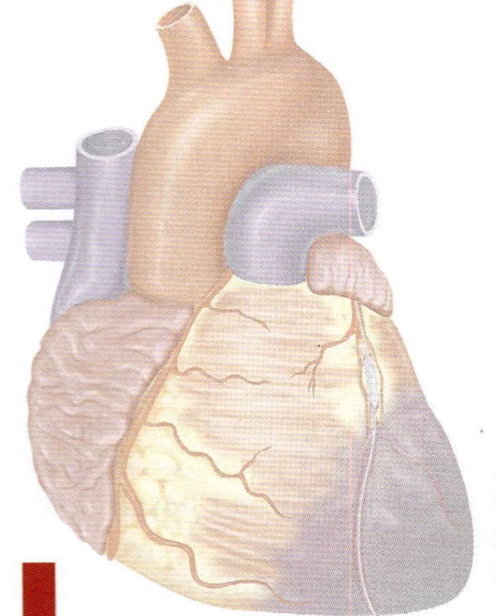

Left Atrial Failure in HFpEF: The Role of SGLT2is, ARNI, Bisoprolol, and MRAs

Harinder K Bali, Navdeep S Sidhu

INTRODUCTION

In recent years, there has been a growing emphasis on the role of left atrium (LA) structure and function in the pathophysiology and the clinical course of heart failure (HF), rather than it being only a passive conduit for the blood flow into the left ventricle (LV).[1] Left atrial volume was the initial parameter used to integrate the severity and duration of LV diastolic dysfunction and an important marker of adverse events. Recently, many studies have explored novel parameters of LA function such as LA strain, LA emptying fraction (LAEF), left atrial sphericity index (LASI), LA ejection force, mitral annular A' velocity, etc., as important determinants of adverse major cardiovascular (CV) events, including death and HF admissions in patients with heart failure with reduced ejection fraction (HFrEF) as well as heart failure with preserved ejection fraction (HFpEF), and have indicated that these may be more strongly associated with adverse outcomes in these patients, as compared to LA volume or dimensions.[2]

On comparing the LA structure/function in HFrEF and HFpEF, it has been suggested that the predominant LA abnormality in HFrEF consists of eccentric LA remodeling and dilatation, whereas in HFpEF it consists of increased LA stiffness and higher LA pressure pulsatility.[3] Although there is less severe impairment of global LA function in HFpEF than in HFrEF, there is stronger association of LA impairment with mortality in HFpEF, implying a greater susceptibility to the loss of LA function in HFpEF patients.[3]

LEFT ATRIAL FUNCTION: FROM ATRIAL REMODELING TO ATRIAL FAILURE

The LA dysfunction or failure were previously viewed as a marker or a consequence of the underlying valvular or ventricular abnormalities, but recently it has been recognized as an important clinical entity which may occur without overt ventricular or valvular pathologies and portend a worse prognosis. Bisbal et al. have recently characterized atrial cardiomyopathy, atrial remodeling, and atrial failure as three different, but interconnected entities.[4]

The atrial remodeling is considered as the cellular, structural, or electrical changes in atrial myocytes in response to various abnormal mechanical, electrical, or metabolic factors (like pressure or volume overload, tachyarrhythmias) resulting in persistent changes in LA structure (enlargement, increased sphericity), function, or electrochemical properties. Atrial cardiomyopathy indicates a diseased state of the atrial myocardium with electrical and/or mechanical dysfunction and exhibiting increased myocardial fibrosis, hypertrophy, or dilatation. The pathophysiological processes of atrial remodeling and atrial cardiomyopathy, result in a diseased and fibrotic atrium and ultimately lead to the development of signs and symptoms of atrial dysfunction or failure. Although these authors define atrial failure as "any atrial dysfunction causing impaired heart performance and symptoms and worsening quality of life or life expectancy, in the absence of significant valvular or ventricular abnormalities," it is important to recognize that these three phenomena

Flowchart 1: Pathogenic pathways for atrial failure.

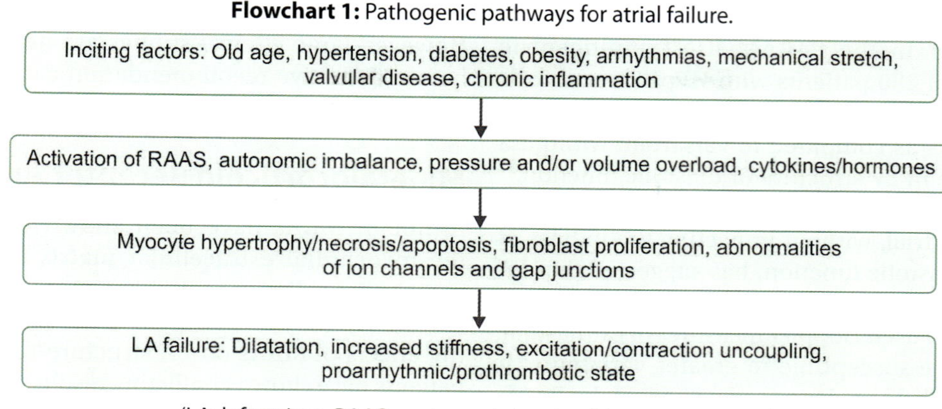

(LA: left atrium; RAAS: renin-angiotensin-aldosterone system)

are intricately intertwined and must be considered as a pathophysiological continuum, with LA remodeling resulting in or being caused by atrial cardiomyopathy and the associated symptoms pointing toward the progression of the disease into the stage of atrial failure **(Flowchart 1)**.

Whether the changes of atrial remodeling or cardiomyopathy occur due to an idiopathic atrial cardiomyopathy or a secondary cause, the resultant perturbations in the mechanical, functional, or electrical functions of LA, ultimately culminating in the clinical manifestations of LA failure such as increased thromboembolic risk (which may be independent of the increased risk of atrial fibrillation), adverse LV hemodynamics (HF), myocardial ischemia, and pulmonary hypertension.[4]

MANAGEMENT OF LEFT ATRIAL FAILURE IN HEART FAILURE WITH PRESERVED EJECTION FRACTION

Till date, the diagnostic and therapeutic strategies for the LA failure in HFpEF have not been standardized. LA may represent an important independent target for a therapeutic approach in HFpEF and reverse LA remodeling is feasible as shown in patients after surgery for mitral valve disease and in hypertensive patients after treatment with angiotensin converting enzyme (ACE) inhibitors.[5] Reverse remodeling of the LA with reduction in its volume and/or pressure may exert a beneficial effect on the LV function and compliance as a result of LA-LV interdependency.[6]

Some of the potential therapies for LA failure include treatment of underlying valvular/ventricular abnormality, decongestive measures (use of diuretics, interatrial shunt devices, LA decompression pumps, etc.), management of atrial fibrillation (consideration for rhythm control, oral anticoagulation), extracellular matrix modulation [mineralocorticoid receptor antagonists (MRAs)], therapies targeting endothelial-cardiomyocyte interactions [angiotensin receptor neprilysin inhibitor (ARNI)], and LA inotropy (cardiac myosin activators).[7] In the following paragraphs, we discuss the effects of sodium-glucose transport protein 2 inhibitors (SGLT2is), ARNI, β-adrenergic antagonists (especially bisoprolol), and MRAs on LA dysfunction or failure in HFpEF.

Sodium-glucose Transport Protein 2 Inhibitors

These drugs have been approved for use in both HFrEF and HFpEF patients, given their salutary CV effects as demonstrated by robust clinical evidence from multiple large randomized controlled trials (RCTs). SGLT2is reduce plasma volume, cardiac preload, afterload, and myocardial oxygen consumption by inducing glycosuria, natriuresis, and osmotic diuresis. As a result, these medications may help to decrease left atrial dilatation.

Empagliflozin effectively reduced the effects of hypertension-related left atrial dilatation, LA, and LV fibrosis and corrected the elevated expression of PPAR, natriuretic peptides, and TNF-α in the atria and ventricles in animal research using a model of HFpEF in hypertensive rats.[8] In the CAMEO-DAPA RCT in patients with HFpEF, treatment with dapagliflozin resulted in significant reduction in pulmonary capillary wedge pressure (PCWP), an important surrogate for LA pressure and function.[9] However, large prospective studies are needed to further elucidate the effects of SGLT2is on LA remodeling and function in patients with HFpEF.

Angiotensin Receptor Neprilysin Inhibitor

The ARNI (sacubitril-valsartan) has revolutionized the treatment of HFrEF and has shown some positive effects on outcomes in female patients with HFpEF and in

HFpEF patients with a lower range of ejection fraction (LVEF: 45–57%).[10] In the PARAMOUNT multicentric RCT comprising of 290 patients with HFpEF, sacubitril-valsartan significantly reduced left atrial volume index (LAVI) at 36 weeks as compared to valsartan, without a significant change in LV structure or diastolic function.[11] The rapid reverse LA remodeling with the use of ARNI in the PARAMOUNT trial, without impacting the indices of LV structure or diastolic function, has suggested that LA remodeling may be a better predictor of LV filling pressures than the commonly used Doppler measures of LV diastolic function which are susceptible to greater variability. It has been postulated that a decreased activity of the RAAS, coupled with an augmented natriuretic peptide activity have incremental benefits in terms of improvement in CV hemodynamics and LA reverse remodeling.[12]

The mechanisms underlying the benefits of sacubitril-valsartan with regard to LA structure and function are probably multifactorial. Many animal studies have demonstrated that sacubitril-valsartan can decrease interstitial fibrosis, decrease myolysis, and contractile protein loss.[13] It has also been demonstrated to shorten the duration of paroxysmal AF and may prevent it from turning into permanent AF. Other beneficial mechanisms include cardiac unloading, improved hemodynamics, and decreased myocardial stress, and myocardial work.[14]

Bisoprolol

β-blockers are an established treatment for HFrEF, however their role in the management of HFpEF is still controversial with lack of sufficient clinical data. Nevertheless, in the real-world practice, β-blockers are commonly prescribed in patients with HFpEF.[15] Many potential pathways for positive effects of β-blockers in HFpEF have been postulated including, the inhibition of detrimental effects of sympathetic overactivation, attenuation of myocardial hypertrophy, and fibrosis, antioxidant and anti-inflammatory effects of some β-blockers such as bisoprolol and carvedilol. It is plausible that these drug may reduce the occurrence of de novo atrial fibrillation (AF) in patients with HFpEF, similar to that seen in patients with HFrEF.[16] β-blockers may also aid in the improvement of LA cardiomyopathy by prolonging the relative refractory period of atrial myocytes, in addition to lowering heart rates and enabling an extended LV filling time.[17]

Bisoprolol has been shown to favorably alter the collagen metabolism in the myocardial extracellular matrix, thus potentiating cardiac reverse-remodeling.[18] In a rat model of diastolic HF, bisoprolol especially at high doses resulted in improved survival, probably related to its antioxidative and anti-inflammatory properties.[19] However, large clinical studies are needed in this field before definitive recommendation can be made for the clinical practice.

Mineralocorticoid Receptor Antagonists

Although MRAs have been shown to favorably alter the myocardial extracellular matrix and decrease the myocardial collagen matrix, a major contributor toward the LA myopathy/failure; the clinical studies evaluating the effects of MRAs on LA structure/function in HFpEF patients have shown conflicting results.

In an RCT by Mak et al. in 44 HFpEF patients, treatment with eplerenone for 12 months did not result in any significant effect on LAVI as compared to placebo.[20] A similar RCT by Deswal et al. in 44 HFpEF patients, eplerenone therapy for 6 months did not differ from placebo in terms of changes in LA volume.[21] In an echocardiographic substudy consisting of 239 HFpEF patients in the "Treatment of Preserved Cardiac Function Heart Failure With an Aldosterone Antagonist (TOPCAT)" trial, spironolactone therapy did not lead to meaningful improvements in LA and LV structure or function; however an overall decrease in LA volume was independently associated with a lower risk of CV death, hospitalization for HF, or aborted cardiac arrest.[22]

The possible mechanisms responsible for this lack of effect on LA structure/function may be the lesser susceptibility of the LA myocardium to modification by MRAs in advanced stages of HFpEF, or the requirement of a longer time period for the antifibrotic effects of MRAs to manifest in terms of meaningful changes in LA structure or function.[12,22]

CONCLUSION

Left atrial structure and function are important determinants of clinical outcomes in patients with HFpEF and represent an emerging target for new therapies. However, given the lack of robust clinical data in this field, large well designed clinical trials are necessary before definite recommendations can be made for the clinical practice.

REFERENCES

1. Triposkiadis F, Pieske B, Butler J, et al. Global left atrial failure in heart failure. Eur J Heart Fail. 2016;18(11): 1307-20.
2. Pellicori P, Zhang J, Lukaschuk E, et al. Left atrial function measured by cardiac magnetic resonance imaging in patients with heart failure: clinical associations and prognostic value. Eur Heart J. 2015;36(12):733-42.

3. Melenovsky V, Hwang SJ, Redfield MM, et al. Left atrial remodeling and function in advanced heart failure with preserved or reduced ejection fraction. Circ Heart Fail. 2015;8(2):295-303.
4. Bisbal F, Baranchuk A, Braunwald E, et al. Atrial failure as a clinical entity: JACC review topic of the week. J Am Coll Cardiol. 2020;75(2):222-32.
5. Rossi A, Gheorghiade M, Triposkiadis F, et al. Left atrium in heart failure with preserved ejection fraction: structure, function, and significance. Circ Heart Fail. 2014; 7(6):1042-9.
6. Inciardi RM, Rossi A. Left atrium: a forgotten biomarker and a potential target in cardiovascular medicine. J Cardiovasc Med (Hagerstown). 2019;20(12):797-808.
7. Peigh G, Shah SJ, Patel RB. Left atrial myopathy in atrial fibrillation and heart failure: clinical implications, mechanisms, and therapeutic targets. Curr Heart Fail Rep. 2021;18(3):85-98.
8. Lee HC, Shiou YL, Jhuo SJ, et al. The sodium-glucose co-transporter 2 inhibitor empagliflozin attenuates cardiac fibrosis and improves ventricular hemodynamics in hypertensive heart failure rats. Cardiovasc Diabetol. 2019;18(1):45.
9. Borlaug BA, Reddy YNV, Braun A, et al. Cardiac and metabolic effects of dapagliflozin in heart failure with preserved ejection fraction: The CAMEO-DAPA trial. Circulation. 2023;148(10):834-44.
10. Solomon SD, McMurray JJV, Anand IS, et al. PARAGON-HF Investigators and Committees. Angiotensin-Neprilysin Inhibition in Heart Failure with Preserved Ejection Fraction. N Engl J Med. 2019;381(17):1609-20.
11. Solomon SD, Zile M, Pieske B, et al. Prospective comparison of ARNI with ARB on Management Of heart failUre with preserved ejectioN fracTion (PARAMOUNT) Investigators. The angiotensin receptor neprilysin inhibitor LCZ696 in heart failure with preserved ejection fraction: a phase 2 double-blind randomised controlled trial. Lancet. 2012;380:1387-95.
12. Inciardi RM, Bonelli A, Biering-Sorensen T, et al. Left atrial disease and left atrial reverse remodelling across different stages of heart failure development and progression: a new target for prevention and treatment. Eur J Heart Fail. 2022;24(6):959-75.
13. Li LY, Lou Q, Liu GZ, et al. Sacubitril/valsartan attenuates atrial electrical and structural remodelling in a rabbit model of atrial fibrillation. Eur J Pharmacol. 2020;881:173120.
14. Dong Y, Zhai Z, Wang J, et al. Angiotensin receptor-neprilysin inhibitor delays progression from paroxysmal to persistent atrial fibrillation. Sci Rep. 2023;13(1):3140.
15. Xu X, Wang DW. The progress and controversial of the use of beta blockers in patients with heart failure with a preserved ejection fraction. Int J Cardiol Heart Vasc. 2019; 26:100451.
16. Kotecha D, Flather MD, Altman DG, et al. Heart rate and rhythm and the benefit of beta-blockers in patients with heart failure. J Am Coll Cardiol. 2017;69(24):2885-96.
17. Kotecha D, Holmes J, Krum H, et al. Efficacy of β blockers in patients with heart failure plus atrial fibrillation: an individual-patient data meta-analysis. Lancet. 2014; 384(9961):2235-43.
18. Fukui M, Goda A, Komamura K, et al. Changes in collagen metabolism account for ventricular functional recovery following beta-blocker therapy in patients with chronic heart failure. Heart Vessels. 2016;31(2):173-82.
19. Nishio M, Sakata Y, Mano T, et al. Beneficial effects of bisoprolol on the survival of hypertensive diastolic heart failure model rats. Eur J Heart Fail. 2008;10(5):446-53.
20. Mak GJ, Ledwidge MT, Watson CJ, et al. Natural history of markers of collagen turnover in patients with early diastolic dysfunction and impact of eplerenone. J Am Coll Cardiol. 2009;54(18):1674-82.
21. Deswal A, Richardson P, Bozkurt B, et al. Results of the randomized aldosterone antagonism in heart failure with preserved ejection fraction trial (RAAM-PEF). J Card Fail. 2011;17(8):634-42.
22. Shah AM, Claggett B, Sweitzer NK, et al. Prognostic importance of changes in cardiac structure and function in heart failure with preserved ejection fraction and the impact of spironolactone. Circ Heart Fail. 2015;8(6): 1052-8.

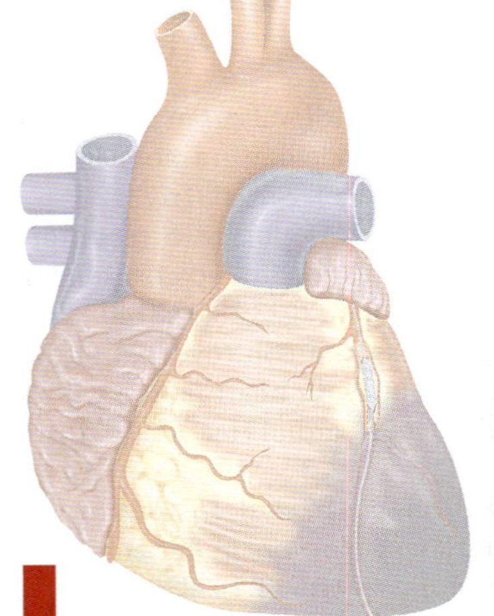

Development of Treatment Selection Algorithm for SGLT2 Inhibitors in HFpEF

Devesh Kumar, Nirmal Ghati

INTRODUCTION

Heart failure (HF) is a life-threatening syndrome characterized by significant morbidity, poor functional capacity, and high mortality rates. It affects >64 million people worldwide.[1] The global prevalence of HF is gradually increasing due to the easy availability of guideline-directed therapy to prolong the survival of ischemic heart disease patients and the increasing prevalence of the aged population. Almost half the patients with HF have an ejection fraction of >50% and these are classified as heart failure with preserved ejection fraction (HFpEF).[1,2] The last 2 decades have witnessed a renaissance in the drug treatment of patients with heart failure with reduced ejection (HFrEF) fraction. However, there is a big lacuna in the pharmacological treatment of patients with HFpEF with no drugs having a proven mortality benefit besides SGLT2 inhibitors.

Thus, SGLT2 inhibitors form the core therapy for patients with HFpEF with recent evidence from randomized control trials showing a significant reduction in both morbidity and mortality. In this chapter, we aim to review the mechanism of action, evidence, current guidelines, and precautions while using SGLT2 inhibitors in patients with HFpEF.

MECHANISM OF ACTION

The SGLT2 inhibitors act on multiple diverse pathways and regulate key steps to produce dramatic cardio-metabolic effects **(Flowchart 1)**. Therefore, any single mechanism with the most clinical impact is difficult to elucidate. They inhibit the reabsorption of sodium and glucose from the proximal convoluted tubules in the kidney and subsequently cause natriuresis, diuresis, and glucosuria. As a consequence, systolic blood pressure decreases by 3 mm Hg and HbA1c reduces by 0.6–1%.[3] As increased sodium and glucose reach distally to the renal tubules, it results in the activation of tubuloglomerular feedback leading to vasoconstriction of the afferent arteriole, a decrease in intraglomerular pressure, and a decrease in proteinuria.[4]

The cardiometabolic effects of SGLT2 inhibitors outnumber the minuscule benefits produced by the mechanisms mentioned above as these drugs impact multiple pathways of inflammation and regulate the autonomic nervous system **(Flowchart 1)**. They inhibit inflammatory pathways involved in HF by promoting autophagy and lysosomal degradation, increasing the circulating burden of vascular progenitor cells, promoting vascular function; promote the release of EPO by the kidneys; and cause excretion of uric acid in urine.[5] They enhance cardiac metabolism by promoting the use of ketones, helping the energy-deprived myocytes with an additional fuel.[6] By lowering HbA1c, they decrease the oxidative damage due to free radical injury. Further, they lower weight by 2–3 kilograms and positively modulate the lipid profile by increasing HDL cholesterol and decreasing triglyceride levels.[7]

Besides these well-known mechanisms, various newer mechanisms have recently been discovered that help to improve the overall cardiac diastolic function. SGLT2 inhibitors decrease the epicardial adipose tissue and alter adipocyte signaling, thus decreasing the oxidative stress

Flowchart 1: Mechanisms of action of SGLT2 inhibitors in patients with HFpEF.

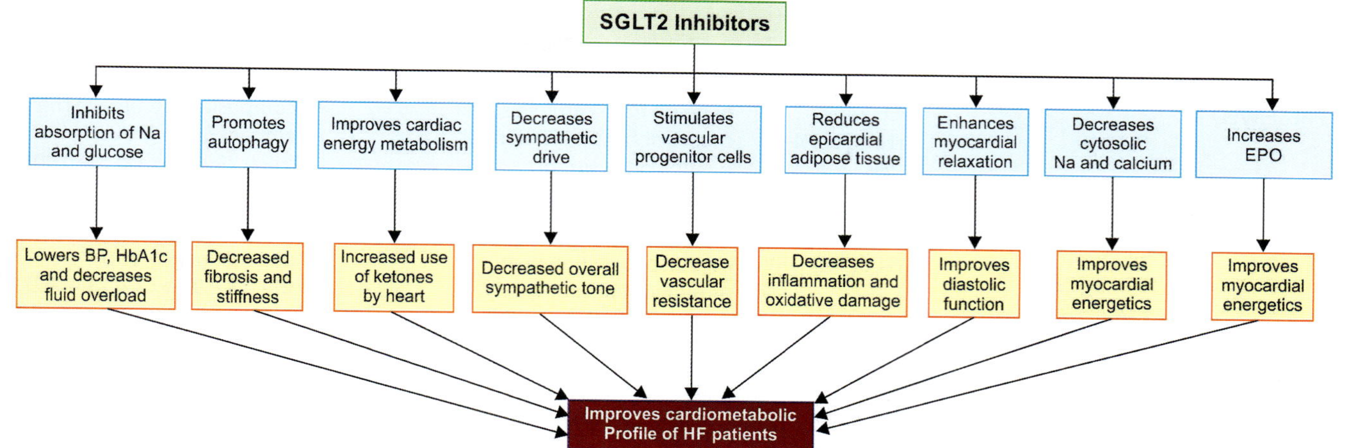

(BP: blood pressure; EPO: erythropoietin; HF: heart failure)

and overall inflammation.[8,9] These drugs also augment myofilament relaxation and reduce extracellular matrix remodeling, thus decreasing fibrosis and improving diastolic function.[10] SGLT2 inhibitors impact cardiomyocyte ionic homeostasis by lowering the cytosolic sodium and calcium in the myocytes, thus improving cardiac energetics.[11] Lastly, they have been shown to improve cardiac energetics and function by inducing a nutrient-deprived and hypoxic-like transcriptional paradigm in addition to increasing ketosis, erythropoietin, and autophagic flux.[12,13]

Therefore, SGLT2 inhibitors work through various novel mechanisms to improve myocardial relaxation, decrease inflammation, and improve myocardial energetics and truly are the first novel class of disease-modifying drugs in patients with HFpEF.

EVIDENCE FOR USE IN HFpEF

The EMPA-REG OUTCOME trial was the first trial that highlighted the benefits of SGLT2 inhibitors when used for patients with diabetes and high cardiovascular risk and showed a significant decrease in HF hospitalizations.[14] This was further highlighted in other trials, namely, CANVAS, CREDENCE, and DECLARE-TIMI-58. The results of these trials gave rise to two clinical questions: (1) Will they be beneficial in patients already diagnosed with heart failure, and (2) will they have the same impact on nondiabetics as they had in the diabetic populations in the trials mentioned above?

The SGLT2 inhibitors were initially tested in patients with heart failure with reduced ejection fraction (HFrEF) in the EMPEROR-REDUCED and the DAPA-HF trial and showed a significant reduction in mortality, morbidity, and HF hospitalization.[15,16] The findings of both these studies were concordant and clinically significant with a significant reduction in mortality as well as morbidity resulting in SGLT2 inhibitors becoming one of the major pillars for the management of HFrEF.

Having shown promising results in the HFrEF population, they were subsequently tested in a population with HFpEF. HFpEF is a unique disease where no drugs had a proven mortality benefit or improvement in hospitalizations. These patients with HFpEF account for half of the total population living with HF, and hence, efforts were underway to develop a drug that reduces morbidity and mortality in this population.

The EMPEROR–PRESERVED AND DELIVER **(Table 1)** were two subsequent trials that included patients with ejection fraction >40% and NYHA Class II–IV. Both trials showed a significant reduction in the primary endpoint (composite of cardiovascular death and HF hospitalization) in the treatment arm as compared to the placebo arm, which was due to a profound reduction in HF hospitalizations.[17,18]

The SOLOIST-WHF and EMPULSE trials showed the positive impact of these drugs when tested in patients with acute HF. Both these trials showed a significant reduction in deaths and hospitalization when applied to patients with acute HF.[19,20] Most clinicians now begin SGLT2 inhibitors once the patient is decongested and in the hospital to optimize the drug therapy at discharge.

The compelling results from these trials have motivated the European Society of Cardiology (ESC) to recommend SGLT2 inhibitors in all patients with HFpEF and heart failure with mid-range ejection fraction (HFmrEF) in NYHA Class II–IV symptoms as a class 1 indication. These are the only class of drugs along with loop diuretics

TABLE 1: Summary of the evidence from randomized trials showing benefits in patients with HFpEF and acute heart failure.

Study	*Drug*	*Patient*	*Inclusion criteria*	*Primary endpoints*	*Follow-up (months)*	*Outcomes*
EMPEROR-PRESERVED	Empagliflozin	5,988	>18 years LVEF >40% NYHA Class II–IV	Primary composite outcome of death from cardiovascular causes or hospitalization for HF (first or recurrent)	26	*Reduction* in the primary composite outcome in the empagliflozin group (HR 0.79; 95% CI, 0.69–0.90)
DELIVER	Dapagliflozin	10,584	>18 years LVEF >40% NYHA Class II–IV	Primary composite outcome of worsening HF (hospitalization or an urgent visit resulting in IV therapy for HF) or death from cardiovascular causes	28	*Reduction* in the primary composite outcome in the dapagliflozin group (HR 0.82; 95% CI, 0.73–0.92)
SOLOIST-WHF	Sotagliflozin	1,222	18–85 years with DM and admitted for AHF	Total number of deaths from cardiovascular causes, hospitalizations, and urgent visits	9	*Reduction* in the primary end-point events in the sotagliflozin group (HR 0.67; 95% CI, 0.52–0.85
EMPULSE	Empagliflozin	530	>18 years, hospitalized with worsening HF with volume overload	Hierarchical composite outcome of time to all-cause death, the number of HF exacerbations, time to first HF exacerbation, and a 5-point or greater difference in change from baseline in KCCQ-TSS after 90 days of treatment	3	*Empagliflozin was superior* in 53.9% of paired comparisons and placebo was superior in 39.7%, whereas 6.4% of comparisons were tied (win ratio 1.36, 95% CI 1.09–1.68)

that have class 1 indication in all patients with HFpEF. Therefore, irrespective of the ejection fraction, SGLT 2 inhibitors should be prescribed to all patients with HF.

SIDE EFFECTS

The SGLT2 inhibitors are unique with a wide spectrum of side effects like orthostatic hypotension and genitourinary infections. Euglycemic ketoacidosis, amputations, and bone fractures are rare but amount the most dreaded complications. A meta-analysis of 77 trials with more than 52,000 patients showed that the risk of urinary infections was minuscule (1.05 times that of the control population), and hence, the actual risk, if any, was very nonsignificant.[21] On the other hand, genital infections (RR 1.29) are more frequent in this population. Most genital infections are very mild and need topical treatment or a single dose of oral fluconazole.

Limb amputations (2.7/1,000 person-years) and bone fractures (15.4/1,000 person-years) are rare complications unique and limited to canagliflozin (CANVAS trial), and hence, use should be abstained in any high-risk patient.[22] Another rare, yet fatal complication is euglycemic ketoacidosis (1.3/1,000 person-years) as these drugs favor lipolysis, thus mobilizing ketones. So, any patient on an SGLT2 inhibitor with a decreased intake of food or suffering from acute illness should transiently withhold these medications.[23]

CONTRAINDICATIONS

Absolute contraindications to SGLT2 inhibitors are pregnancy, end-stage renal disease (eGFR <15 mL/min/1.73 m^2), type-1 diabetes mellitus, history of anaphylaxis to SGLT2 inhibitor, acute kidney injury, shock, and hemodynamic instability.[24]

GUIDELINES

The SGLT2 inhibitors have been given a class 1 recommendation by ACC and ESC for use in patients with HFpEF as they are the only family of drugs that have shown a reduction in mortality, morbidity, and HF hospitalization.[25,26]

CONCLUSION

The SGLT2 inhibitors are the cornerstone for therapy in patients with HF across the entire spectrum of ejection fraction. Randomized trials have shown a significant reduction in both morbidity and mortality and a significant reduction in HF hospitalizations in patients with both

HFrEF and HFpEF. They may cause postural hypotension and genitourinary infections and may transiently worsen renal function once initiated; hence, they should be used with utmost caution, especially in the geriatric population. Cost is a major obstacle in the uptake of these drugs in the Indian context; however, they are being used more commonly with decreasing clinical inertia and increasing patient awareness. Appropriate implementation of SGLT2 inhibitor therapy in HFpEF patients across the widespread spectrum of T2DM and chronic kidney disease is very crucial to improve event-free survival and reduce associated healthcare costs.

REFERENCES

1. Braunwald E. The war against heart failure: The Lancet lecture. Lancet. 2015;385(9970):812-24.
2. Pfeffer MA, Shah AM, Borlaug BA. Heart Failure with preserved ejection fraction in perspective. Circ Res. 2019; 124(11):1598-617.
3. Mazidi M, Rezaie P, Gao HK, et al. Effect of sodium-glucose cotransport-2 inhibitors on blood pressure in people with type 2 diabetes mellitus: A systematic review and meta-analysis of 43 randomized control trials with 22,528 patients. J Am Heart Assoc. 2017;6(6):e004007.
4. Ferrannini E, Baldi S, Frascerra S, et al. Renal handling of ketones in response to sodium-glucose cotransporter 2 inhibition in patients with type 2 diabetes. Diabetes Care. 2017;40(6):771-6.
5. Mazer CD, Hare GMT, Connelly PW, et al. Effect of empagliflozin on erythropoietin levels, iron stores, and red blood cell morphology in patients with type 2 diabetes mellitus and coronary artery disease. Circulation. 2020;141(8):704-7.
6. Ferrannini E, Mark M, Mayoux E. CV protection in the EMPA-REG OUTCOME Trial: A "Thrifty Substrate" Hypothesis. Diabetes Care. 2016;39(7):1108-14.
7. Cai X, Yang W, Gao X, et al. The association between the dosage of SGLT2 inhibitor and weight reduction in type 2 diabetes patients: A meta-analysis. Obesity (Silver Spring). 2018;26(1):70-80.
8. Kalman E, Chan J, Goel V, et al. SGLT2 inhibitors reduce epicardial adipose tissue: A meta-analysis. Heart Lung Circ. 2022;31:S179-80.
9. Wu P, Wen W, Li J, et al. Systematic review and meta-analysis of randomized controlled trials on the effect of SGLT2 inhibitor on blood leptin and adiponectin level in patients with type 2 diabetes. Horm Metab Res. 2019; 51(8):487-94.
10. Pabel S, Wagner S, Bollenberg H, et al. Empagliflozin directly improves diastolic function in human heart failure. Eur J Heart Fail. 2018;20(12):1690-700.
11. Uthman L, Baartscheer A, Bleijlevens B, et al. Class effects of SGLT2 inhibitors in mouse cardiomyocytes and hearts: Inhibition of Na^+/H^+ exchanger, lowering of cytosolic Na^+ and vasodilation. Diabetologia. 2018;61(3):722-6.
12. Hoong CWS, Chua MWJ. SGLT2 inhibitors as calorie restriction mimetics: Insights on longevity pathways and age-related diseases. Endocrinology. 2021;162(8).
13. Packer M. Autophagy stimulation and intracellular sodium reduction as mediators of the cardioprotective effect of sodium-glucose cotransporter 2 inhibitors. Eur J Heart Fail. 2020;22(4):618-28.
14. Zinman B, Wanner C, Lachin JM, al.; EMPA-REG OUTCOME Investigators. Empagliflozin, cardiovascular outcomes, and mortality in type 2 diabetes. N Engl J Med. 2015;373(22):2117-28.
15. McMurray JJV, Solomon SD, Inzucchi SE, et al.; DAPA-HF Trial Committees and Investigators. Dapagliflozin in patients with heart failure and reduced ejection fraction. N Engl J Med. 2019;381(21):1995-2008.
16. Petrie MC, Verma S, Docherty KF, et al. Effect of dapagliflozin on worsening heart failure and cardiovascular death in patients with heart failure with and without diabetes. JAMA. 2020;323(14):1353-68.
17. Anker SD, Butler J, Filippatos G, et al. Empagliflozin in heart failure with a preserved ejection fraction. N Engl J Med. 2021;385(16):1451-61.
18. Solomon SD, McMurray JJV, Claggett B, et al.; DELIVER Trial Committees and Investigators. Dapagliflozin in heart failure with mildly reduced or preserved ejection fraction. N Engl J Med. 2022;387(12):1089-98.
19. Bhatt DL, Szarek M, Steg PG, et al.; SOLOIST-WHF Trial Investigators. Sotagliflozin in patients with diabetes and recent worsening heart failure. N Engl J Med. 2021; 384(2):117-28.
20. Voors AA, Angermann CE, Teerlink JR, et al. The SGLT2 inhibitor empagliflozin in patients hospitalized for acute heart failure: A multinational randomized trial. Nat Med. 2022;28(3):568-74.
21. Liu J, Li L, Li S, et al. Effects of SGLT2 inhibitors on UTIs and genital infections in type 2 diabetes mellitus: A systematic review and meta-analysis. Sci Rep. 2017;7(1):2824.
22. Neal B, Perkovic V, Mahaffey KW, et al. Canagliflozin and cardiovascular and renal events in type 2 diabetes. N Engl J Med. 2017;377(7):644-57.
23. Goldenberg RM, Berard LD, Cheng AYY, et al. SGLT2 inhibitor-associated diabetic ketoacidosis: Clinical review and recommendations for prevention and diagnosis. Clin Ther. 2016;38(12):2654-64.e1.
24. Simes BC, MacGregor GG. Sodium-glucose cotransporter-2 (SGLT2) inhibitors: a clinician's guide. Diabetes Metab Syndr Obes. 2019;12:2125-36.
25. McDonagh TA, Metra M, Adamo M, et al.; ESC Scientific Document Group. 2023 focused update of the 2021 ESC guidelines for the diagnosis and treatment of acute and chronic heart failure. Eur Heart J. 2023;44(37): 3627-39.
26. Heidenreich PA, Bozkurt B, Aguilar D, et al. 2022 AHA/ACC/HFSA Guideline for the Management of Heart Failure: A Report of the American College of Cardiology/American Heart Association Joint Committee on Clinical Practice Guidelines. Circulation. 2022;145(18): e895-1032.

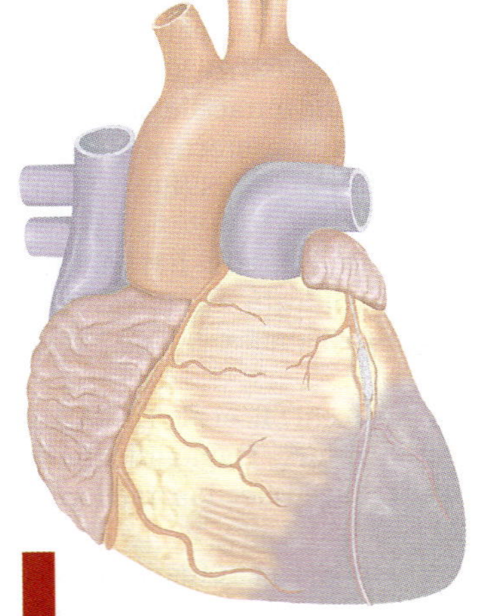

Role of SGLT2 Inhibitors in Cardiac Remodeling Reversal: Beyond Glycemic Control in HFpEF

Mukesh Sharma, Piyush Tak, SK Kaushik

INTRODUCTION

Cardiac remodeling is defined as molecular, cellular, and interstitial changes that manifest clinically as changes in the mass, geometry (e.g., wall thickness and shape), size, and function of the heart, and it is an important determinant of the development and progression of heart failure (HF).

In adverse cardiac remodeling (ACR), LV loses its ellipse, elongated, bullet-like contour and becomes more spherical. There is anatomical remodeling (LV hypertrophy and dilatation), molecular remodeling (proinflammatory proteins activation), histological remodeling (interstitial myocardial fibrosis, capillary paucity, and hypertrophy of cardiomyocytes), neurohormonal remodeling (RAAS activation), and metabolic remodeling (myocardial energy level switching).[1] ACR is the primary mechanism of HF characterized by increased apoptosis and necrosis, increased metabolic errors, and blunted mitophagy. If prolonged, this ACR can result in myocardial fibrosis promoting ventricular stiffness and impair ventricular contraction, leading to both systolic and diastolic HF. Diastolic dysfunction is mainly caused by defects in myocardial relaxation, ventricular filling, and distensibility.

The RAAS inhibitors, beta-blockers, and aldosterone blockers reverse cardiac remodeling but no drug till now has promising results because the molecular mechanism of ACR is incompletely understood. As a result, HF incidence remains very high and the 5-year mortality still exceeds 50%. Currently, treatment of HF with reduced ejection fraction (HFrEF) is based on alteration of the RAAS and sympathetic system, which are not so beneficial in HF with preserved ejection fraction (HFpEF). Sodium-glucose cotransporter 2 inhibitors (SGLT2is) are originally applied to treat type 2 diabetes mellitus (T2DM) but are known to have cardiovascular benefits in population with HF of all types and atherosclerotic diseases. SGLT2 receptors are found in the kidneys whereas SGLT1 receptors are expressed in the cardiomyocytes and small intestine with some receptors in the kidneys as well.[2] SGLT2i inhibit the coupled reabsorption of sodium and glucose from proximal tubules in the kidney.

TRIAL EVIDENCE OF SGLT2 INHIBITORS ON CARDIAC REMODELING

Starting their role in animal studies and later in human studies, SGLT2i have shown promising results in reversing ACR. Empagliflozin has been proven to reduce blood pressure (BP) and LV hypertrophy and volume in rodents successfully, resulting in improved diastolic function.[3] In another study, sotagliflozin significantly decreased enlarged left atrium in HFpEF. In the EMPA-HEART CardioLink-6 trial in patients with stable coronary artery disease and T2DM without HF, empagliflozin resulted in good reduction of LV mass index measured on Cardiac MRI.[4]

Impact of dapagliflozin on left ventricular diastolic dysfunction in patients with T2DM (IDDIA) trial showed significant improvement in diastolic function.[5] In DAPA-LVH RCT[6] on 66 patients, dapagliflozin reduced LV mass, body weight, and 24-hour systolic BP in patients with

T2DM without HF. DAPA-HF[7] and EMPEROR Reduced[8] trials on SGLT2i showed CV benefits in HFrEF.

MOLECULAR MECHANISM OF SGLT2 INHIBITOR ACTION IN HFpEF

Cardiac Mechanism

Artificial neural networks (ANN) identify relationships between the drug targets and clinical elements. In this AI model, empagliflozin reverses 59% of the protein alterations in patients of HFpEF by inhibition of Na^+/H^+ exchanger 1 (NHE1) while other SGLT2 played minor role. After 12 months of empagliflozin treatment, decrease in oxidative stress, stiffness of cardiomyocytes, LV hypertrophy, and ECM remodeling were noticed. Empagliflozin has the greatest (2,500-fold) selectivity for SGLT2 over SGLT1.[9] As per AI model, "NHE1 is the only target protein of empagliflozin (10 mg/day dose used) expressed in vascular cells and cardiomyocytes". It acts by directly reducing cytoplasmic oxidative stress. Inhibition of NEH1 leads to decreased mitochondrial swelling by Ca^{2+} and decrease in reactive oxygen species (ROS) in cardiomyocytes. Clinical impact of the previously mentioned findings has been shown that in the EMPEROR-Preserved trial, which included ~6,000 patients with NYHA class II–IV and preserved EF, empagliflozin reduced the combined risk of CV death, hospitalization for heart failure, and emergency hospital visit requiring intravenous treatment.[10] Above benefits are mediated via multiple mechanisms, including enhanced weight loss, better glucose control, raising erythropoietin and thereby hemoglobin levels, natriuresis, optimizing cardiac ATP metabolism and reducing uric acid levels, and lowering of BP and intravascular/intraventricular volume.

Limitations of AI model are: It included small number of ambulatory patients in NYHA class I or II with HFpEF and diabetes, which is indication for use of empagliflozin and pharmacological effects of SGLT2i on oxidative stress can be affected by other minor signaling molecules.

Empagliflozin showed significant reductions in HF admissions and CV mortality by 38% (EMPA-REG OUTCOME), likely mechanisms are indirect effects of empagliflozin on reduction of afterload (via reduction in BP), preload (via natriuresis/diuresis), or via increasing fatty acid and glucose oxidation).[11]

Molecular-level involvement in cardiac remodeling is given in **Table 1**.

TABLE 1: Molecular-level involvement in cardiac remodeling.

Parameters	*Major molecules involved*
Cardiomyocyte oxidative stress	NHE1 via AKTs, NFATs, and NOS2
ECM remodeling, cardiomyocyte stiffness, and concentric hypertrophy	VEGF-A, CO1A1, TGF-B1, NFATs, and IL-10
Systemic inflammation	TNF-A, IL-1B, ICAM-1, NACHT, LRR, NLRP-3, and inflammasomes

Extracardiac Mechanism

The SGLT2 inhibitors have direct or indirect action on many organs leading to various benefits. They are:

- 80% patients of end-stage renal disease on hemodialysis are having ACR. Its progression is reduced by use of SGLT2i.[12]
- SGLT2i, by improving erythropoietin, improve systolic and diastolic dysfunction by reversing ventricular remodeling.[13]
- In myocardial-IRON trial in patients with stable HF, LVEF <50%, and iron deficiency,[14] treated with ferric carboxymaltose (FCM) and SGLT2i (empagliflozin 10 mg/d) showed significant clinical improvement on CMR at 30th day compared with the FCM–without empagliflozin group. the EMPATROPISM trial also suggested similar results.[15]
- Chronic hypertension is known to cause ACR. SGLT2i decrease BP up to 9–10 mm Hg in patients with high BP at the onset as in CKD.[16]
- Some HFpEF patients have diastolic dysfunction due to hepatic steatosis. Metanalysis suggested that SGLT2i can reverse hepatic steatosis.[17]
- A meta-analysis of RCTs concluded that SGLT2i decrease atrial fibrillation.[18]

EFFECT OF SGLT2 INHIBITORS ON CARDIAC REMODELING AND FUNCTION: META-ANALYSIS OF RANDOMIZED CONTROLLED TRIALS

In 15 RCTs with 1,343 patients with HF and T2DM, 663 received SGLT2i therapy and rest were in control group. In 7 studies using empagliflozin, dapagliflozin, canagliflozin, etc. with follow-up ranging from 1.5 to 12 months, SGLT2i significantly improved left atrial volume index (LAVi), left ventricular ejection fraction (LVEF), left ventricular mass index (LVMi), heart rate (HR), left ventricular end-systolic volume (LVESV) and E/e', and prognosis of patients with HF independent of the presence of T2DM. Subgroup analysis showed that compared with other SGLT2i, empagliflozin significantly decreased LVESV, E/e', LVMi, LVEDV, LAVi, and increased LVEF. Benefits may be due to multifactorial mechanisms, including BP control, weight loss, and cardiac energy metabolism modulation.[1] Empagliflozin was associated with reduced adverse events and improved cardiometabolic parameters.[19] Meta-analysis by Fan et al.[20] included studies with Jadad score ranging from 5 to 7, which indicated their high quality.

Previous published meta-analyses by Dhingra revealed that SGLT2i were not associated with statistical changes in LVMi, LVESV, LVEDV, or LVEF compared to placebo.[21] A metanalysis on the impact of SGLT2 inhibition on imaging markers of cardiac function by Theofilis et al. also proved that SGLT2i have no effect on LVEDV, but slightly improved LVEF.[22] Recently published meta-analysis by Nan Zhang found that compared with other SGLT2i, empagliflozin shows a greater improvement in LVM, LVMi, LVEDV, and LVESV.[23] Several strengths of this meta-analysis are: (1) they only included RCTs that guaranteed the data quality and assessed cardiac function by echocardiography or cardiac MRI, which may reduce heterogeneity; (2) They evaluated the effect of SGLT2i on heart rate, left atrium volume index, and other cardiac function parameters and this is the first study that showed that compared to other SGLT2i, empagliflozin exerts greater improvement in cardiac remodeling and function.

The SGLT2 inhibitors have significant cardiovascular benefits. The molecular mechanism may be due to activated autophagy, reduced ROS, attenuated inflammation, and enhanced mitochondria homeostasis by SGLT2i.[24] Since LAVi and E/e' are compared to assess diastolic function of heart, results revealed that SGLT2i decrease LAVi and E/e' and improve diastolic dysfunction.

RECENT TRIAL-BASED RECOMMENDATIONS

As per recent update (2023) on HF by European Society of Cardiology,[25] SGLT2i (dapagliflozin or empagliflozin) are recommended in patients with HFpEF to reduce the risk of HF hospitalization or CV death as class 1 recommendation with level of evidence A. These recommendations are based on the following trials:

- EMPULSE trial in the year 2022 tested the efficacy of the early initiation of empagliflozin in patients hospitalized for acute HF. The primary endpoint was "clinical benefit", defined by composite of death from any cause, time to first HF event, number of HF events, or a ≥5-point difference in change from baseline in the Kansas City Cardiomyopathy Questionnaire total symptoms at 90 days. The primary endpoint was achieved in more patients treated with empagliflozin compared with placebo ($p = .0054$). The efficacy was independent of LVEF and diabetes status and the rate of adverse events was similar between the two treatment groups.[26]
- DAPA-CKD (results published in the year 2023) was a multicenter, double-blind, placebo-controlled, randomized control trial including both diabetic and nondiabetic patients with an eGFR of 25–75 mL/min/1.73m^2 and urinary albumin-to-creatinine ratio ≥200 mg/g, and these patients were randomly assigned 1:1 to dapagliflozin 10 mg once daily or placebo. Among 468 of the 4,304 patients, CV death was reduced by 39% by dapagliflozin compared with placebo ($p < .001$), and the risk of the secondary outcome of HF hospitalization or CV death was decreased by dapagliflozin compared with placebo ($p = .009$).[27]
- EMPA-KIDNEY (results published in the year 2023) enrolled a broader group of patients with CKD, compared to DAPA-CKD, including patients with an eGFR of 45–90 mL/min/1.73 m^2 and a urinary albumin-to-creatinine ratio ≥200 mg/g or eGFR 20–45 mL/min/1.73 m^2, even in the absence of albuminuria. Patients were randomized 1:1 to empagliflozin 10 mg once daily or placebo. 658 of the 6,609 patients enrolled (10%) had a history of HF. During a median follow-up of 2.0 years, reduction in the primary composite endpoint of progression of kidney disease or CV death was observed.[28]

CONCLUSION

Reversal of ACR is a central mechanism of the cardiovascular benefits of SGLT2i. SGLT2i play a beneficial role in HFpEF by optimizing cellular cardiac energy metabolism, reducing inflammatory process, uptitrating cellular homeostasis (e.g., autophagy), reducing oxidative stress, counteracting vascular remodeling of coronary microcirculation, and causing inhibition of the sympathetic nervous system. These mechanisms along with other extracardiac processes (e.g., improvement of kidney function and hemodynamics) can reverse cardiac remodeling. This seems to be the underlying mechanism for various benefits of SGLT2i, primarily in HF hospitalization in HFpEF patients.

REFERENCES

1. Salah HM, Verma S, Santos-Gallego CG, et al. Sodium-glucose cotransporter 2 inhibitors and cardiac remodeling. J Cardiovasc Transl Res. 2022;15(5):944-56.
2. Vrhovac I, Balen Eror D, Klessen D, et al. Localizations of Na(+)-D-glucose cotransporters SGLT1 and SGLT2 in human kidney and of SGLT1 in human small intestine, liver, lung, and heart. Pfugers Arch. 2015;467(9):1881-98.
3. Connelly KA, Zhang Y, Visram A, et al. Empagliflozin improves diastolic function in a nondiabetic rodent model of heart failure with preserved ejection fraction. JACC Basic Transl Sci. 2019;4(1):27-37.

4. Verma S, Mazer CD, Yan AT, et al. Effect of empagliflozin on left ventricular mass in patients with type 2 diabetes mellitus and coronary artery disease: The EMPA-HEART CardioLink-6 Randomized Clinical Trial. Circulation. 2019;140(21):1693-702.
5. Shim CY, Seo J, Cho I, et al. Randomized, controlled trial to evaluate the effect of dapagliflozin on left ventricular diastolic function in patients with type 2 diabetes mellitus: The IDDIA Trial. Circulation. 2021;143(5):510-2.
6. Brown AJM, Gandy S, McCrimmon R, et al. A randomized controlled trial of dapagliflozin on left ventricular hypertrophy in people with type two diabetes: The DAPA-LVH trial. Eur Heart J. 2020;41(36):3421-32.
7. Kaplinsky E. DAPA-HF trial: Dapagliflozin evolves from a glucose-lowering agent to a therapy for heart failure. Drugs Context. 2020;9:2019-11-3.
8. Špinar J, Špinarová L, Vítovec J. [EMPEROR reduced-empagliflozin in patients with heart failure and reduced ejection fraction]. Vnitr Lek. 2021;67(1):43-7.
9. Zelniker TA, Braunwald E. Cardiac and renal effects of sodium-glucose cotransporter 2 inhibitors in diabetes. J Am Coll Cardiol. 2018;72(15):1845-55.
10. Anker SD, Butler J, Filippatos GS, et al.; EMPEROR-Preserved Trial Committees and Investigators. Evaluation of the effects of sodium-glucose cotransporter 2 inhibition with empagliflozin on morbidity and mortality in patients with chronic heart failure and a preserved ejection fraction: Rationale for and design of the EMPEROR-Preserved Trial. Eur J Heart Fail. 2019;21(10):1279-87.
11. Sattar N, McLaren J, Kristensen SL, et al. SGLT2 inhibition and cardiovascular events: Why did EMPA-REG outcomes surprise and what were the likely mechanisms? Diabetologia. 2016;59(7):1333-9.
12. Heerspink HJL, Stefánsson BV, Correa-Rotter R, et al. Dapaglifozin in patients with chronic kidney disease. N Eng J Med. 2020;383(15):1436-46.
13. Mazer CD, Hare GMT, Connelly PW, et al. Effect of empagliflozin on erythropoietin levels, iron stores, and red blood cell morphology in patients with type 2 DM and coronary artery disease. Circulation. 2020;141(8):704-7.
14. Núñez J, Miñana G, Cardells I, et al. Noninvasive imaging estimation of myocardial iron repletion following administration of intravenous iron: The Myocardial-IRON Trial. J Am Heart Assoc. 2020;9(4):e014254.
15. Angermann CE, Santos-Gallego CG, Requena-Ibanez JA, et al. Effects of empagliflozin on iron metabolism in non-diabetic patients with heart failure. Sub-study of the EMPATROPISM Randomized Trial. Late-breaking science abstracts and featured science abstracts from the American Heart Association's Scientific Sessions 2021. Circulation. 2021;144:e564-93.
16. Kario K, Okada K, Kato M, et al. Twenty-four-hour blood pressure-lowering effect of a sodium-glucose cotransporter 2 inhibitor in patients with diabetes and uncontrolled nocturnal hypertension: Results from the Randomized, Placebo-Controlled SACRA Study. Circulation. 2019;139(18):2089-97.
17. Xing B, Zhao Y, Dong B, et al. Effects of sodium-glucose cotransporter 2 inhibitors on nonalcoholic fatty liver disease in patients with type 2 diabetes: A meta-analysis of randomized controlled trials. J Diabetes Investig. 2020;11(5):1238-47.
18. Li WJ, Chen XQ, Xu LL, et al. SGLT2 inhibitors and atrial fibrillation in type 2 diabetes: A systematic review with meta-analysis of 16 randomized controlled trials. Cardiovasc Diabetol. 2021;19(1):130.
19. Yang AY, Chen HC. Study comparing the efficacy and renal safety for patients with diabetes switching from dapagliflozin to empagliflozin. Int J Clin Pharm. 2021;43(4):1015-23.
20. Fan G, Guo DL. The effect of sodium-glucose cotransporter-2 inhibitors on cardiac structure remodeling and function: A meta-analysis of randomized controlled trials. Eur J Intern Med. 2023;114:49-57.
21. Dhingra NK, Mistry N, Puar P, et al. SGLT2 inhibitors and cardiac remodelling: A systematic review and meta-analysis of randomized cardiac magnetic resonance imaging trials. ESC Heart Fail. 2021;8(6):4693-700.
22. Theofilis P, Antonopoulos AS, Katsimichas T, et al. The impact of SGLT2 inhibition on imaging markers of cardiac function: A systematic review and meta-analysis. Pharmacol Res. 2022;180:106243.
23. Hammoudi N, Jeong D, Singh R, et al. Empagliflozin improves left ventricular diastolic dysfunction in a genetic model of type 2 diabetes. Cardiovasc Drugs Ther. 2017;31(3):233-46.
24. Heerspink HJL, Perco P, Mulder S. Canaglifozin reduces inflammation and fibrosis biomarkers: A potential mechanism of action for beneficial effects of SGLT2i in diabetic kidney disease. Diabetologia. 2019;62(7):1154-66.
25. McDonagh TA, Metra M, Adamo M, et al; ESC Scientific Document Group. 2023 Focused Update of the 2021 ESC Guidelines for the diagnosis and treatment of acute and chronic heart failure: Developed by the task force for the diagnosis and treatment of acute and chronic heart failure of the European Society of Cardiology (ESC) With the special contribution of the Heart Failure Association (HFA) of the ESC. Eur Heart J. 2024;26(1):5-17.
26. Biegus J, Voors AA, Collins SP, et al. Impact of empagliflozin on decongestion in acute heart failure: The EMPULSE trial. Eur Heart J. 2023;44(1):41-50.
27. Wheeler DC, Stefánsson BV, Jongs N, et al; DAPA-CKD Trial Committees and Investigators. Effects of dapagliflozin on major adverse kidney and cardiovascular events in patients with diabetic and non-diabetic chronic kidney disease: A prespecified analysis from the DAPA-CKD trial. Lancet Diabetes Endocrinol. 2021;9(1):22-31.
28. EMPA-KIDNEY Collaborative Group. Impact of primary kidney disease on the effects of empagliflozin in patients with chronic kidney disease: Secondary analyses of the EMPA-KIDNEY trial. Lancet Diabetes Endocrinol. 2024;12(1):51-60.

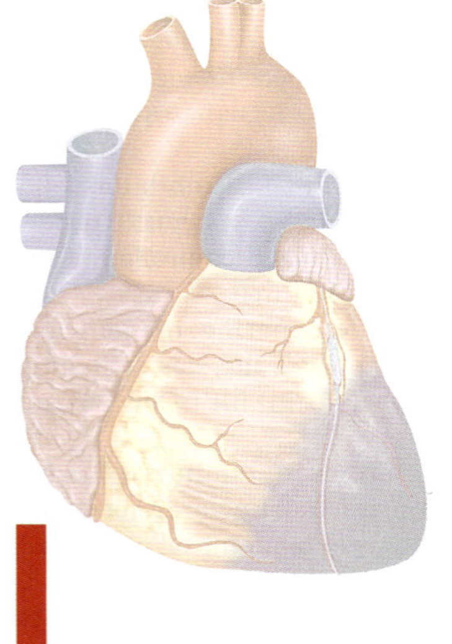

Role of SGLT2i in all Spectrum of HFpEF Management

Arati Dave Lalchandani

INTRODUCTION

The standard definition of heart failure (HF), i.e., inability to pump blood to various organs of the body to fulfill its needs or the heart is able to do so only at high filling pressures, has served well till now, but with the advent of modern diagnostic machines and technology, the ejection fraction has become an important parameter during consideration of prognosis, mortality, and treatment.

There has been a paradigm shift in the understanding of HF, so now we have in the spectrum, heart failure with reduced ejection fraction (HFrEF), which is used to be an essential criterion for the diagnosis of HF. Moreover, we now have evidence that there is a significantly increased risk of mortality and morbidity and hospitalization in patients with HF even without reduction of ejection fraction.

The role of sodium-glucose cotransporter 2 inhibitors (SGLT2i) in HF, especially with preserved ejection fraction, is a moot point, which shall be debated in this chapter.

CONTENT AND DESCRIPTION

Sodium-glucose cotransporter 2 inhibitors are a new class of antihyperglycemic drugs which by blocking the SGLT in proximal tubule of the kidney increases urinary excretion of glucose as well as sodium. Along with this, there is reduction in body weight and blood pressure which together with loss of sodium and water results in improvement in HF symptoms, along with improved outcomes such as reduced cardiovascular (CV) mortality and reduced hospitalization.

GUIDELINES

The EMPA-REG OUTCOME (Empagliflozin Cardiovascular Outcome Event Trial in Type 2 Diabetes Mellitus Patients) showed that empagliflozin reduced mortality rate from CV causes by 38%, hospitalization in HF by 35%, and terminal kidney failure in patients with type 2 diabetes mellitus (DM) with CV disease.[1]

In DAPA-HF, dapagliflozin and empagliflozin in EMPEROR-Reduced trials, it was seen that there was significant improvement in HF and reduction in CV death in the NYHA class II–IV HF patients.[2] The primary outcome was a composite of CV death or deterioration of HF. The primary outcome was similar in patients with or without diabetes. The patients in EMPEROR-Reduced had more severe HF than those in DAPA-HF, suggesting that SGLT2i is less effective in reduced EFHF.

There are sparse studies of SGLT2i in heart failure with preserved ejection fraction (HFpEF). Neither the ACC/AHA/HFSA guidelines nor European HF guidelines have included SGLT2i recommendations in HFrEF or HFpEF. However, random studies and shared experiences of cardiologists and communications and exchanges from deliberations over use of SGLT2i in HFpEF strongly suggest that SGLT2i may give benefits of clinical improvement with regard to symptoms and signs; so, it could be worthwhile using it as an additional drug in the management of HFpEF.

The CANVAS program used SGLT2i canagliflozin or placebo. There was a significant risk reduction in HF hospitalization with canagliflozin.[3]

In the multicenter trial to evaluate effect of dapagliflozin on incidence of CV events (DECLARE-TIMI 58), there was a 27% reduction in risk of HF hospitalization.[4]

Other SGLT2i used in trials, ertugliflozin and sotagliflozin, also showed reduction in CV death and hospitalization for HF.

CONCLUSION

In the quest for search and research on improving survival and reducing symptoms and give a better quality of life to patients of HF, the cardiologists tend to grab at any new medicine or therapy, which could reduce the fluid load without having a negative inotropic effect on the heart or any adverse effect on the circulatory system; therefore, the cardiologists are keeping a vigil on any new drug in the pharmacologic coffers for the management of disorders of the kidney, liver, hypertension, or DM.

REFERENCES

1. Inzucchi SE, Zinman B, Fitchett D, et al. How does empagliflozin reduce cardiovascular mortality? Insights from a mediation analysis of the EMPA-REG OUTCOME trial. Diabetes Care. 2018;41:356-63.
2. Inzucchi SE, Kosiborod M, Fitchett D, et al. Improvement in cardiovascular outcomes with empagliflozin is independent of glycemic control. Circulation. 2018;138:1904-7.
3. Neal B, Perkovic V, Mahaffey KW, et al. Canagliflozin and cardiovascular and renal events in type 2 diabetes. N Engl J Med. 2017;377:644-57.
4. Wiviott SD, Raz I, Bonaca MP, et al. Dapagliflozin and cardiovascular outcomes in type 2 diabetes. N Engl J Med. 2019;380:347-57.

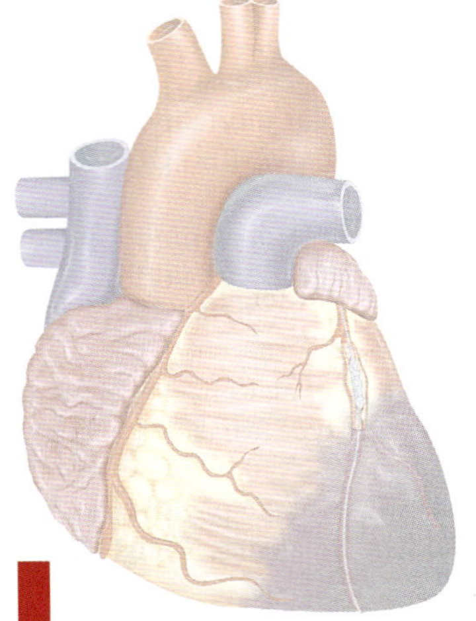

ACC/AHA Guidelines on Beta-blocker Use in HFpEF

Ruman Kugashiya, Upendra Kaul

INTRODUCTION

Beta-blockers are core therapeutic agents for the treatment of heart failure with reduced ejection fraction (HFrEF) with multiple studies consistently showing a reduction in morbidity and mortality; however, a clinical randomized trial data on use of beta-blockers in patients with heart failure with preserved ejection fraction (HFpEF) is lacking. A meta-analysis of 11 randomized trials suggested that the benefits of beta-blockers extend to patients with heart failure with mildly reduced ejection fraction (HFmrEF), data on beta-blockers in HFpEF remain limited to observational studies and a small number of less well-phenotyped trials with inconclusive results.[1-3] Given the limited evidence from randomized trials, the latest European Society of Cardiology and American Heart Association (AHA)/American College of Cardiology (ACC)/Heart Failure Society of America (HFSA) guidelines do not recommend the use of beta-blockers for the treatment of HFpEF.[4]

Flowchart 1: Treatment of HFpEF.

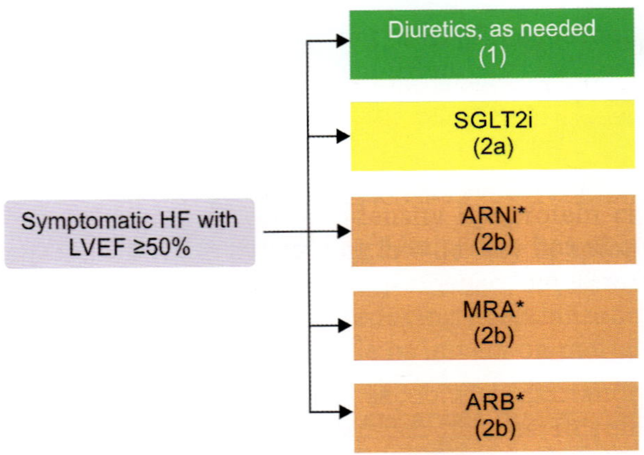

*Greater benefit in patients with LVEF closer to 50%.
(ARB: angiotensin receptor blocker; ARNi: angiotensin receptor–neprilysin inhibitors; HF: heart failure; MRA: mineralocorticoid receptor antagonist; SGLT2i: sodium–glucose cotransporter-2 inhibitor)

CONTENTS AND DESCRIPTION

Current ACC/AHA guidelines provide a Class IIb recommendation for beta-blocker use in patients with HFmrEF based on the rationale that such patients are pathophysiologically similar to those with HFrEF and rescinded the previous Class IIa recommendation for beta-blocker use in patients with HFpEF.

The treatment of HFpEF is given in **Flowchart 1**.

Beta-blocker is widely used in patients of HFpEF with comorbidities like hypertension, ischemic heart disease, and atrial fibrillation.[5-9] In various large clinical trials in patients of HFpEF, the use of beta-blockers has been found to range between 30 and 86%. The major indications for use of beta-blockers in these patients were:

- Hypertension
- Atrial fibrillation and atrial flutter
- Ischemic heart disease
- Previous HFrEF and HFmrEF But in recent years, many observational studies have suggested that beta-blockers may be potentially harmful in patients with HFpEF,[1,2,10] likely caused by a number of mechanisms

such as relatively fixed stroke volume, chronotropic incompetence, or prolongation of diastolic filling that increases ventricular pressures.[2,11,12] A meta-analysis in 2014 demonstrated that the beta-blockers treatment reduced all-cause mortality in HFpEF patients with EF >40%, while it did not affect hospitalization.[13]

In recent study, patients with HFpEF with hypertension, left ventricular hypertrophy, and possible diastolic dysfunction without clinical signs of heart failure (HF) on long-term treatment with beta-blocker were protected against new-onset symptomatic HF and its progression and diastolic dysfunction.[14]

The TOPCAT (Aldosterone Antagonist Therapy for Adults with Heart Failure and Preserved Systolic Function) trial and a recent analysis of the US National Cardiovascular Data Registry PINNACLE (Practice Innovation and Clinical Excellence) suggested that beta-blocker use may be associated with a potentially increased risk of hospitalizations for HF in patients with HFpEF.[10,15]

Similarly, the PRESERVE-HR (beta-blockers Withdrawal in Patients with HFpEF and Chronotropic Incompetence: Effect on Functional Capacity) trial showed that the withdrawal of beta-blockers may improve functional capacity and chronotropic incompetence in patients with HFpEF.[2]

LIMITATION OF BETA-BLOCKER USE

Beta-blocker use is more common in patients with HFrEF, HFmrEF, and patients with hypertension, coronary artery disease, and atrial arrhythmias. Clinical studies described highly significant interactions between beta-blocker use and LVEF for both HF hospitalization and death. In patients with HFmrEF, beta-blockers appeared to be protective, but in patients with higher LVEF, particularly >60%, beta-blocker use was associated with no mortality benefits and a higher risk of HF hospitalization. These associations were also similar in patients with hypertension, coronary artery disease, and atrial fibrillation/flutter. These findings suggest that beta-blocker use in patients with HFpEF may carry some risk. There is biochemical evidence of increased cardiac sympathetic activation in HFpEF,[16] which could indicate a potential beneficial target for beta-blockers; clinical evidence has generally shown beta-blockers to exert either neutral or negative effects on outcomes in these patients.

The summary of evidence for beta-blocker versus risk according to LVEF is given in **Figure 1**.

DISCUSSION

Beta-blockers are most commonly used agents in various clinical cardiac diseases, such as hypertension, ischemic heart disease, arrhythmias, and HF, and even in noncardiac disease, like tremors, portal hypertension, and migraines. There has been evidence for benefit of beta-blockers in patients with HF for nearly 50 years, and the 1995 ACC/AHA Guidelines for the Evaluation and Management of Heart Failure included beta-blockers as a class II indication for patients with HF and dilated cardiomyopathy and for patients with HFpEF to augment ventricular relaxation and improve ventricular compliance.[17]

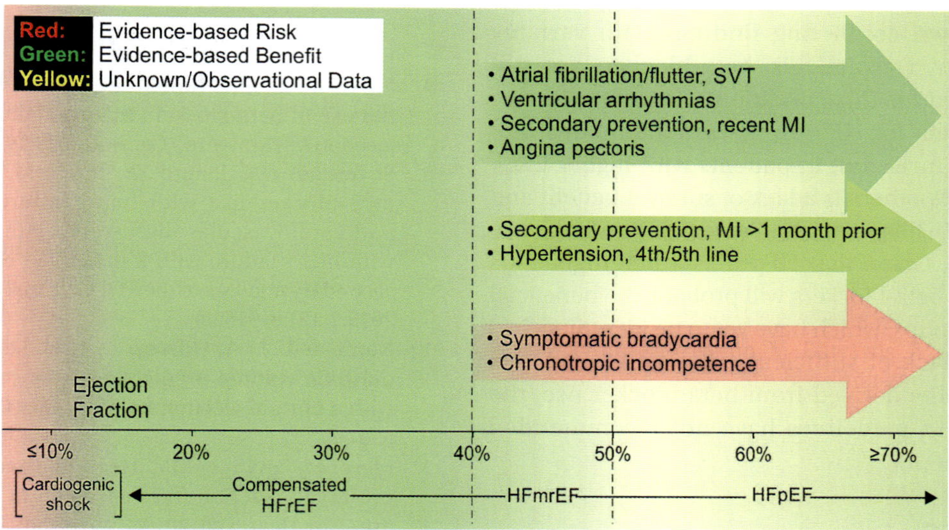

Fig. 1: Summary of evidence for beta-blocker versus risk according to LVEF. (HFmrEF: heart failure with mildly reduced ejection fraction; HFpEF: heart failure with preserved ejection fraction; HFrEF: Heart failure with reduced ejection fraction; LVEF: left ventricular ejection fraction; MI: myocardial infarction; SVT: supraventricular tachycardia)

Beta-blockers were class I indication for HFrEF in 2001 and have remained there since, with benefits only increasing over time. However, the evidence base for beta-blocker use in the treatment of HFpEF, and the more recently defined HFmrEF, has been lacking, and thus, there has been limited guidance on whether or how beta-blockers fit into the treatment of patients with LVEF ≥40%. Beta-blockers were changed to a Class IIb recommendation for HFpEF in 2001 (defined at that time as LVEF ≥40%)[18] and subsequently to a Class IIa recommendation for HFpEF with hypertension in 2013.[19] In the most recent 2022 guideline, beta-blockers were not mentioned as part of the treatment pathway for HFpEF (now defined as LVEF ≥50%) except for treatment of concomitant arrhythmias, and they were given a Class IIb recommendation in HFmrEF (LVEF 40–49%), as are all other guideline-directed medical therapies for HFrEF.[6]

For treatment of hypertension along with HFpEF, medications such as mineralocorticoid receptor antagonists[20,21] and sodium–glucose cotransporter 2 inhibitors[22,23] should be considered because both have benefits in patients with HFpEF and lower blood pressure. The recommendation for beta-blockers use in ischemic heart disease has also weakened over time. Although beta-blockers have mortality benefits in the immediate period after myocardial infarction,[24] there does not appear to be any mortality benefit beyond 1–2 years after myocardial infarction or in patients with chronic coronary disease who have normal LVEF.[25]

CONCLUSION

The evidence of beta-blocker therapy in patients with HFpEF has shown conflicting findings with variably reported efficacy. Despite this, beta-blockers are still widely prescribed for this condition. There is evidence of potential benefit for HF hospitalization and death in patients with HFmrEF, but in patients with higher LVEF (particularly >60%), there is a lack of survival benefit and a higher risk of HF hospitalization associated with the use of beta-blockers. Given that HFpEF is a heterogeneous entity, the use of beta-blockers will probably be beneficial in selected subgroups, which have yet to be identified.

So far with lack of sufficient convincing evidence in favor of benefits derived from beta blocker use, the current ACC/AHA guidelines have not recommended it in patients of HFpEF.

REFERENCES

1. Cleland JGF, Bunting KV, Flather MD, et al. Beta-blockers for heart failure with reduced, mid-range, and preserved ejection fraction: An individual patient-level analysis of double-blind randomized trials. Eur Heart J. 2018;39(1):26-35.
2. Meyer M, Du Fay Lavallaz J, Benson L, et al. Association between β-blockers and outcomes in heart failure with preserved ejection fraction: Current insights from the Sweden HF Registry. J Card Fail. 2021;27(11):1165-74.
3. Flather MD, Shibata MC, Coats AJ, et al. Randomized trial to determine the effect of nebivolol on mortality and cardiovascular hospital admission in elderly patients with heart failure (SENIORS). Eur Heart J. 2005;26(3):215-25.
4. Heidenreich PA, Bozkurt B, Aguilar D, et al.; ACC/AHA Joint Committee Members. 2022 AHA/ACC/HFSA guideline for the management of heart failure: A Report of the American College of Cardiology/American Heart Association Joint Committee on Clinical Practice Guidelines. Circulation. 2022;145(18):e895-1032.
5. McDonagh TA, Metra M, Adamo M, et al. 2021 ESC guidelines for the diagnosis and treatment of acute and chronic heart failure: Developed by the Task Force for the Diagnosis and Treatment of Acute and Chronic Heart Failure of the European Society of Cardiology (ESC). With the special contribution of the Heart Failure Association (HFA) of the ESC. Eur J Heart Fail. 2022;24:4-131.
6. Heidenreich PA, Bozkurt B, Aguilar D, et al.; ACC/AHA Joint Committee Members. 2022 AHA/ACC/HFSA guideline for the management of heart failure: A report of the American College of Cardiology/American Heart Association Joint Committee on Clinical Practice Guidelines. JACC. 2022;79(17):e263-421.
7. Shah SJ, Heitner JF, Sweitzer NK, et al. Baseline characteristics of patients in the treatment of preserved cardiac function heart failure with an aldosterone antagonist trial. Circ Heart Fail. 2013;6(2):184-92.
8. Solomon SD, Rizkala AR, Lefkowitz MP, et al. Baseline characteristics of patients with heart failure and preserved ejection fraction in the PARAGON-HF trial. Circ Heart Fail. 2018;11(7):e004962.
9. Musse M, Lau JD, Yum B, et al. Physician perspectives on the use of beta blockers in heart failure with preserved ejection fraction. Am J Cardiol. 2023;193:70-4.
10. Silverman DN, Plante TB, Infeld M, et al. Association of β-blocker use with heart failure hospitalizations and cardiovascular disease mortality among patients with heart failure with a preserved ejection fraction: A secondary analysis of the TOPCAT trial. JAMA Netw Open. 2019;2(12):e1916598.
11. Nambiar L, Li A, Howard A, et al. Left ventricular end-diastolic volume predicts exercise capacity in patients with a normal ejection fraction. Clin Cardiol. 2018;41(5):628-33.
12. Meyer M, LeWinter MM. Heart rate and heart failure with preserved ejection fraction: Time to slow beta-blocker use? Circ Heart Fail. 2019;12(8):e006213.
13. Liu F, Chen Y, Feng X, et al. Effects of beta-blockers on heart failure with preserved ejection fraction: A meta-analysis. PLoS ONE. 2014;9(3):e90555.

14. Gu J, Fan YQ, Bian L, et al. Long-term prescription of beta-blocker delays the progression of heart failure with preserved ejection fraction in patients with hypertension: A retrospective observational cohort study. Eur J Prev Cardiol. 2016;23(13):1421-8.
15. Harolds JA. Quality and safety in health care, part XXXIV: The PINNACLE registry. Clin Nucl Med. 2018;43(4): 246-7.
16. Kaye DM, Nanayakkara S, Wang B, et al. Characterization of cardiac sympathetic nervous system and inflammatory activation in HFpEF patients. JACC Basic Trans Sci. 2022;7(2):116-27.
17. Guidelines for the evaluation and management of heart failure. Report of the American College of Cardiology/ American Heart Association task force on practice guidelines (committee on evaluation and management of heart failure). Circulation. 1995;92(9):2764-84.
18. Hunt SA, Baker DW, Chin MH, et al. ACC/AHA guidelines for the evaluation and management of chronic heart failure in the adult: Executive summary. A report of the American College of Cardiology/American Heart Association task force on practice guidelines (committee to revise the 1995 guidelines for the evaluation and management of heart failure). J Am Coll Cardiol. 2001; 38(7):2101-13.
19. Yancy CW, Jessup M, Bozkurt B, et al. 2013 ACCF/AHA guideline for the management of heart failure: A report of the American College of Cardiology Foundation/American Heart Association task force on practice guidelines. J Am Coll Cardiol. 2013;62(16):e147-239.
20. Pitt B, Pfeffer MA, Assmann SF, et al. Spironolactone for heart failure with preserved ejection fraction. N Engl J Med. 2014;370(15):1383-92.
21. Fernet M, Beckerman B, Abreu P, et al. Antihypertensive effect of the mineralocorticoid receptor antagonist eplerenone: A pooled analysis of patient-level data from comparative trials using regulatory-approved doses. Vasc Health Risk Manag. 2018;14:233-46.
22. Anker SD, Butler J, Filippatos G, et al. Empagliflozin in heart failure with a preserved ejection fraction. N Engl J Med. 2021;385(16):1451-61.
23. Ferdinand KC, Lee J, Meng L, et al. Empagliflozin improves blood pressure as well as glycemic control in African American patients with type 2 diabetes and hypertension: A 24-week randomized controlled trial. J Am Coll Cardiol. 2018;71(11):A1750 (Suppl March 2018).
24. Hjalmarson A, Elmfeldt D, Herlitz J, et al. Effect on mortality of metoprolol in acute myocardial infarction: A double-blind randomised trial. Lancet. 1981;2(8251): 823-7.
25. Bangalore S, Steg G, Deedwania P, et al. Beta-blocker use and clinical outcomes in stable out-patients with and without coronary artery disease. JAMA. 2012;308(13): 13409.

CHAPTER

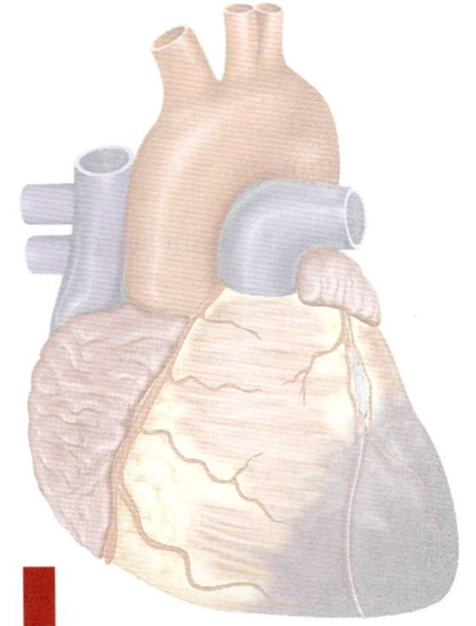

Role of Bisoprolol in HFpEF with AF, Stroke, and Hypertension

Pradeep Jain, Himanshu Jain, SN Pathak

INTRODUCTION

The incidence and prevalence of heart failure with preserved ejection fraction (HFpEF) continue to rise in tandem with the increasing age and burdens of obesity, sedentariness, and cardiometabolic disorders. During the past 20 years, the diagnostic approach to HFpEF has markedly evolved in parallel with our scientific understanding of this complex clinical syndrome.[1] Recent efforts have garnered consensus around a new universal definition, anchored clinically to the syndrome of heart failure (HF) caused by structural and/or functional cardiac abnormalities, with HFpEF defined as a left ventricular ejection fraction (LVEF) 50% or more further corroborated by either elevated natriuretic peptide (NP) levels or other evidence of congestion.[2] Using pooled data from the Cardiovascular Health Study (CHS) and Multi-Ethnic Study of Atherosclerosis (MESA), the estimated lifetime risk of HFpEF at age 45 years is >10% in both men and women.[3] Although the incidence of HFpEF is similar among men and women, the prevalence of HFpEF is higher in women compared with men.[4,5] In addition, physical inactivity was associated with higher risk of HFpEF compared with HFrEF in a dose-dependent manner.[6] Excess body fat leads to development of HFpEF.

DIAGNOSTIC EVALUATION OF HEART FAILURE WITH PRESERVED EJECTION FRACTION (FLOWCHART 1)

In patients with unexplained dyspnea and normal EF, the probability of underlying HFpEF can be estimated by the H_2FPEF score or HFA-PEFF score. Patients with intermediate probability scores should undergo additional hemodynamic exercise stress testing to establish the diagnosis.

TREATMENT OF HEART FAILURE WITH PRESERVED EJECTION FRACTION

Once HFpEF has been diagnosed and alternate diagnoses have been excluded, systematic treatment of HFpEF, which includes management of comorbidities and pharmacologic and nonpharmacologic therapies, should be instituted.

COMORBIDITY MANAGEMENT

Blood pressure control in accordance with clinical practice guidelines (target <130/80 mmHg) is important in the management of HFpEF, with selection of antihypertensive agents driven by the presence of other comorbidities and other indications.[7] Among all β-blockers, bisoprolol is most cardioselective β-blocker that provide superior dynamic HR reduction and noninferior dynamic BP reduction versus metoprolol CR. As per CIBIS-ELD trial compared to carvedilol the pulmonary adverse effect is less in Bisoprolol.[8] Bisoprolol is an effective antihypertensive drug with no detrimental effects on sexuality in newly diagnosed men with hypertension.[9]

Atrial fibrillation (AF) is highly prevalent in HFpEF and is associated with more advanced disease, poorer exercise capacity, and increased mortality.[10,11]

Flowchart 1: Diagnostic evaluation of heart failure with preserved ejection fraction.

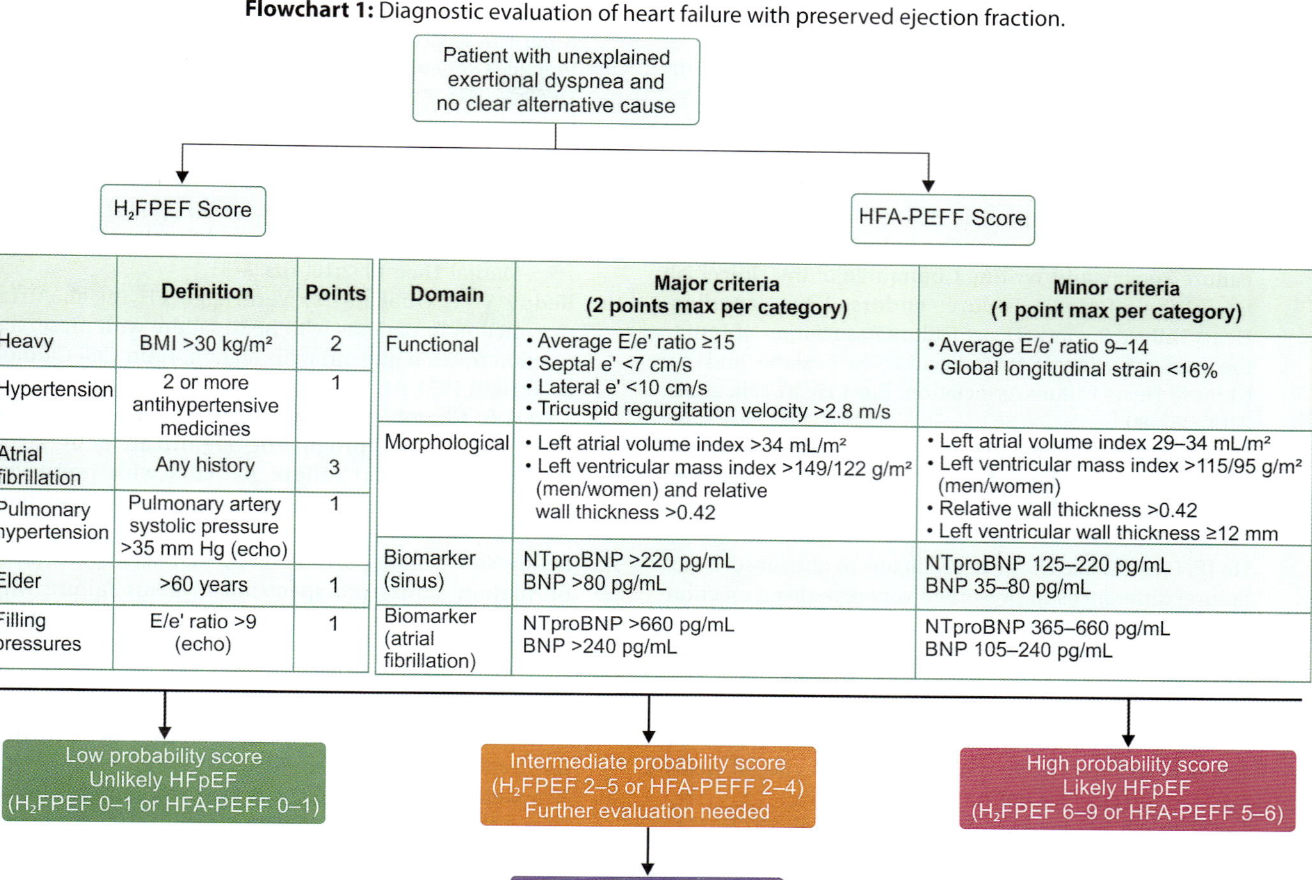

	Definition	Points
Heavy	BMI >30 kg/m²	2
Hypertension	2 or more antihypertensive medicines	1
Atrial fibrillation	Any history	3
Pulmonary hypertension	Pulmonary artery systolic pressure >35 mm Hg (echo)	1
Elder	>60 years	1
Filling pressures	E/e' ratio >9 (echo)	1

Domain	Major criteria (2 points max per category)	Minor criteria (1 point max per category)
Functional	• Average E/e' ratio ≥15 • Septal e' <7 cm/s • Lateral e' <10 cm/s • Tricuspid regurgitation velocity >2.8 m/s	• Average E/e' ratio 9–14 • Global longitudinal strain <16%
Morphological	• Left atrial volume index >34 mL/m² • Left ventricular mass index >149/122 g/m² (men/women) and relative wall thickness >0.42	• Left atrial volume index 29–34 mL/m² • Left ventricular mass index >115/95 g/m² (men/women) • Relative wall thickness >0.42 • Left ventricular wall thickness ≥12 mm
Biomarker (sinus)	NTproBNP >220 pg/mL BNP >80 pg/mL	NTproBNP 125–220 pg/mL BNP 35–80 pg/mL
Biomarker (atrial fibrillation)	NTproBNP >660 pg/mL BNP >240 pg/mL	NTproBNP 365–660 pg/mL BNP 105–240 pg/mL

Emerging data suggest a greater role for more aggressive rhythm control, although prospective trial data is required.[12] Notably, aggressive rate control may be deleterious in HFpEF patients with AF due to significant LA dysfunction resulting in low stroke volume and inability to increase stroke volume during exertion. β-blockers are among the most frequently used drugs in patients with AF. They are often used for ventricular rate control, acutely in emergency situations and chronically, in patients with persistent or permanent AF.

Systemic hypertension is the most common underlying disorder associated with AF. Hypertension is present in between 50 and 75% of patients with AF. In patients with hypertension, and particularly left ventricular hypertrophy (LVH), new persistent AF occurs in 1–2% of patients per year, even when blood pressure is controlled. In patients with heart rates >84 beats per minute during follow-up, this incidence is as high as 2.1% per year.[13] Overall, β-blocker therapy is associated with a reduced incidence of new onset AF. In a large randomized study, the **Ra**te **C**ontrol **E**fficacy in Permanent Atrial Fibrillation **II** (RACE II) study, "strict" rate control aiming to achieve a resting heart rate of <80 beats per minute, was not superior to "lenient" rate control aiming to achieve a resting heart rate of <110 beats per minute, on either morbidity, mortality, or quality of life.[14] β-blockers especially bisoprolol were most effective at reducing ventricular rates at rest and with exercise.

CONCLUSION

HFpEF is one of the most pressing diagnostic and therapeutic challenges in clinical medicine today, given its increasing prevalence, underdiagnosis, poor prognosis, limited therapeutic options, and substantial burden on the healthcare system worldwide.

Despite these challenges, the success of recent SGLT2i trials has shown that HFpEF is treatable and the most important point in HFpEF treatment is management of comorbidities.

REFERENCES

1. Pfeffer MA, Shah AM, Borlaug BA. Heart failure with preserved ejection fraction in perspective. Circ Res. 2019; 124(11):1598-617.
2. Bozkurt B, Coats AJS, Tsutsui H, et al. Universal definition and classification of heart failure: a report of the Heart Failure Society of America, Heart Failure Association of the European Society of Cardiology, Japanese Heart Failure Society and Writing Committee of the Universal Definition of Heart Failure: endorsed by Canadian Heart Failure Society, Heart Failure Association of India, the Cardiac Society of Australia and New Zealand, and the Chinese Heart Failure Association. Eur J Heart Fail. 2021; 23(3):352-80.
3. Pandey A, Omar W, Ayers C, et al. Sex and race differences in lifetime risk of heart failure with preserved ejection fraction and heart failure with reduced ejection fraction. Circulation. 2018;137(17):1814-23.
4. Ho JE, Lyass A, Lee DS, et al. Predictors of new-onset heart failure: differences in preserved versus reduced ejection fraction. Circ Heart Fail. 2013;6(2):279-86.
5. Dunlay SM, Roger VL, Redfield MM. Epidemiology of heart failure with preserved ejection fraction. Nat Rev Cardiol. 2017;14(10):591-602.
6. Pandey A, LaMonte M, Klein L, et al. Relationship between physical activity, body mass index, and risk of heart failure. J Am Coll Cardiol. 2017;69(9):1129-42.
7. Heidenreich PA, Bozkurt B, Aguilar D, et al. 2022 AHA/ACC/HFSA Guideline for the Management of Heart Failure: a report of the American College of Cardiology/American Heart Association Joint Committee on Clinical Practice Guidelines. J Am Coll Cardiol. 2022;79:e263-e421.
8. Düngen HD, Apostolovic S, Inkrot S, et al. Titration to target dose of bisoprolol vs. carvedilol in elderly patients with heart failure: the CIBIS-ELD trial. Eur J Heart Fail. 2011;13(6):670-80.
9. Broekman CP, Haensel SM, Van de Ven LL, et al. Bisoprolol and hypertension: effects on sexual functioning in men. J Sex Marital Ther. 1992;18(4):325-31.
10. Reddy YNV, Obokata M, Verbrugge FH, et al. Atrial dysfunction in patients with heart failure with preserved ejection fraction and atrial fibrillation. J Am Coll Cardiol. 2020;76(9):1051-64.
11. Zakeri R, Chamberlain AM, Roger VL, et al. Temporal relationship and prognostic significance of atrial fibrillation in heart failure patients with preserved ejection fraction: a community-based study. Circulation. 2013;128(10):1085-93.
12. Reddy YNV, Borlaug BA, Gersh BJ. Management of atrial fibrillation across the spectrum of heart failure with preserved and reduced ejection fraction. Circulation. 2022;146(4):339-57.
13. Okin PM, Wachtell K, Kjeldsen SE, et al. Incidence of atrial fibrillation in relation to changing heart rate over time in hypertensive patients: the LIFE study. Circ Arrhythm Electrophysiol. 2008;1(5):337-34.
14. Van Gelder IC, Groenveld HF, Crijns HJ, et al. Lenient versus strict rate control in patients with atrial fibrillation N Engl J Med. 2010;362(15):1363-73.

CHAPTER 150

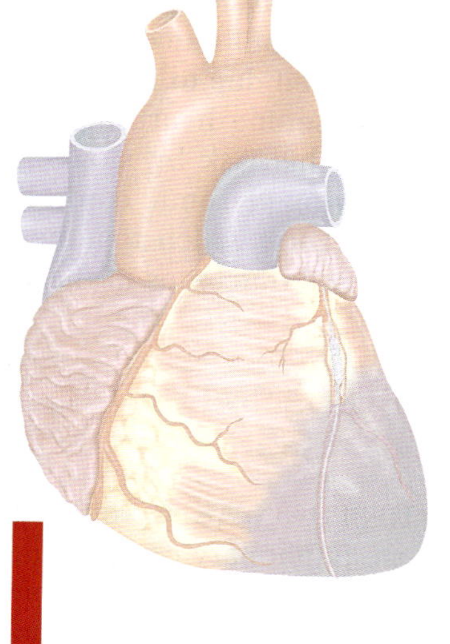

Morbidity and Mortality Benefits of SGLT2i, ARNI, and Bisoprolol in HFpEF with Atrial Fibrillation

Dhiman Kahali

INTRODUCTION

Atrial fibrillation (AF) and heart failure with preserved ejection fraction (HFpEF) are frequently coexisting cardiovascular conditions that are strongly interconnected, with each condition significantly increasing the risk of developing the other. AF, the most common cardiac arrhythmia, and HFpEF, characterized by impaired myocardial relaxation and abnormal intracardiac hemodynamics, are linked through progressive left atrial myopathy and shared cardiovascular risk factors. Studies, including the *Framingham Heart Study*[1] and the *PREVEND study*[2], show that AF significantly raises the risk of HFpEF, and HFpEF similarly increases the likelihood of developing AF. This review examines the morbidity and mortality benefits of combining sodium-glucose co-transporter-2 (SGLT-2) inhibitors, angiotensin receptor-neprilysin

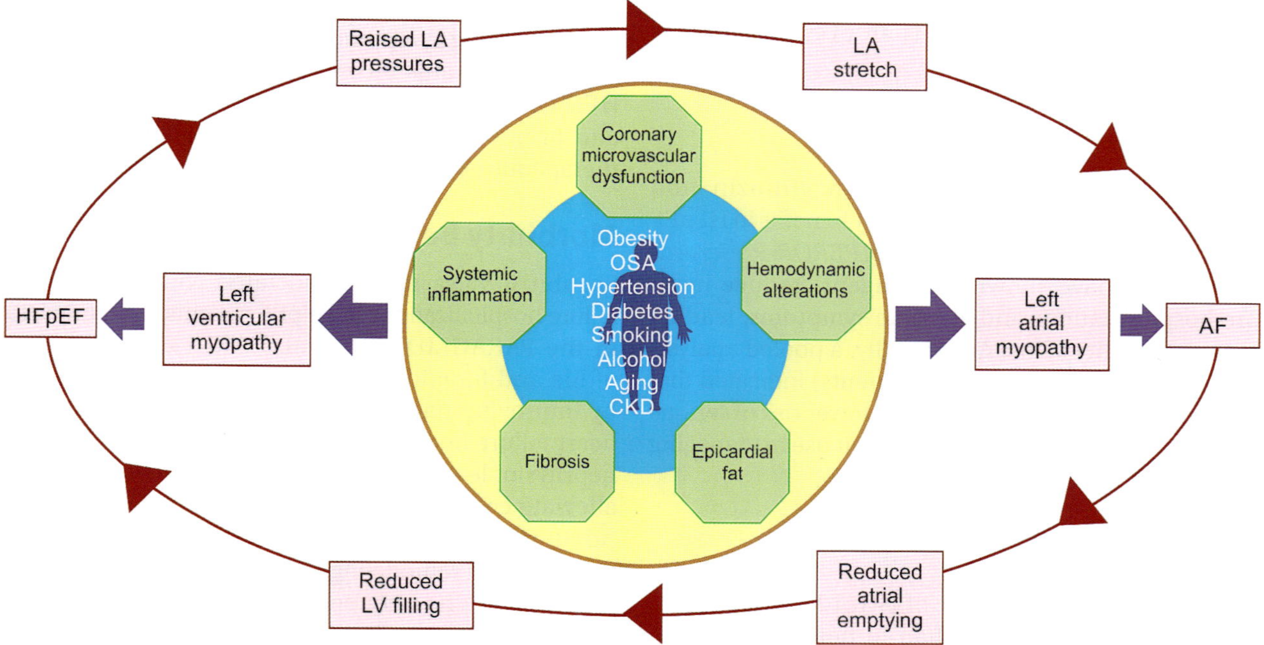

Fig. 1: Mechanisms underlying coexisting atrial fibrillation and heart failure with preserved ejection fraction (AF-HFpEF).[5]
(LA: left atrial; LV: left ventricular)

inhibitors (ARNI), and bisoprolol in managing HFpEF with AF, a complex yet synergistic therapeutic approach.

HEART FAILURE WITH PRESERVED EJECTION FRACTION AND ATRIAL FIBRILLATION

Systemic inflammation, hemodynamic changes, microvascular dysfunction, epicardial adiposity, and myocardial fibrosis are key consequences of cardiovascular risk factors and contribute significantly to the atrial and ventricular myopathies involved in both AF and HFpEF. These mechanisms do not act independently; instead, they form a complex, interrelated network.[3] Furthermore, AF and HFpEF each promote the onset and progression of the other, establishing a vicious cycle that, if untreated, leads to rapid advancement of both conditions. The development of left atrial (LA) disease appears to be the final common pathway linking these mechanisms and is increasingly recognized as a crucial factor in the interplay between AF and HFpEF **(Fig. 1)**.[4]

SODIUM-GLUCOSE COTRANSPORTER-2 IN HEART FAILURE WITH PRESERVED EJECTION FRACTION WITH ATRIAL FIBRILLATION

The SGLT2 inhibitors have shown significant benefits in reducing morbidity and mortality in patients with HFpEF, including those with AF.[6] Here is an overview of their effects.

Morbidity Benefits

The SGLT2 inhibitors, such as empagliflozin and dapagliflozin, offer significant morbidity benefits in HFpEF patients with AF. Studies such as *EMPEROR-Preserved*[7] and *DELIVER*[8] have shown these agents reduce heart failure hospitalizations and alleviate symptoms, leading to improved quality of life. Additionally, a pooled analysis of 31 trials[9] (involving over 75,000 patients) indicated that SGLT2 inhibitors are associated with a lower risk of serious AF/flutter events, further supporting their use in managing HFpEF with comorbid AF.

Mortality Benefits

While the mortality benefits of SGLT2 inhibitors in HFpEF are less pronounced than in heart failure with reduced ejection fraction (HFrEF), these agents still provide important cardiovascular advantages, including reductions in all-cause and cardiovascular mortality across both groups. In patients with HFpEF and comorbid AF, the risk of mortality is heightened due to increased thromboembolic events and worsening heart failure. SGLT2 inhibitors may mitigate this risk by slowing heart failure progression, improving glycemic control, and reducing inflammatory markers, which together contribute to better overall survival outcomes in these high-risk patients.

Key Mechanisms Supporting Sodium-Glucose Cotransporter-2 Benefits[10]

The SGLT2 inhibitors benefit HFpEF with AF by providing a mild diuretic effect to reduce pulmonary congestion, helping manage symptoms. They also reduce inflammation and fibrosis, potentially slowing left atrial enlargement and AF progression, which improves morbidity and mortality. Additionally, their renal protective effects support kidney function, further alleviating symptoms and enhancing survival.

ANGIOTENSIN RECEPTOR-NEPRILYSIN INHIBITORS IN HEART FAILURE WITH PRESERVED EJECTION FRACTION WITH ATRIAL FIBRILLATION

The ARNI, specifically sacubitril/valsartan has shown notable morbidity benefits in HFpEF patients, including those with AF, primarily by reducing hospitalizations and improving symptoms. While its impact on mortality in HFpEF remains inconclusive and less robust than in HFrEF, the drug significantly enhances quality of life and promotes atrial remodeling, making it a valuable therapeutic option for this patient population.

Morbidity Benefits

Sacubitril/valsartan is associated with reduced heart failure hospitalizations in HFpEF patients, as demonstrated in the PARAGLIDE-HF trial.[11] ARNI enhances quality of life and functional status in HFpEF patients with AF by improving patient-reported outcomes and reducing heart failure hospitalizations. Mechanistically, it inhibits neprilysin, leading to increased natriuretic peptides that alleviate congestion by reducing preload and afterload. Additionally, ARNI therapy reduces myocardial fibrosis and left atrial remodeling, helping to slow AF progression and decrease its frequency. The renal protective effects of ARNI are particularly beneficial for HFpEF patients with AF, as improved renal function can mitigate the exacerbation of heart failure and AF symptoms.

Mortality Benefits

While the PARAGON-HF trial did not show a statistically significant reduction in cardiovascular mortality for the overall HFpEF population, certain subgroups, particularly those with lower ejection fractions or high-risk features like AF, may benefit from decreased cardiovascular events and mortality. ARNIs mechanisms, which enhance hemodynamics and reduce atrial stretch, may further lower the mortality risk in HFpEF patients with AF, who are particularly susceptible to thromboembolic events and cardiovascular death.

BISOPROLOL IN HEART FAILURE WITH PRESERVED EJECTION FRACTION WITH ATRIAL FIBRILLATION

Bisoprolol, a β-1 selective blocker, is beneficial for managing HFpEF with AF by effectively controlling heart rate, reducing hospitalizations, and improving quality of life. Though its mortality benefits in HFpEF are less established, it offers significant morbidity benefits by minimizing HF symptoms and potentially lowering the risk of AF-related complications, making it a valuable option for managing HFpEF with AF.[12]

Morbidity Benefits

In HFpEF patients with AF, bisoprolol provides morbidity benefits by effectively controlling heart rate, which reduces symptoms such as dyspnea and fatigue, improves exercise tolerance, and enhances quality of life. It may also lower HF-related hospitalizations by stabilizing symptoms and reducing AF exacerbations, contributing to better functional status and symptom management. In HFpEF patients with AF, bisoprolol offers morbidity benefits by lowering sympathetic overactivity to improve heart rate control and reduce myocardial oxygen demand. Its rate-slowing effect aids diastolic filling, supporting diastolic function, while reducing atrial remodeling and ventricular strain, potentially decreasing AF episodes and slowing disease progression.

The RATE-HF trial[13] demonstrated that in patients primarily with HFpEF, β-blockers offered no advantage over digoxin for rate control in those with permanent AF. Additionally, overly stringent rate control in HFpEF may lead to chronotropic incompetence, potentially reducing activity tolerance. In stable HFpEF patients (38.5% with a history of AF), discontinuing β-blockers led to improvements in symptoms and functional status.[14]

Mortality Benefits

In HFpEF with AF, bisoprolol's mortality benefits are modest but may reduce risks indirectly. By controlling AF, bisoprolol can help lower complications such as thromboembolism, stroke, and HF exacerbations. Additionally, its heart rate reduction can lower adverse cardiac events, potentially reducing fatal episodes of acute decompensated HF. There is no direct trial regarding role of bisoprolol in HFpEF patient with AF.

CONCLUSION

In HFpEF patients with AF, the combination of SGLT2 inhibitors, ARNI, and bisoprolol offers complementary and synergistic morbidity and mortality benefits, although with varying degrees of evidence. SGLT2 inhibitors have demonstrated robust morbidity benefits, particularly in reducing heart failure hospitalizations and enhancing quality of life, with modest indications of mortality reduction. ARNI therapy, primarily sacubitril/valsartan, has shown reductions in hospitalization rates and symptom relief, especially in high-risk HFpEF patients, though its mortality impact remains inconclusive. Bisoprolol provides valuable rate control, reducing AF symptoms and possibly lowering hospitalization risk, though mortality benefits in HFpEF are not well established. Together, these therapies target critical pathophysiological mechanisms—volume overload, inflammation, and sympathetic overactivity—making them essential tools in the multifaceted management of HFpEF with AF.

REFERENCES

1. Santhanakrishnan R, Wang N, Larson MG, et al. Atrial fibrillation begets heart failure and vice versa. Circulation. 2016;133(5):484-92.
2. Vermond RA, Geelhoed B, Verweij N, et al. Incidence of atrial fibrillation and relationship with cardiovascular events, heart failure, and mortality. J Am Coll Cardiol. 2015;66(9):1000-7.
3. Packer M. HFpEF is the substrate for stroke in obesity and diabetes independent of atrial fibrillation. JACC Heart Fail. 2020;8(1):35-42.
4. Bisbal F, Baranchuk A, Braunwald E, et al. Atrial failure as a clinical entity. J Am Coll Cardiol. 2020;75(2):222-32.
5. Ariyaratnam JP, Elliott AD, Mishima RS, et al. Heart failure with preserved ejection fraction: An alternative paradigm to explain the clinical implications of atrial fibrillation. Heart rhythm. 2021;2(6Part B):771-83.
6. Van Gelder IC, Rienstra M, Bunting KV, et al. 2024 ESC Guidelines for the management of atrial fibrillation developed in collaboration with the European Association

for Cardio-Thoracic Surgery (EACTS). Eur Heart J. 2024;45(36):3314.

7. Anker SD, Butler J, Filippatos G, et al. Empagliflozin in heart failure with a preserved ejection fraction. N Engl J Med. 2021;385(16):1451-61.
8. Solomon SD, McMurray JJV, Claggett B, et al. Dapagliflozin in heart failure with mildly reduced or preserved ejection fraction. N Engl J Med. 2022;387(12):1089-98.
9. Pandey AK, Okaj I, Kaur H, et al. Sodium-Glucose Co-Transporter Inhibitors and Atrial Fibrillation: A Systematic Review and Meta-Analysis of Randomized Controlled Trials. J Am Heart Assoc. 2021;10(17):e022222.
10. Lytvyn Y, Bjornstad P, Udell JA, et al. Sodium Glucose Cotransporter-2 Inhibition in Heart Failure: Potential Mechanisms, Clinical Applications, and Summary of Clinical Trials. Circulation. 2017;136(17):1643-58.
11. Vaduganathan M, Mentz RJ, Claggett JA, et al. Sacubitril/valsartan in heart failure with mildly reduced or preserved ejection fraction: a pre-specified participant-level pooled analysis of PARAGLIDE-HF and PARAGON-HF. Eur Heart J. 2023;44(31):2982-93.
12. Hyun J. Heart Failure With Preserved Ejection Fraction and Atrial Fibrillation: Are Beta-Blockers Still Relevant? Int J Heart Failure. 2024;6(3):127-8.
13. Kotecha D, Bunting KV, Gill SK, et al. Effect of Digoxin vs Bisoprolol for Heart Rate Control in Atrial Fibrillation on Patient-Reported Quality of Life: The RATE-AF Randomized Clinical Trial. JAMA. 2020;324(24):2497-508.
14. Dye C, Dela Cruz M, Larsen T, et al. A review of the impact, pathophysiology, and management of atrial fibrillation in patients with heart failure with preserved ejection fraction. Am Heart J Plus. 2023;33:100309.

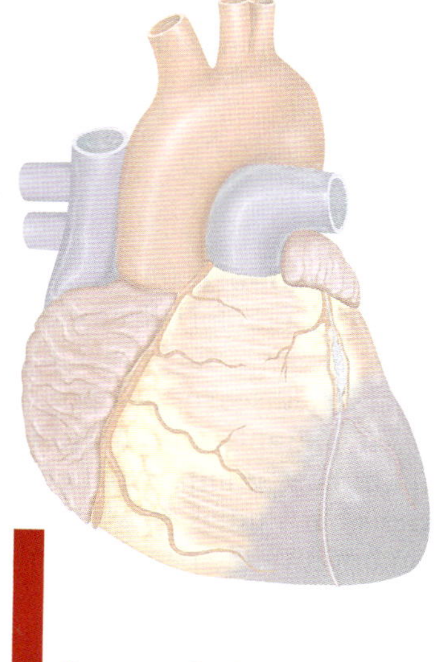

Promise of Bisoprolol in HFpEF: Present Status

Ameet G Sattur

INTRODUCTION

Heart failure (HF) is the leading cardiovascular disease in the world. In the last three to four decades, the knowledge regarding the pathophysiology of this complex clinical syndrome has developed to a very great extent, thus leading to the use of drugs that can significantly improve the morbidity and mortality of HF patients, called "HF modifying drugs."[1]

Among the HF modifying drugs, the benefits of β-blockers (BBs) are well established in patients with heart failure with reduced ejection fraction (HFrEF). All guidelines (ACC/AHA, ESC, and others) recommend BBs in the treatment of patients with chronic HFrEF.[2,3]

The present management for heart failure with preserved ejection fraction (HFpEF) focuses on symptom relief usually with the use of diuretics, treating of underlying etiologies (amyloidosis), and managing comorbid conditions such as hypertension, chronic kidney disease, arrythmias, and others.[2,4] However, the beneficial effects of BBs in HFpEF remains unclear and uncertain. There is no current consensus on the efficacy of BBs on mortality and rehospitalization among patients with HFpEF.

PATHOGENESIS AND MECHANISM

The pathogenesis of HF is multifactorial:

- *Sympathetic nervous system (SNS) overactivity* leads to short LV diastolic filling time, increased blood pressure, and increased propensity to develop arrhythmias. Persistent stimulation of BBs results in cardiac myocyte apoptosis, hypertrophy, and fibrosis.[5]
- *Renin-angiotensin-aldosterone system (RAAS) overactivation* causes retention of salt and water, constriction of peripheral arteries, and increased myocardial contractility.

To counteract the effects of SNS, BBs are proposed. HFpEF patients are usually elderly who are at risk or already have cardiovascular disease, atrial fibrillation, and hypertension where BBs are indicated. On the other hand, there are concerns that BBs, by slowing the heart rate, could cause chronotropic incompetence and could aggravate the symptoms of HF.

Another potential benefit of BB use in HFpEF is direct myocardial protection from catecholamine toxicity. Catecholamines are oversecreted in patients with HFpEF as a counterregulation to a reduction in cardiac output. Prolonged duration of catecholamine exposure also worsens the physical and psychological outcomes, affecting the quality of life (QoL) in these patients.[6]

DISCUSSION

The first study showing beneficial effect of BBs in HFpEF was by Bavishi et al.,[7] which reported reduced mortality in patients with HFpEF and old myocardial infarction with propranolol. The first and probably only prospective randomized trial to report the effect of carvedilol in patients with HFpEF was the Japanese Diastolic Heart Failure (J-DHF) trial. In this trial, carvedilol did not improve a composite of cardiovascular death and hospitalization.[8] But the J-DHF study was criticized for not having achieved the expected number of events due to poor enrollment and high follow-up loss of patients.

The SENIORS (Study of Effects of Nebivolol Intervention on Outcomes and Rehospitalization in Seniors with Heart Failure) trial showed a beneficial effect and reduction in the composite endpoints of all-cause mortality and hospital admissions with nebivolol. In this trial, there were only 15% of patients who had HFpEF.[9]

Another meta-analysis of 10 randomized studies in patients with HFpEF showed a significant decrease in all-cause mortality and hospitalization for HF.[10]

A Korean Acute Heart Failure registry,[11] which was a prospective observational multicenter cohort study that included 2,152 patients with HFpEF, showed a 14% reduced all-cause death with use of BBs but not with reduced rehospitalizations.

Another systematic review and meta-analysis of BB therapy in HFpEF by Kaddoua et al., which included 27,188 patients, showed a significant 19% reduction in all-cause mortality, whereas rehospitalization for HF was similar between the BBs and control groups.[12]

New techniques such as use of global longitudinal strain (GLS) have shown that in patients with HF and GLS <14, BB therapy improved survival.[13]

Use of BBs in cardiovascular and noncardiovascular comorbidities:

- *Respiratory comorbidity:* Severe asthma and not severe chronic obstructive pulmonary disease (COPD) is a relative contraindication to BB therapy. COPD is present in 30% of HF patients. Bisoprolol is the first choice, followed by nebivolol, and should be preferred in HFpEF patients with COPD.[14]
- *Diabetes mellitus:*[15] Diabetics have higher sympathomimetic activity, and BBs are thus helpful. Higher doses of bisoprolol may provide higher mortality benefits in HFpEF, and the subset of HFpEF patients with T2DM is particularly likely to derive higher mortality benefits from high-dose bisoprolol.
- Others are shown in **Figure 1**.

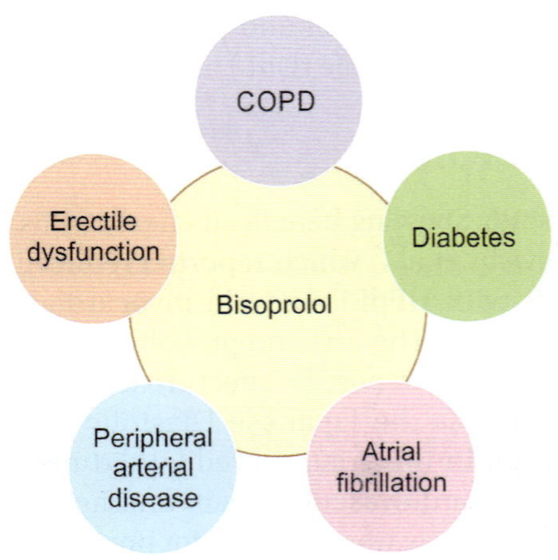

Fig. 1
(COPD: chronic obstructive pulmonary disease)

CONCLUSION

Heart failure with preserved ejection fraction is a heterogenous entity, and the use of bisoprolol will be more beneficial in selected subgroups such as atrial fibrillation, hypertension, and coronary artery disease. Bisoprolol reduces all-cause mortality in patients with HFpEF; rehospitalizations due to HF in these group of patients have mixed results and need further studies. It is a well-tolerated drug, and its use can improve the patient's QoL in HFpEF.

REFERENCES

1. Komajda M, Böhm M, Borer JS, et al. Incremental benefit of drug therapies for chronic heart failure with reduced ejection fraction: a network meta-analysis. Eur J Heart Fail. 2018;20(9):1315-22.
2. McDonagh TA, Metra M, Adamo M, et al. 2021 ESC guidelines for the diagnosis and treatment of acute and chronic heart failure. Euro Heart J. 2021;42(36):3599-726.
3. Heidenreich PA, Bozkurt B, Aguilar D, et al. 2022 AHA/ACC/HFSA guideline for the management of heart failure: a report of the American College of Cardiology/American Heart Association Joint Committee on Clinical Practice Guidelines. J Am Coll Cardiol. 2022;79(17):e263-421.
4. Heidenreich PA, Bozkurt B, Aguilar D, et al. 2022 AHA/ACC/HFSA guideline for the management of heart failure: a report of the American College of Cardiology/American Heart Association Joint Committee on Clinical Practice Guidelines. Circulation. 2022;145(18):e895-1032.
5. Fukuta H, Goto T, Wakami K, et al. Effects of drug and exercise intervention on functional capacity and quality of life in heart failure with preserved ejection fraction: a meta-analysis of randomized controlled trials. Eur J Prev Cardiol. 2016;23(1):78-85.
6. Henning RJ. Diagnosis and treatment of heart failure with preserved left ventricular ejection fraction. World J Cardiol. 2020;12(1):7-25.
7. Bavishi C, Chatterjee S, Ather S, et al. Beta-blockers in heart failure with preserved ejection fraction: a meta-analysis. Heart Fail Rev. 2015;20(2):193-201.
8. Yamamoto K, Origasa H, Hori M, et al. Effects of carvedilol on heart failure with preserved ejection fraction: the Japanese Diastolic Heart Failure Study (J-DHF). Eur J Heart Fail. 2013;15(1):110-8.
9. van Veldhuisen DJ, Cohen-Solal A, Böhm M, et al. Beta-blockade with nebivolol in elderly heart failure patients with impaired and preserved left ventricular ejection

fraction: data from SENIORS (study of effects of nebivolol intervention on outcomes and rehospitalization in seniors with heart failure). J Am Coll Cardiol. 2009;53(23):2150-8.

10. Wu M, Ni D, Huang LL, et al. Association between the beta-blockers, calcium channel blockers, all-cause mortality and length of hospitalization in patients with heart failure with preserved ejection fraction: a meta-analysis of randomized controlled trials. Clin Cardiol. 2023;46(8):845-52.
11. Kim SH, Yun SC, Park JJ, et al. Beta-blockers in patients with heart failure with preserved ejection fraction: results from the Korean Acute Heart Failure (KorAHF) registry. Korean Circ J. 2019;49(3):238-48.
12. Kaddoura R, Madurasinghe V, Chapra A, et al. Beta-blocker therapy in heart failure with preserved ejection fraction (B-HFpEF): a systemic review and meta-analysis. Curr Probl Cardiol. 2024;49(3):102376.
13. Park JJ, Choi HM, Hwang IC, et al. Myocardial strain for identification of β-blocker responders in heart failure with preserved ejection fraction. J Am Soc Echocardiogr. 2019;32(11):1462-9.
14. Sinagra G, Corrà U, Contini M, et al. Choosing among β-blockers in heart failure patients according to β-receptors' location and functions in the cardiopulmonary system. Pharmacol Res. 2020;156:104785.
15. Witte KK, Drozd M, Walker AMN, et al. Mortality reduction associated with β-adrenoceptor inhibition in chronic heart failure is greater in patients with diabetes. Diabetes Care. 2018;41(1):136-42.

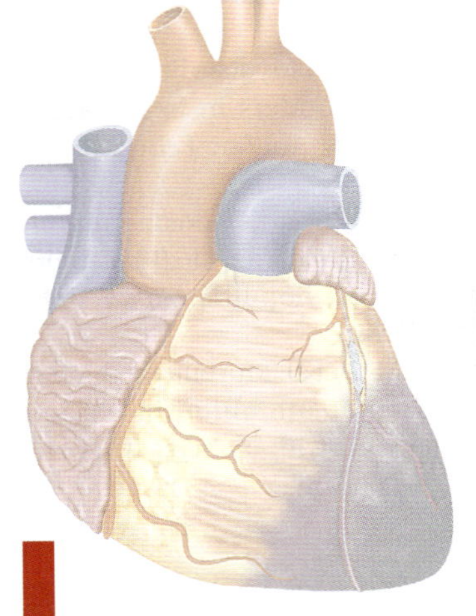

Role of Bisoprolol in Patients with HFpEF

Kiron Varghese

INTRODUCTION

Heart failure with preserved ejection fraction (HFpEF) is a complex clinical syndrome characterized by symptoms of heart failure (HF) despite a "preserved" left ventricular ejection fraction (LVEF). The first challenge in the diagnosis of HFpEF is to define the threshold of ejection fraction. Based on the universal definition of HF and consensus from the US HF Collaboratory and Academic Research Consortium, HFpEF is defined as a clinical diagnosis of HF with LVEF of 50% or greater.[1] HFpEF is increasingly recognized as a significant contributor to morbidity and mortality in the aging population, and its prevalence is rising due to the increasing incidence of comorbid conditions such as hypertension, obesity, and diabetes mellitus. Traditional HF treatments have primarily focused on patients with heart failure with reduced ejection fraction (HFrEF), leading to a relative lack of evidence-based therapies for HFpEF. Bisoprolol, a selective beta-1 adrenergic antagonist and other beta-blockers (BBs), may constitute a potential treatment option in selected patients.

Bisoprolol being a highly selective BB has advantages over other selective BBs such as metoprolol and atenolol as well as carvedilol, a nonselective BB.[2]

This chapter reviews the role of bisoprolol in HFpEF, focusing on its efficacy, safety, and mechanism of action, supported by relevant literature.

UNDERSTANDING HEART FAILURE WITH PRESERVED EJECTION FRACTION

Heart failure with preserved ejection fraction is a heterogeneous condition with a multifactorial etiology. It is often associated with diastolic dysfunction, where the heart's ability to relax and fill with blood is impaired. Key clinical features include exertional dyspnea, fatigue, and fluid retention. Comorbidities such as hypertension, obesity, diabetes mellitus, coronary artery disease (CAD), and atrial fibrillation are frequently present, complicating the management of these patients.[1]

CURRENT MANAGEMENT STRATEGIES

Management strategies for HFpEF have traditionally been symptomatic, focusing on diuretics to alleviate congestion. However, unlike HFrEF, where BBs, angiotensin-converting enzyme (ACE) inhibitors, neprilysin inhibitors, and mineralocorticoid receptor antagonists have been established as foundational therapies, evidence supporting the use of these agents in HFpEF is limited.[1]

ROLE OF BETA-BLOCKERS IN HEART FAILURE WITH PRESERVED EJECTION FRACTION

Beta-blockers, including bisoprolol, have been the subject of investigation for their potential benefits in HFpEF. While these medications are well established for managing HFrEF, their role in HFpEF has been less clear, and there is no clear consensus on the benefits of bisoprolol or other BB in patients with HFpEF.[3] Many guidelines recommend against the use of BB in HFpEF[4] or suggest their use only in selected patients with comorbidities.[1]

MECHANISM OF ACTION

The mechanisms by which bisoprolol may exert benefits in HFpEF involve several physiological pathways given as follows:

- *Heart rate reduction:* Bisoprolol like other BBs reduces heart rate, allowing for longer diastolic filling times, which may improve cardiac output despite impaired relaxation.[5]
- *Improved exercise tolerance:* By decreasing heart rate and improving myocardial oxygen supply–demand balance, especially in patients with underlying CAD, bisoprolol may enhance exercise tolerance, a key concern for HFpEF patients.[5]
- *Neurohormonal modulation:* BBs may also exert beneficial effects on neurohormonal activation, which is often upregulated in HF. By blocking excessive adrenergic stimulation, bisoprolol can reduce cardiac stress and prevent further deterioration of heart function.
- *Management of comorbidities:* Bisoprolol is effective in managing hypertension and atrial fibrillation, both common in HFpEF, which can indirectly improve HF symptoms.

The pathogenesis of HFpEF is multifactorial in most patients, and sympathetic overactivation is noted in several patients, often leading to tachycardia, hypertension, tachyarrhythmias, and abbreviated LV filling time. Conceptually, BB therapy should be beneficial by countering the sympathetic nervous system-induced detrimental neurohormonal effects. Additionally, the majority of patients with HFpEF are elderly or have multiple comorbidities such as atrial fibrillation, hypertension, and CAD for which BB is often indicated.[3]

ROLE OF BETA-BLOCKERS AFTER ACUTE MYOCARDIAL INFARCTION WITH PRESERVED EJECTION FRACTION

Coronary artery disease is common in patients with HFpEF, with epicardial disease prevalent in over 50% of patients and microvascular dysfunction in up to 75% of patients.[6] An early study of a BB (atenolol) for 1 week after acute myocardial infarction (MI) demonstrated a reduction in vascular mortality in the first 7 days after treatment.[7] However, HF was not a prerequisite for enrollment in the trial, and only 0.7% previously had HF. A more recent study (REDUCE-AMI) that randomized patients with acute MI documented obstructive CAD and LVEF ≥50% to BB therapy with metoprolol or bisoprolol. In this study, long-term BB treatment with either metoprolol or bisoprolol did not lead to a lower risk of the composite primary end point of death or new MI compared to no BB use.[8]

The Korean Acute Heart Failure (KorAHF) prospective, observational, multicenter cohort study evaluated the role of BB therapy in 2,152 patients hospitalized for acute HF syndrome. In the propensity score-matched population, BB therapy was associated with reduced all-cause death [HR 0.80; 95% confidence interval (CI) 0.69–0.94] but not with reduced rehospitalization.[9]

One of the limitations of this study was the cutoff for defining HFpEF was LVEF ≥40% unlike the current definition of LVEF ≥50%. It should also be noted that this was not a randomized controlled trial, and these findings need to be replicated in randomized clinical trials.

In the light of such conflicting evidence, the routine use of BBs such as bisoprolol after acute MI and LVEF ≥50% is probably not justified in the absence of other compelling indications.

Safety is a critical concern when considering bisoprolol for HFpEF patients, particularly those with comorbid conditions such as asthma and chronic obstructive pulmonary disease (COPD). Bisoprolol is a highly selective BB and, thus, less likely to cause bronchospasm compared to nonselective BBs. In a study that evaluated the impact of BB selectivity on long-term outcomes in congestive heart failure (CHF) patients with COPD, bisoprolol significantly reduced the incidence of CHF and/or COPD exacerbation compared with carvedilol.[10]

CLINICAL GUIDELINES AND RECOMMENDATIONS

Current clinical guidelines provide limited support for the use of BBs in HFpEF. The 2017 American College of Cardiology/American Heart Association (ACC/AHA) guidelines suggest that BBs may be considered in patients with HFpEF who have comorbid conditions such as hypertension or atrial fibrillation.[10] However, they emphasize that the evidence remains less robust compared to HFrEF.[11]

The more recent 2023 ACC Expert Consensus on HFpEF states that BBs may be used in patients with HFpEF who have specific indications, such as atrial fibrillation, angina, or previous MI (for up to 3 years). However, since BBs may contribute to chronotropic incompetence, exercise tolerance should be monitored.[1]

The RATE-AF randomized clinical trial studied the effects of digoxin versus bisoprolol in patients with atrial fibrillation and symptoms of HF. This was a small trial (160 subjects) primarily to assess the effects on quality of life and heart rate. Approximately 80% of the patients had

HFpEF. The study failed to show a significant difference in the quality of life between the two groups. Although NT-proBNP levels were significantly reduced in the digoxin group, there was an increase in the bisoprolol group, suggesting a limited role for BBs in patients with atrial fibrillation and HFpEF.[12]

Beta-blockers are widely used in various conditions, and it is pertinent to note that 83, 86, 78, and 80%, respectively, of patients enrolled in the DELIVER, EMPEROR-Preserved, TOPCAT, and PARAGON-HF clinical trials of patients with HFpEF had a background usage of BBs.[1] Given the high background usage of BB in such patients, it may prove difficult to assess the benefit of BB in HFpEF.

Meta-analyses of BB therapy in HFpEF are complicated by varying definitions of HFpEF, which has earlier been variously defined as patients with HF and LVEF >40, 45, or 50%. One large recent meta-analysis, the first to include studies that recruited patients with HFpEF defined as LVEF of ≥50% as per the recent guidelines, evaluated the efficacy of BB in HFpEF. This study, which included cohort studies of variable follow-up durations, demonstrated a significant reduction in all-cause mortality by 19% [odds ratio (OR) 0.81; 95% CI 0.65–0.99, $p = 0.044$]. However, there was no difference in rehospitalization for HF between the BB and control groups.[3]

FUTURE DIRECTIONS IN RESEARCH

The role of bisoprolol and other BBs in HFpEF is an evolving field of research. It must be emphasized that large-scale randomized trials are required to clarify the current uncertainty regarding BB therapy in HFpEF and to evaluate whether some subsets of HFpEF patients may benefit most from BB therapy. Investigations into the effects of BBs on clinical end points, quality of life, and hospitalizations are particularly critical.

CONCLUSION

Bisoprolol may represent a promising option for managing patients with HFpEF, particularly those with comorbid conditions such as hypertension and atrial fibrillation. While evidence supporting its use in this population is still developing, some studies indicate potential benefits. As the understanding of HFpEF evolves, bisoprolol may play a more central role in the therapeutic landscape, especially as more data emerge from ongoing and future studies. Until then, clinicians should consider individual patient characteristics and comorbidities when incorporating bisoprolol into HFpEF management.

REFERENCES

1. Kittleson MM, Panjrath GS, Amancherla K, et al. 2023 ACC Expert Consensus Decision Pathway on Management of Heart Failure with Preserved Ejection Fraction: A report of the American College of Cardiology Solution Set Oversight Committee. J Am Coll Cardiol. 2023;81(18): 1835-78.
2. Chopra HK, Nair T, Wander GS, et al. Role of bisoprolol in Heart Failure Management: A Consensus Statement from India. J Assoc Physicians India. 2023;71(12): 77-88.
3. Kaddoura R, Madurasinghe V, Chapra A, et al. Beta-blocker therapy in heart failure with preserved ejection fraction (B-HFpEF): a systematic review and meta-analysis. Curr Probl Cardiol. 2024;49:102376.
4. Heidenreich PA, Bozkurt B, Aguilar D, et al. 2022 AHA/ACC/HFSA guideline for the management of heart failure: a report of the American College of Cardiology/American Heart Association Joint Committee on clinical practice guidelines. Circulation. 2022;145(18):e895-1032.
5. Fukuta H, Goto T, Kamiya T. Effects of beta-blocker withdrawal in patients with heart failure with preserved ejection fraction: a protocol for systematic review and meta-analysis. PLoS One. 2023;18(11):e0294347.
6. Rush CJ, Berry C, Oldroyd KG, et al. Prevalence of coronary artery disease and coronary microvascular dysfunction in patients with heart failure with preserved ejection fraction. JAMA Cardiol. 2021;6:1130-43.
7. Randomised trial of intravenous atenolol among 16,027 cases of suspected acute myocardial infarction: ISIS-1. Lancet. 1986;2(8498):57-66.
8. Yndigegn T, Lindahl B, Mars K, et al. Beta-blockers after myocardial infarction and preserved ejection fraction. N Engl J Med. 2024;390(15):1372-81.
9. Kim SH, Yun SC, Park JJ, et al. Beta-blockers in Patients with Heart Failure with Preserved Ejection Fraction: Results from the Korean Acute Heart Failure (KorAHF) Registry. Korean Circ J. 2019;49(3):238-48.
10. Kubota Y, Asai K, Furuse E, et al. Impact of β-blocker selectivity on long-term outcomes in congestive heart failure patients with chronic obstructive pulmonary disease. Int J Chron Obstruct Pulmon Dis. 2015;10: 515-23.
11. Yancy CW, Jessup M, Bozkurt B, et al. 2017 ACC/AHA/HFSA focused update of the 2013 ACCF/AHA guideline for the management of heart failure: a report of the American College of Cardiology/American Heart Association Task Force on clinical practice guidelines and the Heart Failure Society of America. Circulation. 2017;136(6): e137-61.
12. Kotecha D, Bunting KV, Gill SK, et al. Effect of Digoxin vs Bisoprolol for Heart Rate Control in Atrial Fibrillation on Patient-reported Quality of Life. The RATE-AF Randomized Clinical Trial. JAMA. 2020;324(24):2497-508.

Beta-blockers in the Management of HFpEF: What is the Consensus?

M Somasundaram, GV Senthilnathan, R Divya

INTRODUCTION

Heart failure with preserved ejection fraction (HFpEF) is a syndrome marked by the heart's inability to fill properly during diastole despite a normal ejection fraction, and it accounts for nearly half of all heart failure cases, particularly affecting older adults with comorbidities such as hypertension, diabetes, and obesity.[1,2] The increasing prevalence of HFpEF presents a significant public health challenge due to its high morbidity, frequent hospitalizations, and reduced quality of life. Unlike heart failure with reduced ejection fraction (HFrEF), where treatments such as beta-blockers have clear benefits, the management of HFpEF is complicated by its heterogeneous nature, involving multiple pathophysiological mechanisms such as diastolic dysfunction, systemic inflammation, and vascular stiffness. While beta-blockers are well established in HFrEF, their role in HFpEF remains unclear and controversial due to these differing underlying mechanisms. This paper aims to review the current consensus on beta-blocker use in HFpEF by examining clinical evidence, guidelines, and expert opinions to clarify their potential role and highlight areas for further research.[1,3,4]

PATHOPHYSIOLOGY OF HFpEF AND MECHANISM OF ACTION OF BETA-BLOCKERS

Understanding HFpEF

Heart failure with preserved ejection fraction is characterized by a normal left ventricular ejection fraction (LVEF) but abnormal diastolic function, where the heart muscle becomes stiff or less compliant, resulting in impaired filling during diastole. This condition is complex and involves several interrelated pathophysiological mechanisms. As discussed in the publication by Borlaug et al., the primary hallmark of HFpEF is diastolic dysfunction, which is the heart's inability to relax and fill efficiently during diastole. This can be due to increased myocardial stiffness or altered relaxation dynamics, often compounded by elevated filling pressures that contribute to symptoms such as dyspnea and exercise intolerance. In addition to diastolic dysfunction as discussed in the study by Borovac et al., HFpEF is associated with systemic inflammation, endothelial dysfunction, and vascular stiffness, which further complicate its pathophysiology. Systemic inflammation, often driven by comorbid conditions such as obesity, diabetes, and hypertension, can promote myocardial fibrosis and stiffness, exacerbating diastolic dysfunction. Vascular stiffness, characterized by reduced compliance of the large arteries, increases afterload and further impairs cardiac filling. Together, these mechanisms create a vicious cycle that leads to the progressive nature of HFpEF, making its management particularly challenging.[2,5,6]

Mechanism of Action of Beta-blockers in HFpEF

Beta-blockers, which are commonly used in the management of HFrEF, have a different potential role in HFpEF due to the distinctive pathophysiological characteristics of this condition.[7] The primary mechanism of beta-blockers involves blocking beta-adrenergic receptors, thereby reducing the effects of sympathetic nervous system activation, which is often heightened in heart failure. By reducing heart rate and myocardial oxygen demand, beta-blockers can potentially improve symptoms and prevent further cardiac remodeling.[8] In the context of HFpEF, beta-blockers may offer several theoretical benefits. For instance, by lowering heart rate, they can increase diastolic filling time, which may be beneficial in a condition characterized by impaired diastolic relaxation. Moreover, the reduction in sympathetic nervous system activity could help alleviate systemic inflammation and endothelial dysfunction, both of which are implicated in the pathophysiology of HFpEF.[3,4,9]

However, the evidence supporting these potential benefits remains limited and inconclusive. Unlike in HFrEF, where the reduction of sympathetic stimulation directly addresses the underlying problem of systolic dysfunction, the benefits of beta-blockers in HFpEF are less clear due to the complex interplay of diastolic dysfunction, vascular stiffness, and systemic inflammation. Some studies suggest that beta-blockers may improve symptoms in certain HFpEF patients, particularly those with high heart rates or significant ischemic heart disease, but these benefits have not been consistently observed across all patient populations. Consequently, the role of beta-blockers in HFpEF remains a matter of debate, and their use is often guided by individual patient characteristics and comorbidities rather than by strong, universally accepted clinical guidelines.[10,11]

EVIDENCE OF THE USE OF BETA-BLOCKERS IN HFpEF

Several clinical trials and studies have explored the use of beta-blockers in the management of HFpEF with mixed and often inconclusive results. The J-DHF trial, for example, evaluated the impact of the beta-blocker carvedilol in Japanese patients with HFpEF and found no significant reduction in mortality or hospitalization rates compared to placebo, although some improvement in left ventricular diastolic function was noted.[12] Similarly, the SENIORS trial, which included a broader heart failure population, showed that the beta-blocker nebivolol reduced mortality and hospital admissions, but these benefits were not clearly differentiated between patients with preserved versus reduced ejection fraction. The variable results in these studies reflect the complex pathophysiology of HFpEF and raise questions about the uniform efficacy of beta-blockers across different patient populations.[13,14]

The key findings from these studies are limited by several factors. Most trials have involved small sample sizes and heterogeneous patient groups, making it difficult to draw definitive conclusions. Additionally, there is a lack of large-scale, high-quality randomized controlled trials (RCTs) specifically focused on beta-blocker use in HFpEF. This has resulted in mixed evidence regarding their impact on critical outcomes such as mortality, hospitalization rates, and quality of life. Consequently, while beta-blockers may offer potential benefits for certain subgroups of HFpEF patients, the overall evidence remains insufficient to support their widespread use, highlighting the need for more targeted research.[12,15]

GUIDELINES AND CURRENT RECOMMENDATIONS

Major cardiovascular societies, including the American Heart Association (AHA), American College of Cardiology (ACC), and the European Society of Cardiology (ESC), provide limited and somewhat inconsistent recommendations regarding the use of beta-blockers in the management of HFpEF. The AHA/ACC guidelines do not give a strong endorsement for beta-blocker use in HFpEF primarily due to the lack of robust evidence demonstrating a clear mortality or morbidity benefit.[16] They suggest beta-blockers may be considered for managing comorbid conditions such as hypertension or atrial fibrillation, which are common in HFpEF patients, but they are not specifically recommended for improving heart failure outcomes.[16,17]

In contrast, the ESC guidelines recognize that while beta-blockers may help control symptoms such as tachycardia and manage comorbid conditions, they do not recommend their routine use for all HFpEF patients due to the variability in clinical trial results. The ESC also highlights the absence of conclusive data supporting a reduction in mortality or heart failure hospitalizations with beta-blockers in this patient population.[17] Overall, there is a consensus among these guidelines that beta-blockers should not be universally prescribed for HFpEF and that their use should be tailored to individual patient needs, particularly for those with specific comorbidities such as atrial fibrillation or hypertension. However, there is some controversy due to the lack of high-quality evidence, with different guidelines varying in their emphasis on beta-blockers' potential symptomatic benefits versus their unclear impact on clinical outcomes. This reflects the broader uncertainty in the field and highlights the need for more focused research to clarify the role of beta-blockers in HFpEF management.

CLINICAL PRACTICE AND EXPERT OPINIONS

Expert opinions and consensus statements reflect a cautious stance on the use of beta-blockers in HFpEF. Many experts agree that while beta-blockers might be beneficial in managing certain symptoms or comorbidities, there is insufficient evidence to recommend their widespread use for all HFpEF patients. Some consensus statements, such as those from the Heart Failure Society of America (HFSA), suggest that beta-blockers may be considered for HFpEF patients with specific indications, such as atrial fibrillation or high heart rates, but emphasize that they should not be viewed as a primary therapy for HFpEF itself. Overall, expert opinions converge on the need for personalized treatment approaches, acknowledging that beta-blockers may offer some benefits in selected patients but are not universally effective for HFpEF management **(Flowchart 1)**.[7,9,18-20]

INITIATION AND TITRATION TO TARGET DOSES IN HFpEF

Since the evidence does not strongly support specific target doses in HFpEF, the goal is to achieve the highest tolerated

Flowchart 1: Initiation, titration steps, and target doses of beta blockers in stages C and D HFrEF.

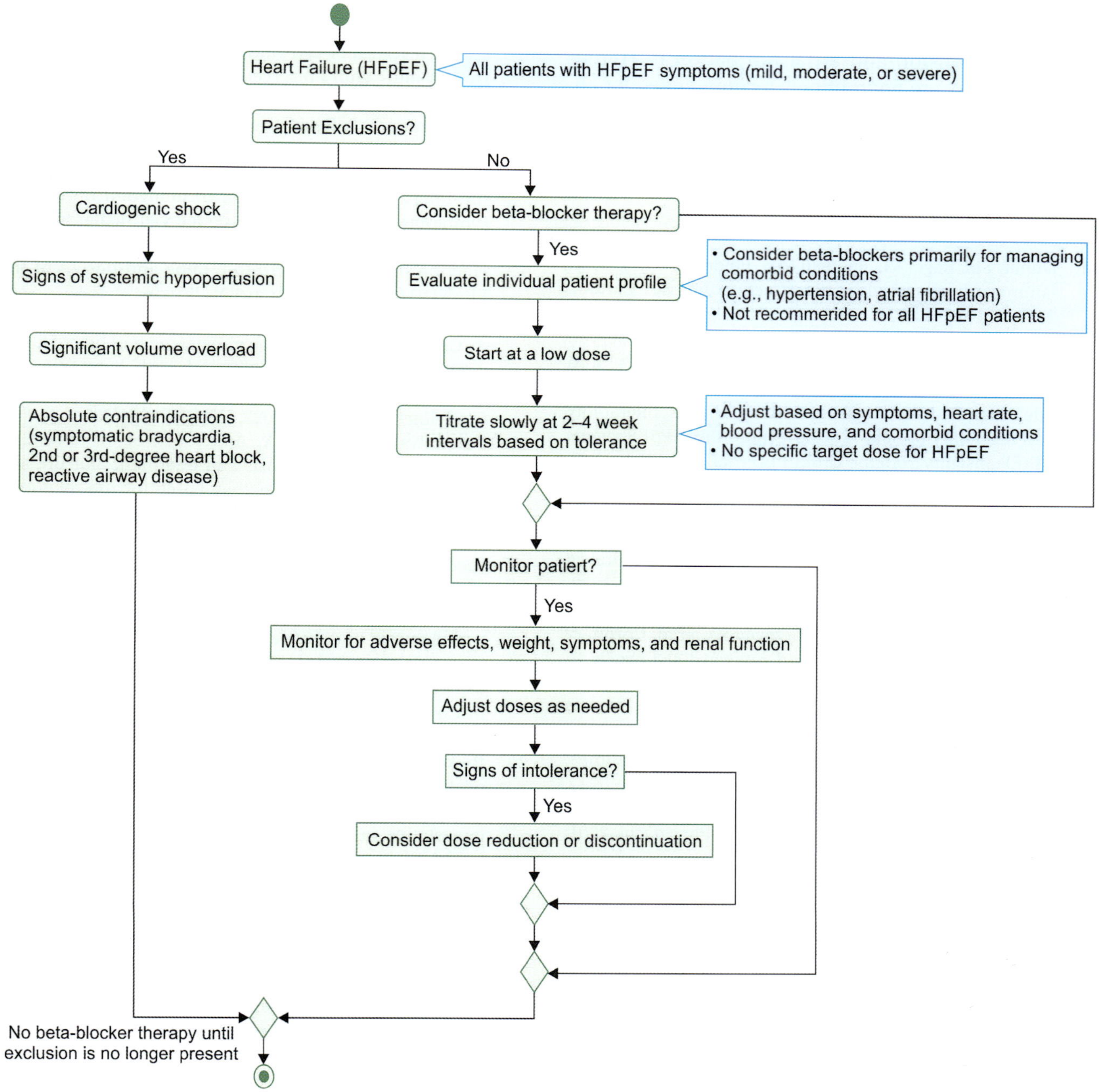

dose that effectively controls symptoms and manages comorbidities. Abrupt discontinuation should be avoided to prevent potential rebound effects or worsening symptoms; instead, dose adjustments should be closely monitored, focusing on changes in clinical parameters such as heart rate, blood pressure, renal function, and electrolytes.[21,22]

CONCLUSION

In conclusion, while beta-blockers are a cornerstone in the management of HFrEF, their role in HFpEF remains uncertain due to mixed and inconclusive evidence. Current guidelines and expert opinions suggest that beta-blockers may offer benefits in managing comorbidities such as hypertension and atrial fibrillation in HFpEF patients, but they are not routinely recommended for all. The variability in clinical trial results and lack of large-scale, high-quality studies highlight the need for a more individualized approach to beta-blocker use in HFpEF.

REFERENCES

1. Dunlay SM, Roger VL, Redfield MM. Epidemiology of heart failure with preserved ejection fraction. Nat Rev Cardiol. 2017;14(10):591-602.
2. Borlaug BA, Paulus WJ. Heart failure with preserved ejection fraction: pathophysiology, diagnosis, and treatment. Eur Heart J. 2011;32(6):670-9.
3. Edelmann F, Musial-Bright L, Gelbrich G, et al. Tolerability and feasibility of beta-blocker titration in HFpEF versus HFrEF: insights from the CIBIS-ELD trial. JACC Heart Fail. 2016;4(2):140-9.
4. Waagstein F, Caidahl K, Wallentin I, et al. Long-term beta-blockade in dilated cardiomyopathy. Effects of short- and long-term metoprolol treatment followed by withdrawal and readministration of metoprolol. Circulation. 1989; 80(3):551-63.
5. Mohammed SF, Hussain S, Mirzoyev SA, et al. Coronary microvascular rarefaction and myocardial fibrosis in heart failure with preserved ejection fraction. Circulation. 2015;131(6):550-9.
6. Cai Z, Wu C, Xu Y, et al. The NO-cGMP-PKG axis in HFpEF: from pathological mechanisms to potential therapies. Aging Dis. 2023;14(1):46-62.
7. Bouzamondo A, Hulot JS, Sanchez P, et al. Beta-blocker treatment in heart failure. Fundam Clin Pharmacol. 2001; 15(2):95-109.
8. Xu X, Wang DW. The progress and controversial of the use of beta blockers in patients with heart failure with a preserved ejection fraction. Int J Cardiol Heart Vasc. 2019;26:100451.
9. Fonarow GC, Abraham WT, Albert NM, et al. Influence of beta-blocker continuation or withdrawal on outcomes in patients hospitalized with heart failure: findings from the OPTIMIZE-HF program. J Am Coll Cardiol. 2008; 52(3):190-9.
10. Palau P, Seller J, Domínguez E, et al. Effect of β-blocker withdrawal on functional capacity in heart failure and preserved ejection fraction. J Am Coll Cardiol. 2021; 78(21):2042-56.
11. Gheorghiade M, Colucci WS, Swedberg K. Beta-blockers in chronic heart failure. Circulation. 2003;107(12):1570-5.
12. Yamamoto K, Origasa H, Suzuki Y, et al. Relation of risk factors with response to carvedilol in heart failure with preserved ejection fraction: a report from the Japanese Diastolic Heart Failure Study (J-DHF). J Cardiol. 2014;63(6):424-31.
13. Flather MD, Shibata MC, Coats AJS, et al. Randomized trial to determine the effect of nebivolol on mortality and cardiovascular hospital admission in elderly patients with heart failure (SENIORS). Eur Heart J. 2005;26(3):215-25.
14. Australian New Zealand Clinical Trials Registry (ANZCTR). (2019). Investigator Led Study of Intravenous Milrinone in Heart Failure with Preserved Ejection Fraction (HFpEF). [online] Available from https://www.anzctr.org.au/Trial/Registration/TrialReview.aspx?id=366475. [Last accessed January, 2025].
15. Kamp O, Metra M, De Keulenaer GW, et al. Effect of the long-term administration of nebivolol on clinical symptoms, exercise capacity and left ventricular function in patients with heart failure and preserved left ventricular ejection fraction: background, aims and design of the ELANDD study. Clin Res Cardiol. 2010;99(2):75-82.
16. Heidenreich PA, Bozkurt B, Aguilar D, et al. 2022 AHA/ACC/HFSA guideline for the management of heart failure: a report of the American College of Cardiology/American Heart Association Joint Committee on Clinical Practice Guidelines. Circulation. 2022;145(18):e895-1032.
17. Ponikowski P, Voors AA, Anker SD, et al. 2016 ESC guidelines for the diagnosis and treatment of acute and chronic heart failure: the Task Force for the diagnosis and treatment of acute and chronic heart failure of the European Society of Cardiology (ESC) developed with the special contribution of the Heart Failure Association (HFA) of the ESC. Eur Heart J. 2016;37(27):2129-200.
18. The Cardiac Insufficiency Bisoprolol Study II (CIBIS-II): a randomised trial. Lancet. 1999;353(9146):9-13.
19. Effect of metoprolol CR/XL in chronic heart failure: Mmetoprolol CR/XL Randomised Intervention Trial in Congestive Heart Failure (MERIT-HF). Lancet. 1999; 353(9169):2001-7.
20. Packer M, Fowler MB, Roecker EB, et al. Effect of carvedilol on the morbidity of patients with severe chronic heart failure: results of the carvedilol prospective randomized cumulative survival (COPERNICUS) study. Circulation. 2002;106(17):2194-9.
21. Peikert A, Bart BA, Vaduganathan M, et al. Contemporary use and implications of beta-blockers in patients with HFmrEF or HFpEF: the DELIVER trial. JACC Heart Fail. 2024;12(4):631-44.
22. Kaddoura R, Madurasinghe V, Chapra A, et al. Beta-blocker therapy in heart failure with preserved ejection fraction (B-HFpEF): a systematic review and meta-analysis. Curr Probl Cardiol. 2024;49(3):102376.

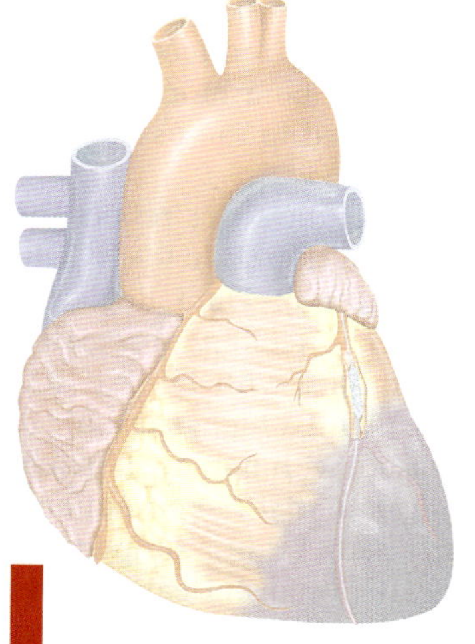

Use of Beta-blockers in Patients with HFpEF and Comorbidities

Abdullah AS Majumder, AKM Monwarul Islam

INTRODUCTION

In contrast to universal recommendation for the therapeutic management of heart failure with reduced ejection fraction (HFrEF), the role of beta blockers in heart failure with preserved ejection fraction (HFpEF) is debatable and controversial.[1-3] This is well understood considering the different pathophysiology of the two, though both present with the same clinical features of heart failure. In HFrEF, beta blockers are used to fight back the increased sympathetic tone that results from the compensatory mechanism, which is initially beneficial but later self-defeating. In contrast, chronotropic incompetence exists in many cases of HFpEF, thus raising fear of the use of beta blockers.[4] The observational studies, randomized controlled trials (RCTs), and meta-analyses have so far yielded conflicting results in this regard. The issue has become even more complex because of the evolving criteria for the definition of HFpEF; the cutoff of left ventricular (LV) ejection fraction (LVEF) has been reset from 40% through 45% to the current 50%. The LVEF between 40 and 49% has now been classified as heart failure with mildly reduced ejection fraction (HFmrEF).[2,3]

PATHOPHYSIOLOGY OF HFpEF IN THE CONTEXT OF ROLE OF BETA BLOCKERS

Heart failure with preserved ejection fraction is often accompanied by comorbidities such as hypertension, diabetes mellitus, atrial fibrillation (AF), chronic kidney disease, chronic obstructive pulmonary disease, obesity, and obstructive sleep apnea. Concomitant comorbidities often initiate a systemic proinflammatory state that leads to coronary microvascular endothelial inflammation.[5] Endothelial inflammation, in turn, promotes myocyte hypertrophy and interstitial fibrosis. Consequently, LV diastolic stiffness increases, diastolic relaxation slows, diastolic filling pressure increases, cardiac output decreases, and symptomatic heart failure manifests.[5,6]

In HFpEF, overactivation of sympathetic nerve activity (SNA) and LV diastolic dysfunction occur.[7,8] Overactivation of SNA increases the rate of impulse generation (heart rate), velocity of conduction of impulse, force of contraction of myocardium, and myocardial relaxation. Beta blockers can calm down this sympathetic overactivity by means of their sympatholytic effect mediated by blocking the beta-1 adrenoceptors, which translates into lowering of heart rate and blood pressure (BP), enhancing relaxation, increasing diastolic filling, decreasing myocardial oxygen demand, augmenting myocardial perfusion, reducing ischemia, preventing arrhythmia, and improving ventricular remodeling.[7,9-13] Beta blockers also block the renin–angiotensin–aldosterone system activity by blocking the beta-1 receptors of the juxtaglomerular cells of the kidney.[14]

Beta blockers improve diastolic dysfunction by multiple mechanisms including reduction of heart rate and BP and increasing diastolic filling time and myocardial perfusion. Beyond this, these drugs may prevent left ventricular hypertrophy (LVH) and myocardial fibrosis. The third-generation beta blockers with vasodilator properties, such as nebivolol, improve endothelial dysfunction, thereby, exerting a favorable effect on diastolic dysfunction.[15]

On the other hand, beta blockers are a heterogenous group of drugs having both "class effects" and individual properties. The first-generation beta blockers, the prototype of which is propranolol, block both beta-1 and beta-2 adrenoceptors nonselectively. They decrease heart rate and BP and increase diastolic filling time, but at the same time, they decrease exercise capacity, which may be undesirable in the context of HFpEF. The second-generation beta blockers such as atenolol, metoprolol, and bisoprolol are more selective blockers of beta-1 adrenoceptors and may have less deleterious effect on exercise capacity. The third-generation beta blockers include labetalol, carvedilol, and nebivolol. Carvedilol nonselectively blocks beta-1, beta-2, and alpha-1 adrenoceptors and has no intrinsic sympathomimetic activity (ISA). It has pleiotropic effect, may be associated with less bradycardia, may improve cardiac remodeling, and improves significantly some parameters of LV diastolic dysfunction, for example, mitral E/A ratio.[16,17] Nebivolol is the unique beta blocker that highly selectively blocks the beta-1 adrenoceptors, exerts ISA against beta-2 adrenoceptors, and releases nitric oxide in endothelium. Compared with the other beta blockers, it reduces heart rate less and is associated with less chronotropic incompetence, causes peripheral vasodilation, and improves LV filling.[12,17] It appears a promising beta blocker for HFpEF.

CURRENT EVIDENCE FOR THE ROLE OF BETA BLOCKERS IN HFpEF

So far, studies in relation to the use of beta blockers in HFpEF have produced conflicting results. RCTs are few, in fact, the Japanese Diastolic Heart Failure (J-DHF) study is the only dedicated RCT that was specifically designed to evaluate the effect of a beta blocker in HFpEF. Here, carvedilol was tested for heart failure with an LVEF >40% (not >50%). Compared with the control group without carvedilol, carvedilol did not reduce the composite outcome of cardiovascular (CV) death and heart failure hospitalization.[18] In the SENIORS (Study of the Effects of Nebivolol Intervention on Outcomes and Rehospitalization) trial, nebivolol was not associated with worse outcomes in patients with LVEF >35%.[19] The TOPCAT (Treatment of Preserved Cardiac Function Heart Failure with an Aldosterone Antagonist) trial and its post hoc analysis found that beta blocker use was associated with an increased risk of HF hospitalization in patients with LVEF ≥50% but not in those with LVEF between 45 and 49%.[20,21] In the DELIVER (Dapagliflozin Evaluation to Improve the Lives of Patients With Preserved Ejection Fraction Heart Failure) trial, beta blocker use was not associated with a higher risk of worsening HF or CV death in patients with heart failure with LVEF >40%, and dapagliflozin consistently and safely reduced clinical events, irrespective of background beta blocker use.[22] **Table 1** shows selected RCTs related to the use of beta blockers in HFpEF.

The observational studies and registries reflect the real-world effect of beta blockers on HFpEF. In the NCDR-PINNACLE (National Cardiovascular Data Registry–Practice Innovation and Clinical Excellence) registry, older outpatients with heart failure with LVEF ≥40%, beta blocker use was associated with a higher risk of HF hospitalization as LVEF increased, with potential benefit in patients with HFmrEF and potential risk in patients with higher LVEF (particularly >60%).[23] In a propensity-matched analysis of the SwedeHF (Swedish Heart Failure) registry, in patients with heart failure and LVEF ≥50%, beta blockers were neither associated with nor did they modify the risk for heart failure hospitalization or CV death.[24]

The results of meta-analyses published so far are also inconclusive **(Table 2 and Fig. 1)**. An updated Cochrane review of 10 RCTs involving 3,087 heart failure patients with LVEF >40% found possible reduction of the risk of CV mortality with beta blocker treatment.[25] A recently published meta-analysis of 16 observational studies involving 27,188 patients with HFpEF and LVEF ≥50% showed potential reduction of all-cause mortality with beta-blocker therapy; however, there was no effect on rehospitalization for heart failure or composite with all-cause mortality.[1] Another very recent systematic review and network meta-analysis of RCTs including patients with HF and LVEF >40% found no reduction of mortality and rehospitalization with beta blockers (also renin-angiotensin system inhibitors and digoxin).[26]

BETA BLOCKERS IN HFpEF AND COMORBIDITIES

Current heart failure management guidelines emphasize treatment of comorbidities as the first-line strategy for HFpEF.[2,3,27,28] In fact, until recent past, except for the use of diuretics for relief of congestion, control of comorbidities was only given the class I recommendation in HFpEF.

Hypertension

Hypertension is a common association of HFpEF. Exaggerated BP response to exercise and development of acute pulmonary edema are common. Optimum control of BP helps prevention of heart failure and episodes of decompensation. Angiotensin receptor blockers (ARBs), angiotensin-converting enzyme inhibitors (ACEi), and calcium channel blockers (CCBs) may help the regression of LVH. BP should be optimally controlled to systolic BP

TABLE 1: RCTs on beta blocker use in HFpEF.

Study; author	*Objectives*	*Sample size; LVEF cutoff*	*Beta blocker used*	*Primary outcomes*	*Follow-up*	*Main findings*
J-DHF study; Yamamoto et al.[18]	To assess effects of carvedilol in HFpEF	*n* = 245; LVEF >40%	Carvedilol vs. placebo	Composite of CV death and unplanned hospitalization for HF	3.2 years	Carvedilol did not reduce composite of CV death and HF hospitalization
SENIORS study; Flather et al.[19]	To assess effects of nebivolol in ≥70 years, regardless of LVEF	*n* = 2,128; LVEF ≤ 35%	Nebivolol vs. placebo	Composite of all-cause mortality or CV hospitalization	21 months	Nebivolol was not associated with worse outcomes in LVEF >35%
TOPCAT trial, post hoc analysis; Silverman et al.[20]	To determine association of beta blocker with HF hospitalizations and CV mortality, overall and in LVEF ≥50% or <50%	*n* = 1,761; LVEF ≥50%	Any beta blocker	Incident HF hospitalization and CV mortality	3.3 years	For LVEF ≥50%, beta blocker was associated with increased risk of HF hospitalizations but not CV mortality. For LVEF 45–49%, no such association
DELIVER trial, post hoc analysis; Peikert et al.[22]	To determine contemporary use and implications of beta blockers in HFmrEF or HFpEF	*n* = 6,263, 5,177 on beta blocker; LVEF >40%	Any beta blocker	CV death or worsening HF	2.3 years	Beta blocker was not associated with a higher risk of worsening HF or CV death

(CV: cardiovascular; HF: heart failure; HFmrEF: heart failure with mildly reduced ejection fraction; HFpEF: heart failure with preserved ejection fraction; LVEF: left ventricular ejection fraction; RCTs: randomized controlled trials)

TABLE 2: Metanalyses on beta blocker use in HFpEF.

Author	*Included studies; sample size*	*LVEF cutoff*	*Beta blocker used*	*Main findings*
Martin et al.[25]	10 RCTs, 3,087 patients	LVEF >40%	Any beta blocker	Possible reduction of risk of CV mortality with beta blockers
Kaddoura et al.[1]	16 observational studies, 27,188 patients	LVEF ≥50%	Any beta blocker	Potential reduction of all-cause mortality, no effect on rehospitalization for HF or composite with all-cause mortality
Zafeiropoulos et al.[26]	13 RCTs, 29,875 patients	LVEF >40%	Any beta blocker	No reduction of mortality and rehospitalization for HF with beta blockers

(CV: cardiovascular; HF: heart failure; HFpEF: heart failure with preserved ejection fraction; LVEF: left ventricular ejection fraction)

<130 mm Hg. Diuretics, angiotensin receptor–neprilysin inhibitors (ARNIs), ARBs, and mineralocorticoid antagonists (MRAs) are recommended to treat hypertension.[28] So, beta blockers are not the first-line antihypertensive agent. In the presence of tachycardia or ischemic background, vasodilatory beta blockers such as nebivolol may be used.

Atrial Fibrillation

Atrial fibrillation is highly prevalent in HFpEF, and its presence indicates more advanced disease with poorer exercise capacity along with increased mortality.

Rhythm control may be more beneficial than rate control in HFpEF with AF; beta blockers and non-dihydropyridine CCBs are recommended as first-line agents with the addition of digoxin if required.[28] In the RATE-AF (Rate Control Therapy Evaluation in Permanent Atrial Fibrillation) study, both digoxin and bisoprolol were effective in rate control; however, digoxin was more well tolerated than bisoprolol.[29]

For rhythm control strategy, ablation may be better than antiarrhythmics. In refractory cases, atrioventricular node ablation and permanent pacemaker implantation may be done; for LVEF >50%, cardiac resynchronization therapy is not superior to right ventricular pacing.[2]

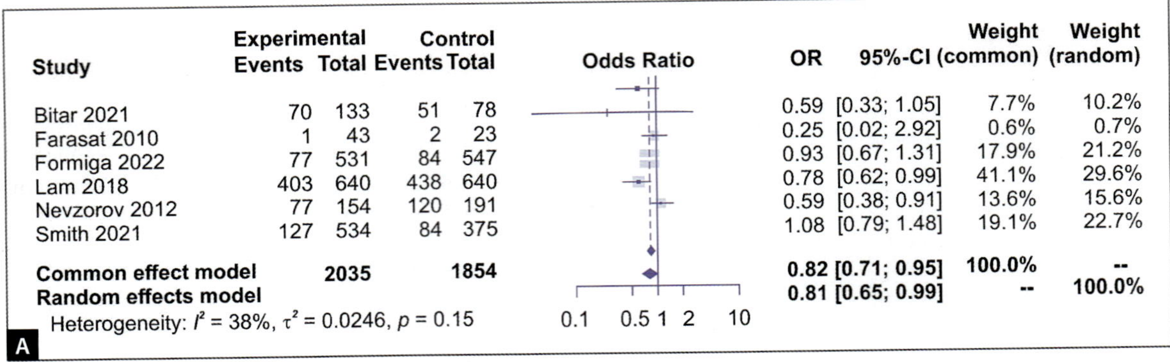

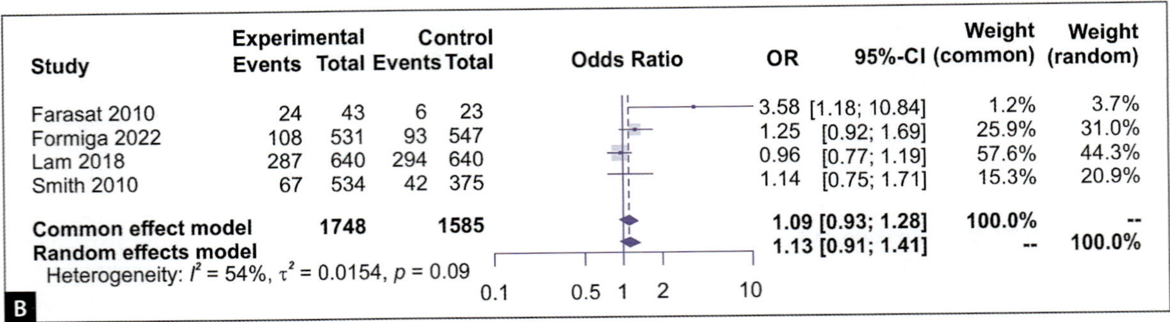

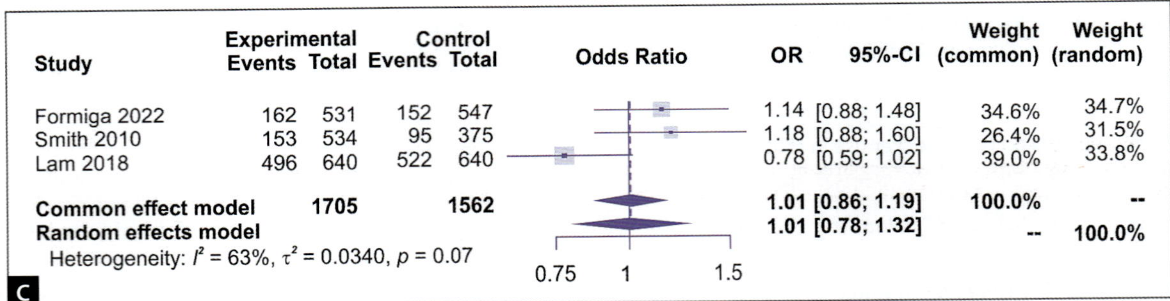

Figs. 1A to C: (A) Forest plot showing all-cause mortality of any duration; (B) Rehospitalization for heart failure of any duration; (C) Mortality or rehospitalization for heart failure of any duration.[1]

Chronic Coronary Syndrome

Coronary artery disease (CAD) is common in HFpEF. Patients with HFpEF commonly tolerate exercise poorly and are prone to the development of pulmonary edema. Exercise tolerance test may be less suitable for them for noninvasive documentation of myocardial ischemia. Rather, coronary computed tomography angiography may be a better choice for those with low-to-intermediate probability of CAD. For those with intermediate-to-high probability of CAD, invasive coronary angiography may be the optimum choice.[3] Myocardial ischemia should be addressed pharmacologically or by coronary revascularization as per the general guidelines.[3] Beta blockers may be useful in the presence of CAD.

GUIDELINE RECOMMENDATIONS FOR BETA BLOCKERS IN HFpEF

Unlike for HFrEF, current guidelines do not recommend the routine use of beta blockers in HFpEF.[2,3,27,28] In the 2022 AHA/ACC/HFSA Guideline for the Management of Heart Failure, diuretics are the only drugs having class I recommendation in HFpEF.[2] On the other hand, the 2023 Focused Update of the 2021 ESC Guidelines for the diagnosis and treatment of acute and chronic heart failure recommends diuretics and SGLT2 inhibitors (dapagliflozin and empagliflozin) as the class I agents.[27] Beta blockers are preferred in patients with a history of myocardial infarction or AF.[28]

CONCLUSION

The role of beta blockers in HFpEF is in evolution at present. In general, beta blockers' use in HFpEF is on the negative side till now. They may be beneficial, if at all, at the lower end of LVEF. However, they are recommended in presence of comorbidities like ischemic heart disease and AF. Selected beta blockers with vasodilatory properties, particularly nebivolol, have shown promise in HFpEF.

REFERENCES

1. Kaddoura R, Madurasinghe V, Chapra A, et al. Beta-blocker therapy in heart failure with preserved ejection fraction (B-HFpEF): a systematic review and meta-analysis. Curr Probl Cardiol. 2024;49(3):102376.
2. Heidenreich PA, Bozkurt B, Aguilar D, et al. 2022 AHA/ACC/HFSA guideline for the management of heart failure: a report of the American College of Cardiology/American Heart Association Joint Committee on Clinical Practice Guidelines. J Am Coll Cardiol. 2022;79(17):e263-421.
3. McDonagh TA, Metra M, Adamo M, et al. 2021 ESC guidelines for the diagnosis and treatment of acute and chronic heart failure. Eur Heart J. 2021;42(36):3599-726.
4. Hernandez AF, Hammill BG, O'Connor CM, et al. Clinical effectiveness of beta-blockers in heart failure: findings from the OPTIMIZE-HF (Organized Program to Initiate Lifesaving Treatment in Hospitalized Patients with Heart Failure) registry. J Am Coll Cardiol. 2009;53(2):184-92.
5. Paulus WJ, Tschöpe C. A novel paradigm for heart failure with preserved ejection fraction: comorbidities drive myocardial dysfunction and remodeling through coronary microvascular endothelial inflammation. J Am Coll Cardiol. 2013;62(4):263-71.
6. Pieske B, Tschöpe C, de Boer R, et al. How to diagnose heart failure with preserved ejection fraction: the HFA-PEFF diagnostic algorithm: a consensus recommendation from the Heart Failure Association (HFA) of the European Society of Cardiology (ESC). Eur Heart J. 2019;40(40):3297-317.
7. Mittal N, Shafiq N, Reddy S, et al. Evaluation of efficacy of metoprolol in patients having heart failure with preserved ejection fraction: a randomized, double-blind, placebo-controlled pilot trial. Perspect Clin Res. 2017;8(3):124-31.
8. Farasat SM, Bolger DT, Shetty V, et al. Effect of beta-blocker therapy on rehospitalization rates in women versus men with heart failure and preserved ejection fraction. Am J Cardiol. 2010;105(2):229-34.
9. Formiga F, Chivite D, Nuñez J, et al. Beta-blocker use in patients with heart failure with preserved ejection fraction and sinus rhythm. Rev Port Cardiol. 2022;41(10):853-61.
10. Bitar S, Thilly N, Agrinier N. Prognostic association of medication trajectories with 3-year mortality in heart failure and preserved ejection fraction: findings from the EPICAL2 cohort study. Eur J Clin Pharmacol. 2021;77(10):1569-81.
11. Lund LH, Benson L, Dahlström U, et al. Association between use of β-blockers and outcomes in patients with heart failure and preserved ejection fraction. JAMA. 2014;312(19):2008-18.
12. Conraads VM, Metra M, Kamp O, et al. Effects of the long-term administration of nebivolol on the clinical symptoms, exercise capacity, and left ventricular function of patients with diastolic dysfunction: results of the ELANDD study. Eur J Heart Fail. 2012;14(2):219-25.
13. Dobre D, van Veldhuisen DJ, DeJongste MJ, et al. Prescription of beta-blockers in patients with advanced heart failure and preserved left ventricular ejection fraction. Clinical implications and survival. Eur J Heart Fail. 2007;9(3):280-6.
14. do Vale GT, Ceron CS, Gonzaga NA, et al. Three generations of β-blockers: history, class differences and clinical applicability. Curr Hypertens Rev. 2019;15(1):22-31.
15. Nevzorov R, Porath A, Henkin Y, et al. Effect of beta blocker therapy on survival of patients with heart failure and preserved systolic function following hospitalization with acute decompensated heart failure. Eur J Intern Med. 2012;23(4):374-8.
16. Domagoj M, Branka JZ, Jelena M, et al. Effects of carvedilol therapy in patients with heart failure with preserved ejection fraction: results from the Croatian heart failure (CRO-HF) registry. Med Clin (Barc). 2019;152(2):43-49.
17. Wernhart S, Papathanasiou M, Rassaf T, et al. The controversial role of beta-blockers in heart failure with preserved ejection fraction. Pharmacol Ther. 2023;243:108356.
18. Yamamoto K, Origasa H, Hori M, et al. Effects of carvedilol on heart failure with preserved ejection fraction: the Japanese Diastolic Heart Failure Study (J-DHF). Eur J Heart Fail. 2013;15(1):110-8.
19. Flather MD, Shibata MC, Coats AJ, et al. Randomized trial to determine the effect of nebivolol on mortality and cardiovascular hospital admission in elderly patients with heart failure (SENIORS). Eur Heart J. 2005;26(3):215-25.
20. Silverman DN, Plante TB, Infeld M, et al. Association of β-blocker use with heart failure hospitalizations and cardiovascular disease mortality among patients with heart failure with a preserved ejection fraction: a secondary analysis of the TOPCAT trial. JAMA Netw Open. 2019;2(12):e1916598.
21. Lewis EF, Kim HY, Claggett B, et al. Impact of spironolactone on longitudinal changes in health-related quality of life in the treatment of preserved cardiac function heart failure with an aldosterone antagonist trial. Circ Heart Fail. 2016;9(3):e001937.
22. Peikert A, Bart BA, Vaduganathan M, et al. Contemporary use and implications of beta-blockers in patients with HFmrEF or HFpEF: the DELIVER trial. JACC Heart Fail. 2024;12(4):631-44.
23. Arnold SV, Silverman DN, Gosch K, et al. Beta-blocker use and heart failure outcomes in mildly reduced and preserved ejection fraction. JACC Heart Fail. 2023;11(8 Pt 1):893-900.

24. Meyer M, Du Fay Lavallaz J, Benson L, et al. Association between β-blockers and outcomes in heart failure with preserved ejection fraction: current insights from the SwedeHF registry. J Card Fail. 2021;27(11):1165-74.
25. Martin N, Manoharan K, Davies C, et al. Beta-blockers and inhibitors of the renin-angiotensin aldosterone system for chronic heart failure with preserved ejection fraction. Cochrane Database Syst Rev. 2021;5(5):CD012721.
26. Zafeiropoulos S, Farmakis IT, Milioglou I, et al. Pharmacological treatments in heart failure with mildly reduced and preserved ejection fraction: systematic review and network meta-analysis. JACC Heart Fail. 2024;12(4):616-27.
27. McDonagh TA, Metra M, Adamo M, et al. 2023 focused update of the 2021 ESC guidelines for the diagnosis and treatment of acute and chronic heart failure. Eur Heart J. 2023;44(37):3627-639.
28. Kittleson MM, Panjrath GS, Amancherla K, et al. 2023 ACC expert consensus decision pathway on management of heart failure with preserved ejection fraction: a report of the American College of Cardiology solution set oversight committee. J Am Coll Cardiol. 2023;81(18):1835-78.
29. Kotecha D, Bunting KV, Gill SK, et al. Effect of digoxin vs bisoprolol for heart rate control in atrial fibrillation on patient-reported quality of life: the RATE-AF randomized clinical trial. JAMA. 2020;324(24):2497-508.

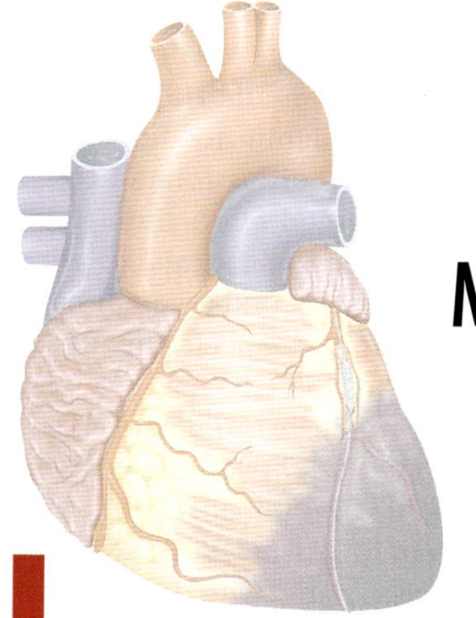

Mineralocorticoid Receptor Antagonist in HFpEF and Atrial Fibrillation

Esha Chaudhary, Karishma Suri, Rohit Walia

INTRODUCTION

Atrial fibrillation (AF) is a common comorbidity in patients with symptomatic heart failure with preserved ejection fraction (HFpEF), and heart failure (HF) is also a risk factor for new-onset AF and recurrence of AF.[1] It is associated with an increased risk of stroke and death. Enhanced activation of the renin–angiotensin–aldosterone system (RAAS) and subsequent aldosterone production plays an important role in AF causation in HF.[1,2]

TYPES OF MINERALOCORTICOID RECEPTOR ANTAGONIST

Mineralocorticoid receptor antagonist (MRA) drugs come in steroidal and nonsteroidal forms. **Table 1** describes their properties.[3,4]

TABLE 1: Mineralocorticoid receptor antagonist—drugs and their properties.

	Spironolactone	*Eplerenone*	*Finerenone*
Structural properties	Flat (steroidal)	Flat (steroidal)	Bulky (nonsteroidal)
MR affinity	+++	+	+++
MR selectivity	+	++	+++
Sex hormone-related side effects	++	+	–
CNS penetration	+	+	–
Plasma $t½$	>20 hours	4–5 hours	2–5 hours
Effect on BP	+++	++	+
Kidney versus heart	Kidney > Heart	Kidney > Heart	Kidney = Heart

HOW IS ATRIAL FIBRILLATION RELATED TO HEART FAILURE WITH PRESERVED EJECTION FRACTION?

Aldosterone competitively binds to the mineralocorticoid receptor, initiating structural cardiac remodeling, a process driven by fibrosis formation.[3,4] Both HF and AF are characterized by structural atrial remodeling due to atrial fibrosis.[5] Thus, MRAs may reduce HF symptoms and the risk of AF.

Mineralocorticoid receptor antagonist is a first-line therapy in patients with HFrEF (RALES, EMPHESUS).[6] Multiple HFpEF phenotypes have been specified including an older vascular aging type, a metabolic obese type, and a relatively younger natriuretic peptide deficient phenotype.

The older vascular aging phenotype depends on noncardiac factors such as vascular stiffness or chronic kidney disease (CKD)-associated renal factors responsible for cardiac hypertrophy, left atrial myopathy, and RV dysfunction.

Metabolic obese phenotype is provoked by noncardiac factors such as systemic fat accumulation during obesity and impaired insulin glucose metabolism and direct alteration of cardiac metabolism. Disturbances of cardiac metabolism in HFpEF include impaired mitochondrial structure and function.[7]

Diabetes, CKD, hypertension (HTN), and increasing age are associated with an increasing incidence of AF. Fluctuations in blood glucose levels occurring in diabetes, inflammatory processes, and oxidative stress lead to structural, electromechanical, electrical, and autonomic remodeling processes in the myocardium that promote AF.[7,8]

Cardiac metabolic flexibility is lost in HFpEF which goes along with increased rates of anaerobic glycolysis, a shift toward the hexosamine pathway and increased fatty uptake paralleled by impaired fatty acid oxidation resulting in enhanced cardiac triacylglycerol, diacylglycerol, and ceramide storage.

Younger natriuretic peptide-deficient phenotype is characterized by its reduced clearance and might be driven by perturbations in the cell matrix compartment.

Thus, aldosterone regulates inflammation, fibrosis, and cardiac hypertrophy which results in structural cardiac remodeling, CKD progression, and increased risk. Finerenone has anti-inflammatory, antifibrotic, and antihypertensive effects in preclinical studies and FIDELIO-DKD (Finerenone in Reducing Kidney Failure & Disease Progression in Diabetic Kidney Disease) study.[8]

EVIDENCE

Mineralocorticoid receptor antagonists were found to be effective in reducing new-onset AF or recurrence of pre-existing AF in patients with HF. The EMPHASIS-HF (Eplerenone in Mild Patient Hospitalization & Survival Study in Heart failure) trial showed that eplerenone significantly reduced new-onset AF in HFrEF.[6]

TOPCAT (Treatment of Cardiac Function with an Aldosterone Antagonist), a phase III, multicenter international, randomized, double-blind placebo-controlled trial, assessed the influence of AF at baseline on HF outcomes. Patients with AF had a higher cardiovascular risk than patients without AF independent of spironolactone use. Patients with symptomatic HF and LVEF >45% combined with either a hospitalization for HF within 12 months before inclusion or an elevated natriuretic peptide level. The patient had to be aged >50 years and have controlled systolic blood pressure <140 mm Hg (or <160 mm Hg if the patient was taking three or more medications to control BP and a serum K level <5 mmol/L). Patients with life expectancy < 3 years, estimated glomerular filtration rate <30 mL/min/1.73 m^2 BSA, or serum creatinine >2.5 mg/dL were excluded.[7]

TOPCAT found that spironolactone did not reduce the risk of the primary composite outcome of death from cardiovascular causes, aborted cardiac arrest, or reduced hospitalization for the management of HF in patients either with or without a history of AF at baseline. Spironolactone did not reduce new-onset AF or recurrence of AF compared with placebo in patients with symptomatic HFpEF. Also, subgroup analysis did not reveal any significant differences separately in patients with comorbidities related to an increased risk of AF such as enlarged left atrium (LA), HTN, and obesity. These findings are in contrast to prior findings in patients with HFrEF. In a secondary analysis of the EMPHASIS-HF trial, eplerenone reduced new-onset AF by 42% compared with placebo.[6,7]

Patients with HFrEF tend to have prevalent CAD. Patients included in the TOPCAT trial reflect the characterization of patients with HFpEF with a very high prevalence of HTN. The incidence of AF in HFpEF is higher than HFrEF.[7] HFrEF has been associated with degradation and focal fibrosis formation, whereas fibrosis formation with HFpEF is less obvious which may explain the absence of reduction of AF incidence by MRAs in HFpEF. HFpEF is characterized by increased left atrial stiffness and pressure overload, which is thought to contribute to the high burden of AF in HFpEF which MRA may not particularly affect. This, in turn, may lead to both cardiac and noncardiac comorbidities, involving myocardial microvascular dysfunction, leading to myocardial remodeling and dysfunction.[9-12]

Dabrowski et al. randomized patients with paroxysmal AF without HF and with a mean EF of 69% to spironolactone and no spironolactone. The recurrence of AF was significantly less frequent in patients treated with spironolactone. Importantly, systolic and diastolic blood pressure did not differ between treatment arms. Thus, although an indirect effect of spironolactone on AF via treatment of HF may well be possible, an additive effect on the AF substrate seems unlikely. RAAS activity has been suggested to play a larger role in HFrEF than in HFpEF.[13]

Mineralocorticoid receptor antagonist alters the risk of AF by reducing profibrotic pathways in the atrial wall which are triggered by RAAS activation and aldosterone production in the setting of HFrEF, and there was a decrease in the markers of cardiac fibrosis in both types of HF. The transition from paroxysmal to persistent AF commonly occurs through the evolution of an arrhythmogenic atrial substrate characterized by structural remodeling processes consisting of atrial dilatation, fibrosis, and altered cellular ultrastructure which led to conduction disturbances that maintain AF. Activation of the RAAS, in particular angiotensin II (Ang II), promotes structural remodeling and is upregulated in AF.[10,11]

Takemoto et al. investigated the benefits of the eplerenone on AF burden and structural and electrical remodeling in an ovine model with AF induced by continuous atrial pacing. Three principal findings are as follows:

1. AF inducibility, burden, and complexity were reduced with eplerenone in addition to a significant delay in the onset of persistent AF.
2. Structural remodeling as reflected by the degree of atrial dilatation, fibrosis, and myocyte hypertrophy was blunted in animals who receive eplerenone.
3. There was little effect on electrical remodeling, including action potential duration, dominant frequency, ion channel currents, and protein expression. Thus, MR blockade as an upstream therapy reduced AF burden through the prevention of atrial structural but not electrical remodeling.[14]

Finerenone significantly reduced the risk of cardiovascular events in patients with CKD and diabetes mellitus type 2 (DM2) in the FIDELLO DKD (Finerenone in Reducing Kidney Disease) phase III trial. In preclinical models, finerenone reduced mineralocorticoid receptor-mediated myocardial remodeling including prevention of left atrial dilatation and left atrial fibrosis. Finerenone lowers the incidence of new-onset AF in patients with CKD and DM2.[8] A similar observation was reported in the EMPHASIS-HF trial in which the incidence of new-onset AF was decreased by treatment with steroidal MRA. Eplerenone in a different population of patients with symptomatic HF with reduced ejection fraction who were excluded from the FIDELIO DKD trial. In contrast, the post hoc analysis of the TOPCAT trial showed that spironolactone did not reduce the risk of either new-onset AF or AF recurrence in patients with symptomatic HFpEF.[8]

In FINE ARTS-HF (Finerenone Trial to Investigate Efficacy & Safety Superior to Placebo in patients with Heart Failure) trial conducted in patients with mildly reduced or preserved ejection fraction, finerenone significantly reduced the rate of composite of total worsening HF events and death from cardiovascular causes over placebo.[15]

A potential mechanism explaining the benefit of finerenone on new-onset AF is the attenuation of adverse atrial remodeling associated with CKD or DM2 by inhibition of aldosterone activity. DM2 may further predispose patients to AF through atrial electrical and structural remodeling triggered by increased reactive oxygen species or advanced glycation end products. In cardiac fibroblasts, finerenone prevented aldosterone-induced myocardial remodeling and fibrosis. Furthermore, finerenone attenuated left atrial and left ventricular dilatation and significantly reduced mineralocorticoid receptor overactivation and fibrosis in transgenic mice with cardiac-specific overexpression in the development of cardiac fibrosis and remodeling.[8]

Diabetes mellitus and AF show a steady increase in their prevalence. Diabetes mellitus is a relevant risk factor for the development and maintenance of AF. Fluctuations in blood glucose levels occurring in diabetes, inflammatory processes, and oxidative stress lead to structural, electromechanical, and electrical and autonomic remodeling processes in the myocardium that promote AF. The increasing burden of AF is at least in part related to the increase in age-associated predisposing conditions such as CKD and DM2. One limitation of TOPCAT trial is the possibility that clinically silent or asymptomatic cases of new-onset AF may have been missed because history of AF was determined by the investigators at the start of the trial and 12-lead ECGs were only performed annually after the start of the trial unless there was a clinical need.

The process of atrial electrical, structural, and functional remodeling, collectively called atrial disease or atrial myopathy, provides the substrate for the development of AF and seems to be triggered by different cardiac and extracardiac morbidities including HF with reduced EF, DM, and CKD. This may partly explain the reduction in the incidence of AF that was observed in the FEDELIO-DKD trial.[16-18]

In patients with HFmrEF/HFpEF, finerenone reduced the risk of cardiovascular death and worsening HF events, irrespective of LVEF. In this regard, atrial disease has been proposed as the intersection of the pathogenetic process leading to AF, HFpEF, and perhaps thromboembolism which coexist frequently. As a result, targeting atrial derangement at an early stage of development with drugs such as finerenone may result in the prevention of downstream conditions and the improvement of overall outcomes in high-risk patients.[15]

FIDELITY study concluded that finerenone reduced the risk of clinically important cardiovascular and kidney outcomes across the spectrum of CKD patients in DM. Finerenone improved HF-related outcomes in patients with CKD and DM2 with consistent benefit across estimated glomerular filtration rate (eGFR). Finerenone gives cardiorenal protection in patients with CKD and DM2 to reduce the risk of kidney function decline, kidney failure, cardiovascular death, nonfatal heart attacks, and hospitalization for HF.[19]

CONCLUSION

Finerenone has shown promising results in reducing AF burden in diabetic and kidney disease-related patients with HFpEF. Future studies are required to explore the beneficial effects of MRA in other subsets of patients with HFpEF and its effect in AF prevention.

REFERENCES

1. Kirchhof P, Benussi S, Kotecha D, et al. 2016 ESC Guidelines for the management of atrial fibrillation developed in collaboration with EACTS. Eur Heart J. 2016;37(38):2893-962.
2. Ponikowski P, Voors AA, Anker SD, et al. 2016 ESC Guidelines for the diagnosis and treatment of acute and chronic heart failure: the Task Force for the diagnosis and treatment of acute and chronic heart failure of the European Society of Cardiology (ESC) developed with the special contribution of the Heart Failure Association (HFA) of the ESC. Eur Heart J. 2016;37(27): 2129-200.
3. Kotecha D, Chudasama R, Lane DA, et al. Atrial fibrillation and heart failure due to reduced versus preserved ejection fraction: a systematic review and meta-analysis of death and adverse outcomes. Int J Cardiol. 2016;203: 660-6.
4. Lavall D, Selzer C, Schuster P, et al. The mineralocorticoid receptor promotes fibrotic remodeling in atrial fibrillation. J Biol Chem. 2014;289(10):6656-68.
5. Parviz Y, Iqbal J, Pitt B, et al. Emerging cardiovascular indications of mineralocorticoid receptor antagonists. Trends Endocrinol Metab. 2015;26(4):201-11.
6. Swedberg K, Zannad F, McMurray JJ, et al. Eplerenone and atrial fibrillation in mild systolic heart failure: results from the EMPHASIS-HF (Eplerenone in Mild Patients Hospitalization And SurvIval Study in Heart Failure) study. J Am Coll Cardiol. 2012;59(18):1598-603.
7. Cikes M, Claggett B, Shah AM, et al. Atrial fibrillation in heart failure with preserved ejection fraction: the TOPCAT trial. JACC Heart Fail. 2018;6(8):689-97.
8. Filippatos G, Bakris GL, Pitt B, et al.; FIDELIO-DKD Investigators. Finerenone Reduces New-Onset Atrial Fibrillation in Patients With Chronic Kidney Disease and Type 2 Diabetes. J Am Coll Cardiol. 2021;78(2): 142-52.
9. Lv R, Xu L, Che L, et al. Cardiovascular-renal protective effect and molecular mechanism of finerenone in type 2 diabetic mellitus. Front Endocrinol (Lausanne). 2023;14:1125693.
10. Nattel S, Burstein B, Dobrev D. Atrial remodeling and atrial fibrillation: mechanisms and implications. Circ Arrhythm Electrophysiol. 2008;1(1):62-73.
11. Neefs J, van den Berg NW, Limpens J, et al. Aldosterone pathway blockade to prevent atrial fibrillation: a systematic review and meta-analysis. Int J Cardiol. 2017;231:155-61.
12. Zannad F, McMurray JJ, Krum H, et al. Eplerenone in patients with systolic heart failure and mild symptoms. N Engl J Med. 2011;364(1):11-21.
13. Dabrowski R, Borowiec A, Smolis-Bak E, et al. Effect of combined spironolactone-beta-blocker +/− enalapril treatment on occurrence of symptomatic atrial fibrillation episodes in patients with a history of paroxysmal atrial fibrillation (SPIR-AF study) Am J Cardiol. 2010;106(11):1609-14.
14. Takemoto Y, Ramirez RJ, Kaur K, et al. Eplerenone Reduces Atrial Fibrillation Burden Without Preventing Atrial Electrical Remodeling. J Am Coll Cardiol. 2017;70(23):2893-905.
15. Bakris GL, Agarwal R, Anker SD, et al.; FIDELIO-DKD Investigators. Effect of Finerenone on Chronic Kidney Disease Outcomes in Type 2 Diabetes. N Engl J Med. 2020;383(23):2219-29.
16. Chimura M, Petrie MC, Schou M, et al. Finerenone Improves Outcomes in Patients with Heart Failure with Mildly Reduced or Preserved Ejection Fraction Irrespective of Age: A Prespecified Analysis of FINEARTS-HF. Circ Heart Fail. 2024;17(11):e012437.
17. Docherty KF, Henderson AD, Jhund PS, et al. Efficacy and Safety of Finerenone Across the Ejection Fraction Spectrum in Heart Failure with Mildly Reduced and Preserved Ejection Fraction: a Prespecified Analysis of The FINEARTS-HF Trial. Circulation. 2025;151(1):45-58.
18. Solomon SD, McMurray JJV, Vaduganathan M, et al.; FINEARTS-HF Committees and Investigators. Finerenone in Heart Failure with Mildly Reduced or Preserved Ejection Fraction. N Engl J Med. 2024;391(16):1475-85.
19. Agarwal R, Filippatos G, Pitt B, et al.; FIDELIO-DKD and FIGARO-DKD investigators. Cardiovascular and kidney outcomes with finerenone in patients with type 2 diabetes and chronic kidney disease: the FIDELITY pooled analysis. Eur Heart J. 2022;43(6):474-84.

Global Data on Ferric Carboxymaltose in HFpEF

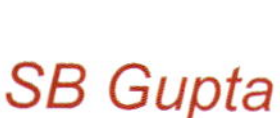

SB Gupta

INTRODUCTION

There is enough evidence that exists both clinically and data wise, regarding the correlation of iron deficiency with an increased incidence of heart failure. Existing data demonstrate that iron supplementation in patients of heart failure with reduced ejection fraction (HFrEF) have beneficial effects. Data regarding the beneficial effects of iron supplementation in patients with heart failure with preserved ejection fraction (HFpEF) is emerging.

Iron deficiency (ID) as such is a major public health issue, especially in developing nations and contributes to the poor outcome in many disease states, including myocardial dysfunction. Persons may be iron deficient and may not be anemic and only 50% of anemia cases are clearly correlated with ID. Different pathophysiological conditions lead to ID with or without anemia. Reduced iron stores in heart failure (HF) are a consequence of inflammation and oxidative stress, which lead to inappropriate iron absorption. Iron deficiency is a common morbidity in patients of HFpEF, affecting up to 50% of the individuals suffering from this condition, leading to fatigue, reduced exercise capacity, and impaired quality of life (QoL). Worse clinical outcomes including increased hospitalizations and higher mortality has been reported in HFpEF patients who are iron-deficient.[1]

Initially, 2012 European Society of Cardiology (ESC) guidelines suggested that intravenous iron may be considered for patients with HF and ID.[2] Subsequently in 2021 ESC guidelines recommended routine use of IV FCM in the treatment of HF and ID to improve the QoL and functional status.[3] There is reduction in long-term hospitalizations in patients of decompensated HF after IV FCM administration. The safety profile of FCM is good as far as cardiovascular, renal, respiratory or nervous system are concerned and fewer adverse reactions after administering higher doses for a shorter duration of infusion as compared to other IV iron preparations, making FCM is therapeutic choice for replenishing iron stores in HF patients.

Intravenous administration of a single bolus of ferric carboxymaltose (FCM) in patients with ID and HF with or without anemia with an EF of <40–45% has shown improvement in exercise capacity, irrespective of the presence of anemia.[4] Another trial, CONFIRM-HF also showed the improvement in the QoL and reduction in rate of hospitalizations in patients with HFrEF with iron supplementation.[5]

Iron-deficient HFpEF patients have similar health-related QoL as of HFrEF patients, as shown in various studies.[6] Concomitant ID in HFpEF patients, irrespective of anemia have shown similar prognosis in terms of increased mortality from all causes as in HFrEF patients.[7] In a single-blind, randomized clinical trial, no beneficial effects were noted either on submaximal exercise capacity or QoL when patients of HFpEF with anemia were treated with epoetin alfa or oral iron.[8]

However, a recent multicentric, double-blind, randomized, placebo-controlled study done on 64 subjects of HFpEF with ID, detected based on ferritin levels [serum ferritin levels of <100 µg/L or serum ferritin levels of 100–299 µg/L with transferrin saturation (TSAT), 20%]. The degree anemia was defined as <13 g/dL for men and <12 g/dL for women. A 6-minute walking test

(6MWT) along with echocardiographic features of left ventricular diastolic function (LVDD) were evaluated. Serum malondialdehyde (MDA) was estimated to study the oxidative stress biomarkers. One arm received placebo (100 mL normal saline IV over 10 minutes; $n = 32$) and the other arm received 500 mg IV infusion of FCM at 0 and at 4 weeks; $n = 32$). Patients with ID were frequently associated with impaired diastolic dysfunction, reduced 6MWT, and endothelial dysfunction depicted by elevated MDA levels. Treatment with FCM improved ferritin levels with improvement in 6MWT, better cardiac diastolic dysfunction, and a significant reduction in MDA levels.

Patients with severe LVDD had basal ferritin levels 60.3 ± 13.3 ng/mL in the treatment arm, 62.3 ± 12.4 ng/mL in the placebo arm and treatment with FCM led to increase in ferritin levels to 129.1 ± 13.9 ng/mL ($p < 0.05$). 6MWT improved from 291.1 ± 22.6 m to 354.4 m ($p < 0.05$) and MDA levels dropped from 1.1 ± 0.1 µg/dL to 0.7 ± 0.1 µg/dL ($p < 0.05$) at 8 weeks. The study confirmed that ID is a frequent comorbidity in HFpEF patients and is associated with reduced exercise capacity and endothelial dysfunction and supplementation with intravenous FCM corrected the ferritin levels and led to improvement in diastolic dysfunction, increase in exercise capacity and improved endothelial dysfunction.[9]

Another retrospective study[10] included 484 patients finally for analysis—288 patients of HFrEF and 196 patients with HFpEF [LVEF ≥50%, elevated levels of natriuretic peptides (BNP >35 pg/mL or NT-proBNP >125 pg/mL)] and one additional criterion of either relevant structural heart disease or diastolic dysfunction). FCM was administered in dosage of 500–1,000 mg IV (depending upon weight and basal hemoglobin level) diluted in normal saline over 15–30 minutes. All follow-up evaluations were done at 2 months (range 1–3 months) after FCM administration. As compared to patients with HFrEF, more increase in ferritin and TSAT levels were found in HFpEF patients (4.4-fold and 1.6-fold in HFrEF patients vs. 6-fold and 2-fold in HFpEF patients, respectively). Majority of patients of HFpEF showed improvement in NYHA Class from III to Class II-III. However, there were no significant reduction NT-proBNP levels. There was absence of clinically significant negative effects at renal or hepatic level in this study.

Another study, a retrospective, unicentric and observational registry included 235 patients, 51.5% females with mean age of 73 years and 50.8% >75 years of age. All consecutive HF patients of all range of EF were part of the study—96 patients of HFrEF (40.8%), 41 patients of HF of mid-range EF (HFmrEF 17.4%), and 98 patients of HFpEF (41.7%). The study concluded that: (1) ID is effectively corrected by FCM irrespective of LVEF, (2) functional status is less likely to improve in HFpEF patients, (3) after 3 months of administration, FCM resulted in reduction in NT-ProBNP levels even in HFpEF patients, and (4) FCM is safe in all group of patients with HF.[11]

The most recent trial, the FAIR-HFpEF trial, a prospective, multicenter, 1:1 randomized, double-blind, placebo-controlled trial studying the effects of IV FCM in patients of HFpEF with ID on exercise capacity, and QoL. The trial was terminated prematurely as 39 patients could only be enrolled for final analysis (21 patients in placebo arm and 18 patients in FCM arm). 6MWTD improved in FCM group from 308 meters median at base line to 403 meters at 24 weeks ($p = 0.014$). No significant changes were noted in QoL or NYHAclass.[12]

The editorial on the above trial concluded that "We have walked a long way in understanding the benefits of IV iron therapy in HFrEF, but the journey to uncover its potential in HFpEF is just beginning".[13]

CONCLUSION

Iron deficiency and heart failure are common associations and insufficient levels of iron are not capable to meet the physiological demands. Iron deficiency in heart failure is associated with increased morbidity and mortality and it is modifiable comorbidity and treating iron deficiency in heart failure can have significant impact on the functional status, exercise tolerance, symptoms and overall QoL. Robust data for the outcome in HFpEF and iron deficiency treated with iron is insufficient on date and future studies will tell us the path for management of iron deficiency in HFpEF patients.

REFERENCES

1. Shabeer H, Samore N, Ahsan S, et al. Safety and efficacy of ferric carboxymaltose in heart failure with preserved ejection fraction and iron deficiency. Curr Probl Cardiol. 2024;49(1 Pt C):102125.
2. McMurray JJ, Adamopoulos S, Anker SD, et al. ESC Guidelines for the diagnosis of and treatment of heart failure 2012: the Task Force for the Diagnosis and Treatment of Acute and Chronic Heart Failure2012 of the European Society of Cardiology. Developed in collaboration with Heart Failure Association (HFA) of the ESC. Eur Heart J. 2012;33:1787-847.
3. McDonagh TA, Metra M, Adamo M, et al. 2021 ESC Guidelines for the diagnosis and treatment of acute and chronic heart failure. Eur Heart J. 2012;42:3599-726.
4. Anker SD, Comin-Colet J, Filippatos G, et al. FAIR-HF Trial Investigators. Ferric carboxymaltose in patients with heart failure and iron deficiency. N Eng J Med. 2009;361: 2436-48.

5. Ponikowski P, van Veldhuisen DJ, Comin-Colet J, et al. CONFIRM-HF Investigators. Beneficial effects of long-term intravenous iron therapy with ferric carboxymaltose in patients with symptomatic heart failure with iron deficiency. Eur Heart J. 2015;36:657-68.
6. Zusman O, Itzhaki BZO, Gafter-Gvilli A. Management of iron deficiency in heart failure. Acta Haematol. 2019; 142:51-6.
7. Jankowaska EA, Rozentryt P, Witkowska A, et al. Iron deficiency: an ominous sign in patients with systolic chronic heart failure. Eur Heart J. 2010;31:1872-80.
8. Vullaganti S, Goldsmith J, Teruya S, et al. Cardiovascular effects of haemoglobin response in patients receiving epoetin alfa and oral iron in heart failure with preserved ejection fraction. J Geriatr Cardiol. 2014; 11: 100-105.
9. Mollace A, Macrì R, Mollace R, et al. Effect of Ferric Carboxymaltose Supplementation in Patients with Heart Failure with Preserved Ejection Fraction: Role of Attenuated Oxidative Stress and Improved Endothelial Function. Nutrients. 2022;14:5057.
10. López-Vilella R, Lozano-Edo S, Martin PA, et al. Impact of intravenous ferric carboxymaltose on heart failure with preserved and reduced ejection fraction. ESC Heart Fail. 2022;9:133-45.
11. Esteban-Fernández A, Méndez-Bailón M, Pérez-Serrano M, et al. Ferric carboxymaltose for patients with heart failure in all-range ejection fraction. CardioClinics. 2023;58(4):281-8.
12. Von Haehling S, Doehner W, Evertz R, et al. Ferric carboxymaltose and exercise capacity in heart failure with preserved ejection fraction and iron deficiency: the FAIR-HFpEF trial. Eur Heart J. 2024;45(37): 3789-3800.
13. Kittipibul V, Mentz RJ. Intravenous iron therapy in heart failure with preserved ejection fraction: how far have we walked? Eur Heart J. 2024;45(37):3801-3.

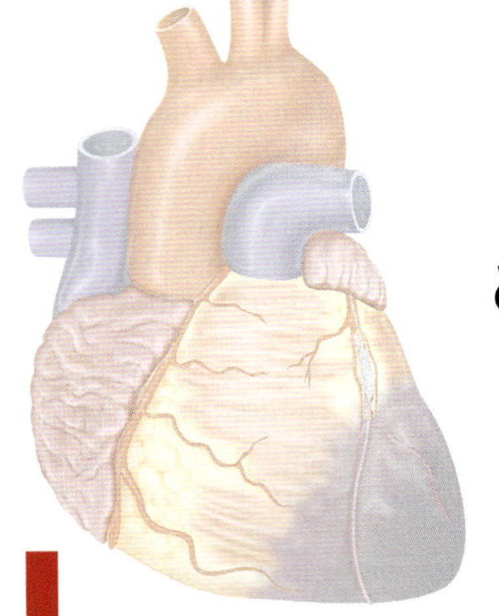

Semaglutide in Patients with Obesity and HFpEF with or without Diabetes and Prespecified Pooled Analysis of STEP-HFpEF and STEP-HFpEF-DM Trials

AK Pancholia, HK Chopra

INTRODUCTION

More than 50% of all cases of heart failure (HF) are having heart failure with preserved ejection fraction (HFpEF) with rising prevalence.[1-3] The majority of these patients are overweight or obese. Evidence now confirms that obesity and excess adiposity play an important role in the development and progression of HFpEF.[4-8] Obesity-associated HFpEF is responsible for more adverse hemodynamics and greater symptom burden, worse functional capacity, and more severely impaired quality of life (QoL) than those who do not have obesity.[9-12] Recently, pharmacotherapy to specifically target obesity has been tested to see its impact on symptoms and physical limitations in these subsets of patients. Once weekly semaglutide, which is a potent glucagon-like peptide 1 receptor agonist approved for long-term weight management, at a dose of 2.4 mg administered subcutaneously has shown a larger reduction in HF-related symptoms and physical limitations, greater improvements in exercise function, and greater weight loss than placebo in patients with HFpEF and obesity in two randomized, placebo-controlled trials—STEP-HFpEF (in patients with or without diabetes)[13] and STEP-HFpEF DM (in patients with diabetes).[14] Very recently in the prespecified pooled analysis of these two trials, semaglutide also showed a reduction in inflammation, regardless of either baseline CRP or magnitude of weight loss during the trials.[15] Semaglutide also reduced NT-proBNP, those with higher baseline NT-proBNP had a similar degree of weight loss but experienced larger reductions in HF-related symptoms and physical limitations than those with lower NT-proBNP.[16] The magnitude of semaglutide-mediated improvements in HF-related symptoms and physical limitations was more pronounced in those with AF versus those without AF at baseline[17] and the benefit is consistent in all diuretic-use categories with a reduction in loop diuretic use and dose between baseline and 52 weeks.[18]

SEMAGLUTIDE TREATMENT EFFECT IN PEOPLE WITH OBESITY AND HEART FAILURE WITH PRESERVED EJECTION FRACTION—STEP-HFpEF TRIAL[13]

This study was conducted on 529 patients to see the effect of semaglutide 2.4 mg once weekly on function and symptoms in subjects with obesity-related HFpEF, a randomized placebo-controlled trial. A larger reduction in HF-related symptoms and physical limitations, greater improvements in exercise function, and greater weight loss than placebo have been observed **(Figs. 1 to 3)**.

SEMAGLUTIDE TREATMENT EFFECT IN PEOPLE WITH OBESITY AND HFpEF AND DIABETES MELLITUS—STEP-HFpEF DM TRIAL[14]

The STEP-HFpEF study was done in 310 type 2 diabetes patients with similar protocols and goals. Semaglutide treatment in the dose of dose of 2.4 mg weekly was given and patients were followed up to 52 weeks. Semaglutide was superior to placebo in improving body weight (~6.4% greater weight loss) **(Fig. 4)** and patient-oriented QoL outcomes including KCCQ-CSS and 6MWD at 52 weeks **(Fig. 5)**.

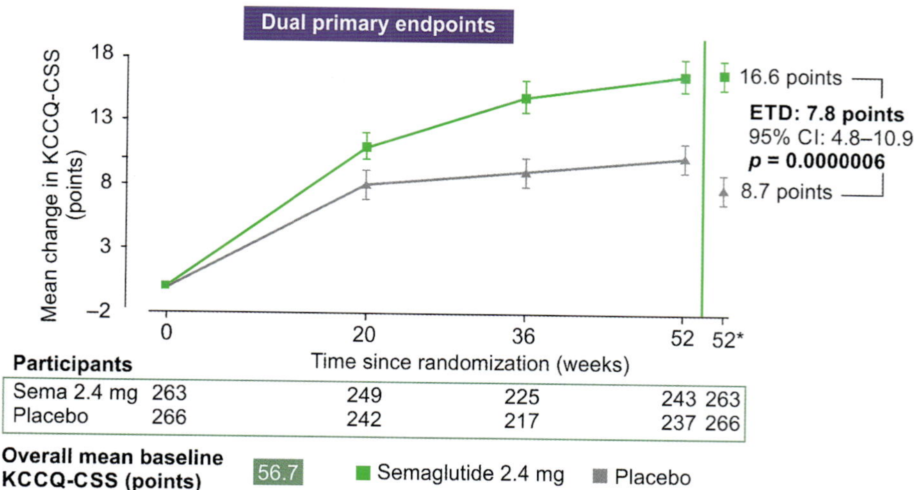

Fig. 1: Change in baseline to week 52 in KCCQ-CCS.
*Data are estimated mean changes from baseline to week 52 for the treatment policy estimated using ANCOVA and an imputation approach for missing data.
Source: Kosiborod et al. (2023).

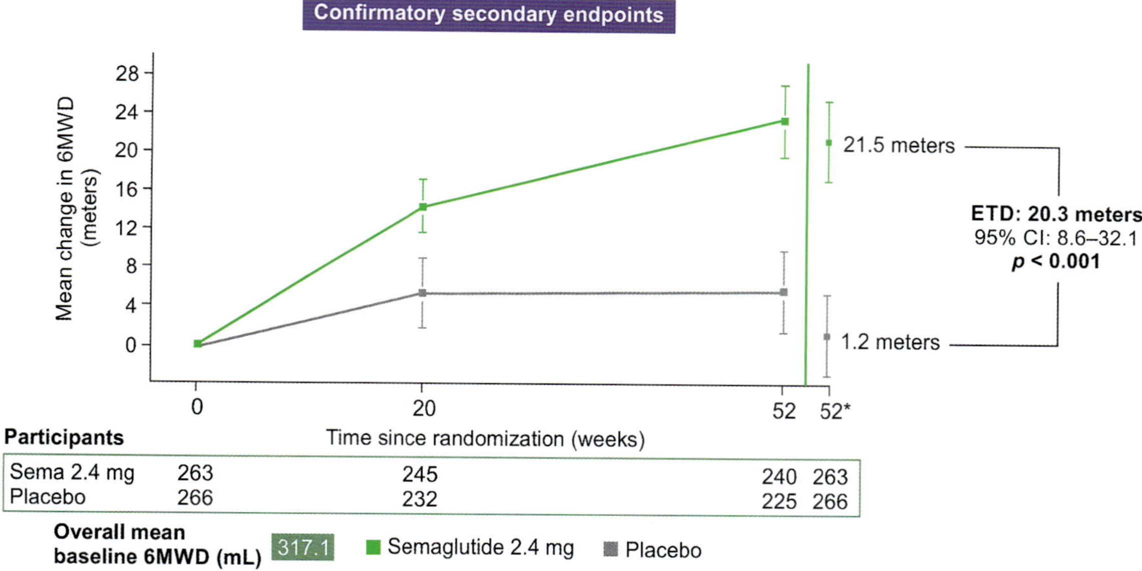

Fig. 2: Change in baseline to week 52 in 6MWD.
*Data are estimated mean changes from baseline to week 52 for the treatment policy estimated using ANCOVA and an imputation approach for missing data.
Source: Kosiborod et al. (2023).

PRESPECIFIED POOLED ANALYSIS OF STEP-HFpEF AND STEP-HFpEF DIABETES MELLITUS TRIALS

In the STEP-HFpEF and STEP-HFpEF DM trials, the GLP-1 receptor agonist semaglutide improved symptoms, physical limitations, body weight, and exercise function in people with obesity-related HFpEF with or without diabetes. A more definitive assessment of the effects of semaglutide across a range of outcomes and to test whether these effects were consistent across key patient subgroups, a prespecified pooled analysis of the STEP-HFpEF and STEP-HFpEF DM trials has been done recently. These are mainly focused on:

- Inflammation
- NT-proBNP
- Diuretic use
- Baseline AF

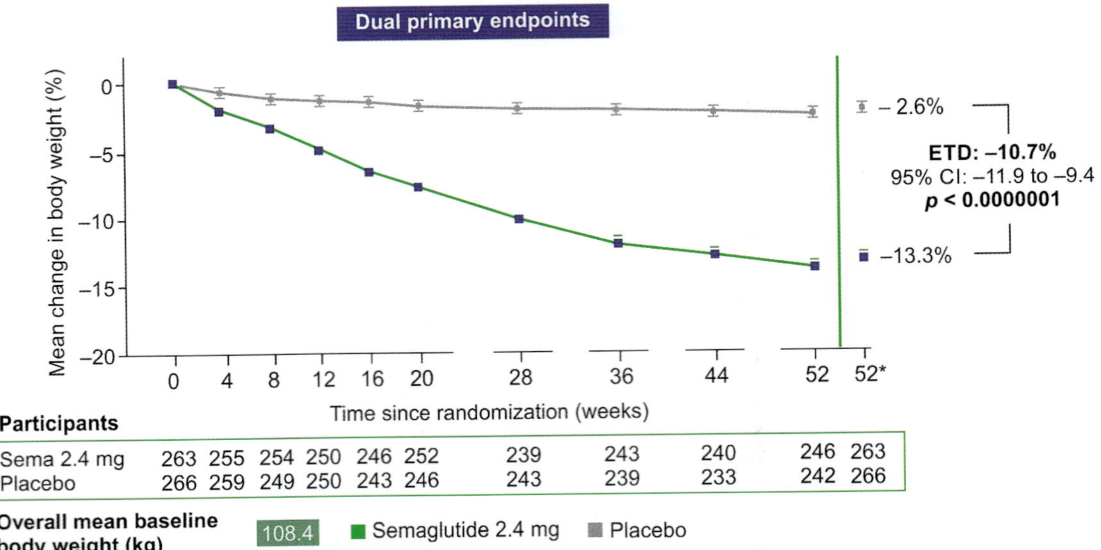

Fig. 3: Change in baseline to week 52 in body weight.
*Data are estimated mean changes from baseline to week 52 for the treatment policy estimated using ANCOVA and an imputation approach for missing data.
Source: Kosiborod et al. (2023).

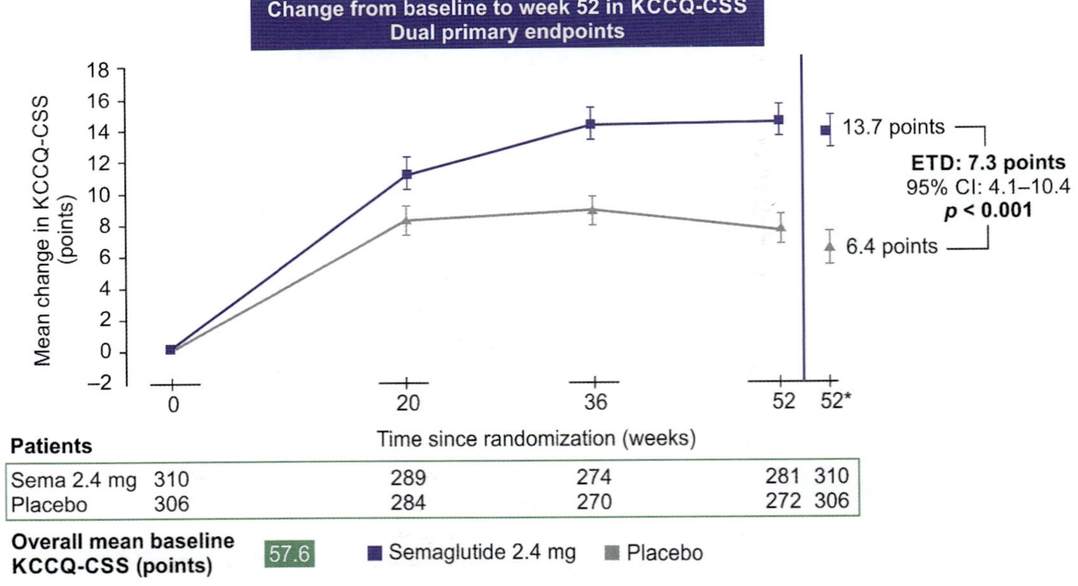

Fig. 4: STEP-HFpEF DM.
*Data are estimated mean changes from baseline to week 52 for the treatment policy estimated using ANCOVA and an imputation approach for missing data.
Source: Kosiborod et al. (2024).

SEMAGLUTIDE AND INFLAMMATION IN OBESITY-RELATED HFpEF[15]

There has been an increasing recognition that obesity causes adipose tissue expansion and local and systemic inflammation, which consequently exacerbates cardiac remodeling and leads to the development of obese HFpEF. There is high prevalence of inflammation in obesity-related HFpEF. Semaglutide also reduced inflammation, regardless of either baseline CRP or magnitude of weight loss during the trials. Semaglutide consistently improved HF-related symptoms, physical limitations, and exercise function, and reduced body weight across the categories of baseline CRP **(Fig. 6)**.

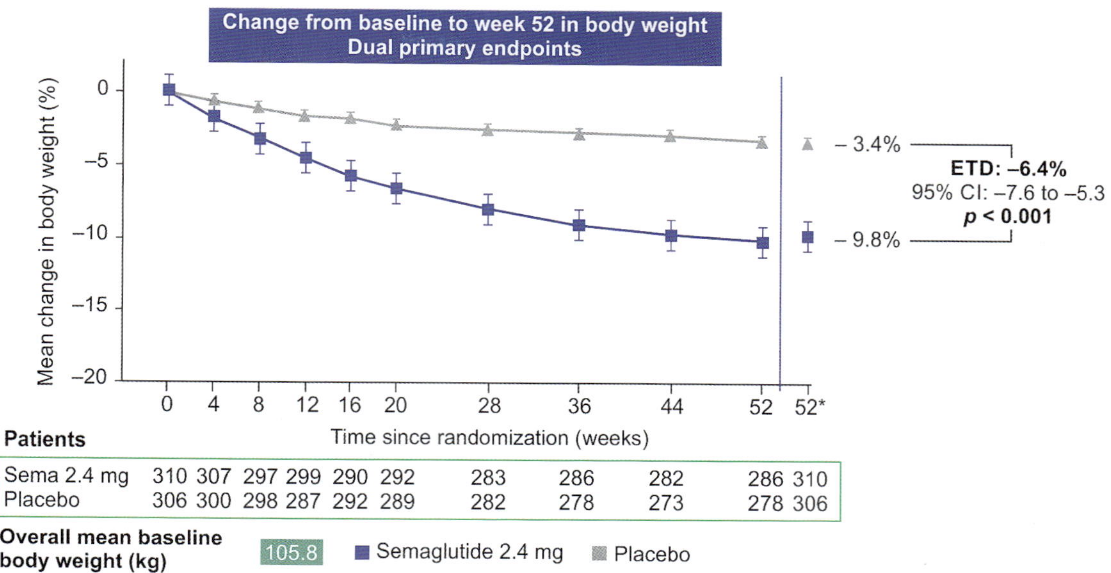

Fig. 5: STEP-HFpEF -DM.
*Data are estimated mean changes from baseline to week 52 for the treatment policy estimated using ANCOVA and an imputation approach for missing data.
Source: Kosiborod et al. (2024).

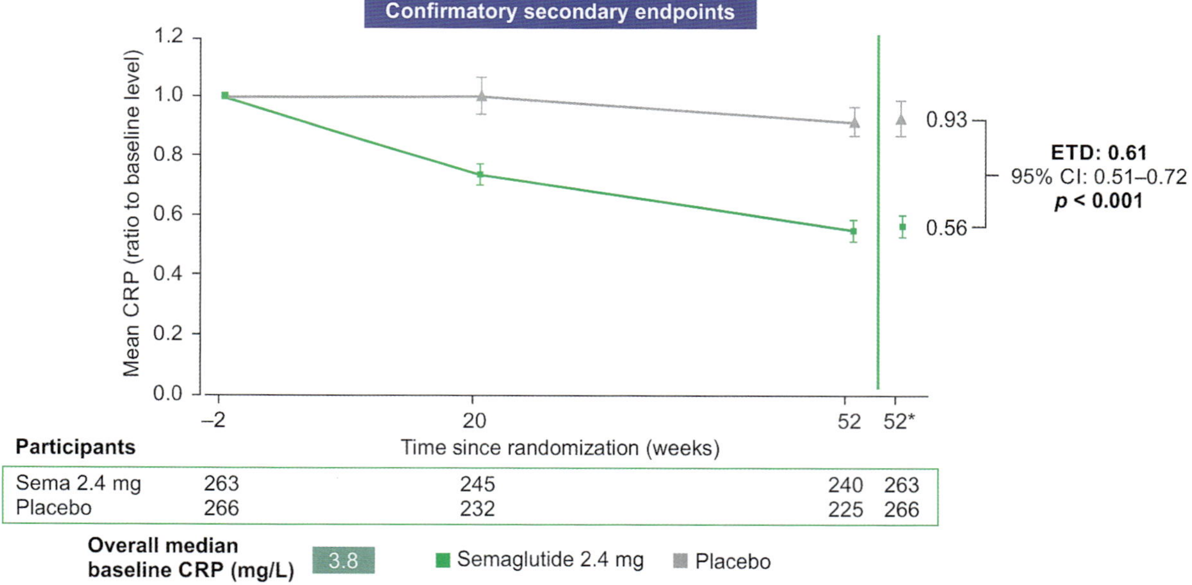

Fig. 6: Change from baseline to week 52 in CRP.
*Data are estimated mean changes from baseline to week 52 for the treatment policy estimated using ANCOVA and an imputation approach for missing data.
Source: Verma et al. (2024).

SEMAGLUTIDE AND NT-proBNP IN OBESITY-RELATED HFpEF[16]

Prespecified secondary analysis of pooled data from these two randomized trials (STEP-HFpEF and STEP-HFpEF DM) showed substantial reduction in NT-proBNP at 52 weeks and change in the dual primary endpoints of KCCQ-CCS and body weight by baseline NT-proBNP **(Figs. 7A and B)**. Participants with higher baseline NT-proBNP had a similar degree of weight loss but experienced larger reductions in HF-related symptoms and physical limitations with semaglutide than those with lower NT-proBNP.

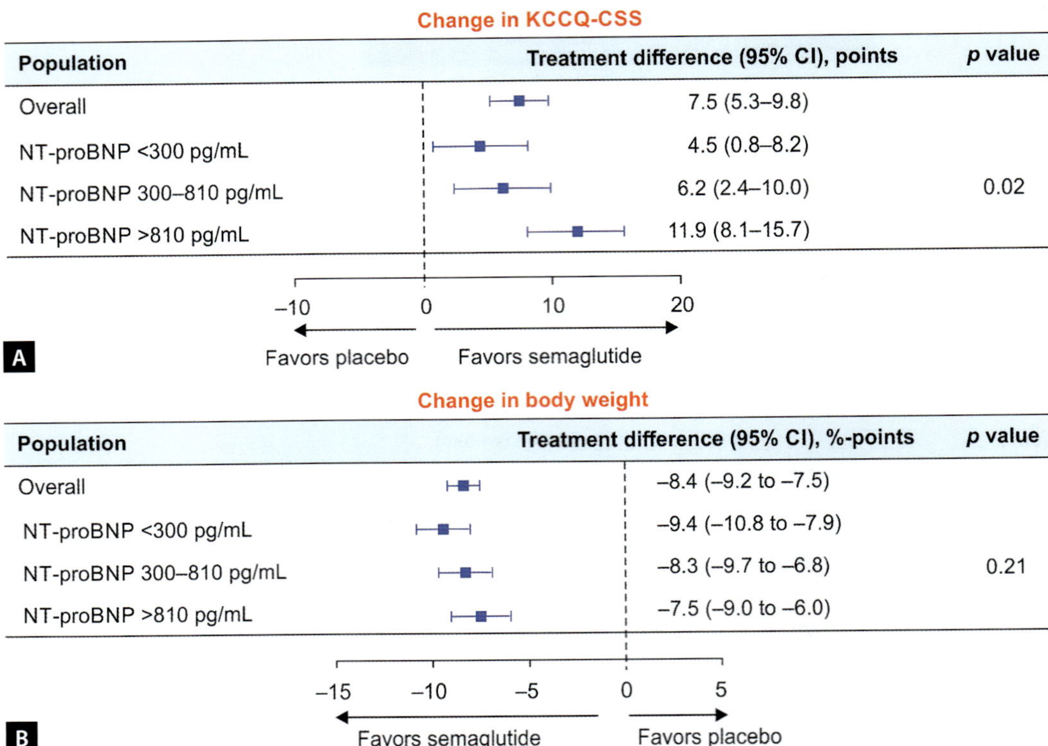

Figs. 7A and B: Effect of semaglutide on primary endpoint according to baseline NT-proBNP tertile.
Source: Petrie et al. (2024).

ATRIAL FIBRILLATION AND SEMAGLUTIDE EFFECTS IN OBESITY-RELATED HEART FAILURE WITH PRESERVED EJECTION FRACTION[17]

This was again a secondary analysis of pooled data from the STEP-HFpEF and STEP-HFpEF DM trials. Treatment with semaglutide showed significant improvements in HF-related symptoms, physical limitations, and exercise function, as well as reductions in weight, CRP, and NT-proBNP in people with and without AF and across AF types. The magnitude of semaglutide-mediated improvements in HF-related symptoms and physical limitations was more pronounced in those with AF versus those without AF at baseline **(Figs. 8A and B)**.

SEMAGLUTIDE AND DIURETIC USE IN OBESITY-RELATED HFpEF: A POOLED ANALYSIS OF STEP-HFpEF AND STEP-HFpEF-DM TRIALS[18]

This prespecified analysis of pooled data from the STEP-HFpEF and STEP-HFpEF-DM trials is to see the efficacy of semaglutide with baseline diuretic use and also to see its effect on the diuretic dose in patients with obesity-related HFpEF. Over 52 weeks of treatment, semaglutide showed benefit in change in body weight across diuretic use categories and Kansas City Cardiomyopathy Questionnaire clinical summary score. Patients on loop diuretics showed better improvement compared to those not on loop diuretics. Dose of loop diuretic has also decreased by 17% in the semaglutide group, while it has increased by 2.4% in placebo group (p <0.0001) **(Fig. 9)**.

CONCLUSION

In patients with HFpEF and obesity, treatment with semaglutide (2.4 mg) in both STEP HFpEF and STEP-HFpEF DM trials led to substantial reductions in symptoms and greater improvements in exercise function with more weight loss than placebo. In the pooled analysis of these two trials, semaglutide also reduced inflammation regardless of either baseline CRP or magnitude of weight loss. Semaglutide also showed a reduction in NT-proBNP; those with higher baseline NT-proBNP experienced larger reductions in HF-related symptoms and physical limitations than those with lower NT-proBNP. In patients with AF, the magnitude of semaglutide-mediated

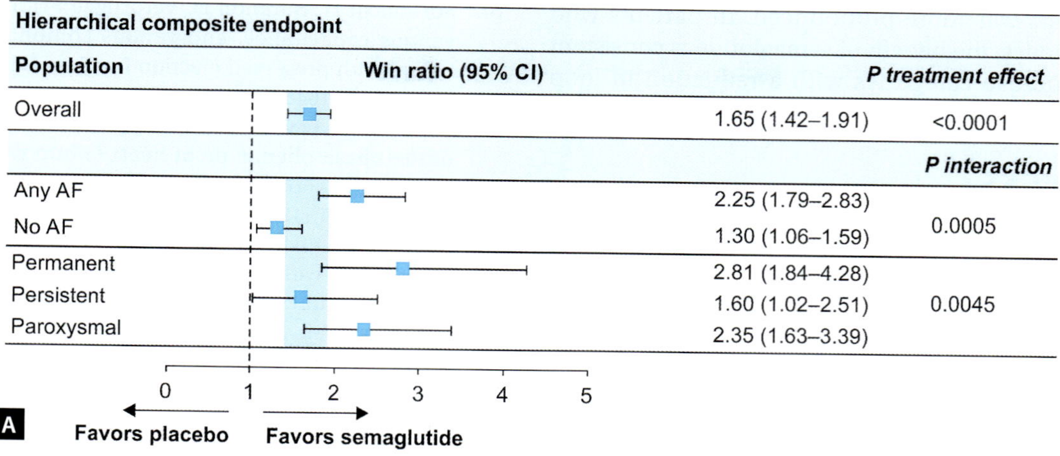

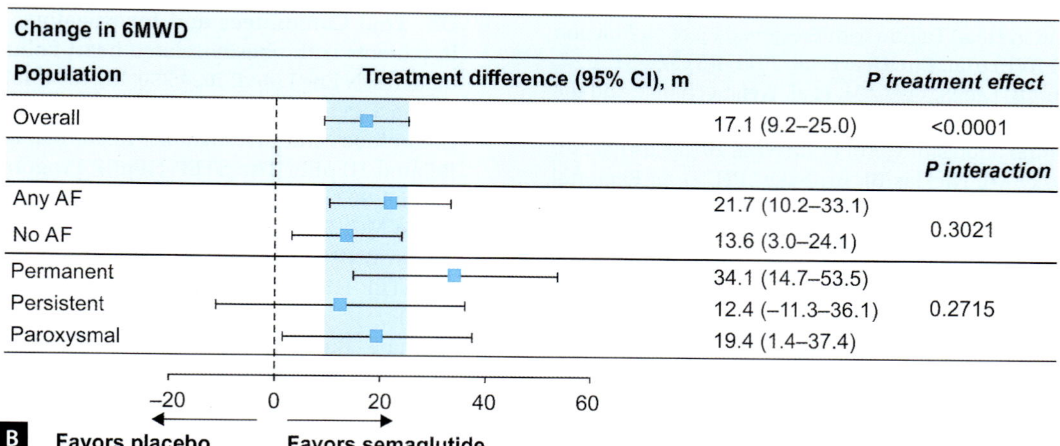

Figs. 8A and B: Semaglutide effects on 6MWD and hierarchical composite endpoint by AF history.
Source: Verma et al. (2024).

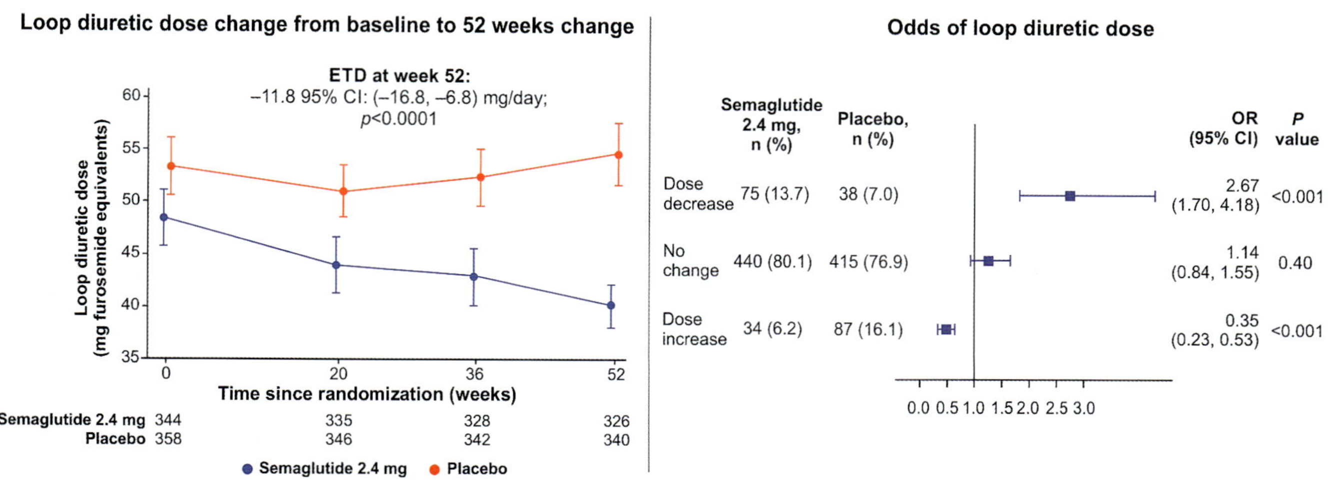

Fig. 9: Effect on loop diuretic dose changes from baseline to week 52.
Source: Shah et al. (2024).

improvements was more pronounced. In patients who were on diuretics, the benefit of semaglutide is consistent in all diuretic use categories with a reduction in loop diuretic use and dose between baseline and 52 weeks.

REFERENCES

1. Roger VL. Epidemiology of heart failure: a contemporary perspective. Circ Res. 2021;128(10):1421-34.
2. Redfield MM, Borlaug BA. Heart failure with preserved ejection fraction: a review. JAMA. 2023;329:827-38.
3. Borlaug BA. Evaluation and management of heart failure with preserved ejection fraction. Nat Rev Cardiol. 2020; 17(9):559-73.
4. Haass M, Kitzman DW, Anand IS, et al. Body mass index and adverse cardiovascular outcomes in heart failure patients with preserved ejection fraction: Results from the Irbesartan in Heart Failure with Preserved Ejection Fraction (I-PRESERVE) trial. Circ Heart Fail. 2011;4(3):324-31.
5. Newman AB, Lee JS, Visser M, et al. Weight change and the conservation of lean mass in old age: the health, aging, and body composition study. Am J Clin Nutr. 2005;82(4):872-8.
6. Haykowsky MJ, Nicklas BJ, Brubaker PH, et al. Regional adipose distribution and its relationship to exercise intolerance in older obese patients who have heart failure with preserved ejection fraction. JACC Heart Fail. 2018; 6(8):640-9.
7. Kitzman DW, Nicklas BJ. Pivotal role of excess intra-abdominal adipose in the pathogenesis of metabolic/obese HFpEF. JACC Heart Fail. 2018;6:1008-10.
8. Borlaug BA, Jensen MD, Kitzman DW, et al. Obesity and heart failure with preserved ejection fraction: new insights and pathophysiological targets. Cardiovasc Res. 2023;118(18):3434-50.
9. Obokata M, Reddy YNV, Pislaru SV, et al. Evidence supporting the existence of a distinct obese phenotype of heart failure with preserved ejection fraction. Circulation. 2017;136(1):6-19.
10. Sorimachi H, Burkhoff D, Verbrugge FH, et al. Obesity, venous capacitance, and venous compliance in heart failure with preserved ejection fraction. Eur J Heart Fail. 2021;23(10):1648-58.
11. Reddy YNV, Lewis GD, Shah SJ, et al. Characterization of the obese phenotype of heart failure with preserved ejection fraction: a RELAX trial ancillary study. Mayo Clin Proc. 2019;94:1199-209.
12. Reddy YNV, Rikhi A, Obokata M, et al. Quality of life in heart failure with preserved ejection fraction: importance of obesity, functional capacity, and physical inactivity. Eur J Heart Fail. 2020;22(6):1009-18
13. Kosiborod MN, Abildstrøm SZ, Borlaug BA, et al. Semaglutide in patients with heart failure with preserved ejection fraction and obesity. N Eng J Med. 2023;389(12): 1069-84.
14. Kosiborod MN, Petrie MC, Borlaug BA, et al.; STEP-HFpEF DM Trial Committees and Investigators. Semaglutide in patients with obesity-related heart failure and type 2 diabetes. N Eng J Med. 2024;390(15):1394-407.
15. Verma S, Petrie MC, Borlaug BA, et al.; STEP-HFpEF Trial Committees and Investigators. Inflammation in Obesity-Related HFpEF: The STEP-HFpEF Program. J Am Coll Cardiol. 2024;84(17):1646-62.
16. Petrie MC, Borlaug BA, Butler J, et al. Semaglutide and NT-proBNP in Obesity-Related HFpEF Insights From the STEP-HFpEF Program. Am Coll Cardiol. 2024;84(1): 27-40.
17. Verma S, Butler J, Borlaug BA, et al.; STEP-HFpEF and STEP-HFpEF DM Investigators. Atrial Fibrillation and Semaglutide Effects in Obesity-Related Heart Failure With Preserved Ejection Fraction: STEP-HFpEF Program. J Am Coll Cardiol. 2024;84(17):1603-14.
18. Shah SJ, Sharma K, Borlaug BA, et al. Semaglutide and diuretic use in obesity-related heart failure with preserved ejection fraction: A pooled analysis of the STEP-HFpEF and STEP-HFpEF-DM trials. Eur Heart J. 2024;45: 3254-69.

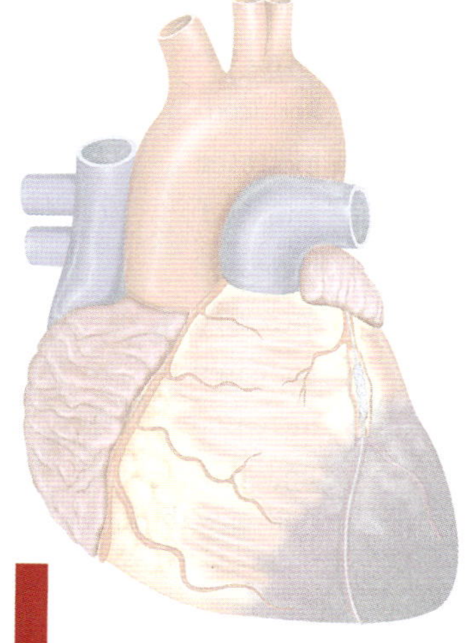

Semaglutide in Obesity, HFpEF, and Diabetes Mellitus: STEP-HFpEF Trial

Sanjay Mittal, Aparajita Kumar

INTRODUCTION

The burden of heart failure with preserved ejection fraction (HFpEF) is increasing globally, attributed to greater life expectancy along with the global epidemic of obesity and type 2 diabetes mellitus (T2DM). Over half of patients with HFpEF have comorbidities such as obesity and/or T2DM and another 15–20% have prediabetes. In contrast to heart failure with reduced ejection fraction (HFrEF), therapeutic options for HFpEF have been limited. Till a few years back, the treatment of HFpEF was largely symptomatic, including diuretics for decongestion and cardiometabolic risk factor control. All commonly used HFrEF disease-modifying therapies, including beta blockers, renin-angiotensin-aldosterone (RAAS) inhibitors, and even angiotensin receptor-neprilysin inhibitors (ARNIs), failed to show any outcome benefit in HFpEF studies. However, on the basis of two recent positive outcome trials—EMPEROR-Preserved and DELIVER—sodium-glucose cotransporter 2 inhibitors (SGLT2i), namely empagliflozin and dapagliflozin, have become class I approved drugs for the management of HFpEF patients.

There is now growing evidence that semaglutide, a glucagon-like peptide-1 receptor agonist (GLP-1 RA) approved for use in T2DM as well as obesity management, may also be effective in improving outcomes in HFpEF patients. The STEP-HFpEF-DM (Semaglutide Treatment Effect in People with Obesity and HFPEF and Diabetes Mellitus) trial showed that semaglutide improved body weight, systemic inflammation, and heart failure (HF) symptoms in people with obesity-related HFpEF and T2DM. By addressing both metabolic and cardiovascular risks, semaglutide is a promising therapeutic option for HFpEF in addition to SGLT2i.

HEART FAILURE WITH PRESERVED EJECTION FRACTION BURDEN

Heart failure is a burgeoning healthcare burden with high mortality and morbidity, impaired functional capacity and quality of life, and a prognosis worse than many malignancies. HFpEF accounts for nearly 50% of HF, and its prevalence is increasing relative to HFrEF. It is estimated that HFpEF affects more than 4.9% of the general population over 60 years. Data gathered from the second 25-year Framingham Heart Study epoch has demonstrated that the lifetime risk of HFpEF is approximately 19.3%, which exceeds the lifetime risk of HFrEF, which is approximately 11.4%.

Heart failure with preserved ejection fraction is a complex syndrome often associated with multiple comorbidities such as diabetes, hypertension, chronic kidney disease, and obesity. HFpEF-associated cardio-renometabolic syndrome frequently causes microvascular inflammation, endothelial dysfunction, and poor cardiac reserve.

PATHOPHYSIOLOGY: THE OMINOUS CONUNDRUM OF HEART FAILURE WITH PRESERVED EJECTION FRACTION, OBESITY, AND DIABETES

Obesity, diabetes, and HFpEF are often associated and adversely impact the clinical outcomes of each other. More than 30% of those overweight or obese individuals have concomitant T2DM. As many as 88% diabetics on the other hand are overweight or obese. More than two third of the deaths in overweight/obese people happen to be due to a cardiovascular cause, which is almost twice of that seen in the general population.

Obesity has been implicated as a strong and specific causal factor of HFpEF, adversely affecting the quality of life and mortality in these patients. It is estimated that more than 1 billion people worldwide are obese, and its prevalence in adults has more than doubled since 1990.

Approximately 40–50% of patients with HFpEF have DM, and about 15–20% have prediabetes. The diabetic subset of HFpEF has increased inflammatory markers, endothelial dysfunction and fibrosis, leading to reduced exercise capacity, and higher mortality. In obese people, excess fat is deposited in various parts of the body, either subcutaneously (subcutaneous adiposity) including the abdominal wall or excess adipocytes deposited around the viscera (visceral adiposity).

There are various mechanisms by which adiposity/obesity potentiates the development of HFpEF. These effects could be mediated through mechanical effects, excessive neurohormonal stimulation, and promotion of inflammation.

- *Hemodynamic effects:* Excessive weight along with the associated cardiovascular comorbidities lead to a number of observed hemodynamic effects responsible for cardiac overload and predisposing to HF. Various hemodynamic abnormalities commonly encountered in obese individuals are given in **Table 1**. The systemic arterial resistance increases causing increased afterload. This leads to left ventricular hypertrophy along with impaired diastolic function. The preload increases due to fluid retention causing increased plasma volume and elevated left ventricular filling pressures. The epicardial visceral adiposity leads to pericardial restraint contributing to low cardiac output and high filling pressures **(Fig. 1)**.
- *Neurohormonal effects:* The various hemodynamic impacts of obesity and visceral adiposity, especially reduced cardiac output and increased filling pressure, lead to increased activity of the renin-angiotensin-aldosterone system (RAAS) and autonomic imbalance, which is characterized by increased sympathetic drive and vagal withdrawal. The elevated RAAS activity leads to increased aldosterone levels, thus enhancing sodium and fluid retention. The paradoxical reduction of natriuretic peptides in obesity is related to excessive degradation of BNP due to an increase in neprilysin activity as well as increased uptake by adipocytes due to high natriuretic peptide density. The various neurohormonal changes in obesity identified in various studies are summarized in **Table 2**.

TABLE 1: Hemodynamic effects of obesity leading to HFpEF.

Arterial resistance	Increased
Cardiac output	Reduced
Plasma volume	Increased
LV diastolic function	Impaired
Filling pressures	Increased
Chamber size	Increased
LV hypertrophy	Increased
Pericardial restraint	Increased
RV function	Reduced

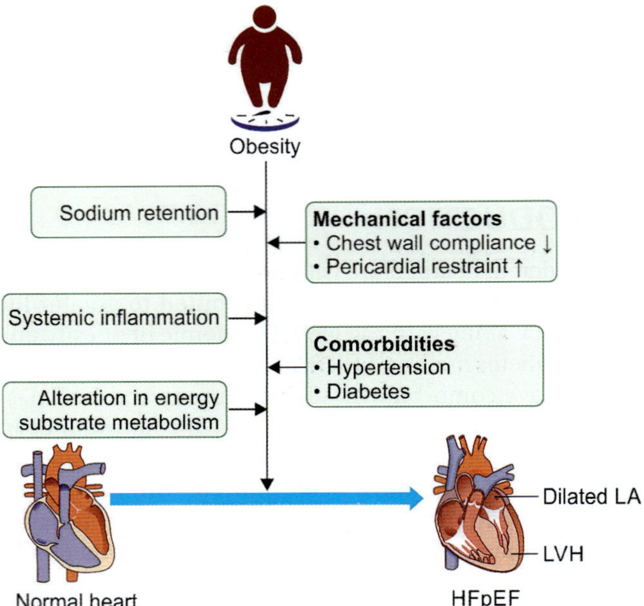

Fig. 1: Pathophysiology of obesity-related heart failure with preserved ejection fraction.

TABLE 2: Neurohormonal effects of obesity leading to HFpEF.

Renin angiotensin activity	Increased
Sympathetic activity	Increased
Sodium retention	Increased
Natriuretic peptides	Reduced
Neprilysin	Increased
Leptin	Increased

- *Inflammatory effects:* Obesity leads to a biological transformation of the adipose tissue toward an inflammatory state, which has deleterious effects on the structure and function of most visceral organs and vasculature. Moreover, coronary microvascular

TABLE 3: Inflammatory effects of obesity leading to HFpEF.

Inflammatory adipokines	Increased
Local inflammation	Increased
Coronary microvascular dysfunction	Increased
Systemic inflammation	Increased
Endothelial dysfunction	Increased
Cardiac fibrosis	Increased
Nitric oxide bioavailability	Reduced

dysfunction and endothelial dysfunction due to myocardial ischemia and injury have a causal role in the pathophysiology of HFpEF. Ischemia may occur due to a supply–demand mismatch on account of elevated left ventricle filling pressure, epicardial disease, and coronary microvascular dysfunction. Cardiac reserve limitations are caused by abnormalities in nitric oxide-cyclic guanosine monophosphate (CGMP) signaling, related to systemic inflammation. Elevated inflammatory biomarkers predict development of incident HFpEF. Increased inflammation leads to alterations in titin content, phosphorylation, and fibrillar collagen in the myocardium, thereby leading to increase in diastolic stiffness causing HFpEF. Other mechanisms include exaggerated senescence, deranged autophagy, and lipotoxicity **(Table 3)**.

CURRENT STRATEGIES IN THE MANAGEMENT OF HEART FAILURE WITH PRESERVED EJECTION FRACTION

There is a paucity of effective therapy in HFpEF, possibly due to phenotypic heterogenicity. Moreover, the obese phenotype of HFpEF is often excluded from clinical trials, either due to body mass index (BMI) eligibility cutoffs or indirectly due to the requirement of elevated natriuretic peptides, whose values are characteristically lower in obesity. There is an increasing need to address the trinity of obesity, diabetes, and cardiovascular disease which culminate in adverse clinical outcomes and mortality.

The only disease-modifying agents recommended to be used in HFpEF today are SGLT2i, namely dapagliflozin and empagliflozin. Both ACC/AHA and European Society of Cardiology (ESC) guidelines recommend the use of SGLT2i use in HFpEF as class IA indication based on data from the clinical trials DELIVER and EMPEROR-Preserved. SGLT2is, however, offer modest weight reduction at best.

The recent data on glucagonGLP-1 RA drug semaglutide on the basis of STEP-HFpEF and SELECT trials show encouraging results, making GLP-1 RA an emerging treatment option for diabetic patients with obesity phenotype of HFpEF.

Glucagon-like Peptide-1 Receptor Agonists: Mechanism of Action

Glucagon-like peptide-1 receptor agonists mimic the action of endogenous GLP-1, activating GLP-1R, thereby enhancing insulin secretion, inhibiting glucagon release, delaying gastric emptying, and reducing food intake through central appetite suppression. These mechanisms make GLP-1 RAs powerful tools for controlling blood glucose and improving metabolic syndrome. Furthermore, their multifaceted mechanisms of action suggest potential applications beyond traditional metabolic disorders.

Glucagon-like peptide-1 is produced and secreted from the L cells of the small intestine in response to nutrients. It then binds to specific GLP-1 receptors, expressed in various tissues, and brings about a battery of effects. The tissues and their respective effects include the following **(Fig. 2)**:

- *Pancreatic beta cells:* GLP-1 exerts its main effect by stimulating glucose-dependent insulin release from the pancreatic islets. It regulates glucagon secretion. In addition, GLP-1 RAs increase beta-cell survival and beta-cell proliferation.
- *Kidney:* GLP-1 RAs have natriuretic effects through the receptors in the kidneys. Thus, they may contribute to decongestion in HFpEF.
- *Liver:* GLP-1 RAs reduce glucose production in liver, thereby reducing blood sugar levels.
- *Heart:* GLP-1 receptor stimulation in the heart leads to reduction in blood pressure and increase in myocardial contractility although a slight increase in heart rate. GLP-1 RAs are cardioprotective.
- *Brain:* By stimulating brain GLP-1 receptors, GLP-1 RAs reduce appetite and increase satiety, thus reducing calorie intake and contributing to weight loss. Moreover, the energy expenditure increases, leading to overall metabolic improvement.
- *Gastric mucosa:* GLP-1 RAs increase acid secretion, thus aiding in digestion. The GI motility and gastric emptying are reduced. This may lead to reduced appetite.
- *Adipose tissue:* GLP-1 increases lipolysis in the adipose tissue and facilitates free fatty acid synthesis. This also contributes to reduction in visceral adiposity.
- *Muscles:* Facilitate glycogen synthesis and glucose oxidation

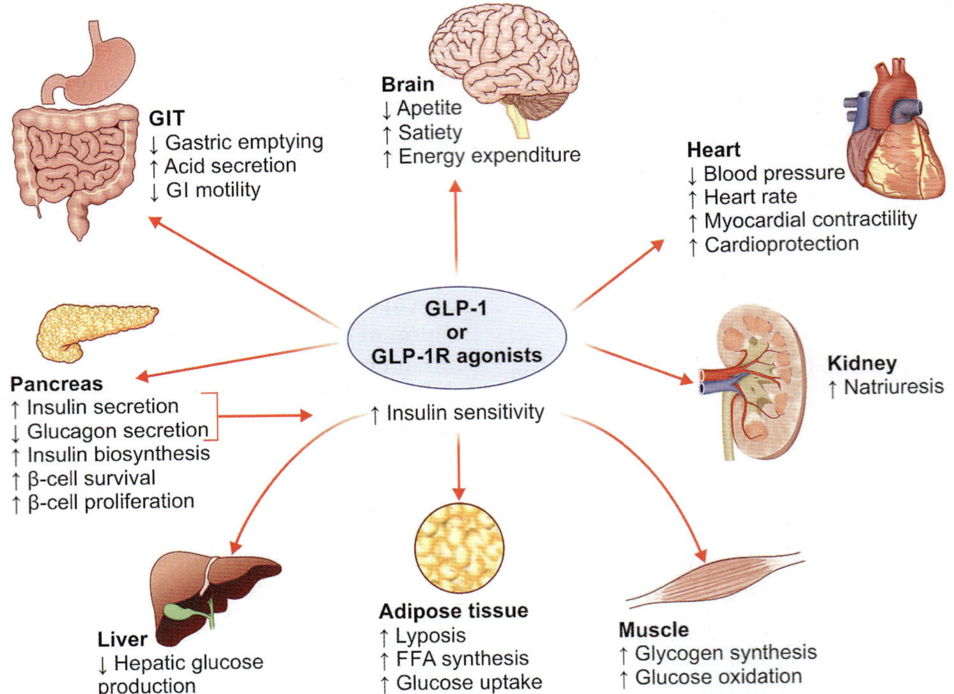

Fig. 2: Pleiotropic effects of GLP-1 or GLP-1R agonists.

Given its effects on slowed gastric emptying and on appetite centers in the hypothalamus, therapy with GLP-1 and its RAs is associated with weight loss.

Synthetic GLP-1 RAs are variably resistant to degradation by the enzyme dipeptidyl peptidase 4 and therefore have a longer half-life, with consequent favorable pharmacological effects. They bind to the GLP-1 receptor and stimulate glucose-dependent insulin release from the pancreatic islets. They do not usually cause hypoglycemia in the absence of therapies that otherwise can cause it. Apart from reduction in glycemic levels, GLP-1 RAs produce weight loss, activate cAMP protein kinase A pathway, inhibit RAAS activation, and exert antihypertensive, antiatherosclerotic, anti-inflammatory, and renoprotective effects.

Semaglutide in Obesity and Heart Failure: The Evidence

Glucagon-like peptide-1 RAs fall under two broad categories: Human GLP-1 backbone agents and exendin-4 backbone agents. The Food and Drug Administration (FDA)-approved GLP-1 agonists include the following:

- *Human GLP-1 backbone:*
  - Dulaglutide
  - Albiglutide—discontinued
  - Liraglutide
  - Semaglutide
- *Exendin-4 backbone:*
  - Exenatide
  - Lixisenatide—discontinued
  - Tirzepatide—GIP analog that activates both GLP-1 and GIP receptors

Results in Patients with Type 2 Diabetes Mellitus

Glucagon-like peptide-1 RAs in various cardiovascular outcome trials (CVOTs) were found to reduce the risk of myocardial infarction (MI), stroke, and CV death in patients with T2DM. GLP-1 RAs with proven cardiovascular benefits in various randomized controlled trials (RCTs) are liraglutide and once-weekly subcutaneous injections of semaglutide, dulaglutide, and albiglutide. GLP-1 RAs such as lixisenatide, extended-release exenatide, and oral semaglutide have shown a neutral effect.

Results in Patients with Heart Failure

Hospitalization for HF did not represent the primary endpoint of the main RCTs, yet GLP-1 RAs were found to slightly reduce the risk of hospitalization for HF by approximately 11%. HF events were reduced in diabetic patients with no HF at baseline, whereas they were generally not changed in the RCTs enrolling patients with HF. A subanalysis of the data suggests a possible increased risk of HF events in the patients with HFrEF at baseline and the converse, i.e., a beneficial effect in patients with HFpEF, especially those with concomitant obesity. Given the results derived from RCTs, international scientific societies currently recommend the use of GLP-1 RAs as part of a comprehensive strategy to reduce the risk of CV events in patients with T2DM, though not yet for the prevention of HF in patients with DM.

Results in Patients with Obesity

Along with the benefits on CV outcome, it has been shown that the administration of GLP-1 RA is associated with weight loss regardless of the diabetic status. Liraglutide has been shown to be effective for weight loss in nondiabetic patients with obesity or overweight when given as an adjunctive therapy to diet and exercise. Injectable semaglutide is also highly effective in patients both with and without T2DM. Moreover, its efficacy was greater compared with other agents. In the SUSTAIN trials, a slightly greater weight loss was observed with subcutaneous once-weekly semaglutide, compared with exenatide, dulaglutide, or liraglutide. Similarly, a secondary analysis of PIONEER-4 showed a greater weight loss with once-daily oral semaglutide compared with subcutaneous liraglutide.

TREATMENT OF PATIENTS WITH HEART FAILURE WITH PRESERVED EJECTION FRACTION

With the recent exception of SGLT2i, trials in patients with HFpEF have failed to show significant results so no specific treatment was recommended in the 2023 ESC guidelines for HF. It can be, however, hypothesized that similar to the beneficial effects of caloric restriction and physical activity leading to weight loss, treatment with weight-reducing GLP-1 RA may be effective for patients with the obese HFpEF phenotype.

STEP TRIALS PROGRAM (SEMAGLUTIDE TREATMENT EFFECT IN PEOPLE WITH OBESITY)

The "STEP Program" trial is a series of 12 trials designed to test the efficacy of semaglutide, at a higher dose of 2.4 mg/wk, for weight loss in patients with or without T2DM having different clinical phenotypes. The STEP 1 trial showed an average 14.9% reduction in body weight with semaglutide 2.4 mg plus a lifestyle intervention, compared with a 2.4% reduction in the placebo plus lifestyle intervention group (treatment difference of 12.4%; $p < 0.001$), among obese or overweight participants with related comorbidities, but not T2DM. The STEP 2 trial showed an average body weight reduction of 9.6% and 6.9% with semaglutide 2.4 and 1.0 mg versus 3.4% with placebo ($p < 0.001$) among participants with T2DM and overweight or obesity. The higher dose also achieved slightly better glycemic control, reductions in cardiometabolic risk, and improved physical function relative to the standard dose. In STEP 3 trial, a weight-reduction treatment difference of 10.3% was observed when treating overweight or obese people with related comorbidities, but not T2DM, with semaglutide 2.4 mg compared with placebo. Patients who continued to take semaglutide after the first 20 weeks lost an additional 7.9% of their body weight in the STEP 4 trial. Consistent results have been observed in other STEP trials **(Table 4)**.

STEP-HFpEF TRIALS: TREATMENT WITH SEMAGLUTIDE IN PATIENTS WITH OBESITY AND HFpEF

As an extension of STEP program, semaglutide injections were tried in patients with DM (STEP-HFpEF-DM) or without DM (STEP-HFpEF) having concomitant obesity and HFpEF.

The STEP-HFpEF-DM trial was a landmark study for optimizing care of people with obesity-related HFpEF and T2DM. A total of 616 adults were recruited from 16 countries in North and South America, Europe, and Asia with specific inclusion criteria:

- Left ventricular ejection fraction >45%
- BMI >30 kg/m^2
- Type 2 diabetes [glycated hemoglobin (HbA1c) <10%]
- New York Heart Association Functional Classification of II–IV
- 6-minute walk distance (6MWD) >100 m
- Kansas City Cardiomyopathy Questionnaire Clinical Summary Score (KCCQ-CSS) <90
- In addition, one of the following: Elevated left ventricular filling pressures, elevated NT-pro B-type natriuretic peptide (NT-proBNP) and structural echocardiographic abnormalities, or a history of HF hospitalization within the past year and ongoing diuretics and/or echocardiographic abnormalities

The participants (median age 69 years; 84% white; 44% female; median BMI 37 kg/m^2; median NT-proBNP 493 pg/mL) were randomized in a 1:1 ratio to receive either 2.4 mg of semaglutide (administered subcutaneously) once per week or placebo for 52 weeks. Use of key medications at baseline included 81% on diuretics, 33% on SGLT2i, 21% on insulin, and 17.5% on sulfonylureas.

TABLE 4: Summary of STEP (semaglutide treatment effect in people with obesity) trials.

Trial	*Trial population*	*Intervention and comparator*	*Primary outcomes*
STEP 1	Obese or overweight, related comorbidities, no diabetes	Semaglutide 2.4 mg or placebo for 68 weeks	14.9% vs. 2.4% average bodyweight reduction from baseline 86.5% of the semaglutide group lost at least 5% of their bodyweight
STEP 2	Obesity and overweight, type 2 diabetes	Semaglutide 2.4 mg vs. 1.0 mg vs. matched placebo for 68 weeks	9.64% vs. 6.99% vs. 3.43% average bodyweight reduction from baseline. Semaglutide 2.4 mg produced slightly better glycemic control, reductions in cardiometabolic risk, and improved physical function than semaglutide 1
STEP 3	Obesity and overweight, related comorbidities, no diabetes	Intensive behavioral therapy plus semaglutide 2.4 mg or placebo for 68 weeks	16% vs. 5.7% average bodyweight reduction from baseline 86.6% vs. 47.6% lost at least 5% of their bodyweight
STEP 4	Obesity and overweight, related comorbidities, no diabetes	Semaglutide 2.4 mg for 20 weeks and then semaglutide 2.4 mg vs. placebo for 48	17.4% vs. 5.0% average bodyweight reduction from baseline Average 7.9% additional weight loss for semaglutide vs. 6.95% weight gain for placebo
STEP 5	Obesity and overweight, related comorbidities, no diabetes	Semaglutide 2.4 mg vs. placebo for 2 years	Average placebo-corrected weight loss of 12.6 percentage points at 104 weeks
STEP 6	East Asian, obesity or overweight, related comorbidities, with or without diabetes	Semaglutide 2.4 mg vs. 1.7 mg vs placebo for 68 weeks	13.2% vs. 9.6% vs. 2.1% average bodyweight reduction from baseline
STEP 7	East Asian, obesity or overweight, with or without type 2 diabetes	Semaglutide 2.4 mg vs. placebo for 44 weeks	12.1% vs. 3.6% mean reduction in bodyweight from baseline 85% vs. 31% of participants lost at least 5% of their bodyweight
STEP 8	Obesity and overweight, with type 2 diabetes	Semaglutide 2.4 mg vs. daily injectable liraglutide 3.0 mg vs. placebo for 68 weeks	15.8% vs. 6.4% average bodyweight reduction from baseline
STEP 9	Obesity, pain due to knee osteoarthritis, no diabetes	Semaglutide 2.4 mg vs. placebo for 68 weeks	Assessing change in bodyweight and change in WOMAC pain score
STEP 10	Obesity, with prediabetes	Semaglutide 2.4 mg or placebo for 52 weeks	Assessing percentage change in bodyweight and change to normoglycemia
STEP 12	BMI of ≥24 kg/m^2 and <28 kg/m^2, at least one weight-related comorbidity, with or without diabetes, or BMI of ≥28 kg/m^2 and <30 kg/m^2, with or without weight-related comorbidities	Semaglutide 2.4 mg vs. placebo for 44 weeks	Assessing change in bodyweight from baseline and the number of participants achieving ≥5% bodyweight reduction from baseline

The STEP-HFpEF trial, on the contrary, excluded patients with DM. The trial randomized 529 patients with otherwise similar inclusion and exclusion criteria. The randomization chart of both the trials is shown in **Figure 3**.

Both STEP-HFpEF and STEP-HFpEF-DM trials had the same co-primary endpoints, which were a change from baseline in body weight and KCCQ-CSS.

In STEP-HFPEF-DM, subcutaneously administering 2.4 mg of semaglutide once per week was superior to placebo in:

- Improving KCCQ-CSS [13.7- vs. 6.4-point change; estimated treatment difference (ETD) 7.3 (95% CI 4.1, 10.4])
- Weight loss [–9.8% vs. –3.4%; ETD –6.4% (95% CI –7.6, –5.2]) at 52 weeks, with no evidence of attenuation of benefits

Further analysis also reported the superiority of semaglutide versus placebo in key secondary endpoints **(Table 5)**, namely:

- Change in 6MWD [12.7 m vs. –1.6 m; ETD 14.3 (95% CI 3.7, 24.9)]
- A hierarchical composite endpoint that included HF events, mortality, and differences in the change in KCCQ-CSS and 6WMD [win ratio 1.58 (95% CI 1.29, 1.94)]

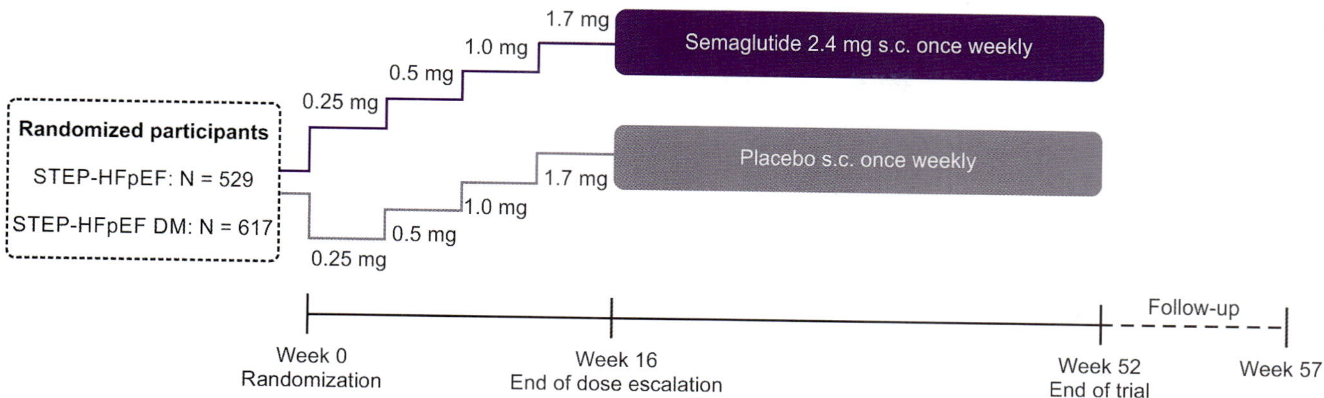

Fig. 3: Randomization chart of STEP-HFpEF and STEP-HFpEF-DM trials.

TABLE 5: Comparison between STEP-HFpEF and STEP-HFpEF DM trials.

	STEP-HFpEF	*STEP-HFpEF DM*
Trial population	Obese or overweight, with heart failure with preserved ejection fraction, no T2DM	Obese or overweight, with heart failure with preserved ejection fraction, with T2DM
Number of patients	529	616
Intervention and comparator	Semaglutide 2.4 mg vs. placebo for 52 weeks	Semaglutide 2.4 mg vs. placebo for 52 weeks
Primary outcomes	16.6 point vs. 8.7 point mean change in KCCQ clinical summary score 13.3% vs. 2.6% mean bodyweight reduction from baseline	13.7 point vs. 6.4 point mean change in KCCQ clinical summary score 9.8% vs. 3.4% mean bodyweight reduction from baseline
Secondary outcomes	Change in 6MWD from baseline to week 52% 21.5 m vs. 1.2 m [95% CI, 8.6–32.1]	Change in 6MWD from baseline to week 52% 12.7 for semaglutide and 1.6 for placebo

- Change in HbA1C [–0.7% vs. 0.1%; ETD –0.8% (95% CI –1.0, –0.6)]
- Change in C-reactive protein (CRP) levels [–42% vs. –12.8%; estimated treatment ratio 0.67 (95% CI 0.55, 0.80)]
- Change in NT-proBNP levels [–23.2% vs. –4.6%; estimated treatment ratio 0.8 (95% CI 0.7, 0.9)]

These findings mirrored those of the similarly designed STEP-HFpEF trial that excluded people with DM. In line with prior studies of antiobesity medications, weight loss in STEP-HFpEF-DM was lower than STEP-HFpEF (6.4% vs. 10.7%), perhaps due to reduced incretin effects among people with T2DM. There could also be attenuation of effects from SGLT2i, in which the use of SGLT2i at baseline was higher in STEP-HFpEF-DM than in STEP-HFpEF (33% vs. 3.6%). Despite similar KCCQ-CSS improvement, people with T2DM had fewer improvements in exercise capacity compared to those without DM in STEP-HFpEF (6MWD: 14.3 m vs. 20.3 m). However, people with T2DM have been reported to have poorer 6MWD performance than those without DM. Considering that this was not a head-to-head comparison, median 6MWD was already lower at baseline in STEP-HFpEF-DM than in STEP-HFpEF (280 m vs. 320 m). Finally, semaglutide was well tolerated without an increased risk of acute pancreatitis, severe hypoglycemia, and diabetic retinopathy, which are the adverse events of interest in people with DM. The risk-mitigation strategies in this trial would be useful in routine practice such as reducing the dose of sulfonylureas and insulin when initiating potent incretin-based therapy, as well as delaying their use until unstable diabetic retinopathy and maculopathy are treated.

The SELECT (Semaglutide Effects on Heart Disease and Stroke in Patients With Overweight or Obesity) trial showed durability of clinically meaningful weight loss with good safety profiles for up to 4 years in people with obesity but not DM (66% with prediabetes). This trial was conducted in patients ≥45 years of age with preexisting cardiovascular disease and BMI ≥27 kg/m^2, but without DM showed that weekly subcutaneous semaglutide was superior to placebo in reducing the incidence of death from cardiovascular causes, nonfatal MI, or nonfatal stroke.

Recently, the FDA approved semaglutide injection 2.4 mg once weekly for chronic weight management in adults with obesity or overweight with at least one weight-related condition (such as high blood pressure, T2DM, or high cholesterol), for use in addition to a reduced calorie diet and increased physical activity. Semaglutide is the first drug approved for chronic weight management in adults with general obesity or overweight since 2014. Although tirzepatide is at an earlier stage of development, it has shown a similar, if not greater, efficacy for weight loss.

IMPLICATIONS

With worsening epidemiological trends for both the incidence and the prevalence of HF worldwide, it is critical to implement optimal prevention and treatment strategies for patients with or without comorbidities as T2DM. Consensus statements and guidelines have recommended GLP-1 RA and SGLT2i as additions to lifestyle interventions with or without metformin in those at a high atherosclerotic disease risk.

Changes in quality of life (QOL) and functional capacity in patients with chronic diseases are often underemphasized as primary endpoints. Though these measures may not necessarily correlate with mortality and morbidity, it may be relevant in HFpEF, which manifests as impaired effort tolerance causing dyspnea and limiting independence. As HFpEF trials have not achieved mortality or morbidity endpoints till date, focusing on symptomatic improvement may improve QOL end points, reflecting a paradigm shift.

From this perspective, GLP-1 RA could represent a cornerstone treatment to modify the natural history of HFpEF. This could potentially lead to a breakthrough in the treatment of HF, which is constantly evolving, especially if we consider the high prevalence and adverse prognosis of patients affected by HFpEF.

CONCLUSION

The number of patients with HFpEF is expected to grow, given the increased life expectancy and the increasing prevalence of risk factors predisposing to HFpEF. It is well known that obesity is one of the most common and clinically relevant phenotypes of HFpEF with specific pathophysiological mechanisms. Therapies targeting body weight reduction are therefore promising. Trials with GLP-1 RA in obese patients, with or without T2DM, have shown their efficacy in weight loss. Future well-designed studies with longer durations of event-driven outcomes are required to define the role of novel therapies to target weight loss and other sequelae of obesity in HFpEF.

SUGGESTED READING

1. Aldawsari M, Almadani FA, Almuhammadi N, et al. The Efficacy of GLP-1 Analogues on Appetite Parameters, Gastric Emptying, Food Preference and Taste Among Adults with Obesity: Systematic Review of Randomized Controlled Trials. Diabetes Metab Syndr Obes. 2023; 16:575-95.
2. Amaro A, Sugimoto D, Wharton S. Efficacy and safety of semaglutide for weight management: evidence from the STEP program. Postgrad Med. 2-22;134(suppl 1):5-17.
3. Anker SD, Usman MS, Anker MS, et al. Patient phenotype profiling in heart failure with preserved ejection fraction to guide therapeutic decision making. A scientific statement of the Heart Failure Association, the European Heart Rhythm Association of the European Society of Hypertension. Eur J Heart Fail. 2023;25(7):936-55.
4. Heidenreich PA, Bozkurt B, Aguilar D, et al. 2022 AHA/ACC/HFSA guideline for the management of heart failure: A report of the American College of Cardiology/American Heart Association Joint Committee on Clinical Practice Guidelines. J Am Coll Cardiol. 2022;79(17):e263-e421.
5. Kenchaiah S, Evans JC, Levy D, et al. Obesity and the risk of heart failure. N Engl J Med. 2002;347(5):305-13.
6. Obokata M, Reddy YNV, Pislaru SV, et al. Evidence supporting the existence of a distinct obese phenotype of heart failure with preserved ejection fraction. Circulation. 2017;136 (1):6-19.
7. Parikh SK, Sharma K, Fiuzat M, et al. Heart Failure with preserved ejection fraction Expert Panel Report: Current controversies and implications for clinical trials. JACC Heart Fail. 2018;6(8):619-32.
8. Pfeffer AM, Shah MA, Borlaug AB. Heart Failure with Preserved Ejection Fraction in perspective. Circ Res. 2019;124(11):1598-617.
9. Sabbah MS, Fayyaz AU, de Denus S, et al. Obese-inflammatory phenotypes in heart failure with preserved ejection fraction. Circ Heart Fail. 2020;13(8):e006414.
10. Saraiva FK, Sposito AC. Cardiovascular effects of GLP1 receptor agonists Cardiovasc Diabetol. 2014;13:142.
11. Savarese G, Becher PM, Lund LH, et al. Global burden of heart failure: a comprehensive and updated review of epidemiology. Cardiovasc Res. 2023;118(17):3272-87. [Erratum in: Cardiovasc Res. 2023:119(6):1453].

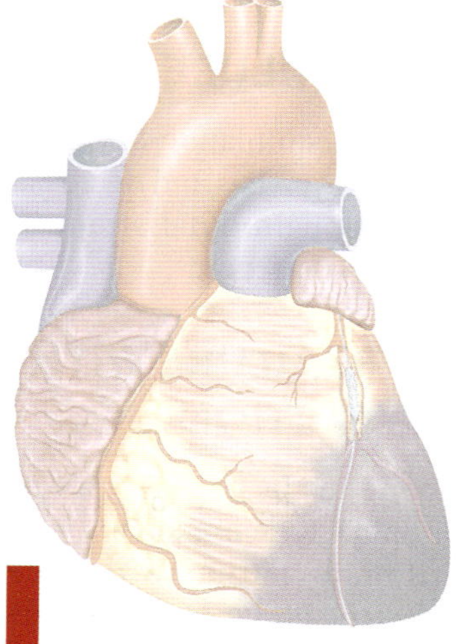

Finerenone in HFpEF with Chronic Kidney Disease: Hope or Hype

Himanshu Verma, Pallavi Prasad

INTRODUCTION

Mineralocorticoid receptors (MRs) are intracellular steroid hormone receptors present in epithelial and nonepithelial cells. Although first described in the kidney and colon for regulation of sodium and water content, they are also present in the cardiovascular (CV) system.

HEART FAILURE WITH PRESERVED EJECTION FRACTION

Heart failure with preserved ejection fraction (HFpEF) is a functional abnormality of the heart associated with decreased compliance of the left ventricle and decreased diastolic relaxation. It accounts for >50% of heart failure (HF) patients worldwide.[1] It is presumed to occur due to risk factors such as hypertension, diabetes mellitus, obesity, and chronic kidney disease, causing MR activation, inflammation, and endothelial dysfunction.

Mineralocorticoid receptor stimulation leads to downstream activation of multiple pathways causing inflammation and fibrosis via plasminogen activator inhibitor, transforming growth factor beta, interleukin-6, monocyte chemoattractant protein 1, and release of reactive oxygen species via NADP mediated pathway.[2] These pathways promote fibrogenesis and inflammation both in the heart and the kidneys. In the myocardium, it can cause left ventricular (LV) stiffness, decreased relaxation, and hence HFpEF.

Heart Failure with Preserved Ejection Fraction in Chronic Kidney Disease

Chronic kidney disease (CKD) itself is a risk factor for HFpEF since it is a state of chronic inflammation associated with hypertension and impaired natriuresis. Increased production of FGF-23 and acidosis also contribute to the profibrotic signals worsening HFpEF. MR overactivation is a known risk factor for the progression of both renal and cardiac disease. Between 26 and 50% of patients of HFpEF have low estimated glomerular filtration rate (eGFR) and can be classified as CKD.[2]

STEROIDAL VERSUS NONSTEROIDAL MINERALOCORTICOID RECEPTOR ANTAGONISTS

Steroidal MRA is now the first-line therapy in heart failure with reduced ejection fraction (HFrEF). The two steroidal MRA spironolactone and eplerenone have a similar binding mode to the MR and function as partial agonists. Spironolactone has a high affinity but low selectivity for MR with a plasma half-life of >20 hours. Eplerenone has a lower MR affinity but higher selectivity with a half-life of 4–6 hours.[3] Despite the differing characteristics, sex steroid-related side effects are seen with both agents and can lead to gynecomastia, breast pain, impotence, and menstrual irregularities.[4] Dose-dependent hyperkalemia is another major limiting factor for the use of MRA in HF, especially in CKD.

Nonsteroidal MRA was developed to overcome the inherent properties of MRA. There are three nonsteroidal MRA in various phases of clinical studies: Finerenone, esaxerenone, and balcinrenone.[4] They have greater potency, higher selectivity, and reduced risk of hyperkalemia compared to steroidal MRA. They have a bulky structure and function as inverse agonists or partial antagonists as compared to steroidal MRA. Amongst these agents, finerenone is one of the most studied drugs—it has a short half-life, with high MR selectivity and affinity along with low risk of hyperkalemia and sex steroid-related adverse effects.[4]

ROLE OF MINERALOCORTICOID RECEPTOR ANTAGONIST IN HEART FAILURE

Mineralocorticoid receptor antagonists have long been used in heart HFrEF. Landmark trials such as RALES,[5] EMPHASIS-HF,[6] and EPHESUS[7] have demonstrated the benefit of steroidal MRA in HFrEF (decreased mortality and hospitalization for HF). However, the use of MRA in HFpEF or HFmrEF has not been clearly established.

The TOPCAT study[8] was a double-blind randomized controlled study that enrolled 3,445 patients with HFpEF. Study subjects were randomized to spironolactone versus placebo. There was no difference in the primary outcome (composite of death from CV causes, aborted cardiac arrest, or hospitalization for HF) or death from CV causes at 3.3 years. However, there was a lower risk of hospitalization for HF in patients in the spironolactone arm (HR = 0.83, p = 0.04). Post hoc analysis of TOPCAT[9] demonstrated that in those in the Americas (who had better compliance as evidenced by drug levels), there was a significant benefit of using spironolactone vs. placebo in the primary outcome.

The Aldo-DHF study[10] randomized 422 patients with HFpEF to spironolactone versus placebo. Spironolactone was seen to improve the E/e' ratio and reduce LV mass index without any effect on patient symptoms, exercise capacity, or quality of life.

The BARACK-D randomized stage 3b CKD patients to spironolactone versus placebo, 24.3% of whom had diabetes, 17.4% had ischemic heart disease, and 2.3% had HF. There was no difference in the primary endpoint (composite of hospitalization for or new onset heart disease, HF, stroke, transient ischemic attack (TIA), or peripheral arterial disease). 67% of patients randomized to spironolactone had treatment withdrawn due to side effects including the drop in eGFR and hyperkalemia.[11]

PRECLINICAL STUDIES OF FINERENONE IN HEART FAILURE

Finerenone is seen to reduce the accumulation of CD68-positive macrophages in the cardiomyocytes and decrease cardiac hypertrophy and global longitudinal strain in various animal models of cardiac dysfunction.[3]

FINERENONE IN HEART FAILURE WITH REDUCED EJECTION FRACTION

In a phase II study of finerenone in HF, finerenone was compared to placebo and spironolactone in patients with HFrEF and CKD. It decreased brain natriuretic peptide (BNP) levels and albuminuria to a similar extent versus spironolactone but with smaller mean rise in potassium levels and lower incidence of hyperkalemia (5.3 and 12.7%, respectively, p = 0.048).[12]

The ARTS-HF study[13] compared different doses of finerenone to eplerenone in patients with either type 2 diabetes mellitus (T2DM) or CKD with left ventricular ejection fraction (LVEF) <40% and worsening HF requiring hospitalization. The primary outcome was efficacy [percentage responders defined as >30% decrease in N-terminal pro-brain natriuretic peptide (NT-proBNP)]. Finerenone was seen to decrease NT-proBNP to a similar extent compared to eplerenone. Additionally, the finerenone 10–20 mg arm was seen to decrease a composite end point of death from any cause, CV hospitalizations, or emergency presentation for worsening HF until day 90 [HR = 0.56, confidence interval (CI): 0.35–0.90, p = 0.02). Hyperkalemia incidence was comparable between the two groups.

FINERENONE IN DIABETIC KIDNEY DISEASE

Finerenone has been extensively studied in diabetic kidney disease.

The FIGARO DKD[14] randomized 7,437 diabetic patients with moderate albuminuria or decreased GFR to finerenone (maximum 20 mg) or placebo. The primary outcome was a composite of CV death, nonfatal myocardial infarction (MI), nonfatal stroke, or hospitalization for HF. During a median follow-up of 3.4 years, a primary outcome event occurred in 12.4% of the finerenone group versus 14.2% in the placebo group (HR = 0.87, CI = 0.76–0.98, p = 0.03). Importantly, this benefit was mainly driven by a lower incidence of hospitalization for HF events (HR = 0.71, CI = 0.56–0.90). The percentage of patients with HFpEF was not known but the cohort had risk factors for

HFpEF including T2DM and CKD in all patients, HT (96% of patients), and obesity (mean BMI: 31.4 kg/m^2). 45.3% of patients had a history of CV disease and 7.8% had a history of HF overall.

The incidence of hyperkalemia was higher with finerenone (10.8%) versus 5.8% with placebo but only 1.2% in the finerenone arm required discontinuation. Also, the mean between-group differences in serum potassium level was 0.16 mmol/L at month 1 and remained stable throughout the trial.

The FIDELIO DKD trial[15] analyzed the efficacy of finerenone on kidney composite outcome (a sustained decrease of at least 40% in the eGFR from baseline, or death from renal causes) in T2DM with CKD with a key CV endpoint (death from CV causes, nonfatal MI, nonfatal stroke, or hospitalization for HF) as a secondary outcome. It enrolled 5,734 patients with either urine albumin creatinine ratio >300 mg or eGFR between 25 and 60 mL/min/1.73 m^2. Both the primary outcome and key secondary CV outcome were significantly lower in patients in the finerenone arm. In the subgroup analysis, though not adequately powered, patients without CV disease at baseline were not seen to have significant benefits versus those with prior CV disease.

FINEARTS HF:[16] This recently published trial is the only dedicated trial of finerenone in HFpEF. The trial recruited 6,016 patients over 37 countries. The trial was designed to analyze the effect of finerenone (10 mg, 20 mg, and 40 mg; maximum dose 20 mg if eGFR <60 mL/min/1.73 m^2) in patients with HF with EF >40% and evidence of structural heart disease and diuretic requirement in 30 days before enrollment. All patients were required to have elevated BNP or NTpro-BNP levels. This included patients at any level of care (hospitalized, recently hospitalized, or ambulatory). Patients with eGFR <25 mL/min/1.73 m^2 or serum potassium >5 mEq/L were excluded from the trial. The primary outcome was a composite of CV death and total HF events. A total of 2,375 primary outcome events were targeted for trial completion. Over a follow of 32 months, the number of primary outcome events was significantly lower in the finerenone arm when compared to placebo (1,083 vs. 1,283 events, rate ratio = 0.84, CI = 0.71–0.94, p = 0.007). This was consistent across all prespecified subgroup analyses (including EF less than or >60%, sodium-glucose cotransporter-2 inhibitor (SGLT2i) use or not, eGFR < or >60 mL/min/1.73 m^2).

Secondary outcome included the number of worsening HF events, which was also significantly lower in the finerenone arm (rate ratio = 0.82, CI = 0.71–0.94) but death from CV causes was comparable between the two groups (HR = 0.93, CI = 0.78–1.11). Kidney composite outcome (sustained decrease in eGFR >50%, eGFR <15 mL/min/1.73 m^2, or initiation of renal replacement therapy) was comparable between the two groups (HR = 1.33, CI = 0.94–1.89). Although the number of hyperkalemia events (K >5.5 meq/l) was more frequent in the finerenone arm (14.3% vs. 6.9%), hyperkalemia leading to hospitalization was rare (0.5%).

The FINE-HEART pooled analysis[17] was a prespecified analysis of three trials FIDELIO-DKD, FIGARO-DKD, and FINEARTS-HF. The three trials included 18,991 patients. At a follow-up of 2.9 years, the primary outcome of CV death was lower in the finerenone arm although it did not reach statistical significance (4.4% vs. 5.0%, HR = 0.89, CI = 0.78–1.01). Death from any cause (HR = 0.91, CI = 0.84–0.99), risk of HF hospitalization (HR = 0.83, CI = 0.75–0.92), and composite kidney outcome (HR = 0.80, CI = 0.72–0.90) was significantly lower in the finerenone arm vs. placebo. **Figure 1** outlines HF outcomes in various trials of finerenone.

UPCOMING STUDIES OF FINERENONE IN HEART FAILURE WITH PRESERVED EJECTION FRACTION

- *REDEFINE HF:* It is an ongoing study in which patients with eGFR >25 mL/min/1.73 m^2 with HFpEF (EF >40%) will be randomized to finerenone and placebo. This study will include patients hospitalized with acute decompensated HF or recently discharged after the same.
- *CONFIRMATION-HF:* It is another ongoing trial to analyze the efficacy of combination therapy of finerenone and empagliflozin over standard of care in patients of acute HF, irrespective of ejection fraction.

LIMITATIONS

- Trials have not assessed the effect of combination therapy of SGLT2i and nonsteroidal MRA in HFpEF and in CKD.
- There are no head-to-head trials of steroidal MRA versus nonsteroidal MRA in HFpEF and CKD are needed.

GUIDELINES

The American Heart Association (AHA)/American College of Cardiology (ACC)/Heart Failure Society of America (HFSA) guidelines suggest that in patients with HFpEF, MRAs may be considered to decrease hospitalizations, particularly amongst patients with LVEF on the lower end of the spectrum (Class 2b).

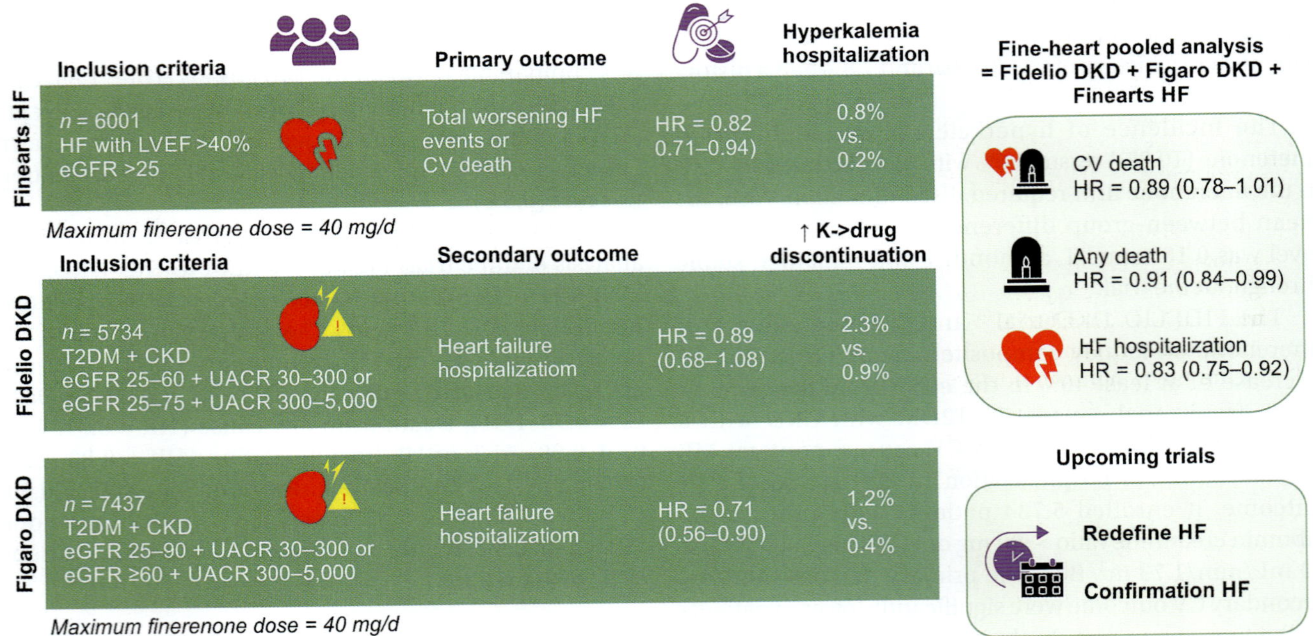

Fig. 1: Heart failure outcomes in trials of finerenone.
(CV: cardiovascular; eGFR: estimated glomerular filtration rate; HF: heart failure; LVEF: left ventricular ejection fraction; MI: myocardial infarction; UACR: urine albumin-creatinine ratio)
↑K = hyperkalemia

Kidney Disease: Improving Global Outcomes (KDIGO) 2022 Clinical Practice Guidelines for Diabetes Management suggest a nonsteroidal MR antagonist with proven kidney or CV benefit for patients with T2D, an eGFR ≥25 mL/min/1.73 m^2, normal serum potassium concentration, and albuminuria (>30 mg/g) despite a maximum tolerated dose of renin-angiotensin system inhibitor (RASi) (Class 2A).

CONCLUSION

Recent trials demonstrate the benefit of finerenone in patients with T2DM with CKD and in HFpEF. The use of finerenone in a patient having both CKD and HFpEF needs to be individualized. Although finerenone has less frequent side effects compared to steroidal MRA, close monitoring of serum potassium should be done at the time of dose initiation or change in patients on finerenone. With SGLT2i becoming the standard of care both in CKD and HF, the role of finerenone in combination with SGLT2i needs to be studied further.

REFERENCES

1. Gronewegen A, Rutten FH, Mosterd A, et al. Epidemiology of heart failure. Eur J Heart Failure. 2020;22(8):1342-56.
2. Patel RN, Sharma A, Prasad A, et al. Heart Failure With Preserved Ejection Fraction With CKD: A Narrative Review of a Multispecialty Disorder. Kidney Med. 2023;5(12):100705.
3. Kintscher U, Edelmann F. The non-steroidal mineralocorticoid receptor antagonist finerenone and heart failure with preserved ejection fraction. Cardiovasc Diabetol. 2023;22(1):162.
4. Chang J, Ambrosy AP, Vardeny O, et al. Mineralocorticoid Antagonism in Heart Failure: Established and Emerging Therapeutic Role. JACC Heart Fail. 2024;12(12):1979-93.
5. Pitt B, Zannad F, Remme WJ, et al. The effect of spironolactone on morbidity and mortality in patients with severe heart failure. Randomized Aldactone Evaluation Study Investigators. N Engl J Med. 1999;341(10):709-17.
6. Zannad F, McMurray JJ, Krum H, et al for EMPHASIS-HF Study Group. Eplerenone in patients with systolic heart failure and mild symptoms. N Engl J Med. 2011;364(1):11-21.
7. Pitt B, Remme W, Zannad F, et al. Eplerenone, a selective aldosterone blocker, in patients with left ventricular dysfunction after myocardial infarction. N Engl J Med. 2003;348(14):1309-21.
8. Pitt B, Pfeffer MA, Assmann SF, et al. Spironolactone for heart failure with preserved ejection fraction. N Engl J Med. 2014;370(15):1383-92.
9. Pfeffer MA, Claggett B, Assmann SF, et al. Regional variation in patients and outcomes in the Treatment of Preserved

Cardiac Function Heart Failure With an Aldosterone Antagonist (TOPCAT) trial. Circulation. 2015;131(1): 34-42.

10. Edelmann F, Wachter R, Schmidt AG, et al. Effect of spironolactone on diastolic function and exercise capacity in patients with heart failure with preserved ejection fraction: the Aldo-DHF randomized controlled trial. JAMA. 2013;309(8):781-91.
11. Hobbs FDR, McManus RJ, Taylor CJ, et al. Low-dose spironolactone and cardiovascular outcomes in moderate stage chronic kidney disease: a randomized controlled trial. Nat Med. 2024;30(12):3634-45.
12. Pitt B, Kober L, Ponikowski P, et al. Safety and tolerability of the novel non-steroidal mineralocorticoid receptor antagonist BAY 94-8862 in patients with chronic heart failure and mild or moderate chronic kidney disease: a randomized, double-blind trial. Eur Heart J. 2013;34(31):2453-63.
13. Filippatos G, Anker SD, Böhm M, et al. A randomized controlled study of finerenone vs. eplerenone in patients with worsening chronic heart failure and diabetes mellitus and/or chronic kidney disease. Eur Heart J. 2016;37(27): 2105-14.
14. Filippatos G, Anker SD, Agarwal R, et al. Finerenone Reduces Risk of Incident Heart Failure in Patients With Chronic Kidney Disease and Type 2 Diabetes: Analyses From the FIGARO-DKD Trial. Circulation. 2022;145(6): 437-47.
15. Bakris GL, Agarwal R, Anker SD, et al. Effect of Finerenone on Chronic Kidney Disease Outcomes in Type 2 Diabetes. N Engl J Med. 2020;383(23):2219-29.
16. Solomon SD, McMurray JJV, Vaduganathan M, et al. Finerenone in heart failure with mildly reduced or preserved ejection fraction. N Engl J Med. 2024;391(16): 1475-85.
17. Vaduganathan M, Filippatos G, Claggett BL, et al. Finerenone in Heart Failure and Chronic Kidney Disease with Type 2 Diabetes: the FINE-HEART pooled analysis of cardiovascular, kidney and mortality outcomes. Nat Med. 2024;30(12):3758-64.

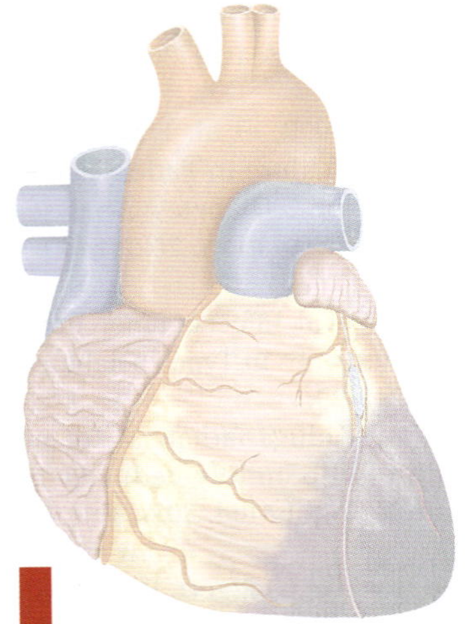

Heart Support Devices in HFpEF

Atul Kaushik, Manbir Singh, Vivudh Pratap Singh

INTRODUCTION

Heart failure (HF) is a complex clinical syndrome with symptoms and signs resulting from any structural or functional impairment of ventricular filling or ejection of blood.[1] It is one of the leading causes of death worldwide.[2] Traditionally, HF has two main types: (1) Heart failure with reduced ejection fraction (HFrEF) with LVEF ≤40% and (2) heart failure with preserved ejection fraction (HFpEF) with LVEF ≥50%. The AHA guidelines have enlisted third type of heart failure with LVEF between ≥40% and 49% called heart failure with mildly reduced ejection fraction (HFmEF).[1] Patients with HFmEF have similar risk of developing atrial fibrillation and diabetes mellitus as the patients with HFpEF, which is higher than patients with HFrEF.[3-5] It has become the dominant type of HF phenotype and accounts for approximately 50% of all cases of HF.[6] The reduction in quality of life (QoL), functional limitation, and overall survival of HFpEF patients are similar to those of HFrEF.[3-6] Hypertension and obesity are major risk factors for HF as they induce proinflammatory state leading to cardiac remodeling and left ventricular (LV) hypertrophy.[7-8] Progressive decrease in left atrial (LA) compliance and LV relaxation causes higher LA pressure and pulmonary capillary wedge pressure (PCWP), especially while exercising.[6-8]

Despite significant increase in understanding of the disease pathophysiology, pharmacological treatments are still not as effective. Atrial shunts, LV expanders, electrical and neurostimulators, and mechanical circulatory support (MCS) devices constitute the four main categories of device-based solutions for the treatment of HFpEF.[7,8]

ATRIAL SHUNT DEVICES

Atrial shunt devices are designed to lower LA pressure by creating a conduit between left atrium and other chambers of heart. Though most of the devices are based on interatrial shunting, new approaches have now emerged to shunt blood from LA to coronary sinus to overcome risks of atrial arrhythmia and paradoxical embolism with interatrial shunt devices (IASDs). These devices have been evaluated in large clinical trials and hold promise for improving symptoms of exercise capacity, pulmonary congestion, and QoL for patients with HFpEF. Patients with elevated PCWP at rest or exercise, a positive left atrium to right atrium pressure gradient, and a history of exercise intolerance are required as inclusion by most of these trials. These devices are also not suitable for patients with right ventricular (RV) dysfunction, valvular defects, or severe restrictive or obstructive lung disease as atrial shunting imposes extra stress on the right heart and significantly affects cardiac and pulmonary hemodynamics. All IASDs can be inserted percutaneously via femoral access under general anesthesia and transesophageal echocardiography guidance, and trans-septal puncture is performed in the middle of interatrial septum.

Interatrial Shunt Device

The IASD (IASD II, Corvia Medical Inc., Tewksbury, MA) is a bare metal nitinol self-expanding frame with an outer diameter of 19 mm, which can create an 8 mm shunt. Patients who have the IASD implanted are treated with lifelong aspirin and short-term (usually 3–6 months) clopidogrel.[9] The feasibility of the IASD was first reported in a pilot trial involving 11 patients (LVEF >45%, PWCP ≥15 mm Hg at rest, or PWCP ≥25 mm Hg during exercise), with one or more hospitalizations for HF within the 12 months before the beginning of the study or persistent NYHA functional class III/IV for at least 3 months.[10] The device was successfully implanted in all patients and showed promising hemodynamic and functional results on 30-day follow-up, including a reduction in LV filling pressure ($p = 0.005$), associated NYHA functional class of HF, and QoL improvements in most of the patients.[10] These findings were corroborated with a 1-year follow-up study conducted on 64 patients, which showed stable reduction in the LV end-diastolic volume ($p < 0.001$) and work-indexed PWCP ($p < 0.01$), alongside sustained improvements in NYHA functional class ($p < 0.001$), QoL ($p < 0.001$), and 6-minute-walking distance ($p < 0.01$). A pooled analysis from 2 trials[10,11] showed that implantation of an IASD in patients with LVEF ≥40% is associated with significant improvements in pulmonary vascular function, with increased pulmonary flow and pulmonary artery compliance during both rest and exercise.

V-Wave Device

The V-wave, Caesarea, Israel, is an hourglass-shaped nitinol self-expanding prosthesis covered with a polytetrafluoroethylene polymer on the left side and a trileaflet porcine pericardium valve on the right side to prevent right-to-left flow and paradoxical embolism and early closure. After implantation, the patient receives anticoagulation with warfarin for 3 months, and aspirin (81–100 mg/day) is administered indefinitely[12,13] This device underwent a prospective multicenter-single-arm open-label trial[14] in which 8 HFpEF patients and 30 HFrEF patients were enrolled and implanted with a V-wave shunt device. 5 of 36 case patients (14%) had total occlusions and 13 (36%) had shunt restenosis due to pannus formation 1 year after device insertion. The device improved NYHA functional class (class I and II in 60% of the patients; $p < 0.001$), QoL (improvements ≥5 points in 73% of the patients; $p < 0.001$), and 6-minute-walking distance (mean increase 28 ± 83 m; $p = 0.012$), whereas no significant changes were observed in laboratory parameters, echocardiographic variables, or hemodynamic status. In the RELIEVE-HR trial,[15] 97 patients with Ventura shunt were followed up for 12 months for safety, effectiveness, and TEE outcomes. They found that KCCQ's overall summary score was improved by 12–16 points at all follow-up time points (all $p < 0.004$), with similar outcomes in patients with reduced and preserved LVEF. At 12 months, LV end-systolic and end-diastolic volumes were reduced ($p = 0.020$ and $p = 0.038$, respectively), LVEF improved ($p = 0.009$), RV end-systolic and end-diastolic areas were reduced ($p = 0.001$ and $p = 0.030$, respectively), RV fractional area changed ($p < 0.001$), and tricuspid annular plane systolic excursion ($p < 0.001$) improved.

Atrial Flow Regulator

The atrial flow regulator (AFR) (Occlutech, Istanbul, Turkey) is a nitinol self-expandable double-disk wired device. The opening can have various diameters (6, 8, and 10 mm) and is designed to allow interatrial bidirectional flow mesh with a central penetration that enables interatrial bidirectional flow.[16] Antiplatelets were usually given to the patients after implantation of an AFR.[17-20] Results from the PRELIEVE [Pilot Study to Assess Safety and Efficacy of a Novel Atrial Flow Regulator (AFR) in Heart Failure Patients] trial[18], which evaluated device safety and feasibility in patients with both HFrEF and HFpEF, confirmed device patency in 92% of the cases at both 3 and 12 months, as well as a 5 mm Hg drop in PCWP ($p = 0.0003$) during rest at the 3-month follow-up.[19] Improvements in PCWP were more significant in the HFpEF cohort than in the HFrEF cohort. However, changes in NYHA functional class, 6-minute-walking distance, and QoL lacked significance, and 2 major adverse events were reported, namely device embolization and postprocedural bleeding and syncope.

TRANSCATHETER ATRIAL SHUNT SYSTEM

To overcome some of the risks associated with interatrial shunts, including right-to-left shunting and systemic embolization, a novel approach was developed to reduce the PWCP through a shunt from the left atrium to the coronary sinus.[21] The transcatheter atrial shunt system (Edwards Lifesciences) is a bare-nitinol implant with 4 arms and an internal shunting diameter of 7 mm. The device is deployed between the left atrium and the coronary sinus through a percutaneous atriotomy, a procedure involving coronary sinus cannulation from the right internal jugular vein and coronary sinus-to-LA puncture under coronary sinus angiography and balloon dilation of the LA wall.[21] The first study of this device was conducted on 11 patients (7 with HFpEF and 4 with HFrEF) with a median of 1 HF hospital admission in the year before implantation, NYHA functional class III or ambulatory class IV, and elevated PWCP. Of the 8 patients who underwent successful implantation, 87.5% improved their NYHA functional class to I or II, 42.9% experienced clinically significant improvements in the 6-minute-walking distance (>32 m), and PCWP was reduced by 9 mm Hg at a median follow-up of 100 days. In addition, follow-up echocardiography exhibited stable LVEF, LA volume index, and RV function, whereas patency of all devices was confirmed by computed tomographic assessment.[21]

LEFT VENTRICULAR EXPANDERS

The LV expanders are spring-like devices that apply outward forces to the left ventricle to enhance filling performance, which is typically diminished in HFpEF. By storing elastic energy during cardiac contraction and transferring it to the LV wall in the diastolic phase, these devices seek to assist in early diastolic recoil of the LV chamber.[22,23]

- *Imcardia* is an elastic self-expanding device made of biocompatible Conichrome FWM 1058 to be implanted on the epicardial surface of the heart. It is made of series of springs, with free lengths ranging from 35 to 46 mm, which are connected to attachment elements and screwed into the epicardium of LV free wall 17–28 mm apart.[24] In an open-label, parallel, nonrandomized clinical trial in 19 patients with HFpEF, the safety and functionality of Imcardia were evaluated. All patients in the device group were shown to maintain systolic function, and improvements in LV mass (38% vs. 21% decrease; $p = 0.08$) and LA area (17% decrease vs 7% increase; $p = 0.02$) were observed relative to control.[25]
- *CORolla assist device* is an elastic self-expanding device that is attached to endocardium and enhances LV diastolic expansion, improves LV filling, and lowers LV end-diastolic pressure and LAP. The patients showed a significant improvement in LV mass, LA-indexed volume, and consistent LV remodeling at 6 months, which might suggest a certain efficacy and safety of device.[9]

ELECTRICAL THERAPY FOR HEART FAILURE WITH PRESERVED EJECTION FRACTION

- *Cardiac contractility modulation (CCM)* is a pacemaker-like therapy for HF that involves applying relatively high-voltage, long-duration, biphasic electric signals to the RV septum during the absolute myocardial refractory period.[26] CCM delivers non-excitatory electrical signals and improves the contraction of the heart. Various studies have demonstrated the benefit of CCM on QoL and exercise tolerance for HFpEF patients.[27,28]
- *LA permanent pacing:* Atrial electrical dyssynchrony following reduced LA function has become an essential target of treatment of HFpEF patients. Laurent et al.[29] conducted a study on six patients with HFpEF and evaluated the difference between the active coronary sinus pacing group and the inactive pacing group. After 3 months, the active pacing group showed significant improvement in their 6-minute walk (190 ± 15 m to 240 ± 25 m, $p < 0.05$), mitral A-wave duration (104 ± 8 to 158 ± 25 ms, $p = 0.002$), and E/A and E/e′ ratio (3.4 ± 1.3 to 1.8 ± 0.9, $p = 0.009$ and 22.6 ± 4.6 to 15.3 ± 4.3, $p = 0.006$, respectively). After 1 week of pacing inactivation, a significant decrease of the 6-minute walk was observed with an on/off response.
- *Baroreceptor activation therapy (BAT)* is an electrical technology that stimulates the carotid sinuses with an implanted pacemaker-like device. Funakosi et al.[30] reported that baroreflex failure might be an important pathogenesis of acute HF, especially in HFpEF models using arterial baroreflex failure models in rats. The largest clinical study of BAROSTIM NEO, an international, randomized, open-label study by Abraham et al.,[31] compared two groups of HFrEF patients: One with 70 patients with BAT and the other with 76 patients without BAT. The results showed that the major adverse event-free rate of BAT was 97.2%, and there were improvements in 6-minute-walk (59.6 ± 14 m vs. 1.5 ± 13.2 m, $p = 0.004$), New York Heart Association class ranking ($p = 0.002$), and QoL score ($p < 0.001$) in the BAT group.

LEFT VENTRICULAR ASSIST DEVICE

The left ventricular assist device (LVAD) is a standard and essential option for end-stage HF patients with dilated or ischemic cardiomyopathy and has been demonstrated to improve morbidity and mortality in HFrEF patients. There are limited reports of LVAD being implanted in HFpEF patients because of the typical feature of a remarkably small LV.[32,33]

- *Heart mate II:* Eight patients with advanced RCM or HCM underwent implantation with a continuous-flow axial LVAD (Heart-Mate II, Abbott, Abbott Park, IL) and were compared with 75 patients with dilated or ischemic cardiomyopathy. Because the inflow cannula of the LVAD needed to be placed at the LV apex to drain blood from the LV, they performed an additional LV myectomy as needed to create enough space in the LV for the inflow cannula. The 1-year survival rate of patients with RCM or HCM was no different from that of patients with dilated or ischemic cardiomyopathy.

Notably, this report mentioned the "suck-down event of the LA", which was observed in one patient among the eight.[32]

- *HVAD:* Muthiah et al.[33] reported outcomes of HCM patients implanted with a centrifugal continuous-flow LVAD (HeartWare HVAD, Medtronic, Minneapolis, MN).

Three HCM patients underwent the HVAD implantation; they were compared with 36 dilated cardiomyopathy patients who received the HVAD. In both groups, an improvement in the mean pulmonary arterial and right atrial pressures was observed. In that study, although myomectomy was not performed in any HCM patients, they did not have suction events. One patient experienced inlet obstruction with an intraventricular clot and died after the antiplatelet therapy was modified due to a transient ischemic attack a week before.[33]

CONCLUSION

The Synergy system (Medtronic, Minneapolis, MN) is a micropump-based form of circulatory support in which pump inflow is derived from the left atrium, implanted through a right, mini thoracotomy procedure without a sternotomy or cardiopulmonary bypass. The outflow graft is attached to the subclavian artery. The body of the micropump is then placed in a subcutaneous pacemaker-like pocket. Burkhoff et al.[34] analyzed the hemodynamic effects of the synergy system in HFpEF patients in the same way as HFrEF patients and suggested that this system may also provide a viable option for end-stage HFpEF patients by reducing LA pressure and decompressing the LA and pulmonary circulation while improving systemic blood flow, as is observed in HFrEF patients.

REFERENCES

1. Heidenreich PA, Bozkurt B, Aguilar D, et al. 2022 AHA/ACC/HFSA Guideline for the Management of Heart Failure: A Report of the American College of Cardiology/American Heart Association Joint Committee on Clinical Practice Guidelines. Circulation. 2022;145(18):e895-1032.
2. World Health Organization. (2021). Cardiovascular Diseases. [online] Available from https://www.who.int/news-room/fact-sheets/detail/cardiovascular-diseases-(cvds) [Last accessed January, 2025].
3. Ponikowski P, Voors AA, Anker SD, et al. 2016 ESC Guidelines for the diagnosis and treatment of acute and chronic heart failure: The Task Force for the diagnosis and treatment of acute and chronic heart failure of the European Society of Cardiology (ESC). Developed with the special contribution of the Heart Failure Association (HFA) of the ESC. Eur Heart J. 2016;37(27):2129-200.
4. Albakri A. Heart failure with mid-range ejection fraction: a review of clinical status and meta-analysis of clinical management methods. Trends Res. 2018;1(4).
5. Owan TE, Hodge DO, Herges RM, et al. Trends in prevalence and outcome of heart failure with preserved ejection fraction. N Engl J Med. 2006;355(3):251-9.
6. Oktay AA, Rich JD, Shah SJ. The emerging epidemic of heart failure with preserved ejection fraction. Curr Heart Fail Rep. 2013;10(4):401-10.
7. Borlaug BA. Evaluation and management of heart failure with preserved ejection fraction. Nat Rev Cardiol. 2020;17(9):559-73.
8. Paulus WJ, Tschöpe C. A novel paradigm for heart failure with preserved ejection fraction: Comorbidities drive myocardial dysfunction and remodeling through coronary microvascular endothelial inflammation. J Am Coll Cardiol. 2013;62(4):263-71.
9. Burlacu A, Simion P, Nistor I, et al. Novel percutaneous interventional therapies in heart failure with preserved ejection fraction: An integrative review. Heart Fail Rev. 2019;24(5):793-803.
10. ClinicalTrials.gov. (2020). Feasibility Trial of the DC Devices Interatrial Septal Device (IASD) System. [online] Available from https://clinicaltrials.gov/study/NCT01570517 [Last accessed January, 2025].
11. ClinicalTrials.gov. (2020). REDUCE LAP-HF TRIAL (REDUCE LAP-HF [online] Available from https://clinicaltrials.gov/ct2/show/ NCT01913613 [Last accessed January, 2025].
12. Amat-Santos IJ, Nombela-Franco L, García B, et al. The V-Wave Device for the treatment of heart failure. Initial experience in Europe. Rev Esp Cardiol (Engl Ed). 2015;68(9):808-10.
13. Amat-Santos IJ, Bergeron S, Bernier M, et al. Left atrial decompression through unidirectional left-to-right interatrial shunt for the treatment of left heart failure: First-in-man experience with the V-Wave device. EuroIntervention. 2015;10(9):1127-31.
14. Rodés-Cabau J, Bernier M, Amat-Santos IJ, et al. Interatrial shunting for heart failure: Early and late results from the first-in-human experience with the V-Wave System. JACC Cardiovasc Interv. 2018;11(22):2300-10.
15. Rodés-Cabau J, Lindenfeld J, Abraham WT, et al. Interatrial shunt therapy in advanced heart failure: Outcomes from the open-label cohort of the RELIEVE-HF trial. Eur J Heart Fail. 2024;26(4):1078-89.
16. Patel MB, Samuel BP, Girgis RE, et al. Implantable atrial flow regulator for severe, irreversible pulmonary arterial hypertension. EuroIntervention. 2015;11(6):706-9.
17. Rajeshkumar R, Pavithran S, Sivakumar K, et al. Atrial septostomy with a predefined diameter using a novel Occlutech atrial flow regulator improves symptoms and cardiac index in patients with severe pulmonary arterial hypertension. Catheter Cardiovasc Interv. 2017;90(7):1145-53.
18. ClinicalTrials.gov. (2022). The Prelieve Trial-Pilot Study to Assess Safety and Efficacy of a Novel Atrial Flow

Regulator (AFR) in Heart Failure Patients (PRELIEVE). [online] Available from https://clinicaltrials.gov/study/NCT03030274?intr=Prelieve%20Trial&rank=1[Last accessed January, 2025].
19. Paitazoglou C, Bergmann MW, Özdemir R, et al. One-year results of the first-in-man study investigating the Atrial-Flow-Regulator for left atrial shunting in symptomatic heart failure patients: The PRELIEVE study. Eur J Heart Fail. 2021;23(5):800-10.
20. ClinicalTrials.gov. (2018). Flow Regulation by Opening the Septum in Patients With Heart Failure Trial (FROST-HF). [online] Available from https://clinicaltrials.gov/ct2/show/NCT03751748 [Last accessed January, 2025].
21. Simard T, Labinaz M, Zahr F, et al. Percutaneous atriotomy for levoatrial-to-coronary sinus shunting in symptomatic heart failure: First-in-human experience. JACC Cardiovasc Interv. 2020;13(10):1236-47.
22. Feld Y, Dubi S, Reisner Y, et al. Future strategies for the treatment of diastolic heart failure. Acute Cardiac Care. 2006;8(1):13-20.
23. Nussinovitch U, Topaz G, Landesberg A, et al. Novel treatments for diastolic heart failure. In: Emerging Technologies for Heart Diseases. Amsterdam: Elsevier; 2020. pp. 95-127.
24. ClinicalTrials.gov. (2011). ImCardiaTM for DHF to Treat Diastolic Heart Failure (DHF) Patient a Pilot Study (ImCardia). [online] Available from https://clinicaltrials.gov/ct2/show/ NCT01347125 [Last accessed January, 2025].
25. Feld Y, Reisner Y, Meyer-Brodnitz G, et al. The CORolla device for energy transfer from systole to diastole: A novel treatment for heart failure with preserved ejection fraction. Heart Fail Rev. 2023;28(2):307-14.
26. Borggrefe M, Mann DL. Cardiac contractility modulation in 2018. Circulation. 2018;138(24):2738-40.
27. Kadish A, Nademanee K, Volosin K, et al. A randomized controlled trial evaluating the safety and efficacy of cardiac contractility modulation in advanced heart failure. Am Heart J. 2011;161(2):329-37.e1-2.
28. Abraham WT, Kuck KH, Goldsmith RL, et al. A randomized controlled trial to evaluate the safety and efficacy of cardiac contractility modulation. JACC Heart Fail. 2018;6(10):874-83.
29. Laurent G, Eicher JC, Mathe A, et al. Permanent left atrial pacing therapy may improve symptoms in heart failure patients with preserved ejection fraction and atrial dyssynchrony: A pilot study prior to a national clinical research programme. Eur J Heart Fail. 2013;15(1):85-93.
30. Funakoshi K, Hosokawa K, Kishi T, et al. Striking volume intolerance is induced by mimicking arterial baroreflex failure in normal left ventricular function. J Card Fail. 2014;20(1):53-9.
31. Abraham WT, Zile MR, Weaver FA, et al. Baroreflex activation therapy for the treatment of heart failure with a reduced ejection fraction. JACC Heart Fail. 2015;3(6):487-96.
32. Topilsky Y, Pereira NL, Shah DK, et al. Left ventricular assist device therapy in patients with restrictive and hypertrophic cardiomyopathy. Circ Heart Fail. 2011;4(3):266-75.
33. Muthiah K, Phan J, Robson D, et al. Centrifugal continuous-flow left ventricular assist device in patients with hypertrophic cardiomyopathy: A case series. ASAIO J. 2013;59(2):183-7.
34. Burkhoff D, Maurer MS, Joseph SM, et al. Left atrial decompression pump for severe heart failure with preserved ejection fraction: Theoretical and clinical considerations. JACC Heart Fail. 2015;3(4):275-82.

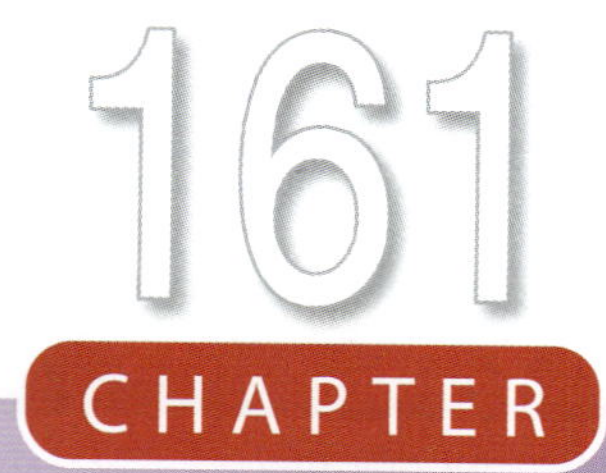

CHAPTER

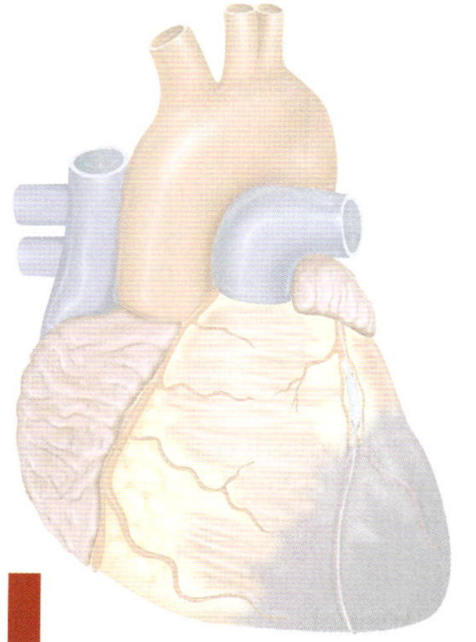

MitraClip in Heart Failure in Patients on Angiotensin Receptor Neprilysin Inhibitors: When and How?

Ramesh Daggubati, Abdul Subhan Talpur, Mustafa Sajjad Cheema

INTRODUCTION

Overview of Heart Failure: Defining the Disease and Its Clinical Burden

Heart failure (HF) is a widespread global health issue that impacts a minimum of 26 million individuals across the globe and is exhibiting an upward trend in terms of its prevalence. Healthcare expenditures in high-income countries are substantial and are projected to experience a significant surge due to the demographic shift toward an aging population. Despite the considerable progress made in the field of therapies and preventive measures, there remains a substantial burden of mortality and morbidity, accompanied by a diminished quality of life.[1]

Significance of Secondary Mitral Regurgitation in the Context of Heart Failure

Mitral regurgitation (MR) is the predominant valvular heart disease observed in individuals suffering from HF, with a prevalence of approximately one-third among those with chronic HF and approximately half among those with acute HF. Therefore, it has been identified as a therapeutic objective in patients with HF.[2] The most common etiology of MR in HF is tethering of leaflets causing posterior/centrally directed get due to cardiomyopathy related changes in subvalvular apparatus.[3]

Brief Glimpse of MitraClip and Angiotensin Receptor Neprilysin Inhibitors

The Transcatheter MitraClip edge-to-edge repair (TEER) uses the surgical Alfieri giving it a “double orifice” mitral valve appearance by closing the gap between leaflet tips.[3] The MitraClip system uses a cobalt chromium clip covered in polypropylene to grasp both the anterior and posterior mitral valve leaflets, reducing MR by increasing coaptation. Occasionally, a second clip may be needed to achieve a final regurgitant severity of ≤2+.[4] New cardiovascular agents called angiotensin receptor-neprilysin inhibitors (ARNIs) act on the renin-angiotensin system (RAS) and natriuretic peptide (NP) systems. Clinical trials have shown that sacubitril/valsartan, an ARNI, is a first-line treatment for HF, especially in patients with reduced ejection fraction.[5]

When to Perform MitraClip?

Multidisciplinary heart teams should evaluate and treat transcatheter mitral valve repair (TMVR) candidates, including cardiologists (general and interventional), cardiac surgeons, valve and HF specialists, imaging specialists, and cardiac anesthesiologists **(Boxes 1 to 3)**.[6]

Other Investigational Devices

Transcatheter mitral valve repair devices are in development, but the MitraClip is the only the Food and

BOX 1: General indications and echocardiographic criteria to perform Mitraclip.

General indications[7,8]

- Chronic moderate-to-severe or severe (3–4+) mitral regurgitation (MR)
- Severely symptomatic (New York Heart Association Class III or IV) heart failure despite medical therapy
- Favorable anatomy for the repair procedure
- Reasonable life expectancy (e.g., ≥2 years)
- Prohibitive surgical risk due to comorbidities

Echocardiographic criteria

(We use the following criteria for moderate-severe (3+) or severe (4+) MR as specified in the EVEREST II trial. At least three of the following criteria should be met).[9]

1. Color flow jet may be central and large (>6 cm^2 or >30% of left atrial area) or smaller if eccentric, encircling the left atrium
2. Pulmonary vein flow may show systolic blunting or systolic flow reversal
3. Vena contracta width ≥0.5 cm measured in the parasternal long axis view
4. Regurgitant volume of ≥45 mL/beat
5. Regurgitant fraction ≥40%
6. Regurgitant orifice area ≥0.30 cm^2

In order to evaluate the viability of transcatheter mitral valve replacement, it is necessary to examine various anatomical characteristics of the mitral valve, in addition to assessing its severity.

The anatomic criteria encompass the following:

7. Planimetered mitral valve area (in parasternal short axis view at tips of the mitral valve) ≥4.0 cm^2
8. Minimal leaflet calcification in the grasping area
9. If leaflet flail is present, width of the flail segment <15 mm and flail gap of <10 mm

BOX 2: Inclusion and exclusion criteria.

Inclusion criteria[10]

The primary regurgitant jet originates from malcoaptation of the A2 and P2 scallops of the mitral valve (MV)

Exclusion criteria[10]

- MV orifice area <4.0 cm^2
- Width of the flail segment ≥15 mm or flail gap ≥10 mm
- Coaptation depth >11 mm or vertical coaptation length is <2 mm
- Severe mitral annular calcification
- Evidence of calcification in the grasping area of the A2 and/or P2 scallops
- Presence of a significant cleft of A2 or P2 scallops
- Prior MV surgery or valvuloplasty
- Echocardiographic evidence of intracardiac mass, thrombus, or vegetation
- History of or active endocarditis or rheumatic heart diseases
- History of atrial septal defect or patent foramen ovale associated with clinical symptoms

BOX 3: Contraindications to MitraClip.

- Patients who cannot tolerate procedural anticoagulation or antiplatelet agents postprocedure
- Active endocarditis of the mitral valve
- Rheumatic mitral valve disease or other causes of mitral stenosis
- Thrombus of the femoral vein, inferior vena cava, or intracardiac thrombus

Drug Administration (FDA)-approved one. Multiple mechanisms power experimental mitral valve repair devices.[9,11]

- To reduce the severity of MR, alter the mitral valve annulus geometry through direct or indirect annuloplasty. A nitinol device in the coronary sinus indirectly cinches the mitral annulus in the CARILLON mitral contour system.[12,13]
- Chordal replacement.
  A redesign of the ventricle can reduce the severity of secondary MR.
- Attach mid-anterior and posterior mitral valve leaflets to a small spacer using PASCAL TMVR.[14]
- Many severe MR patients don't meet MitraClip repair anatomic criteria.[15] PASCAL simplified TMVR anatomy.
- Transcatheter mitral valve replacement with bioprosthetic valves may be an alternative to TMVR.[16,17]

Each technology in MR treatment must be carefully assessed for risk/benefit and durability.

HOW TO DO?

Preprocedural: Preprocedural planning requires transthoracic and transesophageal echocardiography with real-time three-dimensional imaging. Careful, quantitative echocardiographic, or cardiac magnetic resonance imaging assessment should determine MR severity and etiology.

Procedural technique: The procedure of TMVR utilizing the MitraClip device is conducted within the cardiac catheterization laboratory, employing a combination of fluoroscopic and transesophageal echocardiographic (TEE) guidance. Due to the necessity of TEE guidance and meticulous device manipulation, it is customary for the procedure to be conducted under general anesthesia. Access is achieved by utilizing the femoral vein, and subsequently, a transseptal puncture is executed to traverse the interatrial septum and gain entry into the left atrium. Subsequently, the MitraClip steerable catheter is introduced into the left atrium, and the process involves employing echocardiographic guidance to properly position the MitraClip device in alignment with the valve leaflets responsible for regurgitation, ultimately reaching the left ventricle. The MitraClip is subsequently retracted, with its clip arms in an open position, to securely grasp the leaflets at the location where regurgitation occurs. Subsequently, the arms are brought together, and Doppler echocardiography is employed to ascertain the ensuing decrease in MR. In the event that the decrease in MR is deemed insufficient, it is possible to reopen the clip arms and make adjustments to the placement before the device is ultimately deployed. In approximately 40% of instances, an additional MitraClip may be inserted to effectively mitigate MR.[4]

The procedure involves the utilization of real-time two- and three-dimensional TEE to assist in the accurate placement of the transseptal puncture, positioning of the mitral clip, and evaluation of the mitral valve morphology, and severity of regurgitation subsequent to the placement of the clip.[18,19]

COMPLICATIONS OF TRANSCATHETER MITRAL VALVE REPAIR

Transcatheter mitral valve repair has a 15–19% 30-day complication rate.[20,21] Late complications are caused by HF or patient comorbidities, while early (30-day) complications are caused by periprocedural blood transfusion.[21]

Bleeding: As a result of the considerable sheath dimensions, transcatheter mitral valve replacement presents a potential hazard of access site bleeding.

Device embolization or partial clip detachment: The occurrence of device embolization following MitraClip placement is an extremely infrequent complication. It is more frequently observed that the clip may experience partial detachment, a complication that typically necessitates surgical intervention for treatment. Studies have reported a prevalence of clip detachment that is relatively low.

Mitral stenosis: TMVR results in an elevation of the diastolic pressure gradient across the mitral valve. The occurrence of clinically significant mitral stenosis is a possible albeit infrequent complication associated with the implantation of MitraClip.

Infective endocarditis: The available data on the risk of infective endocarditis following MitraClip implantation is limited, as it is primarily based on sporadic case reports.[22]

ANTITHROMBOTIC THERAPY IN MITRACLIP[23]

Prior to transcatheter mitral valve repair: Anticoagulants should be stopped before TMVR to allow normal coagulation to return. During the procedure, vitamin K antagonists (warfarin) should be stopped 3 days prior and an international normalized ratio ≤1.7 verified. Discontinue direct oral anticoagulants like dabigatran before the procedure. Heparin may be used if individual risk of thrombosis and bleeding warrants it while long-term anticoagulation is subtherapeutic before TMVR. The last dose of subcutaneous low molecular heparin should be given 24 hours before the procedure in the last 12 hours. At least 4 hours before the procedure, stop intravenous unfractionated heparin.

During the procedure: Heparin is given to maintain an activated clotting time >250 seconds, especially after transseptal puncture.

Postprocedure: Patients should receive anticoagulation or antiplatelet therapy for at least 6 months after the procedure:

In patients with anticoagulation indications, vitamin K antagonist or oral anticoagulant is restarted.

Aspirin and/or clopidogrel are used as antiplatelet therapy for patients without an indication for anti-coagulation. A loading dose of 325 mg aspirin can be followed by 81 mg daily. A loading dose of 300 mg of clopidogrel within 24 hours of the procedure or immediately afterward is recommended, followed by 75 mg daily. One of these antiplatelet agents should be used for 6 months or more. These recommendations are extrapolated from device endothelialization studies.

OUTCOMES AND BENEFITS OF TRANSCATHETER MITRAL VALVE REPAIR

Reduction in MR: TMVR reduces MR severity to ≤2+ on echocardiography. Transcatheter repair has been shown to reduce MR severity over time, with 21% of patients experiencing 3–4+ MR at 4 years in the EVEREST II trial.[20,24] However, 24.8% required surgery for mitral valve dysfunction. The high-risk and continued access registry of the EVEREST II trial found 16.4% of patients with MR grades of 3+–4+ at 12 months.[21] No mitral valve surgery was performed.

The survival benefit of MitraClip repair is inconclusive. Two randomized trials, RESHAPE in Europe and COAPT in the US, are enrolling functional mitral regurgitation (FMR) patients. These trials compare MitraClip System percutaneous mitral repair to optimal medical therapy. Swaans et al. recently conducted a retrospective comparison study of 139 high-risk MitraClip patients, 53 surgery patients, and 59 conservative medical patients.[25] The study examined all possible causes of the condition, including FMR at 77%, degenerative at 18%, and mixed at 5%. The MitraClip intervention group had an average follow-up duration of 1.7 ± 1.1 years.

After 1 year, transcatheter repair and surgery groups had similar survival rates of 85.8% and 85.2%, respectively. Conservative treatment only saved 67.7% of patients. Both the transcatheter repair ($p=0.006$) and surgical ($p=0.014$) groups had better survival outcomes than the conservatively treated group after adjusting for propensity score and risk factors. In contrast, MitraClip and surgical survival rates were similar ($p = 0.430$). Due to their high risk, including extreme-risk cases, transcatheter mitral repair patients are difficult to observe and demonstrate a survival benefit. This is because these patients have a shorter life expectancy due to advanced cardiac disease in FMR and advanced age and comorbidities in degenerative mitral regurgitation (DMR). Thus, symptoms and quality of life improvement as primary endpoints in these patient subgroups raise legitimate concerns. A randomized trial comparing surgical intervention to optimal medical therapy has not been done.

FOLLOW-UP AFTER MITRACLIP PROCEDURE

Studies have revealed clinical follow-up at 1 week, 1, 6, 12, 18, and 24 months following the implantation procedure and the control group was required to undergo ongoing clinical follow-up following a consultation with the site heart-failure specialist (either of which would take place within 14 days of randomization). Annual clinical follow-up was then required for 5 years.[10] Subsequent evaluations encompass recurring echocardiography, 6-minute walk tests (where greater distances signify greater preserved functional capacity and a 10% relative alteration from the initial value denotes a minimally significant distinction), and evaluations of quality-of-life metrics, such as the NYHA functional class and the Kansas City Cardiomyopathy Questionnaire (KCCQ) score (ranging from 0 to 100, with higher scores denoting improved quality of life, and a 5-point discrepancy indicating a minimally significant difference). The evaluation of the primary efficacy endpoint was intended to be conducted over a period of 2 years, with a mandatory minimum of 1 year of follow-up for all participants. The allowance of crossover was prohibited until a minimum of 2 years of follow-up had been completed.

PROGNOSIS

The COAPT trial demonstrated that the use of MitraClip treatment in patients with HF and moderate-to-severe or severe secondary mitral regurgitation (SMR) was both safe and effective. This treatment approach resulted in a reduction in the combined risk of death or HF hospitalization over a 2-year period, as well as improvements in overall survival and quality of life. These positive outcomes were observed across all age groups, indicating that age did not impact the efficacy of the treatment when compared to guideline-directed medical therapy alone. While the MitraClip treatment led to a decrease in heart failure hospitalization (HFH) rates across all age groups, the extent of reduction in HFH following TEER was found to be more pronounced in younger patients compared to the elderly population. However, both young and elderly patients diagnosed with HF and severe SMR experienced significant advantages from TEER using the MitraClip device. Therefore, it is imperative to recognize that age should not serve as a barrier when considering the timely referral of specific patients with HF and severe SMR for MitraClip treatment.

CONCLUSION

The expansion of available devices and procedural advancements in recent years has broadened the pool of patients who can benefit from TEER. However, ongoing research is exploring several other minimally invasive transcatheter therapies with the aim of providing safer and more effective treatment options for patients with MR. Ongoing trials investigating transcatheter mitral valve replacement devices include the MISCEND trial, which focuses on the Evoque device developed by Edwards Lifesciences, the SUMMIT trial, which examines the Tendyne device developed by Abbott, and the APPOLO trial, which investigates the Intrepid device developed by Medtronic. The Carillon Mitral Contour System, developed by Cardiac Dimensions, is an additional device that focuses on the mitral valve. It is currently being studied in the EMPOWER trial. This newly created device replicates the ring annuloplasty procedure by inserting a transcatheter device through the coronary sinus. Although there are promising preliminary results, it is important to note that none of these devices have received approval from the FDA. Moreover, it is worth noting that existing recommendations advocate for the use of TEER in cases where surgical intervention is not feasible. However, ongoing clinical trials such as PRIMARY and REPAIR MR are actively examining the comparative clinical outcomes of TEER and surgical repair in patients with primary mitral regurgitation (PMR) who meet the criteria for both surgical and transcatheter interventions.[26]

REFERENCES

1. Savarese G, Lund LH. Global Public Health Burden of Heart Failure. Card Fail Rev. 2017;3(1):7-11.
2. Pagnesi M, Adamo M, Sama IE, et al. Impact of mitral regurgitation in patients with worsening heart failure: insights from BIOSTAT-CHF. Eur J Heart Fail. 2021;23(10):1750-8.
3. Maisano F, La Canna G, Colombo A, et al. The evolution from surgery to percutaneous mitral valve interventions: the role of the edge-to-edge technique. J Am Coll Cardiol. 2011;58(21):2174-82.
4. Armstrong EJ, Rogers JH, Swan CH, et al. Echocardiographic predictors of single versus dual MitraClip device implantation and long-term reduction of mitral regurgitation after percutaneous repair. Catheter Cardiovasc Interv. 2013;82(4):673-9.
5. Yamamoto K, Rakugi H. Angiotensin receptor-neprilysin inhibitors: Comprehensive review and implications in hypertension treatment. Hypertens Res. 2021;44(10): 1239-50.
6. O'Gara PT, Calhoon JH, Moon MR, et al. Transcatheter therapies for mitral regurgitation: a professional society overview from the American College of Cardiology, the American Association for Thoracic Surgery, Society for Cardiovascular Angiography and Interventions Foundation, and the Society of Thoracic Surgeons. J Am Coll Cardiol. 2014;63(8):840-52.
7. Nishimura RA, Otto CM, Bonow RO, et al.; American College of Cardiology/American Heart Association Task Force on Practice Guidelines. 2014 AHA/ACC guideline for the management of patients with valvular heart disease: a report of the American College of Cardiology/American Heart Association Task Force on Practice Guidelines. J Am Coll Cardiol. 2014;63(22):2489.
8. Baumgartner H, Falk V, Bax JJ, et al.; ESC Scientific Document Group. 2017 ESC/EACTS Guidelines for the management of valvular heart disease. Eur Heart J. 2017;38(36):2739-91.
9. Feldman T, Young A. Percutaneous approaches to valve repair for mitral regurgitation. J Am Coll Cardiol. 2014;63(20):2057-68.
10. Stone GW, Lindenfeld J, Abraham WT, et al.; COAPT Investigators. Transcatheter Mitral-Valve Repair in Patients with Heart Failure. N Engl J Med. 2018;379(24):2307-18.
11. Nielsen SL. Current status of transcatheter mitral valve repair therapies - From surgical concepts towards future directions. Scand Cardiovasc J. 2016;50(5-6):367-76.
12. Schofer J, Siminiak T, Haude M, et al. Percutaneous mitral annuloplasty for functional mitral regurgitation: results of the CARILLON Mitral Annuloplasty Device European Union Study. Circulation. 2009;120(4):326-33.
13. Siminiak T, Wu JC, Haude M, et al. Treatment of functional mitral regurgitation by percutaneous annuloplasty: results of the TITAN Trial. Eur J Heart Fail. 2012;14(8):931-8.
14. Praz F, Spargias K, Chrissoheris M, et al. Compassionate use of the PASCAL transcatheter mitral valve repair system for patients with severe mitral regurgitation: a multicentre, prospective, observational, first-in-man study. Lancet. 2017;390(10096):773-80.
15. Feldman T, Kar S, Elmariah S, et al.; EVEREST II Investigators. Randomized Comparison of Percutaneous Repair and Surgery for Mitral Regurgitation: 5-Year Results of EVEREST II. J Am Coll Cardiol. 2015;66(25):2844-54.
16. Regueiro A, Granada JF, Dagenais F, et al. Transcatheter Mitral Valve Replacement: Insights From Early Clinical Experience and Future Challenges. J Am Coll Cardiol. 2017;69(17):2175-92.
17. Muller DWM, Farivar RS, Jansz P, et al.; Tendyne Global Feasibility Trial Investigators. Transcatheter Mitral Valve Replacement for Patients With Symptomatic Mitral Regurgitation: A Global Feasibility Trial. J Am Coll Cardiol. 2017;69(9):1213.
18. Wunderlich NC, Siegel RJ. Peri-interventional echo assessment for the MitraClip procedure. Eur Heart J Cardiovasc Imaging. 2013;14(10):935-49.
19. Altiok E, Hamada S, Brehmer K, et al. Analysis of procedural effects of percutaneous edge-to-edge mitral valve repair by 2D and 3D echocardiography. Circ Cardiovasc Imaging. 2012;5(6):748-55.
20. Feldman T, Foster E, Glower DD, et al.; EVEREST II Investigators. Percutaneous repair or surgery for mitral regurgitation. N Engl J Med. 2011;365(2):189.
21. Glower DD, Kar S, Trento A, et al. Percutaneous mitral valve repair for mitral regurgitation in high-risk patients: results of the EVEREST II study. J Am Coll Cardiol. 2014;64(2):172-81.
22. Frerker C, Kuck KH, Schmidt T, et al. Severe infective endocarditis after MitraClip implantation treated by cardiac surgery. EuroIntervention. 2015;11(3):351-4.
23. Calabrò P, Gragnano F, Niccoli G, et al. Antithrombotic Therapy in Patients Undergoing Transcatheter Interventions for Structural Heart Disease. Circulation. 2021;144(16):1323-43.
24. Mauri L, Foster E, Glower DD, et al.; EVEREST II Investigators. 4-year results of a randomized controlled trial of percutaneous repair versus surgery for mitral regurgitation. J Am Coll Cardiol. 2013;62(4):317-28.
25. Swaans MJ, Bakker AL, Alipour A, et al. Survival of transcatheter mitral valve repair compared with surgical and conservative treatment in high-surgical-risk patients. JACC Cardiovasc Interv. 2014;7(8):875-81.
26. Song C, Madhavan MV, Lindenfeld J, et al. Age-Related Outcomes After Transcatheter Mitral Valve Repair in Patients With Heart Failure: Analysis From COAPT. JACC Cardiovasc Interv. 2022;15(4):397-407.

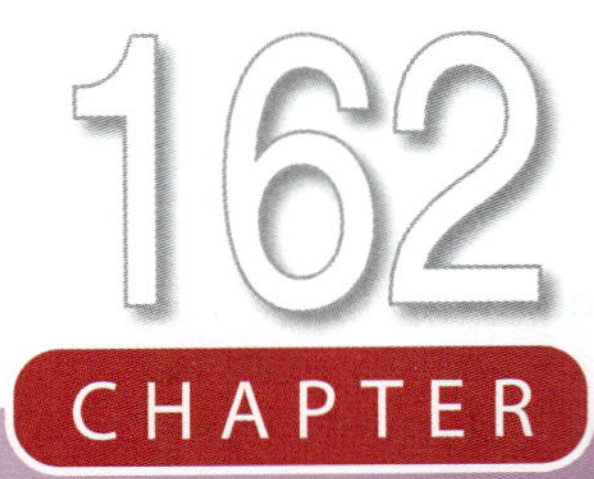

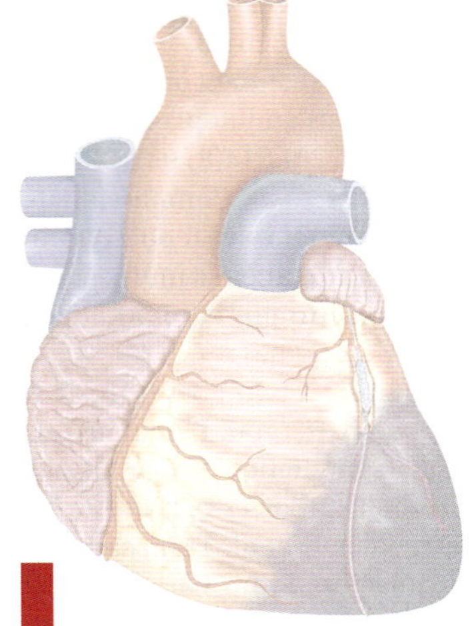

Stage D HFpEF, Heart Transplantation, and Mechanical Circulatory Support

Bhawna Mathur, Ratna Malika Kumar, Rajneesh Malhotra

INTRODUCTION

Threshold for heart failure with preserved ejection fraction (HFpEF), as per the 2022 ACC/AHA and 2023 ESC guidelines,[1] is an LVEF ≥50%. Some of these patients do not have entirely normal LVEF and also do not have major reduction in systolic function, thus the term preserved EF has been used.[2] The patients have evidence of spontaneous or provokable increased left ventricular filling pressures (LVFPs), characterized by elevated natriuretic peptides or hemodynamic measurements.[3]

Stage D HFpEF is defined as the presence of progressive and/or persistent severe signs and symptoms of HF despite optimized medical and surgical therapy in a patient with LVEF ≥50%. It is generally accompanied by recurrent hospitalizations, limited exertional tolerance, and poor quality of life. The true prevalence of Stage D HF in the HFpEF subgroup is unknown. Estimated theoretical number of patients with advanced HFpEF ranges between 110,500 and 325,000.[4]

PATHOPHYSIOLOGY[3]

Risk factors, etiology, and pathophysiology of HFpEF and HFrEF differ significantly; HFpEF is a heterogeneous clinical syndrome. Increasing age is the most significant risk factor, others being female sex, type-2 diabetes, obesity, sleep apnea, systemic and pulmonary hypertension, COPD, iron deficiency, coronary artery disease, atrial fibrillation, and dysrhythmias.

The "HFpEF mimics" are when secondary heart failure occurs in a clinical condition, causing the heart to fail. These include restrictive and hypertrophic cardiomyopathies, constrictive pericarditis, and left-sided valvular heart disease, especially aortic stenosis.

Acute decompensation of HFpEF occurs in the setting of various clinical conditions requiring increased cardiac output, leading to acute pulmonary and systemic venous congestion. These cardiovascular and noncardiovascular conditions include acute kidney injury, worsening chronic kidney disease, anemia, exacerbation of chronic pulmonary disease, tachyarrhythmia, especially new-onset atrial fibrillation, infection, ischemia, increased salt intake, water retention, medication noncompliance, and poorly controlled hypertension.[3]

Today, HFpEF is recognized as a syndrome comprising multiple cardiometabolic entities with cellular and inflammatory mechanisms, leading to diastolic dysfunction, including biventricular systolic impairment and loss of atrial compliance.[5]

SURGICAL ANATOMY OF HFpEF HEART

Commonly, HFpEF has left ventricular diastolic dysfunction secondary to a stiff, hypertrophied left ventricle causing elevated left ventricular filling pressure. In longstanding hypertension, there is severe LVH, leading to relative myocardial ischemia, in turn causing fibrosis and stiffness of the left ventricle. These patients have a smaller left ventricular cavity due to concentric hypertrophy. This results in a decreased stroke volume despite a deceptively normal ejection fraction. Severe aortic stenosis also produces LVH in a similar fashion to longstanding severe systemic hypertension.[6]

MANAGEMENT

Approach to patients with HFpEF requires symptoms and/or signs caused by structural/functional cardiac abnormalities and either elevated natriuretic peptides or objective evidence of cardiogenic pulmonary or systemic congestion.[7]

The HFpEF diagnostic scoring systems:[7,8] The H_2FPEF and HFA-PEFF algorithms use a scoring system to help determine the likelihood that HFpEF is the underlying etiology in a dyspneic person.

Treatment

Goals of therapy:[9] Historically, medical therapy for HFpEF was discouraging; however, recent clinical trials have demonstrated the benefit of guideline-directed medical therapy (GDMT) and initiation of key agents improves symptoms and functional capacity, reduces recurrent hospital admission, and reduces the morbidity and mortality associated with HF.[7]

The HFpEF hearts have small LV cavity (smaller LVEDD and LVEDV) compared to HFrEF[10] and elevated LA pressure leading to pulmonary congestion. Definitive and surgical aim should be to overcome these anatomical and physiological problems. Patients are older and have multiple comorbidities, hence surgical intervention has to be planned accordingly.

Recently, studies in advanced heart failure management with durable mechanical circulatory support (DMCS) devices and heart transplantation have been started for management of stage D HFpEF.

Heart Transplantation

Heart transplantation is generally not considered for patients with HFpEF, it is reserved for patients with end-stage heart failure[11]/bi-ventricular pathology, who remain symptomatic despite other treatments and is recommended to improve survival and quality of life in select cases with advanced HF despite optimal medical therapy.[12]

Prior to 2018, patients with stage D HFpEF in the US were not included in the transplant list following which a system was developed in which noninotrope-dependent patients with stage D HFpEF were assigned to status 4, same as those with LVAD or inotrope support, and those with advanced HFpEF who were active on the heart transplant list and who deteriorated further were assigned higher statuses by exemption, giving them similar access to donor's hearts.[4]

Mechanical Circulatory Support

Temporary mechanical circulatory support (TMCS) involves the use of artificial blood pumps to provide hemodynamic assistance for hours to weeks.[13] They include IABP, ECMO, etc. They are used to resuscitate patients in cardiogenic shock and act as a bridge to myocardial recovery, bridge to durable mechanical circulatory support (DMCS), including ventricular assist device (VAD) implantation and total artificial heart (TAH), or bridge to heart transplantation.[14]

Durable mechanical circulatory support are implantable devices intended for patient discharge and long-term support.

At present DMCS could be:[13]

- Ventricular assist devices (VAD) for patients having only LV pathology (Jarvik, Heartmate II, Heartmate III)
- Total artificial heart (TAH) for hearts involving both ventricular chambers; either BiVAD/TAH implantation or heart transplantation is the treatment option.

A study reported three patients who underwent DMCS as bridge to transplant. In two with hypertrophic cardiomyopathy, the hypertrophic papillary muscles and myocardium were resected to allow for left ventricular assist device implantation. The third with restrictive cardiomyopathy underwent Berlin Heart EXCOR BVAD implantation with left atrial cannulation.[10]

Different types of mechanical support devices are given in **Figure 1**.

DEVELOPMENT AND RESULTS OF VARIOUS VENTRICULAR ASSIST DEVICE TECHNOLOGIES

There is great need to develop novel types of durable MCS for patients with advanced HFpEF, specifically pumps or similar technologies that will accommodate smaller LV cavity sizes,[4] which challenges left-sided pressure unloading, and new anatomical entry points need to be explored for mechanical pressure and volume unloading. LV unloading is not suitable for the HFpEF group due to the small LV cavity size.

The ideal MCS device for the HFpEF population would be a low-risk, long-term durable, and easily implantable device for an older and sicker population where destination therapy (DT) is most likely.

The higher gradient between inflow and outflow will require more energy to maintain forward flow through the MCS. The side effects of LVADs, including systemic thromboembolism, bleeding, infections, and lack of pulse pressure, would have to be addressed to optimize MCS support in an elderly multimorbid HFpEF population.

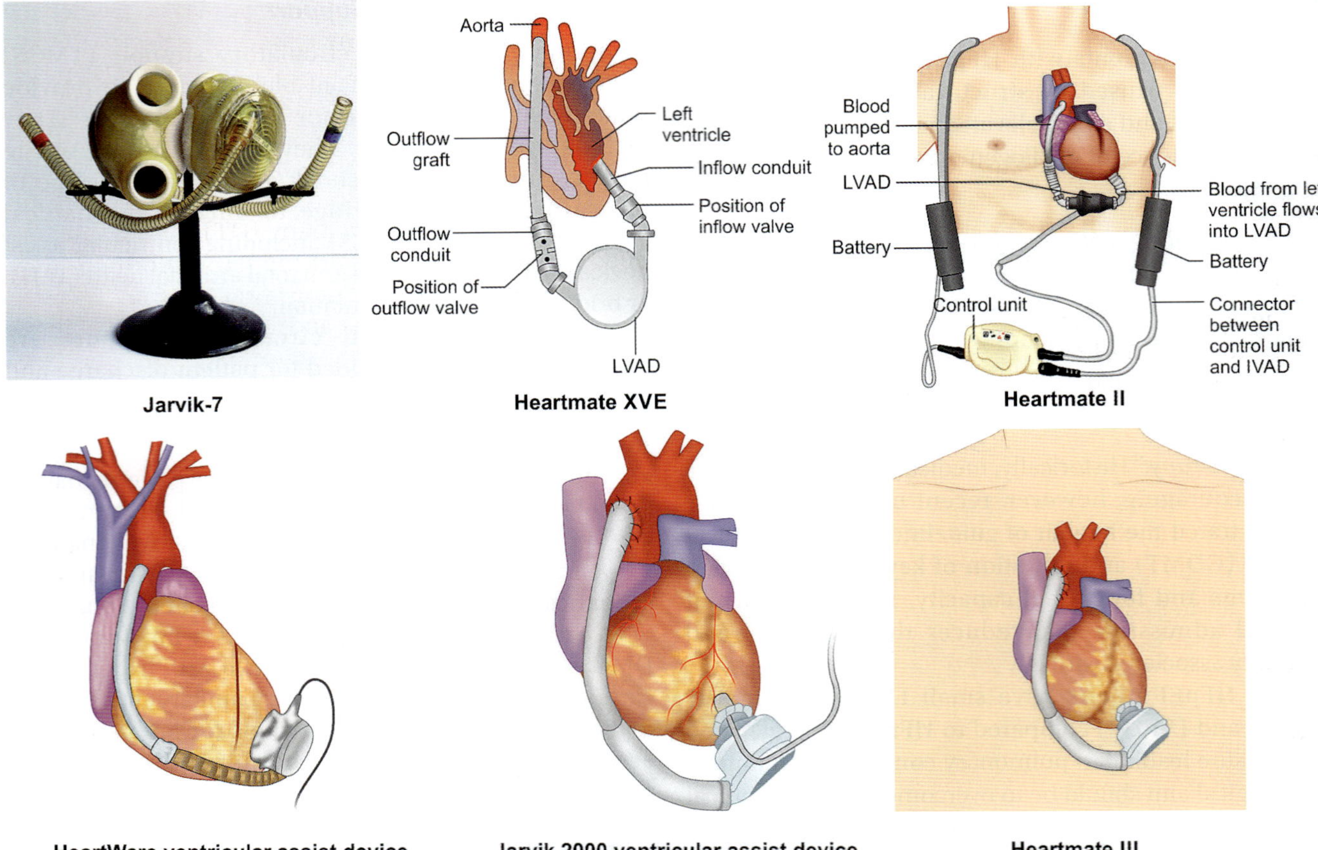

Fig. 1: Different types of mechanical support devices.[15]

A new adaptive mechanical circulatory device has been tested in animal model with inflow from the LA and outflow to descending aorta, indicating that this approach may represent an effective long-term treatment for HFpEF patients with the potential to reduce filling pressures and increase cardiac output, and thereby confer a positive effect on quality of Life.[5]

Mechanical circulatory support provides hemodynamic support to the underperforming left or right ventricles in HFrEF in the terminal phase; however, there are no clinical studies to evaluate their efficacy and safety in HFpEF. Preclinical animal studies have been done for:[16]

- *Left atrial decompression pumps:* Synergy continuous-flow micropump (HeartWare), (pumps from left atrium or left ventricle, eject into the proximal aorta) concluded that in HFpEF, it increases cardiac output, systolic blood pressure, and reduces left atrial and pulmonary pressures.
- *CoPulse:* Valveless pulsatile pump implanted at the apex of the heart, it has a blood and an air chamber divided by a polyurethane membrane. Blood flow enters during diastole and is expelled by displacement of the separating membrane during systole and showed reduced left atrial pressure and increased cardiac output.
- *Left atrial assist device:* First animal-tested MCS device, it is a continuous pump implanted at the mitral valve, transferring blood from left atrium to left ventricle, increasing cardiac output and mean aortic pressure, and decreasing left atrial pressure. LVEDP, CVP, and heart rate remained stable without causing LVOTO.

Long-term MCS devices are being developed for HFpEF patients with atrial unloading, leading to significant reduction of filling pressure, maintenance of pulse pressure, and increase in CO, such as:

- *Pulse VAD:* Unloading from the LA into different outflow sites in the arterial system[5]
- PReduction pump (Pumpinheart Limited, Dublin, Ireland), is a durable partial support pump, deployed across the mitral valve, transcatheter and functions as a diastolic support device.[15]
- *The Tandem Heart device (Cardiac Assist Inc., Pittsburg, PA, USA):* LA to femoral artery and centrifugal pump[5]

- *Partial support LVAD CircuLite Synergy Micro:* Pump device for longer term—LA to the right axillary artery[5]
- *Impeller device:* In the mitral position, to decrease LA pressure and increase LV preload, tested in a mock loop[5]
- Nonpulsatile pump in the mitral position to unload the LA in diastole[5]
- *Pneumatic pulsatile pump (CoPulse):* By unloading from LV into the pump in diastole, demonstrated the pump's potential to unload the LA and increase CO for the four HFpEF phenotypes.[5,17]

A study with HeartMate 3 (HM 3) in 16 virtual cases where simulation of HFpEF hearts was done to overcome smaller left ventricular cavities, which pose challenges for utilizing ventricular assist devices (VADs). In vitro assessment revealed that the HM3 in an LA to AO configuration unloads LA, thus decreasing the LAP and MPAP relieving pulmonary congestion at the cost of increased LVP and AOP, therefore unloading the LA but increasing afterload in rest and exercise conditions. It also showed that HM3 can fit into HFpEF patients without interfering with rigid anatomy but interfered with the aorta, pulmonary veins, or right atrium in 57% of the assessed patients.[18]

LIMITATIONS

The ideal DMCS has not been developed and only a few studies have been done. All these are still in preclinical phase. Heart transplantation as a treatment option stays an indication in stage D. Evidence has not been established due to lack of numbers and clinical trials have not been done yet to see the outcome.

CONCLUSION

Heart failure with preserved ejection fraction is a syndrome comprising multiple cardiometabolic entities with a clinical diagnosis of HF and LVEF ≥50%.[7] The patients are older with comorbidities like diabetes, hypertension, kidney disease, COPD, and obesity. Stage D HFpEF is persistence of symptoms of failure despite medical management, requiring recurrent hospitalization. HFpEF hearts have small, stiff LV cavities and elevated LA pressure, thereby leading to pulmonary congestion. Thus, the definitive and surgical aim should be to overcome these anatomical and physiological problems. There is need to develop new DMCS, which can easily be accommodated in these small LVs.[4] Studies suggest a pump designed for LA cannulation may be beneficial for unloading LA pressures of HFpEF patients and reducing their HF symptoms.[18] Most of these studies are preclinical, and thus, have not yet been accepted and adapted into any specific guidelines. Heart transplantation is the option for these hearts, but on time heart availability remains a problem. Thus, DMCS should be considered as destination therapy.

The need of the hour, for stage D of this silent pandemic, is an ideal MCS device that is low-risk, durable, easily implantable, and for a more senior and frail population, it would be destination therapy (DT). Likely the most effective circulatory support model would unload the LA with outflow to descending aorta, with the potential to reduce filling pressures and increase cardiac output thereby conferring a positive effect on quality of life.

Heart failure with preserved ejection fraction prevails in an aging, frail population with multiple comorbidities, medical management remains the mainstay at present and there is little and less studied role of heart transplant and MCS for long-term benefit. All the above MCS devices discussed here are still preclinical and are based on animal studies with no proven efficacy. There are no prescribed guidelines yet for heart transplant and DMCS in stage D HFpEF.

REFERENCES

1. McDonagh TA, Metra M, Adamo M, et al. 2023 Focused Update of the 2021 ESC Guidelines for the diagnosis and treatment of acute and chronic heart failure. Eur Heart J. 2023;44(37):3627-39.
2. Heidenreich PA, Bozkurt B, Aguilar D, et al. 2022 AHA/ACC/HFSA Guideline for the Management of Heart Failure: A Report of the American College of Cardiology/American Heart Association Joint Committee on Clinical Practice Guidelines. Circulation. 2022;145(18):e895-1032.
3. Golla MSG, Shams P. Heart failure with preserved ejection fraction (HFpEF). In: StatPearls [Internet]. Treasure Island (FL): StatPearls Publishing; 2024. Available from https://www.ncbi.nlm.nih.gov/books/NBK599960/ [Last accessed January, 2025].
4. Gorodeski EZ, Yaranov DM, Starling R, et al. Stage D heart failure with preserved ejection fraction, heart transplantation, and mechanical circulatory support. Diastology. Philadelphia: Elsevier; 2021. pp. 276-89.
5. Gude E, Fiane AE. Can mechanical circulatory support be an effective treatment for HFpEF patients? Heart Fail Rev. 2023;28(2):297-305.
6. Naing P, Forrester D, Kangaharan N, et al. Heart failure with preserved ejection fraction: A growing global epidemic. Aust J Gen Pract. 2019;48(7):465-71.
7. Kittleson MM, Panjrath GS, Amancherla K, et al. 2023 ACC Expert Consensus Decision Pathway on Management of Heart Failure with Preserved Ejection Fraction: A Report of the American College of Cardiology Solution Set Oversight Committee. J Am Coll Cardiol. 2023;81(18):1835-78.
8. Chiorescu RM, Lazar RD, Ruda A, et al. Current insights and future directions in the treatment of heart failure

with preserved ejection fraction. Int J Mol Sci. 2023;25(1): 440.

9. Borlaug BA, Colucci WS. (2024). Treatment and prognosis of heart failure with preserved ejection fraction. In: Gotlieb SS, Dardas TF (Eds). UpToDate. [online] Available from https://www.uptodate.com/contents/treatment-and-prognosis-of-heart-failure-with-preserved-ejection-fraction/print [Last accessed January, 2025]. Treatment and prognosis of heart failure with preserved ejection fraction: Aug 21,2024
10. Lanmueller P, Eulert-Grehn JJ, Schoenrath F, et al. Durable mechanical circulatory support in patients with heart failure with preserved ejection fraction. Interact Cardiovasc Thorac Surg. 2021;33(4):628-630.
11. Saeed D, Feldman D, Banayosy AE, et al. The 2023 International Society for Heart and Lung Transplantation Guidelines for Mechanical Circulatory Support: A 10-Year Update. J Heart Lung Transplant. 2023;42(7):e1-e222.
12. Al Habeeb W, Tash A, Elasfar A, et al. 2023 National Heart Center/Saudi Heart Association Focused Update of the 2019 Saudi Heart Association Guidelines for the Management of Heart Failure. J Saudi Heart Assoc. 2023; 35(1):71-134.
13. Haft J, Cleveland JC. Short-term uses of mechanical circulatory support devices and long-term uses of mechanical circulatory support devices. In: Gravelee GP, Davis RF, Hammon J, Kussman B (Eds). Cardiopulmonary Bypass and Mechanical Support Principles and Practice. Philadelphia: Lippincott Williams & Wilkins; 2015.
14. Nifong W and Chitwood WR. Cardiopulmonary bypass for minimally invasive cardiac surgery. In: Gravelee GP, Davis RF, Hammon J, Kussman B (Eds). Cardiopulmonary Bypass Principles and Practice. Philadelphia: Lippincott Williams & Wilkins; 2015.
15. Dual SA, Cowger J, Roche E, et al; The future of durable mechanical circulatory support: Emerging technological innovations and considerations to enable evolution of the field. J Card Fail. 2024;30(4):596-609.
16. Parra-Lucares A, Romero-Hernández E, Villa E, et al. New opportunities in heart failure with preserved ejection fraction: from bench to bedside and back. Biomedicines. 2022;11(1):70.
17. Samson R, Jaiswal A, Ennezat PV, et al. Clinical phenotypes in heart failure with preserved ejection fraction. J Am Heart Assoc. 2016;5(1):e002477.
18. Langer N, Stephens AF, Šeman M, et al. HeartMate 3 for heart failure with preserved ejection fraction: In vitro hemodynamic evaluation and anatomical fitting. Ann Biomed Eng. 2024;52(12)3208-18.

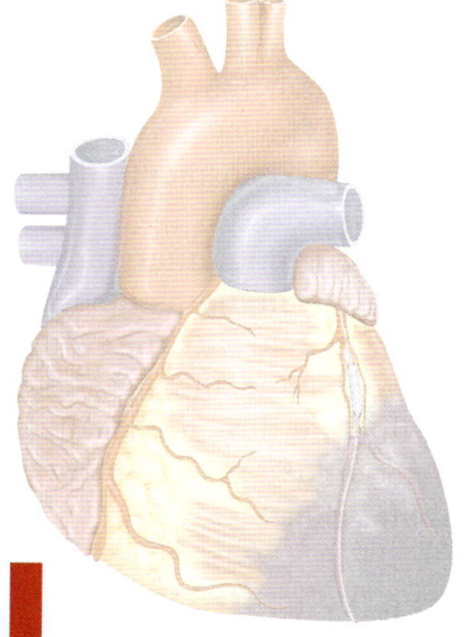

Drug Switch or Device: How do I Decide in HFpEF?

Sabarish Sankaran, Meemansa Kashyap Buch, Bagirath Raghuraman

INTRODUCTION

According to reports from the Framingham Heart Study, Cardiovascular Health Study (CHS), and MESA reports (Multi-ethnic study of atherosclerosis); the lifetime risk of heart failure with preserved ejection fraction (HFpEF) is estimated to be >10% in both males and females at 45 years.[1] The Kerala Heart Failure Registry reported 14.9%[2] patients having HFpEF, which could be an under-representation of the true burden. Global registries account for HFpEF for ~50% of the total HF visits.[3] In the coming decades, HFpEF might be the most dominant or representative phenotype of heart failure and thus merit better treatment. Though this document emphasizes drug and device therapy, it is worth mentioning that in the real world, the management of HFpEF lies in identifying and treating the comorbidities.

PHARMACOLOGICAL MANAGEMENT FOR HEART FAILURE WITH PRESERVED EJECTION FRACTION

- *Sodium-glucose cotransporter-2 inhibitors (SGLT2i):* Based on results of EMPEROR-PRESERVED,[4] PRESERVED HF,[5] DELIVER HF,[6] SCORED,[7] and SOLOIST HF,[8] the only class of drugs that showed improvement in MACE events is SGLT2i. They scored higher than placebo in major primary endpoints such as reduction in cardiovascular mortality, worsening heart failure symptoms, and heart failure hospitalizations (HFHs) including the first HFH. Also, they provide benefits regardless of the status of diabetes mellitus, thus exhibiting a true disease-modifying effect. The use of SGLT2i in HFpEF is now a class IIa recommendation[9] and should be added once the patient is clinically stable. Additionally, the EMPULSE trial[10] showed positive outcomes with empagliflozin in acute decompensated heart failure (ADHF) patients with left ventricular ejection fraction (LVEF) >40% including de novo HFpEF. There was no evidence of dehydration or ketoacidosis with a more thorough decongestion on day 90. Thus, early initiation of SGLT2i is strongly recommended in the armamentarium of HFpEF.
- *Diuretics:* Diuretics continue to remain the principal therapy (Class I)[9] to control acute decompensation when accompanied by congestion.
- *Mineralocorticoid receptor antagonists (MRA):* The landmark TOPCAT trial[11] did not reduce mortality rates with Spironolactone but showed benefits by reducing HFH. It is currently a Class IIb[9] recommendation since it also helps control blood pressure by a balanced diuretic effect via sequential nephron blockade over and above loop diuretics. Recently, the investigators of FINEARTS-HF trial[12] showed a significant reduction in the composite outcome of worsening events and cardiovascular mortality with finerenone. Although it has already received approval for cardiovascular and renal protection in subjects with Type II DM and chronic kidney disease (CKD) based on the FIGARO-DKD study,[13] Food and Drug Administration (FDA) approval for use in HFpEF, is awaited.
- *RAAS blockade:* The results of PARAMOUNT-HF[14] showed a decline in NT-proBNP levels at 12 weeks and PARAGON-HF failed to reduce CV mortality or HFH. ARNI therapy is now given a Class-IIb

recommendation for females and subjects with lower values of LVEF (below median values of 45–57%) based on a subanalysis of the PARAGON-HF cohort.[15] The Candesartan arm of CHARM-PRESERVED showed a modest reduction in primary composite events.[16] Hence, it is reasonable to use angiotensin 2 receptor blockers (ARBs) in patients who are intolerant to angiotensin receptor-neprilysin inhibitors (ARNIs) due to symptomatic hypotension or history of angioedema.

- *Beta blockers:* The SENIORS trial[17] reported a declining trend towards HFH and CV mortality with nebivolol (vs. placebo) but only 15% of these patients had HFpEF. The ELANDD trial[18] failed to show improvement in exercise capacity with Nebivolol. Finally, J-DHF[19] concluded that Carvedilol only when used in standard dose (vs. low dose) reduced unplanned hospitalizations, CV, and all-cause mortality. Current guidelines suggest reserving beta blockers only to specific indications in HFpEF due to their negative chronotropic effects.
- *Nitrates:* The NEAT-HFpEF study[20] showed unfavorable outcomes with decreased daily physical activity measures and QOL with dose-dependent isosorbide mononitrate. Thus, nitrates were found to be detrimental in HFpEF management.
- *Phosphodiesterase inhibitors:* The RELAX-HF trial[21] that studied sildenafil, did not show any improvement in exercise capacity in patients with HFpEF.
- *GLP-1 analogs:* Since the recognition of obesity as a major driver in the pathophysiology of HFpEF, GLP-1 analogs has garnered significant attention. The STEP-HFPEF trial concluded that semaglutide once weekly was superior to placebo in weight reduction (–13.3% vs. –2.6%), HF-related symptom reduction, improved QOL measures, and 6-min walk distance (6MWD) (21.5 m vs. 1.2 m) at 52 weeks.[22] However, it did not demonstrate effects on HF visits, HF rehospitalizations, and time to first HFH.
- *Nonpharmacological:* Continuous pulmonary artery (PA) pressure recording with CardioMems device[23] and invasive cardiac catheterization to aid drug switch is best used for subjects who cannot tolerate either initiation or titration of guideline-directed medical therapy (GDMT). PA catheter-guided management is as such a Class IIb recommendation.[9]

DEVICE-BASED THERAPY FOR HEART FAILURE WITH PRESERVED EJECTION FRACTION (FLOWCHART 1)

Atrial Shunt Devices

- It aims at lowering the left atrial pressure and is well suited in treating type 4 phenotype heart failure **(Table 1)**
- Shunting between the two atria can increase the risk of atrial arrhythmias and paradoxical embolism
- Shunting can be done from the left atrium to the coronary sinus to mitigate the aforementioned risks.
- Since these devices require anticoagulation, patients who have contraindications to long-term anticoagulation, atrial fibrillation, or a history of thromboembolic events are not suitable candidates.

Flowchart 1: Device options for HFpEF.

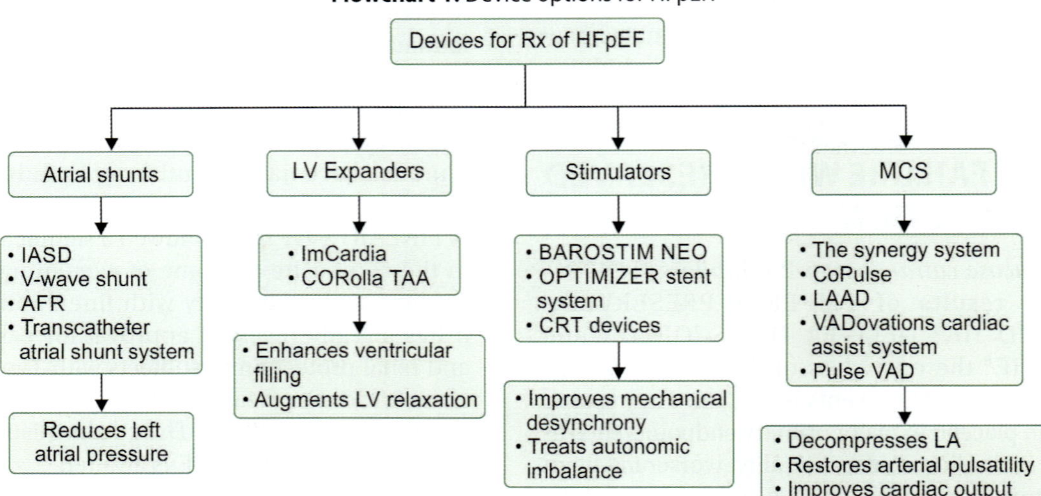

(AFR: atrial flow regulator; CRT: cardiac resynchronization therapy; HFpEF: heart failure with preserved ejection fraction; IASD: interatrial shunt device; LAAD: left atrial assist device; LV: left ventricle; RV: right ventricle; TAA: thoracic aortic aneurysm; VAD: ventricular assist device)

- There can be extraload on the right heart and hence patients with poor RV function, valvular heart disease, or severe lung disease are also not suitable for this device.
- The available devices include an interatrial shunt device (IASD),[25] v-wave shunt, atrial flow regulator (AFR), and transcatheter left atrial to coronary sinus shunt system. Evidence from various studies is depicted in **Table 2**.

TABLE 1: Phenotype of heart failure by Burkhoff et al.[24]

Type	*Features*
1	Hypertrophic cardiomyopathy—diastolic dysfunction
2	Infiltrative cardiomyopathy—diastolic dysfunction and restrictive physiology
3	Non-LVH without significant CV disease—diastolic dysfunction
4	Underlying CV disease—chronic neurohormonal activation, volume overload

(CV: cardiovascular; LVH: left ventricular hypertrophy)

Left Ventricular Expanders

- The ImCardia device was tested in patients with HFpEF undergoing aortic valve replacement. However, the observed improvement in cardiac function could not be attributed to the ImCardia device per se and since this requires invasive implantation the trial was terminated.[35]
- Animal studies with the CORolla transapical approach have shown an increased incidence of mitral regurgitation and mitral valve endocarditis.[36]

NEUROMODULATION THERAPY

- *BAROSTIM NEO:* It increases the parasympathetic tone and diminishes the sympathetic drive thereby offering benefits to patients with heart failure and resistant hypertension.[37]
- *Cardiac contraction modulation therapy:*
  - Stimulus given to the cardiac myocyte results in an enhanced influx of calcium ions thereby

TABLE 2: Evidence across several trials for device therapy for HFpEF.

REDUCE LAP-HF[26]	Phase 1, open-label, single-arm trial (n = 68) • Symptomatic HF • EF ≥40% • PCWP during rest ≥15 mm Hg and exercise ≥ 25 mm Hg	IASD produced a reduction in PCWP in 58% of participants at 6 months with no periprocedural or device-related complications
REDUCE LAP-HF I[27]	Phase 2, randomized, parallel-group, blinded, sham-controlled trial (*n* = 94) • Symptomatic HF • EF ≥ 40% • PCWP during exercise ≥25 mm Hg • PCWP-RA gradient ≥5 mm Hg	IASD produced a greater reduction in PCWP during all stages of exercise compared with sham with no complications at 1 month follow up
REDUCE LAP-HF II[28]	Phase 3, randomized, sham-controlled trial (*n* = 626) • Included patient with: • Age ≥40 years • Symptomatic HF • EF ≥40% • PCWP during exercise ≥25 mm Hg • PCWP-RA gradient ≥5 mm Hg	No differences between groups (IASD vs. sham) in the primary composite end point of CV death, nonfatal ischemic stroke at 12 months, rate of HF events up to 24 months, and change in KCCQ score at 12 months
First in the human V-wave system[29]	Single arm, open-label study (*n* = 38) • Included patients with both HFrEF and HFpEF • Symptomatic HF	• Follow-up at 3 and 12 months showed Improvements in NYHA class, quality of life, 6 min walking distance without changes in left or right-sided function • 14% of devices were occluded and another 36% were stenotic at the valve by 12 months
RELIEVE-HF[30]	Prospective, randomized, double-blind, controlled study (*n* = 605) • Included patients with both HFrEF and HFpEF • Symptomatic HF	Follow-up at 2 years showed no benefit between 2 arms (V-wave system plus standard medical care vs. medical care only)

Contd...

Contd...

PRELIEVE[31]	Prospective, nonrandomized, multicenter study (*n* = 109) • Included patients with both HFrEF and HFpEF • PCWP ≥15 at rest and ≥25 mm Hg with exercise	Follow-up at 3 months showed good AFR device patency in most of the patients with a decrease in resting PCWP with no stroke or reduction in right heart function. Few patients showed improvement in NYHA class, 6 min walking distance, and KCCQ score. One device embolization and one device-related bleeding and syncope were reported
PROLONGER study, AFteR registry, FROST-HF[32,33]	Currently enrolling patients in a multicenter registry/study to assess the safety and efficacy of Occlutech AFR in patients with HF	
In the human experience of the Transcatheter Atrial Shunt System	Included 11 patients with a median of 1 HF admission in the past year, NYHA III/ambulant IV, elevated PCWP	87.5% of patients had improvement in NYHA Class, 42.9% had improvement in 6MWT, and an average reduction of PCWP by 9 mm Hg at a median follow-up of 100 days without any fall in LV or RV function
• *ALT FLOW early feasibility study*[34] • *For APTURE transcatheter atrial shunt system*	Single arm, open-label study (*n* = 87) • Included patients with symptomatic HFpEF • PCWP ≥15 at rest and ≥25 mm Hg with exercise	• Successful device implantation was achieved in 90% • Follow up at 3 and 6 months showed improvement in NYHA class, KCCQ score, and PCWP without change in RV function

(HFpEF: heart failure with preserved ejection fraction; IASD: interatrial shunt device; LV: left ventricle; LVEF: left ventricular ejection fraction; KCCQ: Kansas City Cardiomyopathy Questionnaire; MRA: mineralocorticoid receptor antagonists; NYHA: New York Heart Association; PCWP: pulmonary capillary wedge pressure; RV: right ventricle)

augmenting the cardiac contractility without increasing myocardial oxygen consumption.

- However, this system cannot be used in patients with atrial fibrillation, mechanical tricuspid valve, lack of venous access, and 100% VVI pacing.
- FIX-HF-5 and FIX-HF-5C trials observed that at 2 years follow up cardiac contractility modulation (CCM) improves exercise tolerance, New York Heart Association (NYHA) class, and quality of life and reduces HF hospitalization rates.[38]
- CCM-HFpEF is an ongoing trial in patients with HFpEF to evaluate the safety and efficacy of the device in these patients.

▪ *Cardiac resynchronization therapy:*
  - Subgroup analysis from the PROSPECT trial revealed the benefit of CRT in patients with LVEF > 35%.[39]
  - Biatrial resynchronization therapy has been shown to be associated with improvements in the 6-minute walking test (6MWT) and mitral flow dynamics.
  - His-bundle pacing following AV node ablation has also been shown to improve NYHA functional class and bring down the use of diuretics.
  - Biventricular fusion pacing is currently under evaluation to assess its efficacy in patients with HFpEF.

▪ *Mechanical circulatory support:*
These devices are suitable especially for HFpEF1 phenotype/associated with reduced cardiac output:
  - *Left atrial decompression pumps:*
    - It increases cardiac output by improving LV end-systolic volume and lowering the rate of atrial suction.
    - Retaining pulsatile flow is essential since nonpulsatile continuous flow is associated with increased gastrointestinal bleeding and aortic wall degeneration.[40]
  - *Valveless pulsatile pump (CoPulse):*
    - It consists of two chambers divided by a flexible polyurethane membrane.
    - It is implanted into the apex of the heart and works by improving diastolic flow dynamics.
    - Animal studies have shown improved cardiac output and reduced left atrial pressure with the use of this device[41]
  - *LA assist device (LAAD):*
    - It is a continuous pump designed for implantation at the level of the mitral valve.
    - Animal studies have shown increases in cardiac output and mean aortic pressure with a reduction in left atrial pressure.
    - However, there are unanswered questions regarding the level of implantation of the device and its impact on the LV diastolic function.[42]

Flowchart 2: Algorithm to manage HFpEF at the HF clinic.

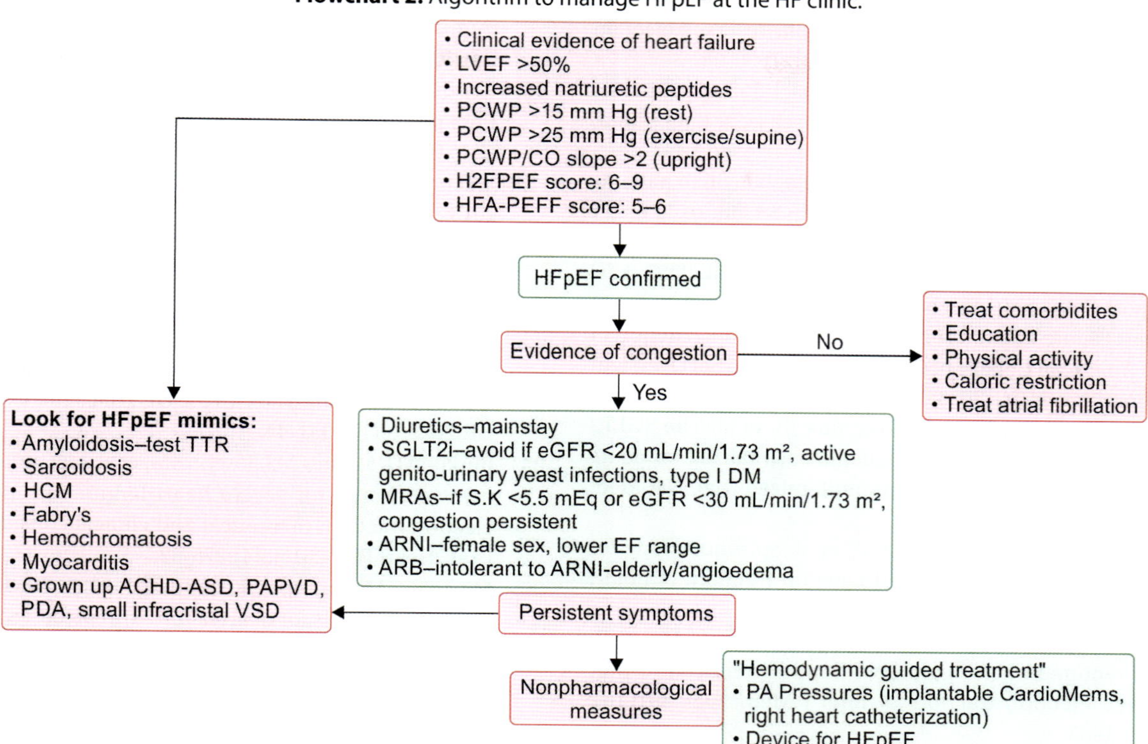

(ARB: angiotensin receptor blocker; ARNI: angiotensin receptor-neprilysin inhibitor; ASD: atrial septal defect; ACHD: adult congenital heart disease; eGFR: estimated glomerular filtration rate; HCM: hypertrophic cardiomyopathy; HFpEF: heart failure with preserved ejection fraction; LVEF: left ventricular ejection fraction; PAPVD: partial anomalous pulmonary venous drainage; PCWP: pulmonary capillary wedge pressure; PDA: patent ductus arteriosus; SGLT2i: sodium-glucose cotransporter-2 inhibitors; VSD: ventricular septal defect)

CONCLUSION

Deciding between pharmacologic treatment and device therapy in heart failure with HFpEF involves several considerations:

- Symptom severity
- Underlying conditions
- Response to medical therapy
- Device therapy options
- Patient preference
- Risk of hospitalization
- Guideline recommendations
- Multidisciplinary approach

Ultimately, the decision should be individualized, considering both clinical evidence and the patient's unique situation. Regular follow-up and reassessment are key to managing HFpEF effectively.

Flowchart 2 discusses the management of HFpEF at the HF clinic.

REFERENCES

1. Borlaug BA, Sharma K, Shah SJ, et al. Heart Failure With Preserved Ejection Fraction: JACC Scientific Statement. J Am Coll Cardiol. 2023;81(18):2023.
2. Joseph S, Panniyammakal J, Abdullakutty J, et al. CSI-KHFR Investigators, The Cardiology Society of India-Kerala Acute Heart Failure Registry: poor adherence to guideline-directed medical therapy. Eur Heart J. 2022;43(9):908-15.
3. Joseph P, Dokainish H, McCready T, et al. G-CHF Investigators. A multinational registry to study the characteristics and outcomes of heart failure patients: The global congestive heart failure (G-CHF) registry. Am Heart J. 2020; 227:56-63.
4. Anker SD, Butler J, Filippatos G, et al. Empagliflozin in heart failure with a preserved ejection fraction. N Engl J Med. 2021;385(16):1451-61.
5. Nassif ME, Windsor SL, Borlaug BA, et al. The SGLT2 inhibitor dapagliflozin in heart failure with preserved ejection fraction: a multicenter randomized trial. Nat Med. 2021;27(11):1954-60.

6. Solomon SD, McMurray JJV, Claggett B, et al. Dapagliflozin in heart failure with mildly reduced or preserved ejection fraction. New Engl J Med. 2022;387(12):1089-98.
7. Bhatt DL, Szarek M, Pitt B, et al. Sotagliflozin in patients with diabetes and chronic kidney disease. N Engl J Med. 2021;384(2):129-39.
8. Bhatt DL, Szarek M, Steg PG, et al. Sotagliflozin in patients with diabetes and recent worsening heart failure. N Engl J Med. 2021;384(2):117-28.
9. Kittleson M, Panjrath G, Amancherla K, et al. 2023 ACC Expert Consensus Decision Pathway on Management of Heart Failure With Preserved Ejection Fraction: A Report of the American College of Cardiology Solution Set Oversight Committee. JACC. 2023;81(18):1835-78.
10. Voors AA, Angermann CE, Teerlink JR, et al. The SGLT2 inhibitor empagliflozin in patients hospitalized for acute heart failure: a multinational randomized trial. Nat Med. 2022;28():568-74.
11. Pitt B, Pfeffer MA, Assmann SF, et al. Spironolactone for heart failure with preserved ejection fraction. N Engl J Med. 2014;370(15):1383-92.
12. Solomon SD, McMurray JJV, Vaduganathan M, et al. Finerenone in heart failure with mildly reduced or preserved ejection fraction. N Engl J Med. 2024;391(16): 1475-1485.
13. Pitt B, Filippatos G, Agarwal R, et al. Cardiovascular events with finerenone in kidney disease and type 2 diabetes. N Engl J Med. 2021;385(24):2252 63.
14. Solomon SD, Zile M, Pieske B, et al. The angiotensin receptor neprilysin inhibitor LCZ696 in heart failure with preserved ejection fraction: a phase 2 double-blind randomised controlled trial. Lancet. 2012;380(9851): 1387-95.
15. Solomon SD, McMurray JJ, Anand IS, et al. Angiotensin-neprilysin inhibition in heart failure with preserved ejection fraction. N Engl J Med. 2019;381(17):1609-20.
16. Yusuf S, Pfeffer MA, Swedberg K, et al. Effects of candesartan in patients with chronic heart failure and preserved left-ventricular ejection fraction: the CHARM-Preserved Trial. Lancet. 2003;362(9386):777-81.
17. Flather MD, Shibata MC, Coats AJ, et al. SENIORS Investigators. Randomized trial to determine the effect of nebivolol on mortality and cardiovascular hospital admission in elderly patients with heart failure (SENIORS). Eur Heart J. 2005;26(3):215-25.
18. Conraads VM, Metra M, Kamp O, et al. Effects of the long-term administration of nebivolol on the clinical symptoms, exercise capacity, and left ventricular function of patients with diastolic dysfunction: results of the ELANDD study. Eur J Heart Fail. 2012;14(2):219-25.
19. Yamamoto K, Origasa H, Hori M. J-DHF Investigators. Effects of carvedilol on heart failure with preserved ejection fraction: the Japanese Diastolic Heart Failure Study (J-DHF). Eur J Heart Fail. 2013;15(1):110-8.
20. Redfield MM, Anstrom KJ, Levine JA, et al. Isosorbide mononitrate in heart failure with preserved ejection fraction. N Engl J Med. 2015;373(24):2314-24.
21. Redfield MM, Chen HH, Borlaug BA, et al. Effect of Phosphodiesterase-5 Inhibition on Exercise Capacity and Clinical Status in Heart Failure With Preserved Ejection Fraction: A Randomized Clinical Trial. JAMA. 2013;309(12):1268-77.
22. Kosiborod MN, Petrie MC, Borlaug BA, et al. Semaglutide in patients with obesity-related heart failure and type 2 diabetes. N Engl J Med. 2024;390(15):1394-407.
23. Zile MR, Mehra MR, Ducharme A, et al. Hemodynamically-Guided Management of Heart Failure Across the Ejection Fraction Spectrum: The GUIDE-HF Trial. J Am Coll Cardiol HF. 2022;10(12):931-44.
24. Burkhoff D, Maurer MS, Joseph SM, et al. Left atrial decompression pump for severe heart failure with preserved ejection fraction: theoretical and clinical considerations. JAAC Heart Fail. 2015;3(4):275-82.
25. Miyagi C, Miyamoto T, Karimov JH, et al. Device-based treatment options for heart failure with preserved ejection fraction. Heart Fail Rev. 2021;26(4):749-62.
26. Hasenfuß G, Hayward C, Burkhoff D, et al. A transcatheter intracardiac shunt device for heart failure with preserved ejection fraction (REDUCE LAP-HF): a multicentre, open-label, single-arm, phase 1 trial. Lancet. 2016;387(10025): 1298-1304.
27. Feldman T, Mauri L, Kahwash R, et al. Transcatheter Interatrial Shunt Device for the Treatment of Heart Failure With Preserved Ejection Fraction (REDUCE LAP-HF I [Reduce Elevated Left Atrial Pressure in Patients With Heart Failure]): A Phase 2, Randomized, Sham-Controlled Trial. 2018;137(4):364-75.
28. Patel RB, Silvestry FE, Komtebedde J, et al. Atrial Shunt Device Effects on Cardiac Structure and Function in Heart Failure With Preserved Ejection Fraction: The REDUCE LAP-HF II Randomized Clinical Trial. JAMA Cardiol. 2024;9(6):507-22.
29. The V-Wave Shunt: FIM Safety and Feasibility Study (VW-SP-1). https://clinicaltrials.gov/ct2/ show/NCT01965015 [Last accessed January, 2025].
30. ClinicalTrials.gov. (2006). Reducing Lung congestion symptoms in advanced heart failure (RELIEVE-HF). [Online] Available from https:// clinicaltrials.gov/show/NCT03499236 [Last accessed January, 2025].
31. Clinicaltrials.gov. (2008). The Prophet Trial -Pilot Study to Assess Safety and Efficacy of a Novel Atrial Flow Regulator (AFR) in Patients With Pulmonary Hypertension (AFR-Prophet). [Online] Available from https://clinicaltrials.gov/ct2/ show/NCT03030274 [Last accessed January, 2025].
32. Clinicaltrials.gov. (2017). The AFteR Registry - Follow-up Study to Monitor the Efficacy and Safety of the Occlutech

AFR in Heart Failure Patients. [Online] Available from https://clinicaltrials.gov/ct2/show/NCT04405583 [Last accessed January, 2025].

33. Clinicaltrials.gov. (2001). Flow Regulation by Opening the Septum in Patients With Heart Failure Trial (FROST-HF). [Online] Available from https://clinicaltrials.gov/ct2/show/NCT03751748 [Last accessed January, 2025].
34. Early Feasibility Study-Transcatheter Atrial Shunt System (ALt FLOW US). https://clinicaltrials.gov/ct2/show/NCT03523416 [Last accessed January, 2025].
35. Feld Y, Dubi S, Reisner Y, et al. Energy transfer from systole to diastole: a novel device-based approach for the treatment of diastolic heart failure. Acute Card Care. 2011;13(4):232-42.
36. Feld Y, Reisner Y, Meyer-Brodnitz G, Hoefler R. Heart Fail Rev. 2021;1:3.
37. Bisognano JD, de Leeuw P, Bach DS, et al. J Card Fail. 2009;15:S62.
38. FIX-HF-5C (FIX-HF-5C). [Online] Available from https://clinicaltrials.gov/ct2/show/ NCT01381172 [Last accessed January, 2025].
39. Chung ES, Katra RP, Ghio S, et al. PROSPECT trial substudy. Eur J Heart Fail. 2010;12(6):581-7.
40. Healy AH, McKellar SH, Drakos SG, et al. J Surg Res. 2016;202(2):363-71.
41. Granegger M, Dave H, Knirsch W, et al. Car diovasc Eng Technol. 2019;10(1):69-79.
42. Fukamachi K, Horvath DJ, Karimov JH, et al. J Thorac Cardiovasc Surg. 2020;162(1):120-6.

CHAPTER

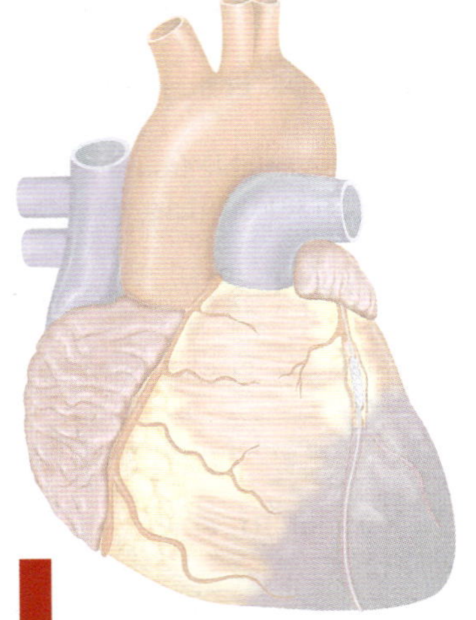

Implant or No-implant, Interatrial Shunt for HFpEF Patients

Ajay M Naik, Aarya A Naik, Aditi A Naik

INTRODUCTION

Guideline-directed medical therapy (GDMT) for heart failure with reduced ejection fraction (HFrEF) is now well established. It includes four pillars: (1) ARNI, (2) beta blockers, (3) MRAs, and (4) SGLT2 inhibitors, with vericiguat probably emerging as the fifth pillar. On the other hand, for heart failure with preserved ejection fraction (HFpEF), the pharmacologic options are limited to SGLT2 inhibitors and further individualization with diuretics, ARNI, or beta blockers. Coexisting morbidities such as diabetes mellitus and hypertension require to be addressed with additional medications. Despite these, the symptomatic and clinical benefit of medications is limited in HFrEF. Device therapy in the form of interatrial shunt (IAS) creation or pacemakers with special algorithms are also being studied to address this problem.[1]

The basic premise of the IAS procedures is decompressing the left atrium (LA). In HF, LA pressures are high. In HFpEF, stiff ventricles and diastolic dysfunction contribute to it. IAS created without or with devices can dynamically unload the LA and reduce the LA pressure at rest and during exertion.[1] Although intuitively this hypothesis may appear attractive, it needs to be proved in clinical outcomes in randomized controlled trials (RCTs). There are a multitude of devices designed and studied in trials with limited number of patients. The benefit–risk data need to be analyzed well before the therapy can be brought into routine practice. Multiple parameters need to be taken into consideration, such as size of shunt, without or with shunt device, design of device, timing of procedure, type of HF, and patient who would benefit the most.

PATHOPHYSIOLOGY OF INTERATRIAL SHUNT IN HIGH LEFT ATRIAL PRESSURE

- Decompression of LA with an IAS to RA may reduce symptoms of pulmonary congestion.
- Reducing chronically high LA pressure also reduces the load in the pulmonary vasculature. This may prevent pathologic progression in the pulmonary venous and arterial walls, thus delaying the onset or reducing the severity of pulmonary hypertension (PH).
- A large LA to RA shunt may result in increased flow to the right-sided chambers, dilated RA and right ventricle (RV), tricuspid regurgitation (TR), RV dysfunction, and right-sided failure.
- Further progression of this pathological process may cause high RA pressures, right to left atrial shunt, hypoxemia, cyanosis, hypoxemic pulmonary vasoconstriction, and PH.
- Atrial dilatation (either or both LA and RA) can predispose to atrial arrhythmias, further worsening the hemodynamics in HF, where atria contribute significantly to ventricular filling and maintaining cardiac output.

BASIC STEPS OF ATRIAL SHUNT THERAPY[1]

1. The procedure is performed percutaneously via common femoral vein access.
2. Transseptal puncture is performed, guided by transesophageal echocardiogram (TEE) or intracardiac echocardiogram.

3. IAS is created by removal of septal tissue or by radiofrequency ablation (RFA) of the tissue.
4. An IAS device (IASD) is placed across the interatrial septum.
5. Shunt may also be created between the LA and the coronary sinus (CS), which would then drain into the RA.

ADVANTAGES OF A SHUNT WITHOUT DEVICE

- Lower incidence of device embolization, infection, device-related thrombosis, or thromboembolism.
- Transseptal access is still possible for future procedures.
- It is possible to close the shunt with closure devices in the future if the need arises.

DISADVANTAGES OF A NONDEVICE SHUNT

- Shunt narrowing or closure due to tissue ingrowth
- Cardiac cycle contractile phases may affect the orifice patency.

INTERATRIAL SHUNT DEVICES IN USE OR UNDER INVESTIGATION (TABLE 1)

Corvia Device

Corvia medical device is a nitinol-based double-disk, 8-mm atrial shunt device. Placement involves a 16F catheter system introduced into the LA after transseptal puncture.

REDUCE LAP-HF I trial was the first RCT conducted in the atrial shunt therapy field. It was a mechanistic study aimed at determining the initial efficacy and safety of the Corvia atrial shunt device.[2] Forty-four patients with HF, EF >40%, elevated exercise PCWP >25 mm Hg, and PCWP to RA pressure gradient >5 mm Hg were randomized 1:1 to the IASD or a sham-control procedure. Patients in the IASD group had a statistically significant ($p = 0.028$) greater reduction in exercise PCWP compared with the sham group at 1-month follow-up.

REDUCE LAP-HF[3] was conducted in patients with HF and EF >40% using rigorous noninvasive screening followed by invasive exercise hemodynamic testing to confirm a peak exercise PCWP >25 mm Hg. This is the largest therapeutic interventional HF trial in HFpEF

TABLE 1: Interatrial shunt devices currently under investigation.

	Corvia	*V-Wave*	*Occlutech*	*Edwards*	*Alleviant*	*NoYA*	*InterShunt*
Device/procedure							
Type	Implant	Implant	Implant	Implant	Procedure	Procedure	Procedure
Description	Nitinol stent	Nitinol/PTFE hourglass	Nitinol braid with central orifice	Tubular nitinol device with retention arms	Coring catheter	RF catheter	Cutting catheter
Shunt flow	LA → RA	LA → RA	LA → RA	LA → CS	LA → RA	LA → RA	LA → RA
Shunt size	8 mm	5.1 mm	4, 6, 8, 10 mm	7 mm	6 mm	4–12 mm	6 mm
Development stage	Pivotal RCT complete, follow-up confirmatory RCT in responder subgroup ongoing	Pivotal RCT enrollment complete, follow-up ongoing	Pivotal RCT enrollment ongoing	Phase 2 feasibility/ mechanistic RCT ongoing	Pivotal RCT enrollment ongoing	Open-label trial ongoing	Small pilot studies in humans

(LA: left atrium; PTFE: polytetrafluoroethylene; RA: right atrium; RCT: randomized controlled trial; RF: radiofrequency)
Source: Adapted from Jagadeesan et al.[1]

to date, with 626 patients randomized. There was a statistically significant increase in major adverse cardiac events in the shunt group compared with the sham group (4 vs. 1%). There were no between-group differences in the primary hierarchical composite endpoint (CV death or nonfatal ischemic stroke at 12 months, followed by HF events up to 24 months, and finally change in KCCQ at 12 months), with a win ratio of 1.0, signifying a "tie" between groups with no overall benefit or harm with IASD versus sham treatment.[4]

Post hoc analyses identified peak exercise PVR <1.74 WU and no cardiac rhythm management (CRM) device (i.e., no pacemaker or implantable cardioverter-defibrillator) at baseline as characteristics that differentiated responders (those with the greatest beneficial treatment response in response to IASD) compared with nonresponders.[5]

RESPONDER-HF (Reevaluation of Atrial Shunt Device in a Precision Medicine Trial to Determine Efficacy in Mildly Reduced or Preserved Ejection Fraction Heart Failure) in patients with the responder phenotype (peak exercise PVR <1.75 WU and no CRM device) is currently underway to validate these findings.

V-Wave Ventura Interatrial Shunt System

This is an hourglass-shaped nitinol skeleton covered with polytetrafluoroethylene. The funnel shape in the central part of the device is designed to provide adequate shunt flow (based on a Venturi effect). The central shunt size has a smaller diameter of 5.1 mm, which theoretically could lower the risk of paradoxical emboli and excessive RV overload by restricting flow.

V-Wave FIH study was an open-label study of 38 HF patients. The original V-Wave device (with a one-way valve to prevent right-to-left shunting) was used. Over one-third of patients had stenosis of the shunt at 12 months due to pannus formation, probably owing to the valve.

Reducing Lung Congestion Symptoms in Advanced Heart Failure trial (*RELIEVE-HF*) is a larger, randomized, sham-controlled pivotal trial with a second iteration of the device without a valve.

Occlutech Atrial Flow Regulator

The atrial flow regulator (Occlutech) is a dual-disk nitinol IASD available in three orifice sizes of 6, 8, and 10 mm.

AFR-PRELIEVE trial studied the device in a prospective, nonrandomized FIH study that enrolled 53 HF patients.

Flow Regulation by Opening the SepTum in Patients with Heart Failure (*FROST-HF*), is the pivotal, prospective, randomized, double-blind, sham-controlled trial currently underway with the goal of randomizing 700 HF patients.

Alleviant

The Alleviant system (Alleviant Medical) utilizes RFA technology to cauterize the interatrial septum and excise a precise disk of septal tissue 7 mm in diameter.

ALLEVIATE-HF 1 and 2 (*Evaluation of the Safety and Feasibility of a Percutaneously Created Interatrial Shunt to Alleviate Heart Failure Symptoms in Patients With Chronic Heart Failure and Preserved or Mid-Range Left Ventricular Ejection Fraction*) included 31 HFpEF patients. The procedure success rate was 100%, there was 100% 6-month shunt patency by TEE and safety events were minimal.

ALLAY-HF (*Safety and Efficacy of the Alleviant System for No-Implant Interatrial Shunt Creation in Patients With Chronic Heart Failure*), a large, multicenter, sham-controlled pivotal RCT of the Alleviant atrial shunt system in patients with HF and EF >40%, is currently underway

Edwards Lifesciences APTURE Shunt

The APTURE shunt (Edwards Lifesciences) uses a nitinol-based frame to create a shunt between the LA and CS with an internal shunt diameter of 7 mm. Theoretical advantages of this approach include preservation of the interatrial septum for future interventions (e.g., AF ablation, LA appendage occlusion, and mitral valve procedures).

The implantation procedure is performed under general anesthesia with TEE guidance and uses a transjugular approach. A 20F guide sheath is inserted into the RA through which a guidewire is inserted into the distal CS. An atriotomy is performed with a solid core needle from the CS into the LA, after using an anchoring balloon to stabilize the system, and a supportive 0.035″ wire to allow placement of the distal end of the shunt into the LA. Balloon dilatation with a 6–8 mm angioplasty balloon is then performed to facilitate the delivery of the device.

ALT-FLOW (*Early Feasibility Study of the Edwards Transcatheter Atrial Shunt System*) was an open-label early feasibility study for this potentially advantageous approach to LA decompression; however, there were some significant adverse safety events, including requirement for emergent surgery.

ALT-FLOW II (*A Randomized, Sham-controlled Trial of the Edwards APTURE Transcatheter Shunt System*) is also underway.

NoYA

The NoYA IAS (NoYA MedTech) is an adjustable RFA-based atrial shunt procedure system. It allows for the creation of an IAS with a waist diameter that ranges from 4 to 12 mm.

Adona

Adona combines an adjustable IAS design with biatrial shunt sensors. The adaptability of the IAS orifice size allows for fine-tuning shunt flow both during the initial procedure and later as needed clinically as per the requirement of each individual patient's hemodynamic requirements.

Intershunt

The InterShunt Percutaneous Atrial Shunt Catheter System (Inter-Shunt Technologies, Inc.) is another deviceless atrial shunt procedure system that excises a 6-mm circular section of tissue in the atrial septum.

OVERVIEW OF CURRENTLY AVAILABLE EVIDENCE

In view of the fact that these are early stages of new device development process, the data are limited. There are >30 prior and active studies involving at least eight different companies in the atrial shunt field. At present, only two RCTs have been completed, both with the Corvia device. The current status of the field remains reliant on single-arm, open-label studies with limited patient numbers.

WHICH PATIENTS WOULD LIKELY BENEFIT FROM INTERATRIAL SHUNT THERAPY?

Evidence for atrial shunt therapeutics is still limited and challenged by different HF presentations and trial designs. Intuitively, if HFrEF patients have a higher prevalence of or are at an increased risk for right heart dysfunction, atrial shunt therapy in these patients could lead to worse outcomes.

The importance of PCWP-RA pressure gradient at rest and/or during exercise for the identification of patients most likely to benefit from atrial shunt therapy remains unknown. The results of pivotal RCTs of other atrial shunt therapies may provide some evidence.

The ability to either maintain a low PVR during exercise (without exercise-induced pulmonary vasoconstriction) or appropriately vasodilate the pulmonary vasculature during exercise (in patients with higher PVR at rest) may be necessary to derive benefit from atrial shunting.[6]

During exercise, if PVR increases to (or remains elevated above) a threshold of 1.75–1.80 WU, blood flow through the pulmonary vasculature is impeded, thereby leading to a greater increase in RA pressure relative to LA pressure. If RA pressure rises to a greater extent than LA pressure during exertion, the LA cannot decompress across the atrial shunt into the RA and systemic veins. The exaggerated rise in RA pressure relative to LA pressure could lead to an intermittent reversal of shunt flow from the RA to LA, resulting in hypoxemia and further increases in PVR (due to hypoxic pulmonary vasoconstriction).

CONTRAINDICATIONS TO INTERATRIAL SHUNT THERAPY

Patients with HF who had significant RV dysfunction, RA pressure elevation, significant TR, or severe PVD would not benefit from atrial shunt therapies due to the following:

- Inability to unload the LA (due to a low LA–RA pressure gradient at rest and during exertion)
- Increased susceptibility to right-sided HF (due to a sicker RV)
- The potential for reversal of the shunt (RA to LA shunt flow), which would be deleterious.

OPTIMAL SIZE OF ATRIAL SHUNTS

The orifice size needs to be optimal to balance adequate LA decompression while avoiding excessive right heart overload and right-sided HF. An 8–9 mm diameter orifice size appeared to be an appropriate size on computer simulation modeling, with less LA decompression at smaller sizes and a greater chance for RV overload at larger sizes.[7]

FUTURE CLINICAL TRIAL DESIGNS

A more comprehensive assessment of patient health status that includes symptom burden, physical/mental/emotional/social status, and health-related QOL (discrepancy between actual and desired well being) may reveal the true benefit of a given therapy. HF patients are also known to willingly concede longevity for an improvement in functional health status ("time trade-off"). A substantial persistent symptomatic or functional improvement would be an acceptable endpoint for drug/device approval as per a 2019 USFDA statement.[8] This is pertinent in HFpEF due to the relative paucity of treatments compared with HFrEF.

LIMITATIONS

Open-label, single-arm studies have demonstrated promising safety and feasibility results with cautiously optimistic clinical endpoints. In trial settings, there is always potential for significant placebo effects and optimized GDMT.

Initial RCT data with a single device and shunt size suggested that a specific responder group with low peak exercise PVR and no CRM device may derive the most benefit.

More robust RCT data will be essential to elucidate the efficacy and safety of the several atrial shunt sizes and designs currently in development. These studies will assist in the identification of the ideal HF subtype that will benefit most from dynamic decompression of the LA with an atrial shunt.

CONCLUSION

Significant advances over the last two decades have improved morbidity and mortality in HF, more so in HFrEF compared with HFpEF.

Suboptimal QOL, persistent symptom burden, adverse side effects, and polypharmacy remain challenges in HF. Atrial shunt therapeutics for HF is a new and exciting frontier that may serve an important role in addressing therapeutic gaps for certain HF patients.

REFERENCES

1. Jagadeesan V, Gray WA, Shah SJ. Atrial shunt therapy for heart failure: an update. J Soc Cardiovasc Angiogr Interv. 2023;2(6 Part B):101203.
2. Feldman T, Komtebedde J, Burkhoff D, et al. Transcatheter interatrial shunt device for the treatment of heart failure: rationale and design of the randomized trial to REDUCE Elevated Left Atrial Pressure in Heart Failure (REDUCE LAP-HF I). Circ Heart Fail. 2016;9(7):e003025.
3. Berry N, Mauri L, Feldman T, et al. Transcatheter interatrial shunt device for the treatment of heart failure: rationale and design of the pivotal randomized trial to REDUCE Elevated Left Atrial Pressure in Patients with Heart Failure II (REDUCE LAP-HF II). Am Heart J. 2020;226:222-31.
4. Shah SJ, Borlaug BA, Chung ES, et al. Atrial shunt device for heart failure with preserved and mildly reduced ejection fraction (REDUCE LAP-HF II): a randomised, multicentre, blinded, sham-controlled trial. Lancet. 2022; 399(10330):1130-40.
5. Borlaug BA, Sharma K, Shah SJ, et al. Heart failure with preserved ejection fraction: JACC scientific statement. J Am Coll Cardiol. 2023;81(18):1810-34.
6. Oakland HT, Shah SJ. Comprehensive investigation of latent pulmonary vascular disease: an important exercise for a novel HFpEF phenotype. JACC Heart Fail. 2023;11(10):1439-42.
7. Kaye D, Shah SJ, Borlaug BA, et al. Effects of an interatrial shunt on rest and exercise hemodynamics: results of a computer simulation in heart failure. J Card Fail. 2014; 20(3):212-21.
8. United States Food and Drug Administration (FDA). Patient-reported outcome measures: use in medical product development to support labeling claims. [online] Available from https://www.fda.gov/regulatory-information/search-fda-guidance-documents/patient-reported-outcome-measures-use-medical-product-development-support-labeling-claims [Last accessed January, 2025].

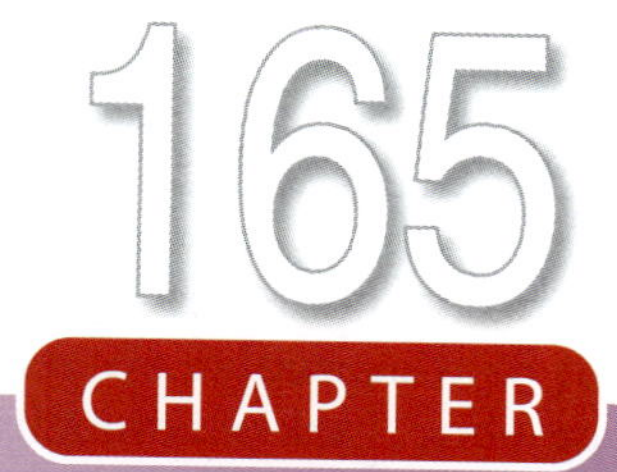

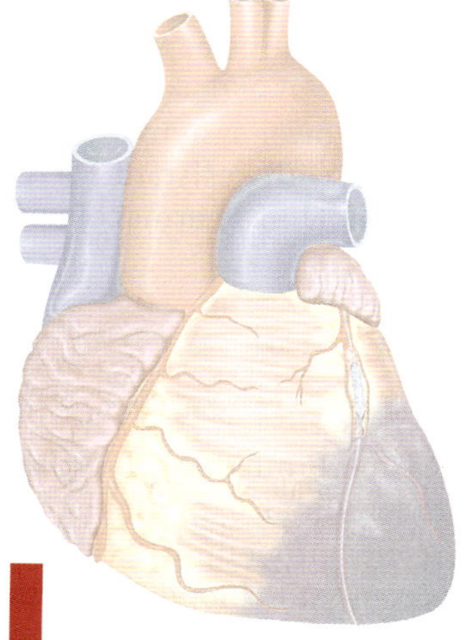

Renal Denervation: A Novel Treatment for Hypertension

Viveka Kumar, Sangeeta Dhir, Mitendra Yadav

INTRODUCTION

Hypertension (HTN), also known as high blood pressure (HBP), is a common cardiovascular condition in which the force of the blood pushing against the walls of the arteries is consistently too high. This condition can strain the heart, damage blood vessels, and increase the risk of health problems such as heart attack, stroke, and kidney disease. Blood pressure is measured in two ways: (1) *Systolic blood pressure (SBP)*, which represents the pressure when the heart beats; the highest pressure is achieved when the heart contracts to pump blood to the body. (2) *Diastolic blood pressure (DBP)*, which represents the pressure when the heart rests between beats, lowest pressure occurring when the heart relaxes after contraction.

A reading of 140/80 mm Hg or higher is generally considered HTN. While it may not cause noticeable symptoms initially, HTN requires careful management through lifestyle changes, regular monitoring, and possibly medication to reduce the risk of serious complications.[1]

TYPES OF HYPERTENSION

Primary HTN has a prevalence of 90–95%, primary causes include genetics, lifestyle, and environmental factors. Secondary HTN has prevalence of 5–10% and causes include cardiovascular, kidney disease, pregnancy, obesity, revascular disease, endocrine disease, mechanical compressions, and others.

GLOBAL CHALLENGE OF HYPERTENSION CONTROL

Hypertension is a leading risk factor for cardiovascular and global health crisis. The average statistics are: Untreated hypertensives are 30%, treated and controlled hypertensives are 35%, treated but uncontrolled hypertensives are 35%, and worldwide hypertensives are 1.1 billion. <20% hypertensive patients have their blood pressure under control. 1.6 billion people to have hypertension by 2025.

Hypertension is estimated to have added $18.6 billion in avoidable cost to the US healthcare system alone. Post pandemic control rates are declining and COVID-19 pandemic accelerated the declining rate of HTN—according to a report from US National Health and Nutritional Examination Survey 2009–2012. Burden of HTN is not borne equally and communities of color are affected disproportionately (Black Americans experience five times more mortality from HTN and related diseases than white Americans).

HYPERTENSION: INDIA PERSPECTIVE

Hypertension is an Indian health crisis, and scaling HTN treatment and control can prevent millions of lives in next decade. Uncontrolled HTN dramatically increases the risk of heart attack, heart failure, stroke, and kidney failure. 53% treated HTN patients do not have their blood pressure under control. HTN is leading preventable cause of heart attack, stroke, and death and reducing SBP by 10 mm Hg leads to clinically meaningful reduction in chances of cardiovascular events regardless of blood pressure baseline. Lack of adherence to medication is recognized as big factor in blood pressure control and is not an easy one to fix in routine practice.

RENAL DENERVATION

Renal denervation (RDN) is an emerging therapeutic approach primarily designed to treat patients with *resistant HTN*, a form of HBP that is difficult to control using conventional medications and lifestyle modifications. RDN targets the sympathetic nervous system, specifically the renal nerves, which play a significant role in the regulation of blood pressure. This chapter will explore the mechanism of action, procedure, indications, clinical evidence, risks, and future directions of RDN.

Anatomy and Physiology of Renal Sympathetic Nerves

The kidneys are vital organs not only for filtration of waste products but also for the regulation of systemic blood pressure. The renal arteries are richly innervated by sympathetic nerves, which are part of the autonomic nervous system. These nerves play a crucial role in the regulation of blood pressure by modulating renal blood flow, salt and water retention, and the release of hormones such as *renin*.

The sympathetic nervous system regulates vascular tone and cardiac output by releasing neurotransmitters such as *norepinephrine*. Overactivation of these renal sympathetic nerves contributes to sustained increases in blood pressure. In patients with HTN, these nerves are often found to be hyperactive, leading to excessive activation of the renin-angiotensin-aldosterone system (RAAS) and sodium retention, which collectively elevate blood pressure.

Mechanism of Action of Renal Denervation

Renal denervation aims to interrupt the sympathetic nerve signals to the kidneys, effectively "quieting" the overactive nerves and reducing their influence on blood pressure regulation. The procedure involves applying ablative energy (such as radiofrequency, ultrasound, or laser energy) to the renal arteries, which causes destruction or modification of the renal sympathetic nerves. By reducing sympathetic nervous system overactivity, *vasodilation* occurs in the renal vasculature, improving renal blood flow. *Reduced renin secretion* leads to decreased activation of the RAAS system. *Decreased sodium retention* and reduced fluid volume contribute to lower blood pressure.

The ultimate goal of RDN is to lower systemic blood pressure, particularly in patients with resistant HTN, who have not responded adequately to pharmacologic treatments.

Procedure

The procedure involves the following:

- *Patient preparation:* RDN is performed in a hospital setting by a skilled interventional cardiologist or vascular surgeon. Before the procedure, patients undergo standard assessments for blood pressure measurement, blood tests (renal function and electrolytes), and angiography to visualize the renal arteries. Patients are typically sedated and local anesthesia is administered at the catheter insertion site.
- *Catheter insertion:* A catheter is inserted through the femoral artery and guided to the renal arteries using fluoroscopic guidance. The catheter contains electrodes or other energy-delivery mechanisms to apply energy to the renal arteries.
- *Energy application:* Once the catheter reaches the renal arteries, it delivers energy to the walls of the arteries where the sympathetic nerves are located. The most commonly used energy sources are: *Radiofrequency ablation (RFA)* that delivers heat to the renal arteries, disrupting the nerves; *ultrasound* that are high-frequency sound waves used to achieve similar effects as RFA; and *cryoablation that* uses freezing temperatures to damage the nerves (less commonly used).

The procedure may target several sites along the renal artery to ensure comprehensive treatment. It is usually completed in 30–60 minutes and patients may be discharged the same day.

Indications for Renal Denervation

The indications for RDN are as follows:

- *Resistant HTN:* It is defined as HBP that remains above target levels despite the use of three or more antihypertensive medications, including a diuretic. Resistant HTN is often characterized by hyperactivity of the sympathetic nervous system and underlying conditions, for example, obesity, diabetes, or chronic kidney disease.
- *Sympathetic nervous system overactivity:* RDN may also be indicated in patients with sympathetic

nervous system-mediated HTN. In this condition, the sympathetic nervous system is overactive and there is little or no response to standard pharmacologic treatments.

- *Secondary HTN:* In some cases, RDN may be explored for secondary forms of HTN, such as primary hyperaldosteronism or pheochromocytoma, where sympathetic nerve overactivity contributes to elevated blood pressure.

CLINICAL EVIDENCE AND EFFECTIVENESS OF RENAL DENERVATION ON CONTROLLING THE HYPERTENSION

The clinical evidence supporting RDN has evolved over the years. Initial studies and early-stage trials demonstrated promising results, showing significant reductions in blood pressure following the procedure. However, the subsequent large-scale clinical trials have yielded mixed results.

- *Symplicity HTN-1 and HTN-2 trials:* These studies suggested that RDN could lead to a substantial reduction in blood pressure in patients with resistant HTN, even in the absence of significant changes in medication.[2]
- *Symplicity HTN-3:* This pivotal trial, however, failed to demonstrate a significant difference in blood pressure reduction between the RDN and control groups, sparking debates regarding its overall effectiveness.
- *SPYRAL HTN-OFF MED pivotal trial* assessed the efficacy of catheter-based RDN in patients with HTN who were not taking any antihypertensive medications. The study demonstrated that RDN resulted in significant and sustained reductions in office-based blood pressure in the absence of pharmacological treatment. Over a period of 3 months, patients who underwent RDN experienced a notable decrease in both SBP and DBP compared to the sham procedure group. These results suggest that RDN can effectively lower blood pressure in patients without relying on medication, providing a promising alternative for managing HTN, particularly for those who are unable to tolerate or do not wish to take antihypertensive drugs. However, further long-term studies are needed to confirm the durability and broader applicability of these findings.
- *SPYRAL HTN-ON MED trial* evaluated the long-term efficacy and safety of RDN in patients with HTN who were already on antihypertensive medications. The study found that RDN when combined with continued medication, resulted in significant and sustained reductions in blood pressure over a period of 3–12 months.[3] Importantly, the procedure was well tolerated, with a safety profile comparable to that of a placebo. These results suggest that RDN can be an effective adjunctive therapy for patients with resistant HTN,[4] offering additional blood pressure control alongside ongoing pharmacologic treatment. However, long-term data is still needed to fully understand the durability and broader implications of this approach.
- *Ongoing trials and studies:* Despite the challenges faced in some trials, RDN remains an area of active research. Newer studies have focused on refining patient selection, improving the technique, and better understanding the long-term benefits of the procedure.

RISKS AND COMPLICATIONS

Risks and complications of RDN are as follows:

- *Vascular complications:* There is a risk of vascular complications, such as bleeding, hematoma, or injury to the renal arteries
- *Kidney injury:* There is a risk of damage to the renal arteries or kidneys, which can impair renal function.
- *Infection:* As with any catheter-based procedure, there is a risk of infection at the catheter insertion site.
- *Hypotension:* A drop in blood pressure after the procedure can occur, thus requiring careful monitoring.

FUTURE DIRECTIONS

Renal denervation is still a developing treatment, and further refinement is needed. Some future considerations include:

- *Improved patient selection:* More precise identification of the patients who will benefit most from RDN (e.g., patients with specific forms of sympathetic overactivity) is needed.
- *Technological advancements:* Newer, more effective energy delivery methods, such as ultrasound or cryoablation, may improve the safety and efficacy of the procedure.
- *Long-term outcomes:* More long-term studies are needed to assess the durability of blood pressure control post-RDN and its effects on cardiovascular outcomes.

CONCLUSION

Renal denervation offers a novel approach to managing resistant HTN, particularly in patients with sympathetic nervous system overactivity. While the procedure shows promise, ongoing research and clinical trials are essential to determine its long-term efficacy, optimal patient selection, and safety profile. As technology improves and understanding of the underlying mechanisms expands, RDN may become an integral part of the HTN treatment landscape.

REFERENCES

1. Mahfoud F, Kandzari DE, Kario K, et al. Long term efficacy and safety of renal denervation in the process of antihypertensive drugs (SPYRAL HTN-ON MED): a randomized sham-controlled trial. Lancet 2022;399:1401-10.
2. Mahfoud F, Mancia G, Schmieder R, et al. Outcomes following radiofrequency renal denervation according to antihypertensive medications: subgroup analysis of the global SYMPLICITY Registry DEFINE. Hypertension. 2023;80(8):1759-70.
3. Kandzari DA, Böhm M, Mahfoud F, et al. Effect of renal denervation on blood pressure in the presence of antihypertensive drugs: 6-month efficacy and safety results from the SPYRAL HTN-ON MED proof-of-concept randomised trial. Lancet. 2018;391(10137):2346-55.
4. Mahfoud F, Mancia G, Schmieder R, et al. Renal denervation in high-risk patients with hypertension. J Am Coll Cardiol. 2020;75(23):2879-88.

SECTION 20

HFpEF and Rehabilitation

166. Exercise Training and Rehabilitation in HFpEF

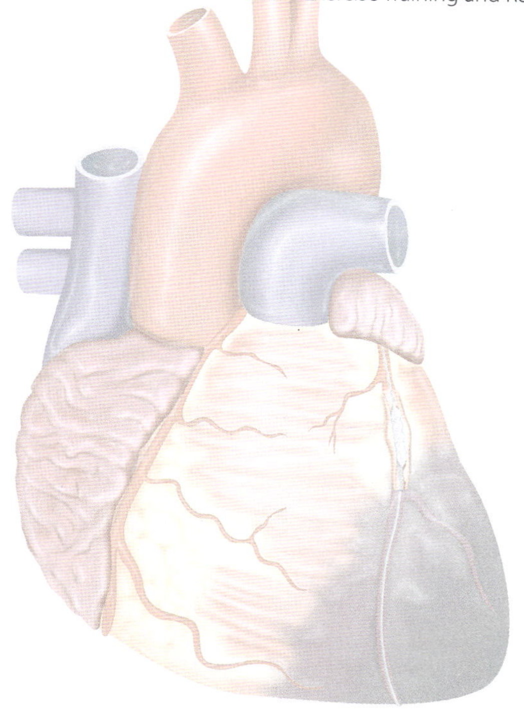

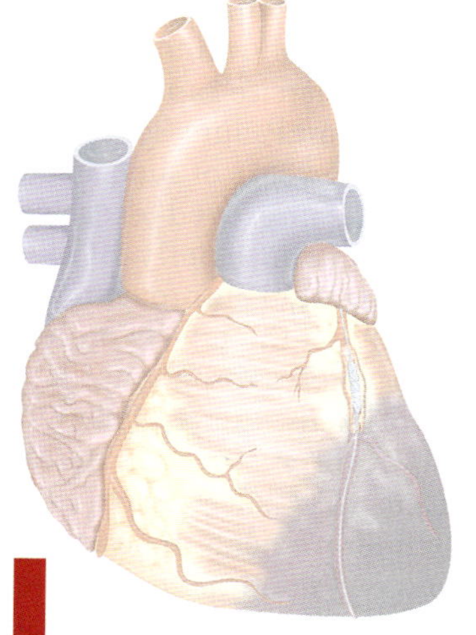

Exercise Training and Rehabilitation in HFpEF

Kushal Madan, Kavita Tyagi, JPS Sawhney

INTRODUCTION

Heart failure with preserved ejection fraction (HFpEF) is characterized by normal left ventricular ejection fraction but impaired ventricular relaxation and filling, leading to elevated filling pressures. This condition accounts for approximately 50% of heart failure (HF) cases, with a high prevalence in elderly, hypertensive, and obese populations. Exercise training has emerged as a promising intervention, with evidence suggesting improvements in functional capacity and quality of life (QoL).

EXERCISE INTOLERANCE IN HEART FAILURE WITH PRESERVED EJECTION FRACTION

Exercise intolerance is a key feature of HFpEF and is associated with poor QoL, a higher incidence of hospitalization, and poor outcomes.[1] Exercise intolerance in HFpEF is due to several factors, including impaired cardiac output, endothelial dysfunction, and skeletal muscle abnormalities. The pathophysiology of HFpEF involves systemic inflammation, endothelial dysfunction, and myocardial fibrosis, leading to increased ventricular stiffness. The result is impaired diastolic filling and reduced cardiac output, particularly during exertion. Additionally, comorbid conditions such as hypertension, obesity, and diabetes contribute to the disease burden.

Aerobic exercise capacity can be quantified objectively and reproducibly in patients with HFpEF as peak oxygen uptake (VO_2) by expired gas analysis. The most commonly used practical alternative for assessing exercise performance in HFpEF is the 6-minute-walk test demonstrating values that are comparable to those in patients with heart failure with reduced ejection fraction (HFrEF) and markedly reduced relative to control subjects.

ROLE OF EXERCISE IN HEART FAILURE WITH PRESERVED EJECTION FRACTION

Exercise for Prevention of Heart Failure with Preserved Ejection Fraction

Physical activity prevents HFpEF through two main mechanisms: (1) By reducing the negative effect of many conventional risk factors for HFpEF (e.g., LDL cholesterol, obesity, and insulin sensitivity) and (2), by exerting beneficial effects on heart structure and cardiovascular performance (e.g., cardiac remodeling and cardiopulmonary performance).[2]

A recent study demonstrated the association between exercise, body mass index, and HF in a cohort of >50,000 patients. It was shown that, among HF subtypes, the cumulative incidence of HFpEF was significantly lower across the higher physical activities subtype as compared to the association between higher levels of physical exercise and the cumulative risk of HFrEF, which was not statistically significant.[3]

In another study involving >20,000 subjects, it was shown that, after adjustment for HF risk factors (i.e., age, blood pressure, diabetes mellitus, body mass index, smoking status, and total cholesterol), a 1-unit greater fitness level in metabolic equivalents reached in midlife was associated with a lower risk HF hospitalization after the age of 65, but with only a modest effect on the risk of coronary diseases.[4]

However, low fitness and physical inactivity also negatively impact through direct effects on the HFpEF risk; specifically, it has been shown that low fitness is associated with a higher prevalence of cardiac remodeling and diastolic dysfunction,[5] suggesting that exercise may lower HF risk through its effect on favorable cardiac remodeling and the prevention of diastolic dysfunction; as a result, inactivity is correlated with diastolic dysfunction, determining a higher risk of HFpEF.

Exercise training has been shown to improve these factors by enhancing peripheral vascular function, increasing skeletal muscle oxidative capacity, and improving autonomic regulation. The primary outcome of interest in exercise interventions is often peak VO_2, a key determinant of exercise capacity and an independent predictor of mortality in HFpEF patients.

EVIDENCE FROM CLINICAL TRIALS

Systematic Reviews and Meta-analyses

A systematic review and meta-analysis conducted by Baral et al. (2024)[6] evaluated the efficacy of exercise training on functional, physiological, and QoL outcomes in HFpEF patients. The analysis included 14 randomized controlled trials (RCTs) with a total of 629 participants, predominantly female, with a mean age of 68.1 years. The findings demonstrated that exercise training significantly improved peak VO_2 [mean difference (MD) 1.96 mL/kg/min, 95% confidence interval (CI) 1.25–2.68; $p < 0.00001$] and Minnesota Living with Heart Failure (MLWHF) score (MD -12.06, 95% CI -17.11 to -7.01; $p < 0.00001$), indicating enhanced exercise capacity and QoL.

Subgroup analyses revealed that high-intensity interval training (HIIT) was associated with a small but significant improvement in peak VO_2 compared to moderate-intensity continuous training (MCT) (MD 1.25 mL/kg/min, 95% CI 0.41–2.08, $p = 0.003$). However, these improvements in exercise capacity did not translate into significant changes in diastolic function markers, such as E/A ratio, deceleration time, or E/e′ ratio, suggesting that while exercise improves functional outcomes, its effects on cardiac structure and function may be limited.

TYPES OF EXERCISE TRAINING

Exercise interventions in HFpEF typically include aerobic training, resistance training, or a combination of both. Aerobic training, which can be delivered as continuous moderate-intensity exercise or HIIT, aims to improve cardiovascular endurance and peripheral oxygen utilization. Resistance training focuses on increasing muscle strength and endurance, which is crucial in combating the skeletal muscle abnormalities observed in HFpEF.

- *Aerobic training:* The most studied form of exercise in HFpEF, aerobic training, has been shown to improve peak VO_2, a critical measure of exercise capacity. The Exercise Training in Diastolic Heart Failure (Ex-DHF)[7] pilot study demonstrated that 16 weeks of supervised aerobic training significantly improved exercise capacity and reduced symptoms in elderly HFpEF patients. The study also suggested improvements in endothelial function, although the effects on left ventricular diastolic function were less pronounced.
- *HIIT:* It involves short bursts of intense exercise followed by periods of lower-intensity recovery. Several studies, including the OptimEx-Clin trial,[8] have shown that HIIT may provide superior improvements in peak VO_2 compared to moderate-intensity continuous exercise in HFpEF patients. However, the benefits of HIIT must be balanced against the potential challenges such as patient adherence, the intensity of the exercise, etc.
- *Resistance training:* While less studied in HFpEF compared to aerobic training, resistance training is increasingly recognized for its benefits in improving muscle strength, endurance, and overall physical function. Resistance training can be particularly beneficial in HFpEF patients who may have reduced muscle mass and strength due to aging and comorbidities.
- *Inspiratory muscle training (IMT):* IMT targets the respiratory muscles, which can be weakened in HFpEF and contribute to dyspnea and reduced exercise capacity. Studies have shown that IMT can improve inspiratory muscle strength, reduce dyspnea, and enhance exercise capacity in HFpEF patients, although the overall impact on cardiac function remains unclear.

IMPACT OF EXERCISE ON QUALITY OF LIFE

Quality of life (is a critical outcome for HFpEF patients. Exercise training has consistently been shown to improve QoL in HFpEF, as measured by tools such as the MLWHF questionnaire. Improvements in QoL are likely mediated through enhanced physical function, reduced symptoms, and psychological benefits associated with regular physical activity. Additionally, exercise may help mitigate the impact of comorbid conditions, such as obesity and diabetes, which are prevalent in the HFpEF population.

MECHANISMS UNDERLYING EXERCISE BENEFITS IN HFpEF

The beneficial effects of exercise in HFpEF are mediated through several mechanisms:

- *Peripheral adaptations:* Exercise training enhances endothelial function and increases skeletal muscle capillary density, which improves oxygen delivery and utilization during physical activity. These peripheral adaptations are crucial in HFpEF, where cardiac output is often insufficient to meet the metabolic demands of exercise.

- *Cardiovascular remodeling:* Although the effects of exercise on left ventricular remodeling in HFpEF are less clear, some studies suggest that regular exercise may reduce ventricular stiffness and improve diastolic function. These effects may be more pronounced with longer durations of training or higher intensity protocols, although more research is needed to confirm these findings.
- *Autonomic regulation:* HFpEF is associated with autonomic dysfunction, characterized by increased sympathetic activity and reduced parasympathetic tone. Exercise training has been shown to improve autonomic balance, reduce resting heart rate, and improve heart rate variability, which are associated with better outcomes in HF.
- *Metabolic benefits:* Exercise improves insulin sensitivity and reduces inflammation, both of which are important in the pathophysiology of HFpEF. These metabolic benefits may help to reduce the progression of HFpEF and improve overall cardiovascular health.

CURRENT GUIDELINES FOR EXERCISE TRAINING IN PATIENTS WITH HEART FAILURE

A recent update to the American College of Cardiology and American Heart Association guidelines for heart failure (HF) management endorse exercise training as a Class 1 recommendation (Level of Evidence A) for HF patients. While this recommendation does not differentiate between HFpEF and (HFrEF, the evidence primarily derives from studies on supervised exercise training in chronic HFrEF patients. Furthermore, the guidelines emphasize the importance of managing comorbidities in the treatment of HFpEF, suggesting that individuals with conditions such as hypertension, obesity, and diabetes may also gain from supervised exercise training.[9]

CONSIDERATIONS IN EXERCISE PRESCRIPTION FOR HFpEF

The following are the considerations in exercise prescription for HFpEF:

- Adherence to exercise programs can be challenging for HFpEF patients, particularly those with comorbidities or severe symptoms.
- HFpEF patients are often elderly and may have multiple comorbid conditions, making safety a key consideration in exercise prescription. It is essential to tailor exercise intensity and duration for the individual's fitness level and to monitor for any adverse events during exercise.
- While short-term improvements in exercise capacity and QoL have been demonstrated, the long-term sustainability of these benefits is less certain.
- Not all HFpEF patients respond equally to exercise training. Factors such as baseline fitness level, severity of HFpEF, and presence of comorbidities may influence the extent of benefit from exercise.

CARDIAC REHABILITATION AND EXERCISE TRAINING GUIDELINES

For patients with clinically stable HFpEF who do not have contraindications to exercise, it is advisable to engage in endurance exercises. Exercises should target large muscle groups, such as cycling and walking. These exercises should be performed for 45–60 minutes, 3–5 days per week, at moderate-to-high intensity to enhance peak VO_2. The intensity of endurance training can be tailored based on the maximal heart rate reserve (HRR), percentage of VO_2peak, or the rate of perceived exertion (RPE). In cases where a maximal cardiopulmonary exercise test (CPX) has been conducted, the initial training intensity during the first few sessions should be set at 40–50% of VO_2peak, gradually increasing to 70–80% as the individual improves in exercise tolerance. If peak heart rate is assessed, the recommended training intensity can be expressed as 40–70% of HRR, calculated using the formula: HRR = 40–70% (peak HR – resting HR) + resting HR. If measuring VO_2 peak or peak heart rate is not feasible or reliable (e.g., due to beta-blocker therapy), the training intensity can instead be guided by the Borg RPE scale, targeting a range of 10–14 out of 20.

The literature on the efficacy and safety of HIIT in HFpEF patients is limited, recent literature offers guidance for its implementation and monitoring in clinical settings. HIIT should ideally include high-intensity intervals of large muscle exercises lasting 10–20 minutes, alternating with active recovery periods, totaling 25–35 minutes of exercise three times per week. These intervals can be structured either as shorter bursts (15–60 seconds of activity at 80–100% of peak power output, followed by equal periods of recovery) or longer intervals (4 minutes at 90–95% peak heart rate, with 3 minutes of active recovery at 50–70% peak heart rate). It is recommended that patients begin their exercise training with shorter intervals, progressively increasing the duration as their tolerance improves. Additionally, training sessions should be supervised to monitor heart rate and RPE. Ensure making necessary adjustments to workload (such as speed or incline) to facilitate continued progress. A brief warm-up and cool-down period, lasting 3–5 minutes each, at light-to-moderate intensity, is recommended before and after endurance or HIIT sessions.

Individuals with HFpEF often present with issues related to both skeletal muscle quantity and quality, which can hinder exercise tolerance and overall physical function. Consequently, resistance training serves as a beneficial approach to enhance muscle strength, quality, and physical function in HF patients. The ideal intensity for resistance training should align with the patient's specific goals. For those aiming to increase muscular endurance, lower-intensity exercises [30–40% of one-repetition maximum (1-RM_, with 10–25 repetitions]should be performed 2–3 times a week. In contrast, for those focused on building strength, higher intensities (40–60% of 1-RM, with 8–15 repetitions) are recommended, also 2–3 times a week. To promote safety and effective progression in muscular strength, a lower starting intensity is advisable, with gradual increases over time to avoid injury and maximize skeletal muscle adaptations.

SAFETY DURING EXERCISE TRAINING IN HFpEF

In a recent meta-analysis conducted by Dieberg et al.,[10] which reviewed seven exercise intervention studies primarily set in cardiac rehabilitation (CR) environments, no fatalities were linked to exercise training among 258 patients with HFpEF. Over a total of 3,744 hours of monitored exercise, these findings indicate a minimal risk of serious or fatal incidents occurring during supervised exercise sessions.

CONCLUSION

Larger RCTs with longer follow-up periods are needed to confirm the benefits of exercise training in HFpEF and to explore the long-term effects on morbidity and mortality. Further research into the mechanisms by which exercise improves outcomes in HFpEF is essential. This includes studying the effects of different types of exercise on cardiac function, vascular health, and metabolic regulation. The use of technology, such as wearable devices and mobile health applications, offers opportunities to enhance exercise adherence, monitor progress, and provide real-time feedback to patients and healthcare providers.

Exercise training is a valuable intervention for patients with HFpEF, offering significant improvements in exercise capacity and QoL. While high-intensity exercise may provide additional benefits over moderate-intensity exercise, the optimal exercise regimen for HFpEF remains to be fully elucidated. As the evidence base grows, exercise should become an integral component of the management strategy for HFpEF, alongside pharmacological treatments and lifestyle modifications.

REFERENCES

1. Salzano A, De Luca M, Israr MZ, et al. Exercise intolerance in heart failure with preserved ejection fraction. Heart Fail Clin. 2021;17:397-413.
2. Kondamudi N, Haykowsky M, Forman DE, et al. Exercise training for prevention and treatment of heart failure. Prog Cardiovasc Dis. 2017;60:115-20.
3. Pandey A, LaMonte M, Klein L, et al. Relationship between physical activity, body mass index, and risk of heart failure. J Am Coll Cardiol. 2017;69:1129-42.
4. Berry JD, Pandey A, Gao A, et al. Physical fitness and risk for heart failure and coronary artery disease. Circ Heart Fail. 2013;6:627-34.
5. Brinker SK, Pandey A, Ayers CR, et al. Association of cardiorespiratory fitness with left ventricular remodeling and diastolic function: The Cooper Center Longitudinal Study. JACC Heart Fail. 2014;2:238-46.
6. Baral R, Ho JSY, Soroya AN, et al. Exercise training improves exercise capacity and quality of life in heart failure with preserved ejection fraction: a systematic review and meta-analysis of randomized controlled trials. Eur Heart J Open. 2024;4(4):oeae033.
7. Edelmann F, Bobenko A, Gelbrich G, et al. Exercise training in Diastolic Heart Failure (Ex-DHF): Rationale and design of a multicentre, prospective, randomized, controlled, parallel group trial. Eur J Heart Fail. 2017; 19(8):1067-74.
8. Mueller S, Winzer EB, Duvinage A, et al.; OptimEx-Clin Study Group. Effect of high-intensity interval training, moderate continuous training, or guideline-based physical activity advice on peak oxygen consumption in patients with heart failure with preserved ejection fraction: A randomized clinical trial. JAMA. 2021;325(6):542-51.
9. Heidenreich PA, Bozkurt B, Aguilar D, et al. 2022 AHA/ACC/HFSA guideline for the management of heart failure: a report of the American College of Cardiology/American Heart Association Joint Committee on Clinical Practice Guidelines. J Am Coll Cardiol. 2022;79(17):e263-421.
10. Dieberg G, Ismail H, Giallauria F, et al. Clinical outcomes and cardiovascular responses to exercise training in heart failure patients with preserved ejection fraction: a systematic review and meta-analysis. J Appl Physiol. 2015;119(6):726-33.

SECTION 21

HFpEF and Future Direction

167. Recent Advances in HFpEF
168. Ongoing Drugs and Device Trials in HFpEF
169. Emerging Epidemic of HFpEF: Issues and Challenges in 2025 and Beyond

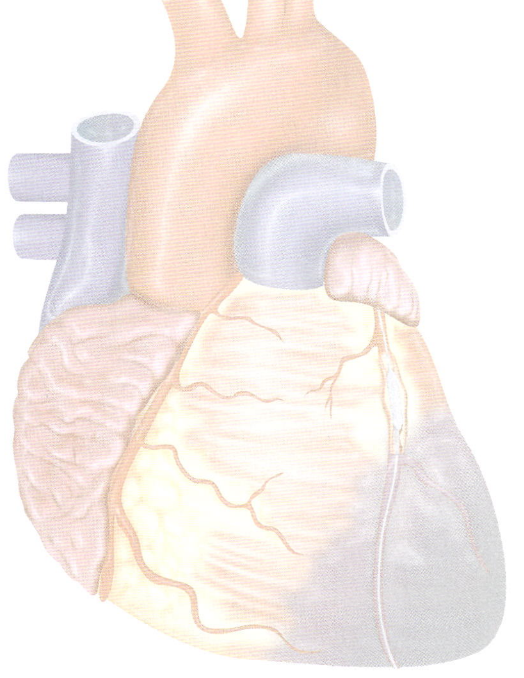

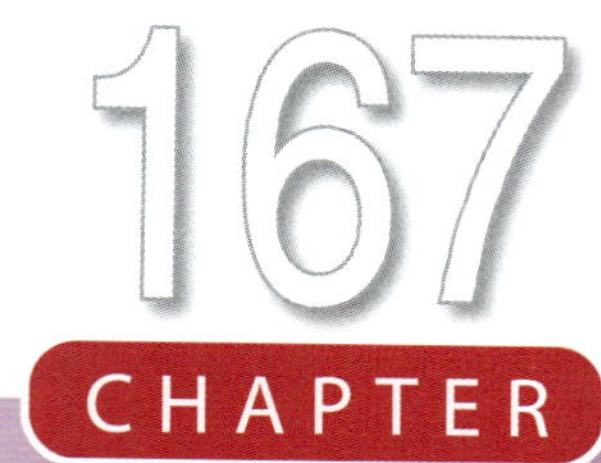

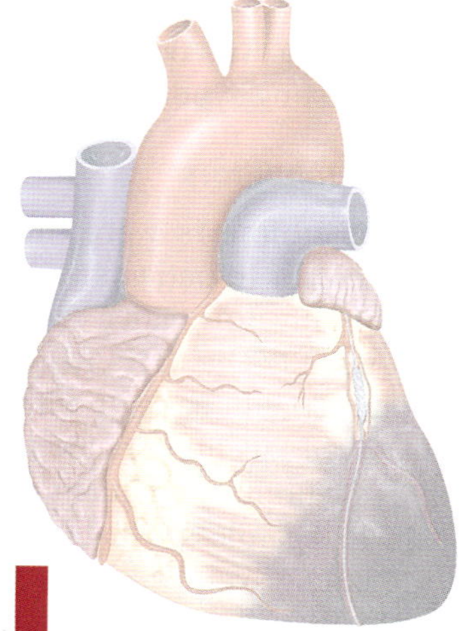

Recent Advances in HFpEF

Aatish Rengan, Sourabh Agstam, Atit A Gawalkar, Sandeep Seth

INTRODUCTION

Heart failure (HF) affects nearly 23 million people worldwide with an estimated prevalence of symptomatic HF ranging from 0.4% to 2%.[1,2] The prevalence of HF rises exponentially with age and affects 4–8% of people over the age of 65 years.[3]

The distribution of ejection fraction (EF) across unselected populations of HF patients is bimodal with peaks centered around 35% and 55%.[4] Approximately half of patients have heart failure with preserved ejection fraction (HFpEF), defined as left ventricular ejection fraction (LVEF) greater than 50%, while the remaining have heart failure with reduced ejection fraction (HFrEF).[4] The prevalence of HFpEF increases dramatically with age and is much more common in women than in men at any age. The prevalence of HFpEF appears to be increasing, perhaps as a result of increasing aging population and increased recognition of the diagnosis.

The 5-year mortality rates for HFrEF range between 53% and 74%, which are comparable to or slightly lower than that of HFrEF.[5,6] The Meta-Analysis Global Group in Chronic Heart Failure (MAGGIC) meta-analysis, reported that patients with HFpEF had lower risk of death from any cause compared to those with HFrEF independent of age, sex, and etiology.[7] As expected, with older age and greater prevalence of comorbidities, the proportion of deaths from non-CV causes is generally higher in HFpEF than in HFrEF. Importantly, cardiovascular (CV) causes still comprise one of the predominant causes of death even in HF patients with LVEF above 40%. Sudden death accounted for up to 43% of CV mortality (~25–30% of total deaths) in clinical trials that included patients with HF and LVEF >40%, with HF deaths accounting for another 20–30% of CV deaths.[8,9]

The rate of hospitalization in HFpEF is high. Following the new diagnosis of HFpEF, patients were hospitalized an average of 1.39 times per year in Olmsted County, Minnesota, with hospitalizations for noncardiovascular causes being more common (0.88 per person-year) than CV hospitalizations (0.46 per person-year).[10] The rate of hospitalization, duration of hospitalization, and quality of life are similar in HFrEF and HFpEF.[10,11]

Considering the significantly high burden of HFpEF and the dismal outcomes comparable to HFrEF, it is alarming that several therapies that have proven to be beneficial in HFrEF have shown no benefit in patients with HF and higher LVEF.

This is primarily due to multifactorial pathophysiology and the heterogeneity in the presentation of this clinical entity, which may entail a more phenotype-specific approach for these patients as compared to the empirical four-pillar approach in HFrEF patients.

RECENT ADVANCES

Multifactorial Pathophysiology

The pathophysiology of HFpEF has been an area of intense research over the past decade. A multitude of factors have been studied and implicated in the pathophysiology of HFpEF and form the primary distinguishing feature between HFrEF, which is primarily a cardiac structural impairment, and HFpEF, which is a condition due to secondary myocardial injury caused by various systemic afflictions like obesity, skeletal muscle dysfunction, renal dysfunction, atrial fibrillation, and systemic microvascular dysfunction.

The comorbidity–inflammation–endothelial dysfunction paradigm has garnered recent attention in HFpEF because patients with HFpEF often have multiple comorbidities, and markers of systemic inflammation are more potent risk factors for incident HFpEF compared with incident HFrEF. Endothelial inflammation causes increased reactive oxygen species, reduced nitric oxide (NO) bioavailability, increased inducible NO synthase (iNOS), and production of peroxynitrite, resulting in reduced soluble guanylate cyclase activity, lower cGMP content, and reduced protein kinase G (PKG). Decreased PKG leads to increased cardiomyocyte hypertrophy, cardiomyocyte stiffness (due to changes in titin phosphorylation), pulmonary vasoconstriction, impaired renal and skeletal muscle function, and increased adiposity.

The pathophysiological role of epicardial adipose tissue (EAT) is also being increasingly recognized. EAT shares a common microcirculation with the heart and can serve as a source of adipocytokines through its anatomical intimacy with the myocardium, contributing to focal and systemic inflammation.[12] Pugliese et al. studied the association of EAT with clinical biomarkers, comprehensive exercise testing, and outcomes in 393 patients with HF. It was found that EAT thickness was significantly increased in patients with HFpEF relative to controls. In HFpEF, thicker EAT (EAT >5 mm) was associated with higher concentrations of troponin T, hs-CRP, and IL-6. Thicker EAT was associated with a decreased VO_2 max and increased risk for CV death or HF hospitalization (HFH).[13] This provides us with evidence of a pathophysiological role of EAT in HFpEF, which may serve as a potential target as well. Because aldosterone can promote the accumulation of EAT, mineralocorticoid receptor antagonists (MRAs) might be beneficial in reducing EAT.[14] Finally, a study in patients with type 2 diabetes mellitus (T2DM) showed that sodium–glucose cotransporter 2 (SGLT2) inhibitors might decrease the quantity of visceral and epicardial fat and reduce the secretion of inflammatory adipokines.[15] Further studies are warranted to determine the beneficial role of MRAs and SGLT2 inhibitors through EAT modulation.

Pharmacological Therapies

There were no available pharmacological therapies with demonstrated benefit in the outcomes of patients with HFpEF until 2021. However, in the past three exciting years of our evolving understanding of the disease, new drugs have demonstrated their benefits and potential future targets have been identified. Also, retrospective analysis of the past trials in this subset of patients with our current understanding has led to some interesting hypotheses.

Sodium–Glucose Cotransporter-2 Inhibitors

Sodium–glucose cotransporter-2 inhibitors were the first class of drugs to improve outcomes in patients with HFpEF, and to this date, remain the only drug with a class I indication for the treatment of HFpEF. The EMPEROR-Preserved (Empagliflozin Outcome Trial in Patients with Chronic Heart Failure with Preserved Ejection Fraction) trial demonstrated a reduction in the primary endpoint of CV death or HFH with empagliflozin regardless of diabetes (13.8% vs. 17.1%, HR 0.79, $p < 0.001$) driven by reduced HFH (8.6% vs. 11.8%, HR 0.71). Death from CV causes did not differ significantly between the two groups.[16]

Similarly, the DELIVER (Dapagliflozin in Heart Failure with Mildly Reduced or Preserved Ejection Fraction) trial showed a significant reduction in the primary composite endpoint of worsening HF event or CV death with dapagliflozin (16.4% vs. 19.5%, HR 0.82, $p < 0.001$), irrespective of T2DM.[17] This was again, driven by reduction in worsening HF events.

GLP1 Analogs

With evolving understanding of the causative role of obesity in the pathophysiology of HFpEF, the effect of semaglutide, a GLP1 analog with proven efficacy in weight reduction, was studied in an obese patient population (BMI ≥30 kg/m^2) with HFpEF with or without T2DM in the STEP-HFpEF and the STEP-HFpEF DM trials, respectively. Treatment with once-weekly injectable semaglutide (2.4 mg) showed a statistically significant reduction in the primary endpoints of change from baseline in the Kansas City Cardiomyopathy Questionnaire clinical summary score (KCCQ-CSS) and change in body weight, irrespective of the presence of diabetes. The studies also showed significant improvement in the six-minute-walk distance (6MWD) and reduction in the C-reactive protein (CRP) levels in the semaglutide arm.[18,19]

An interesting insight from these trials was that the benefits with respect to HF were consistent in the two trials despite the 40% lower weight reduction observed in patients with diabetes compared to the patients without diabetes. This may suggest that the mechanisms of benefit with semaglutide may extend beyond weight loss and may include direct effects on decongestion; vascular, skeletal muscle, and mitochondrial function; epicardial adipose tissue; inflammation; and insulin resistance—factors that (unlike weight loss) may be more pronounced in patients with T2DM than in those without T2DM.

Mineralocorticoid Receptor Antagonists

The data on the effects of use of MRAs in HFpEF, until recently, has been suggestive at best. The TOPCAT (Treatment of Preserved Cardiac Function Heart Failure with an Aldosterone Antagonist) trial showed that the primary endpoint of CV death, chronic HF (CHF) hospitalization, or resuscitated cardiac arrest over 6 years was similar between the spironolactone and placebo arms (18.6% vs. 20.4%, HR 0.89, 95% CI 0.77–1.04) in HF patients with LVEF ≥45%. However, on looking at the individual endpoints, HFH was lower in the spironolactone arm (12% vs. 14.2%, $p = 0.042$).[20]

An interesting post-hoc analysis identified possible regional differences in the effect of aldosterone antagonists.[21]

Finerenone, a nonsteroidal MRA, was evaluated recently in the FINEARTS-HF trial and showed a significant reduction in the primary composite endpoint of total worsening HF events and CV deaths compared with placebo (HR 0.84, $p = 0.007$).[22]

And now that there is conclusive evidence of benefit with MRAs in HFpEF, spironolactone is also currently being tested in two additional large outcomes trials in HFpEF (SPIRRIT and SPIRIT trials) in an effort to validate the findings in TOPCAT-Americas.

Angiotensin Receptor Neprilysin Inhibitors

The PARAGON-HF trial tested sacubitril/valsartan compared with valsartan in 4,822 patients with NYHA Class II–IV HF and LVEF ≥45%. It showed a 13% reduction in total HFH and CV death (HR 0.87, 95% CI 0.75–1.01), which just missed statistical significance.[23] Nevertheless, several secondary endpoints, including measures of functional status, QoL, and renal function were strongly suggestive of a true benefit. Moreover, there was evidence of substantial heterogeneity, with a treatment effect that was most pronounced in patients with LVEF that was at or below the median of 57%, and in women, with women appearing to derive greater benefit than men to a higher EF. These findings have led to an FDA-expanded approval for the use of sacubitril/valsartan in patients with chronic HF, noting that benefit was most evident in those with EF below normal.

Interventional Therapies

Atrial Shunt Device

Elevated LA pressures at rest or with exertion are the principal hemodynamic element of HFpEF. Inspired by the hemodynamic consequences of Lutembacher physiology, there is a huge contemporary interest in the creation of an interatrial shunt large enough to allow for effective LA decompression, thereby leading to a clinically meaningful reduction in pulmonary capillary wedge pressures (PCWP) while avoiding too large a shunt that could lead to right heart overload and consequently, right-sided HF.

The Corvia IASD system II, a nitinol-based double-disc 8 mm atrial shunt device, has the largest volume of evidence to date. The REDUCE LAP-HF study looked at HF patients with EF >40% and exercise PCWP ≥25 mm Hg and demonstrated 2–3 mm Hg reductions in exercise PCWP, with an average shunt fraction (Qp:Qs) of 1.27 and with no reduction in cardiac output at the 3-month follow-up.[24] Subsequently, the REDUCE LAP-HF II trial, a sham-controlled RCT, was conducted to look at the clinical outcomes of the intervention. The trial excluded patients with severe HF (cardiac index <2 L/min/m^2), evidence of right heart enlargement/dysfunction (including moderate or greater TR, RA pressure >14 mm Hg or PVR >3.5 WU at rest), and recent thromboembolic event. The primary endpoint was a hierarchical composite of CV death or nonfatal ischemic stroke at 12 months followed by HF events up to 24 months and change in KCCQ at 12 months showed no between-group differences. From a safety standpoint, there appeared to be an early increase in MACE rates in the shunt group compared with the sham group (4% vs. 1%, $p = 0.025$).[25] PA systolic pressure at 20 W exercise >70 mm Hg emerged as the most significant prespecified subgroup that showed a treatment effect. Subsequent post-hoc analyses identified peak exercise PVR <1.74 WU and no cardiac rhythm management device (pacemaker or ICD) at baseline as the characteristics that differentiated the responders from the nonresponders.[26] However, given the post-hoc nature of these analyses, a follow-up RCT (RESPONDER-HF) is underway to validate these findings in the responder phenotype.

POTENTIAL FUTURE TARGETS

Vagus Nerve Stimulation

Chronic microcurrent stimulation of the vagus nerve has been shown to attenuate the proinflammatory milieu seen in patients with HFpEF. A study evaluating effects of chronic low-level transcutaneous vagus nerve stimulation reported significantly reduced inflammation and improved QoL and cardiac functions.[27] The ANTHEM-HFpEF study (Autonomic Neural Regulation Therapy to Enhance Myocardial Function in Patients with Heart Failure and Preserved Ejection Fraction) showed that cervical vagus nerve stimulation, improved QoL, NYHA class, T-wave alternans, and T-wave heterogeneity on chronic therapy. It also established the safety and tolerability of the chronic autonomic regulation therapy.[28]

Anti-inflammatory Drugs

There are many new exciting targets currently under investigation for therapy in HFpEF. One such target is the inflammatory enzyme myeloperoxidase (MPO) that stems from our evolving understanding of the role of systemic inflammation in the unique pathophysiology of HFpEF. In patients with HF, plasma MPO levels are elevated, associated with worse cardiac function, and have been reported to be predictors of outcome.[29] In preclinical studies, MPO inhibitors have been shown to reduce free radical production, systemic inflammation, and vascular dysfunction.[30] The SATELLITE trial assessed the proteomic patterns associated with clinical outcomes in observational HFpEF cohorts and the changes observed with mitiperstat (formerly AZD4831). The study demonstrated downregulation of the biomarker pathways most associated with clinical outcomes in the patients treated with MPO inhibition and showed safety of the drug.[31] The drug is currently undergoing a dose-finding phase 2b trial (ENDEAVOR trial).

A novel IL6 inhibitor, ziltivekimab, is also being investigated in HFpEF and HFmrEF patients with evidence of systemic inflammation (hsCRP ≥2 mg/dL) in the HERMES trial.[32]

Myosin Inhibitor

The EMBARK-HFpEF trial was a phase-2a proof-of-concept study that evaluated the role of myosin inhibition with mavacamten in HFpEF patients with LVEF 60% or greater. Patients treated with mavacamten showed significant reductions in NTProBNP, hsTnI, and hsTnT levels, which returned toward baseline levels 8 weeks after drug discontinuation. Treatment with mavacamten also demonstrated improvement in NYHA class and echocardiographic parameters of LV diastolic function with no sustained reductions in LVEF observed.[33]

CONCLUSION

There is scarcity of effective therapy that can significantly reduce hospitalization and mortality in patients with HFpEF compared to HFrEF. However, recent progress has been promising and multiple potential targets and therapies are being explored to treat the disease with gradually increasing burden in the population.

REFERENCES

1. Roger VL. Epidemiology of heart failure. Circ Res. 2013;113(6):646-59.
2. Guha K, McDonagh T. Heart failure epidemiology: European perspective. Curr Cardiol Rev. 2013;9(2):123-7.
3. Virani SS, Alonso A, Benjamin EJ, et al. Heart disease and stroke statistics-2020 update: A report from the American Heart Association. Circulation. 2020;141(9):e139-596.
4. Writing Group Members; Mozaffarian D, Benjamin EJ, Go AS, et al. Executive summary: Heart disease and stroke statistics—2016 update: A report from the American Heart Association. Circulation. 2016;133(4):447-54.
5. Owan TE, Hodge DO, Herges RM, et al. Trends in prevalence and outcome of heart failure with preserved ejection fraction. N Engl J Med. 2006;355(3):251-9.
6. Bhatia RS, Tu JV, Lee DS, et al. Outcome of heart failure with preserved ejection fraction in a population-based study. N Engl J Med. 2006;355(3):260-9.
7. Meta-analysis Global Group in Chronic Heart Failure (MAGGIC). The survival of patients with heart failure with preserved or reduced left ventricular ejection fraction: An individual patient data meta-analysis. Eur Heart J. 2012;33(14):1750-7.
8. Vaduganathan M, Patel RB, Michel A, et al. Mode of death in heart failure with preserved ejection fraction. J Am Coll Cardiol. 2017;69(5):556-69.
9. Solomon SD, Anavekar N, Skali H, et al. Influence of ejection fraction on cardiovascular outcomes in a broad spectrum of heart failure patients. Circulation. 2005; 112(24):3738-44.
10. Gerber Y, Weston SA, Redfield MM, et al. A contemporary appraisal of the heart failure epidemic in Olmsted County, Minnesota, 2000 to 2010. JAMA Intern Med. 2015;175(6):996-1004.
11. Nichols GA, Reynolds K, Kimes TM, et al. Comparison of risk of re-hospitalization, all-cause mortality, and medical care resource utilization in patients with heart failure and preserved versus reduced ejection fraction. Am J Cardiol. 2015;116(7):1088-92.
12. Packer M. Epicardial adipose tissue may mediate deleterious effects of obesity and inflammation on the myocardium. J Am Coll Cardiol. 2018;71(20):2360-72.
13. Pugliese NR, Paneni F, Mazzola M, et al. Impact of epicardial adipose tissue on cardiovascular haemodynamics, metabolic profile, and prognosis in heart failure. Eur J Heart Fail. 2021;23(11):1858-71.
14. Guo C, Ricchiuti V, Lian BQ, et al. Mineralocorticoid receptor blockade reverses obesity-related changes in expression of adiponectin, peroxisome proliferator-activated receptor-gamma, and proinflammatory adipokines. Circulation. 2008;117(17):2253-61.
15. Sato T, Aizawa Y, Yuasa S, et al. The effect of dapagliflozin treatment on epicardial adipose tissue volume. Cardiovasc Diabetol. 2018;17(1):6.
16. Anker SD, Butler J, Filippatos G, et al. Empagliflozin in heart failure with a preserved ejection fraction. N Engl J Med. 2021;385(16):1451-61.
17. Solomon SD, McMurray JJV, Claggett B, et al. Dapagliflozin in heart failure with mildly reduced or preserved ejection fraction. N Engl J Med. 2022;387(12):1089-98.
18. Kosiborod MN, Abildstrøm SZ, Borlaug BA, et al. Semaglutide in patients with heart failure with preserved

ejection fraction and obesity. N Engl J Med. 2023;389(12):1069-84.

19. Kosiborod MN, Petrie MC, Borlaug BA, et al. Semaglutide in patients with obesity-related heart failure and type 2 diabetes. N Engl J Med. 2024;390(15):1394-407.
20. Pitt B, Pfeffer MA, Assmann SF, et al. Spironolactone for heart failure with preserved ejection fraction. N Engl J Med. 2014;370(15):1383-92.
21. Pfeffer MA, Claggett B, Assmann SF, et al. Regional variation in patients and outcomes in the treatment of preserved cardiac function heart failure with an aldosterone antagonist (TOPCAT) trial. Circulation. 2015;131(1):34-42.
22. Solomon SD, McMurray JJV, Vaduganathan M, et al. Finerenone in heart failure with mildly reduced or preserved ejection fraction. N Engl J Med. 2024;391(16):1475-85.
23. Solomon SD, McMurray JJV, Anand IS, et al. Angiotensin-neprilysin inhibition in heart failure with preserved ejection fraction. N Engl J Med. 2019;381(17):1609-20.
24. Feldman T, Mauri L, Kahwash R, et al. Transcatheter interatrial shunt device for the treatment of heart failure with preserved ejection fraction (REDUCE LAP-HF I [Reduce Elevated Left Atrial Pressure in Patients With Heart Failure]): A phase 2, randomized, sham-controlled trial. Circulation. 2018;137(4):364-75.
25. Shah SJ, Borlaug BA, Chung ES, et al. Atrial shunt device for heart failure with preserved and mildly reduced ejection fraction (REDUCE LAP-HF II): A randomised, multicentre, blinded, sham-controlled trial. Lancet. 2022;399(10330):1130-40.
26. Borlaug BA, Sharma K, Shah SJ, et al. Heart failure with preserved ejection fraction: JACC Scientific Statement. J Am Coll Cardiol. 2023;81(18):1810-34.
27. Stavrakis S, Elkholey K, Morris L, et al. Neuromodulation of inflammation to treat heart failure with preserved ejection fraction: A pilot randomized clinical trial. J Am Heart Assoc. 2022;11(3):e023582.
28. Kumar HU, Nearing BD, Mittal S, et al. Autonomic regulation therapy in chronic heart failure with preserved/mildly reduced ejection fraction: ANTHEM-HFpEF study results. Int J Cardiol. 2023;381:37-44.
29. Tromp J, Khan MA, Klip IT, et al. Biomarker profiles in heart failure patients with preserved and reduced ejection fraction. J Am Heart Assoc. 2017;6(4):e003989.
30. Eiserich JP, Baldus S, Brennan ML, et al. Myeloperoxidase, a leukocyte-derived vascular NO oxidase. Science. 2002;296(5577):2391-4.
31. Lam CSP, Lund LH, Shah SJ, et al. Myeloperoxidase inhibition in heart failure with preserved or mildly reduced ejection fraction: SATELLITE trial results. J Card Fail. 2024;30(1):104-10.
32. Petrie M, Borlaug B, Buchholtz K, et al. HERMES: Effects of ziltivekimab versus placebo on morbidity and mortality in patients with heart failure with mildly reduced or preserved ejection fraction and systemic inflammation. J Card Fail. 2024;30(1):126.
33. Shah SJ, Rigolli M, Javidialsaadi A, et al. Cardiac myosin inhibition in heart failure with normal and supranormal ejection fraction: Primary results of the EMBARK-HFpEF Trial. JAMA Cardiol. 2024.

CHAPTER

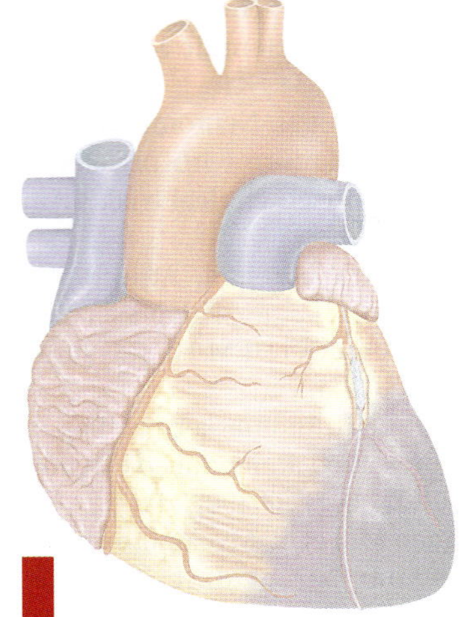

Ongoing Drugs and Device Trials in HFpEF

Rajeev Garg, Vardhini Vijaykumar

INTRODUCTION

Heart failure with preserved ejection fraction (HFpEF) is a multifactorial condition characterized by clinical heart failure with diastolic dysfunction. The term "preserved ejection fraction" was initially used in the CHARM study for defining the LVEF as determined by echocardiography.[1] This chapter reviews current advancements in device and drug trials aimed at improving outcomes in HFpEF patients.

Ongoing research targeting the HFpEF pathophysiological pathways is given in **Figure 1**.

DEVICE TRIALS IN HFpEF

Device therapy for HFpEF primarily targets structural and neurohormonal abnormalities that would not be feasible with pharmacologic approaches.

Cardiac Contractility Modulation

The CCM-REG is a prospective registry that found that cardiac contractility modulation (CCM) was more beneficial in patients with the upper LVEF range (35–45%) and had a greater three-year survival benefit.[2] Hence, it is possible that CCM is appropriate for HFpEF. A prospective pilot research CCM HFpEF (NCT03240237) found that CCM significantly improved the health status in older patients (mean age: 74 years) with NYHA class II or III as determined by the KCCQ overall score, post 24 weeks following implantation of CCM device. In addition, CCM was generally safe, with 93.6% of patients experiencing no device-related complications.[3] The ongoing randomized, multicentric, AIM HIGHER (NCT05064709)[4] study examines the safety and effectiveness of CCM therapy via the OPTIMIZER Smart Mini System in people with symptomatic heart failure and LVEF between 40 and 60%. The device has cables, which are attached to electrodes that track the heart's electrical activity in order to determine the precise moment at which pulses should be given **(Fig. 2)**. This is a quadruple-blind, sham-controlled, two-part integrated experiment. The study aims at determining the safety endpoint in part 1 with the incidence of complications associated with the OPTIMIZER device or procedure during the first year following implantation. Based on clinical outcome data at 18 months, the part 2 efficacy endpoint will evaluate the safety and efficacy of CCM therapy in the trial population.

Vagal Nerve Stimulation

The ANTHEM-HFpEF is the first trial to test the autonomic neural control treatment using the LivaNova VNS Therapy® system in order to enhance myocardial function in patients with HFpEF. The LivaNova® system **(Fig. 3)**, which surrounds the right cervical vagus nerve with an electrical lead, was successfully implanted in all patients who were stable on GDMT. In patients with HFpEF or HFmrEF, ART seemed safe and well-tolerated. Chronic ART was linked to improvements in exercise tolerance, autonomic tone, cardiac electrical stability, and heart failure symptoms but did not affect mechanical function assessments.[5]

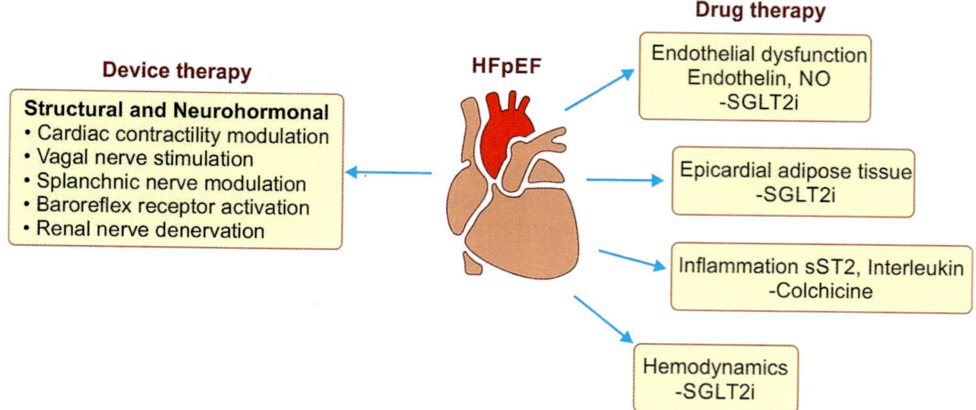

Fig. 1: Ongoing research targeting the HFpEF pathophysiological pathways.

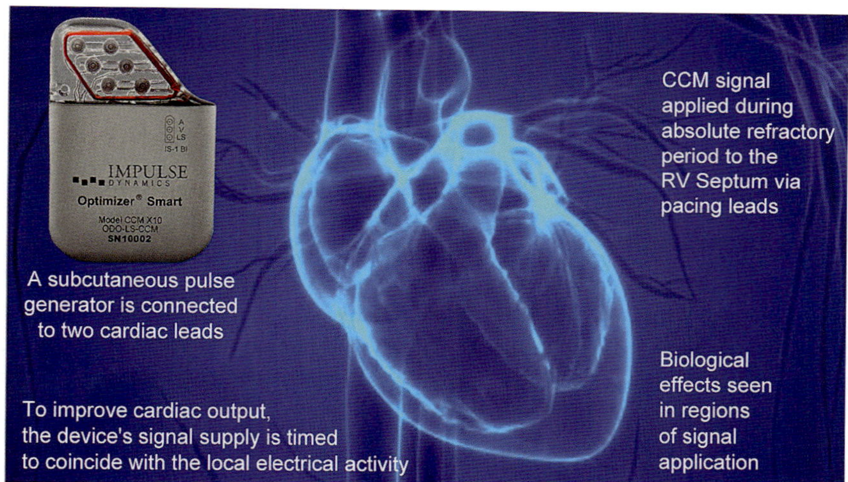

Fig. 2: OPTIMIZER smart mini system.

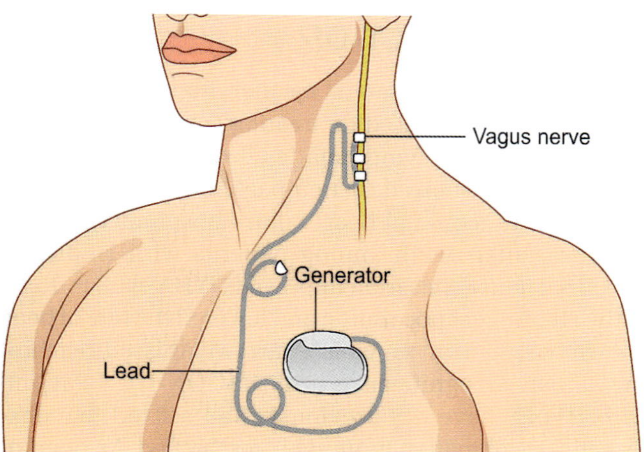

Fig. 3: LivaNova VNS Therapy® system.

Catheter Ablation

Heart failure is commonly associated with AF and RFCA has become the first-line therapy in the symptomatic AF patients. RFCA was found to be superior to antiarrhythmic drugs (AAD) in HFrEF with AF. It is still unknown whether RFCA has favorable effects in HFpEF than long-term AAD despite few nonrandomized retrospective trials.[6] The STABLE-SR IV (NCT06125925)[4] aims to investigate whether RFCA could better improve the clinical outcome of AF patients with HFpEF than long-term AAD's use. The sham-controlled Rebalance-HF trial (NCT04592445) evaluated the safety and effectiveness of unilateral catheter-based ablation of the right greater splanchnic nerve in individuals with HFpEF.[7] More than half of the trial population had a greater reduction in PCWP with legs up and 20W exercise than seen in the overall cohort, although neither difference was significant compared with the sham group. There was, however, a significantly greater drop in work index PCWP (by 18 mm Hg/W/kg) and a greater increase by 95 seconds in exercise duration after ablation. Another prospective, multicentric, randomized, blinded, sham-controlled study (NCT05715697)[4] aims to explore the potential of renal denervation as a therapy for HFpEF.

Interatrial Shunts

Interatrial left-to-right creation is becoming a crucial treatment option when heart failure patients with intact to mid-range ejection fraction, experience dyspnea as a result of elevated left atrial pressure and pulmonary congestion. The RAISE trial treated individuals with HFpEF by creating an interatrial shunt using radiofrequency ablation. The therapy improved clinical markers of cardiac function and was both viable and safe.[8] This work describes a revolutionary nonimplantable system-based radiofrequency ablation-based interatrial shunt construction technique that is a fresh and distinctive form of therapy.

Interatrial Shunt Device System II Implant

The first randomized trial of interatrial shunting was RELIEVE-HF which included HFrEF and HFpEF patients. Despite not meeting its primary goal, the trial advances the field by indicating that the risks and benefits of interatrial shunts may differ depending on the kind of heart failure.[9]

Ventura Interatrial Shunt System

The V-wave technology for interatrial shunting in HFrEF and HFpEF patients proved to be a safe and feasible procedure. Despite shunt patency attenuating in half of the patients, improvements in clinical and functional status were noted early on and at 12 months. Patients who had their shunt patency restored are likely to continue to benefit clinically. It is probably worthwhile to modify the device in a way that increases patency and durability. A predetermined analysis indicated that the shunt may worsen outcomes in individuals with HFpEF and be advantageous in people with HFrEF. This discrepancy might be explained by the heart muscle's increased compliance or flexibility in cases of HFrEF, which might make it easier for the heart to pump more blood into the right atrium. All groups, including those who underwent a placebo operation, showed a surprisingly significant improvement in quality of life (QoL) as measured by KCCQ. This finding raises the possibility that the metric may not be a valid predictor of quality-of-life outcomes in this particular situation. However, the experiment was not powered to demonstrate differences between the two types of heart failure, but the observed disparities in outcomes among individuals with various types of heart failure may guide future research and development for interatrial devices. Therefore, these findings ought to be regarded as exploratory. Also, these results may not be applicable to other interatrial shunts beyond the Ventura shunt.

The RESPONDER-HF (NCT05425459)[4]

It aims to evaluate the Corvia Atrial shunt device in a precision medicine trial to determine efficacy in HFmrEF or HFpEF for patients who are symptomatic despite GDMT. ALLAY HF (NCT05685303)[4] is an ongoing, randomized, double-blind, sham-controlled trial that is being conducted to assess the safety and effectiveness of an interatrial shunt created percutaneously using the Alleviant ALV1 System in patients with HFpEF/HFmrEF who have LVEF >40% and show no signs of latent PVD (peak exercise PVR <1.75 WU).

Baroreflex Activation Therapy

The Hope Heart Failure Study (HOPE4HF) and Baroreflex Activation for Heart Failure (BeAT-HF) trials showed that BAT with the Barostim Neo system plus GDMT significantly improved the 6MWD, MLWHFQ-rated QoL, NYHA functional class, and NT-proBNP in HFrEF patients with NYHA class III and were associated with a trend of reduced hospital days for HF.[10] The BAROSTIM THERAPY in HFpEf (NCT02876042)[4] is an ongoing registry to evaluate the feasibility and effectiveness of BAT in patients with HFpEF combined with refractory hypertension.

ONGOING DRUG TRIALS IN HEART FAILURE WITH PRESERVED EJECTION FRACTION

Heart failure with preserved ejection fraction treatments have historically focused on treating concomitant conditions and offering symptomatic alleviation. EMPEROR-Preserved trial showed that empagliflozin decreased the composite outcome of heart failure hospitalization and cardiovascular death among patients with HFpEF by 21%.[11] Sacubitril–valsartan improved NYHA class in 15.0% of the HFpEF trial population and lowered the rate of heart failure hospitalization, which narrowly missed reaching the statistical significance in PARAGON-HF.[12] Patients with HFpEF have not previously had a fixed low dose diuretics combination thoroughly researched. An ongoing randomized trial (NCT05129722)[4] will determine if a fixed low-dosage combination polypill comprising bumetanide 0.5 mg, eplerenone 25 mg, and empagliflozin 10 mg is more feasible for patients with HFpEF than empagliflozin 10 mg monotherapy. The goal of this study is to further the therapeutic paradigm for this patient population.

Improving Exercise Capacity

The CAMEO-DAPA proved that dapagliflozin reduced PCWP and improved hemodynamics by reducing plasma volume.[13] Another study (NCT06401343)[4] is assessing the effect of empagliflozin on the ability to exercise, heart failure symptoms, cardiac function, myocardial remodeling, and overall QoL in patients with nonobstructive heart failure who have HFpEF. A prospective, randomized, placebo-control trial (NCT04945707) will evaluate the effect of a single dose of IV ferric derisomaltose on exercise capacity following iron repletion in heart failure patients with maintained ejection fraction and functional iron deficit.[4]

Targeting HFpEF Pathways with SGLT2 Inhibitors

A paradigm shift in the pathogenesis of HFpEF paved the way for investigations into medications that could potentially treat HFpEF endothelial dysfunction. Dapagliflozin has been linked to improved diastolic function in rats, possibly as a result of a decrease in the expression of endothelial activation, cardiac inflammation, and cardiac fibrosis markers.[14] In the meantime, it was demonstrated that empagliflozin preserved cardiomyocyte contraction and relaxation by raising nitric oxide production and lowering oxidative stress in a cellular model of endothelial dysfunction.[15] In these lines, the SAK HFpEF Trial (NCT05138575)[4] will evaluate if participants with HFpEF on empagliflozin, with or without potassium nitrate, have improved submaximal exercise endurance, skeletal muscle oxidative phosphorylation capacity, intramuscular perfusion, and changes in the skeletal muscle metabolome and proteome.

Two clinical trials have reported the clinical advantages of dual inhibition of SGLT 1 and 2. While the SCORED study focused on T2DM patients with CKD, the SOLOIST study examined the effects of sotagliflozin in T2DM patients hospitalized for worsening HF. It is noteworthy that the event curves split within the first week of treatment, and that sotagliflozin's effects on outcomes related to heart failure were observed irrespective of LVEF values. Unlike empagliflozin and sacubitril/valsartan, these effects did not appear to diminish with increasing LVEF. The mechanism behind sotagliflozin's favorable effects is unknown. The SOTA-P-CARDIA[4] intends to explore the possible (nonglucose dependent) "cardio-renal" pleiotropic effects of sotagliflozin in nondiabetic HFpEF patients. The trial will analyze the LV mass using CMR, peak VO_2, myocardial mechanics, interstitial myocardial fibrosis, and QoL.

Heart Failure with Preserved Ejection Fraction and Gut Microbiome

An ongoing research-FERMENT HFpEF Trial (NCT06337812)[4] is examining the potential effects of dietary fiber addition in HFpEF patients with T2DM. The research team hopes to find out if supplementing with potato starch encourages increase in short-chain fatty acid production and its effect on the gut microbiome. The safety of an investigational molecule LY3540378 is being evaluated in a phase II clinical trial (NCT05592275)[4] in adults with worsening chronic HFpEF.

Anti-inflammatory Drug Targets

In response to myocardial stress, the soluble suppression of tumorigenicity 2 (sST2), a member of the interleukin (IL)-1 receptor family, is expressed in cardiomyocytes, fibroblasts, and endothelial cells of cardiac microvessels, counteracting the cardioprotective effects of the IL-33/ST2 system. In patients with HFpEF, sST2 is linked to worsening clinical manifestations, fibrosis biomarkers, and neurohormonal activation.[16] Colchicine is thought to lower sST2 levels and lessen inflammation in HFpEF, hence this molecule is being tested in HFpEF (NCT05637398).[4] Although hypertension is clinically significant in HFpEF, little is known about how common antihypertensive medications, especially β-blockers and CCBs, affect the pathophysiologic mechanisms of HFpEF. NCT04434664[4] aims to investigate the mechanism of action of dihydropyridine CCBs in HFpEF, with a comparison to β-blockers, which are routinely used antihypertensive medications in clinical practice. An assessment of the safety and tolerability of MYK-224 in patients with HFpEF is being conducted in phase 2A, randomized, placebo-controlled study.[4]

Obesity and Heart Failure with Preserved Ejection Fraction

Obesity is an establishing risk factor for HFpEF and a number of mechanisms contribute, including hemodynamic, neurohormonal, and inflammatory factors. Obese patients with HFpEF have a distinct phenotype, including impaired LV diastolic function, high filling pressures, and increased ventricular interaction. There is growing contribution of epicardial adipose tissue (EAT) in the pathophysiology of obesity-related HFpEF, even though generalized and visceral adiposity plays a significant role.[17] A novel strategy to ascertain whether a patient with HFPEF who receives 10 mg of dapagliflozin would see a reduction in the volume of their EAT is being currently analyzed (NCT06510270). The CAMEO-SEMA (NCT05371496)[4] is an ongoing trial with the goal to determine if individuals with the obese phenotype of HFpEF may have PCWP improvement with an aggressive weight-loss regimen using semaglutide 2.4 mg SC once weekly for 12 months.

LIMITATIONS

In contrast to HFrEF, HFpEF patients have limited therapeutic options to treat outcomes such as heart failure hospitalization due to the associated phenotypes. In this regard, the HFPEF project (NCT06465043) deals with deep phenotyping to characterize the HFpEF patients. It aims at developing new prognostic markers and prospective monitoring of a cohort of HFpEF patients to evaluate CV outcomes and QoL. Further, the project will identify HFpEF traits that are abnormally identified for genetic research. The heterogeneity of HFpEF requires a personalized approach to treatment, and the efficacy of new interventions must be validated across diverse patient populations. Additionally, long-term safety and effectiveness data are crucial to establish the clinical benefits of novel therapies.

CONCLUSION

The landscape of HFpEF treatment is evolving rapidly with ongoing advancements in both device and drug therapies. Novel pharmacological approaches, including antifibrotic agents, neurohormonal modulators, and new diuretics and vasodilators, are being rigorously tested. Collectively, these trials represent a significant step forward in addressing the unmet needs of HFpEF patients and hold promise for improving QoL and clinical outcomes. Continued research and clinical trials will be crucial in advancing the management of HFpEF and ultimately transforming patient care.

REFERENCES

1. Yusuf S, Pfeffer MA, Swedberg K, et al.; CHARM Investigators and Committees. Effects of candesartan in patients with chronic heart failure and preserved left-ventricular ejection fraction: The CHARM-Preserved Trial. Lancet. 2003;362:777-81.
2. Anker SD, Borggrefe M, Neuser H, et al. Cardiac contractility modulation improves long-term survival and hospitalizations in heart failure with reduced ejection fraction. Eur J Heart Fail. 2019;21:1103-13.
3. Linde C, Grabowski M, Ponikowski P, et al. Cardiac contractility modulation therapy improves health status in patients with heart failure with preserved ejection fraction: a pilot study (CCM-HFpEF). Eur J Heart Fail. 2022;24(12):2275-84.
4. Kumar HU, Nearing BD, Mittal S, et al. Autonomic regulation therapy in chronic heart failure with preserved/mildly reduced ejection fraction: ANTHEM-HFpEF study results. Int J Cardiol. 2023;381:37-44.
5. Qiao Y, Zhao Z, Cai X, et al. Long-Term prognosis of radiofrequency catheter ablation for atrial fibrillation with different subtypes of heart failure in the era of ablation index guidance. Front Cardiovasc Med. 2022;9:922910.
6. Fudim M, Litwin SE, Borlaug BA, et al. Endovascular ablation of the right greater splanchnic nerve in heart failure with preserved ejection fraction: Rationale, design and lead-in phase results of the REBALANCE-HF Trial. J Card Fail. 2024;30(7):877-89.
7. Sun W, Zou H, Yong Y, et al. The RAISE Trial: a novel device and first-in-man trial. Circ Heart Fail. 2022;15(4):e008362.
8. Rodés-Cabau J, Bernier M, Amat-Santos IJ, et al. Interatrial shunting for heart failure: early and late results from the first-in-human experience with the V-wave system. JACC Cardiovascular Interv. 2018;11(22):2300-10.
9. Zile MR, Lindenfeld J, Weaver FA, et al. Baroreflex activation therapy in patients with heart failure with reduced ejection fraction. J Am Coll Cardiol. 2020;76(1):1-13.
10. Anker SD, Butler J, Filippatos G, et al.; EMPEROR-Preserved Trial Investigators. Empagliflozin in heart failure with a preserved ejection fraction. N Engl J Med. 2021;385(16):1451-61.
11. Solomon SD, McMurray JJV, Anand IS, et al.; PARAGON-HF Investigators and Committees. Angiotensin–neprilysin inhibition in heart failure with preserved ejection fraction. N Engl J Med. 2019;381:1609-20.
12. Borlaug BA, Reddy YNV, Braun A, et al. Cardiac and metabolic effects of dapagliflozin in heart failure with preserved ejection fraction: The CAMEO-DAPA Trial. Circulation. 2023;148(10):834-44.
13. Cappetta D, De Angelis A, Ciuffreda LP, et al. Amelioration of diastolic dysfunction by dapagliflozin in a non-diabetic model involves coronary endothelium. Pharmacol Res. 2020;157:104781.
14. Juni RP, Kuster DWD, Goebel M, et al. Cardiac microvascular endothelial enhancement of cardiomyocyte function is impaired by inflammation and restored by empagliflozin. JACC Basic Transl Sci. 2019;4(5):575-91.
15. Shi Y, Liu J, Liu C, et al. Diagnostic and prognostic value of serum soluble suppression of tumorigenicity-2 in heart failure with preserved ejection fraction: a systematic review and meta-analysis. Front Cardiovasc Med. 2022;9:937291.
16. Tromp J, Bryant JA, Jin X, et al. Epicardial fat in heart failure with reduced versus preserved ejection fraction. Eur J Heart Fail. 2021;23(5):835-8.

Emerging Epidemic of HFpEF: Issues and Challenges in 2025 and Beyond

Abhishek Garg, Gautam Singal, Gurpreet Singh Wander

INTRODUCTION

Heart failure with preserved ejection fraction (HFpEF) accounts for nearly half of all heart failure cases. Diagnosing HFpEF can be particularly challenging, especially in elderly patients, as it often involves a combination of cardiac and noncardiac abnormalities and shares characteristics with other conditions that mimic HFpEF. Furthermore, the absence of effective treatments brings out a significant unmet clinical need. The inconclusive results from randomized clinical trials suggest that our understanding of this syndrome remains incomplete. In this chapter, we will review the growing prevalence of HFpEF, discuss the current issues in diagnosis, and address the therapeutic difficulties faced in clinical practice.

EMERGING EPIDEMIC OF HFpEF

The increasing prevalence of HFpEF has led to its classification as an epidemic. Recent studies reveal that, under a common definition, HFpEF encompasses a variety of clinical phenotypes with distinct pathophysiological characteristics and mechanisms.[1] HFpEF is a systemic syndrome involving multiple organs, leading to various cardiac and extracardiac pathophysiological alterations. Substantial variations can be seen in the prevalence of HFpEF, ranging from 13–74%, due to differences in diagnostic criteria and research population.[1-3] The prevalence of HFpEF has generally increased over the years, now accounting for 50% of all HF cases.[1] Epidemiological data show that the prevalence of HFpEF, compared to heart failure with reduced ejection fraction (HFrEF), is rising by 1% annually, suggesting that HFpEF is on track to become the most common form of heart failure.[4]

DRIVERS OF THE HFpEF EPIDEMIC

The I-PREFER multiregional cross-sectional study showed that HFpEF constitutes a significant portion of heart failure cases in non-Western countries.[5] There was notable regional variation, with HFpEF prevalence being higher in Latin America (69%) and North Africa (75%) compared to the Middle East (41%).[5] In India, the prevalence of HFpEF was reported to be 12.7 and 21% in the national heart failure registry (NHFR-HF)[6] and ASIAN-HF registry[7], respectively. However, it remains underdiagnosed in India due to lower awareness and the higher prevalence of valvular heart disease in the population.

The three key epidemiological characteristics of HFpEF are its rising prevalence with increasing age, its higher occurrence in females, and the presence of comorbidities.[4] These comorbidities either contribute to myocardial stiffness (metabolic and inflammatory conditions) or worsen the functional abnormalities (atrial fibrillation) **(Fig. 1)**.[4] The relationship between age and the prevalence of HFpEF was highlighted by the Prevention of Renal and Vascular End-stage Disease (PREVEND) study,[8] a community-based epidemiological investigation conducted in Europe. The study found that the age- and sex-specific prevalence of HFpEF was just 1% in women aged 25–49 years, but it rose significantly to 8–10% in women aged 80 years and older. Additionally, the PREVEND study[8] indicated that the increasing prevalence of HFpEF with age correlates with higher rates of hypertension, atrial fibrillation, and diabetes—a pattern not observed in HFrEF. Type 2 diabetes affects 30–40% of HFpEF patients and is an independent predictor of heart failure, with the risk increasing more than twofold in men

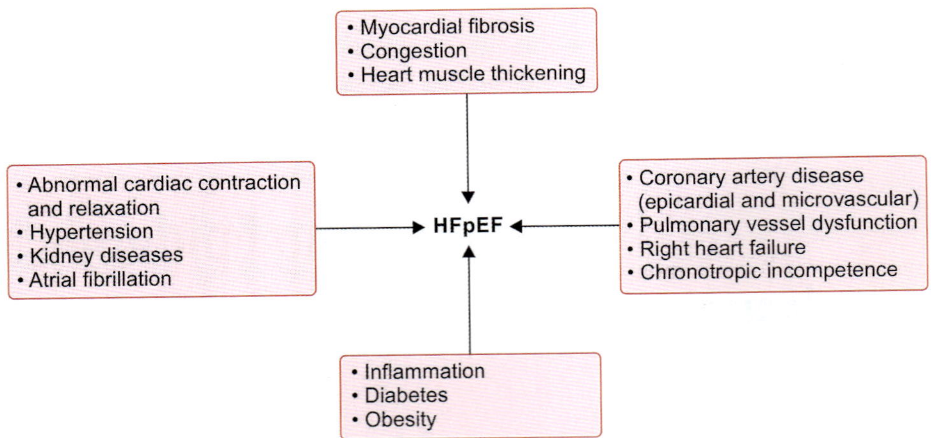

Fig. 1: Interacting causes and contributors of HFpEF reflecting the complex and heterogeneous underlying pathophysiology.

and over fivefold in women.[9] The coexistence of diabetes and HFpEF exacerbates morbidity and mortality rates. Obesity, a growing public health crisis, has seen alarming increases in recent years.[9] Given the strong link between HFpEF and excess body fat, the obesity epidemic is steadily contributing to the rising incidence of HFpEF.[9]

ISSUES IN DIAGNOSIS OF HFpEF

Clinical Symptoms and Signs

For HFrEF, diagnosis typically hinges mainly on the presence of symptoms and signs of heart failure with EF of <40%.[9] In contrast, the diagnosis of HFpEF requires several components, including clinical symptoms of heart failure, biochemical parameters (natriuretic peptides level), and the identification of structural and functional cardiac abnormalities, which can be assessed through echocardiography.[9] The clinical features of HFpEF are similar to those of general heart failure.[9] It is essential to distinguish HFpEF from other conditions causing heart failure with LVEF ≥50%, as these require different management approaches, including valvular heart disease, constrictive pericarditis, storage disorders, high-output heart failure, and cardiac amyloidosis.[9]

Biochemistry Parameters to Aid the Diagnosis of HFpEF

According to American[10] and European guidelines,[11] the measurement of natriuretic peptides, such as BNP or NT-proBNP, is recommended in the diagnostic process of HFpEF. Typically, natriuretic peptide levels are lower in HFpEF compared to HFrEF. However, caution is necessary when interpreting these levels, given potential confounding factors such as atrial fibrillation, pulmonary hypertension, renal failure, or obesity.[9] Since natriuretic peptide levels are often reduced in obese individuals—and obesity is commonly associated with HFpEF—low levels must be carefully evaluated before excluding the diagnosis of HFpEF.[9]

Imaging Criteria

Doppler echocardiography is the primary diagnostic tool for HFpEF.[9] The examination should start by evaluating cardiac abnormalities (such as pathological left ventricular hypertrophy and left atrial dilation) as well as assessing left ventricular systolic dysfunction (including reduced ejection fraction, mitral annulus systolic velocities, and global left ventricular longitudinal strain).[9] Although invasive hemodynamic assessment is the gold standard for analyzing diastolic function, left ventricular filling pressure (LVFP) is considered elevated if the left ventricular atrial pressure (LVAP) is ≥16 mm Hg and the pulmonary capillary wedge pressure (PCWP).[9] In practice, echocardiographic estimates of diastolic function are predominantly utilized.[9]

A variety of echocardiographic parameters can help differentiate between normal and elevated LVFP, and their combinations can assist in assessing the severity of diastolic dysfunction.[9] A challenging aspect is the definition of pathological threshold values, as aging can affect many diastolic function parameters, complicating both diagnosis and screening in older adults.[9] Nonetheless, the severity of diastolic dysfunction remains linked to prognosis. Furthermore, it is important that isolated asymptomatic left ventricular diastolic function abnormalities are much more prevalent than HFpEF and carry a significant risk of progression to HFpEF.[9] In 2016, the American Society of Echocardiography[12] established the following criteria for assessing patients with normal LVEF: Mean E/e'>14, septal e' velocity <7 cm/s or lateral e' velocity <10 cm/s, tricuspid regurgitation (TR) >2.8 m/s, and left atrial volume index >34 mL/m^2. Diastolic dysfunction is diagnosed when more than 50% of these criteria are met. One significant limitation of these guidelines is their inapplicability to patients with atrial fibrillation. Moreover, these parameters may also be ineffective in obese individuals.[12]

A diastolic stress test should be considered for patients with suspected heart failure who exhibit normal resting LVFP, as LVFP may rise only during exercise.[9] Measurements of the *E/e'* ratio and maximal TR velocity during physical activity are feasible for most patients and have been invasively validated for estimating LVFP during exertion.[9]

HFpEF Risk Scoring

In approximately 20% of HFpEF cases where NT-proBNP levels are normal but there is still a high suspicion of the condition, HFpEF risk scores can be useful.[9] Two heart failure scores are the Heart Failure Association Pre-test Assessment, Echocardiography, and Natriuretic Peptide, Functional Testing, Final Aetiology (HFA-PEFF) score (ranging from 0 to 6) and the Heart Failure with Preserved Ejection Fraction (H2FPEF) score (ranging from 0 to 9).[13,14] The variables are shown in **Table 1**. A diagnostic approach to HFpEF is shown in **Flowchart 1**.

This diagnostic approach highlights the complexity of diagnosing HFpEF. Clinicians must focus on a comprehensive diagnostic strategy, including advanced imaging and laboratory testing, to accurately confirm the diagnosis and exclude potential mimics.

CHALLENGES IN MANAGEMENT OF HFpEF

Management of Comorbidities

Unlike the management of HFrEF, there is a lack of large, evidence-based trials that show a clear morbidity and mortality benefit for HFpEF treatment **(Table 2)**. In patients with symptomatic HFpEF, diuretics are recommended to alleviate symptoms caused by volume overload, although the most effective diuretic dosing regimens remain unclear.[11] The core strategies of management of HFpEF include diagnosis and management of comorbidities. HFpEF is commonly associated with multiple cardiac and noncardiac conditions, including hypertension, CAD, diabetes, obesity, CKD, sleep apnea, anemia, AF, and chronotropic incompetence.[15] These comorbidities can accelerate disease progression and contribute to functional intolerance. Blood pressure control, following clinical practice guidelines, plays a crucial role in managing HFpEF. The choice of antihypertensive agents is influenced by the presence of comorbidities and other clinical indications. AF is highly prevalent in HFpEF and

TABLE 1: HFpEF risk scores.

H_2FPEF score[14]			*HFA-PEFF score*[13]		
	Definition	*Points*	*Domain*	*Major criteria (2 points max per domain)*	*Minor criteria (1 point max per category)*
Heavy	BMI >30 kg/m^2	2	Functional	• Average *E/e'* ratio ≥ 15 • Septal *e'* <7 cm/s • Lateral *e'* <10 cm/s • TR velocity >2.8 m/s	• Average *E/e'* ratio 9–14 • GLS <16%
Hypertension	Two or more antihypertensive medicines	1	Morphological	• LAVI >34 mL/m^2 • LVMI >149/122 g/m^2 (men/women) and RWT >0.42	• LAVI 29–34 mL/m^2 • LVMI >115/95 g/m^2 (men/women) • RWT >0.42 • LVWT ≥12 mm
AF	Any history	3	Biomarker (sinus)	• NT-proBNP >220 pg/mL • BNP >80 pg/mL	• NT-proBNP 125–220 pg/mL • BNP 35–80 pg/mL
Pulmonary hypertension	PASP >35 mm Hg (echo)	1	Biomarker (AF)	• NT-proBNP >660 pg/mL • BNP >240 pg/mL	• NT-proBNP 365–660 pg/mL • BNP 105–240 pg/mL
Elderly	>60 years	1	Low probability score—unlikely HFpEF • *H_2FPEF-0-1 or HFA-PEFF 0-1*		
Filling pressure	*E/e'* >9 (echo)	1	Intermediate probability score—further evaluation • *H_2FPEF-2-5 or HFA-PEFF-2-4* High probability score—highly HFpEF • *H_2FPEF-6-9 or HFA-PEFF 5-6*		

(LAVI: left atrial volume index; LVMI: left ventricular mass index ; LVWT: left ventricular wall thickness; RWT: relative wall thickness; TR: tricuspid regurgitation)

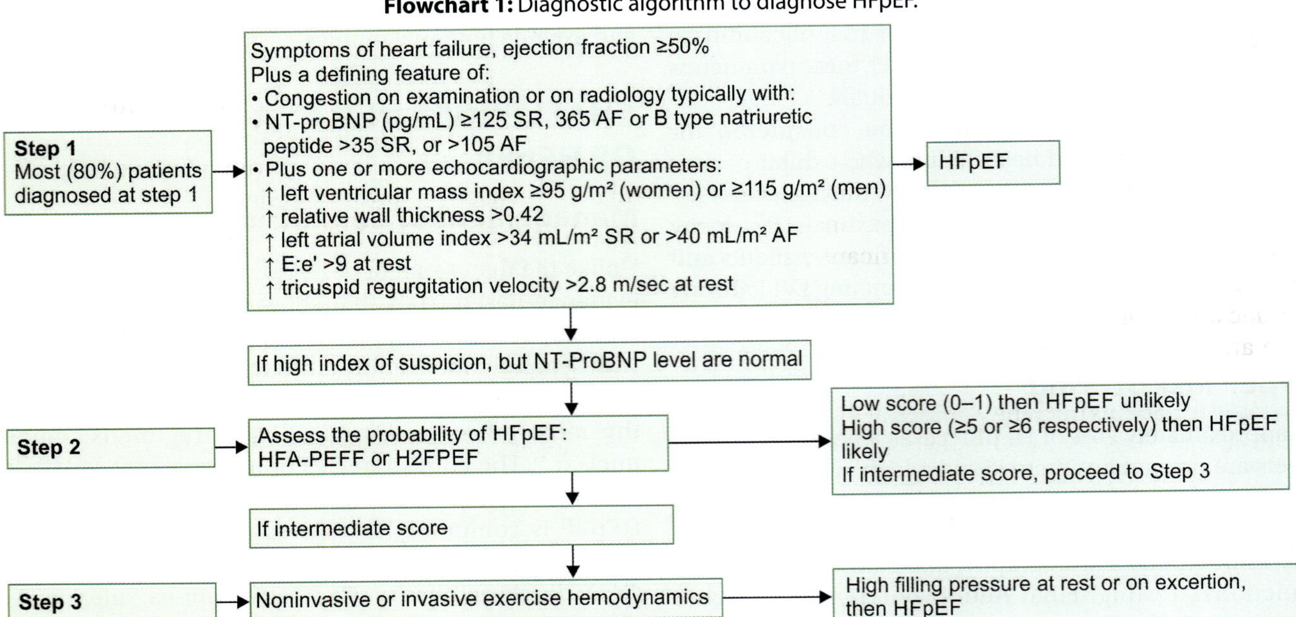

Flowchart 1: Diagnostic algorithm to diagnose HFpEF.

TABLE 2: Main data from the major trials on HFpEF.

Trials	*Drug*	*Year*	*n*	*Primary endpoints*
PEP-CHF[9]	ACEi: Perindopril	2006	850	0.69 (0.47–1.01)
CHARM-preserved[9]	ARB: Candesartan	2003	3,023	0.89 (0.77–1.03)
I-Preserve[9]	ARB: Irbesartan	2008	4,128	0.95 (0.86–1.05)
TOPCAT[18]	MRA: Spironolactone	2014	3,445	0.89 (0.77–1.04)
PARAGON-HF[16]	ARNi: Sacubitril–valsartan	2019	4,822	0.87 (0.75–1.01)
EMPEROR-preserved[20]	SGTL2i: Empagliflozin	2021	5,988	0.79 (0.69–0.90)
DELIVER[21]	SGTL2i: Dapagliflozin	2022	6,273	0.82 (0.73–0.92)

(CHARM-preserved: Effects of candesartan in patients with chronic heart failure and preserved left-ventricular ejection fraction; DELIVER: Dapagliflozin in Heart Failure with Mildly Reduced or Preserved Ejection Fraction; EMPEROR-preserved: Empagliflozin in Heart Failure with a Preserved Ejection Fraction; I-Preserve: Irbesartan in Patients with Heart Failure and Preserved Ejection Fraction; PARAGON-HF: Angiotensin–Neprilysin Inhibition in Heart Failure with Preserved Ejection Fraction; PEP-CHF: perindopril in elderly people with chronic heart failure; TOPCAT: Spironolactone for Heart Failure with Preserved Ejection Fraction)

is linked to more advanced disease, reduced exercise capacity, and increased mortality.[15]

Previous Trials on Pharmacotherapy

Therapies for HFpEF may be considered in line with the 2022 American College of Cardiology (ACC) and American Heart Association (AHA) treatment guidelines.[10] These include angiotensin-receptor blockers (ARBs), ARNI inhibitors, and MRAs. While none of these drugs demonstrated a reduction in primary outcomes in key randomized controlled trials for HFpEF, subsequent analyses have indicated potential benefits in select patient groups **(Table 2)**.

In the PARAGON-HF trial,[16] sacubitril/valsartan, compared to valsartan alone, showed a modest yet statistically nonsignificant reduction in the primary composite outcome of total (first and recurrent) hospitalizations for heart failure and cardiovascular death (rate ratio 0.87; 95% CI 0.75–1.01; $p = 0.06$). However, improvements were observed in secondary endpoints, including quality of life, NYHA class, and a composite of renal events in patients receiving sacubitril/valsartan. Subgroup analyses suggested that women and patients with an LVEF at or below the median value of 57% experienced greater benefit.[16] ARNI has been included in the 2022 AHA heart failure guidelines with a class 2b recommendation for the treatment of HFpEF.[10]

Theoretically, slowing heart rate could extend the diastolic filling period, potentially allowing greater filling of an abnormally stiff left ventricle. However, there is no current consensus on the effect of beta-blockers in HFpEF. According to the OPTIMIZE-HF registry,[17] the use of beta-blockers at discharge did not significantly impact 1-year mortality or hospitalization rates in HFpEF patients.

In the TOPCAT trial,[18] the MRAs spironolactone, compared to placebo, did not significantly reduce the primary outcome of time to cardiovascular death, aborted cardiac arrest, or heart failure hospitalization in patients with an ejection fraction of 45% or more (HR 0.89; 95% CI 0.77–1.04). However, a favorable treatment effect was observed in patients from the Americas, where recruitment criteria included elevated natriuretic peptide levels (HR for the primary composite: 0.82; 95% CI 0.69–0.98), possibly reflecting a true HFpEF population. Treatment benefits were particularly evident in patients with lower-range ejection fractions.[18] MRAs again are included in the 2022 AHA guidelines with a class 2b recommendation for HFpEF treatment.[10]

In the STEP-HFpEF trial,[19] the GLP-1 receptor agonist semaglutide significantly improved health status and reduced weight in patients with HFpEF. It also resulted in a 15% greater reduction in NT-proBNP levels compared to placebo, suggesting reduced LVFP and decreased C-reactive protein levels. Further studies are necessary to determine whether these findings translate into improvements in hard endpoints, which will help clarify the role of GLP-1 agonists in HFpEF management.

After demonstrating the efficacy of SGLT2i in HFrEF, empagliflozin and dapagliflozin were tested in HFpEF through two double-blind, randomized controlled trials. The EMPEROR-Preserved trial[20] was a landmark study for SGLT2 inhibitors in patients with HFpEF and LVEF >40%. Over a median follow-up of 26 months, empagliflozin reduced the primary composite endpoint of cardiovascular death or heart failure hospitalization by 21%.[20] A meta-analysis[21] of the DELIVER, EMPEROR-Preserved, DAPA-HF, EMPEROR-Reduced, and SOLOIST-WHF trials, encompassing a total of 21,947 participants, showed that SGLT2i reduced the composite risk of cardiovascular death or hospitalization for heart failure [RR 0.77 (0.72–0.82)], cardiovascular death [RR 0.87 (0.79–0.95)], first hospitalization for heart failure [RR 0.72 (0.67–0.78)], and all-cause mortality [RR: 0.92 (0.86–0.99)]. These benefits were consistently observed in trials involving both HFpEF and HFmrEF and across all 14 subgroups analyzed, including those with varying LVEF levels.[21]

The pharmacologic management of HFpEF has been largely based on effective treatments for HFrEF and targeting severe neurohormonal abnormalities. However, these neurohormonal imbalances are less pronounced in HFpEF. This disparity adds to the complexity of managing HFpEF, as no pharmacologic agents have yet demonstrated clear mortality benefits in randomized controlled trials for this condition. Consequently, treatment strategies for HFpEF remain challenging, with a focus on symptom management and addressing comorbidities.

Status of Various Device Therapies in HFpEF

Since pharmacologic treatments have not shown mortality benefits in managing HFpEF, attention has shifted toward more understanding of its underlying mechanisms. One key aspect of HFpEF pathophysiology is elevated LVFP, which contributes significantly to disease progression. With this knowledge, several device-based therapies have been developed and assessed to reduce LVFP, thereby potentially decreasing the incidence and severity of HFpEF. Which includes, the REDUCE LAP-HF II trial[22] (randomized trial to REDUCE Elevated Left Atrial Pressure in Patients with Heart Failure II) evaluated the efficacy of an atrial shunt device but found no significant effect on the primary composite outcome, which included cardiovascular death, stroke, heart failure events, and changes in health status. In the RAPID-HF trial[23] (Rate-Adaptive Atrial Pacing in Diastolic Heart Failure), the implantation of a rate-adaptive atrial pacemaker intended to improve heart rate responses to exercise in patients with HFpEF and chronotropic incompetence did not lead to significant enhancements in exercise performance or quality of life.

Monitoring pulmonary artery pressure has proven beneficial in the management of HFpEF, as illustrated by the CHAMPION trial[24] (CardioMEMS Heart Sensor Allows Monitoring of Pressure to Improve Outcomes in NYHA Class III Heart Failure Patients). This study demonstrated a 50% reduction in heart failure hospitalizations compared to standard care over an 18-month follow-up period, with an overall number needed to treat being 2 to prevent a single hospitalization for heart failure.

THE WAY FORWARD AND BEYOND 2025

Despite the extensive trials conducted on various pharmacologic agents and device-based therapies for HFpEF, none has demonstrated significant mortality benefits thus far. Nevertheless, research continues to explore the underlying mechanisms of HFpEF, aiming to develop new drugs or interventions that could reduce its incidence and potentially reduce the growing epidemic.

Ongoing trials are focused on improving our understanding of the disease and discovering innovative treatment strategies.

The SPIRIT-HF trial[25] (Spironolactone in the Treatment of Heart Failure) and the SPIRRIT trial[25] (Spironolactone Initiation Registry Randomized Interventional Trial in Heart Failure with Preserved Ejection Fraction) are currently in progress to enhance our understanding of spironolactone's role in managing HFpEF. Additionally, the ongoing FINEARTS-HF trial[25] is investigating the effects of the nonsteroidal MRA finerenone.

Likewise, the STEP-HFpEF DM trial[25] (Semaglutide Treatment Effect in People with Obesity and HFpEF and Type 2 Diabetes) is also being conducted. The SUMMIT trial[25] is evaluating tirzepatide (LY3298176) for its efficacy and safety in patients with HFpEF and obesity, focusing on the dual action of glucose-dependent insulinotropic polypeptide and GLP-1 receptor agonists.

Furthermore, the HERMES trial[25] is examining the impact of the novel therapeutic monoclonal antibody ziltivekimab, which targets the IL-6 ligand, in patients with HFpEF who also experience inflammation. The ongoing trials are shown in **Table 3**.

CONCLUSION

Numerous key differences between HFpEF and HFrEF suggest that they are two distinct syndromes. Over the past two decades, significant progress has been made in understanding the epidemiology, pathophysiology, molecular mechanisms, diagnosis, and treatment of HFpEF. The prevalence of HFpEF continues to rise, often

TABLE 3: Ongoing trials on HFpEF.[25]

Trial name	*Therapy*	*Enrolment criteria*	*Primary outcome*
Cardiometabolic drug trials			
SUMMIT	Tirzepatide vs. placebo	EF ≥50% and NYHA II–IV BMI ≥30 kg/m²	*Composite:* All-cause mortality, HF events, 6-minute walk distance, KCCQ
STEP HFpEF and STEP HFpEF-DM	Semaglutide vs. placebo	• EF ≥45% and NYHA II–IV • BMI ≥30 kg/m² without or with T2DM	Change in KCCQ and change in body weight at 12 months
Neurohormonal drug trials			
FINEARTS-HF	Finerenone vs. placebo	• EF >40% and NYHA II–IV • Structural heart disease • Elevated NT-proBNP	Total number of CV deaths and HHF
SPIRRIT	Spironolactone vs. standard of care	• EF ≥40% and NYHA II–IV • NT-proBNP >300 ng/L or >750 ng/L in AF	Time to CV death or first HHF
SPIRIT-HF	Spironolactone vs. placebo	• EF ≥40% and NYHA II–IV • NT-proBNP >300 ng/L or >900 ng/L in AF	Total number of CV deaths and HHF
Trials targeting left atrial myopathy and atrial fibrillation			
RESPONDER	Atrial shunt device vs. sham	• LVEF ≥40% and NYHA functional class II–IV • Elevated PCWP during exercise, without high PVR or pacemaker device	Composite of HF event rates and KCCQ at 12 months
RELIEVE-HF	Atrial shunt device vs. sham	• HFpEF and HFpEF, NYHA functional classes II–IV • HHF and/or elevated NP levels	Composite of death, transplant or LVAD, HHF, worsening outpatient HF events, and change in KCCQ
Trials targeting inflammation			
Myeloperoxidase (MPO) inhibitor with exercise in HFpEF	MPO inhibitor vs. placebo	• EF ≥50% and NYHA functional classes II–IV • PCWP ≥15 at rest or PCWP ≥25 with exercise	Exercise PCWP
HERMES	Ziltivekimab vs. placebo	EF ≥40% and NYHA functional classes II–IV, NT-proBNP >300 or >600 in AF, C-reactive protein >2 mg/L	Time to HF hospitalization, cardiovascular death, or urgent outpatient HF visit

going undiagnosed, and even when identified, it is linked to high rates of hospitalization and readmission. After years of neutral trial results, only proven therapy SGLT2i has emerged. However, substantial unmet needs and knowledge gaps still exist. The advancements in HFpEF treatment offer hope for a future with reduced prevalence, mortality, and morbidity associated with this condition, marking a significant advancement in population health.

REFERENCES

1. Hogg K, Swedberg K, McMurray J. Heart failure with preserved left ventricular systolic function: epidemiology, clinical characteristics, and prognosis. J Am Coll Cardiol. 2004;43(3):317-27.
2. Owan TE, Redfield MM. Epidemiology of diastolic heart failure. Prog Cardiovasc Dis. 2005;47(5):320-32.
3. Vasan RS, Benjamin EJ, Levy D. Prevalence, clinical features, and prognosis of diastolic heart failure: an epidemiologic perspective. J Am Coll Cardiol. 1995;26(7):1565-74.
4. Campbell P, Rutten FH, Lee MM, et al. Heart failure with preserved ejection fraction: everything the clinician needs to know. The Lancet. 2024;403(10431):1083-92.
5. Magaña-Serrano JA, Almahmeed W, Gomez E, et al. Prevalence of heart failure with preserved ejection fraction in Latin American, Middle Eastern, and North African Regions in the I PREFER study (Identification of Patients With Heart Failure and PREServed Systolic Function: an epidemiological regional study). Am J Cardiol. 2011; 108(9):1289-96.
6. Harikrishnan S, Bahl A, Roy A, et al. Clinical profile and 90 day outcomes of 10,851 heart failure patients across India: National Heart Failure Registry. ESC Heart Fail. 2022;9(6):3898-908.
7. Tromp J, Tay WT, Ouwerkerk W, et al. Multimorbidity in patients with heart failure from 11 Asian regions: a prospective cohort study using the ASIAN-HF registry. PLoS Med. 2018;15(3):e1002541
8. Brouwers FP, de Boer RA, van der Harst P, et al. Incidence and epidemiology of new-onset heart failure with preserved vs. reduced ejection fraction in a community-based cohort: 11-year follow-up of PREVEND. Eur Heart J. 2013;34(19):1424-31.
9. Logeart D. Heart failure with preserved ejection fraction: new challenges and new hopes. La Presse Méd. 2024; 53(1):104185.
10. Chairy V. 2022 AHA/ACC/HFSA guideline for the management of heart failure. J Am Coll Cardiol. 2022; 79(17):e895-e1032.
11. McDonagh TA, Metra M, Adamo M, et al. 2021 ESC Guidelines for the diagnosis and treatment of acute and chronic heart failure: developed by the Task Force for the diagnosis and treatment of acute and chronic heart failure of the European Society of Cardiology (ESC) with the special contribution of the Heart Failure Association (HFA) of the ESC. Eur Heart J. 2021;42(36):3599-726.
12. Almeida JG, Fontes-Carvalho R, Sampaio F, et al. Impact of the 2016 ASE/EACVI recommendations on the prevalence of diastolic dysfunction in the general population. Eur Heart J Cardiovasc Imaging. 2018;19(4):380-6.
13. Pieske B, Tschöpe C, de Boer RA, et al. How to diagnose heart failure with preserved ejection fraction: the HFA-PEFF diagnostic algorithm: a consensus recommendation from the Heart Failure Association (HFA) of the European Society of Cardiology (ESC). Eur Heart J. 2019;40(40): 3297-317.
14. Reddy YNV, Carter RE, Obokata M, et al. Evidence-based approach to help guide diagnosis of heart failure with preserved ejection fraction. Circulation. 2018; 138(9): 861-70.
15. Upadhya B, Haykowsky MJ, Kitzman DW. Therapy for heart failure with preserved ejection fraction: current status, unique challenges, and future directions. Heart Fail Rev. 2018;23:609-29.
16. Solomon SD, Rizkala AR, Gong J, et al. Angiotensin receptor neprilysin inhibition in heart failure with preserved ejection fraction: rationale and design of the PARAGON-HF trial. JACC Heart Fail. 2017;5(7):471-82.
17. Fonarow GC, Abraham WT, Albert NM, et al. Organized program to initiate lifesaving treatment in hospitalized patients with heart failure (OPTIMIZE-HF): rationale and design. Am Heart J. 2004;148(1):43-51.
18. Pfeffer MA, Claggett B, Assmann SF, et al. Regional variation in patients and outcomes in the Treatment of Preserved Cardiac Function Heart Failure With an Aldosterone Antagonist (TOPCAT) trial. Circulation. 2015;131(1):34-42.
19. Petrie MC, Borlaug BA, Butler J, et al. Semaglutide and NT-proBNP in obesity-related HFpEF: insights from the STEP-HFpEF Program. J Am Coll Cardiol. 2024;84(1):27-40.
20. Packer M, Butler J, Zannad F, et al. Effect of empagliflozin on worsening heart failure events in patients with heart failure and preserved ejection fraction: EMPEROR-preserved trial. Circulation. 2021;144(16):1284-94.
21. Täger T, Atar D, Agewall S, et al. Comparative efficacy of sodium-glucose cotransporter-2 inhibitors (SGLT2i) for cardiovascular outcomes in type 2 diabetes: a systematic review and network meta-analysis of randomised controlled trials. Heart Fail Rev. 2020;26(6):1421-35.
22. Shah SJ, Borlaug BA, Chung ES, et al. Atrial shunt device for heart failure with preserved and mildly reduced ejection fraction (REDUCE LAP-HF II): a randomised, multicentre, blinded, sham-controlled trial. Lancet. 2022;399(10330):1130-40.
23. Reddy YN, Koepp KE, Carter R, et al. Rate-adaptive atrial pacing for heart failure with preserved ejection fraction: the RAPID-HF randomized clinical trial. JAMA. 2023;329(10):801-9.
24. Schmier JK, Ong KL, Fonarow GC. Cost-effectiveness of remote cardiac monitoring with the CardioMEMS heart failure system. Clin Cardiol. 2017;40(7):430-6.
25. Borlaug BA, Sharma K, Shah SJ, et al. Heart failure with preserved ejection fraction: JACC scientific statement. J Am Coll Cardiol. 2023;81(18):1810-34.

Index

Page numbers followed by *b* refer to box, *f* refer to figure, *fc* refer to flowchart, and *t* refer to table.

A

Abdominal discomfort 622
Abdominal fat tissue 672
Abdominal obesity 86
Abdominal wall 950
Ablation procedure 424
Accelerate contraction 526
Access site selection 484
Acetazolamide 171
Achondroplasia, full-term pregnant 568*f*
Acroparesthesias 111
Activated immune cells 77
Activated partial thromboplastin time 816
Activated T cells, nuclear factor of 827, 828
Activin receptor 710
Acute cardiorenal syndrome 609
Acute cardiovascular events 23
Acute coronary syndrome 260, 276, 277, 779
  setting of 780*fc*
Acute heart failure 195, 259, 260, 261*b*, 277, 815*f*, 858, 862, 900*t*
  current management of 261
Acute illness 874
Acute kidney injury 380, 629, 862, 875
  risk of 585
Acute lung injury 813
Acute myocardial infarction 6, 489, 491*t*, 923
Acute pulmonary edema 654
Acute respiratory distress syndrome 813
Acutely decompensated heart failure 862
Acylcarnitines 778
Adenosine
  receptor agonist 637
  triphosphate 54
    synthesis 634
Adenyl cyclase 54
Adherence challenges 107
Adipocytes 950
Adipokines 865
  activation of 95
  signaling 394
Adiponectin 280
Adipose tissue 676, 677, 743, 951
  dysfunction 193
Adjunctive tolvaptan 171
Adona 987
Adrenalin 723
Adrenomedullin 280
Adult congenital heart disease 981
Advanced fibrosis 87
Advanced glycation end products 582, 699, 864
  inhibitors of 640
Advanced glycation, formation of 102
Advanced heart failure trial 986
Adverse cardiac remodeling 902
Adverse drug reactions 874
Aerobic capacity 401
Aerobic exercise 106, 154
Aerobic training 996
Aggressive blood pressure control 157, 160
Aircraft noise 723
Albiglutide 952
Albuminuria 584
Alcohol abuse 874
Aldosterone 148, 280, 834
  antagonist 184, 686, 745
Alleviant 422, 985, 986
  system 986
Alogliptin 892
Alpha-blockers 881
Alpha-linolenic acid 793
Altered adipokine regulation 521
Altered cellular ultrastructure 936
Altered gene expression 753
Amber trial 841
Ambulation 819
American College of Cardiology 34, 182, 418, 567
  guidelines 453, 625, 908
American Diabetes Association guidelines 599
American Heart Association 34, 182, 418, 533, 567, 926
  guidelines 453, 908
Amyloid cardiomyopathy 336
Amyloid-beta 826
Amyloidosis 111, 182, 336*f*, 339, 562, 919
  role of 115
Amyotrophic lateral sclerosis 210
Anderson Fabry disease 562, 402
Anemia 4, 60, 181, 210, 280, 380, 634*f*, 744, 786*f*
  management 602
Angiotensin 826
Angiotensin-converting enzyme 50, 51,144, 173, 268, 509, 649, 826, 872
  inhibitors 4, 123, 126, 136, 184, 189, 238, 239, 269, 277, 298, 459, 496, 516, 547, 548, 563, 564, 589, 590, 619-621, 685, 730, 731, 817, 826, 839, 930
Angiotensin-receptor 761, 826, 828
  blocker 49-51, 123, 126, 141-145, 150, 173, 183, 184, 238, 239, 256, 266, 269, 298, 386, 387, 429, 509, 516, 533, 547, 548, 589, 590, 619, 620, 625, 626, 649, 651, 686, 730, 731, 758, 829, 872, 908, 930, 978, 981, 1014
    pathophysiological basis of 825
    role of 832
Angiotensin-receptor neprilysin inhibitors 49, 119, 126, 127, 141-145, 150, 179, 180, 183, 184, 196, 218, 239, 256, 262, 266, 269, 327, 330, 351, 355, 386, 387, 394, 402, 403, 406, 408, 409, 409*t*, 419, 429, 450, 459, 460, 499, 509, 547, 548, 576, 599, 604, 618, 619, 621, 625, 626, 647, 649, 709, 730, 745, 749, 758, 799, 800, 817, 825, 826, 828, 831, 834, 839, 845-847, 849, 871, 872, 895, 908, 915, 916, 931, 949, 967, 969, 981, 1003
  contraindications of 876
  current role of 500
  drug 499
  effect of 295, 296*t*, 406, 539
  efficacy of 604
  impact of 351, 359
  indication of 875
  mechanisms of action in 407
  meta-analysis of 845
  metabolic benefit of 876
  pathophysiological basis of 827
  pleiotropic effects of 827
  renal benefits of 876
  renal safety and efficacy of 604
  role of 499, 539, 647, 659, 660, 835, 836
  therapy 649*fc*
    role of 648
  uniqueness of 876
  use of 817
Ankle edema 371
Antagonist receptor neprilysin inhibitors 120, 123, 240
Anthracycline 804
  cardiotoxicity, risk factors for 800*b*
  chemotherapy agents, side effect of 799
  induced cardiotoxicity 799
    prevention of 802
  treatment 804
Anthropometric indicators 587

Anthropometry 790
Antialdosterone drugs 225
Antiarrhythmic drugs 1007
Antifibrotic 612
  effects 147
  molecules 639
  therapies 162
Antihyperkalemic drugs 622, 622*t*, 623*t*
Antihypertensive
  drugs 680
  lower doses of 534
Anti-inflammatory agents 162, 638
Anti-inflammatory drugs 1004, 1009
Anti-inflammatory effects 147, 149, 154, 584, 854, 874
Anti-inflammatory properties 612, 896
Anti-inflammatory therapies 750
  testing for 132
Antiobesity medications 745
Antioxidant effects 874
Antithrombotic therapy 969
Anti-tumor necrosis factor-alpha therapy 638
Anxiety 210, 588
Aorta 373*f*
  coarctation of 568*f*
Aortic anatomy, accurate assessment of 481
Aortic annulus 482
  diameter of 482*f*
  measurements 481
Aortic regurgitation 480
Aortic root
  assessment 482
  calcification 482
Aortic stenosis 480, 546
Aortic valve
  calcification, quantification of 481
  replacement 480
Apoptosis 684, 801, 827
Arachidonic acid 793
Arrhythmias 260, 513, 564, 829
  risk of 718
Arrhythmogenic right ventricular cardiomyopathy 48, 267
Arterial access site, calcification of 485*f*
Arterial conduits, use of 505
Arterial hypertension 119*f*, 226, 567, 723
Arterial stiffness 81, 87, 119*f*, 536, 874
Arterial switch operation 546
Artificial heart 973
Artificial intelligence 64
Artificial neural networks 903
Ascending aorta, assessment of 484
Asian sudden cardiac death 777
Aspirin 243, 969
Association of Heart Failure with Preserved Ejection Fraction and Hypothyroidism 753
Atherosclerosis, multi-ethnic study of 912
Atherosclerotic cardiovascular disease 145, 588-590, 779
Atherosclerotic vascular diseases 587
Atrial cardiomyopathy 894
Atrial dysfunction 411
  early detection of 366
Atrial electrical dyssynchrony 964
Atrial failure 894
  pathogenic pathways for 895*fc*
Atrial fibrillation 17, 24, 37, 50, 51, 60, 62, 73, 74, 90, 111, 116, 118, 126, 128, 141, 158, 159, 181, 182, 186, 203, 212, 225, 227, 241, 260, 268, 307, 319-321, 322*f*, 324, 342, 345, 349, 355, 375, 399, 407, 414, 417, 420, 447, 471, 498, 515, 522, 564, 609, 659, 672, 679, 684, 705, 713, 715, 744, 760, 785, 786, 786*f*, 787, 896, 908, 912, 915-917, 929, 931, 935, 946
  care 517
  clinical significance of 51*f*
  drugs therapy for 36*f*
  echocardiographic evaluation of 319
  management of 750, 831
  predicting 365
  presence of 307
Atrial fibrosis 344, 406
Atrial flow regulator 206, 228, 228*f*, 243, 640, 963, 978
Atrial flutter 715, 908
Atrial function 414, 465
  echocardiographic evaluation of 300
Atrial kick 571
Atrial myocardium 894
Atrial natriuretic peptide 189,, 649, 826
Atrial pacing, rate-adaptive 661
Atrial pressure 155
Atrial remodeling
  and ventricular strain, reducing 917
  pathophysiological processes of 894
Atrial secondary mitral regurgitation 301
Atrial septal defect 981
Atrial shunt devices 205, 205*t*, 962, 978, 1003, 1016
Atrial shunt therap
  types of 421
  basic steps of 984
Atrial strain 360, 361, 365
  clinical implications of 366
  prognostic significance of 366
  role of 365
Atrial volume 465
Atriopathy 319
Atrioventricular block 346
Atrioventricular node ablation 517
Autoantibody, binding of 638
Autofluorescence 700
Autonomic dysfunction 77, 102
Autonomic imbalance 82, 950
Autonomic nervous system 723
Autonomic regulation 997
Autophagy 521, 904
Autosomal recessive disorder 562

B

Background therapy 126
Backward expansion wave 37
Balanced diet 105
Balanced steady-state free precession 473
Balloon atrial septostomy 820*f*
Bariatric surgery 677, 745
Baroreceptor activation therapy 229, 964
Baroreflex activation therapy 107, 186, 243, 247, 257, 1008
Barostim Neo system 641
Baseline cardiovascular assessment 806
Behavioral modifications 154
Bempedoic acid 780
Bendopnea 85
Benoarterial extracorporeal membrane oxygenation 819
Beta-adrenergic receptors 54, 925
Beta-adrenoreceptor agonists 710
Beta-blockers 126, 128, 136, 145, 186, 256, 175, 351, 392, 393, 496, 526, 527, 548, 563, 576, 600, 621, 686, 749, 766, 825, 834, 840, 879, 881, 896, 908, 909, 912, 913, 917, 922, 924-926, 929, 930, 931*t*, 932, 949, 978
  benefit of 919
  evidence of 909*f*
  first-generation 930
  mechanism of action of 925
  primary mechanism of 925
  role of 922, 923, 929, 930, 933
  selective 599
  therapy 241, 391, 831
  use 908, 926, 929, 931, 932
    limitation of 909
Bilateral carpal tunnel syndrome 111
Biochemical markers kidney injury 608
Biochemistry parameters 1012
Biomarker 27, 55, 67, 308, 361, 376, 385, 618, 749, 790, 866
  development 410
  driven treatment 162
  score 573
Biopsy 39
Biplane Simpson's method 320*f*
Bisoprolol 600, 896, 912, 915, 917, 922, 923
  promise of 919
  role of 912, 922, 924
Biventricular fusion pacing 980
Bladder cancer 875
Bleeding 969
  tamponade 820*f*

Blood
- conservation strategy 816*fc*
- glucose 876
- pressure 13, 50, 51, 127, 145, 150, 172, 173, 191, 268, 589, 592, 684, 899, 929
  - control 608, 912
  - low 58
  - reduction 854, 874
  - regulation 189
- sugar 172
- tests 33, 755
- urea nitrogen 570

Body
- mass index 8, 62, 111, 139, 140, 342, 375, 588, 589, 679, 683, 741, 790, 792, 951
- surface area 355, 841
- weight 762

Bone fracture 875
Booster strain 351*t*
Bradycardia 930
Bradykinin 826, 835
Brain 951
- development, membrane phospholipids for 793
- natriuretic peptide 56, 61, 260, 275, 280, 736, 826
  - N-terminal prohormone of 74

Breast pain 957
Breath, shortness of 260, 361
Breathlessness quantification 85
Bronze skin 112
B-type natriuretic peptide 62, 119, 139, 140, 223, 239, 376, 649
- level 360

Bundle branch blocks 347

C

Calcium 570, 899
- channel
  - blockers 145, 188, 195, 210, 526, 527, 547, 548, 563, 639, 749, 834, 930
  - nifedipine 637
- dynamics 637, 639
- gluconate 602
- hemostasis 664
- polystyrene sulfonate 622

Caloric restriction 154, 226
Canagliflozin 583, 584, 614, 740, 778
Cancer 806
- diagnostics 432
- therapy-related
  - cardiac dysfunction 432, 799
  - risk factors 434

Candesartan 184
Capillary rarefaction 41
Carbon dioxide production 708
Carboxyethyl lysine 700
Cardiac abnormalities 452, 484, 1011
Cardiac amyloidosis 115, 116, 173, 402, 825
- proposed pathway for excluding 116

Cardiac anatomy, assessment of 453
Cardiac biomarkers 608
Cardiac calcium signaling 25
Cardiac catheterization 30, 575, 576
Cardiac comorbidities 241, 268*t*
Cardiac complications 435
Cardiac computed tomography 482*f*, 573
- angiography 452, 453

Cardiac conditions 865
Cardiac contractility modulation 121, 176, 186, 229, 246, 257, 641, 964, 1006
Cardiac coronary coupling 37, 38
Cardiac cycle 421, 559
- stages of 560*f*

Cardiac death, causes of 209
Cardiac diseases 477
Cardiac dysfunction during breast cancer therapy, prevention of 802
Cardiac fibrosis 25, 801, 951
- different types of 21
- presence of 281

Cardiac fibrous tissue 22
Cardiac function 576
- assessment of 453

Cardiac functional impairment, chronic phase of 695
Cardiac hemochromatosis 402
Cardiac hypertrophy 25, 873, 935
Cardiac injury markers 55
Cardiac insufficiency bisoprolol study 526
Cardiac lipid accumulation, role of 779*fc*
Cardiac magnetic resonance 40, 140, 141, 204, 473, 477, 495, 503, 760
- assessment 476
- evaluation 459, 460, 471
- imaging 46, 101, 459, 472, 473, 554, 778
  - techniques 468
- sequence 473

Cardiac mechanism 903
Cardiac metabolic flexibility 936
Cardiac metabolism, direct alteration of 935
Cardiac myocyte 64
Cardiac output 176, 199, 599, 811, 950
- strategies to 609

Cardiac pathophysiological alterations 1011
Cardiac power 819
- output infraction 811

Cardiac rehabilitation 107, 997
- environments 998
- programs 450

Cardiac remodeling 280, 460, 520, 886, 902, 962
- mechanism of 327
- reversal 460

Cardiac resynchronization therapy 127, 155, 239, 419, 641, 686, 817, 978, 980
- mechanism of action of 156
- potential benefits of 156

Cardiac sarcoidosis 173, 402
Cardiac specific antigens 638
Cardiac stiffness 162, 576, 827
Cardiac surgery, radiation and prior 112
Cardiac troponins 161
Cardiodermatology 697
Cardiodiabetes 727
Cardiogenic pulmonary, evidence of 138, 598
Cardiogenic shock 811, 814, 815, 815*f*, 816*f*, 817
Cardiohelp machine 814*f*
Cardiolipidology 775, 777
Cardiolipin 640
Cardiology Society of India 12
Cardiometabolic benefits 489
Cardiometabolic parameters 904
Cardiometabolic syndrome 739
- management of 740

Cardiomyocyte 221, 638, 826, 827
- alterations 21
- cell death 21, 24, 25
- hypertrophy 1002
- ionic homeostasis 899
- membranes 602
- stiffness 1002

Cardiomyopathy 48, 182, 267, 552, 561, 881
Cardionutrition 783
Cardio-oncology 797
Cardio-ophthalmology 689
Cardioprotective strategies 806
Cardiopulmonary disease 703
Cardiopulmonary exercise 805
- test 46, 708

Cardiopulmonary interaction 714*f*
Cardiorenal cluster 119
Cardiorenal iron deficiency syndrome 635
Cardiorenal syndrome 57, 607, 608*t*, 609, 610, 612
- precipitating factors of 609*f*

Cardio-selective beta-1 blocker 600
Cardiotoxicity 799, 800
- early detection of 806
- monitoring 806

Cardiovascular care, preventive 807
Cardiovascular comorbidities 171, 806
Cardiovascular death 174, 179, 210, 349, 584, 871
- composite of 854, 884*f*
- endpoint of 1015
- risk of 732
- specific cause of 6

Cardiovascular disease 138, 188, 582, 587, 588, 590, 604, 617*f*, 706, 722, 769, 779, 792, 889
- risk factors of 792*f*
- trajectories of 663

Cardiovascular events, risk of 755
Cardiovascular function 152
Cardiovascular health 681, 700
  study 912, 977
Cardiovascular kidney metabolic syndrome 188, 587, 617
Cardiovascular medicine 744
Cardiovascular morbidity 888*f*
Cardiovascular mortality 88*f*, 629, 906, 977
  reduction 614
Cardiovascular outcome 867
  studies 772
Cardiovascular remodeling 997
Cardiovascular risk factors 434, 496, 915
Cardiovascular structure 87, 471
  abnormalities in 471*fc*
Cardiovascular system 77*fc*, 663*fc*, 889*fc*, 891, 957
  receptor agonists on 736
Cardiovascular-kidney-metabolic
  identification 588*b*
  syndrome 589, 590, 590*f*, 617
    management of 589, 589*f*
    risk of 590
    stages of 588*f*, 617*f*
Cardioverter defibrillator 817
Carotenes 794
Carvedilol 527
  effect of 919
Catecholamine-mediated vasoconstriction 684
Catecholamines 834
Catheter ablation 1007
  role of 517
Cell
  apoptosis 434
  therapy 640
  turnover 684
Cellular levels 30
Center for Disease Control and Prevention 791
Central aortic stiffness, measurement of 299
Central blood pressure 890
Central nervous system 722
  inflammation 723
Central retinal arterial equivalent 691
Central venous pressure 573
  elevation of 607
Ceramides 778
Chemokines 102
Chemotherapy 563, 778, 804
  induced cardiomyopathy 685
  related cardiac toxicity 684
Cheops bundle 655
  items of 656
Cherry-on-top pattern 336*f*
Chest
  ultrasound 656
  X-ray 33, 60, 74
Chlorthalidone 534
Chordal replacement 968
Chronic cardiorenal syndrome 609
Chronic coronary syndrome 186, 780, 780*fc*, 932
Chronic heart failure 277, 862
Chronic hyperglycemia 864
Chronic hyperkalemia 842
Chronic hypoperfusion 194
Chronic hypoxemia 546
Chronic inflammation 588, 668
Chronic inflammatory state 668
Chronic kidney disease 8, 24, 37, 50, 51, 54, 77, 80, 87, 119*f*, 123, 160, 173, 186, 188, 211, 215, 217, 268, 380, 570, 581, 581*t*, 583, 584, 587-589, 592-595, 598, 599, 604, 611, 612, 616-621, 625, 629, 630, 634, 634*f*, 635, 637, 681, 705, 713, 744, 759, 779, 819, 825, 839, 846, 919, 929, 935, 957
  management of 581, 584
  mild 595
  moderate 595
  pathophysiology of 593*f*
  progression of 853
  risk factors of 593*f*
Chronic liver diseases 210
Chronic low-grade inflammation 81, 864
Chronic lung disease 712, 713
Chronic myeloid leukemia 805
Chronic obstructive
  airway disease 60
  pulmonary
    disease 37, 38, 45, 54, 77, 80, 123, 181, 277, 328, 420, 498, 593, 659, 705, 713, 744, 759, 920, 923, 929
    disorder 760
Chronic pulmonary disease 380
Chronic renal disease 210
Chronic thromboembolic pulmonary hypertension 379, 429, 707, 712, 713
Chronic uncontrolled hypothyroidism 754
Chronotropic incompetence 50, 51, 64, 90, 225, 226, 268
Cinacalcet 640
Colchicine 638
Collagen
  accumulation 472
  crosslinking 25
  deposition 372, 825
  formation 670
  metabolism 896
Collider bias 746
Color scalograms 285, 285*t*
  basics of 286*f*
Combination therapy 149, 151, 409
Comorbidity 372, 814
  management of 49, 98, 112, 144, 171, 173*t*, 609, 750, 912, 923, 1013
Comparator arm 829
Complex clinical syndrome 391, 962
Computed tomography 46
  angiography 33, 452
    role of 452
Concentric hypertrophy 21
Conduit function 363
Conduit strain 356
Congenital cardiomyopathies 705
Congenital cyanotic heart diseases 545
Congenital heart
  anomalies 182
  disease 545, 551, 563
Congestion 266
Congestive heart failure 504, 587, 789, 923
Constipation 622
Constrictive cardiomyopathy 335
Constrictive pericarditis 173, 339, 379, 402, 454, 575
Constrictive physiology, hallmark features of 336
Continuous positive airway pressure 106, 145, 534, 719
Contractile strain 356
Contrast-induced nephropathy 457
Corolla assist device 964
Coronary artery
  bypass graft 502, 504, 505, 508
    techniques of 504
  calcium 590
  disease 24, 46, 40-51, 60, 112, 123, 123*f*, 158, 160, 173, 182, 215, 226, 268, 276, 277, 379, 402, 420, 477, 487, 498, 502, 567, 659, 669, 673, 679, 684, 825
    detection of 484
    evaluation of 452
    higher prevalence of 777
    phenotype 744
    prognosis of 276
    severity of 135
  number of diseased 135
Coronary blood flow 40
Coronary flow reserve 40
Coronary heart disease 588
Coronary ischemia 546
Coronary microvascular dysfunction 37, 39, 40, 50, 268, 472, 951
  impact of 39
  prevalence of 37, 39
Coronary microvascular endothelial
  cells 372
  dysfunction 665
  inflammation 929
Coronary ostia
  height, measurement of 483*f*
  measurements 483

Coronary sinus 422, 985
Coronary vessel caliber 684
Coronavirus disease-2019 (COVID-19) 76, 77, 77*f*
  effect of 77*fc*
  infection 78
  pandemic 76
Cortisol 723
Corvia 422, 985
  device 985
C-reactive protein 280, 669
Critical vasoactive peptides 835
Current heart failure management guidelines 930
Cyclic adenosine monophosphate 54, 64, 221, 709, 828
Cyclic guanosine monophosphate signaling 673
Cytoskeleton 664
Cytosolic sodium 899

D

Daily living, activities of 91
Damaged cells 20
Danon disease 562
Dapagliflozin 128, 180, 184, 359, 394, 489, 583, 614, 638, 716, 736, 773, 778, 859, 872, 886, 889, 902, 904, 932, 949, 1002, 1010, 1015
  administration of 394*f*
  emerging role of 886
  heart failure, pooled analysis of 855
  impact of 902
  reduction with 869*f*
Dark blood imaging 476
Dasatinib 805
Dead cardiomyocytes 827
Deaths, proportion of 791*f*
Decompress left atrium 820*f*
Deep vein thrombosis 210
Degenerative mitral regurgitation 970
Degrade extracellular matrix 20
Dehydration 614
  signs of 585
Delayed gadolinium imaging 475
Delayed relaxation 343
Deliver trial 854, 867, 883
  visual abstract 613*f*
Depression 588
Device embolization 969
Device therapy 113, 179, 641*f*, 682, 750, 815
Device-based adjunct therapies, recent advances in 186
Diabetes 4, 17, 50, 51, 112, 158, 185, 215, 216, 242, 287*f*, 520, 609, 611, 614, 734, 744, 819, 825, 829, 864, 865, 866, 886
  current management of 735
  impact of 735
  management 960
  mellitus 20, 26, 37, 38, 73, 90, 100, 119*f*, 142, 160, 181, 182, 192, 498, 583, 587, 588, 620*f*, 672, 731, 734, 739, 740, 769, 778, 879, 889, 906, 949, 952, 953, 1002
    combination of 611
    control of 564
    higher prevalence of 502
    management of 853
    trials 943
  pathophysiology of 734
  presence of 735
  prevalence of 734
Diabetic heart 103
Diabetic ketoacidosis 873, 874
Diabetic kidney disease 589, 629, 630, 958
Diabetic macular edema 695
Diabetic nephropathy 582
Diabetic retinopathy 695
  impact of 695
  stages of 695
Diacylglycerols 778
Diamond trial 841
Diarrhea 622
Diastolic blood pressure 989
Diastolic dysfunction 15, 72, 179*fc*, 182, 287*f*, 339, 347, 471, 373*fc*, 480, 496, 567, 568, 572*f*, 654*f*, 656, 668, 753, 754, 864
  assessment of 339*fc*, 345
  clinical implications of 654
  diagnosis of 285*fc*, 341
  echocardiographic indices of 660*b*
  evaluation of 452, 472
  grades of 339, 384*f*, 392*f*
  presence of 825, 834
Diastolic exercise echocardiography 364
  role of 364
Diastolic function 872, 1012
  controlling factors of 560*f*
  improvement 153
  limited assessment of 457
  normal 333*f*
  parameters 329
Diastolic heart failure 567, 679, 996
  diagnosis of 659*t*
  diastolic dysfunction of 234*f*
  etiology of 659*b*
  hypothesis of mechanisms of 660*b*
  pathophysiological mechanisms of 659
Diastolic mitral regurgitation 341
Diastolic pressure 859
Diastolic stress 287*f*
  test 65, 288, 1013
Diastolic ventricular strain 343
Diastology, echocardiographic assessment of 332
Diet 153, 792
Dietary approaches to stop hypertension diet 154
Dietary sodium restriction 108*t*
Dietary strategies 730
Diffuse fibrosis 471
Diffuse myocardial fibrosis 476
Digoxin 563, 639, 686, 834
Dilated cardiomyopathy 552, 561
Dipeptidyl peptidase-4 888
  inhibitors 889*fc*, 891, 892
    beneficial roles of 888*f*
    role of 891
Direct oral anticoagulants 418, 516
Directed medical therapy 183*fc*
Disease-modifying therapy 139, 184
Diuresis 407, 521, 612, 740
Diuretic 98, 112, 129, 171, 180, 183, 195, 225, 599, 731, 749
  therapy 131, 608
Dobutamine stress echocardiography 503
Docosahexaenoic acid 793
Doppler echocardiography 715
Doppler method 413
Doppler study, E-wave of 391
Doxorubicin-induced cardiotoxicity 799
  mechanism of 800*fc*
Drugs 180, 330, 387, 408, 548, 564, 669, 900, 1014
  class 142-144, 184
  studied 740, 741
  switch 977
  therapy 637
Dual-lumen cannula 819
Dulaglutide 952
Durable mechanical circulatory support 973
Dysautonomia 111, 112
Dyselectrolytemia 622
Dysfunctional fatty tissue 587
Dysfunctional renin-angiotensin-aldosterone axis 664
Dysglycemia 50
Dyskalemia 839
Dyslipidemia 587, 829
  management of 779
Dyspnea 18, 60, 119*f*, 262, 372, 547, 551, 684
  cardiopulmonary causes of 70
  differential diagnosis of 56*t*
  noncardiac causes of 65, 69, 210
  severe 88
  symptoms, reduction in 155
Dyssynchrony 156

E

Eccentric hypertrophy 21
Echocardiographic guided therapy 332

Echocardiography 61, 343, 361, 372, 375, 376, 391, 399, 472, 608, 714, 715, 749, 865
  aids 818
  role of 334, 371, 378, 379, 432
Edema 546, 684
  differential diagnosis of 56*t*
Edwards lifesciences apture shunt 986
Eicosapentaenoic acid 793
Ejection fraction 18, 49, 56, 127, 141, 399, 520, 590, 736, 761, 762, 767, 872
  conceptualization of 31*f*
  cut-off 669
  heart failure, preserved 122*f*
  preserved 36*f*, 50*b*, 51, 72, 76, 94, 95, 157, 221, 332, 411, 426, 594, 748, 799, 995, 1006
  reduced 33, 275
  role of 150
  spectrum of 150, 900
Elamipretide 640
Electrical synchrony 156
Electrical therapy 964
Electrocardiogram 46, 60, 74, 588, 715
  color scalogram representation of 285*f*
Electrocardiography 13, 496
Electrodes 1006
Electrolyte
  disturbances 608
  imbalance 612
Elevated blood
  glucose levels 587
  pressure, pathophysiology of 189
Elevated jugular venous pressure 60, 849, 865
Elevated left ventricular filling pressure 363, 371, 406, 825
Elevated natriuretic peptide levels 138, 598, 632, 912, 1015
Elevated serum markers 178
Embolization 421
Emmy trial 490
Empagliflozin 128, 142, 148, 180, 184, 359, 583, 614, 638, 716, 736, 740, 745, 761, 772, 778, 859, 867, 868, 902-904, 932, 949, 1002, 1008, 1015
  effects 585, 1009
Emperor-preserved trial 854, 867, 883
  visual abstract 613*f*
End-diastolic pressure 654, 654*f*, 760
End-diastolic volume 547
Endocardial fibroelastosis 575
Endomyocardial biopsy 33
Endomyocardial fibrosis 562
Endothelial cells 826
Endothelial dysfunction 21, 24, 25, 54, 80, 101, 105, 280, 607, 691, 748, 752, 814, 864, 882, 940, 951
  mechanisms of 81
Endothelial function 193, 854
Endothelial inflammation 827, 929
Endothelial reactive oxygen species 38
Endothelin 280, 539
  receptor
    A 709
    antagonists 707, 709
    B 709
Endothelium 64, 664
End-stage heart disease 489
End-stage kidney disease 584, 587
End-stage renal disease 900
  hemodialysis 595
Energy-dense fatty acids, oxidation of 778
Enrolment criteria 1016
Enzyme 835
Epicardial adipose tissue 455, 1002
  pathophysiological role of 1002
Epicardium 737
Epithelial sodium channels 826
Eplerenone 148, 534, 935
Ertugliflozin 614, 778, 907
Erythropoiesis-stimulating agents 635
Erythropoietin 899
Essential fatty acids 793
Estimated glomerular filtration rate 119, 144, 145, 736, 740, 862, 873, 960, 981
Estrogen 664, 666
  deficiency 663
  mediated mechanistic pathways 664*f*
  receptors, subtypes of 663*fc*
Euglycemic diabetic ketoacidosis 614, 875, 900
European Association of Cardiovascular Imaging 332, 366
European Society of Cardiology 712
Exacerbate capillary rarefaction 677
Exenatide 952
Exendin-4 backbone 952
Exercise 39, 256, 268
  capacity 155, 156, 677, 682, 940, 1009
  evaluation, pretreatment 806
  function 612
  induced left atrial hypertension, management of 200
  integration 154
  intolerance 995
  monitoring during 153
  oscillatory ventilation 708
  prescription 806
  pulmonary capillary wedge pressure 762
  tolerance 153, 923
    reduced 754
  training 106, 107, 152, 256, 564, 995, 996, 998
    types of 996
Exertional shortness of breath, symptoms in 260
Extracardiac morbidities 221, 222*fc*
Extracardiac pathophysiological alterations 1011
Extracardiac structures, evaluation of 454
Extracellular fluid 260
Extracellular matrix 472, 664, 665, 886
  related stiffness 522
  remodeling 102, 899
Extracellular volume 474
Extracorporeal membrane oxygenation 420, 809, 811, 812*t*, 813-815, 816*f*, 817, 818, 821*f*
  advantages of 816*b*
  clinical outcomes of 814
  complications 820*f*
  manual of 814*f*
  recent advances in 819
  system 812*f*, 813
  thrombosis on 820*f*
  types of 816
Ezetimibe 780

F

Fabry disease 111, 379
Fasting blood sugar 588
Fasting plasma glucose 588
Fat 94, 96, 793
Fatigue 547
  clinical characteristic of 96
Fatty acid
  binding protein 55, 280
  composition 794*f*
Fatty liver disease 587
  metabolic-associated 188
Femoral artery 812, 813, 819
Femoral vein 243, 812, 819
Ferric carboxymaltose 786, 903, 939
  single bolus of 939
Fibrillar collagen deposition 886
Fibroblast 826
  growth factor 593
  hypertrophy 825
Fibrosis 41, 103, 203, 275, 279, 319, 426, 583*f*, 630, 715, 752
  reduction in 407
Fibrotic signaling 25
Fidelity 631
Filling pressure 73, 337, 342, 950, 1013
Finerenone 120, 185, 599, 601, 629, 630, 637, 935, 957, 958, 1016
  safety profile of 632
First heart failure, prediction of 700*f*
Fluid
  homeostasis 592
  intake, monitoring 106
  management 106
  removal 656
  retention 95, 718, 867

Fluorodeoxyglucose-positron emission tomography 141, 173
Focal fibrosis 471, 477
Fontan surgery 547
Four-dimensional left ventricular strain 307
Frailty 744
Framingham Heart Study 668, 977
Free thyroxine 755
Free triiodothyronine 755
Fuel energetics, shift in 874
Functional capacity 956, 995
Functional mitral regurgitation 970
Furosemide 749

G

Galectin-3 55, 61, 161, 163
  inhibitors 639
Gastric mucosa 951
Gastrointestinal malabsorption 635
Gene
  activation of 630
  therapy 750
Genetic disorders leading 551
Genital infections 614
Geographic variability 149
Geriatric nutritional risk index 790
Gestational diabetes 684
  consideration 588
Gliflozins 736*f*
Global Burden of Disease Study 125
Global circumferential strain 330
Global longitudinal strain 27, 308, 330, 376, 379, 385, 547, 553
Glomerular filtration rate 581, 588, 604, 669
  reduced 625
Glucagon-like peptide 50, 51, 173, 268, 592, 739, 951
  agonists 121
  analogs 978, 1002
  mechanism of action of 736
  receptor 594
    agonists 98, 129, 145, 178, 185, 256, 589, 590, 618-620, 730, 731, 949, 951
    antagonists 173
Glucose
  dependent insulinotropic polypeptide 113
  levels 583
  plasma concentration of 102
Glycemic control 158, 521
  improvement of 871
Glycemic effects 614
Glycogen storage 152
  disorders 562
Glycosuria 767
Glycosylated hemoglobin 145
Good-quality proteins 793
Gradient echo-echo planar imaging 473
Great arteries, transposition of 546
Greater splanchnic nerve ablation 186
Growing public health crisis 1012
Growth differentiation factor 61, 55, 280
Guanosintrifosphate 709
Guanylate cyclase stimulator 402
Guideline-directed medical therapy 49, 112, 138, 139, 141, 142, 144, 183, 184, 285, 351, 459, 589, 618-620, 649, 682, 745, 758, 984
  benefits of 973
  use of 706
Gut microbiome 1009
Guyton's classic concept 191
Gynecomastia 629, 957

H

Hazard ratio 128, 868
Health, social determinants of 588
Healthcare expenditures 967
Heart 592, 612, 951
  blocks 112
  disease 955
    left-sided 705
    radiation-induced 563
    right-sided 402
  electrical activity 1006
  failure 3, 6, 16, 17, 18*f*, 24, 30, 36*f*, 39, 51*f*, 56, 74, 90, 91, 94, 125, 127, 130, 131, 131*b*, 134, 137-139, 139*f*, 141, 155, 158-160, 188, 194, 199, 211, 238*f*, 239, 255, 266, 275, 276, 284, 295, 355, 362*f*, 371, 383, 386, 387, 391, 408, 414, 419, 437, 447, 452, 459, 460, 495, 502, 515, 520, 545, 552, 559, 581, 583*f*, 584, 588, 592, 598, 600*fc*, 602, 616, 619*f*, 620, 620*f*, 621, 629, 630, 632, 634*f*, 636, 649, 663, 675, 680*f*, 683, 693, 715, 718, 735, 736, 740, 743, 752, 761, 762, 767, 768, 777, 778, 786, 786*f*, 790, 811, 815, 817, 818, 825, 829, 836, 844-847, 849, 859, 862, 864, 876, 883, 889, 891, 899, 908, 915-917, 919, 929, 931, 939, 942, 952, 958, 960, 960*f*, 962, 967, 997, 1001, 1002, 1008
    acute decompensated of 8, 815, 816*b*, 977
    changing landscape of 44
    classification of 34*t*, 56*t*, 94, 137, 137*t*, 284, 371, 831
    clinic 981*fc*
    clinical syndrome of 371
    clusters of 32*f*
    co-management of 617
    context of 967
    device-based therapies of 248*f*
    diagnosis of 125, 618
    different classes of 498*t*
    drug treatment for 180*t*
    epidemiology of 15, 125
    establish diagnosis of 265
    etiology of 15, 684
    events 1015
    hospitalization 871, 970, 977
      benefit 149
      reduction in 149
    incidence of 37, 165
    left atrial strain in 351
    life-prolonging medications of 126*t*
    management 651, 109*t*, 387*f*, 778
    mechanisms of 676*fc*
    monitoring 245*f*
    mortality, prognostic score of 92*t*
    neural cardiac therapy for 248
    noncardiovascular cause of 50*b*
    obesity-related 157, 741*t*, 946
    overview of 967
    pathogenesis of 675
    pathology of 221
    pathophysiology of 648, 779*fc*
    pathway in 395*fc*
    phenotype of 719, 979*t*
    phenotypic spectrum of 520*f*
    population prevalence of 16*t*
    portion of 1011
    powerful predictor of 349
    precursor of 560
    presence of 785
    prevalence of 864
    preventing 737
    primary prevention of 685
    promising treatment for 879
    rates for 892
    reduce risk of hospitalizations for 762
    registry 13, 673
    rehospitalization 17, 932*f*
    risk factors with 777
    scoring system 341
    signs of 18, 53, 56, 178, 211, 339, 367*f*, 547, 582, 871
    spectrum of 906
    stable chronic 858
    stages of 138, 138*fc*
    strain parameters in 296*t*
    symptomatic 693
    symptoms of 18, 53, 56, 85, 178, 211, 367*fc*, 547, 871, 912
    syndrome 15
    therapeutic management of 929
    threshold for 972
    treatment of 625
    trial, preserved 855
    type of 137, 679
    unique aspect of 8*b*

health 721
leads, interstitium of 472
mate 964
rate 392, 903
influence of 525
lowering of 929
reduction 923
resting 684
support devices 962
transplantation 686, 972, 973
Heart Failure Association 266
Heart Failure Association of European Society of Cardiology 342
Heart Failure Association Pre-Test Assessment 1013
Heart Failure Society of America 182, 927
Heart failure with preserved ejection fraction 6t, 1-7, 10, 10t, 11, 12, 13f, 18, 20, 23-26, 37, 38, 46, 47fc, 50, 53, 62, 64, 72, 74, 76-78, 80, 85, 87, 90, 94, 100, 101, 105, 112, 115, 121, 123, 125, 131, 134, 139-142, 147, 148, 156, 158-160, 175, 176, 178-180, 181b, 183, 183fc, 184, 200, 202, 203, 206, 209, 221, 233, 235f, 236, 240, 241, 255, 256, 259, 265, 266, 269, 272, 275, 279, 289, 300, 305, 328, 330, 330t, 332, 360, 361, 362f, 371, 375, 376, 378, 385-387, 399, 402, 406, 407, 408t, 411, 425, 432, 437, 447-449, 451, 453t, 454, 464, 471, 473, 476, 477, 480, 487, 494, 495, 498, 500, 515, 520, 522, 526, 527, 531, 539, 543, 545, 548t, 561, 567, 576, 579, 581, 582, 584, 592, 593, 595, 609f, 611, 612, 614, 625, 629, 640, 645, 649, 657, 669, 677, 679, 681, 681f, 682, 689, 695, 697, 699, 701, 703, 705-707, 721, 727, 734, 735, 736, 739-741, 744, 745, 752, 753, 755, 758, 760, 760f, 762, 772, 779, 785, 787, 789, 801, 804, 806, 811, 814, 811f, 814, 815, 825, 829, 829t, 833f, 834, 844, 849, 853, 864, 865, 872, 872fc, 873, 875, 882, 883, 886, 888, 894, 895, 899, 909, 916, 925, 926, 931, 944f, 950t, 957, 964, 978, 980, 981, 995, 1001, 1006, 1009, 1014t
acute decompensation of 380b
advanced 68fc
assessment of 291
basic cellular pathophysiology of 54f
benefits, multifaceted mechanisms underlying 759
beta-blocker use in 931t
biomarker-based diagnosis of 55t
burden 949
cardiometabolic 730fc
care 653
causative factors of 11f
causes of 101f
classification of 223, 224fc
clinical diagnosis of 44
clinical features of 18
clinical presentation phenotypes 225t
clinical spectrum 1
cluster model of 118f
comorbidities 145fc, 180fc
interplay of 49f
coronary microvascular disease 560
development of 82
devices of 243t, 244f
diagnosis of 46f, 53, 60, 74fc, 97, 126, 138, 165, 178, 255, 266fc, 267fc, 339, 347, 367fc, 387, 561, 562t, 648, 679, 714, 735, 1012, 1014f
diagnostic algorithms for 182
diagnostic evaluation of 561, 912, 913fc
diagnostic scoring systems 57, 57t, 138, 139t
differential diagnosis of 48f, 267fc, 379t
disease 123f
respiratory to 123f
drugs therapy for 34fc, 35fc, 236
echocardiographic evaluation of 180f, 371, 425, 432
effect of 887f
etiology of 182, 561fc
exacerbation 754
exercise training in 998
function in 312t, 471
grading of 568
heart, surgical anatomy of 972
hemodynamics of 237f, 525
hypertensive 157
in emergency, risk stratification with 279
incidence of 137, 1015
management of 32, 43, 48, 139, 167, 182, 210, 214, 227, 233, 255, 334, 402, 594, 615t, 637, 651, 656, 748, 749, 760, 925, 951, 1013
masquerader 115
mechanisms of 100, 520, 575, 813
medical management of 626f
medical therapy for 761f
medications in 402
menopause-associated 665
mimics 138, 140, 141, 211
monitoring therapy in 334
mortality with 12
myocardial signaling in 222f
new guidelines 165
newer management strategies 221
nonpharmacological intervention of 106t
nonpharmacological therapies for 105
obesity and 236, 743, 744, 1009
ongoing trials on 1016t
pathology 221
pathophysiologic mechanism of 280t
pathophysiological basis of 827
pathophysiology of 44, 87, 105, 182, 279, 372, 383, 419, 568, 592, 611, 638f, 680f, 748, 758, 759f, 813, 826fc, 827, 828fc, 873fc, 925, 929
pediatric 550
pharmacological management for 977
pharmacotherapy 137
phenotypes of 11, 170, 259, 569f, 744fc
phenotypic clustering 234
prevalence of 43, 519, 637, 912
prevention of 559, 995
primary diagnostic tool for 1012
primary prevention of 168
probable pharmacotherapy of 563t
prognosis for 88
progression of 83, 306t
recent advances in 1001
risk factors for 77f, 88, 805fc
risk scoring 1013
score 62t, 68, 72, 73, 73t, 140f, 166, 308, 341, 375, 375t, 1013, 1013t
chart 401t
clinical application of 309t
severity of 1015
shared mechanism for 417
signs of 18t
splanchnic ablation for 246f
symptoms in 18t
therapy 126
tool box 285
transitions of 260
treatment of 119, 131, 171, 178, 223, 908fc, 912,
types of 200t
umbrella concept of 402t
updates on 118
Heart failure with reduced ejection fraction 10, 12, 20, 21, 23-26, 77, 91, 131, 139, 147, 170, 239, 295, 306t, 371, 425, 761, 769, 785, 801, 872, 888, 906, 909, 949, 957, 958, 984, 1011
current management of 598
development of 24f, 26f
emerging epidemic of 1011
epidemic, drivers of 1011
evaluation of 43, 44
pathophysiology of 827
pharmaceutical armamentarium for 509f
role of drugs for 536
treatment of 127fc, 204, 908
trials, contemporary 116
Hematopoietic cell transplantation 805
Hemodynamic 656
benefits 155, 156
congestion 266
congestion, mechanisms of 546f
effects 583, 950
Hemoglobin 280
A1C 13, 588, 589

Hemolytic anemia 562
Hemopoietic stem cell 26
Hemorrhage 691
Heparin 969
Hepatomegaly 546
Hepcidin 785, 787
levels 785
Hereditary hemochromatosis gene 141
Hereditary hypertrophic cardiomyopathies 551
Heterogenous disorder 361, 825
Heterozygous familial hypercholesterolemia 779
High blood pressure 865, 989
High left ventricular filling pressure 567
High pulmonary pressures 715
High sensitive cardiac troponin 280
High-density lipoprotein cholesterol 779-781
Higher baseline blood pressures 150
Higher kidney perfusion pressure 191
High-intensity interval training 106
High-output heart failure 173
High-sensitivity C-reactive protein 161, 618
Holistic impact 152
Hormone replacement therapy 666
Hospitalizations, reduced 151
Hourglass-shaped nitinol self-expanding prosthesis 963
Human immunodeficiency virus 588
Hydralazine 129, 239
Hydroxytyrosol 794
Hypercholesterolemia 753
Hyperfiltration 873
Hyperglucagonemia 875
Hyperglycemia 587
role of 101
triggers glomerular hyperfiltration 582
Hyperinflammatory responses 665
Hyperinsulinemia 192, 882
Hyperkalemia 601, 621, 632, 839, 840, 840*t*, 842, 877, 960
incidence of 959
increased risks of 629
leading 959
management of 621
related RAAS inhibitor discontinuation 840
risk factors for 621
Hyperlipidemia 587
Hypersensitivity reactions 877
Hypertension 4, 17, 24, 37, 38, 49, 73, 111, 159, 182, 185, 189, 191, 191*f*, 192, 193*fc*, 202, 215, 216, 287*f*, 407, 420, 471, 498, 520, 531, 587, 589, 608, 609, 659, 664, 671, 684, 718, 721-723, 752, 778, 806, 825, 827, 865, 908, 919, 930, 989, 991, 1013
control, global challenge of 989
development of 575
management of 153, 564, 679
novel treatment for 989
obesity-related 193, 194
secondary 991
severe 840
types of 989
Hypertensive 73, 659, 989
cluster 118
heart disease 778
Hyperthyroidism, subclinical 754, 755
Hypertriglyceridemia 588
management of 781*fc*
Hypertrophic cardiomyopathy 138, 173, 209, 211, 266, 277, 334, 379, 402, 454, 477, 552, 561, 981
Registry of National Heart Lung and Blood Institute 209
Hypertrophic obstructive cardiomyopathy 276
medical management of 335
severe 335*f*
Hypertrophy 520, 664, 827
Hypoglycemia 875
Hypomagnesemia 622
Hypotension 846, 991
Hypothalamus-pituitary-adrenal axis 723
Hypothyroidism 210, 752-755
correction of 756*f*
subclinical 754, 755
Hypovolemic states 874
Hypoxia 713
Hypoxia-inducible factor alpha 786

I

Iatrogenic atrial septal defect 243, 420
Immune
pathways, activation of 102
system 668
Impaired natriuresis, prognostic implications of 196
Impaired systemic vasodilatory reserve 64
Impaired vasodilatory capacity 37
Impaired ventricular relaxation 152
Impella 819
device placement 816*f*
Implantable cardiac defibrillator 127, 298, 402, 686
Implantable heart failure monitor 244, 245*f*
Implantable hemodynamic monitors 106
Implantable pulmonary artery pressure monitors 186
Impulse generation, rate of 929
Inclusion criteria 829, 900
Inconclusive noninvasive stress tests 33
Indapamide 534
Indian Heart Failure Registries 10
Ineffective therapies 50
Infection 380, 827, 874, 991
Infective endocarditis 969
Inferior vena cava 379, 813
dimension 427
Infiltrative cardiomyopathy 138, 681
Infiltrative disorders 182, 339
Inflammation 24, 25, 81, 105, 162, 193, 194, 279, 406, 520, 583*f*, 607, 611, 630, 664, 668, 721, 722, 943, 1002
and fibrosis, reduce 916
reduction in 407
resulting in 587
Inflammatory adipokines 951
secretion of 1002
Inflammatory cytokines 676
Inflammatory diseases 552
Inflammatory effects 950
Inflammatory enzyme myeloperoxidase 1004
Inflammatory factors 718
Inflammatory markers 55, 916
Inflammatory mediators 722
Inflammatory processes 406
Infundibulum 311
In-hospital heart failure diagnosis, incidence of 16*f*
Inorganic nitrite 225, 226
Inotrope therapy 608, 818
Inspiratory muscle training 996
Insulin 770
glucose metabolism 935
resistance 192, 587, 611, 864, 1002
secretion, suppression of 766
sensitivity 882
Insulin-like growth factor binding protein 280
Intensive care unit 653
Interatrial septostomy 661
Interatrial septum 715, 985
Interatrial shunt 244*f*, 1008
creation 984
device 154, 186, 205, 206, 228*f*, 243, 640, 710, 962, 978, 980, 985, 985*t*
system 1008
no-implant 423*f*
pathophysiology of 984
therapy 422*t*, 987
V-wave technology for 1008
Intercommissural distance, measurement of 483*f*
Interleukin 55, 193, 828
receptor 1009
Internal jugular vein 812
Intershunt 422, 985, 987
percutaneous atrial shunt catheter system 987
Interstitial fibrosis 25, 41, 64, 472
Interstitial myocardial fibrosis 551
Interstitial volume, reduction in 147
Interventional therapies 113, 1003

Intra-abdominal
mass 210
pressure, elevation of 607
Intra-aortic balloon pump 815, 819
Intracellular accumulation 551
Intracellular steroid hormone receptors 957
Intracranial hemorrhage 818
Intraglomerular pressure 873
Intraretinal microvascular anomalies 695
Intravenous immunoglobulin 638
Intravenous iron infusion 129
Intraventricular dyssynchrony 503
Intrinsic abnormalities 551
Intrinsic sympathomimetic activity 930
Invasive hemodynamic assessment 111, 866, 749
Invasive nature 108
Invasive testing 401
Ion channel currents 937
Ionic homeostasis 521
Ionic imbalance 520
Irbesartan 832
Iron
overload 562
stores 939
supplementation 640, 939
Iron deficiency 581, 636, 785, 786*f*, 788
anemia 516, 635, 673
treatment of 635
pathophysiology of 785
Ischemia 39, 380, 378, 502
Ischemic background 931
Ischemic cardiomyopathy 504*fc*
testing for 503
Ischemic cardiovascular diseases 587
Ischemic heart disease 15, 123*f*, 241, 259, 587, 722, 777, 908, 926
phenotype 886
Isolated right heart failure 116
Isosorbide dinitrate therapy 129, 239
Isovolumetric relaxation time 550, 553
Istaroxime 639
Ivabradine 129, 527, 563, 834

J

Japanese Acute Decompensated Heart Failure Syndromes Registry 673
Japanese diastolic heart failure 930
Jugular vein distention 18
Jugular venous pressure 13, 546

K

Kansas city cardiomyopathy clinical summary score 127
Kansas city cardiomyopathy questionnaire 120, 121, 206, 423, 669, 862
clinical summary 736
score 121, 732, 767, 946, 953, 1002
score 130, 970
total symptom score 740, 741, 762, 767
Kaplan-Meier
curves 850*f*
estimates 505*f*
Kawasaki disease 561
Kawasaki shock syndrome 552
Ketones 854
utilization of 612
Kidney 189, 882, 951
dysfunction 280
failure 587, 630
function 596
health 612
injury 991
molecule 280
work 592
Kidney disease 111, 588, 619*f*, 960
progression
attenuation of 172
low risk of 632
severe 884
chronic 595
Korean acute heart failure 923
Kussmaul's sign 112
Kyphoscoliosis 210

L

Large left atrial thrombus 322*f*
Large-scale epidemiological studies 787
Late cardiovascular effects 807
Late diastolic mitral inflow velocity 434
Late gadolinium enhancement 461, 464, 475, 554
Late iodine enhancement, evaluation of 453
Late mitral filling velocity 553
Latter attracts leukocytes 827
Leaflet length, measurement of 483*f*
Left atrial 360
assist device 230, 230*f*, 641, 974, 978
atriopathy 203, 447, 449, 451
therapeutic strategies and management of 450
cardiomyopathy 202
contractile strain 437
decompression pumps 641, 974, 980
dilatation 319
echocardiographic parameters 357*t*
emptying fraction 356
enlargement 72, 128, 415, 454, 484, 829
evaluation 355, 465
filling index 345
hypertension, exercise-induced 199
hypertrophy 715
myocardial deformation 413
myopathy 365, 935
pacing therapy 186, 205*t*, 207, 246
permanent pacing 229
phases of 437
pressure 90, 356, 383, 654, 712
reservoir strain 179, 321, 346*f*, 414
size 320, 355, 411
sphericity index 894
structure 836
Left atrial appendage 516
assessment 322
flow pattern 324*f*
occlusion devices 516
scanning of 323*f*
Left atrial dysfunction 65, 203, 406, 451
biomarker of 204
pathophysiology of 448
phenotype 376
Left atrial failure 894
management of 895
Left atrial function 344, 413, 846, 894
assessment of 349, 437
evaluation of 375
quantifying 350*f*
Left atrial stiffness 408
index 345, 346*f*, 406, 437
echocardiographic evaluation of 437
pathophysiology of 406
Left atrial strain 320, 321, 321*f*, 322, 328*f*, 344*f*, 349, 350, 350*f*, 356, 360, 437
clinical implications of 439
clinical utility of 321
components of 361, 362*f*
echocardiography evaluation of 349
imaging 337
measurement of 375*f*
technical aspects of 438
role of 367
Left atrial volume 320, 330, 343, 355, 412
index 27, 39, 62, 140, 332, 376, 385, 903, 1012, 1013
measurement of 320*f*
three-dimensional 355
utility of 320
Left atrium 56, 74, 80*f*, 293, 306, 349, 357, 417, 422, 429, 715, 737, 819, 895, 985
anatomy of 449
atriopathy
clinical implications of 449
prognostic significance of 450
central role of 447
dysfunction 204
clinical implications of 202
diagnosis of 203
diagnostic role of 203
prognostic role of 203
echocardiographic
assessment of 319
evaluation of 355
function 313*t*
physiology of 449

reservoir function of 375*f*
role of 894
strain 345*f*
components, normal values of 344*t*
normal values for 438*t*
three-dimensional evaluation of 311
Left bundle branch
block 127, 708, 715
pacing 641
Left heart
disease 705-708, 712, 713
phenotype 708*t*
failure 441
Left ventricle 38, 56, 80*f*, 330, 373, 379, 425, 715, 819, 820*f*, 978, 980
diastolic function of 327, 465
ejection fraction of 391, 862
end-diastolic volume 373
examination of 305
function assessment 305
hypertrophy 778
Left ventricular aneurysm surgery 507
Left ventricular assist device 230, 239, 815, 881, 964
CircuLite synergy micro, partial support 975
Left ventricular atrial pressure 1012
Left ventricular cavities 574*f*
Left ventricular diastolic dysfunction 25, 101, 391, 432, 433, 433*f*, 551, 653, 705, 748
in cancer patients, prognostic significance of 434
incidence of 433
mechanism of 434
pathogenesis of 551
temporary 552
Left ventricular diastolic function 452, 600, 695, 940
evaluation of 339
Left ventricular distension 818, 819*f*
Left ventricular dysfunction 78, 504
Left ventricular ejection fraction 8, 23, 34*t*, 48, 49, 56*t*, 73, 74, 91, 105, 126, 126*t*, 137, 137*t*, 141, 170, 182, 206, 239, 266, 295, 305, 306, 327, 339, 339*fc*, 340, 360, 372, 386, 387, 406, 447, 504, 547, 550, 582, 626, 632, 659, 669, 683, 736, 740, 741, 748, 804, 829, 849, 879, 882, 891, 903, 909, 912, 922, 931, 953, 960, 977, 980, 981
classification of 32*f*
criteria 386
cutoff 931
measurement of 777, 856
presence of 118
preserved 111
preserved 811
Left ventricular end-diastolic pressure 62, 74, 391, 420, 526, 547, 553, 707
ratio of 407
volume index 64
Left ventricular end-systolic volume 373, 903
Left ventricular expander devices 640, 964, 979
Left ventricular filling pressure 53, 411, 576, 654, 1012
chronic elevation of 300
reduced 153
Left ventricular function 460
assessment 316
evaluation of 484
Left ventricular geometry 61
Left ventricular heart failure 714*f*
Left ventricular hypertrophy 72, 119*f*, 128, 339, 379, 454, 464, 708, 715, 718, 745, 752, 829, 913, 929, 962, 979
risk of 495
Left ventricular mass index 27, 39, 62, 140, 376, 385, 684, 696, 903, 1013
Left ventricular myocardial dysfunction 432
Left ventricular outflow tract 379, 481, 819
width 483
Left ventricular pressure 550
Left ventricular regional function, three-dimensional evaluation of 310
Left ventricular remodeling 471
Left ventricular stiffness 25, 957
Left ventricular systolic dysfunction 26, 705
Left ventricular volumes 291
Left ventricular wall thickness 62, 376, 1013
Leptin 193, 280, 950
Levosimendan 710, 716
Life-saving pharmacological treatments 825
Life-threatening syndrome 898
Light physical activity 681
Limb
amputations 900
ischemia 818
Limbic system 723
Linoleic acid 793
Lipid
lowering agents 563
management 780*fc*
goals 779*fc*
profile 564, 570, 755
Lipoprotein 779
cholesterol 564
Lipotoxicity 778
Liraglutide 952
Livanova VNS therapy system 1007*f*
Liver 951
function tests 570
Lixisenatide 952
Longitudinal strain 343, 361, 415*f*
Long-term blood pressure control 153
Look-locker technique 474
Loop diuretics 171, 619, 749
dose 947*f*
use of 599
Low renal perfusion pressure 194
Low-density lipoprotein 50, 51, 173, 268
cholesterol 779-781
Lower left atrial pressures 155
Lower limb amputation 614, 875
Lower peak oxygen consumption 744
Low-grade vascular inflammation 718
Low-intensity pulsed ultrasound 175, 176*fc*
Low-level tragus stimulation 248, 257
Lung
congestion 225
symptoms, reducing 986
diseases 210
injury, ventilator-induced 813
ultrasound 60
water quantification 454

M

Machine learning, use of 281
Magnesium 570
Magnetic resonance imaging 473
Main current therapeutic options 402
Major adverse cardiovascular events, rate of 879
Major heart failure trials 685*t*
Major public health problem 30
Malabsorption 785
Malignancy 677
Malnutrition 789
prevalence of 790
Matriuresis 521
Matrix metalloproteinase, median levels of 281
Maximal cardiopulmonary exercise test 997
Maximal exercise capacity 600
Maximal heart rate reserve 997
Maximal left atrial volume index 846
Mean arterial pressure 599
Mean blood pressure 811
Mean peak exercise pulmonary capillary wedge pressure 424
Mean pulmonary arterial pressure 705
Mechanical circulatory support 972-974, 980
devices 641, 817, 818*f*, 819*t*, 962
temporary 973
Mechanical support
devices, types of 974*f*
elective use of 506
Mechanical synchrony 156
Mechanical ventilation 655
Mechanisms behind exercise benefits 152
Medical devices 661

Medical management strategies 555
Medical therapy, benefit of 126
Mediterranean diet 154
Membrane-bound particulate guanylate cyclase 827
Mendelian randomization 96
Menopause
pathophysiology of 663
stimulates 670
Menstrual irregularities 957
Mental health disorders 588
Metabolic abnormalities 100
Metabolic adaptations 152
Metabolic benefits 997
Metabolic conditions 1011
Metabolic disease 727
Metabolic disorder 582, 611
Metabolic dysfunction 587
Metabolic effectiveness enhanced myocardial energetics 612
Metabolic effects 584, 614, 676, 867
Metabolic modulation 162
Metabolic phenotype 119
Metabolic shifts 854
Metabolic syndrome 181, 202, 420, 520, 589, 675, 729
stimulate sympathetic nervous system 592
Metabolism disorders 242
Metformin 638, 766
coutilization 589
initiation 589
Microaneurysms 691
Microischemia, subclinical episodes of 41
Microvascular coronary
disease 705, 713
dysfunction 403
Microvascular disease 865
Microvascular dysfunction 27, 37-39, 81, 101, 611, 865
pathophysiology of 37, 38
phenotype 378
Microvascular flow 575
Microvascular inflammation 54
Microvascular resistance, index of 40
Midregional proatrial natriuretic peptide, use of 61
Milrinone 548
Mind-body interventions 107
Mineralocorticoid antagonist 49, 98, 142 931
drugs 402
Mineralocorticoid receptor 239, 592, 593, 957
activation 593*fc*
antagonist
role of 958
types of 935
antagonists 4, 13, 97, 113, 119, 126, 127, 136, 141, 144, 145, 148, 174, 180, 180, 183, 196, 218, 240, 255, 269, 386, 387, 419, 450, 496, 509*f*, 536, 563, 576, 592, 594, 599, 619, 621, 625, 629, 669, 731, 749, 761, 831, 839, 849, 872, 879, 896, 908, 935, 935*t*, 936, 958, 977, 980, 1002, 1003
nonsteroidal 625
steroidal 625
strategic use of 618
Mini nutritional assessment 790
Minimal albuminuria 632
Minimal leaflet calcification 968
Minimally invasive approach 155
Mini-nutritional assessment short form 790
Mitochondrial density 152
Mitochondrial dysfunction 102, 677
Mitochondrial function 1002
Mitochondrial genetics 668
Mitochondrial membrane 640
Mitochondrial therapies 637, 639
Mitogen-activated protein kinase 26, 54, 192
MitraClip 967, 968
procedure 970
system percutaneous mitral repair 970
treatment 970
Mitral annular
A velocity 894
calcification 347
plane systolic excursion 358, 572
relaxation velocities 356
tissue 346*f*
Doppler 332, 384*f*
velocity 367
Mitral annulus
echocardiographic evaluation of 355
evaluation 356
Mitral E wave deceleration time 547
Mitral flow dynamics 980
Mitral inflow
pattern 413*f*
assessment 466
velocity, ratio of 367
Mitral l wave 340
Mitral regurgitation 45, 507, 546, 967
primary 971
reduction in 969
secondary 831
significance of 967
Mitral stenosis 969
cause 575
Mitral transcatheter edge-to-edge repair 130
Mitral valve, systolic anterior motion of 212
Modified look-locker
imaging 473
sequence 474
Molecular abnormalities 171
Monitor exercise tolerance 806
Monounsaturated fatty acids 793
Morbidity 27, 260
benefits 916, 917
Morphological score 573
Mortality 27, 260
benefits 916, 917
regional variation of 3
trends 17
Motivation 153
Multibiomarker strategy 280
Multidisciplinary approach 108
Multidisciplinary car 618
Multifactorial pathophysiology 1001
Multimorbidities disease 255
Multiorgan failure 814
Multiple comorbidities 884
Multiple plasma biomarkers 279
Multiple registries 817, 886
Multisourced edible oils 793
proven health benefits of 794
Multisystem inflammatory syndrome 552
Multitargeted therapy 599
Multivariable analysis 135
Muscle 951
strength and function 152
Muscular dystrophies 210
Musculoskeletal disorders 210
Myeloperoxidase 806
Myocardial acceleration 428
Myocardial alterations 495
Myocardial contractility 919
Myocardial contraction 525
Myocardial coronary blood flow 37
Myocardial damage 275, 718
Myocardial deformation measurements 344
Myocardial disease
evidence of 373*fc*
treatment of 288*f*
Myocardial dysfunction 655, 827
Myocardial energetics 407, 521, 614, 879
Myocardial energy
efficiency 147
level switching 902
substrate utilization 854
use 882
Myocardial extracellular matrix 896
Myocardial fatty acid oxidation 778
Myocardial fibrosis 87, 101, 148, 162, 225, 402, 426, 472, 495, 522, 561, 718, 753, 854, 879, 882, 929
assessment of 477
inhibition of 148
mechanisms of 101*b*
pathophysiology of 472
reduction of 407
Myocardial flow reserve 40
Myocardial hypertrophy 64

Myocardial infarction 135, 349, 502, 520, 909, 960
- risk of 952

Myocardial ionic homeostasis 521
Myocardial ischemia 655
Myocardial mechanics, parameters of 328*f*
Myocardial metabolic modulation 750
Myocardial oxygen demand 917
Myocardial performance index 428
Myocardial perfusion reserve 40
Myocardial recovery 973
Myocardial relaxation 151, 577, 929
Myocardial revascularization 504
Myocardial stiffness 101, 160, 472, 577, 718, 1011
Myocardial stress 277, 280
Myocardial stretch and injury 280
Myocardial tissues 864
Myocardial turgor 575
Myocarditis 173, 561
Myocardium
- contraction of 929
- in jeopardy 503
- increased stiffness of 864
- stiffness of 420
- thickness of 503

Myocyte hypertrophy 575
Myofibroblast activation 64
Myofilament
- function 873
- stiffness 520, 583*f*

Myosin heavy chain 756
Myosin
- inhibitor 1004
- types of 81

N

Nagueh formula 384
National Cardiovascular Data Registry 930
National databases 817
National Health Service 16
National Heart Failure Registry 10, 12, 1011
Native T1 mapping 474
Natriuresis 190, 192, 193, 407, 612, 740, 767, 874
Natriuresis-guided diuretic therapy 195
Natriuretic peptide 27*t*, 58, 60, 61, 94, 401, 440, 539, 545, 801, 828, 835, 846, 950, 1013
- associated effects 664
- elevated levels of 471
- elevation 846
- function 826
- levels 64
- receptors 826, 828
- score 343
- system 598, 967
- testing for 165

Near-normal left ventricular ejection fraction 332
Nebivolol 527, 930
Neck vein distension 371
Neladenoson 640
Nephrotic syndrome 210
Neprilysin 801, 826, 827, 950
- inhibitor 98, 150, 609, 651, 731, 761, 825, 827

Nervous system 190
Neurohormonal activation 102, 280, 406, 426, 581, 607, 825
Neurohormonal antagonism 174, 238
Neurohormonal effects 950
Neurohormonal modulation 407, 608, 923
Neurohormonal pathway, activation of 634
Neurohormonal regulation 153, 575
Neurohormonal systems, activation of 102
Neurohumoral devices 641
Neuromodulation therapy 979
Neuronal cells 826
Neutral endopeptidase 801
Neutrophil 20
- gelatinase associated lipocalin 280

Neutrophil-lymphocyte ratio 55
Newer antihyperkalemic drugs 623
Nicotinamide adenine dinucleotide phosphate oxidase isoform 2 103
Nifedipine inhibits calcium entry 639
Nilotinib 805
Nintedanib 639
Nitrate 225, 978
Nitric oxide 54, 64, 80, 100, 151, 191, 372, 827, 873
- bioavailability 951
- cyclic guanosine monophosphate 951
- deprivation of 221
- donors 639
- pathway modulation 749
- signaling 82, 151
- synthase 54
- synthase, dysfunction of 101

Noise 721, 722
- effect of 721
- pollution 721
  - prevention of 723

Nonalcoholic fatty liver disease 587
Noncardiac abnormalities 1011
Noncardiac comorbidities 268*t*
Noncardiac dyspnea, etiology of 360
Noncardiovascular comorbidities 171
Noncommunicable diseases 791
- burden of 791
- prevalence of 792*f*
- risk factors of 791, 792*b*

Nondevice shunt, disadvantages of 985
Nondevice therapies 130
Nonfatal stroke 595
Nonglyceride components 794, 794*t*
Nonhemorrhagic cerebrovascular diseases 587
Nonhigh-density lipoprotein 564
Nonimplant atrial shunting methods, advantages of 421
Nonimplant interatrial communication 421
Noninsulin-dependent glucose loss 875
Nonmyocardial etiologies 68
Nonpharmacological approaches 628
Nonpharmacological management 97, 175
Nonpharmacological therapies 152, 749
- limitations of 107
- play 109

Nonproliferative retinopathy 695
Non-ST-elevation myocardial infarction 135
Nonsteriodial mineralocorticoid receptor antagonists 629
Nonsteroidal anti-inflammatory drugs 144, 534
Nonsteroidal mineralocorticoid receptor antagonists 261, 620, 957
Noradrenalin 723
Norepinephrine 990
Novel drug therapies 637, 637*t*
N-terminal b-type natriuretic peptide 376
N-terminal pro-B-type natriuretic peptide 13, 27, 56, 139, 140, 161, 239, 280, 385, 740, 829, 862
- n-terminal fragment of 275

N-terminal prohormone B-type natriuretic peptide 736, 547
Nuclear factor kappa B 26
Nuclear myocardial perfusion imaging 503
Nutritional interventions 154
Nutritional risk
- index 790
- screening 790

Nutritional status control 790
Nutritional supplements 107

O

Obese heart failure, pathophysiology of 95
Obese phenotype 119
Obese-diabetic cluster 119
Obesity 24, 50, 51, 73, 90, 181, 202, 210, 215, 217, 268, 280, 339, 372, 471, 640, 659, 672, 705, 743, 748, 825, 865, 929, 949, 952-955, 1012
- causes metabolic syndrome 87
- global epidemic of 949
- in women 675
- management 564
- paradox 96, 729
- pathogenesis of 675
- phenotype 95, 377, 886
- presence of 399
- prevalence of 661

Obesity-related survival advantage 677

Objective physical activity 681
Obstructed sleep apnea 520
Obstructive coronary artery disease 879
Obstructive sleep apnea 50, 51, 95, 145, 159, 210, 534, 588, 659, 718, 744, 929
Occlutech atrial flow regulator 986
Ocular electrophysiology 692
Off-pump bypass surgery 504
Omecamtiv mecarbil 131
Omega-3 polyunsaturated fats 780
Oncological treatment 805*fc*
Ongoing drug
- and device trials 1006
- trials 1008

Ongoing trials and studies 991
On-pump bypass surgery 504
Optical coherence tomography 692
- angiography 692

Optimal projection curve 485
Optimizer smart mini system 1007*f*
Optimum medical therapy 503
Oral anticoagulants 786
Oral fluconazole, single dose of 900
Oral sodium bicarbonate 842
Organ protection, kidney heart connection for 582*f*
Orlistat 745
Orthopnea 85
Oryzanol 794
Osmotic diuresis 767, 882
- and natriuresis 147, 854

Ostmenopausal and hormone replacement therapy 675
Outflow tract 311
- obstruction 705

Overt hyperthyroidism 754, 755
Overweight 955
Oxidative endothelial damage and dysfunction 723
Oxidative injury 563, 607
Oxidative radical formation 664
Oxidative stress 81, 82, 100, 105, 193, 194, 280, 520, 581, 587, 611, 718, 753, 827, 865, 879
- and inflammation 394
- from metabolic syndrome 715
- inhibits glyceraldehyde-3-phosphate dehydrogenase 102
- originates 827
- reduced 583*f*

Oxygen
- diffusion 676
- saturation 261

P

Pacemakers 984
Palliative care 90, 92*f*
Pamrevlumab 639
Pancreatic beta cells 951
Pancreatic deficiency 770
Paradox 746
Paraglide-heart failure trial 150, 605, 649, 650
Parallax-heart failure 605
Paramount-heart failure trial 605
Paravalvular regurgitation 481
Paricalcitol 640
Paroxysmal nocturnal dyspnea 18, 60, 85, 88, 399
Partial anomalous pulmonary venous drainage 981
Partial cardiopulmonary bypass 812
Particulate guanylate cyclase 828
Patent ductus arteriosus 981
Pathogen recognition receptor 26
Patiromer 601, 622, 840
Peak atrial contraction strain 363
Peak atrial longitudinal strain 321, 321*f*, 363
Peak oxygen consumption 152, 401, 450
Perceived exertion, rate of 997
Percutaneous atriotomy 963
Percutaneous coronary intervention 494, 496, 508, 811
Percutaneous pulmonary artery denervation 710
Perhexiline 639
Pericardial constriction 472
Pericardial disease 138, 182
Pericardial disorders 575
Pericardial effusion 484, 574*f*, 575
- mild 574*f*

Pericardial resection 177
Pericardial restraint 950
Periorbital ecchymoses 112
Peripartum cardiomyopathy 684
Peripheral adaptations 996
Peripheral arterial
- disease 588
- stiffness 858

Peripheral circulation 670
Peripheral edema 865
Peripheral oxygen extraction, reduced 152
Peripheral skeletal muscle vasodilatation 222
Peripheral vascular disease 200, 519, 522
Perivascular fibrosis 25
Permanent pacemaker implantation 517
Peroxynitrite 54
- production of 1002

Persistent myocardial damage provokes fibrosis 560
Personal care worker 51
Personalized nutrition plans 154
Phagocytose 20
Pharmacological evidence 526
Pharmacological facets 13
Pharmacological interventions 450
Pharmacological management 97, 171, 218
Pharmacological therapies 147, 268, 526, 749, 1002
- optimization of 496

Pharmacological treatment 731
Pharmacotherapy 508, 536
Phase-sensitive inversion recovery 473
- sequence 475

Phasic left atrial strain 351
Phenolic acid 794
Phenotype 223, 261, 705
Phenotype-guided therapy 162
Phentermine 745
Phlebitis syndrome 210
Phosphodiesterase inhibitors 638, 978
Phosphodiesterase-5 429, 709
- inhibitors 638, 708
  - trials of 715

Phosphokinase G 828
Phospholamban 54
Phospholipase C 54
Phrenic nerve palsy 210
Physical activity 516, 682, 730
- moderate-to-vigorous 681

Physical fitness, lack of 284
Physiological accelerated pacing 229
Physiological stress 39
Pioglitazone 210
Pirfenidone 163, 637, 639
Placebo 868
Planimetered mitral valve area 968
Plant sterols 794
Plasma
- natriuretic peptides, measurement of 260
- renin activity, elevated levels of 834
- volume 762, 950

Pleural diseases 210
Pneumatic pulsatile pump 975
Point-of-care viscoelastic tests 816
Polycystic ovary disease 587
Polymorbidity 261
Polymyositis 210
Polytetrafluoroethylene 422, 985
Polyunsaturated fatty acids 793
Ponatinib 805
Poor dietary 635
Poorer exercise capacity 744
Population 669
- characteristics 740, 741, 860-862
- sample 16
- size 860-862

Portal hypertension 210
Positive airway pressure, effect of 719
Positive end-expiratory pressure 656
Positron emission tomography 40, 46, 402, 503
Postcardiotomy cardiogenic shock 817
Postdischarge management 262
Posterolateral coronary territory 508
Postmyocardial infarction 827

Postoperative congenital cardiac repair 817
Postpercutaneous coronary intervention 499
Postprandial blood sugar 588
Postprocedure evaluation 485
Post-thrombotic syndrome 210
Potassium 570
  selectivity for 622
Potential cardiac remodeling 867
Potential iatrogenic contribution 261
Potential mechanistic insights 409
Powerful vasoconstrictors, array of 676
Precipitating cause 261
Precision medicine 162
Precordial auscultation 865
Preeclampsia 675, 684
Pregnancy 671, 675
Preocclusion brachial artery 83*f*
Preprocedural computed tomography evaluation 481
Preprocedural planning requires transthoracic echocardiography 968
Preserved ejection fraction causes, nonheart failure with 111
Pressure natriuresis 191
  curves 190*f*
  mechanism of 189
  relationship, modulation of 189
Pressure-volume loop 858
Primary care physician 873
Primary composite endpoint 216, 217
PRKG2 syndrome 562
Pro-b-type natriuretic peptide 116
Profibrotic pathways, hyperglycemia-induced activation of 101
Prognostic nutritional index 790
Proinflammatory cytokines 102
Proinflammatory pathway, activation of 634
Proinflammatory state 372
Proliferative diabetic retinopathy 695
Proprotein convertase subtilisin 590
Prostaglandin E2 189
Protective ventilation protocols 813
Protein
  expression 937
  kinase
    A 54
    C 54
    G 54, 176, 593
    G activity 827
    G, reduced 1002
Proteinuria 873
Prothrombotic pathway activation 723
Prothrombotic state, promotion of 418
Prussian helmet appearance 568*f*
Pseudo-hyperkalemia 842
Pseudonormal filling 340
Pseudoxanthoma elasticum 562
Psychosocial benefits 152
Pulmonary artery 62, 127, 131, 180, 712, 715, 817
  compliance 715
  denervation 176, 710
  hypertension 77, 302, 379, 671, 705, 713
    phenotype 886
  pressure 427, 573
    monitoring 1015
  systolic pressure 27, 62, 126, 140, 376, 385, 440
  wedge pressure 420, 705, 707, 712
Pulmonary capillary 53
  wedge pressure 74, 176*f*, 200, 266, 391, 467, 553, 576, 670, 705, 962, 980, 981, 1003, 1012
Pulmonary edema 371
Pulmonary embolism 277
Pulmonary flow 413
Pulmonary function 152
Pulmonary hemodynamic profiles 552, 553
Pulmonary hypertension 26, 64, 73, 78, 86, 90, 126, 211, 225, 227, 293, 342, 376, 420, 426, 429, 472, 503, 552, 659, 705-707, 712, 713*t*, 714, 714*t*, 715, 748, 814, 815, 1013
  clinical characteristics of 712
  management 750
  pathobiology of 713, 714*f*
  presence of 302
  pretest probability of 706
  related heart failure 158
Pulmonary pressure
  management 152
  reduction 151
Pulmonary rales 865
Pulmonary vascular
  disease 376*f*
  phenotype 376
  remodeling 426
  resistance 450
Pulmonary vasculature 455
Pulmonary vasoconstriction 1002
Pulmonary vasodilators 715
Pulmonary vein isolation 46*f*
Pulmonary venous
  congestion 65
  flow 414*f*
  flow pattern 467
  hypertension 503
  pressure 90, 471
  systolic-diastolic ratio 572
Pulse
  pressure 890
  ventricular assist device 974
  wave Doppler of pulmonary flow 376*f*
Pump
  blood 906
  failure 391
Pump-assisted protection 813*b*

Q

Quadruple foundational therapy, rapid optimization of 844
Quality of life 183, 262, 419, 515, 563, 574, 675, 853, 919, 939, 962, 1014

R

Radial strain 343, 361
Radiation effects, monitoring for 806
Radiofrequency ablation
  based interatrial shunt 423
  therapy 424
Radiofrequency generator 424
Radiotherapy induced cardiomyopathy 778
Rail traffic 723
Raised ventricular filling pressures 111
Randomized clinical trial 422
Randomized controlled trials 762, 767, 931, 985
Ranolazine 639
Reactive oxygen species 26, 54, 779, 828
  formation of 102
  production of 102, 372
Recombinant high-density lipoprotein 640
Red blood cell 786
Refractory edema 171
Refractory hypertension 533, 536
Regional mortality differences 5
Regional wall motion abnormalities 503
Regular echocardiographic monitoring 359
Regurgitant lesion 259
Rehabilitation 152, 546, 993, 995
Relative wall thickness 376, 1013
Relaxation disorders 552
Renal artery stenosis 877
Renal denervation 176, 186, 196, 243, 247, 257, 986, 990
  effectiveness of 991
  mechanism of action of 990
Renal disease 17, 520, 579
Renal dysfunction 78, 90, 102, 339, 748
Renal effects 854
Renal end-stage disease, prevention of 1011
Renal failure 181
Renal function 150, 602, 858, 928
  assessment 595
  preservation 121
Renal impairment 827
  resulting 858
Renal injury, modes of 608*f*
Renal interstitial hydrostatic pressure 189
Renal outcomes 614
Renal protection 160, 867
  reduced intraglomerular pressure, mechanisms of 612
Renal replacement therapy 608, 621

Renal safety 604
Renal sodium
reabsorption 190
retention 194
Renal sympathetic nerves
anatomy of 990
physiology of 990
Renin-angiotensin
activity 950
aldosterone system 386, 546
inhibitors 500
Renin-angiotensin system 145, 500, 534, 535, 604, 786, 967
contributes 575
function supports 189
inhibitor 97, 126, 298
role of 648
Renin-angiotensin-aldosterone
blockade 879
derived potent vasoconstrictors 664
inhibitors 949
Renin-angiotensin-aldosterone system 148, 189, 190, 280, 395, 539, 583, 592, 593*f*, 598, 608, 648*fc*, 669, 670, 718, 730, 825, 826, 832, 895, 950, 990
activation of 193, 194, 406, 865, 929, 935
blockade 977
inhibitors 113, 123, 186, 496, 608, 832, 840
overactivation 919
Renoglomerulosclerosis, reduce 873
Replacement fibrosis, type of 22
Reproductive health 671
Reservoir strain 356
Resistance training 106, 996
Resistant hypertension 533, 539, 540, 719, 990
management of 534, 535*fc*
secondary causes of 192
Resistin 193
Respiratory symptoms, causes of 165
Restore tubuloglomerular feedback 873
Restrictive cardiomyopathy 379, 454, 551, 561, 681
Restrictive phenotype 864
Resveratrol 639
Retinal artery narrowing 693
Retinal microaneurysms 691
Retinal microvascular
function 692
impairment 691
structure, assessment of 691
Retinopathies 693
prognosis of 696
Revascularization, benefits of 504*fc*
Reverse cardiac remodeling 576
Reversing ventricular remodeling 903
Rheumatoid arthritis 588
Rhythm control 158, 931
Right atrial
emptying fraction 302
enlargement 454
function, rationale for assessment of 442
strain 442
clinical implications of 443
measurement, technical aspects of 442
Right atrium 306, 422, 985
augmented overload of 420
volume 427
Right greater splanchnic nerve, endovascular ablation of 268
Right heart catheterization 61, 706, 707
Right renal angiogram, selective 569*f*
Right ventricle 293, 373, 420, 425, 454, 715, 978, 980
Right ventricular
cavities 574*f*
diastolic function 427
ejection fraction 379
failure 814
hypertrophy 745
outflow tract 379, 427
pulmonary artery 441
structure, echocardiographic evaluation of 426
systolic pressure 13, 379
volume assessment 316
wall thickness 427
Right ventricular dysfunction 420, 472, 819, 884
phenotype 377
prognostic implications of 428
severe 821*f*
Right ventricular function
normalization of 821*f*
prevalence of 425
rationale for assessment of 440
three-dimensional evaluation of 310
Right ventricular strain 427, 440, 441*f*
assessment 441
clinical implications of 441
measurement, technical aspects of 441
Rituximab 638
Road traffic 723
Robust biomarker 277
Rotem machine 817*f*

S

Sacubitril 184, 225, 403, 600, 649, 719, 801, 802, 827, 828, 835, 844-846, 871, 1008, 1014
cardiovascular benefits of 876
efficacy of 500*f*
inhibits neprilysin 835
mechanism of action of 499*f*
stimulates 599
Sacubitril-valsartan 113, 299, 500, 639
use 731
Salinomycin 639
Salt and water restriction 256
Salt-sensitive hypertension 181
Sarcoidosis 112, 563
Saturated fatty acid 781, 793
Saturation recovery single-shot acquisition 473
Saturation recovery-based t1 mapping techniques 474
Saxagliptin 892
Scar quantification 476
Semaglutide 178, 640, 739-741, 944-946, 949, 952, 956, 1016
effects 946, 955
role of 741*t*
studies 745
subcutaneous injections of 952
treatment 942, 953
Sepsis 277, 655
Septal myectomy 335
Serine phosphorylation 100
Serum
creatinine 570
electrolytes 570
ferritin 787
levels 635
fibrinogen levels 816
glucose 570
potassium levels 596
Severe acute respiratory syndrome coronavirus 2 561
Severe valvular obstructive 259
Sex hormone-related side effects 935
Sex-specific differences 143
Sex-specific risk enhancers 588
Short-term mortality 12
Shunt
advantages of 985
diameter 243
flow 422, 985
size 422, 985
Sildenafil 637
Single photon emission computed tomography 503
Sinotubular junction 482
diameter of 484*f*
measurements 483
Sinus of Valsalva 483
measurements 483
width 483*f*
Sinus rhythm 62, 128
Sitagliptin 638, 889
Six-minute walk
distance 206, 862
test 176, 298, 762, 767, 980, 1002
Skeletal muscle 1002
function 1002
weakness 225

Skin autofluorescence 699, 700*f*, 701
  clinical relevance of 701
Skinfold thickness 790
Sleep apnea 516
  syndrome 339
Sleep disorders 588
Smoking 564
Smooth muscle 81
Snoring 718
Society of thoracic surgeons 505
Sodium 570
  channel 637
  polystyrene sulfonate 622
  pump 637
  reabsorption 95
  restriction 105
  retention 194, 225, 950
    leading 622
    prevention of 149
  zirconium cyclosilicate 601, 622, 840
Sodium-dependent glucose-cotransport inhibitors 858, 859
  mechanistic effects of 858
Sodium-glucose
  cotransport protein 2 inhibitors 831
  cotransporter 761*f*
    benefits 916
    inhibitor 408*t*, 615*t*, 626*f*
    inhibitor beneficial effects of 890
    mechanism of action of 760*f*, 767
  cotransporter-1 inhibitors 172, 184
  cotransporter-2 50, 51, 131, 172, 173, 180, 184, 239, 268, 681, 768, 872, 916
  linked transporter protein 2 inhibitors 419
  transport protein 2 inhibitors 589, 590, 895
  transporter-2 inhibitors 576
Sodium-glucose cotransporter-2
  growing role of 853
  morbidity benefits of 915
  mortality benefits of 915
  uniqueness of 872
Sodium-glucose cotransporter-2 inhibitors 13, 49, 98, 112, 116, 119, 123*f*, 126, 128, 142, 144, 147, 149, 158, 160, 178, 180, 184, 195, 218, 225, 233, 238, 255, 261, 266, 268, 329, 330, 352, 355, 359, 386, 387*f*, 393, 406, 408, 409, 450, 489, 516, 520, 522, 563, 581, 584, 585, 592, 599, 609, 611, 614, 619, 620*f*, 625, 638, 673, 709, 716, 719, 731, 736*f*, 739, 745, 763, 766, 772, 825, 831, 858, 866*f*, 872, 875, 879, 883, 886, 889*fc*, 891, 898, 902, 906, 915, 949, 977, 981, 1002
  action of 490*b*, 740*b*
  administration of 614*t*
  cause osmotic diuresis 854
  clinical advantages of 614
  clinical effects of 521*b*, 761
  composite benefits of 239*f*
  contraindications of 874
  effect of 406, 583*f*, 766, 872, 873, 903
  efficacy of 855
  glucosuric effects of 874
  mechanisms of action of 407, 853, 882, 887*f*, 899*fc*
  metabolic effects of 874
  molecular mechanism of 903
  pooled analysis of 773
  principal effect of 394
  promote 854
  renal protective effects of 873
  role of 583, 660, 739, 740*t*, 758, 853, 864, 866, 867, 879, 902, 906
  therapy 615, 831
  trial evidence of 902
Sodium-glucose-linked cotransporter-2 inhibitor 127
Sodium-hydrogen exchanger-3 195, 582*f*, 883
  inhibition 882
Sodium-myoinositol cotransporter-1 103
Soluble guanylate cyclase 54, 176, 709*f*, 828
  activity 1002
  stimulators 151, 163, 638
Soluble transferrin 787
Sotagliflozin 128, 773, 778
Sound 721
Specialized equipment 368
Specific mortality rates 5*f*
Speckle tracking echocardiography 293, 295, 321, 356, 361, 573
Sphygmomanometer tube 340
Spironolactone 113, 120, 142, 148, 184, 225, 402, 534, 547, 548, 594, 595, 600, 637, 639, 719, 834, 837, 935, 936, 1016
  counteracts 592
  dosing of 595
  efficacy of 592
  monitoring, protocols for 595
  safety of 592
Splanchnic ablation 246, 257
Standard biochemical markers 55
Standard deviation thresholding 476
Standard echocardiographic parameters 411
Standard late gadolinium enhancement sequences 475
Statins 98, 225, 226, 780
ST-elevation myocardial infarction 494, 495, 499
  coexistence of 494
  management of 495, 496*fc*
Stem cell therapy 637
Stenotic aortic valve 568*f*
Sterile inflammation 20
Steroidal mineralocorticoid receptor antagonist 261, 957
  use of 629
Stiff cardiomyocytes 372
Stiff left ventricle 1015
Strain
  clinical applications of 443
  component 344
  parameters 296-298
  rate 343
  values 362
Stress 275
  analysis 384*fc*
  cardiomyopathy 684
  echocardiography 61
  echocardiography, use of 334
  test 401
Stress-hormone-mediated metabolic syndrome 723
Stress-induced cardiomyopathy 879, 881
Stroke 519, 587, 952, 955, 1015
  and heart failure, risk of 417
Stronger receptor-binding affinity 630
Structural heart disease 178
Subcutaneous adiposity 950
Sudden cardiac death 134, 209
  mechanisms of 135
  risk stratification of 134, 135
Sudden death 1001
Sudden nighttime breathlessness 88
Sulfonylurea 892
Superior vena cava 813
Supine bicycle test 334
Supraventricular tachycardia 909*f*
Surgical ventricular reconstruction, role of 507
Swedish heart failure 8, 930
Sympathetic activity 950
Sympathetic nerve activity, overactivation of 929
Sympathetic nervous system 95, 190*f*, 539, 608, 826, 904, 919
  activation of 194, 598
  overactivity 990
Sympathetic-adrenal-medulla axis 723
Sympathoadrenal axis, activation of 722
Synergy pump 641
Systemic congestion 138
Systemic embolism 319, 321
Systemic endothelial inflammation 64
Systemic inflammation 225, 275, 420, 426, 581, 612, 748, 864, 882, 903, 916, 951
Systemic inflammatory biomarker concentration 661

Systemic microvascular inflammation, causes of 95
Systemic peripheral resistance 191
Systemic thromboembolism 324
Systemic vascular stiffness 152
Systolic anterior motion 379
Systolic blood pressure 989
Systolic dysfunction 343
Systolic heart failure 679

T

Tachycardia 334
  presence of 931
  prevention of 392
Tailored exercise intervention 806
Tailored programs 153
Tailored therapy 366
  phenotyping for 234
Takotsubo cardiomyopathy 879, 880
  management of 881
  pathophysiology of 880*f*
Takotsubo syndrome 879
Tamponade 575
Tandem heart device 974
Target blood pressure 539
Targeted patient populations 151
Targeting left atrium dysfunction 450
Technological advancements 991
Telemonitoring 34
Therapeutic implications 275
Therapeutic intervention 386*fc*
Therapeutic value 276
Thoracic aortic aneurysm 978
Three-dimensional echocardiography 305, 428
  role of 291
Three-dimensional vector cardiography 285
Thyroid 753*f*
  abnormalities 754*t*
  disorders 210
  function test 13
  hormone 752
    levels 754
    replacement therapy 755
Thyroid-stimulating hormone 755
Thyrotoxicosis 85
Tirzepatide 640, 741, 952, 1016
Tissue
  characterization 467
  Doppler 414*f*
    imaging 204, 356, 358*f*
  radiofrequency ablation of 985
Titin phosphorylation 1002
Tocotrienols 794
Toxic agents 827
Tragus stimulation 248
Transcatheter aortic valve implantation 480
  planning computed tomography protocol 481
Transcatheter atrial shunt system 243, 640, 963
Transcatheter heart valve 482
Transcatheter interatrial shunt device 121, 175, 176*f*, 227
Transcatheter MitraClip edge-to-edge repair 967
Transcatheter mitral valve repair 967, 969
  complications of 969
Transesophageal echocardiogram 323*f*, 819*f*, 968
Transfatty acid 781
Transferrin saturation 280, 635, 786, 787, 939
Transforming growth factor beta 26, 77, 175, 760*f*
Transmitral Doppler imaging 358
Transmitral flow 413
Transoral robotic surgery 719
Transseptal access 985
Transthoracic echocardiography 33, 553
Transthyretin amyloid cardiomyopathy 116
Transthyretin cardiac amyloidosis 35*fc*
Transunsaturated fatty acids 793
Treadmill testing 334
Tricuspid annular plane systolic excursion 379, 425, 502
Tricuspid annulus, tissue Doppler imaging of 427
Tricuspid regurgitation 13, 27, 45, 62, 74, 140*f*, 179, 266, 373, 376, 384, 385, 420, 442, 1012, 1013
  peak velocity 355
Tricuspid valve 426
  interventions 132
Trigger cardiomyocyte autophagy 827
Triggers peripheral vasodilation 635
Triglyceride 589
Triiodothyronine 756
Trivandrum heart failure registry 10
Troponin 61
Tube-crimping roller pumps 819
Tumor necrosis factor 280
  alpha 193, 281, 786, 828
Tumorigenesis-2, soluble suppression of 55, 61, 1009
Tumorigenicity-2
  protein, soluble suppression of 280
  suppression of 161
Two-dimensional left atrial volume 355
Two-dimensional speckle tracking echocardiography 204
Two-dimensional transthoracic echocardiography 291
Tyrosine phosphorylation, instead of 100

U

Udenafil 637
Ultrafiltration 609
Ultra-wide-field imaging 692
Upper airway
  collapse 719
  obstruction 210
Upper arm circumference 790
Upper body hypoxemia 420
Uric acid 55
Urine albumin-creatinine ratio 588, 589*f*, 605, 828, 904, 960

V

Vagal nerve 248
  stimulation 175, 175*fc*, 186, 257, 430, 1003, 1006
Valsalva procedure 339
Valsalva technique 340
  hemodynamic basis of 340*f*
Valsartan 121, 184, 329, 403, 500*f*, 600, 649, 719, 801, 802, 828, 835, 844-846, 871, 1008, 1014
  cardiovascular benefits of 876
  mechanism of action of 499*f*
Valveless pulsatile pump 974, 980
Valvular disease 138
Valvular heart disease 173, 182, 276, 277, 379, 407, 679, 705
Valvular obstructive, moderate 259
Vascular cell adhesion molecule 828
Vascular compliance 151
Vascular complications 991
Vascular derangements 280
Vascular disease 819
Vascular dysfunction 82, 83, 1004
  pathogenesis of 80*f*
  therapeutic implications of 83
Vascular effects 147
Vascular end-stage disease, prevention of 1011
Vascular health 152
Vascular hypertrophy 194
Vascular inflammation 82
Vascular permeability 826
Vascular proliferation 664
Vascular remodeling 715
Vascular resistance 753, 754
Vascular smooth muscle cells 826
Vascular stiffness 162, 607, 925, 935
  reduction in 149
Vascular wall, elastic property of 81
Vasoactive substances, imbalance of 418
Vasoconstriction 873
Vasoconstrictor endothelin-1, produce 192
Vasodilators 609

Vasodilatory beta-blockers 931
Vasopressin 539
Venoarterial extracorporeal membrane oxygenation 812, 817
Venous
  congestion 581
  disorders 210
Venovenous extracorporeal membrane oxygenator 812
Ventricles, capacity of 559
Ventricular arrhythmias 24, 112
Ventricular arterial
  coupling 748
  stiffening 64, 526
Ventricular assist device 686, 973, 978
  implantation 973
  technologies 973
Ventricular dyssynchrony 156
Ventricular end-diastolic pressure, estimation of 553
Ventricular filling, functional impairment of 962
Ventricular geometry 337
Ventricular hypertrophy, moderate-to-severe 259
Ventricular interdependence 426
Ventricular myocardium 503
Ventricular relaxation 571
Ventricular remodeling 737, 748
  predominate 134
Ventricular septal defect 981
Ventricular stiffness 332, 550, 679
Ventura interatrial shunt system 1008
Vericiguat 129, 151
  mechanism of action of 151
Viability testing, role of 503
Vibrational shear waves, measurement of 477
Visceral obesity 193
Visual analog scale 859, 862
Vitamin E 794
Volumetric methods 413
V-wave 228*f*, 422, 985
  device 206, 227, 963
  shunt 243, 244, 640

W

Wall motion score index 310
Weight loss 515, 521, 745, 874, 954
  interventions 153, 154
  measures 745
Weight management 105, 153
  benefits of 153
Workstation software computes area 482
Worsening heart failure, incidence of 762

Y

Yoga 107

Z

Ziltivekimab 1016
Zinc-dependent metalloproteinase 801